COMPREHENSIVE
GYNECOLOGY

COMPREHENSIVE GYNECOLOGY

FOURTH EDITION

MORTON A. STENCHEVER, M.D.
Professor and Chairman Emeritus
Department of Obstetrics and Gynecology
University of Washington School of Medicine
Seattle, Washington

WILLIAM DROEGEMUELLER, M.D.
Clinical Professor and Chairman Emeritus
Department of Obstetrics and Gynecology
University of North Carolina School of Medicine
Chapel Hill, North Carolina

ARTHUR L. HERBST, M.D.
Joseph Bolivar DeLee Distinguished Service Professor and Chairman
Department of Obstetrics and Gynecology
University of Chicago
Chicago, Illinois

DANIEL R. MISHELL, JR., M.D.
The Lyle G. McNeile Professor and Chairman
Department of Obstetrics and Gynecology
Keck School of Medicine
University of Southern California
Los Angeles, California

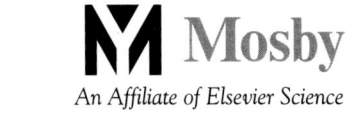

Mosby
An Affiliate of Elsevier Science
St. Louis • London • Philadelphia • Sydney • Toronto

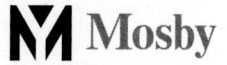

An Affiliate of Elsevier Science

Mosby Inc.
An Affiliate of Elsevier Science
11830 Westline Industrial Drive
St. Louis, Missouri 63146

Printed in the United States of America

Library of Congress Cataloging in Publication Data

Comprehensive gynecology / Morton A. Stenchever ... [et al.]. — 4th ed.
    p. cm.
  Includes bibliographical references and index.
  ISBN 0-323-01402-X
    1. Gynecology. I. Stenchever, Morton A.

  RG101.C726 2001
  618.1–dc21   00-052541

Last digit is print number: 9 8 7 6 5 4 3

DEDICATION

The authors wish to dedicate this edition to the memory
of Diane H. Stenchever, wife of Morton Stenchever,
who passed away in April 1999 after a long battle with cancer.

Contributors

Dee E. Fenner, M.D.
Associate Professor and Vice Chair, Department of Obstetrics and Gynecology,
University of Washington, Seattle, Washington
Anatomic Defects of the Abdominal Wall and Pelvic Floor, Rectal Incontinence

Vern Katz, M.D.
Clinical Associate Professor, Oregon Health Sciences University;
Director, Perinatal Services, Sacred Heart Medical Center, Eugene, Oregon
Diagnostic Procedures

Jacob Rotmensch, M.D.
Professor, Section Head Gynecologic Oncology,
Department of Obstetrics and Gynecology, University of Chicago,
Chicago, Illinois
Principles of Radiation Therapy and Chemotherapy in Gynecologic Cancer

Fidel A. Valea, M.D.
Director, Division of Gynecologic Oncology, Director, Residency Program
in Obstetrics and Gynecology, Associate Professor, State University of New York
at Stony Brook, Stony Brook, New York
Breast Diseases

Steven E. Waggoner, M.D.
Associate Professor, Division of Gynecologic Oncology,
Department of Obstetrics and Gynecology, University of Chicago,
Chicago, Illinois
Immunology and Molecular Oncology in Gynecologic Cancer

Carolyn Westhoff, M.D., M.Sc.
Professor of Obstetrics and Gynecology; Professor of Public Health,
Joseph Mailman School of Public Health and College of Physicians and Surgeons;
Attending Physician, Director, Division of Prevention and Ambulatory Care,
Medical Director, Family Planning, New York Presbyterian Hospital,
New York, New York
Evidence-Based Medicine and Clinical Epidemiology

Preface

The fourth edition of *Comprehensive Gynecology* continues the tradition of being the work of the four authors, but in five of the chapters of this edition the authors have collaborated with colleagues who are experts in specific areas of the specialty. It is intended that such collaboration will broaden the scope of these chapters. In addition, a chapter on evidence-based medicine and clinical epidemiology has been added. As always, the authors have critically reviewed each chapter.

All four of the authors have served long tenures as chairs of departments of obstetrics and gynecology at major schools of medicine, and all have had extensive experience in academic and clinical gynecology. The book is designed to offer comprehensive knowledge of gynecology to students, residents, and practicing physicians. This edition has been extensively revised with considerable new information added. As with previous editions, however, the unique teaching features of the key terms at the beginning of each chapter, the key points summarizing important areas of information at the end of each chapter, and an updated bibliography have been retained, as has the two- color format that was introduced in the third edition.

The authors wish to thank our wives, families, and support staff for their help and understanding during the preparation of this edition. As we have worked together through these four editions, we have become a close extended family.

Morton A. Stenchever
William Droegemueller
Arthur L. Herbst
Daniel R. Mishell, Jr.

Contents

Part Three   General Gynecology

Part Four   Gynecologic Oncology

PART ONE

Basic Sciences

Fertilization and Embryogenesis

Meiosis, Fertilization, Implantation, Embryonic Development, Sexual Differentiation

KEY TERMS AND DEFINITIONS

Acrosome Reaction. The process by which the cap over the head of the sperm, the acrosome, is removed to expose the portion of the sperm head containing the hydrolytic enzymes, which makes it possible for the sperm to penetrate the cells and structures investing the egg. This process is involved in capacitation but is not necessarily the same response as capacitation.

Anlage. The cell mass that gives rise to a specific organ or structure.

Bivalent. Homologous chromosomes that become paired during meiosis.

Blastocyst. The stage of the conceptus that follows the morula stage. It consists of a fluid-filled cavity surrounded by trophoblasts with embryonic cells at one pole.

Blastula. The stage of embryonic development that follows the morula stage. At this stage a cyst (blastocyst) forms within the cell mass, and early differentiation begins.

Capacitation. The morphologic, physiologic, and biochemical changes that a sperm goes through to be capable of penetrating the cumulus oophorus, corona radiata, and zona pellucida of the egg. It involves the sequentially timed release of a series of hydrolytic enzymes, which allows the sperm to digest a passage through the aforementioned structures.

Chemotaxis. The attraction of the sperm to the ova.

Chemokinesis. The stimulation of sperm motility.

Chiasmata. Points of attachment of homologous chromosomes during meiosis, where the exchange of genetic material occurs.

Cleavage. The first cell division of the fertilized ovum (zygote).

Conceptional Age. The age of the conceptus from the time of fertilization.

Conceptus. The fertilized oocyte and its derivatives at all stages of development from fertilization until birth and including all extraembryonic membranes.

Cumulus Oophorus. The cell mass that invests the egg. It is a remnant of the primitive sex cords of the embryonic ovary.

Embryo. The developmental stage of the conceptus after the development of the primitive streak and until all major organs are developed. In the human, it begins at about conceptional day 14 and ends when organ development is complete. The definition of the end of the embryonic period is not entirely agreed upon by authorities but is probably between postconceptional days 36 and 50.

Fertilization. The point at which one spermatozoon penetrates the oocyte. This is the stage before the pronuclei are formed.

Gartner's Duct. Remnants of the mesonephric (wolffian) duct system often found in the broad ligament and beside the uterus, cervix, and vagina of the adult woman.

Gestational Age. The stage of the embryo counting from the first day of the last menstrual period. On average, it is about 2 weeks longer than conceptional age, assuming a 28-day menstrual cycle.

H-Y Antigen. A cell surface antigen that leads to male differentiation of the gonad.

Implantation. The process by which the early embryo burrows within the endometrial lining of the uterus.

Mesonephros. The mesodermal anlage of the male sexual duct system.

Metanephros. The anlage of the adult kidney.

Morula. A ball of cells composing the early embryo that produces both the embryo and the placenta and membranes. Each cell is totipotential.

Oogenesis. The development of the ovum from an oogonium by meiosis.

Paramesonephric (Müllerian) Duct. The anlage of the female sex duct system that gives rise to the fallopian tube, uterus, and cervix in the adult woman.

Polar Body. The daughter cell produced during oogenesis at first and second meiotic division (first and second polar body); it contains a nucleus and minimal cytoplasm. For each polar body the nuclear material is similar to the nucleus of the ovum at the same stage.

Primordium. An early embryonic structure that further differentiates into an adult structure.

Sister Chromatid Exchange. The exchange of chromosomal material between the homologous arms of a chromosome that has already divided all of its structure except its centromere.

Spermatogenesis. The development of mature sperm from spermatogonia by meiosis.

Synapsis. The pairing process that brings together homologous chromosomes of maternal and paternal origin during meiosis.

Syngamy. The active union of the sperm and the egg to form a zygote.

Teratogen. An endogenous or exogenous substance that causes the formation of an anomaly.

Teratogenesis. The process of developing an anomaly of an organ or organs.

Zona Pellucida. The translucent belt consisting of a noncellular layer of mucopolysaccharide that is deposited at the periphery of the ovum while it is in the ovary and continues to surround the egg, the conceptus, and the morula until the stage of implantation.

Zygote. The one-cell stage of the fertilized ovum after pronuclear membrane breakdown but before first cleavage occurs.

Two areas of investigation within the field of gynecology have refocused attention on the process of fertilization and embryonic development: teratology and assisted reproductive technology. The process under which eggs and sperm are produced and fertilization occurs is gaining close scrutiny. Likewise, the preimplantation, implantation, and embryonic stages of development in the human can be studied because of the development of newer techniques and pursuits. This chapter considers the processes of oocyte meiosis, fertilization and early cleavage, implantation, development of the genitourinary system, and sex differentiation.

OOCYTE MEIOSIS

The oocyte is a unique and extremely specialized cell. During the process of oocyte meiosis, genetic variability of the species is ensured. Later the oocyte develops the ability to facilitate fertilization and to provide the energy system to support the early embryonic development of the new individual.

Primordial germ cells in both males and females are large eosinophilic cells derived from endoderm in the wall of the yolk sac. These cells migrate to the germinal ridge by way of the dorsal mesentery of the hindgut by ameboid action. Here they undergo a period of intense mitotic activity in which their numbers increase to 6 to 7 million. By 20 weeks' gestation, this rapid multiplication has ended, and indeed the numbers rapidly fall off, being about 2 to 4 million at birth and about 400,000 at menarche. By 5 months' gestation, surviving oocytes enter the process of meiosis and progress to the prophase of the first meiotic division before entering an arrest period that lasts many years. After puberty a few oocytes mature during each ovarian cycle. The numbers vary from species to species, being one or two in the human. Maturation then continues to the second meiotic metaphase, when once again arrest of meiosis occurs unless the oocyte is activated by fertilization.

Figure 1-1 illustrates the steps of meiosis through both the first and second meiotic divisions. Prophase of the first meiotic division is divided into several phases. The earliest, the leptotene stage, is associated with condensation of the chromatin, which becomes visible as single elongated, threadlike structures. The next stage, zygotene, features the migration of these single threadlike chromosomes toward the equatorial plate of the nucleus. Homologous chromosomes arrange themselves close to one another to form bivalents. At the end of this

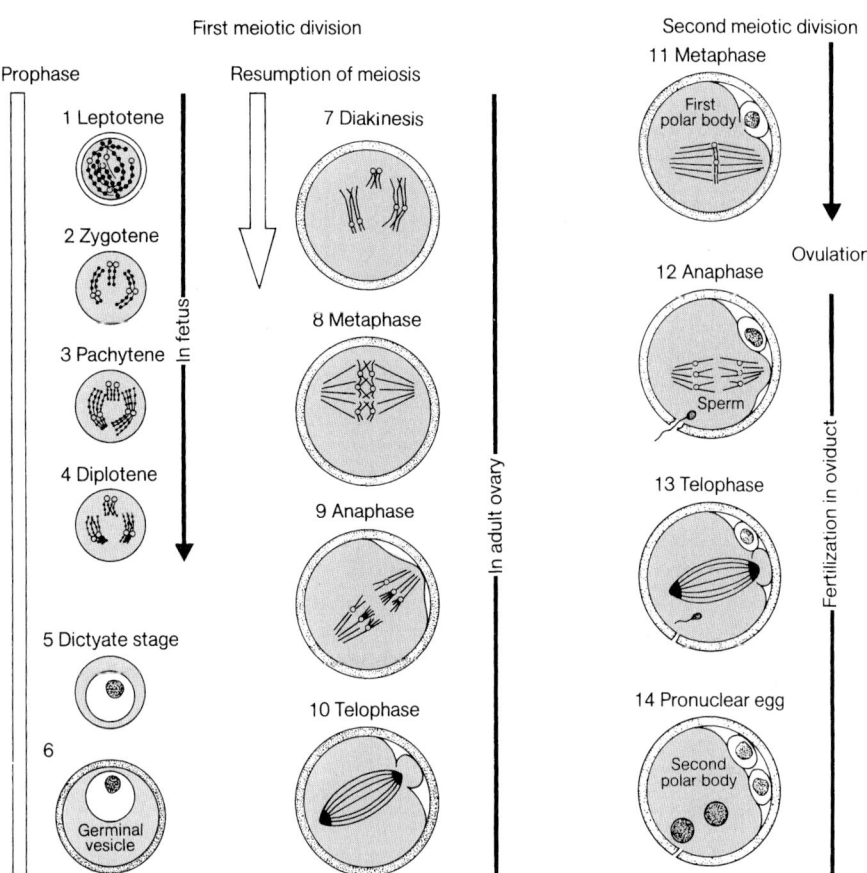

First meiotic division

Prophase

Resumption of meiosis

1 Leptotene

2 Zygotene

3 Pachytene

4 Diplotene

5 Dictyate stage

6

Germinal vesicle

In fetus

7 Diakinesis

8 Metaphase

9 Anaphase

10 Telophase

In adult ovary

Second meiotic division

11 Metaphase

First polar body

Ovulation

12 Anaphase

Sperm

13 Telophase

14 Pronuclear egg

Second polar body

Fertilization in oviduct

FIGURE 1-1 Diagram of oocyte meiosis. For simplicity, only three pairs of chromosomes are depicted. *1–4*, Prophase stages of the first meiotic division, which occur in most mammals during fetal life. The meiotic process is arrested at the diplotene stage ("first meiotic arrest"), and the oocyte enters the dictyate stages *(5–6)*. When meiosis is resumed, the first maturation division is completed *(7–11)*. Ovulation occurs usually at the metaphase II stage *(11)*, and the second meiotic division *(12–14)* takes place in the oviduct only after sperm penetration. (From Tsafriri A: Oocyte maturation in mammals. In Jones RE, ed: The vertebrate ovary, New York, 1978, Plenum Publishing Corp.)

stage, tight pairing of the chromosomes along their entire length, synapsis, takes place. The pachytene stage follows, during which the chromosome pairs contact one another and become shorter and thicker. During this stage each chromosome splits longitudinally, and two chromatids are produced that are united at the centromere. Thus the bivalent is now a structure composed of four closely opposed chromatids, or tetrads. The human ovum at pachytene demonstrates 23 tetrads. In the next stage, diplotene, the member chromosomes of the bivalents are held together only at certain points. At these terminal bridges, called chiasmata, the crossing over of genetic material takes place. The sister chromatids are still joined at the centromere, and crossing takes place only between the chromatids of homologous chromosomes and not between identical sister chromatids. The ovum then enters the dictyate stage, and meiosis is arrested. Ova at this stage usually form germinal vesicles. Initiation of the meiotic process occurs because of stimulation by meiotic-inducing substance,

which originates in the rete cords derived from the developing mesonephric tubules. Meiosis-preventing substance, probably produced by the granulosa cells of the differentiated ovarian follicle, acts as a countersubstance to inhibit meiosis. Apparently the interaction of these two substances regulates meiosis in the developing gonad. Once the ovum at the dictyate stage is encapsulated in granulosa cells, oogenesis is arrested because of the interruption of contact with the rete ovarii, and the meiosis-preventing substance becomes dominant.

After puberty, with follicle ripening, meiosis resumes in a few follicles during each cycle with the formation of the diakinesis stage. Here the bivalents contract, and the chiasmata move toward the end of the chromosomes. The homologs pull apart, and the nuclear membrane disappears, ending prophase I. Metaphase I then occurs. The bivalents, which are highly contracted, align themselves along the equatorial plate of the cell. Chromosomes derived from paternal and maternal sources line up completely at random to one another, and in the following stage, anaphase I, the homologous chromosomes of the bivalent pairs separate. Telophase I is similar to telophase in the mitotic process except that one daughter cell receives the majority of the cytoplasm and the second daughter cell becomes the first polar body. Both the oocyte and the polar body are present within the zona pellucida covering. The oocyte then advances immediately to metaphase II of the second meiotic division, during which time ovulation occurs. The remaining steps of the second meiotic division take place in the oviduct after sperm penetration takes place.

FERTILIZATION AND EARLY CLEAVAGE

In humans and most other mammals, the egg is released from the ovary in the metaphase II stage. At the time it enters the fallopian tube, it is surrounded by a cumulus of granulosa cells (cumulus oophorus) and intimately surrounded by a clear zona pellucida. Within the zona pellucida are both the egg and the first polar body. Meanwhile, spermatozoa are transported through the cervical mucus and the uterus and into the fallopian tubes. During this transport period they undergo two changes, capacitation and acrosome reaction, which essentially activate enzyme systems within the sperm head and make it possible for the sperm to transgress the cumulus oophorus and the zona pellucida.

Recent studies have shed light on how a sperm are attracted to an egg. The process known as chemotaxis seems to be related to capacitation of the sperm, which is aided by the binding of progesterone to a surface receptor on the sperm. This allows an increase in intracellular calcium ion, which increases sperm motility (chemokinesis). Oeheniger et al. noted that only 11% of sperm from fertile men had this progesterone combining capacity, but this response was far lower in infertile men. Villanueva-Diaz et al. have demonstrated that progesterone is a chemotoxic agent for spermatozoa. Ralt et al. have demonstrated that fluid from human follicles attract sperm and that follicular fluid from ova that were fertilized in vitro attracted sperm better than follicular fluid from ova that were not fertilized. They also showed that the fluid from the follicles of the ova that were fertilized caused sperm hypermobility.

Once the sperm has passed the barrier of the zona pellucida, it attaches to the cell membrane of the egg and enters the cytoplasm. When the sperm enters the cytoplasm, intracytoplasmic structures, the coronal granules, arrange themselves in an orderly fashion around the outermost portion of the cytoplasm just beneath the cytoplasmic membrane, and the sperm head swells and gives rise to the male pronucleus. The egg completes its second meiotic division, casting off the second polar body to a position also beneath the zona pellucida. The female pronucleus swells as well. In most mammals the male pronucleus can be recognized as the larger of the two. The pronuclei, which contain the haploid sets of chromosomes of maternal and paternal origin, do not fuse in mammals. However, the nuclear membranes surrounding them disappear, and the chromosomes contained within each membrane arrange themselves on the developing spindle of the first mitotic division. In this way the diploid complement of chromosomes is reestablished, completing the process of fertilization.

Cell division (cleavage) then occurs, giving rise to the two-cell embryo. The first division takes about 20 hours to complete, and the actual phase of fertilization generally occurs in the ampulla of the fallopian tube. A significant number of fertilized ova do not complete cleavage for a number of reasons, including failure of appropriate chromosome arrangement on the spindle, specific gene defects that prevent the formation of the spindle, and environmental factors. Teratogens acting at this point are usually either completely destructive or cause little or no effect. Twinning may occur by the separation of the two cells produced by cleavage, each of which has the potential to develop into a separate embryo. Twinning may occur at any stage until the formation of the blastula, since each cell is totipotential. Both genetic and environmental factors are probably involved in the causation of twinning.

Morula and Blastula Stage:
Early Differentiation

After the first mitotic division the cells continue to divide as the embryo passes along the fallopian tube and enters the uterus. This process takes 3 to 4 days after fertilization in the human, and the embryo may arrive at the uterus in any form, from 32 cells to the early blastula stage. In the human, implantation generally takes place 3 days after the embryo enters the uterus.

Implantation depends on the development of early trophoblastic cells during the blastula stage. These cells digest away the zona pellucida and allow the embryo to fix to the wall of the uterus and subsequently to burrow within the endometrium. The development of the blastula and the separation of the embryonic disk cells from the developing trophoblastic cells together make up the first stage of differentiation in the embryo. Again, at this stage of development, teratogens are generally either completely destructive or have little or no effect, since each of the cells of the early embryonic disk is multipotential. Differentiation within the embryonic disk, however, proceeds fairly rapidly, and if separation of cells and twinning occur at this point, the twins are frequently conjoined in some fashion. Figure 1-2 presents photomicrographs of several fresh human embryos obtained during in vitro fertilization. Various early cleavage stages are depicted as well. Figure 1-3 schematically demonstrates the process of

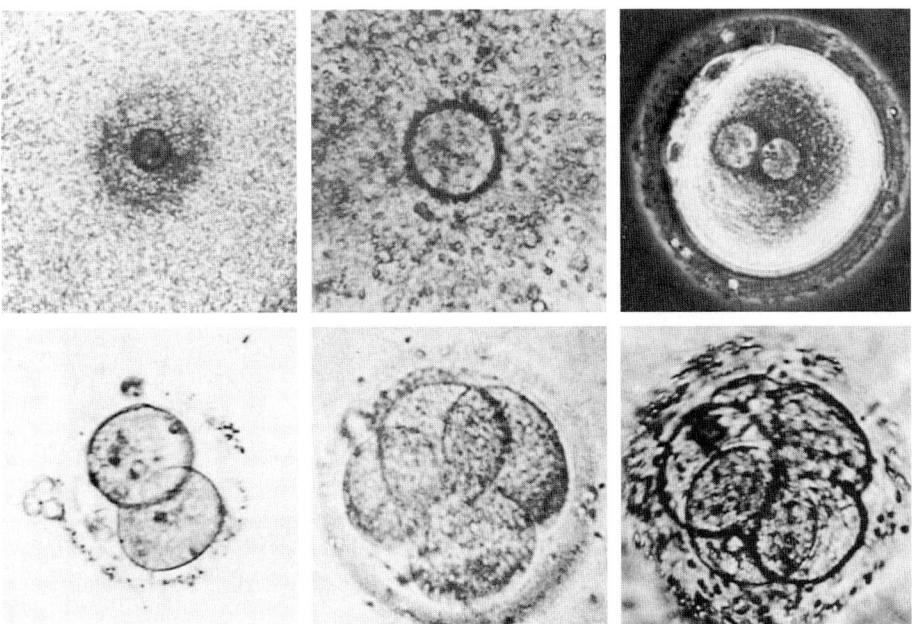

FIGURE 1-2 Six photomicrographs of fresh, unmounted human eggs and embryos. **A,** Early maturing oocyte. **B,** Mature oocyte surrounded by granulosal cells, zona pellucida visible. **C,** Fertilized oocyte demonstrating male and female pronuclei and both polar bodies. **D,** Two-cell zygote. **E,** Four-cell embryo. **F,** Eight-cell embryo.

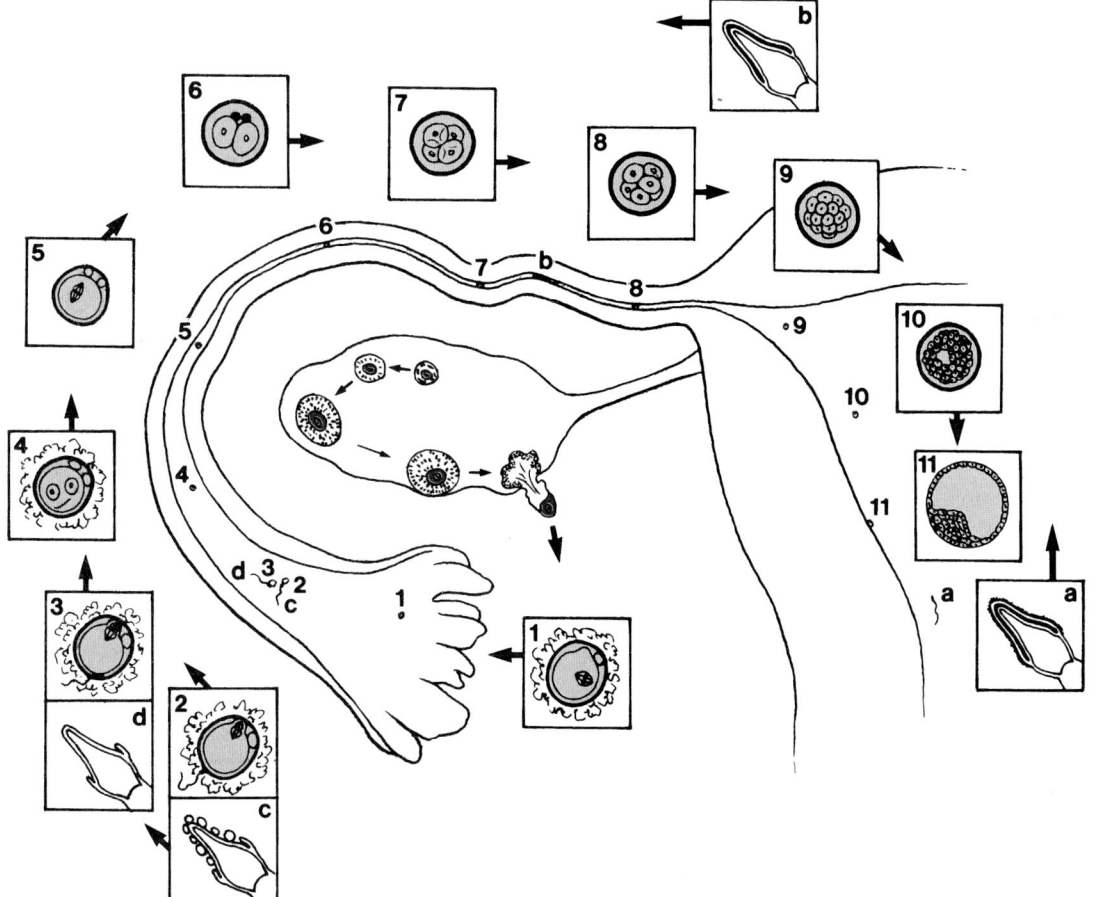

FIGURE 1-3 Diagrammatic representation of follicle growth, ovulation, sperm migration and maturation, fertilization, and preimplantation. *a–d,* Demonstrate sperm during migration through female tract accomplishing capacitation and acrosome reaction. *1,* Egg in meiosis enters fallopian tube after ovulating. *2,* Capacitated sperm penetrates cumulus cells and zona pellucida. *3,* Fertilization occurs; second meiotic division is complete. *4,* Male and female pronucleui are seen within the cytoplasm of egg; both polar bodies are present beneath the zona pellucida. *5,* First mitotic division takes place. *6,* Cleavage is complete. *7,* Four-cell stage. *8,* Eight-cell stage. *9,* Morula. *10,* Early blastocyst formation. *11,* Blastocyst formation; implantation occurs.

follicle growth, ovulation, sperm capacitation, fertilization, and preimplantation.

IMPLANTATION

Implantation has been noted to occur in the human embryo as early as day 6 after ovulation. For implantation to take place, the zona pellucida must be removed from the developing blastocyst, which occurs because of enzyme action produced either by cells of the blastocyst or by some endometrial enzymes. Endometrial capillaries in contact with the invading syncytiotrophoblast are engulfed to form venous sinuses at or about 7½ days after conception and are seen abundantly by day 9. Endometrial spiral arteries are not invaded at this point. The endoplasmic reticulum of the syncytiotrophoblast is probably responsible for the synthesis of chorionic gonadotrophin, which is well developed by 11 days after ovulation. Transfer is probably through the venous sinuses before intact circulation to the developing embryo has been established. It is important that chorionic gonadotrophin be transmitted to maternal circulation by one means or another, since it is responsible for maintaining the corpus luteum. Chorionic gonadotrophin has been detected in the peripheral blood of the mother as early as 6 days after ovulation but is always seen by the twelfth day. The concentration doubles every 1.2 to 2 days, reaching its highest point at 7 to 9 weeks of pregnancy.

Discussion of implantation is not complete without at least considering why the fetus is not immunologically rejected by the mother. Although it is not completely understood why rejection does not occur, some theories have been advanced. One theory suggests that some substance or substances suppress lymphocyte transformation in the mother. Such substances could be any that are produced by the embryo, including chorionic gonadotrophin, or by the decidua. Other theories include the production of suppressor T lymphocytes by the fetus, which could inhibit maternal lymphocyte transformation by secreting an inhibitory substance that crosses the placenta. One possibility is that an enzyme, indoleamine 2, 3-dioxygenase (IDO), is produced by the fetus, which destroys tryptophan needed by the mother's T cells to respond to the fetus. Alternatively, the phenomenon of enhancement, which states that weakly antigenic sites on the trophoblast are blocked by maternal antibodies, thereby rendering them unavailable to circulating T cells, is also a possibility. Finally, the trophoblast may prevent entry of maternal lymphocytes to the fetus by virtue of features of its cell membrane molecular structure or by substances secreted by it to block the action of maternal antibodies.

Table 1-1 describes the events of implantation.

TABLE 1-1
Events of Implantation

Event	Days After Ovulation
Zona pellucida disappears	4–5
Blastocyst attaches to epithelial surface of endometrium	6
Trophoblast erodes into endometrial stroma	7
Trophoblast differentiates into cytotrophoblastic and syncytial trophoblastic layers	7–8
Lacunae appear around trophoblast	8–9
Blastocyst burrows beneath endometrial surface	9–10
Lacunar network forms	10–11
Trophoblast invades endometrial sinusoids, establishing a uteroplacental circulation	11–12
Endometrial epithelium completely covers blastocyst	12–13
Strong decidual reaction occurs in stroma	13–14

Early Organogenesis in the Embryonic Period

During the third week after fertilization, the primitive streak forms in the caudal portion of the embryonic disk, and the embryonic disk begins to grow and change from a circular to a pear-shaped configuration. At that point the epithelium facing superiorly is considered ectoderm and will eventually give rise to the developing central nervous system, and the epithelium facing downward toward the yolk sac is endoderm. During this week the neuroplate develops with its associated notochordal process. By the sixteenth day after conception the third primitive germ layer, the intraembryonic mesoderm, begins to form between the ectoderm and endoderm. Early mesoderm migrates cranially, passing on either side of the notochordal process to meet in front in the formation of the cardiogenic area. The heart soon develops from this area. Later in the third week extraembryonic mesoderm joins with the yolk sac and the developing amnion to contribute to the developing membranes. An intraembryonic mesoderm develops on each side of the notochord and neural tube to form longitudinal columns, the paraxial mesoderm. Each paraxial column thins laterally into the lateral plate mesoderm, which is continuous with the extraembryonic mesoderm of the yolk sac and the amnion. The lateral plate mesoderm is separated from the paraxial mesoderm by a continuous tract of mesoderm called the intermediate mesoderm. By the twentieth day, paraxial mesoderm begins to divide into paired linear bodies known as somites. About 38 pairs of somites form during the next 10 days. Eventually a total of 42 to 44 pairs will develop, and these will give rise to body musculature.

Angiogenesis, or blood vessel formation, can be seen in the extraembryonic mesoderm of the yolk sac by day 15 or 16. Embryonic vessels can be seen about 2 days later and develop when mesenchymal cells known as angioblasts aggregate to form masses and cords called blood islands. Spaces then appear within these islands, and the angioblasts arrange themselves around these spaces to form primitive endothelium. Isolated vessels form channels and then grow into adjacent areas by endothelial budding. Primitive blood cells develop from endothelial cells as the vessels develop on the yolk sac and allantois. However, blood formation does not begin within the embryo until the second month of gestation, occurring first in the developing liver and later in the spleen, bone marrow, and lymph nodes. Separate mesenchymal cells surrounding the primitive endothelial vessels differentiate into muscular and connective tissue elements. The primitive heart forms in a similar manner from mesenchymal cells in the cardiogenic area. Paired endothelial channels called heart tubes develop by the end of the third week and fuse to form the primitive heart. By the twenty-first day, this primitive heart has linked up with blood vessels of the embryo, forming a primitive cardiovascular system. Blood circulation starts about this time, and the cardiovascular system becomes the first functioning organ system within the embryo.

From the fourth to the seventh week of gestation all the organ systems are formed. Only the genitourinary system is considered in detail later in this chapter.

A teratogenic event that takes place during the embryonic period gives rise to a constellation of malformations related to the organ systems that are actively developing at that particular time. Thus cardiovascular malformations tend to occur because of teratogenic events early in the embryonic period, whereas genitourinary abnormalities tend to occur because of events that occur later. Figure 1-4 demonstrates the malformations that were seen when thalidomide was applied to a human population during gestational days 35 to 50. Teratogenic effects before implantation often cause death but not malformations.

In general, the effects of a given teratogen depend on the genetic makeup of the individual, other environmental factors in play at the time, the stage during embryonic development that the teratogen is applied, and in some cases the dose of the teratogen and the duration that it is allowed to act. Some teratogens in and of themselves are harmless, but their metabolites cause the damage. Teratogens may be chemical substances and their by-products, or they may be physical entities, such as temperature elevation and irradiation. Teratogenic agents applied after the forty-ninth day of gestation may injure or kill the embryo or cause developmental and growth retardation but usually will not be responsible for specific malformations. The period of embryonic development is said to be complete when the embryo attains a crown-rump length of 30 mm. It corresponds in most cases to day 49 after conception.

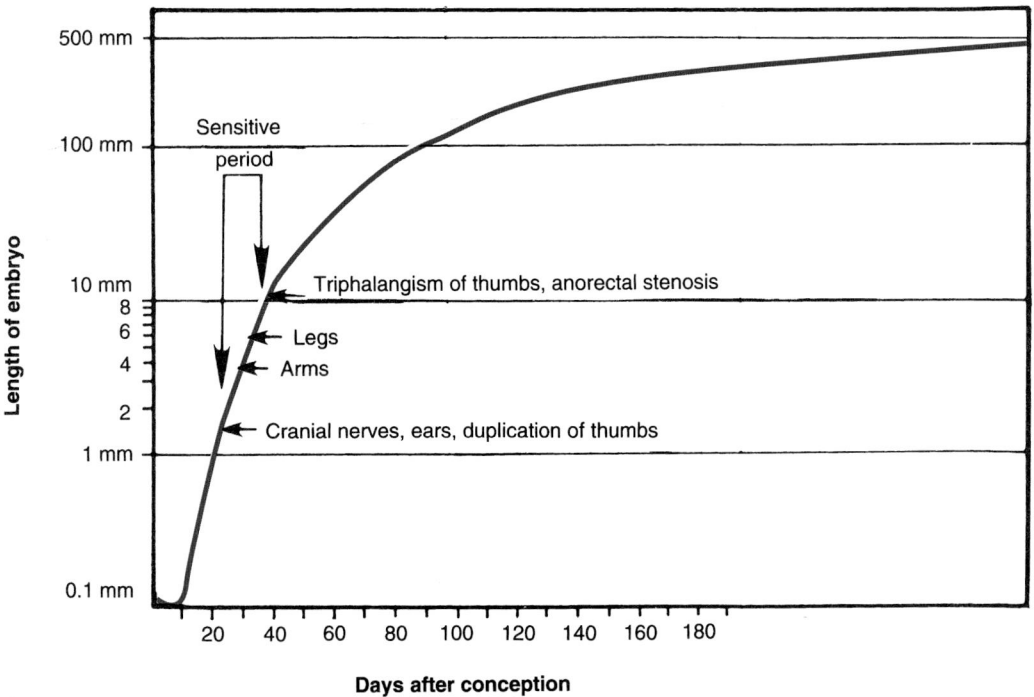

FIGURE 1-4 Schematic drawing of sensitive period for teratogenic effect of thalidomide with corresponding length of embryo. (From Lenz W: Chemicals and malformations in man. In Fishbein M, ed: Second International Conference on Congenital Malformations, New York, 1964, International Medical Congress.)

DEVELOPMENT OF THE GENITOURINARY SYSTEM

Excretory System

Nephrogenic cords develop from the intermediate mesoderm as early as the 2 mm embryo stage, beginning in the more cephalad portions of the embryo. Three sets of excretory ducts and tubules develop, each bilaterally. The first, the pronephros, with its pronephric ducts, forms in the most cranial portion of the embryo at about the beginning of the fourth week after conception. The tubules associated with the duct probably have no excretory function in the human. Late in the fourth week a second set of tubules, the mesonephric tubules, and their accompanying mesonephric ducts begin to develop. These are associated with tufts of capillaries, or glomeruli, and tubules for excretory purposes. Thus the mesonephros functions as a fetal kidney, producing urine for about 2 or 3 weeks. As new tubules develop, those derived from the more cephalad tubules degenerate. Usually about 40 mesonephric tubules function on either side of the embryo at any given time.

The metanephros, or permanent kidney, begins its development early in the fifth week of gestation and starts to function late in the seventh or early in the eighth week. The metanephros develops both from the metanephrogenic mass of mesoderm, which is the most caudal portion of the nephrogenic cord, and from its duct system, which is derived from the metanephric diverticulum (ureteric bud). It is a cranially growing outpouching of the mesonephric duct close to where it enters the cloaca. The latter gives rise to the ureter, the renal pelvis, the calyces, and the collecting tubules of the adult kidney. A critical process in the development of the kidney requires that the cranially growing metanephric diverticulum meet and fuse with the metanephrogenic mass of mesoderm so that formation of the kidney can take place. Originally the metanephric kidney is a pelvic organ, but by differential growth it becomes located in the lumbar region.

The fetus produces urine throughout all the periods of gestation, but the placenta handles the excretory functions of the fetus. The urine produced by the fetus contributes to the amniotic fluid. The fetus may swallow the amniotic fluid and recirculate it through the digestive system. This seems to be an important factor in regulating the amount of amniotic fluid present in the fetus. Agenesis of the kidneys generally results in little or no amniotic fluid, and gastrointestinal malformations or the inability of the fetus to swallow the amniotic fluid may lead to hydramnios.

Bladder and Urethra

The embryonic cloaca is divided by the urorectal septum into a dorsal rectum and a ventral urogenital sinus. The urogenital sinus, in turn, is divided into three parts: the cranial portion—the vesicourethral canal, which is continuous with the allantois; a middle pelvic portion; and a caudal urogenital sinus portion, which is closed over externally by the urogenital membrane. The epithelium of the developing bladder is derived from the endoderm of the vesicourethral canal. The muscular layers and serosa of the bladder develop from adjacent splanchnic mesenchyme. As the bladder develops, the caudal portion of the mesonephric ducts is incorporated into its dorsal wall. The portion of the mesonephric duct distal to the points where the metanephric duct is taken up into the bladder becomes the trigone of the bladder. Although this portion is mesoderm in origin, it is probably epithelialized eventually by endodermal epithelium from the urogenital sinus. In this way the ureters, derived from the metanephric duct, come to open directly into the bladder.

In the male the mesonephric ducts open into the urethra as the ejaculatory ducts. Also in the male, mesenchymal tissue surrounding the developing urethra where it exits the bladder develops into the prostate gland, through which the ejaculatory ducts traverse. Figure 1-5 demonstrates graphically the development of the male and female urinary systems.

The epithelium of the female urethra is derived from endoderm of the vesicourethral canal.

Bourdelat et al. described the development of the urethral sphincter. In a morphologic study carried out on 25 human embryos with crown-rump lengths of 3 to 60 mm and 20 human fetuses, ages 15 to 40 weeks, these authors demonstrated that a mesenchymal condensation forms around the urethra after the division of the cloaca in the 12- to 15-mm embryo. Then, following the opening of the anal membrane at the 20- to 30-mm stage, the pubo-rectalis muscle appears. At 15 weeks' gestation, striated muscle can be seen, and a smooth muscle layer thickens at the level of the developing bladder neck, forming the inner part of the urethral musculature. Thus the urethral sphincter is composed of both central smooth muscle and peripheral striated muscle. These authors and Kokoua et al. have demonstrated that the sphincter develops primarily in the anterior wall of the urethra in a horseshoe or omega shape.

Genital Duct System

Early in embryonic life, two sets of paired genital ducts develop in each sex: the mesonephric (wolffian) ducts and the paramesonephric (müllerian) ducts. The mesonephric duct development precedes the paramesonephric duct development. The paramesonephric ducts develop on each side of the mesonephric ducts from the evaginations of the coelomic epithelium. The more cephalad ends of the ducts open directly into the peritoneal cavity, and the distal ends grow caudally, fusing in the lower midline to form the uterovaginal primordium. This tubular structure joins the dorsal wall of the urogenital sinus and produces an elevation, the müllerian tubercle. The mesonephric ducts enter the urogenital sinus on either side of the tubercle.

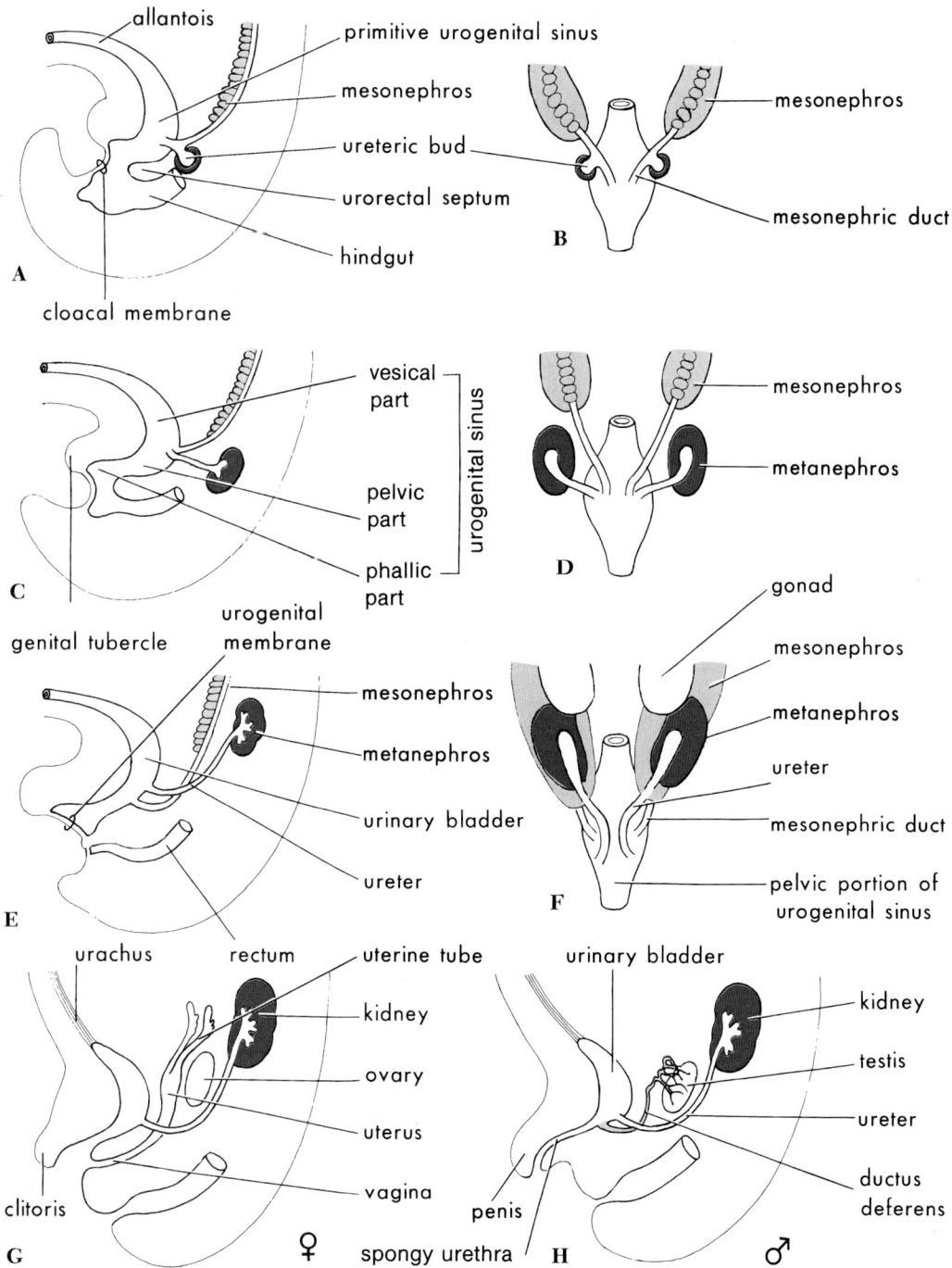

FIGURE 1-5 Graphic development of the urinary system in the male and female. Diagrams showing (1) division of the cloaca into urogenital sinus and rectum, (2) absorption of the mesonephric ducts, (3) development of the urinary bladder, urethra, and urachus, and (4) changes in the location of the ureters. **A,** Lateral view of the caudal half of 5-week-old embryo; **B, D,** and **F,** dorsal views; **C, E, G,** and **H,** lateral views. The stages shown in **G** and **H** are reached at about 12 weeks. (From Moore KL: The developing human: clinically oriented embryology, ed 3, Philadelphia, 1982, Courtesy WB Saunders Co.)

Male Genital Ducts

Some seminiferous tubules are produced in the fetal testes during the seventh and eighth weeks after conception, and in the eighth week interstitial (Leydig) cells differentiate and begin to produce testosterone. At this point the mesonephric duct differentiates into the vas deferens, epididymis, and seminal vesicles, and the müllerian anlage is suppressed by the action of a substance known as antimüllerian hormone (AMH). This has also been called müllerian inhibiting factor (MIF), produced by the Sertoli cells of the testes. The development of the prostate gland was referred to earlier. The bulbourethral glands, which are small structures that develop from outgrowths of endodermal tissue from the membranous portion of the urethra, incorporate stroma from the adjacent mesenchyme.

The most distal portion of the paramesonephric duct remains, in the male, as the appendix of the testes. The most proximal end of the paramesonephric duct remains as a small outpouching within the body of the prostate gland, known as the prostatic utricle. Occasionally the prostatic utricle is developed to the point where it will excrete a small amount of blood and cause hematuria in adult life.

Female Genital Ducts

In the presence of ovaries or of no gonads at all, the mesonephric ducts regress, and the paramesonephric ducts develop into the female genital tract. This process begins at about 6 weeks and proceeds in a cephalad and caudal fashion. The more cephalad portions of the paramesonephric ducts, which open directly into the peritoneal cavity, form the fallopian tubes. The fused portion, or uterovaginal primordium, gives rise to the epithelium and glands of the uterus and cervix. Endometrial stroma and myometrium are derived from adjacent mesenchyme.

Failure of development of the paramesonephric ducts leads to agenesis of the cervix and the uterus. Failure of fusion of the caudal portion of these ducts may lead to a variety of anomalies of the uterus, including complete duplication of the uterus and cervix or partial duplication of a variety of types, which are outlined in Chapter 11.

Peritoneal reflections in the area adjacent to the fusion of the two paramesonephric ducts give rise to the formation of the broad ligaments. Mesenchymal tissue here develops into the parametrium.

Pietryga and Wózniak studied the development of uterine ligaments in 12 human embryos and 76 fetuses. They noted the development of the round ligament at the eighth week, the cardinal ligaments at the tenth week, and the broad ligament at week 19. From weeks 8 to 17, the round ligament is connected to the uterine tube. Beginning at week 18, it arises separately to the border of the uterus.

The vagina develops from paired solid outgrowths of endoderm of the urogenital sinus, the sinovaginal bulbs. These grow caudally as a solid core toward the end of the uterovaginal primordium. This core constitutes the fibromuscular portion of the vagina. The sinovaginal bulbs then canalize to form the vagina. However, abnormalities in this process may lead to either transverse or horizontal vaginal septa. The junction of the sinovaginal bulbs with the urogenital sinus remains as the vaginal plate, which forms the hymen. This remains imperforate until late in embryonic life, although occasionally, perforation does not take place normally (imperforate hymen).

Failure of the sinovaginal bulbs to form leads to agenesis of the vagina. The precise boundary between the paramesonephric and urogenital sinus portions of the vagina has not been established.

Auxiliary genital glands in the female form from buds that grow out of the urethra. The buds derive contributions from the surrounding mesenchyme and form the urethral glands and the paraurethral glands (Skene's glands). These glands correspond to the prostate gland in males. Similar outgrowths of the urogenital sinus form the vestibular glands (Bartholin's glands), which are homologous to the bulbourethral glands in the male.

The remnants of the mesonephric duct in the female include a small structure called the appendix vesiculosa, a few blind tubules in the broad ligaments, the epoophoron, and a few blind tubules adjacent to the uterus collectively called the paroophoron. Remnants of the mesonephric duct system are often present in the broad ligaments or are adjacent to the uterus or the vagina as Gartner's duct cysts. The epoophoron or paroophoron may develop into cysts. Cysts of the epoophoron are known as paraovarian cysts.

Remnants of the paramesonephric duct in the female may be seen as a small, blind cystic structure attached by a pedicle to the distal end of the fallopian tube, the hydatid of Morgagni. Table 1-2 categorizes the adult derivatives and residual remnants of the urogenital structures in both the male and female. Figure 1-6 outlines schematically the development of the internal sexual organs in both sexes.

External Genitalia

In the fourth week after fertilization, the genital tubercle develops at the ventral tip of the cloacal membrane. Two sets of lateral bodies, the labioscrotal swellings and urogenital folds, develop soon after on either side of the cloacal membrane. The genital tubercle then elongates to form a phallus in both males and females. By the end of the sixth week, the cloacal membrane is joined by the urorectal septum. The septum separates the cloaca into the urogenital sinus ventrally and the anal canal and rectum dorsally. The point on the cloacal membrane where the urorectal septum fuses becomes the location of the perineal body in later development. The cloacal membrane is then divided into the ventral urogenital membrane and the dorsal anal membrane. These membranes then rupture, opening the vulva and the anal canal. Failure of the anal membrane to rupture gives rise to an imperforate anus. With the opening of the urogenital membrane, a urethral groove forms on the undersurface of the phallus, completing the undifferentiated portion of external genital development. Differences between male and female embryos can be noted as early as the ninth week, but the distinct final forms are not noted until 12 weeks.

TABLE 1-2
Male and Female Derivatives of Embryonic Urogenital Structures

Embryonic Structure	Derivatives	
	Male	**Female**
Labioscrotal swellings	Scrotum	Labia majora
Urogenital folds	Ventral portion of penis	Labia minora
Phallus	Penis	Clitoris
	Glans, corpora cavernosa penis, and corpus spongiosum	Glans, corpora cavernosa, bulb of the vestibule
Urogenital sinus	Urinary bladder	Urinary bladder
	Prostate gland	Urethral and paraurethral glands
	Prostatic utricle	Vagina
	Bulbourethral glands	Greater vestibular glands
	Seminal colliculus	Hymen
Paramesonephric duct	Appendix of testes	Hydatid of Morgagni
		Uterus and cervix
		Fallopian tubes
Mesonephric duct	Appendix of epididymis	Appendix vesiculosis
	Ductus of epididymis	Duct of epoophoron
	Ductus deferens	Gartner's duct
	Ejaculatory duct and seminal vesicle	—
Metanephric duct	Ureter, renal pelvis, calyces, and collecting system	Ureter, renal pelvis, calyces, and collecting system
Mesonephric tubules	Ductuli efferentes	Epoophoron
	Paradidymis	Paroophoron
Undifferentiated gonad	Testis	Ovary
Cortex	Seminiferous tubules	Ovarian follicles
Medulla	—	Medulla
	Rete testis	Rete ovarii
Gubernaculum	Gubernaculum testis	Round ligament of uterus

Androgens produced by the testes are responsible for the masculinization of the undifferentiated external genitalia. The phallus grows in length to form a penis, and the urogenital folds are pulled forward to form the lateral walls of the urethral groove on the undersurface of the penis. These folds then fuse to form the penile urethra. Defects in fusion of various amounts give rise to various degrees of hypospadias. The skin at the distal margin of the penis grows over the glans to form the prepuce (foreskin). The vascular portion of the penis (corpora cavernosa penis and corpus cavernosum urethrae) arises from the mesenchymal tissue of the phallus. Finally, the labioscrotal swellings grow toward each other and fuse in the midline to form the scrotum. Later in embryonic life, usually at about the twenty-eighth week, the testes descend through the inguinal canal guided by the gubernaculum.

Kalloo et al. in 1993 demonstrated the presence of androgen receptors in the corpus cavernosum and the stroma of the inner prepuce, scrotum, and periphery of the glans penis. The corpus spongiosum was not yet developed at this fetal age, but its primordium, the peri-urethral mesenchyme, was very rich in androgen receptors. The epithelium of the preputial skin, penile shaft skin, and scrotal skin were androgen receptor negative. No estrogen receptors were noted in these regions, suggesting that there was no direct influence of maternal estrogen on male genital development. Female external genital structures contained androgen receptors, and the distribution of androgen receptors resembled that of the male. This would explain why female genitalia can be masculinized if exposed to high androgen levels early in gestation.

In the absence of androgen stimulation, feminization of the undifferentiated external genitalia occurs. The embryonic phallus does not demonstrate rapid growth and becomes the clitoris. Urogenital folds do not fuse except in front of the anus. The unfused urogenital folds form the labia minora. The labioscrotal folds fuse posteriorly in the area of the perineal body but laterally remain as the labia majora. The labioscrotal folds fuse anteriorly to form the mons pubis. A portion of the urogenital sinus between the level of the hymen and the labia develops into the vestibule of the vagina, into

☐ Urogenital sinus   ■ Mesonephric duct   ▨ Paramesonephric duct

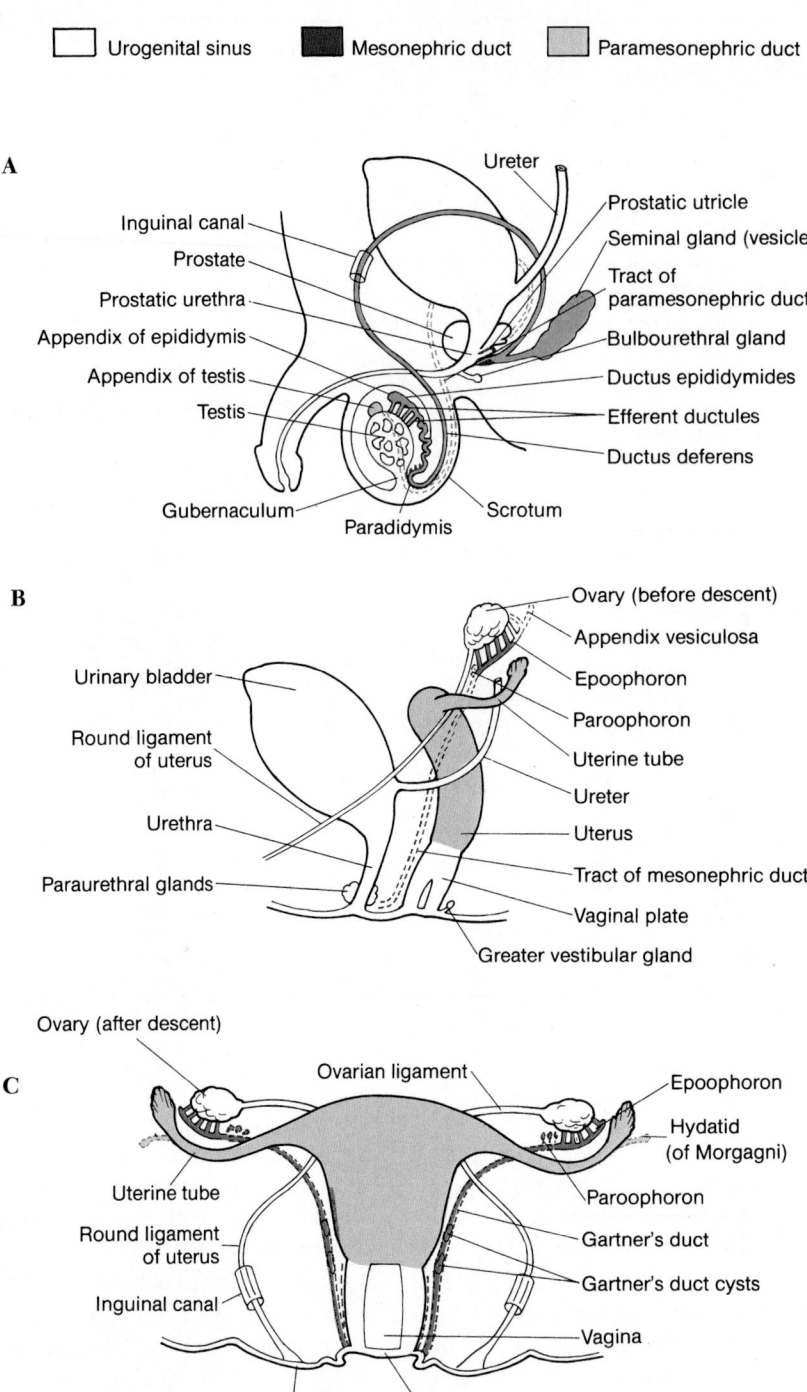

FIGURE 1-6 Schematic drawings illustrating development of male and female reproductive systems from the primitive genital ducts. Vestigial structures are also shown. **A,** Reproductive system in a newborn male. **B,** Reproductive system in a female fetus at 12 weeks. **C,** Reproductive system in a newborn female. (From Moore KL: The developing human: clinically oriented embryology, Philadelphia, 1973, WB Saunders Co.)

which the urethra, the vagina, and the ducts of Bartholin's glands enter. The work of Kalloo et al. demonstrated that the female external genitalia were also intensely estrogen receptor positive compared with the genitalia of the male. These receptors were seen primarily in the stroma of the labia minora and in the periphery of the glans and interprepuce. The presence of such receptors suggests that there may be a direct role of maternal estrogens in the development of female external genitalia. This is in contrast to the long-held belief that female genital development was passive and occurred in the absence of androgens.

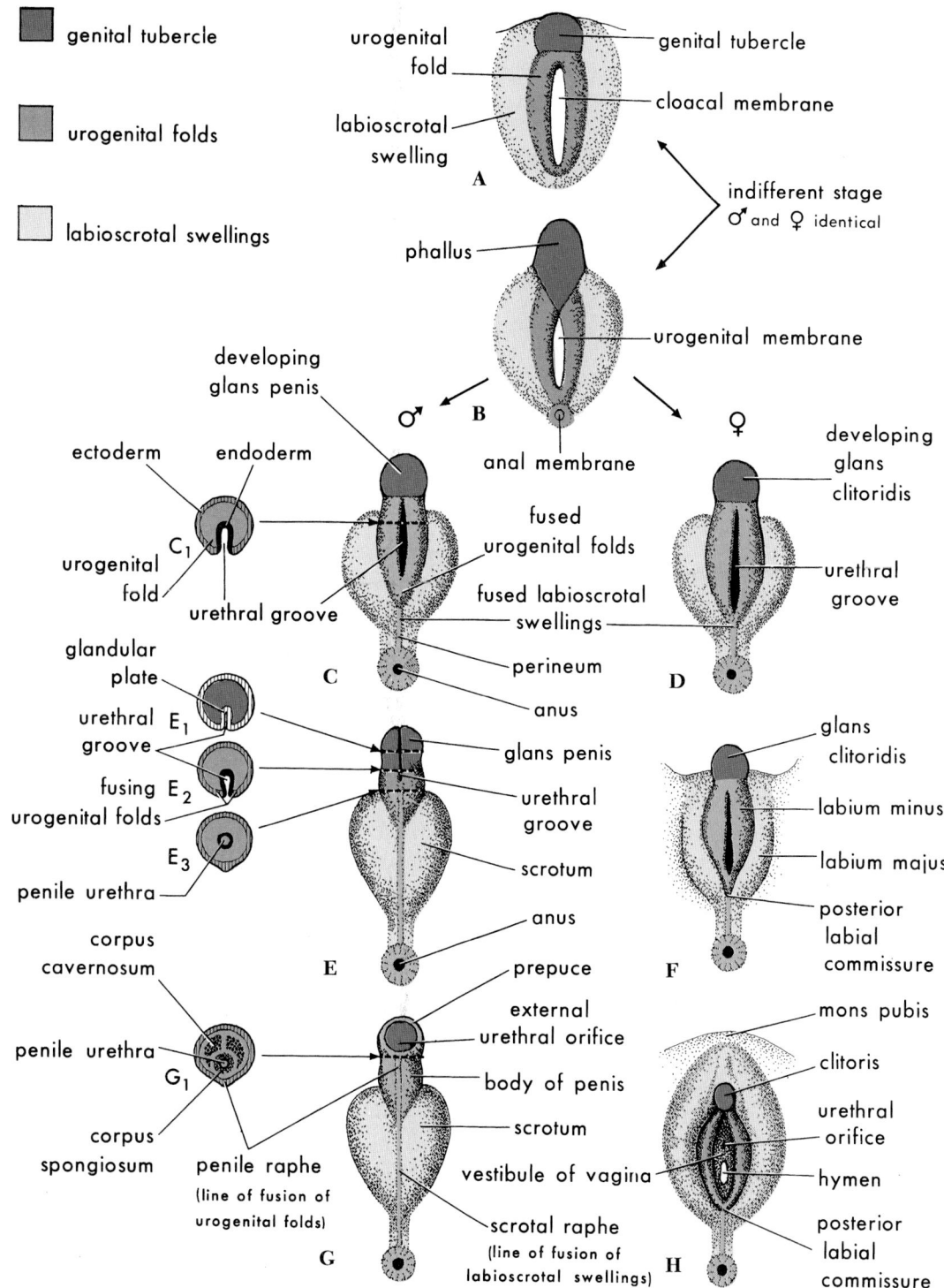

FIGURE 1-7 **A** and **B,** Development of the external genitalia in different stages (4 to 7 weeks). **C, E,** and **G,** Stages in the development of the external male genitalia at about 9, 11, and 12 weeks, respectively. To the left are schematic transverse sections (*C1, E1* to *E3,* and *G1*) through the developing penis, illustrating formation of the penile urethra. **D, F,** and **H,** Stages in the development of the female external genitalia at 9, 11, and 12 weeks, respectively. (From Moore KL: The developing human: clinically oriented embryology, ed 3, Philadelphia, 1982, Courtesy WB Saunders Co.)

The ovaries do not descend into the labioscrotal folds. A structure similar to the gubernaculum develops in the inguinal canal, giving rise to the round ligaments, which suspend the uterus in the adult. Figure 1-7 summarizes the development of the external genitalia in each sex.

SEX DIFFERENTIATION

Genetic sex is determined at the time of conception. In general, a Y chromosome is necessary for the development of the testes, and the testes are responsible for the organization of the sexual duct system to a male configuration and for the suppression of the paramesonephric system. In the absence of a Y chromosome, indeed, in the absence of a gonad, development will be female in nature. General phenotypic development of the female seems to be a neutral event or perhaps one related to maternal estrogen activity.

One theory on sex differentiation is that genes coded on the Y chromosome are responsible for the development of a cell-specific protein, the H-Y antigen. In rare cases a Y chromosome may be absent, but the H-Y antigen may express itself. In theory, one could speculate that in such cases the H-Y antigen was indeed present on another chromosome, most likely the X chromosome, and that either an activator gene or some other gene that acts as an activator is capable of stimulating its response. A gene very similar to H-Y has been found on the X chromosome.

Recently Amice et al. noted H-Y-positive lymphocytes in women with both idiopathic hirsutism and hirsute women with polycystic ovaries. These authors concluded that women can produce H-Y antigen in the same way as men and that hirsutism is associated with an increase in H-Y antigen.

New evidence suggests an alternative theory, which uses evidence that at least two genes are involved. The first is a testis-determining gene probably coded on the Y chromosome and designated TDF (testis-determining factor). The second is an ovary-determining gene present on either the X chromosome or an autosome and designated Od. These genes are believed to interact and initiate either testis or ovary development, depending on their presence and time of expression in development. Thus in a normal XY male the TDF gene is probably expressed earlier than the Od gene and may be responsible for Od inactivation. With a lack of TDF in the normal XX female, the Od gene is expressed, and the ovary develops. Sinclair et al. have described a 35-kilobase region on the human Y chromosome necessary for the male sex determination. This gene shows homology with other mammals, including the mouse, and is a candidate to be the TDF gene. In 1991 Koopman et al. demonstrated in the mouse that a gene Sry (sex-determining region Y) not only was involved in testes determination but also was the only gene on the Y chromosome required for this to occur. This gene is present in other mammals, including humans. It is a relatively small gene and qualifies as the testes-determining gene. Evidence for the association of mutations within the DNA-binding domain of this gene with male to female sex reversal in humans and also male sex reversal seen when a small fragment including this gene was transgenetically placed into an XX mouse embryo supports the thesis that this is probably the case. The transgene experiment carried out by Koopman therefore showed that Sry not only was involved in testes determination but also that it was the only gene on the Y chromosome required for this process.

Lovell-Badge in 1993 reviewed the action of this gene and concluded that it acted during the critical period of gonadal differentiation to divert the normal or default pathway of gene activity that would otherwise lead to the development of ovaries into one that leads to the development of testes. It was postulated that it acts on the precursor cells that would give rise to Sertoli cells in the testis or follicle cells in the ovary, forcing the rest of the cells in the gonad to follow its determined pathway. It was concluded that the process depended on cell-cell interaction, since it is not required within the non-Sertoli cells for their differentiation. Sry is a gene that produces proteins necessary for DNA binding, permitting other factors to interact, which, in turn, can either activate or repress transcription. Thus the gene seems to influence cell fate rather than direct it. The means by which the gene actually works is not known. Lovell-Badge speculates that it may be a repressor acting on the female pathway of gonad differentiation long enough to allow the male pathway of gene activity to operate.

An interesting bit of evidence for the importance of the Sry gene in the development of male sexual differentiation is seen in the 45,X/47, XYY mosaics. Hsu reviewed the phenotypes of 15 postnatally diagnosed cases and found that 8 were female, 3 male, and 4 intersex. He postulated that the sex reversal occurred because of deletion or mutation of the Sry gene. To date, more than 30 mutations of the Sry gene have been reported and all are associated with sex reversals (female phenotype). Takagi et al. reported a case of a 45,X/47,XYY female who demonstrated a single nucleotide deletion, which led to a frame shift mutation. The mutation was apparently a new mutation, since it was not found in the father's DNA.

During the fifth week after conception, coelomic epithelium, later known as germinal epithelium, thickens in the area of the medial aspect of the mesonephros. As germinal epithelial cells proliferate, they invade the underlying mesenchyme, producing a prominence known as the gonadal ridge. In the sixth week the primordial germ cells, which have formed at about week 4 in the wall of the yolk sac, migrate up the dorsal mesentery of the hindgut and enter the undifferentiated gonad. For the formation of a testis, H-Y antigen must be activated. The somatic cells of the primitive gonadal ridge then differentiate into interstitial cells (Leydig cells) and Sertoli cells. As they do so, the primordial germ cells and Sertoli cells become enclosed within seminiferous tubules, and the interstitial cells remain outside these tubules. H-Y antigen can be demonstrated in Sertoli cells at this stage but not in the developing germ cells. However, the H-Y antigen activity is passed to the germ cells by Sertoli cells when they are encased in the seminiferous tubules in the seventh and eighth weeks. In the eighth week Leydig cells differentiate and begin to produce testosterone.

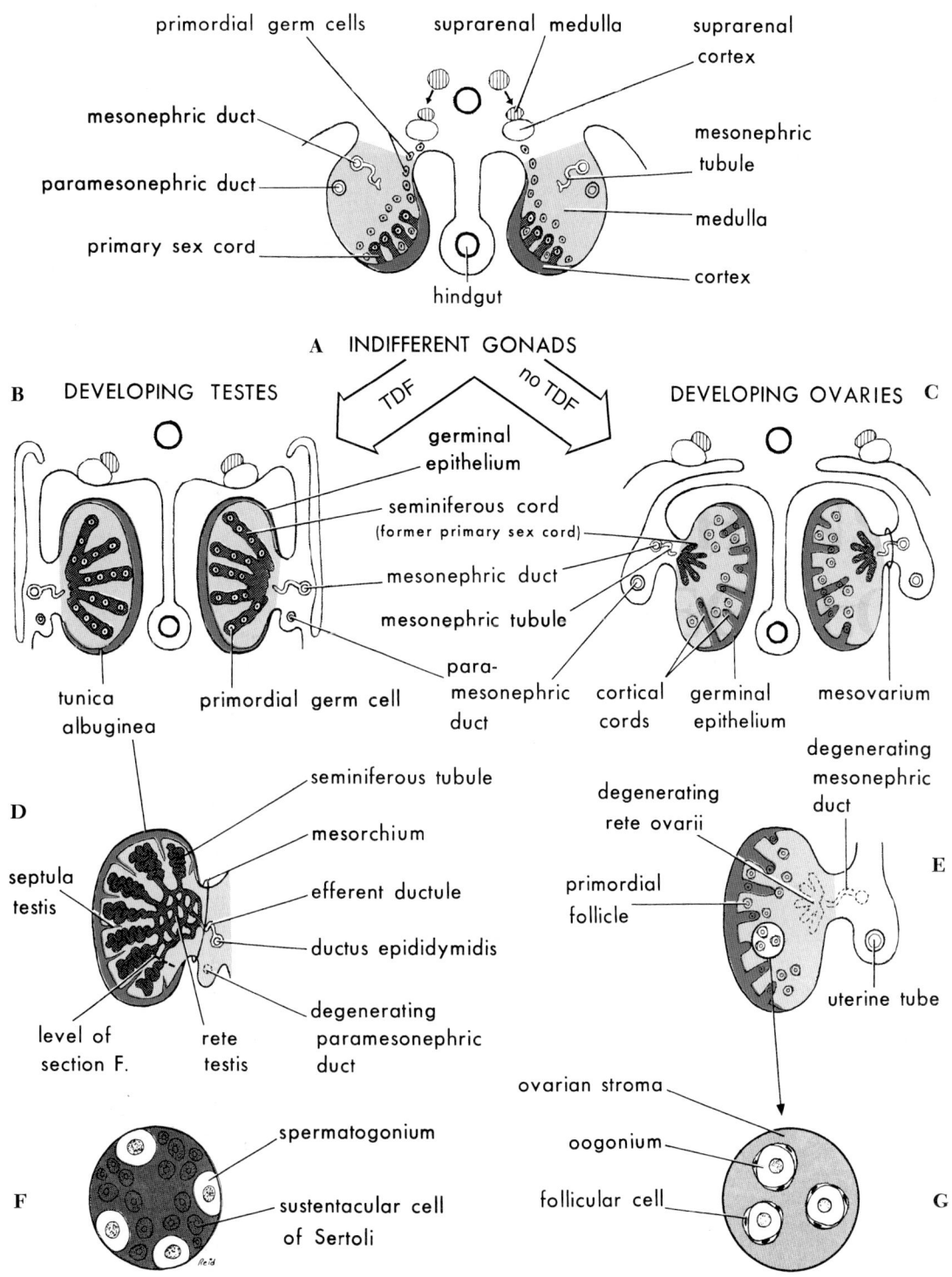

FIGURE 1-8 Differences in development in gonads of each sex. TDF = Testicular development factor. (From Moore KL: The developing human: clinically oriented embryology, ed 5, Philadelphia, 1993, Courtesy WB Saunders Co.)

At this point the mesonephric (wolffian) duct differentiates into the vas deferens, epididymis, and seminal vesicles while the paramesonephric duct is suppressed because of the action of anti-müllerian hormone (AMH).

Primary sex cords, meanwhile, have condensed and extended to the medullary portion of the developing testes. They branch and join to form the rete testis. The testis therefore is primarily a medullary organ, and eventually the rete testis connects with the tubules of the mesonephric system and joins the developing epididymal duct.

In specific androgen target areas, testosterone is converted to 5-α-dihydrotestosterone by the microsomal enzyme Δ-4-5-α-reductase. Data suggest that two androgens, testosterone and its metabolite, dihydrotestosterone, are involved in sexual differentiation in the male fetus, with selective roles for each hormone during embryogenesis; that is, dihydrotestosterone stimulates the testes and scrotum, and testosterone stimulates the prostate gland.

Androgen action must be initiated at the target areas. Testosterone enters the cell and either is bound to a cytoplasmic receptor or, in certain target tissue, is converted to dihydrotestosterone. Dihydrotestosterone in such cells would then bind to a cytoplasmic receptor. Afterward, the androgen-receptor complex gains access to the nucleus, where it binds to chromatin and initiates the transcription of messenger ribonucleic acid. This leads to the metabolic process of androgen action.

For normal male development in utero, the testes must differentiate and function normally. At a critical point, AMH, produced by Sertoli cells, and testosterone, secreted by Leydig cells, must be produced in sufficient amounts. AMH acts locally in suppressing the müllerian duct system, and testosterone acts systemically, causing differentiation of the mesonephric duct system and affecting male development of the urogenital tubercle, urogenital sinus, and urogenital folds. Thus the masculinization of the fetus is a multifactorial process under a variety of genetic controls. Genes on the Y chromosome are responsible for testicular differentiation. Enzymes involved in testosterone biosynthesis and conversion to dihydrotestosterone are regulated by genes located on autosomes. The ability to secrete AMH is a recessive trait coded on either an autosome or the X chromosome, and genes for development of cytoplasmic receptors of androgens seem to be coded on the X chromosome.

Development of the ovary occurs at about the eleventh or twelfth week. Two functional X chromosomes seem necessary for optimal development of the ovary. The effect of an X chromosome deficiency is most severe in species in which there is a long period between the formation and use of oocytes (i.e., the human). Thus in 45,X and 46,XY females, the ovaries are almost invariably devoid of oocytes. On the other hand, germ cells in the testes do best when only one X chromosome is present; rarely do they survive in the XX or XXY condition.

When non-Y-bearing oocytes enter the differentiating gonad, the primary sex cords do not become prominent but, instead, break up and encircle the oocytes in the cortex of the gonad. This occurs at about 16 weeks, and the isolated cell clusters derived from the cortical cords that surround the oocytes are called primordial follicles. No new oogonia form after birth, and many of the oogonia degenerate before birth. Those that remain grow and become primary follicles to be stimulated after puberty. Figure 1-8 illustrates the differences in development in the gonads of each sex.

KEY POINTS

- Oocyte meiosis is arrested at prophase I from the fetal period until the time of ovulation.

- Fertilization occurs in the ampulla of the fallopian tube before the second polar body is cast off.

- After fertilization, first cell division leading to the two-cell embryo takes 20 hours.

- The human embryo enters the uterus somewhere between 3 and 4 days after conception. At this point it will be between the 32-cell and blastocyst stages of development.

- Implantation occurs when trophoblastic cells contact endometrium and burrow beneath the surface by enzymatic action. This generally takes place 3 days after the embryo enters the uterus.

- Twinning may occur at any time until the formation of the blastula, after which time each cell is no longer multipotential.

- The earliest fetal epithelium to develop is the ectoderm; the second is the endoderm; and the third is the mesoderm.

- Chorionic gonadotrophin is secreted by the syncytiotrophoblast at about the time of implantation. It doubles in quantity every 1.2 to 2 days until 7 to 9 weeks of gestation.

- Angiogenesis is seen by day 15 or 16. Embryonic heart function begins in the third week of gestation.

- Organogenesis is complete by day 49.

- The mesonephric duct system gives rise in the male to the epididymis, vas deferens, and seminal vesicles. Remnants of the mesonephric duct system in the female remain as parovarian cysts and Gartner's duct.

- The paramesonephric duct system develops in the female to give rise to the fallopian tube, uterus, and cervix. Remnants give rise to the hydatid of Morgagni at the end of the fallopian tubes. Remnants in the male remain as the appendix of the testes and prostatic utricle. This duct system is suppressed in the male by the action of anti-müllerian hormone (AMH).

- The vagina develops from the sinovaginal bulbs, which are outgrowths of the urogenital sinus. Failure of these bulbs to form leads to agenesis of the vagina.

- The adult kidney develops from the metanephros, and its collecting system (ureter and calyceal system) develops from the metanephric (ureteric) bud from the mesonephric duct.

- The urinary bladder develops from the urogenital sinus.

- A Y chromosome is responsible for the development of testes. Without the presence of a Y chromosome, the gonadal development is usually that of an ovary or is undifferentiated. If no testicular tissue is present, the paramesonephric duct system develops into a phenotypic female configuration, and the mesonephric duct system is suppressed.

- The genital tubercle elongates to form the penis in the male and the clitoris in the female.

- Two functional X chromosomes are necessary for optimal development of the ovary.

BIBLIOGRAPHY

Amice B, Bercovic JP, Nahoul K, et al: Increase in H-Y antigen-positive lymphocytes in hirsute women: effects of cyproterone acetate and estradiol treatment, J Clin Endocrinol Metab 68:58, 1989.

Billington WD: Maternal immune response in pregnancy, Reprod Fertil Dev 1:183, 1989.

Blackmore P, Beebe S, Danforth D, Alexander N: Progesterone and 19-alpha-hydroxyprogesterone level stimulators of calcium influx in human sperm, J Biol Chem 265:1376, 1990.

Bourdelat D, Barbet JP, and Butler-Browne GS: Fetal development of the urethral sphincter, Eur J Pediatr Surg 2:35, 1992.

Cohen-Dayag A, Ralt D, Tur-Kaspa I, Manor M, Mahler A, Dor J, et al: Sequential acquisition of chemotactic responsiveness by human spermatozoa, Biol Reprod 50:786, 1994.

Feckner P: The role of Sry in mammalian sex determination, Acta Paediatr Jpn 38:380, 1996.

Hartman CG: Science and the safe period: a compendium of human reproduction, Huntington, NY, 1972, RE Krieger Publishing Co.

Harvey VR, Jackson DI, Hextal PJ, et al: DNA binding activity of recombiant SRY from normal males and XY females, Science 225:453, 1992.

Heap RV, Flint AP, and Gadsby JE: Role of embryonic signals in the establishment of pregnancy, Br Med J 35:129, 1979.

Hsu L: Phenotype/karyotype correlations of Y chromosome aneploidy with emphasis on structural aberrations in postnatally diagnosed cases, Am J Med Genet 53:108, 1994.

Kalloo NB, Gearhart JP, and Barrack ER: Sexually dimorphic expression of estrogen receptors, but not of androgen receptors in human fetal external genitalia, J Clin Endocrinol Metab 77:692, 1993.

Kokoua A, Homsy Y, Lavigne JF, et al: Maturation of the external urinary sphincter: a comparative histotopographic study in humans, J Urol 150:617, 1993.

Koopman P, Gubbay J, Vivian N, et al: Male development of chromosomally female mice transgenic for Sry, Nature 351:117, 1991.

Lenz W: Chemicals and malformations in man. In Fishbein M, ed: Second International Conference on Congenital Malformations, New York, 1964, International Medical Congress.

Lovell-Badge R: Sex determining gene expression during embryogenesis, Philos Trans R Soc Lond B Biol Sci 27:339, 1993.

Mohr LR, Trounson AO, Leeton JF, and Wood C: Evaluation of normal and abnormal human embryo development during procedures in vitro. In Beier HM and Lindner HR, eds: Fertilization of human egg in-vitro, Berlin, 1983, Springer-Verlag.

Moor RM and Warnes RM: Meiosis in mammalian oocytes, Br Med Bull 35:97, 1979.

Moore KL: The developing human: clinically oriented embryology, Philadelphia, 1973, WB Saunders Co.

Moore KL: The developing human: clinically oriented embryology, ed 3, Philadelphia, 1982, WB Saunders Co.

Moore KL and Persaud TVN: The developing human: clinically oriented embryology, ed 5, Philadelphia, 1993, WB Saunders Co.

Oeheninger S, Blackmore P, Morshedi M, Sueldo C, Acosta A, Alexander NJ: Defective calcium influx and acrosome reaction (spontaneous and progesterone-induced) in spermatozoa of infertile men with severe teratozoospermia, Fertil Steril 61:349, 1994.

Parhar RS, Yagel S, and Lala PK: PGE-2-mediated immunosuppressive by first trimester: human decidual cells block activation of maternal leukocytes in the decidua with potential antitrophoblast activity, Cell Immunol 120:61, 1989.

Patton HD, Fuchs AF, Hill EB, et al: Textbook of physiology, vol 2, Philadelphia, 1989, WB Saunders Co.

Pietryga E and Wózniak W: The development of the uterine ligaments in human fetuses, Folia Morphol 51:181, 1992.

Ralt D, Goldenberg M, Fetterolf P, Thompson D, Dor J, Mashiach S, et al: Sperm attraction of follicular factor(s) correlated with human egg fertilizability, Proc Natl Acad Sci USA 88:2840, 1991.

Ralt D, Manor M, Cohen-Dayag A, Tur-Kaspa I, Ben-Shlomo I, Makler A, et al: Chemotaxis and chemokinesis of human spermatozoa to follicular factor, Biol Reprod 50:774, 1994.

Short RV: Sex determination in differentiation, Br Med Bull 35:121, 1979.

Sinclair AH, Berta P, Palmer MS, et al: A gene from the human sex-determining region encodes a protein with homology to a conserved DNA-binding motif, Nature 346:240, 1990.

Thomas P, Meiezel S: Phosphatidylimositol 4,5-bisphosphate hydrolysis in human sperm stimulated with follicular fluid on progesterone is dependent on Ca++ influx, Biochem J 264:539, 1989.

Tsafriri A: Oocyte maturation in mammals. In Jones RE, ed: The vertebrate ovary, New York, 1978, Plenum Publishing Corp.

Tsafriri A, Bar-Ami S, and Lindner HR: Control of the development of meiotic competence in an oocyte maturation in mammals. In Beier HM and Lindner HR, eds: Fertilization of human egg in-vitro, Berlin, 1983, Springer-Verlag.

Villanueva-Diaz C, Arias-Martinez J, Bernejo-Martinez L, Vadillo-Ortega F: Progesterone indices human sperm chemotaxis. Fertil Steril 64:1183, 1995.

Whittingham DG: In-vitro fertilization, embryo transfer and storage, Br Med Bull 35:105, 1979.

Yang J, Seres C, Philibet D, Robel P, Baulieu EE, Jouarnet P: Progesterone and RU 486: Opposing effects on human sperm, Proc Natl Acad Sci USA 91:529, 1994.

Reproductive Genetics

Gene Action, Mutation, Types of Inheritance, Counseling Issues, Oncogenes

KEY TERMS AND DEFINITIONS

Allele. Any different form of a gene that occupies the same position on homologous chromosomes and has a similar function.

Centromere. A region of a chromosome known as a primary constriction forming a point at which the chromatids are held together during meiosis and mitosis. It is also the point that attaches to the spindle and has been called the *kinetochore*. It is the dynamic center for disjunction in both meiosis and mitosis.

Chimerism. The presence of two different cell populations derived from two separate conceptuses within the same individual.

Chromatid. A constituent strand of chromosome seen in prophase, after division of the chromosomes.

Chromatid Break. Separation in chromatin material in one chromatid arm only.

Chromosome. A nuclear structure containing genes in linear arrangements. Short arms are designated "p," and long arms are designated "q." The loss of all or a portion of the arm is designated by a –. Additions to arms are designated by a +. For example, 5p– indicates that all or a portion of the short arm of chromosome 5 is missing.

Codon. A sequence of three purine or pyrimidine bases representing the code for a specific amino acid.

Deletion. The loss of a chromosome or part of a chromosome (partial deletion).

Deoxyribonucleic Acid (DNA). A molecule composing the basic chemical constituents of the chromosome arranged in the form of a double helix, each strand containing a sugar (deoxyribose), a phosphate, and a purine

(adenine, guanine) or a pyrimidine (thymine, cytosine) base. The sequence of these bases determines the code of the genetic message.

Expressivity. The degree to which a phenotypic change occurs in a specific individual.

Fragment. A small piece of chromosome separated from its centromere.

Gene. A unit of genetic information, a sequence of nucleotides that forms the code for the production of a specific protein.

Gene Cloning. The process by which a segment of the DNA molecule is isolated and stimulated to produce multiple copies (amplification). This produces large amounts of identical copies that can be more easily studied.

Genome. A complete complement of genes found in a haploid set of chromosomes.

Genotype. The gene assortment of an individual.

Insertion. A condition occurring when a fragment of one chromosome is inserted into another chromosome; the final product is a chromosome with a new piece inserted into its midposition.

Inversion. A condition occurring when a chromosome suffers two breaks with a 180-degree rotation of the fragments. If the centromere is involved in the inversion, the condition is called a *pericentric inversion*. If the centromere is not included, it is called a *paracentric inversion*.

Isochromosome. An abnormal chromosome that is produced by a transverse split instead of the usual longitudinal split of the centromere. The daughter chromosome formed will have either the two long arms or the two short arms of the parent chromosome.

Karyotype. An arrangement of all the chromosomes of a cell at metaphase in descending order of size.

Locus. The specific site on a chromosome of a given gene.

Mosaicism. The presence of two or more genetically different cell types within the same individual.

Mutation. An alteration in DNA leading to a phenotypic change. A dominant characteristic is one expressed phenotypically when the gene on only one chromosome of the pair is affected. A recessive characteristic requires the same mutant gene on both paired chromosomes for expression.

Nondisjunction. The failure of a pair of chromosomes to separate during meiosis or mitosis. In meiosis, if one daughter cell receives both members of the chromosome pair, after fertilization a triple number of the chromosome, or a trisomic state, exists in each cell.

Oncogene. A gene normally important in cell skeleton structure or vital cell functions that when mutated may convert the cell to a cancer cell.

Penetrance. The percentage of individuals in a population with a mutation that actually demonstrates a phenotypic change.

Polymerase Chain Reaction (PCR). The process by which a small segment of DNA may be amplified to produce larger amounts of materials for analysis.

Polymorphism. Alterations within genes that may lead to variations in the expression of that particular gene. This is often due to point mutation or deletion within the genetic material.

Restriction Endonucleases. Bacterial enzymes that recognize and cut specific nucleotide sequences in the double-stranded DNA molecule at specific sites. More than 200 different ones are known.

Restriction Fragment Length Polymorphism (RFLP). The study of DNA fragments produced by restriction endonucleases has demonstrated that normal individuals may have variations in the DNA sequences without the presence of an abnormality. In addition, differences are often seen in individuals with specific diseases, such as sickle cell anemia. Thus polymorphism exists with respect to the presence or absence of restriction sites, and this has been defined as restriction fragment length polymorphism.

Ribonucleic Acid (RNA). A single-helix nuclear protein that serves several purposes in the cell. It is composed of a sugar (ribose), a phosphate, and a purine or pyrimidine base.

Translocation. The rearrangement of two chromosomes involving the exchange of chromosome material. Balanced translocation is one in which no active genetic material is lost.

A number of illnesses and conditions have a genetic basis. In some cases the problem arises from a single-point mutation within a gene, whereas others may involve changes in multiple genes or in an interreaction of genes and environmental factors. Finally, some conditions are the result of chromosome abnormalities of a variety of types. Although this chapter cannot provide a complete course in genetics, it attempts to offer an understanding of the genetic basis of conditions of particular interest to the gynecologist.

GENES AND GENE ACTION

Genes consist of deoxyribonucleic acid (DNA) molecules, which are made up of a linear sequence of nucleotides, each of which is composed of a pentose sugar, a phosphate, and a nitrogenous base. Four such bases are found in a DNA molecule. They are two purines, adenine (A) and guanine (G), and two pyrimidines, thymine (T) and cytosine (C). It has been shown that the total amount of purine in DNA molecules equals the total amount of pyrimidine, and the pairings of A to T and G to C always occur in the two strands of the double helix. These associations allow for accuracy both in the replication of the DNA molecule and in the translation of a genetic message from the DNA molecule to the development of a single-strand ribonucleic acid (RNA) molecule known as messenger RNA. The message is transmitted in such a fashion that a configuration with three bases in sequence (codon) represents a code, known as the *genetic code*, for an amino acid. With the message of the gene encoded on the messenger RNA, the latter leaves the nucleus of the cell, attaches to a cytoplasmic structure (the ribosome), and then attracts amino acids by means of smaller RNA molecules known as *transfer RNA*. Transfer RNA molecules each carry a specific amino acid and have three bases, which match the code of the messenger RNA, following the A to T and G to C pairings. In the RNA molecule, uracil (U) is substituted for thymine. When all segments of the message are covered, the amino acids are spliced together and the protein determined by the message is

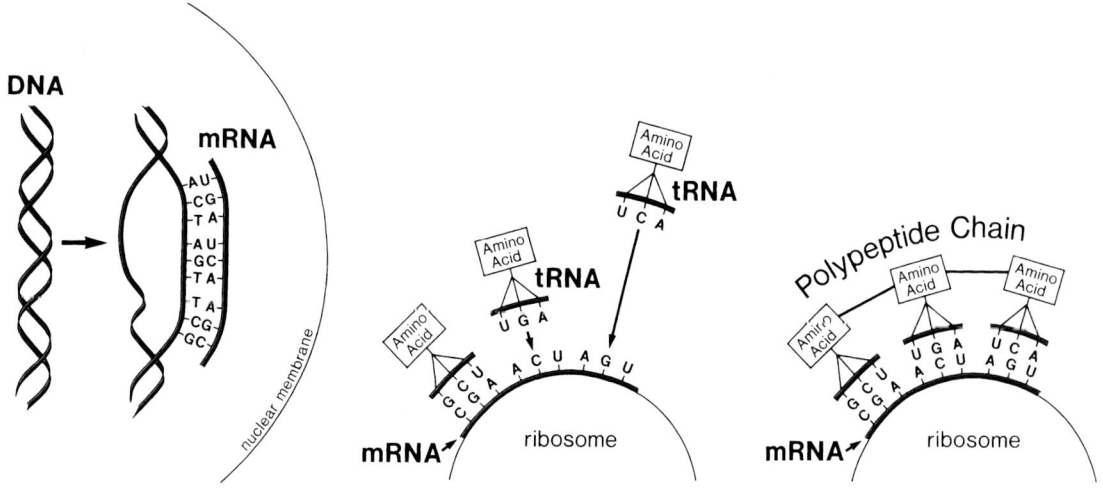

FIGURE 2-1 Schematic representation of protein production from genetic message on the DNA molecule to the final product.

complete and free for use in the cell and for transport from the cell. Figure 2-1 schematically demonstrates this process.

GENE MUTATION

Conditions that change the sequence of bases in the genetic code may cause a mutation. The mutation may involve a single point, that is, the changing of a single base, or a larger segment, in which the bases are removed or replaced. Mutation may occur spontaneously by the accidental replacement of one base with another during replication of DNA, by the incorporation of an inappropriate base during repair of a DNA molecule, or by an intermediate replacement with a substance similar to a usual base but capable of entering the DNA molecule and later attracting an inappropriate base in the next replication. Agents such as x-rays or other forms of irradiation may break a DNA strand, leading to the loss of one or more bases and a complete change in the sequence or to a replacement with an inappropriate base during healing. Even a single-point mutation will lead to the production of a modified protein that may be responsible for an abnormal expression of a trait. Figure 2-2 demonstrates such an occurrence for a group of hemoglobinopathies caused by the substitution of a single base at a single point.

Recent studies using molecular genetic techniques have made it possible not only to isolate and amplify genes responsible for specific characteristics but also to evaluate the biochemical nature of a mutation. The key to the localization of genetic information on the DNA molecule has been the discovery of a group of more than 200 bacterial enzymes, restriction endonucleases, that recognize and cut specific nucleotide sequences in the double-stranded DNA molecule. The sites of their action are known as restriction sites. Each enzyme recognizes a unique sequence of

	Possible Mutation 1	Possible Mutation 2
Hgb A (glutamic acid)	CTT	CTC
Hgb S (valine)	C A T	C A C
Hgb C (lysine)	T TT	T TC

FIGURE 2-2 Point mutation in a DNA molecule causing a single amino acid substitution and conversion of hemoglobin A to hemoglobin S or hemoglobin C.

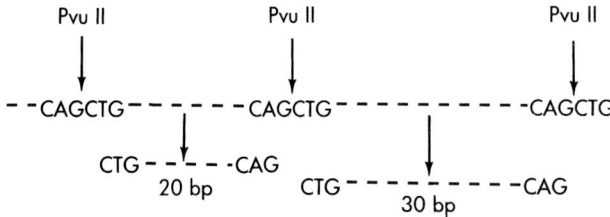

FIGURE 2-3 Simplified diagram illustrating the manner in which a restriction endonuclease cuts DNA at a specific nucleotide sequence. Pvu II recognizes only the sequence CAGCTG. DNA is separated into fragments of different lengths on the basis of distances between restriction enzyme recognition sites. The farther between sites, the longer the intervening DNA (i.e., 20 versus 30 base pairs). Shorter DNA fragments (e.g., 20 base pairs) show greater mobility and migrate farther in an agarose cell. (From Simpson JL: Genetic counseling and prenatal diagnosis. In Gabbe SG, Niebyl JR, and Simpson JL, eds: Obstetrics: normal and problem pregnancies, New York, 1986, Churchill Livingstone.)

nucleotides. Figure 2-3 demonstrates the action of one such enzyme, Pvu II, to separate the nucleotide junction GC in the sequence CAGCTG. Using these techniques it has been possible to define the specific genetic material related to many disease states, such as sickle cell anemia, the thalassemias, and cystic fibrosis. Identification of an affected individual or carrier may be accomplished by specifically identifying the mutant gene or by identifying a closely linked gene known to be associated with the mutant gene in one of the parents. This linkage study is an indirect means of identifying whether the mutant gene is present and is based on the fact that closely linked genes rarely separate during the process of meiotic crossover. These techniques have been helpful in the prenatal diagnosis of several conditions and in the identification of carrier states.

Often in genetic analysis, it is important to increase the amount of genetic material available for study. This can be accomplished by cloning of genes. After cleavage is brought about by a restriction enzyme, the specific fragment of DNA may be joined with a vector, frequently a bacterial plasmid. The vector is then capable of autonomous replication allowing for the production of up to several milligrams of DNA, making the study of the mutant gene possible. This process is known as polymerase chain reaction (PCR).

The study of DNA fragments produced by restriction endonucleases has identified a number of normal individuals with variations in DNA sequences but without any specific abnormality. Likewise, DNA fragment differences have been discovered in different individuals with the same condition. Therefore it is known that polymorphism exists with respect to the presence or absence of restriction sites, referred to as *restriction fragment length polymorphism (RFLP)*. A number of genetic diseases have been identified as associated with RFLPs (Table 2-1). One example is noted with respect to the gene for cystic fibrosis. This is a common autosomal recessive condition seen in Caucasian populations of European background. It occurs in 1:2500 births in such populations but is found in the carrier state in 1:25 Caucasian Americans. More than 230 alleles of the single gene responsible have been discovered. The gene, known as the cystic fibrosis transmembrane conductance regulator (CFTR), most commonly has

---

TABLE 2-1

Genetic Diseases Associated with Restriction Fragment Length Polymorphism (RFLP)

Disease	Chromosome	Disease	Chromosome
Huntington's disease	4	Duchenne's muscular dystrophy	X
Cystic fibrosis	7	Becker-type muscular dystrophy	X
Polycystic kidney disease	16	Emery-Dreifuss muscular dystrophy	X
Familial Alzheimer's disease	21	Hemophilia A	X
Myotonic muscular dystrophy	19	Hemophilia B (factor IX deficiency)	X
Wilm's tumor	11	Ornithine transcarbamoylase deficiency	X
Sickle cell anemia	11	Lesch-Nyhan syndrome	X
Thalassemia	11	Choroideremia	X
Acute intermittent porphyria	11	Lowe's oculocerebrorenal syndrome	X
Retinoblastoma	13	Wiskott-Alderich syndrome	X
von Recklinghausen's neurofibromatosis	17	Coffin-Lowry syndrome	X
Bilateral acoustic neurofibromatosis	22	Andersen-Fabry disease (alpha-galactosidase A deficiency)	X
Systemic amyloidosis in juvenile arthritis	1	Adrenoleukodystrophy	X
Osteogenesis imperfecta	7	Fragile X syndrome (X-linked mental retardation)	X
Multiple endocrine neoplasia type 2A	10	Steroid sulphatase deficiency (X-linked ichthyosis)	X
Familial adenomatous polyposis (colon cancer)	5	Charcot-Marie-Tooth disease (X-linked neuropathy)	X
Manic-depressive illness	11	X-linked spinal muscular atrophy	X
Tuberous sclerosis	9	X-linked anhidrotic ectodermal dysplasia	X
Phenylketonuria	12	X-linked retinitis pigmentosa	X
von Willebrand's disease	12	X-linked retinoschisis	X
Alpha-antitrypsin deficiency	14	X-linked chronic granulomatous disease	X
Spinocerebellar ataxia	6	X-linked hypophosphatemia	X
Congenital and adrenal hyperplasia (steroid 21-hydroxylation deficiency)	6	X-linked nephrogenic diabetes insipidus	X
		X-linked spastic paraplegia	X
		X-linked cleft palate	X
		X-linked myotubular myopathy	X
		X-linked dysplasia gigantism syndrome	X

From Watkins PC: Restriction fragment length polymorphism (RFLP): applications in human chromosome mapping and genetic disease research, Biotechniques 6:310, 1988.

delta F508 as its mutation. Delta F508 accounts for about 70% of all mutations seen of this gene; however, along with it, five other specific point mutations comprise more than 85% of cases. Any mutation of the gene, however, will lead to the trait being present in the carrier state, and when two genes of a pair are mutated, the individual will have cystic fibrosis, regardless of the point on the gene at which the mutation occurred.

These molecular techniques continue to be useful tools in the prenatal diagnosis of an increasing number of conditions but will also aid in the development of our understanding of many disease states and conditions. Eventually they will play a role in our ability to find therapies for conditions whose roots are in genetic mutation.

TYPES OF INHERITANCE

Autosomal Dominant Trait

If only one gene of a pair is mutated and if the altered protein produced by the mutated gene brings about a phenotypic change, the condition is said to be *autosomal dominant*. If both genes of a pair must carry the mutation for the phenotypic characteristic to occur, the condition is said to be *autosomal recessive*. Usually, if 50% of the protein produced by the gene pair is enough to give the usual phenotype, the condition is dominant. However, phenotypic expression of a mutation may occasionally occur under unusual circumstances. For example, a patient with sickle cell trait usually does not experience red blood cell sickling at sea level with normal oxygen saturation but may do so at high altitudes or in cases of decreased oxygen saturation, which may occur with pneumonia. Thus the presence of hemoglobin S in the red blood cell in equal proportions to hemoglobin A does not usually lead to the expression of sickling unless oxygen saturation is decreased.

With respect to autosomal dominant conditions, the concept of *penetrance* and *expressivity* must be introduced to explain some variations noted. Penetrance is the percentage of individuals in a population with the mutation that actually demonstrates the phenotypic change. Expressivity is the degree to which the phenotypic change occurs in the affected individual, that is, the degree to which the gene expresses itself. Penetrance and expressivity are dependent on the action of other genes and on environmental factors that may modify the action of the mutated gene.

The following general statements can be made about autosomal dominant mutations:

1. Phenotypic expression appears with equal frequency in both sexes.
2. For inheritance to take place, at least one parent must be affected unless a new mutation has occurred.
3. When an individual who is homozygous for the

mutation (mutation occurs on both genes of the pair) is mated with a normal individual, all offspring will demonstrate the trait. When a heterozygous individual is mated with a normal individual, 50% of the offspring will demonstrate the trait.
4. If the trait is rare in the population, most individuals demonstrating it will be heterozygous.

The following is a list of a number of autosomal dominant conditions:

Achondroplasia
Angioedema, hereditary
Craniofacial dysostosis
Dupuytren's contracture
Ehlers-Danlos syndrome
Facial palsy, congenital
Huntington's chorea
Intestinal polyposis
Keloid formation
Marfan's syndrome
Mitral valve prolapse
Muscular dystrophy
Neurofibromatosis (von Recklinghausen's disease)
Night blindness
Otosclerosis
Pectus excavatum
Renal disease, polycystic, adult type
Tuberous sclerosis
von Willebrand's disease
Wolff-Parkinson-White syndrome (some cases)

When one parent demonstrates one of these conditions, appropriate counseling would be that 50% of future offspring could be expected to demonstrate the condition as well. When neither parent demonstrates the condition but when a child is born with such a condition, it can be assumed that the problem is caused by a new mutation. In such cases, future progeny of the couple would be expected to be no more likely to have the condition than would occur by chance mutation.

Autosomal Recessive Trait

The following general statements can be made about an autosomal recessive trait:

1. The characteristic will occur equally in both sexes.
2. For the characteristic to be present, both parents must demonstrate or be carriers of the recessive trait.
3. If both parents are homozygous for the trait, all offspring will demonstrate it.
4. If both parents are heterozygous (carrier) for the trait, 25% of the offspring will have the trait and 50% will be carriers. The remaining 25% will be free of the trait.

5. Consanguinity is often present in families demonstrating frequent occurrences of rare recessive traits.

The following is a list of a number of common autosomal recessive conditions:

Acid maltase deficiency
Alkaptonuria
Ataxia-telangiectasia
Bloom's syndrome
Color blindness (total)
Cystic fibrosis
Cystinosis
Cystinuria
Deafness (many variants)
Dysautonomia
Galactosemia
Gaucher's disease
Glaucoma (congenital)
Homocystinuria
11β-hydroxylase deficiency
21-hydroxylase deficiency
Maple syrup urine disease
Mucolipidosis I, II, III
Mucopolysaccharidosis I-H, I-S, III, IV, VI, VII
Muscular dystrophy (autosomal recessive)
Niemann-Pick disease
Phenylketonuria
Sickle cell anemia
Tay-Sachs disease
Wilson's disease

In counseling a couple who has produced a child with such a characteristic, it is appropriate to tell them that 25% of future offspring will have the condition and 50% will be carriers. If a prenatal diagnostic test is available, it should be offered. One autosomal recessive condition, Tay-Sachs disease, is the subject of a large national screening program to determine carriers. Because the condition usually occurs in Jews of Eastern European origin, such individuals should certainly be offered screening. Another major screening program is aimed at discovering sickle cell anemia in blacks.

X-Linked Trait

Most X-linked conditions are recessive in type, since female carriers do not demonstrate the trait. A few conditions belie this rule, however, and are really X-linked dominant conditions. For the X-linked recessive trait the following statements are true:

1. The condition is more common in males.
2. If both parents are free of the trait and a male is produced with the trait, it must be assumed that the mother is a carrier.
3. If the father is affected and an affected male is produced, it must be assumed that the mother is at least a carrier of the trait.

4. If a female is produced who exhibits the X-linked trait, she may do so for one of two reasons. First, she may have received the mutant gene from both the mother and father and thereby is homozygous for the trait. Generally this would imply the father is affected and the mother is a carrier. Second, she may exhibit the trait as a function of the Lyon hypothesis, which states that in a female heterozygous for the trait, each cell of the developing embryo from about the time of implantation selects and uses one X chromosome only. Thereafter all developing cells from these particular cells use the same X chromosome. Thus a female is mosaic for her two X chromosomes, with some cells using the paternal X chromosome and some using the maternal X chromosome. Because this selection occurs on a random basis, some females will be produced who use an X chromosome predominantly from one parent. If the X chromosome has the mutation, the female will exhibit the trait because of the quantitative influence of that chromosome. Thus the female may be genotypically heterozygous but still exhibit the trait.

In the case of X-linked dominant traits the following may be said:

1. They occur in both males and females with equal frequency.
2. An affected male mated to a normal female will produce offspring with the trait 50% of the time, but all female offspring will be affected.
3. An affected homozygous female mated to a normal male will produce offspring with the trait 100% of the time.
4. Occasional heterozygous females will not exhibit the trait on the basis of the Lyon hypothesis.

The following is a list of several X-linked recessive conditions:

Agammaglobulinemia, X-linked, infantile
Androgen resistance syndrome, complete
Androgen resistance syndrome, incomplete
Color blindness, several varieties
Diabetes insipidus, some varieties
Fabry's disease
Glucose-6-phosphate dehydrogenase deficiency
Gonadal dysgenesis, XY type (probable)
Gout, some types
Factor VIII disease
Factor IX disease
Lesch-Nyhan syndrome
Mucopolysaccharidosis II
Muscular dystrophy, Duchenne type

Some X-linked dominant conditions are as follows:

Aeroosteolysis, dominant type
Cervicooculoacoustic syndrome

Hyperammonemia
Orofaciodigital syndrome I
Tubular stenosis (possible)

Multifactorial Inheritance

Multifactorial inheritance is defined as traits or characteristics produced by the action of several genes, with or without the interplay of environmental factors. A number of structural abnormalities such as cleft palate and harelip, open neural tube disease (including anencephaly and spina bifida), and several orthopedic and cardiac defects are examples of such conditions. When both parents are normal and an affected child is produced, the chance of recurrence is generally between 2% and 5% for any given pregnancy. These risk rates, however, are modified when one or both parents are affected with the condition or when close relatives are also affected. Many multifactorial diseases and conditions are more common in offspring when transmitted via the mother, and in general, when more than one offspring is affected in a family, the chances that subsequent offspring will be affected are greater.

Open neural tube disease (NTD) is a good example of a multifactorial defect. When a couple produces a child with such a defect, appropriate counseling is important. In this condition the observation that alpha-fetoprotein is increased both in the amniotic fluid and in the maternal serum in affected offspring is helpful in making a prenatal diagnosis of the condition. Ultrasound examination is also helpful in making a specific diagnosis. Although the diagnosis can be made prenatally if sought, 9 of 10 cases occur spontaneously in the offspring of couples who have no family or personal history. This observation has led to the suggestion that all pregnancies be screened with maternal serum alpha-fetoprotein determinations to uncover such cases antenatally. At present, screening programs are common. In fact, California has developed a statewide screening program for all pregnancies. Patients should be offered the option of being studied even if there is no family history of open neural tube disease.

The screening of 1000 pregnant women will uncover about 50 who have maternal serum alpha-fetoprotein determinations in excess of 2.5 times the mean for values considered normal for their specific week of gestation. Although a number of instances of multiple gestation, Turner syndrome, other anomalies, and fetal demise may be uncovered, only about 1 of these 50 women will actually prove to be carrying a fetus with NTD.

Chromosome Abnormalities

A variety of chromosome abnormalities may occur during meiosis or mitosis (see Chapter 1). They fall into several general categories, and many clinical conditions are associated with each type. Although it is impossible within the scope of this chapter to discuss every clinical condition associated with a known chromosome abnormality, an attempt is made to categorize the specific types of anomalies and the more common problems seen by obstetricians and gynecologists that relate to these anomalies. Several conditions are dealt with in more detail in other chapters of this book.

Nondisjunctional Events and Deletion

A nondisjunctional event is the faulty separation of chromosome pairs at anaphase in either meiosis or mitosis. The result in meiosis is that the daughter cell receives either both chromosomes of the pair or neither. At the time of fertilization, with the addition of another haploid set of chromosomes, the resulting individual will have either three chromosomes at that particular position or only one (Figure 2-4). In normal mitosis, after division of the chromosomes at anaphase, a complete pair goes to each daughter cell. If nondisjunction occurs, three chromosomes go to one daughter cell and one to the other.

Deletion is the simple loss of a chromosome at anaphase because of either anaphase lag or nondisjunction. In this instance the new cell receives only one chromosome of the pair and is essentially monosomic for that chromosome. Monosomic states involving autosomes are extremely rare and generally lethal. With respect to the

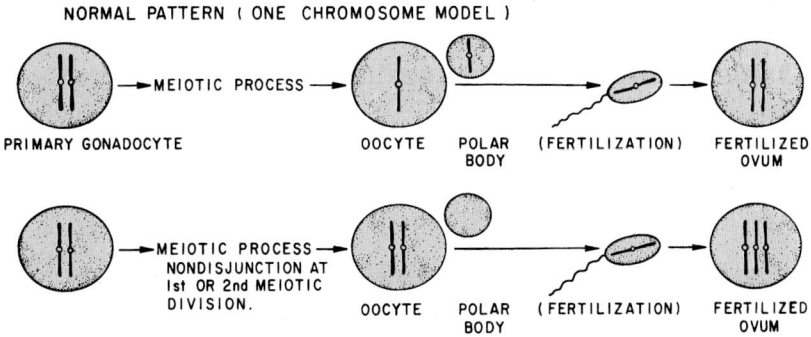

FIGURE 2-4 Meiotic nondisjunction, graphic representation. (From Stenchever MA: Human cytogenetics: a workbook in reproductive biology, Chicago, 1973, Mosby-Year Book, Inc.)

sex chromosomes, monosomy of the Y chromosome without the presence of an X chromosome is likewise lethal and has never been seen in a clinical situation or even in an abortus. Monosomy of the X chromosome, however, is the typical finding in the condition known as *Turner syndrome*. This condition is likewise lethal, with as many as 24 of each 25 of such conceptuses being aborted. When an infant is born alive with a 45,X karyotype (Figure 2-5), the common denominators of shortness of stature and sexual infantilism are seen, and many abnormalities involving most of the organ systems may likewise occur. One frequent occurrence (about 50% of cases) is webbing of the neck, which is the end product of hygromas seen during embryologic development (Figure 2-6).

Nondisjunctional events involving the autosomes have been seen in abortus material in all but chromosomes 1 and 17. However, in infants born alive, only trisomic states of chromosomes 13, 18, 21, and 22 and an occasional C group chromosome have been seen. Trisomy of chromosome 13 (Patau's syndrome) results in gross multiple structural defects that are usually incompatible with extended life. Trisomy of chromosome 18 likewise leads to a syndrome (Edwards' syndrome) that has a characteristic group of structural abnormalities, again generally not compatible with long life. Trisomy 21 is classic Down syndrome, and trisomy 22 has been seen in a few live-born individuals but is associated with severe retardation.

Trisomy involving the sex chromosomes has been seen in circumstances relating to both the X and the Y chromosome. Nondisjunctional events involving both oogenesis and spermatogenesis can be responsible, as in autosomal trisomy.

If trisomy X is the result, a female with a reasonably normal phenotype is produced. Mild mental retardation is occasionally present, but fertility is present in at least 50% of such individuals. Although most of the offspring produced are normal chromosomally, there is a slight increase of offspring with nondisjunctional events involving both the sex chromosomes and the autosomes.

Individuals with a 47,XXY karyotype are likewise produced as the result of a nondisjunctional event involving the sex chromosomes that may occur by an error in either oogenesis or spermatogenesis. This leads to the clinical state of Klinefelter syndrome. The classic finding in these individuals is that they are usually tall and have azoospermia caused by sclerosis of the seminiferous tubules. Other mild phenotypic anomalies may be present, such as gynecomastia, which is present in about one third of the cases. Men with Klinefelter syndrome have primary infertility.

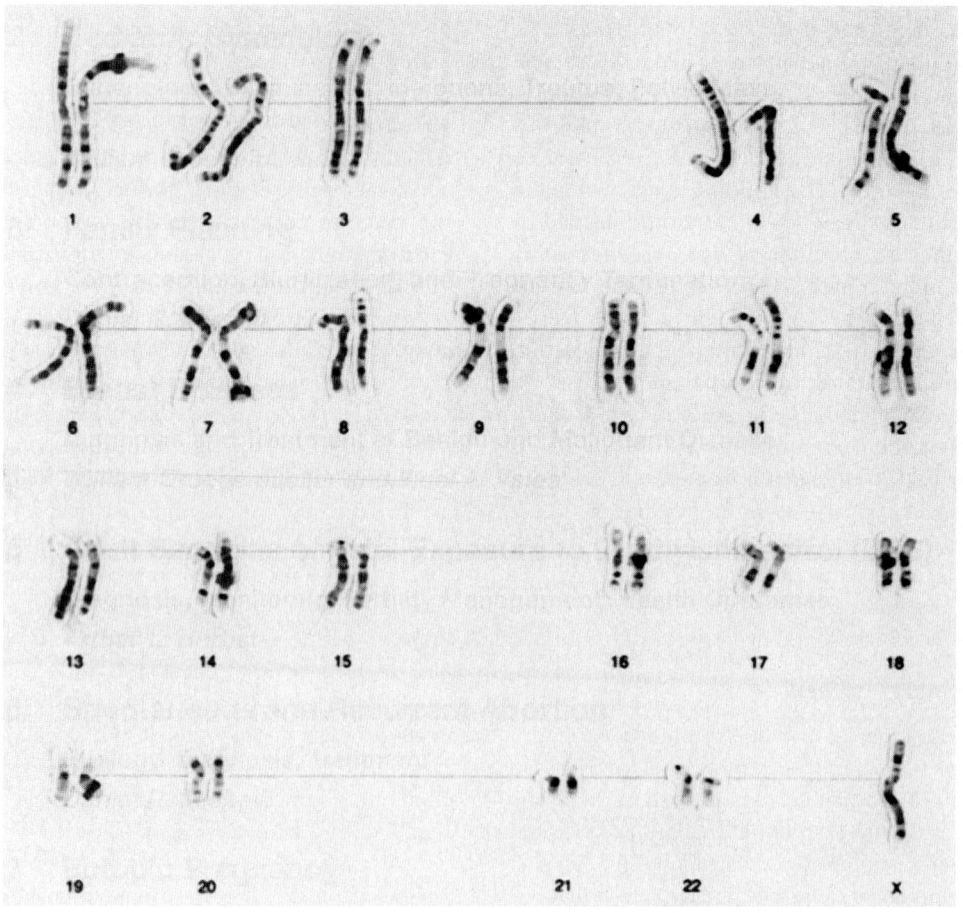

FIGURE 2-5 Example of a karyotype from a newborn patient with Turner syndrome showing the presence of a single X chromosome (45,X).

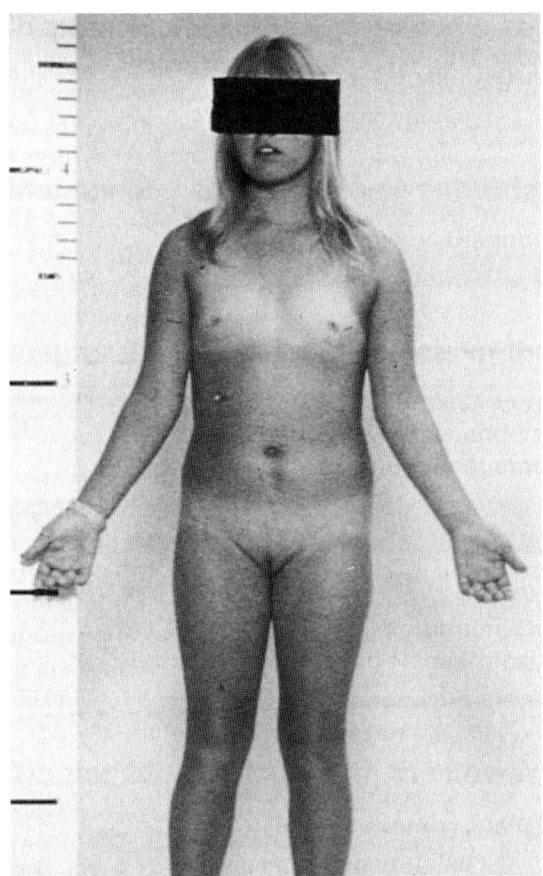

FIGURE 2-6 A 17-year-old patient with Turner syndrome demonstrating short stature, poor sexual development, and increased carrying angles at elbows. Patient also has webbing of the neck.

TABLE 2-2
Karyotypes Discovered in Patients with Phenotypic Characteristics of Turner Syndrome

Karyotype	Error
45,X	Deletion X
45,Xi (Xq)	Deletion Xp, Isochromosome Xq
45,X,Xq	Deletion Xp
45,X/46,XX	Mosaicism
45,X/46,XX/47,XXX	Mosaicism
45,X/46,XY	Mosaicism
45,X/46,XY/47,XYY	Mosaicism
45,XringX	Ring chromosome
46,XX	Phenotype with normal karyotype

Turner syndrome has afforded an excellent opportunity to evaluate the various chromosomal mechanisms that can lead to the same (or similar) phenotypic finding. Table 2-2 summarizes many of the karyotypes that have been detected in patients with the clinical findings of Turner syndrome. Thus the clinical picture can occur because of an error in meiosis or mitosis or because of chromosome rearrangements.

Chromosome Breaks and Rearrangements

Chromosome breaks and rearrangements may be brought about by damage to the chromosome caused by irradiation of many different types, by viruses, or by other changes within the cell or within its environment that can damage the chromosome structure or the DNA molecule within the chromosome. When these breaks occur, a number of things can happen. The break may simply heal, with or without a point mutation at the point of breakage. If a segment of the chromosome is lost during this healing process, partial deletion of chromatin material may take place. If two chromosomes break, they may exchange chromosome arms and give rise to a translocation. In karyotypes, translocations have been seen involving various combinations of all the chromosomes. Although they are probably a chance occurrence, there may be some active areas on various chromosomes that make such events more common. Rearranged chromosomes at first are generally balanced with respect to gene complement, and the individual so affected is referred to as a *carrier* of the translocation and can expect in most cases to be phenotypically normal. About 10% of new translocations, even though balanced, are associated with mental retardation and other mild anomalies. These carrier individuals, however, have difficulty when meiosis occurs in gametogenesis. With the production of the gametes, the stage might be set for reassortment of chromosomes in such a way that normal chromosomes pair with abnormal chromosomes, leading to partial trisomy or partial monosomy of various chromatin materials. Such individuals are

Nondisjunction during spermatogenesis involving the Y chromosome can lead to the karyotype 47,XYY. Such individuals may be entirely normal phenotypically but generally are tall, and many have aggressive personalities. For this reason a number of these individuals have been found in prisons and mental hospitals, but just as many have been found among the normal population. Although such men are fertile, their female partners often have repetitive abortion and other reproductive wastage problems, and this may be the means of identifying such cases. In addition, they often produce offspring with normal karyotypes but may produce conceptuses with trisomic problems involving both autosomes and the sex chromosomes.

Nondisjunctional events during mitosis in the early embryo frequently produce individuals with cell populations containing different chromosome numbers. This condition, known as *mosaicism,* may involve any of the members of the autosome complement or the sex chromosomes. The actual phenotype produced depends on the number of cells present with an abnormal complement and on the tissue in which these cells have the opportunity to express themselves.

said to be unbalanced and generally have severe phenotypic abnormalities. Roughly 3% to 4% of all abortuses have unbalanced chromosome rearrangements, and some live-born infants have unbalanced translocations.

Figure 2-7 demonstrates two possible ways that such translocations can come about. The first involves the fusion of two acrocentric chromosomes in which the short arms of both and the centromere of one are lost, with the production of a chromosome that essentially has the long arm of each of these two chromosomes and an overall reduction of the chromosome number by one. Thus the balanced carrier has 45 chromosomes with the loss of one normal chromosome from each pair involved and the formation of one translocated chromosome, which is known as *Robertsonian fusion*. Gametes produced by such an individual are normal in chromosome configuration, balanced as in the parent, unbalanced because the translocated chromosome and one or the other of the normal chromosomes of the pairs involved are included, or monosomic because only one of the chromosomes is present and not the translocated chromosome. After fertilization, the following are possible: 25% of the offspring should be normal; 25%, carriers; 25%, unbalanced and affected; and 25%, monosomic and probably aborted. In actual experience with reproduction in such carriers, the unbalanced karyotype in offspring seems to occur less frequently than would be expected by chance with the carrier state, and normal karyotype occurs more frequently. This is particularly true if the father is the carrier.

The other means of translocation is the reciprocal translocation, in which chromatin material is exchanged between chromosomes but the chromosome number does not change. In this case, two new chromosomes are essentially produced, and with gamete formation one can expect a normal gamete, a gamete with the two balanced translocated chromosomes, or two possibilities in which a normal chromosome of one pair is matched with one of the translocated chromosomes. About 25% of the offspring could be expected to be normal, 25% balanced carriers, and 50% unbalanced and abnormal. Indeed, women with the carrier state of reciprocal translocation are frequently found among those with recurrent abortions. Although it is difficult to ascertain the percentage of such conceptuses with unbalanced karyotypes that end in abortion, the preponderance of conceptions that are live born favor the normal or carrier state.

If one chromosome breaks at two points, the broken segment may turn on its axis, leading to an *inversion*. If the centromere is present in the broken segment, a *pericentric inversion* is seen. Although this, too, will allow the individual to be phenotypically normal, problems involved in meiosis are such that infants with unbalanced chromosome components may be produced.

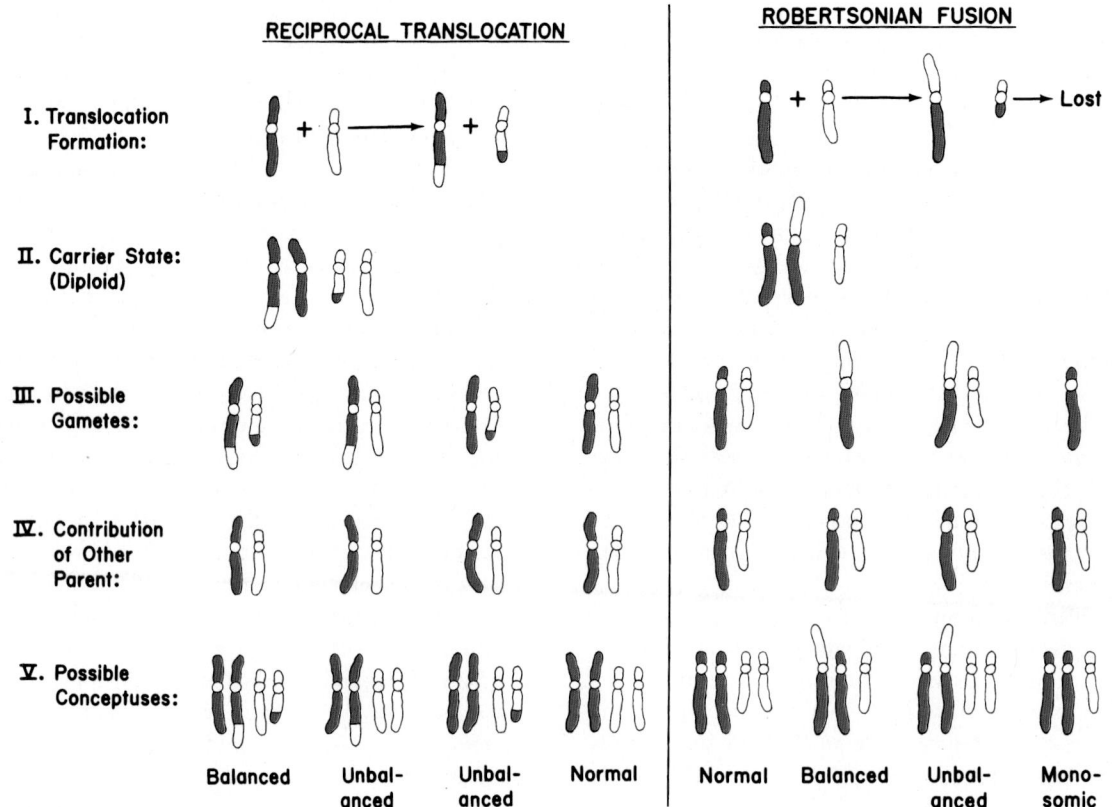

FIGURE 2-7 Schematic representation of translocation formation, including reciprocal translocation and Robertsonian fusion. (From Stenchever MA: Contemp OB/GYN 16:24, 1980.)

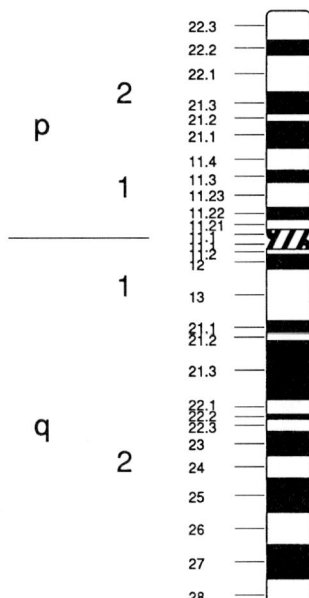

FIGURE 2-8 Diagram showing the banding of the X chromosome at the 550-band level. The short and long arms are designated "p" and "q," respectively, and the band designation is shown at the left. (Diagram derived from the ISCN nomenclature, as prepared by D. Adler, Arrowpoint, Bainbridge Island, Wash.)

Finally, a break may lead to the actual loss of a small segment of the chromosome, a *partial deletion*. With the loss of the genes on that segment, the infant produced usually is extremely abnormal. A few such partial deletions have been seen in individuals born alive. The resulting abnormalities include Wolf's syndrome, with the deletion of a portion of the short arm of chromosome 4, which leads to severe retardation problems; cri-du-chat syndrome, which involves the loss of a portion of the short arm of chromosome 5, again leading to gross retardation in an individual in whom laryngeal changes result in a cry that sounds like the plaintive cry of a cat; and gross abnormalities resulting from the deletion of the short arm of chromosome 18.

Partial deletions of both the X and Y chromosomes have been seen. With the loss of part or all of the short arm (Xp−) of the X chromosome, many of the findings of Turner syndrome, including shortness of stature, have been noted. With the loss of all or part of the long arm of the X chromosome (Xq−), some of the findings of Turner syndrome have been seen but not shortness of stature. Figure 2-8 depicts the X chromosome divided by arms and bands.

Chromosome Abnormalities and Abortion

Hertig and Rock observed, as early as 1949, that many early gestations were obviously defective and that a genetic defect might be responsible. When it became possible to karyotype these abortuses, a number of investiga-

tors verified this theory by finding specific chromosome anomalies of a variety of types. Now with banding techniques, specific chromosomes can be identified, and the abnormalities can be more accurately categorized.

With the use of the data from a number of different studies, it has been estimated that about 15% of ova penetrated by sperm fail to divide. Another 15% fail to implant, and 25% to 30% are aborted spontaneously at previllous stages. Of the roughly 40% of fertilized ova that survive the first missed menstrual period, as many as one fourth are aborted spontaneously, so that only about 30% to 35% of all ova penetrated by sperm actually result in live-born infants.

From the work of many, it has been estimated that between 30% and 60% of early pregnancy losses that are recognizable as having been gestations are associated with chromosome abnormalities and many of the rest probably have other genetic defects.

Of those abortuses with chromosome abnormalities, roughly 50% have autosomal trisomy. Trisomies have been defined in abortus material for all autosomes except chromosomes 1 and 17. A trisomy of chromosome 16 has been noted in about one third of the cases, and since this has never been seen in living individuals, it must be considered universally lethal. Autosomal trisomies such as those of chromosomes 13, 18, and 21 do occur in live-born babies but may be seen in abortus material as well. It is of interest that as many as 80% of trisomy 21 fetuses are aborted. The error itself is that of nondisjunction of the chromosome pair at anaphase in either the first or the second meiotic division. Because the risk of repeating a nondisjunctional event is greater than in the general population, a woman who is known to have produced a trisomic abortus should be offered prenatal diagnosis by amniocentesis or chorionic villus sampling in much the same fashion as she would be if she had previously produced a live-born infant with a trisomy. In women who have produced a conceptus that is trisomic, the risk of subsequent trisomy is 1% to 2%, being somewhat less for women under the age of 35 and higher for women over the age of 35.

Roughly 20% of the chromosomally aborted abnormal fetuses have the karyotype 45,X. Only about 5% of such conceptuses are born alive, and these have the characteristic findings of Turner syndrome. The mechanism responsible for this condition seems to be the loss of a sex chromosome at zygote formation, but the loss of a chromosome via the mechanism of nondisjunction is also possible. The error leading to the problem may occur in either male or female meiosis, and a variety of mosaic patterns have been seen, indicating that errors in mitosis after fertilization may also occur. Data obtained from studies using as a marker the Xg blood group, which is coded on the X chromosome, suggest that about three fourths of living 45,X individuals use the X chromosome derived from the mother.

Sex chromosome trisomies such as 47,XXX, 47,XXY, and 47,XYY are rarely found in abortus material. The relative lethality of such karyotypes is probably minor, and most individuals are born alive. Each birth occurs about once per thousand live births of infants of the appropriate sex.

Triploidy occurs in between 14% and 19% of abortuses with chromosome abnormalities and apparently results from errors in meiosis or from double fertilization of a single ovum. It has been seen in live-born infants only as a mosaic when a normal cell line is also present. Using special chromosome banding techniques, Kajii and Nikawa demonstrated that triploidy occurs by a variety of mechanisms. This phenomenon has been seen in artificially bred cattle and in other animals as well and is thought to be the result of late insemination in some cases. In such situations, double fertilization in an egg that has lost its selectivity for penetration by normal sperm may be the mechanism. Triploid abortuses frequently are associated with multiple anomalies as well as hydropic degeneration of the placenta (Figure 2-9). Some hydatidiform moles therefore have a triploid karyotype.

Tetraploidy, or a mean chromosome count of 92, occurs in 3% to 6% of all chromosomally abnormal abortuses. This condition is undoubtedly lethal, since it

has never been seen in living individuals. It probably occurs when chromosome division is not followed by cytoplasmic division in the initial cell division of the zygote.

Rearrangements, primarily translocations and inversions, are noted in about 3% of all chromosomally abnormal abortuses. According to Creasy and associates, most but definitely not all of these are unbalanced translocations. Although most unbalanced translocations in conceptuses result in abortion, some individuals are born alive.

A discussion of chromosome abnormalities among early abortuses is not complete without mentioning the findings in a series of stillbirths. Shepard and Fantel noted that of 283 stillborn infants, 17 had chromosome abnormalities, a rate of 6%. Trisomies occurred in 58.8% of these chromosomally abnormal fetuses. Sex chromosome abnormalities occurred in 29.4%, but none had a karyotype of 45,X. There was one instance of translocation and one of triploidy among the stillborn infants.

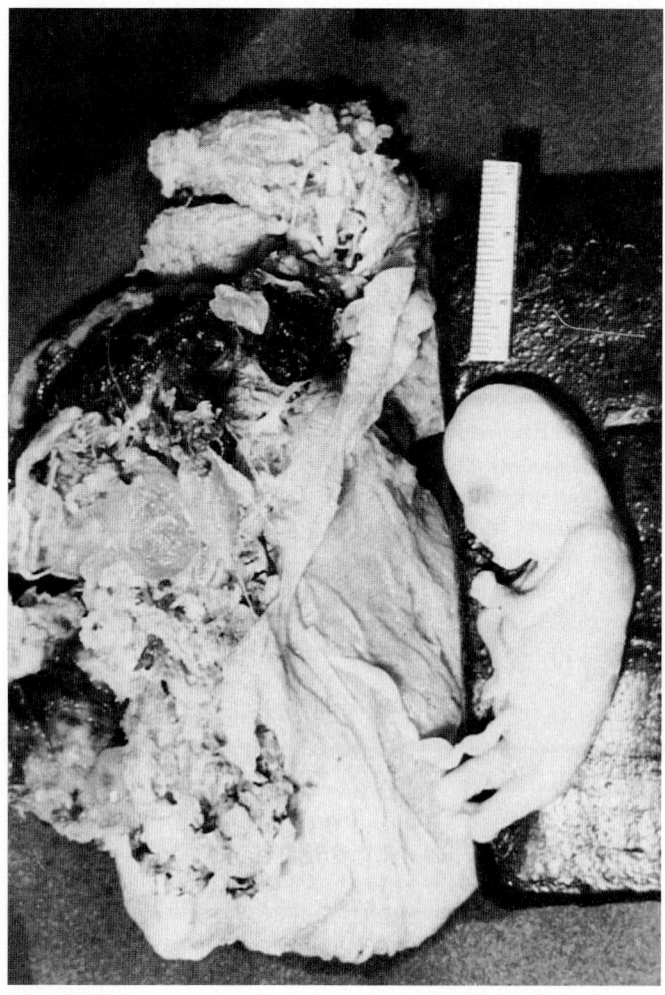

FIGURE 2-9   Abortus with triploid karyotype. Note hydropic degeneration of the placenta. (From Stenchever MA: Contemp OB/GYN 17:38, 1981.)

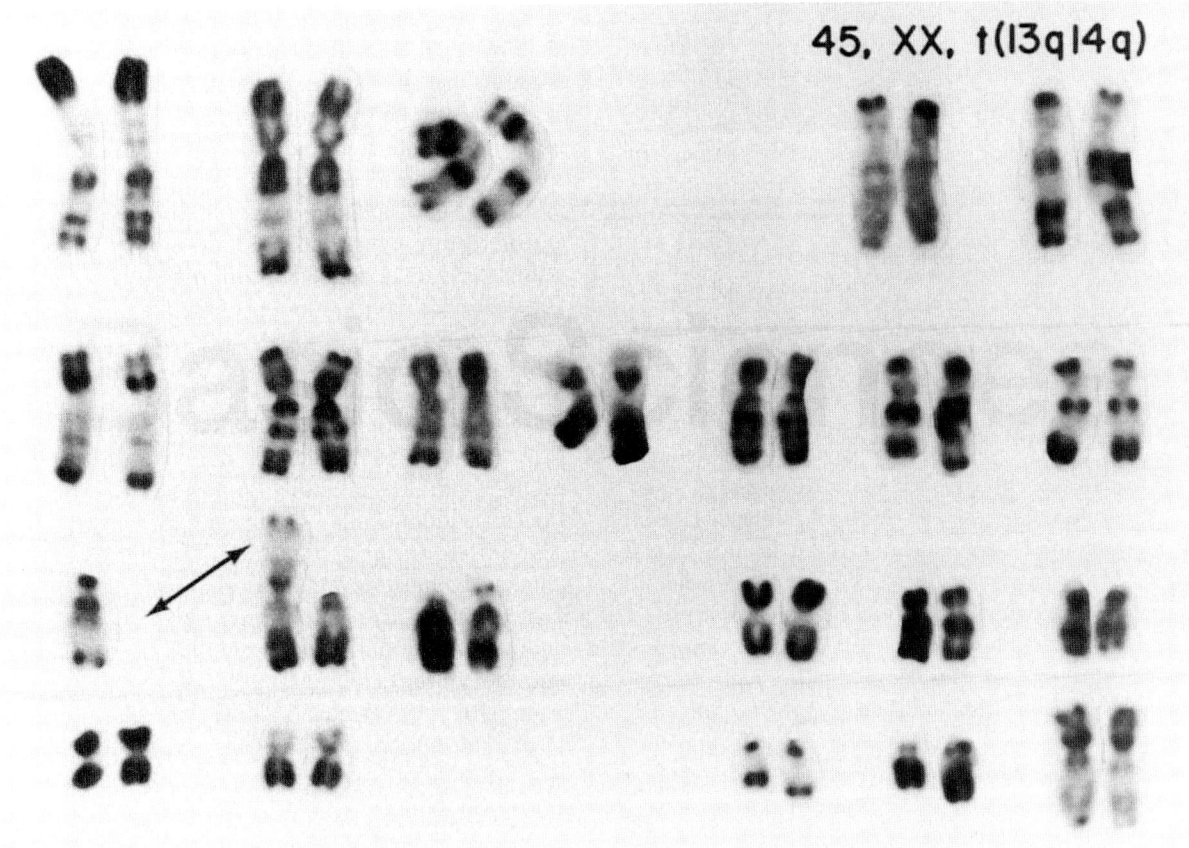

FIGURE 2-10   Karyotype of patient with 13 to 14 translocations (45,XX,+[13q 14q]) who had a history of three spontaneous first-trimester abortions. (From Stenchever MA: Contemp OB/GYN 17:38, 1981.)

It is interesting to compare the findings of chromosome abnormalities among spontaneous abortuses with those among live-born infants. In a series of 43,558 live-born infants reported by Ratcliffe, 247 (0.56%) had chromosome abnormalities. Of these, two (0.8%) had a karyotype of 45,X, 36.8% had other sex chromosome abnormalities, and 21.1% had autosomal trisomies of chromosomes 13, 18, and 21. The latter abnormality was by far the most common. Balanced chromosomal translocations were found in 32.4% of chromosomally abnormal individuals, and unbalanced translocations were present in 3.2%. The remaining abnormalities were classified as miscellaneous. In a comparison of chromosome abnormalities in live-born infants with those in abortuses and stillborn infants, a concept of lethality can be noted.

Recurrent Abortion

Roughly 1% to 2% of couples have multiple abortions or multiple pregnancy wastage. A review of the world literature by Simpson revealed that the prevalence of chromosome abnormalities in women with chronic spontaneous abortion problems was about twice that in men (4.8% versus 2.4%). Stephenson, in a study of 197 couples who experienced 843 spontaneous abortions (average 4.1, range 3-12), found a structural chromosome anomaly in 7 (3.5%), of which 5 were in the female and 2 in the male. Although occasional sex chromosome abnormalities such as 47,XXX and 47,XYY, as well as a variety of mosaic representations, are seen among such couples, the majority demonstrate either balanced reciprocal translocations or Robertsonian fusion problems (Figure 2-10).

Fortuny et al. studied the karyotypes of 445 couples who demonstrated repetitive (two or more) abortions and detected a balanced translocation in 19 (4.7%) of the couples, pericentric inversions in 8 (1.8%) of the couples, and polymorphisms in 52 (11.4%) of the couples. Significantly higher frequencies of translocations and polymorphism were found in these couples than in a control group of 600 consecutively delivered live-born infants (0.33% and 2.3%, respectively). No differences were noted in the incidence of inversions. Of the translocations in the study group, 16 were reciprocal and 3 were Robertsonian. Of the couples with chromosome rearrangements, 17 underwent subsequent prenatal testing. Of 11 fetuses with parent carriers of a Robertsonian-type translocation, 9 were carriers of the balanced translocation, 2 were normal, and none were unbalanced. Of the 4 who had a carrier parent with a reciprocal translocation, 3 fetuses had a balanced translocation and 1 had a normal karyotype. Again, no unbalanced karyotypes were noted in offspring. Two carriers of inversions underwent prenatal diagnosis; one fetus carried the inversion and the other was normal. Although balanced carriers and normals seem to have the advantage over the unbalanced state, it is still not known whether there are fewer conceptions of fetuses with unbalanced karyotypes or that such conceptuses frequently end in early abortion.

In a large collaborative study of 71 European prenatal diagnosis centers reported by Boue and Gallano, when parents carried Robertsonian translocations, all unbalanced fetuses were detected when the mother was the carrier of the translocation. When the translocation involved chromosome 21, the risk that the fetus would have Down syndrome was 10% to 15%. In contrast, when the mother is a carrier of a Robertsonian translocation that does not include a chromosome 21 or when the father is the carrier of any type of Robertsonian translocation, the risk of producing a fetus with an unbalanced karyotype is low. This work is supported by the observations of several other investigators. Table 2-3 summarizes the risk of Down syndrome based on specific risk factors and is an example of the risks for producing chromosomally abnormal fetuses when risk factors are known.

The diagnosis of a chromosome abnormality in couples with chronic pregnancy wastage is important for two reasons. The first is to rule out an abnormality incompatible with normal gestation. Examples are homologous translocations between identical members of the same group of chromosomes, such as 13-13, 14-14, 15-15, 21-21, and 22-22. Individuals with other types of reciprocal translocations or Robertsonian fusion may have a normal pregnancy in which the chromosome makeup reflects either a normal karyotype or a balanced carrier state. However, such individuals may produce a conceptus with an unbalanced translocation, which would not be normal. In addition, chromosomally abnormal individuals are more likely to produce offspring with chromosome abnormalities. In some cases in which the father is the carrier of a chromosome abnormality, particularly when the abnormality is incompatible with normal gestation, artificial insemination with donor sperm may be offered. The techniques of ovum donation or embryo transplant may offer potential help to the woman with such a chromosomal problem.

Hydatidiform Mole

The two most common karyotypes noted in hydatidiform moles, and indeed in other trophoblastic disease, are 46,XX and triploidy. The use of Q and R banding techniques has shown that most moles have a karyotype of 46,XX, and all homologous chromosomes are homozygous for banding polymorphism. Thus although the moles are diploid in number, the chromosomes arise from a haploid set from one parent. In each case that parent proved to be the father. Some moles have been found to have a karyotype of 46,XY, but in all cases both haploid sets of chromosomes have been found to be of paternal origin. Even the occasional tetraploid mole has also been noted to be derived from a diploid set of chromosomes, all of which are of paternal origin. Thus it appears that in the formation of a hydatidiform mole, the female nucleus is lost and all chromosomes are of paternal origin either by the duplication of a haploid set or by the presence of two separate haploid sets of paternal origin. Therefore all of the genetic material of the mole is foreign to the mother (Figure 2-11).

The other type of chromosome abnormality seen in hydatidiform moles is triploidy. Frequently a fetus is present, and the problem is represented by a hydropic degeneration of the placenta. Although most choriocarcinomas are derived from 46,XX moles, triploidy has occasionally been seen. Triploidy may occur because of extra haploid chromosome sets from either parent, but molar degeneration seems to occur when at least two haploid sets are of paternal origin.

Genetic Abnormalities in Cancer

A number of tumors have demonstrated aneuploidy, and many have been seen with marker chromosomes specific for that particular tumor. The best example is the Philadelphia chromosome, seen in chronic myelogenous leukemia. This minute chromosome disappears from peripheral circulation and from the bone marrow when therapy is effective and the patient's cancer is in remission. Space does not allow a categorization of each tumor that can occur in the human and its chromosome experience. It should be noted, however, that premalignant (dysplastic) cells of the cervix are generally aneuploid, as are the cells that compose invasive squamous cell carcinomas. This aneuploid distribution has been observed in cancers that arise in other organs as well but frequently is not observed in tumors arising in endocrine organs (including endometrium, breast, and thyroid).

TABLE 2-3
Risk of Producing a Down Syndrome Offspring by Specific Risk Factors

Risk Factor	Risk (%)
Previous trisomy-21, normal parental karyotypes	1–2
D-G (21) Robertsonian translocation	
Mother is carrier	10–15
Father is carrier	1–2
G-G heterologous translocation (21–22)	15
G-G homologous translocation (21–21)	100

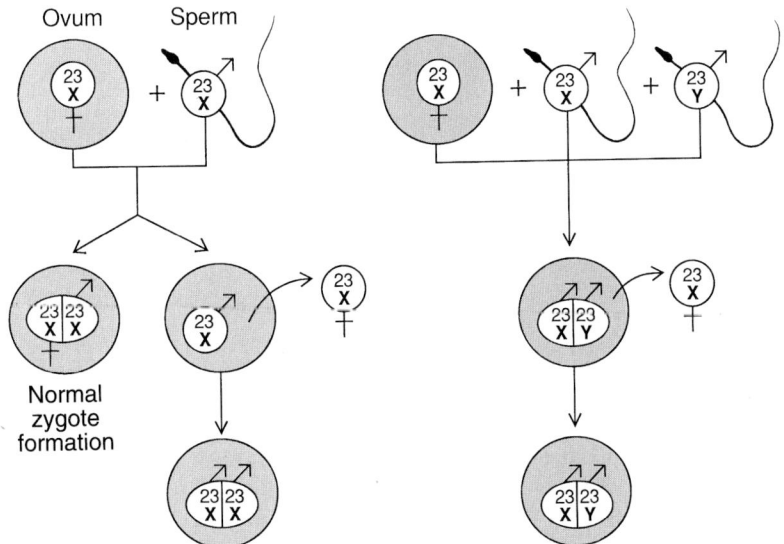

FIGURE 2-11 Diagram demonstrating potential mechanisms for developing a hydatidiform mole. All genetic material is derived from the father.

A variety of cancers occur in individuals who have fragile chromosomes and may be associated with chromosome breaks and rearrangements or with mutations that occur when breaks take place and healing is faulty. Such conditions are seen in families with Bloom's syndrome, Fanconi's anemia, and ataxia-telangiectasia. In each case there is an increased percentage of individuals with a variety of cancers, and chromosome breaks are commonly seen in the cells of these individuals.

Current theories suggest that the majority of human cancers arise from a genetic change in a single cell. Such genetic alterations may be of a variety of types but essentially involve either (1) the somatic activation of cell oncogenes through point mutations, rearrangements, or amplifications or (2) the inactivation of tumor-suppressor genes by point mutation or deletion in either germ or somatic cells. For example, Fearon et al., using cloning techniques, have identified an allelic deletion in a gene on chromosome 18q (long arm) in 70% of studied colorectal tumors. This gene, thought to be a tumor-suppressor gene, may play a role in the pathogenesis of the cancer, perhaps through the alteration of normal cell-cell interactions controlling growth.

An oncogene that is probably involved in the initial phases of neoplastic disease and its progression is the breast ovarian cancer gene (BRCA1). Seen in families with a strong tendency for this disease, the gene has several mutant alleles and is located on the short arm of chromosome 17. In 1994 Miki et al. demonstrated predisposing mutations in five of eight families presumed to segregate BRCA1 susceptibility alleles. Mutations include an 11-base pair deletion, a 1-base pair insertion, a stop codon, a missense substitution, and an inferred regulatory mutation. These authors found the gene to be expressed in a number of different tissues, including breast and ovary, and coding for a protein of 1863 amino acids. Mutation of this gene

seems to account for approximately 45% of families with significant high breast cancer incidences and at least 80% of families with increased incidence of both early onset breast cancer and ovarian cancer. A second gene, BRCA2, was recently mapped on the long arm of chromosome 13. It appears to account for a portion of early onset breast cancer equal to that resulting from BRCA1. Remaining individuals with susceptibility to early onset breast cancer may have mutations of, until now, unmapped genes or mutations that encode tumor suppressor protein p53.

Oncogenes seem to fall into two general categories: those related to the structure of the cell's skeleton and those related to the transmission and transduction of growth regulatory signals. Watson et al. demonstrated that a nuclear-associated protein product of the C-myc gene, $P62^{C-myc}$, is of a significantly higher level in serous papillary carcinomas of the ovary than in normal ovarian tissue. Borderline tumors demonstrated levels between normal and cancer cell levels. The levels between normal cells and borderline cancer cells were significantly different, but no significant differences were noted between the cells of the borderline and frank tumors. The majority of these carcinomas were also noted to be aneuploid. The C-myc gene seems to be related to DNA synthesis. Another oncogene whose protein product is thought to function as a receptor for a growth regulating molecule is HER-2/neu. This gene has been identified on the long arm of chromosome 17 and amplification of it has been reported in breast, ovarian, endometrial, cervical, and fallopian tube cancers. Overexpression of this gene has been found to be a poor prognostic factor for survival in advanced-stage ovarian cancer, breast cancer with positive nodes, and endometrial cancer. It is currently the focus of research for new therapies.

It is likely that the methods of molecular biology now available will make it possible to identify the genetic systems that, when altered, lead to cancer transformation and may eventually offer clues to therapy.

Hermaphroditism

TRUE HERMAPHRODITISM. True hermaphroditism, which involves the presence of both male and female gonads within the same individual, is frequently associated with the karyotype 46,XX. However, a variety of other chromosome findings have been noted. One of these, 46,XX/46,XY, is a condition that most likely occurs when the fertilization of two eggs is followed by their fusion, resulting in chimerism within the individual. Chimerism is defined as the presence of two different cell populations from two separate conceptuses within the same individual. Uehara et al. recently performed molecular biologic analyses for chimerism in a true hermaphrodite with a 46,XX/46,XY karyotype using RFLP analyses of the pseudoautosomal region of the X chromosome. They discovered that this individual had four bands—two of maternal origin and two of paternal origin—whereas a normal diploid individual would have only two bands. They concluded that two separate cell lineages compose the individual originating from two separate maternal haploids and two different spermatozoa.

Other chromosome anomalies associated with true hermaphroditism include various mosaicisms involving 45,X/46,XY and 45,X/47,XYY karyotypes, as well as karyotypes with various translocations and deletions of the X and Y chromosomes. The influence of these chromosomes in the development of hermaphroditism is discussed in detail elsewhere.

PSEUDOHERMAPHRODITISM. Female pseudohermaphroditism occurs when a female is androgenized during embryonic life. The most common such case is associated with congenital adrenal hyperplasia, which may come about because of a number of enzyme defects transmitted as autosomal recessive characteristics. The most common is 21-hydroxylase deficiency, but 11-β-hydroxylase deficiency may also cause the syndrome. A third and rarer defect is the 18-hydroxysteroid dehydrogenase deficiency, which leads to aldosterone deficiency but no genital tract anomalies. In every case, such individuals have a 46,XX karyotype unless other conditions are associated by chance. These are discussed in detail elsewhere.

Male pseudohermaphroditism occurs when the individual has a 46,XY karyotype and is genetically and gonadally male but phenotypically and psychologically female. The most common condition in which this is found is the androgen resistance syndrome (testicular feminization syndrome).

In this condition the genetic error is transmitted as an X-linked recessive characteristic leading to a faulty androgen receptor on the cell membranes, preventing the cell from transporting testosterone or dihydrotestosterone into the cell. Both complete and incomplete forms exist. A related condition, 5α-reductase deficiency, prevents the conversion of testosterone to dihydrotestosterone. Because the latter is the form of testosterone that enters most cells, a defect of the enzyme mimics the findings of androgen resistance.

KEY POINTS

- Base pairing in DNA molecules is always A-T and G-C, and in RNA molecules is always A-U and G-C.

- Endonuclease enzymes cleave specific nucleotide pairs, making DNA fragment evaluation and gene cloning possible. More than 200 different endonucleases exist.

- Through a process known as polymerase chain reaction (PCR), small fragments of DNA may be cloned to produce larger amounts of the same material suitable for analysis.

- When a heterozygous individual who has an autosomal dominant trait mates with a normal individual, 50% of their offspring will have the trait.

- When two individuals who carry an autosomal recessive trait mate, 25% of their offspring will demonstrate the trait and 50% will be carriers.

- X-linked recessive characteristics are transmitted from maternal carriers to male offspring and will affect 50% of such male offspring.

- In general, if a couple produces an offspring with a multifactorial defect and the problem has never occurred in the family, it can be expected to be repeated in 2% to 5% of subsequent pregnancies.

- The findings always present in 45,X Turner syndrome are shortness of stature and sexual infantilism.

- A variety of different karyotypes have been discovered in individuals with the phenotype of Turner syndrome.

- Nondisjunctional events have been described in every autosome except chromosomes 1 and 17. The risk of producing a second conceptus with a nondisjunctional event is 1% to 2%.

- Conditions always seen in individuals with Klinefelter syndrome (47,XXY) are tallness of stature and azoospermia. One third of these individuals have gynecomastia.

- Of ova penetrated by sperm, 15% fail to implant and 25% to 30% are aborted spontaneously at a previllous stage. Of the 40% that survive the first missed menstrual period, as many as one fourth abort spontaneously. From 30% to 35% of ova penetrated by sperm end in live-born individuals.

- Between 30% and 60% of known aborted conceptuses have chromosome abnormalities. Half of these have autosomal trisomies; 20%, 45,X; 14% to 19%, triploidy; 3% to 6%, tetraploidy; and 3% to 4%, chromosome rearrangements.

- Of live-born infants with chromosome abnormalities, about 0.8% to 1% have 45,X; 36.8% have other sex chromosome abnormalities; 21% have autosomal trisomies; and balanced chromosome translocations occur in 32.4%. About 3.2% have unbalanced translocation abnormalities.

- One in 200 women has recurrent (three or more) abortions, with chromosome abnormalities occurring in about 4.8% of the mothers and 2.4% of the fathers.

- When chromosome 21 is present as part of a Robertsonian translocation with a D group chromosome, the chance of transmission of an unbalanced karyotype (leading to a Down syndrome offspring) is 10% to 15% if the mother is the carrier and 1% to 2% if the father is the carrier.

- Hydatidiform moles are either diploid (46,XX or 46,XY) or triploid. The chromosomes of the diploid type, usually seen in true moles, are completely derived from paternal chromosomes. Triploidy moles have at least two haploid sets derived from paternal origin.

- Oncogenes fall into two general categories: those related to the cell skeleton and those related to the transmission or transduction of growth-regulating signals. Mutations in these genes by a variety of genetic mechanisms may lead to loss of normal cell controls, resulting in transformation of the cell to cancer.

BIBLIOGRAPHY

American College of Obstetricians and Gynecologists. Technical Bulletin 208: Genetic technologies, July 1995, Washington, DC.

Berchuck A, Kohler MF, Marks JR, et al: The p53 tumor suppressor gene frequently is altered in gynecologic cancers, Am J Obstet Gynecol 170:246, 1994.

Borresen AL: Oncogenesis in ovarian cancer, Acta Obstet Gynecol Scand Suppl 155:25, 1992.

Boue J, Boue A, and Lazar P: Retrospective and prospective epidemiological studies of 1500 karyotyped spontaneous human abortions, Teratology 12:11, 1975.

Boue A and Gallano P: A collaborative study of segregation of inherited chromosome structural rearrangements in 1356 prenatal diagnoses, Prenat Diagn 4:45, 1984.

Bowcock AM, Anderson LA, Friedman LS, et al: THRA1 and P17S183 flank an interval of <4cM for the breast-ovarian cancer gene (BRCA1) on chromosome 17q21, Am J Hum Genet 52:718, 1993.

Cirisano FD and Karlan BY: The role of the HER-2/neu oncogene in gynecologic cancers, J Soc Gynecol Investig 3:99, 1996.

Creasy MR, Crolla JA, and Alberman ED: A cytogenetic study of human spontaneous abortion using banding techniques, Hum Genet 31:177, 1976.

Dewhurst J: Fertility in 47,XXX and 45,X patients, J Med Genet 15:132, 1978.

Easton DF, Bishop DT, Ford D, and Crockford BP: Breast cancer linkage consortium, Am J Hum Genet 52:718, 1993.

Erlich A, Gelfand DH, and Saiki RK: Specific DNA amplification, Nature 331:46, 1988.

Evans HJ and Prosser J: Tumor-suppressor genes: cardinal factors in inherited predisposition to human cancers, Environ Health Perspect 98:25, 1992.

Fearon ER, Cho KR, Nigro JM, et al: Identification of a chromosome 18q gene that is altered in colorectal cancers, Science 247:49, 1990.

Feunteun J, Narod SA, Lynch HT, et al: A breast-ovarian cancer susceptibility gene maps to chromosome 17q21, Am J Hum Genet 52:736, 1993.

Ford EHR: Human chromosomes, New York, 1973, Academic Press.

Fortuny A, Carrio A, Soler A, et al: Detection of balanced chromosome rearrangements in 445 couples with repeated abortion and cytogenetic prenatal testing in carriers, Fertil Steril 49:774, 1988.

Futreal PA, Liu Q, Shattuck-Eidens D, et al: BRCA1 mutations in primary breast and ovarian carcinomas, Science 266:120, 1994.

Hamerton JL, Canning N, Ray M, and Smith S: A cytogenetic survey of 14,069 newborn infants. I. Incidence of chromosome abnormalities, Clin Genet 8:223, 1975.

Harnden DG and Klinger HP, eds: An international system for human cytogenetic nomenclature, published in collaboration with Cytogenet Cell Genet, Basel, Switzerland, 1985, S Karger Medical and Scientific Publishers.

Jones HW Jr and Scott WM: Hermaphroditism: genital anomalies and related endocrine disorders, Baltimore, 1971, Williams & Wilkins.

Kajii T and Nikawa N: Origin of triploidy and tetraploidy in man: cases with chromosome markers, Cytogenet Cell Genet 18:109, 1977.

Kajii T and Ohama K: Androgenetic origin of hydatidiform mole, Nature 268:633, 1977.

Kerem B-S, Rommens JM, Buchanan JA, et al: Identification of the cystic fibrosis gene: genetic analysis, Science 245:1073, 1989.

King CR: Prenatal diagnosis of genetic disease with molecular genetic technology, Obstet Gynecol Surv 43:493, 1988.

Lubinsky MS: Female pseudohermaphroditism and associated anomalies, Am J Med Genet 6:123, 1980.

Malkin D, Li FP, Strong LC, et al: Germ line p53 mutations in a familial syndrome of breast cancer, sarcomas, and other neoplasms, Science 250:1233, 1990.

McKusick VA: Mendelian inheritance in man, Baltimore, 1978, The Johns Hopkins Press.

Miki Y, Swensen J, Shattuck-Eidens P, et al: A strong candidate for the breast and ovarian cancer susceptibility gene BRCA1, Science 266:66, 1994.

Raskin S, Phillips JA, Kaplan G, et al: Cystic fibrosis genotyping by direct PCR analysis of Guthrie blood spots, PCR Methods Appl 2:154, 1992.

Ratcliffe S: Postnatal chromosome abnormalities. In Boyce HJ, ed: Chromosome variations in human evolution, London, 1975, Taylor & Francis.

Roman E: Fetal loss rates and their relation to pregnancy order, J Epidemiol Community Health 38:29, 1984.

Schmike RN: Genetics and cancer in man, Edinburgh, 1980, Churchill Livingstone.

Shepard TH and Fantel AG: Embryonic and early fetal loss, Clin Perinatol 6:219, 1979.

Simpson JL: Disorders of sexual differentiation: etiology and clinical delineation, New York, 1976, Academic Press.

Simpson JL: True hermaphroditism: etiology and phenotypic considerations, Birth Defects 14:9, 1978.

Simpson JL: Repeated suboptimal pregnancy outcome, Birth Defects 17:113, 1981.

Simpson JL, Globus MS, Martin AO, and Sarto GE: Genetics in obstetrics and gynecology, New York, 1982, Grune & Stratton.

Stene J, Stene E, and Mikkelsen M: Risk for chromosome abnormality at amniocentesis following a child with a non-inherited chromosome aberration, Prenat Diagn 4:81, 1984.

Stephenson MD: Frequency of factors associated with habitual abortion in 197 couples, Fertil Steril 66:24, 1996.

Uehara S, Nata M, Nagae M, et al: Molecular biologic analyses of tetragemetic chimerism in a true hermaphrodite with 46,XX/46,XY, Fertil Steril 63:189, 1995.

Vejerslev LO, Fisher RA, Surti U, and Walke N: Hydatidiform mole: cytogenetically unusual cases and their implications for the present classification, Am J Obstet Gynecol 157:180, 1984.

Watkins PC: Restriction fragment length polymorphism (RFLP): applications in human chromosome mapping and genetic disease research, BioTechniques 6:310, 1988.

Watson EJ, Hernandez E, and Miyazawa K: Partial hydatidiform moles: a review, Obstet Gynecol Surv 42:540, 1987.

Watson JD, Hopkins NH, Roberts WJ, et al: Molecular biology of the gene, ed 4, Menlo Park, Calif, 1987, Benjamin-Cummings Publishing Co.

Watson JV, Curling OM, Munn CF, and Hudson CN: Oncogene expression in ovarian cancer: a pilot study of C-myc oncoprotein in serous papillary ovarian cancer, Gynecol Oncol 28:137, 1987.

Wooster R, Neuhausen SL, Mangion J, et al: Localization of a breast cancer susceptibility gene, BRCA2, to chromosome 13q12-13, Science 265:2088, 1994.

Reproductive Anatomy
Gross and Microscopic, Clinical Correlations

KEY TERMS AND DEFINITIONS

Auerbach's Plexus. A network of twin vessels within the tunica muscularis of the ureters.

Apocrine Gland. A gland that produces secretions formed partially from the secreting cells of the gland itself.

Bladder Neck. That part of the bladder that is continuous with the urethra.

Canal of Nuck. A tubular process of peritoneum that accompanies the round ligament into the inguinal canal. It is generally obliterated in the adult but sometimes remains patent.

Carunculae Myrtiformes. Small nodules of fibrous tissue at the vaginal orifice that are remnants of the hymen.

Cornua. The superolateral aspects of the uterine cavity; the anatomic areas where the oviducts enter the uterine cavity.

Cul-de-sac of Douglas. A deep pouch formed by the most caudal extent of the parietal peritoneum. It is anterior to the rectum, separating the uterus from the large intestine.

Eccrine Gland. A simple sweat-producing gland in which the secreting cells are maintained intact during production of secretions.

Fimbria Ovarica. One of the largest fingerlike projections of the distal end of the oviducts. The fimbria ovarica usually attaches the oviducts to the ovary.

Frankenhäuser's Plexus. An extensive concentration of both myelinated and nonmyelinated nerve fibers located in the uterosacral ligaments and supplying primarily the uterus and the cervix.

Fundus. The dome-shaped top of the uterus.

Genitocrural Fold. The skin line dividing the external female genitalia and the medial aspects of the thigh.

Isthmus. The short area of constriction in the lower uterine segment.

Parametria. The extraperitoneal fatty and fibrous connective tissue immediately adjacent to the uterus. The parametria lie between the leaves of the broad ligament and in the contiguous area anteriorly between the cervix and the bladder.

Pelvic Diaphragm. A thin, muscular layer of tissue that forms the inferior border of the abdominal pelvic cavity. The primary muscles of the pelvic diaphragm are the levator ani and coccygeus muscles.

Perineum. The region between the thighs bounded anteriorly by the vulva and posteriorly by the anus.

Plexus. A mixture of preganglionic and postganglionic fibers; small, inconsistently placed nerve ganglia; and afferent sensory fibers. In the female pelvis a plexus also may be termed a *nerve*.

Plicae Palmatae. Longitudinal folds in the mucous membrane of the endocervical canal. The secondary branching folds are called *arbor vitae*.

Posterior Fourchette. The fold of skin that joins the labia minora at their inferior margins.

Presacral Nerves. A midline plexus of nerves that contains the most important components of the pelvic autonomic nerves. The presacral nerves are located in the retroperitoneal connective tissue from the fourth lumbar vertebra to the hollow over the sacrum. (Also termed the *superior hypogastric plexus*.)

Rugae. Numerous transverse folds of the vagina in women of reproductive age.

Space of Retzius. The area lying between the bladder and symphysis pubis, bounded laterally by the obliterated hypogastric arteries.

Urachus. The adult remnant of the embryonic allantois.

Urogenital Diaphragm. A strong, muscular membrane that occupies the area between the symphysis pubis and the ischial tuberosities. Posteriorly, the urogenital diaphragm inserts into the central point of the perineum.

Vestibular Bulbs. Two elongated masses of erectile tissue situated on either side of the vaginal orifice. They are homologous to the bulb of the penis in the male.

The organs of the female reproductive tract are classically divided into the external and the internal genitalia. The external genital organs are present in the perineal area and include the mons pubis, clitoris, urinary meatus, labia majora, labia minora, vestibule, Bartholin's glands, and periurethral glands. The internal genital organs are located in the true pelvis and include the vagina, uterus, cervix, oviducts, ovaries, and surrounding supporting structures. This chapter integrates the basic anatomy of the female pelvis with clinical situations.

Embryologically the urinary, reproductive, and gastrointestinal tracts develop in close proximity. This relationship continues throughout a woman's life span. In the adult the reproductive organs are in intimate contact with the lower urinary tract and large intestines. Because of the anatomic proximity of the genital and urinary systems, altered pathophysiology in one organ often produces symptoms in an adjacent organ. The gynecologic surgeon should master the intricacy of these anatomic relationships to avoid major surgical complications.

This chapter does not duplicate the completeness of anatomic texts or surgical atlases; it concentrates on the norms of human anatomy. The reader must appreciate that wide individual differences in anatomic detail exist among patients. Understanding these variations is one of the greatest challenges of clinical medicine.

EXTERNAL GENITALIA

Vulva

The vulva, or pudendum, is a collective term for the external genital organs that are visible in the perineal area. The vulva consists of the following: the mons pubis, labia majora, labia minora, hymen, clitoris, vestibule, urethra, Skene's glands, Bartholin's glands, and vestibular bulbs (Figure 3-1).

The boundaries of the vulva extend from the mons pubis anteriorly to the rectum posteriorly and from one lateral genitocrural fold to the other. The entire vulvar area is covered by keratinized, stratified squamous epithelium. The skin becomes thicker, more pigmented, and more keratinized as the distance from the vagina increases.

Mons Pubis

The mons pubis is a rounded eminence that becomes hairy after puberty. It is directly anterior and superior to the symphysis pubis. The hair pattern, or escutcheon, of most women is triangular. Genetic and racial differences produce a variety of normal hair patterns, with approximately one in four women having a modified escutcheon that has a diamond (malelike) pattern.

Labia Majora

The labia majora are two large, longitudinal, cutaneous folds of adipose and fibrous tissue. Each labium majus is approximately 7 to 8 cm in length and 2 to 3 cm in width. The labia extend from the mons pubis anteriorly to become lost in the skin between the vagina and the anus in the area of the posterior fourchette. The skin of the outer convex surface of the labia majora is pigmented and covered with hair follicles. The thin skin of the inner surface does not have hair follicles but has many sebaceous glands. Histologically the labia majora have both sweat and sebaceous glands (Figure 3-2). The apocrine glands are similar to those of the breast and axillary areas. The size of the labia is related to fat content. Usually the labia atrophy after menopause. The labia majora are homologous to the scrotum in the male.

Labia Minora

The labia minora, or nymphae, are two small, red cutaneous folds that are situated between the labia majora and the vaginal orifice. They are more delicate, shorter, and thinner than the labia majora. Anteriorly, they divide at the clitoris to form superiorly the prepuce and inferiorly the frenulum of the clitoris. Histologically they are composed of dense

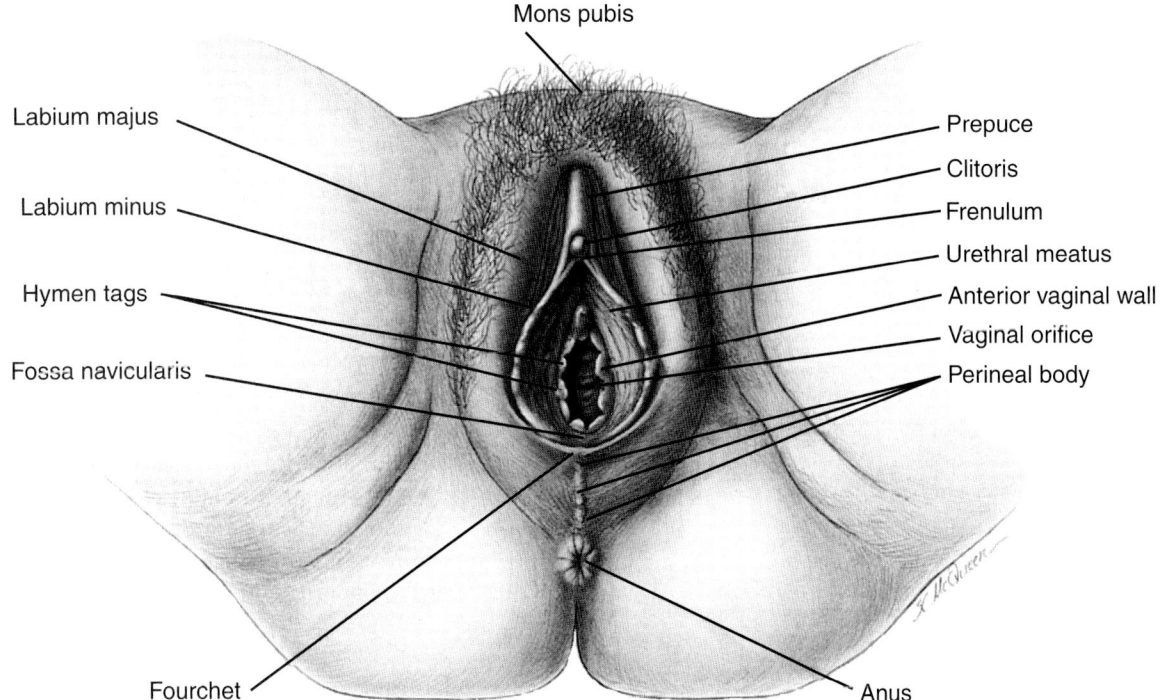

FIGURE 3-1 The structures of the external genitalia that are collectively called the *vulva*. (Redrawn from Pritchard JA, MacDonald PC, and Gant NF: Williams' obstetrics, ed 17, New York, 1985, Appleton-Century-Crofts, p. 8.)

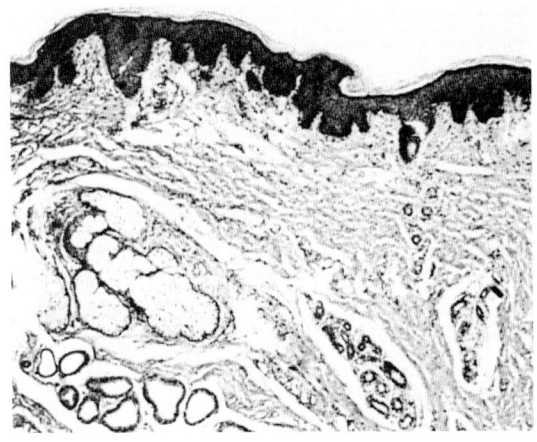

FIGURE 3-2 A histologic section from the labium majus. A cornified squamous epithelium covers the dermis, which contains eccrine, apocrine, and sebaceous glands. (H&E stain; ×77.) (Reproduced with permission from Kaufman RH: Anatomy of the vulva and vagina. In Gardner HL and Kaufman RH, eds: Benign disease of the vulva and vagina, ed 2, Chicago, 1981, Mosby–Year Book, Inc.)

connective tissue with erectile tissue and elastic fibers, rather than adipose tissue. The skin of the labia minora is less cornified and has many sebaceous glands but no hair follicles or sweat glands. The labia minora and the breasts are the only areas of the body rich in sebaceous glands without hair follicles. Among women of reproductive age, there is considerable variation in the size of the labia minora. They are relatively more prominent in children and postmenopausal women. The labia minora are homologous to the penile urethra and part of the skin of the penis in males.

Hymen

The hymen is a thin, usually perforated membrane at the entrance of the vagina. There are many variations in the structure and shape of the hymen. The hymen histologically is covered by stratified squamous epithelium on both sides and consists of fibrous tissue with a few small blood vessels. Small tags, or nodules, of firm fibrous material, termed *carunculae myrtiformes*, are the remnants of the hymen identified in adult females.

Clitoris

The clitoris is a short, cylindrical, erectile organ at the superior portion of the vestibule. The normal adult glans clitoris has a width less than 1 cm, with an average length of 1.5 to 2 cm. Previous childbearing may influence the size of the clitoris, but age, weight, and oral contraceptive use do not change the anatomic dimensions. Usually, only the glans is visible, with the body of the clitoris positioned beneath the skin surface. The clitoris consists of a base of two crura, which attach to the periosteum of the symphysis pubis. The body has two cylindric corpora cavernosa composed of thin-walled, vascular channels that function as erectile tissue. The distal one third of the clitoris is the glans, which has many nerve endings. The clitoris is the female homologue of the penis in the male.

Vestibule

The vestibule is the lowest portion of the embryonic uro-genital sinus. It is the cleft between the labia minora that is visualized when the labia are held apart. The vestibule extends from the clitoris to the posterior fourchette. The orifices of the urethra and vagina and the ducts from Bartholin's glands open into the vestibule. Within the area of the vestibule are the remnants of the hymen and numerous small mucinous glands.

Urethra

The urethra is a membranous conduit for urine from the urinary bladder to the vestibule. The female urethra measures 3.5 to 5 cm in length. The mucosa of the proximal two thirds of the urethra is composed of stratified transitional epithelium, whereas the distal one third is stratified squamous epithelium. The distal orifice is 4 to 6 mm in diameter, and the mucosal edges grossly appear everted.

Skene's Glands

Skene's glands, or paraurethral glands, are branched, tubular glands that are adjacent to the distal urethra. Usually Skene's ducts run parallel to the long axis of the urethra for approximately 1 cm before opening into the distal urethra. Sometimes the ducts open into the area just outside the urethral orifice. Skene's glands are the largest of the paraurethral glands; however, many smaller glands empty into the urethra. Skene's glands are homologous to the prostate in the male.

Bartholin's Glands

Bartholin's glands are vulvovaginal glands that are located beneath the fascia at about 4 and 8 o'clock, respectively, on the posterolateral aspect of the vaginal orifice. Each lobulated, racemose gland is about the size of a pea. Histologically the gland is composed of cuboidal epithelium (Figure 3-3). The duct from each gland is lined by transitional epithelium and is approximately 2 cm in length. Bartholin's ducts open into a groove between the hymen and the labia minora. Bartholin's glands are homologous to Cowper's glands in the male.

Vestibular Bulbs

The vestibular bulbs are two elongated masses of erectile tissue situated on either side of the vaginal orifice. Each bulb is immediately below the bulbocavernosus muscle. The distal ends of the vestibular bulbs are adjacent to Bartholin's glands. They are homologous to the bulb of the penis in the male.

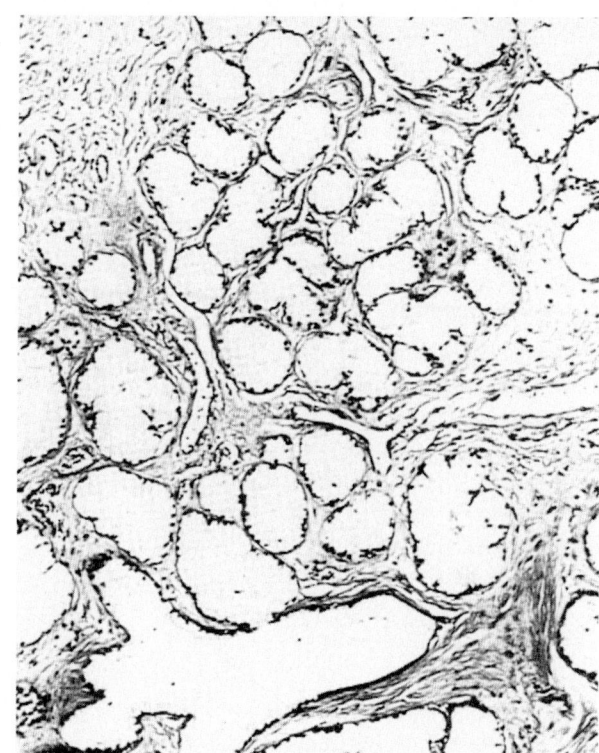

FIGURE 3-3 A histologic section of a Bartholin's gland, showing cuboidal epithelium lining acinar structures. (H&E stain; ×117.) (Reproduced with permission from Kaufman RH: Anatomy of the vulva and vagina. In Gardner HL and Kaufman RH, eds: Benign diseases of the vulva and vagina, ed 2, Chicago, 1981, Mosby–Year Book, Inc.)

Clinical Correlations

The skin of the vulvar region is subject to both local and general dermatologic conditions. The intertriginous areas of the vulva remain moist, and obese women are particularly susceptible to chronic infection. The vulvar skin of a postmenopausal woman is sensitive to topical cortisone and testosterone but insensitive to topical estrogen. The most common large cystic structure of the vulva is a Bartholin's duct cyst. This condition may become painful if the cyst develops into an acute abscess. Chronic infections of the periurethral glands may result in one or more urethral diverticula. The most common symptoms of a urethral diverticulum are similar to the symptoms of a lower urinary tract infection: urinary frequency, urgency, and dysuria.

Vulvar trauma frequently results in a large hematoma or profuse external hemorrhage. The richness of the vascular supply and the absence of valves in vulvar veins contribute to this complication. The abundant vascularity of the region promotes rapid healing, with an associated low incidence of wound infection in episiotomies or obstetric tears of the vulva.

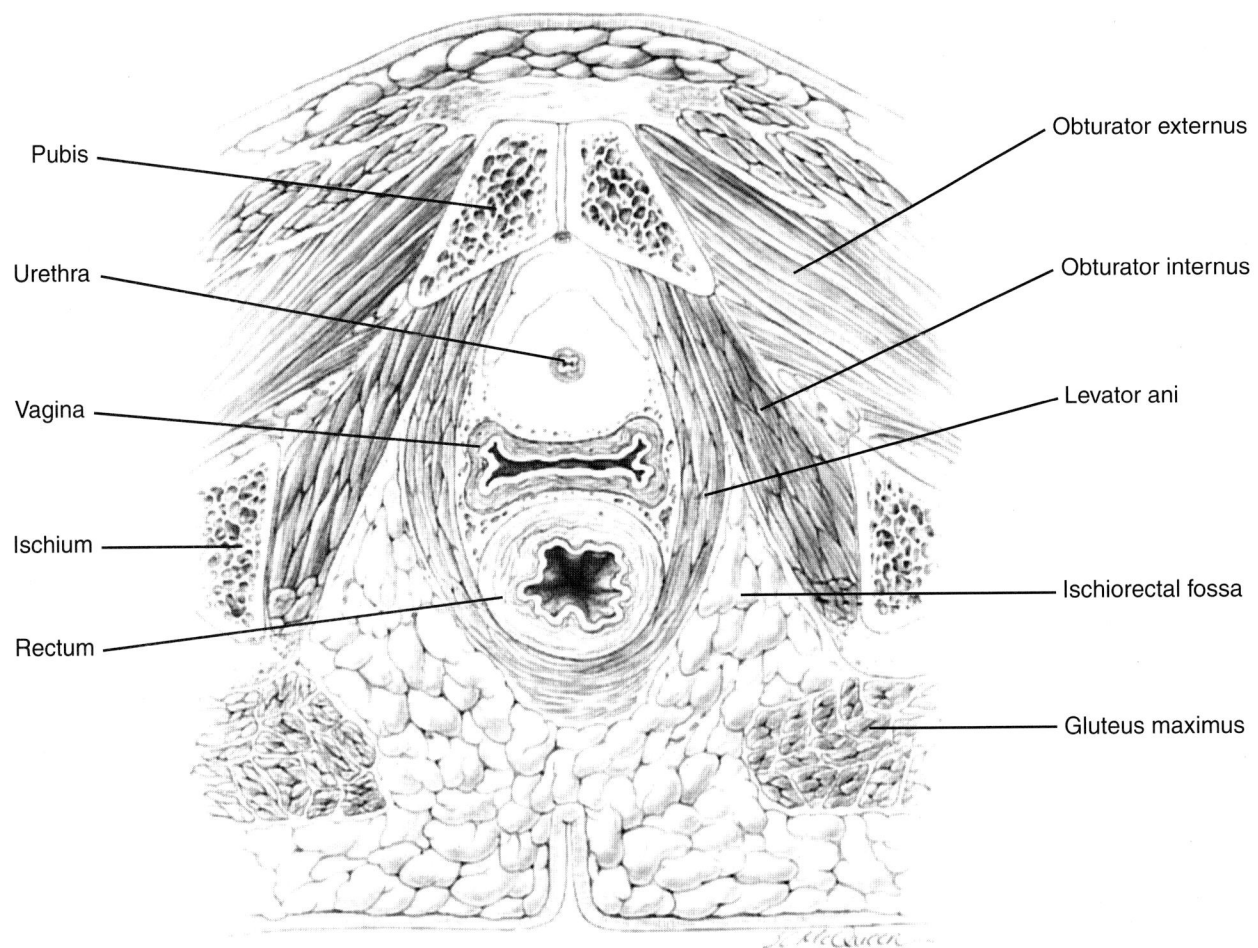

Pubis

Urethra

Vagina

Ischium

Rectum

Obturator externus

Obturator internus

Levator ani

Ischiorectal fossa

Gluteus maximus

FIGURE 3-4 A schematic drawing of a cross section of the female pelvis, demonstrating the H shape of the vagina. Note the surrounding levator ani muscle. (Redrawn from Pritchard JA, MacDonald PC, and Gant NF: Williams' obstetrics, ed 17, New York, 1985, Appleton-Century-Crofts, p. 12.)

VAGINA

The vagina is a thin-walled, distensible, fibromuscular tube that extends from the vestibule of the vulva to the uterus. The potential space of the vagina is larger in the middle and upper thirds. The walls of the vagina are normally in apposition and flattened in the anteroposterior diameter. Thus the vagina has the appearance of the letter H in cross section (Figure 3-4).

The axis of the upper portion of the vagina lies close to the horizontal plane when a woman is standing, with the upper portion of the vagina curving toward the hollow of the sacrum. In most women an angle of at least 90 degrees is formed between the axis of the vagina and the axis of the uterus. The vagina is held in position by the surrounding endopelvic fascia and ligaments.

The lower third of the vagina is in close relationship with the urogenital and pelvic diaphragms. The middle third of the vagina is supported by the levator ani muscles and the lower portion of the cardinal ligaments. The upper third is supported by the upper portions of the cardinal ligaments and the parametria.

The vagina of reproductive-age women has numerous transverse folds, termed *rugae*. They help provide accordion-like distensibility and are more prominent in the lower third of the vagina. The cervix extends into the upper part of the vagina. The spaces between the cervix and attachment of the vagina are called *fornices*. The posterior fornix is considerably larger than the anterior fornix; thus the anterior vaginal length is approximately 6 to 9 cm in comparison with a posterior vaginal length of 8 to 12 cm.

Histologically the vagina is composed of four distinct layers. The mucosa consists of a stratified, nonkeratinized squamous epithelium. If the environment of the vaginal mucosa is modified, as in uterine prolapse, then the epithelium may become keratinized. The squamous epithelium is similar microscopically to the exocervix, although the vagina has larger and more frequent papillae that extend into the connective tissue. The normal vagina does not have glands. The next layer is the lamina propria, or tunica. It is composed of fibrous connective tissue. Throughout this layer of collagen and elastic tissue is a rich supply of vascular and lymphatic channels. The density of the connective tissue in the endopelvic fascia varies throughout the longitudinal axis of the vagina. The muscular layer has many interlacing fibers. However, an inner circular layer and an outer longitudinal layer can be identified. The fourth layer consists of cellular areolar connective tissue containing a large plexus of blood vessels.

The vascular system of the vagina is generously supplied with an extensive anastomotic network throughout its length. The vaginal artery originates either directly from the uterine artery or as a branch of the internal iliac artery arising posterior to the origin of the uterine and inferior vesical arteries. The vaginal arteries may be multiple arteries on each side of the pelvis. There is an anastomosis with the cervical branch of the uterine artery to form the azygos arteries. Branches of the internal pudendal, inferior vesical, and middle hemorrhoidal arteries also contribute to the interconnecting network and the longitudinal azygos arteries.

The venous drainage is complex and accompanies the arterial system. Below the pelvic floor the principal venous drainage occurs via the pudendal veins. The vaginal, uterine, and vesical veins, as well as those around the rectosigmoid, all provide venous drainage of the venous plexuses surrounding the middle and upper vagina.

The nerve supply of the vagina comes from the autonomic nervous system's vaginal plexus, and sensory fibers come from the pudendal nerve. Pain fibers enter the spinal cord in sacral segments 2 to 4. There is a paucity of free nerve endings in the upper two thirds of the vagina.

The lymphatic drainage is characterized by its wide distribution and frequent crossovers between the right and left sides of the pelvis. In general the primary lymphatic drainage of the upper third of the vagina is to the external iliac nodes, the middle third of the vagina drains to the common and internal iliac nodes, and the lower third has a complex and variable distribution, including the common iliac, superficial inguinal, and perirectal nodes.

Clinical Correlations

In clinical practice anatomic descriptions of pelvic organs are derived from Latin roots, such as "vagina," from the Latin word for sheath. In contrast, the names for surgical procedures of pelvic organs are derived from Greek roots. *Colpectomy, colporrhaphy,* and *colposcopy* are derived from *kolpos* (fold), the Greek word for the vagina.

Clinicians should consider the H shape of the vagina when they insert a speculum and inspect the walls of the vagina. The posterior fornix is an important surgical landmark, since it provides direct access to the cul-de-sac of Douglas. The distal course of the ureter is an important consideration in vaginal surgery. Ureteral injury has occurred as a result of vaginally placed sutures to obtain hemostasis with vaginal lacerations. The anatomic proximity and interrelationships of the vascular and lymphatic networks of the bladder and vagina are such that inflammation of one organ can produce symptoms in the other. For example, vaginitis sometimes produces urinary tract symptoms, such as frequency and dysuria.

Gartner's duct cyst, a cystic dilation of the embryonic mesonephros, is usually present on the lateral wall of the vagina. However, in the lower third of the vagina these cysts are present anteriorly and may be difficult to distinguish from a large urethral diverticulum.

An interesting phenomenon is the source of vaginal lubrication during intercourse. For years there was speculation on how an organ without glands is able to "secrete" fluid. Vaginal lubrication occurs from a transudate produced by engorgement of the vascular plexuses that encircle the vagina. Many drugs readily enter the systemic circulation when placed in the vagina.

The anatomic relationship between the long axis of the vagina and other pelvic organs may be altered by pelvic relaxation resulting primarily from the trauma of childbirth. Atrophy or weakness of the endopelvic fascia and muscles surrounding the vagina may result in the development of a cystocele, rectocele, and/or enterocele. One of the popular operations for vaginal vault prolapse is fixation of the apex to the vagina to the sacrospinous ligament. A rare complication of this operation is massive hemorrhage. The arterial bleeding is usually from the inferior gluteal or pudendal arteries.

CERVIX

The lower, narrow portion of the uterus is the cervix. The word *cervix* originates from the Latin word for neck. The Greek word for neck is *trachelos,* and when the cervix is removed, the surgical procedure is termed *trachelectomy.* The cervix may vary in shape from cylindrical to conical. It consists of predominantly fibrous tissue in contrast to the primarily muscular corpus of the uterus.

The vagina is attached obliquely around the middle of the cervix; this attachment divides the cervix into an upper, supravaginal portion and a lower segment in the vagina called the *portio vaginalis* (Figure 3-5). The supravaginal segment is covered by peritoneum posteriorly and is surrounded by loose, fatty connective tissue, the parametrium, anteriorly and laterally.

The canal of the cervix is fusiform, with the widest diameter in the middle. The length and width of the endocervical canal varies; it is usually 2.5 to 3 cm in length and 7 to 8 mm at its widest point. The width of the canal varies with the parity of the woman and changing hormonal lev-

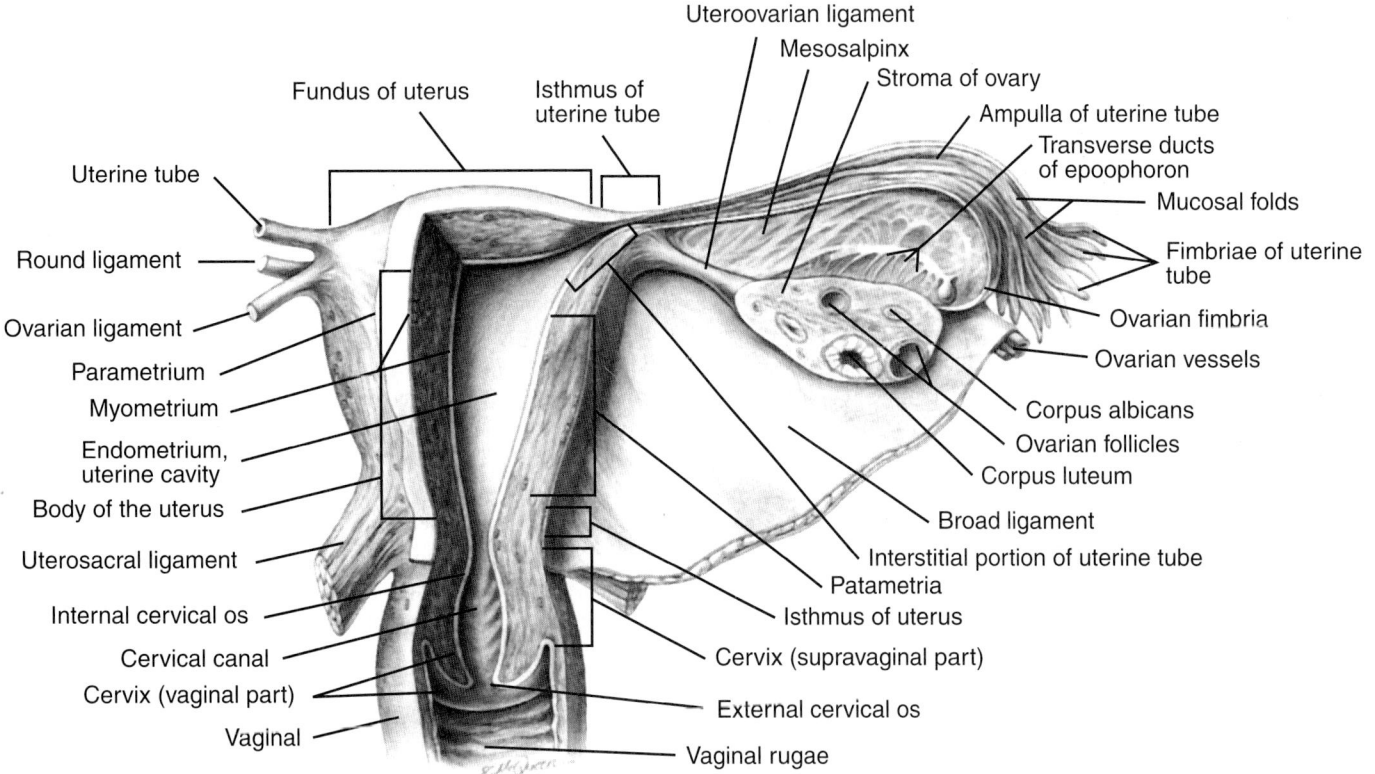

Uteroovarian ligament
Mesosalpinx
Stroma of ovary
Fundus of uterus
Isthmus of uterine tube
Ampulla of uterine tube
Transverse ducts of epoophoron
Mucosal folds
Uterine tube
Fimbriae of uterine tube
Round ligament
Ovarian fimbria
Ovarian ligament
Ovarian vessels
Parametrium
Corpus albicans
Myometrium
Ovarian follicles
Endometrium, uterine cavity
Corpus luteum
Body of the uterus
Broad ligament
Uterosacral ligament
Interstitial portion of uterine tube
Patametria
Internal cervical os
Isthmus of uterus
Cervical canal
Cervix (supravaginal part)
Cervix (vaginal part)
External cervical os
Vaginal
Vaginal rugae

FIGURE 3-5 A schematic drawing of a posterior view of the cervix, uterus, fallopian tube, and ovary. Note that the cervix is divided by the vaginal attachment into an external portio segment and a supravaginal segment. Note that the uterus is composed of the dome-shaped fundus, the muscular body, and the narrow isthmus. Note the fimbria ovarica, or ovarian fimbria, attaching the oviduct to the ovary. (Redrawn from Clemente CD: Anatomy: a regional atlas of the human body, ed 3, Baltimore-Munich, 1987, Urban & Schwarzenberg.)

els. The cervical canal opens into the vagina at the external os of the cervix. In the majority of women the external os is in contact with the posterior vaginal wall. The external os is small and round in nulliparous women. The os is wider and gaping following vaginal delivery. Often lateral or stellate scars are residual marks of previous cervical lacerations.

The mucous membrane of the endocervical canal of nulliparous women is arranged in longitudinal folds, plicae palmatae, with secondary branching folds, the arbor vitae (Figure 3-6). These folds, which form a herringbone pattern, disappear following vaginal delivery.

A single layer of columnar epithelium lines the endocervical canal and the underlying glandular structures. This specialized epithelium secretes mucus, which facilitates sperm transport. An abrupt transformation usually is seen at the junction of the columnar epithelium of the endocervix and the nonkeratinized stratified squamous epithelium of the portio vaginalis (Figure 3-7). The stratified squamous epithelium of the exocervix is identical to the lining of the vagina.

The dense, fibromuscular cervical stroma is composed primarily of collagenous connective tissue and mucopolysaccharide ground substance. The connective tissue con-

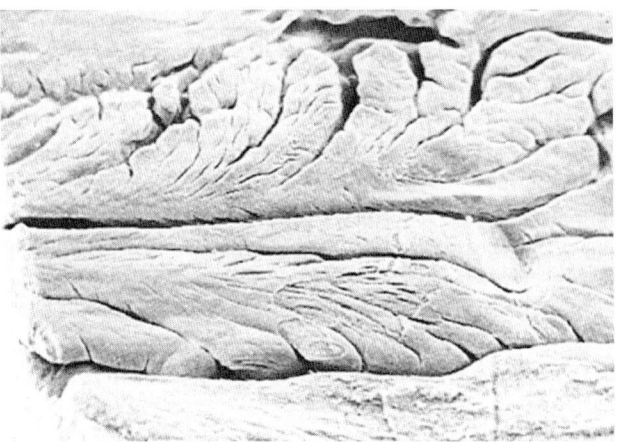

FIGURE 3-6 An electron micrograph of the endocervical canal, demonstrating the "arbor vitae." These folds and crypts provide a reservoir for sperm. (From Singer A and Jordan JA: The anatomy of the cervix. In Jordan JA and Singer A, eds: The cervix, Philadelphia, 1976, WB Saunders Co., p. 18.)

tains approximately 15% smooth muscle cells and a small amount of elastic tissue. However, there are few muscle fibers in the distal portions of the cervix.

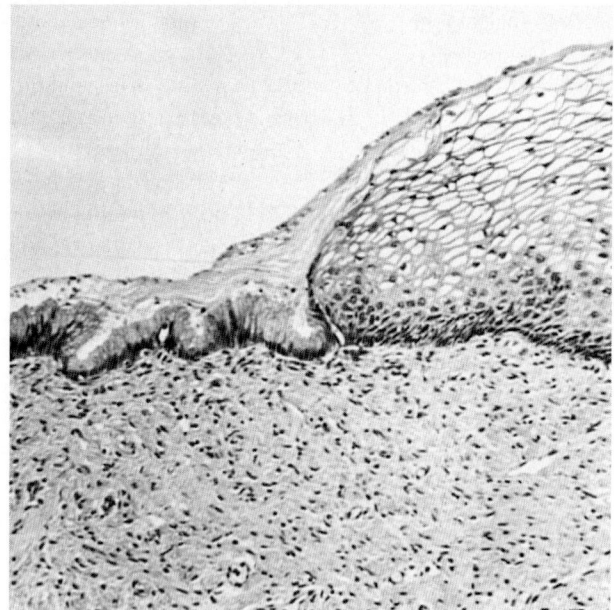

FIGURE 3-7 A histologic section through the squamocolumnar junction of the cervix. Note the abrupt transformation from squamous to columnar epithelium. (From Ferenczy A: Anatomy and histology of the cervix. In Blaustein A, ed: Pathology of the female genital tract, ed 2, New York, 1982, Springer-Verlag, p. 127.)

It is not surprising that the cervical and uterine vascular supplies are interrelated. The arterial supply of the cervix arises from the descending branch of the uterine artery. The cervical arteries run on the lateral side of the cervix and form the coronary artery, which encircles the cervix. The azygos arteries run longitudinally in the middle of the anterior and posterior aspects of the cervix and the vagina. There are numerous anastomoses between these vessels and the vaginal and middle hemorrhoidal arteries. The venous drainage accompanies these arteries. The lymphatic drainage of the cervix is complex, involving multiple chains of nodes. The principal regional lymph nodes are the obturator, common iliac, internal iliac, external iliac, and visceral nodes of the parametria. Other possible lymphatic drainage includes the following chains of nodes: superior and inferior gluteal, sacral, rectal, lumbar, aortic, and visceral nodes over the posterior surface of the urinary bladder. The stroma of the endocervix is rich in free nerve endings. Pain fibers accompany the parasympathetic fibers to the second, third, and fourth sacral segments.

Clinical Correlations

The major arterial supply to the cervix is located on the lateral cervical walls at the 3 and 9 o'clock positions, respectively. Therefore a deep figure-of-eight suture through the vaginal mucosa and cervical stroma at 3 and 9 o'clock helps to reduce blood loss during procedures such as cone biopsy. If the gynecologist is overzealous in placing such a hemostatic suture high in the vaginal fornix, it is possible to compromise the course of the distal ureter.

The transformation zone of the cervix is an important anatomic landmark for clinicians. This area encompasses the transition from stratified squamous epithelium to columnar epithelium. Dysplasia of the cervix develops within this transformation zone. The position of a woman's transformation zone, in relation to the long axis of the cervix, depends on her age and hormonal status.

The endocervix is rich in free nerve endings. Occasionally, women experience a vagovagal response during transcervical instrumentation of the uterine cavity. Serial cardiac monitoring during insertion of intrauterine devices demonstrates a reflex bradycardia in some women. The sensory innervation of the exocervix is not as concentrated or sophisticated as that of the endocervix or external skin. Therefore, usually the exocervix may be cauterized by either cold or heat without major discomfort to the patient.

UTERUS

The uterus is a thick-walled, hollow, muscular organ located centrally in the female pelvis. Adjacent to the uterus are the urinary bladder anteriorly, the rectum posteriorly, and the broad ligaments laterally (Figure 3-8). The uterus is globular and slightly flattened anteriorly; it has the general configuration of an inverted pear. The short area of constriction in the lower uterine segment is termed the *isthmus* (see Figure 3-5). The dome-shaped top of the uterus is termed the *fundus*. The lower edge of the fundus is described by an imaginary line drawn between the site of entrance of each oviduct. The size and weight of the normal uterus depend on previous pregnancies and the hormonal status of the individual. The uterus of a nulliparous woman is approximately 8 cm long, 5 cm wide, and 2.5 cm thick and weighs 40 to 50 g. In contrast, in a multiparous woman, each measurement is approximately 1.2 cm larger, and normal uterine weight is 20 to 30 g heavier. The upper limit for weight of a normal uterus is 110 g. The capacity of the uterus to enlarge during pregnancy results in a 10- to 20-fold increase in weight at term. After menopause the uterus atrophies in both size and weight.

The cavity of the uterus is flattened and triangular. The oviducts enter the uterine cavity at the superolateral aspects of the cavity in the areas designated the cornua. In the majority of women, the long axis of the uterus is both anteverted in respect to the long axis of the vagina and anteflexed in relation to the long axis of the cervix. However, a retroflexed uterus is a normal variant found in approximately 25% of women.

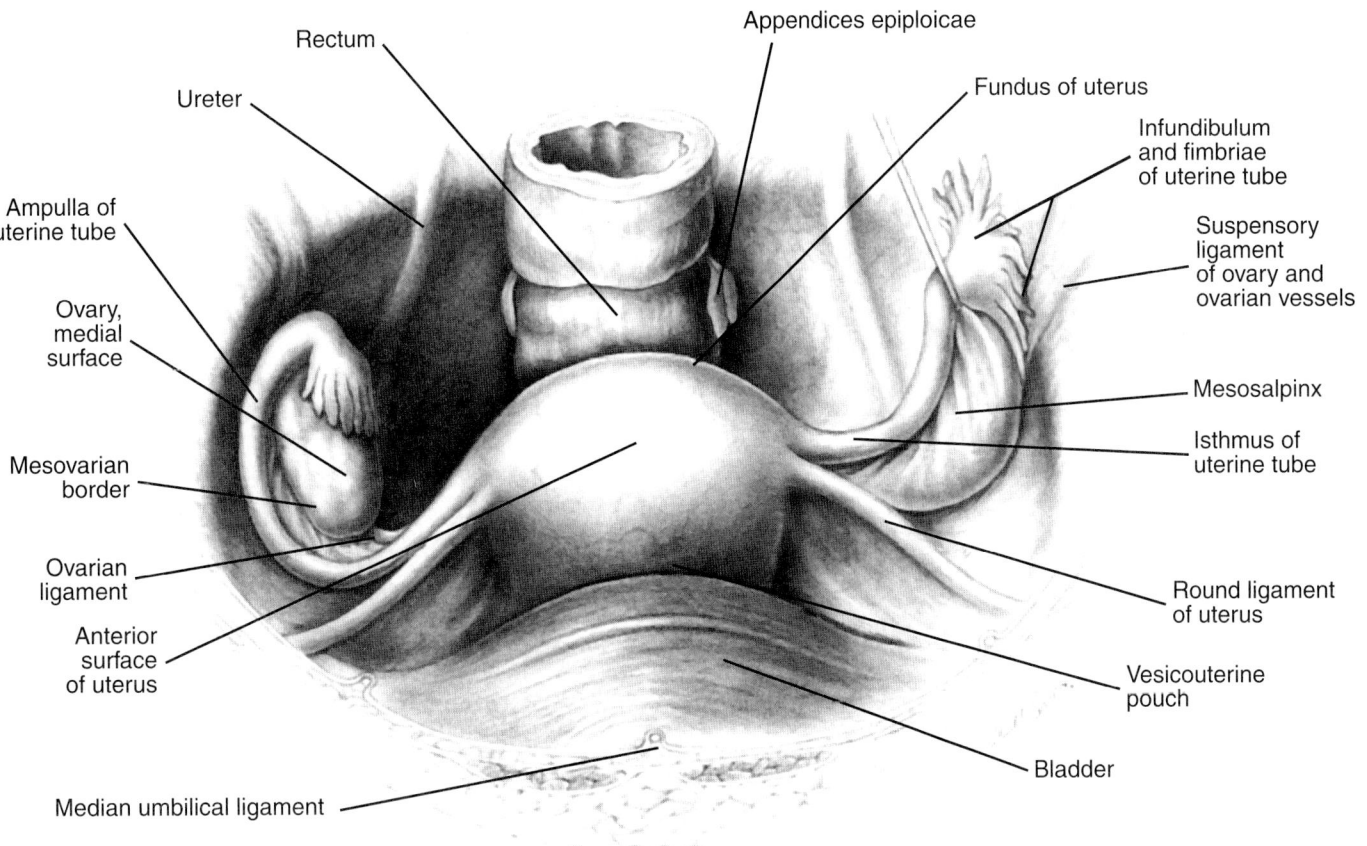

FIGURE 3-8 The organs of the female pelvis. The uterus is surrounded by the bladder anteriorly, the rectum posteriorly, and the folds of the broad ligaments laterally. (Redrawn from Clemente CD: Anatomy: a regional atlas of the human body, Baltimore-Munich, 1987, Urban & Schwarzenberg.)

The uterus has three layers, similar to other hollow abdominal and pelvic organs. The thin, external serosal layer is comprised by the visceral peritoneum. The peritoneum is firmly attached to the uterus in all areas except anteriorly at the level of the internal os of the cervix. The wide middle muscular layer is composed of three indistinct layers of smooth muscle. The outer longitudinal layer is contiguous with the muscle layers of the oviduct and vagina. The middle layer has interlacing oblique, spiral bundles of smooth muscle and large venous plexuses. The inner muscular layer is also longitudinal. The endometrium is a reddish mucous membrane that varies from 1 to 6 mm in thickness, depending on hormonal stimulation. The uterine glands are tubular and composed of tall columnar epithelium. The cells of the endometrial stroma resemble embryonic connective tissue with scant cytoplasm and large nuclei (Figure 3-9). The endometrium may be divided into an inner stratum basale and an outer stratum functionale. The stratum functionale may be further subdivided into an inner compact stratum and a more superficial spongy stratum. Only the stratum functionale responds to fluctuating hormonal levels.

The arterial blood supply of the uterus is provided by the uterine and ovarian arteries. The uterine arteries are large branches of the hypogastric arteries, whereas the ovarian arteries originate directly from the aorta. The veins accompany the arteries. Therefore venous drainage from the fundus goes to the ovarian veins, and blood from the corpus exits via the uterine veins into the iliac veins. The lymphatic drainage of the uterus is complex. The majority of lymphatics from the fundus and the body of the uterus go to the aortic, lumbar, and pelvic nodes surrounding the iliac vessels, especially the internal iliac nodes. However, it is possible for metastatic disease from the uterus to be found in the superior inguinal nodes transported via lymphatics in the round ligament.

In contrast to other pelvic organs, the afferent sensory nerve fibers from the uterus are in close proximity to the sympathetic nerves. Afferent nerve fibers from the uterus enter the spinal cord at the eleventh and twelfth thoracic segments. The sympathetic nerve supply to the uterus comes from the hypogastric and ovarian plexus. The parasympathetic fibers are largely derived from the pelvic nerve and from the second, third, and fourth sacral segments.

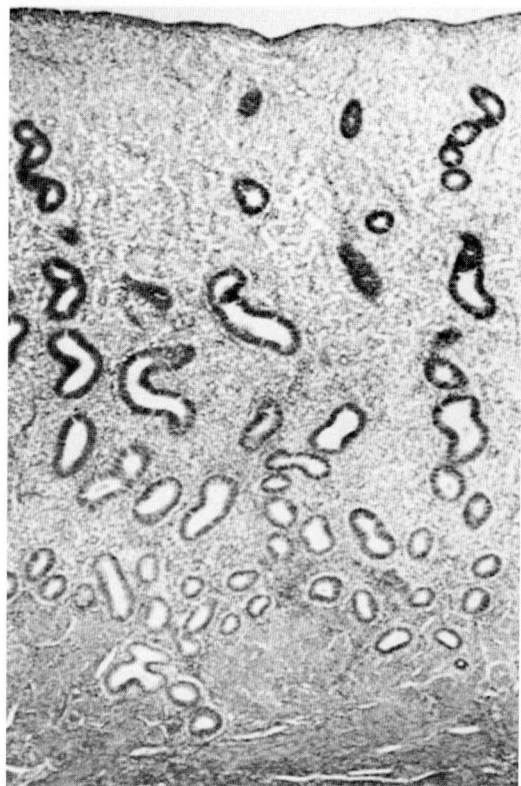

FIGURE 3-9 A histologic view of the endometrium during the proliferative phase. (From Demopoulos RI: Normal endometrium. In Blaustein A, ed: Pathology of the female genital tract, ed 2, New York, 1982, Springer-Verlag, p. 216.)

Clinical Correlations

Removal of the uterus is termed *hysterectomy,* which is derived from the Greek word *hystera,* meaning womb. The symptoms of primary dysmenorrhea are treated successfully in most women by prostaglandin synthetase inhibition. Rarely is a woman's pain not controlled by oral medication. However, it is possible to alleviate uterine pain by cutting the sensory nerves that accompany the sympathetic nerves. This operation is termed a *presacral neurectomy.* During the operation the gynecologist must be careful to avoid injuring the ureters and also careful to control hemorrhage from vessels in the retroperitoneal space.

The position of the fundus of the uterus in relation to the long axis of the vagina is quite variable. Not only are there differences between individual women but also in the same woman secondary to normal activity. In some women the uterus is anteflexed or anteverted, whereas in others the normal position is retroflexed or retroverted. In the 1930s and 1940s a retroflexed uterus was believed to be one of the primary causes of pelvic pain. To alleviate this condition many women underwent an anterior uterine suspension. Modern gynecologists have abandoned the suspension operation as a treatment for pelvic pain.

The arterial blood supply enters the uterus on its lateral margins. This relationship allows morcellation of an enlarged uterus to facilitate removal of multiple myomas without appreciably increasing blood loss during vaginal hysterectomy.

Methods of transcervical female sterilization designed to occlude the tubal ostia at the uterine cornua have been attempted for many years. Procedures that blindly inject caustic solutions into the uterine cornua have a high percentage of failure. Individual differences in size and shape of the uterine cavity and muscular spasm of this region are the primary reasons that sufficient amounts of the caustic chemicals do not reach the fallopian tubes in up to 20% of patients.

OVIDUCTS

The paired uterine tubes, more commonly referred to as the *fallopian tubes* or *oviducts,* extend outward from the superolateral portion of the uterus and end by curling around the ovary (see Figure 3-5). The tubes are contained in a free edge of the superior portion of the broad ligament. The mesentery of the tubes, the mesosalpinx, contains the blood supply and nerves. The uterine tubes connect the cornua of the uterine cavity and the peritoneal cavity. The ostia into the endometrial cavity are 1.5 mm in diameter, whereas the ostia into the abdominal cavity are approximately 3 mm in diameter.

The oviducts are between 10 and 14 cm in length and slightly less than 1 cm in external diameter. Each tube is divided into four anatomic sections. The uterine intramural, or interstitial, segment is 1 to 2 cm in length and is surrounded by myometrium. The isthmic segment begins as the tube exits the uterus and is approximately 4 cm in length. This segment is narrow, 1 to 2 mm in inside diameter, and straight. The isthmic segment has the most highly developed musculature. The ampullary segment is 4 to 6 cm in length and approximately 6 mm in inside diameter. It is wider and more tortuous in its course than other segments. Fertilization normally occurs in the ampullary portion of the tube. The infundibulum is the distal trumpet-shaped portion of the oviduct. From 20 to 25 irregular fingerlike projections, termed *fimbriae,* surround the abdominal ostia of the tube. One of the largest fimbriae is attached to the ovary, the fimbria ovarica (see Figure 3-5).

The tube contains numerous longitudinal folds, plicae, of mucosa and underlying stroma. Plicae are most prominent in the ampullary segment (Figure 3-10). The mucosa of the oviduct has three different cell types. Columnar ciliated epithelial cells are most prominent near the ovarian end of the tube and overall compose 25% of the mucosal cells. Secretory cells, also columnar in shape, compose 60% of the epithelial lining and are more prominent in the isthmic segment. Narrow peg cells are found between secretory and ciliated cells and are believed to be a morphologic

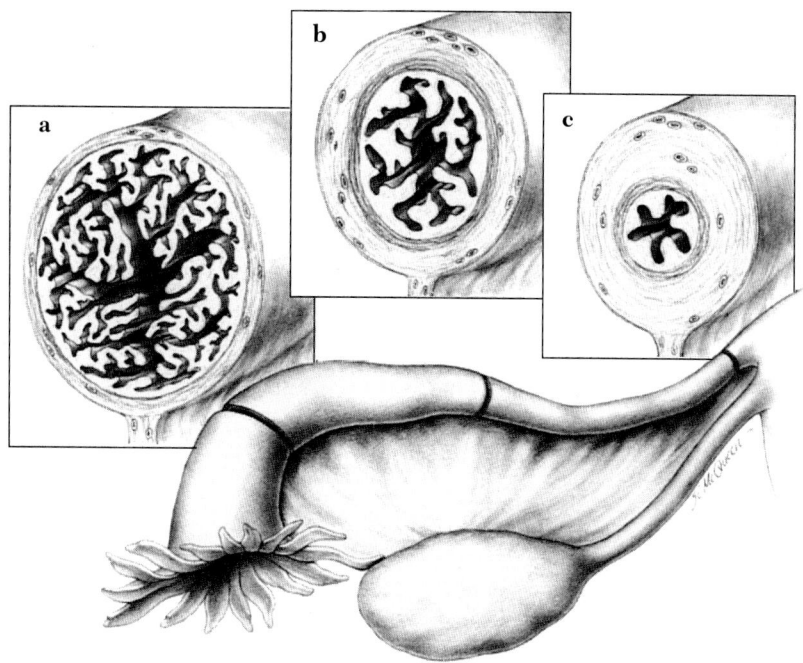

FIGURE 3-10 The longitudinal folds of the oviduct seen in cross section. **a,** Infundibulum. **b,** Ampulla. **c,** Isthmus. (Redrawn from Pritchard JA, MacDonald PC, and Gant NF: Williams' obstetrics, ed 17, New York, 1985, Appleton-Century-Crofts, p. 24.)

variant of secretory cells. The stroma of the mucosa is sparse. However, there is a thick lamina propria with vascular channels between the epithelium and muscular layers. The smooth muscle of the tube is arranged into inner circular and outer longitudinal layers. Between the peritoneal surface of the tube and the muscular layer is an adventitial layer that contains blood vessels and nerves.

The arterial blood supply to the oviducts is derived from terminal branches of the uterine and ovarian arteries. The arteries anastomose in the mesosalpinx. Blood from the uterine artery supplies the medial two thirds of each tube. The venous drainage runs parallel to the arterial supply. The lymphatic system is separate and distinct from the lymphatic drainage of the uterus. Lymphatic drainage includes the internal iliac nodes and the aortic nodes surrounding the aorta and the inferior vena cava at the level of the renal vessels.

The tubes are innervated by both sympathetic and parasympathetic nerves from the uterine and ovarian plexuses. Sensory nerves are related to spinal cord segments T11, T12, and L1.

Clinical Correlations

The vast majority of ectopic pregnancies occur in the oviduct. The acute abdominal and pelvic pain that women with an ectopic pregnancy experience is believed to be caused by hemorrhage. The most catastrophic bleeding associated with ectopic pregnancy occurs when the implantation site is in the intramural segment of the tube.

During insertion of the laparoscope, one should adjust for the caudal deviation in the vertical axis of the umbilicus in extremely obese women with a large panniculus.

The isthmic segment of the oviduct is the preferred site to apply an occlusive device, such as a clip, for female sterilization. The right oviduct and appendix are often adjacent. Clinically it may be difficult to differentiate inflammation of the tube from acute appendicitis. Accessory tubal ostia are discovered frequently and always connect with the lumen of the tube. These accessory ostia are usually found in the ampullary portion of the tube.

The wide mesosalpinx of the ampullary segment of the tube allows torsion of the tube, which occasionally results in ischemic atrophy of the ampullary segment. Paratubal or paraovarian cysts can reach 5 to 10 cm in diameter and occasionally are confused with ovarian cysts before surgery.

Although a definitive anatomic sphincter has not been identified at the uterotubal junction, a temporary physiologic obstruction has been identified during hysterosalpingography. Sometimes clinicians may alleviate this temporary obstruction by giving the patient intravenous sedation, a paracervical block, or intravenous glucagon.

OVARIES

The paired ovaries are light gray, and each one is approximately the size and configuration of a large almond. The surface of the ovary of adult women is pitted and indented from previous ovulations. The ovaries contain approximately 1 to 2 million oocytes at birth. During a woman's reproductive lifetime, about 8000 follicles begin development. The growth of many follicles is blunted in various stages of development, however approximately 300 ova eventually are released. The size and position of the ovary depend on the woman's age and parity. During the reproductive years, ovaries weigh 3 to 6 g and measure approximately 1.5 cm × 2.5 cm × 4 cm. As the woman ages, the ovaries become smaller and firmer in consistency.

In a nulliparous woman who is standing, the long axis of the ovary is vertical. The ovary in nulliparous women rests in a depression of peritoneum named the ovarian fossa. Immediately adjacent to the ovarian fossa are the external iliac vessels, the ureter, and the obturator vessels and nerves.

There are three prominent ligaments that determine the anatomic mobility of the ovary (see Figure 3-5). The posterior portion of the broad ligament forms the mesovarium, which attaches to the anterior border of the ovary. The mesovarium contains the arterial anastomotic branches of the ovarian and uterine arteries, a plexus of veins, and the lateral end of the ovarian ligament. The ovarian ligament is a narrow, short, fibrous band that extends from the lower pole of the ovary to the uterus. The infundibular pelvic ligament, or suspensory ligament of the ovary, forms the superior and lateral aspect of the broad ligament. This ligament contains the ovarian artery, ovarian veins, and accompanying nerves. It attaches the upper pole of the ovary to the lateral pelvic wall.

The ovary is subdivided histologically into an outer cortex and an inner medulla (Figure 3-11). The ovarian surface is covered by a single layer of cuboidal epithelium, termed the *germinal epithelium*. The latter term is a misnomer because the cells are similar to those of the coelomic mesothelium, which forms the peritoneum, and because the germinal epithelium is not related to the histogenesis of graafian follicles. If the ovary is transected, numerous transparent, fluid-filled cysts are noted throughout the cortex. Microscopically these are graafian follicles in various stages of development, active or regressing corpus luteum, and atretic follicles. The stroma of the cortex is composed primarily of closely packed cells around the follicles. These specialized connective tissue cells form the theca. The medulla contains the ovarian vascular supply and a loose stroma. The specialized polyhedral hilar cells are similar to the interstitial cells of the testis.

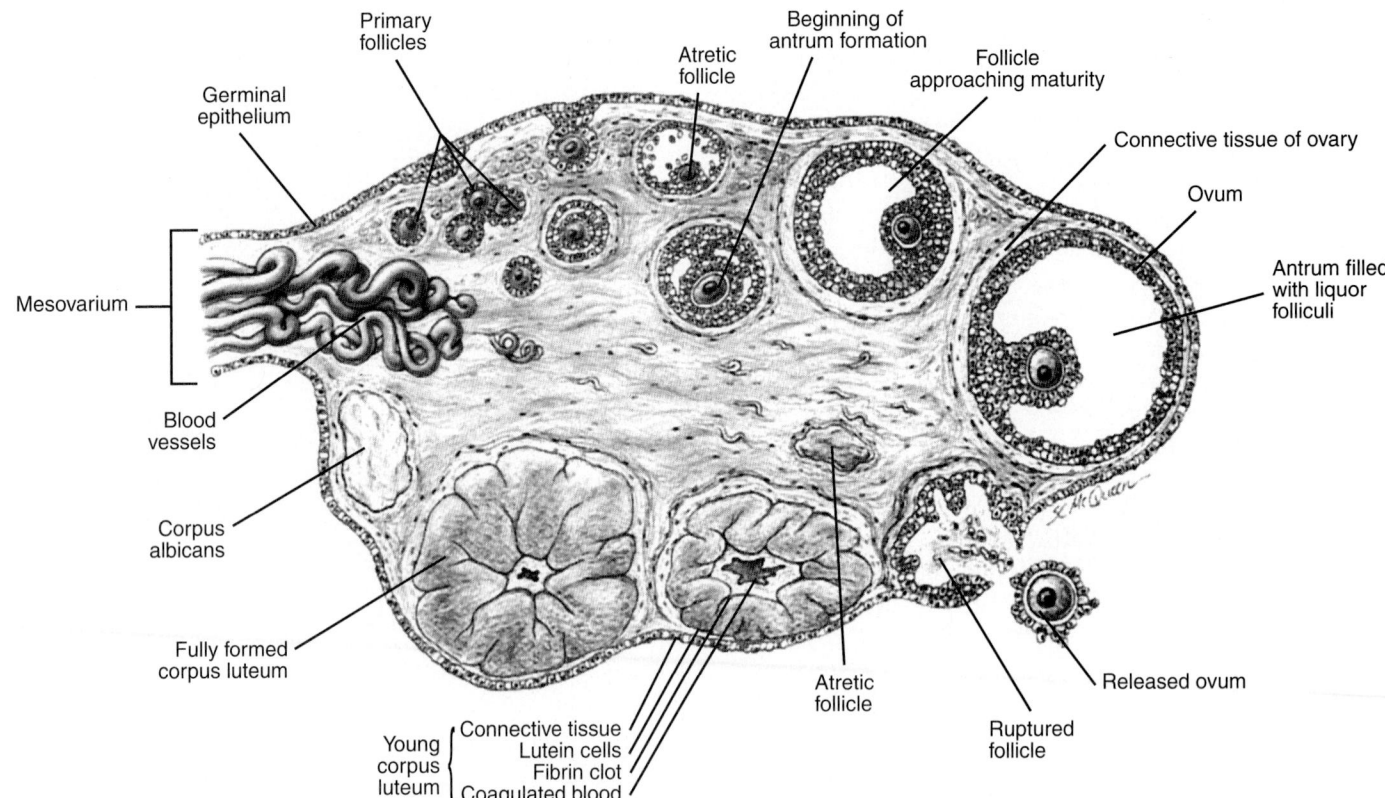

FIGURE 3-11 A schematic drawing of the ovary. Note the single layer of cuboidal epithelium called the *germinal epithelium*. Note the graafian follicles in different stages of development. Note the inner medullary region of stroma and blood vessels. (Adapted from Gray's anatomy of the human body, ed 35, Philadelphia, 1973, Lea & Febiger. Redrawn from Blaustein A: Anatomy and histology of the human ovary. In Blaustein A, ed: Pathology of the female genital tract, ed 2, New York, 1982, Springer-Verlag, p. 417.)

Each of the ovarian arteries arises directly from the aorta just below the renal arteries. They descend in the retroperitoneal space, cross anterior to the psoas muscles and internal iliac vessels, and enter the infundibulopelvic ligaments, reaching the mesovarium in the broad ligament. The ovarian blood supply enters through the hilum of the ovary. The venous drainage of the ovary collects in the pampiniform plexus and consolidates into several large veins as it leaves the hilum of the ovary. The ovarian veins accompany the ovarian arteries, with the left ovarian vein draining into the left renal vein, whereas the right ovarian vein connects directly with the inferior vena cava.

The lymphatic drainage of the ovaries is primarily to the aortic nodes adjacent to the great vessels at the level of the renal veins. Metastatic disease from the ovary occasionally takes a shorter course to the iliac nodes. The autonomic and sensory nerve fibers accompany the ovarian vasculature in the infundibulopelvic ligament. They connect with the ovarian, hypogastric, and aortic plexuses.

Clinical Correlations

The size of the "normal" ovary during the reproductive years and the postmenopausal period is important in clinical practice. Before menopause a "normal" ovary may be up to 5 cm in length. Thus a small physiologic cyst may cause an ovary to be 6 to 7 cm in diameter. In contrast, the "normal" atrophic postmenopausal ovary usually cannot be palpated during pelvic examination.

It is important to emphasize that the ovaries and surrounding peritoneum are not devoid of pain and pressure receptors. Therefore it is not unusual for a woman during a routine pelvic examination to experience discomfort when normal ovaries are palpated bimanually.

Attempts have been made to alleviate chronic pelvic pain by performing an ovarian denervation operation by cutting and ligating the infundibulopelvic ligaments. This operation has been abandoned because of the high incidence of cystic degeneration of the ovaries, which resulted from the interruption of their primary blood supply that was associated with the neurectomy procedure.

The close anatomic proximity of the ovary, ovarian fossa, and ureter is emphasized in surgery for severe endometriosis or pelvic inflammatory disease. It is important to identify the course of the ureter in order to facilitate removal of all of the ovarian capsule that is adherent to the peritoneum and surrounding structures so as to avoid immediate ureteral injury and residual retroperitoneal ovarian remnants in the future. Prophylactic oophorectomy is performed at the time of pelvic operations in postmenopausal women. Sometimes bilateral oophorectomy is technically more difficult when associated with a vaginal procedure in contrast to an abdominal hysterectomy. Vaginal removal of the ovaries may be facilitated by identifying the anatomic landmarks similar to the abdominal approach and separately clamping the round ligaments and infundibular pelvic ligaments.

VASCULAR SYSTEM OF THE PELVIS

Several generalizations should be made in describing the network of arteries that bring blood to the female reproductive organs. The arteries are paired, are bilateral, and have multiple collaterals (Figure 3-12). The arteries enter their respective organs laterally and then unite with anastomotic vessels from the other side of the pelvis near the midline. There is a long-standing teaching generalization that the pelvic reproductive viscera lie within a loosely woven basket of large veins with numerous interconnecting venous plexuses. The arteries thread their way through this interwoven mesh of veins to reach the pelvic reproductive organs, giving off numerous branching arcades to provide a rich blood supply.

Arteries

Inferior Mesenteric Artery

The inferior mesenteric artery, a single artery, arises from the aorta approximately 3 cm above the aortic bifurcation. It supplies part of the transverse colon, the descending colon, the sigmoid colon, and the rectum and terminates as the superior hemorrhoidal artery. The inferior mesenteric artery is occasionally torn during node dissections performed in staging operations for gynecologic cancer. Because of the rich collateral circulation from the middle and inferior hemorrhoidal arteries, the inferior mesenteric artery can be ligated without compromise of the distal portion of the colon.

Ovarian Artery

The ovarian arteries originate from the aorta just below the renal vessels. Each one courses in the retroperitoneal space, crosses anterior to the ureter, and enters the infundibulopelvic ligament. As the artery travels medially in the mesovarium, numerous small branches supply the ovary and oviduct. The ovarian artery unites with the ascending branch of the uterine artery in the mesovarium just under the suspensory ligament of the ovary.

Common Iliac Artery

The bifurcation of the aorta occurs at the level of the fourth lumbar vertebra, forming the two common iliac arteries. Each common iliac artery is approximately 5 cm in length before the vessel divides into the external iliac and hypogastric arteries.

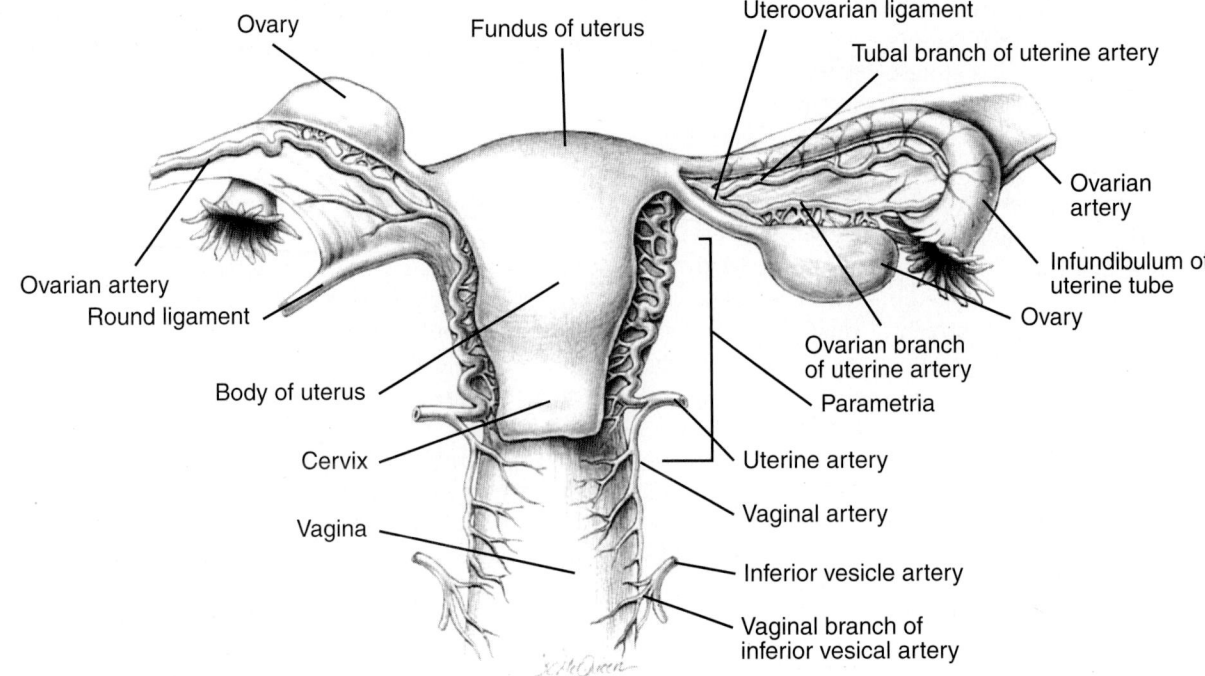

FIGURE 3-12 The arteries of the reproductive organs. Note the paired arteries entering laterally and freely anastomosing with each other. (Redrawn from Clemente CD: Anatomy: a regional atlas of the human body, Baltimore-Munich, 1987, Urban & Schwarzenberg.)

Hypogastric Artery (Internal Iliac Artery)

The hypogastric arteries are short vessels, each approximately 3 to 4 cm in length. Throughout their course they are in close proximity to the ureters, which are anterior, and to the hypogastric veins, which are posterior. Each hypogastric artery branches into an anterior and a posterior division (or trunk). The posterior trunk gives off three parietal branches: the iliolumbar, lateral sacral, and superior gluteal arteries. The anterior trunk has nine branches. The three parietal branches are the obturator, internal pudendal, and inferior gluteal arteries. The six visceral branches include the umbilical, middle vesical, inferior vesical, middle hemorrhoidal, uterine, and vaginal arteries. The superior vesical artery usually arises from the umbilical artery. The individual branches of the hypogastric artery may vary from one woman to another.

Uterine Artery

The uterine artery arises from the anterior division of the hypogastric artery and courses medially toward the isthmus of the uterus. Approximately 2 cm lateral to the endocervix, it crosses over the ureter and reaches the lateral side of the uterus. The ascending branch of the uterine artery courses in the broad ligament, running a tortuous route to finally anastomose with the ovarian artery in the mesovarium (Figure 3-13). Through its circuitous route in the parametrium, the uterine artery gives off numerous branches that unite with arcuate arteries from the other side. This series of arcuate arteries develops radial branches that supply the myometrium and the basalis layer of the endometrium. The arcuate arteries also form the spiral arteries of the functional layer of the endometrium. The descending branch of the uterine artery produces branches that supply both the cervix and the vagina. In each case the vessels enter the organ laterally and anastomose freely with vessels from the other side.

Vaginal Artery

The vaginal artery may arise either from the anterior trunk of the hypogastric artery or from the uterine artery. It supplies blood to the vagina, bladder, and rectum. There are extensive anastomoses with the vaginal branches of the uterine artery to form the azygos arteries of the cervix and vagina.

Internal Pudendal Artery

This artery is the terminal branch of the hypogastric artery and supplies branches to the rectum, labia, clitoris, and perineum.

Veins

The venous drainage of the pelvis begins in small sinusoids that drain to numerous venous plexuses contained within or immediately adjacent to the pelvic organs. Invariably there are numerous anastomoses between the

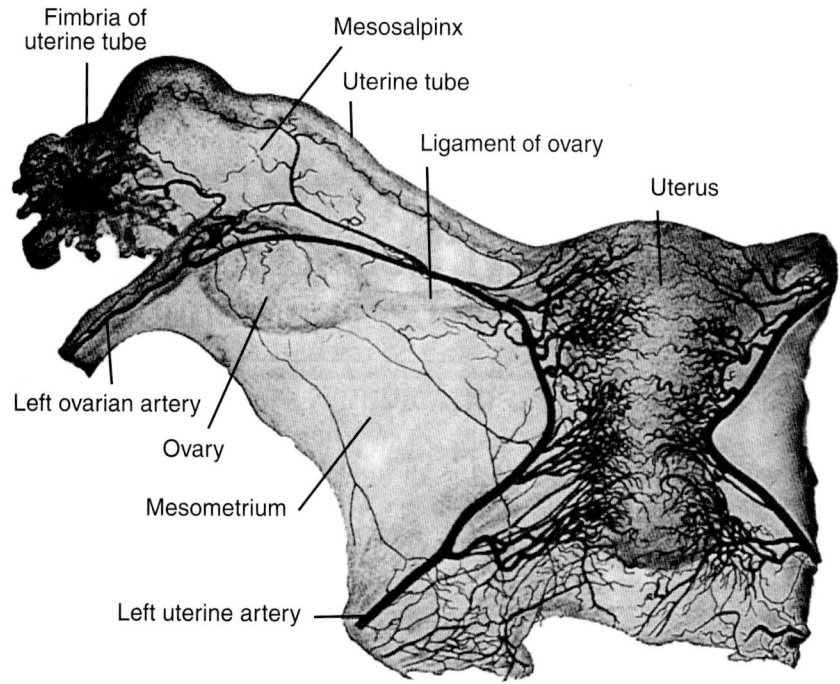

Fimbria of
uterine tube

Mesosalpinx

Uterine tube

Ligament of ovary

Uterus

Left ovarian artery

Ovary

Mesometrium

Left uterine artery

FIGURE 3-13 A photograph of an injected specimen demonstrating the rich anastomoses of the uterine and ovarian arteries. (From Warwick R and Williams PL: Gray's anatomy, ed 35, Edinburgh, 1973, Churchill Livingstone, p. 1361.)

parietal and visceral branches of the venous system. In general the veins of the female pelvis and perineum are thin walled and have few valves.

The veins that drain the pelvic plexuses follow the course of the arterial supply. Their names are similar to those of the accompanying arteries. Often multiple veins run alongside a single artery. One special exception is the venous drainage of the ovaries. The left ovarian vein empties into the left renal vein, whereas the right ovarian vein connects directly with the inferior vena cava.

Clinical Correlations

Although the external iliac artery and its branches do not supply blood directly to the pelvic viscera, they are important landmarks in surgical anatomy. The fact that the external iliac artery gives rise to the obturator artery in 15% to 20% of women must be considered in radical cancer operations with associated node dissections of the obturator fossa. The external iliac artery also gives rise to the inferior epigastric artery. The inferior epigastric artery should be avoided when performing laparoscopic operative procedures.

In certain clinical situations associated with profuse hemorrhage from the female pelvis, hypogastric ligation is performed. Because of the extensive collateral circulation, this operation does not produce hypoxia of the pelvic viscera but reduces hemorrhage by decreasing the pulse pressure. The extent of collateral circulation after hypogastric artery ligation depends on the site of ligation and may be divided into three groups (Table 3-1).

TABLE 3-1
Collateral Arterial Circulation of the Pelvis

Branches from aorta

Ovarian artery—anastomoses freely with uterine artery
Inferior mesenteric artery—continues as superior hemorrhoidal artery to anastomose with middle and inferior hemorrhoidal arteries from hypogastric and internal pudendal
Lumbar and vertebral arteries—anastomose with iliolumbar artery of hypogastric
Middle sacral artery—anastomoses with lateral sacral artery of hypogastric

Branches from external iliac artery

Deep iliac circumflex artery—anastomoses with iliolumbar and superior gluteal of hypogastric
Inferior epigastric artery—gives origin to obturator artery in 25% of cases, providing additional anastomoses of external iliac with medial femoral circumflex and communicating pelvic branches

Branches from femoral artery

Medial femoral circumflex artery—anastomoses with obturator and inferior gluteal arteries from hypogastric
Lateral femoral circumflex artery—anastomoses with superior gluteal and iliolumbar arteries from hypogastric

Reprinted with permission from Mattingly RF and Thompson JD: Te Linde's operative gynecology, ed 6, Philadelphia, 1985, JB Lippincott Co.

In cases of intractable pelvic hemorrhage, it may be necessary to supplement the effects of bilateral hypogastric artery ligation with ligation of the anastomotic sites between the ovarian and uterine vessels. Ligation of the terminal end of the ovarian artery preserves the direct blood supply to the ovaries, and there is no fear of the subsequent cystic degeneration of the ovaries that may occur after ligation of the vessels in the infundibulopelvic ligaments. An alternative approach to ligation is to insert a catheter via fluoroscopy and inject small particulate material to produce hemostasis in the bleeding vessels. A rare condition that presents an interesting challenge to the clinician is a congenital arterial-venous malformation in the female pelvis. Most of these A-V fistulas are treated with preoperative embolization and subsequent operative ligation.

One of the treatments for repetitive embolization from the female pelvis is the placement of a vascular umbrella into the inferior vena cava. Collateral circulation exists between the portal venous system of the gastrointestinal tract and the systemic venous circulation through anastomosis in the pelvis, especially in the hemorrhoidal plexus. The pelvic veins also anastomose with the presacral and lumbar veins. Therefore patients may develop trophoblastic emboli to the brain without the trophoblast being filtered by the capillary system in the lungs.

LYMPHATIC SYSTEM

External Iliac Nodes

The external iliac nodes are immediately adjacent to the external iliac artery and vein (Figures 3-14 and 3-15). There are two distinct groups, one situated lateral to the vessels and the other posterior to the psoas muscle. The distal portion of the posterior group is enclosed in the femoral sheath. The majority of lymphatic channels to this group of nodes originates from the vulva, but there are also channels from the cervix and lower portion

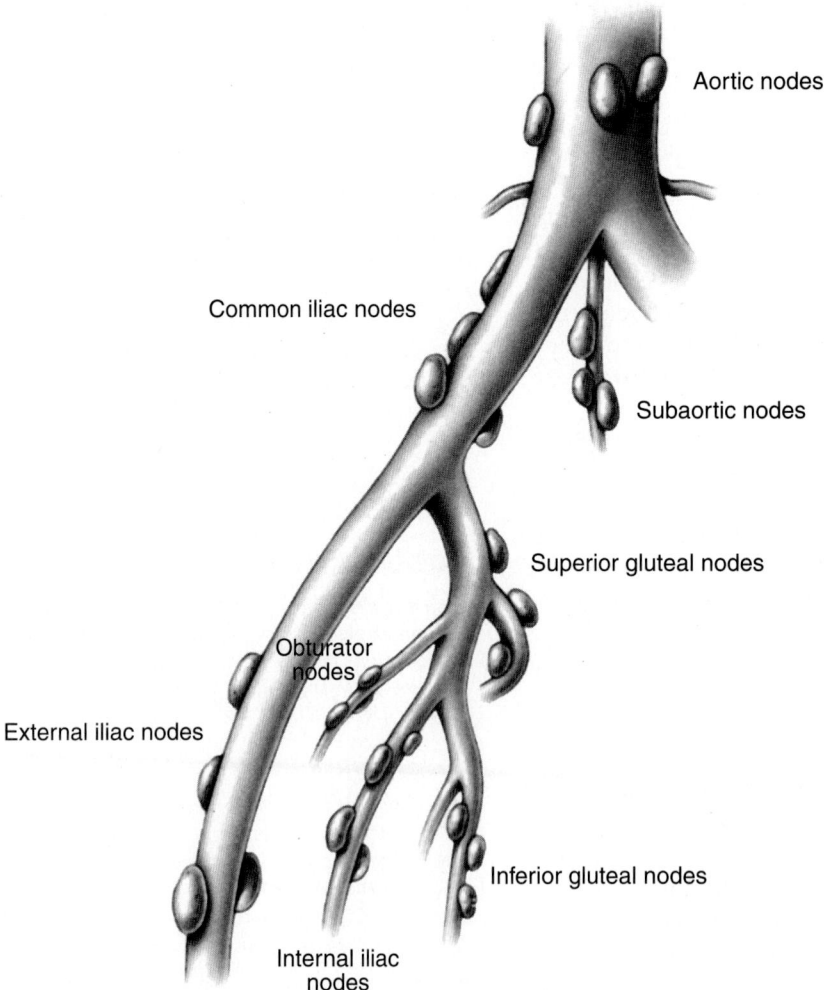

FIGURE 3-14 Schematic view of the pelvic lymph nodes. (From Plentl AA and Friedman EA: Lymphatic system of the female genitalia, Philadelphia, 1971, WB Saunders Co., p. 13.)

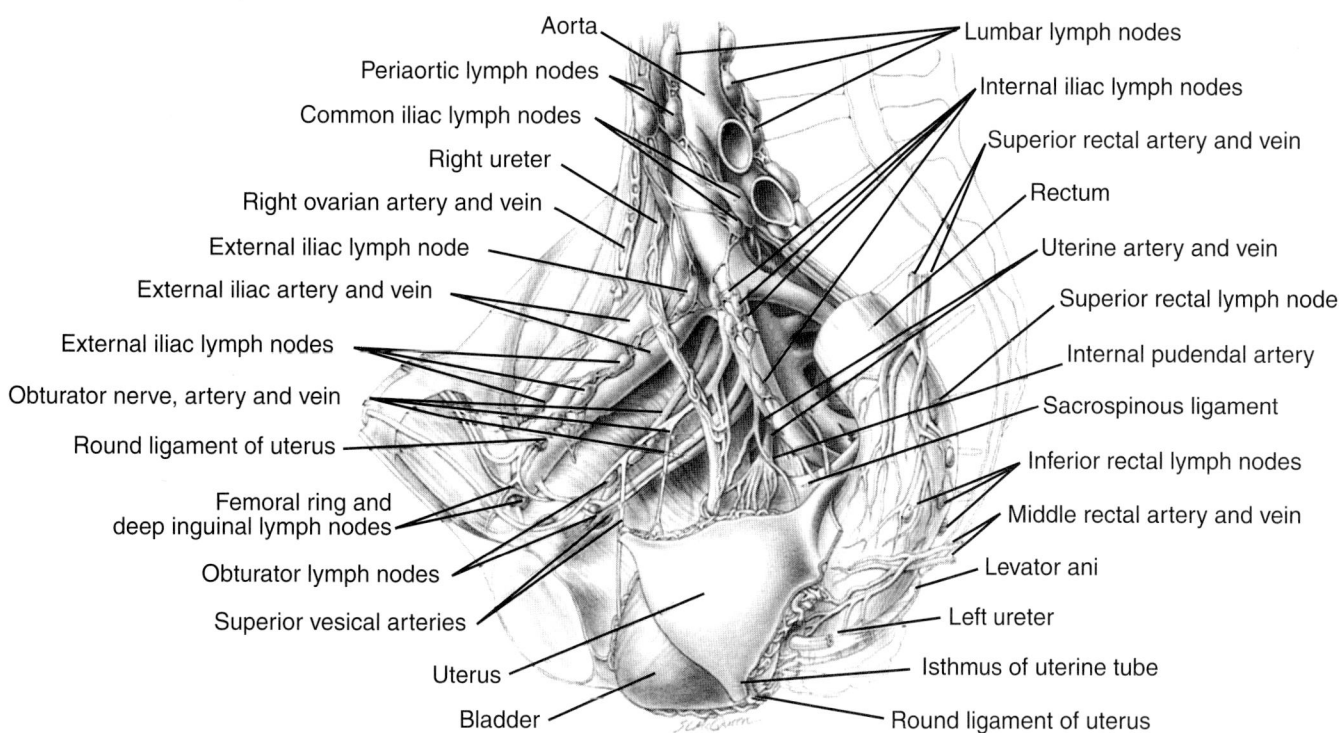

Aorta
Periaortic lymph nodes
Common iliac lymph nodes
Right ureter
Right ovarian artery and vein
External iliac lymph node
External iliac artery and vein
External iliac lymph nodes
Obturator nerve, artery and vein
Round ligament of uterus
Femoral ring and
deep inguinal lymph nodes
Obturator lymph nodes
Superior vesical arteries
Uterus
Bladder

Lumbar lymph nodes
Internal iliac lymph nodes
Superior rectal artery and vein
Rectum
Uterine artery and vein
Superior rectal lymph node
Internal pudendal artery
Sacrospinous ligament
Inferior rectal lymph nodes
Middle rectal artery and vein
Levator ani
Left ureter
Isthmus of uterine tube
Round ligament of uterus

FIGURE 3-15 A lateral view of the female pelvis demonstrating the extensive lymphatic network. Note that most of the lymphatic channels follow the courses of the major vessels. (Redrawn from Clemente CD: Anatomy: a regional atlas of the human body, Baltimore-Munich, 1987, Urban & Schwarzenberg.)

of the uterus. The external iliac nodes receive secondary drainage from the femoral and internal iliac nodes.

Internal Iliac Nodes

The internal iliac nodes are found in an anatomic triangle whose sides are composed of the external iliac artery, the hypogastric artery, and the pelvic sidewall. Included in this clinically important area are nodes with special designation, including the nodes of the femoral ring, the obturator nodes, and the nodes adjacent to the external iliac vessels. This rich collection of nodes receives channels from every internal pelvic organ and the vulva, including the clitoris and urethra.

Common Iliac Nodes

The common iliac nodes are a group of nodes located adjacent to the vessels that bear their name and are between the external iliac and aortic chains. Most of these nodes are found lateral to the vessels. To remove this chain, it is necessary to dissect the common iliac vessels away from their attachments to the psoas muscle. This group receives lymphatics from the cervix and the upper portion of the vagina. Secondary lymphatic drainage from the internal iliac, external iliac, superior gluteal, and inferior gluteal nodes flows to the common iliac nodes.

Inferior Gluteal Nodes

A small group of lymph nodes, the inferior gluteal nodes, are located in anatomic proximity to the ischial spines and are adjacent to the sacral plexus of nodes. It is difficult to remove these nodes surgically. The nodes receive lymphatics from the cervix, the lower portion of the vagina, and Bartholin's glands. This group of nodes secondarily drains to the internal iliac, common iliac, superior gluteal, and subaortic nodes.

Superior Gluteal Nodes

The superior gluteal nodes are a group of nodes found near the origin of the superior gluteal artery and adjacent to the medial and posterior aspects of the hypogastric vessels. The superior gluteal nodes receive primary lymphatic drainage from the cervix and the vagina. Efferent lymphatics from this chain drain to the common iliac, sacral, or subaortic nodes.

Sacral Nodes

The sacral nodes are found over the middle of the sacrum in a space bounded laterally by the sacral foramina. These nodes receive lymphatic drainage from both the cervix and the vagina. Secondary drainage from these nodes runs in a cephalad direction to the subaortic nodes.

Subaortic Nodes

The subaortic nodes are arranged in a chain and are located below the bifurcation of the aorta, immediately anterior to the most caudal portion of the inferior vena cava and over the fifth lumbar vertebra. The primary drainage to this chain of nodes is from the cervix, with a few lymphatics from the vagina. This group is the first secondary chain to receive the efferent lymphatics as lymph flow progresses in a cephalad direction from the majority of other pelvic nodes.

Aortic Nodes

The many aortic nodes are immediately adjacent to the aorta on both its anterior and lateral aspects, predominantly in the furrow between the aorta and inferior vena cava. Primary lymphatics drain from all the major pelvic organs, including the cervix, uterus, oviducts, and especially the ovaries. The aortic chain receives secondary drainage from the pelvic nodes. In general, primary afferent lymphatics drain into the nodes over the anterior aspects of the aorta, whereas secondary efferent drainage from other pelvic nodes is found in those nodes situated lateral and posterior to the aorta.

Rectal Nodes

The rectal nodes are found subfascially and in the loose connective tissue surrounding the rectum. Primary drainage from the cervix flows to the superior rectal nodes, and drainage from the vagina appears in the rectal nodes in the anorectal region. Secondary drainage from the rectal nodes goes to the subaortic and aortic groups.

Parauterine Nodes

The number of lymph nodes in the group of parauterine nodes is small; most frequently there is a single node immediately lateral to each side of the cervix and adjacent to the pelvic course of the ureter. Though anatomists frequently do not comment about the parauterine nodes, the group receives special attention in radical surgical operations for uterine or cervical malignancy. Primary drainage to this node originates in the vagina, cervix, and uterus. Secondary drainage from this node is to the internal iliac nodes on the same side of the pelvis.

Superficial Femoral Nodes

The superficial femoral nodes are a group of nodes found in the loose, fatty connective tissue of the femoral triangle between the superficial and deep fascial layers. These lymph nodes receive lymphatic drainage from the external genitalia of the vulvar region, the gluteal region, and the entire leg, including the foot. Efferent lymphatics from this group of nodes penetrate the fascia lata to enter the deep femoral nodes. Plentl and Friedman have stated that this area undoubtedly represents the greatest concentration of lymph nodes in the female (Figure 3-16).

Deep Femoral Nodes

The deep femoral nodes are located in the femoral sheath, adjacent to both the femoral artery and the vein within the femoral triangle. The femoral triangle is the anatomic space lying immediately distal to the fold of the groin. The boundaries of the femoral triangle are the sartorius and adductor longus muscles and the inguinal ligament. Each space contains, from medial to lateral, the femoral vein, femoral artery, and femoral nerve. This chain receives the primary lymphatics for the lower extremity and receives secondary efferent lymphatics from the superficial lymph nodes and thus the vulva. This group of lymph nodes is in direct continuity with the iliac and internal iliac chains.

Clinical Correlations

A precise knowledge of pelvic lymphatics is important for the gynecologic oncologist who is surgically determining the extent of spread of a pelvic malignancy. Aortic and pelvic lymphadenectomy operations require precise knowledge of normal anatomy and possible anomalies in both the urinary and vascular systems. The fact that most lymphatic metastatic spread from ovarian carcinoma occurs in a cephalad direction should be emphasized. This explains the importance of sampling aortic and subaortic nodes during second-look operations for ovarian cancer. In carcinoma of the vulva, lymphatic drainage may occur to either side of the pelvis. Thus bilateral node dissections are important. Pelvic hemorrhage is the most common acute complication of a lymph node dissection because most pelvic lymph nodes are in anatomic proximity to major pelvic vessels. Lymphocysts in the retroperitoneal space are the most common chronic complication associated with radical node dissections.

For many years it was believed that all the superficial femoral nodes drained to a sentinel node called *Cloquet's node*. Cloquet's node, by the present classification system, would be one of the most proximal and medial of the nodes in the external iliac chain. Cloquet's node is only of historical interest, since the assumption is neither anatomically nor clinically correct.

INNERVATION OF THE PELVIS

Internal Genitalia

The innervation of the internal genital organs is supplied primarily by the autonomic nervous system. The sympathetic portion of the autonomic nervous system originates

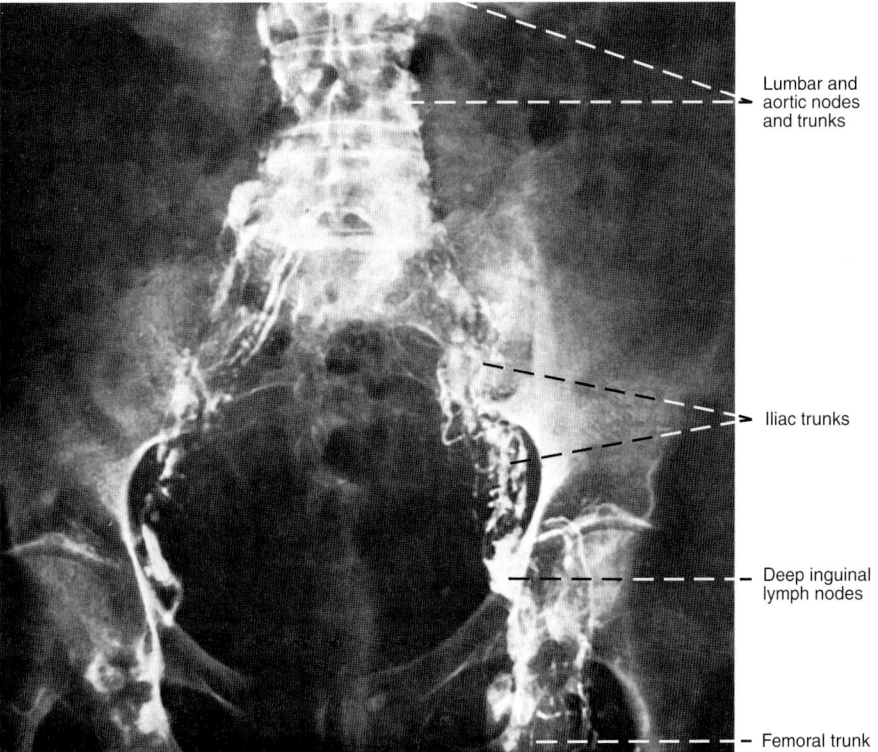

Lumbar and
aortic nodes
and trunks

Iliac trunks

Deep inguinal
lymph nodes

Femoral trunk

FIGURE 3-16 A lymphangiogram of the pelvis and lumbar areas. This x-ray film shows the course of the lymphatics from the deep femoral nodes into the iliac nodes. Note the extensive network of nodes in the inguinal region. (From Clemente CD: A regional atlas of the human body, ed 3, Baltimore-Munich, 1987, Urban & Schwarzenberg.)

in the thoracic and lumbar portions of the spinal cord, and sympathetic ganglia are located adjacent to the central nervous system. In contrast, the parasympathetic portion originates in cranial nerves and the middle three sacral segments of the cord, and the ganglia are located near the visceral organs. Although the fibers of both subdivisions of the autonomic nervous system frequently are intermingled in the same peripheral nerves, their physiologic actions are usually directly antagonistic. As a broad generalization, sympathetic fibers in the female pelvis produce muscular contractions and vasoconstriction, whereas parasympathetic fibers cause the opposite effect on muscles and vasodilation.

The semantics of pelvic innervation are confusing and imprecise. A plexus is a mixture of preganglionic and postganglionic fibers; small, inconsistently placed ganglia; and afferent (sensory) fibers. Throughout both the anatomic and surgical literature, a plexus may also be termed a *nerve.* For example, the superior hypogastric plexus is also called the *presacral nerve.*

Although autonomic nerve fibers enter the pelvis by several routes, the majority are contained in the superior hypogastric plexus, which is a caudal extension of the aortic and inferior mesenteric plexuses. The superior hypogastric plexus is found in the retroperitoneal

connective tissue. It extends from the fourth lumbar vertebra to the hollow over the sacrum. In its lower portion the plexus divides to form the two hypogastric nerves, which run laterally and inferiorly. These nerves fan out to form the inferior hypogastric plexus in the area just below the bifurcation of the common iliac arteries. The nerve trunks descend farther into the base of the broad ligament, where they join with parasympathetic fibers to form the pelvic plexus. Both motor fibers and accompanying sensory fibers reach the pelvic plexus from S2, S3, and S4 via the pelvic nerves, or nervi erigentes. From the pelvic plexus secondary plexuses are adjacent to all pelvic viscera, namely, the rectum, anus, urinary bladder, vagina, and Frankenhäuser's plexus in the uterosacral ligaments. Frankenhäuser's plexus is extensive and contains both myelinated and nonmyelinated fibers passing primarily to the uterus and cervix, with a few fibers passing to the urinary bladder and vagina. The ovarian plexus, like the blood supply to the ovaries, is not part of the hypogastric system. The ovarian plexus is a downward extension of the aortic and renal plexuses.

It is impossible to separate afferent, sensory fibers from pelvic organs into morphologically independent tracts. The majority of fibers accompany the vascular system from the organ and then enter plexuses of the autonomic nervous system before eventually entering white rami communicates to the cell bodies in dorsal root ganglia of the spinal column. The major sensory fibers from the uterus accompany the sympathetic nerves, which enter the nerve roots of the spinal cord in segments T11 and T12. Thus referred uterine pain is often located in the lower abdomen. In contrast, afferents from the cervix enter the spinal cord in nerve roots of S2, S3, and S4. Referred pain from cervical inflammation is characterized as low back pain in the lumbosacral region.

External Genitalia

The pudendal nerve and its branches supply the majority of both motor and sensory fibers to the muscles and skin of the vulvar region. The pudendal nerve arises from the second, third, and fourth sacral roots. It has an interesting course in which it initially leaves the pelvis via the greater sciatic foramen. Next, it crosses beneath the ischial spine, running on the medial side of the internal pudendal artery. The pudendal nerve then reenters the pelvic cavity and travels in Alcock's canal, which runs

along the lateral aspects of the ischial rectal fossa. As the nerve reaches the urogenital diaphragm, it divides into three branches: the inferior hemorrhoidal, the deep perineal, and the superficial perineal (Figure 3-17). The dorsal nerve of the clitoris is a terminal branch of the deep perineal nerve.

The skin of the anus, clitoris, and medial and inferior aspects of the vulva is supplied primarily by distal branches of the pudendal nerve. The vulvar region receives additional sensory fibers from three nerves. The anterior branch of the ilioinguinal nerve sends fibers to the mons pubis and the upper part of the labia majora. The genital femoral nerve supplies fibers to the labia majora, and the posterior femoral cutaneous nerve supplies fibers to the inferoposterior aspects of the vulva.

Clinical Correlations

An unusual but troublesome postoperative complication of gynecologic surgery is injury to the femoral nerve. During abdominal hysterectomy the femoral nerve may be compromised by pressure from the lateral blade of a

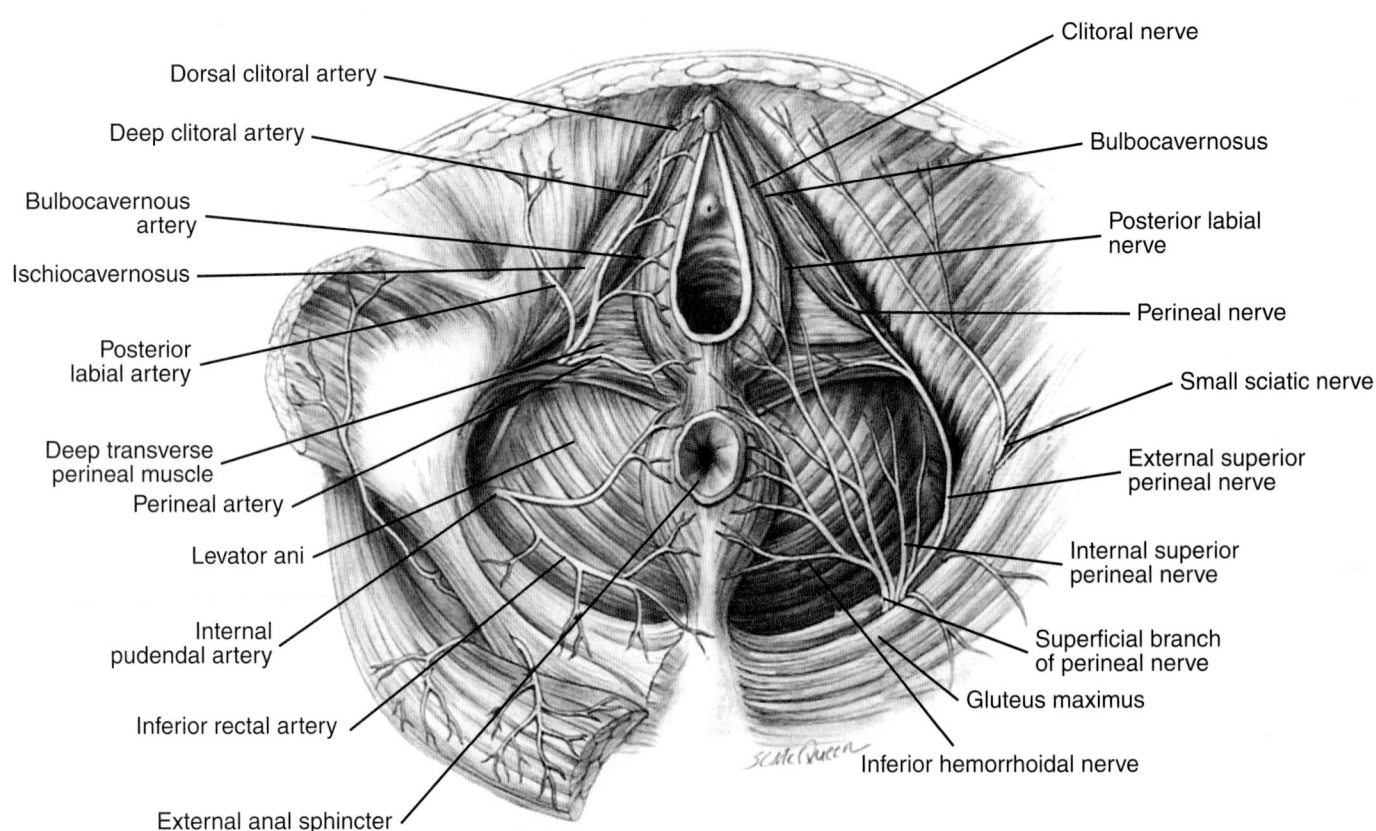

FIGURE 3-17 A posterior view of the female perineum demonstrating the pudendal nerve emerging externally. The nerve divides into three segments as it passes out of the pelvis: the inferior hemorrhoidal nerve and the deep and superficial perineal nerves. The clitoral nerve is the terminal branch of the deep perineal nerve. (Redrawn from Mattingly RF and Thompson JD: Te Linde's operative gynecology, ed 6, Philadelphia, 1985, JB Lippincott Co., p. 49.)

self-retaining retractor in the area adjacent to where the femoral nerve penetrates the psoas muscle. During vaginal hysterectomy the femoral nerve may be injured from exaggerated hyperflexion of the legs in the lithotomy position, since hyperflexion produces stretching and compression of the femoral nerve as it courses under the inguinal ligament.

Because of the low density of nerve endings in the upper two thirds of the vagina, women are sometimes unable to determine the presence of a foreign body in this area. This explains how a "forgotten tampon" may remain unnoticed for several days in the upper part of the vagina until its presence results in a symptomatic discharge, abnormal bleeding, or odor. Infrequent but serious complications of pudendal nerve block are hematomas from trauma to the pudendal vessels and intravascular injection of anesthetic agents. The vessels or nerves are in close anatomic proximity to the ischial spine.

The fallopian tube is one of the most sensitive of the pelvic organs when crushed, cut, or distended, a fact that is appreciated in performing tubal ligations with the patient under local anesthesia. Damage to the obturator nerve during radical pelvic operations does not affect the pelvis directly. Although the nerve has an extensive pelvic course, its motor fibers supply the adductors of the thigh and its sensory fibers innervate skin over the medial aspects of the thigh.

DIAPHRAGMS AND LIGAMENTS

Pelvic Diaphragm

The pelvic diaphragm is a wide but thin muscular layer of tissue that forms the inferior border of the abdominopelvic cavity. Composed of a broad, funnel-shaped sling of fascia and muscle, it extends from the symphysis pubis to the coccyx and from one lateral sidewall to the other. The primary muscles of the pelvic diaphragm are the levator ani and the coccygeus (Figure 3-18). This structure is the evolutionary remnant of the tail-wagging muscles in lower animals.

The muscles of the pelvic diaphragm are interwoven for strength, and a continuous muscle layer encircles the terminal portions of the urethra, vagina, and rectum. The levator ani muscles constitute the greatest bulk of the pelvic diaphragm and are divided into three components, which are named after their origin and insertion: pubococcygeus, puborectalis, and iliococcygeus. Some refer to the pubococcygeus muscles by a more descriptive name— the "pubovisceral muscle." The coccygeus is a triangular muscle that occupies the area between the ischial spine and the coccyx.

The paired levator ani muscles act as a single muscle and functionally are important in the control of urination, in parturition, and in maintaining fecal continence. Zacharin has proposed that these muscles function as a "pelvic trampoline." The pelvic diaphragm is important in

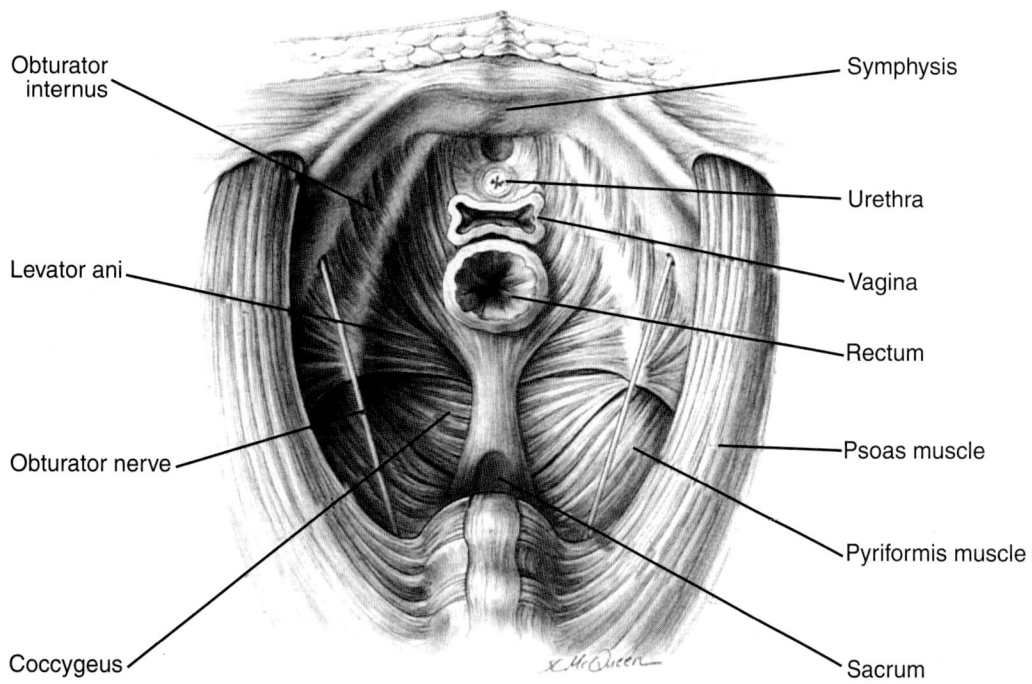

FIGURE 3-18　A superior view of the pelvic diaphragm of the pelvic floor. The primary muscles that compose this funnel-shaped sling are the coccygeus and the levator ani. (Redrawn from Mattingly RF and Thompson JD: Te Linde's operative gynecology, ed 6, Philadelphia, 1985, JB Lippincott Co., p. 41.)

supporting both abdominal and pelvic viscera and facilitates equal distribution of intraabdominal pressure during activities such as coughing.

Urogenital Diaphragm

The urogenital diaphragm, also called the *triangular ligament*, is a strong, muscular membrane that occupies the area between the symphysis pubis and ischial tuberosities

(Figure 3-19) and stretches across the triangular anterior portion of the pelvic outlet. The urogenital diaphragm is external and inferior to the pelvic diaphragm. Anteriorly, the urethra is suspended from the pubic bone by continuations of the fascial layers of the urogenital diaphragm. The free edge of the diaphragm is strengthened by the superficial transverse perineal muscle. Posteriorly, the urogenital diaphragm inserts into the central point of the perineum. Situated farther posteriorly is the ischiorectal

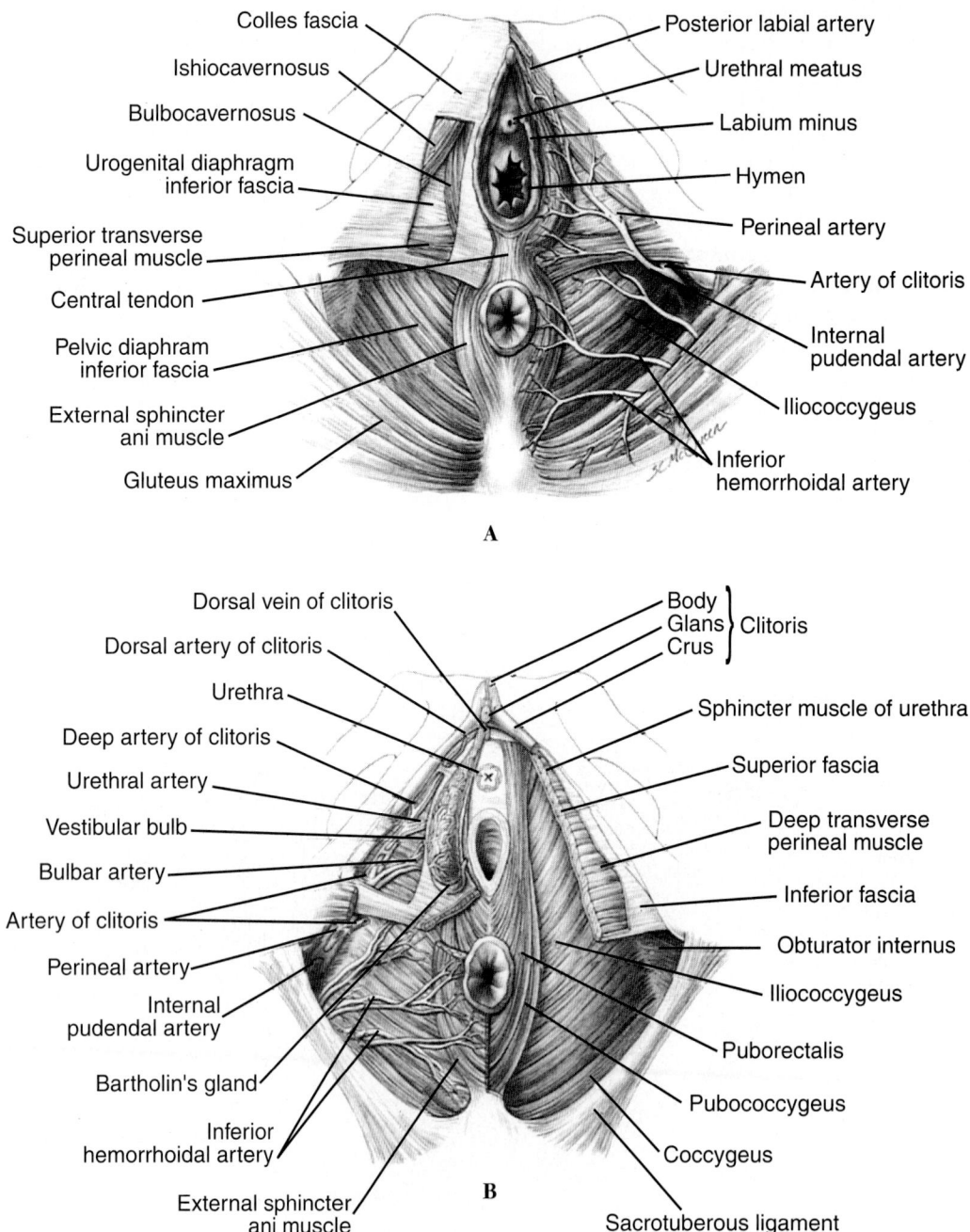

FIGURE 3-19 **A,** Schematic views of the perineum demonstrating superficial structures. Note the two layers of the urogenital diaphragm enfolding the deep transverse perineal muscle. **B,** Schematic views of the perineum demonstrating superficial structures and deeper structures. Note the pelvic diaphragm deep to the perineum, composed primarily of the levator ani and the coccygeus muscles. (Redrawn from Pritchard JA, MacDonald PC, and Gant NF: Williams' obstetrics, ed 17, New York, 1985, Appleton-Century-Crofts, p. 14.)

fossa. Located more superficially are the bulbocavernosus and ischiocavernosus muscles.

The urogenital diaphragm has two layers that enfold and cover the striated, deep transverse perineal muscle. The latter muscle surrounds both the vagina and the urethra, which pierce the diaphragm. The pudendal vessels and nerves, the external sphincter of the membranous urethra, and the dorsal nerve to the clitoris are also found within the urogenital diaphragm. The deep transverse perineal muscle is innervated by branches of the pudendal nerve. The major function of the urogenital diaphragm is support of the urethra and maintenance of the urethrovesical junction.

Ligaments

The pelvic ligaments are not classic ligaments but are thickenings of retroperitoneal fascia and consist primarily of blood and lymphatic vessels, nerves, and fatty connective tissue. Anatomists call the retroperitoneal fascia *subserous fascia,* whereas surgeons refer to this fascial layer as *endopelvic fascia.* The connective tissue is denser immediately adjacent to the lateral walls of the cervix and the vagina.

Broad Ligaments

The broad ligaments are a thin, mesenteric-like double reflection of peritoneum stretching from the lateral pelvic sidewalls to the uterus (Figure 3-20). They become contiguous with the uterine serosa, and thus the uterus is contained within two folds of peritoneum. These peritoneal folds enclose the loose, fatty connective tissue termed the *parametrium.* The broad ligaments afford minor support to the uterus but are conduits for important anatomic structures. Within the broad ligaments are found the following structures: oviducts; ovarian and round ligaments; ureters; ovarian and uterine arteries and veins; parametrial tissue; embryonic remnants of the mesonephric duct, and wolffian body, and secondary two ligaments; the mesovarium; and the mesosalpinx. The round ligament is composed of fibrous tissue and muscle fibers. It attaches to the superoanterior aspect of the uterus, anterior and caudal to the oviduct, and runs via the broad ligament to the lateral pelvic wall. It, too, offers little support to the uterus. The round ligament crosses the external iliac vessels and enters the inguinal canal, ending by inserting into the labia majora in a fanlike fashion. In the fetus a small, fingerlike projection of the peritoneum, known as *Nuck's canal,* accompanies the round ligament into the inguinal canal. Generally it is obliterated in the adult woman.

Cardinal Ligaments

The cardinal, or Mackenrodt's, ligaments extend from the lateral aspects of the upper part of the cervix and the vagina to the pelvic wall. They are a thickened condensation of the

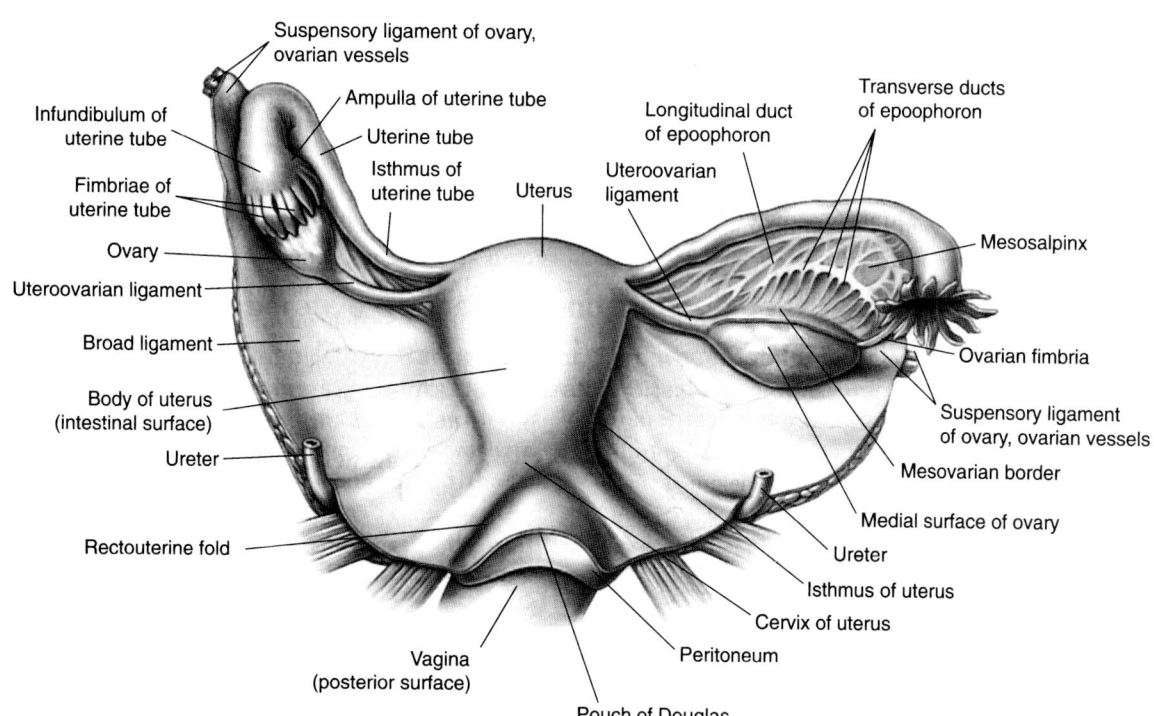

FIGURE 3-20 A schematic drawing of the broad ligament, posterior view. Note the many structures contained within the broad ligament. Note the posterior aspect of the rectouterine fold, called the cul-de-sac, or pouch, of Douglas. (Redrawn from Clemente CD: Anatomy: a regional atlas of the human body, Baltimore-Munich, 1987, Urban & Schwarzenberg.)

subserosal fascia and parametria between the interior portion of the two folds of peritoneum. The cardinal ligaments form the base of the broad ligaments, laterally attaching to the fascia over the pelvic diaphragm and medially merging with fibers of the endopelvic fascia. Within these ligaments are found blood vessels and smooth muscle. The cardinal ligaments help to maintain the anatomic position of the cervix and the upper part of the vagina and provide the major support of the uterus and cervix.

Uterosacral Ligaments

The uterosacral ligaments extend from the upper portion of the cervix posteriorly to the third sacral vertebra. They are thickened near the cervix and then run a curved course around each side of the rectum and subsequently thin out posteriorly. The external surface of the uterosacral ligaments is formed by an inferoposterior fold of peritoneum at the base of the broad ligaments. The middle of the uterosacral ligaments is composed primarily of nerve bundles. The uterosacral ligaments serve a minor role in the anatomic support of the cervix.

Clinical Correlations

The posterior fibers of the levator ani muscles encircle the rectum at its junction with the anal canal, thereby producing an abrupt angle that reinforces fecal continence. Surgical repair of a displacement or tear of the rectovaginal fascia and levator ani muscles resulting from childbirth is important during posterior colporrhaphy. Normal position of the female pelvic organs in the pelvis depends on mechanical support from both fascia and muscles. Vaginal delivery sometimes results in anal sphinction dysfunction. Etiology of this problem may be direct injury to the striated muscles of the pelvic floor or damage to the pudendal and presacral nerves during labor and delivery.

The round ligament is an important surgical landmark in making the initial incision into the parietal peritoneum to gain access to the retroperitoneal space. Direct visualization of the retroperitoneal course of the ureter is an important step in many pelvic operations, including dissections in women with endometriosis, pelvic inflammatory disease, large adnexal masses, broad ligament masses, and pelvic malignancies. A cyst of Nuck's canal may be confused with an indirect inguinal hernia. When a large amount of fluid is placed in the abdominal cavity, postoperative bilateral labial edema may develop in some women because of patency of the canal of Nuck.

During pelvic surgery, traction on the uterus makes the uterosacral and cardinal ligaments more prominent. There is a free space approximately 2 to 4 cm below the superior edge of the broad ligament. In this free space there are no blood vessels, and the two sides of the broad ligament are in close proximity. Often gynecologic surgeons utilize this area to facilitate clamping of the anastomosis between the uterine and ovarian arteries.

NONGENITAL PELVIC ORGANS

Ureters

The ureters are whitish, muscular tubes, 28 to 34 cm in length, extending from the renal pelves to the urinary bladder. The ureter is divided into abdominal and pelvic segments. The diameters vary. The abdominal segment is approximately 8 to 10 mm in diameter. The pelvic segment is approximately 4 to 6 mm. A congenital anomaly of a double, or bifid, ureter occurs in 1% to 4% of females. Ectopic ureteral orifices may occur in either the urethra or the vagina.

The abdominal portion of the right ureter is lateral to the inferior vena cava. Four arteries and accompanying veins cross anterior to the right ureter. They are the right colic artery, the ovarian vessels, the ileocolic artery, and the superior mesenteric artery. The course of the left ureter is similar to its counterpart on the right side in that it runs downward and medially along the anterior surface of the psoas major muscle.

The iliopectineal line serves as the marker for the pelvic portion of the ureter. The ureters run along the common iliac artery and then cross over the iliac vessels as they enter the pelvis. There is a slight variation between the two sides of the female pelvis. The right ureter tends to cross at the bifurcation of the common iliac artery, whereas usually the left ureter crosses 1 to 2 cm above the bifurcation.

The ureters follow the descending, convex curvature of the posterolateral pelvic wall toward the perineum. Throughout its course the ureter is retroperitoneal in location. The ureter can be found on the medial leaf of the parietal peritoneum and in close proximity to the ovarian, uterine, obturator, and superior vesical arteries (Figure 3-21). The uterine artery lies on the anterolateral surface of the ureter for 2.5 to 3 cm. At approximately the level of the ischial spine, the ureter changes its course and runs forward and medially from the uterosacral ligaments to the base of the broad ligament. There the ureter enters into the cardinal ligaments. In this location the ureter is approximately 1 to 2 cm lateral to the uterine cervix and is surrounded by a plexus of veins. The ureter then runs upward and medially in the vesical uterine ligaments to obliquely pierce the bladder wall. Just before entering the base of the bladder, the ureter is in close contact with the anterior vaginal wall.

The ureter has a rich arterial supply with numerous anastomoses from many small vessels that form a longitudinal plexus in the adventitia of the ureter. Parent vessels that send branches to this arterial plexus surrounding the ureter include the renal, ovarian, common iliac, hypogastric, uterine, vaginal, vesical, middle hemorrhoidal, and superior gluteal arteries. The ureter is

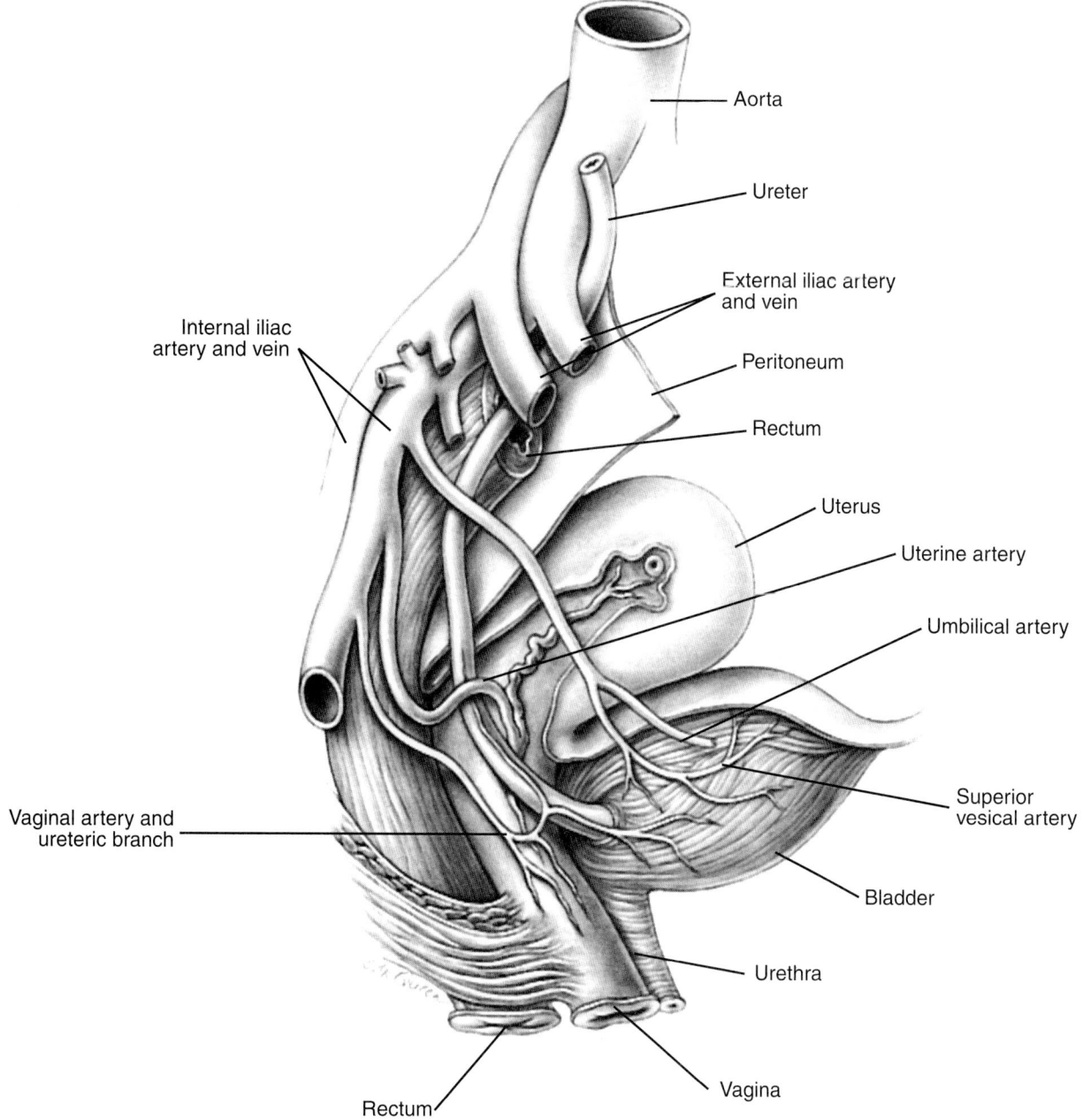

FIGURE 3-21 A schematic drawing of the female pelvis, lateral view, demonstrating the ureter's relation to the major arteries. Note the uterine artery crossing over the ureter. (From Buchsbaum HJ and Schmidt JD: Gynecologic and obstetric urology, Philadelphia, 1978, WB Saunders Co., p. 24.)

resistant to injury resulting from devascularization unless the surgeon strips the adventitia from the muscular conduit.

Urinary Bladder

The urinary bladder is a hollow muscular organ that lies between the symphysis pubis and the uterus. The size and shape of the bladder vary with the volume of urine it contains. Similarly, the anatomic proximity to other pelvic organs depends on whether the bladder is full or empty. The superior surface of the bladder is the only surface covered by peritoneum. The inferior portion is immediately adjacent to the uterus. The urachus is a fibrous cord extending from the apex of the bladder to the umbilicus. The urachus, which is the adult remnant of the embryonic allantois, is occasionally patent for part of its length. The base of the bladder lies directly adjacent to the endopelvic fascia over the anterior vaginal wall. The bladder neck and connecting urethra are attached to the symphysis pubis by fibrous ligaments. The prevesical or retropubic space of Retzius is the area lying between the bladder and symphysis pubis and is bounded laterally by the obliterated hypogastric arteries. This space extends from the fascia covering the pelvic diaphragm to the umbilicus between the peritoneum and transversalis fascia.

The mucosa of the anterior surface of the bladder is light red and has numerous folds. The inferoposterior surface delineated by the two ureteral orifices and the urethral orifice is the trigone. The trigone is a darker red than the rest of the bladder mucosa and is free of folds. When the bladder is empty, the ureteral orifices are approximately 2.5 cm apart. This distance increases to 5 cm when the bladder is distended. The muscular wall of the bladder, the detrusor muscles, is arranged in three layers. The arterial supply of the bladder originates from branches of the hypogastric artery: the superior vesical, inferior vesical, and middle hemorrhoidal arteries. The nerve supply to the bladder includes sympathetic and parasympathetic fibers, with the external sphincter supplied by the pudendal nerve.

Rectum

The rectum is the terminal 12 to 14 cm of the large intestine. The rectum begins over the second or third sacral vertebra, where the sigmoid colon no longer has a mesentery. After the large intestine loses its mesentery, its anatomic posterior wall is in close proximity to the curvature of the sacrum. Anteriorly, peritoneum covers the upper and middle thirds of the rectum. The lowest one third is below the peritoneal reflection and is in close proximity to the posterior wall of the vagina.

The rectum empties into the anal canal, which is 2 to 4 cm in length. The anal canal is fixed by the surrounding levator ani musculature of the pelvic diaphragm (see Figure 3-4). The external sphincter of the anal canal is a circular band of striated muscle. Recent studies of the cross-sectional anatomy of the external anal sphincter by both ultrasound and magnetic resonance imaging have identified two distinct layers of the external anal sphincter. They are a subcutaneous and a deep layer. The rectum, unlike other areas of the large intestine, does not have teniae coli or appendices epiploicae. The arterial supply of the rectum is rich, originating from five arteries: the superior hemorrhoidal artery, which is a continuation of the inferior mesenteric; the two middle hemorrhoidal arteries; and the two inferior hemorrhoidal arteries. Approximately 10% of carcinomas of the large bowel occur within the rectum. Therefore during rectal examination special emphasis to palpate the entire circumference of the rectum, not just the area of the rectovaginal septum, is an important part of screening for colon cancer.

Clinical Correlations

The anatomic proximity of the ureters, urinary bladder, and rectum to the female reproductive organs is a major consideration in most gynecologic operations. Surgical compromise of the ureter may occur during clamping or ligating of the infundibulopelvic vessels, clamping or ligating of the cardinal ligamentsor wide suturing in the endopelvic fascia during an anterior repair. Operative injuries to the bladder or ureter occur in approximately 1 out of 100 major gynecologic operations. Bladder injuries are approximately five times more common than ureteral injuries. Two of the classic ways to differentiate a ureter from a pelvic vessel are (1) visualization of peristalsis after stimulation by a surgical instrument and (2) visualization of Auerbach's plexuses, which are numerous, wavy, small vessels that anastomose over the surface of the ureter. Injury to the ureter or bladder during urethropexy operations for genuine stress incontinence are common. Therefore, most urogynecologists routinely give indigo carmine intramuscularly and either open the bladder or perform cystoscopy near the end of the operative procedure.

For years teachers have referred to the area in the base of the broad ligament near the cervix where the uterine artery crosses the ureter as the area where "water flows under the bridge."

The urinary bladder, if properly drained, will heal rapidly after a surgical insult if the blood supply to the bladder wall is not compromised. This capacity allows the gynecologist to use a suprapubic cystostomy tube without fear of fistula formation.

One of the surgical approaches for urinary stress incontinence is to suspend the periurethral tissue to either the symphysis pubis or Cooper's ligaments. Occasionally, this surgical approach is complicated by a significant amount of postoperative venous bleeding. A subfascial hematoma may extend as high as the umbilicus in the space of Retzius. One of the most common etiologies of female urinary incontinence is defective connective tissue, especially in the periurethral connective tissue, the pubourethral ligaments, and pubococcygeus muscles.

Rectal injury may occur during vaginal hysterectomy with associated posterior colporrhaphy. In the middle third of the vagina the distance between vaginal and rectal mucosa is only a few millimeters, and usually the connective tissue is densely adherent and should be separated by sharp dissection. The rectum bulges anteriorly into the vagina in this area producing a further challenge during the operative procedure.

OTHER STRUCTURES

Cul-de-sac of Douglas

The cul-de-sac of Douglas is a deep pouch formed by the most caudal extent of the parietal peritoneum. The cul-de-sac is a potential space and is also called the *rectouterine pouch* or *fold* (see Figure 3-20). It is anterior to the rectum, separating the uterus from the large intestine. The parietal peritoneum of the cul-de-sac covers the cervix and upper part of the posterior vaginal wall, then reflects to cover the anterior wall of the rectum. The pouch is bounded on the lateral sides by the peritoneal folds covering the uterosacral ligaments.

Parametria

The parametria are the coats of extraperitoneal fatty and fibrous connective tissues adjacent to the uterus. The parametria lie between the leaves of the broad ligament and in the contiguous area anteriorly between the cervix and bladder. This connective tissue is thicker and denser adjacent to the cervix and vagina, where it becomes part of the connective tissue of the pelvic floor. The parametria may also thicken in response to radiation, pelvic cancer, infection, or endometriosis.

Clinical Correlations

The parametria and cul-de-sac of Douglas are important anatomic landmarks in advanced pelvic infection and neoplasia. Intrauterine infection, cervical carcinoma, and endometrial carcinoma may penetrate the endocervical stroma or the myometrium and secondarily may invade the loose connective tissue of the parametria.

The pouch of Douglas is easily accessible in performing transvaginal surgical procedures. Vaginal tubal ligation may be the procedure of choice in massively obese women. Posterior colpotomy is frequently chosen for drainage of a pelvic abscess occurring in the cul-de-sac of Douglas.

Many women with uterine prolapse have an associated enterocele, which is a hernia that protrudes between the uterosacral ligaments. Occasionally the cul-de-sac of Douglas is obliterated by the inflammatory process associated with either endometriosis or advanced malignancy.

KEY POINTS

- The labia majora are homologous to the scrotum in the male. The labia minora are homologous to the penile urethra and a portion of the skin of the penis in males.

- The clitoris is the female homologue of the penis in the male. Skene's glands are homologous to the prostate gland in the male.

- The average length of the clitoris is 1.5 to 2 cm. Clinically, in determining clitoromegaly width is more important and should be less than 1 cm, for it is difficult to actually measure the length of the clitoris.

- The female urethra measures 3.5 to 5 cm in length. The mucosa of the proximal two thirds of the urethra is composed of stratified transitional epithelium, and the distal one third is stratified squamous epithelium.

- When a woman is standing, the axis of the upper portion of the vagina lies close to the horizontal plane, with the upper portion of the vagina curving toward the hollow of the sacrum.

- The lower third of the vagina is in close anatomic relationship to the urogenital and pelvic diaphragms.

- The middle third of the vagina is supported by the levator ani muscles and the lower portion of the cardinal ligaments.

- The primary lymphatic drainage of the upper third of the vagina is to the external iliac nodes, the middle third of the vagina drains to the common and internal iliac nodes, and the lower third has a wide lymphatic distribution, including the common iliac, superficial inguinal, and perirectal nodes.

- Descriptive terms for pelvic organs are derived from the Latin root, whereas terms relating to surgical procedures are derived from the Greek root.

- The length and width of the endocervical canal vary. The width of the canal varies with the parity of the woman and changing hormonal levels. It is usually 2.5 to 3 cm in length and 7 to 8 mm at its widest point.

- The fibromuscular cervical stroma is composed primarily of collagenous connective tissue and ground substance. The connective tissue contains approximately 15% smooth muscle cells and a small amount of elastic tissue.

- The major arterial supply to the cervix is located in the lateral cervical walls at the 3 and 9 o'clock positions.

- The pain fibers from the cervix accompany the parasympathetic fibers to the second, third, and fourth sacral segments.

- The transformation zone of the cervix encompasses the border of the squamous epithelium and columnar epithelium. The location of the transformation zone changes on the cervix depending on a woman's hormonal status.

- The uterus of a nulliparous woman is approximately 8 cm long, 5 cm wide, and 2.5 cm thick and weighs 40 to 50 g. In contrast, in a multiparous woman each measurement is approximately 1.2 cm larger and normal uterine weight is 20 to 30 g heavier. The maximal weight of a normal uterus is 110 g.

- In the majority of women, the long axis of the uterus is both anteverted in respect to the long axis of the vagina and anteflexed in relation to the long axis of the cervix. However, a retroflexed uterus is a normal variant found in approximately 25% of women.

- The arterial blood supply of the uterus is provided by the uterine and ovarian arteries. The uterine arteries are large branches of the anterior division of the hypogastric arteries, whereas the ovarian arteries originate directly from the aorta.

- Afferent nerve fibers from the uterus enter the spinal cord at the eleventh and twelfth thoracic segments.

- The oviducts are 10 to 14 cm in length and are composed of four anatomic sections. Closest to the uterine cavity is the interstitial segment, followed by the narrow isthmic segment, then the wider ampullary segment, and distally the trumpet-shaped infundibular segment.

- The right oviduct and appendix are often anatomically adjacent. Clinically it may be difficult to differentiate inflammation of the upper portion of the genital tract and acute appendicitis.

- During the reproductive years the ovaries measure approximately 1.5 cm × 2.5 cm × 4 cm.

- The ovary in nulliparous women rests in a depression of peritoneum named the *fossa ovarica*. Immediately adjacent to the ovarian fossa are the external iliac vessels, the ureter, and the obturator vessels and nerves.

- Three prominent ligaments determine the anatomic mobility of the ovary: the mesovarian, the ovarian ligament, and the infundibulopelvic ligament.

- The arterial supply of the pelvis is paired, bilateral, and has multiple collaterals and numerous anastomoses.

- The extent of collateral circulation after hypogastric artery ligation depends on the site of ligation and may be divided into three groups: branches from the aorta, branches from the external iliac arteries, and branches from the femoral arteries.

- The internal iliac nodes are found in an anatomic triangle whose sides are composed of the external iliac artery, the hypogastric artery, and the pelvic sidewall. This rich collection of nodes receives channels from every internal pelvic organ and the vulva, including the clitoris and urethra.

- The femoral triangle is the anatomic space lying immediately distal to the fold of the groin. The boundaries of the femoral triangle are the sartorius and adductor longus muscles and the inguinal ligament.

- The pudendal nerve and its branches supply the majority of both motor and sensory fibers to the muscles and skin of the vulvar region.

- The femoral nerve may be compromised by pressure on the psoas muscle during abdominal surgery and by hyperflexion of the leg during vaginal surgery.

- The pelvic diaphragm is important in supporting both abdominal and pelvic viscera and facilitates equal distribution of intraabdominal pressure during activities such as coughing. The levator ani muscles constitute the greatest bulk of the pelvic diaphragm.

- The major function of the urogenital diaphragm is support of the urethra and maintenance of the urethrovesical junction.

- Contained within the broad ligaments are the following structures: oviducts; ovarian and round ligaments; ureters; ovarian and uterine arteries and veins; parametrial tissue; embryonic remnants of the mesonephric duct and wolffian body, and two secondary ligaments; the mesovarian; and the mesosalpinx.

- The cardinal ligaments provide the major support to the uterus.

- A congenital anomaly of a double, or bifid, ureter occurs in 1% to 4% of females.

- When the urinary bladder is empty, the ureteral orifices are approximately 2.5 cm apart. This distance increases to 5 cm when the bladder is distended.

- The distal ureter enters into the cardinal ligament. In this location the ureter is approximately 1 to 2 cm lateral to the uterine cervix and is surrounded by a plexus of veins.

- Two ways of distinguishing the ureter from pelvic vessels are (1) identification of peristalsis after stimulation with a surgical instrument and (2) identification of Auerbach's plexuses.

- Surgical compromise of the ureters may occur during clamping or ligating of the infundibulopelvic vessels, clamping or ligating of the cardinal ligaments, or wide suturing in the endopelvic fascia during an anterior repair.

- Three important axioms that should be in the forefront of decision making during difficult gynecologic surgery are (1) do not assume that the anatomy of the left and right side of the pelvis are invariably identical mirror images; (2) during difficult operations with multiple adhesions operate from known anatomic areas into the unknown; and (3) from the sage advice of a distinguished Canadian gynecologist, Dr. Henry McDuff:

> If the disease be rampant and the anatomy obscure,
> And the planes of dissection not pristine and pure,
> Do not be afraid, nor faint of heart,
> Try the retroperitoneum, it's a great place to start.

BIBLIOGRAPHY

Aronson MP, Bates SM, Jacoby AF, et al: Periurethral and paravaginal anatomy: an endovaginal magnetic resonance imaging study, Am J Obstet Gynecol 173:1702, 1995.

Beckmann CRB, Lipscomb GH, Murrell L, et al: Instruction in surgical anatomy for gynecology residents using prosected human cadavers, Am J Obstet Gynecol 170:148, 1994.

Benedetti-Panici P, Maneschi F, Scambia G, et al: Anatomic abnormalities of the retroperitoneum encountered during aortic and pelvic lymphadenectomy, Am J Obstet Gynecol 170:111, 1994.

Benedetti-Panici P, Scambia G, Baiocchi G, et al: Anatomical study of para-aortic and pelvic lymph nodes in gynecologic malignancies, Obstet Gynecol 79:498, 1992.

Burchell RC: Physiology of internal iliac artery ligation, J Obstet Gynaecol Br Commnw 75:642, 1968.

Clemente CD: Gray's anatomy, ed 30, Philadelphia, 1985, Lea & Febiger.

Cruikshank SH and Stoelk EM: Surgical control of pelvic hemorrhage: method of bilateral ovarian artery ligation, Am J Obstet Gynecol 147:724, 1983.

DeLancey JOL: Anatomy and biomechanics of genital prolapse, Clin Obstet Gynecol 36:897, 1993.

DeLancey JOL: Structural anatomy of the posterior pelvic compartment as it relates to rectocele, Am J Obstet Gynecol 180:815, 1999.

Fenner DE, Kriegshauser JS, Lee HH, et al: Anatomic and physiologic measurements of the internal and external anal sphincters in normal females, Obstet Gynecol 91:369, 1998.

Grant JCB: An atlas of anatomy, ed 9, Baltimore, 1991, Williams & Wilkins.

Hahn L: Clinical findings and results of operative treatment in ilioinguinal nerve entrapment syndrome, Br J Obstet Gynaecol 96:1080, 1989.

Hoffman MS, Lynch C, Lockhart J, and Knapp R: Injury of the rectum during vaginal surgery, Am J Obstet Gynecol 181:274, 1999.

Jelen I and Bachmann G: An anatomical approach to oophorectomy during vaginal hysterectomy, Obstet Gynecol 87:137, 1996.

Koelbl H, Strassegger H, Riss PA, and Gruber H: Morphologic and functional aspects of pelvic floor muscles in patients with pelvic relaxation and genuine stress incontinence, Obstet Gynecol 74:789, 1989.

Kurman RJ: Blaustein's pathology of the female genital tract, ed 4, New York, 1994, Springer-Verlag.

Krantz KE: The anatomy of the urethra and anterior vaginal wall, Am J Obstet Gynecol 62:374, 1951.

Krantz KE: Innervation of the human vulva and vagina, Obstet Gynecol 12:382, 1958.

Netter FH: Reproductive system, vol 2, The CIBA collection of medical illustrations, Summit, NJ, 1983, CIBA Pharmaceutical Products.

Nichols DH and Randall CL: Vaginal surgery, ed 4, Baltimore, 1996, Williams & Wilkins.

Novak ER and Woodruff JD: Gynecologic and obstetric pathology, ed 8, Philadelphia, 1979, WB Saunders Co.

Pelosi MA III and Pelosi MA: Alignment of the umbilical axis: an effective maneuver for laparoscopic entry in the obese patient, Obstet Gynecol 92:869, 1998.

Peschers UM, DeLancey JOL, Fritsch H, et al: Cross-sectional imaging anatomy of the anal sphincters, Obstet Gynecol 90:839, 1997.

Plentl AA and Friedman EA: Lymphatic system of the female genitalia: the morphologic basis of oncologic diagnosis and therapy. Philadelphia, 1971, WB Saunders Co.

Richardson AC: The rectovaginal septum revisited: its relationship to rectocele and its importance in rectocele repair, Clin Obstet Gynecol 36:976, 1993.

Shull B: Using videography to teach retropubic space anatomy and surgical technique, Obstet Gynecol 77:640, 1991.

Thakar R and Clarkson P: Bladder, bowel and sexual function after hysterectomy for benign conditions, Br J Obstet Gynaecol 104:983, 1997.

Thompson JR, Gibb JS, Genadry R, et al: Anatomy of pelvic arteries adjacent to the sacrospinous ligament: importance of the coccygeal branch of the inferior gluteal artery, Obstet Gynecol 94:973, 1999.

Ulmsten U and Falconer C: Connective tissue in female urinary incontinence, Curr Opin Obstet Gynecol 11:509, 1999.

Vedantham S, Goodwin SC, McLucas B and Mohr G: Uterine artery embolization: an underused method of controlling pelvic hemorrhage, Am J Obstet Gynecol 176:938, 1997.

Verkauf BS, Von Thron J, and O'Brien WF: Clitorial size in normal women, Obstet Gynecol 80:41, 1992.

Wall LL: The muscles of the pelvic floor, Clin Obstet Gynecol 36:910, 1993.

Wynn RM and Jollie WP: Biology of the uterus, ed 2, New York, 1989, Plenum Publishing Co.

Zacharin RF: The suspensory mechanism of the female urethra, J Anat 97:423, 1963.

Zacharin RF: Pulsion enterocele: review of functional anatomy of the pelvic floor, Obstet Gynecol 55:135, 1980.

Reproductive Endocrinology

Neuroendocrinology, Gonadotrophins, Sex Steroids, Prostaglandins, Ovulation, Menstruation, Hormone Assay

KEY TERMS AND DEFINITIONS

Activin. Peptide with a similar structure to inhibin but an opposite action. Activins stimulate pituitary follicle-stimulating hormone (FSH) release and ovarian estradiol production.

Affinity (K). Degree to which a hormone binds to its receptor. Affinity is determined by the degree to which the hormone structurally fits, or interlocks, with the receptor.

Arcuate Nucleus. A group of nerve cells lying in the medial portion of the hypothalamus just above the median eminence. Nerve cells in the arcuate nucleus are the major source of gonadotrophin-releasing hormone (GnRH) secretion.

Aromatization. Synthesis of a phenolic, or aromatic, benzene ring, as occurs during conversion of testosterone to estradiol.

Atresia. Process of regression of preantral follicles.

Autocrine. Producing hormonal effects by intracellular communication.

Bioassay. Measurement of the amount of hormone present in a substance by determining its effect on a target organ in an animal and comparing it with the effect produced by a known (standard) amount of hormone.

Catechol Estrogens. Steroids that structurally resemble both estrogens and catecholamines and have only a weak estrogenic action.

Coefficient of Variation (CV). Mathematical technique to measure precision of assay after results of measurement of same substance are calculated several times in one assay (intraassay CV) or in several assays (interassay CV).

Cortical Granules. Particles in ooplasm that are released into the surface membrane after one sperm penetrates the ovum. They may act to block further sperm penetration.

Cross-reaction. Interference in immunoassay by a substance that is not being measured but reacts with the antibody to a lesser degree than the hormone being measured. It thus alters the results of the assay.

Desensitization (Down Regulation). The condition wherein a hormone is secreted or administered for a prolonged period and produces an inhibitory instead of a stimulatory response because of saturation of its receptor.

Dominant Follicle. Follicle that enlarges to about 2 cm in diameter and eventually ovulates.

Eicosanoids. Class of fatty acid derivatives containing prostaglandins, thromboxanes, and leukotrienes. Eicosanoids are derived from the unsaturated fatty acid form of eicosanoic acid and have a high degree of biologic activity. The most important precursor of the eicosanoids is arachidonic acid.

β-Endorphin. A potent opioid peptide—more potent than morphine—that is concentrated in the hypothalamus and pituitary. It inhibits luteinizing hormone (LH) secretion.

Extraglandular Conversion. Process whereby one steroid is converted to another steroid in tissue other than endocrine organs.

Follicle-Stimulating Hormone (FSH). A glycoprotein with a molecular weight of 33,000 daltons that is composed of a nonspecific α subunit and a specific β subunit.

The primary action of FSH in the female is to stimulate granulosa cell synthesis.

Germinal Vesicle. Nuclear material that is surrounded by a membrane, visible histologically, and that is present in the primary oocyte.

Gonadotrophin-Releasing Hormone (GnRH). A decapeptide synthesized in and secreted by the hypothalamus at periodic intervals to stimulate gonadotrophin release from the pituitary gland.

Gonadotrophin-Releasing Hormone Analogue (GnRH Analogue). GnRH analogues are proteins composed of the 10 amino acids found in the parent molecule of GnRH, but with substitutions at certain amino acids 6 and 10 to increase potency and half-life.

Growth Factors. Small peptides or polypeptides that interact with cell membrane receptors and usually promote cell proliferation and/or differentiation.

Hormone Receptors. Proteins on the cell membrane or within the cell of the target tissue that bind to a specific molecule of a hormone (ligand) for the purpose of eliciting a biologic response. Hormone receptors bind only to ligands of a specific hormone and thus are hormone specific.

Hypothalamus. Portion of the base of the brain that is located just below the optic chiasm and that has a major role in regulating the hormones involved in reproductive endocrinology.

Inhibin. A polypeptide dimer composed of an α and a β subunit joined by disulfide bonds. This hormone is produced by ovarian granulosa cells and inhibits FSH secretion.

Leptin. A peptide secreted by adipose tissue. It is believed to be a peripheral signal of amount of fat stores.

Leukotrienes. Derivatives of unsaturated eicosanoic acid, particularly arachidonic acid, which do not have a closed ring structure but have a similar system of assignment of letters and numeric subscripts. Their biologic effects are not completely understood but appear to stimulate smooth muscle.

Luteinizing Hormone (LH). A glycoprotein with a molecular weight of 28,000 daltons that is composed of a nonspecific α subunit and a specific β subunit. The primary action of LH in the female is to stimulate ovarian steroid synthesis.

Median Eminence (Infundibulum). The portion of the neurohypophysis lying in the midline at the base of the hypothalamus. It is connected to the infundibular stalk and the posterior (neural) lobe of the pituitary gland.

Metabolic Clearance Rate (MCR). Volume of plasma, serum, or blood that is cleared of the steroid per unit of time (liters per day).

Monoclonal Antibody. Single type of antibody produced by the spleen cell of a mouse that was injected with antigen. The spleen cell is subsequently fused with a myeloma cell to form a hybridoma cell in order to produce large quantities of the antibody.

Neurohypophysis. The portion of the hypothalamus consisting of the median eminence, infundibular stalk, and posterior lobe of the pituitary.

Neuromodulator. A substance that affects the action of a neurotransmitter.

Neurotransmitter. Biogenic amines secreted by a nerve cell that produce an action on another cell.

Nonradioactive Immunoassays. Assays that do not use a radioactive marker but act by the same principle. These include the chemiluminescent immunoassay, fluoroimmunoassay, and enzyme immunoassay, which uses excess antigen, and enzyme-linked immunosorbent assay (ELISA), which uses excess antibody.

Oogonia. Primordial female germ cells with a full chromosomal complement that are present in the fetal ovary.

Paracrine. Producing hormonal effects by diffusion to contiguous cells.

Primary Follicle (Preantral Follicle). Immature oocyte covered by multiple layers of granulosa cells but without an antrum.

Primary Oocyte. Female germ cell in the diplotene stage of first meiotic division.

Primordial Follicle. Immature oocyte covered by a single layer of granulosa cells.

Production Rate. Amount of steroid that enters the circulation per unit of time (usually measured in milligrams or micrograms per day).

Prostaglandins. Prostanoids with a cyclopentane ring and two side chains. The different letters assigned to the various prostaglandins refer to different substitutions in the cyclopentane ring, and the numbers in the subscript of the letter indicate the number of double bonds in the side chain.

Prostanoids. Family of closely related lipids that include prostaglandins and thromboxanes. They have the basic structure of prostanoic acid, which consists of 20 carbon atoms arranged in a ring structure with two side chains.

Radioimmunoassay (RIA). Technique of measurement of hormone using a specific antibody raised against the hormone (antigen). The antigen competes for binding to the antibody with a radioactive-labeled form of the same antigen.

Second Messenger. A substance, usually a cyclic nucleotide, that is activated when a protein hormone attaches to its receptor to induce changes within the cell.

Sex Hormone–Binding Globulin (SHBG). A serum globulin that has a high affinity for dihydrotestosterone, testosterone, and estradiol estrogens and androgens (also called testosterone-estrogen–binding globulin [TeBG]).

Standard Curve. Curved line that results from connecting the endpoints derived from assay of different amounts of known (standard) hormone plotted graphically against the amount of hormone present.

Stratum Basale. Thin, lowermost portion of endometrium that overlies muscularis and consists of primordial glands and densely cellular stroma.

Stratum Functionale. Thick, uppermost portion of endometrium that grows under the influence of estrogen. It is composed of a thin superficial stratum compactum and an underlying broader stratum spongiosum.

Thromboxanes. Prostanoids with an oxane ring instead of a cyclopentane ring. Letters and numeric subscripts are assigned similar to those used with prostaglandins.

Transcription. Generation of messenger RNA from a segment of DNA produced by the hormone-receptor complex in the nucleus.

Transformation. The change in receptor configuration produced by a steroid that allows the receptor-hormone complex to undergo translocation.

Zona Pellucida. Mucopolysaccharide coat surrounding oocyte that allows only sperm of the same species to penetrate the ovum.

INTRODUCTION

The endocrinologic regulation of the reproductive system is extremely complex. Much information has been accumulated in the past three decades, and new information is constantly becoming available. Entire books have been written about each aspect of reproductive endocrinology. In this chapter, only the basic information required for an understanding of this complex process will be presented.

No single organ that secretes hormones involved in the reproductive process acts independently. Nevertheless, for ease of understanding, each organ and its principal hormones will be discussed as a unit. Information in this chapter will include the central nervous system control of gonadotrophin-releasing hormone (GnRH) secretion, GnRH action on gonadotrophin secretion, gonadotrophin effects on the ovary, and ovarian steroid effects on the uterus. The positive and negative feedback control of the various organs involved in human reproduction will be presented. The regulation of prolactin secretion is discussed in Chapter 39. Because of space limitations, even though the adrenal and thyroid hormones have a profound influence on the reproductive system, a discussion of adrenal and thyroid endocrinology will not be included in this text.

NEUROENDOCRINOLOGY OF GnRH SECRETION

The hypothalamic hormone that controls gonadotrophin release is GnRH. GnRH is a decapeptide whose structural formula was first determined by Schally et al. (Figure 4-1). The gene that encodes for GnRH is located on the short arm of chromosome 8. The GnRH receptor has been found to be present in many organs besides the pituitary.

The cell bodies of the hypothalamic neurons that produce GnRH are concentrated mainly in two areas: the anterior hypothalamus and the medial basal (tuberal) hypothalamus. In the latter area, the greatest number of GnRH-producing neurons are in the arcuate nucleus (Figure 4-2). From these areas, GnRH is transported along the axons of these neurons, which terminate in the median eminence around the capillaries of the primary portal plexus. The nerve cells that transport GnRH from the arcuate nucleus to the median eminence are called the *tuberoinfundibular tract*.

The median eminence, or infundibulum, together with the infundibular stalk and posterior (neural) lobe of the pituitary, make up the neurohypophysis. The three components of the neurohypophysis share a common capillary network and have a direct arterial blood supply from the hypophyseal arteries. The capillaries of the median eminence have a fenestrated epithelium similar to that of peripheral tissue, which allows passage of large molecules. These capillaries differ from those present in the brain, and thus the median eminence is outside the blood-brain barrier.

The nerve cell terminals of the tuberoinfundibular tract secrete GnRH directly into the portal circulation, which carries the hormone to the gonadotrophin-containing cells in the anterior lobe of the pituitary. The pars tuberalis of the anterior lobe of the pituitary (adenohypophysis) receives its vascular supply from pituitary portal vessels and is located adjacent to the base of the hypothalamus and the pituitary stalk (Figure 4-2). Unlike the neurohypophysis, the adenohypophysis has no direct

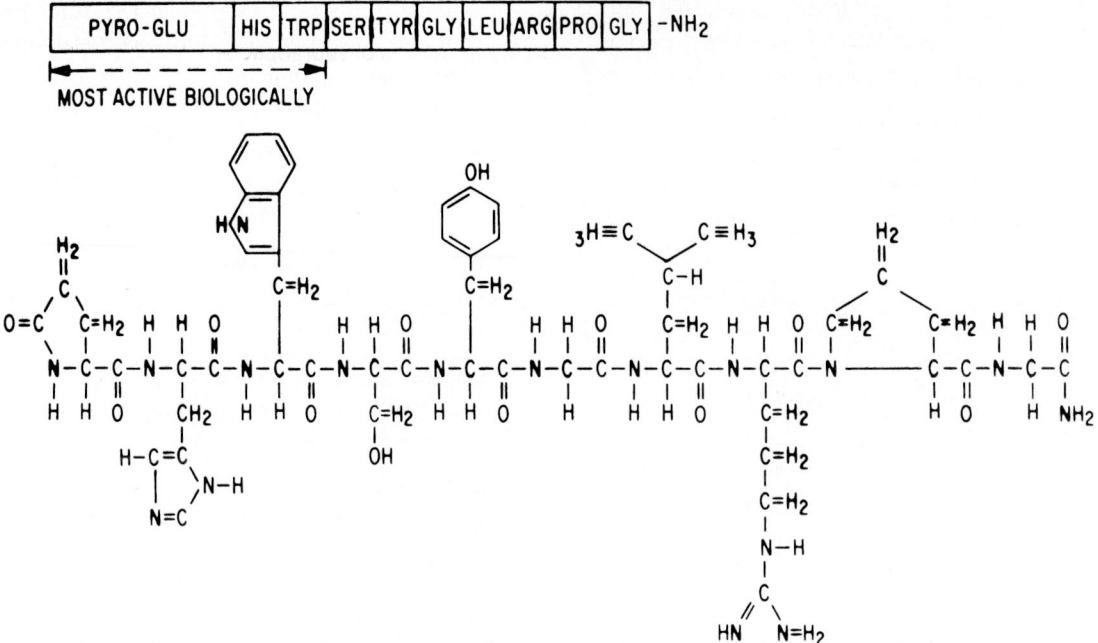

FIGURE 4-1 Amino acid sequence of gonadotrophin-releasing hormone (GnRH). (From Kletzky OA and Lobo RA: Reproductive neuroendocrinology. In Mishell DR Jr, Davajan V, and Lobo RA, editors: Infertility, contraception and reproductive endocrinology, ed 3, Cambridge, Mass, 1991, Blackwell Scientific Publications.)

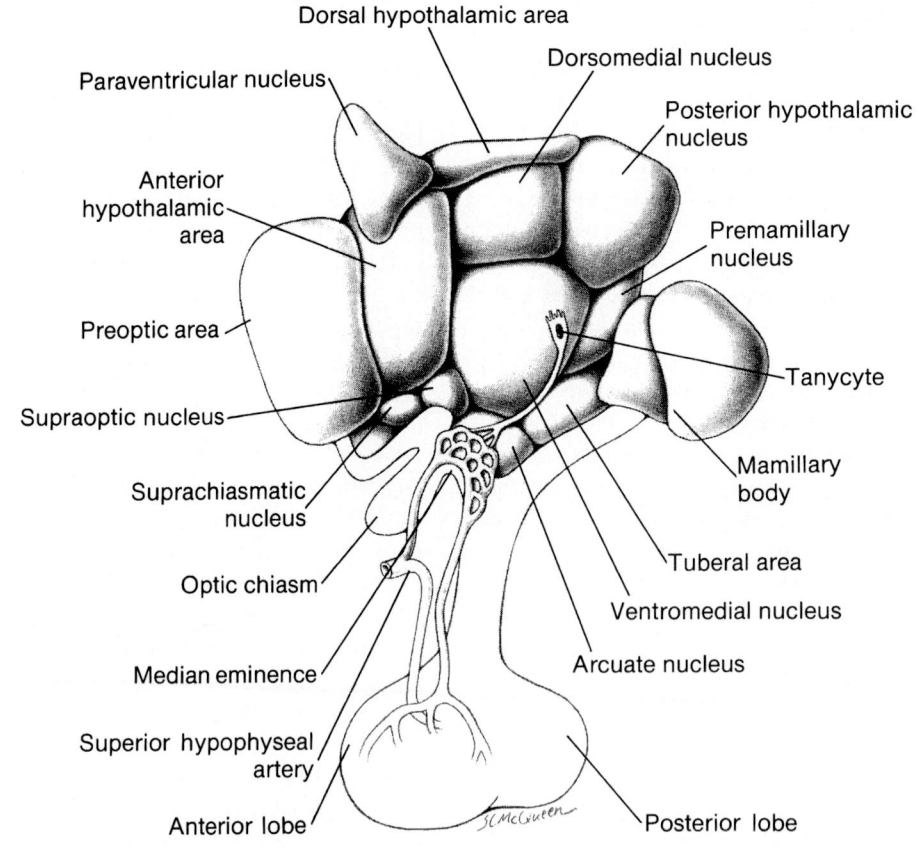

FIGURE 4-2 Nuclear organization of hypothalamus, shown diagrammatically in sagittal plane as it would appear from third ventricle. Rostral area is to left and caudal to right. Pituitary gland is shown ventrally. *AL*, Anterior lobe; *MB*, mamillary body; *ME*, median eminence; *NL*, neural lobe; *OC*, optic chiasm. (Redrawn from Moore RY: Neuroendocrine mechanisms: cells and systems. In Yen SSC and Jaffe R, editors: Reproductive endocrinology: physiology, pathophysiology and clinical management, Philadelphia, 1986, WB Saunders Co.)

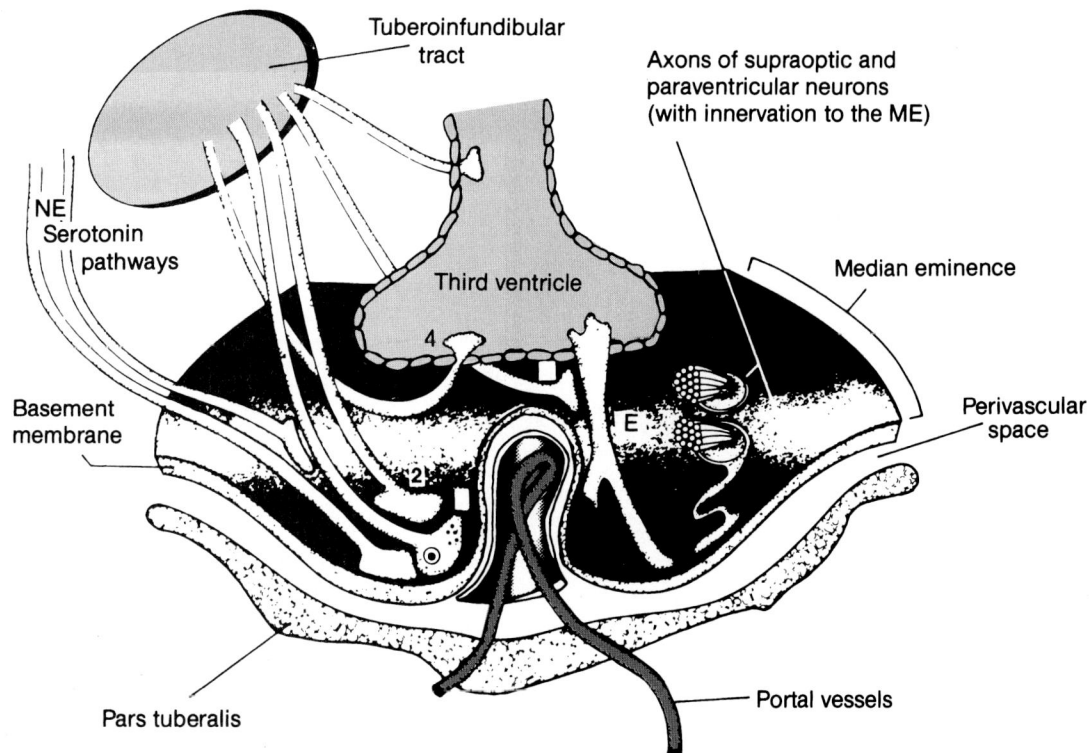

FIGURE 4-3 Schematic diagram showing tanycytes *(E)*, stretching between third ventricle and outer portion of median eminence. (From Reichlin S: Neural control of the pituitary gland: normal physiology and pathophysiologic implications. In Current concepts, Kalamazoo, Mich, 1978, Upjohn Publications.)

arterial blood supply and receives all of its blood from the portal vessels. After leaving the pituitary gland, the circulation returns to the neurohypophyseal capillary plexus, allowing pituitary hormones to help regulate the secretion of GnRH from the median eminence.

In addition to this major route of GnRH transport, an alternative route may exist. Axons of the tuberoinfundibular tract may transport GnRH directly into the third ventricle. A specialized ependymal cell, the tanycyte, extends from the lumen of the third ventricle into the outermost zone of the median eminence (Figure 4-3). Since, when GnRH is administered into the third ventricle, it is transported into the portal system, it has been postulated that transport occurs via the tanycytes and their microvilli. Thus GnRH can be released both in large amounts periodically via the tuberoinfundibular tract (cyclic release) and in a low-grade continuous transependymal manner (tonic release) via the tanycytes.

In humans, GnRH is secreted in a pulsatile manner and has a half-life of only 2 to 4 minutes. The amplitude and frequency of the pulse vary throughout the menstrual cycle, with the frequency being more rapid in the follicular phase, about 1 pulse per hour, and slower in the luteal phase, about 1 pulse in 2 to 3 hours.

Knobil et al. performed a series of elegant experiments using an oophorectomized monkey model in which endogenous GnRH secretion had been abolished by a lesion in the hypothalamus. These investigators showed that altering the interval of GnRH pulses interferes with gonadotrophin secretion. If exogenous GnRH pulses were administered every hour, a midcycle gonadotrophin surge occurred (Figure 4-4). However, when the pulse frequency was increased to five pulses per hour, gonadotrophin secretion was inhibited (Figure 4-5). Decreasing GnRH pulse frequency to once every 3 hours decreased the levels of luteinizing hormone (LH) and increased those of follicle-stimulating hormone (FSH); in addition, no gonadotrophin surge occurred. Decreasing the amount of exogenous GnRH also inhibited gonadotrophin release.

Crowley et al. have demonstrated that some women with anovulation (hypothalamic amenorrhea) and amenorrhea without a known cause have altered pulse frequency or amplitude of GnRH secretion or both. Thus, the control of episodic GnRH secretion is extremely important for the maintenance of normal ovulatory cyclicity. The amplitude and frequency of GnRH secretion by the hypothalamus not only are regulated by the feedback of two ovarian steroids, estradiol and progesterone, but also by gonadotrophins through the humoral input pathway. Amplitude and frequency also are modulated by several neurotransmitters and neuromodulators within the brain through a neural input pathway.

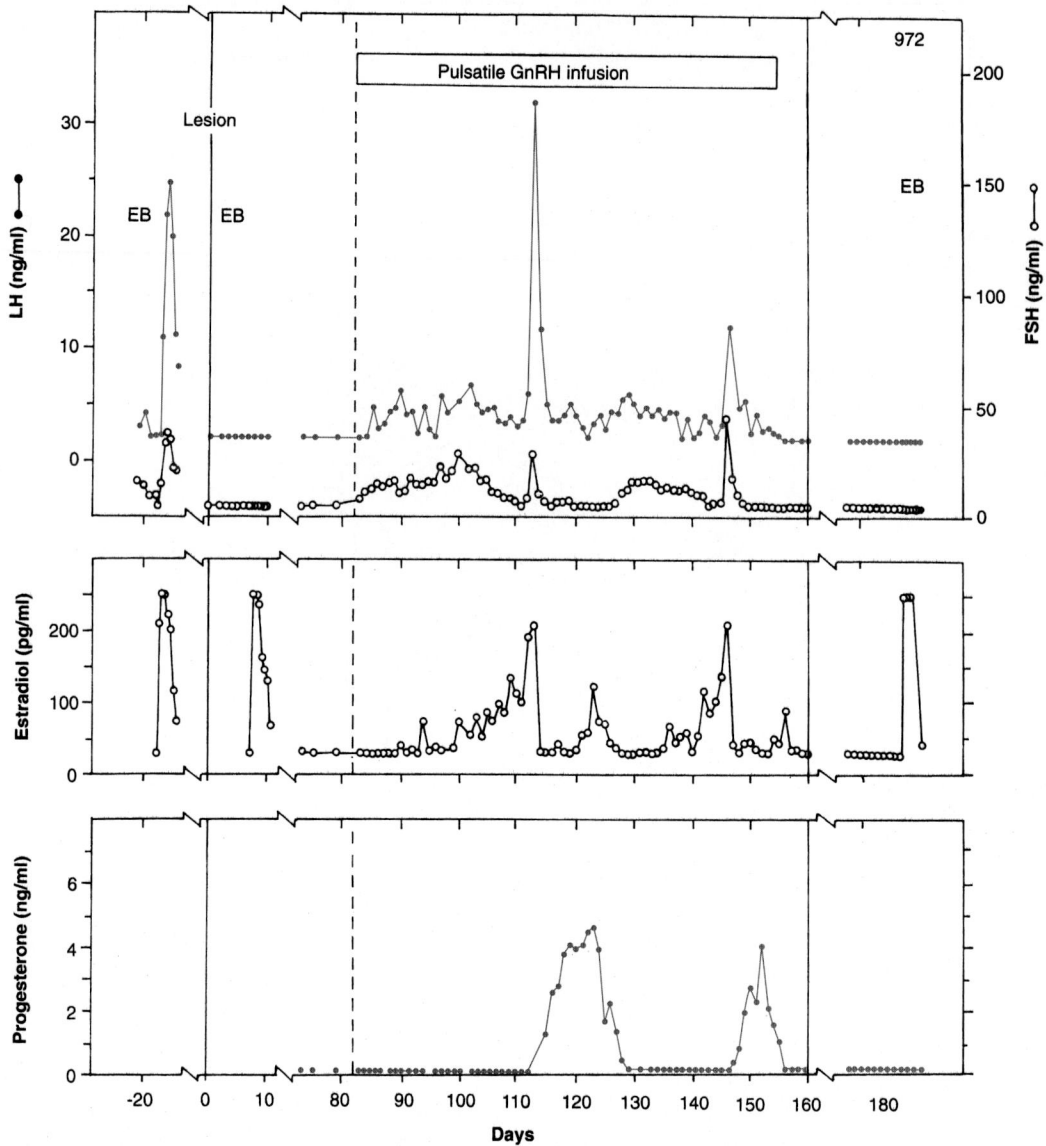

FIGURE 4-4   Induction of two ovulatory menstrual cycles by administration of pulsatile GnRH replacement (1 µg/min for 6 minutes, once every hour) in rhesus monkey with hypothalamic lesion that had abolished endogenous GnRH secretion. Estradiol benzoate *(EB)* elicited gonadotrophin response before placement of lesion but not afterward. (Redrawn from Knobil E, Plant TM, Wildt L, et al: Science 207:1371, 1980.)

Neurotransmitters

The most important neurotransmitters involved in reproductive neuroendocrinology are two catecholamines, dopamine and norepinephrine, as well as an indolamine, serotonin. All three of these neurotransmitters are monoamines. Dopamine and norepinephrine are produced by conversion of tyrosine in the midbrain (Figure 4-6). The enzyme tyrosine hydroxylase converts tyrosine to dopa, which is then decarboxylated to dopamine. Pyridoxine is an important coenzyme in this process. Dopamine oxidase converts dopamine to norepinephrine. Norepinephrine is then converted to epinephrine by the addition of a methyl group by a methyl transferase enzyme.

The precursor of serotonin is tryptophan, which is first converted to 5-hydroxytryptophan by the enzyme tryptophan-hydroxylase (Figure 4-7). This substance is then decarboxylated to form serotonin. The principal metabolite of serotonin is 5-hydroxyindoleacetic acid (5-HIAA), which can be measured in urine. Serotonin has not been shown to affect GnRH release, but it does stimulate the release of prolactin, probably by stimulating the release of the hypothalamic prolactin-releasing factor.

The current concept regarding the action of neurotransmitters is that the biogenic catecholamines modulate GnRH pulsatile release. Norepinephrine is thought to exert stimulatory effects on GnRH, while serotonin exerts

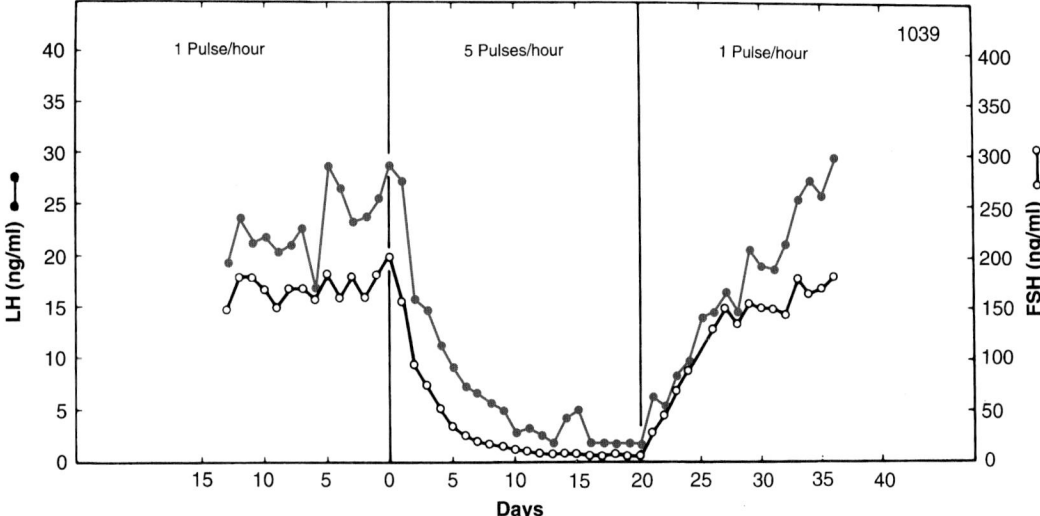

FIGURE 4-5 Same rhesus monkey preparation as in Figure 4-4. Gonadotrophin suppression in which GnRH pulse is increased to five per hour and is restored by returning to the physiologic frequency of one pulse per hour. (From Knobil E: Recent Prog Horm Res 36:53, 1980.)

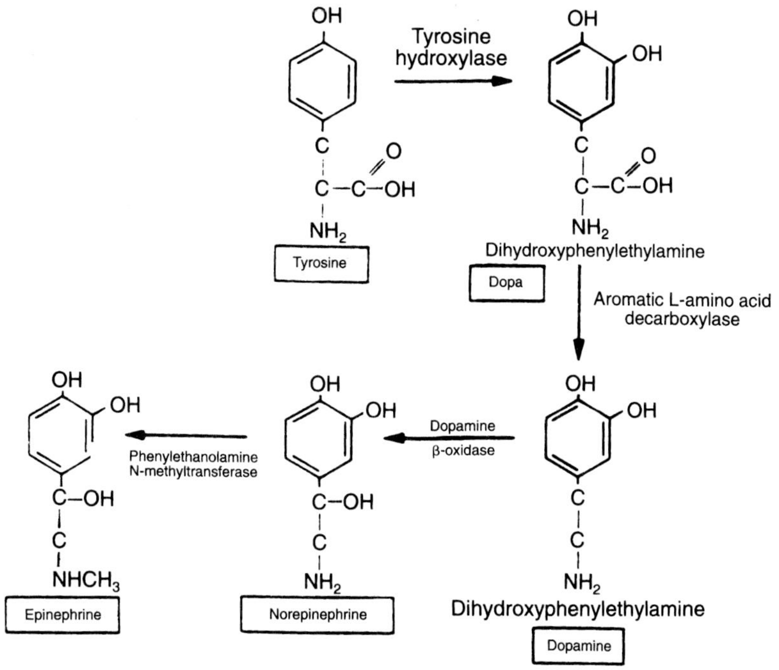

FIGURE 4-6 Metabolic pathways of dopamine, norepinephrine, and epinephrine synthesis. (From Kletzky OA and Lobo RA: Reproductive neuroendocrinology. In Mishell DR Jr, Davajan V, and Lobo RA, editors: Infertility, contraception and reproductive endocrinology, ed 3, Cambridge, Mass, 1991, Blackwell Scientific Publications.)

inhibitory effects. The probable mode of action of catecholamines is to influence the frequency and perhaps the amplitude of GnRH release. Thus pharmacologic or physiologic factors that affect pituitary function probably do so by altering catecholamine synthesis or metabolism, and thus the pulsatile release of GnRH.

The intravenous administration of dopamine to both men and women is associated with a suppression of circulating prolactin and gonadotrophin levels. Dopamine does not exert a direct effect on gonadotrophin secretion by the anterior pituitary; instead its effect is mediated through inhibition of GnRH release in the hypothalamus. Although the exact chemical nature of the endogenous prolactin inhibiting hormone remains unknown, overwhelming evidence indicates that dopamine is the hypothalamic inhibitor of prolactin secretion. Thus dopamine may directly suppress hypothalamic GnRH activity and pituitary prolactin secretion.

Mechanism of Action and Pharmacologic Effects

The effects of neurotransmitters on the secretion of hypothalamic hormones probably are exerted by different mechanisms. One possible mechanism is through a direct cell-to-cell connection or a multisynaptic communication whereby the neurotransmitter is released by the terminal nerve and depolarizes the receptor site on a hypothalamic cell (Figure 4-8). Depolarization results in the release of a specific hormone from the hypothalamic cell.

These specific effects of neurotransmitters on hypo-

thalamic cells can be altered by the systemic administration of certain drugs. For example, methyldopa and α-methyl-*p*-tyrosine can block dopamine and norepinephrine synthesis by inhibiting tyrosine hydroxylase. Reserpine and chlorpromazine interfere with norepinephrine, dopamine, and serotonin binding and storage. Finally, and clinically important, the frequently prescribed tricyclic antidepressants inhibit the reuptake of neurotransmitters, whereas other medications such as propranolol, phentolamine, haloperidol, and cyproheptadine act by blocking the receptors at the level of the hypothalamus.

As a consequence of receiving such medications, many patients develop disorders such as galactorrhea and oligoamenorrhea. These clinical entities are a result of either hyperprolactinemia or alterations in GnRH-gonadotrophin secretion.

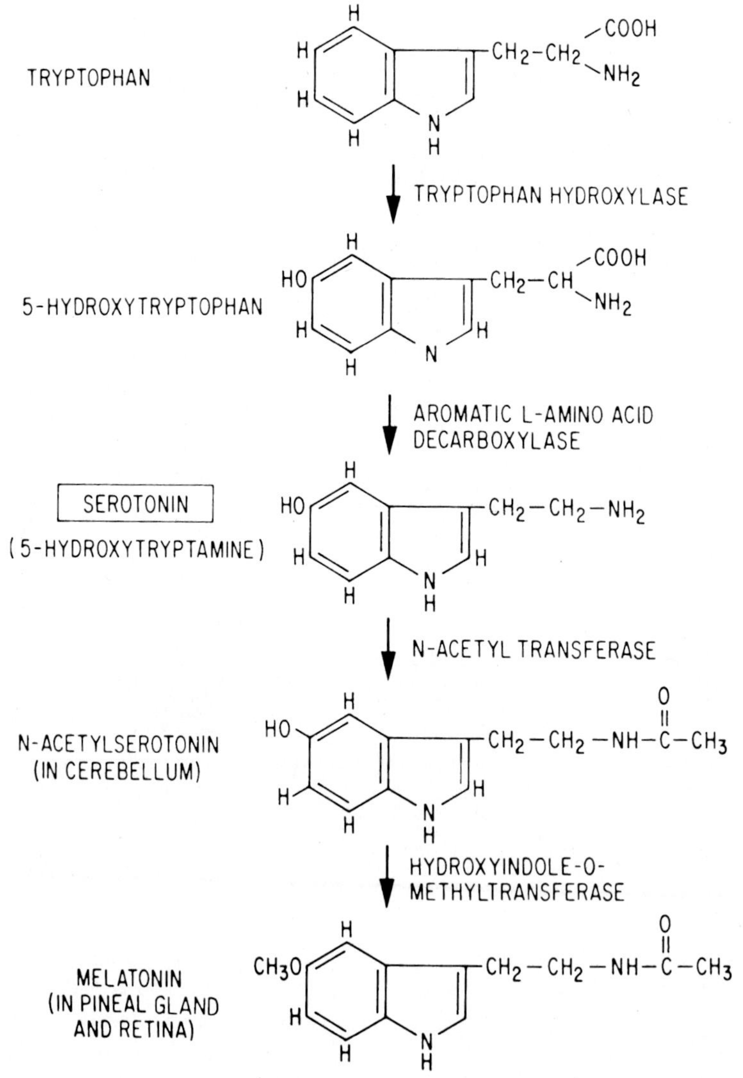

FIGURE 4-7   Metabolic pathway of serotonin synthesis. (From Kletzky OA and Lobo RA: Reproductive neuroendocrinology. In Mishell DR Jr, Davajan V, and Lobo RA, editors: Infertility, contraception and reproductive endocrinology, ed 3, Cambridge, Mass, 1991, Blackwell Scientific Publications.)

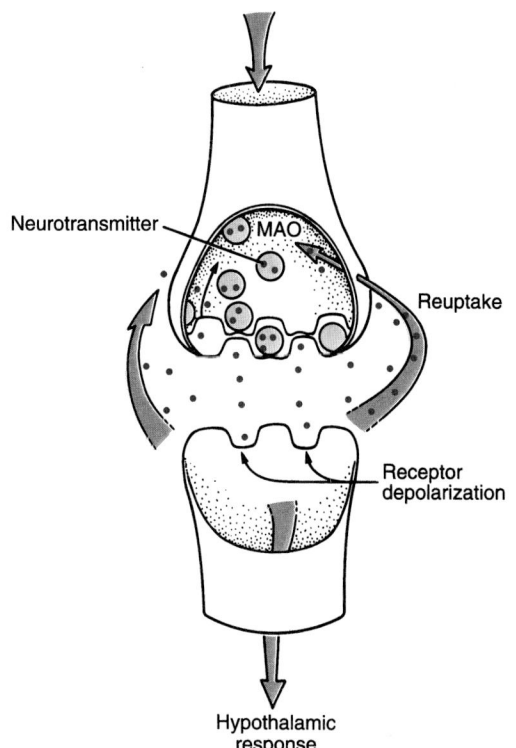

FIGURE 4-8 A stimulus induces release of stored neurotransmitter by exocytosis. Most of it is taken up again; the rest binds to a specific receptor, resulting in hypothalamic response. *MAO*, Monoamine oxidase. (From Kletzky OA and Lobo RA: Reproductive neuroendocrinology. In Mishell DR Jr, Davajan V, and Lobo RA, editors: Infertility, contraception and reproductive endocrinology, ed 3, Cambridge, Mass, 1991, Blackwell Scientific Publications.)

Neuromodulators

Opioids

Receptors for the opioid peptides are present in the brain. There are three subgroups of opiates: enkephalins, endorphins (α, β, γ), and dynorphins. β-Endorphin (β-EP) contains 31 amino acids, is 5 to 10 times as potent as morphine, and is concentrated mainly in the arcuate nucleus and median eminence of the hypothalamus, as well as the pituitary gland. β-EP has also been localized in the placenta, pancreas, gastrointestinal (GI) tract, and in seminal fluid. The concentrations of endorphins are about 1000 times higher in the pituitary than in the hypothalamus. Infusion of β-EP results in an increase in prolactin and a decrease in LH, the latter occurring by an inhibitory effect on GnRH neurons in the hypothalamus. It is now believed that the opiates alter GnRH release by modulating synthesis of substances in the catecholamine pathway, principally norepinephrine.

Peripheral measurement of plasma β-EP is difficult to interpret because it does not reflect levels in the central nervous system (CNS) circulation. Specifically, the pituitary and/or peripheral pool of β-EP appears to be separate from the pool within the hypothalamus. Therefore peripheral measurements of β-EP reflect pituitary and non-CNS secretions rather than those from the hypothalamus. Another difficulty results from the low peripheral concentration of β-EP. In addition, cross-reactivity with β-lipotropins occurs in the immunoassays currently used for β-EP.

Therefore, to study β-EP action, experiments are performed using infusions of naloxone, an opioid antagonist. Infusion of greater than 1 mg per hour blocks brain

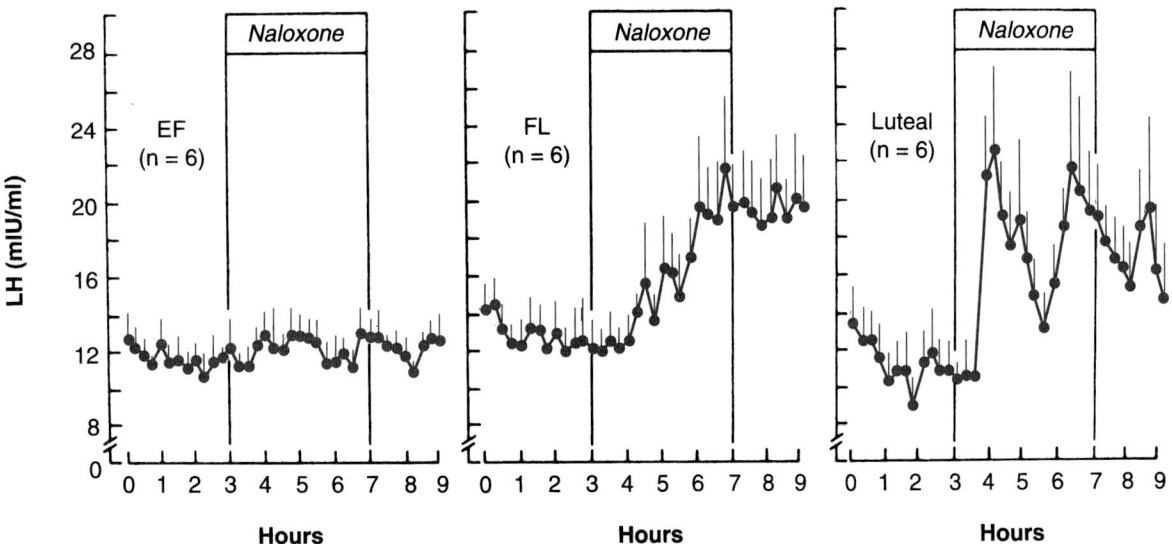

FIGURE 4-9 Infusion of naloxone, an opiate receptor antagonist, elicits incremental change of LH in subjects during late follicular *(LF)* and midluteal phases of cycle (but not in early follicular *[EF]* phase), indicating progressive increase in endogenous opioid inhibition of GnRH secretion, especially during luteal phase. (From Quigley ME and Yen SSC: J Clin Endocrinol Metab 51:179, 1980. © 1980 by The Endocrine Society.)

opioid activity and results in an increase of LH in the late follicular and luteal phases but not in the early follicular phase or postmenopausally. This suggests that both estrogen and progesterone increase levels of β-EP in the brain (Figure 4-9). The increase in β-EP may account for the decreased frequency of GnRH pulses in the luteal phase.

Prostaglandins

Hypothalamic levels of prostaglandins may modulate the release of GnRH. Administration of prostaglandin E_2 significantly increases GnRH levels in the portal blood. Furthermore, a physiologic role of prostaglandins in regulating or modulating the secretion of GnRH is supported by experiments demonstrating that the midcycle surge of LH can be abolished in the rat and ewe by the administration of aspirin or indomethacin, which blocks the synthesis of prostaglandins. No information is available at present concerning the effects of prostaglandins, or of inhibitors of prostaglandin synthesis, on gonadotrophin secretion in the human.

Catechol Estrogens

The compounds 2-hydroxyestradiol and 2-hydroxyestrone, as well as their 3-methoxy derivatives, are present in higher concentrations in the hypothalamus than are prostaglandins E_1 and E_2. It has been hypothesized that these compounds may act as neuromodulators by regulating the function of catecholamines through inhibition of tyrosine hydroxylase and competition for the enzyme catechol-O-methyltransferase. However, the evidence that catechol estrogens have a major effect on neuromodulating reproductive function is insufficient.

Brain Peptides

Many peptides can function as neurotransmitters, but most act locally to regulate autocrine and paracrine functions. Although pituitary hormone synthesis and secretion is largely controlled by classic hormonal messenger systems, considerable local intercellular communications exist as well. Brain peptides that function as neurotransmitters are described below.

Neuropeptide Y

Neuropeptide Y stimulates pulsatile release of GnRH and in the pituitary potentiates gonadotrophin response to GnRH. It thus may facilitate pulsatile secretion of GnRH and gonadotrophins. In the absence of estrogen, neuropeptide Y inhibits gonadotrophin secretion. Because undernutrition is associated with an increase in neuropeptide Y and increased amounts have been measured in cerebrospinal fluid of women with anorexia nervosa and

bulimia nervosa, it has been proposed that neuropeptide Y is one of the factors linking altered nutrition and reproductive function.

Angiotensin II

Several components of the renin-angiotensin system are present in the brain. Receptors for angiotensin II are found in various pituitary cell types, suggesting that angiotensin II affects the secretion of pituitary hormones by local action. In addition, angiotensin II in the hypothalamus appears to influence the effects of norepinephrine and dopamine on the releasing factors that control gonadotrophin and prolactin secretion.

Somatostatin

Somatostatin is a hypothalamic peptide that inhibits the release of growth hormone, prolactin, and TSH from the pituitary.

Activin and Inhibin

Activin and inhibin are produced by the gonads and are peptide members of the transforming growth factor-β family. These peptides have opposing effects on FSH secretion. Inhibin selectively diminishes FSH but not the release of LH, while activin stimulates FSH but not LH release.

Follistatin

Follistatin is an ovarian peptide that has also been called FSH-suppressing protein because of its main action: inhibition of FSH synthesis and secretion and the FSH response to GnRH. Follistatin also binds to activin and in this manner decreases the activity of activin.

Galanin

Galanin is released into the portal circulation in pulsatile fashion. It positively influences LH secretion. Galanin secretion is inhibited by dopamine and somatostatin and stimulated by TRH and estrogen.

GnRH ACTION

When GnRH reaches the anterior lobe of the pituitary, it stimulates the synthesis and release of both LH and FSH from the same cell in the pituitary gland. Thus, whereas the hypothalamic control of prolactin is both inhibitory (dominant) and stimulatory, the hypothalamic control of gonadotrophins is only stimulatory. Peptide hormones, such as GnRH, bind to specific receptors on the surface membrane of the target cell, in contrast to steroid hormones, which pass through the cell membrane to bind to intracellular receptors.

Protein hormone receptors are of high molecular weight (200,000 to 300,000 daltons), and each receptor binds a single molecule of the protein. Polypeptide hormones, including LH, FSH, and prolactin, although highly soluble in aqueous media, have low solubility in lipids and thus do not readily pass the lipid barrier of the target cell's plasma membrane. After the protein hormone binds to its receptor, the hormone receptor complex may be brought through the cell membrane to protect it from other interactions. This process is called *internalization*. In addition to hormone-receptor complex internalization, the hormone message may be transmitted into the cell by transmembrane signaling via at least three known pathways: (1) production of an intracellular second messenger, which increases phosphorylation of regulatory proteins to produce a cellular response; (2) production of a membrane-bound second messenger; or (3) membrane-bound cystosolic phosphorylation activity triggered by hormone binding at the extracellular interface (Figure 4-10).

When a protein hormone binds to its specific receptor, it activates or inhibits the enzyme adenylate cyclase, the second messenger, which in turn changes the concentration of adenosine 3'5'-cyclic monophosphate (cyclic AMP, cAMP). The cAMP then activates protein kinase in the cytoplasm by binding its regulatory subunit thereby dissociating this subunit from its catalytic subunit. When the regulatory subunit of the protein kinase is freed from the catalytic subunit, the latter subunit is able to transfer a phosphate from adenosine triphosphate (ATP) to the protein substrate. This action modifies the biologic function of the protein to produce a cellular response.

At the pituitary gonatrophin cell membrane, GnRH binding is facilitated by the action of calcium and prostaglandin. The hormone-receptor complex activates membrane-bound adenylate cyclase, which stimulates cAMP production and activates a protein kinase by dissociating its regulatory component from the catalytic subunit. The catalytic subunit then phosphorylates the membrane protein to increase calcium permeability. This change allows calcium to enter the cell. Calcium activates the release of stored LH and FSH, producing a stimulus-secretion coupling analogous to muscle excitation-contraction coupling. Enhanced LH and FSH synthesis is also seen and may involve altering ribosomal phosphorylation to increase messenger ribonucleic acid (mRNA) translation. GnRH receptor synthesis is also stimulated by GnRH action. Differential secretion of LH and FSH is attained by feedback of steroid and peptide hormones on the gonadotrophs.

When GnRH is administered to humans in a bolus, a rapid increase occurs in circulating LH, which peaks at 30 minutes, and in FSH, which peaks at 60 minutes. Levels of both LH and FSH return to baseline after 3 hours. With a constant infusion of GnRH, there is a biphasic release of LH but not of FSH. Yen has theorized that the initial rise represents the release of previously synthesized LH (first pool), and the second rise represents the release of newly synthesized LH (second pool) (Figure 4-11). The combined size of both pituitary sensitivity (first pool) and reserve (second pool) has been called the functional capacity of the gonadotrophs. However, if GnRH continues to be infused, gonadotrophin secretion is inhibited, probably because the receptors are saturated and are unable to continue to stimulate release of the second messenger (Figure 4-12). Although maximal hormonal stimulation occurs when only a small percentage of the target cell receptors are bound by hormone, when stimulation is maximal the unoccupied receptors become refractory to hormone binding for 12 to 72 hours. This phenomenon has allowed frequent administration of GnRH analogues to be used clinically.

GnRH analogues are synthesized by substitution of amino acid 6 in the parent molecule with a *d*-amino acid and/or replacement of amino acid 10 with an *N*-ethylamide (Na-CH_2-CH_3) or Aza-Gly (NHNHCO) moiety. The various agonists have greater potencies (15 to 200 times) and longer half-lives (1, 3, 6 hours) than GnRH. The agonists initially simulate gonadotrophic release (flare). This effect lasts from 1 to 3 weeks. After this time, as the GnRH receptors become saturated with the constantly administered analogue, the stimulatory effect of the periodic release of endogenous GnRH on the pituitary gland is blocked. The process is called *desensitization* or *down regulation*. Therefore these analogues are used clinically to treat various steroid hormone–dependent entities (see box on page 83).

Initial attempts to synthesize GnRH antagonists were hindered by allergic reactions induced by histamine release. In 1985 the GnRH agonist leuprolide acetate was approved for the palliative treatment of prostate cancer. Leuprolide is also available in the depot form (7.5 mg), which allows for the monthly intramuscular administration of 3.75 to 7.5 mg for women with endometriosis and leiomyomata uteri. Although therapy has been shown to be effective, bone mineral content has decreased and hot flashes occur as a result of low estradiol levels. Presently, investigators are using combinations of leuprolide with conjugated estrogens or progestins ("add back" therapy) to minimize these side effects.

A potent GnRH-antagonist, Nal-Glu, which does not induce histamine release, has been synthesized. Nal-Glu has been shown to decrease serum LH levels effectively when administered in a single dose (in a dose- and time-dependent manner) in both men and women without a flare effect. Nal-Glu acutely inhibits ovulation and affects LH more than FSH while decreasing estradiol levels at midcycle. Applications of GnRH antagonists have focused primarily in assisted reproductive technologies for down regulation of the hypo-

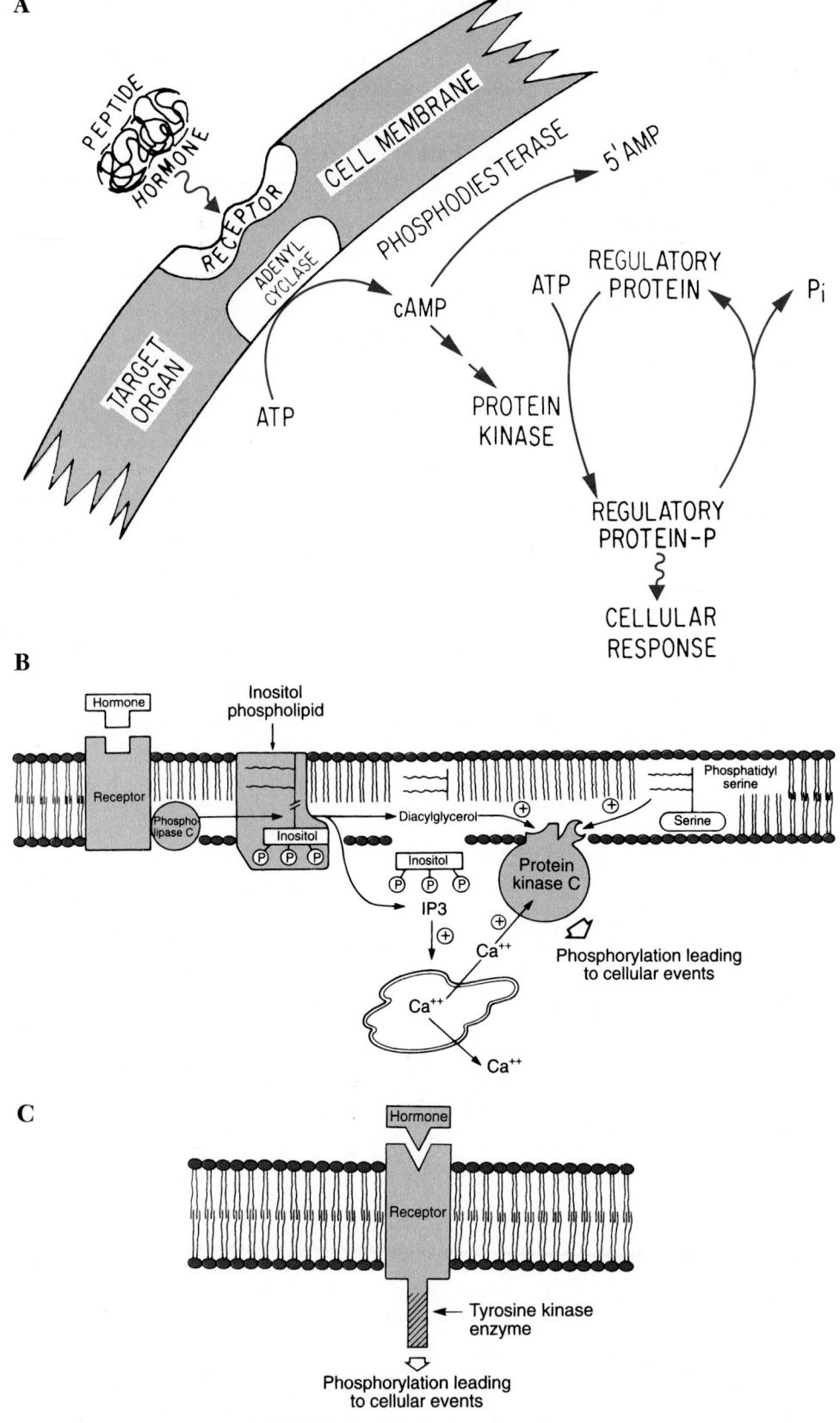

FIGURE 4-10   For legend see opposite page.

thalmic-pituitary axis during ovarian stimulation cycles. Newer applications of GnRH antagonists, including the treatment of uterine leiomyomas, are still under investigation.

Use of GnRH and GnRH Analogues in Gynecology

Stimulation of pituitary-gonadal function (GnRH)
    Delayed puberty
    Induction of ovulation
Suppression of pituitary-gonadal function
    (GnRH analogues)
    Precocious puberty
    Endometriosis
    Breast cancer
    Uterine leiomyomas
    Ovarian androgen excess

GONADOTROPHIN STRUCTURE AND FUNCTION

LH and FSH are glycoproteins of high molecular weight, 28,000 and 37,000 daltons, respectively. They each have the same α subunit (14,000 daltons) of about 90 amino acids, which is similar in structure to the α subunit of thyroid-stimulating hormone and human chorionic gonadotrophin. The β subunits of all these hormones have different amino acids and carbohydrates and provide specific biologic activity. The α and β subunits are joined by disulfide bonds. The sialic acid content of each hormone increases with the duration of biologic action from one or two molecules in LH, which has a half-life of 30 minutes, to five molecules in FSH, which has a half-life of 3.9 hours. In the female, although the two gonadotrophins act synergistically, LH acts primarily on the theca cells to induce steroidogenesis, whereas FSH acts primarily on the granulosa cells to stimulate follicular growth.

FSH release is greater than LH release until puberty, when the normal menstrual cycle is established and LH secretion overtakes that of FSH. After menopause the LH/FSH ratio is again reversed. This preferential inhibition of FSH release during the reproductive years results from increasing levels of both estradiol and inhibin.

Receptors for LH exist on the theca cells at all stages of the cycle; they are on granulosa cells after the follicle matures under the influence of FSH and estradiol, as well as on the corpus luteum. Each gonadal target tissue cell contains between 2000 and 30,000 membrane receptors. Maximal stimulation of hormonal activity occurs when less than 5% of these receptors are bound with hormone. The main action of LH is to stimulate androgen synthesis by the theca cells and progesterone synthesis by the corpus luteum through stimulation of intracellular cAMP production (Figure 4-13). The precise action of LH on granulosa cells has not been determined, but it probably acts synergistically with FSH to help follicular maturation. LH stimulates several other metabolic events in the ovary, such as amino acid transport and RNA synthesis. LH may also induce ovulation by stimulating a plasminogen activator that decreases tensile strength of the follicle wall before follicular rupture occurs.

FSH receptors exist primarily on the granulosa cell membrane. In addition to stimulating LH receptors on this cell membrane, FSH activates the aromatase and the 3β-hydroxysteroid dehydrogenase enzymes within the cell by increasing cAMP. FSH stimulation of isolated granulosa cells in vitro produces only small amounts of estrogen; however, when androgens or theca cells are added, large amounts of estrogen are produced. These data support the two-cell hypothesis of estrogen production. This hypothesis proposes that LH acts on the theca to produce androgens (androstenedione and testosterone), which are then transported to the granulosa cells, where they are aromatized to estrogens (estrone and estradiol) by the action of FSH (see Figure 4-13). The aromatase enzyme catalyzes this conversion.

FIGURE 4-10 **A,** Second messenger model of peptide hormone action. Interaction of hormone with receptor leads to activation of membrane-bound adenylate cyclase, resulting in conversion of adenosine triphosphate *(ATP)* to cyclic AMP (cAMP). cAMP then interacts with cAMP-dependent protein kinase, causing activation of the enzyme and phosphorylation of intracellular regulatory protein substrates, with ATP as phosphate donor. *P,* Phosphate group; P_i, inorganic phosphate. cAMP is inactivated by conversion to 5′-AMP by phosphodiesterase. **B,** Phospholipase C–protein kinase C pathway. Peptide hormone binds to its receptor on external surface, which activates the enzyme phospholipase C within membrane. This enzyme hydrolyzes phosphatidylinositol-4,5-bisphosphate to produce two second messengers: inositol triphosphate *(IP3)* and 1,2-diacyglcerol (DG). IP3 is soluble in cystol, where it binds to receptors on endoplasmic reticulum, causing an opening of Ca^{++} channels and an increase of cytosolic Ca^{++}. DG remains in membrane, where it activates protein kinase C (PKC). Ca^{++} is also necessary for full activation of PKC. Activation of PKC causes phosphorylation and cellular responses. **C,** Receptor-associated tyrosine kinase. Hormone binds to membrane-spanning receptor, causing activation of a cytosolic domain of receptor, which is actually a tyrosine kinase enzyme. Once activated, tyrosine residues on proteins are phosphorylated, resulting in cellular actions. (**A, B,** and **C** from Hylka VW and di Zerega GS: Reproductive hormones and their mechanisms of action. In Mishell DA Jr, Davajan V, and Lobo RA, editors: *Infertility, contraception and reproductive endocrinology,* ed 3, Cambridge, Mass, 1991, Blackwell Scientific Publications.)

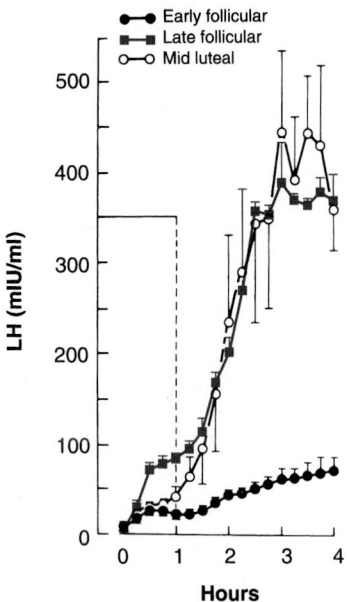

FIGURE 4-11 Quantitative LH release from first and second pool during GnRH infusion. Dotted line separates two pools. (From Hoff JD, Lasley BL, Wang CF, et al: J Clin Endocrinol Metab 44:302, 1977. ©1977 by The Endocrine Society.)

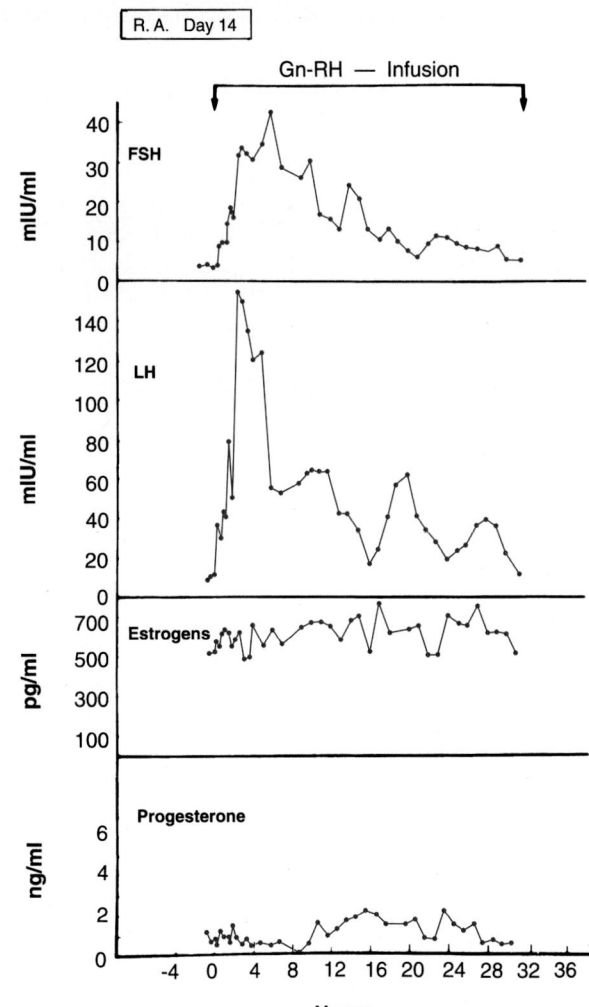

FIGURE 4-12 Mean serum FSH, LH, estrogen, and progesterone levels during 30-hour continuous infusions of GnRH at midcycle phase in three normal women. (From Jewelewicz R, Ferin M, Dyrenfurth I, et al: Long-term LH, RH infusions at various stages of the menstrual cycle in normal women. In Beling CG and Wenitz AC, editors: The LH-releasing hormone, New York, 1980, Masson Publishing.)

Concomitant with increased estrogen production, mitosis is stimulated in granulosa cells, augmenting cell number. Estradiol and FSH receptor production is increased as well, maintaining intracellular cAMP levels as circulating FSH decreases. In granulosa cells primed by exposure to large amounts of estradiol and FSH, LH acts synergistically with FSH to increase LH receptors and induces luteinization of the follicle, increasing progesterone production. Premature delivery of LH will disrupt the process, resulting in premature luteinization, whereas the capacity of the follicle to respond to estrogen appears to determine whether it will mature or become atretic.

LH also stimulates prostaglandin synthesis by intracellular production of cAMP. Prostaglandin may play a role in follicle rupture, since the prostaglandin content of preovulatory follicles increases at the time of the gonadotrophin surge and may stimulate smooth muscle contraction. Progesterone augments the activity of proteolytic enzymes, which act together with prostaglandins to promote follicular degradation and rupture. Plasminogen activator (PA) concentration also increases in the midcycle follicle, and its action is enhanced by LH. Follicle rupture is blocked by administration of PA inhibitors in vivo.

At the level of the ovary, follicular recruitment and initial growth take place independently of gonadotrophic hormones. Animal studies have demonstrated that follicular development can proceed to the antrum stage in the absence of gonadotrophic influence. Although several

hundred follicles probably start to grow, the vast majority will degenerate and no more than about 30 precursor follicles are likely to become gonadotrophic dependent and be present at the beginning of the menstrual cycle. Of these only a few under physiologic conditions, with optimal FSH/LH stimulation, will be selected for further growth and development. It is believed that the rescue of follicles from degeneration by FSH is achieved by reducing androgenicity and by maintaining a predominately estrogenic environment. Initially this is accompanied by FSH indirectly by stimulating activin production and later by directly metabolizing LH-induced thecal androgens to estrogens through stimulation of the aromatizing process

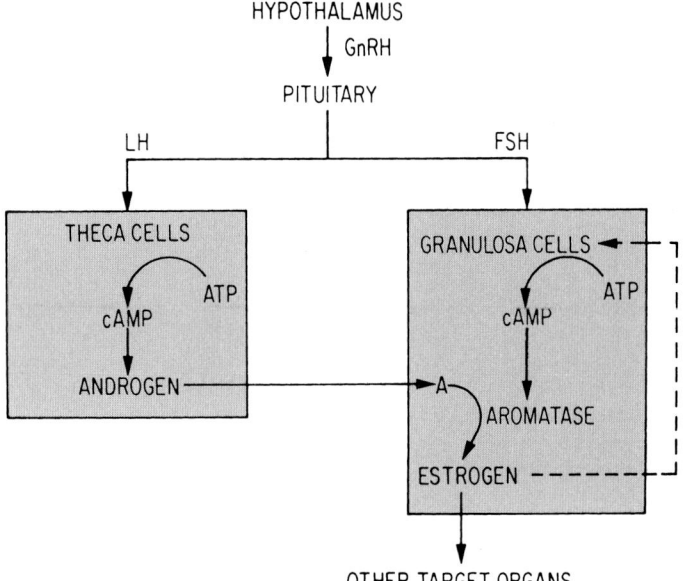

FIGURE 4-13 Action of gonadotrophins on ovary: LH stimulates theca cell to synthesize androgen by cyclic AMP (cAMP)–mediated action. FSH stimulates granulosa cells to activate aromatase via cyclic AMP–mediated action. Aromatase in granulosa cell converts androgen to estrogen, which is then utilized by target organs. Estrogen also stimulates granulosa cell proliferation. (From a concept in Schulster D, Burstein S, and Cooke BA, editors: Control of gonadal steroidogenesis by FSH and LH. In Molecular endocrinology of the steroid hormones, London, 1976, John Wiley & Sons, Ltd.)

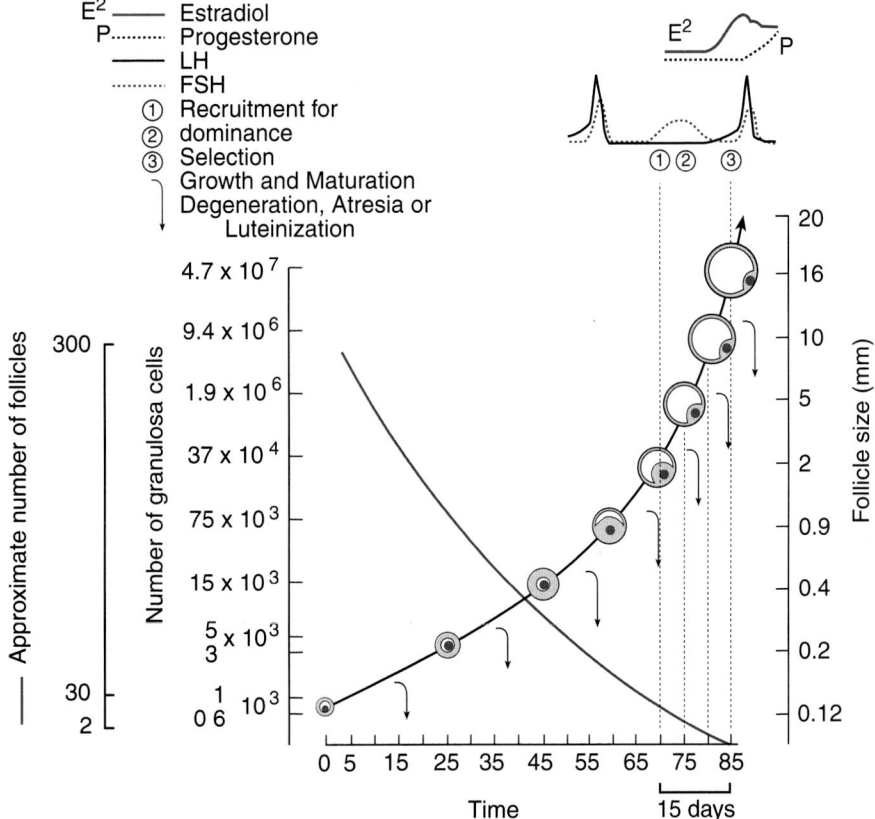

FIGURE 4-14 Time required for oocyte development capable of gonadotrophic responsiveness. (From Lunenfeld B: Aust N Z J Obstet Gynaecol 34:265, 1994.)

TABLE 4-1
Role of Growth Factors in Ovarian Function

Factor	Granulosa Cells	Theca Cells	Corpus Luteum	Other
Insulin	Has receptors Augments basal and HCG-induced P Enhances prostaglandin E_2-stimulated P	Enhances LH/HCG-induced Adione, E_2, P, T Increases basal secretion of E_2, P, T, Adione	Enhances secretion of oxytocin and P	Receptors present in stroma
IGF-I (somatomedin C)	Has type I receptors that are increased by FSH Made here Enhances cAMP-induced P Enhances FSH-induced P, E_2, cAMP, adenylate cyclase, luteinization, LH receptors, proteoglycans Enhances PMSG-induced aromatase and P Stimulated by LH, FSH, cAMP, GH, EGF Enhances HDL-induced P Enhances P and inhibin production	Has type I receptors Increases HCG-induced E_2, P, T, Adione Increases basal secretion of P	Increases secretion of oxytocin and P	Stimulated by GH in whole ovary Enhances aromatase in luteinized granulosa cells Enhances androsterone from theca-interstitial cells Stimulated in ovary by HCG
IGF-II (MSA)	Made here Enhances steroidogenesis Has type II receptors Stimulated by LH and FSH Increases ornithine decarboxylase	Enhances HCG-induced P, T, E_2	Stimulated by GH, HCG, HPL, PRL, and FSH in luteinized granulosa cells	
TGFβ	Inhibits EGF-induced growth Enhances FSH-induced LH receptors, aromatase, EGF receptors, and inhibin Inhibits EGF-induced IGF-I Inhibits basal and FSH-stimulated P Increases production of E_2, cAMP, inhibin Increases growth	Produced here Increases basal and HCG-induced E_2 production Inhibits HCG-induced P, T, Adione Inhibits basal P, Adione		
EGF/TGFα	Inhibits FSH-induced aromatase, E_2 Stimulates growth/mitosis Has receptors Receptors are stimulated by FSH and inhibited by LH Stimulates P and E_2 Enhances FSH-receptor binding Inhibits LH-receptor binding, inhibin secretion	TGFα made here (not EGF) Decreases basal and HCG-stimulated E_2 Stimulates growth		Augments basal and HCG-induced P in luteinized granulosa cells Present in theca-interstitial cells
FGFα	Produced here Inhibits FSH-induced LH receptors Inhibits FSH-induced cAMP, E_2		Produced here	

From Hylka VW and di Zerega GS: Reproductive hormones and their mechanisms of action. In Mishell DR Jr, Davajan V, and Lobo RA, editors: Infertility, contraception and reproductive endocrinology, ed 3, Cambridge, Mass, 1991, Blackwell Scientific Publications.

P, Progesterone; T, testosterone; PMSG, pregnant mare serum gonadotrophins; HDL, high density lipoprotein; HPL, human placental lactogen; Adione, androstenedione; TGF, transforming growth factor; MSA, multiplication stimulating activity; HCG, human chorionic gondotrophin; GH, growth hormone; EGF, epidermal growth factor; FGFa, acidic fibroblast growth factor.

in granulosa cells. Lastly, the selection of the dominant follicle is marked by its increased sensitivity to FSH and its ability to produce a high concentration of estrogen, as well as its ability to modulate gonadotrophin secretion (Figure 4-14). The dominant follicle is usually established by day 7 of the cycle.

GONADAL REGULATION BY GROWTH FACTORS

Growth factors provide traditional hormonal, autocrine, and paracrine effects within the ovary, as summarized in Table 4-1.

Insulin-like Growth Factors (IGFs)

The growth factor family consists of two peptides, namely IGF-I and IGF-II, which have structural homology to proinsulin. The IGFs are produced at multiple sites throughout the body, and serum levels do not vary throughout the menstrual cycle, thus underscoring the importance of their autocrine/paracrine functions. They bind to type I and type II IGF receptors on target cells, with the type I receptor mediating most of their actions. While circulating, the IGFs remain bound to a family of binding proteins (IGFBPs) that regulate IGF action in target tissues.

IGF-I stimulates basal and gonadotrophin-induced steroidogenesis in both theca and granulosa cells. It enhances FSH-induced increases in cAMP, LH receptors, proteoglycan, and basal inhibin synthesis in granulosa cells. While the granulosa cell is the primary site of IGF-I production in the ovary, the receptor is made in both granulosa and theca cells, thus suggesting a plausible regulatory mechanism for the two compartments of ovarian steroidogenesis.

IGF-II is secreted by granulosa cells and enhances steroidogenesis in both theca and granulosa cells. Receptors have been found in the granulosa cell. Although insulin is not produced by the ovary, it may affect ovarian steroidogenesis by several mechanisms. Insulin is known to interact with granulosa cell receptors and may bind to IGF-I receptors at high concentration. Futhermore, insulin is partially responsible for regulating circulating levels of IGFBPs, which are decreased in women with polycystic ovarian syndrome, insulin resistance, and hyperinsulinemia. It is thus plausible that the androgenic characteristics of these syndromes are secondary to insulin acting via the type 1 receptor in ovarian stroma.

Inhibin, Activin, and Follistatin

Substantial evidence exists to suggest that inhibin, activin, and follistatin play critical roles in ovarian steroidogenesis. Inhibin and activin are glycoproteins consisting of two subunits that are connected by disulfide bonds. The subunits are highly conserved evolutionarily, which understates the importance of their roles in ovarian steroidogenesis. Inhibin consists of one type of alpha (alpha) and one of two beta (A-beta and B-beta) subunits, while activin consists of two of the same beta units from inhibin (A-beta/A-beta, A-beta/B-beta, B-beta/B-beta) (Figure 4-15).

The two bioactive inhibins, inhibin A and inhibin B, each have molecular weights of 32,000 daltons and are believed to possess identical biologic functions. The pre-

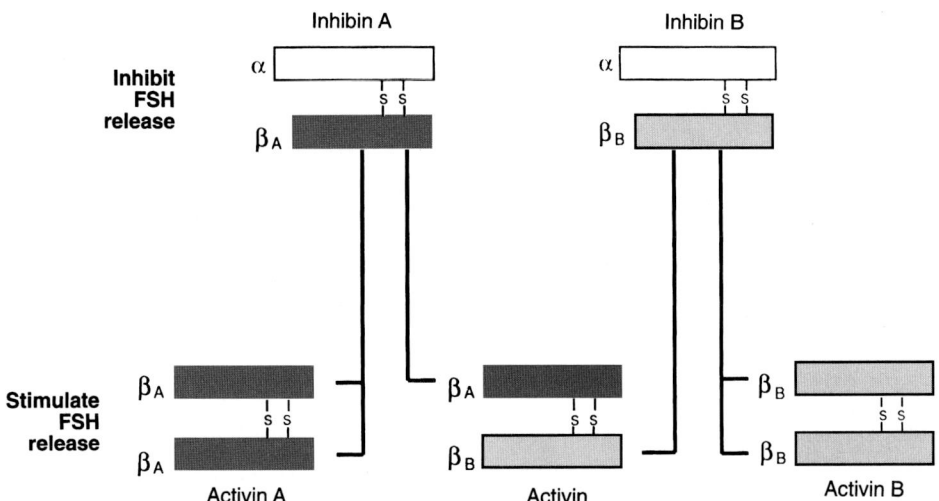

FIGURE 4-15 Chemical relationships of inhibins and activins. *S,* Disulfide bond. (From Hylka VW and di Zerega GS: Reproductive hormones and their mechanisms of action. In Mishell DR Jr, Davajan V, and Lobo RA, editors: Infertility, contraception and reproductive endocrinology, ed 3, Cambridge, Mass, 1991, Blackwell Scientific Publications.)

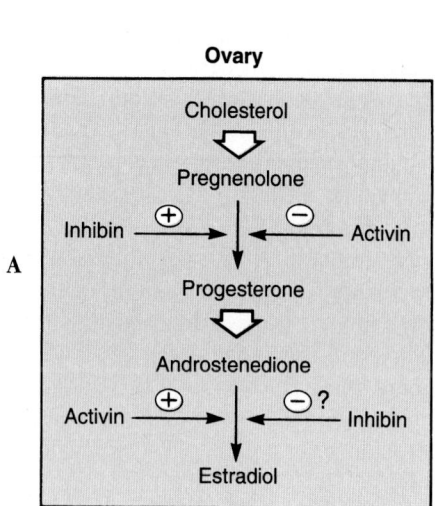
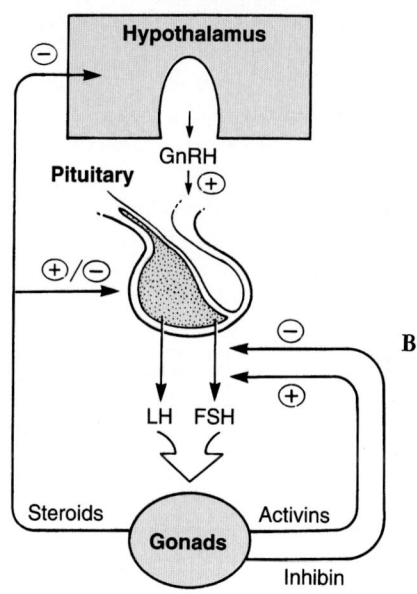

FIGURE 4-16 Generalized schemata showing involvement of activins and inhibins **A,** in hypothalamic-hypophyseal-gonadal axis and **B,** when activins and inhibins regulate steroidogenesis intragonadally. (From Hylka VW and di Zerega GS: Reproductive hormones and their mechanisms of action. In Mishell DR Jr, Davajan V, and Lobo RA, editors: Infertility, contraception and reproductive endocrinology, ed 3, Cambridge, Mass, 1991, Blackwell Scientific Publications.)

dominant sites of production include granulosa cells, testicular Sertoli cells, the corpus luteum, and the placenta. Inhibin production is primarily regulated in a positive fashion by FSH levels, although evidence is emerging that various autocrine and paracrine factors may alter its release. Inhibin is characterized by its ability to preferentially inhibit FSH release over LH release (Figure 4-16). Its local actions within the ovary appear to be confined to stimulation of thecal androgen production and inhibitory effects on oocyte maturation. The menstrual cycle is characterized by low inhibin levels during the early and midfollicular phases, with a rise a few days after the midcycle LH surge, and subsequent peak in the mid to late luteal phase. Their levels decrease dramatically in the perimenopause and menopause and may be the permissive factor that results in elevated FSH levels at this stage of life.

While all three forms of activin are found in humans, activin A (A-beta/A-beta) predominates in women. The bioactive forms of these molecules have a molecular weight of 28,000 daltons. At the levels of the pituitary, the activins stimulate FSH release in opposition to inhibin. Their paracrine/autocrine functions include aromatase activity and progesterone production, promotion of folliculogenesis via its differentiating effects on granulosa cells, and prevention of premature luteinization.

Follistatin is structurally unrelated to inhibin or activin. It is also highly conserved evolutionarily. Follistatin is derived from a single gene and is cleaved and glycosylated, resulting in several bioactive forms.

Functionally, it inhibits FSH release by binding activin, thus preventing activin's bioactivity. Further-more, follistatin inhibits many of activin's para/autocrine functions, but it may also directly affect granulosa cells, that is, acceleration of the rate of oocyte maturation.

Transforming Growth Factor alpha/beta and Epidermal Growth Factor

These growth factors share significant homology with the β-subunit of the inhibin and activin molecules. Within the ovary, they both bind with equal affinity to a common receptor. TGF-α and EGF are potent regulators of granulosa cell proliferation and differentiation. They have been demonstrated to inhibit both gonadotrophin-supported granulosa cell differentiation and follicular cell steroidogenesis. TGF-β promotes growth and cAMP accumulation in granulosa cells and enhances FSH-induced increases in aromatase and LH receptors. TGF-β also inhibits follicular cell growth and thus facilitates follicle cell growth.

Interleukin-1

This polypeptide cytokine is predominately produced and secreted by macrophages, but within the ovary, it is also produced by theca-interstitial cells and granulosa cells following follicular rupture. Regulation within the ovary is primarily determined by local progesterone concentrations. It possesses antigonadotrophic activity as it suppresses the functional and morphologic luteinization of

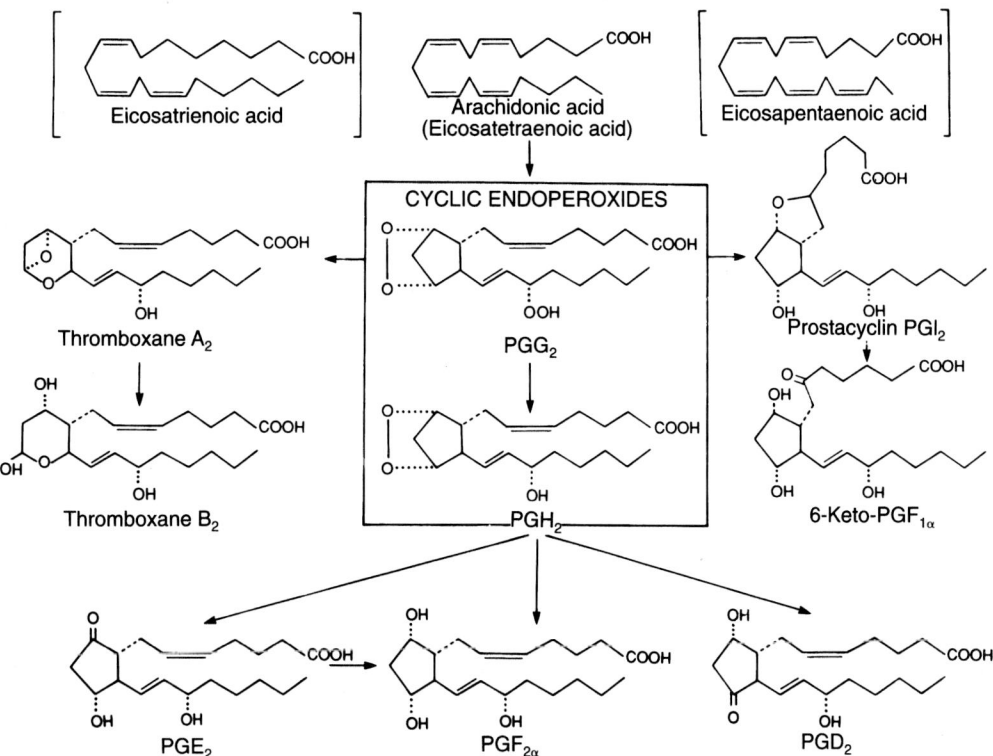

FIGURE 4-17 Biosynthesis of prostanoids. (From Stanczyk FZ: Prostaglandins and related compounds. In Mishell DR Jr, Davajan V, and Lobo RA, editors: Infertility, contraception, and reproductive endocrinology, ed 3, Cambridge, Mass, 1991, Blackwell Scientific Publications.)

granulosa cells. In addition, evidence exists to support that it may play a central role in the preovulation cascade of follicular rupture.

PROSTAGLANDINS AND RELATED COMPOUNDS

Arachidonic acid, the most abundant and important precursor for the biosynthesis of eicosanoids in humans, is formed from linoleic acid and is supplied in the diet. Arachidonic acid is released from membrane phospholipids by lipases, which are activated by various stimuli.

The biosynthesis of prostanoids takes place through the cyclic endoperoxides prostaglandin G (PGG) and prostaglandin H (PGH) (Figure 4-17). PGG, through which all prostanoids are formed, is itself formed from one of the three precursor fatty acids by the microsomal enzyme prostaglandin synthetase. The formation of endoperoxides and their subsequent conversion to prostanoids is very rapid. Since prostanoids are then released immediately from the cell, measurement of tissue or serum levels of prostanoids does not accurately reflect in vivo levels before biopsy or blood collection.

The biosynthesis of prostanoids can be inhibited by several groups of compounds, including the nonsteroidal antiinflammatory drugs (NSAIDs) type 1 (aspirin and indomethacin, which inhibit endoperoxide formation) and type 2 (phenylbutazone), which inhibit action of endoperoxide isomerase and reductase. Corticosteroids can also inhibit prostanoid formation by decreasing precursor phospholipid hydrolysis and release (Figure 4-18).

In contrast to steroid hormones, which are stored and act at target organs distant from their source, prostanoids are produced intracellularly shortly before they are released and generally act locally. Specific prostanoids can have variable effects on different tissues, as well as variable effects on the same organ, even when released in the same concentration (Table 4-2). One important effect is their ability to modulate the responses of endogenous stimulators and inhibitors, such as ovarian stimulation by LH, which is modulated by $PGF_{2\alpha}$, which in turn regulates ovarian receptor availability.

Eicosanoids have a wide variety of biologic effects throughout the body and an important role in reproductive system function. Prostaglandins have an important role in ovarian physiology. They help control early follicular growth by increasing blood supply to certain follicles and inducing FSH receptors on granulosa cells of preovulatory follicles. Both PGE_2 and $PGF_{2\alpha}$ are concentrated in

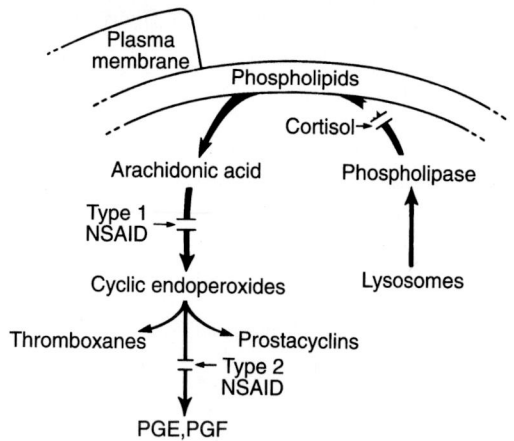

FIGURE 4-18 Inhibition of enzymes involved in biosynthesis of prostanoids. *NSAID,* Nonsteroidal antiinflammatory drug. (From Stanczyk FZ: Prostaglandins and related compounds. In Mishell DR Jr, Davajan V, and Lobo RA, editors: Infertility, contraception and reproductive endocrinology, ed 3, Cambridge, Mass, 1991, Blackwell Scientific Publications.)

TABLE 4-2
Effects of Eicosanoids

Prostaglandins	Effects
PGI_2, PGE_2, PGD_2	Vasodilation Cytoprotection Platelet aggregation Leukocyte aggregation Cyclic AMP formation IL-1 and IL-2 formation
$PGF_{2\alpha}$	Vasoconstriction Bronchoconstriction Smooth muscle contraction
TXA_2	Vasoconstriction Platelet aggregation Lymphocyte proliferation Bronchoconstriction
LTB_4	Vascular permeability Leukocyte aggregation IL-1 formation IL-2 formation Natural killer cell cytotoxicity Chemoattractant
LTC_4, LTD_4	Bronchoconstriction Vascular permeability

PGI_2, Prostacyclin; *PG,* prostaglandin; *TX,* thromboxane; *LT,* leukotriene; *IL,* interleukin.

the follicular fluid of preovulatory follicles and may assist the process of follicular rupture by facilitating proteolytic enzyme activity in the follicular walls. Prostaglandins may help regulate the life span of the corpus luteum. PGE_2 is probably luteotrophic, and $PGF_{2\alpha}$ results in luteolysis.

Prostaglandins also have potent effects on oviductal motility, mediating the stimulatory estrogen effect and the inhibitory progesterone effect on oviductal muscular contractility. They also act to delay passage of the fertilized ovum into the uterus by influencing uterotubal junction activity. In the cervix, PGE_2 relaxes the smooth muscle, whereas $PGF_{2\alpha}$ causes the muscle to contract.

Many prostanoids are produced by the endometrium. These include PGE_2, $PGF_{2\alpha}$, PGI_2, and thromboxane A_2 (TXA_2). Concentrations of PGE_2 and $PGF_{2\alpha}$ increase progressively from the proliferative to the secretory phase. The highest levels are found during menstruation. These prostaglandins help regulate myometrial contractility and appear to be important in regulating the process of menstruation.

OVARIAN STEROIDS

Chemistry

Steroids are lipids that have a basic chemical structure or nucleus. The nucleus consists of three 6-carbon rings (A, B, and C) joined to a 5-carbon atom (D) ring that is called cyclopentanoperhydrophenanthrene, or gonane (Figure 4-19). The molecular weight of most steroid hormones is in the range of 250 to 550 daltons. Ste-

roids such as progesterone and estradiol are insoluble in water but dissolve readily in organic solvents such as diethyl ether and chloroform. In contrast, steroids that have a sulfate or glucuronide group attached (conjugated steroids), such as dehydroepiandrosterone sulfate (DHEAS) and pregnanediol glucuronide, are water soluble.

Steroids are named according to a generally accepted convention that is used to determine their systemic (scientific) names. Most steroid hormones also have common (trivial) names, such as progesterone and estradiol, which are generally used instead of the scientific names. The carbon atoms of steroids are numbered as shown in Figure 4-19. Functional groups above the plane of the molecule are preceded by the β symbol and shown in the structural formula by a solid line, whereas those below the plane are indicated by an α symbol and a dotted line. The symbol Δ indicates a double bond, and those steroids with a double bond between carbon atoms 5 and 6 (cholesterol, pregnenolone, 17-hydroxypregnenolone, and dehydroepiandrosterone) are called Δ^5 steroids, whereas those with a double bond between carbon atoms 4 and 5 (progesterone, 17-hydroxyprogesterone, androstenedione, testosterone as well as all mineralocorticoids and glucocorticoids) are Δ^4 steroids.

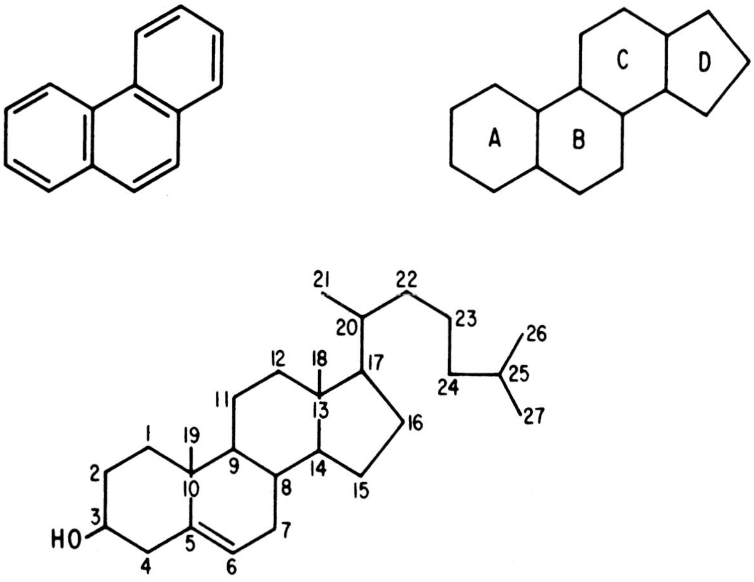

FIGURE 4-19 Phenanthrene *(top left)*. Cyclopentanoperhydrophenanthrene nucleus *(top right)*, in which the three 6-carbon rings *(A, B, and C)* resemble the phenanthrene ring system and the 5-carbon ring *(D)* resembles cyclopentane. Cholesterol *(bottom)* is the common biosynthetic precursor of steroid hormones. Numbers *1* to *27* indicate the conventional numbering system of carbon atoms in steroids. (From Stanczyk FZ: Steroid hormones. In Lobo RA, Mishell DR Jr, Paulson RJ, and Shoupe D, editors: Mishell's textbook of infertility, contraception and reproductive endocrinology, ed 4, Malden, Mass, 1997, Blackwell Science.)

Biosynthesis

All steroids in the body are formed from acetate, a 2-carbon compound. The first step in its conversion to a variety of steroids is the formation of cholesterol, a 27-carbon steroid, via a complex series of reactions (11 steps). All sex steroids and corticosteroids are derived by stepwise degradation of cholesterol. The steroidogenic acute regular l(StAR) protein is thought to be the regulator of acute cholesterol transfer into the mitochondria for adrenal and ovarian steroidogenesis. Corticosteroids, pregnenolone, 17-hydroxypregnenolone, progesterone, and 17-hydroxyprogesterone have 21 carbon atoms. Androgens, DHEA, DHEAS, androstenedione and testosterone have 19 carbon atoms. Estrogens (estrone and estradiol) have 18 carbon atoms and a phenolic or aromatic ring A.

The first step in ovarian steroid biosynthesis is transformation of cholesterol to pregnenolone by hydroxylation of C-20 and C-22 and cleavage between these atoms. This process reduces the C-27 compound cholesterol to the C-21 compound pregnenolone. From pregnenolone, ovarian steroid biosynthesis proceeds along two major pathways under the influence of specific enzymes: (1) the Δ^5 pathway through 17-hydroxypregnenolone and DHEA to Δ^5 androstenediol and (2) the Δ^4 pathway through progesterone and 17-hydroxyprogesterone to androstenedione and testosterone (Figure 4-20). LH stimulates this synthesis. Androstenedione and testosterone are interconverted, and the former can be converted to estrone and the latter to estradiol, respectively, by the aromatase enzyme. This enzymatic process aromatization results in loss of the C-19 methyl group and formation of the aromatic ring in the C-18 steroid.

The ovary secretes three primary steroids: estradiol, progesterone, and androstenedione. These hormones are the chief secretory products of the maturing follicle, corpus luteum, and stroma, respectively. The ovary also secretes, in varying amounts, pregnenolone, 17-hydroxyprogesterone, testosterone, DHEA, and estrone. Because the ovaries lack 21-hydroxylase, 11β-hydroxylase, and 18-hydroxylase activity, they are unable to synthesize mineralocorticoids or glucocorticoids. Each day the ovary secretes between 0.1 and 0.5 mg of estradiol, with the amount being lowest during menses and highest just before ovulation. Daily progesterone production varies from 0.5 mg in the follicular phase to 20 mg in the luteal phase. During the follicular phase, almost all progesterone is secreted from the adrenal gland and very little from the ovary. The ovary secretes between 1 and 2 mg of androstenedione, less than 1 mg of DHEA, and about 0.1 mg of testosterone daily. Androgen metabolism and corticosteroid synthesis are discussed in Chapter 40.

In addition to gonadal steroid biosynthesis, steroid metabolism occurs in extraglandular tissues. Interconversion of androstenedione and testosterone, as well as estrone and estradiol, takes place outside the ovaries, mainly by oxidation of the latter steroids to the former,

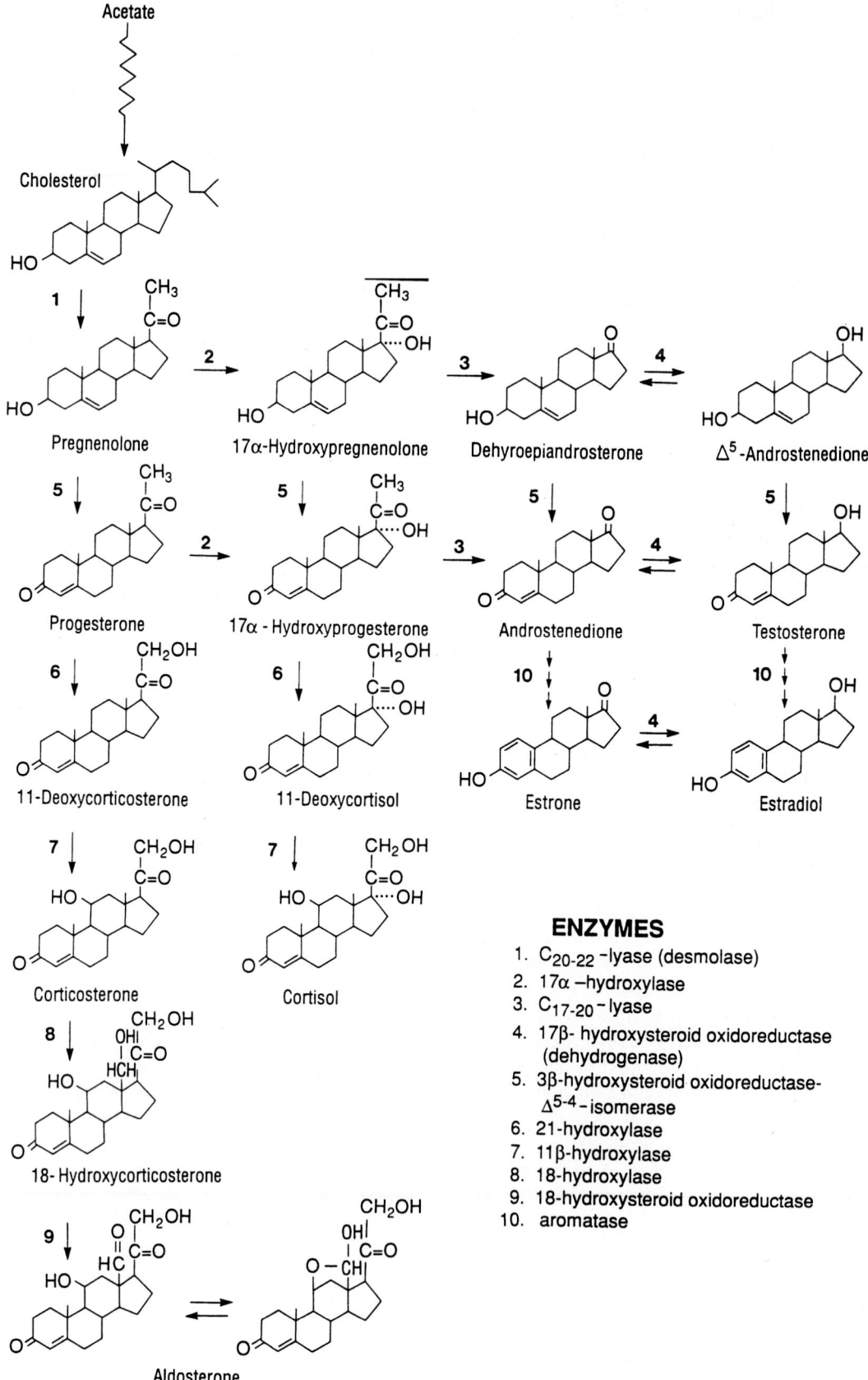

ENZYMES

1. C$_{20-22}$ –lyase (desmolase)
2. 17α –hydroxylase
3. C$_{17-20}$ – lyase
4. 17β- hydroxysteroid oxidoreductase (dehydrogenase)
5. 3β-hydroxysteroid oxidoreductase-Δ$^{5-4}$-isomerase
6. 21-hydroxylase
7. 11β-hydroxylase
8. 18-hydroxylase
9. 18-hydroxysteroid oxidoreductase
10. aromatase

FIGURE 4-20 Biosynthesis of androgens, estrogens, and corticosteroids. (From Stanczyk FZ: Steroid hormones. In Lobo RA, Mishell DR Jr, Paulson RJ, and Shoupe D, editors: Mishell's textbook of infertility, contraception and reproductive endocrinology, ed 4, Malden, Mass, 1997, Blackwell Science.)

thus reducing their biologic potency. Estrone is also converted to estrone sulfate, which has a long half-life and is the largest component of the pool of circulating estrogens (Figure 4-21). Although estrone sulfate is not biologically active, sulfatases in tissues such as the breast and endometrium can readily convert it to estrone, which in turn can be converted to estradiol.

MacDonald et al. showed that androstenedione is peripherally converted to estrone in adipose tissue. The greater the amount of fat tissue present, the greater the percentage of androstenedione that is converted to estrone. In a normal individual about 1.3% of the daily 3000 μg of androstenedione produced is converted to estrone (40 μg), whereas in an obese individual as much as 7% (200 μg) of the 3000 μg is converted.

Transport

After they are secreted into the circulation, steroids bind to either specific proteins, such as sex hormone–binding globulin (SHBG) and corticosteroid-binding globulin (CBG), or to nonspecific proteins, such as albumin. The bound form of a steroid hormone represents approximately 95% of the total circulating concentration of the hormone; the remainder is unbound ("free"). For example, in premenopausal women approximately 65% and 30% of circulating testosterone is bound to SHBG and albumin, respectively; approximately 2% is unbound. SHBG and CBG have a low capacity for steroids but bind them with high affinity ($K_a = 1 \times 10^8$ to 1×10^9), whereas albumin has a high capacity but binds with low affinity ($K_a = 1 \times 10^4$ to 1×10^6). Albumin binds all steroids. SHBG primarily binds dihydrotestosterone, testosterone, and estradiol (in order of decreasing affinity). CBG binds with highest affinity to cortisol, corticosterone, and 11-deoxycortisol, and, to a lesser extent, to progesterone. Circulating levels of each of the globulins are increased by estrogen; SHBG levels are also increased by obesity and hyperthyroidism and lowered by androgens and hypothyroidism.

Metabolism

The liver and, to a small extent, the kidney are the major sites of metabolism of steroids in the body. Transformation mechanisms include hydroxylation of carbons on different sites of the steroid nucleus, reduction of ketone groups and double bonds, and conjugation(formation of sulfates and glucuronides). The process by which steroids are conjugated involves the transformation of lipophilic compounds, which are only sparingly soluble in water, into metabolites that are readily water soluble and can therefore be eliminated in urine. Examples of conjugation include the following: About 10% to 15% of progesterone is transformed to pregnanediol-3-glucuronide, which is the major urinary metabolite of progesterone. Estradiol and estrone are converted in the liver to estriol. These three estrogens are often referred to as the *classic* estrogens because they were the first ones to be isolated. These estrogens are conjugated by the liver and intestinal mucosa into different forms of estrogen sulfates and glucuronides, such as estrone sulfate, estradiol-17-glucuronide, and estriol-16-glucuronide.

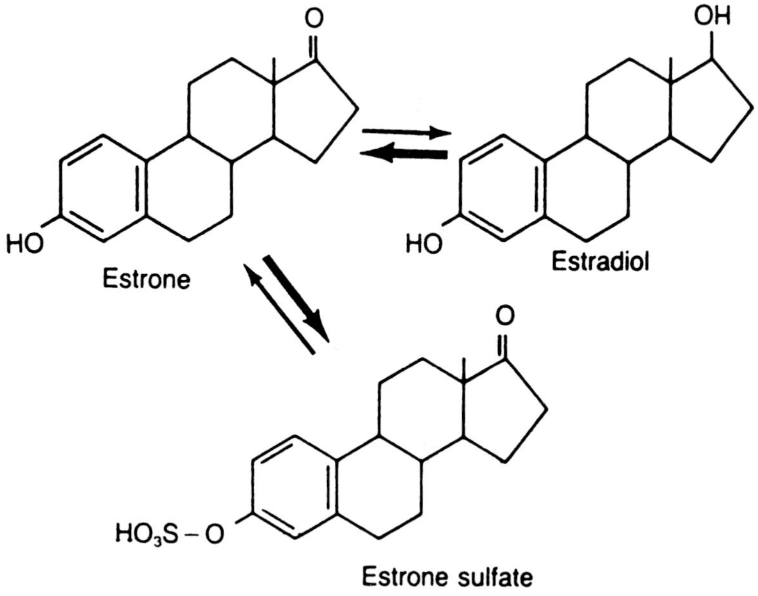

FIGURE 4-21 Interconversion of three principal circulating estrogens. (From Stanczyk FZ: Steroid hormones. In Lobo RA, Mishell DR Jr, Paulson RJ, and Shoupe D, editors: Mishell's textbook of infertility, contraception and reproductive endocrinology, ed 4, Malden, Mass, 1997, Blackwell Science.)

Dynamics of Hormone Production and Metabolism

The concentration of a steroid hormone in serum or plasma is dependent on its production rate (PR) and metabolic clearance rate (MCR). The MCR is determined by infusing a radioactively labeled steroid in tracer amounts at a constant rate over several hours and measuring the tracer concentration at steady state. The MCR is calculated according to the following formula:

$$MCR = \frac{\text{Tracer administered/time}}{\text{Tracer concentration}}$$

$$= \frac{\text{Counts/min/day}}{\text{Counts/min/liter}} = \text{Liters/day}$$

The concentration (C) of steroid can be measured by radioimmunoassay, and when both MCR and C are known, the PR is determined by multiplying the MCR by C: PR = MCR × C = liters/day × amount/liter = amount/day. Normal C, MCR, and PR of androgens, estrogens, and progesterone at different phases of the menstrual cycle have been calculated (Table 4-3).

Hormone Action

In contrast to the membrane receptors of protein hormones, steroid hormone receptors are intracellular. Steroid hormone receptors bind a specific class of steroids. Thus, estrogen receptors will bind natural and synthetic estrogens but not progestins or androgens. The affinity of a receptor for a steroid correlates with steroid potency. For example, the estrogen receptor has a greater affinity for estradiol than for estrone or estriol. After the steroid hormone (S) is bound to its receptor (R), a hormone-receptor (SR) complex forms. Steroid hormone receptors are located in either the cytoplasm or nucleus. They are maintained in an inactive state by association with heat shock proteins. Hormone binding leads to disassociation of the heat shock proteins and conformational changes (transformation) that allow it to bind to the hormone responsive element (HRE) of nuclear DNA. Thereafter, mRNA is generated from a segment of DNA (transcription). The mRNA migrates into the cytoplasm, where it attaches to ribosomes and translates information so that they synthesize new protein (Figure 4-22).

The magnitude of the signal to the cell depends on the concentration of both hormones (S) and receptors (R), as

TABLE 4-3
Plasma Concentrations (C), Metabolic Clearance Rates (MCR), and Production Rates (PR) of Androgens, Estrogens, and Progesterone During Menstrual Cycle

| Steroid Hormone | Phase of Cycle | Plasma Concentration* | | | Metabolic Clearance Rate Plasma* (L/day) | Production Rate (mg/day) (PR = C × MCR) | |
		Mean	Range	Units		Mean	Range
Androstenedione	†	1.4	0.7–3.1	ng/ml	2000	2.8	1.4–6.2
Testosterone	†	0.35	0.15–0.55	ng/ml	700	0.25	0.1–0.4
Dehydroepiandrosterone	†	4.2	2.5–7.8	ng/ml	1600	6.7	4.8–12.5
Dehydroepiandrosterone sulfate	†	1.6	0.8–3.4	µg/ml	7	11.2	5.6–23.8
Estradiol	Follicular	44	20–120	pg/ml	1350	0.059	0.027–0.162
	Preovulatory	250	150–600	pg/ml	1350	0.338	0.203–0.810
	Luteal	110	40–300	pg/ml	1350	0.149	0.054–0.405
Estrone	Follicular	40		pg/ml	2200	0.088	
	Preovulatory	170		pg/ml	2200	0.374	
	Luteal	92		pg/ml	2200	0.202	
Estrone-sulfate	Follicular	470		pg/ml	146	0.069	
	Luteal	890		pg/ml	146	0.130	
Progesterone	Follicular	0.2	0.06–0.37	ng/ml	2300	0.46	0.14–0.85
	Luteal	8.9	4.3–19.4	ng/ml	2300	20.5	9.9–45.0

From Stanczyk FZ: Steroid hormones. In Mishell DR Jr, Davajan V, and Lobo RA, editors: Infertility, contraception and reproductive endocrinology, ed 3, Cambridge, Mass, 1991, Blackwell Scientific Publications.

*These values may vary somewhat depending on investigator and method.

†Unspecified. No major changes during menstrual cycle.

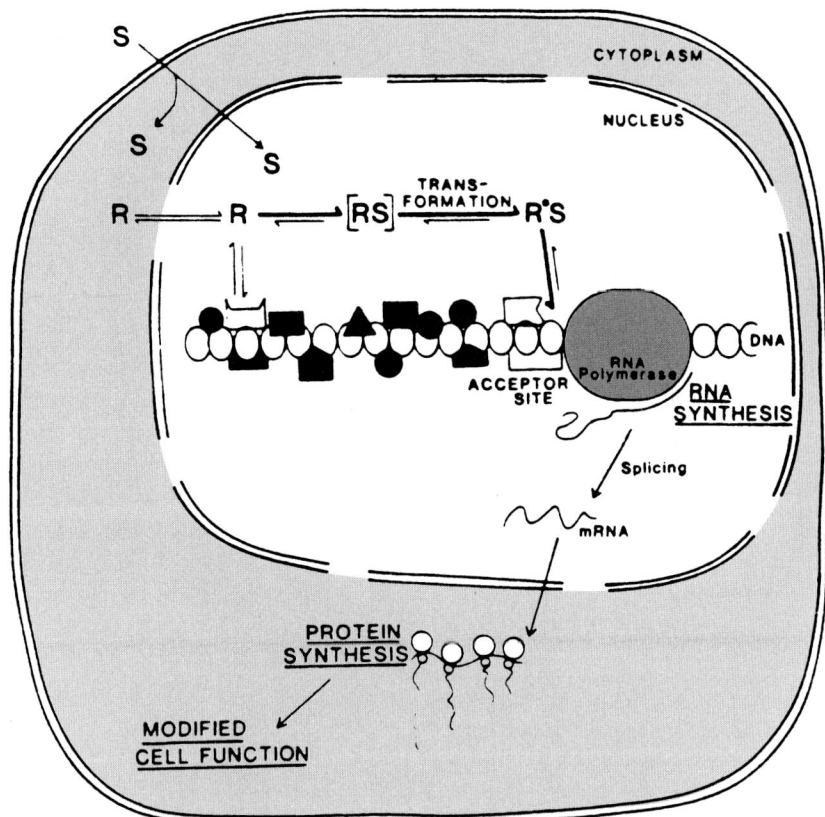

FIGURE 4-22 Revised model of steroid-receptor interaction and induction of cellular response. For simplicity, molecular aspects of receptor structure have been omitted. (From Walters MR: Endocrinol Rev 6:512, 1985.)

well as on the affinity (K) of the receptor for hormone. Thus the hormone effect may be altered by receptor concentration and affinity, as well as by concentration of the hormone in the circulation. Affinity is quantitatively characterized by a constant derived from the law of mass action.

$$S + R \underset{k_d}{\overset{k_a}{\rightleftharpoons}} SR$$

The association constant, K_a, is determined by dividing the rate constant for association, k_a, by the rate constant for dissociation, k_d. The dissociation constant, K_d, is the inverse of K_a; therefore, $K_d = 1/K_a$. K_d is equal to the concentration of the hormone when half the receptor sites are occupied. Steroid hormones are present in concentrations of 10^{-10} to 10^{-8} M, and most steroid receptors have a K_d of 10^{-9}. It should be emphasized that these processes are greatly modulated by numerous other activator and repressor factors. The different tissue response to estrogen and estrogen-like compounds depends on the sum of these various interactions.

Estrogen stimulates the synthesis of both estrogen and

progesterone receptors in target tissues such as the endometrium. Progestins inhibit the synthesis of both estrogen and progesterone receptors. Thus, the estrogen/progesterone receptor content in the endometrium peaks about midcycle and then decreases (Figure 4-23). Mitotic activity and endometrial growth rates, therefore, peak at midcycle. Progestins also increase the intra-cellular synthesis of estradiol dehydrogenase, which converts the more potent estradiol to the less potent estrone, further decreasing estrogenic activity in the target cell.

Antiestrogens, such as clomiphene or tamoxifen, bind to the estrogen receptor but initiate little transcription. Thus, estrogen receptors are depleted without new receptor synthesis or estrogenic action.

EFFECTS OF HORMONES ON SPECIFIC REPRODUCTIVE FACTORS

Ovarian Gametogenesis (Oogenesis)

Oogenesis begins in fetal life when the primordial germ cells migrate to the genital ridge. These germ cells, oogonia, increase in number by mitotic division from

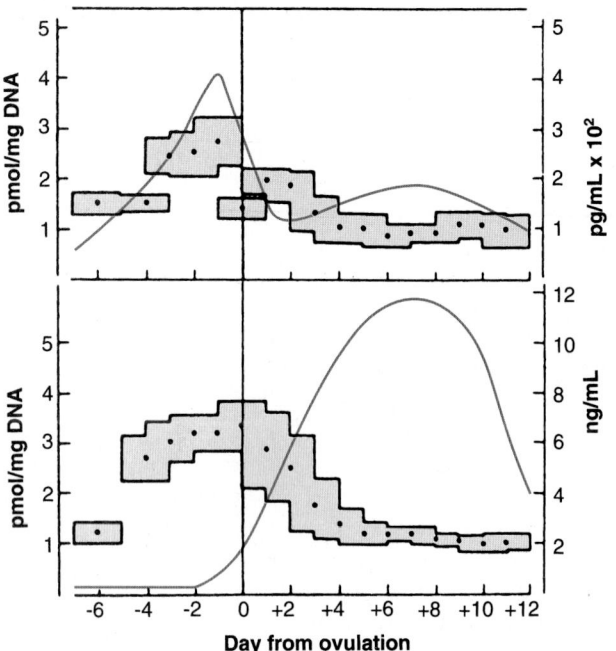

FIGURE 4-23 Estradiol and progesterone receptors in endometrial cells during normal menstrual cycle. Concentrations of estradiol receptor *(upper panel)* and of total progesterone receptor *(lower panel)* for each day of cycle were pooled with those of adjacent days. Each point represents the mean of pooled values. It is surrounded by a rectangle, with its abscissa extending from preceding to following day to account for imprecision of dating and with its ordinate equal to twice the standard error of the mean. Curves represent mean values of plasma estradiol *(upper panel)* and progesterone *(lower panel)*. (From Levy C, Robel P, Gautray JP, et al: Am J Obstet Gynecol 136:646, 1980.)

about 600,000 in the second month to 7 million in the seventh month of fetal life. The oogonia then begin meiotic division and are called primary oocytes. Just prior to birth the primary oocytes, which now number 2 to 4 million, undergo meiosis until they reach the diplotene stage of the prophase, which is also called the germinal vesicle stage (for further details refer to Chapter 1). The oocytes stay quiescent or undergo atresia until puberty, at which time some of the oocytes mature and resume their meiotic division under the stimulatory influence of FSH.

Leptin, a peptide secreted by adipose tissue, is thought to be a peripheral signal of fat stores. Rodent models deficient for leptin or leptin receptor activity demonstrate hyperphagia and obesity. A role for leptin in reproduction is supported by the observation that mice lacking leptin fail to undergo puberty, the presence of leptin in the human ovarian follicle, and a possible role in the hormonal aberrations associated with polycystic ovarian disease. Frisch proposed that a critical weight must be reached in order to elicit menarche and maintain menstruation. Leptin may therefore act as a periph-

eral messenger to the central nervous system in order to elicit the pattern of GnRH secretion necessary for puberty.

The primary oocyte that is still in the diplotene stage of its first meiotic division is covered by a single layer of granulosa cells and constitutes the primordial follicle. Even without gonadotrophin stimulation, some primordial follicles develop into primary (preantral) follicles, which are oocytes covered by multiple layers of granulosa cells (Figure 4-24). This FSH-independent process occurs in all premenopausal women during the nonovulatory states of childhood, pregnancy, and oral contraceptive use, as well as during ovulatory cycles. However, only in the presence of FSH in ovulatory cycles do some of those primary follicles develop to the antrum stage. Without the FSH stimulation, all follicles become atretic.

Under the influence of FSH the number of granulosa cells in the primordial follicle increases dramatically, and the follicle matures into a primary (preantral) follicle. As the number of granulosa cells increases under the influence of LH and FSH, there is a concomitant parallel increase in estradiol production and secretion as FSH stimulates aromatase synthesis. Estradiol stimulates preantral follicle growth, prevents follicle atresia, and increases FSH action on the granulosa cells. Testosterone, on the other hand, increases follicle atresia and prevents preantral follicle growth. Ross et al. suggested that local

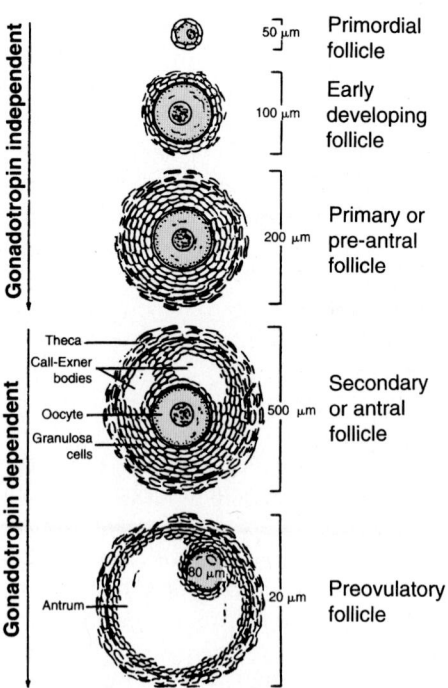

FIGURE 4-24 Follicle development. Progress beyond primary follicle stage depends on FSH stimulation. (From Paulson RJ: Oocytes: from development to fertilization. In Mishell DR Jr, Davajan V, and Lobo RA, editors: Infertility, contraception and reproductive endocrinology, ed 3, Cambridge, Mass, 1991, Blackwell Scientific Publications.)

concentration of estrogens and androgens within the follicle determines whether a specific follicle grows or becomes atretic.

The follicle destined to become dominant secretes the greatest amount of estradiol, which in turn increases the density of FSH receptors. Thus, mitotic activity and the number of granulosa cells also increase. In addition, the rising concentration of estradiol exerts a negative feedback effect of FSH release from the pituitary, which halts development of all the other follicles so that they become atretic. In addition, granulosa cells secrete a glycoprotein substance, inhibin, which also suppresses FSH secretion. The dominant follicle continues to develop because it has a greater density of FSH receptors, and its theca cells become more vascularized than the other follicles, allowing more FSH to reach its receptors.

As the oocyte develops, it becomes surrounded by the zona pellucida, and fluid accumulates in the follicle. The zona pellucida is a mucopolysaccaride coat containing specific protein sites that allow only spermatozoa of the same species to penetrate and fertilize the ovum. Underneath the zona pellucida is the vitelline membrane, which surrounds the ooplasm. Cortical granules form just below this membrane as the oocyte matures. Once the zona pellucida has been penetrated by a single sperm cell, these granules are released and block further sperm penetration (Figure 4-25). The follicular fluid contains estrogens, androgens, and various proteins. Granulosa cells are not just recipients of regulatory protein hormones. As mentioned earlier, granulosa cells have also been shown to secrete various peptides (see Table 4-2), which regulate hormone synthesis in the ovary via autocrine and paracrine mechanisms. Some of those regulatory proteins, such as inhibin, have an endocrinologic influence on the gonadotrophin release from the pituitary gland. Circulating inhibin levels are low during the follicular phase of the cycle but rise in parallel with progesterone levels in the luteal phase. In contrast, plasma levels of free activin remain relatively constant through the cycles (Figure 4-26.) Several of the proteins in follicular fluid are now being characterized, and they, in addition to the steroids, appear to help regulate follicle maturation by acting within the follicle to alter gonadotrophin action. As the granulosa cells proliferate, LH receptors appear on their surface membrane; when LH binds to these receptors, granulosa cell - proliferation ceases and the cells begin to secrete progesterone.

The pattern of follicular growth, as determined by ultrasonography, has been correlated with the endocrine pattern in several studies. Eissa et al., as well as Zegers-Hochschild et al., correlated these parameters in 43 cycles in which conception occurred. Both of these groups found a steady increase in follicular diameter and volume that parallels the rise in estradiol (Figure 4-27).

As determined by ultrasonography, the dominant follicle has a maximal mean diameter of about 19.5 mm, with a range of 18 to 25 mm just before ovulation. The mean maximal follicular volume is 3.8 ml, with a range of 3.1 to 8.2 ml. The investigators just mentioned, as well as others, have shown that the maximal size of the dominant follicle can vary among different women. Lemay et al. have shown that the mean maximal diameter of the preovulatory follicle can vary in the same woman in different cycles.

About 80% of the approximately 500 μg of estradiol produced daily just before ovulation comes from the dominant follicle. The rapidly rising estradiol levels, in combination with a small but significant increase in progesterone produced by the dominant follicle, serve as the signal to the hypothalamic-pituitary axis that the follicle is ready to ovulate. When estradiol levels rise substantially at midcycle, to about 200 pg/ml or higher for 2 or more days, LH secretion is stimulated (positive feedback) (Figure 4-28). Apparently the small preovulatory increase in progesterone also stimulates the release of LH and may be responsible for the midcycle FSH surge. Thus, by a positive feedback, these steroids elicit a surge in LH and FSH release from the pituitary. The midcycle LH surge initiates the ovulatory process.

A task force of the World Health Organization correlated the temporal relation of changes in hormone levels with the time of ovulation as determined by histologic examination of the maturity of the corpus luteum, which had been removed at the time of subsequent laparotomy in 78 women. With the use of those parameters, it was determined that ovulation occurs about 24 hours after the estradiol peak. Ovulation occurs about 32 hours after the initial rise in LH levels and about 12 to 16 hours after the peak of LH levels in serum (Table 4-4). Using ultrasonography to detect the time of ovulation, Lemay et al. reported that ovulation occurs between 18 and 48 hours after the initial rise in LH levels. With serial ultrasound definition and LH measurements, Eissa et al. and Zegers-Hochschild et al. reported that in conception cycles, ovulation usually occurs within 24 hours and always within 48 hours after the LH peak.

The midcycle LH surge initiates germinal vesicle disruption, and metaphase I is completed. As the oocyte enters metaphase II, the first polar body appears. Completion of meiosis and extrusion of the second polar body occur only when a spermatozoon penetrates the ovum. In preparation for follicular rupture, LH stimulates synthesis of both $PGF_{2\alpha}$ and PGE_2 and proteolytic enzymes (collagenase). The rise in FSH levels stimulates production of a plasminogen activator, which converts plasminogen to the proteolytic enzyme plasmin. Plasmin helps to detach the cumulus from the parietal granulosa cells and thus aids in the process of extrusion of the egg and cumulus at the time of follicle rupture.

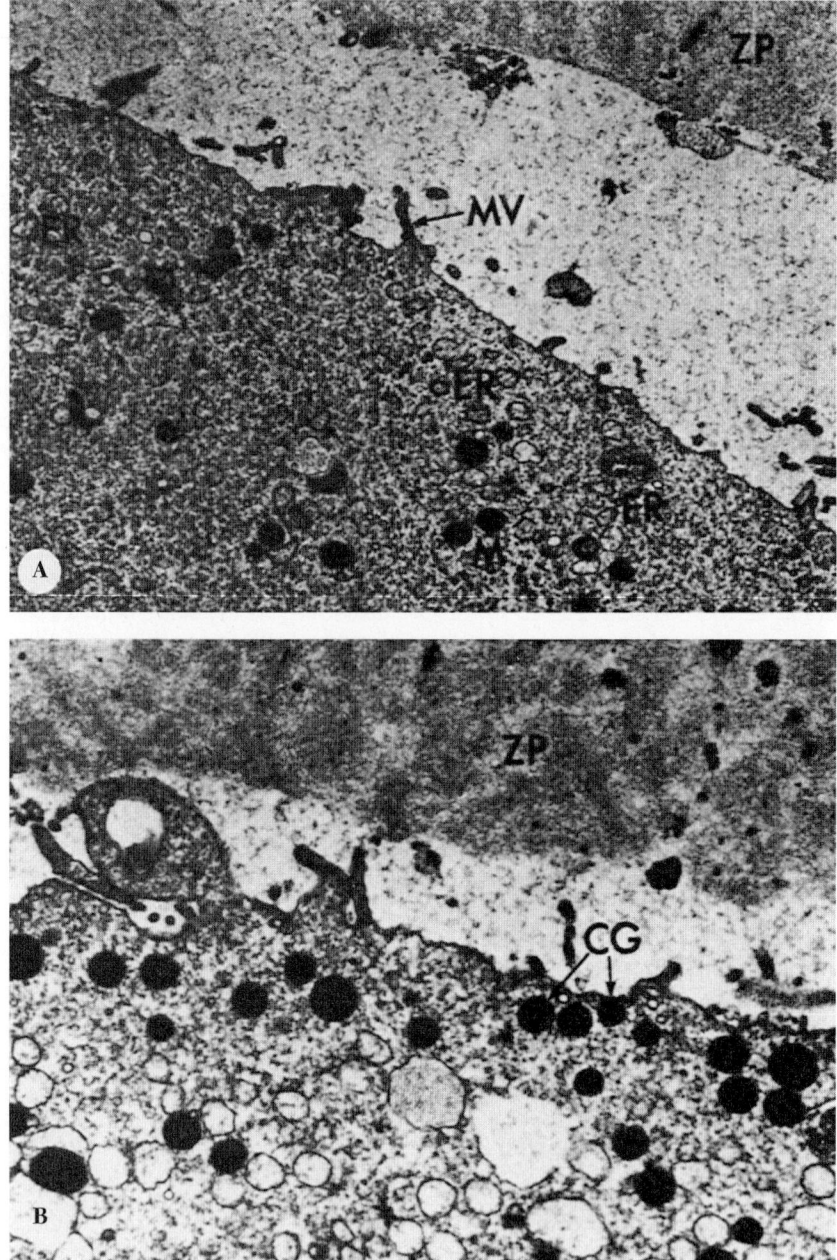

FIGURE 4-25 **A,** Surface of fertilized ovum, showing absence of cortical granules. A few microvilli *(MV)* are projecting into perivitelline space, which has been widened by retraction of ooplasm from zona pellucida *(ZP)*. Dense mitochondria *(M)* and large vesicular components of endoplasmic reticulum *(ER)* are visible in ooplasm. The egg was fixed 3 hours after insemination in vitro. (×15,400.) **B,** Surface of unfertilized ovum that had been inseminated for 3 hours. Numerous extremely electron-dense cortical granules *(CG)* are present beneath vitelline membrane. Zona pellucida *(ZP)* has a fine fibrillar appearance. (×19,600.) (From Lopata A, Sathananthan AM, McBain JC, et al: Fertil Steril 33:12, 1980. Reproduced with permission of the publisher, The American Fertility Society.)

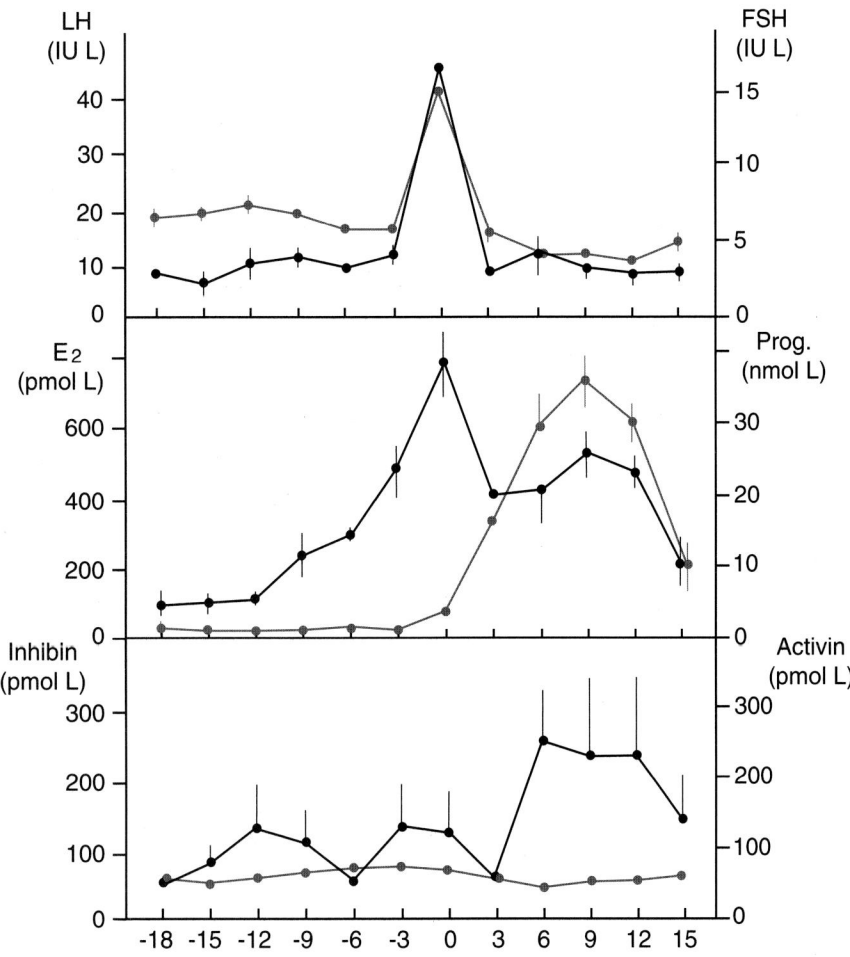

FIGURE 4-26   Hormonal profiles of four normal subjects during menstrual cycle. Day 0 was defined as the day corresponding to a surge of LH and FSH. **A,** Plasma levels of LH *(blue circles)* and FSH *(solid circles)*. **B,** Levels of E_2 *(blue circles)* and progesterone *(solid circles)*. **C,** Plasma levels of inhibin *(blue circles)* and activin *(solid circles)*. Each *point* represents the mean of four subjects, and *horizontal bars* represent the standard error of the mean. (Courtesy of Demura R, Suzuki T, Tajima S, et al: J Clin Endocrinol Metab 76:1080, 1993.)

After the oocyte is extruded, the amount of follicular fluid is markedly reduced, the follicular wall becomes convoluted, and the follicular diameter and volume greatly decrease. These changes are detectable by ultrasonography (Figure 4-29). As the granulosa and theca cells become luteinized, they take up lipids and lutein pigment, giving them a yellow coloration. The granulosa cell layer becomes vascularized only after ovulation. Under the influence of LH, the corpus luteum produces progesterone in amounts of about 20 μg/24 hours and also secretes estradiol. High LH levels are necessary for the support of corpus luteum secretory function. In case of conception, the production of progesterone in the corpus luteum continues under the stimulatory action of human chorionic gonadotrophin secreted by the syncytiotrophoblast.

Levels of progesterone steadily increase in the serum after ovulation and plateau about 1 week later, after which they decline unless pregnancy occurs. The increasing levels of progesterone and estradiol exert a negative feedback on FSH and LH secretion. Estradiol inhibits mainly FSH (negative feedback), whereas progesterone inhibits mainly LH. There is also evidence that luteal estradiol production exerts a local luteolytic action. It is postulated that increased intraovarian progesterone concentration prevents follicle maturation in that ovary in the subsequent cycle.

As luteolysis occurs and estradiol and progesterone levels decline, there is less negative feedback. Therefore, FSH and LH levels begin to rise before the onset of menstruation to stimulate follicular growth for the next cycle.

Estradiol and progesterone exert both a direct inhibitory effect on pituitary gonadotrophin synthesis and secretion, and an effect on GnRH release, altering the fre-

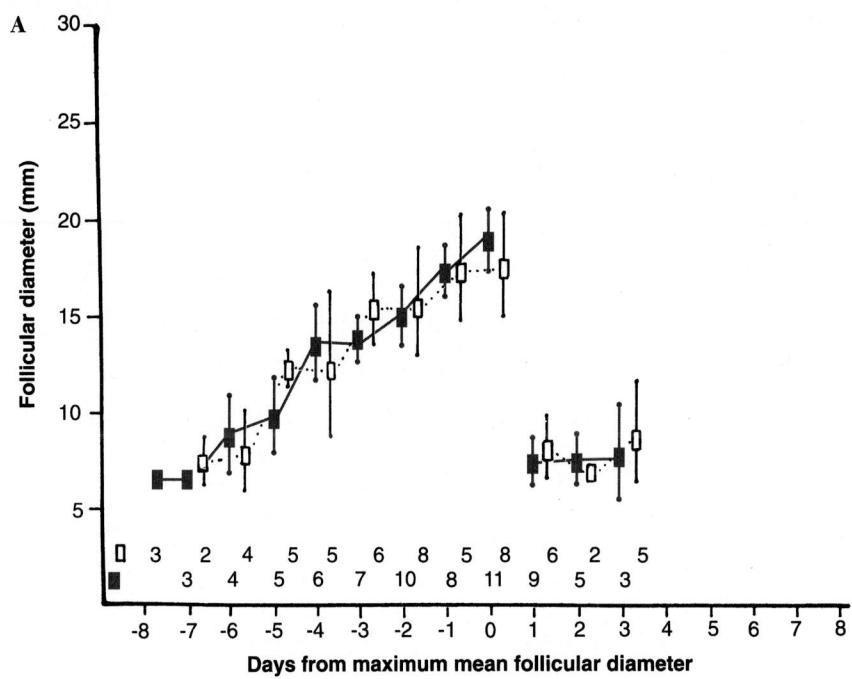

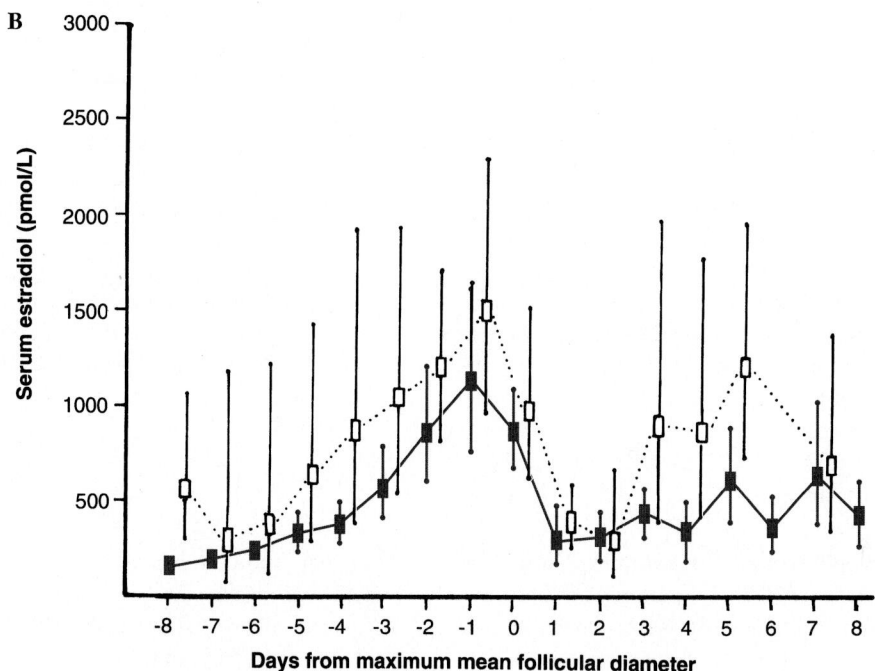

FIGURE 4-27 Correlation of follicular diameter with follicular growth and folllicular volume with estradiol in 11 spontaneous and 8 induced conception cycles. (Redrawn from Eissa MK, Obhrai MS, Docker MF, et al: Fertil Steril 45:191, 1986. Reproduced with permission of the publisher, The American Fertility Society.)

quency as well as the amplitude of GnRH pulses. The steroid feedback on GnRH release occurs by a direct effect on the neurotransmitters (dopamine and norepinephrine) and the neuromodulators (β-endorphin) in the arcuate nucleus.

Three studies by Reame et al., Crowley et al., and Fil-

icori et al. have shown that the frequency of LH peaks, and presumably of GnRH pulses, changes throughout the menstrual cycle when blood sampling was performed every 10 minutes. In sleep, there is a close relationship between the frequency of GnRH pulses in portal blood and the frequency of LH pulses in the peripheral circula-

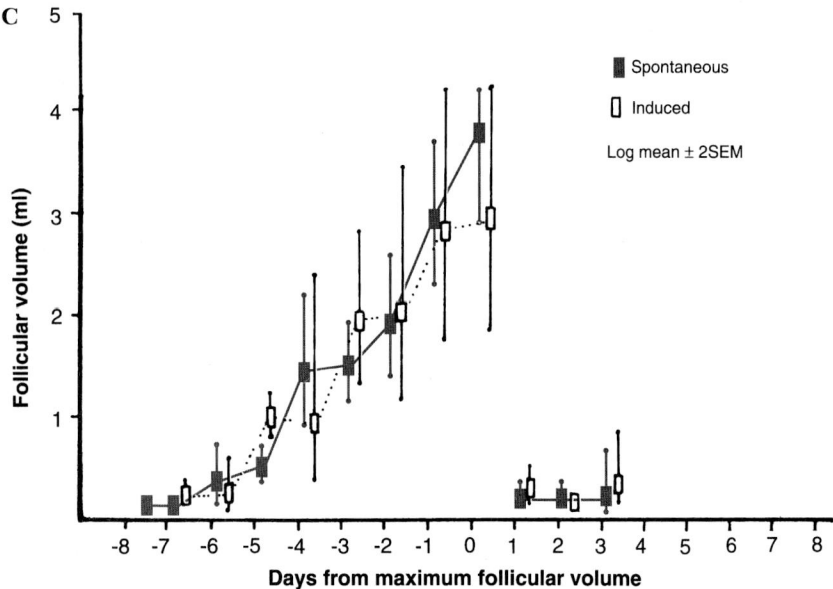

FIGURE 4-27, cont'd. For legend see opposite page.

tion. In the early follicular phase, LH pulses occur about once every 90 minutes, with an absence of pulsation during sleep (Figure 4-30). The frequency of LH pulses significantly increases in the middle and late follicular phases to about one pulse per hour throughout the day and night. The amplitude of LH pulses is low and decreases somewhat between the early and middle follicular phases; however, during the late follicular (preovulatory) phase, LH amplitude significantly increases (Figure 4-31). LH pulse frequency progressively slows in the luteal phase from about one pulse every 90 minutes in the early luteal phase to about one every 3 hours in the late luteal phase (Figure 4-32). The amplitude of LH pulses varies after ovulation, with a bimodal distribution of small and large pulses. Overall mean LH levels are higher in the luteal phase than in the follicular phase (Figure 4-33). Similar changes in FSH pulsation in peripheral blood do not occur, probably because of its longer half-life.

The increase in frequency of LH pulses during the late follicular phase is probably important in stimulating follicular secretion of estradiol, since 80% of LH pulses are followed by a rise in circulating estradiol levels. An increased amplitude of LH pulses is observed during the midcycle LH surge, probably because of either an increased frequency of GnRH pulsations or the positive feedback effect of increasing levels of estradiol and progesterone on increasing gonadotrophin responsiveness to GnRH. Middle to late luteal LH pulses stimulate progesterone production. Bächström et al. and Filicori et al. have shown that beginning in the midluteal phase, progesterone is secreted in a pulsatile manner, with increases

occurring immediately following an LH pulse (Figure 4-32). The variations in LH pulse amplitude and the slower frequency in the midluteal phase are probably caused by the negative feedback effects of progesterone and estradiol. Filicori et al. have postulated that the decrease in LH frequency is due to an action of progesterone on hypothalamic release of GnRH, possibly being mediated through increased levels of β-endorphin, whereas the decrease in amplitude of LH pulses is due to a negative feedback effect of progesterone on the pituitary.

The patterns of FSH and LH levels obtained by radioimmunoassay (RIA) measurements in serum are similar to the patterns observed by bioassay of urinary extracts, except that the midcycle FSH peak occurs 2 days later and is more pronounced, probably because of the longer half-life of FSH in serum (Figure 4-34). The amounts of urinary FSH and LH excretion are about 1 to 10 IU/24 hours, whereas serum levels fluctuate between 1 and 100 mIU/ml.

Excretion of the three classic estrogens, estrone, estradiol, and estriol, is lowest during the early follicular phase, peaks just before LH peaks, decreases shortly thereafter, and rises in the luteal phase, after which it falls again. The luteal-phase rise of these estrogens is of smaller amplitude but longer duration than the preovulatory peak (Figure 4-35). Midcycle peak urinary excretion of all three estrogens is about 50 to 75 μg/24 hours. Serum levels of estradiol follow a similar pattern throughout the cycle, rising from less than 50 pg/ml in the early follicular phase to 200 to 500 pg/ml at midcycle and having a broad luteal-phase peak level of about 100 to 150 pg/ml (Figure 4-28).

The major metabolite of progesterone excreted in the urine is pregnanediol. Levels of pregnanediol are less than 0.9 μg/24 hours before ovulation (mean, 0.4 μg/24 hours) and consistently greater than 1 μg/24 hours (mean, 3 to 4 μg/24 hours) after ovulation (Figure 4-36). Progesterone levels in serum are less than 1 ng/ml before ovulation and reach midluteal levels of 10 to 20 ng/ml. In cycles followed by conception, several investigators have reported that progesterone levels are always greater than 9 ng/ml. However, as progesterone is secreted in a pulsatile manner with wide fluctuations in its serum levels, a single low serum value may not be indicative of a lack of corpus luteum formation or of an inadequate corpus luteum.

Levels of the steroid metabolite 17-hydroxyprogesterone increase concomitantly with the increase of the LH surge, indicating a shift of steroidogenesis from the Δ^5 to the Δ^4 pathway (see Figure 4-28). Levels of 17-hydroxyprogesterone then fall and rise again in the midluteal phase as progesterone and estradiol levels increase. About 4 to 6 days before the onset of menses, levels of estradiol, progesterone, and 17-hydroxyprogesterone all begin to decline.

During midcycle the first event is a rise in estradiol. When estradiol reaches peak levels, there is an abrupt increase (surge) in LH and FSH (Figure 4-37). The increase in LH reaches a peak in about 18 hours, and peak levels plateau for about 14 hours, after which there is a decline. The mean duration of the LH surge is about 24 hours. Beginning about 12 hours before the onset of the LH surge, there is an increase of both progesterone and 17-hydroxyprogesterone. With the occurrence of the LH peak there is a decline in estradiol and a further increase in progesterone. This shift in steroidogenesis in favor of progesterone instead of estradiol production is brought about by the luteinization of the granulosa cells produced by LH.

Levels of numerous other hormones have been measured in serum throughout the cycle and summarized in the excellent review by Diczfalusy and Landgren. Serum levels of androstenedione and testosterone change little during the cycle, but mean levels are slightly higher during the follicular rather than the luteal phase (Figure 4-38). Serum thyroid-stimulating hormone (TSH) levels also remain relatively constant, while adrenocorticotropic hormone (ACTH) and growth hormone (GH) have a preovulatory peak. Prolactin levels appear to be slightly higher in the luteal phase.

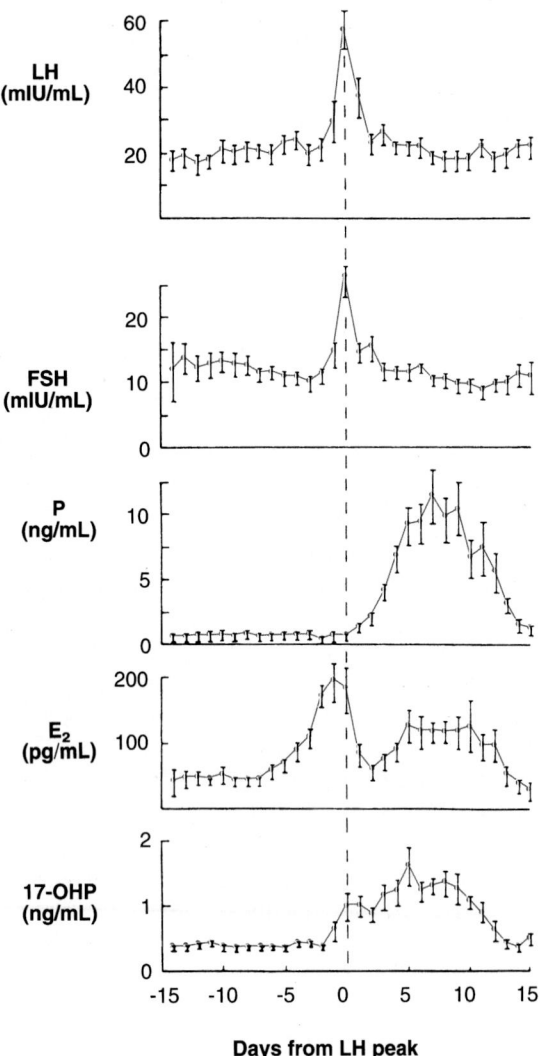

FIGURE 4-28 Means and standard errors of serum *LH, FSH,* progesterone *(P),* estradiol *(E₂),* and 17-hydroxyprogesterone *(17-OHP)* levels measured in nine women daily during entire ovulatory menstrual cycle. Individual daily results were grouped according to day of midcycle LH peak and averaged. (From Thorneycroft IH, Mishell DR Jr, Stone SC, et al: Am J Obstet Gynecol 111:947, 1971.)

TABLE 4-4
Range of Observed Times from Defined Hormonal Events and Time of Ovulation

| | Time of Ovulation (hours) from Rise to Peak | | | |
| | First Significant Rise | | Peak | |
Hormone	Median	Range	Median	Range
17β-Estradiol	82.5	48–168	24.0	0–48
LH	32.0	24–56	16.5	8–40
FSH	21.1	8–24	15.3	8–40
Progesterone	7.8	0–32	—	—

From World Health Organization: Am J Obstet Gynecol 138:383, 1980.

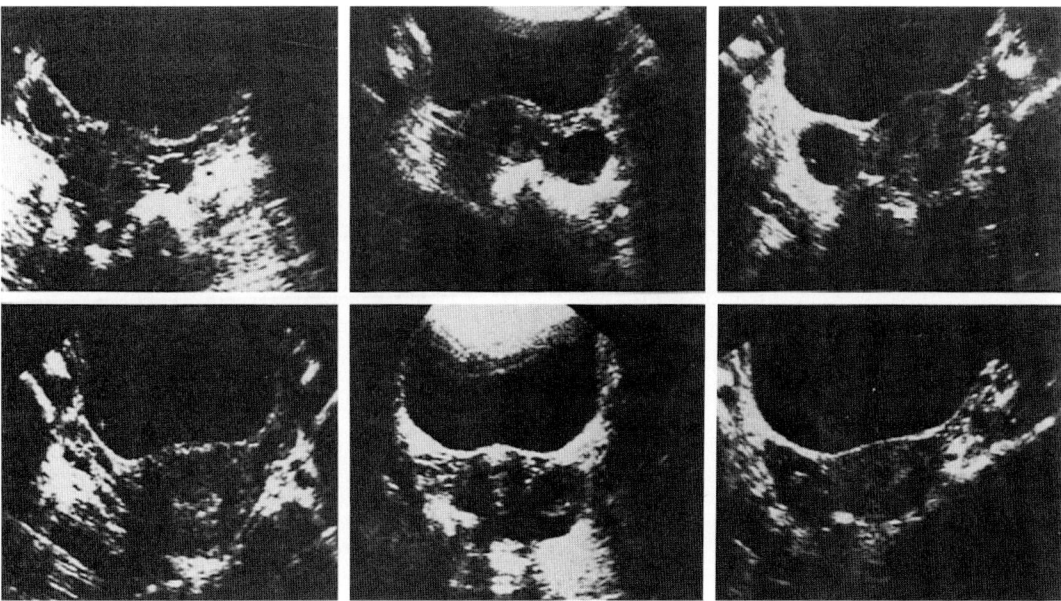

FIGURE 4-29 Ultrasonographic signs of ovulation: complete disappearance *(left)*, loss of volume and thickening of wall *(middle)*, and replacement by irregular spongy area *(right)*. (From Wetzels LCG and Hoogland HJ: Fertil Steril 37:336, 1982. Reproduced with permission of the publisher, The American Fertility Society.)

Menstrual Cycle Length

The mean age of menarche is about 13 years, and the mean age of menopause is about 51 years. Therefore women have menses for a duration of about 38 years. Menstrual cycle length varies among different women and for an individual woman at different times of her life. The most information regarding menstrual cycles comes from the classic study of Treloar et al., who analyzed 275,947 menstrual intervals recorded by more than 2700 women over prolonged periods. Analysis of these data revealed that menstrual cycle length is most irregular in the 2 years after menarche and the 3 years before menopause, times of life during which anovulatory cycles are most frequent (Table 4-5). During these times of life, both shortened and prolonged cycle lengths are common, with the latter being more frequent (Figure 4-39).

Menstrual cycle length is least variable between the ages of 20 and 40 years. During this time there is a gradual decrease of mean cycle length. The follicular phase length defined as the interval from the onset of menstruation up to, but not including, the day of the LH peak decreases with age from 14.2 to 10.4 for women aged 18 to 24 and 40 to 44, respectively. However, between these ages, menstrual cycle length still varies in an individual woman, as recorded by the women, with the most regular duration of menstrual cycles among the several thousand studied by Vollman for many years (Figure 4-40). It is generally accepted

that the mean duration of menstrual cycle length is 28 ± 7 days, with the occurrence of shorter cycles (<21 days) being called polymenorrhea and that of longer cycles (>35 days) being called oligomenorrhea. The mean duration of menstrual flow is 4 ± 2 days.

Endometrial Histology

Human endometrium is made up of two basic layers: the stratum basale, which lies above the myometrium, and the stratum functionale, lying between the stratum basale and the uterine lumen. The stratum basale consists of primordial glands and densely cellular stroma, which changes little throughout the menstrual cycle and does not desquamate at the time of menstruation. The stratum functionale is divided into two layers. The superficial, narrow stratum compactum consists of the necks of the glands and densely populated stromal cells. The underlying, broader stratum spongiosum consists primarily of glands with less densely populated stroma and large amounts of interstitial tissue. The stratum functionale grows during the cycle, and a portion of it desquamates at the time of menses.

After menstruation, the endometrium is only 1 to 2 mm thick and consists mainly of the stratum basale and a portion of the spongiosum. Under the influence of estrogen, the stratum functionale proliferates greatly by multiplication of both glandular and stromal cells. Mitotic figures are abundant. In the late follicular phase, the glands become more tortuous in appearance. As

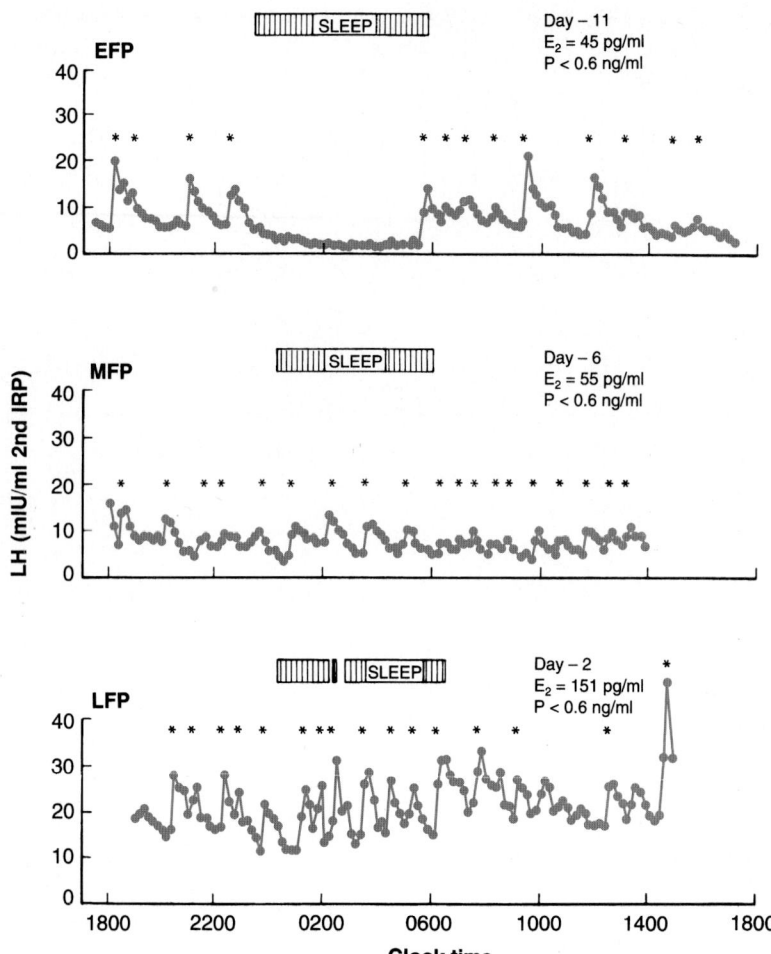

FIGURE 4-30 Patterns of episodic LH secretion throughout follicular phase of menstrual cycle. Representative examples of early follicular phase *(EFP)*, midfollicular phase *(MFP)*, and late follicular phase *(LFP)* series are shown. Stage of follicular phase is indicated from Day 0. LH pulsations are indicated by asterisks. Levels of prostaglandin E_2 and progesterone represent mean of samples obtained at 6-hour intervals. Sleep is indicated by hatched bars. *P*, Progesterone. (From Filicori M, Santoro N, Merriam GR, et al: J Clin Endocrinol Metab 62:1136, 1986.)

estrogen levels peak immediately before ovulation, the cells lining the glandular lumina undergo pseudostratification (Figure 4-41).

Just after ovulation, glycogen-rich subnuclear vacuoles appear in the base of the cells lining the glands (Figure 4-42). This subnuclear vacuolization is the first histologic indication of the effect of progesterone but is not evidence that ovulation has occurred. As progesterone levels increase in the early luteal phase, the glycogen-containing vacuoles ascend toward the gland lumina. Soon thereafter, the contents of the glands are released into the endometrial cavity. The glycogen provides energy to the free-floating blastocyst, which reaches the endometrial cavity about 3½ days after fertilization. Implantation occurs 1 week after fertilization.

In the midluteal phase the glands become increasingly tortuous and the stroma becomes more edematous and vascular (Figure 4-43). During the secretory phase,

several specific proteins are produced by the endometrium. The two major proteins are placental proteins 14 and 12 (PP14 and PP12). The former is also called pregnancy-associated endometrial protein (PEP), and α_2 pregnancy-associated endometrial globulin, as well as glycodelin. PP12 is also called α uterine protein and chorionic α_2 globulin. PP-14 is not actually a placental protein, but rather a major secretory product of glandular epithelium during the secretory phase. Circulating levels of PP14 correlate with serum progesterone levels, but the exact purpose of PP14 has not been determined. In addition, other peptide hormones, growth factors, and prostaglandins are produced by the endometrium and may have roles in the development of the decidualized endometrium. If implantation of the blastocyst does not occur in the late luteal phase and hCG is not produced to maintain the corpus luteum, the glands begin to collapse and fragment. Sub-

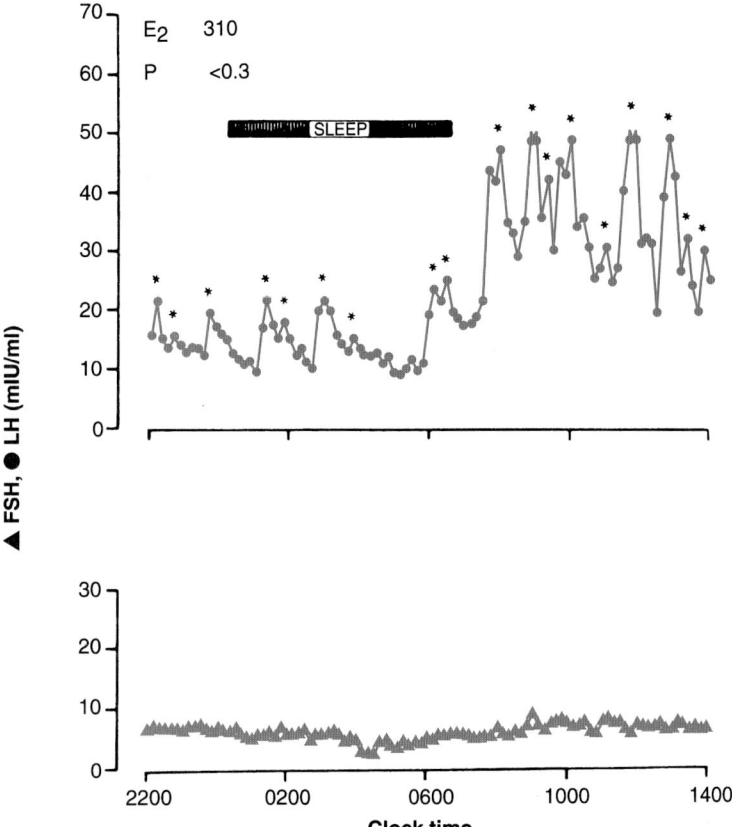

FIGURE 4-31 LH secretory response in normal woman studied on day of LH surge. Note increase in amplitude and frequency of GnRH secretion, absence of any day-night variation, and discernible FSH pulsations. (From Crowley WF, Filicori M, Spratt DI, et al: Recent Prog Horm Res 41:473, 1985.)

sequently, polymorphonuclear leukocytes and monocytes infiltrate the glands and stroma, autolysis of the functional zone of the endometrium occurs, and desquamation begins.

The histologic pattern of the endometrium has been correlated with the phase of the menstrual cycle in the classic study of Noyes et al. (Figure 4-44). This subjective method of correlating the degree of maturation of the endometrium is relatively imprecise. Several blind studies have demonstrated wide variability of both interobserver interpretation and interpretation by the same observer at different intervals. Recently, hormonal levels have been correlated with endometrial indices based on quantitative morphometric analysis. Li et al. noted that this methodology could produce a significant correlation with chronologic dating of the length of the luteal phase when only 5 of 17 morphometric measurements were used. These five measurements were (1) the frequency of mitosis per 1000 gland cells, (2) the amount of secretion in gland lumen, (3) the amount of gland cell pseudostratification, (4) the proportion of glands infused by gland cells, and (5) the amount of predecidual reaction. These authors concluded that use of these objective morphometric criteria resulted in better correlation with the actual length of the luteal phase than did histologic dating by the method of Noyes et al. Numerous authors have now confirmed the day of LH surge is a more appropriate dating correlate than the onset of the next menstrual cycle (Figure 4-45).

With the use of serial vaginal sonography of normal ovulatory women, Bakos et al. reported that the endometrial thickness, including both the anterior and posterior layers, steadily increased from a mean of about 4 mm in the early follicular phase to about 12 mm at the time of ovulation (Figure 4-46). The mean endometrial thickness remained at 12 mm during the luteal phase. Endometrial volume showed a similar pattern.

Menstruation

There has been relatively little research regarding the mechanism of menstruation since the classic studies of Markee and those of Bartelmez in the 1930s and 1940s. In Markee's study, endometria from rhesus monkeys were

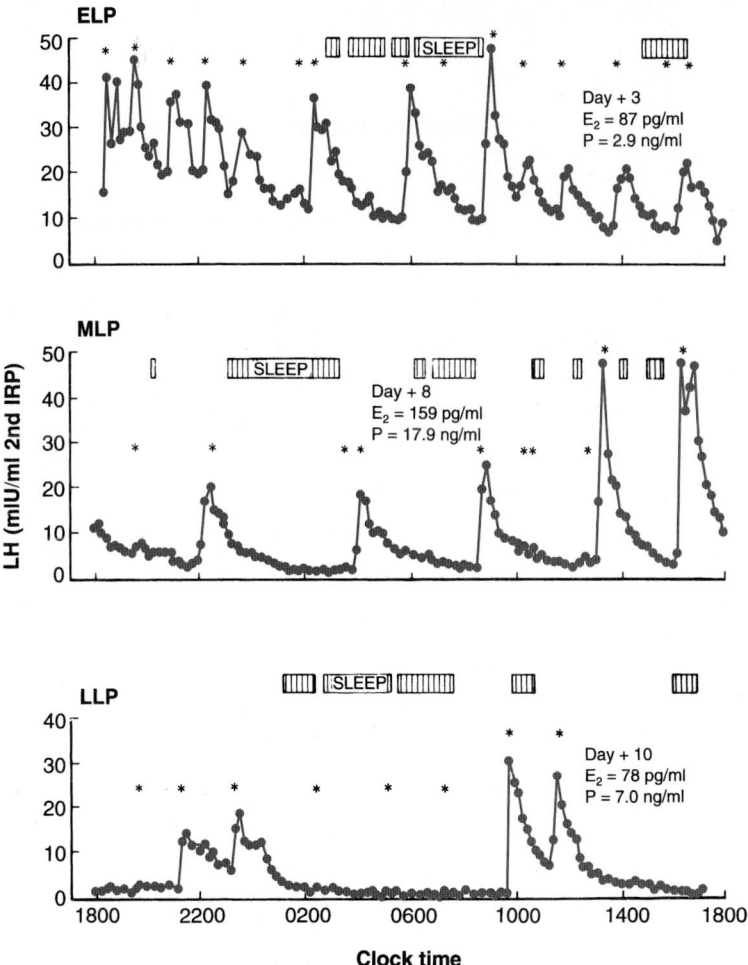

FIGURE 4-32 Patterns of episodic LH secretion throughout luteal phase of menstrual cycle. Representative examples of early *(ELP)*, middle *(MLP)*, and late *(LLP)* series are shown. Stage of luteal phase is indicated as post-Day 0. *P*, Progesterone. (From Filicori M, Santoro N, Merriam GR, et al: J Clin Endocrinol Metab 62:1136, 1986.)

transplanted into the anterior chamber of the eye of the same animal from which the tissue was obtained. He observed that during the cycle the transplants underwent four periods of change: (1) the period of rest (just after menses), (2) the first period of growth, (3) the second period of growth (after ovulation, when the transplants doubled in size again), and (4) the period of regression (when menstruation occurred) (Figure 4-47). Markee noted that as steroid levels fell several days before menstruation, there was regression in the size of the transplants, resulting in coiling of the spiral arteries and slowing of the blood flow within them. Subsequently, vasoconstriction of the coiled arteries occurred. About 4 to 24 hours after vasoconstriction began, the coiled arteries relaxed, blood escaped from them, and menstruation began. Only the spiral arteries that supply the upper two thirds of the endometrium became coiled and constricted.

The straight arteries supplying the stratum basale did not constrict.

Both Markee and Bartelmez, who performed histologic studies on uteri removed by hysterectomy in the 1930s, concluded that menstruation begins in different areas at different times. Although it is classically believed that all tissue of the stratum functionale is exfoliated, leaving only the stratum basale remaining at the end of menstruation, Bartelmez reported that only the entire stratum compactum is uniformly shed, with variable amounts of the stratum spongiosum being desquamated. McLennan and Rydell confirmed this finding in their 1965 study and showed that regeneration of the endometrium comes from cells in the spongiosum that were previously a portion of the secretory endometrium, and not from the stratum basale. These investigators also found extreme variations in the amount of endometrial shedding in different areas

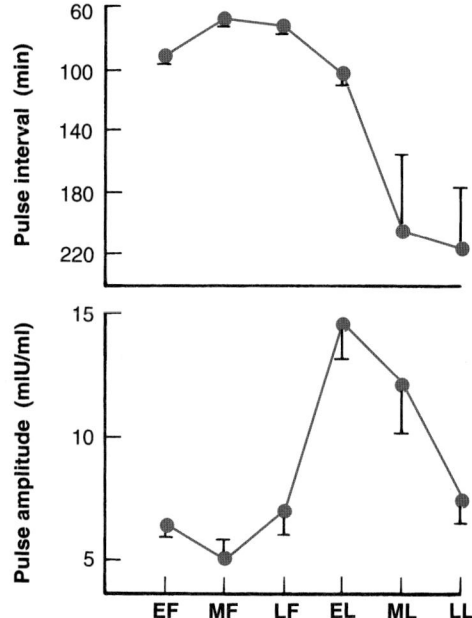

FIGURE 4-33 LH interpulse interval and amplitude during different stages of menstrual cycle. Data shown were obtained by pulse analysis and are expressed as means and standard errors. *EF,* Early follicular phase; *MF,* midfollicular phase; *LF,* late follicular phase; *EL,* early luteal phase; *ML,* midluteal phase; *LL,* late luteal phase. (From Filicori M, Santoro N, Merriam GR, et al: J Clin Endocrinol Metab 62:1136, 1986.)

of the same uterus, as well as variations among different uteri removed by hysterectomy.

Nogales-Ortiz et al. also found extreme variability in the extent of endometrial exfoliation. In their study, they found that usually only the entire compactum and some parts of the spongiosum were shed, but in some areas nearly the entire endometrium was desquamated. Desquamation of the endometrium occurs mainly in the fundus, not in the isthmus or cornual areas. As early as 36 hours after the onset of menses, regeneration of surface epithelium from the glandular stumps begins even as endometrial shedding continues.

Ferenczy, using scanning as well as transmission electron microscopy, reported that the endometrium remained intact in the cervical and isthmic areas. His studies revealed that reepithelialization of the desquamated endometrium began 2 to 3 days after menses began and was completed in 48 hours. Ferenczy and co-workers performed historadioautography studies and concluded that repair of the desquamated endometrium occurred by both epithelial outgrowth from the mouths of the basal glands and by ingrowth from the endometrium in the cervical and isthmic areas that had not been desquamated. They believe that regeneration of the endometrial surface occurs as a local reaction to injury and is not mediated by ovarian

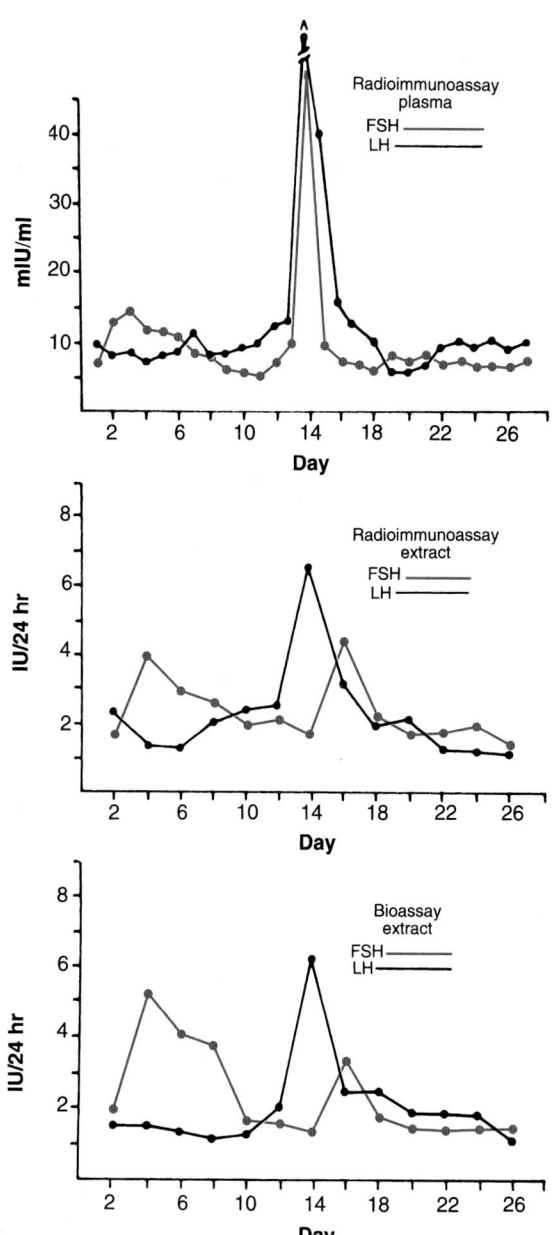

FIGURE 4-34 Serum FSH and LH measured by radioimmunoassay (RIA) and urinary FSH and LH measured by both RIA and bioassay through an entire ovulatory menstrual cycle. (From Stevens VC: J Clin Endocrinol Metab 29:904, 1969. © 1969 by The Endocrine Society.)

steroid hormones, whose levels are very low at this time of the cycle.

In 1978 Flowers and Wilborn performed a histologic, histochemical, and ultrastructural study of endometrial biopsy specimens obtained from a group of menstruating women. In these detailed studies, they also found that the

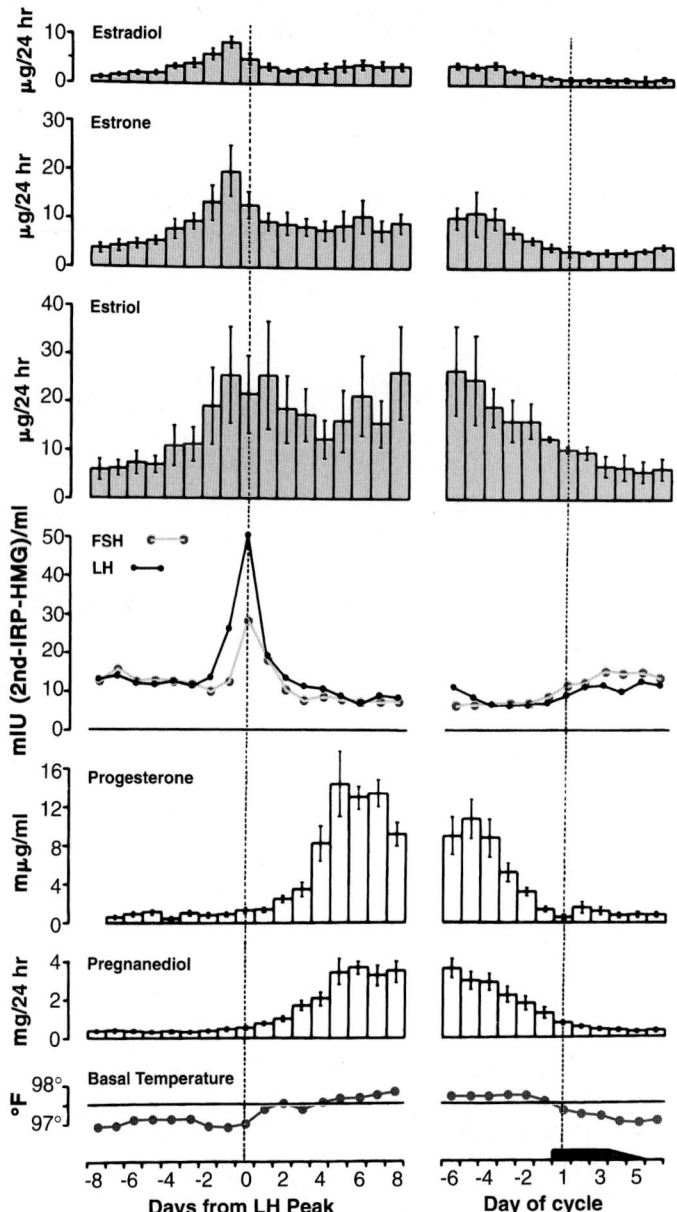

FIGURE 4-35 Mean serum FSH and LH levels, urinary estrogen levels, pregnanediol excretion, and basal body temperatures measured daily in five women during ovulatory menstrual cycle. Bars depict standard errors. Individual results were grouped according to day of midcycle LH surge *(left)* or first day of menstruation *(right)* and averaged. (From Goebelsmann UT, Midgey AR Jr, and Jaffe RB: J Clin Endocrinol Metab 29:1222, 1969. © 1969 by The Endocrine Society.)

only cells desquamated are from the compactum and upper spongiosum layers. In addition, they found that few endometrial cells undergo necrosis. Instead, the majority of cells in the endometrium survive and undergo regression in size by autophagocytosis, heterophagocytosis, and release of enzymes. Endometrial autophagocytosis is carried out by lysosomes, which digest the cytoplasm; heterophagocytosis is performed by macrophages, which phagocytose debris from stromal tissue; enzymes digest the reticular fibers. More recent studies have demonstrated that interleukin-8 (IL-8) levels may be important

in recruitment of these macrophages. IL-8 attracts neutrophils into tissues and causes them to degranulate. Evidence suggests that progesterone may inhibit endometrial production of IL-8. Thus, decreasing progesterone levels in the late luteal phase may allow increased production of IL-8 in the endometrial cells leading to leukocyte immigration and degranulation. Progesterone maintains the stability of the lysosomes, which contain enzymes that degrade the substances providing support for the growing endometrium such as mucopolysaccharides, collagen, and reticulum. Matrix metalloproteinases are a family of

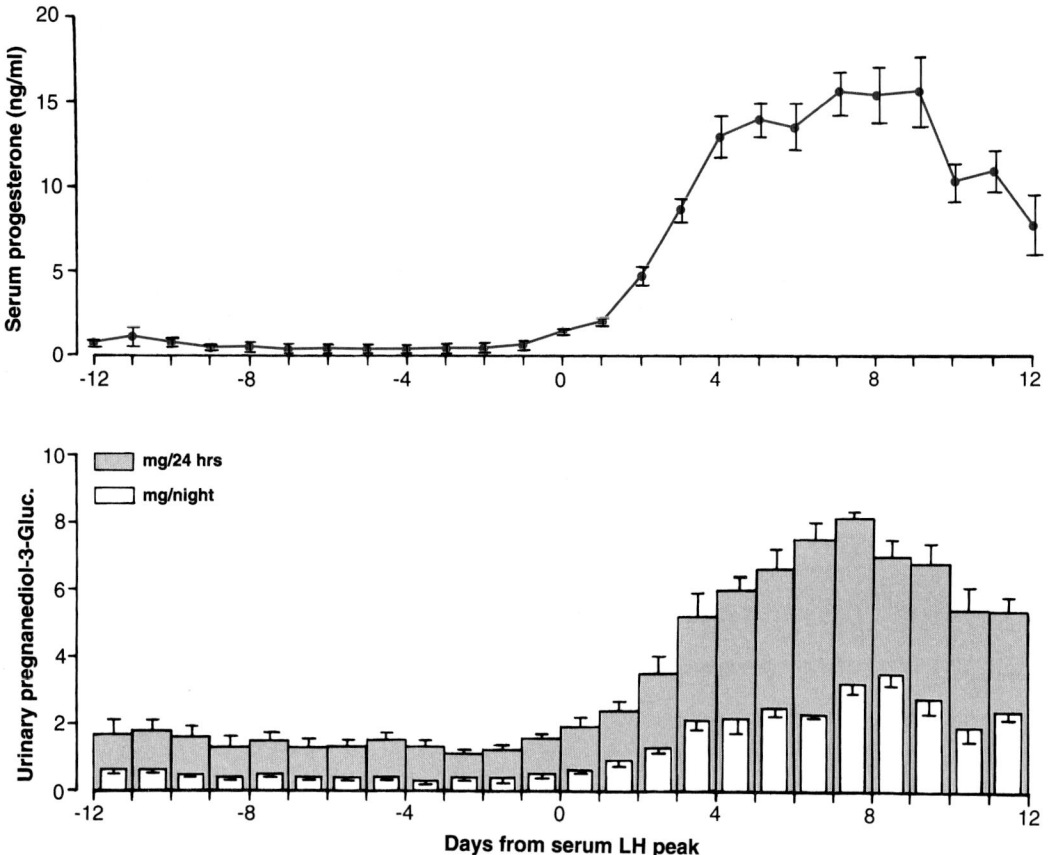

FIGURE 4-36 Means and standard errors of daily 8 AM serum progesterone concentrations and 24-hour (8 AM to 8 AM) and overnight urinary excretion of radioimmunoassayable pregnanediol-3-glucuronide in seven women during entire menstrual cycle. Data obtained in individual subjects were grouped according to day of midcycle LH peak and averaged. (From Stanczyk FZ, Miyakama I, and Goebelsmann UT: Am J Obstet Gynecol 137:443, 1980.)

enzymes that degrade structural elements of the extracellular matrix and basement membrane. Enzymes in the lysosomes degrade the substances that make up the supporting growth substance of the endometrium, the mucopolysaccharides, collagen, and reticulum.

Other changes within the endometrial cells may also contribute to disorganization of the endometrium during menstruation. Recent studies have determined that expression of proteins, important in epithelial cell-cell binding in human endometrium, changes throughout the menstrual cycle. These proteins include E-cadherin, α- or β-catenin, β-actin, and desmoplalkin I/II. Menstrual shedding is associated with disorganization of the site-specific distribution of these proteins. Therefore, menstruation may also be the result of withdrawal of steroid hormones leading to the dissolution of integrity of the tight, gap, intermediate and desmosomal junctions that bind the epithelial, stromal, and glandular cells. These changes have not been observed in the basalis layer, which is not shed during the menstrual phase.

After this sequence of events, the cells are reorganized in structure and participate in the new proliferative process as described earlier, and the same cells that previously formed the secretory endometrium also form the new proliferative endometrium. Thus menstruation in humans is probably a combination of superficial tissue shedding brought about by ischemia, increases in IL-8, lysis from hydrolytic enzymes from macrophages, and loss of cell-cell binding proteins followed by reorganization and regeneration of endometrial cells.

TECHNIQUE OF HORMONE ASSAY

Bioassay

Measurement (assay) of reproductive hormones was initially done by bioassay techniques. Hormones such as the gonadotrophins were measured in urine. Bioassays measure the biologic response (growth) of target organs of certain animals (usually rats, rabbits, or mice), which is produced by administering different concentrations of the substances to be assayed, such as in urinary extracts. First, various dilutions of a known (standard) preparation of hormone are administered. The varying increases in weight of the target organ in the animal are then used to

FIGURE 4-37 Serum FSH, LH, estradiol *(E₂)*, and progesterone *(PROG)* levels around midcycle. (From Thorneycroft IH, Sribyatta B, Tom WK, et al: J Clin Endocrinol Metab 39:754, 1974. © 1974 by The Endocrine Society.)

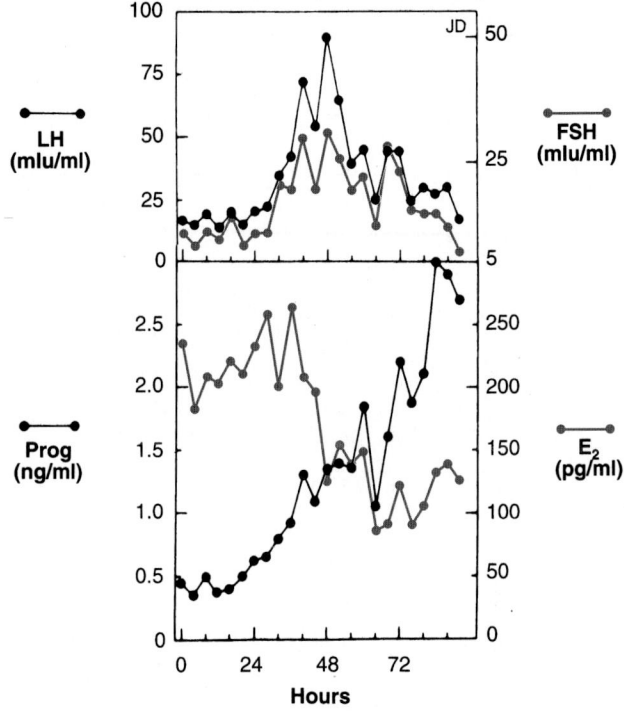

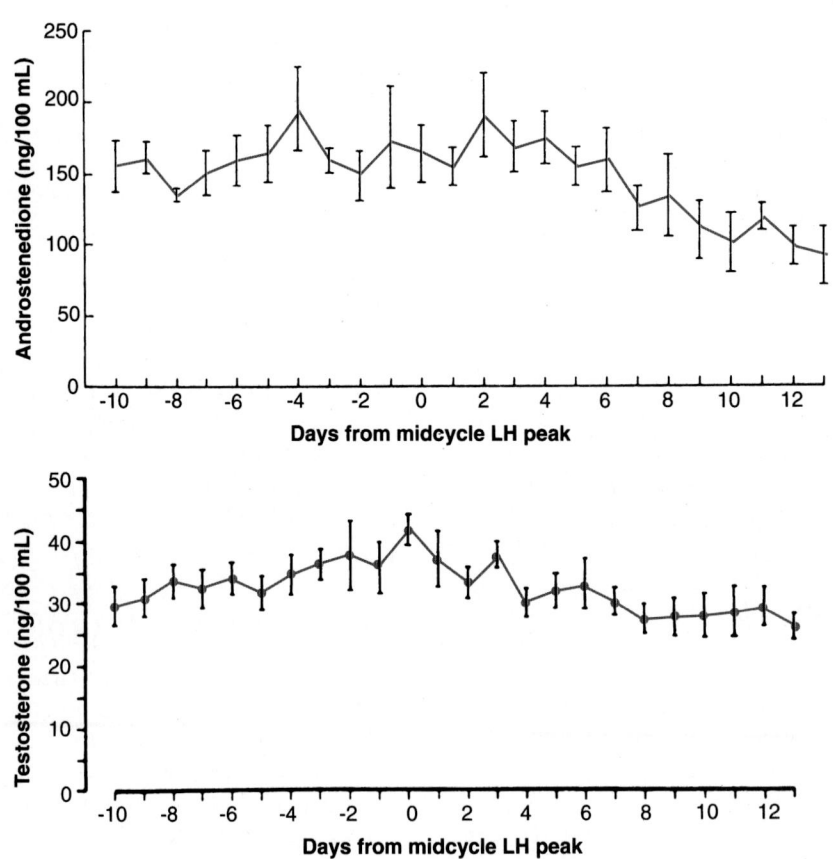

FIGURE 4-38 *Upper panel:* Means and standard errors of serum androstenedione concentrations measured in six women daily during entire ovulatory menstrual cycle. Individual daily results were grouped according to day of preovulatory serum estradiol peak and averaged. *Lower panel:* Means and standard errors of serum testosterone concentrations measured daily in eight women during entire ovulatory menstrual cycle. Individual daily results were grouped according to day of midcycle LH peak and averaged. (From Ribeiro WO, Mishell DR Jr, and Thorneycroft IH: Am J Obstet Gynecol 119:1026, 1974; and Goebelsmann UT, Arce JJ, Thorneycroft IH, et al: Am J Obstet Gynecol 119:445, 1974.)

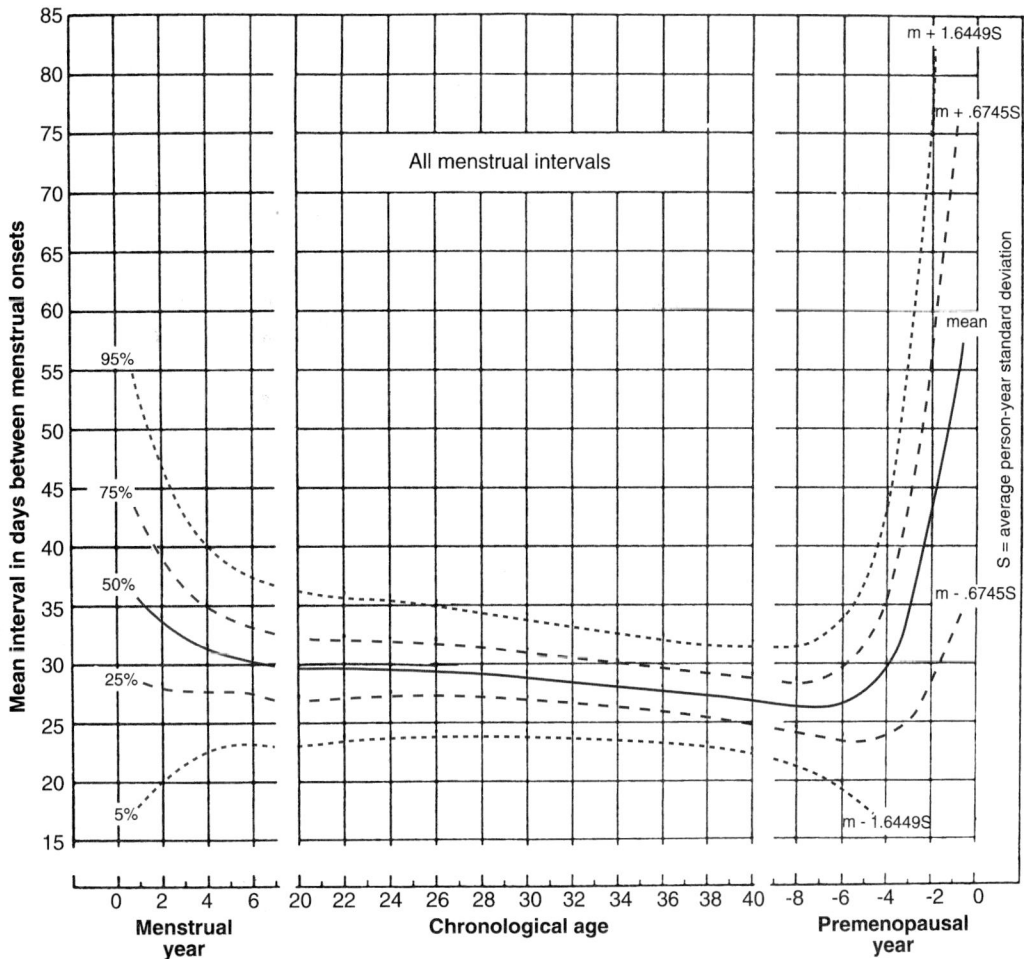

FIGURE 4-39 Normal curve contours for distribution of menstrual intervals in three zones of menstrual life. (From Treloar AE, Boynton RE, Borghild BG, et al: Int J Fertil 12:77, 1967.)

TABLE 4-5
Means and Standard Deviations in Days
for Menstrual Intervals at Selected Ages

Age	Mean (Days)	Standard Deviation (Days)
2 yr after menarche	32.20	8.38
20 yr	30.09	3.94
25 yr	29.84	3.45
30 yr	29.30	3.16
35 yr	28.22	2.67
40 yr	27.26	2.83
3 yr before menopause	33.20	14.24

Data from Treloar AE, Boynton RE, Borghild BG, et al: Int J Fertil 12:77, 1967.

develop a dose-response curve against which the response of the substance being assayed is determined.

Chemical Methods

Chemical assay methods were developed to measure urinary sex steroid levels in women. These assays lack the sensitivity to quantify steroid levels in blood (serum or plasma). Three basic procedural steps are performed in chemical assays of steroids. First, the steroids undergo hydrolysis to remove the conjugate (sulfate or glucuronide group). This is necessary because steroids in urine are present almost entirely in a conjugated form. Second, the steroids are extracted by organic solvents from the urinary hydrolysate. The final basic step is purification of the steroid by column chromatography. The amount of steroid is then quantified by measurement of the color reaction, using either colorimetry or the more sensitive flurometry. A more sensitive chemical method of measurement of steroids is gas chromatography, an extremely tedious procedure.

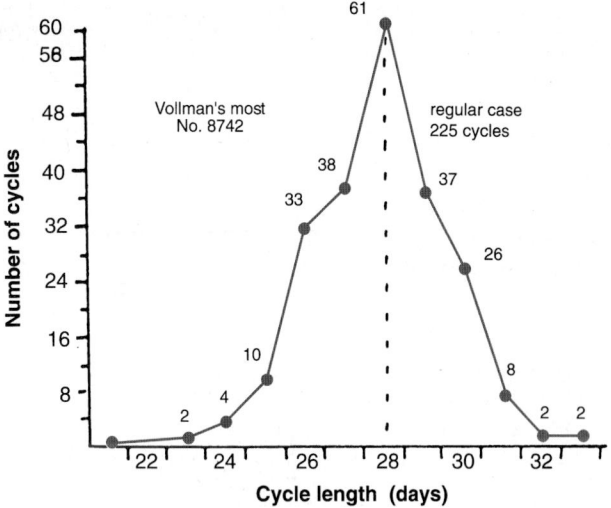

FIGURE 4-40 Frequency distribution of cycle lengths of Vollman's "most regular" subject. (From Hartman CG: The irregularity of the menstrual cycle. In Science and the safe period, Huntington, NY, 1972, RE Krieger Publishing Co.)

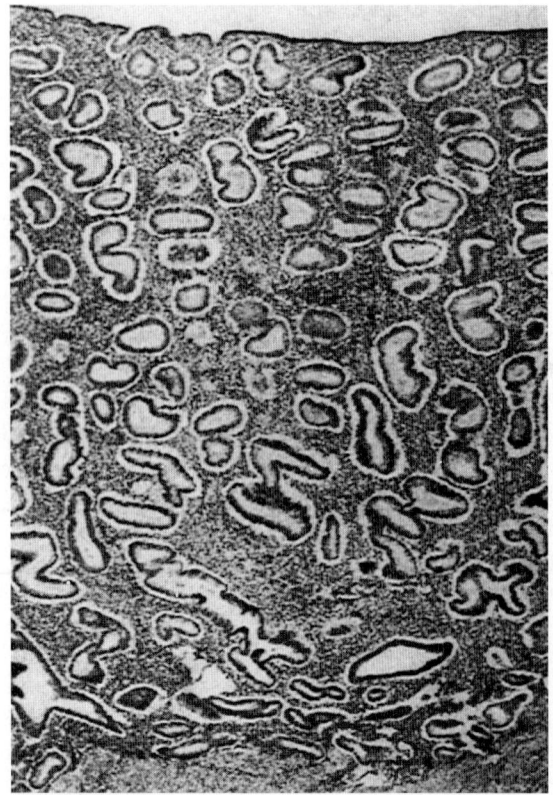

FIGURE 4-41 Early-interval endometrium. (From Novak E and Novak ER, editors: Textbook of gynecology, ed 4, Baltimore, 1952, Williams & Wilkins.)

Radioimmunoassay

In 1959 Yalow and Berson developed the technique of radioimmunoassay, which provided the method of measuring extremely small amounts of hormone in serum or plasma. Use of this technique has greatly increased the knowledge of reproductive endocrinology. Radioimmunoassay allows a much greater number of assays to be performed than does bioassay or chemical assay, in addition to having much greater sensitivity and needing less than 1 ml of serum or plasma for testing. However, this technique measures only the immunologic property of a hormone, not its biologic effects. The two effects frequently differ in magnitude.

The basic principle of radioimmunoassay involves competition between a radioactively labeled and an unlabeled antigen, both of which are present in excess, for binding sites on a limited amount of antibody. To produce a standard curve that permits measurement of a hormone in the serum or plasma, the investigator uses a standard preparation of the hormone to be measured (antigen). Varying known amounts of the unlabeled (cold) antigen and the labeled (hot) antigen are incubated for a time with an antibody raised specifically against the antigen to be measured, and an antigen-antibody complex is formed (Figure 4-48). Since there is always an excess of labeled and unlabeled antigen in the reaction, some of each type of antigen is always bound to the antibody and some always remains free in solution after the incubation. After a predetermined incubation period, the bound complex is separated from the excess free antigen in solution, usually by the addition of an antibody (second antibody) raised against the first antibody, the amount of tracer present in either the bound or free component (usually the bound complex) is measured by a radioactive analyzer (counter). A standard curve is then constructed by plotting the counts per minute measured in the bound components obtained from assaying the various dilutions of the standard preparation, against the mass of antigen used. The type of curve varies with the scale of the abscissa (Figure 4-49).

For measurement of the amount of hormone in the unknown specimen, the same amount of labeled antigen and antibody used for the standard curve preparation are also added to an aliquot of the unknown specimen. After incubation and separation, the amount of tracer that is bound in the antigen-antibody complex is counted. The number of counts per minute measured in the complex is located on the ordinate, and from this point a line is intersected on the standard curve. A perpendicular line is dropped to the abscissa to determine the amount of hormone in the unknown specimen. Rapid calculations of hormone concentrations can be performed by use of a programmed calculator or by a computer.

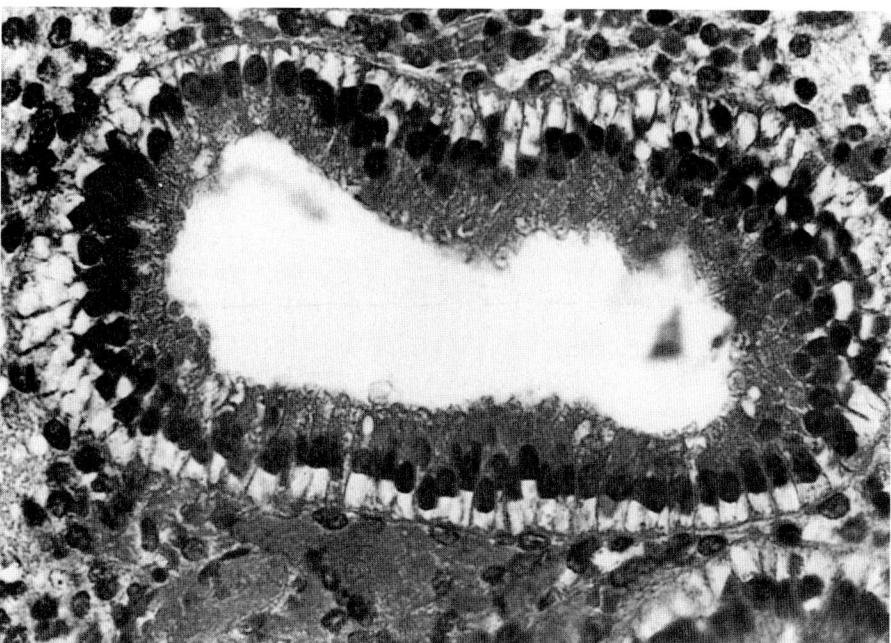

FIGURE 4-42   Subnuclear vacuoles lining base of endometrial gland 2 to 3 days after ovulation. (×500; reduced by 22%.) (From March CM: The endometrium in the menstrual cycle. In Mishell DR Jr, Davajan V, and Lobo RA, editors: Infertility, contraception and reproductive endocrinology, ed 3, Cambridge, Mass, 1991, Blackwell Scientific Publications.)

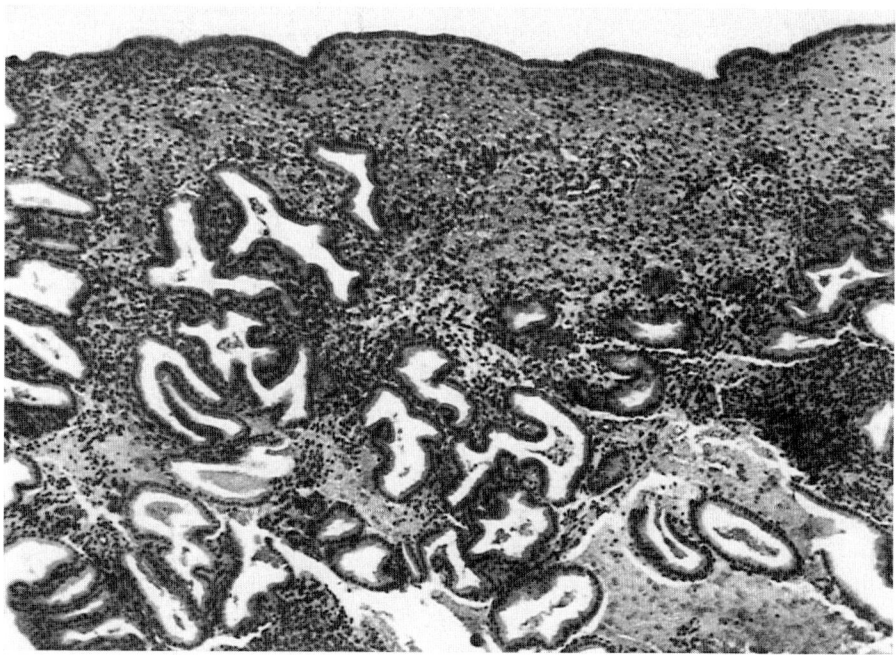

FIGURE 4-43   Maximal secretory activity characteristic of 7 to 8 days after ovulation. (×90; reduced by 22%.) (From March CM: The endometrium in the menstrual cycle. In Mishell DR Jr, Davajan V, and Lobo RA, editors: Infertility, contraception and reproductive endocrinology, ed 3, Cambridge, Mass, 1991, Blackwell Scientific Publications.)

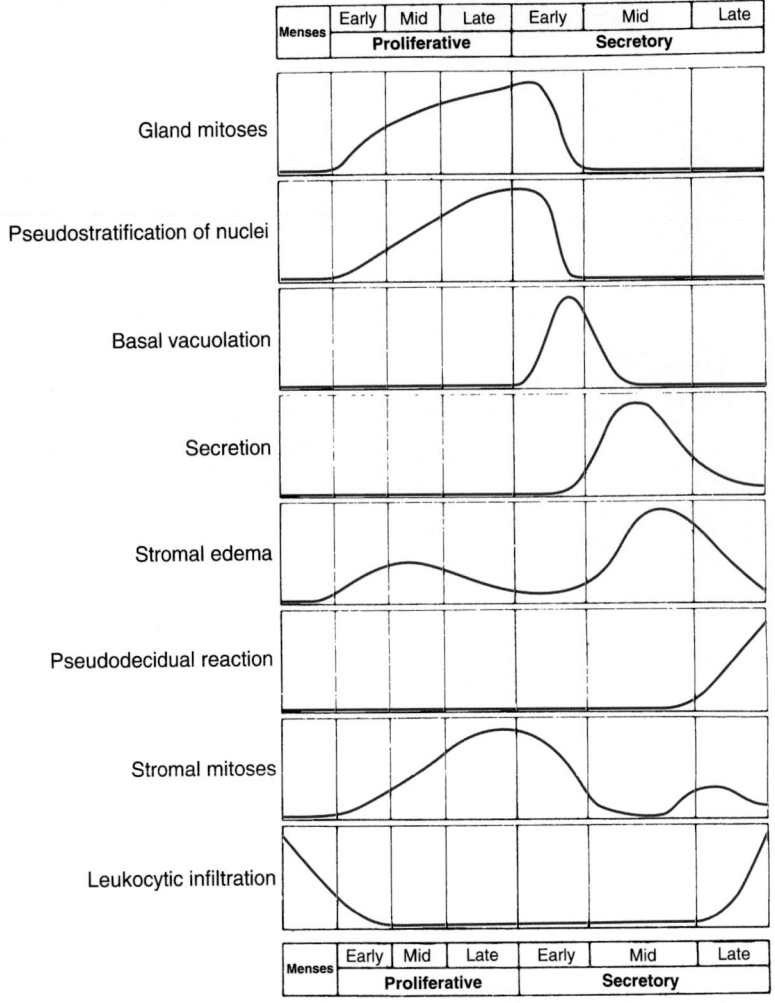

FIGURE 4-44 Patterns of histologic changes throughout menstrual cycle. (Modified from Noyes RW, Hertig AT, and Rock J: Fertil Steril 1:3, 1950. Reproduced with permission of the publisher, The American Fertility Society.)

Antibodies

In contrast to steroid hormones, protein hormones themselves are antigenic and can produce antibody formation. Since steroids are haptens and are not antigenic by themselves, they need to be attached to a carrier protein (usually bovine serum albumin) to induce antibody formation. Even with the injection of purified antigens, there is a degree of cross-reaction of most hormone antibodies (polyclonal) with other hormones. To increase assay specificity, antibodies are now being produced to eliminate the variability and heterogeneity of antibodies produced by several injections of antigen. Monoclonal antibodies are produced by first injecting the antigen into a mouse to induce an immunologic reaction in its spleen (Figure 4-50). The spleen cells are screened to find those particular ones (clones) capable of secreting a single antibody type. These cells are then fused with a myeloma cell from the same species to form a hybrid or hybridoma cell. Because of the immortality of the myeloma cell in culture, the hybridoma continually secretes antibodies characteristic of the selected spleen cell. This clone line is maintained in culture to provide homogenous monoclonal antibody molecules, which are used for sensitive and specific immunoassays of protein hormones.

Antigens

To produce standard curves, varying amounts of known pure preparations of hormone need to be utilized. Since steroid hormones are available as chemically pure preparations, the amount added to form the standard curve and determine the amount in the unknown can be expressed in terms of absolute mass or weight, such as nanograms

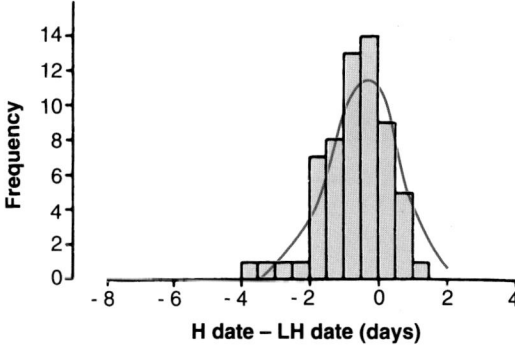

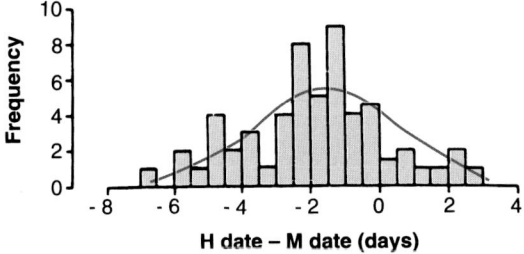

FIGURE 4-45 Frequency distribution of difference between histologic dating *(top)* and chronologic dating *(bottom)* by each method. *H date,* Mean value of histologic dating by two observers. *LH date,* Chronologic dating derived from LH surge. *M date,* Chronologic dating derived from onset of next menstrual period. Normal curve has been fitted to frequency distribution according to bar chart. (From Li TC, Rogers AW, Lenton EA, et al: Fertil Steril 48:928, 1987.)

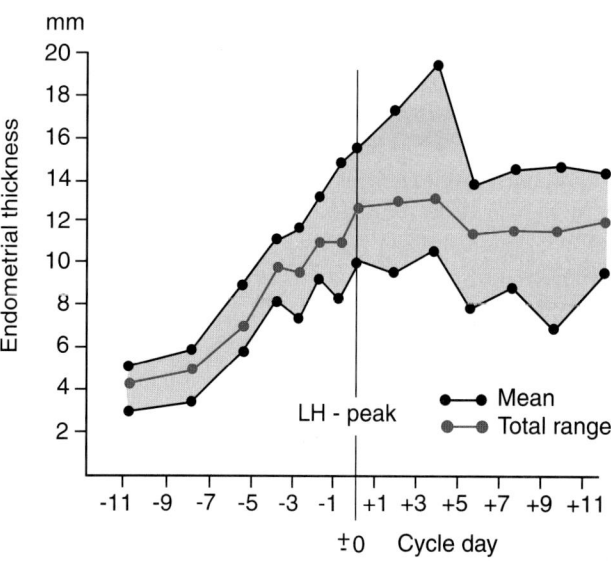

FIGURE 4-46 The endometrial thickness in mm measured by transvaginal ultrasound, presented as the mean and the total range, in 16 women during an ovulatory cycle. Each point on the curve represents a minimum of six observations.

(10^{-9}) or picograms (10^{-12}). Thus, the results obtained from different laboratories should be constant. However, most European laboratories express the results in terms of nanomoles instead of nanograms. For most steroids, about 3 nmol/L is equivalent to 1 ng/ml.

Protein hormones, however, being of high molecular weight, are not available in pure form. Therefore, the results of measuring unknown samples need to be expressed in terms of the amount of a standard reference preparation by use of standard extracts of the hormone obtained from collections of urine, serum, or pituitary glands. Thus, the levels of hormone measured by laboratories using different standards do not always agree, and clinicians should be aware of the normal levels used by these laboratories. The protein standard is frequently an international reference preparation, and the results are usually expressed in international units.

Assay Markers

As described earlier, quantitation in a radioimmunoassay is carried out by measuring the radioactive antigen (assay marker). The use of radioisotopes for radioimmunoassay has become a negative factor in recent years because of the problems associated with radioactive waste disposal. During the past few years, major advances have occurred in both the development of new instruments and the identification of new nonradioactive markers. When coupled to assay antigens, these result in assays whose markers are almost as sensitive as radioimmunoassay and sometimes are as sensitive as the most sensitive radioimmunoassay. Use of these markers has rejuvenated the field of immunoassays by allowing individuals without training in the use of radioisotopes to perform these assays. One can easily extend this use to the home, and "home kits" are becoming readily available. Examples of nonradioactive markers are given in the next section.

Types of Immunoassays

Because of advances made in the development of nonradioactive markers to replace the radioactive markers used in radioimmunoassays, many new types of assays, some related and others not related, to radioimmunoassays, have been established. All these assays, however, use the antigen-antibody interaction and thus are now usually referred to as immunoassays. Immunoassays can be categorized not only on the basis of whether they use excess antigen or excess antibody, but also according to whether they use a radioactive tracer. A categorization of some of the most frequently used types of immunoassays in reproductive endocrinology laboratories is shown in Table 4-6.

The basic principle of the nonradioactive immunoassays that use antigen excess is the same as that of radioimmunoassay (Figure 4-51). The nonradioactive immunoassay uses a nonradioactive tag, such as fluorescein in the fluorometric immunoassay (FIA), luminol in the chemiluminescent immunoassay (CIA), and an alkaline phosphatase conjugate in the enzyme immunoassay (EIA). Quantification of these tags is achieved by use of a fluorometer in the FIA and a luminometer in the CIA. In the EIA, quantification is carried out by addition of a specific substrate. For example, *p*-nitrophenylphosphate isused with alkaline phosphatase, and the product

formed, *p*-nitrophenol, can be measured spectrophotometrically.

Two of the most widely used excess-antibody assays in clinical reproductive endocrinology laboratories are the immunoradiometric assay (IRMA) and the enzyme-linked immunosorbent assay (ELISA). In the IRMA the principle involves the use of excess radiolabeled antibody that binds to the antigen, followed by removal of excess antibody. At present the two-site IRMA (Figure 4-52) is often employed. It requires the addition of a second antibody attached to a solid phase, such as a bead. The second antibody differs from the first one

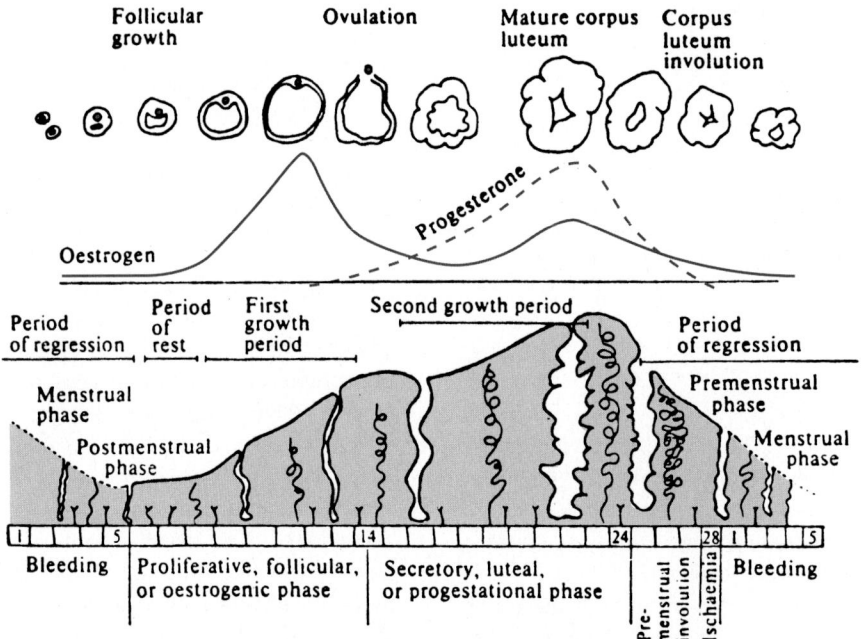

FIGURE 4-47   Diagram of changes in normal human ovarian and endometrial cycles. (From Shaw ST Jr and Roche PC: Menstruation. In Finn CA, editor: Oxford reviews of reproduction and endocrinology, vol 2, London, 1980, Oxford University Press.)

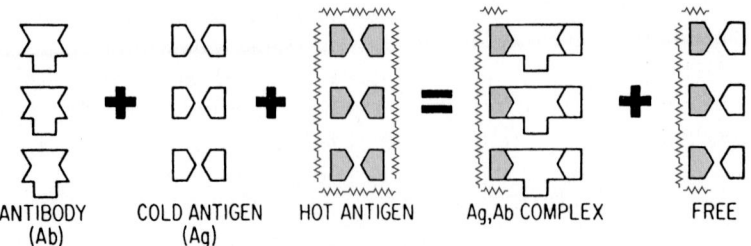

FIGURE 4-48   Schematic representation of antigen-antibody reaction in radioimmunoassay. For final analysis, free component must be separated from the antigen-antibody complex. (From Kletzky OA and Nakamura RM: Measurement of hormones. In Mishell DR Jr, Davajan V, and Lobo RA, editors: Infertility, contraception and reproductive endocrinology, ed 2, Cambridge, Mass, 1986, Blackwell Scientific Publications.)

in that the second is not radioactive and recognizes a different site on the antigen. Since the complex formed is attached to a solid phase, it can be readily separated from the excess radioactive antibody by centrifugation. The amount of radioactivity measured in the final complex is directly proportional to the concentration of standard used to prepare the standard curve and the concentration of analyte in the specimen. This is in contrast to the inverse relationship between the "bound" radioactivity and standard concentrations observed in a radioimmunoassay.

In the ELISA, antigen is bound to an excess of antibody, which is attached to a solid phase, such as a plastic tube or plate (Figure 4-53). Once the antigen-antibody complex is formed, an antibody-enzyme conjugate is added. The antibody in this conjugate is directed against an antigenic site different from that recognized by the first antibody. The result is a "sandwich" type of complex, thus the term *sandwich ELISA*. Following the addition of the appropriate substrate for the enzyme, the resulting product is measured spectrophotometrically. The relationship between the product concentration and concentration of standard or analyte is similar to that obtained by IRMA.

Four characteristics of assays apply to each of these techniques: sensitivity, specificity, accuracy, and precision. Sensitivity is the least amount of substance that can be measured in the assay. Specificity is the ability of the assay to measure only one substance and not allow the measurement to be altered by the presence of other substances (cross-reaction). Accuracy is the ability to measure the exact amount of substance in the sample; thus specimens (quality controls) containing known low and high values of the substance to be mea-

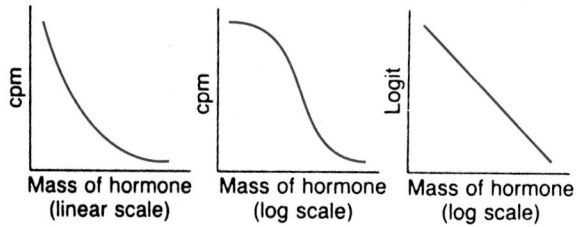

FIGURE 4-49 Standard curve using linear scale *(left)* or log scale *(center and right)* for the abscissa and linear *(left and center)* or logit *(right)* for the ordinate. *cpm,* Counts per minute. (From Nakamura RM and Stanczyk FZ: Immunoassays. In Lobo RA, Mishell DR Jr, Paulson RJ, and Shoupe D, editors: Mishell's textbook of infertility, contraception and reproductive endocrinology, ed 4, Malden, Mass, 1997, Blackwell Science.)

TABLE 4-6
Types of Immunoassays

Assay Type	Examples
Excess antigen	
Radioactive	Radioimmunoassay (RIA)
Nonradioactive	Chemiluminescent immunoassay (CIA)
	Fluoroimmunoassay (FIA)
	Enzyme immunoassay (EIA)
Excess antibody	
Radioactive	Immunoradiometric assay (IRMA)
Nonradioactive	Enzyme-linked immunosorbent assay (ELISA)

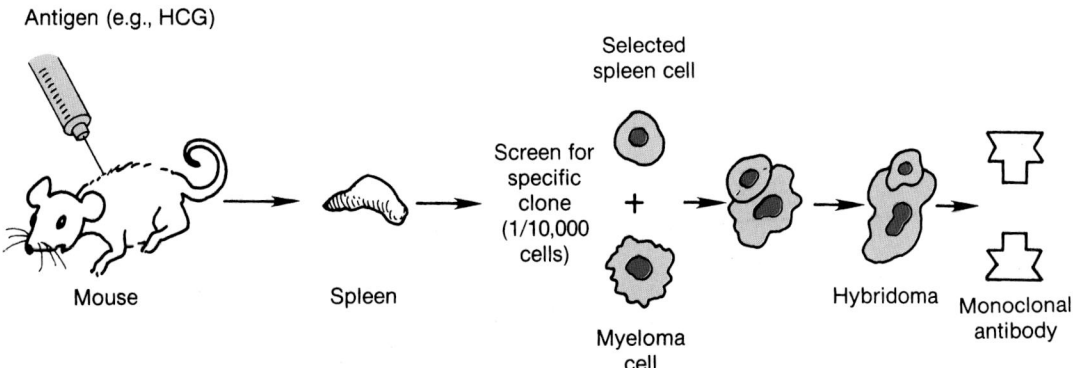

FIGURE 4-50 Schematic representation of monoclonal antibody production. (From Nakamura RM and Stanczyk FZ: Immunoassays. In Lobo RA, Mishell DR Jr, Paulson RJ, and Shoupe D, editors: Mishell's textbook of infertility, contraception and reproductive endocrinology, ed 4, Malden, Mass, 1997, Blackwell Science.)

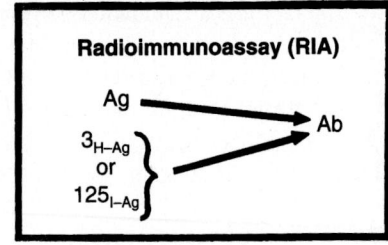

1. **Fluoroimmunoassay (FIA)**

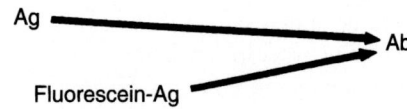

2. **Chemiluminescent assay (CIA)**

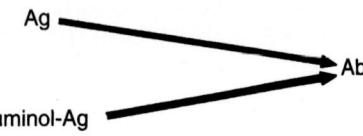

3. **Enzyme immunoassay (EIA)**

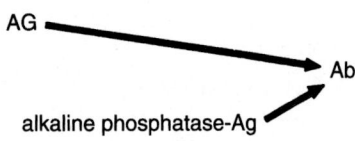

FIGURE 4-51 Competition between excess antigen *(Ag)* (analyte or standard) and excess radioactive or nonradioactive antigen (marker) for a limited amount of antibody *(Ab)*. (From Stanczyk FZ: Immunoassays. In Lobo RA, Mishell DR Jr, Paulson RJ, and Shoupe D, editors: Mishell's textbook of infertility, contraception and reproductive endocrinology, ed 4, Malden, Mass, 1997, Blackwell Science.)

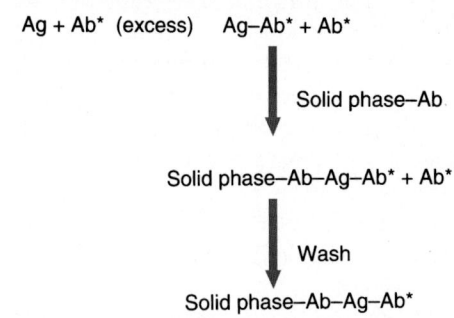

FIGURE 4-52 Principle of the immunoradiometric assay. *Ag,* Antigen; *Ab,* antibody. (From Stanczyk FZ: Immunoassays. In Lobo RA, Mishell DR Jr, Paulson RJ, and Shoupe D, editors: Mishell's textbook of infertility, contraception and reproductive endocrinology, ed 4, Malden, Mass, 1997, Blackwell Science.)

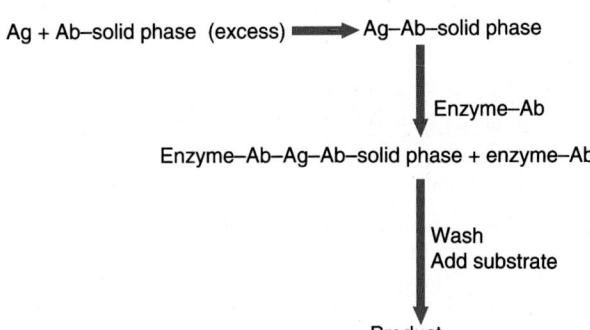

FIGURE 4-53 Principle of the enzyme-linked immunosorbent assay. *Ag,* Antigen; *Ab,* antibody. (From Stanczyk FZ: Immunoassays. In Lobo RA, Mishell DR Jr, Paulson RJ, and Shoupe D, editors: Mishell's textbook of infertility, contraception and reproductive endocrinology, ed 4, Malden, Mass, 1997, Blackwell Science.)

sured are always included in each assay. Precision is the ability of the assay to consistently reproduce the same results. Precision is determined by measuring the within-assay, or intraassay, coefficient of variation (CV) and the between-assay, or interassay, CV. The intraassay CV is calculated by determining the amounts of a known sample measured in about 10 replicates in the same assay.

$$CV = \frac{\text{Standard deviation}}{\text{Mean}} \times 100$$

The interassay CV is determined by measuring the same unknown sample on different days. The intraassay CV should be less than 10%, and the interassay CV should be less than 15% for satisfactory precision of the assay.

The normal range of values of hormones in normal women is frequently expressed in terms of the mean level plus the mathematically calculated 95% confidence limits (±2 SD). However, the distributions of hormone levels in the menstrual cycles of a group of women with normal ovulation have been shown to follow a log-normal distribution instead of a gaussian (normal) distribution. Although results of normal values usually vary from laboratory to laboratory, the 95% confidence limits of measurement of reproductive hormones among women in our laboratory are listed in Table 4-7 as a guide of normality.

TABLE 4-7
95% Confidence Limits of Hormones Used in Reproduction

Hormone	Phase of Menstrual Cycle			
	Follicular	Midcycle	Luteal	Menopause
LH (mIU/ml)	4.0–20.0	43–145	3–18	>40
FSH (mIU/ml)	3.2–9.0	10–18	3–9	>30
Prolactin (ng/ml)	8.0–20.0	0–22	10–30	8–25
Estradiol (pg/ml)	30–140	150–480	50–250	10–30
Progesterone (ng/ml)	0.5–1.0	0.8–2.0	3.0–31	0.5–1.0
Testosterone (ng/dl)	20–85	20–85	20–85	8–30*
Free testosterone (ng/dl)	1.2–9.9	1.2–9.9	1.2–9.9	3–13†
DHEA-S (μg/ml)	0.5–2.8	0.5–2.8	0.5–2.8	0.2–1.5

From Nakamura RM and Stanczyk FZ: Immunoassays. In Mishell DR Jr, Davajan V, and Lobo RA, editors: Infertility, contraception and reproductive endocrinology, ed 3, Cambridge, Mass, 1991, Blackwell Scientific Publications.

*In oophorectomized women the range is 4 to 18 ng/dl.

†In oophorectomized women the range is 1 to 10 ng/dl.

KEY POINTS

- The hypothalamic hormone that controls gonadotrophin release, namely gonadotrophin-releasing hormone (GnRH), is a decapeptide.

- The cell bodies of the hypothalamic neurons that produce GnRH are concentrated mainly in two areas: the anterior hypothalamus and the medial basal (tuberal) hypothalamus.

- GnRH can be released both in large amounts periodically via the tuberoinfundibular tract (cyclic release) and in a low-grade continuous transependymal fashion (tonic release) via the tanycytes.

- GnRH is secreted in a pulsatile manner. The amplitude and frequency of the pulses vary throughout the menstrual cycle. The frequency is rapid in the follicular phase, about one pulse per hour, and slower in the luteal phase, about one pulse every 2 or 3 hours.

- The most important neurotransmitters involved in reproductive neuroendocrinology are two catecholamines, dopamine and norepinephrine, as well as an indolamine, serotonin.

- Infusion of β-endorphin results in an increase in prolactin and a decrease in luteinizing hormone (LH), the latter occurring by an inhibitory effect on GnRH neurons in the hypothalamus.

- Peripheral measurement of plasma β-endorphin levels does not reflect levels in the central nervous system circulation.

- The peptide hormones, such as GnRH, bind to specific receptors on the surface membrane of the target cell, in contrast to steroid hormones, which pass through the cell membrane to bind to intracellular receptors.

- When a protein hormone binds to its specific receptor, it activates or inhibits the enzyme adenyl cyclase, the second messenger, which in turn changes the concentration of adenosine 3′,5′-cyclic monophosphate (cyclic AMP, cAMP).

- The various growth factors provide hormonal effects within the ovary by both autocrine and paracrine mechanisms.

- Inhibin inhibits pituitary follicle-stimulating hormone (FSH) release, whereas in the ovarian follicle inhibin stimulates progesterone and inhibits estradiol production. Activins have an opposite action to inhibins by stimulating pituitary FSH release and opposing ovarian action by inhibiting progesterone and stimulating estradiol.

- Biosynthesis of prostanoids from arachidonic acid and other precursors takes place via the cyclic endoperoxides, prostaglandins G and H (PGG and PGH). Prostanoids are produced intracellularly shortly before they are released and generally act locally, in contrast to steroids.

- Following a single intravenous bolus of GnRH, the LH levels peak in 30 minutes and FSH in 60 minutes.

- With a constant infusion of GnRH there is a biphasic release of LH but not of FSH. The initial increase of LH occurs 30 minutes, and the second, 90 minutes after the start of the infusion.

- When stimulation by hormone is maximal, the unoccupied receptors become refractory to hormone binding for 12 to 72 hours. This phenomenon has allowed frequent administration of GnRH analogues to be used clinically to inhibit FSH and LH levels, and thus decrease steroidogenesis.

- GnRH analogues are synthesized by substitution of amino acids in the parent molecule at the 6 and 10 positions. The various agonists have greater potencies and longer half-lives than the parent GnRH.

- LH and FSH have the same α subunit, which is similar in structure to the α subunit of thyroid-stimulating hormone and human chorionic gonadotrophin (HCG). The β subunits of all these hormones have different amino acids and carbohydrates, which provide specific biologic activity.

- The half-life of LH is more rapid (30 minutes) than that of FSH (3.9 hours).

- LH acts primarily on the theca cells to induce steroidogenesis, whereas FSH acts primarily on the granulosa cells to stimulate follicular growth.

- LH acts on the theca cells to produce androgens, which are then transported to the granulosa cells, where they are aromatized to estrogens.

- After sufficient LH receptors have been produced by the action of FSH and estradiol, LH acts directly on the granulosa cells to cause luteinization and production of progesterone.

- The ovary secretes three principal steroid hormones: estradiol from the follicle, progesterone from the corpus luteum, and androstenedione from the stroma.

- Pregnenolone, 17-hydroxypregnenolone, progesterone, 17-hydroxyprogesterone, and corticosteroids have 21 carbon atoms; androgens (testosterone and androstenedione) have 19 carbon atoms; estrogens have 18 carbon atoms and a phenolic ring A.

- Because the ovaries lack 21-hydroxylase, 11β-hydroxylase, and 18-hydroxylase reductase activity, they are unable to synthesize mineralocorticoids or glucocorticoids.

- Estradiol and estrone are interconverted outside the ovary. Estrone is then converted to estrone sulfate, which has a long half-life and is the largest component of the pool of circulating estrogens.

- The greater the amount of fat tissue present, the greater is the percentage of androstenedione that is converted to estrone. In a normal individual, about 1.3% of the daily 3000 μg of androstenedione produced is converted to estrone (40 μg), whereas in an obese individual as much as 7% of the 3000 μg is converted (200 μg).

- The process by which steroids are conjugated involves the transformation of lipophilic compounds, which are only sparingly soluble in water, into metabolites (sulfates and glucuronides) that are readily water soluble and can therefore be eliminated in urine. Progesterone first undergoes extensive reduction of its double bond and ketone group(s) before it is conjugated. Its major urinary metabolite is pregnanediol glucuronide. The major urinary metabolites of estradiol and estrone are glucuronides and sulfates of estrone, estradiol, and estriol.

- Sex hormone–binding globulin (SHBG) primarily binds dihydrotestosterone, testosterone, and estradiol. About 65% of circulating testosterone is bound to SHBG and 30% to albumin. Approximately 2% remains unbound or free.

- Corticosteroid-binding globulin (CBG) binds with highest affinity to cortisol, corticosterone, and 11-deoxycortisol, and to a lesser extent to progesterone.

- Estrogen stimulates the synthesis of both estrogen and progesterone receptors in target tissues, and progestins inhibit the synthesis of both estrogen and progesterone receptors.

- Just before birth the primary oocytes, which at that time number 2 to 4 million, reach the diplotene stage, also called the germinal vesicle stage of development.

- Estradiol stimulates preantral follicle growth, reduces follicular atresia, and increases FSH action on the granulosa cells. Testosterone increases follicular atresia and prevents preantral follicle growth.

- The follicle destined to become dominant secretes the greatest amount of estradiol, which in turn increases the density of FSH receptors.

- With ultrasound it has been found that there is a steady increase in follicular diameter and volume that parallels the rise in estradiol. The dominant follicle has a maximal mean diameter of about 19.5 mm, with a range of 18 to 25 mm just before ovulation. The mean maximal follicular volume is 3.8 ml, with a range of 3.1 to 8.2 ml.

- Ovulation occurs about 24 hours after the estradiol peak, as well as 32 hours after the initial rise in LH, and about 12 to 16 hours after the peak of LH levels in serum.

- The midcycle LH surge initiates germinal vesicle disruption, and metaphase I is completed. As the oocyte enters metaphase II, the first polar body appears. Completion of meiosis and extrusion of the second polar body occur only when a sperm penetrates the ovum.

- By serial ultrasound observation and LH measurements, ovulation usually occurs within 24 hours and always within 48 hours after the peak in LH.

- Beginning in the midluteal phase, progesterone is secreted in a pulsatile manner, occurring immediately following an LH pulse.

- Serum levels of estradiol rise from less than 50 pg/ml in the early follicular phase to 200 to 500 pg/ml at midcycle and have a broad luteal-phase peak level of about 100 to 300 pg/ml.

- Progesterone levels in serum are less than 1 ng/ml before ovulation and reach midluteal levels of 10 to 20 ng/ml.

- During a normal ovulatory cycle at midcycle, the first event is a rise in estradiol. When estradiol reaches peak levels, there is an abrupt increase (surge) in LH and FSH. The increase in LH reaches a peak in about 18 hours, and peak levels plateau for about 14 hours, after which there is a decline. The mean duration of the LH surge is about 24 hours. Beginning about 12 hours before the onset of the LH surge, there is an increase of both progesterone and 17-hydroxyprogesterone.

- With the occurrence of the LH peak, there is a decline in estradiol and a further increase in progesterone. This shift in steroidogenesis in favor of progesterone instead of estradiol production is brought about by the luteinization of the granulosa cells produced by LH.

- Menstrual cycle length is most irregular in the 2 years after menarche and the 3 years before menopause, times of life during which anovulatory cycles are most frequent.

- The mean duration of menstrual cycle length is 28 ± 7 days, with menstruation in which cycles occur at more frequent intervals (<21 days) being called polymenorrhea, and that in which cycles are less frequent (>35 days) being called oligomenorrhea. The mean duration of menstrual flow is 4 ± 2 days.

- Only the spiral arteries that supply the upper two thirds of the endometrium become coiled and constrict.

- After menstruation, regeneration of the endometrium comes from cells in the spongiosum that were previously a portion of the secretory endometrium and not from the stratum basale, as previously believed.

- The endometrium produces growth factors, prostaglandins, and peptide hormones, including a specific peptide called pregnancy-associated endometrial protein.

- The subjective method of correlating the degree of maturation in the endometrium by histologic visualization is relatively imprecise, and more precise indices based on quantitative morphometric analysis have been developed. To date the endometrium most accurately, the maturation should be correlated with the days after LH peak, not the number of days before the onset of the next menstrual period.

- There are extreme variations in the amounts of endometrial shedding in different areas of the same uterus, as well as variations among different uteri removed by hysterectomy.

- Menstruation in humans is probably a combination of some superficial tissue shedding, brought about by ischemia and the presence of hydrolytic enzymes and possibly relaxin, as well as mainly by tissue regression and reorganization of the endometrial cells.

- Just after ovulation, glycogen-rich subnuclear vacuoles appear in the base of the cells lining the glands. This subnuclear vacuolization is the first histologic indication of the effect of progesterone, but is not evidence that ovulation has occurred.

- Enzyme-linked immunosorbent assay (ELISA), or "sandwich," techniques have been developed to measure protein hormones (e.g., LH, FSH, hCG), with the use of monoclonal antibodies against the α and β subunits. The endpoint is a color reaction and can be read in a spectrophotometer.

- There are four characteristics of hormone assays that establish their reliability: sensitivity, specificity, accuracy, and precision.

BIBLIOGRAPHY

Bächström CT, McNeilly AS, Leask RM, et al: Pulsatile secretion of LH, FSH, prolactin, oestradiol and progesterone during the human menstrual cycle, Clin Endocrinol 17:29, 1982.

Bakos O, Lundkvist O, Wide L, and Bergh T: Ultrasonographical and hormonal description of the normal ovulatory menstrual cycle, Acta Obstet Gynecol Scand 73:790, 1994.

Brzech PR, Jakimiuk J, Agarwal SK, et al: Serum immunoreactive leptin concentrations in women with polycystic ovary syndrome, J Clin Endocrinol Metab 81:4166, 1966.

Chehab FF, Mounzih K, Lu R, and Lim ME: Early onset of reproductive function in normal female mice treated with leptin, Science 275:88, 1997.

Chikasawa K, Araki S, and Tameda T: Morphological and endocrinological studies on follicular development during the human menstrual cycle, J Clin Endocrinol Metab 62:305, 1986.

Clark JR, Dierschke DJ, and Wolf RC: Hormonal regulation of ovarian folliculogenesis in rhesus monkeys. III. Atresia of the preovulatory follicle induced by exogenous steroids and subsequent follicular development, Biol Reprod 25:3320, 1981.

Crowley WF Jr, Filicori M, Spratt DI, et al: The physiology of gonadotropin-releasing hormone (GnRH) secretion in men and women, Recent Prog Horm Res 41:501, 1985.

Diczfalusy E and Landgren BM: Hormonal changes in the menstrual cycle. In Diczfalusy E and Diczfalusy A, editors: Regulation of human fertility, Copenhagen, 1977, Scriptor.

di Zerega GS and Hodgen GD: The interovarian progesterone gradient: a trial and temporal regulator of folliculogenesis in the primate ovarian cycle, J Clin Endocrinol Metab 54:495; 1982.

Eissa MK, Obhrai MS, Docker MF, et al: Follicular growth and endocrine profiles in spontaneous and induced conception cycles, Fertil Steril 45:191, 1986.

Felberbaum RE, Germe U, Ludwig M, et al: Treatment of uterine fibroids with a slow-release formulation of the gonadotropin releasing hormone antagonist Cetrorlix, Human Reprod 13(6):1660, 1998.

Ferenczy A: Studies on the cytodynamics of human endometrial regeneration, Am J Obstet Gynecol 124:64, 1976.

Filicori M, Santoro N, Merriam GR, et al: Characterization of the physiological pattern of episodic gonadotropin secretion throughout the human menstrual cycle, J Clin Endocrinol Metab 62(6):1136, 1986.

Flowers CE and Wilborn WH: New observations on the physiology of menstruation, Obstet Gynecol 51:16, 1978.

Frisch RE: Body fat, menarche, and reproductive ability, Semin Reprod Endocrinol 3:45, 1985.

Knobil E: The neuroendocrine control of the menstrual cycle, Recent Prog Horm Res 36:53, 1980.

Laughlin GA, and Yen SSC: Serum leptin levels in women with

polycystic ovarin syndrome: the role of insulin resistance/hyperinsulinemia, J Clin Endocrinol Metab 82:1692, 1997.

Lemay A, Maheux R, Faure N, et al: Reversible hypogonadism induced by a LH-RH agonist (Buserelin) as a new therapeutic approach for endometriosis, Fertil Steril 41:863, 1984.

Li TC, Dockery P, Rogers AW, et al: How precise is histologic dating of endometrium using the standard dating criteria? Fertil Steril 51:759, 1989.

Li TC, Rogers AW, Lenton EA, et al: A comparison between two methods of chronological dating of human endometrial biopsies during the luteal phase, and their correlation with histologic dating, Fertil Steril 48:928, 1987.

Li TC, Rogers AW, Dockery P, et al: A new method of histologic dating of human endometrium in the luteal phase, Fertil Steril 50:52, 1988.

Lin D, Sugawara T, Strauss JF, III, et al: Role of steroidogenic acute regulatory protein in adrenal and gonadal steroidogenesis, Science 267;1828, 1995.

McLennan CE and Rydell AH: Extent of endometrial shedding during normal menstruation, Obstet Gynecol 26:605, 1965.

Nogales-Ortiz F, Puerta J, and Nogales FF Jr: The normal menstrual cycle, J Obstet Gynecol 51:259, 1978.

Nolan JJ, Olefsky JM, Nyce MR, et al: Effect of troglitazone on leptin production: studies in vitro and in human subjects, Diabetes 45:1276, 1996.

Reame N, Sauder SE, Kelch RP, et al: Pulsatile gonadotropin secretion during the human menstrual cycle: evidence for altered frequency of gonadotropin-releasing hormone secretion, J Clin Endocrinol Metab 59:328, 1984.

Reissman T, Felberbaum R, Diedrich K, et al: Development and applications of luteinizing hormone-releasing hormone antagonists in the treatment of infertility: an overview, Hum Reprod 10(8):1974-81, 1995.

Ross GT, Cagrille CM, Lipsett MB, et al: Pituitary and gonadal hormones in women during spontaneous and induced ovulatory cycles, Recent Prog Horm Res 26:1, 1970.

Treloar AE, Boynton RE, Borghild BG, et al: Variation of the human menstrual cycle through reproductive life, Int J Fertil 12:77, 1967.

Yalow RS and Berson SA: Assay of plasma insulin in human subjects by immunological methods, Nature 184:1648, 1959.

Zegers-Hochschild F, Lira CG, Parada M, et al: A comparative study of the follicular growth profile in conception and nonconception cycles, Fertil Steril 41:244, 1984.

CHAPTER
5

Evidence-Based Medicine and Clinical Epidemiology

Attributable Risk. The excess cases or the fraction of a disease in the population that is due to a particular factor or exposures. Also the population excess rate or the rate difference.

Bias. Any effect at any stage of investigation or inference tending to produce results that depart systematically from the true values (to be distinguished from *random error*). The term *bias* does not necessarily carry an imputation of prejudice or other subjective factor, such as the experimenter's desire for a particular outcome. This differs from conventional usage in which *bias* refers to a partisan point of view.

Case-Control Study. A study that starts with the identification of persons with the disease (or other outcome variable) of interest and a suitable control (comparison, reference) group of persons without the disease. The relationship of an attribute to the disease is examined by comparing the diseased and nondiseased with regard to how frequently the attribute is present or, if quantitative, the levels of the attribute in each of the groups.

Clinical Practice Guideline. A systematically developed statement designed to assist clinician and patient decisions about appropriate health care for specific clinical circumstances.

Cohort. 1. The component of the population born during a particular period and identified by period of birth so that its characteristics (e.g., causes of death and numbers still living) can be ascertained as it enters successive time and age periods. 2. The term *cohort* has broadened to describe any designated group of persons who are followed or traced over a period of time, as in cohort study (prospective study).

Cohort Study. Involves identification of two groups (cohorts) of patients, one that received the exposure of interest and one that did not, and following these cohorts forward for the outcome of interest.

Confidence Interval, Confidence Limits. A range of values determined by the degree of presumed random variability in the data, within which the point estimate is thought to lie, with the specified level of confidence. The boundaries of a confidence interval are the confidence limits. The confidence interval is symmetric around the point estimate. If the confidence interval overlaps 1.0, the change in risk is statistically insignificant.

Confounding. A situation in which the effects of two processes are not separated. The distortion of the apparent effect of an exposure on risk brought about by the association with other factors that can influence the outcome.

Epidemiology. The study of the distribution and determinants of health-related states and events in a population, and the application of this study to control of health problems.

Evidence-Based Medicine. The conscientious, explicit, and judicious use of current best evidence in making decisions about the care of individual patients. The practice of evidence-based medicine means integrating individual clinical expertise with the best available external clinical evidence from systematic research.

Incidence. The proportion of new cases of the target disorder in the population at risk during a specified time interval.

Meta-Analysis. A systematic review that uses quantitative methods to summarize the results. Meta-Analysis is a collection of techniques to produce a pooled effect estimate from several studies.

Observational Study (nonexperimental study, survey). Epidemiologic study in situations where nature is allowed to take its course; changes or differences in one characteristic are studied in relation to changes or differences in other(s), without the intervention of the investigator.

Odds Ratio (cross-product ratio, relative odds). The ratio of two odds. Consider the following notation for the distribution of a binary exposure and a disease in a population or a sample:

	Exposed	**Unexposed**
Disease	a	b
No disease	c	d

The odds ratio (cross-product ratio) is ad/bc. The exposure-odds ratio for a set of case-control data is the ratio of the odds in favor of exposure among the cases (a/b) to the odds in favor of exposure among noncases (c/d). This reduces to ad/bc. With incident cases, unbiased subject selection, and a rare disease (say, under 2% cumulative incidence rate over the study period), ad/bc is an approximate estimate of the risk ratio.

Outcomes. All possible results that may stem from exposure to a causal factor or from preventive or therapeutic interventions; all identified changes in health status arising as a consequence of the handling of a health problem.

Positive Predictive Value. Proportion of people with a positive test who have the target disorder.

Power. Relative frequency with which a true difference of specified size between populations would be detected by the proposed experiment or test. It is equal to 1 minus the probability of type II error. Resolving power is the comparable property of individual measurements.

Precision. The quality of being sharply defined or stated. One measure of precision is the number of distinguishable alternatives from which a measurement was selected, sometimes indicated by the number of significant digits in the measurement. Another measure of precision is the standard error of measurement, the standard deviation of a series of replicate determinations of the same quantity. In statistics, precision is defined as the inverse of the variance of a measurement or estimate.

Random Error (sampling error). Error due to chance, when the result obtained in the sample differs from the result that would be obtained if the entire population ("universe") were studied. Two varieties of sampling error are type I, or alpha error, and type II, or beta error. In an experiment, if the experimental procedures do not in reality have any effect, an apparent difference between experimental and control groups may nevertheless be observed by chance, a phenomenon known as type I error. Another possibility is that the treatment is effective but by chance the difference is not detected on statistical analysis—type II error. In the theory of testing hypothesis, rejecting a null hypothesis when it is incorrect is called "type I error." Accepting a null hypothesis when it is incorrect is called "type II error."

Randomized Control Clinical Trial (RCT). A group of subjects is randomized into an experimental group and a control group. These groups are followed up for the variables/outcomes of interest.

Relative Risk. The ratio of the risk of disease or death among the exposed to the risk among the unexposed; this usage is synonymous with risk ratio. Alternatively, the ratio of the cumulative incidence rate in the exposed to the cumulative incidence rate in the unexposed (i.e., the cumulative incidence ratio). The term *relative risk* has also been used synonymously with *odds ratio* and, in some biostatistical articles, has been used for the ratio of the forces of morbidity. The use of the term *relative risk* for several different quantities arises from the fact that for rare diseases (e.g., most cancers) all the quantities approximate one another. For common occurrences (e.g., neonatal mortality in infants under 1500 g birth weight), the approximations do not hold.

Risk Ratio (RR). The ratio of risk measured in the treated group (ERR) to risk measured in the control group. Used in randomized trials and cohort studies: RR = ERR/CER.

Sensitivity. The proportion of truly diseased persons in the screened population who are identified as diseased by the screening test. Sensitivity is the measure of the probability of correctly diagnosing a case or the probability that any given case will be identified by the test.

Specificity. The proportion of truly nondiseased persons who are so identified by the screening test. It is a measure of the probability of correctly identifying a nondiseased person with a screening test.

Systematic Review. A summary of the medical literature that uses explicit methods to perform a thorough literature search and critical appraisal of individual studies and that uses appropriate statistical techniques to combine these valid studies.

There is an ongoing explosion of knowledge in the basic sciences that forms the basis of the medical sciences. A fundamental of medical science is to take our knowledge of embryology, genetics, anatomy, and endocrinology and then apply this knowledge to clinical problems. The leap from bench to bedside, however, is vast and uncertain, and the results can be inadequate.

Clinical epidemiology comprises a set of methods that

can help us directly at the bedside and inform public health decisions. The results of observational epidemiologic studies help connect the bench and the bedside by generating hypotheses about diseases that can be tested in the laboratory. Similarly, experimental studies in humans, the randomized clinical trials, serve to test ideas that arise in the laboratory to see if they apply to clinical practice as predicted.

This chapter presents the basics of epidemiologic study design and the statistical terminology commonly used to present results of clinical studies; however, statistical methods per se are not covered here. We also discuss approaches for interpreting study results. Finally, we consider new, explicit approaches to combining data from different studies that are used to prepare evidence reviews and clinical guidelines. This information will help the clinician read and interpret the clinical literature.

ESSENTIALS OF STUDY DESIGN

The basic purpose of an epidemiologic study is to estimate the relationship between an exposure and an outcome in order to establish whether a causal relationship exists. An exposure can be a behavior, a genetic factor, a screening program, or any aspect of a treatment. An outcome can be a symptom, a measure of functional status, a new-onset disease, or a change in the course of an existing disease. Some studies are primarily descriptive, providing statistics about incidence, prevalence, and mortality rates of diseases in particular populations. Descriptive studies are important to the clinician in order to provide a context—the most dramatic new research findings always must be interpreted with respect to the frequency and characteristics of the disease in one's own patient population. Descriptive studies can also help generate new hypotheses, but studies with this design do not serve to test hypotheses or answer etiologic questions.

More applicable to evidence-based medical practice are analytic epidemiologic studies that focus on establishing an association between a particular exposure (e.g., hormone replacement therapy) and the risk of a particular disease or outcome (e.g., reduction in the incidence of osteoporotic fractures). Analytical epidemiologic studies can be classified as experimental or observational. In experimental studies, the clinical investigator controls exposure to the factor of interest. Experimental studies, or randomized controlled trials (RCTs), are characterized by the prospective assignment of study participants to a study group (who receive the factor of interest, typically a new treatment) or a placebo, no treatment, and/or standard care group. Study groups, usually two, but often many more, are then followed over time to evaluate differences in outcomes. The outcomes may include prevention or cure of a disease, reduction in severity of the condition, or differences in costs, quality of life, or side effects between the treatments. The great feature of RCTs is that,

through randomizing participants, they can equalize all other factors that might influence the study outcome and leave only the effect of the study treatment itself. RCTs usually provide the best evidence for making clinical decisions. Despite the theoretical superiority of the RCT approach, this is true only if the study has been thoughtfully designed, implemented with extraordinary care, and analyzed appropriately.

Subjects recruited for a trial must receive information about the study purpose, its procedures, the likely risks and benefits, and the available alternatives. Both ethical and practical considerations may limit the use of randomized trials to answer clinical questions. It is clearly unethical to expose anyone to a potential cause of disease simply to learn about etiology; thus we do not randomize our patients to, for instance, smoking in order to learn about the effect of tobacco on the ovary. RCTs are rarely used to address etiologic questions. To study the effect of a treatment, making comparisons with a placebo control group is usually most efficient. However, if an effective and accepted treatment exists, it is not ethical to use a placebo control group for studies of serious conditions where the subject may experience harm due to lack of effective treatment. If the condition is mild, the treatment period is brief, or effective treatment is not generally available, many investigators believe that a placebo control group is ethical. For a clinician to recruit or refer patients into a clinical trial, it is essential the clinician believe, based on current evidence, that the study treatments may be similar or at least balanced in benefits and harms. This belief state is called "therapeutic equipoise." If a clinician believes that evidence already exists to indicate a treatment is superior, then it is not ethical to recruit subjects into a comparative trial. In contrast, if the superior treatment is unclear, then a randomized trial is the most ethical approach for all patients because it provides them with an equal chance to undergo the better treatment, and also may provide an unbiased answer to the clinical question more quickly so all future patients can benefit. Clearly, it is critical to be honest and humble about our current state of knowledge prior to planning any randomized clinical trial.

Practical considerations frequently determine whether a clinical question will be addressed using a randomized trial. Acute clinical problems where every patient has a relevant outcome in a short period of time are ideal to study using clinical trials. Gynecologic examples include comparisons of short-term pain or febrile morbidity following different surgical approaches, comparisons of cure rates or side effects in the treatment of infections, or pregnancy rates following different infertility treatment regimens. For clinical problems like these, clinicians should be able to rely on RCT data. In contrast, RCTs to study long-term or rare outcomes are much more difficult to carry out. If a treatment outcome is rare or takes years to develop (cancer being an excellent example of both), one needs a very large study over years or decades to answer the clinical question. Even when large trials like the Women's Health Initiative are implemented, clinicians usually have to rely on other data for clinical decision making during the many years before study results are available. Finally, because of the time, effort, and expense involved in carrying out an RCT, many questions of great clinical interest have not yet been addressed in this way.

Observational studies, where the investigator does not control the exposure, provide an alternative approach to answering clinical questions. Depending on the data collection process, observational studies are classified as cross-sectional, cohort, or case-control studies. Cross-sectional studies generate prevalence data by examining the relationship between exposure and the outcomes of interest in a defined population at a single point in time. With reference to only a designated moment in time, these studies are not able to provide strong causal evidence. However, cross-sectional studies can highlight associations that deserve additional evaluation whether in clinical experiments or in the laboratory.

Epidemiologic studies that provide stronger evidence are cohort and case-control studies (Figure 5-1). A cohort study selects a group of individuals at risk for the outcome of interest and divides them into subgroups based on the presence or absence of one or more exposures to be studied. Subgroups are then evaluated over time to count the outcomes as they occur. Unlike RCTs, in cohort studies the exposure is selected by the individual subject, not by the investigator. Most studies of the long-term health effects of contraceptive methods have employed a cohort design where the subjects themselves decided which contraceptive method to use. A particular difficulty of this approach is that the subjects almost certainly differ in many characteristics beyond the main exposure of interest. When these other characteristics are related to both the exposure and the risk of experiencing an outcome, they can confound the results of the study. Age, for instance, is nearly always a confounding variable. Advancing age increases the risk of a heart attack and most other diseases and is also associated with very decreased use of oral contraceptives. If age is not accounted for in a statistical analysis, it might appear that oral contraceptives provide enormous protection against heart attacks because all of the (older) women experiencing heart attacks are not oral con-

traceptive users anymore. To the extent that we collect information about known or suspected confounding factors, it is possible to control their effect in the statistical analysis, and precise adjustment for age is needed in most studies. Adjustment techniques can work only for confounding variables that the investigators know about and measure. A reason that RCTs provide stronger evidence than observational studies is that randomization balances confounding variables across the study groups, even confounders that are not recognized to be important at the time the study is performed.

A strength of cohort studies is the possibility of assessing many different outcomes over time, but a weakness is often the need to wait many years until enough outcomes occur to allow an analysis. Thanks to computerized databases of medical information, cohort studies can now sometimes be done historically; that is, the research question is formulated and the analyses are done years after the data have been collected and recorded for routine uses. This approach can be quick and very cost effective, but the value of such studies is completely dependent on the quality of the original data.

Case-control studies are always retrospective. Study participants are selected on the basis of already having the outcome of interest (the case group) or of not having that outcome (the control group). Case status needs to be carefully defined and should include all cases of new-onset disease drawn from an identifiable population. Controls should be sampled from the same population; the purpose of the control group is to estimate the frequency in the population of the exposures being studied if there were no relationship with the disease being studied. In the past, investigators often found it convenient to select controls from among other patients found in the same hospital as the cases, but choosing controls from the general population is highly preferable. After identifying the cases and controls, data are then gathered, usually by interview, concerning past exposures. The exposure information from cases and controls is then compared quantitatively to obtain an estimate of risk. As with cohort studies, statistical adjustment techniques are needed to account for confounding variables. The quality of the results from these studies is very dependent on uniform, meticulous interview techniques when collecting data from cases and controls. The

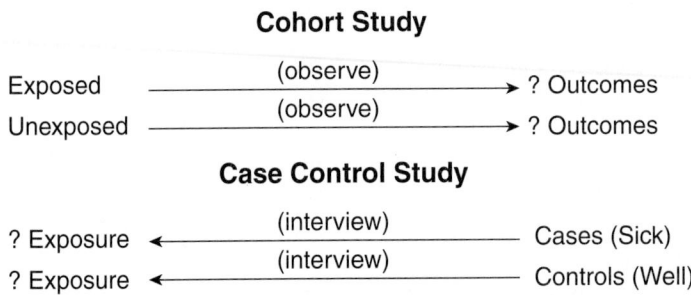

FIGURE 5-1 Schematic diagram of methodology used to estimate risk of exposure to outcome in cohort and case-control studies.

case-control study is often the best approach to study rare diseases. A case-control study including only 8 cases and 31 controls was able to identify the strong association between vaginal adenocarcinoma and in utero exposure to diethylstilbesterol (DES). Although a randomized trial of DES had been performed to evaluate its now-recognized ineffectiveness in preventing spontaneous abortion, that study was not large enough or long enough to identify a rare cancer that was identified in daughters 20 years later.

PRESENTATION OF STUDY RESULTS

Epidemiologic studies use a quantitative approach to describing both exposures and outcomes. Whether RCT, cohort study, or case-control study, all of these studies attempt to present their results as a single number, usually referred to as the point estimate, that quantifies the relationship between the exposure and the outcome. This number is an estimate of the truth rather than the truth itself because each study, however large, includes only a sample of all the people who are affected by the exposure–outcome relationship. The point estimate expresses the strength of the association between the exposure and outcome. In an RCT or a cohort study, the point estimate is the relative risk (RR). Risk in the study subjects is the number of cases or outcomes that occur over time. The relative risk is simply

---

TABLE 5-1
Interpretation of Relative Risk (RR)
and Odds Ratio (OR) Values

RRs and ORs <1.0 indicate protection from outcome.

RRs and ORs >1.0 indicate risk of outcome.

RRs and ORs = 1.0 indicate no association to outcome.

For both RR and OR, the further away the value is from 1.0 the stronger the relationship.

---

the risk of disease (or other outcome) among the exposed or treated subjects divided by the risk in the unexposed subjects. A case-control study does not measure risk directly, but calculates its results as an odds ratio (OR), which is generally equivalent to a relative risk from a cohort study (Table 5-1).

If there is no association at all between the exposure and outcome, then the RR or OR would be 1.0. RRs and ORs greater than 1.0 indicate an increased risk of the outcome. RRs and ORs less than 1.0 indicate a decreased risk of the outcome. For both RRs and ORs the further away the value is from 1.0, the stronger the relationship between the exposure and the outcome (Figure 5-2). Investigators do not limit the presentation of all of their analyses to a single

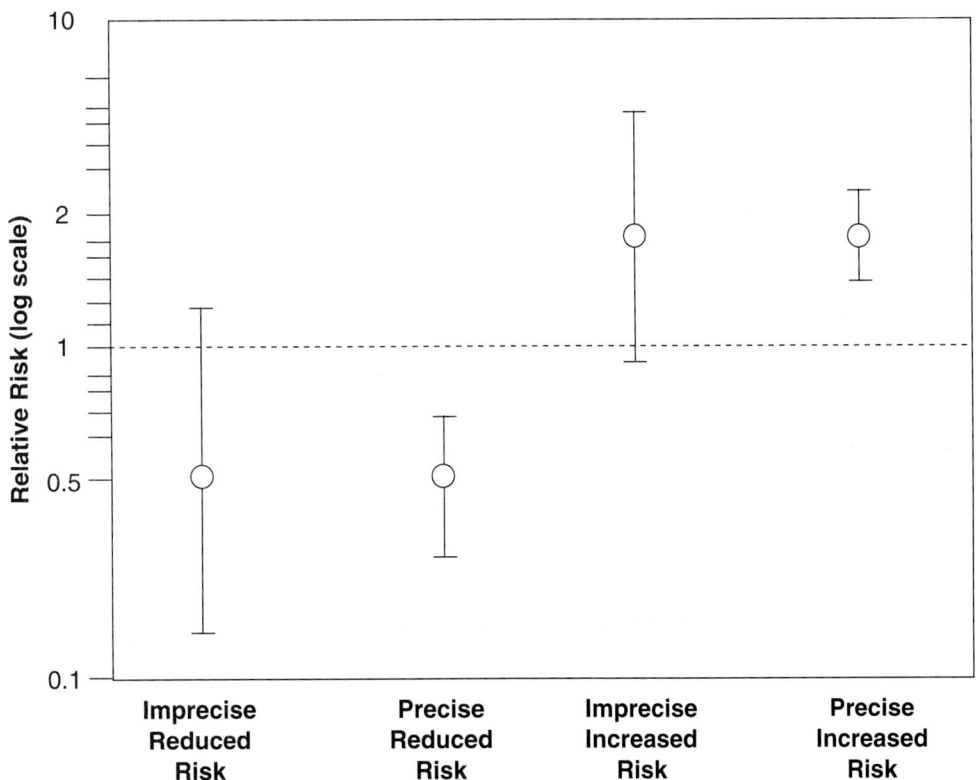

FIGURE 5-2 Examples of point estimates (○) and confidence intervals (Ⅰ) of two studies with reduced risk and two studies with increased risk. If confidence interval overlaps 1.0, the change in risk is statistically insignificant.

point estimate. Usually RRs are presented separately for different doses (e.g., estrogen levels in the oral contraceptive) or durations of exposure (e.g., pack-years of cigarette smoking) or for subgroups of subjects (e.g., those with or without a family history of the outcome).

Because the relative risk is based on results from just the people in one particular study and not the entire universe, there is sampling error; thus the quantitative description of the study results needs to include a measure of this uncertainty. The confidence interval is widely used to express the precision of the point estimate; a wide confidence interval indicates less precision, and a narrow confidence interval indicates more. In general, the larger the study, the narrower the confidence interval. There are several cautions about interpreting confidence intervals correctly. First, the confidence interval indicates only uncertainty that is due to the play of chance; it does not inform us about uncertainty in the results due to other factors such as uncontrolled confounding or peculiarities of the population that was studied or poor study quality. Second, a wide confidence interval does not mean there is no association between the exposure and the outcome; even an imprecise point estimate remains the best answer and the best explanation of the relationship until that estimate is supplanted by results from larger or better studies. Finally, confidence intervals are often drawn as a straight line around the point estimate to show the width of their range; this might seem to suggest that the location of the true point estimate would be equally likely to fall anywhere within that interval. In fact, the confidence interval could better be shown as a bell-shaped curve centering on the point estimate, and the true point estimate thus is most likely to be close to the center of the range.

Relative risk estimates do not take into account the incidence or the importance of the problem being evaluated. A relative risk of 4 says that the outcome increases 400% in exposed individuals compared to unexposed individuals. This increase often causes great worry or excitement, but needs to be interpreted in the context of the frequency of the outcome. For instance, the incidence of venous thromboembolism (VTE) in young women without using oral contraceptives is about 1 in 10,000, and the incidence while using oral contraceptives is 4 in 10,000; thus the relative risk is 4. The absolute risk of VTE is still low in both groups of women with a difference in risk of 3 in 10,000. The risk in the exposed minus the risk in the unexposed is the risk difference. The risk difference describes the size of the effect in absolute terms. This is also called attributable risk, and it is very useful for putting large relative risks into a clinically useful perspective. This is also called the absolute risk reduction when a benefit is identified, and the absolute risk increase when a harm is identified.

For clinicians and patients, even the calculation of absolute risk differences in a population may not seem a very helpful way to assess possible risks and benefits in personal terms. An alternative calculation looks at the complementary concept: how many patients need to be treated to observe one benefit or one adverse event? The number of patients who need to be treated to achieve one additional good outcome is the reciprocal of the absolute risk reduction (the risk difference for good outcomes). The number of patients who, if they received the treatment, would lead to one additional patient being harmed, compared to patients not receiving the treatment, is the reciprocal of the absolute risk increase (the risk difference for bad outcomes). Thus, using the example of oral contraceptives, with a treatment effectiveness of about 97%, and a risk of VTE of 4 in 10,000, the number needed to treat (NNT) to avoid one pregnancy is 1.03 (the reciprocal of 0.97, which is the absolute risk reduction) and the number needed to harm (NNH), that is, to experience one extra VTE, is 3333 (the reciprocal of 3 in 10,000, which is the absolute risk increase). The effectiveness of oral contraceptives and other contraceptives is extraordinarily high, and because pregnancy is extremely common in the absence of contraception, the NNT is close to 1, that is, one treatment yields one good outcome. In contrast, for most preventive services, the outcome to prevent is less common and the treatment is less effective; thus, in providing drug therapy to prevent osteoporotic fractures in menopausal women, the NNT is generally greater than 20. Calculations of NNT and NNH are increasingly being used to calculate the potential benefits and harms of therapies, preventive services, and screening tests. A benefit of these calculations is that they allow us to compare benefits and harms across different treatment strategies.

INTERPRETATION OF STUDY RESULTS

Not every association found in a study is due to cause and effect. We can attempt to assess whether causation is a good explanation of an association based on the quality of the study, the design of the study, and other specific criteria. Making these assessments is a critical part of evidence-based medicine. The design of the study is the simplest criterion to assess; a well-designed and properly controlled randomized trial is the highest level of evidence, and associations identified in this type of study can generally be interpreted as causal. When the available evidence comes from observational studies, it is generally necessary to apply additional criteria to decide whether the reported associations are likely to be causal.

In all studies the process of data collection, analysis, and interpretation can lead to conclusions that are systematically different from the truth. These deviations can occur through study bias or the presence of confounding variables. Selection bias is an error due to systematic differences in characteristics between those selected to participate in the study and those who are not selected. For instance, women without health insurance might never have a chance to enter a study because they cannot be seen at the center where the study is offered; women who are very busy with work and home responsibilities might not have the time to meet study requirements; study results thus may only apply to the subset of women who have an opportunity to enter a study. There are also biases due to diagnostic testing. For instance, women who take oral contraceptives may see their physician more often than women who have undergone tubal ligation. Consequently, women using oral contraceptives may undergo more screening and diagnostic tests, and diseases may be uncovered more often in this group. Recall bias occurs because recall of information is affected by illness, which can be a major problem for retrospective studies. Women with an illness may recall in great detail all events they believe might be associated with the illness, whereas healthy controls may not remember similar exposures. Several other factors can bias the assessment of drug side effects. First, is the intense surveillance of patients who are placed on a new therapy compared to those taking an older, conventional therapy. This often leads to more complete identification of adverse events among those using newer therapy. Conversely, the long-term users of any treatment tend to be unusually healthy and free of side effects because all those who don't tolerate the treatment well will have stopped using it. These biases tend to make new treatments appear more dangerous and old treatments more safe than they really are. Biases are more likely to occur in observational studies than in randomized trials.

Distinguishing whether associations are causal is highly relevant to clinical care. If an association is strong (i.e., the relative risk is far from 1.0) and precise (i.e., narrow confidence intervals), and if the risk or benefit is clinically important based on the context, then it is particularly important to assess causality. For three decades, the Bradford-Hill criteria have been used as one approach to differentiate causality from association (Table 5-2). In the United States these criteria are often referred to as the surgeon general's criteria because of their initial use in interpretation of evidence regarding cigarette smoking and lung cancer. An experiment, in regard to these criteria, is typically a randomized, controlled trial. The investigator has controlled for all differences between two groups except the treatment under study. This kind of evidence can provide the strongest support for a causal relationship. If a relative risk is strong, at least greater than 2.0 or less than 0.5, causality is a more likely explanation. Weaker associations can often be explained instead by confounding variables, and weak associations are frequently overinterpreted by enthusiastic investigators or worried patients. The presence of a dose-response effect or duration-response effect also supports a causal association as when a higher dose or a longer treatment is associated with a better treatment response. In contradistinction, peculiar dose-response effects indicate the need for more study to understand the effect. Biologic plausi-

bility also needs to be considered in evaluating results, especially from observational studies; our knowledge of physiology can often support, refute, or indicate a need for more data. The notion of specificity can be more challenging to apply. One exposure, one outcome is an appealing and parsimonious approach to scientific explanation, and when a relationship is that specific, causality is likely. Conversely, when an exposure is related to a wide range of bad outcomes—or good ones—one must suspect a placebo effect is operating or an unsuspected bias. As a caution against dismissing such relationships too easily, an early argument rejecting the adverse health effects of cigarette smoking was that the very wide range of adverse effects was too nonspecific to be true! It seems obvious that an exposure causes an outcome only if it precedes the outcome. An important weakness of cross-sectional studies is that they often cannot establish the temporality of the relationship being evaluated. Even with stronger study designs, our lack of knowledge about the timing of the preclinical onset of a condition can make it difficult to obtain exposure information for the biologically important interval. Seeking analogies can help clarify a possible cause-and-effect relationship. We need to consider whether similar agents or drugs are known to have similar effects. We also need to consider whether the same exposure is known to cause similar diseases. Finally, coherence of the evidence demands that the criteria listed above be considered in conjunction with all of our other knowledge. Some of the above criteria consider the internal validity of the study; others consider the external validity: how the study relates to the larger population outside of the study. We also need to consider how the study results fit in with our general biologic knowledge including data from animal and laboratory studies.

TABLE 5-2
Bradford-Hill Criteria for Causation

Experiment	Investigator control or laboratory experiments
Strength	Size of RR (>2.0 or <0.5)
Consistency	Similar RR in several studies
Gradient	Dose-response relationship
Biologic plausibility	Physiologic explanation for association
Specificity	Outcome only associated with intervention
Temporality	Exposure precedes outcome
Analogy	Similar association in other related diseases or exposures
Coherence	Evidence from different sources fits together

R, relative risk.

(From Bradford-Hill A: Principles of medical statistics, ed 9, New York, 1971, Oxford University Press, p 309.)

REVIEW AND SYNTHESIS OF THE EVIDENCE

Evidence-based medicine relies on the assessment of our full body of knowledge, which is usually not limited to a single study. The process of evidence-based medicine starts with formulating a specific clinical question and then finding the best research evidence. Research evidence only rarely applies exactly to our own patient population or to the particular clinical problem that has our attention. Therefore, the research evidence must be evaluated for our own context, and integrated with our clinical expertise and with the preferences and values of each patient. The process is motivated by our need for up-to-date and valid information regarding diagnosis, prognosis, therapy, and preventive services. Practicing evidence-based medicine has become possible in large part because of the development of information systems that allow us to search for relevant clinical data. At best, we can look for data using the Internet right at the bedside or in the clinic to address specific questions that apply to our current patient. The bedside practice of evidence-based medicine can be efficient and practical if we learn to find and use sources that synthesize and summarize the effects of the interventions we are interested in.

Because individual studies often have imprecise results, statistical methods to combine the results sometimes can be helpful. Meta-analysis is a collection of techniques to produce a pooled effect estimate from several studies. Meta-analysis at its best involves pooling and reanalyzing raw data from several similar randomized trials to produce a result with a tighter confidence interval. Several statistical approaches are used, but the main purpose of any meta-analysis is to improve precision. There are many meta-analyses that combine data from observational studies (rather than randomized trials), but these must be interpreted with extreme caution because the individual studies always vary in population, entry criteria, case definition, and exposure definitions, and these differences make combining the data problematic. This is particularly true if the analysis combines data from published tables rather than combining the raw data from the original studies. If the results from individual studies disagree in direction or report very different results, then meta-analysis is not appropriate. Often the main value of a meta-analysis proves to be the rigorous approach to collecting, evaluating, and presenting together all of the relevant data regarding a particular problem.

To make the assessment of evidence more uniform, a grading system that rates studies according to quality is often used (Table 5-3). This grading system rates the randomized clinical trial as the highest level of evidence. Following this are controlled trials without randomization. The next level of evidence comes from cohort studies and case-control studies. Although results taken from cross-sectional studies, studies that rely on external control groups, and ecological studies are a lesser level of evidence,

Level	Evidence
I	At least one properly controlled randomized trial.
II-1	Controlled trials without randomization.
II-2	Well-designed cohort and case-control studies.
II-3	Cross-sectional studies, studies with external control groups, or ecological studies.
III	Evidence derived from report of an expert committee, which itself used a scientific approach.

TABLE 5-3
Categorizing the Level of Evidence

The periodic health examination Canadian Task Force on the Periodic Health Examination. Reprinted with permission from the publisher, CMAJ 121:1193, 1979.

they often remain valuable specifically because of the lack of higher levels of evidence. All of these sources of evidence are more valuable than opinion, regardless of the credentials of the individual, committee, or organization that might publish an opinion.

Because of the clinical need for good evidence and the need for evidence synthesis that goes beyond opinion, additional approaches to evidence reviews are being developed and used. Systematic evidence reviews include a comprehensive review and evaluation of the literature and are reported using a standardized format that must include a detailed description of the search strategy used to identify the relevant literature and the results of the search. Systematic reviews also carry out critical appraisal of the studies they evaluate. Critical appraisal employs a rigid standardized assessment of the relevance and quality of each study. The goal of systematic reviews is to synthesize the world literature regarding a specific clinical question and to use an approach that will minimize bias and random error.

Because systematic reviews are so comprehensive, they are typically far too long to be published as regular journal articles. Journal articles may present a summary of an evidence review, but readers generally have to go to sources on the Web to find complete documentation of these reviews. The major source of systematic reviews is the Cochrane Collaboration (*www.cochrane.org*). This collaboration is an international organization that aims to help people make well-informed decisions about health care by preparing, maintaining, and promoting the accessibility of systematic reviews of the effects of health care interventions. There are review groups for more than 50 areas of medicine including several that are relevant to gynecology; the groups in each area prepare and electronically publish systematic reviews. The U.S. Preventive Services Task Force also performs systematic reviews regarding clinical preventive services; these are published in book form and increasingly as electronic publications by the Agency for Healthcare Research and Quality (ARHQ). To help translate these often lengthy reviews into briefer, clinically useful documents, many professional groups have begun to issue practice guidelines to assist clinicians in making patient-care decisions. An electronic collection of such guidelines is now available; to be accepted for electronic publication, the guideline must specify the search strategy that was used to obtain the evidence and must specify the methods of data synthesis (*www.guidelines.gov*).

Recommendations are often graded, but the systems for grading evidence and practice recommendations are continuing to evolve. In general, recommendations for or against clinical interventions need to specify whether they are based on ample or sparse evidence, and whether the evidence comes from randomized trials or from lesser studies. Even with recommendations based on ample evidence from RCTs, clinicians will always need to decide individually whether the available evidence applies to their practice setting and whether it applies directly to their specific patient problem.

KEY POINTS

- Epidemiologic studies link laboratory bench research to the bedside.

- Randomized controlled trials (RTCs) provide the strongest level of evidence to link cause and effect and are used to test hypotheses.

- Randomized trials may not be practical to study outcomes that are extremely rare or take many years to develop.

- Cohort studies are often excellent to study a single exposure that may lead to a wide range of outcomes.

- Case-control studies are excellent to study rare diseases and to evaluate a wide range of exposures.

- Descriptive studies, including cross-sectional and ecological studies, help generate hypotheses and also can illuminate the size and context of a health problem.

- Evidence-based medicine helps provide firm basis for clinical decisions.

BIBLIOGRAPHY

Bradford-Hill A. Principles of medical statistics, ed 9, New York, Oxford University Press, 1971.
Fletcher RH, Fletcher SE, Wagner EH: Clinical epidemiology, the essentials, ed 2, Baltimore, 1988, Williams & Wilkins.
Herbst AL, Poskanzer DC, Robboy SJ, et al: Prenatal exposure to stilbestrol. A prospective comparison of exposed female offspring with unexposed controls, N Engl J Med 13:334, 1975.
Kelsey JL, Whittemore AS, Evans AS, and Thompson WD: Methods in observational epidemiology, ed 2, New York, 1996, Oxford University Press.
Last JM: A dictionary of epidemiology, New York, 1983, Oxford University Press.

Meinert CL and Tonascia S: Clinical trials, design, conduct, and analysis, New York, 1986, Oxford University Press.
Petitti DB: Meta-analysis, decision analysis, and cost-effectiveness analysis: methods for quantitative synthesis in medicine, ed 2, New York, 2000, Oxford University Press.
Sackett DL, Haynes RB, Guyatt GH, and Tugwell P: Clinical epidemiology: a basic science for clinical medicine, ed 2, Boston, 1991, Little, Brown.
Sackett DL, Straus SE, Richardson WS, et al: Evidence-based medicine: how to practice and teach EBM, ed 2, New York, 2000, Churchill Livingstone.
U.S. Preventive Services Task Force: Guide to clinical preventive services, ed 2, Alexandria, Va, 1996, International Medical Publishing.

PART TWO

Comprehensive Evaluation of the Female

History, Physical Examination, and Preventive Health Care

General, Gynecologic and Psychosocial History and Examination, Health Care Maintenance, Disease Prevention

Anovulatory Cycle. Menstrual cycle when ovulation does not occur.

Dyspareunia. Painful intercourse.

Dysuria. Painful urination.

Ectropion. The presence of endocervical (glandular) epithelium on the portio vaginalis of cervix. It may result from scarring of the external os or it may be congenital.

LMP. Last menstrual period.

Menstrual Formula. Age of menarche × number of days of cycle × number of days of menstrual flow (e.g., 13 × 28 × 5).

Metaplasia. The process of covering glandular epithelium or raw areas with squamous epithelium.

Nabothian Cyst. An inclusion cyst of the cervix.

Normal Transformation Zone. Area of columnar epithelium and squamous metaplasia in the vagina or on the cervix that has normal colposcopic patterns.

PMP. Previous menstrual period.

Portio Vaginalis. The portion of the cervix exposed to the vagina.

Sexual Dysfunction. A psychologic or physiologic problem or condition that prevents the usual full participation and enjoyment of coitus.

Total Procedentia. The prolapse of the uterus and cervix through the introitus.

The first contact a physician has with a patient is critical. It allows an initial bond of trust to be developed on which the future relationship may be built. The patient will share sensitive information, feelings, and fears. The physician will gain her confidence and establish rapport by the understanding and nonjudgmental manner in which he or she collects these data.

The first contact generally involves taking a complete history, performing a complete physical examination, and ordering appropriate initial laboratory tests. In such a way the physician gains impressions of the patient's problems and needs and develops a plan for solutions. A gynecologic history includes a complete general history and adds information of gynecologic importance. In like manner the physical examination should be complete; no corners should be cut. The physician practicing obstetrics and gynecology should not assume that the patient's general medical needs are cared for by others but should assume the role of her primary physician.

This chapter focuses on the appropriate manner that a gynecologic physician should use to conduct a history and physical examination and discusses the appropriate ingredients of ongoing health maintenance.

DIRECT OBSERVATIONS BEFORE SPEAKING TO PATIENT (NONVERBAL CLUES)

When meeting a patient it is important to *look* at her even before speaking. Some experienced physicians observe patients sitting in their waiting rooms before actually beginning personal contact. The general demeanor of the patient should be evaluated. Basically five general impressions can be transmitted both by facial expression and by posture, including happiness, apathy, fear, anger, and sadness.

A patient who is happy, self-assured, and in good personal control generally has a relaxed face with a smile and a sparkle in her eyes. She is generally sitting relaxed and will offer the physician a warm and friendly greeting. Many new patients are apprehensive about meeting a new physician, and this apprehension may modify their usual expression of good spirits. Even under these circumstances, however, their warmth shows. Happy patients returning for visits after having established a relationship with a physician are usually warm, relaxed, and responsive.

Apathetic patients generally have a blank facial expression. The eyes lack sparkle, there is little muscular movement of the face, and the mouth is generally thin and in a neutral position, neither turned up nor down. The posture may be somewhat slouched, the handshake may be weak, and answers to verbal questions are short and unemotional. Although apathetic patients may have severe emotional illness, they may also be demonstrating resignation to an imagined or serious condition or they may be responding to multiple problems, which make them feel overwhelmed.

The frightened patient frequently has a tense expression on her face; her mouth is tight and the eyes are darting and narrow. She may be perspiring but have a dry mouth. Her posture demonstrates forward leaning, and there is often endless hand activity. When she reacts, it may be grossly out of proportion to offered stimuli.

The angry patient frequently has narrowed eyes, furrowed brows, and narrow, tight lips. She may be sitting on the edge of her chair, leaning forward as if to pounce. Unlike the frightened patient, whose pose may be defensive, the angry patient radiates aggression. Her voice is usually harsh, and her overreaction to questions usually involves short, threatening phrases.

The sad patient generally sits with slouched shoulders; large, sad eyes; and a turned-down mouth. The eyes may glisten, and there may be tears. This patient is most likely depressed, and her speech reflects remorse and hopelessness.

By observing these nonverbal clues, the physician determines the appropriate style for conducting the interview. Often an opening remark appropriate to the patient's demeanor may be useful, such as, "You seem sad today, Ms. Jones," or, "I detect a note of anger in your voice, Ms. Smith. Can you tell me why that is?" By so doing, the physician projects sensitivity to the patient's feelings and genuine care with respect to her circumstances.

ESSENCE OF THE GYNECOLOGIC HISTORY

Chief Complaint

The patient should be encouraged to tell the physician why she has sought help. Questions such as, "What is the nature of the problem that brought you to me?" or, "How may I help you?" are good ways to begin. The patient should be able to present the problem as she sees it, in her own words, and should be interrupted only for specific clarification of points or to offer direction if she digresses too far. During the interview the physician should face the patient with direct eye contact and acknowledge important points of the history either by nodding or by a word or two. Such an approach allows the physician to be involved in the problem and demonstrates a degree of caring to the patient. When the patient has completed the history of her current problem, pertinent open-ended questions should be asked with respect to specific points made by the patient. This process allows the physician to develop a more detailed database. Directed questions may be asked where pertinent to clarify points. In general, however, the patient should be encouraged to tell her story as she sees it rather than to react with short answers to very specific questions. Under the latter circumstance the physician may get the answers he or she is looking for, but they may not be accurate answers.

A general outline for a gynecologic and general history is given in the box on the facing page. The outline is given in a specific order for general orientation. The information, however, may be collected through any comfortable discussion with the patient that seems appropriate in the circumstances. It is important that all aspects be covered.

Pertinent Gynecologic History

A pertinent gynecologic history can be divided into several parts. It begins with a menstrual history, in which the age of menarche, duration of each monthly cycle, number of days during which menses occur, and regularity of the menstrual cycles should be noted. The dates of the last menstrual period and previous menstrual period should be obtained. In addition, the characteristics of the menstrual flow, including the color, the amount of flow, and accompanying symptoms, such as cramping, sweating, headache, or diarrhea, should be noted. In general, menstruation that occurs monthly (range 21 to 40 days), lasts 4 to 7 days, is bright red, and is often accompanied by cramping on the day preceding and the first day of the period is characteristic of an ovulatory cycle. Menstruation that is irregular, often dark in color, painless, and frequently short or very long may indicate lack of ovulation. The first few cycles in teenagers or cycles in premenopausal women are frequently anovulatory and as a result may come at irregular intervals.

History Outline

I. Observation—nonverbal clues
II. Chief complaint
III. History of gynecologic problem(s)
    A. Menstrual history—LMP, PMP
    B. Pregnancy history
    C. Vaginal and pelvic infections
    D. Gynecologic surgical procedures
    E. Urologic history
    F. Pelvic pain
    G. Vaginal bleeding
    H. Sexual status
    I. Contraceptive status
IV. Significant health problems
    A. Systemic illnesses
    B. Surgical procedures
    C. Other hospitalizations
V. Medications, habits, and allergies
    A. Medications taken
    B. Medication and other allergies
    C. Smoking history
    D. Alcohol usage
    E. Illicit drug usage
VI. Bleeding problems
VII. Family history
    A. Illnesses and causes of death of first-order relatives
    B. Congenital malformations, mental retardation, and reproductive wastage
VIII. Occupational and avocational history
IX. Social history
X. Review of systems
    A. Head
    B. Cardiovascular/respiratory
    C. Gastrointestinal
    D. Genitourinary
    E. Neuromuscular
    F. Psychiatric
    G. Depression
    H. Physical abuse
        1. Sexual abuse
            a. Incest
            b. Rape

The second pertinent point in the gynecologic history is that of previous pregnancies. The patient should be asked specifically to list pregnancies that she has experienced, including the year of the pregnancy; the duration; the type of delivery; the size, sex, and current condition of the baby; any complications that may have occurred; and whether the infant was breastfed and, if so, for how long. Elective terminations of pregnancy and spontaneous abortions should also be noted, including the time of gestation that they occurred and the circumstances under which they took place. Ectopic or molar pregnancies should also be noted, including the type of therapy that was given. When such events have occurred, obtaining old records for review is appropriate. Any pregnancy should be discussed with respect to excessive bleeding, chills, fever, known infection, or other complicating events. It is also appropriate to ask the patient about the individual who fathered each of these pregnancies so that the physician may determine the number of sexual partners the patient has had.

A history of vaginal and pelvic infections should be obtained. The patient should be asked what types of infection she has had, what treatment was received, and what complications were experienced. Risk factors for human immunodeficiency virus (HIV) infection, such as intravenous drug abuse or coitus with drug abusers or bisexual men, should be sought by direct questioning and HIV screening offered where appropriate. All hospitalizations should be reviewed as to cause and outcome.

All instances of gynecologic surgical procedures should be noted, including minor operations, such as endometrial biopsies; vulvar, vaginal, or cervical biopsies; dilation and curettage; laparoscopic examinations; and any major procedure that the patient may have undergone. When such data are elicited, dates, types of procedures, diagnoses, and significant complications should be noted. In cases where pertinent, past records should be sought.

A careful urologic history should be taken. A history of bladder dysfunction, dysuria, loss of urine, acute or chronic bladder or kidney infections, or other urologic problems, such as hematuria or the passage of kidney stones, should be noted.

Symptoms of pelvic pain or discomfort should be discussed fully. The pain should be described, noting the presence or absence of a relationship to the menstrual cycle and its association with other events, such as coitus or bleeding.

Any vaginal bleeding not related to menses should be noted, as well as its relationship to the menstrual cycle and to other events, such as coitus, the use of tampons, or the use of a contraceptive device.

A complete sexual history should be obtained (see box on page 140), and specific problems should be evaluated. The history should include whether the patient is sexually active, the types of relationships she has, whether she is orgasmic, whether she experiences pain or discomfort with coitus (dyspareunia), and whether she or her partner is experiencing problems with sexual performance (sexual dysfunction). It is important that the physician review or rehearse the types of questions that will be asked and consider the response he or she will give to less typical answers (e.g., responses concerning homosexuality or less common sexual practices). This helps prevent the physician from demonstrating surprise and thus transmitting an attitude of disapproval.

Finally, the patient's contraceptive history should be investigated, including methods used, length of time they have been used, and any complications that may have arisen.

Important Points of Sexual History

1. Sexual activity (presence of)
2. Types of relationships
3. Individual(s) involved
4. Satisfaction? Orgasmic?
5. Dyspareunia
6. Sexual dysfunction
   a. Patient
   b. Partner

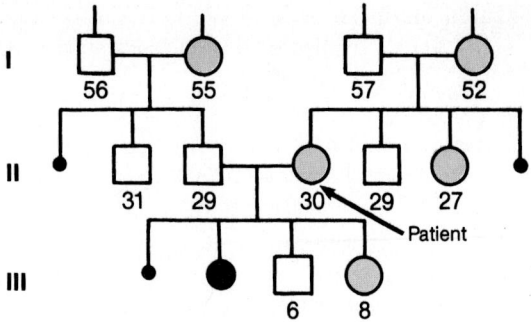

● Spontaneous miscarriage

◯ Living females

▢ Living males

● Female who died neonatally because of prematurity (30 weeks)

FIGURE 6-1 Family tree of typical gynecologic patient.

General Health History

The patient should be asked to list any significant health problems that she has had during her lifetime, including all hospitalizations and operative procedures. It is reasonable for the physician to ask about specific illnesses, such as diabetes, hepatitis, tuberculosis, or rheumatic fever, that seem likely based on what is known about the patient or about the patient's situation. Some physicians use a history checklist of the most common conditions, but a careful physician who questions appropriately can be equally effective.

Medications taken and reasons for doing so should be noted, as should allergic responses to medications. Patients should be encouraged to bring all medications, both prescription and over-the-counter drugs, to subsequent health maintenance visits.

The patient should be questioned for evidence of a bleeding or clotting problem, such as a history of hemorrhage with minor procedures, easy bruisability, or bleeding from mucous membranes.

A history of smoking should be obtained in detail, including amount and length of time she has smoked. She should be questioned about the use of illicit drugs, including marijuana and cocaine. Any affirmative answers should be followed by specific questions concerning length of use, types of drugs used, and side effects that may have been noticed. Her use of alcohol should be detailed carefully, including the number of drinks per day and any history of binge drinking or previous therapy for alcoholism.

Family History

A detailed family history of first-order relatives (mother, father, sisters, brothers, children, and grandparents) should be taken, and a family tree constructed (Figure 6-1). Serious illnesses or causes of death for each individual should be noted. Also, an inquiry should be made about any congenital malformations, mental retardation, or pregnancy wastage in either the patient's or her husband's family. Such information may offer clues to hereditarily determined causes of reproductive problems.

Occupational and Social History

The patient should be asked to detail her and her husband's occupational histories, including jobs held and work performed. It is also useful to elicit a history of hobbies and other avocations that might affect health or reproductive capacity.

A social history should be obtained. This involves where and with whom the patient lives, other individuals in the household, areas of the world where the patient and her husband have lived or traveled, and unusual experiences that either may have had.

Safety Issues

The patient should be questioned about safety matters. She should be asked about the use of seat belts and helmets (if she rides a bicycle or motorcycle or rides a horse). She should be asked whether there are firearms in her household and, if so, whether appropriate safety precautions are taken.

A discussion regarding whether the patient's hearing is adequate to ensure safety while she goes about her usual activities is important, especially in older women who may be suffering hearing loss, but also in younger women who may use Walkman-type recorders while they walk or jog. Appropriate footwear should be encouraged, taking into consideration the woman's usual activities, physical capabilities, and age.

Review of Systems

A complete review of systems is necessary to uncover symptoms from other areas that relate to reproduction and gynecologic problems (e.g., serious headaches, epileptic seizures, dizziness, or fainting spells). Such a history also may indicate exposure to medications that may be injurious should a pregnancy occur.

It is important to obtain a good cardiovascular/respiratory history, as well as a history of hypertension, heart disease, or chest problems, such as asthma. Each of these may have an immediate effect on the patient and may also influence a future pregnancy.

Of importance to the gynecologist is a history of gastrointestinal disorders, such as functional bowel problems, diverticulitis, diverticulosis, or hepatitis. Patients should be asked about any rectal incontinence of gas or stool that they may be experiencing or have experienced in the past. Affirmative answers should be fully investigated with respect to specific illnesses and potential residuals that may affect the patient's current health or well-being.

Questions about the genitourinary system are important both from the standpoint of bladder function and as an indication of whether renal function has been or is impaired.

Neurologic or neuromuscular impairment may be important from the standpoint of the ability of the patient to carry and deliver a child without difficulty.

A history of vascular disease, including thrombophlebitis with or without pulmonary embolism, varicose veins, or other vascular problems, should be sought. If a positive history of thrombophlebitis is obtained, possible relationship to a hormonal exposure, such as pregnancy or oral contraceptive use, should be sought.

The psychiatric history should be detailed carefully for any emotional or mental disease processes. Specifically, evidence for depression and suicidal ideology should be sought. In addition, the patient should be asked specifically whether she has been sexually abused in adult life, in childhood, by a stranger, or incestuously, or raped. This topic is further discussed in Chapter 9. Finally, she should be questioned about the possibility of physical abuse, neglect, or intimidation.

ESSENCE OF COMPLETE PHYSICAL EXAMINATION

The gynecologist should perform a complete physical examination on every patient at the first visit and at each annual checkup, particularly if the gynecologist is the primary physician caring for the patient. Physical examination is a time both to gather information about the patient and to teach the patient information she should know about herself and her body.

The patient should disrobe completely and be covered by a hospital gown that ensures warmth and modesty. During each step of the examination she should be allowed to maintain personal control by being offered options whenever possible. These options begin with the presence or absence of a chaperone. The chaperone, a third party,

usually a woman, serves a variety of purposes. She may offer warmth, compassion, and support to the patient during uncomfortable or potentially embarrassing portions of the examination. She may help the physician to carry out procedures, such as the Papanicolaou (Pap) smear, and in some cases she offers the physician protection from having his or her intentions misunderstood by a naive or suspicious individual. Although the presence of a chaperone is not absolutely imperative in every physician-patient relationship, the availability of one for the specific instance where it is deemed advisable should be ensured. Many clinics insist on the presence of a chaperone, and it is wise for the physician to follow local custom.

The examination should begin with a general evaluation of the patient's appearance and posture. Her weight and her blood pressure should be taken initially, and postmenopausal women should have their height measured routinely to document evidence of osteoporosis, which causes vertebral compression fractures.

The patient's eyes, ears, nose, and throat should be examined. Funduscopic examination should be performed at least annually to inspect the blood vessels of the retina and to observe the lens for evidence of early cataract formation. The gynecologist should either measure intraocular pressures in women over age 40 or suggest that they be seen by an ophthalmologist for this purpose. The patient should be inspected for evidence of upper lip or chin hair, which may indicate increased androgen activity.

The thyroid gland should be palpated for irregularities or increase in size (goiter). Discrete areas of enlargement, hardness, and tenderness should be described. The patient's neck should be palpated for evidence of adenopathy along the supraclavicular and posterior auricular chains.

The chest should be inspected for symmetry of movement of the diaphragm, percussed for areas of consolidation, and auscultated bilaterally for breath and adventitious sounds.

The heart should be examined by palpation for points of maximum impulse, percussed for size, and auscultated for irregularities of rate and evidence of murmurs and other adventitious sounds. An older woman's neck should be auscultated for evidence of vascular bruits. The patient's heart should be auscultated in both the lying and the sitting positions.

A careful breast examination should be carried out in a systematic fashion as described in Chapter 14. At this time the patient should be taught breast self-examination and encouraged to perform this each month.

The abdomen should be systematically examined in the following fashion:

Inspection. The abdomen should be inspected for symmetry; scars, protuberance, or discoloration of the skin; and striations, which may suggest previous pregnancies or adrenal gland hyperactivity. The hair pattern should be noted. The typical female pattern is that of an inverted triangle over the mons pubis. A male pattern involves hair growth between the area of the mons pubis and the umbilicus, also known as a diamond pattern, and may indicate excessive androgen activity in the patient (Figure 6-2).

Palpation. The abdomen should be palpated for organomegaly (enlarged organs), particularly involving the liver, spleen, kidneys, and uterus, and for adnexal masses, which may be palpated abdominally. Palpation also affords the possibility of noting a fluid wave, which would suggest either ascites or hemoperitoneum. Palpation also yields evidence for rigidity of the abdomen, which would imply spasm in the rectus muscles secondary to intraabdominal irritation. Where the irritation is caused by intraabdominal hemorrhage or infection, this rigidity is often evidence of an acute abdomen. During the palpation of the abdomen the physician should elicit the phenomenon of *rebound*, which also signifies intraabdominal irritation, by gently pressing the abdomen and then releasing. The release may cause pain either under the spot (direct rebound) or in a different portion of the abdomen (referred rebound). It should be noted, however, that sudden, rough pressure may cause pain even in a normal patient. Gentle pressure carried out systematically may elicit painful "trigger points."

Percussion. Percussion affords the ability to differentiate fluid waves and to outline solid organs and masses.

Auscultation. The physician should listen for bowel sounds. Hypoactive or absent bowel sounds may imply an ileus caused by peritoneal irritation of the bowel. Hyperactive bowel sounds may imply intrinsic irritation of the bowel or partial or complete bowel obstruction.

The groins should be palpated for adenopathy and inguinal hernias. The physician should also elicit the femoral pulses beneath the groin in the femoral triangles, and when these are present, the differences that may exist between the two femoral areas should be noted.

Legs should be examined for evidence of varicose veins, edema, and other lesions. In addition, it is reasonable to judge arterial circulation to the extremities by palpating pedal pulses on the dorsum of the foot.

PELVIC EXAMINATION

The pelvic examination is conducted with the patient lying supine on the examining table with her legs in stirrups. The patient may or may not desire to be draped with a sheet. Because the physician should be pointing out aspects of the patient's pelvic anatomy where possible, many patients prefer to have the head of the table elevated and to use a small hand mirror to follow the examination with the physician. In such instances, a sheet may be cumbersome. The physician should be sure the patient is as relaxed as possible and should take a few minutes to describe the procedure and allow the shy or nervous patient to prepare herself. Suggesting that the patient allow her legs to fall wide apart and concentrate on relaxing her abdominal muscles may be helpful.

Inspection

The perineum should be carefully inspected beginning with the mons pubis. The quality and pattern of the hair on the mons and the labia majora should be noted. Areas of alopecia should be noted, because they may imply a skin abnormality. In general, as a woman ages, the pubic hair becomes less dense and may turn gray. During the inspection of the pubic hair the physician should look for evidence of body lice (pediculosis). Next, the skin of the perineum is inspected for redness, excoriation, discoloration, or loss of pigment and for the presence of vesicles, ulcerations, pustules, warty growths, or neoplastic growths. In addition, pigmented nevi or other pigmented lesions should be noted, as should varicose veins. Skin scars denoting previous episiotomy or other obstetric lacerations should be noted.

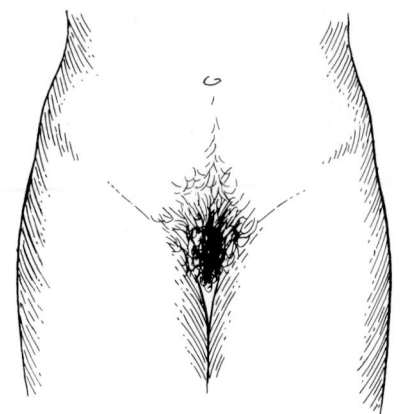 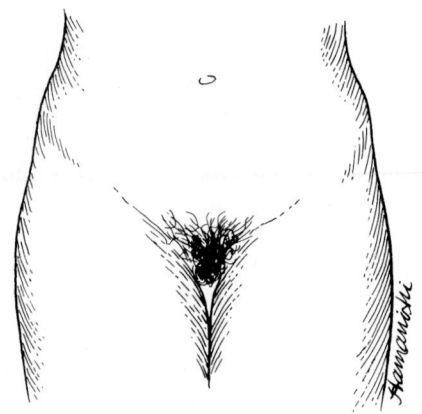

FIGURE 6-2   Normal female pubic hair pattern *(right)* and hair pattern of female showing male (androgenized) pattern *(left)*.

Next, the specific structures of the perineum should be systematically evaluated. The clitoris should be noted and its size and shape described. Normally it is 1 to 1.5 cm in length. Any irregularities or abnormalities of the labia majora or minora should be noted and carefully described. At times these areas are injured by trauma related to coitus, accidental injury, or childbearing. The patient should be questioned about evidence of trauma when appropriate.

The introitus should be observed closely. Whether the hymen is intact, imperforate, or marital and whether the perineum gapes or remains closed in the usual lithotomy position should be noted.

The perineal body, the area at the posterior aspect of the labia where the muscles of the superficial perineal compartment come together, should be inspected. It represents the focal point of support for the perineum and is between the vagina and the rectum. The perianal area is then inspected for evidence of hemorrhoids, sphincter continence, and other lesions (Figure 6-3).

Palpation

The next step in the examination of the perineum involves palpation. With the second and fourth fingers of the gloved hand separating the labia minora, the urethra is inspected and the length of the urethra is palpated and "milked" with the middle finger. In this way, irregularities and inflammation of Skene's glands (periurethral glands),

pus or mucus expressed, or a suburethral diverticulum can be noted. Any pus expressed from the urethra should be submitted to Gram stain and cultured, since it is frequently found to contain gonococci. The gloved hand then palpates the area of the posterior third of the labia majora, placing the index finger inside the introitus and the thumb on the outside of the labium. In this way, enlargements or cysts of Bartholin glands are noted. This exercise should be performed on each side.

With the gloved hand holding the labia apart, the opening of the vagina should be inspected. The presence of a cystocele or a cystourethrocele should be noted. This would be seen as a bulging of vaginal mucosa downward from the anterior wall of the vagina. The presence of this abnormality may be noted either by simply observing or by asking the patient to bear down (Figure 6-4). Likewise, the posterior wall should be noted for a bulging upward, which would represent a rectocele (Figure 6-5). Also, with the patient bearing down, the cervix may become visible, indicating prolapse of the uterus. A cystic bulge in the cul-de-sac may represent an enterocele (Figure 6-6). Each of these observations is evidence for relaxation of the pelvic supports and should be graded 1+ to 4+, with 1+ being a minimum bulge and 4+ being a bulge through the introitus. A prolapse of the cervix and uterus downward into the uterine canal can be graded in stages I, II, and III, with stage I being a minimum descent of the cervix into the vaginal canal,

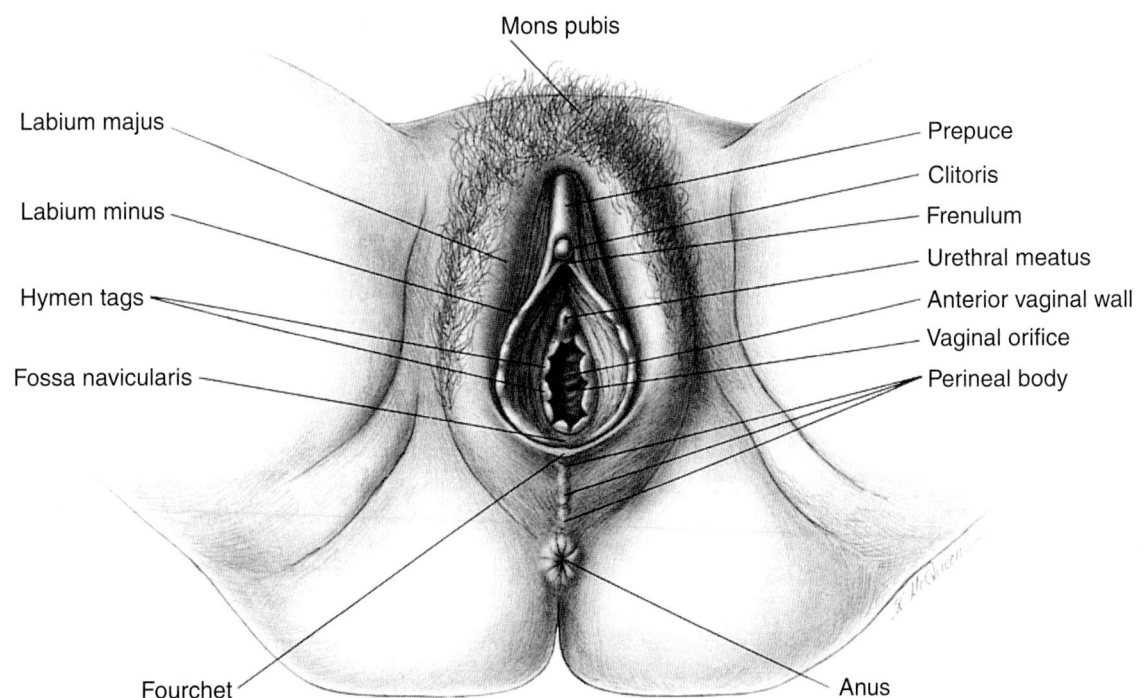

Mons pubis

Labium majus

Labium minus

Hymen tags

Fossa navicularis

Fourchet

Prepuce

Clitoris

Frenulum

Urethral meatus

Anterior vaginal wall

Vaginal orifice

Perineal body

Anus

FIGURE 6-3 Normal female perineum. (Redrawn from Krantz KE: Anatomy of the female reproductive system. In Benson RC, ed: Current obstetric and gynecologic diagnosis and treatment, ed 5, Los Altos, Calif, 1984, Lange Medical Publications.)

stage II being a descent of the cervix to the introitus, and stage III being the prolapse of the cervix or uterus through the introitus (total descensus, total procedentia) (Figure 6-7).

The descriptions and definitions of pelvic floor relaxation problems just listed have been the standard for many years and used by most gynecologists. During the last decade, however, the International Continence Society Committee of Standardization of Terminology, Subcommittee on Pelvic Organ Prolapse and Pelvic Floor Dysfunction has been collaborating with the American Urogynecology Society and the Society of Gynecologic Surgeons to develop a standardized site-specific system for describing, quantitating, and staging pelvic support in women. Its purpose is to enhance clinical and academic communication with respect to individual patients and populations of patients. In 1996 this system was adopted by these organizations. It is discussed and defined in Chapter 20 and Chapter 21.

Speculum Examination

After palpation the physician chooses the appropriate speculum for the patient. The typical Graves speculum generally is of three sizes: small, which is used in young children, women who have undergone tight perineal repair, or occasionally in the aged patient who has undergone severe involution; medium, used for most women; and large, which is often useful in large or obese women or those who are grand multiparas. Also available is the Pederson speculum, which is the length of the Graves speculum but narrow, for women who have not become active sexually, have never become pregnant, or have not used tampons. It is also of value for women who have undergone operations that have narrowed the vaginal diameter. For the majority of women the length of the vagina is similar, approximately 6 to 7 cm, and the Pederson or medium Graves speculum is appropriate (Figure 6-8).

The speculum should be warmed, either by a warming device or by being placed in warm water, and then touched to the patient's leg to determine that she feels the temperature is appropriate and comfortable. The speculum is then inserted by placing the transverse diameter of the blades in the anteroposterior position and guiding the blades through the introitus in a downward motion with the tips pointing toward the rectum. Because the anterior wall of the vagina is backed by the pubic symphysis, which is rigid, pressure upward causes the patient discomfort. This is avoided by following the described method of introducing the speculum. Also, in the resting state the vagina lies on the rectum and actually extends posteriorly from the introitus. The procedure may be facilitated by placing two fingers into the introitus and pressing down.

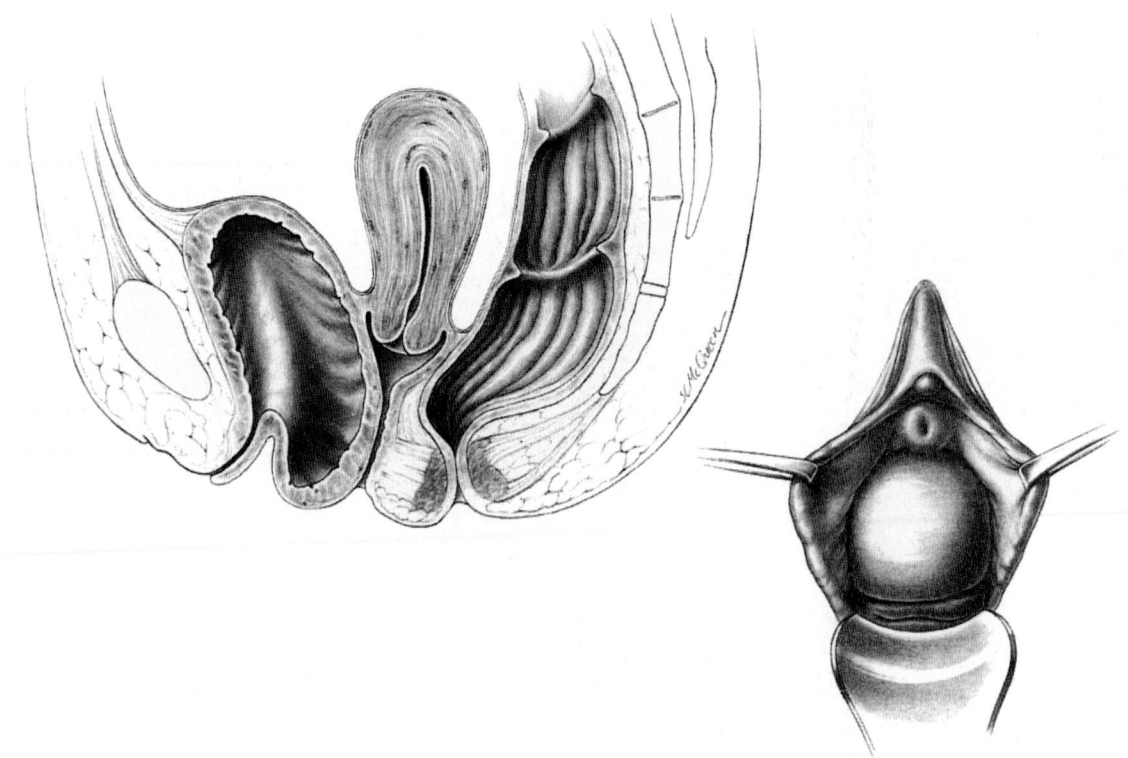

FIGURE 6-4 Side and direct views of cystocele. (Redrawn from Symmonds RE: Anatomy of the female reproductive system. In Benson RC, ed: Current obstetric and gynecologic diagnosis and treatment, ed 5, Los Altos, Calif, 1984, Lange Medical Publications.)

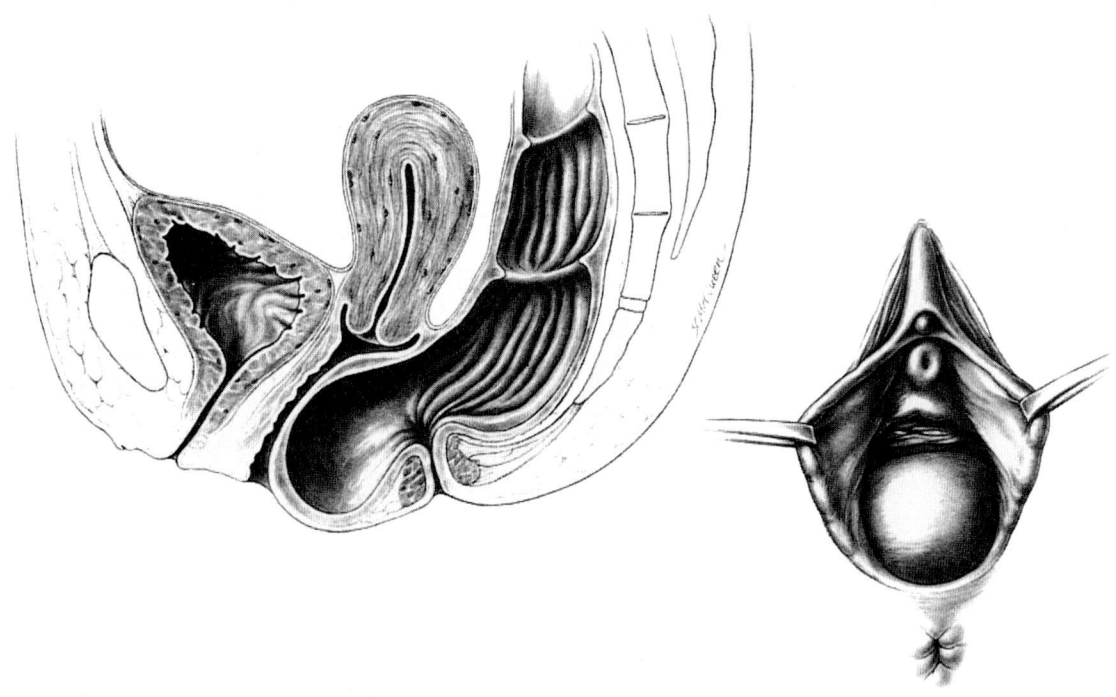

FIGURE 6-5   Side and direct views of rectocele. (Redrawn from Symmonds RE: Relaxations of pelvic supports. In Benson RC, ed: Current obstetric and gynecologic diagnosis and treatment, ed 5, Los Altos, Calif, 1984, Lange Medical Publications.)

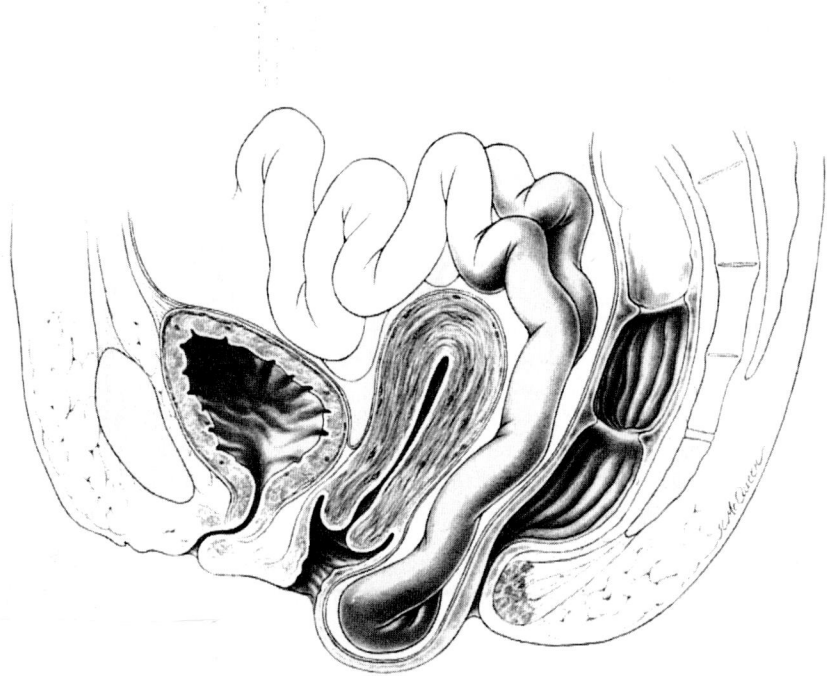

FIGURE 6-6   Lateral view of enterocele. (Redrawn from Symmonds RE: Relaxations of pelvic supports. In Benson RC, ed: Current obstetric and gynecologic diagnosis and treatment, ed 5, Los Altos, Calif, 1984, Lange Medical Publications.)

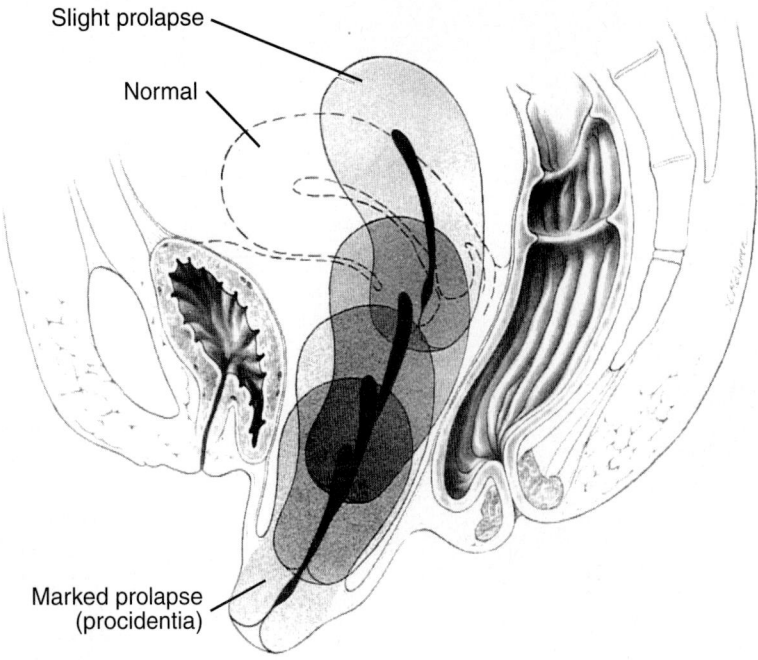

FIGURE 6-7   Depiction of prolapse of uterus. (Redrawn from Symmonds RE: Relaxations of pelvic supports. In Benson RC, ed: Current obstetric and gynecologic diagnosis and treatment, ed 5, Los Altos, Calif, 1984, Lange Medical Publications.)

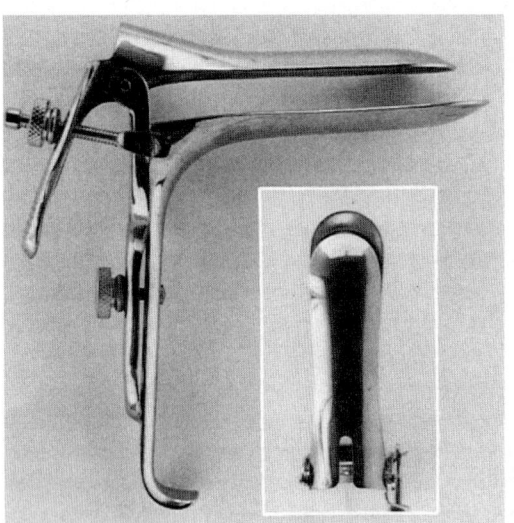 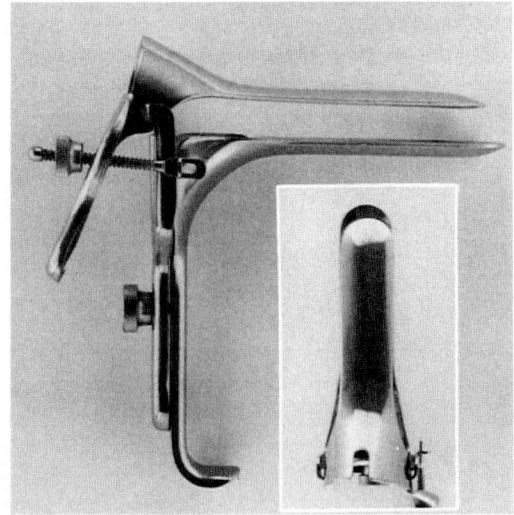

FIGURE 6-8   Graves *(left)* and Pederson *(right)* specula.

Once the blades are inserted, the speculum should be turned so that the transverse axis of the blades is in the transverse axis of the vagina. The blades should be inserted to their full length and then opened so that the physician may inspect for the position of the cervix. The cervix generally fits into the open blades with ease. If this does not occur, the physician should inspect for the position of the cervix with his or her finger and then reinsert the speculum accordingly. Once the blades are inserted and the cervix is visualized, the speculum should be opened and the introitus widened so that the cervix can be adequately inspected and a Pap smear taken. This can be done by using the screw adjustment on the base of the speculum. When inserted properly the speculum generally stays in place.

The physician then inspects the vagina and cervix. The vaginal canal is inspected during the insertion of the speculum or on its removal. The vaginal epithelium should be noted for evidence of erythema or lesions. Fluid discharge

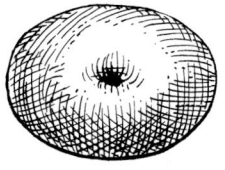 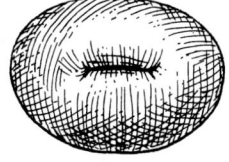 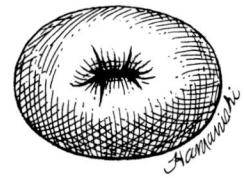

Nulliparous   Parous   Stellate

FIGURE 6-9 Nulliparous, parous, and stellate lacerations of cervix.

should be evaluated on slides prepared by placing one drop of vaginal secretion in one drop of sodium chloride solution, cover-slipping the specimen, and inspecting it for unicellular flagellated protozoa, *Trichomonas vaginalis*. The vaginal epithelial cells should also be inspected. The cells should have sharp borders and normal-appearing nuclei. Any variation from the normal appearance of cells may imply infection (see Chapter 22). A drop of potassium hydroxide is placed on another slide, and a drop of vaginal secretion is placed within this. The potassium hydroxide causes lysis of the epithelial cells and trichomonads but leaves intact the mycelium of *Candida*. Thus the presence of mycelium is helpful in diagnosing vaginal candidiasis. Vaginal lesions, such as areas of adenosis (see Chapter 15), clear cystic structures (Gartner's cysts), or inclusion cysts on the lines of scars or episiotomy incisions, should be noted.

The cervix is inspected next. It should be pink, shiny, and clear. In a nulliparous individual, the external os should be round. When a woman is parous, the external os takes on a fishmouth appearance, and if there have been cervical lacerations, healed stellate lacerations may be noted (Figure 6-9). Normally the transformation zone (i.e., the junction of squamous and columnar epithelium) is just barely visible inside the external os. Occasionally, glandular epithelium may be present on the portio vaginalis, moving the transformation zone onto the portio. This is common in teenage girls, women who have been exposed to diethylstilbestrol in utero, some women with vaginitis, or women immediately postpartum or postabortion. Generally this is cleared by a process of metaplasia, in which squamous epithelium covers the columnar epithelium. This process, however, may leave small areas of irregularities and inclusion cysts, called *nabothian cysts*, which may be seen in various sizes and shapes. They are of no clinical significance. Often after a woman has delivered a baby, there is lateral scarring at the 3 and 9 o'clock positions, causing an eversion of the external os so that the reddened columnar epithelium is visible on the anterior and posterior lips of the cervix. If the observer looks closely, the transitional zone can be seen along the edges of this area of eversion and may be perfectly healthy. This is called an *ectropion* and is not evidence of a pathologic condition.

Any lesions of the cervix should be noted and, where appropriate, a biopsy should be performed. In a patient with acute herpes progenitalis, vesicles or ulcers may be noted. In a patient infected with human papillomavirus, warts (condyloma acuminata) on the cervix may also be observed.

Papanicolaou Smear

At this point in the examination a Pap smear is usually taken. In 1943 Papanicolaou and Trout published their now classic monograph demonstrating the value of vaginal and cervical cytology as a screening tool for cervical neoplasm. With the use of the Pap smear in screening programs, the incidence of invasive cervical cancer has been reduced 50%. Recently, programs focusing on cost effectiveness have suggested that the screening interval may be extended from the usual 1 year to 3 years in certain low-risk individuals. Because low risk is often difficult to define, the American College of Obstetricians and Gynecologists suggested in 1984 that annual screening was appropriate for most American women. Initial screening should begin at age 18 or when the individual becomes sexually active. High-risk women, those with a history of early sexual activity and multiple partners, should be screened annually. Those patients with later exposure to coitus who have only one sexual partner and who have had three successive negative annual smears may be considered low risk and should be screened every 1 to 2 years at the discretion of the physician. A case-control study by Shy et al. questioned the wisdom of extending the screening interval beyond 2 years. Although no significant increase was noted in the incidence of cervical cancer in women screened every 2 years compared with annually, the risk increased 3.9 times if the interval was 3 years and 12.3 times in women not screened for 10 years. The presence of risk factors did not influence these results.

A Pap smear can be performed in a number of ways. The major objective is to sample secretions from the endocervical canal and to scrape the transitional zone. It is also useful to sample the vaginal pool, although this does not usually yield as high an incidence of cervical disease as does sampling of the canal and the transitional zone. One way of performing the Pap smear is as follows:

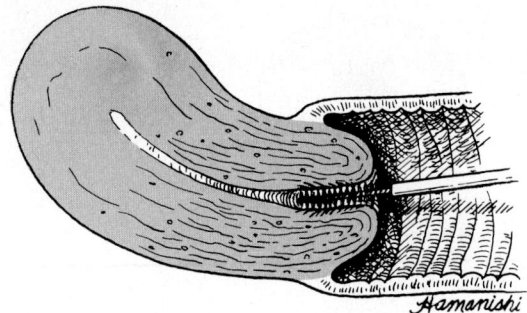

FIGURE 6-10   Obtaining cells from endocervix using a cytobrush.

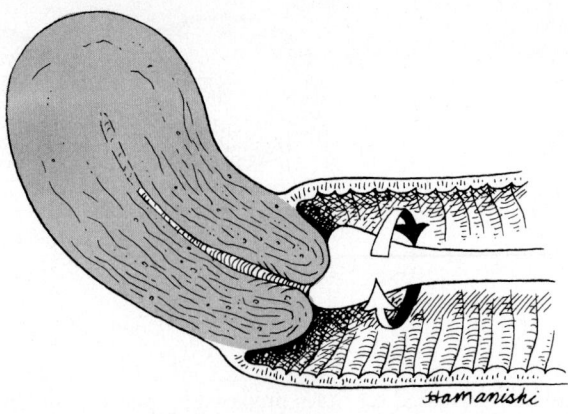

FIGURE 6-11   Obtaining cells from transformation zone using Ayers spatula.

1. After excess mucus is gently removed, the endocervical canal is sampled with either a cotton-tipped applicator or a cytobrush, which is placed into the canal and rotated. Although both instruments generally dislodge adequate numbers of cells for study, the cytobrush appears to give more accurate results and higher yields of positive findings. The material obtained is then smeared thinly on a microscope slide by rotation of the swab or brush on the glass surface. This is labeled *endocervix* and fixed immediately either by use of a spray fixative or by immersion of the slide into a fixative solution (Figure 6-10).

2. With an Ayers spatula or some variation thereof, the entire transformation zone is scraped and smeared thinly on a second slide, which is immediately fixed. If the physician wishes a sample of the vaginal pool, this may be taken with the reverse side of the Ayers spatula and smeared on a third slide or on a second portion of the slide containing the transformation zone material (Figure 6-11).

A number of fixatives are available, but it is important that they be applied immediately before drying and distortion of the cells takes place. Pap smears may be reported using the following descriptive system:

Normal
Atypical
    Inflammation
    Possible dysplasia
Metaplasia
Mild dysplasia
Moderate dysplasia
Severe dysplasia—carcinoma in situ
Invasive cancer

In the past decade the terminology suggested by the Bethesda Conference has been utilized by several laboratories. This is as follows:

Adequacy of smear
Infection type
Squamous abnormalities
    Reaction (inflammatory changes)
    Epithelial cell abnormalities
    Atypical type, undetermined
    Squamous intraepithelial lesion (SIL)
        Low grade: HPV or mild dysplasia (CIN I)
        High grade: Moderate to severe dysplasiaCarcinoma in situ (CIN II-III)
Glandular type
    Atypical and source
    Adenocarcinoma and source

In most instances, particularly with new patients, it is appropriate to culture for gonorrhea and *Chlamydia* using swabs that sample secretions from the endocervical canal. This step may be performed after the Pap smear.

Bimanual Examination

The bimanual examination allows the physician to palpate the uterus and the adnexa. The index and middle fingers of the dominant hand are placed within the vagina, and the thumb is folded under so as not to cause the patient distress in the area of the mons pubis, clitoris, and pubic symphysis. The fingers are inserted deeply into the vagina so that they rest beneath the cervix in the posterior fornix. The physician should be in a comfortable position at this point, generally with the leg on the side of the vaginal examining hand on a table lift and the elbow of that arm resting on the knee. The opposite hand is placed on the patient's abdomen above the pubic symphysis. The flat of the fingers are used for palpation. The physician then elevates the uterus by pressing up on the cervix and deliver-

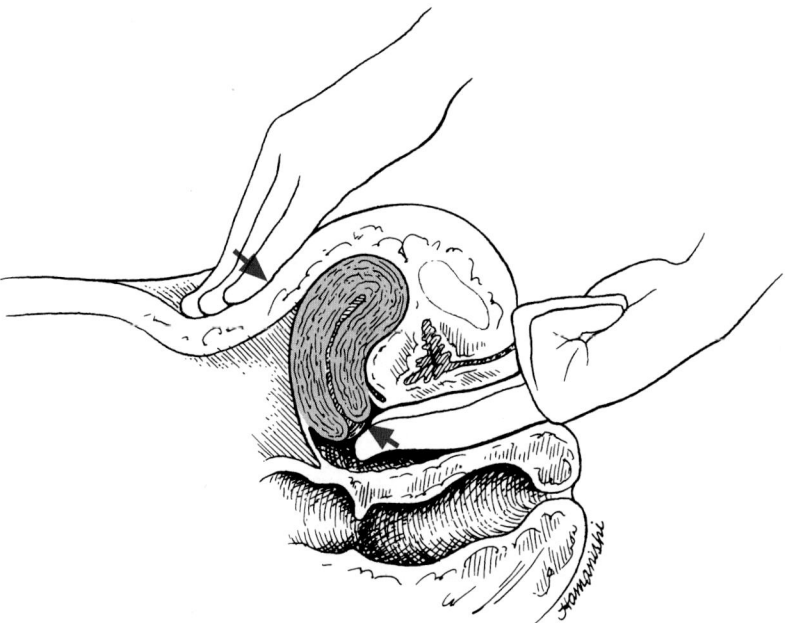

FIGURE 6-12   Bimanual examination of uterus.

ing the uterus to the abdominal hand so that the uterus may be placed between the two hands, thereby identifying its position, size, shape, consistency, and mobility. In the normal and nonpregnant state the uterus is approximately 6 cm by 4 cm and weighs about 70 g. It may be somewhat larger in a woman who has had children (Figure 6-12).

Enlargement of the uterus should be described in detail. Size may be estimated in centimeters or by comparing with weeks of normal gestational age.

The uterus in two thirds of instances is anteflexed so that the abdominal hand is palpating the posterior wall of the uterus and the vaginal fingers the anterior wall. The uterus may be retroverted. If it is positioned in a straight line with the vagina, it is said to be midposition or first-degree retroverted; if it lies backward in the cul-de-sac off the direct line of the vagina, it is said to be second-degree retroverted; if it is flexed deeply into the cul-de-sac pressing toward the rectum, it is third-degree retroverted. A third-degree retroverted uterus that cannot be brought forward by manipulation is best examined by rectovaginal examination, which is described later in the chapter. The general shape of the uterus is that of a pear, with the broadest portion at the upper pole of the fundus. Generally the uterus is mobile, and if it fails to move, it may be fixed by adhesions. The surface should be smooth; irregularities may indicate the presence of uterine leiomyomas (fibroids).

The shape of the uterus should also be described in detail. The consistency of the uterus is generally firm but

not rock-hard, and this should be noted in the examination. Any undue tenderness caused by palpation or movement of the uterus should be noted, since it may imply an inflammatory process.

Attention is then turned to examination of the adnexa. If the right hand is the pelvic hand, the first two fingers of the right hand are then moved into the right vaginal fornix as deeply as they can be inserted. The abdominal hand is placed just medial to the anterior superior iliac spine on the right, the two hands are brought as close together as possible, and with a sliding motion from the area of the anterior superior iliac spine to the introitus, the fingers are swept downward, allowing for the adnexa to be palpated between them. A normal ovary is approximately 3 cm by 2 cm (about the size of a walnut) and will sweep between the two fingers with ease unless it is fixed in an abnormal position by adhesions. When the adnexa is palpated, its size, mobility, and consistency should be described. However, this portion of the examination should be brief, since it causes the patient a mild to moderate sickening sensation. When the right adnexa has been palpated, the left adnexa should be palpated in a similar fashion by turning the vaginal hand to the left vaginal fornix and repeating the exercise on the left side (Figure 6-13). Adnexa are usually not palpable in postmenopausal women because of involution and retraction of the ovary to a position higher in the pelvis. A palpable organ in such an individual should be further investigated for ovarian pathology.

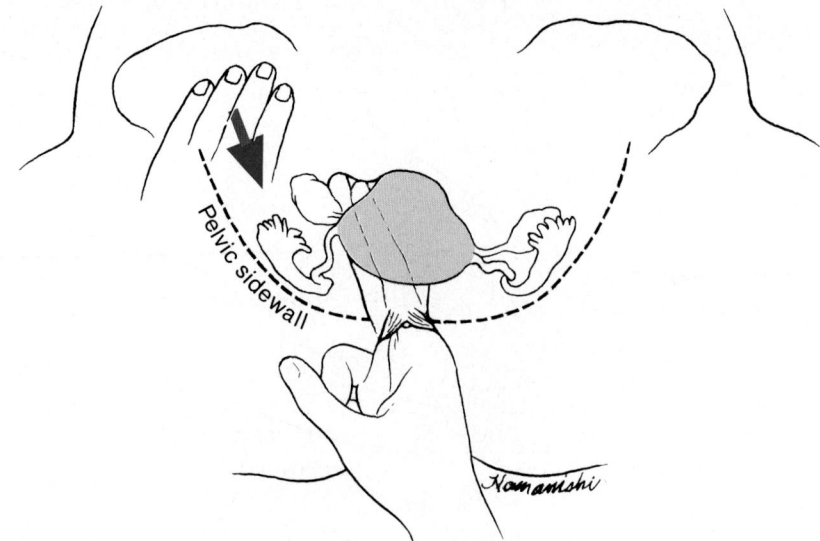

FIGURE 6-13 Bimanual examination of adnexa.

Rectovaginal Examination

After completing the vaginal portion of the bimanual examination, the middle finger is relubricated with a water-soluble lubricant and placed into the rectum. Many physicians think the glove should be changed so as not to contaminate the rectum with vaginal organisms. The index finger is reinserted into the vagina. In this fashion the rectovaginal septum is palpated between the two fingers, and any thickness or mass is noted. The finger should also attempt to identify the uterosacral ligaments, which extend from the posterior wall of the cervix posteriorly and laterally toward the sacrum. Any thickening or beadiness of these structures may imply an inflammatory reaction or endometriosis. If the uterus is retroverted, that organ should be outlined for size, shape, and consistency at this point. It may be examined appropriately using the fingers inserted into the vagina and the rectum, as well as using the abdominal hand (Figure 6-14).

Rectal Examination

The rectum is then palpated in all dimensions with the rectal examining finger. It should be possible to palpate as many as 70% of bowel lesions with the rectal finger. Because bowel cancer is common in women, particularly after the age of 35, this part of the examination should not be overlooked. The physician should also note the tone of the anal sphincter and any other anal abnormalities, such as hemorrhoids, fissures, or masses. Finally, a stool sample is taken on the examining finger and tested for occult blood. This is particularly important in women past the age of 35 who may be at risk for bowel cancer.

At the end of the examination the physician should give the patient some facial tissue so that she may

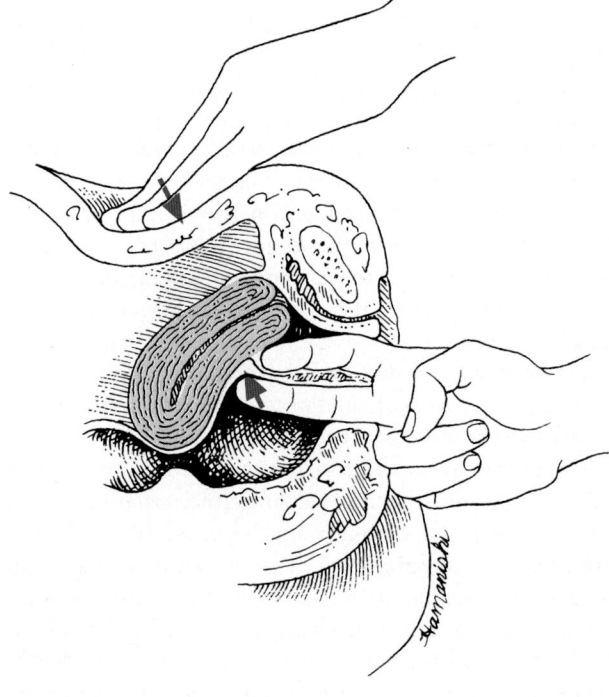

FIGURE 6-14 Rectovaginal examination.

remove the lubricating jelly from her perineum before she dresses.

It is important that each step of the examination be explained to the patient and that she be reassured about all normal findings. Wherever possible, abnormal findings should be pointed out to the patient either by allowing her to palpate the pathologic condition or by demonstrating it to her using a hand mirror. It is also appropriate to demonstrate normal structures to the patient, such as the cervix and portions of the vagina that she may be able to see with her hand mirror. The physician should use the examination as a vehicle for teaching the patient about her body.

THE ANNUAL VISIT

The annual visit is important for both health maintenance and preventive medicine reasons. Although the visit varies in emphasis depending on the patient's age, the long-term goals should be to maintain the patient in the best health and functional status possible and to promote high-quality longevity.

Although the gynecologist is generally the primary physician for women during their reproductive years, until recently this was not necessarily the case for postmenopausal women. However, it has become clear that the gynecologist with appropriate training and motivation can continue being the primary physician for older women as well.

Byyny has pointed out that poor lifestyle is often at least partly responsible for chronic disease, disability, and premature mortality. In 1973 Belloc reported that in a study of women past the age of 45 the life expectancy was 7 years greater for those who routinely practiced six of seven important health habits as compared with those who practiced three or fewer (see box on this page). During the annual visit physicians should therefore discuss nutrition regarding (1) proper caloric intake to maintain the patient's weight near her optimum and avoid obesity, (2) restricting saturated fat and cholesterol, and (3) understanding the need for adequate calcium in the diet (1200–1500 mg/day).

At each checkup the physician should also encourage the patient to develop an exercise program appropriate for her abilities and to avoid smoking and excessive alcohol use (if she has these habits). The physician should discuss possible stressors in the patient's life, such as her relationship with her husband and other family members, her satisfaction or dissatisfaction with her job, and other social problems that she may be experiencing. It is appropriate to ask questions that assess her sexual activity and gratification and questions that detect abuse or intimidation in her life. It is also appropriate to discuss the physical and emotional implications of loss and grief. Everyone suffers loss during his or her lifetime, and the older the patient the more likely that this is the case. Grief may be the result of a loss of a spouse or loved one, a pet, a job, a body part, or the ability to perform activities the patient has enjoyed (see Chapter 8).

The patient should be asked to bring all medications that she is taking. Both prescription and over-the-counter drugs should be included. This will give the physician the opportunity to review with the patient why she is taking each one, and also to assess for possible potential adverse

Good Health Habits
Eat moderately
Eat regularly
Eat breakfast
Avoid smoking
Exercise regularly
Use alcohol in moderation or not at all
Sleep 7 to 8 hours per night

drug interactions. It may also be possible to tie specific drug use to an undesirable symptom the patient may be experiencing.

The annual visit is an opportunity for the physician to screen for a variety of illnesses affecting not only the reproductive organs but all of the organ systems. The visit should include an interim health history and a complete physical examination. The weight, height, and blood pressure measurements and the breast, pelvic, and rectal examinations should all be performed and recorded so that comparisons may be made from year to year. A gross assessment of the patient's hearing ability and visual acuity should be performed annually.

Recently, the American College of Obstetricians and Gynecologists Task Force on Primary Preventive Health Care recommended screening laboratory tests for the annual visit for women in different age groups (Table 6-1). It was recommended that an annual Pap smear be begun at age 18 or at the time a woman becomes sexually active. For women before the age of 18 who are in specific high-risk groups, hemoglobin, urine testing for bacteriuria, testing for sexually transmitted diseases and human immunodeficiency virus (HIV), genetic testing, rubella titer, tuberculosis skin test, lipid profile, and hepatitis C virus testing may be appropriate.

For women between the ages of 19 and 39, an annual Pap smear should be ordered unless the patient is monogamous and has had three consecutive normal tests. After that and at the discretion of the physician and the patient, the testing may be done every 1 to 2 years. Cholesterol testing should be done every 5 years. For women in this age group who are at high risk, cholesterol testing, hemoglobin, bacteriuria, mammography, fasting glucose, testing for sexually transmitted diseases and HIV, rubella titer, tuberculosis skin test, lipid profile, TSH, and hepatitis C virus testing may be indicated.

For women between the ages of 40 and 64, annual Pap smear as noted above, mammography every 1 to 2 years until age 50 and annually after that, cholesterol every 5 years, fasting glucose testing every 3 years after age 45, fecal occult blood test on three occasions annually, and sigmoidoscopy every 3 to 5 years after age 50 are recommended. For women in this age group who are considered high risk, hemoglobin, bacteriuria, fasting glucose, testing

TABLE 6-1
Suggested Laboratory Studies for Annual Health Maintenance Visit

Ages	Routine	High Risk
13–18	Pap test	Hgb Bacteriuria STD, HIV testing Genetic testing Rubella titer TB skin test Lipid profile Fasting glucose testing Cholesterol testing Hepatitis C virus testing
19–39	Pap test Cholesterol (every 5 years)	Hgb Bacteriuria Mammography FBS Cholesterol testing STD, HIV testing Genetic testing Rubella titer TB skin test Lipid profile TSH Hepatitis C virus testing
40–64	Pap test Mammography (as suggested) Cholesterol (every 5 years) Fecal occult blood test Sigmoidoscopy (every 3–5 years after age 50) Fasting glucose testing (every 3 years after age 45)	Hgb Bacteriuria Mammography FBS STD, HIV testing TB skin test Lipid profile TSH Colonoscopy Hepatitis C virus testing
65 and older	Pap test Urinalysis Mammography Cholesterol (every 3–5 years) Fecal occult blood test Sigmoidoscopy (every 3–5 years) TSH (every 3–5 years) FBS (every 3 years)	Hgb FBS STD, HIV testing TB skin test Lipid profile Colonoscopy Hepatitis C virus testing

In addition, urinalysis, mammography, cholesterol (every 3 to 5 years), annual testing for fecal occult blood, sigmoidoscopy every 3 to 5 years, and TSH every 3 to 5 years should be ordered. For women in particular high-risk groups, hemoglobin, fasting glucose, testing for sexually transmitted diseases and HIV, tuberculosis skin test, lipid profile, colonoscopy, and hepatitis C virus testing should be considered.

Women in the youngest age group should be given tetanus-diphtheria booster shots once between the ages of 13 to 16. Measles/mumps/rubella (MMR), hepatitis B vaccine, and fluoride supplementation to prevent tooth decay should be offered to those at risk. Susceptible adolescents *and* adults should be offered varicella vaccination.

For women between the ages of 40 and 64, periodic tetanus-diphtheria boosters every 10 years should be given, and influenza vaccine should be offered annually beginning at age 55. For women in high-risk groups, MMR, hepatitis B vaccine, influenza vaccine, and pneumococcal vaccine should be offered.

For women who are 65 and older, tetanus-diphtheria booster every 10 years should be continued, influenza vaccine should be given annually, and pneumococcal vaccine should be given and repeated every 5 years.

In addition, women in all age groups should be offered appropriate immunizations and vaccinations when they travel to other countries. Hepatitis A vaccine is now available and should be offered to women of all ages.

Physicians should discuss risk behavior annually with their patients. In line with injury prevention, the patient should be reminded to use seat belts and helmets (if she rides bicycles, motorcycles, or horses) and to be aware of recreational hazards such as athletic activities beyond her capabilities. She should be asked if there are firearms in the house and if there are, whether appropriate safety precautions are taken. Hearing problems should be discussed and situations that hinder hearing in at-risk circumstances, such as jogging on a busy thoroughfare while listening to a Walkman, should be discussed. The patient should be informed about the importance of appropriate footwear for activities she may undertake; this is particularly important for women in the older age group.

Exposure of the skin to ultraviolet radiation and proper precautions to avoid overexposure should be discussed. In addition, the patient should be asked about depression and possible suicidal ideology and of destructive habits such as the use of tobacco, alcohol, or drugs. Where indicated, possible remedial suggestions should be given.

Promoting good health is a continuing responsibility for both the physician and the patient. It represents a challenge that includes education and observation on the physician's part and motivation on the patient's part.

for sexually transmitted diseases and HIV, tuberculosis skin test, lipid profile, TSH, colonoscopy, and hepatitis C virus testing should be considered.

For women who are 65 and older, Pap smears should be performed every 1 to 2 years at the discretion of the patient and physician after three consecutive normal tests.

- Five general impressions of patients may be gleaned nonverbally (by observation): happiness, apathy, fear, anger, and sadness.

- Menstrual history includes age of menarche, number of days of cycle, number of days of flow, presence of bleeding between menstrual periods, the date of the last menstrual period, and the date of the previous menstrual period.

- Menstrual cycles occurring just after puberty and just before menopause are frequently anovulatory and may be irregular in frequency.

- Pregnancy history should include the details of term and premature labors, spontaneous abortion, ectopic pregnancies, molar pregnancies, and terminations.

- A complete gynecologic evaluation should always include a sexual history, contraceptive history, and history of physical or sexual abuse.

- A detailed family history includes inquiry about congenital malformations, mental retardation, or pregnancy wastage in the families of the patient and her husband.

- Occupational and avocational activity should be investigated for the presence of potential hazards to the patient's health.

- Pap smears should be performed every 1 to 3 years, depending on the patient's risk level.

- Sexually active women should be evaluated at appropriate intervals for sexually transmitted diseases.

- The physician should use the occasion of the history and physical examination to teach the patient important aspects of self-evaluation.

- Goals of preventive medicine are to maintain good health and function and promote high-quality longevity.

- The physician should maintain an immunization record for each patient and offer appropriate vaccinations as recommended by public health guidelines.

BIBLIOGRAPHY

American College of Obstetricians and Gynecologists: Cervical cytology: evaluation and management of abnormalities, Tech Bull 81, 1984.

American College of Obstetricians and Gynecologists Committee Opinion: Primary and preventive care: periodic assessment. No. 229, December 1999, Washington, DC.

American College of Obstetricians and Gynecologists Committee Opinion: Routine cancer screening. No. 185, September 1997, Washington, DC.

Belloc NB: Relationship of health practices and mortality, Prev Med 2:67, 1973.

Byyny RL: Establishing guidelines for preventive medicine, Contemp Obstet Gynecol 31:43, 1988.

Papanicolaou GN and Trout HF: Diagnosis of uterine cancer by vaginal smears, New York, 1943, The Commonwealth Fund.

Shy K, Chu J, Mandelson M, et al: Papanicolaou smear screening interval and risk of cervical cancer, Obstet Gynecol 74:838, 1989.

Taylor PT, Andersen WA, Barber SR, et al: The screening Papanicolaou smear: contribution of the endocervical bush, Obstet Gynecol 70:734, 1987.

The Obstetricians and Gynecologists and Primary Preventive Health Care. ACOG Task Force in Primary and Preventive Health Care. American College of Obstetricians and Gynecologists, 1993, Washington, DC.

Differential Diagnosis of Major Gynecologic Problems by Age Groups
Vaginal Bleeding, Pelvic Pain, Pelvic Mass

KEY TERMS AND DEFINITIONS

Hematocolpos. Distention of an obstructed vagina (caused by imperforate hymen or transverse septum) with blood and blood products.

Hematometria. A uterus distended with blood, secondary to partial or complete obstruction of any portion of the lower genital tract.

Levator Spasm. Spasm of the levator ani muscles frequently associated with chronic pelvic pain or vaginismus.

Menorrhagia. Heavy or prolonged menstrual flow.

Metrorrhagia. Intermenstrual bleeding.

Pain. An unpleasant sensory or emotional experience associated with actual or potential tissue damage or described in terms of such damage.

Pelvic Congestion Syndrome. Vascular engorgement of the uterus and the vessels of the broad ligament and lateral pelvic walls, which may lead to chronic pelvic pain.

Trigger Points. Painful spasm of local muscle bundles or areas of scar tissue within the abdominal wall, at times associated with chronic pelvic and lower abdominal pain.

The gynecologist will evaluate a variety of women at different periods of life for relatively few specific symptoms and signs. Perhaps the three most common of these are unusual vaginal bleeding, pelvic pain, and pelvic or abdominal mass. Although each of these complaints will be of concern to the individual patient, their diagnostic implications may vary greatly depending on the patient's age. This chapter considers unusual vaginal bleeding, pelvic pain, and pelvic or abdominal mass from the standpoint of differential diagnosis, emphasizing the differences seen at different periods of a woman's life, and includes a detailed consideration of the problem of chronic pelvic pain.

VAGINAL BLEEDING

Abnormal vaginal bleeding includes prepubertal bleeding, menorrhagia, metrorrhagia or postcoital bleeding, and postmenopausal bleeding. Although the cause of the bleeding will frequently determine the characteristics that it exhibits, the physician should develop a systematic approach to the differential diagnosis of abnormal vaginal bleeding. The box on page 156 offers an outline that can be followed in considering a patient with abnormal vaginal bleeding. In addition, Chapter 37 considers this topic in detail.

Pregnancy

The possibility of a pregnancy must be considered in any woman in the reproductive years. This possibility can be rapidly ruled out using a sensitive serum pregnancy test. If the patient is found to be pregnant and vaginal bleeding is noted, the diagnostic possibilities include implantation bleeding; threatened, inevitable, complete, or incomplete abortion; ectopic pregnancy; and molar pregnancy.

Implantation bleeding is quite common. It usually consists of minimal bleeding at about the time of the first missed menstrual period and generally lasts a very short

Etiology of Abnormal Vaginal Bleeding

Pregnancy
   Abortion
      Threatened
      Inevitable
      Complete
      Incomplete
   Ectopic
   Molar—trophoblastic disease
Dysfunctional uterine bleeding
   Postpuberty
   During reproductive years
   Perimenopausal
Neoplastic
   Vulva and vagina
   Cervix
   Uterine corpus
   Fallopian tube
   Ovary
   Other
Inflammatory
   Vulvitis and vaginitis
   Cervicitis
   Endometritis
   Pelvic inflammatory disease
Traumatic
   Foreign body
   Direct trauma
Systemic diseases
   Coagulopathies
   Blood dyscrasias
   Endocrinopathy
   Drug effects
   Others

time. Occasionally it may be present for 1 to 2 days, with a flow similar to that of a menstrual period. Often implantation bleeding is not perceptible to the patient but can be seen by the physician as a brownish-tinged cervical mucus if a pelvic examination is performed. Bleeding in excess of a normal menstrual flow is quite rare, and prolonged bleeding does not usually occur.

Bleeding in the first trimester of pregnancy is not uncommon. About 20% to 25% of all pregnant women spot or bleed in the first trimester. If the bleeding can be observed to be coming from the cervix and the cervix is closed, a diagnosis of threatened abortion can be made (Chapter 16). The size of the uterus should be consistent with what is normal for the dates of the pregnancy, and the uterus may or may not be contracting and tender to the touch. A threatened abortion becomes inevitable when the cervix dilates and products of conception pass through the internal os or when the bleeding is profuse.

A complete abortion is noted when the uterus has expelled its contents, the internal os is closed, the bleeding is minimal, and the uterus has returned to near normal size. It is unusual for a patient who has a complete abortion to experience significant pelvic cramping or to cramp

when a uterotonic agent such as ergonovine maleate (Ergotrate) or methylergonovine maleate (Methergine) is administered.

Incomplete abortion occurs when a part of the products of conception has been expelled but some remains within the uterus. The cervix is generally dilated, and there is usually bleeding, which may be profuse. The uterus is generally enlarged, and the patient may experience cramping pain. Most gestations of 6 weeks or less from the time of the last menstrual period will abort completely. Incomplete abortions become more common after 6 weeks of gestation.

A missed abortion occurs when the embryo dies but the products of conception are not expelled from the uterus. Generally the uterus involutes so that it is smaller than expected by dates. There may be dark red or brown vaginal bleeding, often minimal in amount. Pregnancy tests may remain positive for quite some time in the face of a missed abortion. Such conditions are more common when progestational agents have been given in the hopes of supporting the pregnancy.

Ectopic pregnancies are quite common and seem to be becoming more prevalent (Chapter 17). Currently about 1% of all pregnancies end as ectopic pregnancies, but these figures vary from group to group. An ectopic pregnancy is defined as one that is implanted outside of the endometrial cavity. Thus an ectopic pregnancy may exist in the cervix, within various portions of a fallopian tube, in the ovary, in the peritoneal cavity, and, in some rare instances, within the myometrium or a distant organ such as the spleen. A primary ectopic pregnancy in a specific organ implies that the pregnancy was implanted directly within that organ. A secondary ectopic pregnancy implies that the pregnancy ruptured from the fallopian tube and reimplanted completely or partially on another organ.

Ectopic pregnancies cause vaginal bleeding because of the separation of the decidua from the endometrium as the ectopic pregnancy dies or because of direct bleeding from the site of the ectopic pregnancy, with the blood being transported to the uterus and through the cervix. In most but not all cases the patient misses at least one menstrual period, begins to bleed from scant to significant amounts, and generally experiences pelvic pain. The pain may be limited to one side, in the case of a fallopian tube pregnancy, or may present as a more generalized pelvic pain. The pain may be similar to that experienced with pelvic inflammatory disease, but the patient with an ectopic pregnancy has a low-grade fever or is afebrile.

If the ectopic pregnancy is ruptured, intraperitoneal hemorrhage may occur and the patient may exhibit signs and symptoms of hypovolemia. Such an acute situation requires rapid intervention.

Ectopic pregnancies become a diagnostic problem when they are unruptured. Vaginal bleeding occurs in about 90% of early ectopic pregnancies that are unruptured, and almost all such patients experience pain. The uterus may be slightly enlarged or seem to be normal in size. If the ectopic pregnancy is tubal or ovarian, an adnexal mass may be noted. However, adnexal masses are not uncommon in normal pregnancies, representing the corpus luteum of pregnancy, and this may make the differential diagnosis somewhat more difficult.

With the availability of serum pregnancy tests, rapidly ascertaining that the patient is pregnant is possible. When a pregnancy is diagnosed, it becomes necessary to establish whether it is intrauterine or ectopic. A vaginal ultrasound examination may be of help. If the pregnancy has progressed beyond 6 weeks' gestation, it is frequently possible to see a pregnancy sac within the uterine cavity. Occasionally such a sac may be seen outside the uterine cavity in an adnexa.

Several authors have attempted to compare the levels of human chorionic gonadotrophin (hCG) with the gestational age of the pregnancy and determine from this whether a normal pregnancy is developing. However, it is not yet possible to differentiate with certainty between an intrauterine and an ectopic pregnancy by relating levels of hCG to the presence or absence of a sac. DiMarchi et al. noted that in their series of 131 cases, ectopic pregnancies were identified with hCG levels of 15,000 to 100,000 mIU. A combination of hCG and vaginal ultrasound observations helped make the diagnosis, often because of poor correlation of findings referable to interuterine pregnancy. Tubal rupture rarely occurred if the hCG level was below 100 mIU/ml unless the pregnancy was in a region of the fallopian tube other than the ampulla. Although 83% of their pregnancies were ampullary, the remainder were more difficult to diagnose before rupture because the rupture often occurred with lower levels of hCG and before good ultrasound findings could be obtained. This is discussed more completely in Chapter 17.

In a patient experiencing vaginal bleeding and pelvic pain who has a positive pregnancy test and who does not exhibit a gestational sac within the uterus on ultrasound, the physician should consider the diagnosis of ectopic pregnancy. A gestational sac appearing outside the uterine cavity may be suggestive of an ectopic pregnancy, but frequent error has been noted in such diagnoses and often the gestational sac does turn out to be intrauterine.

If the patient appears to have intraperitoneal bleeding, a culdocentesis may help. The presence of unclotted blood within the peritoneal cavity is evidence for intraperitoneal hemorrhage. Intraperitoneal fluid seen on ultrasound examination is also suggestive of intraperitoneal bleeding.

Several types of patients are at high risk for ectopic pregnancy. These include women who have had previous ectopic pregnancies, those who have undergone tubal reparative procedures, those who have had previous pelvic infections, and those who have been exposed in utero to diethylstilbestrol (DES). Ectopic pregnancy should also be considered in users of intrauterine devices (IUDs), since IUDs only partially protect from tubular implantation. Management of ectopic pregnancy is considered and discussed in Chapter 17.

Another cause of abnormal vaginal bleeding associated with pregnancy is trophoblastic disease (Chapter 35). Most trophoblastic tumors are hydatidiform moles, which occur about once in every 1000 gestations in nonoriental women. Although they may present in a variety of ways, the classic molar pregnancy may include vaginal bleeding and a uterus enlarged beyond the size expected for gestational age. These findings may be associated with the passage of grapelike structures per vaginum, representing hydropic villi. At times hypertension, edema, and proteinuria occur. Some molar pregnancies are associated with uteri that are small or normal for gestational age. In these cases the diagnosis may be suspected by an elevation of quantitative chorionic gonadotrophin greater than 100,000 mIU/ml. Molar pregnancy must be differentiated from normal gestation, multiple gestation, and uterine enlargements caused by other factors, such as uterine myoma. Bleeding that occurs in the second trimester and is associated with hydatidiform mole may also be associated with a uterus that is large for gestational age; this will also need to be differentiated from hydramnios. An ultrasound examination in the late first trimester or early second trimester generally will detect hydatidiform mole and help in the differential diagnosis of other conditions, such as multiple gestation, hydramnios, and other uterine disorders.

Dysfunctional Uterine Bleeding

The endocrinology of dysfunctional uterine bleeding is discussed in Chapter 37. The frequency with which dysfunctional uterine bleeding occurs, however, is such that it is an important consideration in the differential diagnosis of abnormal vaginal bleeding. It is often a diagnosis of exclusion. The common denominator in many patients with dysfunctional uterine bleeding is anovulation or short ovulatory cycle, but this is not always the case. It is most commonly seen in the postpubertal period when normal hypothalamic function is not well established. In most instances, menstrual periods occur irregularly, often with long gaps between menses. When menses occurs, it may vary from very heavy flow to scanty flow and may continue for a number of days. The bleeding in most instances is from a nonsecretory endometrium. Occasionally the bleeding is profuse with associated signs and symptoms of hypovolemia, requiring emergency care. Endometrial sampling will generally yield scanty nonsecretory endometrium. Rarely is any other pathologic condition noted. In a study in Montreal, Falcone et al. noted that in 61 adolescent patients, 93.4% responded to medical management, only 5 (8.2%) required dilation and curettage, and most had normal clotting factor profiles. Two had newly diagnosed hematologic problems (one had immune thrombocytopenic purpura and one had acute promyelocytic leukemia), but 29% gave a past history of some significant medical problem.

Women in the perimenopausal period who are undergoing some early evidence of ovarian failure may also experience dysfunctional uterine bleeding. Again the pattern may be one of irregularity, and the flow may vary from one that is increased in amount with clots to a scant flow with prolonged spotting. Endometrial biopsy or D&C may yield a diagnosis of nonsecretory endometrium, on histologic section, but hyperplasia of the endometrium may also be noted. In perimenopausal women it is important to differentiate dysfunctional uterine bleeding from other intrauterine disease, and endometrial sampling is indicated. An endometrial biopsy is generally sufficient to establish the appropriate diagnosis and rule out more serious conditions.

Dysfunctional uterine bleeding may also occur during the reproductive years. It may be associated with polycystic ovarian disease or as a secondary symptom to stress, excessive weight change, or increased exercise performance. In such instances amenorrhea, oligomenorrhea, menorrhagia, or metrorrhagia may all be seen. Endometrial sampling generally produces nonsecretory endometrium; rarely is specific disease seen. In patients with polycystic ovarian disease, hyperplasticendometrium may be present. In a study of 1033 premenopausal women ages 17 to 50 who were menstruating regularly but who were complaining of abnormal menstrual bleeding, endometrial biopsy revealed normal endometrium in 93%, endometrial polyps in 2.2%, complex hyperplasia in 2.3%, atypical hyperplasia in 0.03%, and endometrial carcinoma in only 0.05%. Fifty-six percent of the patients were over age 40 and 22.1% over age 45. Sixteen percent were nulliparous, 7% complained of infertility, and 3.4% were diabetics. Thirty-two percent complained of menstrual bleeding lasting longer than 7 days and 8% longer than 14 days. Irregular menstrual bleeding was experienced by one-third of the patients.

The diagnosis of polycystic ovarian syndrome was made in 2.3%. Risk factors for the women with hyperplasia were weight equal to or greater than 90 kg, age 45 or older, infertility, nulliparity, and a family history of colon cancer. Dysfunctional uterine bleeding is discussed more fully in Chapter 37.

Neoplastic Conditions

Although vaginal bleeding can be caused by a wide variety of neoplastic lesions, both benign and malignant affecting the various organs of the female reproductive tract, there are specific patterns that are typical of many of these (Table 7-1). In addition, knowledge of occurrence rates of specific neoplasms in various age groups may help the physician in developing a differential diagnosis.

Cancers of the vulva and vagina may present with vaginal bleeding and usually occur in women who are in the latter reproductive years or in the postmenopausal period. Should they occur in women during the reproductive years, the bleeding is generally intermittent and therefore presents as metrorrhagia or postcoital bleeding rather than with any specific relationship to the menstrual cycle. The bleeding is generally minimal, although in advanced cases it can become profuse. An unusual vaginal tumor that may occur in teenage or young women is clear-cell cancer of the vagina, which is most often seen in women who have been exposed in utero to diethylstilbestrol (DES). Since this condition was first described by Herbst et al. in 1971, the actual incidence has been found to be quite low in such women (Chapter 15). In addition, rare cases of clear-cell cancer of the vagina have been found in women who were not exposed to DES.

Tumors of the cervix are most often squamous cell carcinomas, although as many as 10% are adenocarcinomas and may be present within the endocervical canal (Chapter 29). Such lesions will generally bleed eventually, and the bleeding pattern will be one of metrorrhagia or postcoital

---

TABLE 7-1
Bleeding Pattern Seen in Tumors of the Reproductive Tract

Condition	Menorrhagia	Metrorrhagia	Postmenopausal Bleeding
Vulvar cancer	−	++	++
Vaginal cancer	−	++	++
Cervical cancer	−	++	++
Cervical polyp	−	++	+
Uterine myoma	++	+	−
Carcinoma of endometrium	−	−	++
Fallopian tube cancer	−	−	+
Ovarian cancer	−	±	±

++, Usually occurs; +, occasionally occurs; ±, occurs rarely.

staining. With larger lesions the bleeding may be quite profuse. Other cervical lesions, such as endocervical polyps, may also cause metrorrhagia.

The most common lesions of the uterine corpus that cause abnormal bleeding during the reproductive years are leiomyomas (fibroids). Although these are generally benign, they may become quite large and may cause menorrhagia or menometrorrhagia (Chapter 18). Submucous myomas are generally associated with severe menorrhagia. Leiomyomas rarely cause vaginal bleeding in postmenopausal women. Endometrial carcinoma, generally an adenocarcinoma but occasionally a sarcoma, carcinosarcoma, or some intermediate variety, will cause vaginal bleeding (Chapter 30). Most of these occur in postmenopausal women and therefore would present as postmenopausal bleeding. The bleeding may be scant or profuse. Approximately 5% of endometrial adenocarcinomas occur in premenopausal women. These women most often are exposed to continuous endogenous estrogen stimulation and are often found to have polycystic ovarian disease or a functioning ovarian tumor, such as a granulosal cell tumor or a thecoma. When adenocarcinoma occurs in premenopausal women, these diagnostic possibilities should be considered.

Vaginal bleeding in association with fallopian tube cancer is quite rare and generally occurs in the postmenopausal woman. Nonetheless, scant vaginal bleeding associated frequently with a watery discharge, crampy pain, and occasionally with an adnexal mass should alert the physician to the possibility of this condition (Chapter 34).

Ovarian cancers may present with vaginal bleeding, which is most often the result of intraperitoneal blood finding its way through the fallopian tube and through the uterus into the vagina. In the case of functioning ovarian tumors such as granulosal cell tumor or thecoma, the bleeding may be caused by either a hyperplastic endometrium or an endometrial cancer secondary to the estrogen stimulation.

Rarely, other intraperitoneal tumors may cause intraperitoneal bleeding with eventual vaginal bleeding from secondary passage of the blood through the reproductive tract. This is an unusual occurrence but should be considered in the differential diagnosis of unexplained vaginal bleeding.

Inflammatory Conditions

Although bleeding is not common as a symptom in inflammatory conditions, severe inflammation in tissue will often lead to capillary oozing or a small blood vessel erosion. Thus vulvitis, vaginitis, cervicitis, and endometritis may all be associated with vaginal bleeding or spotting, generally without relationship to menses. At times patients with acute salpingitis or tuboovarian abscess may also experience vaginal bleeding. This most likely comes

from endometrial inflammation or abnormal uterine bleeding secondary to ovarian dysfunction. The symptoms and signs of inflammation, including discharge, pain, and tenderness, and generalized signs and symptoms of infection, will help in the differential diagnosis.

Traumatic Conditions

Direct trauma to the female external genitalia and internal reproductive tract may occur secondary to accidental injury, the placement of foreign bodies within the vagina, and traumatic coitus. Direct lacerations secondary to one of these causes may lead to scant or profuse bleeding, depending on the extent of the injury. Often the bleeding is arterial and requires suture ligations. In children the insertion of foreign bodies into the vagina may lead to vaginal discharge with or without bleeding. Pencils, crayons, pieces of chalk, wads of paper, hairpins, and other items may be found. This is discussed more fully in Chapter 12. In adults, bleeding may be secondary to tampons or contraceptive devices. In older women bleeding may occur when a pessary is being used.

Coital lacerations may occur because of rape or as part of normal sexual function. Tears of the hymen or lacerations of the vagina when tissue is rigid may lead to severe vaginal bleeding. Occasionally, bleeding occurs from the vaginal vault after a hysterectomy. Although this often occurs shortly after the operation, there are reports of dehiscence of the upper vault years later.

Systemic Diseases

A number of systemic diseases are associated with clotting defects and therefore may present with vaginal bleeding or have vaginal bleeding associated with the natural history of the disease. These include various coagulopathies, blood dyscrasias, and endocrinopathies. In addition, patients who take medications that interfere with the normal clotting mechanism may suffer vaginal bleeding. Examples of such medications are heparin and sodium warfarin (Coumadin), which may affect the clotting mechanism directly, or agents that interfere with normal platelet function, such as salicylates and other prostaglandin synthetase inhibitors. Many such conditions can be suspected or diagnosed by history and physical examination. General laboratory studies such as complete blood count, cell smear, and assessment of the clotting mechanism will usually help discover such problems if they exist.

Postmenopausal Bleeding

Although postmenopausal bleeding may be associated with a number of different conditions, it must always be investigated because many causes are premalignant or malignant. The most common premalignant and malig-

TABLE 7-2
Benign Conditions Causing Postmenopausal
Bleeding Found in Patients Seen at the
Chelsea Hospital for Women, London

Cause	Number
Atrophic vaginitis	129
Cervical polyps	65
Leiomyomata uteri	24
Endometrial hyperplasia	13
Cervical erosion	5
Trichomoniasis	3
Hematuria	2
Trauma	1
Vaginal endometriosis	1
Hemorrhoids	1
Moniliasis	1
Bartholin gland abscess	1
Vulvar warts	1
Urethral caruncle	1
TOTAL	248

Modified from Dewhurst J: Clin Obstet Gynecol 26:769, 1983.

nant causes are complex hyperplasia with atypia and carcinoma of the endometrium. These disorders are present in as many as one third of the patients evaluated for postmenopausal bleeding in many series.

Dewhurst described the benign causes of postmenopausal bleeding in 249 women seen at the Chelsea Hospital for Women in London. These are listed in Table 7-2. A large variety of lesions were noted, and the commonest single cause proved to be atrophic vaginitis. Dewhurst wisely counsels that even though an apparent benign cause of bleeding is found, women with postmenopausal bleeding deserve a thorough evaluation to rule out a malignancy that may *also* be present.

Although many other lesions of the reproductive tract, both benign and malignant, may be discovered, one fourth to one third of the patients evaluated may demonstrate no obvious pathologic condition other than an atrophic endometrium.

Currently the diagnostic procedures available for investigating postmenopausal bleeding are endometrial biopsy, D&C, vaginal ultrasonography, sonohysterography, and hysteroscopy with directed biopsy. Endometrial biopsy is comparable with D&C in detecting endometrial carcinoma with a sensitivity of between 85% and 95%, but is not accurate in diagnosing endometrial polyps or myomas. Hysteroscopy with directed biopsy offers the best chance of making an accurate diagnosis but is quite costly.

Endometrial biopsy coupled with sono-hysterography was found to correlate well with the findings of hysteroscopy with biopsy in a study by O'Connell et al. These authors found a greater than 95% correlation with a sensitivity of 94% and a specificity of 96%, suggesting that endometrial biopsy coupled with sonohysterography is a reliable office tool for identifying patients that should be considered for surgical intervention.

PELVIC AND ABDOMINAL PAIN

In 1979 the Taxonomy Committee of the International Association for the Study of Pain defined pain as "an unpleasant sensory and emotional experience associated with actual or potential tissue damage or described in terms of such damage." The committee further stated that pain is always subjective, with each individual learning the application of the word through experience related to injury in early life. It is always unpleasant and is, therefore, an emotional experience. They recognize that people may report pain in the absence of tissue damage or any likely pathophysiologic cause and that this may be secondary to psychologic or psychosocial reasons. Blendis points out that most children and adults have experienced abdominal pain that is often short-lived and rarely associated with physical or organic cause. In many cases, both physical and psychogenic elements exist, making it impossible to tell which was the cause.

Acute Abdomen

A number of intraabdominal conditions can lead to the findings of an acute abdomen. These findings include acute pain, generally of sudden onset; tenderness to palpation; rebound tenderness; and diminished or absent bowel sounds. The pain may be caused by infection, hemorrhage, infarction of tissue, or obstruction of bowel. In the case of bowel obstruction, bowel sounds may be hyperactive. It is important to construct a differential diagnosis when signs and symptoms of acute abdomen are noted. Table 7-3 lists the more common causes of an acute abdomen and identifies the quadrant of the abdomen where findings are more likely to be positive. It should be remembered, however, that the abdominal cavity is a continuum and overlap of signs is extremely common. Disease within a tubular viscus, such as the bowel, fallopian tube, or ureter, may cause crampy pain. Frequently patients complain of paroxysms of sharp, crampy pain interspaced with no pain at all or with periods of dull ache. Inflammatory conditions involving the ovary are frequently associated with continuous pain often described as sharp and throbbing.

Acute appendicitis, mesenteric lymphadenitis, and occasionally torsion of an adnexa may be found in preadolescent and adolescent girls. Appendicitis is, of course, a possible differential diagnosis in all age groups. It often

TABLE 7-3
Conditions That May Cause Signs and Symptoms of Acute Abdomen and Abdominal Quadrants in Which They Most Often Occur

Condition	Quadrant			
	Right Upper	Right Lower	Left Upper	Left Lower
Salpingitis	−	+	−	+
Tuboovarian abscess	±	+	±	+
Ectopic pregnancy	−	+	−	+
Torsive adnexa	−	+	−	+
Ruptured ovarian cyst	−	+	−	+
Acute appendicitis	−	+	−	−
Mesenteric lymphadenitis	−	+	−	−
Crohn's disease	−	+	−	−
Acute cholecystitis	+	±	−	−
Perforated peptic ulcer	+	±	+	±
Acute pancreatitis	+	−	+	−
Acute pyelitis	+	±	+	±
Renal calculus	+	+	+	+
Splenic infarct	−	−	+	−
Splenic rupture	−	−	+	−
Acute diverticulitis	−	−	−	+

+, More frequently; ± may occur.

presents initially as periumbilical pain that localizes to the right lower quadrant and is accompanied by anorexia or nausea and vomiting. Salpingitis, tuboovarian abscess, ectopic pregnancy, and ruptured ovarian cysts are common findings in those patients of reproductive age who have an acute abdomen. Patients with salpingitis tend to have a higher fever than those with appendicitis, but great variability may be observed. Although their pain may be severe, they tend to be less ill than those with appendicitis. However, these women may have Crohn's disease, acute cholecystitis, perforated peptic ulcer, acute pyelitis, renal calculi, splenic infarct, and splenic rupture. Occasionally, they may also suffer from acute pancreatitis, which usually presents as epigastric pain often radiating to the back.

Acute abdomen in older women suggests torsion or rupture of an adnexa, acute cholecystitis, perforated ulcer, or acute diverticulitis. Pelvic inflammatory disease is less common in older women, and acute exacerbations are rare in those who have had tubal ligation.

Acute Pelvic Pain

Acute pain of gynecologic origin presents as both pelvic and lower abdominal pain. Diseases and dysfunction of the genitourinary tract, gastrointestinal tract, and muscu-loskeletal system may also cause pain in these regions. The box on page 162 lists a number of gynecologic and nongynecologic conditions that can cause acute onset of pelvic or lower abdominal pain.

Threatened, inevitable, or incomplete abortion generally is accompanied by midline or bilateral lower abdominal pain, usually of a crampy, intermittent nature. In such instances vaginal bleeding is generally present. When infection occurs concurrently (septic abortion), there is generally temperature elevation, systemic symptoms of chills and malaise, and often an elevated white cell count and erythrocyte sedimentation rate (ESR). Rapid serum pregnancy tests are generally positive.

Ectopic pregnancy generally is associated with unilateral, continuous, crampy pain, although there may be some bilaterality to the presentation. Most ectopic pregnancies are associated with vaginal bleeding. Temperature elevation, if present, is usually minimal, and white cell count and ESR are generally normal but may be slightly elevated, particularly if there is intraperitoneal hemorrhage. Serum β-hCG is positive, and ultrasound examination may help in the diagnosis either by revealing a gestational sac in an adnexa or by ruling out the diagnosis through demonstration of a gestational sac within the uterus. Physical examination frequently

Possible Causes of Acute Pelvic and Lower Abdominal Pain

Pregnancy-related
  Abortion
  Ectopic
Disorders of the uterus and cervix
  Cervicitis
  Endometritis
  Degenerating myoma
Disorders of the adnexa
  Salpingitis
  Tuboovarian abscess
  Endometriosis (endometrioma)
  Torsion of adnexa
  Torsion of hydatid of Morgagni
  Rupture of follicle or corpus luteum cyst
  Ovarian hyperstimulation syndrome
  Degenerating ovarian tumor
Nongynecologic disorders
  Appendicitis
  Mesenteric lymphadenitis
  Diverticulitis
  Functional bowel syndrome
  Cystitis
  Trigonitis
  Renal calculus
  Musculoskeletal disorders

demonstrates the presence of a mass in the adnexal region. Intraperitoneal bleeding may be suspected by seeing fluid on ultrasound examination and diagnosed by culdocentesis, with a definitive diagnosis made by laparoscopy.

Acute cervicitis, often caused by *Neisseria gonorrhoeae* or *Chlamydia trachomatis*, may frequently be associated with lower abdominal and pelvic pain. The pain is often of a dull, aching nature and may radiate to the low back or to the upper thighs. There is generally a cervical and vaginal discharge, and there may be a low-grade fever, slight leukocytosis, and slight increase in ESR. Definitive diagnosis is made by specific culture for the organism.

Endometritis is generally transient and occurs in *Neisseria* or *Chlamydia* infections as part of their natural history. Occasionally, vigorous chemical douching will lead to a chemical endometritis. The pain is generally midline, pelvic, or lower abdominal and often aching in type.

Degenerating myoma will frequently cause acute, sharp, or aching pain in the region of the myoma. Diagnosis is aided by the facts that the uterus is irregular and enlarged and that there is tenderness to palpation. There may be a mild leukocytosis, but generally laboratory parameters are normal.

Salpingitis and tuboovarian abscess have been discussed under Acute Abdomen. Endometriosis is discussed in detail in Chapter 19. The pain pattern depends on the location of the endometrial implants and varies from dysmen-

orrhea and dyspareunia to continuous, generalized pelvic discomfort.

Torsion of an adnexa with or without an ovarian cyst or tumor may lead to acute, crampy, or continuous pain and has been discussed under Acute Abdomen. It can be confused with appendicitis or pelvic inflammatory disease (PID). Occasionally a hydatid of Morgagni will undergo torsion and give similar symptoms.

Rupture of an ovarian cyst may cause a sudden onset of pain. Leaking from a corpus luteum cyst generally occurs midcycle and, if it is on the right side, may be misdiagnosed as appendicitis. Ovarian hyperstimulation syndrome is a rare entity that may occur in women being treated with follicle-stimulating hormone (Pergonal) to stimulate ovulation; it is most likely to occur if pregnancy ensues. In such instances the gestation is often found to be multiple. Ovarian hyperstimulation-like conditions may occur in women suffering from trophoblastic disease and, rarely, in women with severe isoimmunization disease such as Rh isoimmunization. It is often seen in women undergoing in vitro fertilization procedures because of the ovulation-stimulating drugs.

Degenerating adnexal tumors that have outgrown their blood supply may also cause acute-onset lower abdominal or pelvic pain.

Appendicitis, mesenteric lymphadenitis, and diverticulitis have all been discussed under Acute Abdomen. Appendicitis and mesenteric lymphadenitis generally present as right lower quadrant or right pelvic pain, and diverticulitis most often presents as a left-sided pain. Young women suffering from functional bowel syndrome will often present with a crampy severe left lower quadrant pain generally made worse by emotional tension and stress. As many as 25% of young women may have this condition.

Patients suffering from cystitis and trigonitis may complain of lower abdominal or pelvic pain, generally midline in nature, accompanied by dysuria. Women suffering from renal calculus will generally have severe, intermittent flank pain on the side of the stone; this pain often radiates toward the lower abdomen.

A variety of musculoskeletal disorders may also present as pelvic pain, lower abdominal pain, or backache. Slocumb has called attention to the presence of "trigger points" discernible by palpation in the abdominal wall, lower back, and in the vaginal vault. Touching or stimulating these may simulate the pain about which the patient is complaining. Slocumb noted relief in several patients after the injection of these points with a local anesthetic such as 0.25% bupivacaine on one or several occasions. He notes that the pain often disappears for longer periods than the drug would be expected to cause. Because of this he speculates that in some instances chronic pelvic pain may be caused by a neurologic reflex that can be interrupted by the injection. Certainly irritation of the musculoskeletal system by exercise or injury can produce pain that can cause the patient to believe she has internal organ disease. Perhaps the injection of "trigger points" contributes to a reassurance that this is not the case.

Pain emanating from the uterus, such as with dysmenorrhea or that associated with adenomyosis and occasionally adnexal disease, may radiate to the anterior thigh. Rarely are the inner or outer aspects of the thigh involved, and the posterior thigh is never involved with such conditions. Pain radiating to the posterior thigh generally denotes sciatic nerve involvement, and this is commonly seen with cervical cancer of an advanced nature. Occasionally, endometriosis may cause such pain by irritating the sciatic nerve.

Most pain that is limited to the lower back but not to the abdominal region is generally of musculoskeletal origin rather than from gynecologic disease.

Chronic Pelvic Pain

Chronic and recurrent pelvic pain is one of the major problems seen by the gynecologist. Dysmenorrhea (see Chapter 35) is perhaps the commonest example of recurrent pelvic pain. In addition, incompletely treated pelvic infections, recurrent pelvic infections, endometriosis, and possibly postoperative pelvic adhesions and diseases of the urinary tract and bowel may all be responsible for recurrent or persistent pelvic pain. Many who complain of chronic pelvic pain have no demonstrable pelvic disorder. Cunanan et al. reviewed 1194 charts of consecutive pelvic pain patients who had undergone diagnostic laparoscopy and discovered that in 355 cases a normal pelvis was found. Interestingly, of the 1194 patients, 749 had a normal pelvic examination before the diagnostic laparoscopy and, of these, 479 (63%) had abnormal findings on diagnostic laparoscopy. Of the 445 patients who had been thought to have an abnormal pelvic examination before laparoscopy, 78 (17.5%) actually had normal findings on diagnostic laparoscopy.

Kresch et al. reported the laparoscopic findings of 100 women who complained of constant pelvic pain in the same location for a minimum of 6 months. These authors compared the findings in this group with those of 50 women who were asymptomatic but who were undergoing laparoscopic tubal ligation. Overall, 83% of the group with pelvic pain had abnormal pelvic findings, whereas only 29% of the asymptomatic group demonstrated such findings. Pelvic adhesions were the most common pathologic finding, accounting for 38% of the abnormalities seen. Pelvic endometriosis accounted for 32% of the abnormal findings in the symptomatic group. These authors pointed out that when chronic pelvic pain exists in the same area for a minimum of 6 months, it is usually associated with specific pathologic conditions. However, even in this group of patients, 17% had no pelvic disorder at the time of diagnostic laparoscopy.

The question of whether pelvic adhesions are a frequent cause of chronic pelvic pain is as yet unanswered. Rapkin reviewed 100 consecutive laparoscopies performed because of chronic pelvic pain and compared the pelvic findings with those noted in 88 laparoscopies performed in infertility patients. A total of 26 (26%) of the pain group and 34 (39%) of the infertility group demonstrated pelvic adhesions as the only pathology seen. However, only 4 of the 34 patients in the infertility group complained of pain. Peters et al. performed a randomized trial of adhesiolysis in 48 patients found by laparoscopy to have ASRM stage II-IV pelvic adhesions. Twenty-four underwent adhesiolysis, and 24 did not. After 9 to 12 months of follow-up, no significant differences with respect to pelvic pain were noted between the two groups. However, eight of nine women in a subgroup who had dense, vascularized (stage IV) adhesions involving bowel showed significant improvement after adhesiolysis, whereas only one of six not given adhesiolysis reported improvement of pain. These authors concluded that pain relief might be obtained by lysing dense adhesions but probably not by lysing light or moderate adhesions.

Patients presenting with chronic pelvic pain deserve an adequate workup. In most cases this would include a laparoscopic examination.

The box on page 164 offers an outline of a workup for a patient with chronic pelvic pain. It is important that the physician determine not only the specific nature of the pain itself but also acquire a good understanding of the patient's basic physical, mental, and social status to determine what factors may be influencing the patient's symptom complex.

A complete physical examination with emphasis on the effects of previous operations, infections, injuries, and, of course, a complete pelvic examination should be carried out. Cervical cultures for gonococcus and *Chlamydia*, as well as a Pap smear, are appropriate.

Laboratory data for patients with chronic pelvic pain should include CBC, ESR, serologic tests for syphilis, urine analysis, and urine culture where appropriate. When indicated by history and physical findings, radiologic or ultrasound evaluation of the gastrointestinal (GI) and genitourinary (GU) tracts should be ordered.

Other studies that may be appropriate, depending on the history and physical examination, include psychiatric evaluation, social work evaluation, psychologic testing, such as the Minnesota Multiphasic Personality Index (MMPI), and biopsies if indicated. Laparoscopic examination is often indicated in such patients to discover or rule out pathologic conditions.

After completing the workup the physician may still be unable to find a cause for the chronic pelvic pain. In the past a variety of explanations were offered, including abnormal positioning of the uterus, laceration of the uterine supports, and vascular congestion of the pelvic organs. However, many of these patients have a psychosomatic disorder and benefit from counseling or treatment for depression.

Workup of a Patient with Chronic Pelvic Pain

History
  Description and timing of pain (menstrual, intermittent, continuous, related to stress, etc.)
  Presence of pain in other parts of the body (headache, backache, etc.)
  Menstrual history and history of abnormal bleeding
  Sexual history
    Dyspareunia
  Work and leisure habits
  Problems involving other organ systems (urinary tract, GI tract)
  Previous pelvic and abdominal infections
  Previous operative procedures or diagnostic procedures
  Other gynecologic disorders (e.g., endometriosis)
  Social history (marital status; children; stresses in life as a child, an adolescent, and an adult; history of physical or sexual abuse or intimidation)
Physical examination
Laboratory evaluation
  CBC
  ESR
  VDRL
  Urinalysis and culture
  Evaluation of GI and GU tracts (where appropriate)
  Pap smear
Other studies (where appropriate)
  Psychiatric evaluation
  Social work evaluation
  Psychologic testing (e.g., MMPI)
  Laparoscopy
  Ultrasound
  CT scan, magnetic resonance imaging
  Biopsies if indicated
  Cultures of cervix

Perhaps as many as 20% of all women demonstrate retroversion or retroflexion of the uterus at any given time. Rarely is the condition pathologic, and in most cases the uterus can be displaced from its posterior position in the pelvis to its normal anterior position by bimanual examination or by positioning the patient in the knee-chest position. When such anterior displacement of the uterus has been effected, the physician may place a Smith-Hodge pessary into the vagina to hold the uterus in an anterior position. If this maneuver alleviates the pain, the patient may continue to wear the pessary or may be offered a uterine suspension procedure. In most cases, however, retrodisplacement of the uterus does not appear to be a cause of pelvic pain, and replacement will make no difference in the patient's symptoms. Occasionally the uterus is fixed in the posterior pelvis by postinflammatory or postoperative adhesions or by endometriosis. In these instances, the primary disease, not the retrodisplacement, may be responsible for the pain.

Allen and Masters defined the problem of traumatic lacerations of the uterine supports in 1955. They theorized that lacerations of the posterior leaf of the broad ligament or of the uterosacral ligament may have occurred at the time of a traumatic obstetric delivery and that with healing a greater rotation was allowed for the uterus. This condition has been called the *universal joint syndrome,* since it was theorized that the uterus could rotate freely, as with a universal joint. Many physicians have attempted to repair these so-called lacerations, and they are visible in some patients on laparoscopic examination. However, it is difficult to demonstrate a cause-and-effect relationship with pelvic pain, and a placebo effect may be responsible for occasional apparently successful outcomes.

Pelvic vascular engorgement has been observed on many occasions. Taylor defined the pelvic congestion syndrome as pain and heaviness in the pelvis that occurs after arising and becomes worse as the day progresses. On laparoscopic examination the uterus usually appears to be dusky blue and mottled, and often varicosities of the veins of the broad ligament are noted. Not all women with such findings complain of pelvic pain, and it is difficult to prove an actual cause. Beard et al. offered some evidence that pelvic varicosities might be a source of chronic pelvic pain. They compared 45 patients with chronic pelvic pain and no obvious pathology with 10 patients with pelvic pathology and 8 who were scheduled for tubal ligations. Each patient underwent a pelvic venogram, and the pelvic vein varicosities were graded by a radiologist blinded to the patients' complaints. A definite difference was noted in the increased diameters of the ovarian veins associated with a slower emptying time in the pelvic pain group. Beard et al. found very good relief of pain in 36 women with demonstrated pelvic congestion, 33 of whom had failed medical management, when total abdominal hysterectomy and bilateral salpingo-oophorectomy was performed. Hormone replacement therapy was utilized, and there was a 1-year follow-up before reevaluation.

Some patients do appear to suffer from psychosomatic disease with pelvic pain as a manifestation. Patients with chronic pelvic pain who do not seem to have obvious pathologic conditions will often reveal chaotic social histories involving both early and present life. Many of these individuals will be depressed and suffer from stress and anxiety, and some will suffer from borderline personality disorders. It is difficult to draw specific conclusions in this respect, however. Renaer demonstrated multiple symptom complaints in 12 of 24 patients with chronic pelvic pain without obvious disease. But only 1 of 22 patients suffering from chronic pelvic pain and endometriosis had such multiple symptoms. However, personality profiles developed by psychometric testing in each group failed to show differences between the two groups. A number of previous authors have pointed out that personality examinations in patients with chronic pain do not differentiate between psychogenic and organic pain.

Some investigators have noted a relationship between a history of childhood and later-life physical and sexual abuse and chronic pelvic pain. Harrop-Griffiths et al. ascertained a greater prevalence of lifetime major depression, current major depression, lifetime substance abuse history, sexual dysfunction, somatization, and an increased incidence of childhood and adult sexual abuse in a group of chronic pelvic pain patients at the time of laparoscopy compared with a group of patients without pain undergoing laparoscopy for tubal ligation or infertility.

Walling et al. studied 64 women with chronic pelvic pain, 42 women with chronic headache, and 46 pain-free women using a structured interview technique. They found that women with chronic pelvic pain had a higher lifetime prevalence of sexual abuse involving penetration or other genital or anal contact (major sexual abuse) than either of the other groups. However, with respect to physical abuse, the chronic pelvic pain group had a higher lifetime prevalence than the pain-free group but not the headache group. The difference between the headache and pain-free group was not significant—thus this study supports a specific relationship between a history of major sexual abuse and chronic pelvic pain and a more general association between physical abuse and chronic pain.

Budura et al. studied 46 women with chronic pelvic pain using a structured interview to assess sexual and physical abuse and somatization. The Dissociative Experience Scale was used to assess dissociation, and an abbreviated COPE scale was used to assess adaptive and maladaptive coping strategies as well as substance abuse. They found that those women in the group with self-reported sexual or physical abuse histories had significantly higher disassociation, somatization, and substance abuse scores than did the patients without such histories.

Physicians should evaluate chronic pelvic pain patients in a holistic fashion, investigating past social and emotional problems along with the physical evaluation. This makes it possible to offer specific multidiscipline therapy without suggesting to the patient that the problem is "all in her head." Placing the pain in the context of the patient's total life situation rather than as a specific isolated entity often makes a holistic approach possible.

Patients with chronic pain who do not demonstrate apparent organic causes will frequently have levator ani muscle spasm or spasm of other groups of muscle within the pelvis. Occasionally, trigger points may be defined in the anterior abdominal wall by deep digital pressure. These probably also represent spasm in local muscle bundles. These patients may also suffer from tenderness of the uterus and adnexa, which conceivably could be caused by vascular engorgement or adenomyosis. They pose difficult and demanding diagnostic and treatment challenges.

If no pathologic condition is evident but pain is persistent, physicians and patients alike have often yielded to the temptation of treating with a total hysterectomy and bilateral salpingo-oophorectomy. There is no evidence that this therapy relieves the pain in such patients and, indeed, failure to relieve the pain may lead to anger and frustration. Slocumb has shown that hysterectomy was successful in relieving pelvic pain only if dysmenorrhea was part of the symptom complex. Therefore patients without obvious pelvic disease who have pelvic pain but not dysmenorrhea should not be offered hysterectomy. In such cases the physician should seek and treat psychosocial problems, depression, or other psychologic disease with medications, counseling, or referral to a psychiatrist or other mental health worker where appropriate.

PELVIC AND LOWER ABDOMINAL MASSES

Pelvic and lower abdominal masses may be cystic or solid and occur in any age group. They may originate from the cervix, the uterus, or the adnexa; from other organs, such as the GU tract or the bowel; or from the musculoskeletal system, vascular-lymphatic system, or nervous system. In this section the relevant incidence of pelvic and lower abdominal tumors in the various age groups will be considered and, where appropriate, means of differential diagnosis will be discussed.

Before discussing relative frequencies and types of abdominal and pelvic tumors found in different age groups, some comparisons of the more common adnexal tumors by age group are appropriate. During the reproductive years the majority of adnexal masses are follicle cysts. These tumors are functional in nature and generally disappear in 1 to 3 months. They vary in size from just a few centimeters to as much as 8 to 10 cm in diameter. They are thin-walled and frequently rupture during pelvic examination. In and of themselves they are of no clinical significance. It is likely that most women develop follicle cysts from time to time, and discovery may be related to the chance of performing a pelvic examination at the time when they exist. They rarely cause symptoms; however, when they do become large, they may cause some heaviness in the lower pelvis or in the leg. Because they are filled with follicular fluid, their rupture rarely causes any pathologic problem. A cystic adnexal mass of 5 to 8 cm that develops in a woman during the reproductive years is usually followed for at least one menstrual cycle, since functional cysts are common and the risk of malignancy is small. Ultrasound studies, particularly using a vaginal probe, can be very helpful in establishing a diagnosis and following the progress of a cyst, and can be reassuring to the patient and the doctor alike. It can help differentiate between a simple and a multiloculated cyst and can rule out a solid tumor. Figure 7-1 is an example of a simple follicle cyst seen with vaginal ultrasound.

Also common during the reproductive years are hemorrhagic corpora lutea. These masses rarely become larger than 5 cm in diameter and frequently are somewhat tender to palpation. If they leak blood, they may mimic an ectopic pregnancy. They generally regress within a few weeks. Figure 7-2 demonstrates a 3.1 cm hemorrhagic corpus luteum on vaginal sonogram. (Courtesy of Dr. Steven R. Goldstein.)

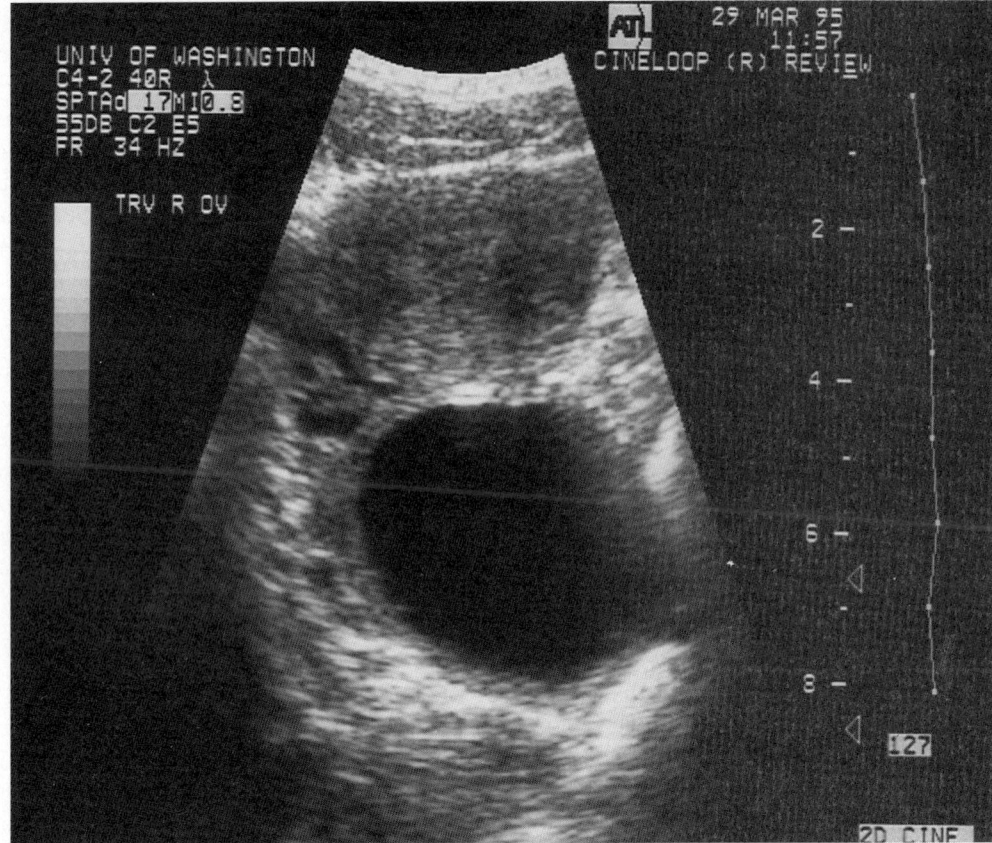

FIGURE 7-1   Large simple follicle cyst detected by vaginal ultrasound examination.

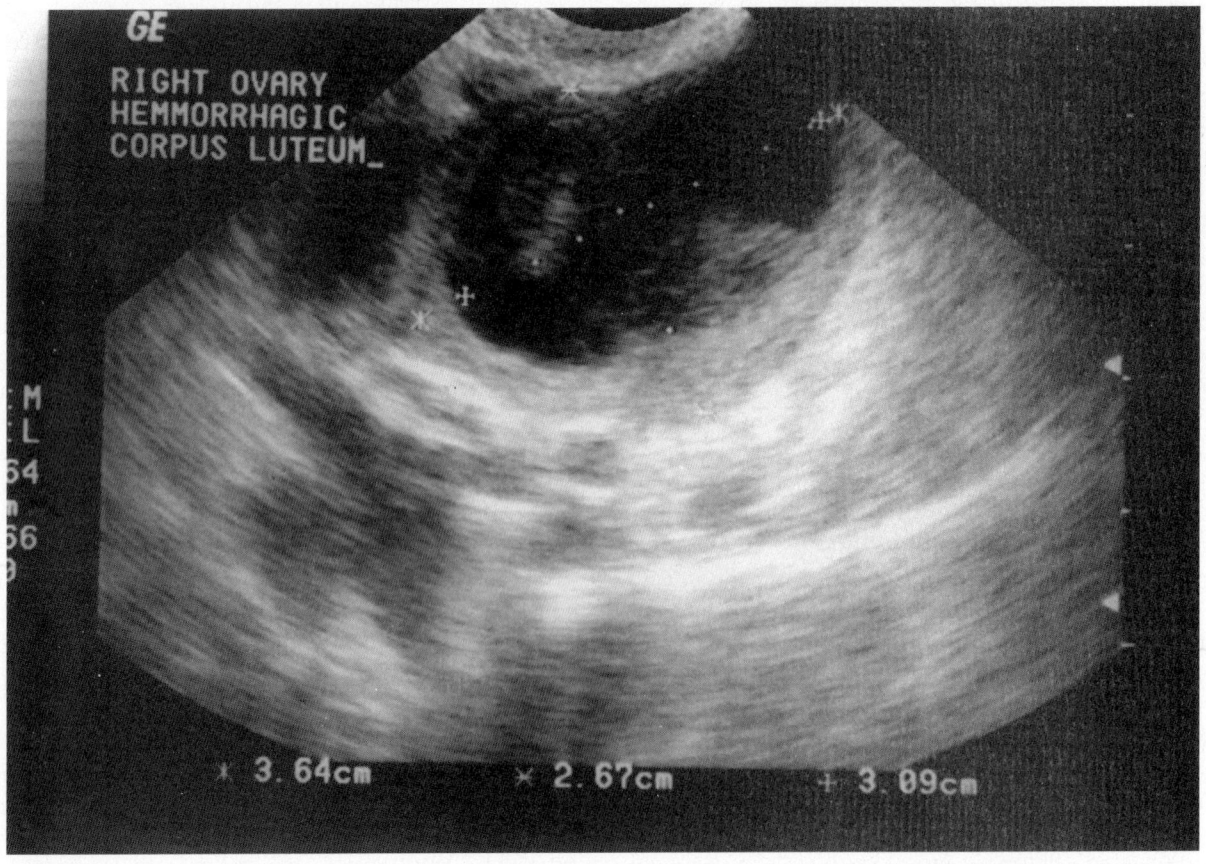

FIGURE 7-2   Transvaginal sonogram depicting a 3.1 cm hemorrhagic corpus luteum. (Courtesy of Dr. Steven R. Goldstein.)

TABLE 7-4
Age Distribution and Laterality of 443 Benign Ovarian Neoplasms

Type	Age						
	0–19	20–44	45–54	55–64	65–74	75+	Total
Serous cystadenoma							
U*	4	124	35	23	10	2	198
B	1	17	3	4	2	0	27
Mucinous cystadenoma							
U	1	42	5	5	1	0	54
B	0	1	0	0	0	0	1
Benign teratoma							
U	8	93	12	7	2	0	122
B	0	9	1	0	0	0	10
Brenner							
U	1	4	1	0	0	0	6
B	0	0	0	0	0	0	0
Thecoma-fibroma							
U	0	11	3	8	1	1	24
B	0	0	0	1	0	0	1
TOTAL							
U	14	274	56	43	14	3	404
B	1	27	4	5	2	0	39

From Bennington JL, Ferguson BR, and Haber SL: Obstet Gynecol 32:627, 1968. Reprinted with permission from The American College of Obstetricians and Gynecologists.

*Location of neoplasm; U, unilateral; B, bilateral.

There are a number of benign and malignant neoplasms of the ovary that occur quite frequently and do have special incident relationships to various age groups (Chapters 18 and 31). In 1968 Bennington et al. reviewed 443 benign and 106 malignant neoplasms of the ovary discovered in a period from 1951 to 1963 at the Oakland Kaiser Foundation Hospital. During those years, between 61,000 and 83,500 women were served annually. Because the Kaiser enrollees represented a cross section of the population in that area of California, this study made it possible to observe the relative frequency of different ovarian neoplasms within the general population. Most other studies were reported by referral institutions, and therefore the data from the standpoint of prevalence was clouded. Thus, although this is a comparatively old study, it still represents useful data because it is an indication of incidence of various tumors in the general population. Bennington et al. noted that serous cystadenoma and benign cystic teratoma (dermoid cyst) were the most commonly observed benign neoplasms of the adnexa. In addition, mucinous cystadenoma, Brenner tumors, thecomas, and fibromas were also seen. Table 7-4 demonstrates the age distribution and occurrence of bilaterality of 443 benign ovarian neoplasms observed by Bennington et al. Although benign ovarian neoplasms were uncommon in the group up to 19 years of age, the most commonly seen

benign neoplasm in this age group was the benign cystic teratoma. In the 20- to 44-year age group, serous cystadenomas were the most common benign neoplasm, with benign cystic teratomas and mucinous cystadenomas next in frequency. The serous cystadenomas occurred in all age groups but less commonly in women over age 75. Mucinous cystadenomas occurred sporadically in all age groups, but none were seen after age 75. The majority of mucinous cystadenomas, however, occurred in women in the reproductive years. Similarly, benign cystic teratomas occurred in all age groups until age 75, but the majority occurred in the reproductive years. Brenner tumors occurred sporadically; however, none were seen after age 55. Thecomas and fibromas occurred in all age groups from 20 to beyond 75, but again the majority were in women between the ages of 20 and 64.

Malignant tumors of the ovary were not seen in the 19- and-younger age group of the Kaiser population except for one tumor that was metastatic to the ovary from another site. Serous cystadenocarcinoma occurred in all age groups from 20 to beyond 75 and was the most common malignant tumor seen in all age groups, but ovarian carcinomas are rare before age 40 (Figure 7-3). Metastatic tumors to the ovary were the second most common ovarian malignant neoplasm seen in this study. Of the serous cystadeno-

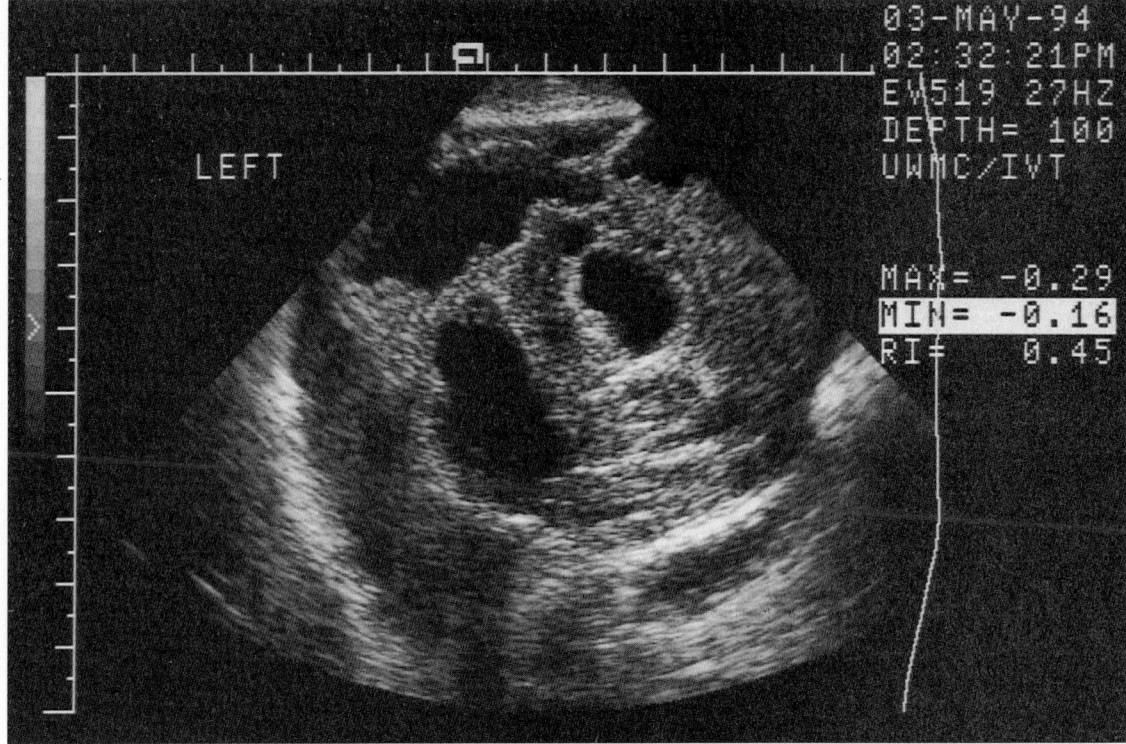

FIGURE 7-3   Multiloculated ovarian cyst detected by vaginal ultrasound. Pathology proved to be serous cystadenocarcinoma.

carcinomas, 40% were bilateral, and roughly 50% of metastatic neoplasms were bilateral in all age groups. Mucinous cystadenocarcinoma was seen in all age groups from 20 to beyond 75. In general the chance of malignancy seemed to be greater in these tumors in the older age groups. Endometrioid carcinoma occurred in a few patients in the series, as did granulosal cell carcinoma. Few other tumors were seen in this study. Table 7-5 summarizes the 106 patients with malignant ovarian neoplasm in the Bennington study by age distribution, laterality, and cell type.

Figure 7-4 plots the incidence of a number of the tumors noted in the Bennington study per 100,000 woman-years. Although their numbers of cases were relatively small, the incidence figures do demonstrate the prevalence by age of these various tumors.

Killackey and Neuwirth evaluated pelvic masses in 540 patients admitted to St. Lukes-Roosevelt Hospital in New York in 1984-85. Of 249 patients admitted with a diagnosis of uterine myomas, 235 (94.4%) diagnoses proved to be correct, whereas benign adnexal masses were found in 7 (2.8%), cancers in 4 (1.6%), and miscellaneous findings in 3 (1.2%). Of 291 patients evaluated for "pelvic mass," benign ovarian or tubal cysts were noted in 98 (33.7%), uterine myoma in 42 (14.4%), cancers in 40 (13.7%), benign cystic teratomas in 38 (13.1%), endometriosis in 28 (9.6%), miscellaneous in 23 (7.9%), and pelvic inflammatory disease in 22 (7.6%). Table 7-6 demonstrates these diagnostic findings by patient age.

Koonings et al. also studied a large group of women (861) who were admitted for adnexal masses over a 10-year period. They wished to clarify the distribution of primary ovarian neoplasms by decade of life. They found that the overall risk for malignancy was 13% in premenopausal women and 45% in postmenopausal women. As seen in other studies, germ cell tumors predominated in women under age 40, and epithelial tumors became more frequent in the decades after age 40.

Masses in Childhood

Occasionally, babies are born with adnexal cysts that present as abdominal masses. These are generally follicular cysts secondary to maternal hormone stimulation of fetal ovaries. The cysts generally regress within the first few months of life. Thereafter cysts and all tumors of the female pelvic organs are quite rare during childhood. Abdominal masses found in the young child are more likely to be Wilms' tumors or neuroblastomas. Tumors of the GI tract, musculoskeletal system, or lymphatic system may also occur occasionally. Solid or mixed solid and cystic adnexal masses are rare, but when they do occur are almost always dysgerminomas or teratomas. Mueller et al. reviewed 427 cases of dysgerminoma in 1950 and noted that 6.89% of the tumors occurred in the 1- to 10-year age group. Asadourian and Taylor, reviewing 105 cases of dysgerminoma in the Armed Forces Institute of Pathology experi-

TABLE 7-5
Age Distribution and Laterality of 80 Primary and 26 Secondary Malignant Ovarian Neoplasms

Type	Age						
	0–19	20–44	45–54	55–64	65–74	75+	Total
Serous cystadenocarcinoma							
U*	0	8	9	10	1	2	30
B	0	7	11	3	2	1	24
Mucinous cystadenocarcinoma							
U	0	1	0	4	1	1	7
B	0	0	0	2	1	0	3
Endometroid carcinoma							
U	0	2	0	0	0	0	2
B	0	0	1	1	1	0	3
Granulose carcinoma							
U	0	2	0	2	1	1	6
B	0	0	0	0	0	0	0
Other							
U	0	1†	4‡	0	0	0	5
B	0	0	0	0	0	0	0
Metastases							
U	1	3	7	1	0	0	12
B	0	7	4	3	0	0	14
TOTAL							
U	1	17	20	17	3	4	62
B	0	14	16	9	4	1	44

From Bennington JL, Ferguson BR, and Haber SL: Obstet Gynecol 32:627, 1968. Reprinted with permission from The American College of Obstetricians and Gynecologists.

*Location of neoplasm: U, unilateral; B, bilateral.

†Squamous carcinoma arising in a cystic teratoma.

‡One arrhenoblastoma, one germinoma, one malignant Brenner tumor, and one mesonephric carcinoma.

ence, noted that only seven of these patients were 9 years of age or younger.

Although benign and malignant teratomas have been reported in childhood, they are quite rare before the age of 10. Caruso et al., reporting on 305 teratomas of the ovary, found none in children under age 10. However, Costin and Kennedy, reviewing 200 ovarian tumors in infants and children, found 25% to be benign cystic teratomas.

Masses in Adolescence (Menarche to 19 Years)

Once menses begins, obstruction of the lower reproductive tract, such as with imperforate hymen, agenesis of the vagina with intact cervix and uterus, or vaginal septum, may give rise to a hematocolpos or a hematometrium. Thus abdominal or pelvic masses may occur secondary to these conditions. Other anomalies of the reproductive tract, such as obstructed uterine horns, may also give rise to a hematometrium and a pelvic mass (Chapter 11). Myomas of the uterus are rare in this age group but have been reported.

The majority of adnexal masses in this age group are functional cysts and vary in size from 3 to 10 cm. Of neoplastic ovarian tumors found, the most common is benign cystic teratoma of the ovary. In Caruso's study of 305 teratomas of the ovary, 8.5% occurred in this age group. These tumors are generally between 5 and 10 cm in diameter, are slow-growing, and are frequently asymptomatic. Some benign cystic teratomas are larger than 10 cm. In Caruso's series of 305 teratomas, 49 measured 10 to 14 cm; 21, 15 to 19 cm; and 11, between 20 and 39 cm. They are generally found because a mass is detected on abdominal or pelvic examination. However, benign cystic teratomas may cause adnexal torsion and present as an acute abdomen. Rarely, the tumor may rupture, spilling oily, irritating contents into the peritoneal cavity and creating evidence of an acute abdomen. These tumors frequently have a thickened capsule, and rupture is unusual. Because benign cystic teratomas may contain bone or teeth, abdominal roentgenograms or ultrasound may identify these. Figure 7-5 demonstrates a transvaginal sonogram of a 4.0 × 3.6 cm dermoid cyst. (Courtesy of Dr. Steven R. Goldstein.)

Solid or solid and cystic adnexal tumors, although rare in adolescence, are almost always dysgerminomas or malignant teratomas.

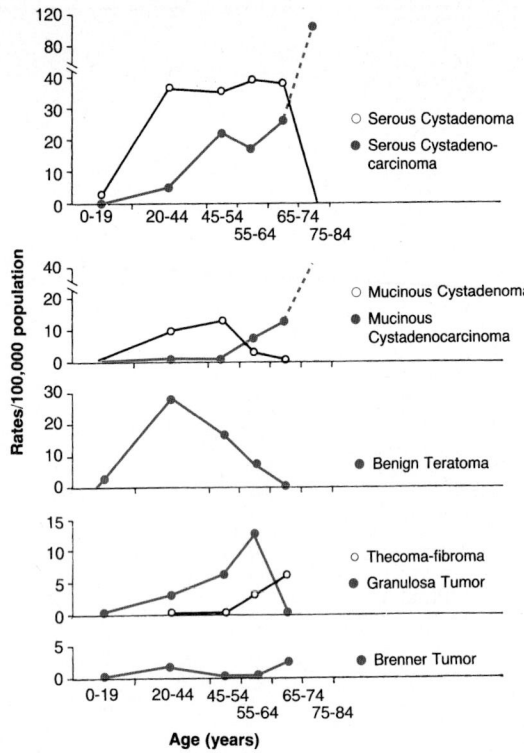

FIGURE 7-4 Incidence rates for ovarian tumors by age group per 100,000 women at each age interval. (From Bennington JL, Ferguson BR, and Haber SL: Obstet Gynecol 32:627, 1968. Reprinted with permission from The American College of Obstetricians and Gynecologists.)

In 137 women younger than 21 years who were found to have ovarian enlargement reported by Diamond et al., 82 had ovarian neoplasms, of which 8 were borderline or malignant. All 6 malignant lesions were germ cell in origin. Likewise, in a study by Norris and Jensen of 353 primary ovarian neoplasms in women younger than 20 years, germ cell tumors represented 58% of cases. Of these 205 patients, 71 had benign cystic teratomas, 54 malignant teratomas, 48 dysgerminomas, and 32 embryonal carcinomas. Of the remaining cases, 67 (19%) were of epithelial origin, 62 (18%) stromal, and 19 (5%) miscellaneous.

Dysgerminomas and teratomas can vary from just a few centimeters to an extremely large size. In 117 dysgerminomas reviewed by Asadourian and Taylor, 12 were found to have other germ cell elements, including embryonal carcinoma, teratocarcinoma, and choriocarcinoma.

Cystic adnexal masses derived from mesonephric elements, such as paraovarian and paratubal cysts, are also seen in this age group. They may vary in size from 1 to 2 cm to quite large. They are thin-walled, benign entities without solid components.

Masses emanating from other organ systems in the pelvis and abdomen also occur in this age group and must be considered.

Masses During the Reproductive Years (20 to 44 Years)

Masses seen in women of reproductive age may develop from the uterus and cervix, the adnexa, and other organ systems. Intrauterine pregnancy, ectopic pregnancy, and trophoblastic disease should always be considered in women of reproductive years who develop such masses. These conditions can often be ruled in or out by use of a serum pregnancy test and ultrasound. Ectopic pregnancy is generally associated with an adnexal mass, vaginal

---

TABLE 7-6
Surgical Findings in 540 Patients Evaluated for Leiomyomata/Pelvic Masses at St. Lukes-Roosevelt Hospital 1984–1985

Surgical Diagnosis	Number of Patients in Each Age Group							
	10–20	21–30	31–40	41–50	51–60	61–70	>70	Total
Leiomyomata	0	13	99	142	19	3	0	276
Benign/functional cysts	1	24	32	23	8	9	7	104
Cancer	2	0	3	11	7	12	9	44
Benign cystic teratoma	4	17	9	3	0	3	1	37
Endometriosis	0	7	16	7	2	0	0	32
Miscellaneous	1	4	11	2	1	4	2	25
Tubo-ovarian abscess/ pelvic inflammatory disease	2	7	9	4	0	0	0	22
TOTAL	10	72	179	192	37	31	19	540

From Killackey MA and Neuwirth RS: Obstet Gynecol 71:319, 1988.

bleeding, and pelvic pain, as discussed earlier in this chapter. Trophoblastic disease may be associated with inappropriate uterine size for menstrual dates, vaginal bleeding, pelvic pain, and symptoms of toxemia of pregnancy. Adnexal enlargements caused by thecalutein cysts of the ovaries may be associated with trophoblastic disease.

Myomas of the uterus, the cervix, the round ligament, or other pelvic organs are quite common in this age group. As many as 30% of women in the reproductive years may develop myomas of the uterus and accessory organs, and by age 50, perhaps as many as 40% will have developed such tumors. These tumors occur three times more frequently in blacks than in whites. The majority are benign and vary in size from very small to large enough to fill the entire abdominal cavity. These tumors are composed of smooth muscle cells in concentric whorls and are generally benign. Leiomyosarcoma occurring in such tumors is rare (0.1% to 0.5%). The tumors are usually solid but with degeneration may give the impression of a cystic consistency. Ultrasound, CT, or MRI scan may be helpful in making a specific diagnosis.

Rarely, myomas of the uterus occur in the cervix or lower uterine segment. They may become quite large and may put pressure on the bladder neck, causing acute urinary retention. Myomas tend to enlarge premenstrually and in pregnancy. Occasionally cervical or lower uterine segment myomas have caused intermittent urinary retention premenstrually or during early pregnancy.

Adnexal masses in the reproductive years may involve any known ovarian tumor, as well as cysts of mesonephric origin. In this age group functional cysts of the ovary are still the most common adnexal masses found, and benign cystic teratomas are the most common neoplastic adnexal masses. During the reproductive years, endometriosis occurs, and ovarian endometrial cysts develop reasonably frequently in this age group. They generally are accompanied by the usual symptoms for endometriosis in association with a tender adnexal mass. Figure 7-6 depicts a bilobed endometrioma on vaginal sonogram. It measures 5.1 × 4.1 cm and 5.1 × 3.9 cm, respectively. (Courtesy of Dr. Steven R. Goldstein.)

Tumors emanating from other organ systems should also be considered in the differential diagnosis as in other age groups. One of the more common of these is not a tumor at all but a pelvic kidney. An intravenous pyelogram should be useful in differentiating this entity from other pathologic conditions.

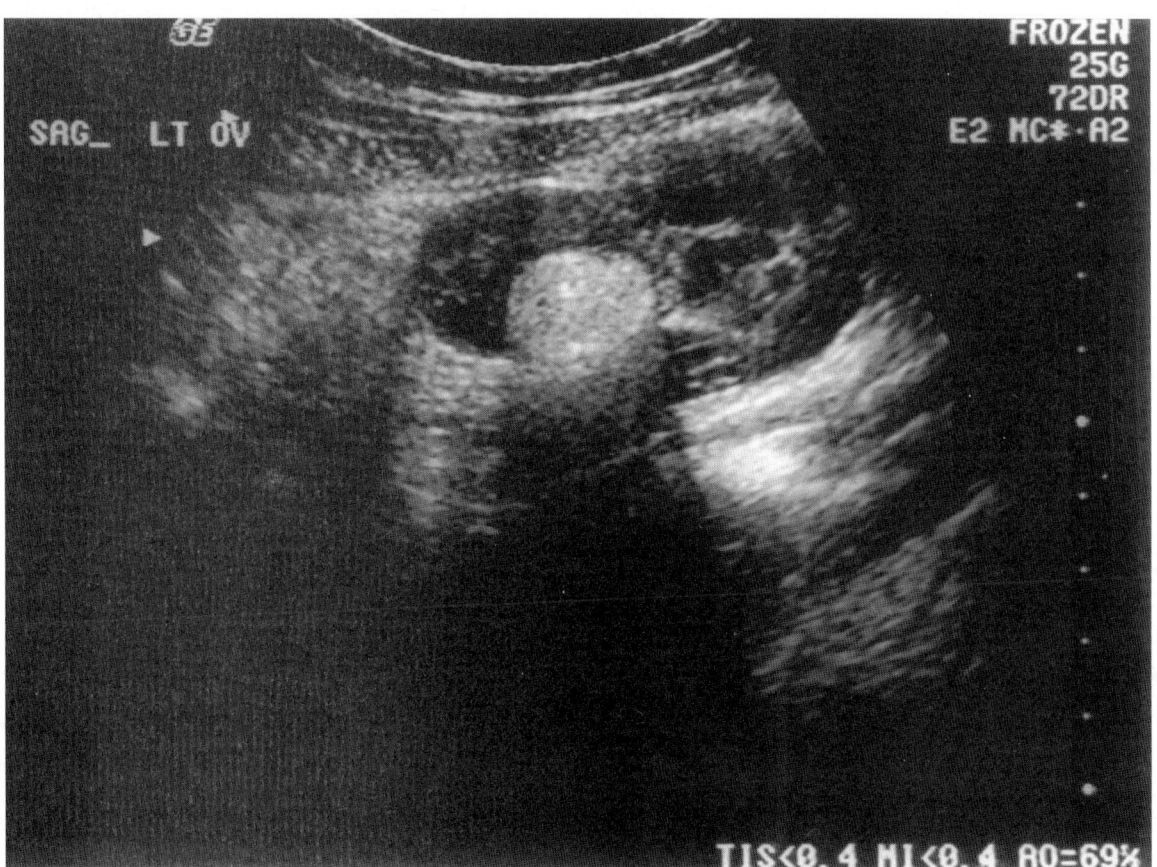

FIGURE 7-5 Transvaginal sonogram of a dermoid cyst. (Courtesy of Dr. Steven R. Goldstein.)

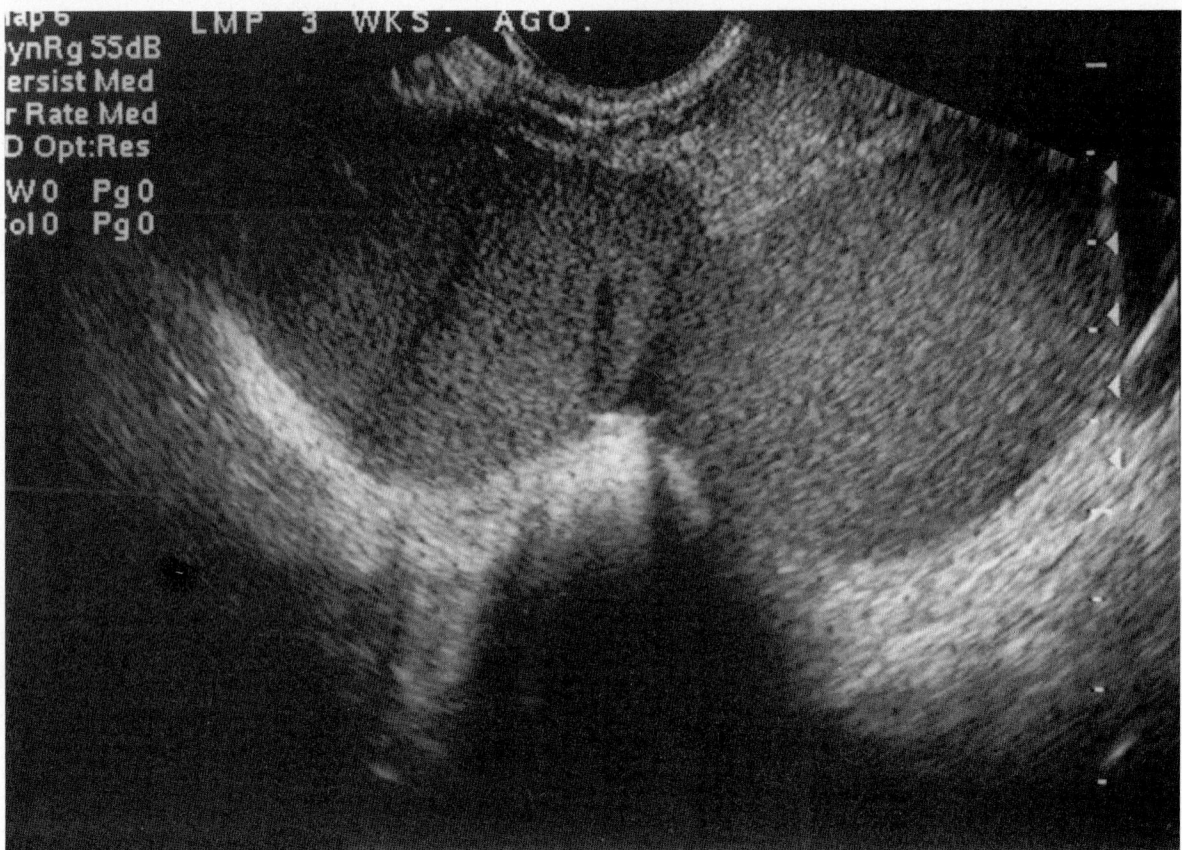

FIGURE 7-6   Transvaginal sonogram of a bilobed endometrioma. (Courtesy of Dr. Steven R. Goldstein.)

Masses in the Perimenopausal and Postmenopausal Years

In this age group it is once again appropriate to consider masses originating from the uterus and cervix, from the adnexa, and from other organ systems. In general, myomas of the uterus regress postmenopausally even in the face of estrogen hormone replacement. Therefore a uterus that is growing in size should be investigated for the possibility of malignancy. Adenocarcinoma of the endometrium, sarcomas, and mixed tumors of the uterus are all more common in the postmenopausal period, and many will be responsible for enlargement of uterine size, as well as postmenopausal bleeding.

Adnexal masses occurring in postmenopausal women may still be benign, but the chance of malignancy increases with age. The presence of ascites and the detection of the tumor bilaterally suggest malignancy. Rulin and Preston analyzed 150 adnexal tumors in women over the age of 50 and noted 103 benign tumors and 47 malignant ones. Table 7-7 summarizes these tumors by size and pathologic findings. Only 1 tumor of 32 that were less than 5 cm proved to be malignant, whereas 6 of 55 tumors 5 to 10 cm and 40 of 63 tumors larger than 10 cm were malignant.

TABLE 7-7
Adnexal Masses in 150 Women ≥50 Years

Pathology	<5 cm	5–10 cm	>10 cm
Benign disease			
Epithelial tumors	12	26	15
Stromal and germ cell tumors	7	12	4
Nonneoplastic ovarian cysts	2	1	0
Uterine myomas	3	3	4
Nonovarian adnexal lesions	2	6	0
Absence of true mass	5	1	0
Malignant disease			
Epithelial carcinomas	1	3	29
Borderline tumors	0	2	2
Other ovarian carcinomas	0	0	4
Nonovarian carcinoma	0	1	5
TOTAL	32	55	63

From Rulin MC and Preston AL: Obstet Gynecol 70:578, 1987.

The majority of the malignant tumors were epithelial in this age group, and most were greater than 10 cm. In a similar study from Tel Aviv, Ovadia and Goldman reported that in 380 postmenopausal women operated on for adnexal masses in a 10-year period, 297 (78.2%) had benign and 83 (21.8%) had malignant tumors. They, too, showed that the chance of malignancy increased with size of tumor and with age. One third of benign adnexal masses were simple cysts.

Endometriosis occurs primarily in women in the reproductive years; however, as many as 5% of cases do occur postmenopausally, particularly in women on hormone replacement therapy. Therefore endometriosis of the ovaries should be part of the differential diagnosis in such women (Chapter 19).

Masses from other organ systems are quite common in this age group. Diverticulitis may be responsible for a painful left adnexal mass. Bowel tumors may present as abdominal masses, as may tumors of the kidney, the musculoskeletal system, and the lymphatic system. Blood dyscrasias and lymphomas are more common in this age group. Lymphomas may present as rapidly growing, firm masses, at times accompanied by ascites. They may develop from any abdominal or pelvic organ, including lymph nodes.

Special Considerations

A number of findings associated with abdominal mass may help direct the physician to the appropriate diagnosis. If ascites is present, as detected by physical examination or ultrasound, a malignant tumor, frequently of the ovary, is strongly suspected. A needle aspiration with cell block of the fluid obtained may be diagnostic. Benign fibromas of the ovary may also be associated with ascites and pleural effusion (Meig's syndrome).

Defeminization or masculinization of the patient may suggest a rare masculinizing tumor of the ovary, such as a Sertoli-Leydig tumor. In the preadolescent female, precocious puberty of a heterosexual type may be the presenting symptom. In the postpubertal girl, cessation of menses and early masculinization may occur. These may also be the presenting symptoms in women in the reproductive years.

Feminizing tumors, such as granulosal cell tumors and thecomas, are more common. In the prepubertal girl they may present as precocious puberty. In the menstruating woman they may cause menometrorrhagia, and in the postmenopausal woman they may present with postmenopausal bleeding. In a granulosal cell tumor a solid or cystic mass is readily detected. Thecomas are solid tumors and are also readily detected. Occasionally other ovarian stromal tumors, such as a Brenner tumor, may produce sex steroids and present in a similar fashion.

Struma ovarii, a teratoma with thyroid elements, may present by developing signs of hyperthyroidism in the patient.

General Diagnostic Considerations

Specific differential diagnosis of abdominal and pelvic masses is often aided by ultrasound, CT, or MRI scan. In addition, special radiographic studies, such as intravenous pyelogram, barium enema, and upper GI series, may be helpful in identifying the site of the tumor. Because metastatic cancer to the ovaries is common, investigation of the patient for another primary source is often fruitful.

Tumor markers may be elevated, such as Ca-125 in epithelial tumors, serum hCG and alpha fetoprotein in germ cell tumors, and androgens or estrogens in specific hormone-producing tumors. These tests have frequent false-positive and false-negative findings and should be used only in conjunction with other diagnostic procedures.

KEY POINTS

- Bleeding in early pregnancy usually implies threatened or inevitable abortion, ectopic pregnancy, or trophoblastic disease.

- Bleeding at the time of the missed menstrual period may represent implantation bleeding.

- About 90% of all ectopic pregnancies are associated with vaginal bleeding.

- Vaginal bleeding in a patient with a positive pregnancy test, lower abdominal pain, adnexal mass, and failure to demonstrate a gestational sac by ultrasound beyond 6 weeks of gestational age should suggest the possibility of an ectopic pregnancy.

- Incidence of ectopic pregnancy is increased in women who have had previous ectopic pregnancies, have undergone tubal reparative procedures, have had previous pelvic infections, wear an IUD, or were exposed to DES in utero.

- Molar pregnancies are suggested by vaginal bleeding, uteri larger than gestational age, and serum hCG levels of 100,000 mIU/ml or greater.

- Molar pregnancy must be differentiated from normal gestation, multiple gestation, uterine enlargement because of uterine pathology, and hydramnios.

- Molar pregnancies are best diagnosed with the aid of ultrasound examination.

- Dysfunctional uterine bleeding is generally associated with anovulation or short ovulatory cycle.

- Dysfunctional uterine bleeding is most commonly seen in the postpubertal period, perimenopausally, or in women during their reproductive years who have undergone excessive weight change, who are under stress, or who have embarked on a strenuous exercise program.

- A patient presenting with symptoms or signs of PID who is afebrile or has a low-grade fever should be suspected of having an ectopic pregnancy.

- Appendicitis is characterized by periumbilical pain that radiates to the right lower quadrant accompanied by loss of appetite, nausea, and vomiting. Patients with PID can have similar pain but usually have a higher fever and mild gastrointestinal symptoms and appear less ill.

- Dysfunctional uterine bleeding is often associated with polycystic ovarian syndrome and functioning ovarian tumors.

- Endometrial biopsy with dysfunctional uterine bleeding in younger women will generally demonstrate nonsecretory endometrium.

- Clear-cell cancer of the vagina is often associated with intrauterine DES exposure.

- Myomas of the uterus often are associated with vaginal bleeding; submucous myomas are most commonly associated with this problem.

- Of all adenocarcinomas of the endometrium, 95% occur in postmenopausal women.

- Adenocarcinoma of the endometrium found in premenopausal women is most often associated with polycystic ovarian syndrome or a functioning ovarian tumor.

- Systemic diseases that cause abnormal vaginal bleeding include coagulopathies, blood dyscrasias, and certain endocrinopathies.

- In a study of 1194 patients with chronic pelvic pain, 749 had normal pelvic examinations.

- In 749 patients with chronic pelvic pain who had normal pelvic examinations, 63% had abnormal findings at diagnostic laparoscopy.

- Of 445 patients who had abnormal pelvic examinations and a history of chronic pelvic pain, 17.5% had normal findings at the time of diagnostic laparoscopy.

- Of 100 women who reported constant pelvic pain in one place for at least 6 months, 83% had abnormal findings at diagnostic laparoscopy. Pelvic adhesions and endometriosis accounted for the majority of abnormalities seen.

- Pelvic adhesions may not be the cause of chronic pelvic pain. Whereas 26% of 100 such patients were found to have adhesions on laparoscopy, 39% of 88 patients undergoing laparoscopy for tubal ligation or infertility also had adhesions, and only 4 of these 34 patients complained of pain. Dense pelvic adhesions, especially those that are vascularized, may cause pelvic pain.

- A total of 20% of all women demonstrate retroversion or retroflexion of the uterus. This anatomic variation usually does not cause symptoms.

- Of patients with chronic pelvic pain, 50% demonstrated multiple symptom complaints.

- Personality examinations in patients with chronic pelvic pain frequently define psychosocial problems, but such testing does not determine whether the pain is psychogenic or organic in nature.

- Chronic pelvic pain patients have been found to have a greater prevalence of lifetime major depression, current major depression, lifetime substance abuse, sexual dysfunction, somatization, and a greater incidence of childhood and adult sexual abuse.

- The majority of adnexal masses in women in the reproductive years are follicle cysts of the ovary.

- The most common benign neoplastic tumors of the ovary are serous cystadenoma and benign cystic teratoma.

- The most common benign cystic neoplasms of the ovary in the 20- to 44-year age group are benign cystic teratoma, serous cystadenoma, and mucinous cystadenoma.

- Serous cystadenocarcinoma is the most common malignant tumor in all age groups from 20 to 75 years but increases in incidence with age.

- Wilms' tumor and neuroblastoma are the most common abdominal tumors in childhood.

- Dysgerminoma and teratoma are the most common solid adnexal tumors in young women.

- Most benign cystic teratomas are 10 cm or less in diameter, but about one sixth will be larger.

- Of women in the reproductive years, 30% develop myoma of the uterus. By age 50, 40% will have developed such tumors.

- A total of 95% of all endometriosis occurs in women in the reproductive years.

- Of 150 adnexal tumors in women over age 50, 103 were benign. Of the malignant tumors in this age group, most were epithelial tumors. Tumors less than 5 cm were usually benign, but 40 of 63 tumors larger than 10 cm were malignant.

- Postmenopausal bleeding may be caused by a premalignant or malignant lesion of the uterus or cervix but is often associated with an atrophic endometrium.

- The most common cause of vaginal bleeding in childhood is foreign bodies in the vagina.

BIBLIOGRAPHY

Allen WM and Masters WH: Traumatic lacerations of uterine support, Am J Obstet Gynecol 70:500, 1955.

Anderson B: Diagnosis of endometrial cancer. Clin Obst Gynecol 13:739-50, 1986.

Asadourian LA and Taylor HB: Dysgerminoma: an analysis of 105 cases, Obstet Gynecol 33:370, 1969.

Badura AS, Reiter RC, Altmaier EM, Rhonberg A, Elos D: Dissociation, somatization, substance abuse, and coping in women with chronic pelvic pain. Obstet Gynecol 90:405, 1997.

Beard RW, Kennedy RG, Gangar KR, et al: Bilateral oophorectomy and hysterectomy in the treatment of intractable pelvic pain associated with pelvic congestion, Br J Obstet Gynecol 98:988, 1991.

Beard RW, Pearce S, Highman JH, and Reginald RW: Diagnosis of pelvic varicosities in women with chronic pelvic pain, Lancet 2:946, 1984.

Bennington JL, Ferguson BR, and Haber SL: Incidence and relative frequency of benign and malignant ovarian neoplasms, Obstet Gynecol 32:627, 1968.

Blendis LM: Abdominal pain. In Wall DP and Melzack R, eds: Textbook of pain, New York, 1984, Churchill Livingstone.

Buttram VC and Reiter RC: Uterine leiomyomata: etiology, symptomatology, and management, Fertil Steril 36:433, 1981.

Caruso PA, Marsh MR, Minkowitz S, and Karten G: An intense clinical pathologic study of 305 teratomas of the ovary, Cancer 27:343, 1971.

Costin ME and Kennedy RLJ: Ovarian tumors in infants and children, Am J Dis Child 76:127, 1948.

Cunanan RG, Courey NG, and Lippes J: Laparoscopic findings in patients with pelvic pain, Am J Obstet Gynecol 146:589, 1983.

Dewhurst J: Postmenopausal bleeding from benign causes, Clin Obstet Gynecol 26:769, 1983.

Diamond MP, Baxter JW, Pennau CG Jr, and Burnett LS: The occurence of ovarian malignancy in childhood and adolescents: a community-wide evaluation, Obstet Gynecol 71:858, 1988.

DiMarchi JM, Kosasa TS, and Hale RW: What is the significance of the human chorionic gonadotropin value in ectopic pregnancy? Obstet Gynecol 74:851, 1989.

Falcone T, Desjardins C, Bourque J, et al: Dysfunctional uterine bleeding in adolescents, J Reprod Med 39:761, 1994.

Farquhar CM, Lethaby A, Soroter M, Verry J, Baranyai J: An evaluation of risk factors for endometrial hyperplasia in premenopausal women with abnormal menstrual bleeding. Am J Obstet Gynecol 181:525-29, 1999.

Fraiz J and Jones RB: Chlamydial infections, Ann Rev Med 39:357, 1988.

Harrop-Griffiths J, Katon W, Walker E, et al: The association between chronic pelvic pain, psychiatric diagnoses, and childhood sexual abuse, Obstet Gynecol 71:589, 1988.

Herbst AL, Ulfelder H, and Poskanzer DC: Adenocarcinoma of the vagina: association of maternal stilbestrol therapy with tumor appearance in young women, N Engl J Med 284:878, 1971.

Hertweck SP: Dysfunctional uterine bleeding, Obstet Gynecol Clin North Am 19:129, 1992.

Killackey MA and Neuwirth RS: Evaluation and management of the pelvic mass: a review of 540 cases, Obstet Gynecol 71:314, 1988.

Koonings PP, Campbell K, Mishell DR Jr., and Grimes DA: Relative frequency of primary ovarian neoplasms: a 10 year review, Obstet Gynecol 74:921, 1989.

Kresch A, Seifer DB, Sachs LD, and Barrese I: Laparoscopy in 100 women with chronic pelvic pain, Obstet Gynecol 64:672, 1984.

Longstreth GF: Irritable bowel syndrome and chronic pelvic pain, Obstet Gynecol Surv 49:7, 1994.

Merskey H, Albe-Fessard DG, Bonica JJ, et al: Definitions and notes on usage recommended by the IASP Subcommittee on Taxonomy, Pain 6:249, 1979.

Mueller CW, Tompkins P, and Lapp WA: Dysgerminoma of the ovary: an analysis of 427 cases, Am J Obstet Gynecol 60:153, 1950.

Norris HJ and Jensen RD: Relative frequency of ovarian neoplasms in childhood and adolescence, Cancer 30:713, 1972.

O'Connell LP, Fries MH, Zerinque E, Brehrn W: Triage of abnormal postmenopausal bleeding: A comparison of endometrial biopsy and transvaginal sonohysterography versus fractional curettage with hysteroscopy. Am J Obstet Gynecol 178:956-61, 1998.

Ovadia J and Goldman GA: Ovarian masses in postmenopausal women, Int J Gynecol Obstet 39:35, 1992.

Paavonen J, Kiviat N, Brunham RC, et al: Prevalence and manifestations of endometritis among women with cervicitis, Am J Obstet Gynecol 152:280, 1985.

Peters AAW, Trimbos-Kemper GCM, Admiraal C, and Trimbos JB: A randomized clinical trial on the benefit of adhesiolysis in patients with intraperitoneal adhesions and chronic pelvic pain, Br J Obstet Gynecol 99:59, 1992.

Peterson WF, Prevost EC, Edmunds FT, et al: Benign cystic teratomas of the ovary: a clinico-statistical study of 1007 cases with review of the literature, Am J Obstet Gynecol 70:368, 1955.

Rapkin AJ: Adhesions and pelvic pain: a retrospective study, Obstet Gynecol 68:13, 1986.

Reiter RC and Gambone JC: Nongynecologic somatic pathology in women with chronic pelvic pain and negative laparoscopy, J Reprod Med 36:253, 1991.

Renaer M: Gynecological pain. In Wall DP and Melzack R, editors: Textbook of pain, New York, 1984, Churchill Livingstone.

Renaer MJ, Vertommen H, Nijs P, et al: Psychic aspects of pelvic pain in women, Am J Obstet Gynecol 134:75, 1979.

Rulin MC and Preston AL: Adnexal masses in postmenopausal women, Obstet Gynecol 70:578, 1987.

Slocumb JC: Neurological factors in chronic pelvic pain: trigger points and the abdominal pelvic pain syndrome, Am J Obstet Gynecol 149:536, 1984.

Slocumb JC: Chronic somatic, myofascial, and neurogenic abdominal pelvic pain, Clin Obstet Gynecol 33:145, 1990.

Stenchever MA: Symptomatic retrodisplacement, pelvic congestion, universal joint, and peritoneal defects: fact or fiction? Clin Obstet Gynecol 33:161, 1990.

Taylor HC: Vascular congestion and hyperemia. I. Physiologic basis in history of the concept, Am J Obstet Gynecol 57:211, 1949.

Taylor HC: Vascular congestion and hyperemia. II. The clinical aspects of congestion-fibrosis syndrome, Am J Obstet Gynecol 57:637, 1949.

Walker EA, Sullivan ND, and Stenchever MA: Use of antidepressants in the management of women with chronic pelvic pain, Obstet Gynecol Clin North Am 20:743, 1993.

Walling MK, Reiter RC, O'Hara MW, Milburn AK, Lilly G, Vincent SD: Abuse history and chronic pain in women: I. Prevalences of sexual abuse and physical abuse. Obstet Gynecol 84:193-99, 1994.

Emotional Aspects of Gynecology

Sexual Dysfunction, Eating Disorders, Substance Abuse, Depression, Grief, Loss

KEY TERMS AND DEFINITIONS

Agitated Depression. A severe and rare grief reaction in which the bereaved develops tension, agitation, insomnia, feelings of worthlessness, and fantasies of the need for punishment, at times including suicide.

Anhedonia. Loss of feelings of joy and pleasure.

Anorexia Nervosa. A psychiatric disease associated with a food aversion, fear of weight gain or obesity, and a distorted body image in which the individual limits caloric intake to starvation levels. In addition to severe weight loss, there is a decreased metabolic rate and amenorrhea.

Behavior Modification. A treatment program using reward and punishment techniques to change behavior.

Binge Drinking. The consumption of five or more drinks on a specific occasion or drinking until intoxicated.

Bulimia. A symptom of anorexia nervosa that features binge eating and self-induced purging using both vomiting and diarrhea as methods.

Cognitive Behavior Therapy. The technique of behavior change that attempts to modify beliefs, assumptions, and thinking styles.

Delayed Grief Reaction. The postponement of the grief reaction for various reasons and for a period from days to years.

Distorted Grief Reaction. The assumption of the characteristics of the deceased by the bereaved for a pro-

longed period and at times in a distorted fashion, during which the bereaved often evidences no sense of loss.

Dyspareunia. Painful intercourse.

Excessive Alcohol Consumption. The consumption of 45 or more alcoholic drinks per month or 5 or more alcoholic drinks on a specific occasion.

Grief Reaction. A group of symptoms associated with loss, which generally resolves in 6 to 18 months.

Obesity. An eating disorder in which the individual's weight is 20% or more above the mean weights for individuals of the same sex and height. Mild obesity is defined as 20% to 40% overweight; moderate obesity as 41% to 100% overweight; and severe obesity as greater than 100% overweight.

Orgasmic Dysfunction. Difficulty or inability in reaching orgasm.

Sexual Dysfunction. A psychologic or physiologic problem or condition that prevents the usual full participation and enjoyment of coitus.

Sexual Response Curve. The graphic expression of sexual response as defined by Masters and Johnson involving four phases: excitement, plateau, orgasm, and resolution.

Vaginismus. Involuntary spasm of vaginal, introital, and levator ani muscles causing painful sexual intercourse or preventing penetration.

During a lifetime the individual faces several tasks and challenges. Perhaps the first is the development of an identity and the building of a self-esteem. This begins in early childhood and continues through adolescence. Such development is aided by positive and nurturing forces. On the other hand, attacks against the young individual's mental or physical well-being may have a distorting influence. The quality of her self-esteem and self-perception will influence the choices she makes in life situations and will affect her personal development.

All individuals experience loss throughout their lifetime. The scope of such loss may be quite varied, including lack of accomplishment or loss of opportunity in career, the loss of a body organ or a body part, the loss of a friend or a loved one through separation or death, the loss of a relationship, or the loss of a physical or mental ability because of illness or accident. In general, loss is managed by a grieving process. The way in which the individual grieves and resolves grief often determines the degree of success in the next stage of life. The inability to handle grief appropriately may lead to lost opportunities, poor choices, and poorly developed future relationships.

The gynecologist is in an important position to help the young woman develop her self-image and to help her manage the losses that she will inevitably face. The gynecologist has the opportunity to participate with the patient in critical life events from adolescence to late in life and to provide or obtain counseling for her as she works her way through these problems.

This chapter will outline the major social problems that can arise during a woman's lifetime and will offer suggestions as to how the physician can aid the patient.

CHILDHOOD COUNSELING PROBLEMS

Self-esteem begins to develop in early childhood and is the result of positive efforts of parents and others in the child's immediate environment. Continuous reinforcement of a child's worth as an individual, by verbal and nonverbal means, should be encouraged. Touching, talking to the child in gentle ways, positively praising the child's actions, and, as the child becomes older, setting limits that are socially acceptable within the framework of the family are all reasonable steps. Punishment should be limited to reinforcing the needs for the limits set. Intimidation by verbal or physical means should be avoided. The physician may have the opportunity to suggest help for parents by offering reading material, discussing the issue directly with them, or referring them to parenting classes. In general, positive reinforcement of the child's worth as an individual mixed with appropriate warmth and love tends to build self-esteem, whereas negative statements or actions tend to tear it down. The child has little with which to compare, and if she is given negative information about herself, the tendency is to believe it.

Physical or sexual abuse in childhood can have serious consequences for the child's development. These are extreme influences and must be handled energetically when they occur or as soon afterward as they are noted. The health care professional must communicate to the child that she is a victim and in no way responsible for what has happened. Any contrary statements may have a lasting effect on the child's developing self-esteem. Issues of abuse are discussed more fully in Chapter 9.

Parental Loss in Childhood

A serious threat to normal emotional development in childhood is the loss of a parent by death or permanent separation. Laajus reviewed a large number of studies addressing this problem. Because the study methodology is complex, it is difficult to draw comparisons between different reports. However, a number of general observations were made. In Laajus's experience parental loss was a common finding in children referred for psychiatric treatment and was associated with a variety of pathologic and behavior disturbances. The period between the loss of a parent and the onset of the disorder is often quite long.

Tennant et al., applying multiple regression analysis, believe that the earlier the separation and the longer its duration, the more maladjustment is likely to occur. The risk of developing a psychiatric disorder seems greatest if the child is younger than 5 years or an adolescent and if the child loses a parent of the same sex. Males seem more susceptible to the loss of a father than to the loss of a mother and seem to be more affected by this loss than are females. In general, their major reaction is to develop antisocial tendencies. On the other hand, loss of a father during adolescence seems to influence the emotional development of females, although the problems may not be manifested for a number of years. Loss of a mother in girls under age 11 seems to significantly affect development.

Some of the difficulty in clarifying the role of the loss of a mother or father in young children relates to the way parent substitutes are developed. Because maternal loss usually necessitates the finding of a care provider, often a female, the effect of maternal loss may be blunted. On the other hand, male substitution after paternal loss may not occur rapidly or at all. Tennant et al. showed a consistent relationship between parental loss and the development of psychiatric illness in all ages. Children between the ages of 5 and 10 years seem to be the most susceptible to behavior changes. But adolescence was also a time of important vulnerability in cases of schizophrenia, depression, and a variety of medical illnesses occurring in adolescence. The loss of a parent early in life was a frequent and significant finding in such patients, with the loss of a father being noted more frequently than the loss of a mother.

Gregory has demonstrated that parental loss is often associated with antisocial disorders, especially delinquency. The highest rates seem to occur among males who have lost their father. One study shows a 3.5-fold increase of severe crimes in a group of males who had lost one or more parents before the age of 5 years. On the other hand, the perpetration of severe crimes was less frequent among males who had experienced parental losses later in life. Anderson compared a group of delinquent and nondelinquent boys who had suffered parental loss between the ages of 4 and 7 years and demonstrated that a father substitution had occurred more frequently in the group that was not delinquent.

Counseling considerations for children and adolescents who have suffered parental loss should include attention to the child's bereavement with active help in working through the acute phase of grief followed by the incorporation of an individual into the child's life who is of the same sex as the lost parent. If the mother is deceased or absent, a loving, nurturing, and supportive female or group of females should be identified to participate in the child's care and development. This may be a grandparent, an aunt, a hired nanny, or an effective childcare program. Eventually it may be a stepmother. If the father is lost, older brothers, grandfathers, uncles, or males volunteering as "big brothers" may all be considered. In addition, surviving parents should be encouraged to protect the child as much as possible from their own grieving process and to maintain the integrity of the family unit.

Similar observations have been made with respect to the loss of a parent through separation or divorce. Hostile marital relationships seem to be more detrimental to child development than does the permanent absence of a parent by divorce or separation. Continuous discord within the family has been shown by Rutter to be associated with an increase of antisocial disorders in boys but not in girls. Tennant et al. investigated individuals with psychiatric disorders and looked at four causes of separation from parents during childhood. These include illness of the individual, wartime evacuation, parental illness, and marital discord. They found that parental illness and marital discord had a statistically significantly greater association with the development of psychiatric diseases than did separation because of the individual's illness or wartime evacuation.

Fergusson et al. performed a 15-year longitudinal study in which a sample of 935 children subjected to parental separation were evaluated at age 15 for measures of adolescent psychopathology and problem behavior. After adjusting for confounding factors, they found increased risks for problems, which included substance abuse or dependency, conduct or behavioral disorders, mood and anxiety disorders, and early-onset sexual activity, occurring at increased odds ratios of 1.07 to 3.32, with a median increase of 1.46. Males and females responded similarly.

Two review articles by Johnston and by Amato demonstrate that high conflict divorce is associated with a two to four times increase in emotional and behavioral problems in children compared with national norms, with boys at greater risk than girls; that joint physical custody or frequent visitations lead to poorer child outcome, especially in girls; and that outcome depends on many variables including quality time spent with the noncustodial parent, the psychologic adjustment and parenting skills of the custodial parent, and the degree of economic hardship. They advise taking these factors into consideration in designing legal and therapeutic interventions.

PROBLEMS IN ADOLESCENCE AND ADULTHOOD

Eating Disorders

Anorexia nervosa, bulimia, and obesity are the major eating disorders affecting adolescents and young adults. On the one hand, eating is one of the major gratifications of life and is also a readily available substitute for other forms of gratification that cannot be achieved. Today a young woman is bombarded by two very different signals stemming primarily from advertising campaigns presented on television and radio and in magazines and books. The first of these involves food. Citizens of the Western world are offered foods of vast variety and unusual quantity presented in an appealing and almost demanding fashion. Stimuli to eat are seductive and almost continuous. On the other hand, the image of the American woman as depicted by the media is one of thinness. Garner and Garfinkel, in discussing the cultural expectations of American women, noted that a definite trend for decrease in body weight was noted between 1959 and 1978 in *Playboy* centerfold models and participants in the Miss America pageant. In both instances these women weighed significantly less than the average American woman. Further, the weights of the finalists in the Miss America pageant were noted to be significantly below those of other contestants during the years 1970 through 1978. Rubenstein and Caballero recently reported a steady statistically significant ($P < .0001$) drop in body mass index (BMI) in contestants from 1920 until the present. In earlier years the BMI was in the range now felt to be normal (20-25 kg/m^2). But there have been an increasing number of winners in the BMI range of less than 18.5 (a level defined by the World Health Organization as undernourished), with some as low as 16.9. The image that these "ideal women" create is in severe contrast to the reality that the average weight of American women increased by several pounds during that same period. Although the ideal of thinness may have lessened during the 1980s, it seems to have been reinstated since then.

Johnson et al. reported that in a survey of 1200 high school girls, 48% believed that they were either overweight or very overweight, whereas only 8% considered themselves underweight. Interestingly, the mean weight of these young women was within the normal range. Because the majority believed they were overweight, 50% of those who were 14 years or older and 70% who were

18 years or older were actively dieting. Many reported the use of diuretics, diet pills, laxatives, and self-induced vomiting to lower their weight. In another survey in 1978, 56% of women between the ages of 24 and 54 were found to be dieting, and 75% of the dieters stated that they did so for cosmetic reasons.

The effects of dieting may bring women to the attention of the gynecologist and may be responsible for symptoms that may not seem readily related to dieting. For instance, Pirke et al. studied 13 healthy women of normal weight who volunteered to lose 1 kg/week on an 800-calorie vegetarian diet for an average weight loss of 4.9 ± 0.7 kg. At the completion of the study, their body mass index was 99% of ideal body weight (Metropolitan Life Insurance standards). During their control cycles, each demonstrated normal gonadal function, but during the dietary cycles only two remained normal. Seven did not develop dominant follicles, and four others who did demonstrated impaired progesterone secretion by the corpus luteum. Dieting altered episodic luteinizing hormone (LH) secretion during the follicular phase, and LH concentrations and the frequency of episodic secretions were significantly reduced during the follicular phase but not during the luteal phase. Follicle-stimulating hormone (FSH) was unaltered by dieting.

Likewise, Kreipe et al. studied two groups of women who had clinical or subclinical eating disorders classified as restrictive anorexia nervosa, bulimic anorexia nervosa, normal weight bulimia nervosa, and other subclinical eating disorders and compared these with control subjects. None had weights above 110% of ideal body weight. Of 48 women with a diagnosed eating disorder, 45 (93.7%) had a menstrual abnormality consisting of amenorrhea or oligomenorrhea. Of the 22 patients with subclinical eating disorders, 21 gave a history of amenorrhea although none had this problem at present. Nine complained of oligomenorrhea. Most of these women reported weight fluctuations of 10% to 20% of ideal body weight in the past. Of the 37 controls, only 1 had a history of amenorrhea and 4 of oligomenorrhea. Thus an eating disorder apparently can present with menstrual abnormalities even in the subclinical stages and can probably affect reproductive efficiency.

Johnson and Schlundt stated that stress on women is accentuated by the double role they must play. Not only are they expected to fill the traditional roles of wives and mothers, but also they are expected to compete in the marketplace for contemporary careers. On the traditional side they must compete with women, whereas on the contemporary side they must compete with men as well.

Anorexia Nervosa and Bulimia

Although anorexia nervosa is quite uncommon in the general population (0.24 to 1.6 per 100,000 people), it is quite common in middle-class adolescent girls, occurring in about 1 in every 100. The incidence in professional ballet dancers varies from 5% to 20% depending on the level of competition of the ballet company, the weight standards imposed, and the number of hours of exercise required. The condition is 9 times more common in women than in men. It does occur among men who must restrict their weights in training for competitive athletic events.

Sundgot-Borgen studied risk factors for eating disorders in 603 elite Norwegian female athletes ages 12 to 35. They used the Eating Disorder Inventory to classify these individuals and with this defined 117 at risk. Of these, 103 were given a structured clinical interview for eating disorders. A control group of 30 athletes chosen from the not-at-risk pool were also interviewed. Ninety-two of the at-risk group met the criteria for anorexia nervosa or bulimia, and the prevalence of these disorders was higher in athletes performing in sports employing leanness compared with controls. Athletes with eating disorders began sports-specific training and dieting earlier and believed that puberty had occurred too early for optimal performance. The onset of eating disorders was often associated with prolonged dieting, frequent weight fluctuation, sudden increase in training, injury, or loss of a coach.

Although various clinical signs and symptoms occur in the patient with anorexia nervosa, it basically concerns food aversion, fear of weight gain or obesity, and a distorted body image. There is often an associated amenorrhea, which frequently disappears with weight gain. The central nervous system and endocrine considerations are discussed in Chapter 38.

Bulimia occurs in about 50% of anorectic patients and is defined as binge eating and self-induced purging. Not all bulimics have low body weight. Bulimic persons may have more severe psychologic problems and be more difficult to treat. In a study by Casper et al. 57% of bulimic patients reported vomiting after meals, in contrast to only 18% of patients with anorexia without bulimia. Bulimic persons in this series tended to be more extroverted and demonstrated symptoms of depression and anxiety, particularly with sleep disturbances. They also were more obsessional about food than were anorectics without bulimia.

Strober et al. looked at the incidence of anorexia nervosa, bulimia, and subclinical anorexia nervosa in first- and second-degree relatives of anorectic patients and demonstrated that eating disorders are familial. They were, however, unable to demonstrate mechanisms responsible for these familial relationships. They suggested that genetically transmitted defects in the neurobiologic processes that control feeding behavior may be present but could not rule out specific psychologic or familial vulnerabilities, common exposure to psychologically determined environmental experiences, cotransmission, or personality traits or psychopathologic disorders that may involve eating disturbances. They also could not rule out some important combinations of all of these factors.

Walters and Kendler studied a population-based sample

of 2163 female twins, and noted that co-twins of twins with anorexia nervosa were at a significantly higher risk of anorexia nervosa, bulimia, major depression, and current low body mass index. Significant association was found between anorexia nervosa and major depression, bulimia, generalized anxiety disorder, alcoholism, phobia, and panic disorders. They concluded that anorexia-like syndromes are familial and share etiologic factors with major depression.

An interesting association between eating disorders and an adverse sexual experience was noted by Oppenheimer et al. Two thirds of /8 patients with eating disorders reported such experiences and stated that thoughts of previous sexual abuse were often stressing and significant to the individuals. A total of 80% of the events occurred in childhood or adolescence, and most involved a significantly older male, usually a person known to the subject. In most cases both social taboo and personal trust were violated. The authors felt that given the nature of their study questionnaire, the incidence of such adverse sexual experience among anorectics may have been underreported.

Pope et al., however, studied the incidence of childhood sexual abuse in three groups of bulimic women in three different countries (the United States, Austria, and Brazil). Although sexual abuse was reported in 24% to 36% of women in these three groups, only 15% to 32% of these women reported the abuse before the onset of bulimia and there was no increase in the incidence of childhood sexual abuse over what was reported for women in the general populations of these countries. They concluded that childhood sexual abuse is not a risk factor for bulimia. Obviously, the potential for a relationship is still not clear.

Johnson and Schlundt in commenting on therapy for anorexia nervosa pointed out that the general modalities have included medication, hospitalization, nutritional support, and behavior therapy. To evaluate any therapy it is important to understand what the spontaneous remission rate might be among untreated patients. Hsu et al. compared three groups of patients with anorexia nervosa who were evaluated between 1968 and 1973 and were followed for 4 to 6 years. Within the group there were those treated as inpatients and as outpatients, and those not treated. Evaluation included weight gain and menstrual function. Good or fair outcomes were observed in 88% of those treated as inpatients, 77% of those treated as outpatients, and 59% of those not treated. In general, inpatient therapy consisted of hospitalization, nutritional support, various medications, and often individual or family counseling and psychotherapy. Most studies report excellent weight gain in such patients. Agres and Kraemer, in reviewing a number of studies, found that the therapy lasted 2½ to 3½ months, with an average weight gain of 4.1 kg per month noted.

A number of medications have been tried with varying success. These medications have included insulin, lithium, tricyclics, and phenothiazides, as well as high-potency vitamins. In many case-control studies these have not been found to be more effective than placebo. It is often difficult to separate the effect of a medication from the effects of counseling and psychotherapy given simultaneously.

In severe cases, patients have been fed intravenously, given total parenteral nutrition, or given nasogastric tube feedings. Generally, these methods are used when normal feeding attempts in inpatient therapy have not been associated with weight gain. Such extreme measures are generally used in the most severe and life-threatening situations.

In the 1960s and 1970s therapy was often tailored to the technique of behavior modification. When controlled studies were carried out, it seemed apparent that hospitalization per se would allow for reasonable weight gain, but when behavior modification was added, the hospital course could be shortened because of accelerated weight gain. Behavior modification was based on the reward and punishment program used for a number of behavior and habituation problems.

More recently, however, cognitive behavior therapy has been used in the treatment of anorexia. This therapy is aimed at bringing to the attention of the individual the fact that her beliefs, assumptions, and style of thinking have brought about distorted body image, food aversion, phobias, and unreasonable fears of weight gain. In short, the therapy is aimed at reshaping patients' thinking processes with respect to themselves and to their body images. No specific studies have been done to compare one method with another, but cognitive behavior therapy appears to be directed toward the specific thinking disorder rather than merely to its effect.

Finally, it is important to consider ultimate outcome in groups of patients with anorexia nervosa and bulimia. Theander, in a discussion of outcome, reviewed three long-term follow-up studies and discussed the results of his own study in Sweden. In three British studies a 5- to 6-year follow-up demonstrated good to intermediate results in 74% of patients. However, 23% of patients experienced a poor outcome, with 3% dying of the disease. In the Swedish study described by Theander with a mean observation time of 33 years, good to fair outcomes were noted in 76% of patients, poor outcomes in 6%, and death in 18%. Deaths were the result of starvation or suicide. Isager et al. analyzed survival data in 151 cases of anorexia nervosa, considering specifically death and relapse rates. Follow-up was from 4 to 22 years. The authors calculated the hazard of death as 0.5% per year and the hazards of relapse at 3% per year. Both hazards, however, declined steadily after therapeutic contact.

Obesity

Obesity is currently defined as a BMI greater than 25 kg/m². Based on this definition, 25.1% of American women were classified as obese during the period 1988 to

1994 with black women at a higher rate (37.6%) than white women (23.5%). Women ages 45 to 54 had a rate of obesity of 32.4% compared with lower rates in younger women and women over 65 years.

Stunkard has suggested a classification for obesity in which mild designates individuals who are 20% to 40% overweight; moderate, 41% to 100% overweight; and severe, greater than 100% overweight (Table 8-1). By these standards, 35% of women in the United States are considered obese. U.S. vital health statistics in 1983 suggest that of women who qualify as obese by these guidelines, 90.5% of the cases are classed as mild, 9% as moderate, and 0.5% as severe. Table 8-2 is the 1983 Metropolitan Life Insurance Company height and weight table.

Severe obesity is a health hazard that carries a twelve-fold increase in mortality for persons between the ages of 25 and 34 years. Often these individuals suffer complicating factors, such as hypertension, diabetes, hyperlipidemias, arthritis, increased operative morbidity and mortality, and compromised pulmonary function. According to Stunkard, severe obesity may also be associated with hypertrophic adipose tissue cells with an increased proliferation of adipose tissue and thus an increasing severity of obesity.

Stunkard suggests that diet and behavior modification provided by lay supervision is appropriate for those suffering from mild obesity; diet and behavior modification under medical supervision is appropriate for those suffering from moderate obesity; and operative intervention is appropriate for those suffering from severe obesity. Patients suffering from severe obesity almost always have medical complications, and these often improve with weight reduction. In previous years jejunoileal bypass procedures were the treatment of choice. These, however, had many complications. Currently procedures that reduce gastric size and narrow the outlet of the stomach seem to be the most appropriate approaches taken.

When dietary and pharmacologic therapy has been used for treating severe obesity, 15% of patients suffer from severe depression and 26% from moderate depression. Depression is much less common in patients who undergo gastric reduction operations. Of these individuals, 75% report elation and a feeling of well-being. In addition, 91% of these patients state that before the operation

they had required a good deal of willpower to keep from overeating, and indeed, 33% stated that they could eat another full meal after eating most of their meals. Only 14% ever felt satisfied after eating. After the operation 10% state that they require willpower to keep from eating more, and only 1% state that they could eat another full meal after eating. On the other hand, 94% feel that they could eat no more after completing the usual meal. Also, Letiexke et al. demonstrated that after successful gastroplasty in eight grossly obese women, normal insulin secretion, clearance, and action on glucose metabolism occurred after body weight was normalized.

Moderately obese patients will lose weight on diets of 1200 to 1500 calories and generally find this approach comfortable. However, weight loss under these circumstances takes a long time. On very low-calorie diets (400 to 700 calories), which consist mostly of protein (fish, fowl, or lean meat), dramatic change in weight can usually be accomplished in 3 months. The patient will lose 1.5 to 2.3 kg per week depending on the amount of body fat at the beginning of dieting. The major problem with such individuals is maintaining weight loss.

Exercise is a useful addition to diet regimens. Several studies have demonstrated that although similar weight loss can be obtained by both diet alone and diet plus exercise programs, the latter will allow for a greater loss of fat stores while maintaining muscle mass. To maintain this advantage, exercise programs must be maintained.

TABLE 8-1
Recommended Therapy in Obesity

Degree of Obesity	Percent Above Normal Weight	Therapy
Mild	20–40	Diet and lay supervision
Moderate	40–100	Low-calorie diet and medical supervision
Severe	>100	Gastric reduction operation

TABLE 8-2
Height and Weight Table for Women*

Height		Weight (lbs)		
Feet	Inches	Small Frame	Medium Frame	Large Frame
4	10	102–111	109–121	118–131
4	11	103–113	111–123	120–134
5	0	104–115	113–126	122–137
5	1	106–118	115–129	125–140
5	2	108–121	118–132	128–143
5	3	111–124	121–135	131–147
5	4	114–127	124–138	134–151
5	5	117–130	127–141	137–155
5	6	120–133	130–144	140–159
5	7	123–136	133–147	143–163
5	8	126–139	136–150	146–167
5	9	129–142	139–153	149–170
5	10	132–145	142–156	152–173
5	11	135–148	145–159	155–176
6	0	138–151	148–162	158–179

From 1983 Metropolitan Height & Weight Tables, Metropolitan Life Insurance Company, Statistical Bulletin.

*Weights at ages 25 to 59 based on lowest mortality. Weight in pounds according to frame (in indoor clothing weighing 3 pounds; shoes with 1-inch heels).

Craighead et al. point out that unless behavior is modified, weight loss is usually not maintained. These workers studied 145 patients who were approximately 60% overweight and divided them into three groups. Treatment continued for 6 months, and there was at least 1 year of follow-up in 99% of those who completed the therapy. Group 1 underwent behavior modification using Ferguson's *Learning to Eat* manual. They lost an average of 11.4 kg and regained only 1.8 kg during the follow-up year. Group 2 received medication therapy with an appetite suppressant, fenfluramine hydrochloride (Pondimin). They lost an average of 14.5 kg but regained 8.6 kg during the follow-up period. The third group was treated with a combination of behavior modification and medication and lost an average of 15.0 kg but regained 9.5 kg during the follow-up period. The authors concluded that behavior modification without medication was the most appropriate therapy for moderate obesity.

Mild obesity seems to respond best to dieting and behavior modification under lay supervision. Such individuals will generally embrace fad diets and look for magic cures. However, if placed on a nutritionally appropriate limited-caloric diet, they will generally do well if their attitudes toward eating and response to various stimuli are modified. Lay groups, such as Weight Watchers or Take Off Pounds Sensibly (TOPS), are usually quite successful for motivated individuals. Currently there are many commercial diet centers available for referral. Most prescribe or sell low-fat foods in an attempt to achieve a diet containing about 20% fat. Because fat represents 9 calories/gram and protein and carbohydrate represent 4 calories/gram, it is possible by changing eating habits to allow a patient a considerable quantity of food without high numbers of calories. Educating patients to change eating habits in this fashion is the key not only to losing weight, but to maintaining the weight loss.

Obesity in adolescence is a variant of the problem in the general population. Because the risk for progression with increasing morbidity and mortality is great, prompt support and behavior modification are most important. School and parental involvement are important aspects of controlling the problem. Where an obese parent is also present, best results seem to be achieved when both the parent and the child undergo therapy but in separate counseling sessions. In a study by Brownell et al. using 16 weeks of treatment of 42 obese adolescents ages 12 through 16, three groups were studied. When the child alone attended group therapy, there was an average 3.3-kg weight loss; when the child and mother were treated together there was an average 5.3-kg weight loss; and when the child and mother were both treated but separately, there was an 8.4-kg weight loss. After 1 year of follow-up the group in which the mother and child were treated separately maintained their weight loss at a mean of 7.7 kg, whereas the other two groups had regained their previous baseline levels.

Obviously, counseling and behavior modification are important in the management of both the adolescent and adult obese patient.

Sexual Function and Dysfunction

Sexual satisfaction is one of the more important human experiences, yet it has been estimated that as many as 50% of all married couples experience some sexual dissatisfaction or dysfunction. Although there is a strong physiologic basis for sexual function, it is impossible to separate sexual response from the many emotional and other contributing factors that may influence a relationship.

In 1966 Masters and Johnson published their now famous book, *Human Sexual Response*, which was a discussion of observations made on the sexual cycles of 700 subjects. It is on this important work that our current understanding of the female sexual response is based. Masters and Johnson described four phases of the sexual response: excitement, plateau, orgasm, and resolution (Figure 8-1).

The excitement or seduction phase may be initiated by a number of internal or external stimuli. As shown in the box on page 186, physiologically this phase is associated with deep breathing, increase in heart rate and blood pressure, a total body feeling of warmth associated often with erotic feelings, and an increase in sexual tension. There is generalized vasocongestion, which leads to breast engorgement and the development of a maculopapular erythematous rash on the breasts, the chest, and the epigastrium, which is called the *sex flush*. There is also engorgement of the labia majora (seen particularly in multiparous women) and of the labia minora. The clitoris generally swells and becomes erect, causing it to be tightly applied to the clitoral hood. The vagina "sweats" a transudative lubricant, and the Bartholin glands may secrete small amounts of liquid. With the increasing deep breathing the uterus may tent up into the pelvis, perhaps as a result of the Valsalva maneuver. There is also a myotonic effect, which is most notable in nipple erection. Much of the response in the excitement phase is caused by stimulation of the parasympathetic fibers of the autonomic nervous system. In some cases anticholinergic drugs may interfere with a full response in this stage.

Next is the plateau stage, which is the culmination of the excitement phase and is associated with a marked degree of vasocongestion throughout the body. Breasts and their areolae are markedly engorged, as are the labia and the lower third of the vagina. The vasocongestion in the lower third of the vagina is such that it forms what has been called the *orgasmic platform*, causing a decrease in the diameter of the vagina by as much as 50% and thus allowing for greater friction against the penis. At this stage the clitoris retracts tightly against the pubic symphysis, and the vagina lengthens, with dilation of the upper two thirds. Uteri in the normal anteflex position tend to tent up more. Retroverted uteri do not.

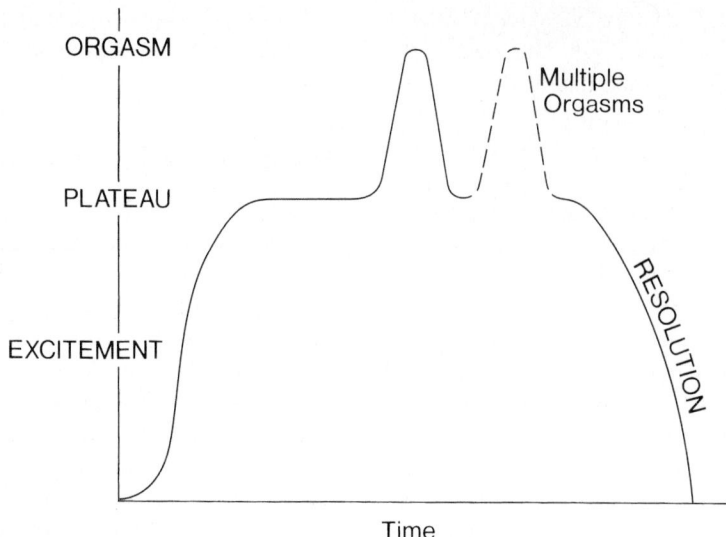

FIGURE 8-1 Sexual response cycle defined by Masters and Johnson. (From Masters WH and Johnson VE: Human sexual response, Boston, 1966, Little, Brown & Co.)

The next stage is orgasm, in which the sexual tension that has been built up in the entire body is released. Characteristics of orgasm are listed in the box on page 187. A myotonic response involves muscle systems of the entire body. Individuals may experience carpal spasm. Rarely, a grand mal type seizure may be observed. There is contraction of the muscles surrounding the vagina, as well as the anal sphincter. The uterus also contracts. Muscle contraction occurs 2 to 4 seconds after the woman begins to experience the orgasm and repeats at 0.8-second intervals. The actual number and intensity of contractions vary from woman to woman. Some women observed to have orgasmic contractions are not aware that they are having an orgasm. Masters and Johnson feel that prolonged stimulation during the excitement phase, during masturbation, or in conjunction with the use of a vibrator may lead to more pronounced orgasmic activity. Whereas the excitement phase is under the influence of the parasympathetic portion of the autonomic nervous system, orgasm seems to be related to the sympathetic portion. Medication such as antihypertensive drugs may affect orgasmic response.

The resolution stage is last and represents a return of the woman's physiologic state to the preexcitement level. Although a refractory period is typical of the sexual response cycle in the male, no such refractory periods have been identified in women. Therefore new sexual excitement cycles may be stimulated at any time after orgasm. During the resolution phase the woman generally experiences a feeling of personal satisfaction and well-being.

Masters and Johnson identified the clitoris as the center of sexual satisfaction in the female. Recently several lay publications have suggested that the cervix plays a role in sexual response, basing this theory on the fact that the cervix has a rich nerve supply. To date, no scientific data

supports this theory. Sexual gratification and orgasmic behavior definitely seem to be associated with nerve endings in the clitoris, mons pubis, labia, and possible pressure receptors in the pelvis. In a study by Andersen et al., 42 women aged 31 to 81 (average 50.3) who had been treated for in situ vulvar carcinoma were compared with a group of comparable women aged 30 to 61 (average 44.3) with respect to sexual function. Six of the women had undergone local therapy with laser or chemotherapy, 26 had wide excision of lesions, 9 had undergone simple vulvectomy, and 1 had undergone a radical vulvectomy. Sexual behavior patterns and desires were maintained after therapy, but a specific disruption of the phases of excitement and resolution, and to a lesser extent orgasm, were noted. There was 2 to 3 times greater incidence of sexual dysfunction in the patient group, and 30% became sexually inactive. Loss or disruption of the clitoris seemed to be the single most important factor.

Characteristics of Excitement Phase of Sexual Response Cycle in the Female

Deep breathing
Increased pulse
Increased blood pressure
Warmth and erotic feelings
Increased tension
Generalized vasocongestion
Skin flush
Breast engorgement
Nipple erection
Engorgement of labia and clitoris
Vaginal transudation
Uterine tenting

Characteristics of Orgasm in the Female
Release of tension
Generalized myotonic contractions
Contractions of perivaginal muscles and anal sphincter
Uterine contractions

Sexual Response and Menopause

The postmenopausal woman who is not on hormone replacement experiences progressive atrophy of vaginal epithelium, a change in vaginal pH, a decrease in quantity of vaginal secretions, and a decrease in the general circulation to the vagina and uterus. She may also have pelvic relaxation, including cystocele, rectocele, or prolapse of the uterus, and a general loss of vaginal tone. Women on replacement hormone therapy have been shown by Semmens and Semmens not to suffer the problems of vaginal atrophy and poor circulation. It is likely that hormone replacement, therefore, prolongs the postmenopausal woman's ability to demonstrate a more normal sexual response.

A postmenopausal woman may experience other sexual problems relating to her partner, or if she is single, widowed, or divorced, to her lack of availability of male partners. In addition, her general health and the general health of her partner will play a role in her ability to respond sexually in a satisfactory manner. Couples with marital or communication problems may find that the menopause is an appropriate excuse to cease sexual activities. A concerned physician can help a couple sort out their needs and desire for sexual compatibility at this stage of life. Frequently counseling aimed at dealing with problems of the relationship will alleviate sexual response difficulties.

Male partners of older women may suffer from medical illnesses or be affected by medications they must take, with resultant decrease in arousal, difficulties in maintaining an erection, or complete impotence. The physician should ask women about sexual function and if male dysfunction is evident, should make suggestions for appropriate referral to physicians or other health care workers who may deal with the male sexual dysfunction problems. Table 8-3 lists several drugs that can affect sexual function.

Sexual Dysfunction

Sexual dysfunction is quite common. Masters and Johnson estimated that it exists in 50% of marriages. Higher percentages of dysfunction are seen in couples presenting for marital therapy. That sexual dysfunction is not necessarily incompatible with a happy marriage was noted in a study by Frank et al. who surveyed couples felt to be well adjusted who were selected from general community groups. Of these couples, 83% rated their marriages as happy or very happy, but 63% of the women and 40% of the men gave a history of sexual dysfunction. A total of 48% of the women stated that they had difficulties becoming sexually excited, and 33% found difficulty in maintaining excitement. Of the total group, 46% of the women experienced difficulty in reaching orgasm, and 15% had never had an orgasm. Finally, 35% of the women expressed disinterest in sex. These workers' experience implies that physicians caring for women should make a special effort to uncover sexual dysfunction or poor sexual response in their patients even when the patients demonstrate general marital satisfaction. Obviously, assembling a careful history by asking general and directed questions is appropriate when dealing with a patient in a gynecologic visit. The patient should be asked if she is sexually active, if intercourse is comfortable and enjoyable (if heterosexual), and if orgasm is experienced. If she answers no to any of these questions, more specific questioning should follow with the objective of outlining the extent of the problem and the basis for it.

Sexual response problems may be the result of a previous negative sexual experience or may be secondary to emotional or physical illness. The problem may also be related to difficulties in the current relationship or to alcohol or drug abuse. Although an occasional alcohol drink may decrease inhibitions and improve sexual response, in general, alcohol is a depressant and decreases the woman's ability to become sexually aroused and to become vaginally lubricated. Drugs with antihypertensive and anticholinergic activity, as well as those active at the alpha and beta receptor sites, may decrease arousal or inhibit sexual interest. Narcotics, sedatives, and antidepressive drugs such as the SSRI group may also depress sexual responsiveness. Finally, decreased arousal or ability to remain aroused may be due to distractions in the woman's life such as concerns for children, job, or other problems that may enter her consciousness during arousal.

Inhibited sexual desire is the most common sexual dysfunction. Because each individual has his or her own libidinal drive, it is not surprising that couples may have some incompatibility of needs. It is important, however, that these needs and desires be discussed openly and that reasons for lack of sexual arousal that may involve experiences or problems inherent in the relationship be resolved. At times the problem may be merely a failure to set aside appropriate time for intimacy. The couple should be encouraged to give sexual activity a high priority within their relationship rather than leaving it last on the list after the 11 o'clock news. Couples should be encouraged to use arousal and seduction techniques that are appropriate for their relationship. Satisfactory foreplay of a mutually enjoyable nature should be encouraged.

TABLE 8-3
Drugs That May Affect Sexual Function

Drug	Adverse Effect	Drug	Adverse Effect
Acetazolamide (Diamox and others)	Loss of libido; decreased potency	Dichlorphenamide (Daranide and others)	Decreased libido; impotence
Alprazolam (Xanax)	Inhibition of orgasm; delayed or no ejaculation	Digoxin	Decreased libido; impotence
Amiloride (Midamor)	Impotence; decreased libido	Disopyramide (Norpace and others)	Impotence
Amiodarone (Cordarone)	Decreased libido	Disulfiram (Antabuse and others)	Impotence
Amitriptyline (Elavil and others)	Loss of libido; impotence; no ejaculation	Doxepin (Adapin Sinequan)	Decreased libido; ejaculatory dysfunction
Amoxapine (Asendin)	Loss of libido; impotence; retrograde, painful, or no ejaculation	Estrogens	Decreased libido in men
Amphetamines and related anorexic drugs	Chronic abuse; impotence; delayed or no ejaculation in men; no orgasm in women	Ethionamide (Trecator-SC)	Impotence
		Ethosuximide (Zarontin)	Increased libido
		Ethoxzolamide (Ethamide)	Decreased libido
Anticholinergics	Impotence	Fenfluramine (Pondimin)	Loss of libido (frequent in women with large doses or long-term use); impotence
Atenolol (Tenormin)	Impotence		
Baclofen (Lioresal)	Impotence; inability to ejaculate	Fluoxetine (Prozac)	Decreased libido
Barbiturates	Decreased libido; impotence	Fluphenazine (Prolixin, Permitil)	Changes in libido; erection difficulties; inhibition of ejaculation
Carbamazepine (Tegretol)	Impotence		
Chlorpromazine (Thorazine and others)	Decreased libido; impotence, no ejaculation; priapism	Guanabenz (Wytensin)	Impotence
Chlorprothixene (Taractan)	Inhibition of ejaculation; decreased intensity of orgasm	Guanadrel (Hylorel)	Decreased libido; delayed or retrograde ejaculation; impotence
Chlorthalidone (Hygroton and others)	Decreased libido; impotence	Guanethidine (Ismelin)	Decreased libido; impotence; delayed, retrograde, or no ejaculation
Cimetidine (Tagamet)	Decreased libido (men and women); impotence		
Clofibrate (Atromid-S)	Decreased libido; impotence	Guanfacine (Tenex)	Impotence
Clomipramine (Anafranil)	Decreased libido; impotence; retarded or no ejaculation (men) or orgasm (women); spontaneous orgasm associated with yawning	Haloperidol (Haldol and others)	Impotence; painful ejaculation
		Hydralazine (Apresoline and others)	Impotence; priapism
		Hydroxyprogesterone caproate (Delalutin and others)	Impotence
Clonidine (Catapres and others)	Impotence; delayed or retrograde ejaculation; inhibition of orgasm (women)	Imipramine (Tofranil and others)	Decreased libido; impotence; painful, delayed ejaculation; delayed orgasm in women
Danazol (Danocrine)	Increased or decreased libido	Indapamide (Lozol)	Decreased libido; impotence
Desipramine (Norpramin and others)	Decreased libido; impotence; difficult ejaculation and painful orgasm	Interferon (Roferon-a)	Decreased libido; impotence
		Isocarboxazid (Marplan)	Impotence; delayed ejaculation; no orgasm (women)
		Ketoconazole (Nizoral)	Impotence
Diazepam (Valium and others)	Decreased libido; delayed ejaculation; retarded or no orgasm in women	Labetalol (Trandate, Normodyne)	Priapism; impotence; delayed or no ejaculation; decreased libido

Vaginismus is a condition that is secondary to involuntary spasm of vaginal introital and levator ani muscles. Because of this spasm penetration is either painful or impossible. Lamont has attempted to classify the degrees of vaginismus and, in a group of 80 patients, noted that 27 (34%) had first-degree vaginismus, defined as perineal and levator spasm relieved by reassurance during pelvic examination. Another 21 (26%) had second-degree vaginismus, defined as perineal spasm maintained throughout the pelvic examination. Another 18 (22.5%) demonstrated third-degree vaginismus, defined as levator spasm and elevation of the buttocks. A total of 10 (12.5%) had fourth-

Drugs That May Affect Sexual Function

Drug	Adverse Effect	Drug	Adverse Effect
Levodopa (Dopar and others)	Increased libido	Phenelzine (Nardil)	Impotence; retarded or no ejaculation; delayed or no orgasm (men and women)
Lithium (Eskalith and others)	Decreased libido; impotence		
Maprotiline (Ludiomil)	Impotence; decreased libido	Phenytoin (Dilantin and others)	Decreased libido; impotence
Mazindol (Sanorex, Mazanor)	Impotence; spontaneous ejaculation; painful testes	Pimozide (Orap)	Impotence; no ejaculation; decreased libido
Mecamylamine (Inversine)	Impotence; decreased libido	Pindolol (Visken)	Impotence
Mepenzolate bromide (Cantil)	Impotence	Prazosin (Minipress)	Impotence; priapism
Mesoridazine (Serentil)	No ejaculation; impotence; priapism	Primidone (Mysoline and others)	Decreased libido; impotence
		Progesterone	Decreased libido; impotence
Methadone (Dolophine and others)	Decreased libido; impotence; no orgasm (men and women); retarded ejaculation	Propantheline bromide (Pro-Banthine and others)	Impotence
Methandrostenolone (Dianabol)	Decreased libido	Propranolol (Inderal and others)	Loss of libido; impotence
Methantheline bromide (Banthine)	Impotence	Protriptyline (Vivactil)	Loss of libido; impotence; painful ejaculation
Methazolamide (Neptazane)	Decreased libido (men and women); impotence; delayed or no ejaculation (men) or orgasm (women)	Rantidine (Zantac)	Loss of libido; impotence
		Reserpine	Decreased libido; impotence; decreased or no ejaculation
Methyldopa (Aldomet and others)	Decreased libido; impotence; delayed or no ejaculation (men) or orgasm (women)	Sertraline (Zoloft)	Decreased libido
		Spironolactone (Aldactone and others)	Decreased libido; impotence
Metoclopramide (Reglan and others)	Impotence; decreased libido	Thiazide diuretics	Impotence
Metoprolol (Lopressor)	Decreased libido; impotence	Thioridazine (Mellaril and others)	Impotence; priapism; delayed, decreased, painful, retrograde, or no ejaculation
Metyrosine (Demser)	Impotence; failure of ejaculation		
Mexiletine (Mexitil)	Impotence; decreased libido	Thiothixene (Navane and others)	Spontaneous ejaculations; impotence; priapism
Molindone (Moban)	Priapism		
Naltrexone (Trexan)	Delayed ejaculation; decreased potency	Timolol (Blocadren, Timolide, Timoptic)	Decreased libido; impotence
Naproxen (Anaprox, Naprosyn)	Impotence; no ejaculation	Tranylcypromine (Parnate)	Impotence
Norethindrone (Norlutin and others)	Decreased libido; impotence	Trazodone (Desyrel)	Priapism; increased libido (women); retrograde ejaculation
Nortriptyline (Aventyl, Pamelor)	Impotence; decreased libido	Trifluoperazine (Stelazine and others)	Decreased, painful, or no ejaculation; spontaneous ejaculations
Paragyline (Eutonyl)	No ejaculation; impotence		
Paroxetine (Paxil)	Decreased libido	Verapamil (Calan and others)	Impotence
Perphenazine (Trilafon)	Decreased or no ejaculation		

From Med Lett Drugs Ther 29:65, 1987.

degree vaginismus, defined as levator and perineal spasm with withdrawal and retreat. Four of the 80 patients refused pelvic examination.

These patients frequently complain not only of pain or fear of pain with coitus or pelvic examination but also of difficulty in inserting a tampon or vaginal medication. The condition may be primary, in which case the individual has never experienced successful coitus. This problem is generally based on either early sexual abuse or aversion to sexuality in general. This leads to a form of conversion hysteria or to a lack of appropriate learning about sex secondary to cultural or familial teaching that sex is evil, painful, or undesirable. Vaginismus may also occur in patients who have been sexually active when an injury or vaginal infection has led to vaginal pain with attempted coitus. This has been seen in rape victims, women who have had painful episiotomy repairs, or severe yeast vaginitis. When the underlying cause for the vaginismus is understood, the matter may be discussed frankly with the patient and her partner to effect a relearning process that is conducive to relieving the symptoms. The actual vaginal spasm then may be relieved by teaching the patient self-dilation techniques, using fingers or dilators, in which she and her partner can participate. The period of therapy is usually short and the results good.

Orgasmic dysfunction is quite common. As many as 10% to 15% of women have never experienced an orgasm through any form of sexual stimulation, and another 25% to 35% will have difficulty reaching an orgasm on any particular occasion. Many women may be orgasmic secondary to masturbation or oral sex but may not be orgasmic with penile intercourse. It is important to discern by history the extent of the patient's problem and to place it into proper perspective. If the patient is anorgasmic during intercourse but has experienced orgasms, communication with her partner may aid in bringing about an orgasm during intercourse by allowing her or her partner to stimulate her clitoral area with the intensity and timing necessary to bring about an orgasm. If the woman is anorgasmic, she may be taught masturbatory techniques to demonstrate an orgasm to her, and then these techniques may be applied to the coital situation, thereby developing the desired response during coitus. Couples should be encouraged to communicate their sexual needs so that appropriate stimulation is offered during the arousal period and during intercourse. Developing this type of dialogue is often difficult but can be aided by counseling with a sensitive physician.

Dyspareunia is a sexual dysfunction that frequently has an organic basis. The physician should obtain a careful history of when the dyspareunia occurs (i.e., on insertion of the penis, at the mid-vagina during thrusting, or with deep penetration of the vault), since facts obtained by this history may point to organic causes, such as poor lubrication, urethritis, cystitis, trigonitis, poorly healed vaginal lacerations or episiotomy, and disease such as pelvic inflammatory disease or endometriosis. When no organic cause can be found for the dyspareunia, techniques similar to those used in evaluating and managing vaginismus are appropriate. Specific pathologic conditions should, of course, be treated. At times dyspareunia can be relieved by changing coital position. Couples should be encouraged to experiment with female-dominant and side-by-side positions to see if the pain can be prevented.

Female Homosexuality (Lesbianism)

Obstetricians and gynecologists will clearly take care of lesbians in their practices and should be prepared to understand and have a sensitivity for their medical problems. Little usable data are available in the literature concerning this issue, and ascertaining a patient's sexual per-suasion is not always easy. Bradford et al. completed a National Lesbian Health Care Survey with implications on mental health. Detailed questionnaires were distributed in all 50 states through a variety of lesbian organizations. The questionnaire was carefully constructed with a good deal of user input, and 1925 lesbians responded. The authors admitted that their means of ascertaining was not and could not be a random sample of the total population of lesbians and therefore did not assume that the results of their study could be generalized. Likewise, no comparable control group of heterosexual women was obtainable given the construction of the study. Therefore, it is not possible to know whether the problems that the homosexual women suffered differed from those suffered by a comparable group of heterosexual women. Nevertheless, the survey does give some insight into the problems that these women face.

The authors discovered that 88% of the sample were open about their sexual orientation to other lesbians and gays but only 27% were open to family members, 28% to heterosexual friends, and 17% to co-workers. Nineteen percent shared their sexual preference with no family members and 29% with no co-workers.

With respect to relationships, 60% of the group were involved in a primary relationship with another woman, 20% were single and uninvolved, and 2% were legally married to men at the time of the survey. With respect to the common concerns held by these women, 57% identified concerns over money, 31% concerns about job or school, 27% concerns about a lover, 23% responsibilities at work, and 21% family problems. Only 12% reported concerns about people knowing that they were homosexual. Many of these women felt unsafe, a third reported having suffered depression and anxiety, with 11% experiencing current depression, and 11% were currently undergoing treatment for depression. Fifty-seven percent stated that they had, at one time or another, entertained thoughts of suicide, and 18% had actually attempted suicide.

Forty-one percent of the patients gave a history of physical abuse at some time during their life, with 37% having been beaten harshly at least once. Twenty-four percent stated they had been physically abused while growing up, 16% had been abused as adults, and 6% as both adults and children.

Forty-one percent reported that they had been raped or sexually abused at least one time in their lives, with 21% reporting such attacks in childhood and 15% in adulthood. Four percent had been raped or sexually attacked in both adult and childhood. Nineteen percent had been victims of incest; of these, 34% were victimized by their brothers, 28% by their fathers, 27% by uncles, 18% by cousins, 9% by stepfathers, 8% by grandfathers, 3% by mothers, and 3% by sisters.

Thirty percent of the sample smoked cigarettes daily, and another 11% smoked occasionally. A third of the sample used alcohol regularly, with 6% using alcohol every day and another 25% using it at least once a week.

Forty-seven percent of the sample used marijuana at least occasionally, and 19% had tried cocaine but only 1% used it more than once a week. Eleven percent of the sample used tranquilizers, but only 1% used them daily.

Two thirds of the sample reported overeating, but only 4% indicated that they used vomiting as a means of weight control.

Seventy-three percent of the sample were in counseling or had received some counseling or mental health support from a professional at some time in the past. In general, the counseling was sought because of feeling sad or depressed (50%), feeling anxious or scared (31%), or because of loneliness (21%).

It can be seen that lesbian women have many social and emotional problems; however, whether these are in every case out of proportion with a comparable group of heterosexual women has not been demonstrated. The physician should be sensitive to these problems and attempt to offer appropriate care when such problems are discovered.

Tobacco, Alcohol, and Drug Use

The use of tobacco, alcohol, marijuana, cocaine, and other drugs is quite common in the United States, and the abuse of these substances is not unusual. The prevalence of their use among women is variable and often age-dependent. In 1970 one third of American women of childbearing age were cigarette smokers. However, only 20% to 25% of pregnant women were actually believed to smoke during their pregnancies. In 1995 the U.S. Department of Health and Human Services reported an overall smoking incidence among females of 22.8%, with rates varying by age: 21.8% in women 18-24, 27.1% in 35-44 age group, and 11.5% in women over 65 years. The overall rate came down gradually from a high of 34% in 1965 but has been fairly stable since 1990.

Alcohol use among American women is quite high with 50.7% being current consumers in 1990, and varying by age group: 58.3% in the 18-44 year group, 47.6% in the 45-64 year group, and 31.3% in women over 65.

Sokol found in a study of pregnant women in Cleveland that only 1.2% would state that they had an alcohol problem; however, on careful questioning about alcohol consumption, 11% were noted to be heavy drinkers.

In a detailed history of marijuana use, Nahas reviewed the work of several other authors and noted that in 1970 between 7% and 20% of college students were using marijuana. In addition, he pointed out that 15% of adolescents between the ages of 12 and 17 in one series were found to be using marijuana, with an incidence of 17% among boys and 14% among girls. Recent data imply that the percentages of users are higher. In 1997 21% of girls ages 12 to 17 were reported to have used marijuana within the past month of being surveyed, and among women ages 18 to

25, the use was 35%. The prevalence of cocaine, heroin, and other drug use is variable from group to group, but overall these uses are quite common.

It is beyond the scope of this book to discuss the health hazards of these various agents, the problems of habituation, or the social and legal considerations. It is appropriate, however, to recognize that each of these agents adversely affects the reproductive process, causes a variety of illness, and influences the health and social relationships of the users.

The obstetrician and gynecologist is in an excellent position to discourage young women from beginning to use these substances by offering educational information at the time of visits for routine check-ups, for treatment of simple problems such as dysmenorrhea or vaginitis, or during consultations for contraception. The obstetrician and gynecologist may also influence women contemplating reproduction by pointing out the potential dangers of these substances to the fetus. As the primary physician for women, the obstetrician and gynecologist has the opportunity to periodically define activities that may be affecting the individual's health and offer education and counseling to modify these activities. Where appropriate, referrals to other health care specialists may be made.

To modify behavior in patients who abuse tobacco, alcohol, and other drugs, the physician must first identify their use. A history at the time of a routine check-up should include the following:

1. Smoking history. Does the patient smoke? For how long has she smoked? What substances are smoked and in what quantity? Moderate cigarette smokers (1 to 10 cigarettes per day) may be influenced to stop by simply discussing health hazards and suggesting that the practice be terminated. If the individual smokes fewer than 10 cigarettes a day, stopping without tapering off is appropriate and if motivated, the individual is usually successful. If the individual smokes more than 10 cigarettes a day, habituation may be a problem. Reducing the number of cigarettes to 10 per day and then stopping may be successful. If not, consultation with health care professionals who may use behavioral modification therapy is appropriate. Organized behavior modification programs to aid individuals to quit smoking are available in most communities. Fiore et al. have demonstrated, however, that 90% of successful quitters and 80% of unsuccessful quitters used individual methods similar to those described above. In their series, 47.5% of individuals who had tried to quit on their own in the previous 10 years were successful, whereas only 23.6% of those who used organized cessation methods were successful. These programs, however, were shown by the authors to aid a small group of smokers who were primarily heavy smokers.

2. Alcohol use. Cahalan defined high-volume alcohol use as the consumption of 45 drinks a month or at least 5 drinks on some occasions (binge drinking). To describe a particular patient's drinking habits it is necessary to take a detailed history of how many drinks per day the patient takes and the type of substance consumed (whiskey, beer, or wine). One ounce of whiskey, a wineglass of wine, and 12 ounces of beer are interchangable. Binge drinking, which is defined as five drinks or more per day or periodic drinking to intoxication, should be noted as should its frequency. If a patient consumes more than 45 drinks per month or is a binge drinker, the physician should attempt to obtain behavior modification help for the patient. Generally, attendance at an Alcoholics Anonymous program with or without other specialized health care is indicated. If the patient does not consume large amounts of alcohol but does drink regularly, educational literature and counseling should be provided.

3. Marijuana use. Marijuana is an illegal substance and has many biologic side effects. Its use should be discouraged among all patients. If marijuana is used daily, the patient's habituation must be recognized and behavior modification therapy offered.

4. Other drug use. Patients are frequently habituated to illegal drugs, such as cocaine and heroin, and often to prescription drugs as well (i.e., tranquilizers, barbiturates, and amphetamines). The physician should identify the quantity and type of drug used by history and should make the appropriate referral to a health care agency. Cocaine is a major problem in the United States at present. It is addicting and gives users a sense of power and strength that they find rewarding. Because of this and the fact that users can often function reasonably well under its influence, stopping its use can be very difficult. Cocaine use and possible addiction should be sought by the physician in all patients and treatment vigorously suggested when it is discovered. For instance, individuals habituated to cocaine are often treated in a fashion similar to alcoholics, using such help groups as Cocaine Anonymous.

Depression

Depression is a common symptom in a variety of conditions. Patients suffering loss or grief are often depressed. However, depression as a symptom is quite common in the general population. In a review, Ripley offered evidence from the world literature to indicate that as many as 10% of all individuals are depressed. For 1998 the National Center for Health Statistics reported 3,037,765 visits to physicians for depression in individuals between the ages of 25 and 44, and 1,943,349 visits for individuals 45 to 64. Depression associated with psychoses such as is seen in manic-depressive (bipolar) psychosis may occur as often as 3 to 4 per 1000 people. Dorpat and Ripley noted that 9.3% of patients suffering from personality disorders, 26.9% of patients suffering from alcoholism, and 12.0% of schizophrenics had depression as a major symptom. Unfortunately, patients who suffer from depression are more prone to suicide, and psychiatric patients who commit suicide are more likely to have a depressive component to their illness.

Depression in infants and young children is frequently the result of deprivation, particularly maternal deprivation. It is frequently characterized by crying and behavior disorders and later by despair and withdrawal. The child may fail to eat and may eventually starve to death. If the child does not die, strong depressive symptomatology may continue into adulthood. Ripley cites the work of several authors who have shown a significantly higher rate of bereavement or broken homes in childhood among adult depressive patients.

It is useful for a gynecologist to understand the way in which depression may present in patients. Early symptoms include chronic fatigue, anxiety and irritability, anhedonia (loss of feelings of joy and pleasure), decreased interest in usual pursuits including sexual activity and personal appearance, and mental changes, including poor concentration and lack of decisiveness. The individual may complain of loss of recent memory; insomnia, especially occurring shortly after falling asleep; a pessimistic outlook about the future, often associated with feelings of guilt; and a number of physical complaints including loss of appetite or a great increase in appetite; change in bowel habits, including constipation or diarrhea; headache; various aches and pains; and general lability.

Late in the disease the patient may experience deep feelings of hopelessness, with difficulty in presenting ideas. The patient may also complain of generalized weakness, fear of impending doom from a serious illness or fear that serious problems will befall a close family member, suicidal thoughts, and occasionally, delusions.

The physician should be alert to patients who have suffered personal loss or grief but who are still deeply depressed after 6 to 18 months of grieving. Although depression is normal in a grief situation, it should not last for a prolonged period.

The diagnosis is often suspected by simply assessing the patient's appearance and asking the usual questions concerning the patient's mood and health. Several psychologic tests have been developed to assess depression and can be used in subtle cases. The physician should assess the degree to which the patient is depressed and whether the reason for the depression is appropriate. If the patient is grieving because of a real life situation, the physician should demonstrate concern and offer appropriate assurance that the problem will be relieved with time.

If the degree of depression is inappropriate for the life

situation, the physician should determine whether the individual has suicidal thoughts and assess whether these thoughts are likely to be put into practice. Such questions as, "Have you considered harming yourself or taking your own life?" are appropriate in this situation. If the patient states that she has had such thoughts, the degree to which she is contemplating them may be assessed by asking if she has considered how she would carry out the suicide or what circumstances deterred her from attempting this act. If the patient seems to be seriously considering suicide, prompt referral to a mental health worker or facility should be made.

Patients who are depressed but give no evidence for psychosis may be helped by medication. Currently, the most effective agents for this purpose are the tricyclic antidepressants (TCAs) and the selective serotonin reuptake inhibitors (SSRIs). Table 8-4 lists the currently available medications by functional group and by generic and trade names. The SSRIs are very effective in alleviating symptoms of depression but may have among their side effects appetite suppression and decrease in libido. Most of the TCAs have an atropine-like effect; therefore, dryness of the mouth, blurred vision, hesitancy of urination or dribbling, some menstrual disorders (i.e., amenorrhea or irregularity), and a decrease in sexual arousal are complaints often associated with their use. Each of these agents causes slightly different undesirable side effects, and a specific patient's symptoms may be alleviated by switching to a different medication. Although patients may note a reduction in symptoms of depression after 1 to 2 weeks of drug use, real improvement may take as long as 1 month and the physician may wish to continue the use of these agents for 6 months to 1 year. Many patients can use antidepressant drugs intermittently when symptomatology warrants. The dosage will need to be varied depending on the patient's response. For patients with serious emotional or social problems, counseling may be necessary along with drug therapy. Often drug therapy is necessary to bring the patient's depression under control to an extent that allows psychotherapy or counseling to be useful.

Lithium salts have been used to treat depression and are most useful in the treatment of bipolar disorder (manic-depressive psychosis). Monoamine oxidase inhibitors are also in common clinical use but frequently have serious side effects and should be administered only by individuals well experienced in their use.

Loss and Grief

Loss is a common human experience and may affect women of all ages. The loss of a child, a spouse, or a close relative should and probably will precipitate an acute grief reaction. However, the physician must remember that a similar reaction will be precipitated by a spontaneous abortion, by the loss of a body part or organ, or by the realization that infertility and childlessness face the couple. It may also occur in women undergoing separation or divorce, losing a job, or losing a pet.

Lindemann points out that acute grief is a definite syndrome with both psychologic and somatic components. In his vast experience with grieving patients he has observed that the syndrome may appear immediately after the loss or be delayed. If it is delayed, grief may appear to be absent only to occur at a future time, often in a more exaggerated fashion. At times the syndrome may occur in a distorted fashion. For successful resolution of grief, the individual must be helped to transform these distorted reactions into normal grief.

Lindemann points out that the symptomatology of normal grief is quite uniform. The individual often complains of tightness in the throat and chest, a choking sensation, a feeling of shortness of breath, and frequent sighing. An empty feeling in the abdomen, muscle weakness, and a feeling of tension and mental pain are often

---

TABLE 8-4
Antidepressants

Functional Group	Generic Name	Trade Names
Selective serotonin reuptake inhibitors (SSRIs)	fluoxetine hydrochloride	Prozac
	sertraline hydrochloride	Zoloft
	paroxetine hydrochloride	Paxil
Tricyclic antidepressants (TCAs)	amitriptyline	Amitril, Elavil, Amitid, Amitriptyline, Endep, SK-Amitriptyline
	amoxapine	Asendin
	desipramine	Norpramin, Pertofrane
	doxepin	Sinequan, Adapin
	imipramine	Tofranil, Antipress, Imavate, Imipramine, Janimine, SK-Pramine, Presamine
	nortriptyline	Pamelor
	protriptyline	Vivactil
	trimipramine	Surmontil

reported. These symptoms frequently come in waves lasting from minutes to an hour and are often dreaded by the sufferer.

Lindemann further points out that the bereaved experience disorders of the sensorium often involving a sense of unreality, a tendency to place emotional distance between themselves and other people, and a preoccupation with imagery of the deceased. At times the bereaved will assume the mannerisms of the deceased or even attempt to perform the work of the lost loved one. If the mother has died, the bereaved daughter may see the mother's face when she looks at herself in the mirror and may assume the mother's mannerisms in her speech and gestures. There is often the perception that the deceased is nearby and can communicate.

In the immediate grief period the bereaved often feels guilt. This may directly involve the events of the death or of tasks left unfinished before the individual died. The bereaved often feels a lack of warmth and may demonstrate feelings of hostility toward others.

The burden of the grief is often so great that the individual can barely handle the maintenance activities of living, and has little energy left over for social contact or growth and development.

Most authorities feel that a normal grief reaction takes 6 to 18 months and ends when the individual has appropriately experienced the pain and suffering, placed the memory of the deceased in a proper place within the bereaved's life, and established new relationships and new life directions. In older women, however, the grieving period may be prolonged because of the limited number of diversions and opportunities available to them.

Lindemann notes, however, that abnormal grief reactions are possible and divides these into several categories. The first is the delay of reaction, which essentially is a postponement of grieving. This may be seen in an individual who is injured in an accident that kills the person to be grieved. The individual may be preoccupied with personal survival and recuperation and may not have the opportunity to grieve until this has passed. In other instances the individual may delay grieving for a long period, often years. There are often psychologic reasons why this occurs, but when the grieving is finally precipitated, it may appear quite pathologic and out of context for current life situations.

A second variant is a distorted reaction. In this situation the bereaved may take on the characteristics of the deceased without evidencing a sense of loss. The bereaved may actually take on the symptoms of the lost person if that individual had experienced a prolonged illness before death.

A third abnormal reaction to grieving may be the development of a psychosomatic condition. Ulcerative colitis, rheumatoid arthritis, and asthma have all been noted to occur in approximation to bereavement. Lindemann points out that some patients suffering from these problems may improve when the grief reaction is resolved.

Other types of abnormal grief reactions include pathologic alterations in relationships with friends and relatives, inappropriate hostility toward others, behavior patterns resembling psychoses, continuing inability to make decisions or to take initiative, and performance of activities that have destructive social and economic outcomes. Finally, Lindemann notes that in the reaction of agitated depression the bereaved develops tension, agitation, insomnia, feelings of worthlessness, and fantasies of a need for punishment. In such situations suicide may be a danger. Fortunately, agitated depression is quite unusual. Lindemann feels that it may be more common in individuals who have experienced a previous depression or in those who have been intensely involved with the deceased, such as mothers who have lost young children.

Loss of a Child by Abortion, Stillbirth, or Neonatal or Infant Death

Obstetricians and gynecologists may need to counsel patients experiencing grief related to several areas of reproduction. Leppert and Pahlka counseled 22 women who had experienced spontaneous abortion. The study format was to hold a counseling session immediately after abortion and again in 4 to 6 weeks. These authors report that all women demonstrated the classic stages of grief, but that guilt was the stage that appeared the most difficult for them and their spouses to resolve. The authors thought that the unexpressed emotions relating to pregnancy loss might affect the relationship of the couple unless they are explored and defused. They suggested that the obstetrician and gynecologist make it a point to add such counseling to his or her practice routines. Bruhn and Bruhn point out that a predictable pattern of grief follows every stillbirth and perinatal death and urge physicians to work with their patients in resolving these feelings.

In addition to the physician's offering understanding and counseling, there are many self-help groups that offer aid to parents who have lost children either in the perinatal period or in infancy. The physician should become aware of the agencies or groups within the community that offer group and self-help therapy in neonatal and infant loss. It is reasonable for the physician to learn the techniques used by these groups and to assess whether their approach fits the needs of the patient before making referrals.

The physician should also be aware of the fact that each member of the couple may grieve differently and, indeed, the style of grieving that one may exhibit may be in conflict with that of the other. Pointing out these differences and helping the couple to express their true feelings to each other may be very beneficial during this process.

An important issue in understanding the management of grief in couples who have lost infants was demonstrated in an evaluation of a group of patients by Estok and Lehman. They found that such individuals wished health care providers to acknowledge the couple's feelings of shock, guilt, and grief and to recognize the importance of their memories of the birth and of the baby. In essence, they wished the health care providers to help them sharpen the reality of the death of the child and provide support through the postloss period rather than focus on other life events, such as the next pregnancy.

Certain aspects of bereavement should be understood by the physician in dealing with patients who are suffering grief. The loss of a child is always a serious problem. Even the loss of an adult child can have long-term sequelae. Shanfield and Swain noted that parents who have lost adult children in traffic accidents continued to grieve intensely for a prolonged period and had a higher than expected level of psychiatric symptoms and health complaints. Families that were unstable and in which problems had existed with these children suffered more guilt and more psychiatric symptoms. In addition, factors that intensified the bereavement experience were a mother losing a daughter, parents losing children who lived at home, the loss of children born early in the birth order, and the loss of multiple children in a single-car, single-driver accident. A protecting factor seemed to be a prior bereavement experience.

These observations were supported by Lundin, who used the Texas Inventory of Grief to study first-degree relatives 8 years after bereavement. He noted that relatives of persons who had died suddenly or unexpectedly suffered a more pronounced grief reaction than those who had lost someone in a death that was expected. He also noted that bereavement was greater in parents after the loss of a child than in widows or widowers who lost a spouse. The current AIDS epidemic is increasing the incidence of adult child loss grief in older women.

Unplanned Pregnancy

A special counseling challenge involves the care of a woman with an unplanned pregnancy. Such individuals often suffer conflicting feelings, which may include shame and guilt for their predicament, a genuine desire to have a child, fear of social consequences, and fear for their own future and physical well-being. In addition, they may suffer from guilt about the destruction of the pregnancy if abortion is considered. Although many such women have good support groups (e.g., family, significant other, friends, and religious counselors), others will rely on the physician entirely for advice and direction. The physician should discuss all possible options with the patient, including having and raising the child, offering it for adoption, or terminating the pregnancy. Issues involving the role of the baby's father, the effect of any decision on the future life of the patient, and the risks of the procedure should be considered. The patient should be aided in reaching the most appropriate decision for her needs and then should be supported in carrying out her plan. Where necessary, appropriate referrals to social agencies (e.g., adoption, abortion counseling, or welfare services) should be made.

Infertility

The inability to reproduce leads to a major life frustration and often generates a series of symptoms similar to the grief reaction. Many sequelae may occur that stress the couple's relationship. Guilt, anger, and shame may be components, depending on the social forces at play in the relationship. Sexual dysfunction may result because of the stresses imposed by the requirements of a treatment regimen or because of general dysfunction within the relationship brought about by the infertility. At times the problems associated with the infertility (e.g., endometrial implants in the cul-de-sac) may cause dyspareunia and lead to sexual dysfunction. External stresses from family and friends who continuously refer to the couple's childlessness may contribute to the tension as well.

The physician must be complete in the medical evaluation of the couple, as well as supportive of their emotional needs. The physician should discuss fully all treatment options and the chances for success. He or she should also continuously help the couple to accentuate the positives of their relationship and to consider referring them to self-help groups for infertile couples or to health care counselors who can help with the maintenance of their relationship and self-images.

Death of a Spouse

Holmes and Rahe rate the death of a spouse as one of the major life stresses among survivors independent of age and cultural background, and state that it may contribute to a decline in physical and mental well-being of the survivor. Gallagher et al. recently reported the effects of acute bereavement on the indicators of mental health in widows and widowers beyond the age of 55. These workers evaluated a group from the standpoint of past grief, present grief, depression, somatic symptomatology, and self-rating of mental health status. They noted that these individuals in the early stages of their bereavement were suffering from considerable psychologic distress compared with individuals of similar age who were not bereaved. They demonstrated that the degree of effect of bereavement on the patient's mental health did not vary by sex. Those conditions that were more likely to occur in one sex rather than the other occurred with incidence equal to those individuals of the same sex in the study group. Thus findings in women, who tend to have a higher incidence of depression in the general population than do men, demonstrated this to be the case in the same proportions among the study group.

CROSS-CULTURAL DIFFERENCES. Eisenbruch has pointed out that there are significant cross-cultural differences in bereavement, whereas there are great similarities in the grief reaction between different ethnic and cultural groups. Individuals from different backgrounds tend to experience difficulty with their grief when they attempt to respond in a fashion specific for the majority within the culture in which they now reside. Specific rituals, attitudes toward widowhood, mores with respect to length and type of grieving, the way in which the deceased is remembered, and the appropriate length of time for grieving and mourning may be quite different in various minority groups when compared with the general white majority of the United States. Physicians dealing with minority groups are urged to consider the points raised by Eisenbruch in his review to be better able to help the minority patients through their grieving period.

Separation and Divorce

Currently the number of divorces occurring annually in the United States is about 40% of the number of marriages. There are many reasons for this increase, including the emerging of women to a level of self-support, changing attitudes toward a desire to remain married, and an increased public awareness of family dysfunction, such as spouse and child abuse. Often one or both members of a divorcing couple will demonstrate evidence of grief, as well as anger, shame, and guilt. Counseling can be very useful in restoration of self-esteem and in helping the individual to emerge from the experience with the ability to survive in new relationships. Although physicians should recognize these needs in their patients who are going through separation and divorce, their primary role should be to make appropriate referrals to counselors who have the time and the skills to deal with the patient in this area.

Loss of an Organ or Body Part

Loss of a body part can be expected to bring about a grief reaction with accompanying symptoms of an emotional and somatic nature. Depression is frequently a strong component. Workers who have investigated the loss of limbs have noted this, and it is reasonable to expect that the loss of such organs as the breast or the uterus would evoke a similar reaction.

Several workers have reported depression among posthysterectomy patients, with an incidence ranging from 4% to as high as 70%. In a review, Drummond and Field point out that the stages of the process of incorporating the loss of a uterus into the individual's self-image is similar to that of the loss of other body parts. They refer to the four stages of incorporation listed by Roberts: impact, retreat, acknowledgment, and reconstruction.

The impact stage occurs when the individual becomes aware that she has a problem with her uterus. If she is symptomatic this may be obvious. If she has been told she must lose her uterus because it is diseased, such as with cancer, she will need to make a mental adjustment to this fact. Steiner and Aleksandrowicz have pointed out that when the disease that requires operation is life-threatening or serious, the likelihood of depression is minimized. Richards has pointed out that when disease of the uterus is absent, depression is more likely to occur.

The second stage of organ loss is retreat. This is the period in which the patient accepts the need for the loss of an organ and depersonalizes it in her thinking. If denial occurs at this period, the depression that she notes later may be quite severe. The desire for a second opinion often occurs in this phase. It is a healthy response and should be encouraged.

The third stage is acknowledgment. The physician will recognize this stage because it involves the woman's repeated discussion of the procedure, the need for the procedure, and the meaning of the loss of the uterus postoperatively. It is the woman's attempt to place the procedure and the need for the procedure within the appropriate context of her life and her self-image.

The final phase is reconstruction. This involves the redefinition of her self-image without the organ. It will require acceptance by her spouse or significant other and by other members of her community of importance in this event. The physician should attempt to discuss the need for and the likely sequelae of the hysterectomy before it is performed. This discussion should include the significant other in the woman's life so that any fantasies or fears that may arise can be discussed at this point. Some men have difficulty continuing an active sexual experience with a woman who has lost her uterus. These points should be discussed ahead of time so that each realizes the implication of the operation. On the other hand, some women feel that sex is for procreation only and after the removal of the uterus may respond quite differently from what the significant other has known in the past. These points, too, should be discussed before the fact.

If the individual cannot work through the four stages of loss of an organ, disruption of relationships and depression may be sequelae. Newton and Baron have noted that between 20% and 40% of couples stop having sexual intercourse after hysterectomy. They do not state whether this is a direct effect of the hysterectomy and the inability to work out feelings related to this procedure or whether other problems may have existed, allowing for the hysterectomy to be an excuse to stop experiencing intercourse. Physicians should consider these points, however, and discuss them with the patient and her significant other before embarking on an operative procedure, particularly if it is elective and the time is available for discussion.

Loss of a Pet

A final bereavement situation often overlooked by physicians but frequently important to patients is the grief associated with the death of a pet. Quackenbush reviewed the subject and concluded that animals play an important role in the human social system and may contribute greatly to the quality of life of many pet owners. In some cases where the individual lives alone and may be elderly, the animal may be the only living thing in close daily contact with the individual. It is, therefore, not unusual that when the pet dies, the owner suffers grief. Quackenbush states that understanding and sensitivity to the feelings and sense of loss that the pet owner experiences will help to facilitate the resolution of the grief.

Counseling the Dying

Elizabeth Kubler-Ross revolutionized our understanding of the death process with her classic book on the subject in 1969. An important paragraph taken from the first chapter describing the fear of death is quite revealing:

> When we look back in time and study old cultures and people, we are impressed that death has always been distasteful to man and will probably always be. From the psychiatrist's point of view this is very understandable and can perhaps best be explained by our basic knowledge that, in our unconscious, death is never possible in regard to ourselves. It is inconceivable for our unconscious to imagine an actual ending of our own life here on earth and if the life of ours has to end the ending is always attributed to a malicious intervention from the outside by someone else. In simple terms, in our unconscious mind we can only be killed; it is inconceivable to die of a natural cause or of old age. Therefore, death in itself is associated with a bad act, a frightening happening, something that in itself calls for retribution and punishment.*

Kubler-Ross describes five stages through which an individual progresses in the acceptance of the inevitability of death. They are denial, anger, bargaining, depression, and acceptance. *Denial* and isolation is a temporary state brought about by the shock of learning that the individual suffers from a problem from which he or she cannot recover. The transition from denial to partial acceptance will depend on the nature of the patient's illness, how long he or she has left before death will occur, and the way in which he or she has prepared throughout life to cope with such serious situations. Kubler-Ross notes that when confronted with multiple health care providers who are likely to express the inevitable in a variety of ways, the dying person often chooses to accept the individual style of presentation that most fits her need. During this period of adjustment, therefore, a number of different opinions may be sought and specific interpretations questioned. Inevitably the individual may be depressed and may isolate herself from those with whom she would normally associate. Frequently the individual may appear confused and in some cases may

deny that any information about the impending death has ever been given. Most patients, according to Kubler-Ross, will go through this period long before death occurs. However, in 3 of 200 patients that she studied, acceptance of the inevitable did not occur until the very time of death.

Hospital personnel must guard against avoiding patients after having given the initial information. They must not interpret the period of the patient's denial as a distasteful circumstance with which they cannot cope. Instead they should help the patient work through this period by patiently repeating information, answering questions, and offering comfort. Terms that remove all hope, such as *terminal* or *hopeless*, should be avoided.

The second stage described by Kubler-Ross is *anger*. Staff and family members find this the most difficult one with which to cope, since the anger felt by the patient may be inappropriately displaced to everyone and everything in the environment. The physician or nurse caring for the patient falls into the unenviable position of the messenger who is hated because of the bad news he or she has brought. The health care worker who tries to make the patient comfortable may be accused of being overly solicitous, whereas the health care worker who attempts to give the patient the privacy that it is believed she seeks may be accused of being uncaring. Likewise, family members who attempt to be cheerful in visiting the patient may be accused of being glib and uncaring, whereas if they are more somber, they may be accused of being depressing. In such cases the health care worker or family member will probably experience guilt and possibly shame, and may adjust to the problem by avoiding the dying person altogether.

During the anger period the dying individual will be irritated by all stimuli. Happiness depicted on television may upset her because she feels that she is not included in it. Discussion of future plans of friends or family members will be equally depressing because the dying individual realizes that she will not be around to participate. The anger period ends when the individual can reconcile the fact that she is different from every healthy person but is still capable of being loved and accepted.

The third stage is *bargaining*. This is an attempt to postpone the inevitable by offering concessions, presumably to God. It is essentially the hope of getting more time for good behavior. In this period the individual may do charitable acts, correct past misdeeds, or reconcile damaged relationships. It is a time for relieving guilt and defusing the feeling of required punishment. It may, in many ways, be an opportunity to "put one's house in order."

The fourth stage described by Kubler-Ross is *depression*. Although symptoms of depression may occur in the earlier stages, depression at this stage may occur because the patient has had to cope with a number of factors associated with the illness. For instance, she may be concerned

---

*From Kubler-Ross E: On death and dying, New York, 1969, Macmillan Co.

about the expenses of her care, loss of wages, and the simple fact that she feels poorly, added to the fact that she now realizes she is going to die. In addition, fears that her death will adversely affect other members of her family who depend on her may also add to her depression. Health care workers should be comfortable in allowing the patient to know that they understand the reasons for the depression. They should do everything possible to eliminate the feelings of guilt that the patient may have because of the conditions in which she finds herself. She should be made to realize that the financial burdens that may be developing or the effect that her death may have on family members and their lives are not a result of specific actions that she may have taken. In other words, she is not responsible for the condition she is in and the resulting circumstances are not legitimate reasons for her to feel guilt. Family members can be helpful by accentuating the positive aspects of the patient's life, the love they feel for her, and the happiness they have experienced with her. They should downplay the burdens that the patient's illness and death will create for them. Essentially the patient is working through a period of grief, in this case, grief for herself.

The fifth and final stage is *acceptance.* At this point the individual has worked through the anger that she has felt for her misfortune and for those healthy individuals who do not have to die at this time and has also passed the period of depression and into a period of accepting her fate. This step will most often be achieved if there is a long enough period for the individual to work through the previous stages. Unfortunately, many die before all of these stages have been reconciled. In a very ill patient acceptance is frequently a giving in to the symptoms she has had to bear and a looking forward to peace from these symptoms that the death will bring. However, Kubler-Ross points out that the acceptance stage is not necessarily this alone, because patients who are not physically suffering also will go through this stage. This is often a time when the individual takes comfort in having quality visits with family members in which positive experiences are remembered. She may also obtain comfort from interacting with representatives of her religious faith.

A new innovation in the care of the terminally ill and their families was introduced with the hospice concept during the 1970s. There are currently many hospice organizations in the United States, offering psychosocial support to both patients and families. The service includes postdeath follow-up with the families to help them through the grieving period. Hospice organizations include free-standing institutions that offer inpatient services; community-based home programs that include both professional and volunteer services; hospital-based hospice teams, which may include physicians, nurses, social workers, chaplains, and volunteers who are in a position to minister to any patient in any bed; and hospital-based hospice units that are geographically separate from other patients and often are coordinated with a home care program.

Godkin et al. studied 58 bereaved spouses and their families whose loved ones had recently died of late-stage cancer after care in a hospital-based hospice service. These families in general rated hospice care significantly better than that received in prior experiences, stating that the hospice services contributed to an improved family function, greater individual well-being, and the ability of family members to cope with the situation. Over three quarters of the families reported that they were emotionally prepared and prepared in a practical sense for the death of the victim. Health problems were reported by these family members in about the same proportion as was experienced in other bereaved groups, but when these problems occurred they were dealt with within the framework of the program.

Physicians who care for chronically ill and terminal patients, particularly those suffering from cancer, should consider availing themselves of the services of such organizations within their geographic area.

KEY POINTS

- The risk of developing a psychiatric disorder seems greatest if the child loses a parent before age 5 or in adolescence.

- The risk of developing a psychiatric disorder is greatest if the child loses a parent of the same sex.

- The highest rate of delinquency seems to occur in males who have lost their fathers unless father substitution occurs.

- Separation from parents in childhood is more likely to cause psychiatric illness when the separation is necessitated by parental illness or marital discord than when it is necessitated by the child's illness or because of wartime evacuation.

- The ideal of thinness for the American woman has increased at the same time that her actual weight has increased.

- More than half of the women between ages 24 and 54 are dieting even though they are not overweight; 75% state they do it for cosmetic reasons.

- Anorexia nervosa occurs in 1% of middle-class adolescent girls.

- Anorexia nervosa occurs in 5% to 20% of ballet dancers.

- When anorexia nervosa occurs in men, it is usually in those individuals training for competitive athletic events.

- Bulimia occurs in about 50% of anorectic patients.

- Vomiting after meals is 3 times as common in bulimics as it is in patients with anorexia nervosa without bulimia.

- Anorexia nervosa and bulimia occur 6 times more frequently in first-degree relatives than in the general population.

- Good to fair outcomes were observed in 88% of anorexia nervosa patients treated as inpatients, 77% of those treated as outpatients, and 59% of those not treated at all.

- Medications have not been useful in treating anorexia nervosa; counseling and behavior modification programs seem to be more effective.

- Long-term follow-ups of patients with anorexia nervosa calculate the hazard of death as 0.5% per year and of relapse as 3% per year. Treatment reduces these.

- Patients between the ages of 25 and 34 who suffer from severe obesity have a mortality 12 times greater than the general population in that age group.

- Of patients with severe obesity who are treated with nonsurgical management, 15% suffer severe depression and 26% suffer moderate depression.

- Behavior modification without medication is the most successful therapy for moderate obesity.

- Diet modification in the treatment of obesity involves lowering fat content to 20%.

- Obesity in adolescence responds best when parents and children are given behavior modification therapy in separate counseling groups.

- Half of all married couples experience some sexual dysfunction or dissatisfaction.

- The sexual response cycle includes excitement, plateau, orgasm, and resolution.

- Sexual arousal is under the control of the parasympathetic portion of the autonomic nervous system.

- Orgasm is under the control of the sympathetic portion of the autonomic nervous system.

- A total of 15% of healthy women have never experienced orgasm.

- A total of 35% of healthy women in a large survey expressed disinterest in sex.

- Inhibited sexual desire is the most common sexual dysfunction.

- Heavy drinking of alcohol among pregnant women may be 10 times higher than that stated in patient histories. In one study, 11% were noted to be heavy drinkers of alcohol.

- Roughly 7% to 20% of college students use marijuana.

- Smoking more than 10 cigarettes per day is evidence for habituation.

- Most smokers who successfully quit do so without behavior modification programs, but such programs seem to benefit heavy smokers.

- High-volume alcohol use is defined as 45 alcoholic drinks per month or 5 drinks or more on specific occasions.

- A total of 10% of all individuals suffer depression.

- Manic depressive (bipolar) psychoses occur in a ratio of approximately 3 to 4 per 1000 people.

- Acute grief reaction lasts 6 to 18 months but may be longer in older patients.

- Currently the number of divorces occurring annually in the United States is about 40% of the number of marriages.

- Posthysterectomy depression occurs in 4% to 70% of women, depending on the indication for the operation and the preparation offered.

- Roberts' four stages of incorporation as an individual response to organ or body part loss are *impact, retreat, acknowledgment,* and *reconstruction.*

- Kubler-Ross defines the stages of individual progress to acceptance of the inevitability of death as *denial, anger, bargaining, depression,* and *acceptance.*

- Hospice programs are support groups for both dying patients and their families.

BIBLIOGRAPHY

Agres WS and Kraemer HC: The treatment of anorexia nervosa: do different treatments have different outcomes? In Stunkard AJ and Stellar E, editors: Eating and its disorders, New York, 1984, Raven Press.

Amato PR: Life-span adjustment of children to their parents' divorce, Future Child 4:143, 1994.

Andersen BL, Turnquist D, LaPolla J, and Turner D: Sexual functioning after treatment of in situ vulvar cancer: preliminary report, Obstet Gynecol 71:15, 1988.

Anderson RE: Where's Dad? Parental deprivation in delinquency, Arch Gen Psychiatry 18:641, 1968.

Barker MG: Psychiatric illness after hysterectomy, Br Med J 2:91, 1968.

Barnes GE and Prosen H: Parental death and depression, J Abnorm Psychol 94:64, 1985.

Birtchnell J: Early parent death in relation to size and constitution of sibship, Acta Psychiatr Scand 47:250, 1971.

Birtchnell J: Early parent death in psychiatric diagnosis, Soc Psychiatry 7:202, 1972.

Bradford J, Ryan C, and Rothblum ED: National Lesbian Health Care Survey: implications for mental health care, J Consult Clin Psychol 62:228, 1994.

Brown GW, Harris T, and Copeland JR: Depression and loss, Br J Psychiatry 130:1, 1977.

Brownell KD: New developments in the treatment of obese children in adolescence. In Stunkard AJ and Stellar E, editors: Eating and its disorders, New York, 1984, Raven Press.

Brownell KD, Kelman JH, and Stunkard AJ: Treatment of obese children with and without their mothers: changes in weight and blood pressure, Pediatrics 71:515, 1983.

Bruhn DF and Bruhn P: Stillbirth: a humanistic response, J Reprod Med 29:107, 1984.

Cahalan D: Quantifying alcohol consumption: patterns and problems, Circulation 64:7, 1981.

Casper RC, Eckert ED, Halmi KA, et al: Bulimia: its incidence and clinical importance in patients with anorexia nervosa, Br J Psychiatry 27:1030, 1980.

Craighead LW, Stunkard AJ, and O'Brien R: Behavior therapy and pharmacotherapy of obesity, Arch Gen Psychiatry 38:763, 1981.

DeGraaf R: New treatise concerning the generative organs of women. In Ladas AK, Whipple B, and Perry JD, editors: The G-spot and other recent discoveries about human sexuality, New York, 1983, Holt, Rinehart & Winston.

Dietrich DR: Psychological health of young adults who experienced early parent death: MMPI trends, J Clin Psychol 40:901, 1984.

Dorpat TL and Ripley HS: A study of suicide in the Seattle area, Compr Psychiatry 1:349, 1960.

Drummond J and Field PA: Emotional and sexual sequelae following hysterectomy, Health Care Women Int 5:261, 1984.

Earls F: The fathers (not the mothers): their importance and influence with infants and young children. In Chess S and Thomas A, editors: Annual progress in child psychiatry and child development, vol 10, New York, 1977, Brunner/Mazel, Inc.

Eisenbruch M: Cross cultural aspects of bereavement. II. Ethnic and cultural variations in the development of bereavement practices, Cult Med Psychiatry 8:315, 1984.

Estok P and Lehman A: Perinatal death: grief support for families, Birth 10:17, 1983.

Fergusson DM, Horwood LJ, and Lynskey MT: Parental separation, adolescent psychopathology, and problem behaviors, J Am Acad Child Adolesc Psychiatry 33:1122, 1994.

Ferguson JM: Learning to eat: leader's manual and patient manual, Palo Alto, Calif, 1975, Bull Publishing Co.

Field AE, Cheung L, Wolf AM, et al: Exposure to mass media and weight concerns among girls, Pediatrics 103:E36, 1999.

Fiore MC, Novotny TE, Pierce JP, et al: Methods used to quit smoking in the United States, JAMA 263:2760, 1990.

Frank E, Anderson C, and Rubinstein D: Frequency of sexual dysfunction in "normal" couples, N Engl J Med 299:111, 1978.

Gallagher DE, Breckenridge JN, Thompson LW, and Peterson JA: Effects of bereavement on indicators of mental health in elderly widows and widowers, J Gerontol 38:565, 1983.

Garner D and Garfinkel P: Sociocultural factors in the development of anorexia nervosa, Psychol Med 10:647, 1980.

Garrow JS: Treat obesity seriously: a clinical manual, New York, 1982, Churchill Livingstone, Inc.

Godkin MA, Krant MJ, and Doster NJ: The impact of hospice care on families, Int J Psychiatry Med 13:153, 1983-84.

Grafenberg E: The role of the urethra in female orgasm, Int J Sexol 3:145, 1950.

Green BL: A clinical approach to marital problems, Springfield, Ill, 1970, Charles C Thomas, Publishers.

Gregory I: Anterospective data following childhood loss of a parent. I. Pathology, performance, and potential among college students, Arch Gen Psychiatry 13:110, 1965.

Halmi KA, Stunkard AJ, and Mason EE: Emotional responses to weight reduction by three methods: diet, jejunoileal bypass and gastric bypass, Am J Clin Nutr 33:446, 1980.

Hamilton LH, Brooks-Gunn J, and Warren MP: Sociocultural influences on eating disorders in professional female ballet dancers, Int J Eat Disord 4:465, 1985.

Hammond DC: Screening for sexual dysfunction, Clin Obstet Gynecol 27:732, 1984.

Health, United States, 1999. US Department of Health and Human Services. Center for Disease Control and Prevention. DHHS 99-1232, 1999.

Holmes TH and Rahe RH: The social adjustment rating scale, J Psychosom Res 11:213, 1967.

Hsu LKG, Crisp AH, and Harding B: Outcome of anorexia nervosa, Lancet 1:61, 1979.

Isager T, Brinch M, Kreiner S, and Tolstrup K: Death and relapse in anorexia nervosa: survival analysis of 151 cases, J Psychiatr Res 19:515, 1985.

Johnson CL, Lewis C, Love S, et al: Incidence and correlates of bulimic behavior in a female high school population, J Youth Adolescence 13:6, 1984.

Johnson WG and Schlundt DG: Eating disorders: assessment and treatment, Clin Obstet Gynecol 28:598, 1985.

Johnston JR: High-conflict divorce, Future Child 4:165, 1994.

Kalucy RC, Crisp AH, Lacy JH, and Harding B: Prevalence and prognosis of anorexia nervosa, Aust N Z J Psychiatry 11:251, 1977.

Kaplan HS: The new sex therapy, New York, 1974, Brunner/Mazel, Inc.

Kendell RE, Hall DJ, Harley A, and Babigan HM: The epidemiology of anorexia nervosa, Psychol Med 2:200, 1973.

Kline NS: From sad to glad, New York, 1974, GP Putnam's Sons.

Kreipe RE, Strauss J, Hodgman CH, and Ryan RM: Menstrual cycle abnormalities and subclinical eating disorders: preliminary report, Psychosom Med 51:81, 1989.

Kubler-Ross E: On death and dying, New York, 1969, Macmillan Publishing Co.

Laajus S: Parental losses, Acta Psychiatr Scand 69:1, 1984.

LaFerla JJ: Inhibited sexual desire and orgasmic dysfunction in women, Clin Obstet Gynecol 27:738, 1984.

Lamont J: Vaginismus, Am J Obstet Gynecol 131:632, 1978.

Leppert PC and Pahlka BS: Grieving characteristics after spontaneous abortion: a management approach, Obstet Gynecol 64:119, 1984.

Letiexhe MR, Scheen AJ, Gèrard PL, et al: Postgastroplasty recovery of ideal body weight normalizes glucose and insulin metabolism in obese women, J Clin Endocrinol Metab 80:364, 1995.

Lindemann E: Symptomatology and management of acute grief, Am J Psychiatry 101:141, 1944.

Lundin T: Long-term outcome of bereavement, Br J Psychiatry 145:424, 1984.

Masters WH and Johnson VE: Human sexual response, Boston, 1966, Little, Brown & Co.

Masters WH and Johnson VE: Human sexual inadequacy. Boston, 1970, Little, Brown & Co.

Melody GF: Depressive reactions following hysterectomy, Am J Obstet Gynecol 83:410, 1962.

MMWR 46 (55-3), 1994.

Moore DC: Body image and eating behavior in adolescents, J Am Coll Nutr 12:505, 1993.

Munro A and Griffiths AB: Some psychiatric nonsequelae of childhood bereavement, Br J Psychiatry 115:305, 1969.

Nahas GG: Marijuana: deceptive weed, New York, 1973, Raven Press.

Nattiv A, Agostini R, Drinkwater B, and Yeager KK: The female athletic triad: the interelatedness of disordered eating, amenorrhea, and osteoporosis, Clin Sport Med 13:405, 1994.

Newton N and Baron E: Reactions to hysterectomy—fact or fiction, Prim Care 3:781, 1976.

Oppenheimer R, Howells K, Palmer RL, and Chaloner DA: Adverse sexual experience in childhood and clinical eating disorders: a preliminary description, J Psychiatr Res 19:357, 1985.

Parker C and Hadzi-Pavlovic D: Modification of level of depression in mother-bereaved women by parental and marital relationships, Psychol Med 14:125, 1984.

Pirke KM, Schweiger U, Strowitzki T, et al: Dieting causes menstrual irregularities in normal weight young women through impairment of episodic luteinizing hormone secretion, Fertil Steril 51:263, 1989.

Pope HG, Jr., Mangweth B, Negrao AB, et al: Childhood sexual abuse and bulimia nervosa: a comparison of American, Austrian, and Brazilian women, Am J Psychiatry 151:731, 1994.

Renshaw DC: When the patient's chief complaint is sexual disinterest, Prim Care Update OB/GYN 1:194, 1994.

Rubinstein S and Caballero B: Is Miss America an undernourished role model? JAMA 283:1549, 2000.

Quackenbush J: The death of a pet: how it can affect owners, Vet Clin North Am Small Anim Pract 15:395, 1985.

Racette SB, Schoeller DA, Kushner RF, and Neil KM: Effects of aerobic exercise and dietary carbohydrate on energy expenditure and body composition during weight reduction in obese women, Am J Clin Nutr 61:486, 1995.

Richards DH: Depression after hysterectomy, Lancet 2:430, 1973.

Richards DH: A posthysterectomy syndrome, Lancet 2:983, 1974.

Ripley HS: Depression and the life span—epidemiology. In Usdin G, editor: Depression: clinical, biological and psychological perspectives, 1977, New York, Brunner/Mazel, Inc.

Roberts SL: Behavioral concepts in the critically ill patient, Englewood Cliffs, NJ, 1976, Prentice-Hall.

Rutter M: Parent child separation: psychological effects on the child, J Child Psychol Psychiatry 12:233, 1971.

Sager CJ: Sexual dysfunction in marital discord. In Kaplan HS, editor: The new sex therapy. New York, 1974, Brunner/Mazel, Inc.

Semmens JP and Semmens EC: Sexual function in the menopause, Clin Obstet Gynecol 27:717, 1984.

Semmens JP and Wagner G: Estrogen deprivation and vaginal function in menopausal women: a study of menopausal vaginal physiology and the effect of exogenous estrogen therapy, JAMA 248:445, 1982.

Shanfield SB and Swain BJ: Death of adult children in traffic accidents, J Nerv Ment Dis 172:533, 1984.

Smith NJ: Excessive weight loss and food aversion in athletes simulating anorexia nervosa, Pediatrics 66:139, 1980.

Sokol RJ: Alcohol in pregnancy: clinical research problems, Neurobehav Toxicol Teratol 2:157, 1980.

Steege JF: Dyspareunia in vaginismus, Clin Obstet Gynecol 27:750, 1984.

Steiner M and Aleksandrowicz DR: Psychiatric sequelae to gynecological operations, Isr Ann Psychiatr Relat Disciplines 8:186, 1970.

Streissguth AP, Darby BL, and Barr HM, et al: Comparison of drinking and smoking patterns during pregnancy over a 6-year interval, Am J Obstet Gynecol 145:716, 1983.

Strober M, Morrell W, Burroughs J, et al: A controlled family study of anorexia nervosa, J Psychiatr Res 19:239, 1985.

Stunkard AJ: Current status of treatment for obesity in adults. In Stunkard AJ and Stellar E, editors: Eating and its disorders. New York, 1984, Raven Press.

Sundgot-Borgen J: Risk and trigger factors for the development of eating disorders in female elite athletes, Med Sci Sports Exerc 26:414, 1994.

Svendsen OL, Hassager C, and Christiansen C: Effect of an energy-restrictive diet, with or without exercise, on lean tissue mass, resting metabolic rate, cardiovascular risk factors, and bone in overweight postmenopausal women, Am J Med 95:131, 1993.

Svendsen OL, Hassager C, and Christiansen C: Six months' follow-up on exercise added to a short-term diet in overweight postmenopausal women—effects on body composition, resting metabolic rate, cardiovascular risk factors and bone, Int J Obes Relat Metab Disord 18:692, 1994.

Tennant C, Bebbington P, and Hurry J: Social experience in childhood and adult psychiatric morbidity: a multiple regression analysis, Psychol Med 12:321, 1982.

Tennant C, Smith A, Bebbington P, and Hurry J: Parental loss in childhood: relationship to adult psychiatric impairment and contact with psychiatric services, Arch Gen Psychiatry 38:309, 1981.

Theander S: Anorexia nervosa, Acta Psychiatr Scand (suppl) 214:1, 1970.

Theander S: Outcome and prognosis in anorexia nervosa and bulimia: some results of previous investigations compared with those of a Swedish long-term study, J Psychiatr Res 19:493, 1985.

The health consequences of smoking, US Department of Health, Education and Welfare, Jan, 1973.

Thompson M: Cultural expectation of thinness of women. Psychol Rep 47:483, 1980.

Wadden TA, Stunkard AJ, and Brownell KD: Very low calorie diets: their efficacy, safety and future, Ann Intern Med 99:675, 1983.

Walters EE and Kendler KS: Anorexia nervosa and anorexic-like syndromes in a population-based female twin sample, Am J Psychiatry 152:64, 1995.

Warren MP: Anorexia nervosa and the related eating disorders, Clin Obstet Gynecol 28:588, 1985.

Weiner L, Rosett HL, Edelin KC, et al: Alcohol consumption by pregnant women, Obstet Gynecol 61:6, 1983.

Weisberg M: Physiology of female sexual function, Clin Obstet Gynecol 27:697, 1984.

CHAPTER

9

Rape, Incest, and Domestic Violence
Discovery, Management, Counseling

KEY TERMS AND DEFINITIONS

Abuse. This may be defined as aggressive behavior including acts of a sexual or physical nature, verbal belittling, or intimidation. The act may be premeditated, as when one individual wishes to gain control over another, or spontaneous, as a spontaneous response to anger or frustration.

Battered Wife Syndrome. A symptom complex occurring as a result of violence in which a woman has at any time received deliberate, severe, or repeated (more than three times) physical abuse from her husband, in which the minimal injury is bruising.

Battered Woman. Any woman over the age of 16 with evidence of physical abuse on at least one occasion at the hands of an intimate male partner.

Cycle of Battering. Three phases in the cycle of battering are noted: The first is tension building; the second is the act of violence; and the third is the apology and forgiveness phase. As cycles are repeated, the second phase tends to become more violent and the third less intensive.

Domestic Violence. Violence occurring between partners in an ongoing relationship regardless of whether they are married.

Incest. Sexual intimacy with or without coitus involving a close family member. The act may include fondling, exposure, or the penetration of an orifice by the phallus.

Rape. Any act of sexual intimacy performed by one person on another without mutual consent by force, by threat of force, or by the inability of the victim to give appropriate consent.

Rape-Trauma Syndrome. A set of behaviors that occur after a rape. The immediate response (acute phase) lasts hours to days and reflects a distortion or paralysis of the individual's coping mechanisms, but the outward responses vary from complete loss of emotional control to an apparently well-controlled behavior pattern. The delayed (or reorganization) phase involves flashbacks, nightmares, and a need for reorganization of thought process. It may occur months to years after the event and may involve major lifestyle adjustments.

Rape, incest, and other forms of physical and sexual abuse are very common. Physicians in general and obstetricians and gynecologists in particular are in a position to detect these problems and offer treatment and counsel when their patients have been found to be victims. In the acute state, a careful history using a compassionate and nonjudgmental approach will often allow an accurate story to be obtained. When the patient seeks medical advice at a time remote from the experience or when the experience is ongoing, the presenting chief complaint may have little to do with the actual problem. For the physician to elicit a clear picture, it is necessary to resort to open-ended questions and interviewing techniques that allow the patient to comfortably discuss truthfully the actual problem.

These patients are at risk for severe physical and emotional distress, and as victims they may suffer psychologic damage to their self-image, which in turn may lead to many long-term poor choices in important life situations. Although rape, incest, and abuse will be discussed separately, there is frequently a relationship in the social pathology involved, as well as in the long-term effects that the patient must endure. In each instance appropriate physician response and physician responsibility will be discussed.

RAPE

Rape, or the sexual assault of children, women, and men, is a common act. It is defined as any sexual act performed by one person on another without that person's consent. Only recently has it become apparent how common a problem this is. In 1987 the U.S. Department of Justice reported that for females the annual incidence of sexual assault was 73/100,000, accounting for 6% of all violent crimes. This type of crime, however, is often underreported, and the actual incidence may be much higher. Victims are often reluctant to report sexual assault to the authorities because of embarrassment, fear of retribution, feelings of guilt, or simply lack of knowledge of their rights. It has been estimated that as many as 44% of women have been victims of actual or attempted sexual assault at some time in their lives and as many as 50% of these on more than one occasion.

In the past, society has held many misconceptions about the rape victim, particularly a female. These included the notion that the individual encouraged the rape by specific behavior or dress and that no person who did not wish to be raped could be raped. Further, the feeling that rape was an indication of basic promiscuity was widely held. In many instances sexual assault victims were accused of lying to cause problems for otherwise innocent men. To some extent many of these societal misconceptions are held today.

Sexual assault happens to people of all ages and races in all socioeconomic groups. The very young, the mentally and physically handicapped, and the very old are particularly susceptible. Although the perpetrator may be a stranger, he or she is often an individual well known to the victim.

Some situations have been defined as variants of sexual assault. These include marital rape, which involves forced coitus or related acts without consent but within the marital relationship, and "date rape." In the latter situation the woman may voluntarily participate in sexual play, but coitus is performed, often forcibly, without her consent. Date rape is often not reported because the victim may believe she contributed by partially participating. This, however, can scar her self-esteem.

Almost all states have statutes that criminalize coitus with females under certain specified ages. Such an act is referred to as *statutory rape*. Consent is irrelevant because the female is defined by statute as being incapable of consenting.

In submitting, the victim loses control over his or her life for that period and frequently experiences anxiety and fear. When the attack is life threatening, shock with associated physical and psychologic symptoms may occur. Burgess and Holmstrom identify two phases of the rape-trauma syndrome.

The immediate or acute phase lasts from hours to days and may be associated with a paralysis of the individual's usual coping mechanisms. Outwardly, the victim may demonstrate manifestations ranging from complete loss of emotional control to a well-controlled behavior pattern. The actual reaction may depend on a number of factors, including the relationship of the victim to the attacker, whether force was used, and the length of time the victim was held against his or her will. Generally, the victim appears disorganized and may complain of both physical and emotional symptoms. Physical complaints include specific injuries or general complaints of soreness, eating problems, headaches, and sleep disturbances. Behavior patterns may include fear, mood swings, irritability, guilt, anger, depression, and difficulties in concentrating. Frequently the victim will complain of flashbacks to the attack. Medical care is often sought during the acute period, and at this point it is the physician's responsibility to assess the specific medical problems and also to offer a program of emotional support and reassurance.

The second phase of the rape-trauma syndrome involves long-term adjustment and is designated the reorganization phase. During this time flashbacks and nightmares may continue, but phobias may also develop. These may be directed against members of the opposite sex, the sex act itself, or nonrelated circumstances, such as a newly developed fear of crowds or heights. During this period the victim may institute a number of important lifestyle changes, including changes of job, residence, friends, and significant others. If major complications such as the contraction of a sexually transmitted disease or a pregnancy occur, resolution may be more difficult. The reorganization period may last from months to years and generally involves an attempt on the part of the victim to regain control over his or her life. During this time medical care and counseling must be nonjudgmental, sensitive, and anticipatory. When the physician realizes that the patient is contemplating a major lifestyle change during this period, it is probably appropriate to point out to the patient the reasons why the change is being contemplated and the complicating effects it may have on the patient's overall well-being.

Physician's Responsibility in the Care of a Rape Victim

Although any individual may become a rape victim, this discussion will be limited to the care of a female, as is appropriate for a gynecology textbook. The physician's responsibility may be divided into three categories: medical, medical-legal, and supportive, as shown in the box on the facing page.

Medical

The physician's medical responsibilities are to treat injuries and to perform appropriate tests for, to prevent, and to treat infections and pregnancies. It is important to obtain informed consent before examining the patient and

Physician's Responsibilities in Caring for Rape-Trauma Victim

Medical
    Treat injuries
    Diagnose and treat STD
    Prevent pregnancy
Medical-legal
    Document history carefully
    Examine patient thoroughly and specifically note injuries
    Collect articles of clothing
    Collect vaginal (rectal and pharyngeal) samples for sperm and acid phosphatase
    Comb pubic hair for hair samples
    Collect fingernail scrapings where appropriate
    Collect saliva for secretion substance
    Turn specimens over to forensic authorities and receive receipts for chart
Emotional support
    Discuss degree of injury, probability of infection, and possibility of pregnancy
    Discuss general course that can be predicted
    Consult with rape-trauma counselor
    Arrange follow-up visit for medical and emotional evaluation in 1 to 4 weeks
    Reassure as far as possible

collecting specimens. In addition to addressing legal requirements, it helps the victim to regain control over her body and her life.

After acute injuries have been determined and stabilized, a careful history and physical examination should be performed. It is important to have a chaperone present during the taking of the history and the performance of the examination and specimen collection to reassure the victim and to provide support. The presence of such a third party probably reduces feelings of vulnerability on the part of the victim. She should be asked to state in her own words what happened; if she knew the attacker, and if not, to describe the attacker; she should also be asked to describe the specific act(s) performed.

A history of previous gynecologic conditions, particularly infections and pregnancy, use of contraception, and the date of last menstrual period, should be recorded. It is necessary to determine whether the patient may have a preexisting pregnancy or be at risk for pregnancy. It is also important to ascertain whether she has had a preexisting pelvic infection.

Experience derived at the Sexual Assault Center in Seattle, Washington, demonstrated that between 12% and 40% of victims who are sexually assaulted have injuries. Most of these, however, are minor and require simple reparative therapy. Only about 1% require hospitalization and major operative repair. Nonetheless the victim will perceive the experience as having been life threatening, as in many cases it may have been. Many injuries occur when the victim is restrained or physically coerced into the sexual act.

Thus the physician should seek bruises, abrasions, or lacerations about the neck, back, buttocks, or extremities. Where a knife was used as a coercive tactic, small cuts may also be found. Erythema, lacerations, and edema of the vulva and/or rectum may occur because of manipulation of these areas with the hand or the penis. These are particularly common in children or virginal victims but may occur in any woman and should be sought. Superficial or extensive lacerations of the hymen and/or vagina may occur in virginal victims or in the elderly. Lacerations may also be noted in the area of the urethra, the rectum, and at times through the vaginal vault into the abdominal cavity. In addition, bite marks may be noted in any of these regions. Occasionally, foreign objects are inserted into the vagina, the urethra, or the rectum and may be found.

In recent years, some authorities have advised close inspection with a magnifying glass or colposcope of the vulva and vagina of infants and children suspected to be victims of rape. Muram and Elias, however, in a study of 130 prepubertal girls (mean age 5.5) identified as victims of sexual abuse, could identify evidence of trauma in 96% with unaided inspection. Four additional cases were identified by colposcopy, but the lesions were obvious on repeat unaided examination. Simple visual examination without the aid of a colposcope should be sufficient to detect signs of trauma in children.

Where oral penetration has been effected, injury of the mouth and pharynx should be sought.

INFECTION. Most victims are concerned about possible infections incurred as a result of the rape, but until recently no careful follow-up studies in victims had been performed. To determine actual risk it is important to know the prevalence of existing sexually transmitted diseases in the victim population. Recently, Jenny et al. examined 204 girls and women within 72 hours of a rape and discovered that 88 (43%) were harboring at least one STD. These included *Neisseria gonorrhoeae* in 13 of 204 (6% of all tested), cytomegalovirus in 13 of 170 (8%), *Chlamydia trachomatis* in 20 of 198 (10.1%), *Trichomonas vaginalis* in 30 of 204 (14.7%), herpes simplex virus in 4 of 170 (2.4%), *Treponema pallidum* in 2 of 199 (1.0%), HIV-I in 1 of 123 (0.8%), and bacterial vaginosis in 70 of 204 (34.3%). In 109 patients (53%) who returned for follow-up (excluding those who were found to be infected on the first visit or who were treated prophylactically), there were 3 of 71 (4%) cases of gonorrhea, 1 of 65 (0.02%) of chlamydia, 10 of 81 (12%) of trichomoniasis, and 15 of 77 (19%) of bacterial vaginosis. These authors concluded that women who were raped have a higher than average prevalence of preexisting STDs but are also at a substantial risk of acquiring such disease as a result of the assault.

Reynolds et al. recently presented a review on the risk of infection in rape victims that was the result of a MEDLINE search of the English language journals. They also noted that it was often difficult to separate new from existing infection, but placed the prevalence of STDs as follows:

N. gonorrhea 0–26.3%, *C. trachomatis* 3.9–17%, *T. pallidum* 0–5.6%, *T. vaginalis* 0–19%, and HPV 0.6–2.3%.

Few studies are available to predict the actual risk of acquiring an STD, but *Chlamydia trachomatis* may be the most commonly acquired infection incurred under these circumstances. Most victims fear acquiring human immunodeficiency virus (HIV) as a result of a sexual attack, but current risks are probably not high depending on the population involved and the sexual acts performed. Some studies place the risk for adult rape victims of acquiring syphilis as high as 3% to 10%. These authors did not believe the risk of acquiring STDs can be quantified, but they note that the acquisition of viral STDs, including HIV, has been reported both in adults and children.

It must be remembered that infection may not be limited to the vagina but may also include the pharynx or the rectum. Specific history to raise a suspicion of this possibility should be sought. Cultures should be performed for *Neisseria gonorrhoeae* and *Chlamydia trachomatis*. In addition, investigation for syphilis, using either dark-field studies and serology at the time the victim is seen and at a follow-up visit or serology alone, should be performed.

Because the victim is also at risk for infection by the herpes virus, hepatitis B virus, cytomegalovirus, HIV, condyloma acuminatum, and a variety of other sexually transmitted diseases, the physician may wish to screen for those that seem appropriate at the time the victim is seen in the acute stage.

Cultures of the cervical mucus for *Neisseria* gonococcus and for *Chlamydia trachomatis* are indicated. In addition, cultures of the rectum and of the oral pharynx are indicated when the history suggests that this would be productive. A wet mount for *Trichomonas vaginalis* and a potassium hydroxide mount for *Candida albicans* are also useful (see box below).

At follow-up visits the patient should again be investigated for signs and symptoms of the sexually transmitted diseases, and appropriate repeat cultures and serologies should be obtained.

Sexually Transmitted Diseases and Tests Available to Physicians Caring for a Rape-Trauma Victim

Should perform
   Gonorrhea—culture for *Neisseria gonorrhoeae*
   Chlamydia trachomatis—culture
   Syphilis—dark-field microscopy, serology
Could perform
   Herpes simplex—culture lesion or serology
   Hepatitis B—screening serology
   HIV—serology
   Cytomegalovirus—serology
   Condyloma virus—study lesion
   Trichomonas—saline preparation
   Candida—potassium hydroxide preparation

Prophylactic antibiotics are useful in acute rape victim management. The patient should be given a single dose of ceftriaxone 250 mg IM plus doxycycline 100 mg PO two times a day for 7 days. An alternative therapy is spectinomycin 2 g IM (single dose) followed by doxycycline. If the patient is pregnant, erythromycin may be substituted for doxycycline. This should prevent gonorrhea, syphilis, and *Chlamydia* infection but will have no effect on herpes, condylomata, or many of the other problems mentioned.

PREGNANCY. The patient's menstrual history, birth control regimen, and known pregnancy status should be assessed. If the patient is at risk for pregnancy at the time of the assault, an appropriate "morning after" prophylaxis can be offered. This is discussed more fully in Chapter 13. In the experience of most sexual assault centers the chance of pregnancy occurring is quite low. It has been estimated to be approximately 2% to 4% of victims having a single, unprotected coitus. However, if the patient has been exposed at midcycle, the risk will be higher.

Holmes et al. estimated the national rape-related pregnancy rate at 5.0% and stated that among adult women 32,101 pregnancies resulted from rape each year in the United States. Many of these pregnancies occurred in women who did not receive immediate medical attention.

Medical-Legal

To be meaningful, medical-legal material must be collected shortly after the assault takes place. Victims should be encouraged to come immediately to a center where they can be evaluated before bathing, urinating, defecating, washing out their mouths, changing clothes, or cleaning their fingernails. In general, evidence for coitus will be present in the vagina for as long as 48 hours after the attack, but in other orifices the evidence may last only up to 6 hours. Appropriate tests should document the patient's physical and emotional condition as judged by her history and physical examination and should include data that document that force was used, evidence for sexual contact, and materials that may help identify the offender. To document that force was used, the physician should carefully describe each injury noted and possibly illustrate with either drawings or photographs. Detail is important, because injuries suffered by sexual assault victims have common patterns. Since rape and sexual assault are legal terms, they should not be stated as diagnoses; rather the physician should report findings as "consistent with use of force."

Documentation of sexual contact must begin with a history of when the patient had intercourse before the attack. If sperm or semen is found in the vagina or cervix of a victim, it must not be confused with such substances deposited during the victim's prior consenting sexual acts. Sexual contact will be verified by analysis of secretions from the vagina or rectum, seeking motile sperm and the presence of acid phosphatase. Nonmotile sperm may be present as well if the attack occurred 12 to 20 hours previously. In some instances, motile sperm will be noted for as long as 2 to 3 days in the endocervix.

It is difficult to ascertain whether ejaculation occurred in the mouth, because residual seminal fluid is rapidly destroyed by bacteria and salivary enzymes, making documentation of such an event difficult after more than a few hours have passed. Seminal fluid may be found staining the skin or the clothing several hours after the attack, and this should be sought. Because acid phosphatase is an enzyme found in high concentrations in seminal fluid, substances removed for analysis should be tested for this enzyme. Table 9-1 demonstrates the survival time of sperm in the pharynx, rectum, and cervix.

In addition to documenting that intercourse has taken place, an attempt should be made to identify the perpetrator. In this regard, all clothing intimately associated with the area of assault should be collected, labeled, and submitted to legal authorities. In addition, smears of vaginal secretions or a Pap smear should be made to permanently document the presence of sperm. Vaginal secretions needed for acid phosphatase reaction and DNA typing should be collected by wet or dry swab and refrigerated until a pathologist can process them. Spot tests are available for identifying acid phosphatase and zinc in vaginal secretions or on clothing. In the near future tests may also be available to identify prostate specific antigen and seminal vesicle specific antigen in vaginal secretions. DNA fingerprinting is now readily available in all areas and is admissible in many jurisdictions. Pubic hair combings should be performed in an attempt to obtain pubic hair of the assaulter. Saliva should be collected from the victim to ascertain whether she secretes an antigen that could differentiate her from substances obtained from the perpetrator. Finally, fingernail scrapings should be obtained for skin or blood if the victim scratched the perpetrator. Specific blood or DNA typing may be conducted to help identify the attacker. All materials collected should be labeled and turned over to the legal authority or pathologist, depending on the system of the unit. A receipt should be obtained, and this should be documented in the patient's chart.

Emotional Support of the Victim

After the physical needs of the patient have been met and after the physician has carefully documented the information concerning the sexual contact, he or she should discuss with the victim the degree of injury, probability of infection or pregnancy, general course that the victim might be expected to follow with respect to these, and how follow-up to aid prevention will be carried out. The physician must allow the victim to give vent to anxieties and to correct misconceptions. The physician should reassure her, insofar as possible, that her well-being will be restored. In doing this the physician may call on other health personnel, such as individuals trained to handle rape-trauma victims, to facilitate counseling and follow-up. The patient should not be released until specific follow-up plans are made and the patient understands what they are. A follow-up visit should be planned within 1 to 4 weeks to reevaluate the patient's medical, infectious disease, pregnancy, and psychologic status. At this point, encouragement for continued follow-up counseling should be emphasized. It is important at each visit to emphasize to the patient *that she was a victim and holds no blame*. At each step she must be allowed to vent her feelings and to discuss her current conceptions of the problem.

It is important that the physician realize that some patients will appear to have excellent emotional control when seen immediately after a rape. This is an acute expression of the patient's defense mechanisms and should not be misinterpreted to indicate that the patient is coping with the circumstances. All the recommendations just listed should be followed *regardless* of the patient's apparent condition. Specific plans for follow-up are equally important in such an individual, because it must be anticipated that she will follow the same post-rape emotional process as anyone else.

Finally, it is important to emphasize and reemphasize that at no time during the management or follow-up care of the rape victim should any comments be made by health care professionals suggesting that the patient was anything other than a victim. These women are sensitive to any

TABLE 9-1
Survival Time of Sperm

Source	Motile Sperm	Sperm	Acid Phosphatase
Vagina	Up to 8 hr	Up to 7–9 days	Variable (Up to 48 hr)
Pharynx	6 hr	Unknown	100 IU*
Rectum	Undetermined	20 to 24 hr	100 IU*
Cervix	Up to 5 days	Up to 17 days	Similar to vagina

From Anderson S: Sexual assault—medical-legal aspects, an unpublished training packet for pediatric house staff, Harborview Medical Center, Seattle, Wash, 1980.
*Minimum detectable.

accusations and insinuations and may even believe that they may have in some way been responsible for the rape. Their future well-being may be severely affected by creating such an impression.

FEMALE GENITAL MUTILATION. A form of sexual abuse only recently observed in the Western world is female genital mutilation. It is a practice growing out of cultural and traditional beliefs dating back several thousand years. The World Health Organization estimates that between 85 and 200 million women undergo these procedures each year. Although they are often performed in parts of Africa, the Middle East, and Southeast Asia, they are rarely performed in the United States or the rest of the Western world. But about 168,000 women who have undergone such procedures currently live in the United States, and physicians may see the results of these procedures in patients who emigrate from countries where they are practiced.

The various forms of female genital mutilation include removal of the clitoral prepuce, excision of the clitoris, or removal of the clitoris and labia minora. Occasionally the labia majora is also partially removed and the vagina partially sutured closed. The procedures are often performed between early childhood and age 14 and frequently without anesthesia under unsterile conditions by untrained practitioners. Therefore a variety of complications often occur including infection, tetanus, shock, hemorrhage, and death. Long-term problems include chronic infection, scar formation, local abscesses, sterility, and incontinence. In addition, depression, anxiety, sexual dysfunction, obstetric complications, and the psychosomatic conditions associated with sexual abuse may be seen. Physicians who care for women with this condition must develop an understanding of the cultural mores that lead to the performance of the procedure and the current implications on these cultural beliefs that remedial surgery may imply. Certainly the patient and her significant other should be involved in all decisions concerning intervention.

INCEST

Incest must be placed within the context of child sexual abuse. The actual overall incidence of such abuse is difficult to estimate, although several authorities claim that about 10% of all child abuse cases involve sexual abuse. Sarafino estimates that roughly 336,000 children are sexually abused each year in the United States. Retrospective historical data derived from adults imply that incestual activity may be experienced in as many as 15% to 25% of all women and approximately 12% of all men. These figures seem appropriate for the population in general but vary from group to group, being higher in young prostitutes.

Sexual abuse of children may be divided into two types, the first in which the child is victimized by a stranger and the second in which a family member is the perpetrator. It has been estimated that about 80% of all sexual abuse cases of children involve a family member. Rimsza and Niggemann found that only 18% of 311 children and adolescents who were evaluated for sexual abuse were assaulted by strangers.

In the case of child sexual abuse involving a stranger, the act is usually a single episode and is usually reported to the authorities. The child is capable in most instances of clearly stating what happened, and the act may involve any form of sexual activity and may have taken place because of enticement, coercion, or physical force. In such instances the child should be interviewed carefully and allowed to tell what happened. The police or protective services should be notified, and, where appropriate, the techniques used in evaluating a rape victim should be applied. Appropriate prophylaxis against infection should be employed, and counseling should be arranged with a mental health care worker, who should see the child immediately and also take the responsibility for planning long-term follow-up. The molester should be apprehended, and if it is an individual living in the home, he or she should be made to leave. Most communities have sexual abuse crisis intervention centers, and these are appropriate in such circumstances.

In each case the child should be carefully told that *he or she was a victim of a wrongful act and that in no way was he or she to blame.* Statements that imply the child might in some way have enticed the perpetrator into performing the act are inappropriate and may lead to serious compromise in the development of the child's self-esteem in the future. The welfare of siblings must also be considered, and an effort to discover the siblings' status should be made.

About 80% of child sexual abuse involves a parent, guardian, other family member, or mother's significant other. Father-daughter incest accounts for about 75% of reported cases, with mother-son, father-son, mother-daughter, brother-sister, or incest involving another close family member comprising the remaining 25%. Brother-sister incest may be the commonest form but may not be reported often.

Different states define incest in different legal terms. In some, intercourse is required; in others, it is not. Incest is noted to occur in all social groups, including cultures in which it is a stated taboo.

Families in which incestual activity is taking place may appear normal, but family members frequently have limited contact with the outside world. Family relationships are often chaotic, including problems such as alcohol and drug abuse and severe mental illness. In father-daughter incestual relationships the father is frequently a passive, introspective person who experiences a weak sexual relationship with the mother. He may therefore turn his attentions to his daughter or daughters out of loneliness, and the sexual activity may be quite affectionate. Frequently the mother is aware of the situation, but both parents agree consciously or subconsciously that the incestuous relationship is more acceptable than an extramarital one. In such situations the daughter may assume more of the role of the wife around the house, fulfilling many homemaker duties.

Children who have been victimized by incest often feel guilty during adolescence. Many may be afraid to withdraw from the relationship out of fear that in so doing they would destroy the family and the security it provides. Such victims frequently feel humiliated and develop a weak ego and self-image. Because of this, these women may have difficulty in developing appropriate relationships with members of the opposite sex and may make poor choices in their interpersonal relationships in the future. They frequently choose chaotic family existences after they leave home. Fewer than 10% of children involved in incestuous relationships have normal psychologic development at the time of evaluation. Usually they exhibit guilt, anger, behavioral problems, unexplained physical complaints, lying, stealing, school failure, running away, and sleep disturbances.

Gynecologists may see such individuals as teenagers or young adults and may note that some or all of these complaints have been fully developed. When such a profile occurs, the gynecologist should seek a history of incest to fully understand the psychopathology of the patient. Appropriate questions such as, "Were you physically or sexually abused or raped as a child or adolescent?" should be asked as part of a routine history. Affirmative answers to any of these questions require specific detailed and discreet questioning of the individual involved and the circumstances of the incestuous act. The physician should assess the kinds of counseling the patient may already have experienced. Questioning should be nonjudgmental, clear, and specific. For example, the patient should be questioned about the sexual activity experienced and whether it included touching, genital manipulation, or intercourse. Often the individual is relieved to tell the health professional about her experience, because it may be something that she has never previously discussed. The knowledge that this is a common human experience and that the individual is blameless can be very helpful. The physician must then determine the necessity for an appropriate referral to a mental health worker.

Incest victims as adults frequently choose partners with inadequate personalities who may be capable of physical and sexual violence. This may be their unconscious desire to gravitate to a familiar relationship. It is equally possible that their poor social self-image may prevent them from achieving a stronger and more normal relationship.

Several studies have looked at the long-term follow-up of incest victims. Two separate studies in the 1970s by Lukianowicz and Meiselman found that daughters in father-daughter incestual relationships demonstrated difficulties in sexual adjustment, including promiscuity and homosexuality. In 28 cases, 11 girls became promiscuous, as well as delinquent, and 4 of these became prostitutes. Of the 11, 5 married and had problems with sexual arousal, and 4 demonstrated psychiatric symptoms of depression, anxiety, and suicidal ideology. Six, however, demonstrated no specific ill effects.

In another study by Browning and Boatman a gradual improvement in symptomatology occurred with time, regardless of whether treatment plans were followed. In specific instances of incestual relationships with uncles, however, there was great anxiety over the possibility of repeat incest when the uncles were left at large. In this same study violence was reported, including suicides in fathers and one murder of a mother by her son.

Earlier studies had suggested that the degree of emotional disturbance was greater the closer the relationship of the relative and that the degree was also related to whether genital contact actually took place. In a 1980 study of 796 college students Finkelhor reported that about one third of the incestual activity occurred only once but that in 27% the activity continued with varying frequency for more than a year. Of the involved individuals, 30% considered their experience positive, 30% negative, and the rest did not feel strongly one way or the other. In this series, women students who had sexual incestuous experiences as children were more likely to be sexually active. Experiences with siblings seemed to have a more positive effect on sexual development as long as the overall experience with the sibling was positive. Men who had sibling sexual experiences did not seem to have a higher current level of frequency of intercourse and seemed to have lower self-esteem. Thus it is difficult to predict what overall long-term potential problems may occur in victims of incestuous experiences.

Whatever the effect childhood sexual abuse and incest may have on the development of psychologic well-being and self-esteem in the victim, it is more and more clear that at least a subset of such victims develops physical complaints involving several organ systems including respiratory, gastrointestinal, musculoskeletal, and neurologic, as well as a variety of chronic pain syndromes. Therefore, physicians who have patients with such chronic problems should consider childhood sexual abuse and incest as a possible contributor and should offer counseling where appropriate as part of the treatment program.

ABUSE

The Battered Woman

Domestic violence, partner abuse, and *spouse abuse* are terms referring to violence occurring between partners in an ongoing relationship even if they are not married. A battered woman is defined as any woman over the age of 16 with evidence of physical abuse on at least one occasion at the hands of an intimate male partner. The battered wife syndrome is defined as a symptom complex occurring as a result of violence in which a woman has at any time received deliberate, severe, or repeated (more than three times) physical abuse from her husband or significant male partner in which the minimal injury is bruising. The actual physical abuse may vary from minimal activity, such as verbal abuse or threat of violence, to throwing an object, throwing an object at someone, pushing, slapping, kicking, hitting, beating, threatening with a weapon, or using a weapon. These acts may be spontaneous or intentionally planned. Most such violence is accompanied by mental abuse and intimidation. Partner abuse is often seen in conjunction with abuse of children and elderly persons in the same household.

It is difficult to ascertain the specific incidence of domestic violence, but it has been estimated that 2 million cases of domestic violence occur in the United States each year, and some authors have stated that at least 50% of family relationships are violent. In a 1984 U.S. Department of Justice study, 57% of 450,000 annual acts of family violence were committed by spouses or ex-spouses, and the wife was a victim in 93% of cases. In at least one fourth of these cases the violent acts had occurred at least three times in the previous 6 months. In 1990 FBI statistics reported similar findings. In addition, it has been estimated that between one third and one half of female homicide victims are murdered by their male partners, whereas only 12% of male homicide victims are killed by their female partners. In 1992 the AMA published guidelines for diagnosis and treatment of domestic violence. They noted that 47% of husbands who beat their wives do so three or more times per year, that 14% of ever-married women reported being raped by their current or former husbands, and that rape is a significant or major form of abuse in 54% of violent marriages. The AMA guidelines also summarized various studies noting that battered women may account for 22% to 35% of women seeking care for any reason in emergency departments (the majority of whom are seen by medical or nontrauma services) and 19% to 30% of injured women seen in emergency departments. They also noted that 14% of women seen in ambulatory care internal medicine clinics have been battered and 28% of such women have been battered at some time. They state that 25% of women who attempt suicide, 25% receiving psychiatric services, and 23% of pregnant women seeking prenatal care have been victims of domestic violence. In addition, 45% to 59% of mothers of abused children have been abused and 58% of women over the age of 30 who have been raped have been abused. Therefore it can be seen that domestic violence and battered women are common in our society today.

The most common sites for injury are the head, neck, chest, abdomen, breast, and upper extremities. The upper extremities may be fractured as the woman attempts to defend herself. In a study from Yale, 84% of the injuries were severe enough to require medical treatment, and in 81% of the cases patients stated that the assailant had beaten them with the fists. In an English study of 100 women brought to a hostel for battered women, 44% suffered from lacerations and 59% stated that they had been kicked repeatedly. All women stated that they had been hit with a clenched fist. Fractures occurred in 32, and 9 of the women had been beaten and taken to the hostel unconscious. Other studies have demonstrated similar findings.

Murder and suicide are frequent components of the domestic violence problem. In a large study from Denver, Walker reported that three quarters of the battered patients felt that the batterer would kill them during the relationship, and almost half felt that they might kill the batterer. Of these victims, 11% stated that they had actually tried to kill the batterer, and 87% believed that they themselves would be the ones to die if someone were killed. One third of these women stated that they seriously considered committing suicide. Walker noted that victims and their attackers frequently are depressed and may move rapidly between suicidal and homicidal intent.

There is a strong relationship between spouse battering and child abuse. In Walker's study, 53% of men who abused their partners were noted also to abuse their children. Another one third had threatened to abuse their children. Interestingly, in the same relationship, 28% of the wives who themselves were abused stated that they had abused their children while living in the violent household, and an additional 6% thought they might abuse their children at the time they were evaluated.

Physical abuse in pregnancy is quite common and may be referred to as prenatal child abuse. The incidence is somewhere between 3% and 8% depending on the study population. In one study, 81 of 742 (10.9%) patients visiting a prenatal clinic stated that they had been victims of abuse at some time in the past, and 29 of these women stated that the abuse had continued into the pregnancy. One fifth of these noted an increase in abuse during pregnancy while one third noted a decrease. Campbell et al., in a study of a group of Medicaid-eligible postpartum women, noted a constellation of factors associated with violence during pregnancy. Of the patients in this study, 7% suffered battering, and significant correlates including anxiety, depression, housing problems, inadequate prenatal care, and drug and alcohol abuse were identified. The women in the study who were battered during pregnancy suffered a more severe constellation of symptoms than did those who were battered only prior to pregnancy. In the case of pregnant patients, most studies note that battering is frequently directed to the breasts and abdomen.

It is important that physicians increase their ability to recognize the signs of domestic violence and spouse abuse. A study by Hilberman and Monson demonstrated that 25% of women treated for injuries in an emergency room were victims of wife battering. The physicians who were treating these patients made the correct diagnosis originally in only 3% of cases. Viken has listed a profile of the characteristics of the abused wife. These include a history of having been beaten as a child, raised in a single-parent home, married as a teenager, and pregnant before marriage. Such women frequently visit clinics and emergency rooms with a variety of somatic complaints, including headaches, insomnia, choking sensation, hyperventilation, gastrointestinal symptoms, and chest, pelvic, and back pain. Noncompliance with the advice of physicians with respect to these complaints is frequent. (See the box below.)

In visits to the physician's office or emergency room the patient often appears shy, frightened, embarrassed, evasive, anxious, or passive and often cries. The batterer may accompany the patient on such visits and stay close at hand to monitor what is said to the physician. Thus the woman may be hesitant to provide information about how she was injured, and the explanation given may not fit the injuries observed. Alcohol or other drug abuse is common in such individuals.

Physicians should become comfortable in asking the patient whether she has been physically abused. Questions such as, "Has anyone hurt you or tried to injure you?" and "Have you ever been physically abused either recently or in the past?" are very appropriate introductory questions. The physician should follow up on any positive answers in a nonjudgmental manner in an attempt to learn what is happening. Physical examinations should be complete with particular attention to bruises, lacerations, burns, and other signs of injury. If the patient is wearing sunglasses, she should be asked to remove them so the physician can determine whether there are eye injuries. If the patient is pregnant, bruises seen on the breasts or abdomen should always be dis-

cussed. Physicians should carefully note evidence for abuse in their patient record.

Battering acts tend to run in cycles consisting of three phases. The first phase is tension building, in which there is a gradual escalation of tension between the couple manifested by discrete acts that cause family friction. Name calling, intimidating remarks, meanness, and mild physical abuse such as pushing are common. Dissatisfaction and hostility are often expressed by the batterer in a somewhat chronic form. The victim may attempt to placate the batterer in hopes of pleasing him or calming him. She may actually believe at this point that she has the power to avoid aggravating the situation. She may not respond to his hostile actions and may even be successful from time to time in apparently reducing tensions. This, of course, will reinforce her belief that she can control the situation. As the tension phase builds, the batterer's anger is less controlled, and the victim may withdraw, fearing that she will inadvertently set off explosive behavior.

Often this withdrawal is the signal for the batterer to become more aggressive. Anything may spark the hostile act, and the acute battering then takes place. This is the cycle's second phase and is represented by an uncontrollable discharge of tension that has built up through the first phase. The attack may take the form of both verbal and physical abuse, and the victim is often left injured. In self-defense the victim may actually injure or kill the batterer. In approximately two thirds of cases reported by Walker, alcohol abuse was involved. However, the alcohol use may have been the excuse rather than the reason for the battering.

After the abuse has taken place, the third phase generally follows. In this situation, the batterer apologizes, asks forgiveness, and frequently shows kindness and remorse, showering the victim with gifts and promises. This gives the victim hope that the relationship can be saved and that the violence will not recur. Batterers are often charming and manipulative, offering the victim justification for forgiveness.

The cycles, however, do repeat themselves, with the first phase increasing in length and intensity, the battering becoming more severe, and the third phase tending to decrease in both duration and intensity. The batterer learns that he can control the victim without obtaining much forgiveness. The victim becomes more demoralized and loses her ability to leave the situation even if she has the means and opportunity to do so.

Batterers, too, tend to have a specific profile in most cases. They are men who refuse to take responsibility for their behavior, blaming their victims for their violent acts. They often have strong controlling personalities and do not tolerate autonomy in their partners. They have rigid expectations of marriage and sexual behavior and consider their wives or partners as chattel. They wish to be cared for in their most basic needs, frequently make

---

Somatic Complaints in Abused Women

Headaches
Insomnia
Choking sensation
Hyperventilation
Chest, back, or pelvic pain
Other signs and symptoms
    Shyness
    Fright
    Embarrassment
    Evasiveness
    Jumpiness
    Passivity
    Frequent crying
    Often accompanied by male partner
    Drug or alcohol abuse (often overdose)
    Injuries

From ACOG Technical Bulletin Number 124: The battered woman, Jan, 1989.

unrealistic demands on their wives, and show low tolerance for stress. Depression and suicidal gestures are often a part of their behavior pattern, but in general they are aggressive and assaultive in most of their behavior, generally using violence to solve their problems. On the other hand, they are often charming and manipulative, especially in their relationships outside the marriage. They often exhibit low self-esteem, feelings of inadequacy, and a sense of helplessness, all of which are generally made worse by the prospects of losing their wives. It is typical behavior for male batterers to exhibit contempt for women in their usual activities. Therapy is usually ineffective and seems to work only when the man can be made to give up violence as his primary means of solving problems.

Once the physician discovers that a woman is living in an abusive relationship, it is important to acknowledge to the patient the seriousness of the situation. To do otherwise is to give the impression that the physician approves or at least accepts the violent condition. It is important to attend to the patient's injuries and to assess the patient's emotional status from the standpoint of a psychiatric condition such as a suicidal tendency, depression, anxiety reaction, or signs of abuse of drugs, alcohol, or other medications. The physician should also attempt to estimate the woman's ability to assess her own situation and her readiness to take appropriate action. If problems involving mental illness are present, a referral to an appropriate mental health worker who is sensitive to the issues of domestic violence should be made.

Physicians should determine community resources available for handling family violence. The acute situation can be helped by the police department, crisis hotline, rape relief centers, domestic violence programs, and legal aid services for abused women. Hospital emergency rooms and shelters for battered women and children are also excellent resources. Counseling and follow-up care can be offered by health care workers in these organizations or by private practitioners who specialize in the care of battered women, their spouses, and their children. Such individuals may be social workers, psychologists, psychiatrists, or other mental health workers trained specifically for this purpose. Many community hospitals, mental health departments, and community mental health services have set up counseling programs for such couples, since the problem is so common. The physician's job is to recognize the problem and either offer counseling or get counseling for the patient so that she understands her rights and alternatives and learns to protect herself and her children from future harm.

The victim of abuse very likely will not wish to leave her home because of economic concerns and a fear that the batterer may continue to pursue her. Although she may have the batterer arrested and served with restraining orders, she may be convinced that she and her children cannot be protected from the batterer. She may also believe that there is a possibility of reconciliation and of change in behavior on the part of the batterer. It is therefore reasonable to discuss an exit plan with the victim to be used should the violence recur. This exit plan should include the following:

1. Have a change of clothes packed for both her and her children including toilet articles, necessary medications, and an extra set of keys to the house and car. These can be placed in a suitcase and left with a friend or family member.
2. Keep some cash, a checkbook, and a savings account book with the friend or family member.
3. Other identification papers, such as birth certificates, Social Security cards, voter registration cards, utility bills, and driver's license, should be kept available, since children will need to be enrolled in school, and financial assistance may have to be sought.
4. Have something special, such as a toy or book, for each child.
5. Have financial records available, such as mortgage papers, rent receipts, and an automobile title.
6. Determine a plan on exactly where to go regardless of the time of day or night. This may be to a friend or relative's house or to a shelter for battered women and children.

Rehearsing an exit plan as one would conduct a fire drill makes it possible for the battered woman to respond even under the stress of the battering.

Long-term aid and referral of the patient, her children, and the batterer to the appropriate resource individuals is an important aspect of the care of such patients. The American College of Obstetricians and Gynecologists has prepared a patient education brochure that physicians can keep in their offices and give to individuals who suffer from this problem. Making the brochures available in the office waiting room may encourage women with these needs to get help.

These women often suffer from severe psychiatric problems, such as anxiety, depression, and other pathologic conditions, that may require psychotherapy. Group counseling or individual counseling may also help them to rebuild their lives as single individuals or single parents. It is frequently necessary to help them develop a skill that will enable them to be employable. Counseling programs take these things into consideration. Children of victims who may be victims as well also require counseling to avoid behavior patterns that will lead to aggressive behavior in their later lives.

Wife battering is a common problem that affects the family unit in particular and society in general. It can occur in all segments of society and reflects the violence that is a part of life today and the behavior of many. Physicians should learn to detect its presence in their patients and offer ways the victim can seek help. The help may include counseling for the victim, batterer, and children or constructing a plan for the woman to exit the relationship and rebuild her life in safety.

If the male batterer has not undergone violence elimination counseling, family counseling or intervention can be extremely dangerous as it often raises issues that exacerbate the violence and increase the risk of serious harm to the woman and her children. Therefore, this should not be advised until such time as the male batterer has addressed and eliminated his violent behavior. In general, success in such attempts with respect to the male partner is usually minimal.

Although all states have requirements for reporting child abuse, not all states require the reporting of domestic violence. However, many states have aggressive programs for intervening in domestic violence cases, and physicians should become aware of the programs in effect in their area. The patient should always be encouraged to leave a violent situation and may need community resources to help with economic and social adjustment, as well as protection for herself and her children from the violent partner.

The Elderly

The Select Committee on Aging in investigating domestic violence against the elderly held hearings before the Subcommittee of Human Services of the House of Representatives in 1980. The committee noted that approximately 500,000 to 2.5 million cases involving abuse of the elderly occur per year in the United States. The committee documented that abuse of the elderly may be as large a nationwide problem as child abuse. Usually the abused person is a woman past the age of 75, often with a physical impairment. She is generally white, widowed, and living with relatives. The abuser is generally an adult child living within the family but may also be a spouse. Counseling issues involve the entire family but particularly the individual causing the abuse. Physicians who care for geriatric patients should be alert for signs and symptoms of this type of domestic abuse; when it is found, community resources should be activated. All 50 states have passed legislation protecting the elderly from domestic violence and neglect. Forty-two states have mandatory reporting laws.

KEY POINTS

- The incidence of sexual abuse of women in the United States was estimated to be 73/100,000, accounting for 6% of all violent crimes.

- Sexual assault happens to people of all ages, races, and socioeconomic groups, but the very young, the mentally and physically handicapped, and the very old are particularly susceptible.

- Two phases of the rape-trauma syndrome occur. The first is the immediate or acute phase and lasts hours to days. The second, the reorganization stage, lasts months to years.

- In caring for rape-trauma victims, the physician's responsibilities are medical, medical-legal, and supportive.

- From 12% to 40% of victims who are sexually assaulted have injuries.

- Rape-trauma victims should always be treated as victims. At no time should guilt be implied.

- About 10% of all child abuse cases involve sexual abuse.

- As many as half a million children are sexually abused each year in the United States.

- Incestuous activity may be experienced by as many as 15% to 25% of all women and approximately 12% of all men.

- Approximately 80% of all cases of sexual abuse of children involve a family member.

- Father-daughter incest accounts for about 75% of reported cases; however, brother-sister incest may be the commonest type, although it may not be reported often.

- As many as 25% of women treated for injuries in an emergency room are likely to be victims of wife battering. Diagnosis of this by a physician is rare.

- An estimated 2 million cases of domestic violence are reported in the United States each year.

- In 93% of the cases, the wife is the victim of the violence.

- More than half of the men who abuse their partners also abuse their children.

- About 10% of antepartum clinic patients may be victims of battering.

- Victims of battering demonstrate multiple somatic complaints.

- Two thirds of batterers who carry out violent acts are under the influence of alcohol, but this may be the excuse rather than the reason.

- If the male batterer has not undergone a violence elimination program, a referral of the family for family counseling should *not* be made because it may raise issues that exacerbate the violence.

- Between 500,000 and 2.5 million cases of abuse of the elderly reportedly occur in the United States each year.

BIBLIOGRAPHY

American College of Obstetricians and Gynecologists: Domestic violence (Technical Bulletin Number 209), Washington, DC, ACOG, 1995.

American College of Obstetricians and Gynecologists: The Abused Woman (ACOG Patient Education Pamphlet APO83), Washington, DC, ACOG, 1989.

American College of Obstetricians and Gynecologists: Sexual Assault (Technical Bulletin Number 172), Washington, DC, ACOG, 1992.

American College of Obstetricians and Gynecologists: Female Genital Mutilation (Committee Opinion Number 151), Washington, DC, ACOG, 1995.

Bachmann GA, Moeller TP, and Bennett J: Childhood sexual abuse and the consequences in adult women, Obstet Gynecol 71:631, 1988.

Barker B: Suicide by patient: criminal charge against physician, JAMA 238(4):305, 1977.

Batten DA: Incest: a review of the literature, Med Sci Law 23:245, 1983.

Behrman S: Hostility to kith and kin, Br Med J 2(5970):538, 1975.

Benward J and Densen-Gerber J: Incest as a causative factor in antisocial behavior: an exploratory study, Contemp Drug Probl 4:322, 1975.

Bowie SI, Silverman DC, Kalick SM, and Edbril SD: Blitz rape and confidence rape: implications for clinical intervention, Am J Psychother 44:180, 1990.

Browning DH and Boatman B: Incest: children at risk, Am J Psychiatry 134:69, 1977.

Burgess AW and Holmstrom LL: Rape: victims of crisis, Bowie, Md, 1974, RJ Brady Co.

Campbell JC, Poland ML, Waller JB, and Ager J: Correlates of battering during pregnancy, R Nurs Health 15:219, 1992.

Chez RA: Elder abuse, the continuum of family violence. Prim Care Update OB/GYN 6:132, 1999.

Council Reports. Violence against women: relevance for medical practitioners, Council on Scientific Affairs, American Medical Association, JAMA 267:3184, 1992.

Davis LD: Beliefs of service providers about abused women and abusing men, Soc Work 29:2, 1984.

Ehrlich P and Anetzberger G: Survey of state public health departments on procedures for reporting elder abuse, Public Health Rep 106:151, 1991.

Elbow M: Theoretical considerations of violent marriages, Soc Casework 58(9):515, 1977.

Elchalal V, Ben-Aut B, Gillis R, and Brzenzinski A: Ritualistic female genital mutilation: current status and future outlook. Obstet Gynecol Surv 92:643, 1997.

Female genital mutilation: A report of the WHO Technical Working Group, Geneva, 1995.

Finkelhor D: Sex among siblings, Arch Sex Behav 9:195, 1981.

Flitcraft AH, Hadley SM, Hendricks-Matthews MK, et al: Diagnostic and treatment guidelines on domestic violence, JAMA, 1992.

Flugel J: Psychoanalytic study of the family, London, 1926, The Hogarth Press.

Frazer M: Domestic violence: a medicolegal review, J Forensic Sci 31(4):1409, 1986.

Galleno H and Oppenheim W: The battered child syndrome revisited, Clin Orthop Rel Res 162:11, 1982.

Gayford JJ: Battered wives: research on battered wives, R Soc Health J 95(6):288, 1975.

Gelles RJ: Violence in the family: a review of research in the seventies, J Marriage Fam 42(4):873, 1980.

Gelles RJ and Cornel CP, eds: International perspectives on family violence, Lexington, Mass, 1983, DC Heath & Co.

Gentry CE: Incestuous abuse of children: the need for an objective view, Child Welfare 58:355, 1978.

Giordano NH and Giordano JA: Elder abuse: a review of the literature, Soc Work 29:232, 1984.

Goldberg WG and Tomlanovich MC: Domestic violence, victims and emergency departments: new findings, JAMA 251(24):3259, 1984.

Helton A: Battering during pregnancy, Am J Nurs 86(8):910, 1986.

Hilberman E: Overview: the "wife-beater's wife" reconsidered, Am J Psychiatry 137(11):1336, 1980.

Hilberman E and Monson K: Sixty battered women, Victimology 2:460, 1977.

Hillard PJ: Physical abuse in pregnancy, Obstet Gynecol 66(2):185, 1985.

Holmes MM, Resnick HS, Kilpatrick DG, and Best CL: Rape-related pregnancy: estimates and descriptive characteristics from a national sample of women. Am J Obstet Gynecol 175:320, 1996.

Jenny C, Hooton TM, Bowers A, et al: Sexually transmitted diseases in victims of rape, N Engl J Med 322:713, 1990.

Jones JG: Sexual abuse of children, Am J Dis Child 136:142, 1982.

Kahn M and Sexton M: Sexual abuse of young children, Clin Pediatr 22:369, 1983.

Kaplan HS: The evaluation of sexual disorders, New York, 1983, Brunner/Mazel, Inc.

Kempe CH: Sexual abuse: another hidden pediatric problem, The 1977 C Anderson Aldrich lecture, Pediatrics 62:382, 1978.

Kerns DL: Child abuse and neglect: the pediatrician's role, J Contin Educ Pediatr 21:11, 1979.

Klaus PA and Rand MR: Family violence. Washington, DC, US Department of Justice, Bureau of Justice Statistics, 1984.

Lechner ME, Vogel ME, Garcia-Shelton LM, et al: Self-reported medical problems of adult female survivors of childhood sexual abuse, J Fam Pract 36:633, 1993.

Lukianowicz N: Incest. I. Paternal. II. Other types, Br J Psychiatry 120:301, 1972.

Meiselman KC: Incest: a psychological study of cases and effects with treatment recommendations, London, 1978, Jossey-Bass, Inc Publishers.

Morgan SM: Conjugal terrorism: a psychological and community treatment model of wife abuse, Palo Alto, Calif, 1982, R&E Research Associates, Inc.

Muram D and Elias S: Child sexual abuse: genital tract findings in prepubertal girls. II. Comparison of colposcopic and unaided examinations, Am J Obstet Gynecol 160:333, 1989.

Nadelson CC, Notman MT, Zackson H, et al: Follow-up study of rape victims, Am J Psychiatry 139:1267, 1982.

Nakashima II and Zakus GE: Incest: review and clinical experience, Pediatrics 60:696, 1977.

Parker B and Schumacher DN: The battered wife syndrome and violence in the nuclear family of origin: a controlled pilot study, Am J Public Health 67(8):760, 1977.

Pedrick-Cornell C and Gelles RJ: Elderly abuse: the status of current knowledge, Fam Rela 31:457, 1982.

Pillemer K and Suitor JJ: Violence and violent feelings: what causes them among family caregivers?, J Gerontol 47:S165, 1992.

Reynolds MW, Peipert JF, and Collins B: Epidemiologic issues of sexually transmitted diseases in sexual assault victims. Obstet Gynecol Surv 55:51, 2000.

Richwald GA and McCluskey TC: Family violence during pregnancy, Adv Int Matern Child Health 5:87, 1985.

Rimsza ME and Niggemann EH: Medical evaluation of sexually abused children: a review of 311 cases, Pediatrics 69:8, 1982.

Rounsaville B and Weissman MM: Battered woman: a medical problem requiring detection, Int J Psychiatry Med 8(2):191, 1977-1978.

Russell D: The prevalence and incidence of forcible rape and attempted rape offenders, Victimology 7:81, 1982.

Sarafino EP: An estimate of nationwide incidence of sexual offenses against children, Child Welfare 58:127, 1979.

Sarles RM: Incest, Pediatrics 2:51, 1980.

Scarinci IC, McDonald-Haile J, Bradley LA, and Richter JE: Altered pain perception and psychosocial features among women with gastrointestinal disorders and history of abuse: a preliminary model, Am J Med 97:108, 1994.

Schwarcz SK and Whittington WL: Sexual assault and sexually transmitted diseases: detection and management in adults and children, Rev Infect Dis 12:S682, 1990.

Select Committee on Aging: Domestic violence against the elderly, Hearings before the Subcommittee of Human Services, House of Representatives, April 21, 1980, Washington, DC, 1980, US Government Printing Office.

Sgroi SM: Sexual molestation of children: the last frontier of child abuse, Child Today 4:18, 1975.

Star B: Patterns of family violence, Social Casework 60:339, 1980.

Steinman G: Rapid spot tests for identifying suspected semen specimens, Forensic Sci Interv 72:191, 1995.

US Department of Health and Human Services; Public Health Service; Health Resources and Services Administration: Surgeon General's Workshop on Violence and Public Health: Report. DHHS Publication No HRS-D-MC 86-1. Washington, DC, 1986, US Government Printing Office.

US Department of Justice: Uniform crime reports for the United States, 1987, Publication No. 14, Washington, DC, 1987, US Government Printing Office.

Viken RM: Family violence: aids to recognition, Postgrad Med 71(5):115, 1982.

Walker LE: The battered woman syndrome, New York, 1984, Springer Publishing Co, Inc.

CHAPTER

10

Diagnostic Procedures

Imaging, Endometrial Sampling, Endoscopy: Indications and Contraindications, Complications

KEY TERMS AND DEFINITIONS

Adhesiolysis. The cutting or lysis of adhesions.

Computed Tomography (CT). An imaging technique to detect soft tissue abnormalities that uses a computer to integrate differences in x-ray beam attenuation resulting from varying densities in adjacent tissue.

Endometrial Sampling. Obtaining a tissue biopsy of the endometrial lining by abrasion and by placing an instrument transcervically into the endometrial cavity.

Endometrial Stripe. A sonographic measurement of the endometrial thickness that correlates with endometrial pathology.

Falloposcopy. Visualization of the lumen of the fallopian tubes usually transcervically with a microendoscope.

Gadolinium. A rare element used as a contrast agent for MR scans because of its magnetically opaque nature.

Hysterosalpingography. An x-ray imaging technique whereby the uterine cavity and lumina of the fallopian tubes are visualized by injecting contrast material through the cervical canal.

Hysteroscopy. The direct visualization of the endometrial cavity using an endoscope, a light source, and a medium to distend the uterus.

Laparoscopy. Examination and inspection of the peritoneal cavity and pelvic organs by means of an endoscope and a light source.

Magnetic Resonance Imaging (MR). An imaging technique using the resonance of hydrogen nuclei within tissue in a static magnetic field exposed to low-frequency radio waves.

Sonohysterography. A technique for ultrasonographic imaging of the uterine cavity by instilling saline transcervically through a small catheter.

Tubal Ring. A circular, clear-appearing ultrasound finding within the area of the adnexa, representing an early ectopic pregnancy.

Ultrasound. A noninvasive imaging technique using acoustic waves; modern equipment includes linear array and sector scan, endovaginal probes, and Doppler.

This chapter will present an overview of frequently used diagnostic procedures in gynecology. Indications, contraindications, and complications are included for each procedure. For those unfamiliar with the procedures, the diagnostic uses are described. Therapeutic uses are introduced, but details of these aspects of these techniques are covered elsewhere. During the past 4 decades there have been significant changes in the use of endoscopy in gynecologic practice. The fiberoptic bundle and more versatile light sources, as well as the incorporation of advances in technology, have dramatically increased the diagnostic and therapeutic capabilities of the hysteroscope and laparoscope. Colposcopy is discussed in Chapter 29. The use of computer technology has enhanced the ability of ultrasound and MR to allow dramatic advances in imaging.

There are two directly conflicting trends in present medical care. One is the increasing use of noninvasive diagnostic imaging. For example, the applications of magnetic resonance imaging appear limitless. The conflicting trend stems from society's emphasis on cost containment, which curtails the impetus for ordering imaging procedures. As we face the future, expense is one of the foremost issues for the consumer and physician alike. The best use of limited resources should be our goal. Most diagnostic techniques have overlapping applications. Thus the physician must choose the most appropriate technique for each patient. For example, it may be rare to order an MR for staging for endometrial cancer, but in a poor surgical candidate, it is the best technique to evaluate myometrial invasion. When evaluating patients, the physician should try not to order "cafeteria style," one ultrasound, one CT, and then an MR, but rather try to order the best test for the situation.

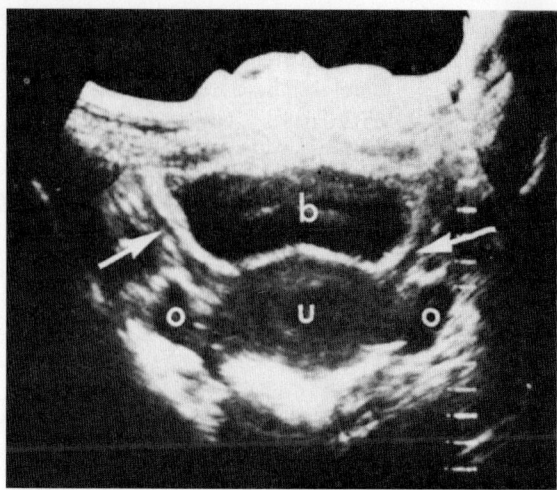

FIGURE 10-1 Normal pelvis on transverse abdominal ultrasonic scan demonstrating uterus (u) lying behind bladder (b). Both ovaries (o) are seen in angle between bladder and pelvic side wall. Round ligaments (arrows) are defined. (From Morley P and Barnett E: The ovarian mass. In Sanders RC and James AE Jr, eds: The principles and practice of ultrasonography in obstetrics and gynecology, ed 2, New York, 1980, Appleton-Century-Crofts.)

ULTRASOUND

Ultrasound, or sonography, is a noninvasive imaging technique utilizing acoustic waves similar to sonar. Endovaginal ultrasound transducers fitted on endovaginal probes are the primary means of gynecologic imaging. The vaginal probes are placed in a sterile sheath, usually a glove or condom, prior to an examination. During the examination the woman is in a dorsal lithotomy position and has an empty bladder. Because the transducer is closer to the pelvic organs than when a transabdominal approach is employed, endovaginal resolution is usually superior. However, if the pelvic structures to be studied have expanded and extend into the patient's abdomen, the organs are difficult to visualize with an endovaginal probe. Most ultrasound machines are equipped with both types of transducers.

For transabdominal gynecologic examinations, a sector scanner is preferable. It provides greater resolution of the pelvis and an easier examination than the linear array. During abdominal pelvic ultrasound examination, it is helpful for the patient to have a full bladder. This serves as an acoustic window for the high-frequency sound waves (Figures 10-1 and 10-2). Ultrasound is approximately 90% accurate in recognizing the presence of a pelvic mass, but does not establish a tissue diagnosis.

Ultrasonography employs an acoustic pulse echo technique. The transducer of the ultrasound machine is made up of piezoelectric crystals that vibrate and emit acoustic pulses. Acoustic echoes return from the tissues being scanned and cause the crystals to vibrate again and release an electric charge. These electric charges are then integrated by a computer within the ultrasound machine to form the image. Present equipment provides resolution of less than 0.5 mm.

Doppler ultrasound techniques assess the frequency of returning echoes to determine the velocity of moving structures. Measurement of diastolic and systolic velocities provide indirect indices of vascular resistance. Muscular arteries have high resistance. Newly developed vessels, such as those arising in malignancies, have little vascular wall musculature and thus have low resistance. Many ultrasound signals per second may be evaluated allowing direct measurement of blood flow. For example, this technique provides a noninvasive method of diagnosing deep vein thrombophlebitis of the legs.

A disadvantage of ultrasound is its poor penetration of bone and air; thus the pubic symphysis and air-filled intestines and rectum often inhibit visualization. Advantages of ultrasound include the real time nature of the image, the absence of radiation, the ability to perform the procedure in the office during or immediately after a pelvic examination, and the ability to describe the findings to the patient while she is watching. One of the most reassuring aspects of sonography is the absence of adverse clinical effects from the energy levels used in diagnostic studies.

The usefulness of ultrasound in gynecology depends largely on the pathologic conditions involved. Ultrasound-directed oocyte retrieval for in vitro fertilization is valuable because it allows for local anesthesia compared with retrieval by laparoscopy, which carries greater operative and anesthetic risks (Figure 10-3). Ultrasound cannot differentiate a benign from a malignant process. However, there are several characteristics of ovarian masses that correlate with malignancy, including septations; internal papillations—echogenic structures protruding into the mass; loculations; solid lesions, or cystic lesions with solid

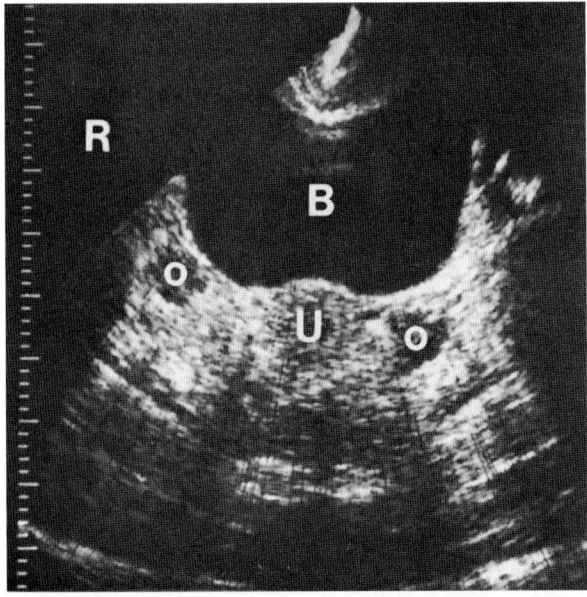

A

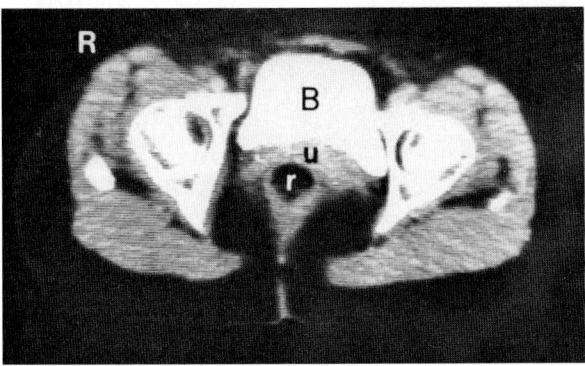

B

FIGURE 10-2 **A,** Transverse abdominal sonogram, and **B,** CT scan of normal female pelvis. In sonogram, normal ovaries (*o*) and uterus (*U*) are seen posterior to bladder. On CT scan gas is seen in the rectum (*r*) posterior to the uterus; ovaries are not imaged (*R,* right; *B,* bladder). (From Sommer FG, Walsh JW, Schwartz PE, et al: J Reprod Med 27:47, 1982.)

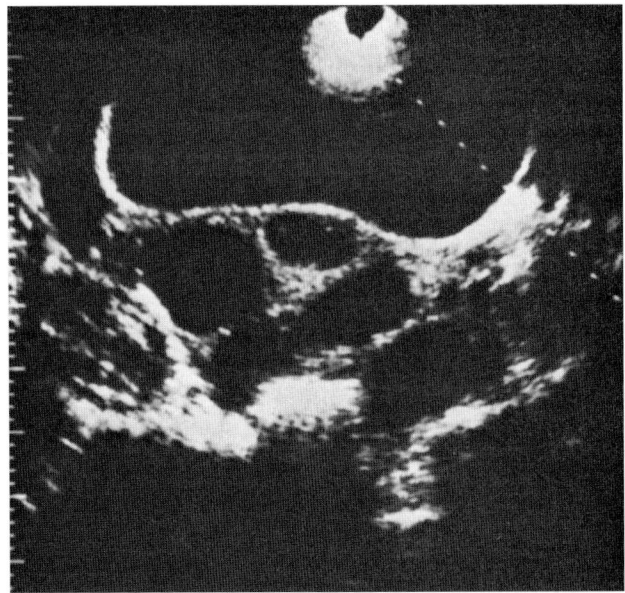

FIGURE 10-3 Transverse abdominal sonogram demonstrating multiple ovarian cysts in Pergonal-induced ovulation. (From DeCherney AH, Romero R, and Polan ML: Ultrasound in reproductive endocrinology, Fertil Steril 37:323, 1982. Reproduced with permission of the publisher, The American Fertility Society.)

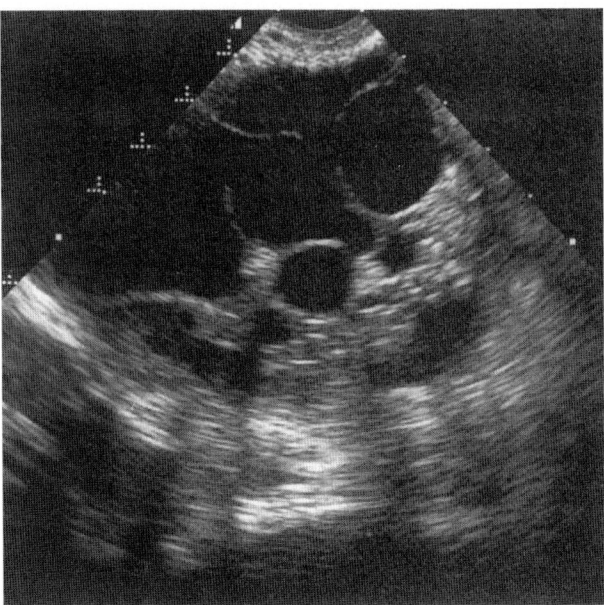

FIGURE 10-4 Transvaginal ultrasound of a large multiseptated mass with cystic and solid components. (From Salem S: The uterus and adnexa. In Rumack CM, Wilson SR, and Charboneau JW, eds: Diagnostic ultrasound, St. Louis, 1998 Mosby–Year Book, Inc.)

components; and smaller cysts adjacent to or part of the wall of the larger cyst—daughter cysts (Figure 10-4). Color flow Doppler is a technique that usually displays shades of red and blue that delineate blood flow within an ovarian neoplasm. Benign ovarian lesions have little color flow. When a color flow Doppler scan does demonstrate vascularity, the vascular resistance can be calculated. Low resistance is associated with malignancy, and high resistance usually is associated with normal tissue or benign disease. Color flow Doppler has been shown to be highly sensitive in evaluating ovarian malignancy.

Ultrasound evaluation of endometrial pathology involves measurement of the endometrial thickness or stripe. The normal endometrial thickness is 4 mm or less in a postmenopausal woman not taking hormones. The thickness varies in premenopausal women at different times of the menstrual cycle (Figure 10-5). The endometrial thickness is measured in the longitudinal plane, from outer margin to outer margin, at the widest part of the endometrium. Ultrasound is not a screening tool in asymptomatic women. However, several studies of postmenopausal women with vaginal bleeding have documented that malignancy is

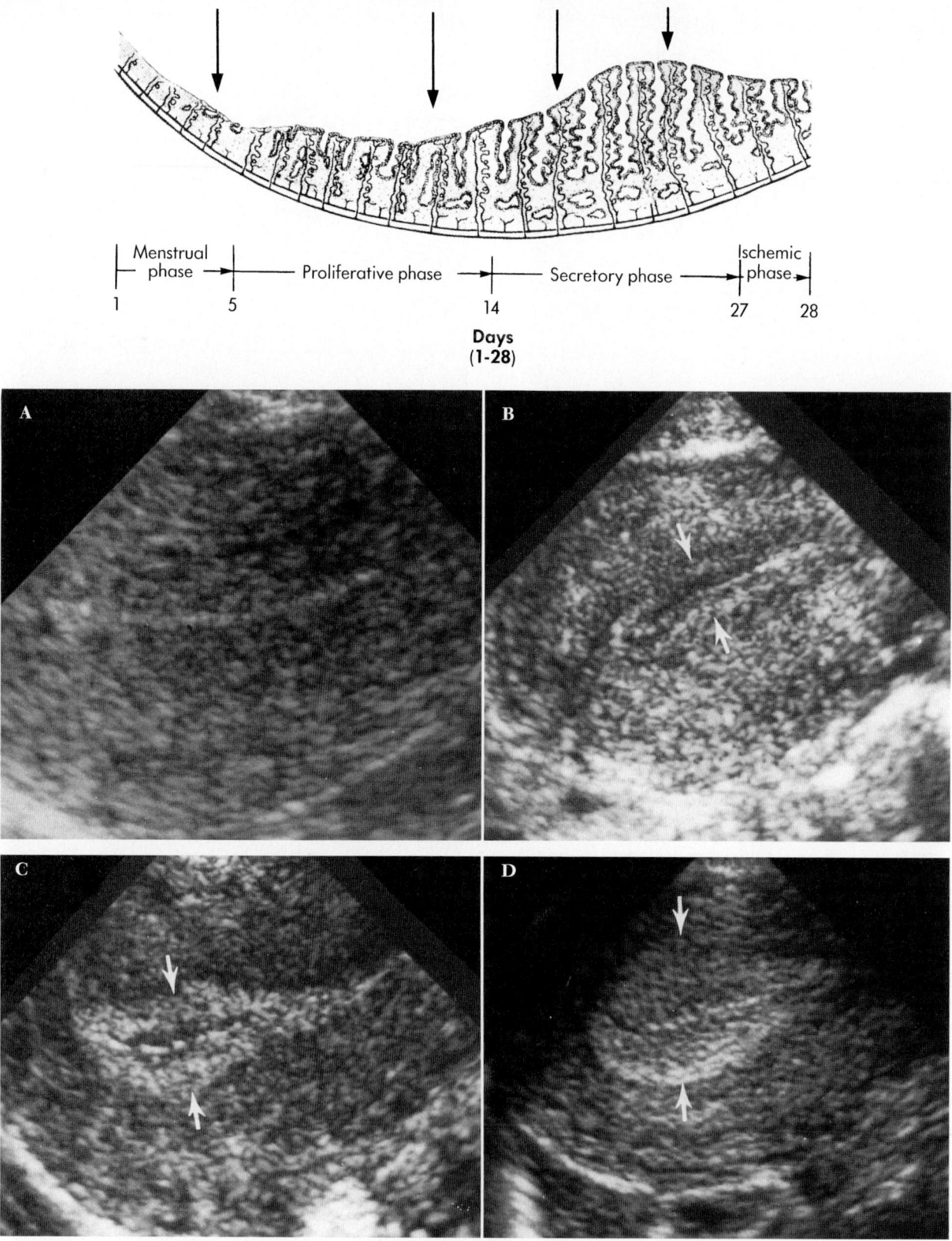

FIGURE 10-5   Variation in endometrium during menstrual cycle. **A,** Early proliferative phase. **B,** Late proliferative phase. **C,** Periovulatory phase. **D,** Late secretory phase. Note increase in endometrial thickness throughout the menstrual cycle. Also, note multilayered appearance in the late proliferative phase. (From Fleischer AC and Kepple DM: Benign conditions of the uterus, cervix, and endometrium. In Nyberg DA, Hill LM, Bohm-Velez M, and Mendelson EB, eds: Transvaginal ultrasound, St. Louis, 1992, Mosby–Year Book, Inc.)

extremely rare in women with an endometrial thickness of 4 mm or less. If an endometrial biopsy obtains inadequate tissue and the endometrial thickness is 5 mm or greater, a repeat biopsy or curettage should be performed (Figure 10-6). In women with abnormal vaginal bleeding, transcervical injection of saline outlines the uterine cavity. The technique of instilling saline in the uterine cavity, called sonohysterography, is an alternative to office hysteroscopy (Figure 10-7). In this procedure, a thin catheter, a pipelle or intrauterine insemination catheter, is inserted through the cervical os and 3 to 10 cc of saline are slowly injected into the uterine cavity (Figure 10-8). Sonohysterography has also been helpful in the evaluation of uterine septae. Importantly, sonohysterography, as with all types of ultrasound, does not make a tissue diagnosis.

Ultrasound not only provides a real time view but also allows scanning in multiple planes and thus has some advantages over CT. Ultrasound demonstrates advanced manifestations of pelvic neoplasm such as ascites and hydronephrosis. Three-dimensional ultrasound is now in its early stages of development. Clinical applications will be evaluated over the next decade.

Ultrasound is clinically useful in the differential diagnosis of abnormalities of early pregnancy. The characteristic "snowstorm" pattern of ill-defined echogenic areas inside the uterus is pathognomonic of hydatidiform mole.

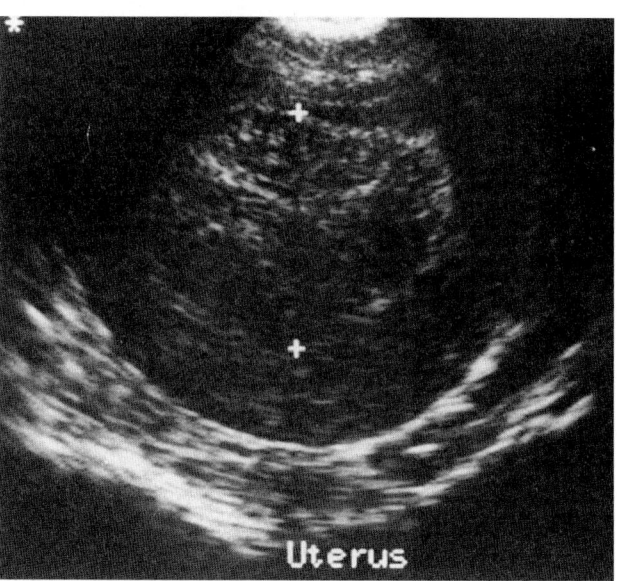

FIGURE 10-6 Endometrial carcinoma. A coronal endovaginal sonogram of a postmenopausal patient with bleeding and proven endometrial carcinoma. The endometrial carcinoma (cursors) has a mass-like effect in the central uterus. (From Hall DA and Yoder IC: Ultrasound evaluation of the uterus. In Callen PW, ed: Ultrasonography in obstetrics and gynecology, ed 3, Philadelphia, 1994, WB Saunders Co.)

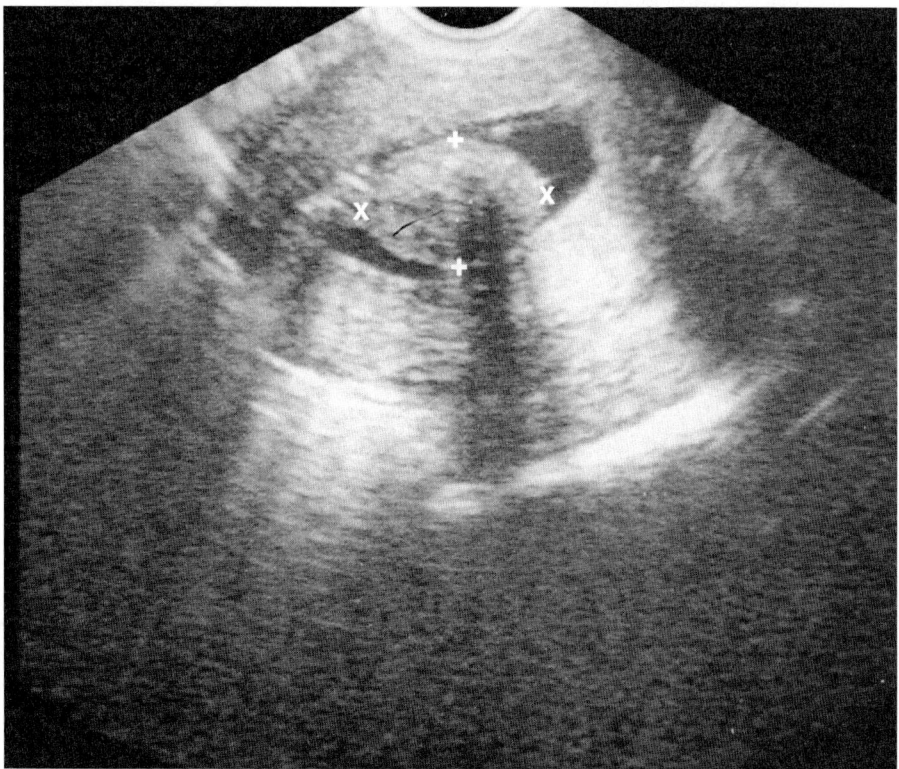

FIGURE 10-7 Endovaginal ultrasound using sonohysterography of an endometrial polyp in a perimenopausal woman with abnormal bleeding and secretory endometrium on endometrial biopsy. (Courtesy Marc A. Fritz, M.D.)

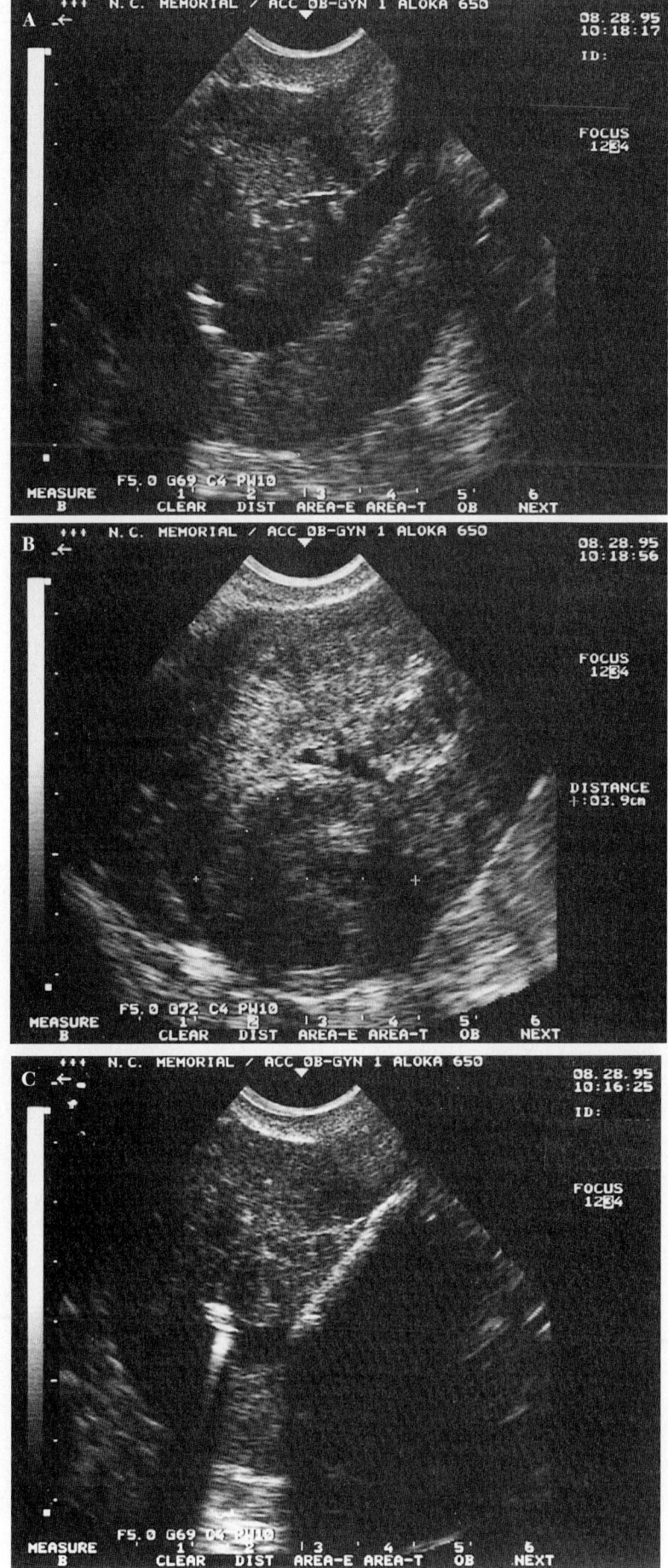

FIGURE 10-8 **A,** Sonohysterography—catheter under polyp in cavity. **B,** Catheter being retracted as fluid is injected (see tip of canal). **C,** Cavity with fluid, myoma post left and polyp to right. (Courtesy Ellen C. Wells, M.D.)

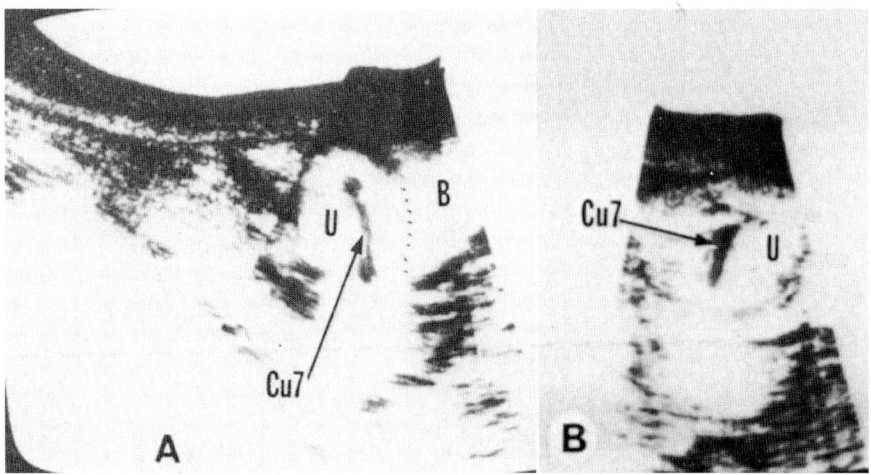

FIGURE 10-9   A, Sonographic longitudinal scan of uterus displaying Copper-7 intrauterine device (IUD) in its longitudinal axis. **B,** Transverse scan through fundus of uterus displaying characteristic "7" configuration of IUD (*B,* bladder; *Cu-7,* Copper-7; *U,* uterus). (From Cochrane WJ: The value of ultrasound in the management of intrauterine devices. In Sanders RC and James AE Jr, eds: The principles and practice of ultrasonography in obstetrics and gynecology, ed 2, New York, 1980, Appleton-Century-Crofts.)

Ultrasound is also of value in differentiating an intrauterine from an ectopic pregnancy. In early pregnancy the single ring inside the uterus may be either a gestational or a pseudogestational sac. The pseudogestational sac is formed by the decidual reaction that accompanies an ectopic pregnancy. Intrauterine pregnancies may be visualized as early as 4 weeks after the last menstrual period with an hCG titer of approximately 1000 mIU/ml. A pregnancy should be routinely visualized by 5 postmenstrual weeks, or when the gestational sac is 4 mm or greater in diameter. Endovaginal scanning can help differentiate the tubal ring or halo, a clear, circular adnexal structure that represents an ectopic gestation, from the corpus luteum.

Sonography is the method of choice to locate a "missing" intrauterine device (IUD) (Figure 10-9). It will help in diagnosing perforation of the uterus or unrecognized expulsion of the device. Endovaginal ultrasound transducers equipped with needle guides are frequently used for oocyte aspiration as part of in vitro fertilization.

The use of ultrasonography in women with pelvic infection has been disappointing. Swayne et al. discovered that acute pelvic inflammatory disease produced images similar to those seen in many other pelvic abnormalities. The lack of specificity in gynecology is a major limitation of ultrasonography. Gas- or fluid-filled intestines are commonly misinterpreted as gynecologic problems.

Ultrasound is often used to follow growth and resolution of myomas. It has been advocated by some in the evaluation of women using tamoxifen. Ultrasound has also been suggested as an adjunctive modality for evaluation of the lower urinary tract and anatomic integrity of the rectal sphincter. Some physicians use ultrasound as a screening method to evaluate the size of the ovaries of postmenopausal women at high risk for ovarian neoplasia.

In summary, ultrasound has become an extremely valuable adjunct to the bimanual examination. In many patients, particularly obese patients, it is superior to bimanual examination alone. An endovaginal ultrasound of an early pregnancy has become a mainstay in the evaluation of the pregnant woman with first-trimester vaginal bleeding. The measurement of endometrial thickness in post- and perimenopausal vaginal bleeding is an important diagnostic test. Whether ultrasound should be used for screening for ovarian cancer is still being investigated.

COMPUTED TOMOGRAPHY

High-resolution computed tomography (CT) is one of the leading examples of advanced technology in gynecology. CT provides detailed, two-dimensional images. The ability to image anatomic areas in a cross section a few millimeters thick has varied clinical applications. CT is popular in studies of the central nervous system, and it has revolutionized the clinical practice of neurology and neurosurgery. The critics of CT cite the expense of the equipment and its impact on cost containment. Proponents counter that CT scans reduce the need for other imaging techniques.

A CT scan identifies gross distortions in local anatomy by using the difference in x-ray beam attenuation that results from different densities in adjacent tissues. For example, this technique is excellent in discovering extension of pelvic cancer into the fat of the retroperitoneal space. It is also helpful in identifying peritoneal implants and abdominal fluid collections. Even so, CT definitely has its limitations. Abnormal masses are visualized, yet a definitive pathologic diagnosis cannot be established until a surgical biopsy is performed, because most masses do not have distinctive enough anatomic shapes or unique density characteristics. The CT scan may recognize a group of enlarged lymph nodes adjacent to pelvic vessels but cannot differentiate between benign hyperplasia or metastatic carcinoma. CT is often used for directed placement of needles or catheters to effect drainage from abdominal fluid collections or abscesses.

There have been several improvements in machinery for CT since its introduction into clinical medicine. The machine rotates the x-ray beam in an arc of 180 degrees perpendicular to the long axis of the body. A group of crystal detectors are directly opposite the narrow beam, only 2 to 10 mm wide. These crystals are capable of photon detection efficiencies of approximately 80%. The detectors measure the amount of tissue absorption, and a computer then develops two-dimensional images of the cross-sectional planes under investigation.

The best images from computed tomography are visualized when there are significant differences in tissue densities. To enhance visualization, contrast medium may be given intravenously, orally, and/or rectally to outline the urinary and upper and lower gastrointestinal tracts. Helical CT is a modification of standard CT that uses movement of the patient combined with rotation of several x-ray registers in a spiraling fashion. Varying speeds of rotation of the x-ray beams and the addition of several x-ray registers has produced several advantages over traditional CT. A tight helix or spiral of images is obtained that may be reconstructed and manipulated by the computer to produce a more detailed image. The distortion from peristalsis may be eliminated and with rapid movement of x-ray registers detailed vascular images are obtained. Helical CT is a reliable and accurate alternative to ventilation-perfusion scans for the diagnosis of pulmonary embolus (Figure 10-10). Helical CT provides two improvements over standard CT. The first is a much faster procedure, only a few minutes in duration. The second is many more images from differing angles. Movement artifact, such as from intestinal peristalsis, is eliminated. Vascular images are of a high enough quality that in many centers, helical CT has replaced pulmonary angiography and ventilation-perfusion scans. The applications for gynecology are still being evaluated.

A common indication in gynecology for a CT scan is the assessment of a prolactin-secreting adenoma of the pituitary gland. CT is superior to standard tomography of the sella turcica in evaluating a woman with elevated serum prolactin levels (Figure 10-11). The scans are used to follow patients with either suprasellar expansion or intrasellar adenomas.

CT is used extensively in gynecologic oncology. In general, it is more useful to the clinician in staging than in diagnosis (Figure 10-12). CT is superior to ultrasound

in the diagnosis of retroperitoneal and intraperitoneal metastases. The lower limit of detectable intraperitoneal implants is between 1 and 5 mm. Nelson et al. summarized several studies and found a detection rate of 50% to 60% of intraperitoneal disease. Often a CT scan helps in the initial evaluation of a pelvic neoplasm. Although imperfect, CT scans are a valuable noninvasive technique to screen patients for retroperitoneal metastatic disease. A CT scan is able to identify an enlarged lymph node when it reaches a diameter of 1.5 to 2 cm (Figure 10-13). Unfortunately, there are many false negative scans. Moldofsky et al. developed a technique of discovering metastatic carcinoma in normal-size retroperitoneal lymph nodes by using monoclonal antibody imaging.

Women with endometrial carcinoma have been studied by CT. Following injection of intravenous contrast material, a hypodense or low-attenuation area in the uterus is specific for endometrial carcinoma. It is possible to predict the depth of penetration of the cancer into the myometrium. However, the reliability of CT is less than that of MR for this indication.

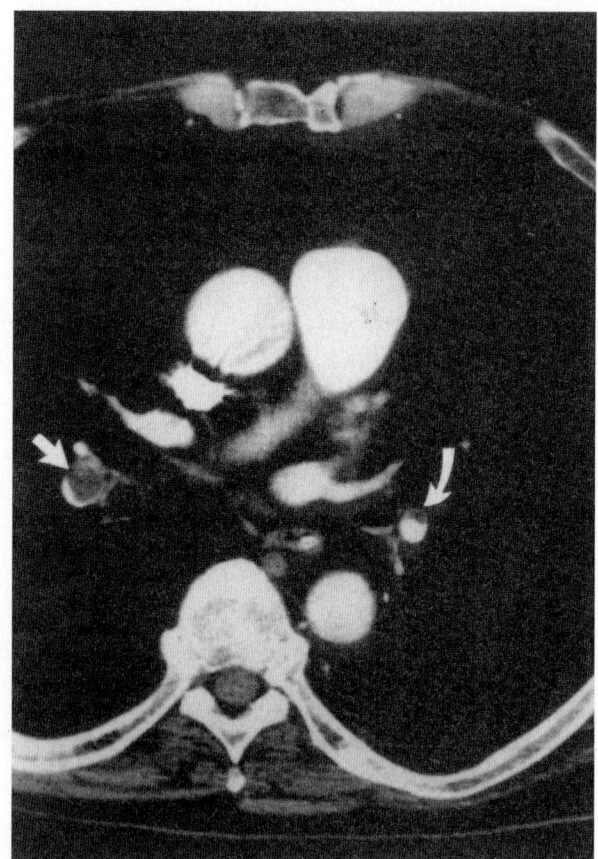

FIGURE 10-10 Bilateral filling defects in the opacified lower lobe pulmonary arteries, central on the right (straight arrow) and peripheral on the left (curved arrow). (From Grenier PA and Beigelman C: Spiral computed tomographic scanning and magnetic resonance angiography for the diagnosis of pulmonary embolism, Thorax 53(Suppl 2):S25, 1998.)

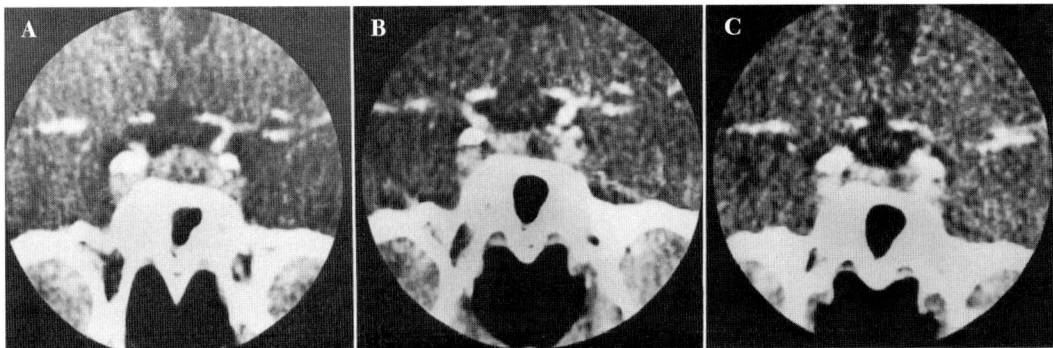

FIGURE 10-11 A 17-year-old woman with amenorrhea, galactorrhea, and hyperprolactinemia. **A,** Coronal CT scan after intravenous injection of contrast medium shows heterogeneous enhancement of pituitary, bulging of sellar diaphragm, and depression of left sellar floor. **B,** Six months after bromocriptine therapy, patient had restoration of ovulatory cycles, disappearance of galactorrhea, and normal prolactin level. CT scan shows decrease in size of content of pituitary fossa; adenoma appears as rounded defect in enhancement, 6 mm in diameter. **C,** One year after initiation of bromocriptine treatment, sellar diaphragm is now in a normal position; adenoma measures less than 4 mm in diameter. (From Bonneville JF, Poulignot D, Cattin F, et al: Radiology 143:454, 1982.)

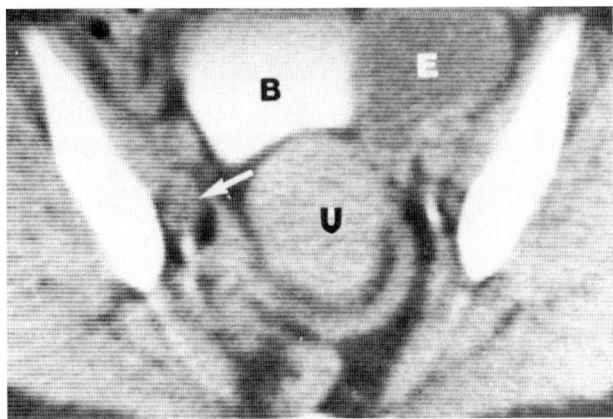

FIGURE 10-12 Stage IIB cervical carcinoma. CT scan through bladder *(B)* and uterine corpus *(U)*. Right obturator lymph node metastasis *(arrow)*, 2 cm in diameter, and left ovarian endometrioma *(E)* confirmed at laparotomy. (From Walsh JW and Goplerud DR: Prospective comparison between clinical and CT staging in primary cervical carcinoma, AJR 137:1000, 1981. Copyright 1981 by American Roentgen Ray Soc.)

In patients with ovarian carcinoma, the primary use of CT scans is in evaluating the extent of the disease. The CT is helpful in that it reduces the need for multiple tests. An abdominal pelvic CT may serve to replace an IVP, barium enema, and liver and spleen scan to assess metastatic disease. It is an excellent technique to discern small collections of ascites (Figure 10-14). CT scans give further information of retroperitoneal involvement and ureteral obstruction. A scan may miss small areas of metastatic spread, especially along serosal surfaces. If the area of carcinoma is less than 5 mm in diameter and is on a visceral surface, it is unlikely to be visualized by this imaging technique. Studies are ongoing as to the use of CT to predict the success of cytoreduction surgery with ovarian malignancy.

CT scans have been used for other intraabdominal and pelvic problems in gynecology (Figure 10-15). CT is valuable in identifying intraabdominal abscesses. CT is the most accurate imaging modality in the diagnosis of appendicitis (Figure 10-16). Using helical CT to avoid the distortion of intestinal activity, CT has been found to be up to 98% sensitive compared to up to 90% for ultrasound. In the postoperative patient with unexplained fever, CT is often helpful in assessing the abdomen and pelvis. After an abscess is localized, it may be possible to aspirate and drain using radiologic imaging techniques. Because of differences between fat, hair, and bone, CT is very accurate in the diagnosis of cystic teratoma. It is an excellent technique to confirm the diagnosis of ovarian vein thrombophlebitis (Figure 10-17). When a linear mass is identified from the adnexal area to the vena cava or renal vein, the diagnosis is established and appropriate medical therapy can be started.

The surface radiation dose for abdominal pelvic CT is between 2 and 10 rads. The dose to the midpelvis is approximately 50% of the surface dose. This radiation exposure is similar to that of a barium enema. Newer CT machines can vary the amount of radiation if there is a particular area of focus. One relative contraindication to the diagnostic use of CT is the inability to tolerate the radiopaque contrast necessary for adequate visualization, usually secondary to allergic reactions to iodine.

In summary, CT scans are useful in evaluating pituitary tumors and in evaluating the spread of malignancy during the evaluation of a woman with a pelvic carcinoma. CT scans also facilitate the drainage of abnormal fluid collections, and are helpful in the evaluation of acute infection processes.

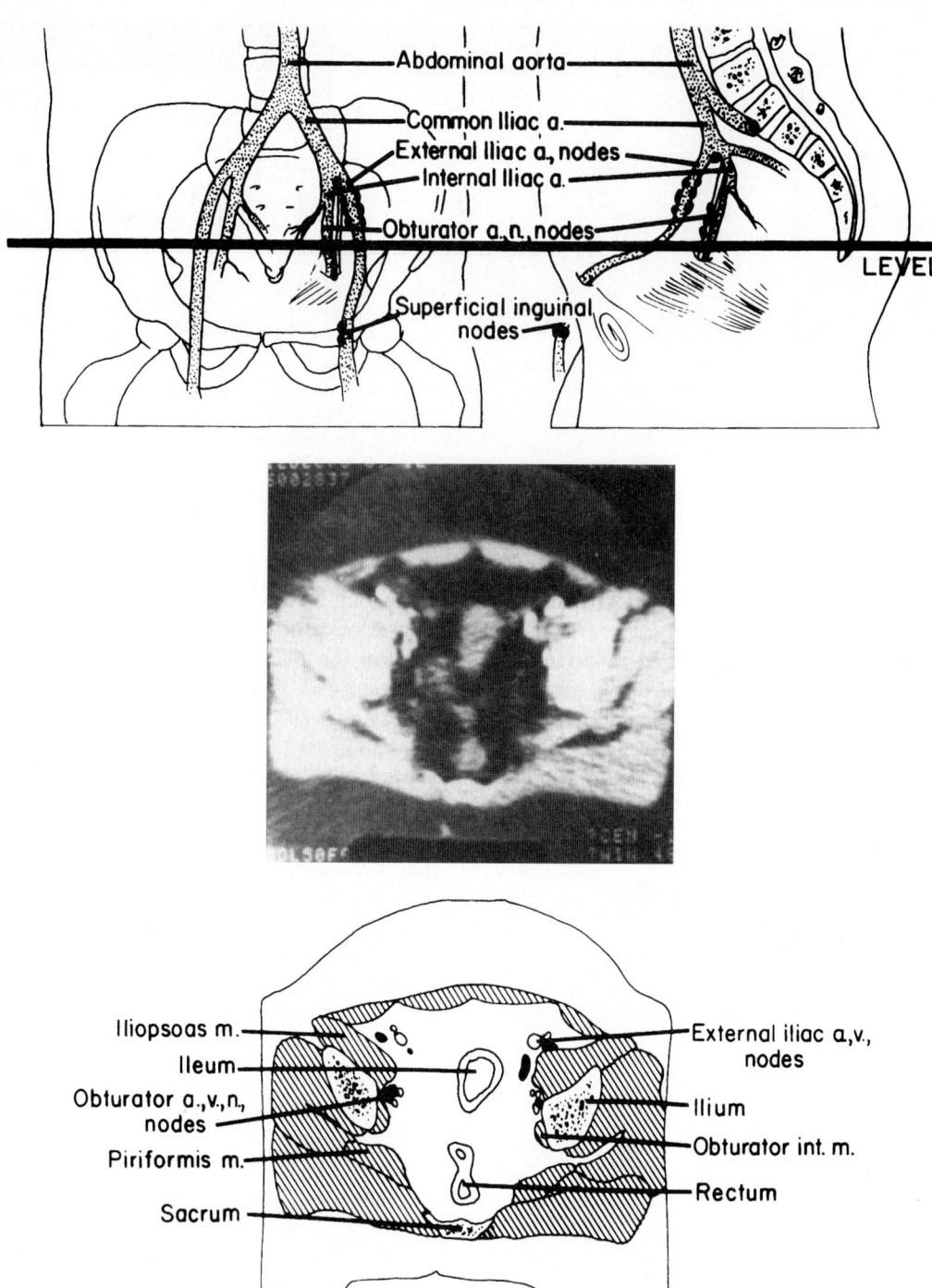

FIGURE 10-13 Illustrations and corresponding CT section after lymphangiography, demonstrating normal anatomic features of pelvic vessels, nerves, and lymph nodes. (From Walsh JW, Amendola MA, Konerding KF, et al: Radiology 137:158, 1980.)

MAGNETIC RESONANCE

Magnetic resonance imaging may be the greatest advance in radiology in the past three decades. The phenomenon of nuclear magnetic resonance was first discovered in 1945 and was renamed magnetic resonance imaging (MR) to avoid misinterpretation of the word *nuclear* by the public.

MR is a technique that uses radio frequency nonionizing radiation and a varying magnetic field. The patient is placed within the machine, and a magnetic field is produced. The image depends on the resonant absorp-

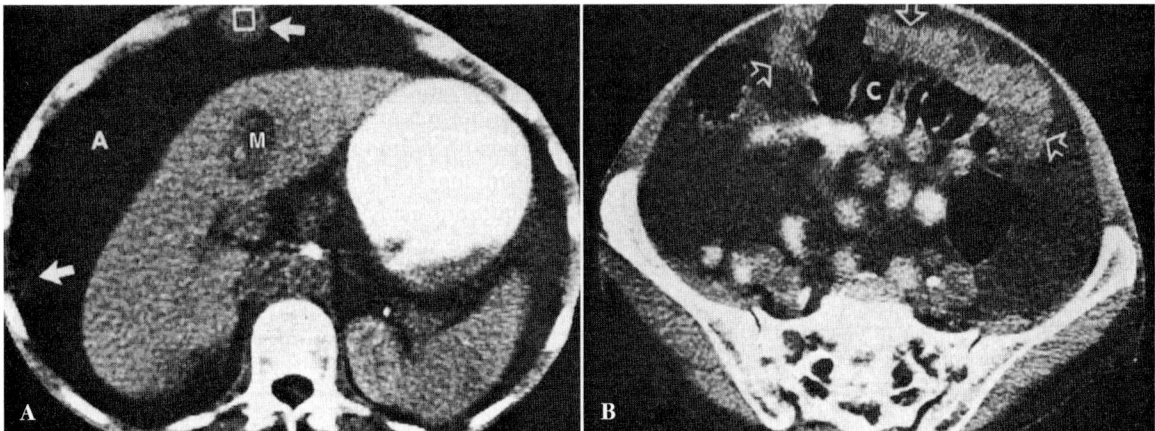

FIGURE 10-14 Metastatic ovarian carcinoma demonstrated by CT scan. **A,** Recurrent carcinoma is evident in this patient by ascites *(A)*, liver metastases *(M)*, and peritoneal metastatic implants *(arrows)*. **B,** Omental metastases are also seen as a flattened mass *(arrows)* lying on top of transverse colon *(C)* in this patient. (From Federle MP: Female Patient 9:45, 1984.)

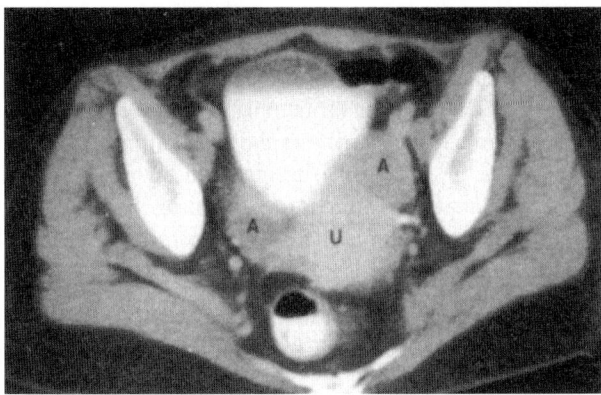

FIGURE 10-15 CT scan of patient with pelvic inflammatory disease with bilateral adnexal masses (*A,* tuboovarian abscesses; *U,* uterus). (From Gross BH, Moss AA, Mihara K, et al: Computed tomography of gynecologic diseases, AJR 141:771, 1983. Copyright 1983 by American Roentgen Ray Soc.)

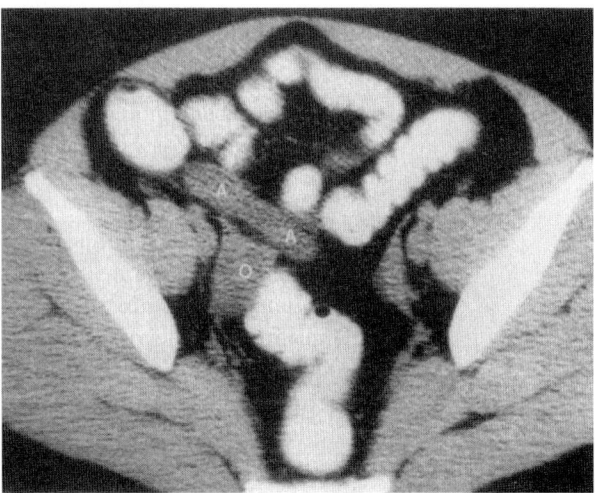

FIGURE 10-16 Computed tomography scan of a 54-year-old woman with an inflamed appendix (A) adjacent to the right ovary (O). (From Rao PM, Feltmate CM, Rhea JT, et al: Helical computed tomography in differentiating appendicitis and acute gynecologic conditions, Obstet Gynecol 93:417, 1999).

tion and emission of radio waves by the atomic nuclei in the various tissues being observed. Because of their intrinsic magnetism, the nuclei act like small bar magnets and are influenced by the machine's magnetic field. The summation of the resonance of the vast number of atomic nuclei in a single thin slice of tissue provides the overall result. Resolution is 0.5 to 1 mm. The intensity of the image can be modified by varying the magnetic field.

Images are tomographic (in thin slices) and may be visualized in multiple planes including coronal, sagittal, or transverse planes. This is particularly valuable in delineating pelvic structures that do not lie in perpendicular planes. The radio waves penetrate bone and air without attenuation. Thus MR allows identification of soft tissue lesions inaccessible to other imaging techniques. Liquid and fat show up quite differently when different types of proton spin (T1 versus T2) are compared. Thus, unlike x-ray, where a tissue density deter-

mines the nature of the image, with MR it is the inherent type of tissue that determines what the image looks like. The addition of computer analysis further increases MR sensitivity by selecting and filtering out particular frequencies such as those from fat, thus allowing further delineation between types of tissue. These differences between MR and CT are why many investigators believe that MR examinations yield more information for the musculoskeletal system and pelvis than CT.

MR uses nonionizing radiation. Extensive basic investigations have demonstrated no evidence of mutagenic effects in studies of bacteria, and no chromosomal changes were produced in human lymphocytes. No adverse or harmful effects have been reported from repetitive examinations. MR is considered safe in pregnancy.

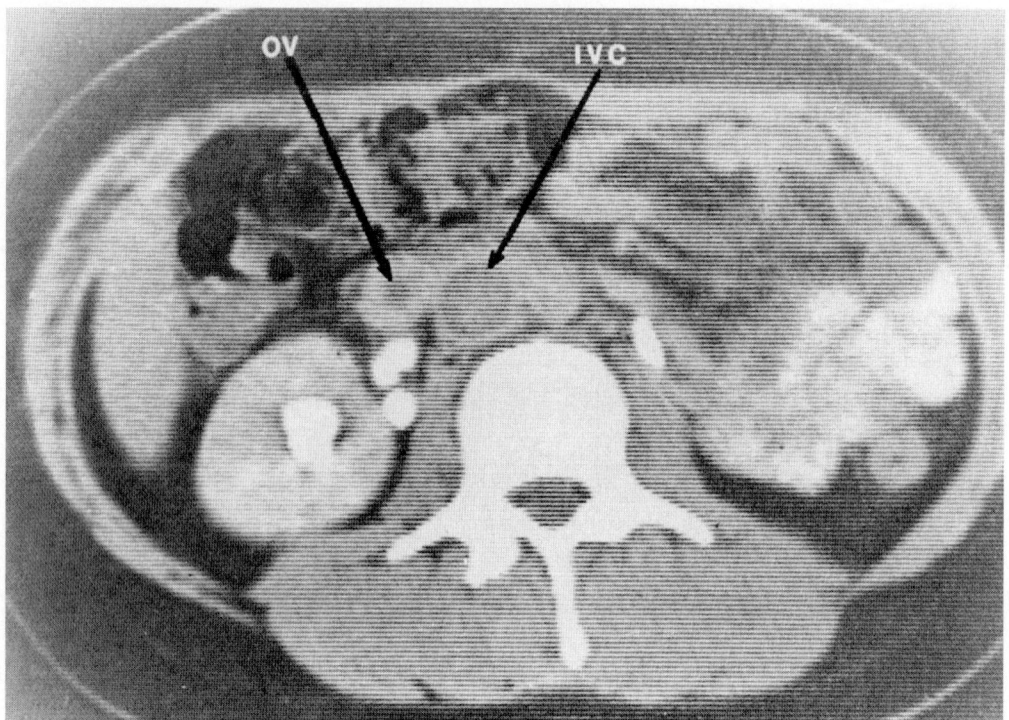

FIGURE 10-17   CT image of abdomen. Note thrombus within lumen of right ovarian (*OV*) and inferior vena cava (*IVC*). Right ovarian vein is markedly enlarged. (From Angel JL and Knuppel RA: Obstet Gynecol 63:62, 1984. Reprinted with permission from The American College of Obstetricians and Gynecologists.)

MR can differentiate normal from malignant tissue and also can identify areas of abnormal tissue metabolism. MR is most specific in the diagnosis of conditions associated with edema. Edema prolongs the spin-spin proton relaxation time (T2), thereby producing a stronger image. Investigators have discovered significant prolonged proton relaxation times or spin lattice relaxation times (T1) for the atoms in most carcinomas.

In an early study of three-dimensional MR, Mann et al. demonstrated that imaging could identify the exact area of a vulvar neoplasm (Figure 10-18). MR correctly identified microscopic tumor at the surgical margin of the vulvectomy incision. Because of the potential of the MR examination to view the pelvis in any plane, it is an excellent modality for evaluating vaginal anatomy and congenital defects of the müllerian system. Chang et al. found MR to have a 95% sensitivity and 90% specificity in evaluating vaginal malignancy. Several reports have documented the advantages of MR in diagnosing and evaluating disease processes of adenomyosis, myomas, endometrial cancer (including myometrial invasion), and cervical carcinoma, both local and distant spread. Kinkel et al., in their recent meta-analysis, concluded that MR is superior to CT or ultrasound for the evaluation of endometrial cancer. Preoperative MR was found to be 93% accurate in predicting ovarian malignancies in a study of 187 adnexal masses by Hricak et al. MR is more accurate than CT in evaluating the spread of uterine and cervical malignancy (Figure 10-19). MR has been employed to evaluate endometriosis and adnexal disease. However, selectivity should be exercised in choosing patients to undergo a preoperative MR.

MR has several distinct advantages over other forms of imaging. It does not use ionizing radiation; therefore there are no known hazards. The x-ray photon has 10 billion times more energy than the radio frequency photon of MR. Radio frequency electromagnetic radiation penetrates calcified material without significant attenuation. Unlike ultrasound, MR can penetrate through gas, thus allowing visualization of the bowel and vagina. In addition, MR does not require the use of radiopaque contrast agents required with CT scans. MR uses gadolinium, a magnetically opaque contrast agent that is given intravenously. Gadolinium is rapidly dispersed into the interstitial spaces and is not nephrotoxic. Glucagon may be given prior to abdominal-pelvic MR to decrease intestinal peristalsis.

The major limitation of MR is patient acceptance. Many patients feel "trapped" in the machine. Meléndez and McCrank reviewed anxiety reactions associated with MR examinations. They found that 4% to 30% of patients experienced some type of psychologic problem, ranging from mild anxiety to severe apprehension necessitating discontinuation of the study. Most complaints focused on anxiety from the claustrophobic reactions and feelings of panic. The need for the patient to remain still

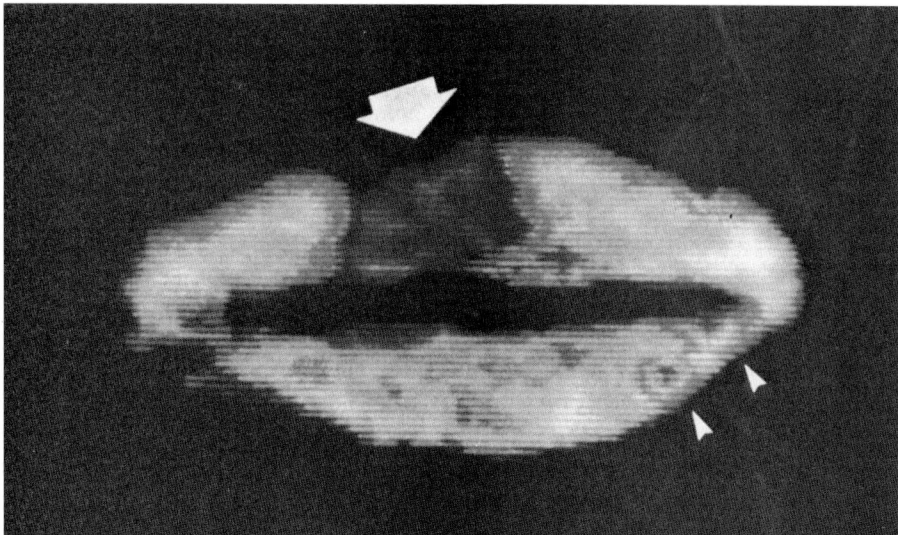

FIGURE 10-18   MR of transverse slice of radical vulvectomy specimen. Large arrow indicates primary vulvar lesion; smaller arrows indicate two nodes containing metastatic disease that measured 0.7 and 1.0 cm in diameter. (From Mann WJ, Mendonca-Dias MH, Lauterbur PC, et al: Am J Obstet Gynecol 148:93, 1984.)

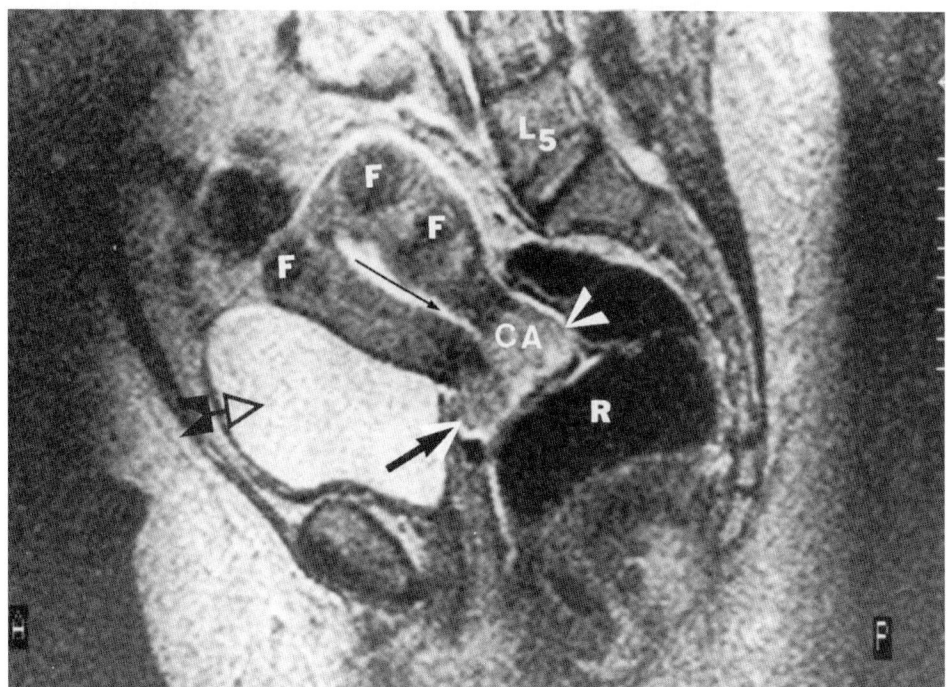

FIGURE 10-19   Sagittal MR of woman with cervical cancer. Cancer *(CA)* is area of higher signal intensity within cervix (between *black arrows* on *white arrowheads*). Rectum *(R)* can be seen immediately posterior and inferior to enlarged cervical mass. Endometrial canal is slightly enlarged and contains fluid *(thin black arrow)*. Three leiomyomata *(F)* can be seen scattered throughout myometrium. Bladder is seen internally as fluid-filled structure *(open black arrow)*. Parameters for this examination were spin echo sequence of TR 2500/TE 80, 256 × 198 matrix, and 1 signal average. (Courtesy Mark L. Schiebler, M.D.)

for the long period of scanning contributed to the anxiety. The authors noted that most patients were fearful prior to the MR examination. Techniques to alleviate anxiety include prescan education programs, music by earphones, antianxiety medications, hypnosis, relaxation techniques, and having family members present. Because patient compliance is essential for successful imaging, attention to patient anxiety prior to the study is important. MR should not be used in patients with cochlear implants or pacemakers. It is safe in women with IUDs, including copper-containing ones, and safe in patients with surgical clips and staples.

In summary, the applications of MR are vast. As an imaging modality it is a nonionizing form of visualization that can help differentiate types of tissue, penetrate bone, provide images in multiple planes, and be used with non-toxic contrast. However, MR is not a screening tool. Examinations require good patient compliance, and need to be individualized by the clinician and radiologist.

ENDOMETRIAL SAMPLING

Endometrial biopsy is one of the diagnostic tests most frequently performed by gynecologists. This rapid, safe, and inexpensive sampling of the endometrial lining is a common procedure in the clinical workup of women with abnormal vaginal bleeding. The renowned gynecologist Howard Kelly was an enthusiast for outpatient endometrial biopsy in the 1920s, and in the past 25 years its popularity has increased, reflecting the emphasis on cost containment in medical practice. Instruments have been developed that abrade, scrape, brush, and aspirate the endometrium.

There are several indications for endometrial sampling. Endometrial sampling is most frequently performed to evaluate dysfunctional uterine bleeding. Another indication is to investigate abnormal bleeding associated with increasing use of hormonal replacement therapy in postmenopausal women. Endometrial biopsy is the standard diagnostic test to confirm a chronic uterine infection such as endometritis. If pelvic tuberculosis is suspected, sampling of the endometrial lining is performed late in the menstrual cycle. This gives the pathologist the best opportunity to discover the classic giant cells and tubercles.

There are only a few contraindications to endometrial biopsy. Profuse bleeding is a relative contraindication.

Endometrial biopsy should not be performed more than 14 to 16 days after ovulation because of the possibility of interfering with an early pregnancy. In contrast, endometrial biopsy 10 to 14 days following the temperature rise does not interfere with implantation during that cycle.

There are many different models and modifications of devices used for endometrial sampling. Most instruments aspirate tissue from the endometrial lining following abrasion or scraping with a small curette or perforated cannula (Figures 10-20 and 10-21).

Endometrial biopsy is performed on an outpatient basis. It is helpful to explain to the patient that she will experience uterine cramping during the short time that the biopsy instrument is inside the uterus. A bimanual examination is performed to note the size of the uterus and direction of the uterine cavity. A single-toothed tenaculum may be used to secure the anterior cervical lip. The exocervix is then cleaned of mucus and bacteria. Many physicians will cleanse the os with an iodine solution prior to sampling. When the indication for the biopsy is to evaluate abnormal bleeding, multiple areas of the endometrial cavity should be sampled. At least four separate areas should be abraded. If copious or necrotic tissue is discovered or the pathology report is inadequate, further evaluation is indicated.

The most frequent problem in performing endometrial sampling is cervical stenosis or spasm. When this is encountered, the optimal method to obtain pain relief and overcome resistance is a paracervical block with 1% Xylocaine. Occasionally the endocervical application of viscous 2% to 4% lidocaine may decrease discomfort. Zupi et al. have described the use of 5 cc of 2% mepivacaine injected transcervically into the uterus to reduce discomfort. Subsequently, the cervix can be dilated painlessly, with narrow metal dilators, and the biopsy completed.

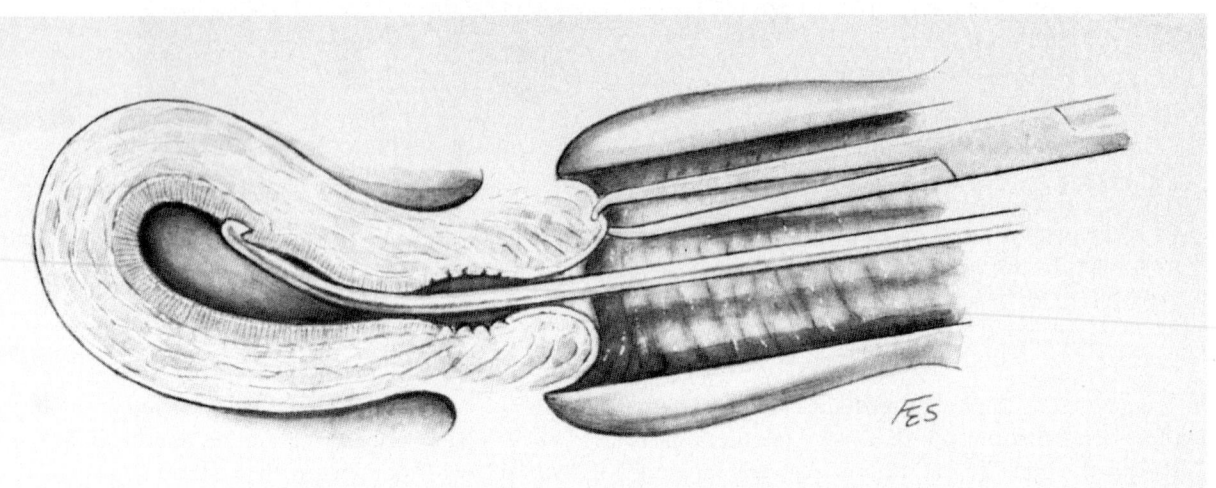

FIGURE 10-20 Office endometrial aspiration with 3-mm Randall suction curette. (From Copenhaver EH: Surgery of the vulva and vagina: a practical guide, Philadelphia, 1981, WB Saunders Co.)

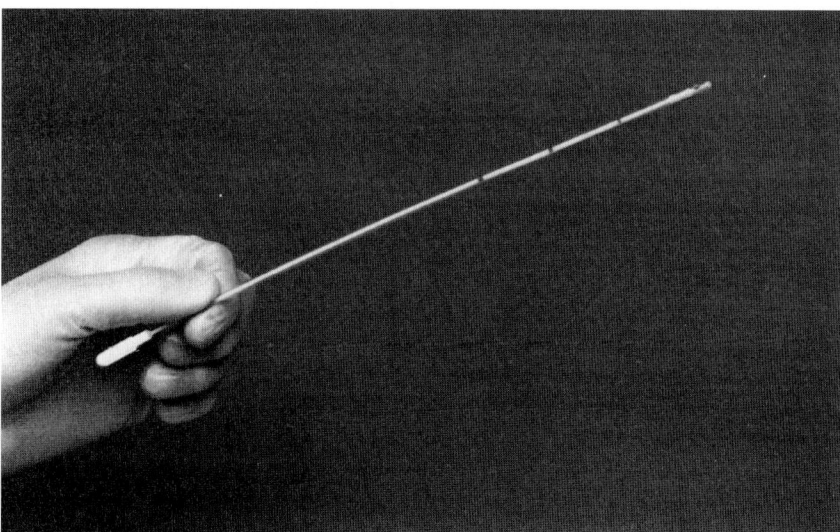

FIGURE 10-21   Pipelle endometrial suction curette. Note small diameter and flexible nature. Suction is produced by partly withdrawing inner stem.

There are many modifications of the original Novak and Randall endometrial biopsy instruments. Most cannulas in current favor are 2 to 4 mm in diameter and are plastic. Aspiration of the endometrium is usually accomplished by a syringe. The thin, flexible polypropylene Pipelle cannula (see Figure 10-21) is as effective as rigid instruments in obtaining endometrial specimens, often with less discomfort. Most clinicians use the Pipelle as the instrument of first choice for endometrial sampling. Other flexible plastic cannulas are equally effective.

Complications following endometrial biopsy are exceedingly rare. The major complication is uterine perforation, with an incidence of 1 or 2 cases per 1000. Infection and post procedure hemorrhage are very rare. Some women develop a severe vasovagal reflex from instrumentation of the uterine cavity. This reflex can be diminished by either giving the patient intravenous atropine or performing a paracervical block. Some clinicians pretreat women with nonsteroidal antiinflammatory agents to decrease the pain associated with this procedure.

The accuracy of endometrial biopsy in diagnosing malignancy is approximately 95% when compared with subsequent findings at hysterectomy. Therefore, if abnormal perimenopausal or menopausal bleeding recurs following an endometrial biopsy, additional diagnostic procedures, such as hysteroscopy or ultrasound, should be performed. Investigators frequently assess the various diagnostic modalities for evaluation of endometrial pathology. Langer et al. studied 448 women. As a screening modality, ultrasound was only 48% specific. Their conclusion was that endometrial biopsy was superior. O'Connell et al. established a triage protocol for postmenopausal women with abnormal uterine bleeding. Endometrial biopsy and sonohysterography were 84% sensitive and 96% specific in correlation with operative findings. Tahir et al. randomized 400 women to ultra-

sound, endometrial biopsy, hysteroscopy, and D&C. They concluded that ultrasound and endometrial biopsy should be the first line of treatment in the evaluation of abnormal bleeding. Feldman et al. evaluated 286 women with perimenopausal bleeding who had had a D&C or an endometrial biopsy. Nine of 86 (10.5%) who had negative findings initially, but continued to bleed, had carcinoma or complex hyperplasia on follow-up biopsy. In a retrospective review of 223 patients, Daniel and Peters found that 16% of tumors had a more advanced grade of endometrial carcinoma at hysterectomy than after office curettage. Thus lesions such as atypical hyperplasia warrant further evaluation. If a hysterectomy is performed, the uterus should be opened and evaluated.

In summary, the major advantages to the patient of the endometrial biopsy over D&C are convenience and cost saving. Multiple instruments have been designed for endometrial biopsy; none is superior. The clinical results obtained depend on two factors: the patient's acceptance and the physician's skill and perseverance. The patient's acceptance is higher with narrow cannulas made of plastic. Liberal use of paracervical block in difficult procedures allows the physician to be successful in obtaining tissue in more than 95% of cases. Routine preoperative endometrial biopsy in asymptomatic women undergoing hysterectomy is an unnecessary procedure and does not improve patient care.

HYSTEROSALPINGOGRAPHY

Hysterosalpingography (HSG) is an x-ray imaging technique in which the uterine cavity and the lumina of the fallopian tubes are visualized by injecting contrast material through the cervical canal. This test was first described by two investigators, Rubin and Cary, working independently in 1914. There have been numerous refinements in techniques. The most important advance has been the addition of image intensification with screen fluoroscopy, which provides more precise visualization and reduces radiation exposure. Spot films have limited value in evaluating infertile patients. HSG is a safe and rapid means of investigating abnormalities in the endometrial cavity and fallopian tubes (Figure 10-22). Often an inference of abnormal function can be postulated from an abnormal HSG. These judgments should not be absolute; for example, approximately 15% of women who have "obstructed" fallopian tubes diagnosed by HSG subsequently become pregnant without further treatment. The etiology of this false reading is thought to be tubal spasm.

The leading indications for HSG are primary and secondary infertility. This imaging technique gives evidence of endometrial irregularities, tubal patency, tubal mobility, and sometimes peritubal disease (Figure 10-23). HSG has an approximate 83% specificity for evaluating tubal patency. Laparoscopy is a more sophisticated and accurate method of diagnosing the tubal factor during an infertility investigation. Chromopertubation with an innocuous dye, such as indigo carmine, demonstrates tubal patency during laparoscopy. Comparative studies have documented that HSG discovers only 50% of the peritubal disease diagnosed by direct visualization via the laparoscope. The study by Hutchins of 409 infertile patients who had sequential HSG and laparoscopy under general anesthesia helped to define our understanding of tubal spasm. In this series, HSG showed 93 women to have blocked tubes, and 30 of these were patent by chromopertubation. Pain relief does not invariably alleviate tubal spasm. Tubal anomalies, including diverticula and accessory ostia, can be diagnosed by HSG. In summary, HSG is useful in diagnosing intrinsic disease of the fallopian tubes, while laparoscopy is more effective in identifying extrinsic disease.

Uterine cavity abnormalities, present in 10% of infertile women, may be discovered by HSG. Congenital müllerian anomalies, such as bicornuate, septate, arcuate, and T-shaped uteri (associated with in utero diethylstilbestrol exposure), may be diagnosed (Figure 10-24). Pathology such as synechiae of the endometrial cavity may also be discovered (Figure 10-25). Hysteroscopy is an alternative technique for evaluating intrauterine pathology. McBean et al. have found, in a retrospective review, that there is a strong correlation between a polypoid-appearing endometrial cavity on HSG and laparoscopically proven endometriosis. HSG is a basic tool in the evaluation of patients with poor reproductive histories. It is specifically applicable for women with repetitive second-trimester losses.

Although HSG has been suggested as a technique to diagnose an incompetent internal cervical os it is rarely used. The maximum normal diameter of the isthmus and internal cervical os is reported to be between 0.7 and 1.0 cm. However, the anatomic changes in the diameter of the internal os in the nonpregnant state have little predictive value for future competency in pregnancy.

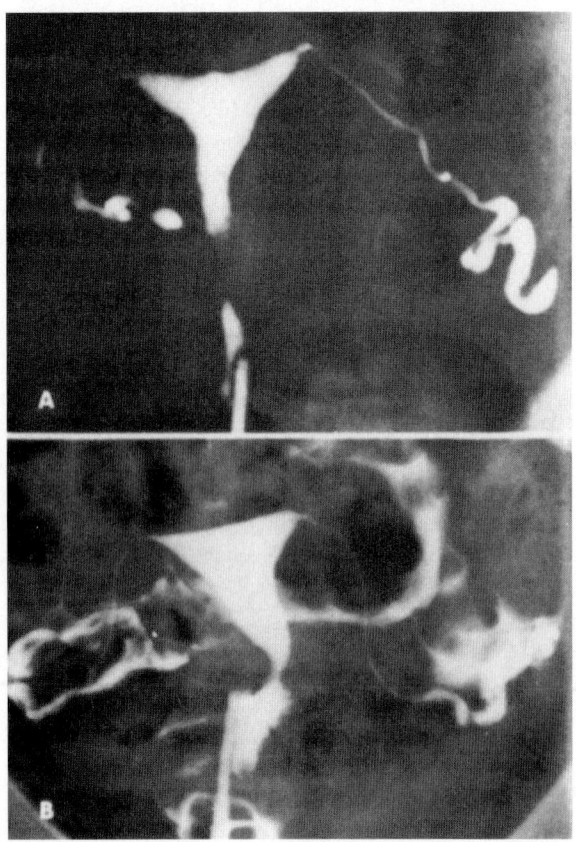

FIGURE 10-22 Two normal hysterosalpingograms. (From Soules MR and Spadoni LR: Oil versus aqueous media for hysterosalpingography: a continuing debate based on many opinions and few facts, Fertil Steril 38:1, 1982. Reproduced with permission of the publisher, The American Fertility Society.)

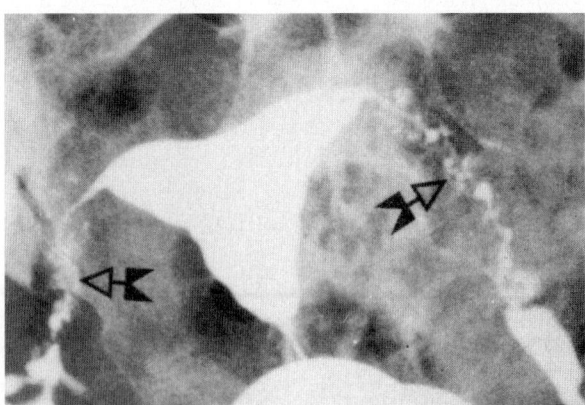

FIGURE 10-23 Hysterosalpingogram from patient with tubal endometriosis. Flecks of contrast material *(arrows)* are seen about isthmus without central linear pattern. Distal ends appear normally patent. (From Siegler AM: Hysterosalpingography, Fertil Steril 40:139, 1983. Reproduced with permission of the publisher, The American Fertility Society.)

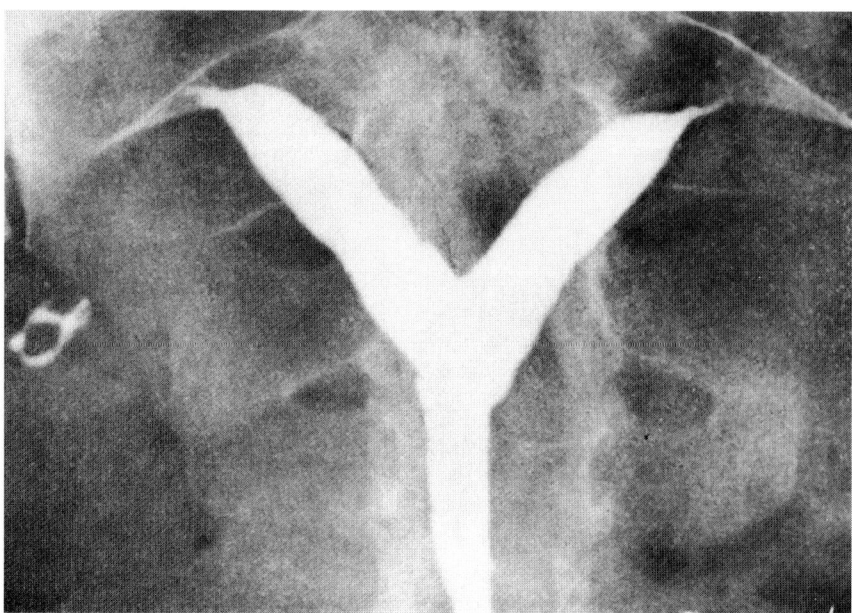

FIGURE 10-24 Hysterosalpingogram from 34-year-old nulliparous woman who had regular menses and no dysmenorrhea. V-shaped fundal defect with single cervix proved to be bicornuate uterus. (From Siegler AM: Hysterosalpingography, New York, 1967, Harper & Row, Publishers, Inc.)

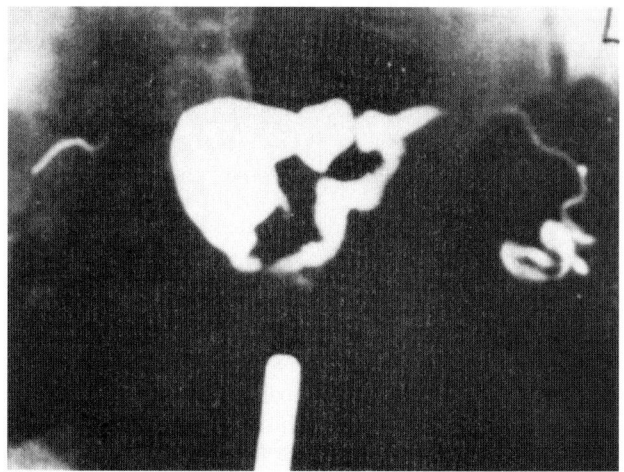

FIGURE 10-25 Hysterosalpingogram demonstrating intrauterine adhesions, grade 3, after repeated curettage for missed abortion. (From Schenker JG and Margalioth EJ: Intrauterine adhesions: an updated appraisal, Fertil Steril 37:593, 1982. Reproduced with permission of the publisher, The American Fertility Society.)

Women with amenorrhea and a history of curettage who do not respond to a hormonal challenge should have an HSG or hysteroscopy. Uterine synechiae are identified by slowly injecting a water-soluble medium. If a woman has synechiae, tubal obstruction, and pelvic calcifications, a diagnosis of pelvic tuberculosis should be strongly suspected. HSG will also discover polyps or small submucous myomas in refractory cases of abnormal uterine bleeding.

Contraindications to HSG include the obvious: acute pelvic infection, active uterine bleeding, pregnancy, and allergy to iodine.

The choice of using a small Foley catheter or an adjustable rubber or plastic acorn and cannula for injection depends on physician preference. This decision does not seem to bias results as long as all air in the system is replaced by the liquid contrast medium. The choice of water-soluble versus oil-based contrast medium depends on the primary indication for the test and physician preference. Water-soluble iodine is preferred for documenting intrauterine filling defects and identifying the severity of mucosal damage in chronic tubal infection. Lipid-based material provides a more distinct and clearer radiographic image. Most investigators report that the pregnancy rate after HSG is 2 to 3 times greater with oil-soluble media. Watson et al. performed a meta-analysis of studies reporting the therapeutic effects of HSG contrast material. They reported a definite therapeutic effect and higher pregnancy rate with lipid-based or oil-soluble contrast. The effect was greatest in women with unexplained infertility. Researchers have speculated that the therapeutic effect may be secondary to a mechanical action on tubal epithelium, tubal debris, and tubal plugs or an inhibition of peritoneal macrophages. In contradistinction, Spring et al. reported from a multicenter randomized study of 666 women that there was no difference between water-soluble contrast and oil-soluble contrast, or both, in rate of term pregnancies at one year.

The endpoint of an x-ray examination for tubal patency is either tubal filling with intraperitoneal spilling or increasing pelvic pain secondary to uterine distention associated with tubal obstruction. Tubal spasm may sometimes be overcome by glucagon (2 mg intravenously), which produces atony of smooth muscle. Glucagon is effective in about one of three women with tubal spasm.

Complications of HSG are rare but serious when they happen. Acute pelvic infection, serious enough to require hospitalization, develops in 0.3% to 3.1% of patients. This incidence of pelvic infection is directly related to the population studied, that is, more common in women with dilated tubes. The use of prophylactic antibiotics may reduce the incidence of acute infection following instrumentation of the uterus. As with any surgical procedure that invades the uterus, pelvic pain, uterine perforation, and vasovagal vasomotor reactions do occur. Allergic reactions, particularly to the iodine dye, are a possibility. Intravasation of the dye into the vascular system occurs with high injection pressures, partial perforation of the cannula, and endometrial defects associated with synechiae (Figure 10-26). Embolic phenomena, pelvic peritonitis, and granuloma formation with oil-based dye are very rare complications.

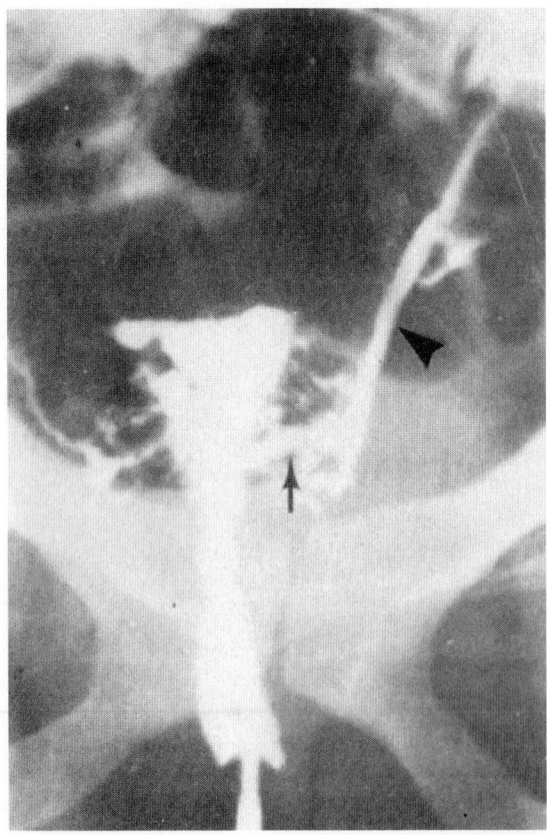

FIGURE 10-26 Hysterosalpingogram showing both lymphatic *(small arrow)* and venous *(large arrow)* intravasation. (From Soules MR and Spandoni LR: Oil versus aqueous media for hysterosalpingography: a continuing debate based on many opinions and few facts, Fertil Steril 38:1, 1982. Reproduced with permission of the publisher, The American Fertility Society.)

In summary, HSG is a relatively safe imaging technique. Its major uses are in the evaluation of patients with infertility or poor pregnancy outcomes. The procedure can diagnose uterine and tubal abnormalities. Both oil- and water-based dyes are used. With a TV screen image intensifier, the average HSG takes 10 minutes to perform. This procedure involves approximately 90 seconds of fluoroscopic time and an average radiation exposure to the ovaries of 1 to 2 rads. Recent advances in hysteroscopy and ultrasound have led to a substantial decrease in the use of HSG.

HYSTEROSCOPY

Hysteroscopy is the direct visualization of the endometrial cavity using an endoscope and a light source. The earliest hysteroscope was nothing more than a hollow tube with an alcohol lamp and mirror for a light source. In 1869 Pantaleoni reported the successful removal of an endometrial polyp through the scope. Modern hysteroscopes are modifications of cystoscopes with channels to introduce light via fiberoptics, uterine cavity distention media, and surgical instruments.

Thirty-five years ago interest in hysteroscopy increased as a result of both improved instrumentation and the use of dextran (Hyskon) as a distending medium. The popularity of hysteroscopy has also been enhanced because it is a simple technique that can be performed in the office. Hysteroscopy has multiple indications, including diagnosis of recurrent abnormal bleeding, repetitive abortion, uterine synechiae, abnormal HSGs, and infertility. Operative procedures, which usually require local or regional anesthesia, performed under hysteroscopic guidance include location and removal of intact or fragmented IUDs, resection of submucous myomas, lysis of synechiae, incision of uterine septa, removal of endometrial polyps, and ablation of the endometrium.

Rigid hysteroscopes vary in diameter (Figure 10-27). The smaller caliber scopes, 3 to 5 mm in diameter, are used for diagnostic purposes. Several are available that have views from 0 to 30 degrees. Similar to that of a cystoscope, the outer sleeve of a rigid hysteroscope contains several channels that extend the full length of the instrument. Large scopes, with diameters of 8 to 10 mm, may be used for high flow of distending media and for procedures. Flexible minihysteroscopic instruments and microendoscopes are also available and may be used in the office for simple operative procedures such as directed biopsies (Figure 10-28). The narrower hysteroscopes, with diameters of 3 to 5 mm, are available for office examinations.

The cavity of the uterus is a potential space. The success of hysteroscopy depends on the medium used to expand this space. The three most popular choices for diagnostic hysteroscopy are 32% dextran, which is highly viscous; 5% dextrose and water, which has low viscosity; and carbon dioxide gas. Another common distending medium is 1.5%

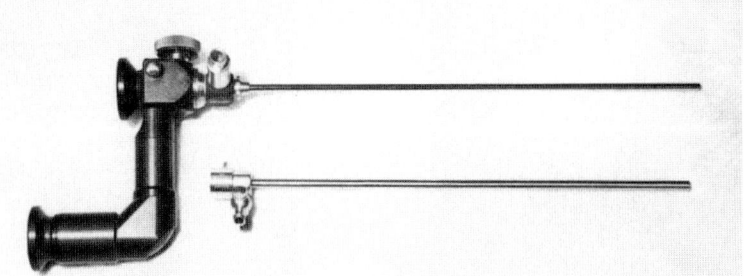

FIGURE 10-27 A 5-mm rigid hysteroscope (Storz Instruments).

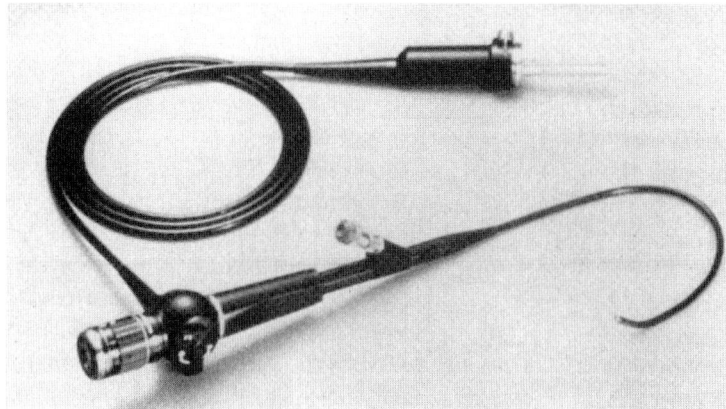

FIGURE 10-28 Small-size steerable fiberoptic hysteroscope offer the advantage of entering hard-to-reach spaces within the uterus and likewise provides excellent operative access to all areas of the uterus. (From: Baggish MS and Valle RF: Future of hysteroscopy. In Baggish MS, Barbot J, and Valle RF, eds, Diagnostic and operative hysteroscopy, ed 2, St. Louis, 1999, Mosby, Inc.)

glycine. High–molecular-weight dextran (average molecular weight, 70,000 Da in 10% glucose) is preferred by the majority of investigators, especially if a surgical procedure is contemplated. This extremely viscous fluid is biodegradable, nontoxic, and nonconductive and has good optical qualities. Most important, dextran is immiscible with blood; this helps to keep the field clear during intrauterine surgery. Dextran has two drawbacks: it is antigenic, and anaphylaxis has been reported. It also rapidly crystallizes; thus endoscopic instruments must be cleaned shortly after the procedure. Rare cases of pulmonary edema and coagulopathies from intravascular dextran have been reported. Carbon dioxide must be infused with special equipment that carefully limits flow to less than 100 ml per minute and maintains the pressure at approximately 60 to 70 mm Hg. The major precaution with 5% dextrose and water is the monitoring of total fluid intake so as not to produce water intoxication.

Diagnostic hysteroscopy is often performed as an office procedure. A local anesthetic is applied to the endocervix, or a paracervical block may be used. Vaginal misoprostol (prostaglandin E_1) has also been used to aid in the transcervical passage of the hysteroscope. Anxious patients may be pretreated with alprazolam, diazepam, and/or nonsteroidal antiinflammatory agents. If extensive resections

are anticipated via hysteroscopy, then the procedure is better performed on an outpatient basis in the surgical suite.

Hysteroscopy is ideal to directly visualize and remove partially perforated or broken IUDs. Women with repetitive abortions should have a diagnostic hysteroscopic procedure. Congenital abnormalities that interfere with the success of early pregnancies, such as septa of the uterus, may be seen (Figure 10-29). Women with recurrent abnormal uterine bleeding may also benefit from this procedure. Often endometrial polyps or small submucous myomas are discovered and may be removed. Women with persistent peri- or postmenopausal bleeding after a negative endometrial biopsy are also candidates for hysteroscopy. Focal lesions, particularly pedunculated structures, are frequently missed by endometrial biopsy or a D&C. The extent and location of the uterine synechiae are best described by hysteroscopic examination.

Hysteroscopy is superior to HSG in discovering intrauterine disease. In comparative studies the use of hysteroscopy revealed synechiae, polyps, or myomas in 40% of patients with normal HSGs (Figure 10-30). These abnormalities were undetected and unsuspected using x-ray techniques. The false positive rate of HSG is 33% when compared with hysteroscopy. One in three women

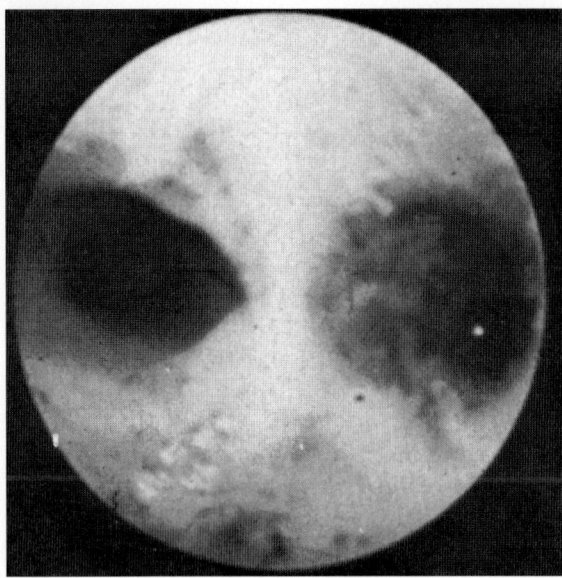

FIGURE 10-29 Intraoperative hysteroscopic view of septate uterus showing inferior point of septum and each uterine horn. (From Israel R and March CM: Am J Obstet Gynecol 149:67, 1984.)

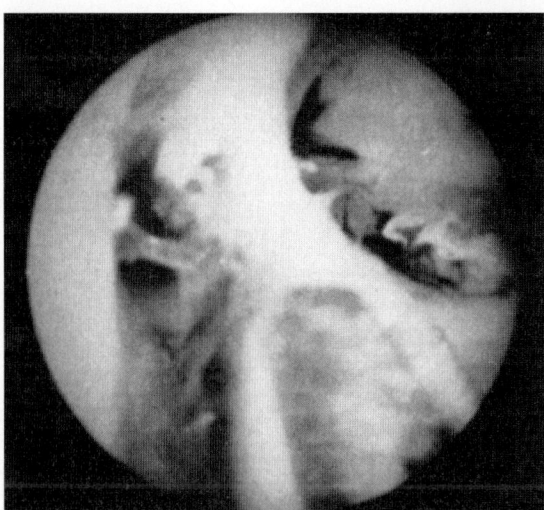

FIGURE 10-30 Hysteroscopic view of intrauterine adhesion in right lateral upper portion of uterus, partially occluding uterotubal junction. (From Valle RF and Sciarra JJ: Hysteroscopic treatment of intrauterine adhesions. In Siegler AM and Lindemann HJ, eds: Hysteroscopy: principles and practice, Philadelphia, 1984, JB Lippincott Co.)

diagnosed as having an intrauterine filling defect by x-ray imaging will have a normal cavity directly visualized with the hysteroscope.

The variety and extent of surgery performed transcervically with the hysteroscope have expanded significantly with technologic advances. Endoscopic procedures have progressed from snaring small polyps to ablating the entire endometrial lining.

Operative hysteroscopy may be performed with mechanical devices such as small operating scissors, electrocautery, and modified resectoscopes and lasers (Figure 10-31). Laser hysteroscopy with carbon dioxide or neodymium:yttrium-aluminum-garnet (Nd:YAG) lasers requires more expensive equipment and expertise. Laser hysteroscopy is less popular and less advantageous than simpler techniques.

The uterine synechiae of a woman with Asherman's syndrome can be cut with microscissors, reestablishing the endometrial cavity. Hysteroscopic metroplasty of intrauterine septa is safer with less complications than laparotomy.

Submucous myomas may be removed with a modified urologic resectoscope using a cutting electric current and shaving the myoma until it is flat with the surrounding endometrial lining. Often an inflatable balloon is inserted into the uterine cavity and left for 12 to 24 hours, facilitating hemostasis. The pregnancy rate is as good or better with hysteroscopic myomectomy versus transabdominal myomectomy.

One of the most popular techniques for endometrial ablation utilizes a roller ball, a wire loop electrode to coagulate and thus destroy the endometrium (Figure 10-32).

In women with abnormal bleeding or menorrhagia who are poor surgical candidates or who wish to preserve their uterus, the endometrial lining may be ablated through the hysteroscope. Lasers may also be used to produce ablation of the endometrium by photovaporizing the epithelium. The operative procedure using laser photovaporization takes longer than electrode resection, and the equipment is more expensive. Hysterograms following treatment have demonstrated contraction, scarring, and dense adhesion formation. Long-term follow-up has documented that endometrial carcinoma may develop in residual foci of endometrium.

Falloposcopy is an innovation using an extension of hysteroscopy. This technique is used to evaluate the lumen of the fallopian tubes by cannulation with a flexible microendoscope through the hysteroscope. Falloposcopy is not as painful to the patient as hysterosalpingography and potentially provides more information about the fallopian tubes in the infertile patient. Several investigators have found it helpful in restoring tubal patency in the case of proximal occlusions.

There are few contraindications to hysteroscopy. Acute pelvic infection is the leading one because of the potential of spreading the disease by the media used for uterine distention. Active bleeding is a relative contraindication. If the bleeding is brisk, the hysteroscopic procedure will be unsatisfactory. Pregnancy is a contraindication as is recent uterine perforation or cervical cancer.

Complications of hysteroscopy are noted in less than 2% of the procedures. Complications include uterine perforation, pelvic infection, bleeding, and fluid overload from absorption of distending media. The potential com-

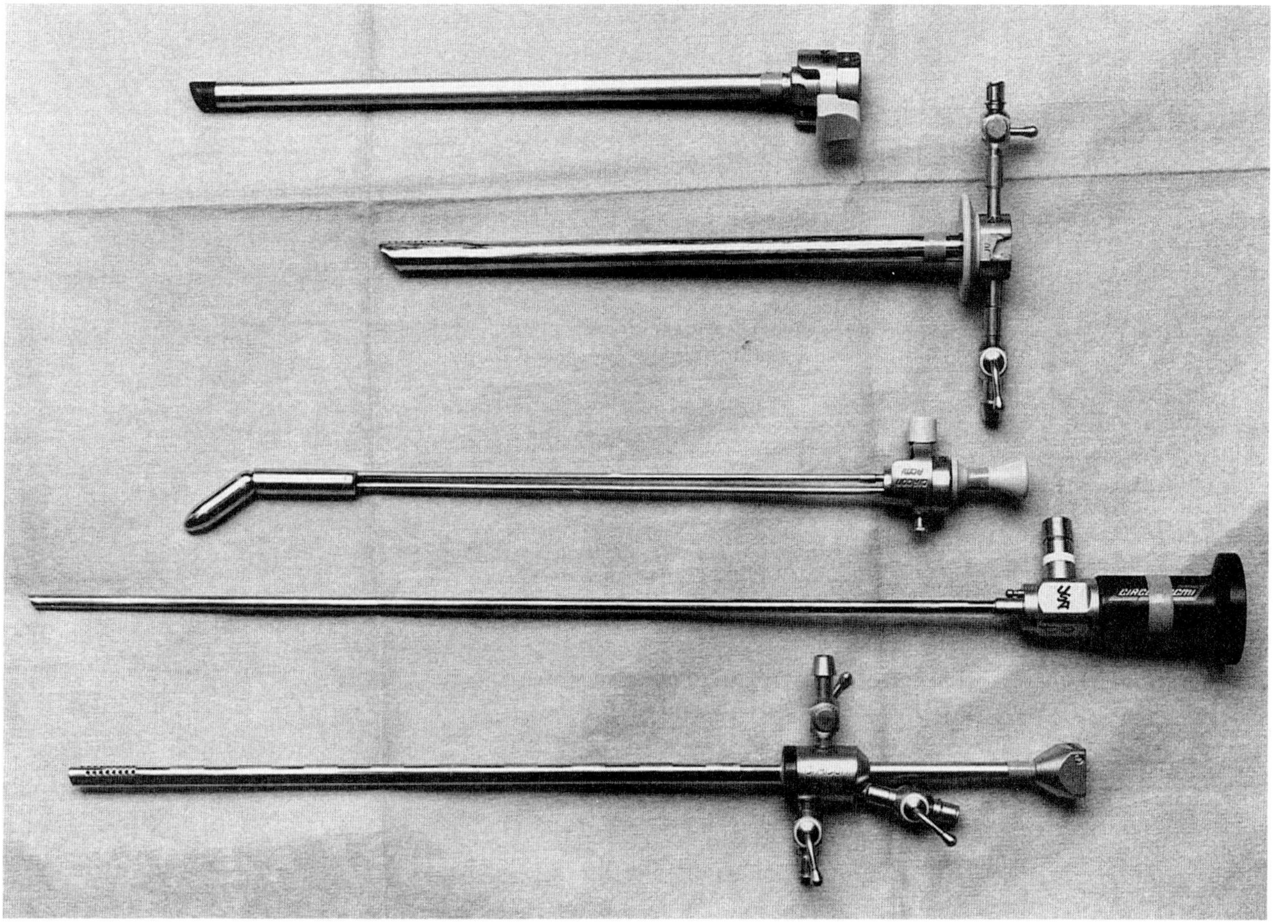

FIGURE 10-31   Operative hysteroscopic equipment.

plications of the distending media include anaphylaxis to dextran, circulatory overload with 5% dextrose and water, pulmonary edema, coagulopathies, hyponatremia, and the potential of gas embolism with carbon dioxide. Monitoring of the patient's fluid status is important because of problems with absorption of distending media, leading to volume overload and electrolyte imbalance. Cardiac arrests have been reported with uterine insufflation with carbon dioxide when unmonitored amounts of gas were used. Thermal injury to surrounding organs may occur with deep resections or perforations with the electrocautery instrument. If injury or perforation is suspected during hysteroscopy, then intraperitoneal evaluation should be performed either by laparoscopy or celiotomy.

In summary, hysteroscopy is a simple technique for the diagnosis and treatment of intrauterine pathology. The indications for intrauterine surgery via the hysteroscope are expanding. Operative hysteroscopic costs vary and depend on the time involved and the specific procedure performed.

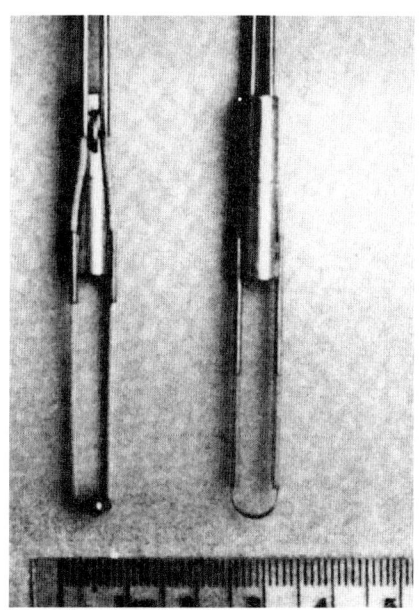

FIGURE 10-32   Ball-end and loop electrodes, side by side. Ball-end electrode is 2 mm in diameter and the loop, 7 mm. (From Vancaillie TG: Obstet Gynecol 74:425, 1989.)

LAPAROSCOPY

Laparoscopy has radically changed the clinical practice of gynecology over the past 30 years. This outpatient surgical technique provides a window to directly visualize pelvic anatomy as well as a technique to perform many operations with less morbidity than laparotomy.

Laparoscopy was first performed in the early 1900s. Two events of the early 1960s renewed interest in this surgical technique, the first being the development of fiberoptic cables and the second the change in society's attitude toward sterilization procedures. Patrick Steptoe is considered the "father" of modern laparoscopy for his work in the mid-1960s with laparoscopic sterilization. By the mid-1970s laparoscopy had been adopted as the method of choice for female sterilization.

The advantages of low cost, convenience, and shorter stay are obvious when laparoscopy is compared with celiotomy (laparotomy). Minilaparotomy in an extremely thin woman may be competitive in time and cost to laparoscopy. However, if a woman is moderately obese, there is no comparison. Postoperative recovery time and the need for hospitalization time are also significantly less when compared with celiotomy. Laparoscopic visualization is excellent because the video camera and endoscope magnify the image.

There are multiple indications for laparoscopy, both diagnostic and therapeutic. The most common indication is female sterilization. Laparoscopy is an essential step in the diagnostic workup of a couple with infertility or a woman with chronic pelvic pain. In the past decade, gynecologists have progressed from using the laparoscope to perform such simple surgical tasks as tubal ligation to more complicated surgery, such as removal of ectopic pregnancies, and treatment of endometriosis, hysterectomy, node dissections, and urogynecologic procedures. The present indications for operative laparoscopy are almost identical to celiotomy.

Laparoscopy has made outpatient sterilization available to women throughout the world. Cumulative 10-year pregnancy rates vary between 8/1000 and 37/1000. Sterilization is accomplished with electric cauterization, or spring-loaded clips. Because of the serious complications with unipolar cautery, most cautery sterilization procedures are performed with bipolar coagulation of approximately 2 cm of the tube without division (Figure 10-33). The clip should be placed on the narrow isthmus so the size of the appliance conforms to the diameter of the fallopian tube (Figure 10-34).

There are both diagnostic and therapeutic indications for laparoscopy in infertile women. Tubal patency and mobility can be directly observed via the laparoscope (Figure 10-35). Laparoscopy is able to confirm or rule out intrinsic pelvic disorders, such as endometriosis or chronic pelvic inflammatory disease. It is possible not only to describe and stage the extent of endometriosis or pelvic adhesions but also to treat them. Adhesions can be lysed, and areas of endometriosis can be ablated by electrocautery or laser.

The management of a patient with pelvic pain has been dramatically changed by the laparoscope. The differential diagnosis of acute pain may be defined by direct visualization of the fallopian tubes, ovaries, and appendix. Several centers include laparoscopy in the management of acute pelvic infection, taking direct bacterial cultures of purulent material from the tubes. These direct transabdominal cultures have changed our opinions concerning the clinical management of polymicrobial pelvic infections. The enigma of chronic pelvic pain may be solved by the findings at laparoscopy and "pain mapping" (Figure 10-36). Following the procedure, a plan for long-term management of the pain can be discussed with the patient.

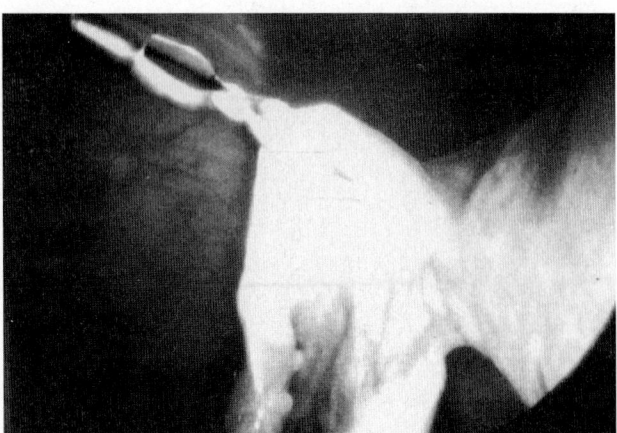

FIGURE 10-33 Laparoscopic view of bipolar coagulation. Kleppinger bipolar forceps has been used to coagulate isthmic-ampullary junction of this tube in three contiguous places. (From Hulka JF: Textbook of laparoscopy, Orlando, Fla, 1985, Grune & Stratton, Inc.)

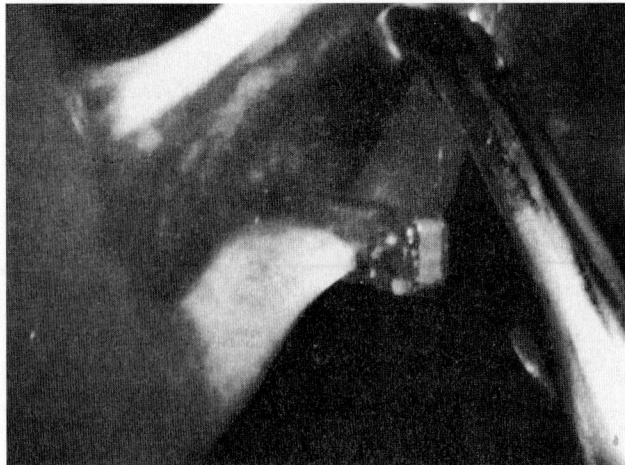

FIGURE 10-34 Laparoscopic view of clip application. Clip has been correctly applied within 1 to 2 cm of uterine fundus. (From Hulka JF: Textbook of laparoscopy, Orlando, Fla, 1985, Grune & Stratton, Inc.)

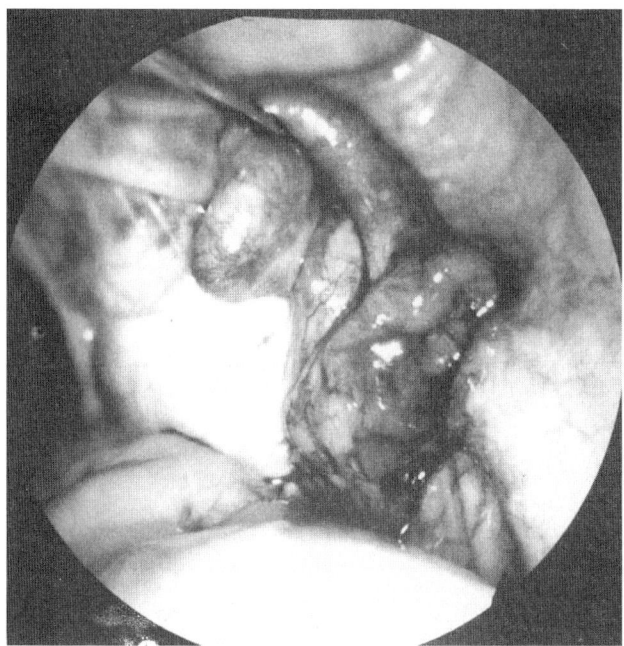

FIGURE 10-35 Laparoscopic view of normal patent tube. (From Hulka JF: Textbook of laparoscopy, Orlando, Fla, 1985, Grune & Stratton, Inc.)

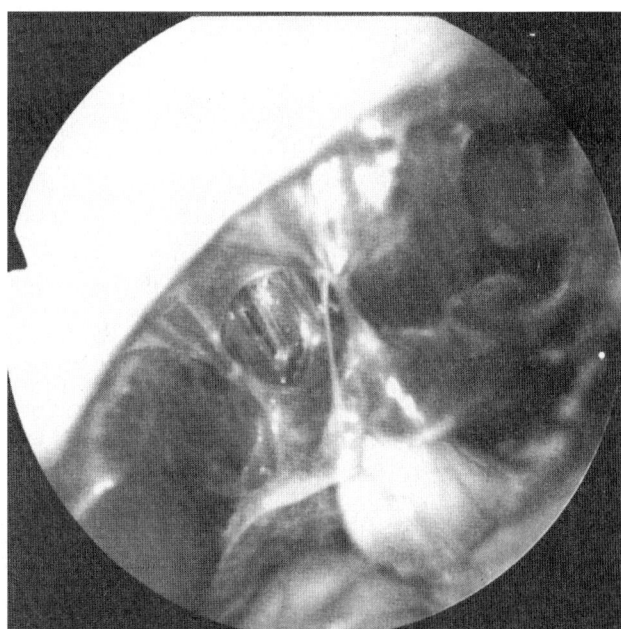

FIGURE 10-36 Laparoscopic view of Fitz-Hugh Curtis syndrome. (From Hulka JF: Textbook of laparoscopy, Orlando, Fla, 1985, Grune & Stratton, Inc.)

The laparoscope is utilized for numerous other therapeutic indications (Figure 10-37). Intraperitoneal intrauterine devices are best retrieved with the laparoscope. Laparoscopic ovarian biopsy (for karyotyping in certain endocrine disorders) is possible. Lysis of adhesions, removal of ectopic pregnancies, and treatment of endometriosis are most frequently performed through the laparoscope. The laparoscope may be used to transform an abdominal hysterectomy into a vaginal hysterectomy, laparoscopically assisted vaginal hysterectomy to sample lymph nodes, and to perform retropubic bladder suspensions. The limits and indications of surgical procedures via the laparoscope depend on the experience and judgment of the gynecologist. At some point, celiotomy is the more reasonable decision. We believe that a procedure should be performed through the laparoscope only if the gynecologist is prepared for the complications that might arise if that procedure were performed through a celiotomy.

Absolute contraindications to laparoscopy include intestinal obstruction, hemoperitoneum that produces hemodynamic instability, anticoagulation therapy, severe cardiovascular disease, and tuberculous peritonitis. Relative contraindications, in which each case must be individualized, include extensive obesity, large hiatal hernia, advanced malignancy, generalized peritonitis, and extensive intraabdominal scarring.

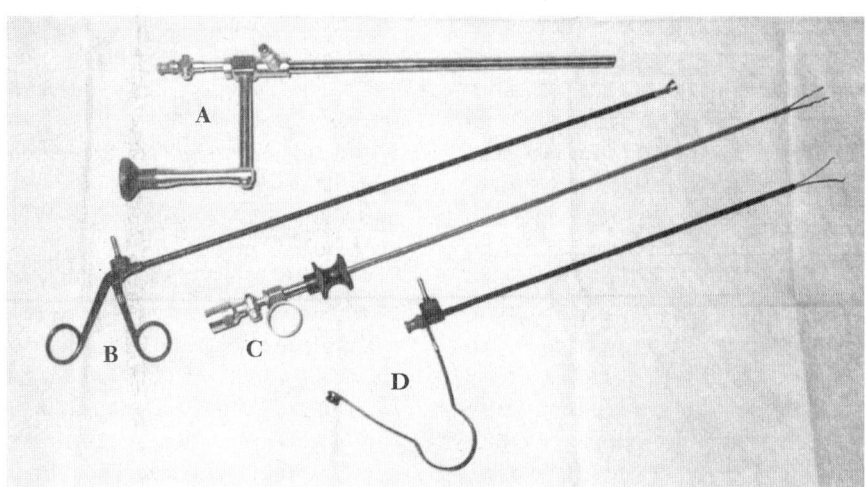

FIGURE 10-37   **A,** Operating laparoscope with instruments: **B,** scissors; **C,** cautery; and **D,** forceps.

Laparoscopy may be performed under local, regional, or general anesthesia. Many prefer local anesthesia for its safety, with the addition of conscious sedation by intravenous medication. The risks associated with general anesthesia are one of the major hazards of laparoscopy. However, when operative laparoscopy is contemplated, general anesthesia is recommended. As Gomel has summarized, the requirements of operative laparoscopy include general anesthesia to ensure adequate muscle relaxation, patient comfort, and the ability to manipulate intraabdominal organs. The standard diagnostic laparoscope is 10 mm in diameter. Secondary puncture trochars vary from 5 mm (bipolar forceps), 7 or 8 mm in width (spring-loaded clip and Silastic band), to 10 mm for pouches to remove specimens. Newer "mini" and "micro" laparoscopes used primarily for diagnostic evaluation are as small as 2 mm in diameter. Most laparoscopes are 30 cm long and provide a field of vision of 60 to 75 degrees. The inferior margin of the umbilicus is the preferred site of entry, as this is the thinnest area of the abdominal wall. Alternative sites are detailed in Figure 10-38. The choice of gas to develop the pneumoperitoneum depends on the choice of anesthesia. Nitrous oxide is preferable with local anesthesia, while carbon dioxide is the choice with general anesthesia. Nitrous oxide is nonflammable but does support combustion. Carbon dioxide quickly forms carbonic acid on the moist parietal peritoneal surface, which results in considerable discomfort to a patient without regional or general anesthesia.

Operative laparoscopy may be performed with mechanical instruments, including an extensive variety of scissors, scalpels, endoscopic syringes, manipulators, suture devices, electrocautery instruments (both unipolar and bipolar), suction, irrigation, and laser instruments. During operative laparoscopy, stabilization of the pelvic organs is essential, such as traction on the edges of an adhesion. Thus third and fourth puncture sites are often required. Because each puncture site is a potential gas leak, high-flow insufflation equipment is necessary. In addition, video cameras are employed so that both the surgeon and assistant can work effectively. Unlike the short time needed for diagnostic laparoscopy, operative laparoscopy may require several hours. Advantages of operative laparoscopy over celiotomy include decreased postoperative adhesion formation, decreased postoperative pain, shorter recovery time, and less, if any, hospital stay.

Laparoscopic treatment of ectopic pregnancy most often involves salpingotomy but also may include salpingectomy or an intra-ectopic injection of methotrexate. HCG titers must be followed after conservative surgery until the titers fall to zero (usually 3 to 4 weeks) to ensure that all trophoblastic tissue has been removed. Tubal patency and subsequent pregnancy rates are comparable between laparoscopic techniques and celiotomy. Laparoscopic treatment of endometriosis includes lysis of adhesions, ablation of endometriomas, and removal of endome-

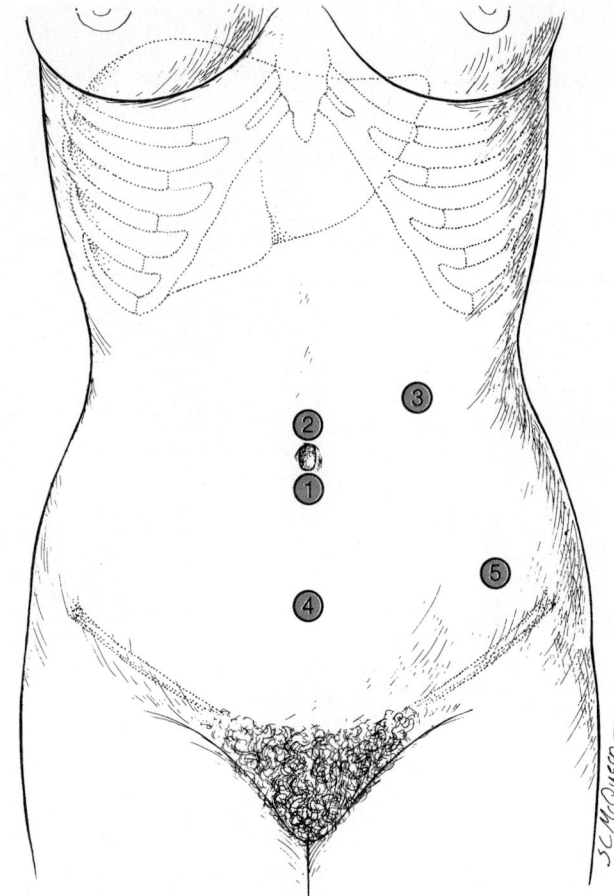

FIGURE 10-38 Usual sites for insertion of insufflating needle in laparoscopy: (1) infraumbilical fold, (2) supraumbilical fold, (3) left costal margin, (4) midway between umbilicus and pubis, and (5) left McBurney's point. (From Corson SL: Operating room preparation and basic techniques. In Phillips JM, ed: Laparoscopy. Copyright 1977 by the Williams & Wilkins Co, Baltimore.)

trial cysts. Operative laparoscopy has been used for myomectomy, ovarian biopsy and wedge resection assisted hysterectomy, salpingo-oophorectomy, salpingostomy and fimbrioplasty, appendectomy, uterosacral ligament ligation, presacral neurectomy, and urogynecologic procedures. The laparoscopic management of ovarian neoplasms is controversial.

The major categories of complications with laparoscopy are laceration of vessels, intestinal and urinary tract injuries, and cardiorespiratory problems arising from the pneumoperitoneum. Since abdominal wall hematomas are usually subfascial in location, care must be taken to avoid the epigastric vessels. For safety, Hurd et al. have recommended that lateral trochars be placed at least 5 cm above the symphysis and at least 8 cm from the midline. Laceration of the aorta, inferior vena cava, or iliac vessels is a surgical emergency. Intestinal injuries may be produced by the Veress needle or the trochar. Complications increase with the age of the patient and the complexity of

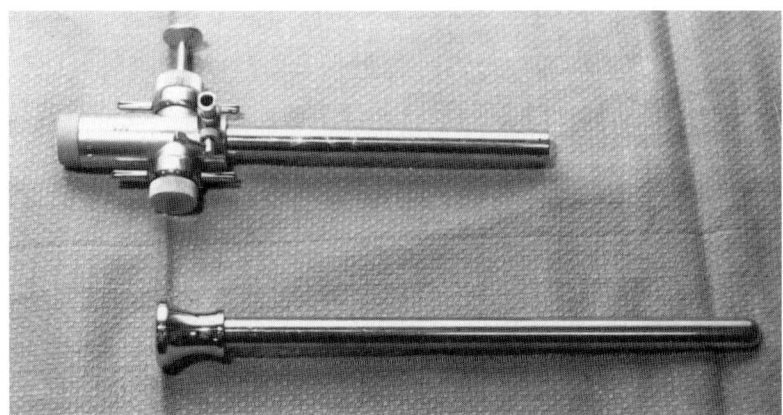

FIGURE 10-39   Open laparoscopy cannula and trochar *(bottom)*. Note blunt end of trochar.

the procedure. Several studies have evaluated the incidence of complications with operative laparoscopy. The incidence of ureteral injuries vary from 1% to 4% with laparoscopic dissection of the cardinal ligaments. The overall rate of complications from large series of operative laparoscopy varies from 0.2% to 2%.

Hasson has advocated open laparoscopy to avoid intestinal injury (Figure 10-39). Instead of blind entry into the peritoneal cavity, a small incision is made in the fascia and parietal peritoneum. The cone is placed in the abdominal cavity under direct visual control. The fascia is secured to the sleeve of the cone to obtain an airtight seal. Open laparoscopy reduces the incidence of both bowel and vascular trauma. It is the procedure of choice if the patient has a history of multiple abdominal operations.

Complications directly related to the pneumoperitoneum include pneumothorax, diminished venous return, gas embolism, and cardiac arrhythmias. It is important not to develop pressures greater than 20 mm Hg in establishing the pneumoperitoneum. High pressures impede venous return and limit excursion of the diaphragm. A rare but life-threatening complication of laparoscopy is gas embolism, which produces hypotension and the classical "mill wheel" murmur, which can be heard over the entire precordium. The patient with this complication should be turned on her left side and the frothy blood aspirated by a central venous catheter directed into the right side of the heart. Other rare complications include incisional hernias at the site of the 10-mm scope. This has been estimated to occur in 1 in 5000 procedures. Metastases from ovarian malignancies to the laparoscopic wound site are also a rare but real problem.

In summary, laparoscopy, more than any other advance, has changed the clinical practice of gynecology over the past 3.5 decades. Today's residents have a difficult time contemplating the practice of the specialty prior to the introduction of the "silver tube." Laparoscopy provides a window for the diagnosis of infertility, pelvic pain, ectopic pregnancy, abdominal and pelvic trauma, staging the extent of pelvic disease, and the visual diagnosis of abnormal anatomy. Therapeutic uses of the laparoscope vary from female sterilization to hysterectomy and node sampling.

KEY POINTS

- Measurement of diastolic and systolic velocities by Doppler ultrasound provide indirect indices of vascular resistance. Muscular arteries have high resistance. Newly developed vessels, such as those arising in malignancies, have little vascular wall musculature and thus have low resistance.

- Advantages of ultrasound include the real time nature of the image, the absence of radiation, the ability to perform the procedure in the office during or immediately after a pelvic examination, and the ability to describe the findings to the patient while she is watching.

- Sonography has not been found to cause adverse clinical effects in humans with the energy levels used in diagnostic studies.

- Several sonographic characteristics of pelvic masses correlate with malignancy including septations; internal papillations—echogenic structures protruding into the mass; loculations; solid lesions; cystic lesions with solid components; and smaller cysts adjacent to or part of the wall of the larger cyst—daughter cysts.

- Ultrasound evaluation of endometrial pathology involves measurement of the endometrial thickness or stripe. The normal endometrial thickness is 4 mm or less in a postmenopausal woman not taking hormones.

- An intrauterine pregnancy should be routinely visualized by endometrial ultrasound by 5 weeks after the last normal menstrual period.

- Helical CT is a modification of standard CT that uses movement of the patient combined with rotation of several x-ray registers in a spiraling fashion. Vascular images are of a high enough quality that in many centers, helical CT has replaced pulmonary angiography and ventilation-perfusion scans.

- Computed tomography (CT) is useful in discovering extension of pelvic cancer into the fat of the retroperitoneal space and the detection of enlarged lymph nodes.

- CT is the most accurate imaging modality in the diagnosis of appendicitis.

- The surface radiation dose from CT scan is between 2 and 10 rads. This radiation exposure is similar to that of a barium enema. Helical CT allows for variations of the radiation dose.

- Magnetic resonance imaging (MR) penetrates bone and air without attenuation. Therefore this technique allows identification of soft tissue disease inaccessible to other imaging techniques.

- Unlike x-ray, where a tissue density determines the nature of the image, in MR the inherent type of tissue determines the nature of the image.

- MR has the capacity to differentiate normal from malignant tissue and also may identify areas of abnormal tissue metabolism.

- MR uses radio frequency radiation, which is nonionizing radiation.

- Techniques to alleviate the anxiety associated with MR include prescan education programs, music by earphones, antianxiety medications, hypnosis, relaxation techniques, and the presence of family members.

- MR should not be used in patients with cochlear implants or pacemakers. It is safe in women with IUDs, including ones containing copper, and safe in patients with surgical clips and staples. Advantages of MR over CT include the use of non–iodine-based contrast material and the ability to obtain images in multiple planes.

- The most frequent problem in performing endometrial sampling is cervical stenosis or spasm.

- Complications following endometrial biopsy are exceedingly rare. The major complication is uterine perforation, with an incidence of 1 to 2 per 1000.

- The diagnostic accuracy of endometrial biopsy is approximately 95% when compared with subsequent findings at hysterectomy.

- Fifteen percent of women who have obstructed fallopian tubes, as determined by hysterosalpingography (HSG), subsequently become pregnant without further treatment.

- The leading indications for HSG are primary and secondary infertility. This imaging technique gives evidence of endometrial irregularities, tubal patency, tubal mobility, and sometimes peritubal disease.

- Acute pelvic infection develops in 0.3% to 3.1% of patients following HSG. As with any surgical procedure that invades the uterus, pelvic pain, uterine perforation, and vasovagal vasomotor reactions do occur. Allergic reactions, particularly to the iodine dye, are a possibility.

- Major indications for diagnostic hysteroscopy include abnormal uterine bleeding, infertility, and recurrent pregnancy loss.

- Operative hysteroscopy may be used to remove polyps, myomas, and synechiae. The endometrial lining may be ablated through the hysteroscope in women with abnormal bleeding or menorrhagia who are poor surgical candidates or who wish to retain their uterus.

- Dextran is an extremely viscous fluid used to distend the uterus during hysteroscopy. Dextran is nontoxic, nonconductive, and immiscible with blood.

- Hysteroscopy is superior to hysterosalpingography in discovering and diagnosing intrauterine pathology.

- Complications of hysteroscopy include uterine perforation, pelvic infection, bleeding, and absorption of the distending media.

- There are both diagnostic and therapeutic indications for laparoscopy in infertile women. Tubal patency and mobility can be directly observed via the laparoscope. It is possible not only to describe and stage the extent of endometriosis or pelvic adhesions but also to treat them. Adhesions can be lysed, and areas of endometriosis can be ablated by electrocautery or laser.

- The enigma of chronic pelvic pain may be solved by the findings at laparoscopy and "pain mapping." Following the procedure, a plan for long-term management of the pain can be discussed with the patient.

- Absolute contraindications to laparoscopy include hemoperitoneum that has produced hemodynamic instability, anticoagulation therapy, advanced malignancy, large abdominal masses, severe cardiovascular disease, and tuberculous peritonitis.

- Patients with ectopic pregnancies treated by laparoscopic salpingotomy should have serial human chorionic gonadotrophin titers until the titers fall to zero.

- Major complications of laparoscopy are laceration of vessels, intestinal and urinary tract injuries, and cardiorespiratory problems arising from the pneumoperitoneum.

- The incidence of complications with operative laparoscopy varies from 0.2% to 2%.

- Laparoscopy provides a window for the diagnosis of infertility, pelvic pain, ectopic pregnancy, abdominal and pelvic trauma, staging the extent of pelvic disease, and the visual diagnosis of abnormal anatomy. Therapeutic uses of the laparoscope vary from female sterilization to hysterectomy and node sampling.

BIBLIOGRAPHY

American College of Obstetricians and Gynecologists: Hysteroscopy, ACOG Tech Bull 191:1, 1994.

American College of Obstetricians and Gynecologists: Operative laparoscopy, ACOG Educ Bull 239:1, 1997.

Auslender R, Bornstein J, Dirnfeld M, et al: Vaginal ultrasonography in patients with postmenopausal bleeding, Ultrasound Obstet Gynecol 3:426, 1993.

Baggish MS, Barbot J, and Valle RF: Diagnostic and operative hysteroscopy: a text and atlas, ed 2, Chicago, 1999, Mosby–Year Book, Inc.

Bateman BG, Kolp LA, and Hoeger K: Complications of laparoscopy—operative and diagnostic, Fertil Steril 66:30, 1996.

Birkett DH: Three-dimensional laparoscopy, J Laparoendosc Surg 5:327, 1995.

Blumenfeld Z, Yoffe N, and Bronshtein M: Transvaginal sonography in infertility and assisted reproduction, Obstet Gynecol Surv 46:36, 1991.

Boike GM, Elfstrand EP, DelPriore G, et al: Laparoscopically assisted vaginal hysterectomy in a university hospital: report of 82 cases and comparison with abdominal and vaginal hysterectomy, Am J Obstet Gynecol 168:1690, 1993.

Brooks PG: Hysteroscopic surgery using the resectoscope: myomas, ablation, septae and synechiae: does pre-operative medication help? Clin Obstet Gynecol 35:249, 1992.

Brooks SE: Preoperative evaluation of patients with suspected ovarian cancer, Gynecol Oncol 55:S80, 1994.

Cacciatore B, Ramsay T, Lehtovirta P, and Ylostalo P: Transvaginal sonography and hysteroscopy in postmenopausal bleeding, Acta Obstet Gynecol Scand 73:413, 1994.

Carlson JA Jr, Arger P, Thompson S, et al: Clinical and pathologic correlation of endometrial cavity fluid detected by ultrasound in the postmenopausal patient, Obstet Gynecol 77:119, 1991.

Carter J, Saltzman A, Hartenbach E, et al: Flow characteristics in benign and malignant gynecologic tumors using transvaginal color flow Doppler, Obstet Gynecol 83:125, 1994.

Castelbaum AJ, Wheeler J, Coutifaris CB, et al: Timing of the endometrial biopsy may be critical for the accurate diagnosis of luteal phase deficiency, Fertil Steril 61:443, 1994.

Chambers JT and Chambers SK: Endometrial sampling: when? where? why? with what? Clin Obstet Gynecol 35:28, 1992.

Chang YCF, Hricak H, Thurnher S, et al: Vagina: evaluation with MR imaging. Part II. Neoplasms, Radiology 169:175, 1988.

Check JH, Chase JS, Nowroozi K, et al: Clinical evaluation of the Pipelle endometrial suction curette for timed endometrial biopsies, J Reprod Med 34:218, 1989.

Chen SS, Rumancik WM, and Spiegel G: Magnetic resonance imaging in stage I endometrial carcinoma, Obstet Gynecol 75:274, 1990.

Childers JM, Aqua KA, Surwit EA, et al: Abdominal-wall tumor implantation after laparoscopy for malignant conditions, Obstet Gynecol 84:765, 1994.

Cooper JM: Hysteroscopic sterilization, Clin Obstet Gynecol 35:282, 1992.

Cooper JM and Brady RM: Hysteroscopy in the management of abnormal uterine bleeding, Obstet Gynecol Clin North Am 26:217, 1999.

Corson SL, Brooks PG, and Soderstrom RM: Gynecologic endoscopic gas embolism, Fertil Steril 65:529, 1996.

Daly DC, Maier D, and Soto-Albors C: Hysteroscopic metroplasty: six years' experience, Obstet Gynecol 73:201, 1989.

Daniel AG and Peters WA III: Accuracy of office and operating room curettage in the grading of endometrial carcinoma, Obstet Gynecol 71:612, 1988.

Daniel JF, Kurtz BR, and Ke RW: Hysteroscopic endometrial ablation using the rollerball electrode, Obstet Gynecol 80:329, 1992.

Diamond MP, Lavy G, and DeCherney AH: Hysteroscopic use of dextran 70, Contemp Obstet Gynecol, 30:29, 1989.

Dijkhuizen FPHLJ, Brölmann HAM, Potters AE, et al: The accuracy of transvaginal ultrasonography in the diagnosis of endometrial abnormalities, Obstet Gynecol 87:345, 1996.

Dunphy B, Taenzer P, Bultz B, et al: A comparison of pain experienced during hysterosalpingography and in-office falloposcopy, Fertil Steril 62:67, 1994.

Duppler DW: Laparoscopic instrumentation, videoimaging, and equipment disinfection and sterilization, Surg Clin North Am 72:1021, 1992.

Edelman RR and Warach S: Magnetic resonance imaging. Part I. N Engl J Med 328:708, 1993.

Edelman RR and Warach S: Magnetic resonance imaging. Part II. N Engl J Med 328:785, 1993.

Eltabbakh GH, Piver MS, Hempling RE, and Recio FO: Laparoscopic surgery in obese women, Obstet Gynecol 94:704, 1999.

Emanuel MH, Verdel MJ, Wamsteker K, and Lammes FB: A prospective comparison of transvaginal ultrasonography and diagnostic hysteroscopy in the evaluation of patients with abnormal uterine bleeding: clinical implications, Am J Obstet Gynecol 172:547, 1995.

Feldman S, Shapter A, Welch WR, and Berkowitz RS: Two-year follow-up of 263 patients with post/perimenopausal vaginal bleeding and negative initial biopsy, Gynecol Oncol 55:56, 1994.

Finikiotis G: Hysteroscopy: a review, Obstet Gynecol Surv 49:273, 1994.

Forstner R, Chen M, and Hricak H: Imaging of ovarian cancer, JMRI 5:606, 1995.

Gleeson NC, Nicosia SV, Mark JE, et al: Abdominal wall metastases from ovarian cancer after laparoscopy, Am J Obstet Gynecol 169:522, 1993.

Goldstein SR: Postmenopausal endometrial fluid collections revisited: look at the doughnut rather than the hole, Obstet Gynecol 83:738, 1994.

Goldstein SR: Saline infusion sonohysterography, Clin Obstet Gynecol 39:248, 1996.

Goldstein SR: Sonohysterography as an office procedure, Contemp Obstet Gynecol 40:9, 1995.

Gomel V: Operative laparoscopy: time for acceptance, Fertil Steril 52:1, 1989.

Goodman SB, Rein MS, and Hill JA: Hysterosalpingography contrast media and chromotubation dye inhibit peritoneal lymphocyte and macrophage function in vitro: a potential mechanism for fertility enhancement, Fertil Steril 59:1022, 1993.

Goodrich MA, Webb MJ, King BF, et al: Magnetic resonance imaging of pelvic floor relaxation: dynamic analysis and evaluation of patients before and after surgical repair, Obstet Gynecol 82:883, 1993.

Grimes DA: Diagnostic dilation and curettage: a reappraisal, Am J Obstet Gynecol 142:1, 1982.

Hardacre JM and Talamini MA: Pulmonary and hemodynamic changes during laparoscopy—are they important? Surg 127:241, 2000.

Härkki-Siren P, Sjöberg J, and Kurki T: Major complications of laparoscopy: a follow-up Finnish study, Obstet Gynecol 94:94, 1999.

Honoré GM, Holden AEC, and Schenken RS: Pathophysiology and management of proximal tubal blockage, Fertil Steril 71:785, 1999.

Hricak H, Chen M, Coakley FV, et al: Complex adnexal masses: detection and characterization with MR imaging—multivariate analysis, Radiol 214:39, 2000.

Hricak H, Quivey JM, Campos Z, et al: Carcinoma of the cervix: predictive value of clinical and magnetic resonance (MR) imaging assessment of prognostic factors, Int J Radiat Oncol Biol Phys 27:791, 1993.

Hulka JF: Textbook of laparoscopy, Philadelphia, Pa, 1998, WB Saunders Co.

Hurd WW, Bude RO, DeLancey JOL, and Newman JS: The location of abdominal wall blood vessels in relationship to abdominal landmarks apparent at laparoscopy, Am J Obstet Gynecol 171:642, 1994.

Hutchins CJ: Laparoscopy and hysterosalpingography in the assessment of tubal patency, Obstet Gynecol 49:325, 1977.

Israel R and March CM: Hysteroscopic incision of the septate uterus, Am J Obstet Gynecol 149:66, 1984.

Istre O, Skajaa K, Schjoensby AP, and Forman A: Changes in serum electrolytes after transcervical resection of endometrium and submucous fibroids with use of glycine 1.5% for uterine irrigation, Obstet Gynecol 80:218, 1992.

Karande VC, Pratt DE, Rabin DS, and Gleicher N: The limited value of hysterosalpingography in assessing tubal status and fertility potential, Fertil Steril 63:1167, 1995.

Karlan BY and Platt LD: The current status of ultrasound and color Doppler imaging in screening for ovarian cancer, Gynecol Oncol 55:S28, 1994.

Karlsson B, Granberg S, Wikland M, et al: Transvaginal ultrasonography of the endometrium in women with postmenopausal bleeding—a Nordic multicenter study, Am J Obstet Gynecol 172:1488, 1995.

Keltz MD, Olive DL, Kim AH, and Arici A: Sonohysterography for screening in recurrent pregnancy loss, Fertil Steril 67:670, 1997.

Kinkel K, Kaji Y, Yu KK, et al: Radiologic staging in patients with endometrial cancer: a meta-analysis, Radiol 212:711, 1999.

Kurjak A, Shalan H, Kupesic S, et al: An attempt to screen asymptomatic women for ovarian and endometrial cancer with transvaginal color and pulsed Doppler sonography, J Ultrasound Med 13:295, 1994.

Langer RD, Pierce JJ, O'Hanlan KA, et al: Transvaginal ultrasonography compared with endometrial biopsy for the detection of endometrial disease, N Engl J Med 337:1792, 1997.

Leonard F, Lecuru F, Rizk E, et al: Perioperative morbidity of gynecological laparoscopy: A prospective monocenter observational study, Acta Obstet Gynaecol Scand 79:129, 2000.

Levine D: Gynaecologic ultrasound, Clin Radiol 53:1, 1998.

Lindequist S, Rasmussen F, Torp HH, et al: Diagnostic quality in hysterosalpingography: comparison between iodixanol and iotrolan, Acta Radiologica 39:730, 1998.

Maly Z, Riss P, and Deutinger J: Localization of blood vessels and qualitative assessment of blood flow in ovarian tumors, Obstet Gynecol 85:33, 1995.

March CM: Hysterectomy, J Reprod Med 37:293, 1992.

Maruri F and Azziz R: Laparoscopic surgery for ectopic pregnancies: technology assessment and public health implications, Fertil Steril 59:487, 1993.

Mayo-Smith WW and Lee MJ: MR imaging of the female pelvis, Clin Radiol 50:667, 1995.

McBean JH, Gibson M, and Brumsted JR: The association of intrauterine filling defects on hysterosalpingogram with endometriosis, Fertil Steril 66:522, 1996.

McCall JL, Sharples K, and Jadallah F: Systematic review of randomized controlled trials comparing laparoscopic with open appendectomy, Br J Surg 84:1045, 1997.

McGonigle KF, Shaw SL, Vasilev SA, et al: Abnormalities detected on transvaginal ultrasonography in tamoxifen-treated postmenopausal breast cancer patients may represent endometrial cystic atrophy, Am J Obstet Gynecol 178:1145, 1998.

McLucas B: Hyskon complications of hysteroscopic surgery, Obstet Gynecol Surv 46:196, 1991.

Meléndez JC and McCrank E: Anxiety-related reactions associated with magnetic resonance imaging examinations, JAMA 270:745, 1993.

Mirhashemi R, Harlow BL, Ginsburg ES, et al: Predicting risk of complications with gynecologic laparoscopic surgery, Obstet Gynecol 92:327, 1998.

Moldofsky PJ, Sears HF, Mulhern CB, et al: Detection of metastatic tumor in normal-sized retroperitoneal lymph nodes by monoclonal-antibody imaging, N Engl J Med 311:106, 1984.

Montz FJ, Holschneider CH, and Munro MG: Incisional hernia following laparoscopy: a survey of the American Association of Gynecologic Laparoscopists, Obstet Gynecol 84:881, 1994.

Mouton WG, Bessell JR, Otten KT, and Maddern GJ: Pain after laparoscopy, Surg Endosc 13:445, 1999.

Nelson BE, Rosenfield AT, and Schwartz PE: Preoperative abdominopelvic computed tomographic prediction of optimal cytoreductin in epithelial ovarian carcinoma, J Clin Oncol 11:166, 1993.

Nelson RC, Chezmar JL, Hoes MJ, et al: Peritoneal carcinomatosis: preoperative CA with intraperitoneal contrast material, Radiology 182:133, 1992.

Neuwirth RS: Hysteroscopic management of symptomatic submucous fibroids, Obstet Gynecol 62:509, 1983.

Nunley WC Jr, Bateman BG, Kitchin JD III, et al: Intravasation during hysterosalpingography using oil-base contrast medium—a second look, Obstet Gynecol 70:309, 1987.

Nurenberg P and Twickler DM: Magnetic resonance imaging in obstetrics and gynecology. In Cunningham FG, MacDonald PC, Gant NF, et al, eds: Williams Obstetrics Supplement, ed 19, Norwalk, Conn, 1995, Appleton & Lange.

O'Connell LP, Fries MH, Zeringue E, and Brehm W: Triage of abnormal postmenopausal bleeding: a comparison of endometrial biopsy and transvaginal sonohysterography versus fractional curettage with hysteroscopy, Am J Obstet Gynecol 178:956, 1998.

Occhipinti KA, Frankel SD, and Hricak H: The ovary: computed tomography and magnetic resonance imaging, Radiol Clin North Am 31:1115, 1993.

Pabuccu R, Atay V, Orhon E, et al: Hysteroscopic treatment of intrauterine adhesions is safe and effective in the restoration of normal menstruation and fertility, Fertil Steril 68:1141, 1997.

Patel VH and Somers S: MR imaging of the female pelvis: current perspective and review of genital tract congenital anomalies, and benign and malignant diseases, Crit Rev Diagn Imaging 36:417, 1997.

Peisner DB: Equipment selection, Clin Obstet Gynecol 39:158, 1996.

Pellerito JS, McCarthy SM, Doyle MB, et al: Diagnosis of uterine anomalies: relative accuracy of MR imaging, endovaginal sonography, and hysterosalpingography, Radiology 183:795, 1992.

Pennehouat G, Risquez F, Naouri M, et al: Transcervical falloposcopy: preliminary experience, Hum Reprod 8:445, 1993.

Perdigon PL: Imaging techniques for diagnosis of serious intraabdominal and pelvic infections, Prim Care Update Ob/Gyn 6:115, 1999.

Peterson HB, Xia Z, Hughes JM, et al: The risk of pregnancy after tubal sterilization: findings from U.S. Collaborative Review of Sterilization, Am J Obstet Gynecol 174:1161, 1996.

Porpora MG and Gomel V: The role of laparoscopy in the management of pelvic pain in women of reproductive age, Fertil Steril 68:765, 1997.

Preutthipan S and Herabutya Y: A randomized controlled trial of vaginal misoprostol for cervical priming before hysteroscopy, Obstet Gynecol 94:427, 1999.

Prömpeler HJ, Madjar H, Sauerbrei W, et al: Diagnostic formula for the differentiation of adnexal tumors by transvaginal sonography, Obstet Gynecol 89, 428, 1997.

Rabin JM, Spitzer M, Dwyer AT, et al: Topical anesthesia for gynecologic procedures, Obstet Gynecol 73:1040, 1989.

Rao PM, Feltmate CM, Rhea JT, et al: Helical computed tomography in differentiating appendicitis and acute gynecologic conditions, Obstet Gynecol 93:417, 1999.

Rasmussen F, Lindequist S, Larsen C, and Justesen P: Therapeutic effect of hysterosalpingography: oil- versus water-soluble contrast media—a randomized prospective study, Radiology 179:75, 1991.

Rock JA and Warshaw JR: The history and future of operative laparoscopy, Am J Obstet Gynecol 170:7, 1994.

Romano F, Cicinelli E, Anastasio PS, et al: Sonohysterography versus hysteroscopy for diagnosing endouterine abnormalities in fertile women, Int J Gynecol Obstet 45:253, 1994.

Rumack CM, Wilson SR, and Charboneau JW, eds: Diagnostic Ultrasound, Vol. 1 & 2, ed 2, St. Louis, 1998, Mosby–Year Book, Inc.

Schutter EMJ, Kenemans P, Sohn C, et al: Diagnostic value of pelvic examination, ultrasound, and serum CA 125 in postmenopausal women with a pelvic mass, Cancer 74:1398, 1994.

Shalev E, Yarom I, Bustan M, et al: Transvaginal sonography as the ultimate diagnostic tool for the management of ectopic pregnancy: experience with 840 cases, Fertil Steril 69, 62, 1998.

Sironi S, Colombo E, Villa G, et al: Myometrial invasion by endometrial carcinoma: assessment with plain and gadolinium-enhanced MR imaging, Radiology 185:207, 1992.

Sladkevicius P, Valentin L, and Marsál K: Endometrial thickness and Doppler velocimetry of the uterine arteries as discriminators of endometrial status in women with postmenopausal bleeding: a comparative study, Am J Obstet Gynecol 171:722, 1994.

Smith DC, Donohue LR, and Waszak SJ: A hospital review of advanced gynecologic endoscopic procedures, Am J Obstet Gynecol 170:1635, 1994.

Spreafico C, Frigerlo L, Lanocita R, et al: Color-Doppler ultrasound in ovarian masses: anatomo-pathologic correlation, Tumori 79:262, 1993.

Spring DB, Barkan HE, and Pruyn SC: Potential therapeutic effects of contrast materials in hysterosalpingography: a prospective randomized clinical trial, Radiol 214:53, 2000.

Stovall TG and Ling FW, eds: Atlas of benign gynecologic and obstetric surgery, 1995, Philadelphia, Mosby-Wolfe.

Stovall TG, Solomon SK, and Ling FW: Endometrial sampling prior to hysterectomy, Obstet Gynecol 73:405, 1989.

Suh-Burgmann EJ and Goodman A: Surveillance for endometrial cancer in women receiving tamoxifen, Ann Intern Med 131:127, 1999.

Sultana CJ, Easley K, and Collins RL: Outcome of laparoscopic versus traditional surgery for ectopic pregnancies, Fertil Steril 57:285, 1992.

Swart P, Mol BWJ, van der Veen F, et al: The accuracy of hysterosalpingography in the diagnosis of tubal pathology: a meta-analysis, Fertil Steril 64:486, 1995.

Swayne LC, Love MB, and Karasick SR: Pelvic inflammatory disease: sonographic-pathologic correlation, Radiology 151:751, 1984.

Tahir MM, Bigrigg MA, Browning JJ, et al: A randomized controlled trial comparing transvaginal ultrasound, outpatient hysteroscopy and endometrial biopsy with inpatient hysteroscopy and curettage, Br J Obstet Gynaecol 106:1259, 1999.

Timbos-Kemper TCM and Veering BT: Anaphylactic shock from intracavitary 32% dextran-70 during hysteroscopy, Fertil Steril 51:1053, 1989.

Togashi K, Nishimura K, Sagoh T, et al: Carcinoma of the cervix: staging with MR imaging, Radiology 171:245, 1989.

Troiano RN and McCarthy S: Magnetic resonance imaging evaluation of adnexal masses, Semin Ultrasound CT MR 15:38, 1994.

Tulandi T and Bugnah M: Operative laparoscopy: surgical modalities, Fertil Steril 63:237, 1995.

Valle RF: Office hysteroscopy, Clin Obstet Gynecol 42:276, 1999.

Valle RF and Sciarra JJ: Intrauterine adhesions: hysteroscopic diagnosis, classification, treatment, and reproductive outcome, Am J Obstet Gynecol 158:1459, 1988.

Van Den Bosch T, Vandendael A, Van Schoubroeck D, et al: Combining vaginal ultrasonography and office endometrial sampling in the diagnosis of endometrial disease in postmenopausal women, Obstet Gynecol 85:349, 1995.

Venezia R, Zangara C, Knight C, and Cittadini E: Initial experience of a new linear everting falloposcopy system in comparison with hysterosalpingography, Fertil Steril 60:771, 1993.

Vercellini P, Rossi R, Pagnoni B, and Fedele L: Hypervolemic pulmonary edema and severe coagulopathy after intrauterine dextran instillation, Obstet Gynecol 79:838, 1992.

Wagner BJ and Woodward PJ: Magnetic resonance evaluation of congenital uterine anomalies, Semin Ultrasound CT MR 15:4, 1994.

Watson A, Vandekerckhove P, Lilford R, et al: A meta-analysis of the therapeutic role of oil soluble contrast media at hysterosalpingography: a surprising result? Fertil Steril 61:470, 1994.

Wieser F, Kurz C, Wenzl R, et al: Atraumatic cervical passage at outpatient hysteroscopy, Fertil Steril 69:549, 1998.

Witz CA, Silverberg KM, Burns WN, et al: Complications associated with the absorption of hysteroscopic fluid media, Fertil Steril 60:745, 1993.

Woodward PJ and Gilfeather M: Magnetic resonance imaging of the female pelvis, Semin Ultrasound, CT, MRI 19:90, 1998.

Worthington JL, Balfe DM, Lee JKT, et al: Uterine neoplasms: MR imaging, Radiology 159:725, 1986.

Wortman M: A guide to hysteroscopic endomyometrial resection, Contemp Obstet Gynecol Dec:61, 1994.

Wortman M and Daggett A: Hysteroscopic endomyometrial resection: a new technique for the treatment of menorrhagia, Obstet Gynecol 83:295, 1994.

Yaziciogulu HF: A clear hysteroscopic view and the use of other diagnostic modalities in addition to hysteroscopy to achieve better diagnostic accuracy, Am J Obstet Gynecol 176:950, 1997.

Zanetta G, Vergani P, and Lissoni A: Color Doppler ultrasound in the preoperative assessment of adnexal masses, Acta Obstet Gynecol Scand 73:637, 1994.

Zupi E, Luciano AA, Valli E, et al: The use of topical anesthesia in diagnostic hysteroscopy and endometrial biopsy, Fertil Steril 63:414, 1995.

PART THREE

General Gynecology

Congenital Abnormalities of the Female Reproductive Tract

Anomalies of the Vagina, Cervix, Uterus, and Adnexa

KEY TERMS AND DEFINITIONS

Accessory Ovary. Excess ovarian tissue near a normally placed ovary and connected to it.

Ambiguous Genitalia. Anatomic modification of the external genitalia, which makes specific determination of gender difficult.

Androgen Resistance Syndrome. An X-linked condition of a testosterone receptor defect in a 46,XY individual with testes and normal male testosterone levels. These individuals have absent uterus, normal female phenotype, and scanty body hair.

Arcuate Uterus. A minimum septate uterus; probably of no clinical importance.

Bicornuate Uterus. A partial lack of fusion of two ßuterine corpora to varying degree. A single cervix is present.

Didelphic Uterus. Complete duplication of the uterus and cervix without fusion of the two cavities. One fallopian tube joins each fundal cavity. This condition may be associated with a septate vagina.

Hematocolpos. Distention of an obstructed vagina (caused by imperforate hymen or transverse septum) with blood and blood products.

Hydrocolpos. Distention of an obstructed vagina (caused by imperforate hymen or transverse septum) with fluid.

Labial Fusion. Fusion of the labia minora in the midline, closing the introitus.

Mucocolpos. A vagina blocked by an imperforate hymen or transverse septum and filled with mucus.

Ovotestes. Gonads that contain both ovarian and testicular remnants.

Repetitive Spontaneous Abortion. The loss of three or more pregnancies before 20 weeks' gestation. Functionally, however, many physicians will do a workup for repetitive spontaneous abortion after two or more pregnancy losses.

Rokitansky-Küster-Hauser Syndrome. A 46,XX female with müllerian failure, usually showing absence of all or most of vagina, cervix, uterus, and fallopian tubes.

Rudimentary Uterine Horn. A structure that develops from one müllerian duct and does not communicate with the uterine cavity. The contralateral fallopian tube communicates with the uterine cavity. The ipsilateral fallopian tube communicates with that horn.

Septate Uterus. The presence of a septum that separates the uterine cavity either partially or completely into two separate cavities.

Supernumerary Ovary. The presence of a third ovary separated from the normally situated ovaries.

Unicolic (Unicornuate) Uterus. A uterus and cervix that develop from a single müllerian duct joined at the top of the fundus by only one fallopian tube. It represents complete arrest of one müllerian duct.

Vaginal Agenesis. Absence of the vagina.

Congenital abnormalities of the female reproductive tract can be caused by a genetic error or by a teratologic event during embryonic development. Minor abnormalities may be of little consequence, but major abnormalities may lead to severe impairment of menstrual and reproductive functions. This chapter categorizes a number of such abnormalities and discusses diagnosis and treatment. For discussion of the etiology of these problems, the reader is referred to Chapter 1.

EXAMINATION OF THE NEWBORN FOR SEXUAL AMBIGUITIES

The first major diagnostic decision of the obstetrician or neonatal physician with respect to the newborn is gender assignment. In most cases the designation is clear. However, in newborns with ambiguous genitalia there is a potentially serious problem for both physician and parents. The female who has been androgenized may appear similar to the male pseudo-hermaphrodite suffering from incomplete androgen resistance syndrome. Also, some vulvar abnormalities may resemble partial androgenization. It is therefore appropriate to systematically evaluate the newborn's genitalia to make the appropriate gender assignment.

The first and probably most important aspect of the examination is inspection. The physician should systematically observe the newborn's perineum, beginning with the mons pubis. The clitoris should be noted for any obvious enlargement, the opening of the urethra should be identified, and the labia should be separated to see if the introitus can be visualized. If the labia are fused, this maneuver will be impossible. At times the labia are joined by filmy adhesions; these generally separate in later childhood or respond to the application of estrogen cream. If it is possible to separate the labia, the hymen may be observed. Generally it is partially perforate, revealing the entrance into the vagina. Posteriorly the labia fuse in the midline at the posterior fourchette of the perineum. Posterior to the perineal body the rectum can be visualized, and it should be tested to be sure that it is perforate. Meconium staining about the rectum is evidence for perforation. If there is doubt, the rectum may be penetrated with a moistened cotton-tipped swab or, if necessary, with the little finger encased in a well-lubricated finger cot.

If the labia are fused and the clitoris is not enlarged, other abnormalities may also be present. For instance, defects of the anterior abdominal wall may exist as well. The infant should be carefully examined for other defects. An enlarged clitoris and fused labia are evidence of androgen effect and may imply congenital adrenal hyperplasia, maternal ingestion of androgens, or increased natural androgen production. A bifid clitoris may be present in and is usually associated with extrophy of the bladder. In such cases, anterior rotation and shortening of the vagina with fused labia are often also present.

In most instances, inspection is all that is necessary. If for any reason, however, the physician wishes to examine the vagina or see the cervix of the newborn, an endoscope, such as a pediatric cystoscope, may be used, since the hymen is generally perforate and will accept this instrument.

If labial fusion is noted, the physician should palpate the groins and labial folds for evidence of gonads. Gonads palpable in the inguinal canal, labioinguinal region, or labioscrotal folds are almost always testes. Thus such a finding implies a male with ambiguous genitalia rather than a virilized female. Conversely, an infant with ambiguous genitalia but without palpable testes in the scrotum is likely to be a virilized female, most often the result of congenital adrenal hyperplasia. Rectal examination may make it possible to palpate a cervix and uterus, thus helping in the sex assignment.

Where ambiguous genitalia are noted, further testing, such as chromosome analysis or buccal smear and blood or urinary studies for androgens and related enzymes, may be required. It is important to order these studies immediately, as gender assignment is an important event that should take place as soon after birth as possible.

SPECIFIC DEFECTS OF THE EXTERNAL AND INTERNAL GENITALIA

In the remaining sections of this chapter, specific defects of each level of the external and internal female genitalia will be discussed.

Perineal and Vaginal Defects

Defects of the Clitoris

The clitoris is generally 1 to 1.5 cm long and 0.5 cm wide in the nonerect state. The glans is partially covered by a hood of skin. The urethra opens near the base of the clitoris. Abnormalities are unusual, although the clitoris may be enlarged because of androgen stimulation. In such circumstances the shaft of the clitoris may be quite enlarged, and partial development of a penile urethra may have occurred. Extreme cases of androgen stimulation are generally associated with fusion of the labia. These findings occur in infants with congenital adrenal hyperplasia and in those exposed in utero to exogenous or endogenous androgens (Figure 11-1).

Bifid clitoris (Figure 11-2) is frequently seen in association with extrophy of the bladder. Extrophy of the bladder occurs rarely (1 per 30,000 births) and has a male predominance (3:1). However, when it occurs in females, it is often associated with bifid clitoris. Stanton noted that 43% of 70 female patients with bladder extrophy had associated reproductive tract anomalies. These included vaginal anomalies and müllerian duct fusion problems. In such cases, an anterior rotation and shortening of the vagina with labial fusion is quite common.

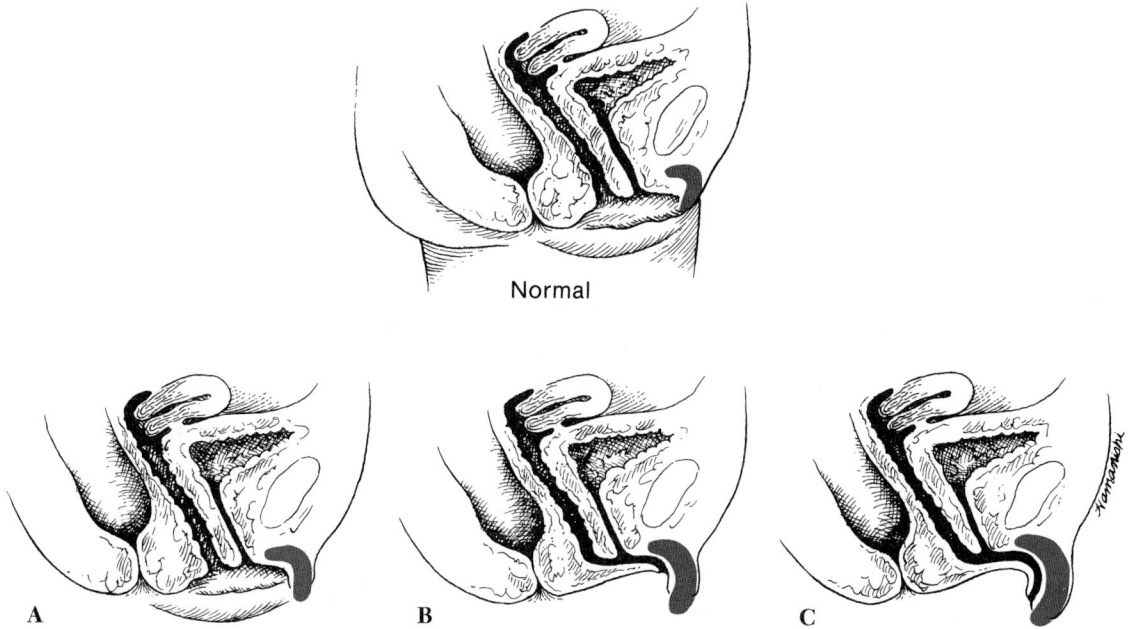

Normal

A   B   C

FIGURE 11-1 Sagittal views of genital deformities seen in female infants who are masculinized. **A,** Minimal masculinization with slight enlargement of the clitoris. **B,** Labial fusion and more marked enlargement of the clitoris. **C,** Complete labial fusion, enlargement of the clitoris, and formation of a partial penial urethra. (Modified from Verkauf BS and Jones HW Jr: South Med J 63:634, 1970.)

Labial Fusion

Although labial fusion may result from exposure to exogenous androgens or be associated with defects of the anterior abdominal wall, the most common cause is congenital adrenal hyperplasia. The most common form is caused by an inborn error of metabolism involving the enzyme 21-hydroxylase. This condition is transmitted as an autosomal recessive gene coded on chromosome 6, and because of the error in 21-hydroxylase metabolism, the major biosynthesis pathway to cortisol is diminished. Homozygous individuals occur at a rate of 1 per 490 to 1 per 67,000 of the population, depending on the community. Heterozygotic carriers are present in the population in a frequency ranging from 1 per 20 to 1 per 250.

The genetically mutated 21-hydroxylase enzyme interferes with cortisol production in such a fashion that plasma 17-hydroxyprogesterone levels are elevated. Two other enzyme defects also transmittable as autosomal recessive traits that may give similar abnormal findings are 11-hydroxylase deficiency and 3-β-hydroxysteroid dehydrogenase deficiency.

Congenital adrenal hyperplasia may be demonstrated at birth by the presence of ambiguous genitalia in genetic females (Figure 11-3). However, a significant proportion of newborns with this condition may develop a life-threatening adrenal crisis as a result of salt loss. Delayed diagnosis may result in accelerated bone maturation, leading ultimately to short stature. The development of premature secondary sexual characteristics in males and further virilization in females may also occur.

In 1977 Pang et al. described a reliable and valid screening test employing capillary blood obtained by heel prick of infants that allowed for the radioimmunoassay determination of 17-hydroxyprogesterone in the serum. This test has been used in screening newborns for 21-hydroxylase deficiency, particularly in known high-risk populations, such as Alaskan Eskimos. Using a 3 mm filter paper disk elution technique to study the presence of 17-hydroxyprogesterone in capillary blood of these day-old newborns, these authors determined levels in normal infants to be less than 40 pg/3 mm disk. Affected infants had 17-OHP levels of 57 to 980 pg/disk.

Treatment of congenital adrenal hyperplasia involves replacement cortisol. This suppresses adrenocorticotropic hormone (ACTH) output and therefore decreases the stimulation of the cortisol-producing pathways of the adrenal cortex.

Imperforate Hymen

The hymen represents the junction of the sinovaginal bulbs with the urogenital sinus and therefore is composed of endoderm from the urogenital sinus epithelium. Ordinarily the hymen is perforated during embryonic life to establish a connection between the lumen of the vaginal canal and the vestibule. If this perforation does not take place, the hymen is imperforate (Figure 11-4).

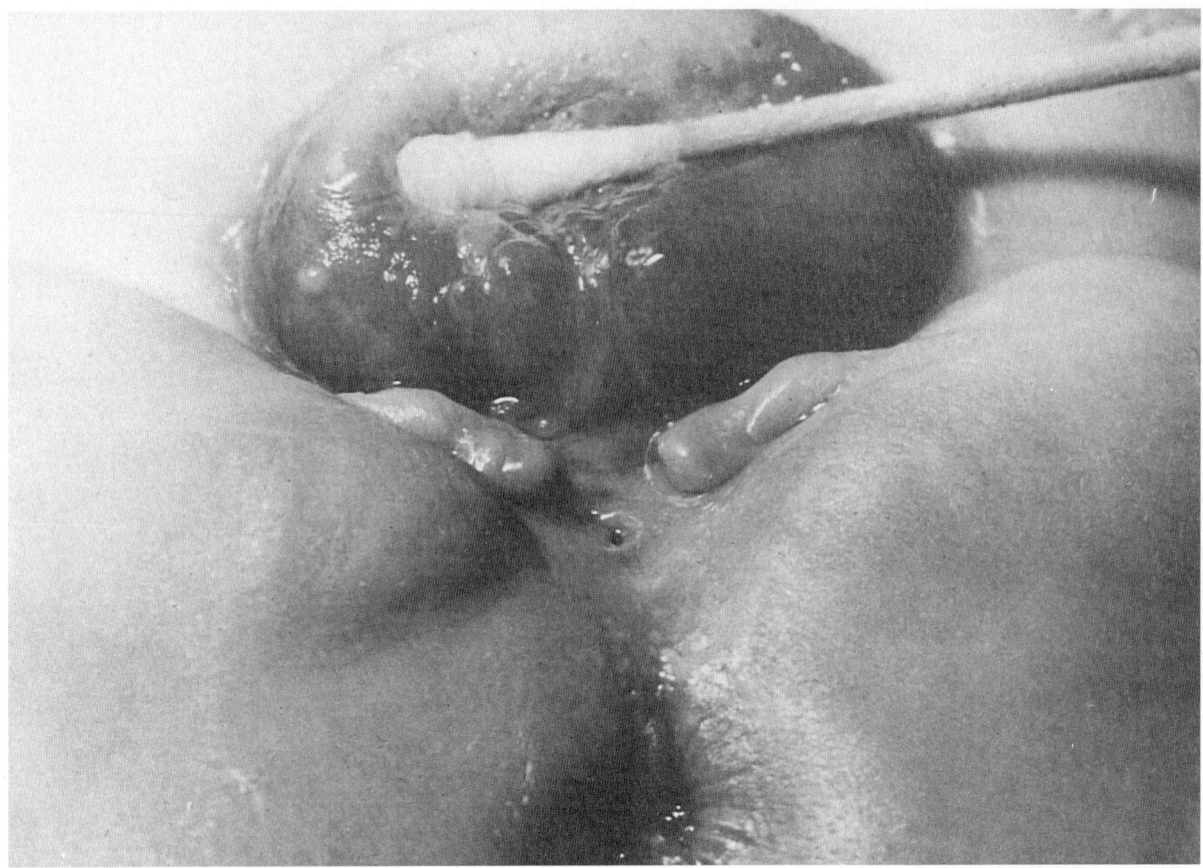

FIGURE 11-2 An example of a bifid clitoris in an infant with extrophy of the bladder. (Courtesy of Julian Ansell, M.D.)

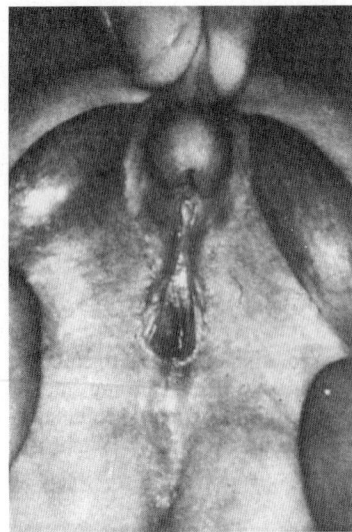

FIGURE 11-3 External genitalia of female with congenital adrenal hyperplasia showing clitoral enlargement and labial fusion. (From Jones HW Jr and Scott WW: Hermaphroditism, genital anomalies and related endocrine disorders, ed 2, Baltimore, 1971, Williams & Wilkins.)

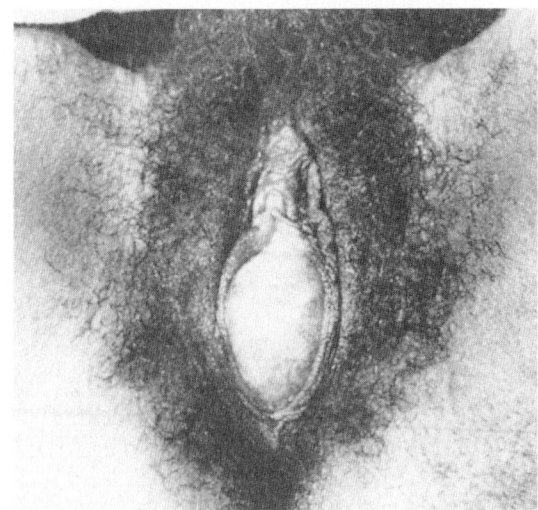

FIGURE 11-4 Imperforate hymen distended by hematocolpos. (From Baramki TA: J Reprod Med 29:376, 1984.)

It is rare to make the diagnosis of imperforate hymen before puberty, at which point primary amenorrhea is the major symptom. Occasionally in childhood a hydrocolpos or mucocolpos may occur. This is caused by a collection of secretions behind the hymen, which in rare cases may build up to form a mass that obstructs the urinary tract. If such is discovered, the hymen should be incised to release the build-up.

At puberty the patient may experience cyclic cramping but no menstrual flow. Over time the patient may develop a hematocolpos and a hematometrium. In more advanced cases the fallopian tubes may be distended with menstrual flow, and the flow may back up through the tubes and form endometrial implants in the peritoneal cavity. Quite surprisingly, many patients are free of symptoms.

The diagnosis can be determined by history and by the presence of a bulging membrane at the introitus. Therapy consists of a cruciate incision into the hymen extending to the 10, 2, and 6 o'clock positions. In dense hymens a triangular section may be excised, although this is rarely necessary. Hemostasis is secured by fine suture, and evolution to normal usually occurs rapidly.

Vaginal Agenesis

Vaginal agenesis is usually associated with the Rokitansky-Küster-Hauser syndrome (Figure 11-5). This syndrome is characterized by congenital absence of the vagina and uterus, although small masses of smooth muscular material resembling a rudimentary bicornuate uterus may be noted. These masses rarely have an epithelial lining and rarely menstruate, although occasionally this does occur, giving rise to monthly cyclic cramping. The ovaries are normal, and the fallopian tubes are usually present. Complete vaginal agenesis is discovered in 75% of patients with Rokitansky-Küster-Hauser syndrome. Approximately 25% of patients have a short vaginal pouch. These individuals have a 46,XX karyotype. The disorder seems to be an accident of development and not an inherited condition.

The androgen resistance syndrome with faulty androgen receptors (testicular feminization syndrome) demonstrates a 46,XY karyotype. While vaginal agenesis or the presence of a short pouch vagina is usually found, these patients have undescended testicles and male sex ducts. They usually exhibit minimal pubic hair after puberty. The testes should be removed after puberty to prevent the development of seminomas. The ovaries of the patient with Rokitansky-Küster-Hauser syndrome are normal and should not be removed.

Phelan et al. reported that of 72 patients with vaginal agenesis, 25% had urologic abnormalities noted on intravenous pyelography. A later study by Baramki demonstrated that 40% of 92 patients had urologic abnormalities. Further, Turunen and Unnerus found that 25 of 200 such patients had skeletal anomalies, usually involving congenital fusion or absence of vertebrae.

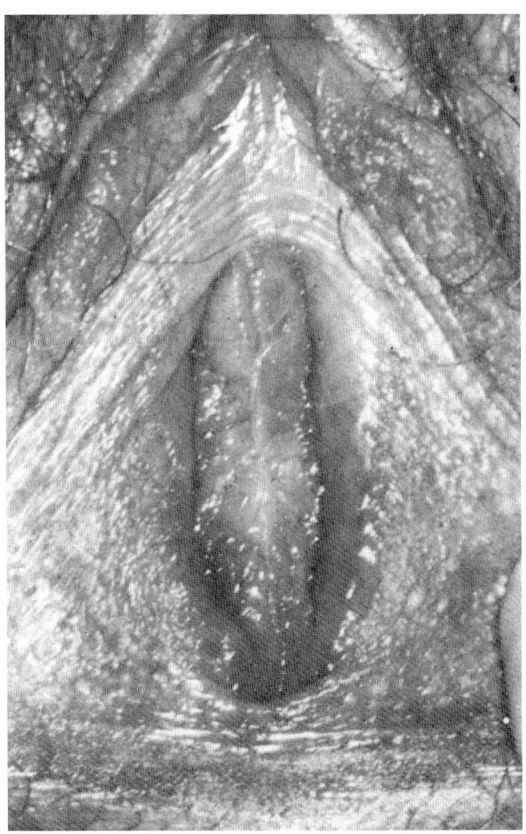

FIGURE 11-5 External genitalia of patient with congenital absence of vagina. (From Baramki TA: J Reprod Med 29:376, 1984.)

Diagnosis of Rokitansky-Küster-Hauser syndrome is demonstrated by the presence of primary amenorrhea at the time of puberty, physical examination that demonstrates the absence of a vaginal opening or the presence of a short vaginal pouch, and failure to palpate a uterus on rectal examination, coupled with the finding of a normal karyotype. Laparoscopic examination may be performed in cases where the diagnosis is not clear or where there is some concern over the presence of a functioning uterus. In most cases, however, laparoscopic diagnosis is not necessary. Ultrasound examination may verify the presence of normal ovaries and the absence of the uterus. Magnetic resonance imaging (MRI) offers an excellent alternative for visualizing congenital anomalies of the internal reproductive organs and may, in many instances, replace laparoscopy and other forms of imaging. Basal body temperature curves and serial progesterone determinations may also be used to verify ovarian function.

Therapy involves the creation of a vagina when the patient wishes to become sexually active. There are several therapeutic choices. The first, which is time consuming but nonsurgical, requires the use of progressive vaginal dilators. This can be accomplished in a well-motivated patient over a period of several months, and functioning vaginas have been achieved in many patients in this manner.

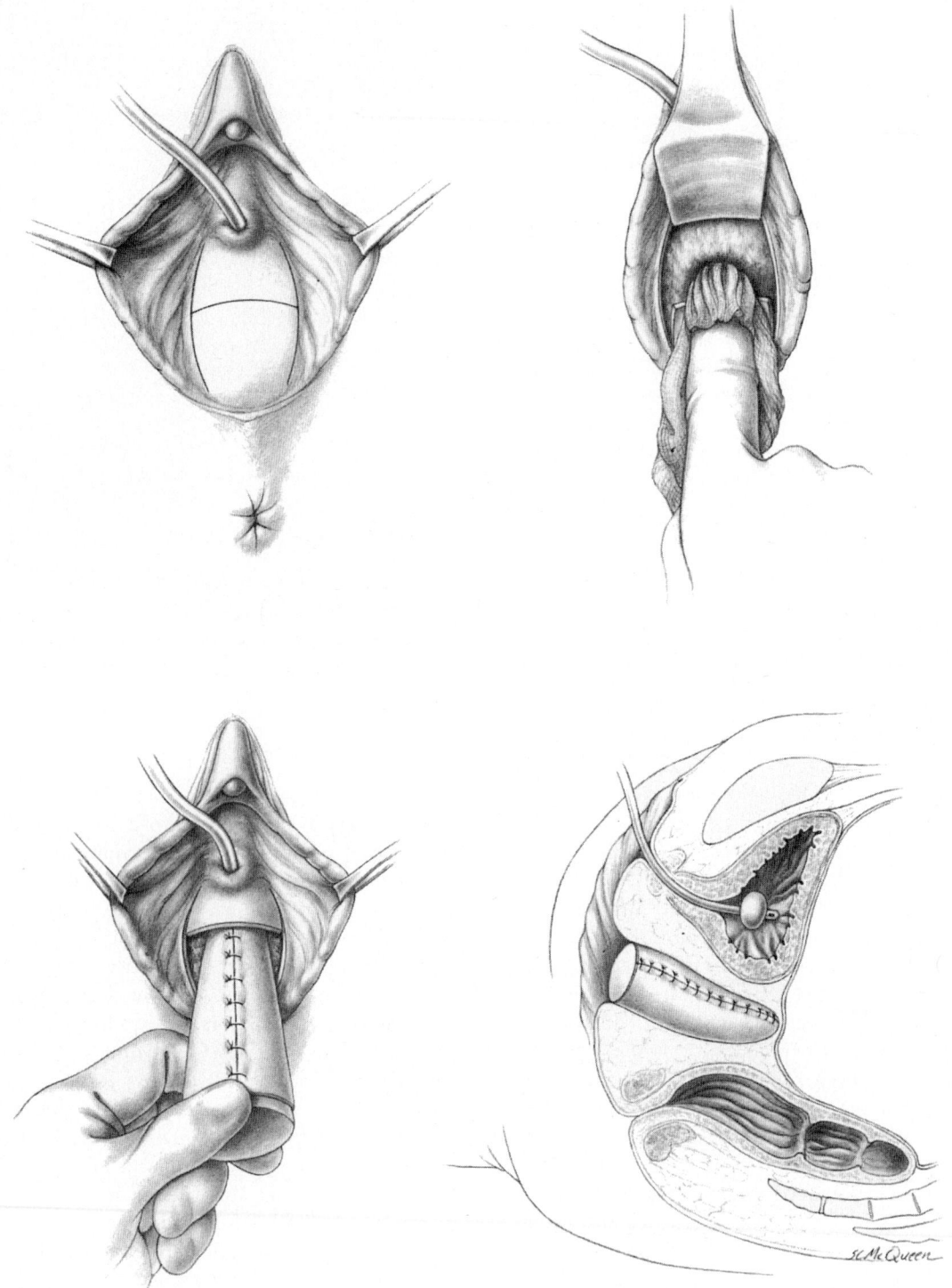

FIGURE 11-6 Construction of vagina (McIndoe-type operation) by means of split-thickness skin graft. (Modified from Durfee RB: Congenital anomalies of female genital tract. In Benson RC, editor: Current obstetric and gynecologic diagnosis and treatment, Los Altos, Calif, 1984, Lange Medical Publishers.)

Using the concept of vaginal dilators, Ingram has devised a useful technique. He used three sets of Lucite dilators. The first set contains 10 that are 1.5 cm in diameter and that increase in length from 1.5 to 10 cm; the second set contains 5 that are 2.5 cm in diameter and that increase in length from 3 to 10 cm; and the third set has 8 dilators, 3.5 cm in diameter and from 3 to 10 cm long. A racing bicycle seat is mounted on a stool and is used to maintain dilator pressure on the introital dimple just posterior to the urethra. The patient holds the dilators in place with a pad or girdle and works through the three sets in progressive fashion, considering length and width as tolerated. The bicycle seat allows continuing pressure against the dilator; pressure is continued for 15 to 30 minutes at a time for a total of at least 2 hours a day. The patient may read or do other activities while sitting. It generally takes 4 to 6 months to develop an adequate neovagina by this technique.

Surgical reconstruction of the vagina has evolved over the years. Each operation has for the most part developed the potential space between the bladder and the rectum and replaced this space with a stent utilizing tissue such as large bowel, small bowel, amniotic membranes, or a split-thickness skin graft (Figure 11-6). The latter procedure, developed by McIndoe, is easy to perform but must be done only when the patient will use the vagina frequently. If she does not and she fails to leave a plastic mold in place, the neovagina will frequently shrivel, scar, and become nonfunctional. Möbus et al. reported that in 24 patients who had undergone operative development of a neovagina, 20 of the 24 were found to be leading a healthy sexual life with unimpaired emotional and sexual responsiveness. They stressed that early and regular postoperative coitus was important for long-term success and was superior to the wearing of a stent. Thus the timing of the operation to coincide with the opportunity for coitus is important.

An alternate procedure has been devised by Williams. This procedure utilizes labial skin and results in a vaginal pouch whose axis is directly posterior. Although it is not as anatomically similar to a normal vagina as is the result of the McIndoe procedure, it does produce a functioning vaginal pouch and is well received by patients; eventually a normal vaginal axis is reported to develop.

Vecchietti has developed a laparoscopic procedure for producing a neovagina. Sutures are placed laparoscopically in the peritoneal fold between bladder and rudimentary uterus. A cutting edge needle then perforates the pseudohymen and an olive is attached to the suture and pulled tightly against the perineum. The sutures (2) are then fixed to a traction device on the anterior abdominal wall and graduated traction applied for 6 to 8 days. The olive is then removed and the patient uses vaginal dilators until sexual intercourse begins 10 to 15 days later. Several authors, including Vecchietti, have reported good success with this procedure.

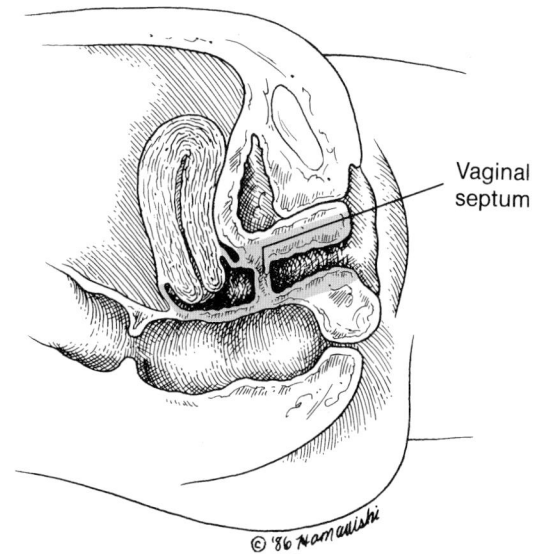

FIGURE 11-7　Diagram of transverse vaginal septum.

Transverse Vaginal Septum

The müllerian ducts join the sinovaginal bulb at a point known as the *müllerian tubercle*. Canalization of the müllerian tubercle and sinovaginal bulb is necessary to give a normal vaginal lumen. If the area of junction between these structures is not completely canalized, a transverse vaginal septum will occur (Figure 11-7). This may be partial or complete and generally lies at the junction of the upper third and lower two thirds of the vagina (Figure 11-8). It occurs in about 1 per 75,000 females. Partial transverse vaginal septa have been reported in diethylstilbestrol (DES)-exposed females (Chapter 15). In the prepubertal state, diagnosis is generally not made unless there is the development of a mucocolpos or mucometrium behind the septum. In such a case an unexplained abdominal mass forms. At puberty, however, if the septum is complete, hematocolpos and hematometrium may occur in a fashion similar to that seen in the imperforate hymen, except that there is no bulging at the introitus. The patient complains of primary amenorrhea with cyclic cramping. The patient with an incomplete transverse septum may bleed somewhat but will still develop hematocolpos and hematometrium over time and may also complain of foul-smelling vaginal discharge.

The septum is usually thin, generally less than 1 cm thick. If an opening is noted, it may be expanded by manual dilation or simple incision, with suturing of the edges of the vagina on either side. Occasionally the septum is thick, and the two areas of the vagina are quite distantly separated. In such a case excision may require the implantation of a split-thickness skin graft in a fashion similar to the McIndoe procedure.

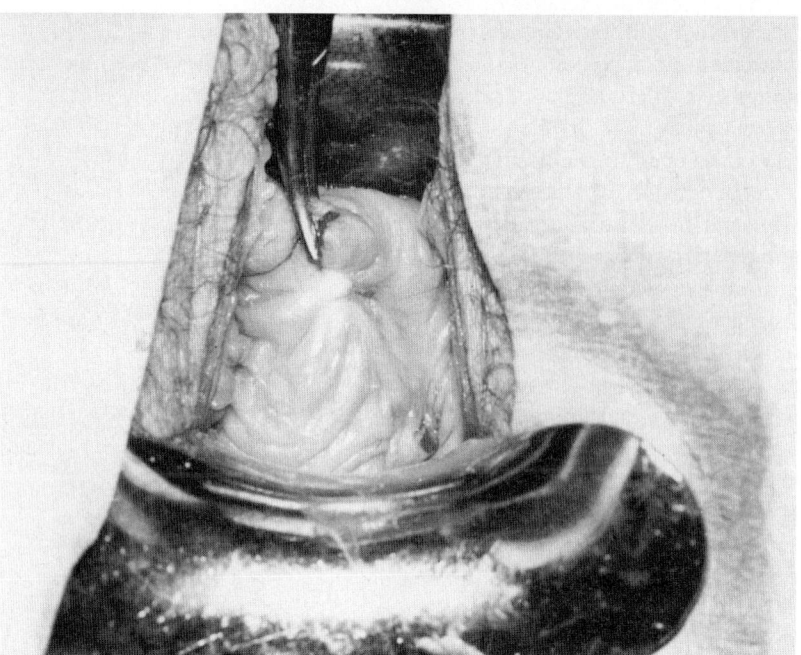

FIGURE 11-8   Patient with complete transverse vaginal septum.

Longitudinal septa of the vagina will be discussed with duplication of the uterus and cervix.

Vaginal Adenosis

In the female exposed to DES in utero the junction between the müllerian ducts and the sinovaginal bulb may not be sharply demonstrated. If müllerian elements invade the sinovaginal bulb, remnants may remain as areas of adenosis in the adult vagina. They are generally palpated submucosally, although they may be observable at the surface. These anomalies are discussed more fully in Chapter 15.

Abnormalities of the Cervix and Uterus

Embryologic Considerations

Between the third and fifth weeks of gestation the metanephric ducts develop and join the cloaca. By the fifth week two ureteric buds develop from the mesonephric ducts close to the distal ends. These grow cephalad toward the mesonephric mass. The müllerian or paramesonephric duct forms from a cleft between the mesonephros and the forming gonad. These ducts are bilateral and grow caudally just lateral to and intimately associated with the mesonephric ducts. The fate of these various elements is therefore closely entwined. Damage to one usually affects the others. The paramesonephric ducts grow caudally, meet in the midline, and descend into the pelvis, reaching the urogenital sinus at an elevation known as the *müllerian tubercle*.

Musset analyzed 133 cases of genitourinary malformation and described a three-stage process for fusion of the two müllerian ducts into the uterus and cervix. The first stage is described as short, taking place at the beginning of the tenth week. The medial aspect of the more caudal portions of the two ducts fuse, starting in the middle and proceeding simultaneously in both directions. In this way a median septum is formed. The second stage continues from the tenth to the thirteenth week and occurs because of a rapid cell proliferation and the filling in of the triangular space between the two uterine cornua. In this way a thick upper median septum is formed. This is wedgelike and gives rise to the usual external contour of the fundus. At the same time the lower portion of the median septum is resorbed, unifying the cervical canal first and then the upper vagina. The third stage lasts from the thirteenth to about the twentieth week. In this stage the degeneration of the upper uterine septum occurs, starting at the isthmic region and proceeding cranially up to the top of the fundus. In this way a unified uterine cavity is formed.

The vagina develops from a combination of the müllerian tubercles and the urogenital sinus. Cells proliferate from the upper portion of the urogenital sinus to form solid aggregates known as the *sinovaginal bulbs*. These cell masses develop into a cord, the vaginal plate, which extends from the müllerian ducts to the urogenital sinus. This plate canalizes, starting at the hymen, which is where the sinovaginal bulb attaches to the urogenital sinus, and proceeding cranially to the developing cervix, which has by this time already canalized. The process is completed at about the twenty-first week of intrauterine life.

Toaff et al. have pointed out from their review of the literature that the type of communicating abnormality of the uterus depends on a teratogenic process active at different stages in the embryonic development. Most symmetric communicating uteri have a normal urinary system, indicating that normal growth of the two mesonephric ducts had taken place before the fusion problem occurred. They point out, however, that all patients with communicating uteri with atretic hemivagina who were studied had ipsilateral renal agenesis. Likewise, in patients with anomalies wherein a hemicervix was absent, ipsilateral renal agenesis occurred. They inferred from these findings that an early teratogenic process active during the fourth week of gestation resulted in arrested growth of one mesonephric duct, agenesis of the ureteric bud, and therefore renal agenesis.

Genetic Studies of Müllerian Fusion Difficulties

Elias et al. reviewed the cases of sisters, mothers, and aunts of 24 women with known müllerian fusion abnormalities. Only 1 sister out of 37 (2.7%) was found to have a similar abnormality. No such abnormalities were found among 24 mothers, 45 maternal aunts, or 50 paternal aunts. However, the data in this study were accumulated by history and medical records and not by direct uterine examination. Nonetheless, Elias et al. concluded that the major genetic transmission mechanism could be only polygenic or multifactorial.

Incidence

It is difficult to estimate the incidence of uterine fusion anomalies because the data in most reports are derived from study groups rather than from the general population. The incidence is reported as 0.1% in retrospective studies and from 2% to 3% in observations of uteri at the time of delivery. Most uteri in the latter study, however, fit into the category of arcuate uterus or subseptate uterus.

Symptoms and Signs

Complete duplication of the vagina, uterus, and cervix may be asymptomatic until the woman begins to menstruate. Frequently the earliest symptom brought to the attention of the gynecologist is the fact that tampons do not obstruct menstrual flow. What occurs is that the patient inserts a tampon into one vagina but the other vagina is still open. The second most common way the diagnosis is made is by observation at the time of the first pelvic examination.

Obstructive vaginal anomalies often lead to cyclic pain at the time of menstruation or to the presence of a mucus-filled or blood-filled mass in the vagina. This may be mistaken for a paravaginal tumor.

A noncommunicating uterine horn may be indicated in one of two fashions. The first may be pain or a mass exacerbated cyclically at the time of menses, which occasionally is associated with symptoms and signs of endometriosis in a teenage woman. The early onset of signs and symptoms of endometriosis should alert the physician to this possibility. A mass is often noted on physical examination. Olive and Henderson noted that 10 of 13 women (77%) with anomalies associated with outflow obstruction had endometriosis, whereas only 16 of 43 (37%) who did not have outflow obstruction had evidence for endometriosis.

The second way such a problem may present is as an ectopic pregnancy. Because sperm may migrate through the patent horn and because the rudimentary horn may have a normal tube attached to it, pregnancy can occur in the rudimentary horn. But because such horns are frequently small, rupture or pain caused by the obstruction may point to the diagnosis.

One of the major presenting symptoms is reproductive wastage. Didelphic uteri are usually not associated with this complaint. Musset estimated that abnormalities of the uterus may occur in as many as 15% to 25% of women with a history of repetitive abortion. Makino et al. studied 1200 habitual aborters with hysterosalpingography and found that 188 had congenital uterine anomalies (15.7%). Most patients with pregnancy wastage, however, had a variation of septate uterus. Whereas pretherapy pregnancy wastage rates were as high as 85% to 90%, in most studies, improvement of pregnancy efficiency to as much as 80% occurred after metroplasty. Table 11-1 summarizes the results of a number of such reports. A recent review of the world literature by Homer et al. found a total of 658 women experiencing 1062 pregnancies of which 88% ended in abortion and 9% in preterm delivery before treatment. Of the 491 pregnancies experienced by these women after hysteroscopic metroplasty, 80% ended in term deliveries, while only 14% were aborted and 6% were preterm births. It is important to thoroughly evaluate such patients before exposing them to an operative procedure, since other problems may cause pregnancy wastage.

Uterine dysfunction and incoordinate uterine action are complicating problems seen in labor in women with septate and bicornuate uteri. Likewise, breech presentations and transverse lies occur more commonly in women with such abnormal uteri.

Diagnosis

Diagnosis of a uterine anomaly may be indicated by a history of spontaneous abortion, especially in the second trimester, but is best proved by hysterosalpingography, hysteroscopy, and at times, laparoscopy. Valdes et al. in 1984 reviewed the use of ultrasound for diagnosing female genital tract anomalies. A group of 64 patients with an ultrasound diagnosis of an anomaly were studied retrospectively to determine the accuracy and usefulness

TABLE 11-1
Results of Studies Evaluating Reproductive Success in Women Who Have Had Repair of Septate Uterus

Author(s) (Year)	Number	Live Births	Abortions	Ectopic Pregnancy
Musich and Behrman (1978)	21	9	2	0
Buttram (1979)	46	23	1	1
Palmer (1981)	100	67	4	0
Rochet and Dargert (1981) (per Audebert, Cittadini, and Cognat [1983])	38	29	2	0
Cardiani and Fedele (1981)	68	31	2	0
Audebert, Cittadini, and Cognat (1983)	54	19	3	0
Perino, Mencaglia, Hamou, and Cittadini (1987)	24	10	1	0
TOTAL	351	188	15	1

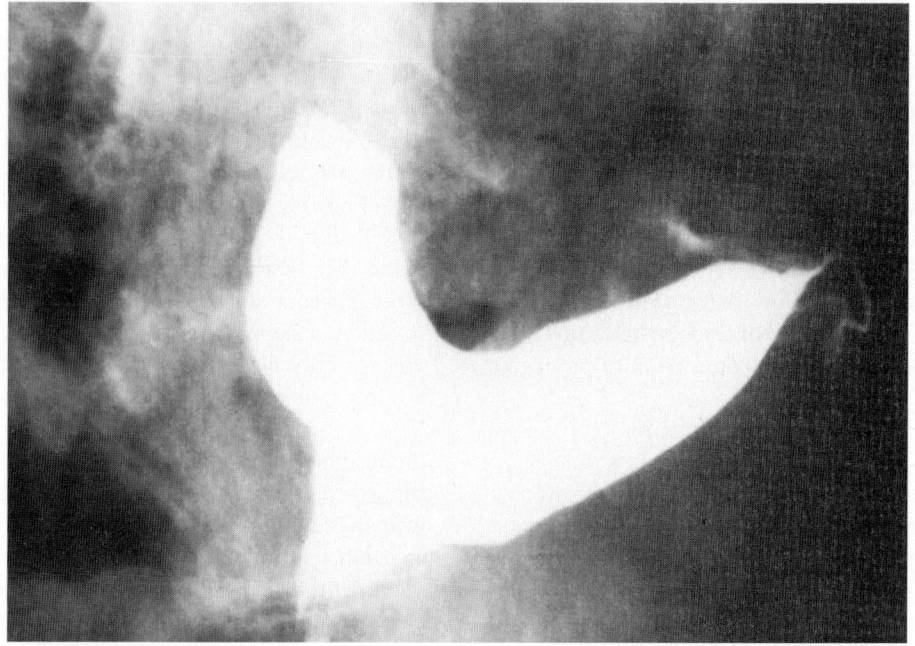

FIGURE 11-9   Hysterosalpingogram of bicornuate uterus seen in patient with repetitive abortions.

of the sonographic examination in such cases. Of these patients, 64% were pregnant; 36% were not. Of 46 patients who had ultrasound diagnoses, 21 cases were diagnosed as bicornuate/septate uterus, 18 cases as didelphia, 3 cases as vaginal and cervical atresia, 2 cases as obstructed lower but normal upper genital tract, and 2 cases as abnormal-appearing uterus. Ultrasound diagnosis was compared with hysterosalpingographic and operative findings in 43 patients and with physical examination in three patients. Scan results were classified as diagnostic in 26%, confirmatory in 63%, and incorrect in 11%.

Fedele et al. studied 43 infertile patients with hysterosalpingographic evidence for bifid uterus, using ultrasound and laparoscopy/hysteroscopy. They were able to ade-

quately visualize the uteri of 39, and they correctly identified with ultrasound: 1 of 2 uteri didelphys, all 11 bicornuate uteri, and all 4 totally and 22 partially septate uteri. In a separate report Fedele et al. studied 14 women with a hysterosalpingographic diagnosis of uterus unicornis. Ultrasound achieved an 85.7% sensitivity and 100% specificity for diagnosing the presence of a rudimentary horn that existed in seven cases.

Ultrasound is a reasonable diagnostic procedure in such cases but should not be considered diagnostic until supplementary studies are performed. Magnetic resonance imaging shows excellent diagnostic promise, but hysterosalpingography and direct observation via hysteroscopy are currently the preferred methods of diagnosis (Figure 11-9). Laparoscopy or laparotomy may be useful in unsual cases.

Specific Anomalies

ABSENCE OF CERVIX AND UTERUS. As discussed under Rokitansky-Küster-Hauser syndrome, the cervix and uterus are often not completely absent; the fallopian tubes and possibly some fibrous tissue are usually present. Absence is frequently associated with urinary tract anomalies.

UNICORNUATE UTERUS. Destruction of one müllerian duct may occur for various embryonic reasons. It is often related to lack of development of the mesonephric system on one side associated with lack of the appropriate development of the müllerian system. When this is the case, there is almost always a missing kidney and ureter on the same side. A single cervix and a single horn of the uterus with the fallopian tube of the side entering it are seen. The ovary may be present on the opposite side. Such a uterus usually supports a pregnancy. Unicornuate uterus may not be diagnosed unless the patient is evaluated with a hysterosalpingogram or is subjected to an operative procedure.

In a review of the literature consisting of 31 patients, Buttram found a 48% spontaneous abortion rate, a 17% prematurity rate, and a 40% live birth rate in patients with this anomaly.

Moutos et al. studied 29 women with unicornuate uteri and 25 women with didelphic uteri. Twenty women with unicornuate uteri produced a total of 40 pregnancies, and 13 women with didelphic uteri produced a total of 28 pregnancies. There was a 33% spontaneous abortion rate in the unicornuate group and a 23% rate in the didelphic group. The unicornuate group produced 9% preterm deliveries, 58% term deliveries, and 61% had living children. The didelphic group produced 32% preterm deliveries, 45% term deliveries, and 60% had living children. None of these differences were statistically different, demonstrating that the pregnancy performance of unicornuate and didelphic uteri are similar.

ANOMALIES OF LATERAL FUSION OF MÜLLERIAN DUCTS. Partial or complete duplication of the vagina, cervix, and uterus may be seen clinically. These may be classified as didelphic, which may involve a complete duplication of the vagina, uterus, and cervix; bicornuate, which consists of a single-chamber vagina and cervix with a complete or partial septate uterus and two uterine bodies (see Figure 11-9); septate, in which the uterus appears as a single organ but contains a midline septum that is either partial or complete; or arcuate, which demonstrates a small septate indentation at the upper end of the fundus. Figure 11-10 graphically depicts these.

Toaff et al. reviewed the subgroup of malformed uteri that includes duplication of the vagina, cervix, and uterus with communication between the horns. Nine subcategories have been described and are depicted in Figure 11-11. Some involve septate uteri and others didelphic uteri. Some involve obstructive areas of the vagina. Because of the structural differences the clinical findings may be quite different from case to case.

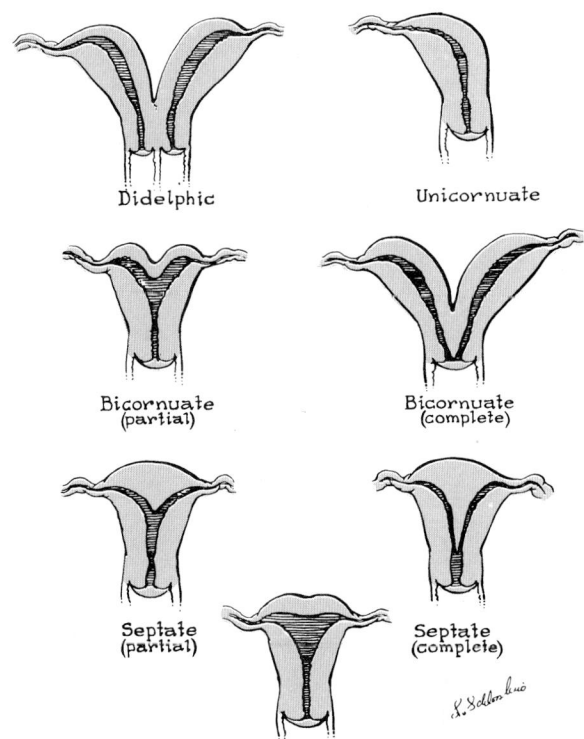

FIGURE 11-10 Nonobstructive maldevelopment of the Müllerian system. (From Baramki TA: J Reprod Med 29:376, 1984.)

Finally, obstructive varieties of duplication may be noted, again involving the uterus or the vagina.

Management

For patients with nonobstructed abnormalities, no therapy may be indicated. This is particularly true for women with unicornuate and didelphic uteri. On the other hand, septate uteri are frequently associated with reproductive wastage problems, and correction may be necessary to relieve these situations. A number of metroplasty procedures are available. The first was described by Strassman and involved the removal of the septum by a wedge incision and the reunification of the two cavities. However, a number of other means have been devised to eliminate the septum. Table 11-2 summarizes some of these and outlines their differences.

Recently septate uteri have been treated by division of the septum through the hysteroscope. To perform this procedure, a laparoscope should first be introduced into the peritoneal cavity so that the uterus can be directly visualized during the procedure. This will also allow differentiation of a septate uterus from a bicornuate or didelphic uterus. An operating hysteroscope is then used to progressively cut the septum with scissors, until a cavity with normal appearing contour is achieved. Other means of dividing the septum may be utilized, including the use of a resectoscope. Vercellini et al. compared two groups of women, one of which had septum separation by microscissors and the other by resectoscope, and could find little difference in morbidity or outcome. Little or no bleeding generally occurs, since the septum is fibrous and poorly vascularized. After the operation some surgeons may insert an IUD for 30 days, and the patient may be treated

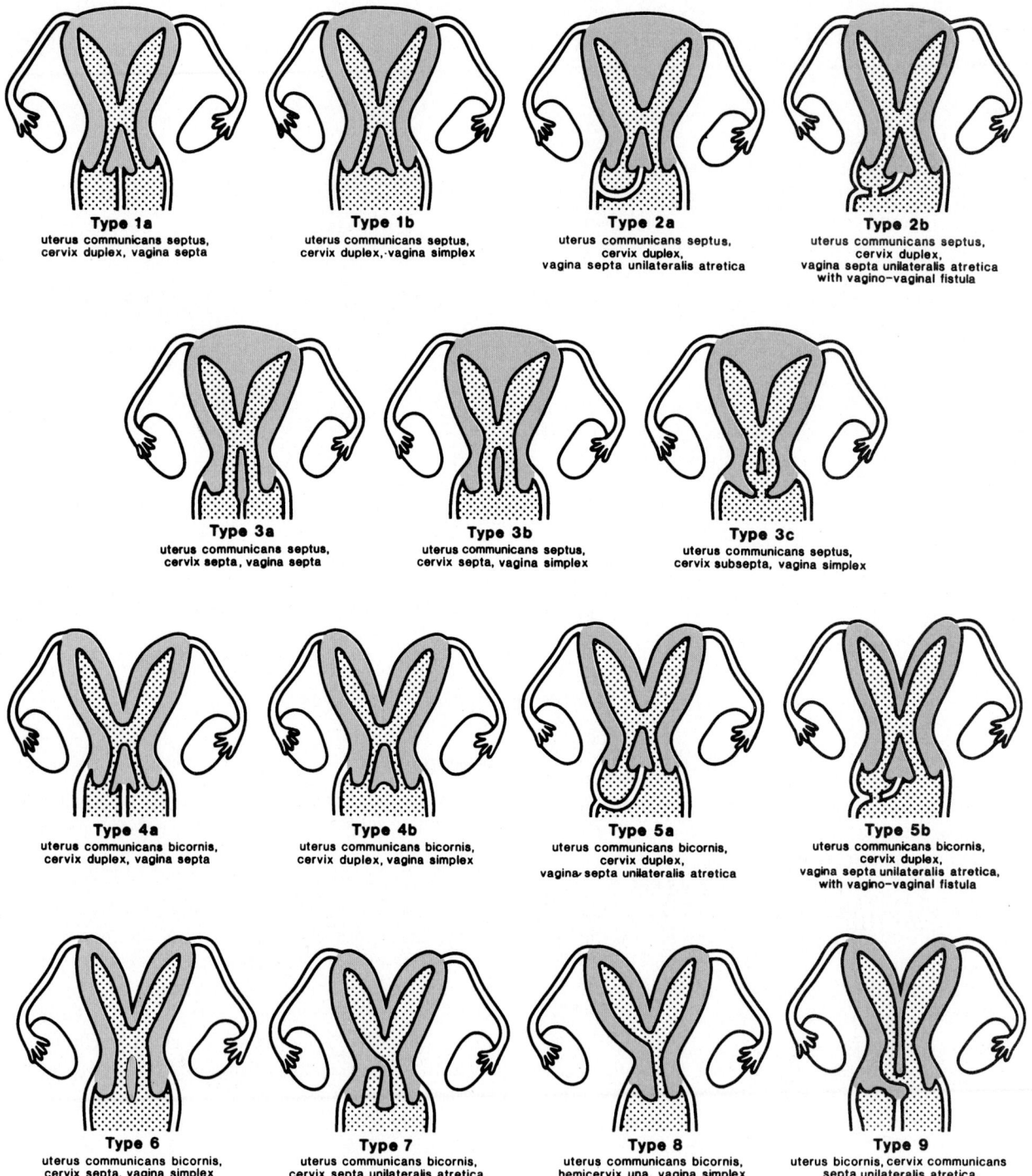

FIGURE 11-11   Morphologic classification of communicating uteri. All have an isthmic communication except type 9, which has a low cervical communication. (From Toaff ME, Lev-Toaff AS, and Toaff R: Fertil Steril 41:661, 1984. Reproduced with permission of the publisher, The American Fertility Society.)

TABLE 11-2
Procedures for Performing Metroplasty
on Uteri with Müllerian Fusion Anomalies

Procedure	Technique
Strassman	Wedge excision of septum—reunification of cavity
Jones	Cone resection of septum
Tompkins Bret Palmer	Sagittal incision with severance of septum
Chervenak Neuwirth Perino	Hysteroscopically controlled severance of septum

with a conjugated estrogen (1.25 mg per day) for 1 month. This step has not been proved to be necessary and often can be withheld. This vaginal approach eliminates the need for an abdominal procedure and thus limits the risk of pelvic adhesions, which may in themselves interfere with fertility. Israel and March noted that no serious complications occurred in 72 such treated patients reported in the world literature.

Although most authors have shown their chronic pregnancy losses reduced after septa are divided or bicornuate uteri are unified, Kirk et al. questioned the efficacy of metroplasty in treating multiple pregnancy loss. These authors identified 146 patients, 23 of whom received metroplasty and 123 who did not. They matched 15 of the nonsurgical patients with 15 of the surgical patients by age, complaint, gravidity, and type of anomaly. The percentage of patients with living children in the nonsurgical group was 67% compared with 73% for patients who underwent metroplasty. This difference was not statistically significant. The authors, however, did note that fetal salvage rates were significantly improved after metroplasty and pointed out that the final outcome was similar in the two groups. They thus question the efficacy of metroplasty in the treatment of multiple pregnancy losses.

Ovarian Abnormalities

Accessory Ovary and Supernumerary Ovary

In 1959 Wharton defined *accessory ovary* and *supernumerary ovary*. The former term is used when excess ovarian tissue is noted near a normally placed ovary and connected to it. Supernumerary ovary occurs when a third ovary is separated from the normally situated ovaries. Printz et al. pointed out that such ovaries may be found in the omentum or retroperitoneally, and Hogan et al. reported the presence of a dermoid cyst in a supernumerary ovary that occurred in the greater omentum. Wharton estimated that the occurrence of either accessory ovary or supernumerary ovary was quite rare, finding approximately 1 case of accessory ovary per 93,000 patients and 1 case of supernumerary ovary in 29,000 autopsies. In fact, only 13 reported cases of supernumerary ovary have been found to date in the world literature. In Wharton's review, 3 of 4 patients with supernumerary ovary and 5 of 19 patients with accessory ovary had additional congenital defects, most frequently abnormalities of the genitourinary tract.

Ovotestes

Ovotestes are present in individuals with ovaries that have an HY antigen present. The majority are true hermaphrodites. The degree to which müllerian and mesonephric development occurs depends on the amount of testicular tissue present in the ovotestes and the proximity to the developing duct system. Where a considerable amount of testicular tissue is present within the organ, there is a tendency for descent toward the labial scrotal area. Thus palpation of the gonad in the inguinal canal or within the labial scrotal area is fairly common. Ovulation and menstruation may occur if the müllerian system is appropriately developed. In a similar fashion, spermatogenesis may occur as well. Where testicular tissue is present, there is an increased risk for malignant degeneration, and these gonads should be removed after puberty. Germ cell tumors, such as dysgerminomas, have been reported in the ovarian portion of ovotestes.

KEY POINTS

- Gender identification in a newborn infant has such emotional impact that it should be considered an emergency procedure.

- Congenital adrenal hyperplasia is an autosomal recessive condition most commonly the result of an inborn error of metabolism involving the enzyme 21-hydroxylase. Homozygous individuals occur in 1 of every 490 to 67,000 births. Heterozygote carriers are present in 1 in 20 to 1 in 250 individuals. Differences depend on ethnic background of people tested.

- The hymen is the junction of the sinovaginal bulb with the urogenital sinuses and is derived from endoderm.

- Vaginal agenesis is most often associated with Rokitansky-Küster-Hauser syndrome. From 25% to 40% of these will have urologic abnormalities. Approximately one eighth will have skeletal abnormalities as well.

- Abnormalities of the uterus and cervix may be transmitted as a polygenic or multifactorial pattern of inheritance. They occur in about 2% to 3% of the female population.

- From 15% to 20% of women with histories of repetitive abortion may be found to have anomalies of the uterus.

- Pretherapy pregnancy wastage rates in women with anomalies of the uterus may be as high as 85% to 90%. After surgical repair the pregnancy efficiency rate may be as high as 80%.

- Accessory ovaries occur in approximately 1 per 93,000 patients. Supernumerary ovaries occur in approximately 1 of every 29,000 women.

BIBLIOGRAPHY

Abrego D and Ibrahim AA: Mesenteric supernumerary ovary, Obstet Gynecol 45:352, 1975.

Audebert AJM, Cittadini E, and Cognat M: Habitual abortion in uterine malformations, Acta Eur Fertil 14:273, 1983.

Baramki TA: The treatment of congenital anomalies in girls and women, J Reprod Med 29:376, 1984.

Beheshti M, Hardy BE, Churchill BM, et al: Gender assignment in male pseudo hermaphrodite children, Urology 22:604, 1983.

Blair RG: Pregnancy associated with congenital malformations of the reproductive tract, J Obstet Gynaecol Br Emp 67:36, 1960.

Buttram VC: Müllerian anomalies and their management, Fertil Steril 40:159, 1983.

Buttram VC, Zanotti L, Acosta AA, et al: Surgical correction of septate uterus, Fertil Steril 25:373, 1974.

Cardiani GB and Fedele L: Clinical management of uterine anomalies, Acta Eur Fertil 12:83, 1981.

Cruikshank SH and VanDrie DM: Supernumerary ovaries: update and review, Obstet Gynecol 60:126, 1982.

Daly DC, Walters CA, Soto-Albers CE, et al: Hysteroscopic metroplasty: surgical technique and obstetric outcome, Fertil Steril 39:623, 1983.

Dapunt O, Sölder E, Moncayo H, and Hohn A: Results of the Strassmann operation at the Innsbruck University Gynecologic Clinic (1976-1991), Gynakol Geburtshilfliche Rundsch 32:134, 1992.

Doyle MB: Magnetic resonance imaging in müllerian fusion defects, J Reprod Med 37:33, 1992.

Dillon WP and Dewey M: A case of accessory ovary, Obstet Gynecol 58:660, 1981.

Elias S, Simpson JL, Carson SA, et al: Genetic studies in incomplete müllerian fusion, Obstet Gynecol 63:276, 1984.

Emans SJ, Grace E, Fleischnick E, et al: Detection of late onset 21-hydroxylase deficiency congenital adrenal hyperplasia in adolescents, Pediatrics 72:690, 1983.

Fedele L, Bianchi S, Tozzi L, et al.: A new laparoscopic procedure for creation of a neovagina in Mayer-Rokitansky-Küster-Hauser syndrome, Fertil Steril 66:854, 1996.

Fedele L, Dorta M, Vercellini P, et al: Ultrasound in the diagnosis of subclasses of unicornuate uterus, Obstet Gynecol 71:274, 1988.

Fedele L, Ferranzzi E, Dorta M, et al: Ultrasonography in the differential diagnosis of "double" uteri, Fertil Steril 50:361, 1988.

Fleischnick E, Rum D, Alosco SM, et al: Extended MHC haplotypes in 21-hydroxylase deficiency congenital adrenal hyperplasia: shared genotypes in unrelated patients, Lancet 1:152, 1983.

Gaucherand P, Awada A, Rudigoz RC, and Dargent D: Obstetrical prognosis of the septate uterus: a plea for treatment of the septum, Eur J Obstet Gynecol Reprod Biol 54:109, 1994.

Greiss FC and Mauzy CH: Congenital anomalies in women: an evaluation of diagnosis, incidence, and obstetric performance, Am J Obstet Gynecol 82:330, 1961.

Hahn-Pedersen J and Larsen PM: Supernumerary ovary, Acta Obstet Gynecol Scand 63:365, 1984.

Hauser GA and Schreiner WE: Das Mayer-Rokitansky-Küster-Syndrom Schweiz Med Wochenschr 91:381, 1961.

Hay D: Uterus unicornis and its relationship to pregnancy, J Obstet Gynaecol Br Emp 68:371, 1961.

Hogan ML, Barber DD, and Kaufmann RH: Dermoid cyst in supernumerary ovary: the greater omentum: report of a case, Obstet Gynecol 29:405, 1967.

Homer HA, Li T-J, and Cooke ID: The septate uterus: a review of management and reproductive outcome, Fertil Steril 73:1, 2000.

Ingram JM: The bicycle seat stool in the treatment of vaginal agenesis and stenosis: a preliminary report, Am J Obstet Gynecol 140:867, 1981.

Israel R and March CM: Hysteroscopic incision of the septate uterus, Am J Obstet Gynecol 149:66, 1984.

Kaufman RH, Noller K, Adam E, et al: Upper genital tract abnormalities and pregnancy outcome in diethylstilbestrol-exposed progeny, Am J Obstet Gynecol 148:973, 1984.

Kelalis P, King L, and Bellman A: Clinical pediatric urology, ed 2, Philadelphia, 1985, WB Saunders Co.

Kirk EP, Chuong CJ, Coulam CB, and Williams GJ: Pregnancy after metroplasty for uterine anomalies, Fertil Steril 59:1164, 1993.

Makino T, Umeuchi M, Nakada K, et al: Incidence of congenital uterine anomalies in repeated reproductive wastage and prognosis for pregnancy after metroplasty, Int J Fertil 37:167, 1992.

Maneschi F, Marana R, Muzil L, and Mancuso S: Reproductive performance in women with bicornuate uterus. Acta Eur Fertil 24:117, 1993.

McIndoe A: Treatment of congenital absence and obliterative conditions of vagina, Br J Plast Surg 2:254, 1950.

Möbus V, Sachweh K, Knapstein PG, and Kreienberg R: Women after surgically corrected vaginal aplasia: a follow-up of psychosexual rehabilitation, Geburtshilfe Frauenheilkd 53:125, 1993.

Moutos DM, Damewood MD, Schlaff WD, and Rock JA: A comparison of the reproductive outcome between women with a unicornuate uterus and women with a didelphic uterus, Fertil Steril 58:88, 1992.

Muller U, Mayerova A, Debus B, et al: Correlation between testicular tissue and HY phenotype in intersex patients, Clin Genet 23:49, 1983.

Musich JR and Behrman SJ: Obstetric outcome before and after metroplasty in women with uterine anomalies, Obstet Gynecol 52:63, 1978.

Musset R: Classification globale des malformations uterines, Gynécol Obstét 66:145, 1967.

Olive D and Henderson DY: Endometriosis and müllerian anomalies, Obstet Gynecol 69:412, 1987.

Palmer R: Anomalies uterines congenitales. In Boury-Heyler C, Maulbeon P, Rochet Y, et al: Uterus et fécondité, vol 1, Paris, 1981, Masson.

Pang S, Hotchkiss J, Drash AL, et al: Microfilter paper method for 17-hydroxyprogesterone radioimmunoassay: its application for rapid screening for congenital adrenal hyperplasia, J Clin Endocrinol Metab 45:1003, 1977.

Pang S, Murphey W, Levine LS, et al: A pilot newborn screening for congenital adrenal hyperplasia in Alaska, J Clin Endocrinol Metab 55:413, 1982.

Perino A, Mencaglia L, Hamou J, and Cittadini E: Hysteroscopy for metroplasty of uterine septa: report of 24 cases, Fertil Steril 48:321, 1987.

Phelan JT, Counseller VS, and Greene LF: Deformities of the urinary tract with congenital absence of the vagina, Surg Gynecol Obstet 97:1, 1953.

Printz JL, Choate JW, Townes PL, et al: The embryology of supernumerary ovaries, Obstet Gynecol 41:246, 1973.

Rock J and Azziz R: Genital anomalies in childhood, Clin Obstet Gynecol 30:682, 1987.

Semens JP: Congenital anomalies of the female genital tract: functional classification based on a review of 56 personal cases and 5 unreported cases, Obstet Gynecol 19:328, 1962.

Stanton S: Gynecologic complications of epispadias and bladder extrophy, Am J Obstet Gynecol 119:749, 1974.

Toaff ME, Lev-Toaff AS, and Toaff R: Communicating uteri: review and classification with introduction of two previously unrecorded types, Fertil Steril 41:661, 1984.

Turunen A and Unnerus CE: Spinal changes in patients with congenital aplasia of the vagina, Acta Obstet Gynecol Scand 46:99, 1967.

Valdes C, Malini S, and Malinak LR: Ultrasound evaluation of female genital tract anomalies: a review of 64 cases, Am J Obstet Gynecol 149:285, 1984.

Vecchietti G: Le neovagin dans le syndrome de Rokitansky-Küster-Hauser, Rev Med Suisse Romande 99:593, 1979.

Vercellini P, Vendola N, Colombo A, et al: Hysteroscopic metroplasty with resectoscope or microscissors for the correction of septate uterus, Surg Gynecol Obstet 176:439, 1993.

Wharton LR: Two cases of supernumerary ovary and one of accessory ovary within an analysis of previously reported cases, Am J Obstet Gynecol 78:1101, 1959.

Pediatric Gynecology
Gynecologic Examination, Infections, Trauma, Pelvic Mass, Precocious Puberty

Adhesive Vulvitis. A self-limiting consequence of chronic vulvitis in which denuded epithelium of adjacent labia minora agglutinates and fuses the two labia together.

Adolescence. A transitional period of life during which an individual matures physiologically and psychologically from a child into an adult.

Factitious Precocious Puberty. The condition that may result when a young girl has ingested medications such as oral estrogens or birth control pills or has used excessive amounts of hormonal creams.

Gelastic Seizures. An unusual neurologic symptom sometimes associated with precocious puberty. It involves seizures with inappropriate laughter.

Heterosexual Precocious Puberty. Premature virilization in a female child, including development of secondary sexual characteristics.

Incomplete or Pseudoprecocious Puberty. Premature female sexual maturation and uterine bleeding without associated ovulation.

McCune-Albright Syndrome (Polyostotic Fibrous Dysplasia). A rare triad of café-au-lait spots, fibrous dysplasia, and cysts of the skull and long bones.

Precocious Puberty. The appearance of signs of secondary sexual maturation at an age more than 2.5 standard deviations below the mean for the population to which the child belongs.

Premature Adrenarche. Isolated early development of axillary hair without other signs of secondary sexual maturation.

Premature Pubarche. Isolated early development of pubic hair without other signs of secondary sexual maturation.

Premature Thelarche. Isolated early unilateral or bilateral breast development without other signs of secondary sexual maturation.

Puberty. The process of biologic and physical development after which sexual reproduction first becomes possible.

Gynecologic diseases are uncommon in children, especially compared with the incidence and prevalence of diseases in women of reproductive age. This chapter considers gynecologic diseases of children from infancy until the completion of puberty. Congenital anomalies and neoplasia of pelvic organs in infants are covered in other chapters. The evaluation of children's gynecologic problems involves considerations of physiology, psychology, and management that are different from those of adult gynecology. The evaluation and treatment of young females is age-dependent. For example, the physical presence of the mother facilitates examining a 4-year-old girl but may inhibit the cooperation of a 14-year-old adolescent.

An outpatient visit by a prepubertal or pubertal child to a

gynecologist should be structured differently from a gynecologic visit by a woman of reproductive age. Considerable time must be devoted to gaining the child's confidence and establishing rapport. If the interaction is poor during the first visit, the negative experience will detract from future physician-patient interactions. Obviously, a child will never allow a physician a second chance to do the first exam. In addition, a child's visit to a gynecologist usually focuses on a perceived problem rather than on preventive medicine, such as occurs with the usual appointment with the pediatrician. Also, the vast majority of children's gynecologic problems are treated by medical rather than surgical means.

The most frequent gynecologic disease of children is *vulvovaginitis*. Vulvitis is the primary problem, with vaginitis of secondary importance unless there is associated vaginal bleeding, a foreign body, sexual abuse, or a sexually transmitted disease.

Adolescence is the period of life during which an individual matures physiologically and psychologically from a child into an adult. This period of transition involves important physical and emotional changes. Before puberty, the child's female organs are in a resting, dormant state. Puberty produces dramatic alterations in both the external and the internal female genitalia. The range of normality of pubertal changes is emphasized in Chapter 38. Because the changes are frequently a cause of concern for adolescent females and their parents, the gynecologist must offer the adolescent female a kind, knowledgeable, and gentle approach. These interactions between the physician and the adolescent female will allow the physician an opportunity to instruct the pubertal teenager about pelvic anatomy and establish a trusting relationship. Subsequently, at the appropriate time, contraceptive counseling may occur.

GYNECOLOGIC EXAMINATION OF A CHILD

A successful gynecologic examination of a child demands that the physician adopt a slow pace, take ample time, and show gentleness and patience. The examination should not be hurried or rushed. The ambiance of the examining room may decrease the anxiety of the child if familiar and friendly objects such as stuffed animals and toys are present. The components of a complete pediatric examination include a history, inspection with visualization of the vagina and cervix, appropriate cultures of the vagina, and a rectal examination if the patient has vaginal bleeding or abdominal or pelvic pain.

To accomplish each step of the examination, the clinician and nurse must establish rapport with the child. A child's reaction will depend on her age, emotional maturity, and previous experience with health care providers. She should be allowed to visualize and handle any instruments that will be used and she should be assured that the instruments are specifically made for young girls. The child's anxiety should be assessed during the general physical examination. Sometimes it is best to defer the pelvic examination until a second visit. This is a difficult decision and is based on the extent of the child's anxiety in relation to the severity of the clinical symptoms. A physician may elect to treat the primary symptoms of vulvovaginitis for 2 to 3 weeks before searching for a foreign body. However, Capraro warned that physicians should not share parents' reluctance to have the female child examined. He emphasized that in the field of pediatric gynecology most errors are errors of omission rather than of commission.

Obtaining a history from a child is not an easy process. Children are not skilled historians and will often ramble, introducing many unrelated facts. Much of the history must be obtained from the parents. However, both the child and the parents are often reluctant to report genital symptoms. Consequently, most gynecologic symptoms in children are chronic before seeking the advice of a physician.

After the history has been obtained, the parents and the child should be reassured that the examination will not hurt. It is important to give the child a sense that she will be in control of the examination process. Emphasize that the most important part of the examination is just "looking" and there will be conversation during the entire process. To successfully examine a child, one needs the cooperation of the patient, her mother, and a skilled nurse with empathy for children. The nurse must be a reassuring influence on the child during the examination.

During the history and most of the general physical examination, the child should sit on the edge of the examination table. A helpful technique is to place the child's hand on top of the physician's hand as the abdominal examination is being performed. This will give the child a sense of control as well as divert the child's attention if she is ticklish or is moving or squirming. For the pelvic examination a young child is best examined on her mother's lap. An older child may be examined in the supine position with her knees apart and her feet together or in the knee-chest position. Draping for the gynecologic examination produces more anxiety than it relieves and should be avoided for the preadolescent child. The most important technique to ensure cooperation is to involve the child as a partner. A handheld mirror helps to involve the child in the examination and facilitates her compliance during it. One should realize that children do not hold still for a long period regardless of the circumstances.

A child should never be restrained for a gynecologic examination. If a child is extremely anxious, mild sedation may be helpful. In rare circumstances it may be necessary to use continuous intravenous conscious sedation or general anesthesia to examine an extremely apprehensive child.

The initial phase of the pelvic examination involves inspection of the vulvar area (Figures 12-1 and 12-2). Many gynecologic conditions in children may be diagnosed by inspection only. The child and the nurse may facilitate inspection of the distal vagina by exerting pressure laterally and posteriorly on the inferior portion of the labia and sur-

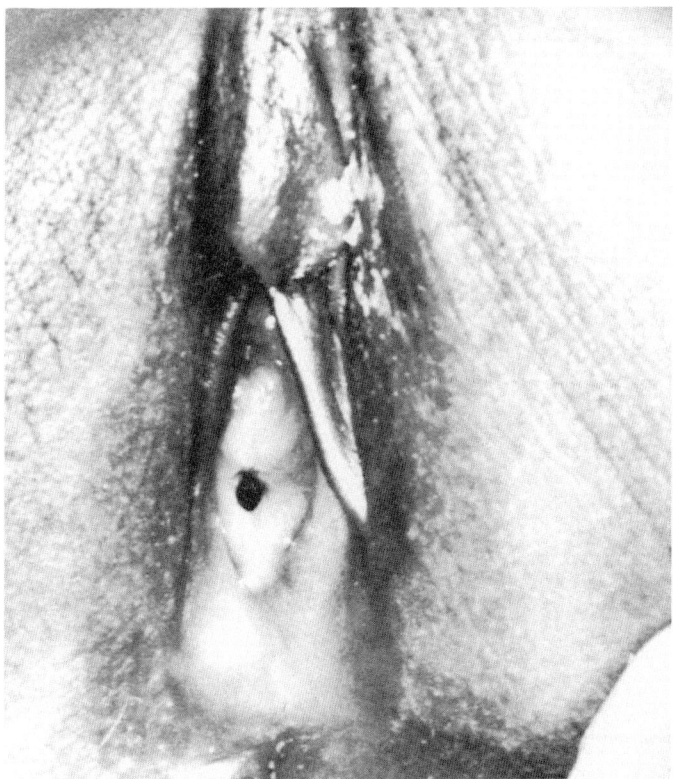

FIGURE 12-1 Appearance of normal external genitalia of a prepubertal female in the supine position using the lateral spread technique. (From Pokorny SF: Pediatric gynecology. In Stenchever MA, ed: Office gynecology, ed 2, St. Louis, Mosby–Year Book, 1996.)

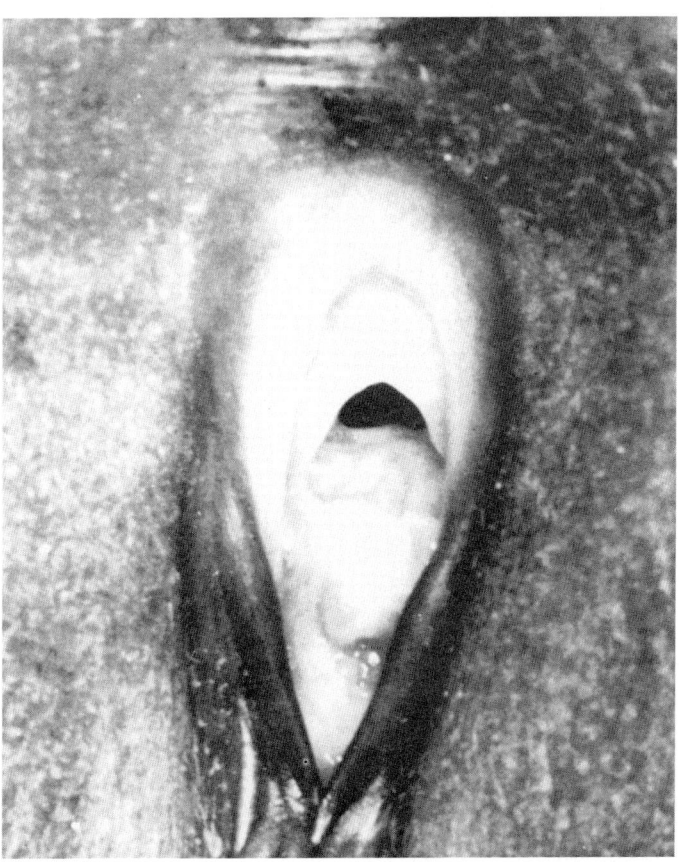

FIGURE 12-2 The same child shown in Figure 12-1 but in the knee-chest position. (From Pokorny SF: Pediatric gynecology. In Stenchever MA, ed: Office gynecology, ed 2, St. Louis, Mosby–Year Book, 1996.)

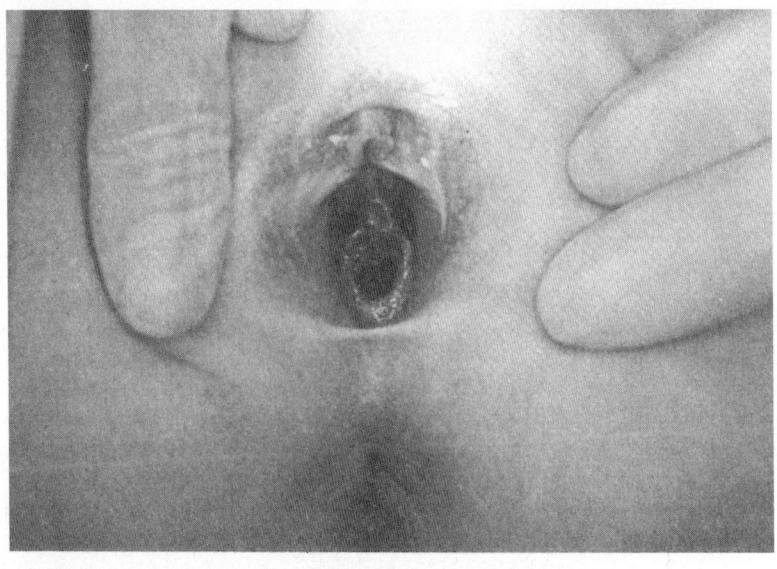

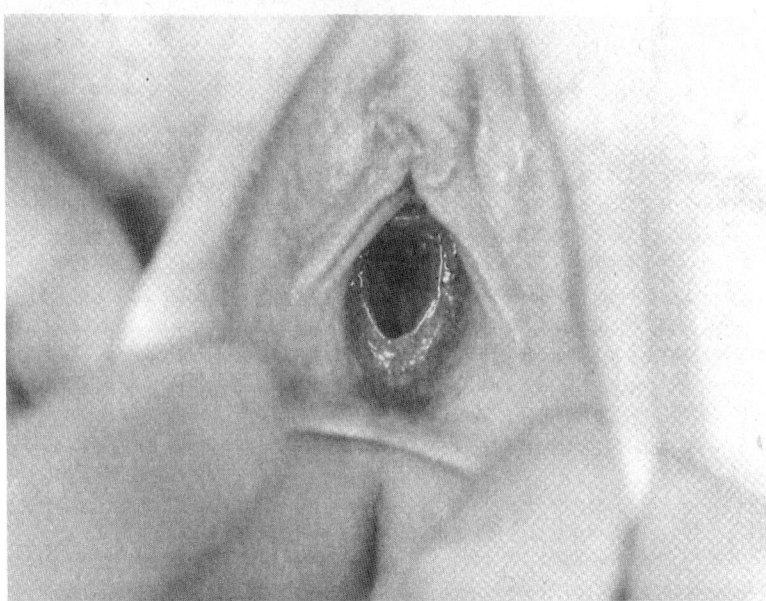

FIGURE 12-3 Examination of the vulva, hymen, and anterior vagina by, **A,** gentle lateral retraction, and **B,** gentle gripping of the labia and pulling anteriorly. (From Emans SJ: Office evaluation of the child and adolescent. In Emans SJ, Laufer MR and Goldstein DP, eds, ed 4, Philadelphia, Lippincott-Raven, 1998.)

rounding skin (Figure 12-3). Asking the child to pretend to blow out candles on a birthday cake may facilitate the process. The hymen of a prepubertal child exhibits a diverse range of normal variations and configurations (Figure 12-4). A detailed understanding of abnormalities of the hymen and vaginal orifice is important in evaluating a child for suspected sexual abuse. The clinical significance of the diameter of the vaginal orifice and its relationship to sexual abuse is controversial. The vaginal epithelium of the prepubertal child appears redder and thinner compared with the vagina of a woman in her reproductive years. The vagina is 4 to 6 cm long, and the secretions have a neutral pH. Emans and Goldstein (1990) have found that the knee-chest

position usually allows the physician to visualize the vagina and cervix of a child after age 2 years without instrumentation. Inspection is facilitated by the vagina being filled with air in the knee-chest position (Figure 12-5). The child is encouraged to lie on her "tummy" with her buttocks in the air. The nurse holds the buttocks apart, and with relaxation of the abdominal muscles and a few deep inspirations, the vaginal orifice opens and the canal fills with air. A bright light helps to illuminate the upper vagina and cervix. The cervix appears as a transverse ridge or pleat that is redder than the vagina. Following inspection of the vagina and cervix, vaginal secretions may be obtained for microscopic examination and culture, with either a plastic medicine

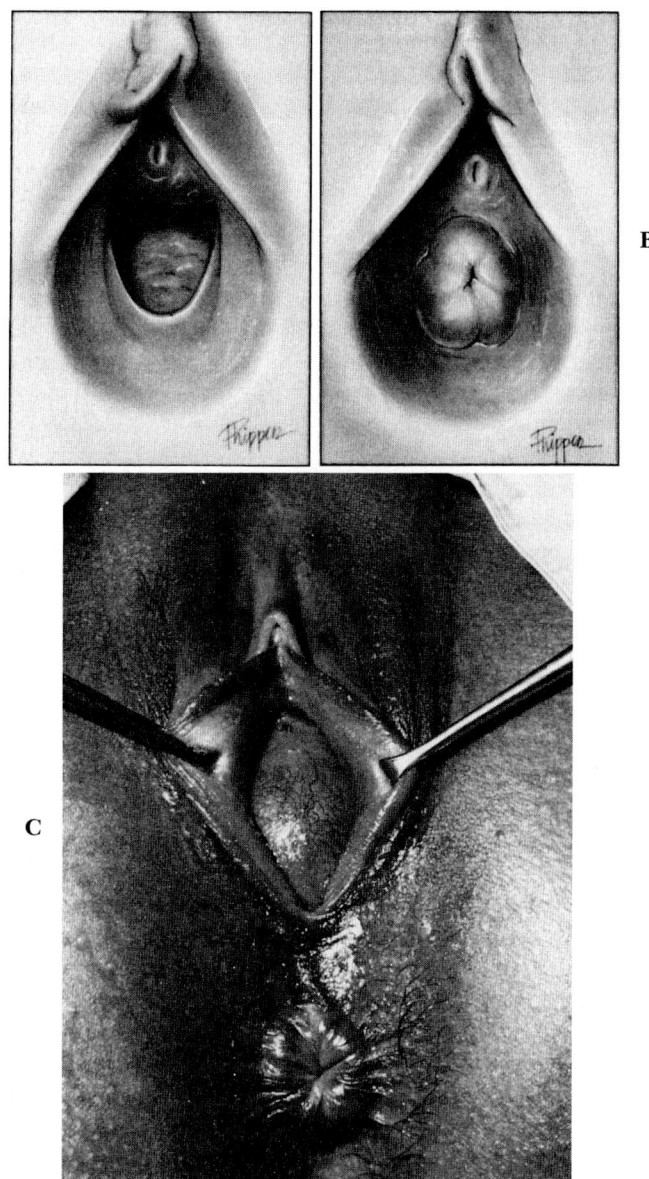

FIGURE 12-4 Types of hymens in prepubertal girls. **A,** Posterior rim of crescentic hymen. **B,** Fimbriated or redundant hymen. **C,** Imperforate hymen. (From Pokorny SF: Configuration of the prepubertal hymen. Am J Obstet Gynecol 157:950, 1987.)

dropper or a saline-saturated, cotton-tipped applicator. Dry cotton-tipped applicators are abrasive and may cause discomfort. Pokorny has described a method for collecting fluid from a child's vagina using a catheter within a catheter. This easily assembled adaptation uses a No. 12 red rubber bladder catheter for the outer catheter and the hub end of an intravenous butterfly catheter for the inner catheter (Figure 12-6). The outer catheter serves as an insulator, and the inner catheter is used to instill a small amount of saline and aspirate the vaginal fluid.

Recurrent vulvovaginitis, persistent bleeding, suspicion of a foreign body or neoplasm, and congenital anomalies are indications for vaginoscopy. Introduction of any instrument into the vagina of a young child takes skillful patience. The prepubertal vagina is narrower, thinner, and lacking in the distensibility of the vagina of a woman in her reproductive years. There are many narrow-diameter endoscopes that will suffice, including the Kelly air cystoscope, contact hysteroscopes, pediatric cystoscopes, small-diameter laparoscopes, plastic vaginoscopes, and special virginal speculums designed by Huffman and Pederson. The ideal pediatric endoscope is a cystoscope or hysteroscope because the accessory channel facilitates lavage of the vagina. A nasal speculum or otoscope is usually too short. Local anesthesia of the vestibule may be obtained with 2% topical viscous Xylocaine. The physician can

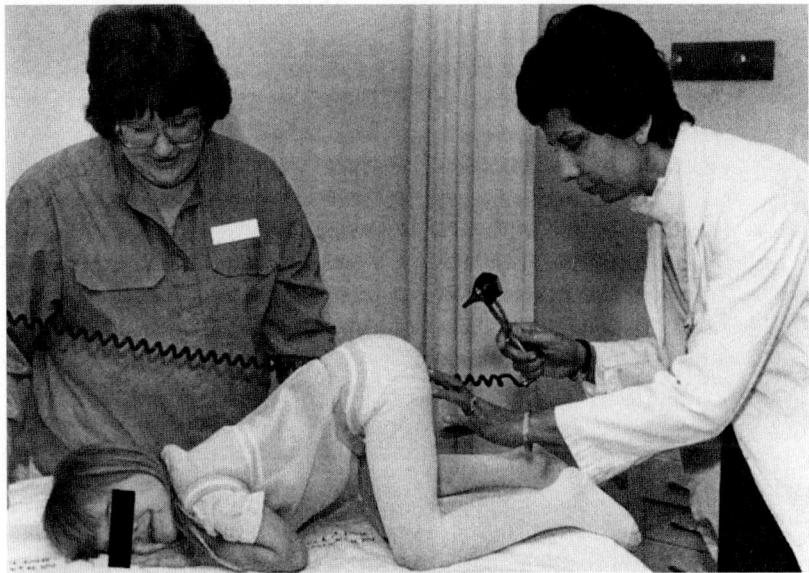

FIGURE 12-5 Knee-chest position used to examine child to visualize cervix and vagina. Otoscope head is usually longer than one shown in photograph. (From Gidwani GP: Clin Obstet Gynecol 30:643, 1987.)

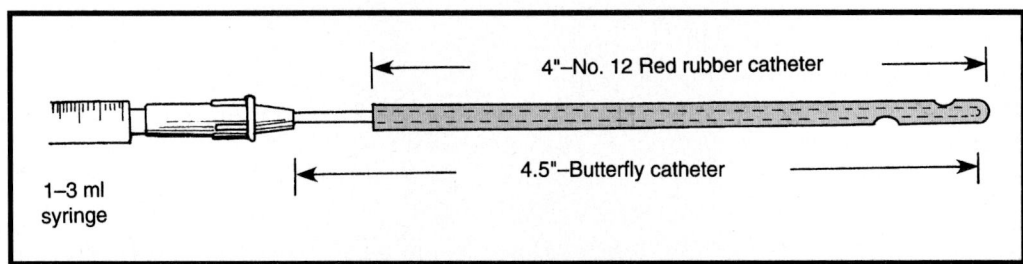

FIGURE 12-6 Assembled catheter within a catheter, as used to obtain samples of vaginal secretions from prepubertal patients. (Redrawn from Pokorny SF and Stormer J: Am J Obstet Gynecol 156:581, 1987.)

divert the child's attention from the endoscope in the vagina by simultaneously gently compressing one of the patient's buttocks.

The last step in the pelvic examination is a rectal examination. This most distressing aspect of the examination may sometimes be omitted, depending on the child's symptoms. Common reasons to perform a rectal examination include genital tract bleeding, pelvic pain, and suspicion of a foreign body or pelvic mass. The child should be warned that the rectal examination will feel similar to the pressure of a bowel movement. The normal prepubertal uterus and ovaries are nonpalpable on rectal examination. The relative size ratio of cervix to uterus is 2 to 1 in a child, in contrast to the opposite ratio of length in the adult. Except for the cervix of an older child, any mass discovered on rectal examination should be considered abnormal. At the conclusion of the rectal examination the child should be praised for her cooperation and mature behavior. The gynecologist should dis-

cuss the findings and proposed treatment with both the child and the mother.

The critical factors surrounding the pelvic examination of a female adolescent are different than examinations of children 2 to 8 years old. Many female adolescents do not want other observers in the examining room. In one study at a university hospital clinic, 24% of inner-city youths did not want a chaperon present. Also 60% to 80% of private adolescent patients request no chaperon, even when the examining gynecologist is a male.

VULVOVAGINITIS

Vulvovaginitis is the most common gynecologic problem of the premenarcheal female. It is estimated that 80% to 90% of outpatient visits of children to gynecologists involve the classic symptoms of vulvovaginitis: introital irritation and discharge. Although the severity of these symptoms varies widely from child to child, usually the parents express great concern. The pathophysiology of the majority of instances of vulvovaginitis in children involves a primary irritation of the vulva with secondary involvement of the lower one third of the vagina. Approximately 75% of children with vulvovaginitis have a nonspecific etiology; that is, cultures are similar to the flora of the gastrointestinal tract. One in four cultures of the discharge from vulvovaginitis will identify a specific organism, such as *Neisseria gonorrhoeae, Trichomonas vaginalis, Chlamydia trachomatis,* herpes simplex virus, *Shigella boydii,* or specific infections such as mycotic or bacterial vaginosis (Table 12-1).

The vulvar irritation may be secondary to a topical allergy, skin or respiratory infection, foreign body, urinary tract infection, vulvar skin disease, ectopic ureter, pinworms, or sexual abuse (see box on p. 276). Positive identification of *Trichomonas,* gonorrhea, or *Chlamydia* in a child with premenarcheal vulvovaginitis often indicates sexual abuse. However, many infants are infected with *Chlamydia trichomatis* during birth and remain colonized for several years in the absence of specific antibiotic therapy. The majority of vulvar and perianal human papillomavirus infections in children, unlike adults, result from nonsexual, indirect transmission of the virus.

There are both physiologic and behavioral reasons why a child is susceptible to vulvar infection. Physiologically, the child's vulva and vagina are exposed to bacterial contamination more frequently than are the adult's. Because the child lacks the labial fat pads and pubic hair of the adult, when a child squats, the lower one third of the vagina is unprotected and open. The vulvar and vaginal epithelium lack the protective effects of estrogen and thus are sensitive to irritation or infection. The labia minora are thin and the vulvar skin is red because the abundant capillary network is easily visualized in the thin skin. The vaginal epithelium of a prepubertal child has a neutral pH, which provides an excellent medium for bacterial growth. The vagina of a child lacks glycogen, lactobacilli, and a sufficient level of antibodies to help resist infection. The normal vagina of a prepubertal child is colonized by an average of nine different species of bacteria—four aerobic and facultative anaerobic species and five obligatory anaerobic species.

The major factor in childhood vulvovaginitis is poor perineal hygiene. This results from the anatomic proximity of the rectum and vagina coupled with the fact that following toilet training, most youngsters are unsupervised when they defecate. Many youngsters wipe their anus from posterior to anterior and thus inoculate the vulvar skin with intestinal flora. A minor vulvar irritation may result in a scratch-itch cycle, with the possibility of secondary seeding because children infrequently wash their hands.

TABLE 12-1
Etiology and Age Distribution for 500 Cases of Vulvovaginitis

Cause	Number	Average Age (Years)
Nonspecific (mixed)	213	8.8
Monilia (Candida)	63	12.5
Foreign body	55	7.2
Streptococcus	45	10.4
Physiologic	33	11.5
Staphylococcus	30	6.9
Gonococcus	24	9.9
Trichomonas	15	11.9
Pinworms	8	6.3
Congenital anomalies	6	6.2
Escherichia coli	5	4.6
Other	2	5.0
4-degree tear	1	14.0

From Capraro VJ: Pediatric gynecology. In Danforth DN, ed: Obstetrics and gynecology, ed 4, Philadelphia, 1981, Harper & Row, Publishers, Inc.

TABLE 12-2
Clinical Features of Children Presenting with Vulvovaginitis

Features	No. (%)
Symptoms:	
Itch	81 (40)
Soreness	108 (54)
Bleeding	37 (19)
Discharge	104 (52)
Signs:	
Genital redness	167 (84)
Visible discharge	66 (33)
Perianal soiling	35 (18)
Specific skin lesion	28 (14)
None	5 (2–4)

From Pierce AM, Hart CA: Arch Dis Child 67:509, 1992.

Similarly, a child with an upper respiratory tract infection may autoinoculate her vulva, especially with group A beta-hemolytic streptococci. Children's clothing is often tight fitting and nonabsorbent, which keeps the vulvar skin warm and moist and prone to vulvovaginitis.

There is nothing specific about the symptoms or signs of childhood vulvovaginitis (Table 12-2). Often the first awareness comes when the mother notices staining of the

Etiologic Factors of Premenarchal Vulvovaginitis

Bacterial

A. Nonspecific
1. Poor perineal hygiene
2. Intestinal parasitic invasion with pruritus
3. Foreign bodies
4. Urinary tract infections with irritation

B. Specific
1. Group A: B-hemolytic streptococcus
2. *Streptococcus pneumoniae*
3. *Haemophilus influenzae/parainfluenzae*
4. *Staphylococcus aureus*
5. *Neisseria meningitidis*
6. *Escherichia coli*
7. *Shigella flexneri/sonnei*
8. Other enterics
9. *Neisseria gonorrhoeae*
10. *Chlamydia trachomatis*

Protozoal-*Trichomonas*

Mycotic
1. *Candida albicans*
2. Other

Helminthiasis-*Enterobius* Vermicularis

Viral/Bacterial Systemic Illness
1. Chicken pox
2. Measles
3. Pityriasis
4. Mononucleosis
5. Scarlet fever
6. Kawasaki disease

Other Viral Illnesses
1. Molluscum contagiosum in genital area
2. Condyloma acuminata
3. Herpes simplex-type II

Physical/Chemical Agents
1. Sandbox
2. Trauma
3. Bubble bath
4. Other

Allergic/Skin Conditions
1. Seborrhea
2. Lichen sclerosus
3. Psoriasis
4. Eczema
5. Contact dermatitis

Tumors

Other
1. Prolapsed urethra
2. Ectopic ureter

From Blythe MJ and Thompson L: Indiana Med 86:237, 1993.

child's underpants. There is a wide range in the quantity of discharge, from minimal to copious. The color ranges from white or gray to yellow or green. Other symptoms associated with vulvovaginitis include irritation, pruritus, pain, and sometimes dysuria. A discharge that is both bloody and foul smelling strongly suggests the presence of a foreign body. The signs of vulvovaginitis are variable and not diagnostic but include vulvar erythema, edema, and excoriation.

The differential diagnosis of persistent or recurrent vulvovaginitis should include considerations of a foreign body, pinworms, primary vulvar skin disease, ectopic ureter, and child abuse. A history of a foul, bloody vaginal discharge is highly indicative of a foreign body; however, the discharge associated with a foreign body is not invariably bloody or foul smelling. If the predominant symptom is pruritus, the most likely diagnosis is pinworms. Approximately 20% of female children infected with pinworms (*Enterobius vermicularis*) develop vulvovaginitis. The classic symptom of pinworms is nocturnal vulvar and perianal itching. At night the milk-white, pin-sized adult worms migrate from the rectum to the skin of the vulva to deposit eggs. They may be discovered by means of a flashlight or by dabbing of the vulvar skin with clear cel-

lophane adhesive tape. The tape is subsequently examined under the microscope. The vulvar skin of children may also be affected by systemic skin diseases, including lichen sclerosus, seborrheic dermatitis, psoriasis, and atopic dermatitis. The classic perianal "figure-of-8" or "hourglass" rash is indicative of lichens sclerosus. An ectopic ureter emptying into the vagina may only intermittently release a small amount of urine; thus this rare congenital anomaly should be considered in the differential diagnosis.

In the period from 6 to 12 months before menarche, children often develop a physiologic vaginal discharge secondary to the increase in circulating estrogen levels. This gray-white discharge is nonirritating. When the physiologic discharge is examined with the microscope, sheets of vaginal epithelial cells are identified. The only treatment necessary is reassurance of both mother and child that this is a normal physiologic process that will subside with time.

The foundation of treating childhood vulvovaginitis is the improvement of local perineal hygiene. Both mother and child should be instructed that the vulvar skin should be kept clean, dry, and cool. For acute weeping lesions, wet compresses of Burow's solution should be prescribed. An alternative is a sitz bath containing 2 tablespoons of baking soda in the water. The child should be instructed to void with her knees spread wide apart and taught to wipe from front to back after defecation. Loose-fitting cotton undergarments should be worn. Chemicals that may produce topical allergies, such as bubble bath, must be discontinued. Harsh soaps and chemicals should be avoided, and dryness of the vulva should be maintained with calamine lotion or a nonirritating cornstarch powder. Approximately one in four episodes of childhood vulvovaginitis is cured by improved local hygiene.

The vast majority of cases of persistent or recurrent nonspecific vulvovaginitis respond to a combination of topical creams and oral antibiotics given for 10 to 14 days. Relief of vulvar irritation may be facilitated by using a bland cream, such as Eucerin, A&D, or Desitin, several times per day. If the initial therapy is not successful, oral antibiotics are continued for 2 more weeks combined with estrogen cream. Estrogen cream is applied to the vulvar area each night. It is not necessary to place hormonal cream into the vagina. The parent should be cautioned that the vulvar skin will become darker and not to use the cream for longer than 3 to 4 weeks because of systemic absorption. If the child has intense pruritus, 0.5% hydrocortisone cream may be applied. Vaginal cultures help to determine the choice of an oral broad-spectrum antibiotic. Dosage of the selected antibiotic depends on the child's weight. The optimal method of obtaining a vaginal culture in a child is to use a nasopharyngeal Calgiswab moistened with saline. The results of the vaginal culture may demonstrate normal flora or an overgrowth of a single organism that is a respiratory, intestinal, or sexually transmitted disease pathogen. The presence of any sexually transmitted organisms in a child is indication that sexual abuse may have taken place and appropriate referral and follow-up is necessary.

Appropriate treatment of pinworms is the anthelmintic agent mebendazole (Vermox). The dosage is one 100-mg chewable tablet for each family member over the age of 2 years (one dose only). Vermox is contraindicated in pregnancy.

Foreign Bodies

Symptoms secondary to a vaginal foreign body are responsible for approximately 4% of pediatric gynecologic outpatient visits. The vast majority of foreign bodies are found in girls between 3 and 9 years of age. The history is usually not helpful because the mother has not witnessed, nor does the child remember, putting a foreign object into the vagina. Many types of foreign bodies have been discovered; however, the most common are small wads of toilet paper. Other common foreign objects include small, hard objects such as hairpins, parts of a toy, crayons, and sand or gravel. The classic symptom is a foul, bloody vaginal discharge. If the foreign body has been in the vagina for a long time, it may be partially embedded in the vaginal mucosa. Large objects may be removed by means of bayonet forceps; small objects such

as sand may be washed out of the vagina by irrigation. It is frustrating to parents and physicians alike that often the child places another foreign body into the vagina several months later.

Vaginal Bleeding

Persistent vaginal bleeding is an extremely rare symptom in a preadolescent female. However, it is important to do a thorough workup because of the serious sequelae of some of the causes of vaginal bleeding. The differential diagnosis of vaginal bleeding in addition to the presence of a foreign body includes neoplasia, precocious puberty, urethral prolapse, trauma, sexual assault, vulvovaginitis, lichen sclerosis, condyloma acuminata, blood dyscrasia, and possible exposure to exogenous estrogens either from oral preparations or skin creams. Neonates may develop a white mucoid vaginal discharge or a small amount of vaginal spotting. Both conditions are secondary to exposure during pregnancy to the high levels of estrogen. The differential diagnosis of a bloody vaginal discharge includes the consideration of two bacterial infections of the vagina: *Shigella* and group A beta-hemolytic streptococcus. The latter usually occurs 7 to 10 days after a sore throat or upper respiratory tract infection. As part of the workup, it is important to adequately visualize the entire lower reproductive tract. Usually, endoscopy for vaginal bleeding is performed in a day-op facility with the child being given continuous intravenous conscious sedation or under general anesthesia.

In a 20-year review of vaginal bleeding, 52 cases were identified in girls 10 years and younger from the Chelsea Hospital for Women. Genital tumors, precocious puberty, vulvar lesions, and urethral prolapse were the four leading causes in this series (Table 12-3). This report by Hill et al. was from a referral center and therefore may not truly represent the cases seen in the practitioner's office. The authors of this series could not explain the absence of the diagnosis of sexual abuse in their study.

TABLE 12-3
Etiology of Vaginal Bleeding

	Number	Percentage
Genital tumors	11	21
Precocious puberty	11	21
Vulval lesions	5	10
Urethral prolapse	5	10
Trauma	4	8
Vulvovaginitis	3	6
Unknown aetiology	13	25

From Hill NCW, Oppenheimer LW, and Morton KE: Br J Obstet Gynaecol 96:467, 1989.

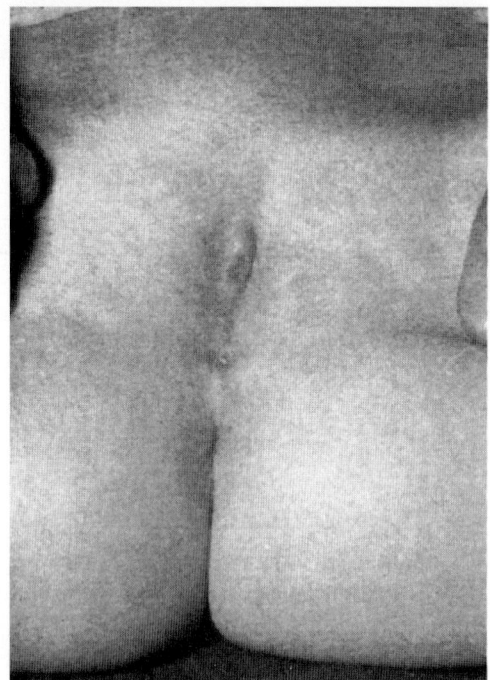
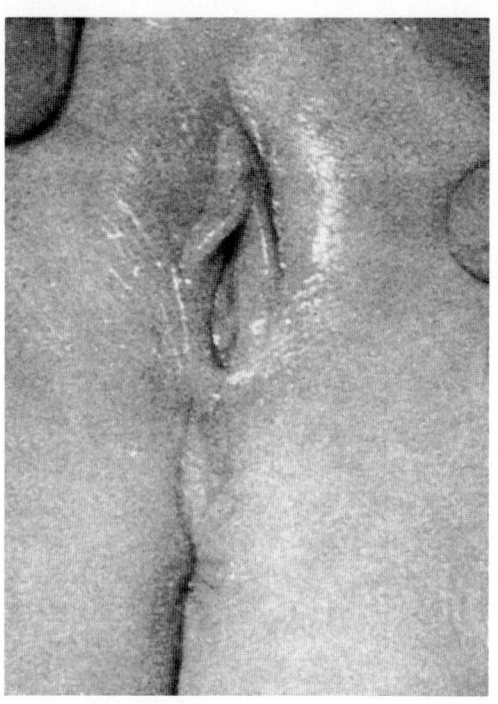

A   B

FIGURE 12-7   A, Labial adhesions in 2½-year-old girl. Two tiny openings exist—one beneath clitoris and another near middle of line of fusion. **B,** Appearance in same child after 10 days of local application of estrogen ointment. (From Dewhurst CJ: Gynaecological disorders of infants and children, Philadelphia, 1963, FA Davis Co.)

ADHESIVE VULVITIS

Adhesive vulvitis is a self-limiting consequence of chronic vulvitis in which denuded epithelium of adjacent labia minora agglutinates and fuses the two labia together creating a "flat appearance" of the vulvar surface. This condition is usually not a serious one; however, it may be mistaken for congenital absence of the vagina. This condition is most common in young girls between 3 and 6 years of age. In one large study the average age of a child with agglutination of the labia was 2½ years; 90% of cases appeared before age 6. The labia minora stick together in the midline, forming a translucent vertical line. This thin, narrow line in an anteroposterior direction is pathognomonic for a diagnosis of adhesive vulvitis. In mild or early stages of the process, agglutination occurs only in the posterior aspects of the labia (Figure 12-7). There is considerable variation in the length of agglutination of the two labia minora. In the most advanced cases, there is fusion over both the urethral and the vaginal orifices. Most children are free of symptoms. If the urethra is covered, there may be difficulty in voiding and associated urinary tract infections.

No treatment is necessary for adhesive vulvitis unless the child has problems in voiding. Jenkinson and Mackinnon published results of a series of 10 girls who had no therapy and noted spontaneous separation of the adhesive vulvitis within 6 to 18 months. Most mothers prefer active treatment of the condition. Topical estrogen cream dabbed onto the labia two times per day will result

in spontaneous separation usually in approximately 2 weeks. Topical estrogen therapy should be continued for a maximum of 3 weeks. Forceful separation is unnecessarily traumatic and should not be done. Recurrent adhesive vulvitis occurs in one of five children. A familial form of true posterior labial fusion has been reported by several authors. Analysis of the pedigrees of these children suggests that this congenital defect may be an autosomal dominant trait with incomplete penetrance. If the labial adhesions are identified early in life and do not resolve with time or estrogen cream, it is appropriate to refer the child to a gynecologic endocrinologist to rule out a congenital anomaly.

McCann et al. (1988) emphasized the association between injuries of the posterior fourchette and labial adhesions in sexually abused children. Labial agglutination alone is so common that suspicion of child abuse is unwarranted. However, the combination of labial adhesions and scarring of the posterior fourchette obligates the gynecologist to consider sexual abuse in the differential diagnosis.

ACCIDENTAL GENITAL TRAUMA

The usual cause of accidental genital trauma during childhood is a fall. Obviously, sexual abuse is an important consideration in the differential diagnosis. Sexual abuse is discussed in Chapter 9. Seventy-five percent of all accidental trauma to the vulva and vagina involves straddle injuries. If the vulva strikes a blunt object, a hematoma usually results. If the object is sharp, such as a fence post, the injury may be a laceration with the potential for penetration of the perineum and injury to internal pelvic organs. Other common causes of vulvar and vaginal trauma include sexual abuse, automobile and bicycle accidents, kicks sustained in a fight, and self-inflicted wounds (Figure 12-8).

The size of vulvar and vaginal hematomas varies widely. Initially there is bleeding into the loose connective tissue. When the pressure from the expanding hematoma exceeds the venous pressure, in most cases the hematoma will stop growing. In lacerations when an artery has been traumatized, bleeding may continue until the artery is ligated.

The diagnosis of a vulvar or vaginal hematoma is straightforward with a history of trauma and the appearance of a bluish red mass. The extent of the hematoma should be determined by both visualization and palpation. The extent of injury with a laceration is more difficult to assess. The depth of most lacerations is usually more extensive than suspected on initial inspection. Vaginal lacerations are almost always associated with corresponding vulvar injuries. The extent of the penetrating injury to the lateral vaginal wall may be more serious than the patient's symptoms indicate, as these injuries are associated with minor symptoms. With penetrating lacerations, trauma to the bladder, intestines, and peritoneal cavity must be ruled out. If gross or microscopic hematuria is discovered, the child should have a CT scan and with gross hematuria the child also should have a voiding cystourethrogram and cystoscopy. General anesthesia is usually required to investigate the extent and depth of all vaginal lacerations and the majority of extensive vulvar lacerations.

The treatment of nonexpanding vulvar hematomas is observation by serial examinations and the use of an ice pack or ice sitz bath. Rarely a hematoma will continue to increase in size, necessitating evacuation and ligation of bleeding vessels. The identification of a bleeding vessel is difficult at best, and conservative therapy is preferable. As stated previously, general anesthesia is usually required for diagnosis of extensive lacerations. During this anesthesia the laceration should be irrigated and débrided, the vessels ligated, and the injuries repaired. Occasionally it is necessary to perform laparoscopy or an exploratory celiotomy for a suspected retroperitoneal hematoma. Children with vulvar trauma should have a booster injection of tetanus toxoid if the last immunization was more than 5 years before the trauma.

In summary, accidental genital trauma often produces extreme pain and overwhelming anxiety for the child and her parents. Because of compassion and empathy, the gynecologist may underestimate the extent of the anatomic injuries. Thus, if in doubt, examine the child under general anesthesia.

OVARIAN TUMORS

Recurrent abdominal pain is a frequent complaint of grammar school children. From 10% to 15% experience this symptom. The young child does not differentiate lower abdominal pain from pelvic pain. Often, because of the smallness of the preadolescent female pelvis, the ovaries are abdominal organs. Thus, increasing abdominal girth is a frequent symptom associated with ovarian enlargement. Ovarian tumors constitute approximately 1% of all neoplasias in premenarcheal children. Thus ovarian neoplasia must be considered in the differential diagnosis of children with persistent or recurrent abdominal pain. Pediatricians used to order an intravenous pyelogram as one of the first diagnostic tests in investigating abdominal pain of unknown origin. Ultrasound, abdominal computed tomography (CT), or magnetic resonance imaging (MR) have been more useful in establishing the diagnosis. Abdominal ultrasonography may be used to establish that the origin of the mass is in the pelvis whether the mass is cystic or solid and the presence of ascites. Calcifications in an ovarian mass indicate a diagnosis of an ovarian teratoma. As part of the preoperative workup, the child should be screened for elevated serum levels of tumor markers such as CA 125, alpha-fetoprotein, human chorionic gonadotropin, inhibin, carcinoembryonic antigen, lactate dehydrogenase, estradiol, and testosterone. The increased use of ultrasound in young females complaining of abdominal pain has led to the discovery of echolucent areas within the ovary. Two to five percent of asymptomatic females have follicular cysts less than 4 cm in diameter discovered by ultrasonography. However, they are clinically unimportant and usually will disappear spontaneously.

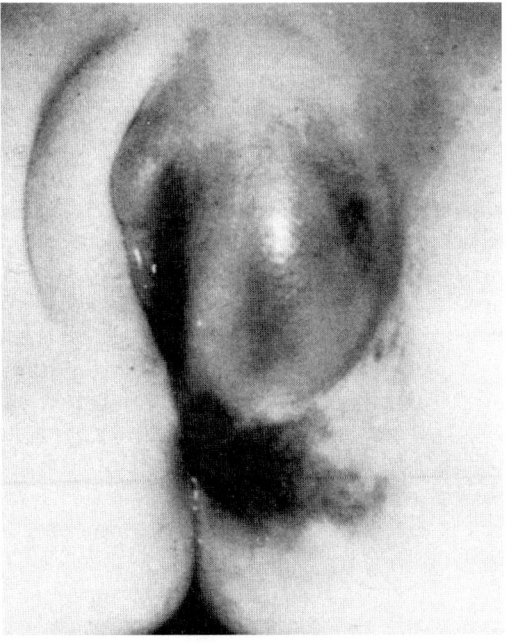

FIGURE 12-8 Vulvar hematoma resulting from a kick in 2-year-old child. (From Huffman JW: The gynecology of childhood and adolescence, ed 2, Philadelphia, 1981, WB Saunders Co.)

Ovarian tumors in preadolescent females, both benign and malignant, are usually unilateral. Thus it is imperative to be conservative in managing the opposite ovary. During surgery the opposite ovary should be carefully inspected and palpated. It is unnecessary and potentially harmful to biopsy a normal-appearing contralateral ovary in a preadolescent female. The most common malignancy in preadolescent females is a germ cell tumor. This neoplasm is highly responsive to platinum-based combination chemotherapy. A recent report of the Pediatrics Oncology Group suggests that surgery alone is curative for most children with resected immature teratomas of the ovary regardless of the grade including those cases with elevated levels of serum alpha-fetoprotein and the findings of microscopic foci of yolk sac tumor. Isosexual GnRH-independent precocious puberty is developed by approximately 75% of prepubertal girls with a granulosa cell tumor.

The most common clinical manifestation of an ovarian tumor is lower abdominal pain or the presence of a mass. Some ovarian tumors in children produce only vague discomfort, such as abdominal fullness or bloating. However, adnexal masses in children are more frequently associated with acute complications, such as torsion, hemorrhage, and rupture, than are similar tumors in adults. Torsion of a normal ovary or fallopian tube is a rare but serious problem in children. Often the symptoms caused by a reduction of the ovarian blood supply produced by torsion is subclinical, with the process progressing to aseptic necrosis of the involved adnexa. The etiology of torsion of normal adnexa in children is not understood. McCrea and other researchers have suggested suspension of the uninvolved ovary to prevent subsequent torsion of the remaining adnexa. Thorp et al. have described a simple surgical technique to limit mobility of the ovary.

Shawis et al. reviewed 71 premenarcheal females with ovarian tumors hospitalized during a 33-year period in Liverpool (Table 12-4). In this series an abdominal mass was palpated in 20 children, and 8 masses were discovered by means of rectal examination. Fifteen of the 71 patients had adnexal torsion. Ten of the tumors (14%) were malignant, with dysgerminoma being the most common malignant neoplasm. Benign teratoma was the most common tumor in children. Conservative surgery, cystectomy, was accomplished in 16 of the 61 benign lesions.

The most common differential diagnosis of an abdominopelvic mass in children that is not an ovarian mass is a benign cyst of the mesentery or omentum. Benign uterine tumors are rare in children. However, functional luteal cysts of the ovary are common in neonates secondary to maternal gonadotrophins. These cysts do not need operative intervention as they will regress spontaneously.

Approximately 75% to 85% of ovarian neoplasms that necessitate surgery, in premenarcheal females, are benign, and approximately 15% to 25% are malignant neoplasms. However, in a review of ovarian masses in children Brown et al. reported that the risk of malignancy was only 3% up

TABLE 12-4
Pathology of Tumors and Cysts of the Ovary

Type	Classification	Number
Benign neoplasms	Teratoma	30
	Cystadenoma	6 (one bilateral)
	Granulosa cell tumor	2
	Brenner's disease	1
Malignant neoplasms	Dysgerminoma	8
	Anaplastic carcinoma	2 (one bilateral)
"Functional" neoplasms	Luteal cysts	8 (one bilateral)
	Follicular cyst	7
Neoplasms of indeterminate histology (hemorrhage or infarction)		8

From Shawis RN, El Gohary AE, and Cook RCM: Ann R Coll Surg Engl 67:28, 1985.

to age 8. Abdominal pain is the most common symptom, and an abdominopelvic mass is the most frequent sign of an ovarian tumor in childhood. In summary, even though ovarian neoplasia is rare in children, this diagnosis must be considered in a young girl with abdominal pain and a palpable mass. The surgical therapy should have two goals: removal of the neoplasia and preservation of future fertility.

PRECOCIOUS PUBERTY

Puberty in the female is the process of biologic change and physical development after which sexual reproduction becomes possible. This is a time of accelerated linear skeletal growth and development of secondary sexual characteristics, such as breast development and the appearance of axillary and pubic hair. The usual sequence of the physiologic events of puberty begins with breast development, the subsequent appearance of pubic and axillary hair, followed by the period of maximal growth velocity, and lastly, menarche. Menarche may occur before the appearance of axillary or pubic hair in 10% of normal females. Normal puberty occurs over a wide range of ages (Chapter 38).

Precocious puberty is arbitrarily defined as the appearance of any signs of secondary sexual maturation at an early specific age more than 2.5 standard deviations below the mean. Five years ago precocious puberty was defined specifically as initiation of secondary sexual characteristics before the age of 8 years or menarche beginning before 9 years. However, data from a recent study of 17,000 healthy 3- to 12-year-old girls demonstrates the onset of puberty in girls is occurring earlier than previous studies in the United States, with breast and pubic hair development appearing on the average of 1 year earlier in Caucasian and 2 years earlier in African American girls (Table

TABLE 12-5
Prevalence of Breast and Pubic Hair Development in White and African-American Girls Between 5 and 10 Years of Age

Age Range in Years	5.00–5.99	6.00–6.99	7.00–7.99	8.00–8.99	9.00–9.99
Prevalence of breast development at Tanner stage 2 or greater (%)					
White	1.6	2.9	5.0	10.5	32.1
African American	2.4	6.4	15.4	37.8	62.6
Prevalence of pubic hair development at Tanner stage 2 or geater (%)					
White	0.4	1.4	2.8	7.7	20.0
African American	3.4	9.5	17.7	34.3	62.6

From Kaplowitz PB, Oberfield SE, and the Drug and Therapeutics and Executive Committees of the Lawson Wilkins Pediatric Endocrine Society: Pediatrics 104:937, 1999.

12-5). In an article by Kaplowitz et al., the Lawson Wilkins Pediatric Endocrine Society proposed that girls with either breast development or pubic hair should be evaluated when these signs occur before age 7 in Caucasian and age 6 in African American girls. Conversely, this panel of experts concluded that in most cases evaluation to find the etiology of precocious puberty in girls with early breast and/or pubic hair development need not be performed for Caucasians older than 7 years of age and for African Americans older than 6 years of age. Precocious puberty is associated with a wide range of disorders. It should be emphasized that regardless of the etiology, precocious puberty is a very rare disease. The incidence of this condition in the United States is estimated to be approximately 1 in 10,000 young girls. When it is diagnosed, the physician should undertake a detailed investigation of the etiology of the condition in order not to overlook a potentially correctable pathologic lesion. The two primary concerns of parents of children with precocious puberty are the social stigma associated with the child being physically different from her peers and the diminished ultimate height caused by the premature closure of epiphyseal growth centers.

Puberty is a time of accelerated growth, skeletal maturation, and resulting epiphyseal closure. Although precocious puberty occurs early in a child's life, it usually develops in the normal sequence. This produces the paradox of precocious puberty. Early in the course of the disease the girls are taller and heavier than their chronologic peers who have not experienced the growth spurt (Figure 12-9). However, although the patient is tall as a child, her eventual adult height will be shorter than normal. Without therapy, approximately 50% of females with precocious puberty will not reach a height of 5 feet. The pathophysiology of this short stature is related to the limited duration of the rapid growth spurt. There is accelerated bone maturation and premature closure of the distal epiphyseal growth centers.

The syndrome of precocious puberty is subdivided into GnRH-dependent (complete, true) or GnRH-independent (incomplete, pseudo) and isosexual and heterosexual disor-

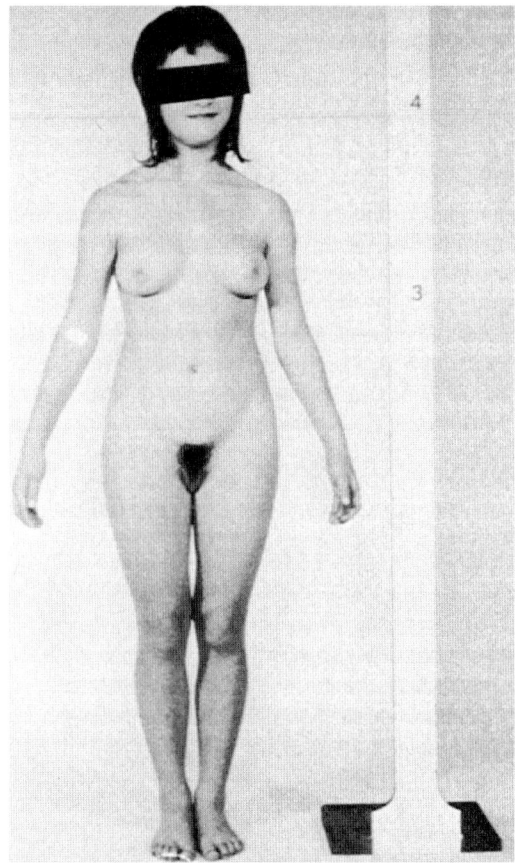

FIGURE 12-9 Child aged 7 years with constitutional precocious puberty. Note increased height for age. (From Dewhurst CJ: Practical pediatric and adolescent gynecology, New York, 1980, Marcel Dekker, Inc. Reprinted courtesy of Marcel Dekker, Inc.)

ders. These categories are of clinical value only after the eventual diagnosis has been established. The pathophysiology and corresponding categories of precocious puberty may change during the course of the disease; for example, congenital adrenal hyperplasia initially is GnRH-independent but subsequently, over many months, eventually becomes a GnRH-dependent form of precocious puberty. The pathophysiology of precocious puberty is divided into two distinct categories: a normal physiologic process occurring at an abnormal time or an abnormal physiologic process independent of an integrated hypothalamic-pituitary-ovarian axis.

GnRH-dependent precocious puberty involves premature maturation of the hypothalamic-pituitary-ovarian axis and includes normal menses, ovulation, and the possibility of pregnancy. GnRH-independent precocious puberty involves premature female sexual maturation and uterine bleeding but without associated ovulation. Both categories have increased circulating levels of estrogen. In the latter syndrome, secretion of estrogens is independent of hypothalamic-pituitary control. Obviously, depending on when the patient is first seen in relationship to the natural history of her disease, it may be necessary to observe her at regular intervals for 2 to 3 years to distinguish one syndrome from another (Table 12-6). Prolonged follow-up is sometimes necessary to rule out subtle, slow-growing lesions of the brain, ovary, or adrenal gland.

The vast majority of females with precocious puberty develop a GnRH-dependent process. The exact etiology of the majority of cases of GnRH-dependent precocious puberty is unknown (constitutional); however, approxi-mately 30% are secondary to central nervous system disease. A definitive diagnosis is established more often for pseudoprecocious puberty, which is usually related to an ovarian or adrenal disorder. If the secondary sex characteristics are discordant with the genetic and phenotypic sex, the condition is termed *heterosexual precocious puberty*. This is premature virilization in a female child and includes development of masculine secondary sexual characteristics. The androgens that cause heterosexual precocious puberty usually come from the adrenal gland.

Premature Thelarche

Premature thelarche is defined as isolated unilateral or bilateral breast development as the only sign of secondary sexual maturation. It is not accompanied by other associated evidence of pubertal development, such as axillary or pubic hair or changes in vaginal epithelium. Breast hyperplasia is a normal physiologic phenomenon in the neonatal period, and it may persist up to 6 months of age. Premature thelarche usually occurs between 1 and 4 years of age. The breast buds enlarge to 2 to 4 cm and sometimes this process is asymmetrical. Nipple development is absent. This is a benign, self-limiting condition that does not require treatment. Often the breast enlargement sponta-

---

TABLE 12-6
Physical Findings Among Patients with Various Syndromes of Precocious Puberty

Findings	Premature Thelarche	Premature Adrenarche	GnRH-Dependent and GnRH-Independent			
			Idiopathic	Central Nervous System Tumor	McCune-Albright Syndrome	Hypothyroid
Breast enlargement	Yes	No	Yes	Yes	Yes	Yes
Pubic hair	No	Yes	Yes	Yes	Yes	Unusual
Vaginal bleeding	No	No	Yes	Yes	Yes	Yes
Virilizing signs	No	No	No	No	No	No
Bone age	Normal	Normal to minimally advanced	Advanced	Advanced	Advanced	Normal or retarded
Neurologic deficit	No	No	No	Yes	Yes	No
Abdominopelvic mass	No	No	Occ'l	No	No	Occ'l

Findings	Isosexual			Heterosexual		
	Ovarian Tumors	Adrenal Tumors	Factitious	Ovarian Tumors	Adrenal Tumors	Adrenal Hyperplasia
Breast enlargement	Yes	Yes	Yes	Yes	Yes	Yes
Pubic hair	Yes	Yes	Yes	Yes	Yes	Yes
Vaginal bleeding	Yes	Yes	Yes	Yes	Yes	Yes
Virilizing signs	No	Yes	No	Yes	Yes	Yes
Bone age	Advanced	Advanced	Advanced	Advanced	Advanced	Advanced
Neurologic deficit	No	No	No	No	No	No
Abdominopelvic mass	Usually	No	No	Occ'l	No	No

From Ross GT: Disorders of the ovary and female reproductive tract. In Wilson JD and Foster DW, eds: Williams textbook of endocrinology, ed 7, Philadelphia, 1985, WB Saunders Co.

neously regresses. It is important to observe these children closely for other signs of precocious puberty. The etiology of premature thelarche is not understood. However, it is postulated to be related to a slight increase in circulating estrogen levels. This condition frequently occurs in female infants who had extremely low birth weights. The child should be seen at regular intervals in follow-up to rule out progression of the symptoms to precocious puberty. However, long-term observation demonstrates that the vast majority of these girls subsequently have normal growth, and puberty occurs in a normal fashion.

Premature Pubarche or Adrenarche

Premature pubarche is early isolated development of pubic hair without other signs of secondary sexual maturation. Premature adrenarche is isolated early development of axillary hair. Neither of these conditions is progressive, and the girls do not have clitoral hypertrophy. However, it is important to differentiate premature pubarche from the virilization produced by the adrenogenital syndrome. Some children with premature pubarche have abnormal electroencephalograms (EEGs) without significant neurologic disease. The bone age should not be advanced. The etiology is poorly understood but believed to be related to increased androgen production by the adrenal glands (DHEA and DHEA-S). Similar to premature thelarche, the child should have periodic follow-up visits to confirm that the condition is not progressive.

GnRH-Dependent Precocious Puberty

Idiopathic development is responsible for approximately 70% of the cases of GnRH-dependent precocious puberty. Some of these children are simply at the earliest limits of the normal distribution of the biologic curve. Most idiopathic cases are sporadic in distribution; however, a few are familial.

A high incidence of abnormal EEGs in children with idiopathic precocious puberty has raised the question of potential central nervous system disease. With increasing use of high-resolution imaging techniques, such as cranial CT scan and magnetic resonance imaging (MR), the number of idiopathic cases is declining.

These girls have no genital abnormality except early development. Occasionally they develop follicular cysts of the ovaries secondary to increased levels of pituitary gonadotrophins (Figure 12-10). In these cases the cysts are a result, not the cause, of precocious puberty. Gonadotrophin levels, sex steroid levels, and response of luteinizing hormone (LH) after administration of gonadotrophin-releasing hormone (GnRH) are similar to those in normal puberty. The cause of premature maturation of the hypothalamic-pituitary-ovarian axis is unknown. The syndrome may appear as early as age 3 to 4 years. When observed for several decades, these women have normal menopausal ages. Emotional problems are a concern

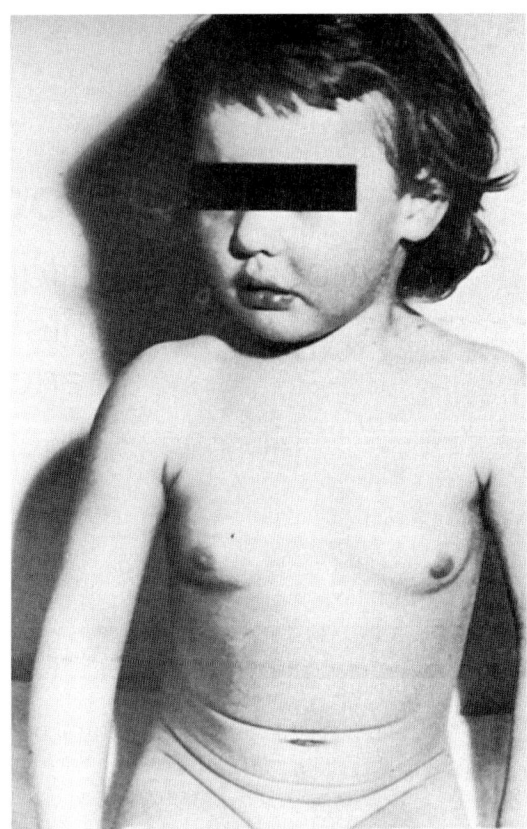

FIGURE 12-10 Precocious puberty in young girl. Child had large lower abdominal swelling, which at operation was shown to be bilateral follicular cysts (result of premature ovarian stimulation and not cause of condition). (From Dewhurst CJ: Practical pediatric and adolescent gynecology, New York, 1980, Marcel Dekker, Inc. Reprinted courtesy of Marcel Dekker, Inc.)

because the young girls suffer from extreme social pressures. The intellectual, behavioral, and psychosocial development of girls with precocious puberty is appropriate for their chronologic age. Most are shy and withdrawn from their peers. The diagnosis of idiopathic or constitutional precocious puberty is made by exclusion.

A wide range of inflammatory, degenerative, neoplastic, or congenital defects that involve the central nervous system may produce GnRH-dependent precocious puberty. Usually, symptoms of a neurologic disease, especially headaches and visual disturbances, precede the manifestations of precocious puberty. A most unusual neurologic symptom that may be associated with precocious puberty is seizures with inappropriate laughter (gelastic seizures). Anatomically, most central nervous system lesions are located near the hypothalamus in the region of the third ventricle, tuber cinereum, or mammillary bodies. Major central nervous system diseases associated with true precocious puberty include tuberculosis, encephalitis, trauma, secondary hydrocephalus, neurofibromatosis, granulomas, hamartomas of the hypothalamus, teratomas, craniopharyngiomas, cranial irradiation, and congenital brain

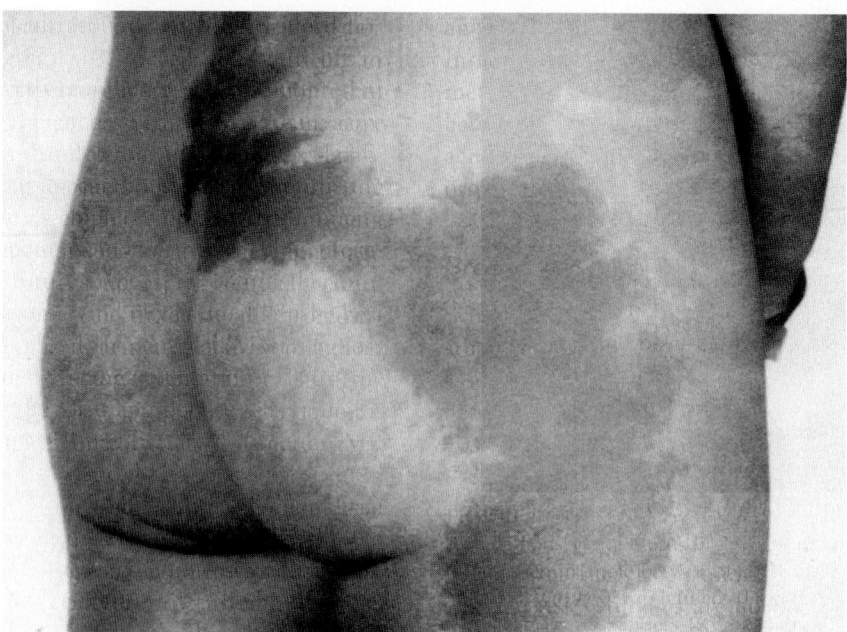

FIGURE 12-11 Large café-au-lait spot in child with precocious puberty as result of McCune-Albright syndrome. (From Dewhurst CJ: Practical pediatric and adolescent gynecology, New York, 1980, Marcel Dekker, Inc. Reprinted courtesy of Marcel Dekker, Inc.)

defects, such as hydrocephalus and cysts in the area of the third ventricle. These children have markedly fluctuating estrogen levels and low gonadotrophin concentrations that are independent of GnRH stimulation. These central nervous system space-occupying masses are most difficult to successfully treat surgically. The pathophysiology by which central nervous system disease produces precocious puberty is poorly understood. It is known that hamartomas may secrete GnRH; this secretion is not subject to the normal physiologic inhibition that occurs during childhood.

GnRH-Independent Precocious Puberty

The most common cause of pseudoprecocious puberty is an estrogen-secreting ovarian tumor. Granulosa cell tumors are the most common type, accounting for approximately 60%. These tumors are usually greater than 8 cm when associated with precocious puberty; 80% can be palpated abdominally. Other ovarian tumors that may be associated with precocious puberty include thecomas, luteomas, teratomas, Sertoli-Leydig tumors, choriocarcinomas, and benign follicular cysts. Thecomas and luteomas are usually much smaller than granulosa tumors and usually cannot be palpated abdominally. Overall, these tumors are rare during childhood; only 5% of granulosa cell tumors and 1% of thecomas occur before puberty. Infrequently, follicular cysts of the ovary enlarge and secrete enough estrogen to be the cause, rather than the result, of precocious puberty. It is speculated that the benign cysts function in an autonomous fashion. The ability of many tumors, including teratomas, choriocarcinomas, and dysgermino-

mas, to secrete human chorionic gonadotrophin (HCG) or estrogen has been established by radioimmunoassay. Rarely do these tumors produce precocious puberty.

McCune-Albright syndrome (polyostotic fibrous dysplasia) is a rare triad of café-au-lait spots, fibrous dysplasia, and cysts of the skull and long bones (Figure 12-11). These patients also have facial asymmetry. Approximately 40% of girls with McCune-Albright syndrome have associated isosexual precocious puberty.

Adrenocortical neoplasms may produce either isosexual or heterosexual precocious puberty. The relationship between congenital adrenal hyperplasia and puberty depends on the time of initial diagnosis and therapy. If the disease is diagnosed in the neonatal period and treated, normal puberty ensues. If the disease is untreated, the girl over time usually develops heterosexual precocious puberty from the adrenal androgens. However, if congenital adrenal hyperplasia is diagnosed late in childhood, isosexual precocious puberty may follow initial treatment of the adrenal disease.

Hypothyroidism most commonly is associated with delayed pubertal development. However, in rare instances untreated hypothyroidism results in either isosexual, GnRH-dependent, or GnRH-independent precocious puberty. The hypothyroidism associated with precocious puberty is due to primary thyroid insufficiency, usually Hashimoto's thyroiditis, and not a deficiency in pituitary thyroid-stimulating hormone (TSH). The pathophysiology of this syndrome is caused by the diminished negative feedback of thyroxine, resulting in an increased production of TSH. There is an associated increase in production

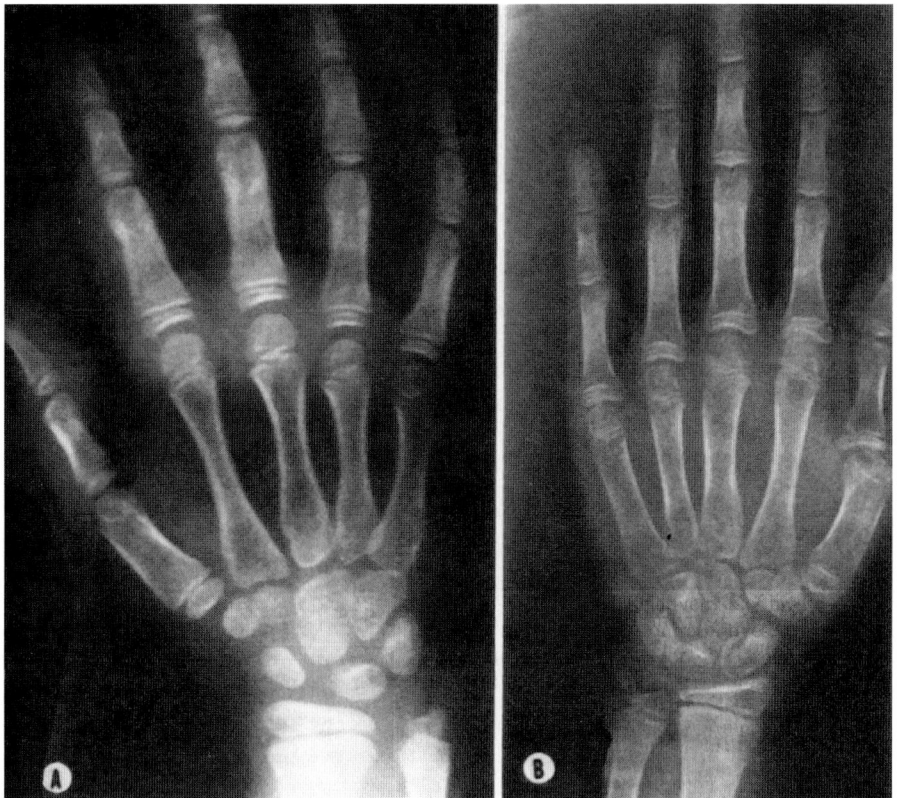

FIGURE 12-12 X-ray films demonstrating bone age. **A,** Normal for 7 years of age. **B,** Advanced bone age in a girl 7 years of age who also shows other signs of isosexual precocity. (From Huffman JW: The gynecology of childhood and adolescence, ed 2, Philadelphia, 1981, WB Saunders Co.)

TABLE 12-7
Laboratory Findings in Disorders Producing Precocious Puberty

	Gonadal Size	Basal FSH/LH	Estradiol or Testosterone	DHAS	GnRH Response
Idiopathic	Increased	Increased	Increased	Increased	Pubertal
Cerebral	Increased	Increased	Increased	Increased	Pubertal
Gonadal	Unilat. incr.	Decreased	Increased	Increased	Flat
Albright	Increased	Decreased	Increased	Increased	Flat
Adrenal	Small	Decreased	Increased	Increased	Flat

From Speroff L, Glass RH, and Kase NG: Clinical gynecologic endocrinology and infertility, ed 6, Baltimore, 1999, Lippincott Williams & Wilkins. p. 396.

of gonadotrophins. Interestingly, hypothyroidism is the only etiology of precocious puberty in which the bone age is retarded. This syndrome is observed usually in girls between the ages of 6 and 8 years.

Iatrogenic or factitious precocious puberty results when a young female has used hormonal cream or ingested adult medication such as oral estrogen or birth control pills. The secondary sexual characteristics regress after discontinuation of the medication.

Diagnosis

The diagnostic workup of a young child with precocious puberty begins with a meticulous history and physical examination. The primary emphasis should be to rule out life-threatening neoplasms of the ovary, adrenal, or central nervous system. The secondary emphasis is to delineate the speed of the maturation process, for this fact is crucial in decisions concerning therapy. The height of the girl and exact stage of pubertal development, including Tanner stage, should be recorded. Similar to other syndromes with a long list of etiologies, a battery of tests, including imaging studies of the brain, serum estradiol levels, FSH levels, and thyroid function tests, may be needed to establish the diagnosis (Table 12-7). Acceleration of growth is one of the earliest clinical features of precocious puberty. Thus bone age should be determined by hand-wrist films and compared with standards for a patient's age (Figure 12-12). Usually these films are repeated at 6-month intervals to evaluate the rate of skeletal maturation and correspondingly the necessity of active treatment of the disease. Advancement of bone age more than 95% of the norm for the child's chronologic age documents a peripheral estrogen effect.

Diseases of the central nervous system should be highlighted during the history such as headaches, seizures, trauma to the head, and encephalitis. These conditions are confirmed or excluded by a series of tests, including neurologic and ophthalmologic examinations, EEGs, skull x-ray films, and subsequent cranial CT and/or MR. Often children who develop precocious puberty had a low birth weight for their gestational age.

Recent improved radiologic diagnosis of subtle central nervous system abnormalities with use of cranial CT, pneumoencephalography, and MR has increased the sensitivity and frequency of discovery of the underlying cause of true precocious puberty. Hypothalamic harmartomas can be classified based on the tumor topology on MR imaging. This classification has been shown to correlate with the clinical manifestations of precocious puberty. Ultrasound and/or CT of the abdomen should be performed to evaluate enlargement of the ovaries (ovarian volume), uterus, or adrenal glands.

Serum levels of FSH, LH, prolactin, TSH, estradiol, testosterone, dehydroepiandrosterone (DHEA) or DHEA-S, HCG, androstenedione, 17-hydroxyprogesterone, triiodothyronine, and thyroxine may be of value in establishing the differential diagnosis. Sometimes a GnRH stimulation test is diagnostic in differentiating incomplete from true precocious puberty, but this test does not specifically identify children with central nervous system lesions.

The LH responses to gonadotrophin stimulation after reaching a basal level are similar in cases of true precocious puberty to the responses of a mature adult. In contrast, a child with precocious puberty secondary to a feminizing ovarian neoplasm does not have a significant elevation in LH response to exogenous gonadotrophins. In summary, a stimulation test with exogenous GnRH is fundamental in helping to delineate the underlying pathophysiology (Table 12-8).

Management

The treatment of precocious puberty depends on the cause, the extent and progression of precocious signs, and whether the cause may be removed operatively. For example, extirpation of a granulosa cell tumor and subtotal removal of a hypothalamic hamartoma are successful treatments because they remove hormone-secreting tumors. Because most cases involve premature maturation of the hypothalamic-pituitary-ovarian axis without a lesion, this discussion focuses on the medical management of this condition. Girls with menarche before age 8 years, progressive thelarche and pubarche, and bone age more than 2 years greater than their chronologic ages definitely should be treated. The goals of therapy are to reduce gonadotrophin secretions and reduce or counteract the peripheral actions of the sex steroids, decrease growth rate to normal, and slow skeletal maturation to allow development of maximal adult height.

The present drug of choice for GnRH-dependent precocious puberty is one of the potent agonists—analogues of GnRH. The development of GnRH agonists was a major advance in the treatment of true precocious puberty, and even conservative endocrinologists have called this type of medication the "ideal drug" for this condition. The long-acting agonists were developed by inserting a D-amino acid in place of the naturally occurring L-amino acid at critical enzyme cleavage sites of the hormone. Presently, these drugs are usually given by monthly injections or, rarely, intranasally. They are

---

TABLE 12-8

Gonadotrophin and Estradiol Levels in Girls with Precocious Puberty Before and After Administration of 100 g GnRH

	Number	LH (IU/L, mean ± SD)		FSH (IU/L, mean ± SD)		Estradiol (pmol/L)	
		Basal	Peak	Basal	Peak	Mean	Range
Idiopathic precocious puberty	18	2.4 ± 2.0	36.9 ± 20.0	3.0 ± 1.8	16.3 ± 7.9	91.2	22–318
Intercranial lesion	9	2.6 ± 2.0	30.7 ± 17.3	4.4 ± 3.0	24.6 ± 5.1	107	22–240

From Lyon AJ, De Bruyn R, and Grant DB: Acta Pediatr Scand 74:953, 1985.

rapid, safe, and effective treatments for children with the disease secondary to disturbances in the hypothalamic-pituitary-ovarian axis. GnRH agonist therapy should be initiated as soon as possible after the diagnosis is established in order to achieve maximal adult height. The effect on adult height depends on the chronologic age at which the GnRH therapy is initiated. The therapy is most effective in 4- to 6-year-olds. Continuous chronic administration of the drug is maintained until the median age of puberty. The optimal dosage of medication may be confirmed by determining that peripheral estradiol levels are in a normal prepubertal range. Medical therapy produces involution of secondary sexual characteristics, with amenorrhea and regression of both breast development and amount of pubic hair. LH and FSH pulsations are abolished. Most importantly the drug not only reverses the ovarian cycle but definitely changes the growth pattern. Growth velocity is usually decreased approximately 50% (Figure 12-13). In one series the predicted adult height increased a mean of 6.5 cm in girls who were age 6 years or less when therapy was initiated. The potent agonists inhibit gonadotrophin secretion by increasing the down regulation of GnRH receptors. This inhibition of the pituitary secretion and release of gonadotrophins through continuous therapy is readily reversible by discontinuing the medication.

Multiple studies have documented that agonist therapy decreases gonadotrophins within 1 week and decreases sex steroids to the prepubertal range within the first 2 weeks of therapy (Figure 12-14). Serial ultrasound examinations have documented that the size of the ovaries and uterus regresses to normal prepubertal shape and size. The most common observed side effect to agonists was cutaneous reaction at the site of injection. However, approximately

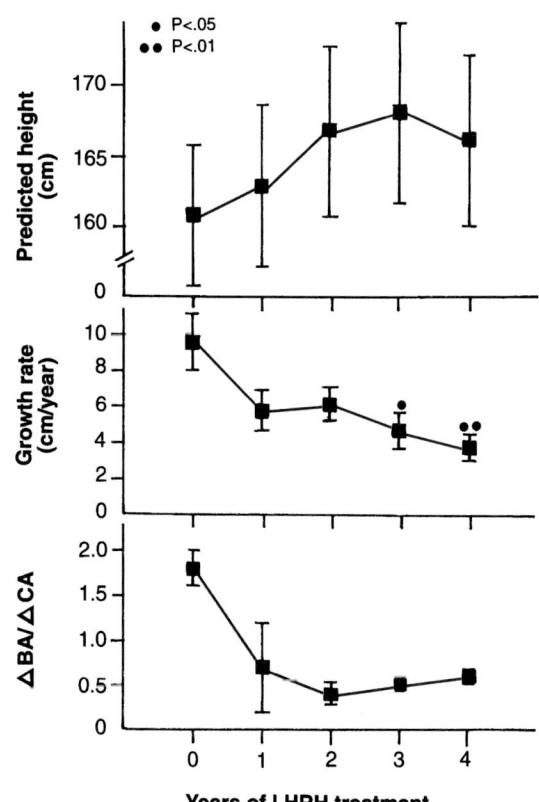

FIGURE 12-13   Predicted height, growth rate, and rate of bone age advancement in six children with central precocious puberty who have received 4 years of therapy with the long-acting analogue of luteinizing hormone releasing hormone (LHRH). Asterisks indicate significant differences compared with pretreatment value. (Redrawn from Comite F, Cassorla F, Barnes KM, et al: JAMA 255:2615, 1986.)

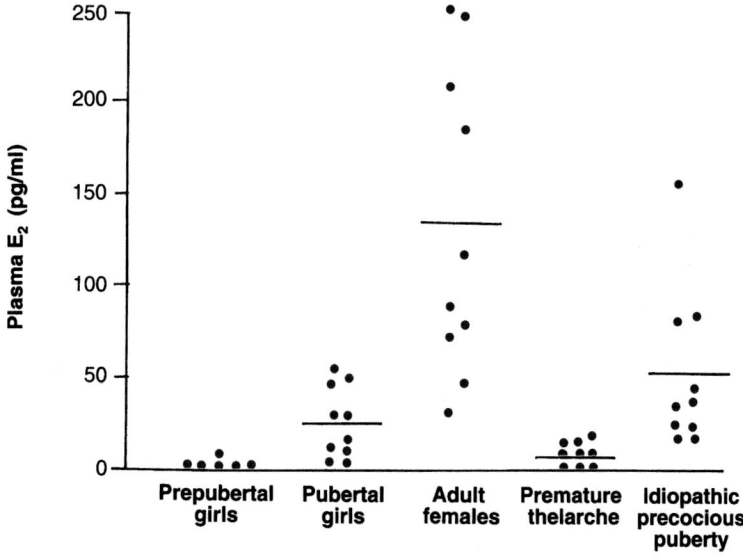

FIGURE 12-14   Estradiol values (x = 1 SD) in normal females and in patients with premature thelarche and idiopathic precocious puberty. (Redrawn from Escobar ME, Rivarola MA, and Bergada C: Acta Endocrinol 81:351, 1976.)

one in four girls experienced recurrent and sometimes prolonged vaginal bleeding while receiving GnRH agonists. The effects of these drugs are quite reversible when the agonists are discontinued after normal height is achieved. The Lawson Wilkins Pediatric Endocrine Society has stated the use of GnRH agonists in 6- to 8-year-old girls with slowly progressing puberty and an accepted predictable adult height based on bone age has not been proven to have a significant effect in improving adult height.

Recently, small studies have suggested a minimal benefit from adding growth hormone to GnRH agonist therapy in girls with suboptimal growth. The initial observations of combination therapy are encouraging, but the clinical data is from small series and of a preliminary nature.

Patients with McCune-Albright syndrome may be treated with testolactone, an aromatase inhibitor, which prevents the conversion of estrogen precursors to biologically active estrogens. This treatment leads to diminished circulating estrogen levels, diminished frequency of menses, and a decreased rate of growth and skeletal maturation.

Both the child with precocious puberty and her family need intensive counseling. The child will have the psychosocial and behavioral maturation of children of her chronologic age, not the age reflected by her physical appearance. She may be exposed to ridicule by her peers and to sexual exploitation. Thus the child needs extensive sex education and help in anticipating and confronting various social experiences. Often it is possible to dress the child in clothes that diminish the recognition of her advanced sexual maturation until the effects of her disease are inhibited by drug therapy.

KEY POINTS

- In the field of pediatric gynecology, most diagnostic errors result from errors of omission during the examination rather than errors of commission.

- It is important to give the child a sense that she will be in control of the examination process. Emphasize that the most important part of the examination is just "looking" and there will be conversation during the entire process.

- Many gynecologic conditions in children may be diagnosed by inspection only.

- The vaginal epithelium of the prepubertal child appears redder and thinner than the vaginal epithelium of a woman in her reproductive years. The prepubertal vagina is also narrower, thinner, and lacking in the distensibility of the vagina of a woman in her reproductive years. The vagina of a child is 4 to 5 cm long and has a neutral pH.

- During the physical examination and rectal examination of the prepubertal child, no pelvic masses except the cervix should be palpated. The normal prepubertal uterus and ovaries are nonpalpable. The relative size ratio of cervix to uterus is 2 to 1 in a child.

- Many female adolescents do not want other observers in the examining room.

- It is estimated that 80% to 90% of outpatient visits of children to gynecologists involve the classic symptoms of vulvovaginitis: introital irritation and discharge.

- Positive identification of *Trichomonas*, gonorrhea, or *Chlamydia* in a child with premenarcheal vulvovaginitis often indicates sexual molestation. However, many infants are infected with *Chlamydia trichomatis* during birth and remain infected for several years in the absence of specific antibiotic therapy.

- The major factor in childhood vulvovaginitis is poor perineal hygiene.

- A vaginal discharge that is both bloody and foul smelling strongly suggests the presence of a foreign body.

- In the period from 6 to 12 months before menarche, children often develop a physiologic discharge secondary to the increase in circulating estrogen levels.

- The foundation of treating childhood vulvovaginitis is the improvement of local perineal hygiene.

- The vast majority of cases of persistent or recurrent nonspecific vulvovaginitis respond to a combination of topical creams and oral antibiotics given for 10 to 14 days.

- The classic symptom of pinworms *(Enterobius vermicularis)* is nocturnal vulvar and perianal itching, the treatment for which is the antihelmintic agent mebendazole (Vermox).

- The most common vaginal foreign body in preadolescent females is a wad of toilet tissue.

- Persistent vaginal bleeding is an extremely rare symptom in a preadolescent female. However, it is important to do a thorough workup because of the serious sequelae of some of the causes of vaginal bleeding.

- Adhesive vulvitis does not require treatment unless voiding is compromised. If necessary, small amounts of daily topical estrogen to the labia may be used for a maximum of 3 weeks.

- If the labial adhesions are identified early in life and do not resolve with time or estrogen cream, it is appropriate to refer the child to a gynecologic endocrinologist to rule out a congenital anomaly.

- The usual cause of genital trauma during childhood is an accidental fall. The majority of such trauma involves straddle injuries.

- Accidental genital trauma often produces extreme pain and overwhelming anxiety for the child and her parents. Because of compassion and empathy, the gynecologist may underestimate the extent of the anatomic injuries. Thus, if in doubt, examine the child under general anesthesia.

- Small follicular cysts are common in preadolescent females and are usually self-limiting.

- Ovarian tumors constitute approximately 1% of all neoplasms in premenarcheal children. In preadolescent females, both benign and malignant ovarian tumors are usually unilateral. It is unnecessary and potentially harmful to biopsy a normal-appearing contralateral ovary in a preadolescent female.

- Approximately 75% to 85% of ovarian neoplasms necessitating surgery are benign, with cystic teratomas being the most common.

- The most common malignancy in preadolescent females is a germ cell tumor. This neoplasm is highly responsive to platinum-based combination chemotherapy.

- Even though ovarian neoplasia is rare in children, this diagnosis must be considered in a young girl with abdominal pain and a palpable mass. The surgical therapy should have two goals: removal of the neoplasia and preservation of future fertility.

- Physiologic development in females with precocious puberty usually follows the normal sequence of changes of secondary sexual characteristics.

- The two primary concerns of parents of children with precocious puberty are the social stigma associated with the child being physically different from her peers and the diminished ultimate height caused by the premature closure of epiphyseal growth centers.

- The exact etiology of the majority of cases of GnRH-dependent (true or complete) precocious puberty is unknown; however, approximately 30% of cases are secondary to central nervous system disease.

- A definitive diagnosis is established more often for GnRH-independent (pseudoprecocious or incomplete) puberty, and it is usually related to an ovarian or adrenal disorder.

- Breast hyperplasia is a normal phenomenon in neonates and may persist up to 6 months of age.

- The most common cause of GnRH-independent precocious puberty is a functioning ovarian tumor. Granulosa cell tumors are the most common type, accounting for approximately 60%.

- The primary emphasis of the diagnostic workup on a child with precocious puberty should be to rule out life-threatening neoplasms of the ovary, adrenal, or central nervous system. The secondary emphasis is to delineate the speed of the maturation process, for this fact is crucial in decisions concerning therapy.

- The goals of therapy of precocious puberty are to reduce gonadotrophin secretions and reduce or counteract the peripheral actions of sex steroids, decreasing growth rate to normal and slowing skeletal maturation. This is best accomplished by GnRH agonists.

- The effect on adult height depends on the chronologic age at which the GnRH therapy is initiated. The therapy is most effective in 4- to 6-year-olds.

- Both the child with precocious puberty and her family need intensive counseling.

BIBLIOGRAPHY

Albright AL and Lee PA: Hypothalamic hamartomas and sexual precocity, Pediatr Neurosurg 18:315, 1992.

Ambrosino MM, Hernanz-Schulman M, Genieser NB, et al: Monitoring of girls undergoing medical therapy for isosexual precocious puberty, J Ultrasound Med 13:501, 1994.

American College of Obstetricians and Gynecologists: Pediatric gynecologic disorders, ACOG Tech Bull 201:1, 1995.

Arita K, Ikawa F, Jurisu K, et al: The relationship between magnetic resonance imaging findings and clinical manifestations of hypothalamic hamartoma, J Neurosurg 91:212, 1999.

Bell TA, Stamm WE, Wang S, et al: Chronic *Chlamydia trachomatis* infections in infants, JAMA 267:400, 1992.

Blake J: Gynecologic examination of the teenager and young child, Obstet Gynecol Clin North Am 19:27, 1992.

Boepple PA, Frisch LS, Wierman ME, et al: The natural history of autonomous gonadal function, adrenarche, and central puberty in gonadotropin-independent precocious puberty, J Clin Endocrinol Metab 75:1550, 1992.

Bonazzi C, Peccatori F, Colombo N, et al: Pure ovarian immature teratoma, a unique and curable disease: 10 years' experience of 32 prospectively treated patients, Obstet Gynecol 84:598, 1994.

Bond GR, Dowd MD, Landsman I, and Rimsza M: Unintentional perineal injury in prepubescent girls: a multicenter, prospective report of 56 girls, Pediatrics 95:628, 1995.

Brenner PF: Precocious puberty in the female. In Lobo R, Mishell DR Jr, Paulson RJ, and Shoupe D, eds: Mishell's textbook of infertility, contraception and reproductive endocrinology, ed 4, Malden, Mass, 1997, Blackwell Science.

Bridges NA, Cooke A, Healy MJR, et al: Standards for ovarian volume in childhood and puberty, Fertil Steril 60:456, 1993.

Brown MF, Hebra A, McGeehin K, and Ross AJ III: Ovarian masses in children: a review of 91 cases of malignant and benign masses, J Pediatr Surg 28:930, 1993.

Buchta RM: Use of chaperons during pelvic examinations of female adolescents, Am J Dis Child 141:666, 1987.

Capraro VJ: Pediatric gynecology. In Danforth DN, ed: Obstetrics and gynecology, ed 4, Philadelphia, 1982, Harper & Row, Publishers, Inc.

Carpenter SE and Rock JA, eds: Pediatric and adolescent gynecology, New York, 1992, Raven Press, Ltd.

Cohen HL, Eisenberg P, Mandel F, and Haller JO: Ovarian cysts are common in premenarchal girls: a sonographic study of 101 children 2-12 years old, AJR 159:89, 1992.

Comite F, Cassorla F, Barnes KM, et al: Luteinizing hormone releasing hormone analogue therapy for central precocious puberty: long-term effect on somatic growth, bone maturation, and predicted height, JAMA 255:2613, 1986.

Cronjé HS, Niemand I, Bam RH, and Woodruff JD: Granulosa and theca cell tumors in children: a report of 17 cases and literature review, Obstet Gynecol Surv 53:240, 1998.

Cushing B, Giller R, Ablin A, et al: Surgical resection alone is effective treatment for ovarian immature teratoma in children and adolescents: a report of the Pediatric Oncology Group and the Children's Cancer Group, Am J Obstet Gynecol 181:353, 1999.

DiMartino-Nardi J: Premature adrenarche: findings in prepubertal African-American and Caribbean-Hispanic girls, Acta Paediatr Suppl 433:67, 1999.

DiMartino-Nardi J, Wu R, Varner R, et al: The effect of luteinizing hormone-releasing hormone analog for central precocious puberty on growth hormone (GH) and GH-binding protein, J Clin Endocrinol Metab 78:664, 1994.

Ehren IM, Mahour GH, and Isaacs H: Benign and malignant ovarian tumors in children and adolescents, Am J Surg 147:339, 1984.

Ehrhardt AA and Meyer-Bahlburg HFL: Psychosocial aspects of precocious puberty, Horm Res 41(S2):30, 1994.

Emans SJ and Goldstein DP: The gynecologic examination of the prepubertal child with vulvovaginitis: use of the knee-chest position, Pediatrics 65:758, 1980.

Emans SJH and Goldstein DP: Pediatric and adolescent gynecology, ed 4, Philadelphia, 1998, Lippincott-Raven.

Emans SJ, Woods ER, Allred EN, and Grace E: Hymenal findings in adolescent women: impact of tampon use and consensual sexual activity, J Pediatr 125:153, 1994.

Farrington PF: Pediatric vulvo-vaginitis, Clin Obstet Gynecol 40:135, 1997.

Feuillan PP, Foster CM, Pescovitz OH, et al: Treatment of precocious puberty in the McCune-Albright syndrome with the aromatase inhibitor testolactone, N Engl J Med 315:1115, 1986.

Freud E, Golinsky D, Steinberg RM, et al: Ovarian masses in children, Clin Pediatr 38:573, 1999.

Galatzer A and Laron Z: Behavior in girls with true precocious puberty, J Pediatr 108:790, 1986.

Goff CW, Burke KR, Rickenback C, and Buebendorf DP: Vaginal opening measurement in prepubertal girls, Am J Dis Child 143:1366, 1989.

Goodpasture JC, Ghai K, Cara JF, and Rosenfield RL: Potential of gonadotropin-releasing hormone agonists in the diagnosis of pubertal disorders in girls, Clin Obstet Gynecol 36:773, 1993.

Hairston L: Physical examination of the prepupertal girl, Clin Obstet Gynecol 40:127, 1997.

Hammerschlag MR: Sexually transmitted diseases in sexually abused children: medical and legal implications, Sex Trans Inf 74:167, 1998.

Handley J, Dinsmore W, Maw R, et al: Anogenital warts in prepubertal children: sexual abuse or not? Int J STD AIDS 4:271, 1993.

Hill NCW, Oppenheimer LW, and Morton KE: The aetiology of vaginal bleeding in children: a 20-year review, Br J Obstet Gynaecol 96:467, 1989.

Hintz RL, Attie KM, Baptista J, and Roche A for the Genentech Collaborative Group: Effect of growth hormone treatment on adult height of children with idiopathic short stature, N Engl J Med 340:502, 1999.

Huffman JW: The gynecology of childhood and adolescence, ed 2, Philadelphia, 1981, WB Saunders Co.

Ibáñez L, Potau N, Francois I, and de Zegher F: Precocious pubarche, hyperinsulinism, and ovarian hyperandrogenism in girls: relation to reduced fetal growth, J Clin Endocrinol Metab 83:3558, 1998.

Ibáñez L, Potau N, and de Zegher F: Endocrinology and metabolism after premature pubarche in girls, Acta Paediatr Suppl 433:73, 1999.

Jabra AA, Fishman EK, and Taylor GA: Primary ovarian tumors in the pediatric patient: CT evaluation, Clin Imaging 17:199, 1993.

Jay N, Mansfield MJ, Blizzard RM, et al: Ovulation and menstrual function of adolescent girls with central precocious puberty after therapy with gonadotropin-releasing hormone agonists, J Clin Endocrinol Metab 75:890, 1992.

Jenkinson SD and Mackinnon AE: Spontaneous separation of fused labia minora in prepubertal girls, Br Med J 289:160, 1984.

Kao SCS, Cook JS, Hansen JR, and Simonson TM: MR imaging of the pituitary gland in central precocious puberty, Pediatr Radiol 22:481, 1992.

Kaplowitz PB, Oberfield SE, and the Drug and Therapeutics and Executive Committees of the Lawson Wilkins Pediatric Endocrine Society: Reexamination of the age limit for defining when puberty is precocious in girls in the United States: implications for evaluation and treatment, Pediatr 104:936, 1999.

King LR, Siegel MJ, and Solomon AL: Usefulness of ovarian volume and cysts in female isosexual precocious puberty, J Ultrasound Med 12:577, 1993.

Klein VR, Willman SP, and Carr BR: Familial posterior labial fusion, Obstet Gynecol 73:500, 1989.

Kletter GB and Kelch RP: Effects of gonadotropin-releasing hormone analog therapy on adult stature in precocious puberty, J Clin Endocrinol Metab 79:331, 1994.

Kreiter M, Burstein S, Rosenfield RL, et al: Preserving adult height potential in girls with idiopathic true precocious puberty, J Pediatr 117:364, 1990.

Layman LC: Mutations in human gonadotropin genes and their physiologic significance in puberty and reproduction, Fertil Steril 71:201, 1999.

Lee PA: Laboratory monitoring of children with precocious puberty, Arch Pediatr Adolesc Med 148:369, 1994.

Lee PA, Page JG, and the Leuprolide Study Group: Effects of leuprolide in the treatment of central precocious puberty, J Pediatr 114:321, 1989.

Leung AKC and Robson WLM: Labial fusion and asymptomatic bacteriuria, Eur J Pediatr 152:250, 1993.

Leung AKC, Robson WLM, and Tay-Uyboco J: The incidence of labial fusion in children, J Paediatr Child Health 29:235, 1993.

Liapi C and Evain-Brion D: Diagnosis of ovarian follicular cysts from birth to puberty: a report of twenty cases, Acta Paediatr Scand 76:91, 1987.

Mansfield MJ, Beardsworth DE, Loughlin JS, et al: Long-term treatment of central precocious puberty with a long-acting analogue of luteinizing hormone–releasing hormone, N Engl J Med 309:1286, 1983.

McCann J, Voris J, and Simon M: Labial adhesions and posterior fourchette injuries in childhood sexual abuse, Am J Dis Child 142:659, 1988.

McCann J, Voris J, Simon M, and Wells R: Comparison of genital examination techniques in prepubertal girls, Pediatr 85:182, 1990.

McCrea RS: Uterine adnexal torsion with subsequent contralateral recurrence, J Reprod Med 25:123, 1980.

Meffert JJ, Davis BM, and Grimwood RE: Lichen sclerosus, J Am Acad Derm 32:393, 1995.

Miller WL: The molecular basis of premature adrenarche: an hypothesis, Acta Paediatr Suppl 433:60, 1999.

Millar DM, Blake JM, Stringer DA, et al: Prepubertal ovarian cyst formation: 5 years' experience, Obstet Gynecol 81:434, 1993.

Muram D: Child sexual abuse—genital tract findings in prepubertal girls. I. The unaided medical examination, Am J Obstet Gynecol 160:328, 1989.

Muram D and Elias S: Child sexual abuse—genital tract findings in prepubertal girls. II. Comparison of colposcopic and unaided examinations, Am J Obstet Gynecol 160:333, 1989.

Muram D and Laufer MR: Limitations of the medical evaluation for child sexual abuse, J Reprod Med 44:993, 1999.

Pacheco BP, Di Paola G, Ribas JMM, et al: Vulvar infection caused by human papilloma virus in children and adolescents without sexual contact, Adolesc Pediatr Gynecol 4:136, 1991.

Pasquino AM, Tebaldi L, Cives C, et al: Precocious puberty in the McCune-Albright syndrome, Acta Paediatr Scand 76:841, 1987.

Pescovitz OH, Comite F, Hench K, et al: The NIH experience with precocious puberty: diagnostic subgroups and response to short-term luteinizing hormone releasing hormone analogue therapy, J Pediatr 108:47, 1986.

Pescovitz OH, Hench KD, Barnes KM, et al: Premature thelarche and central precocious puberty: the relationship between clinical presentation and the gonadotropin response to luteinizing hormone–releasing hormone, J Clin Endocrinol Metab 67:474, 1988.

Pokorny SF: Prepubertal vulvovaginopathies, Obstet Gynecol Clin North Am 19:39, 1992.

Pokorny SF: Long-term intravaginal presence of foreign bodies in children: a preliminary study, J Reprod Med 39:931, 1994.

Pokorny SF: Genital trauma, Clin Obstet Gynecol 40:219, 1997.

Pokorny SF, Pokorny WJ, and Kramer W: Acute genital injury in the prepubertal girl, Am J Obstet Gynecol 166:1461, 1992.

Robinson AJ: Sexually transmitted organism in children and child sexual abuse, International J STD AIDS 9:501, 1998.

Rosenfield RL: Normal and almost normal precocious variations in pubertal development, premature pubarche and premature thelarche revisited, Horm Res 41(S2):7, 1994.

Rosenfield RL: Selection of children with precocious puberty for treatment with gonadotropin releasing hormone analogs, J Pediatr 124:989, 1994.

Sanfilippo JS, ed: Pediatric and adolescent gynecology, Philadelphia, 1994, WB Saunders Co.

Sankila R, Olsen JH, Anderson H, et al: Risk of cancer among offspring of childhood-cancer survivors, N Engl J Med 338:1339, 1998.

Shawis RN, El Gohary AE, and Cook RCM: Ovarian cysts and tumors in infancy and childhood, Ann R Coll Surg Engl 67:17, 1985.

Siegel MJ: Pediatric gynecologic sonography, Radiology 179:593, 1991.

Siegel MJ, Carel C, and Surratt S: Ultrasonography of acute abdominal pain in children, JAMA 266:1987, 1991.

Siegel MJ and Surratt JT: Pediatric gynecologic imaging, Obstet Gynecol Clin North Am 19:103, 1992.

Siegel SF, Finegold DN, Urban MD, et al: Premature pubarche: etiological heterogeneity, J Clin Endocrinol Metab 74:239, 1992.

Sonis WA, Comite F, Pescovitz OH, et al: Biobehavioral aspects of precocious puberty, J Am Acad Child Psychiatry 25:674, 1989.

Speroff L, Glass RH, and Kase NG: Clinical gynecologic endocrinology and infertility, ed 6, Philadelphia, 1999, Lippincott Williams & Wilkins.

Thorp JM, Wells SR, and Droegemueller W: Ovarian suspension in massive ovarian edema, Obstet Gynecol 76:912, 1990.

Valerie E, Gilchrist BF, Frischer J, et al: Diagnosis and treatment of ureteral prolapse in children, Urology 54:1082, 1999.

Vance ML and Mauras N: Growth hormone therapy in adults and children, N Engl J Med 341:1206, 1999.

Van Winter JT, Simmons PS, and Podratz KC: Surgically treated adnexal masses in infancy, childhood, and adolescence, Am J Obstet Gynecol 170:1780, 1994.

Walvoord EC and Pescovitz OH: Combined use of growth hormone and gonadotropin-releasing hormone analogues in precocious puberty: theoretic and practical considerations, Pediatrics 104:1010, 1999.

Yeshaya A, Kauschansky A, Orvieto R, et al: Prolonged vaginal bleeding during central precocious puberty therapy with a long-acting gonadotropin-releasing hormone agonist, Acta Obstet Gynaecol Scand 77:327, 1998.

Zalel Y, Piura B, Elchalal U, et al: Diagnosis and management of malignant germ cell ovarian tumors in young females, Int J Gynaecol Obstet 55:1, 1996.

Zitsman JL, Cirincione E, and Margossian H: Vaginal bleeding in an infant secondary to sliding inguinal hernia, Obstet Gynecol 89:840, 1997.

Family Planning

Contraception, Sterilization, and Pregnancy Termination

KEY TERMS AND DEFINITIONS

Contraception. The temporary avoidance of pregnancy.

Contraceptive Failure Rate. Pregnancy rates with various types of contraceptives at different intervals, usually years. This rate is frequently expressed as number of pregnancies per 100 women at 1 year or per 100 woman-years.

Induced Abortion. Intentional medical or surgical termination of pregnancy before 20 weeks' gestation. Also called *elective pregnancy termination* if performed for the woman's desires or *therapeutic abortion* if performed for reasons of maintaining the mother's health.

Intrauterine Device (IUD). A small foreign body, usually made of plastic with or without copper or a progestin, placed into the endometrial cavity to provide an effective method of contraception.

IUD Event Rates. Incidence of adverse events, such as expulsion, removal for medical reasons, and pregnancy, at various times after insertion of an IUD.

Life Table Method. An actuarial technique for determining rates of occurrence of events, such as pregnancy and discontinuation, at various intervals after starting any type of contraceptive.

Method Effectiveness. The rate of effectiveness when the contraceptive method is always used correctly. Now called *perfect use.*

Natural Family Planning. Periodic abstinence from intercourse during the periovulatory time of the cycle. Also known as *rhythm.*

Norplant. Polysiloxane capsules containing levonorgestrel that are implanted subdermally and release relatively constant amounts of levonorgestrel continuously. This method provides excellent contraceptive effectiveness for at least 5 years.

Oral Contraceptive Steroids (OCs). Formulations of various synthetic progestins usually combined with a synthetic estrogen that are ingested orally to prevent conception.

Pearl Index. A nonactuarial method used for determining the pregnancy (failure) rate of any contraceptive technique:

$$\text{Pregnancy rate} = \frac{\text{No. of pregnancies} \times 1200}{\text{Woman-months of use}}$$

Postcoital Contraception. Administration of steroids or insertion of an IUD within 3 days after a single episode of unprotected, midcycle sexual intercourse.

Progestin. A class of sex steroids having progestational activity. The terms *progestagen* and *gestagen* are synonymous.

Spermicide. A local contraceptive containing the agent nonoxynol 9, which is toxic to sperm.

Sterilization. Permanent prevention of pregnancy by vasectomy or tubal interruption. This method of contraception should be considered permanent.

Use Effectiveness. Overall effectiveness rate in actual use for a specific contraceptive method. Now called *typical use.*

Reversible contraception is defined as the temporary prevention of fertility and includes all the currently available contraceptive methods except sterilization. Sterilization should be considered a permanent prevention of fertility even though both vasectomy and tubal interruption can usually be reversed by a meticulous surgical procedure. The reversible methods are also called *active methods,* while sterilization is also called a *terminal method.* A perfect method of contraception for all individuals is not currently available and probably will never be developed. Each of the various methods of contraception currently available has certain advantages and disadvantages. Therefore, when giving advice about contraception, the clinician should explain to the couple the advantages and disadvantages of each method, so they will be fully informed and can rationally choose the method most suitable for them. Because no contraceptive method other than the condom has yet been developed for use by the male, the contraceptive provider generally counsels the female partner and should inform her if there are medical reasons that contraindicate the use of certain methods and offer her alternatives.

CONTRACEPTIVE USE IN THE UNITED STATES

In 1994 there were about 6.2 million pregnancies in the United States. About two thirds of these pregnancies, 3.9 million, ended in births of children, and about one fourth,

1.4 million, were terminated by elective abortion. The remainder ended in spontaneous abortion or ectopic pregnancy. According to Henshaw's review of the 1995 National Survey of Family Growth, about half the 6 million pregnancies were unintended and 54% of these unintended pregnancies were terminated by elective abortion. The remainder were frequently associated with unwanted children. According to the survey, about half of the women with unwanted pregnancies were using a method of contraception in the cycle in which they conceived. Unintended pregnancies are most likely to occur among young, unmarried, black and Hispanic women and women with low income. According to Piccinino and Mosher's analyses of the 1995 National Survey of Family Growth, the latest survey to be analyzed, of the 60 million women of reproductive age in the United States in 1995, 64%, 3.9 million, were using a method of contraception. Among the group using no method of contraception, about half had a prior hysterectomy or were pregnant, infertile, or trying to conceive. The other half either were not sexually active or were having infrequent episodes of coitus or otherwise did not believe there was a need for contraception. A total of 5% of women of reproductive age were sexually active and not using a method of contraception. Of the contraceptive users nearly 40% were sterilized, 27.7% by female methods and 10.9% by vasectomy (Table 13-1). Almost 27% used oral contraceptives and 20% the male condom. The progestin injection was used by 3%, the diaphragm by 2%, periodic abstinence by 2%, withdrawal by 3%, and the

---

TABLE 13-1

Percentage Distribution and Number (in 000s) of Contraceptive Users Aged 15–44, by Current Method, 1982–1995

Method	1982 %	1982 No.	1988 %	1988 No.	1995 %	1995 No.
Sterilization	34.1	10,295	39.2	13,686	38.6	14,942
Female	23.2	6998	27.5	9614	27.7	10,727
Male	10.9	3298	11.7	4069	10.9	4215
Pill	28.0	8431	30.7	10,734	26.9	10,410
Implant	NA	NA	NA	NA	1.3	515
Injectable	NA	NA	NA	NA	3.0	1146
IUD	7.1	2153	2.0	703	0.8	310
Diaphram	8.1	2436	5.7	2000	1.9	720
Male condom	12.0	3608	14.6	5093	20.4	7889
Foam	2.4	711	1.1	371	0.4	161
Per. abstinence	3.9	1166	2.3	806	2.3	883
Withdrawal	2.0	588	2.2	778	3.0	1178
Other†	2.5	754	2.1	733	1.3	508
Total	100.0	30,142	100.0	34,912	100.0	38,663
Sample n	NA	4242	NA	5176	NA	7145

†"Other" consists of douche, sponge, jelly or cream alone, and other methods. *Note:* NA = not applicable.

From Piccinino LJ, Mosher WD: Trends in contraceptive use in the United States: 1982–1995, Fam Plann Perspect 30:4, 1998.

implant and IUD by about 1%. Thus of women using contraception, about 70% used the very effective methods of sterilization, oral contraceptives, injection, implant, and IUD, and 30% used the less effective methods.

CONTRACEPTIVE EFFECTIVENESS

It is difficult to determine the actual effectiveness of a contraceptive method because of the many factors that affect contraceptive failure. The terms *method effectiveness* and *use effectiveness* (or *method failure* and *patient failure*) were previously used to describe conception occurring while the contraceptive method was being used correctly or incorrectly. These terms have now been replaced by the terms *typical use* and *perfect use*. In general, methods used at the time of coitus, such as the diaphragm, condom, spermicides, and withdrawal, have much greater perfect use effectiveness than typical use effectiveness. There is less difference between perfect and typical use effectiveness among methods not related to the time of coitus, such as OCs, implants, injections, and intrauterine devices. Because less motivation is required with these latter four methods than with coitus-related methods, the four noncoitus-related methods have greater typical use effectiveness than coitus-related methods. Women should be counseled that these four methods are the most effective reversible methods of contraception currently available in the United States. Women should always be informed about perfect use failure rates so that they know what is the percentage of contraceptive failure that will occur when each method is used correctly and consistently.

The U.S. Food and Drug Administration (FDA) has two different centers to regulate drugs and medical devices. The Center for Drug Evaluation and Research has allowed perfect use failure rates to be included in contraceptive product labeling for several years. The Center for Devices and Radiologic Health now allows manufacturers of barrier-method contraceptives to include perfect use failure rates in the product labeling of these methods.

The overall value of the various contraceptive methods as used by a couple (correctly or incorrectly) over a specific period, sometimes called *extended use effectiveness*, is determined by calculating the actual effectiveness and the continuation rate. Actuarial methods should be used to determine the various contraceptive failure rates.

Even with use of these excellent statistical techniques, it is difficult to determine the effectiveness of a contraceptive method in actual practice. Most studies undertaken for this purpose are performed in carefully controlled clinical trials. During these studies, frequent contact with supportive clinic personnel results in lower failure rates and higher continuation rates than actually occur in field use. Furthermore, these clinical trials are infrequently performed in a comparative randomized manner. Therefore,

clinicians cannot accurately compare results of a trial of one type of contraceptive method with those of another.

Several other factors also influence contraceptive failure rates. One of the most important is motivation. Contraceptive failure is more likely to occur in couples seeking to delay a wanted birth compared with those seeking to prevent any more births, especially for coitus-related methods. The woman's age has a strong negative correlation with failure of a contraceptive method, as does socioeconomic status and level of education. Failure rates for most methods usually are lower among populations of married rather than unmarried women. Failure rates reported in prospective studies are also consistently lower than those of retrospective interview studies because of recall bias. Finally, for all methods, failure rates are greater during the first year of use than in subsequent years, yet most studies report only first-year-use failure rates. Thus many variables must be considered when evaluating the effectiveness of any method of contraception for an individual woman.

Trussell et al. have calculated percentage failure rates with the first year of use for the various methods of contraceptives available in the United States (Table 13-2). In this table they have also included an estimate of the percentage of women continuing to use the method after 1 year has elapsed since starting to use the method.

The percentage of actual use failure rates for durations more than 1 year are available for certain methods of long-acting contraceptives. The failure rate for 5 years of use of the 6 progestin implants, Norplant, in clinical trials is 1.1%. The cumulative failure rate of the Copper T380 IUD was 1.0, 1.4, and 1.6 per 100 women after 3, 5, and 7 years of use, respectively, in a large World Health Organization study and only rises to 1.7 per 100 women after 12 years of use.

The failure rate of all types of tubal sterilization is 1.31 after 5 years and 1.85 per 100 women after 10 years, being highest for tubal fulguration and lowest for segmental resection in the 10 years following the procedure. Clinicians counseling women about long-term failure rates should inform them about the high incidence of ectopic pregnancies that occur when conception occurs using progestin-only methods, the IUD, and female sterilization.

Ectopic pregnancy rates for women conceiving while using these methods range from about 30% with tubal sterilization failure to 25% with implant failure and 5% with copper IUD failure.

CONTRACEPTIVE COST

In addition to preventing unwanted pregnancy, all contraceptive methods reduce health care costs. Trussell et al. developed an economic model to compare the effectiveness and costs per person of 15 methods of contraceptives, including both permanent and reversible methods. To

TABLE 13-2

Percentage of Women Experiencing an Unintended Pregnancy During the First Year of Typical Use and the First Year of Perfect Use of Contraception and the Percentage Continuing Use at the End of the First Year: United States

Method (1)	% of Women Experiencing an Unintended Pregnancy within the First Year of Use		% of Women Continuing Use at One Year[3] (4)
	Typical Use[1] (2)	Perfect Use[2] (3)	
Chance [4]	85	85	
Spermicides[5]	26	6	40
Periodic abstinence	25		63
Calendar		9	
Ovulation method		3	
Symptothermal[6]		2	
Postovulation		1	
Cap[7]			
Parous women	40	26	42
Nulliparous women	20	9	56
Sponge			
Parous women	40	20	42
Nulliparous women	20	9	56
Diaphragm[7]	20	6	56
Withdrawal	19	4	
Condom[8]			
Female (Reality)	21	5	56
Male	14	3	61
Pill	5		71
Progestin only		0.5	
Combined		0.1	
IUD			
Progesterone T	2.0	1.5	81
Copper T380A	0.8	0.6	78
LNg 20	0.1	0.1	81
Depo-Provera	0.3	0.3	70
Norplant and Norplant-2	0.05	0.05	88
Female sterilization	0.5	0.5	100
Male sterilization	0.15	0.10	100

Emergency Contraceptive Pills: Treatment initiated within 72 hours after unprotected intercourse reduces the risk of pregnancy by at least 75%.[9]

Lactational Amenorrhea Method: LAM is a highly effective, *temporary* method of contraception.[10]

Source: Updated from Trussell and Kost (1987) and Trussell et al. (1990b). See text.

[1]Among *typical* couples who initiate use of a method (not neccessarily for the first time), the percentage who experience an accidental pregnancy during the first year if they do not stop use for any other reason.

[2]Among couples who initiate use of a method (not necessarily for the first time) and who use it *perfectly* (both consistently and correctly), the percentage who experience an accidental pregnancy during the first year if they do not stop use for any other reason.

[3]Among couples attempting to avoid pregnancy, the percentage who continue to use a method for one year.

[4]The percentages becoming pregnant in columns (2) and (3) are based on data from populations where contraception is not used and from women who cease using contraception in order to become pregnant. Among such populations, about 89% become pregnant within one year. This estimate was lowered slightly (to 85%) to represent the percentage who would become pregnant within one year among women now relying on reversible methods of contraception if they abandoned contraception altogether.

[5]Foams, creams, gels, vaginal suppositories, and vaginal film.

[6]Cervical mucus (ovulation) method supplemented by calendar in the preovulatory and basal body temperature in the postovulatory phases.

[7]With spermicidal cream or jelly.

[8]Without spermicides.

[9]The treatment schedule is one dose within 72 hours after unprotected intercourse, and a second dose 12 hours after the first dose. The Food and Drug Administration has declared the following brands of oral contraceptives to be safe and effective for emergency contraception: Ovral (1 dose is 2 white pills), Alesse (1 dose is 5 pink pills), Nordette or Levlen (1 dose is 4 light-orange pills), Lo/Ovral (1 dose is 4 white pills), Triphasil or Tri-Levlen (1 dose is 4 yellow pills).

[10]However, to maintain effective protection against pregnancy, another method of contraception must be used as soon as menstruation resumes, the frequency or duration of breastfeeds is reduced, bottle feeds are introduced, or the baby reaches 6 months of age.

determine effectiveness the model calculated the number of pregnancies avoided with typical use of each method of contraception compared with the number of pregnancies expected to occur if no contraceptive method was used by the woman. To determine the cost of each contraceptive the direct medical costs of the method itself, costs due to mistimed pregnancies, as well as those incurred or avoided by adverse and beneficial side effects of the contraceptive method, were calculated. The costs of unintended pregnancies because of method failure included the costs of term deliveries as well as spontaneous and induced abortion and ectopic pregnancies. Because the costs of unintended pregnancy when no method of contraception is used are substantial, use of all 15 contraceptives was less costly than use of no method. Costs were calculated for contraceptive use for 1 and 5 years' duration. Although male and female sterilization had high initial costs, they became very cost effective over time for couples wishing no more children. However, these data were calculated before the nearly 2% 10-year failure rate of tubal ligation reported by Peterson et al. was published. The most cost-effective method for 5 years of use were the copper T IUD, vasectomy, the progestin implant, and progestin injection (Figure 13-1). Use of each of these methods for 5 years saved about $14,000 per person and prevented about 4.1 pregnancies per person. Barrier methods and periodic abstinence saved between $9000 and $12,000 over 5 years, while oral contraceptives prevented 4.1 pregnancies and saved nearly $13,000 per year. This study indicated that initial acquisition costs do not predict the economic value of various contraceptives and that the most effective contraception methods provided the greatest cost savings.

SPERMICIDES: FOAMS, CREAMS, AND SUPPOSITORIES

All spermicidal agents contain a surfactant, usually nonoxynol 9, that immobilizes or kills sperm on contact. They also provide a mechanical barrier and need to be placed into the vagina before each coital act. The effectiveness of these agents increases with increasing age of the woman and is similar to that of the diaphragm in all age and income groups.

Marketing of the contraceptive sponge, a cylindric piece of soft polyurethane impregnated with 1 mg of nonoxynol 9, was discontinued by the manufacturers in 1994. Unlike other spermicides, the sponge did not have to be inserted into the vagina before each act of intercourse and was effective for 24 hours. It may again become available for use by women in the United States.

Although a few early studies linked the use of a spermicide at the time of conception with an increased risk of some congenital malformations, these studies were probably flawed by recall bias. Several well-performed studies have shown no increased risk of congenital malformation

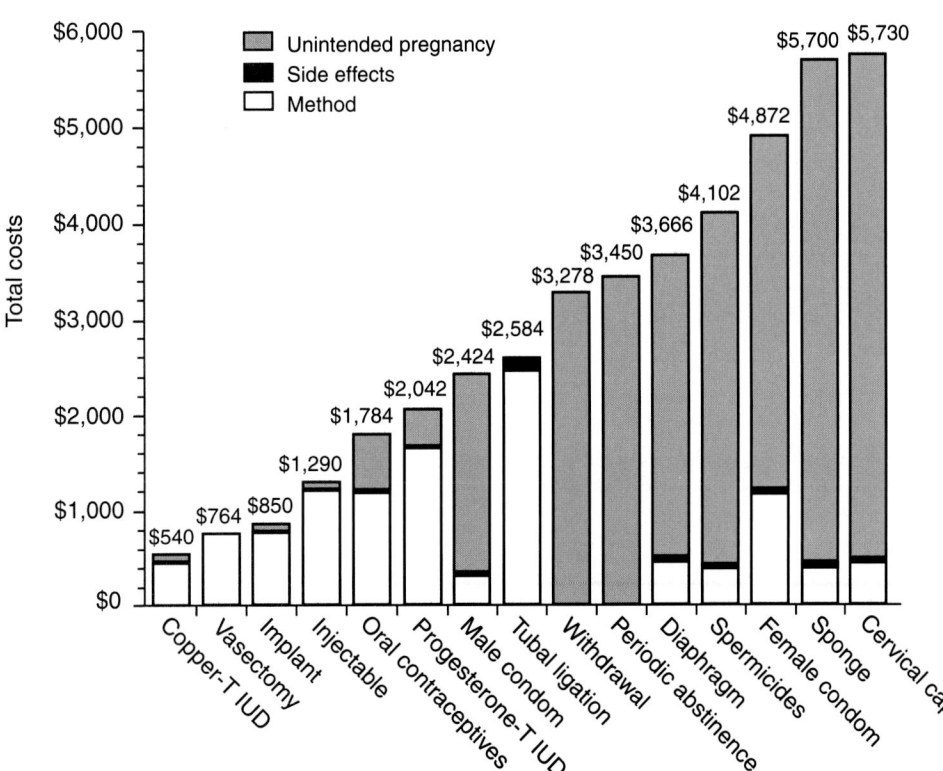

FIGURE 13-1 Five-year costs associated with contraceptive methods in the managed payment model. (From Trussell J, Leveque JA, and Koenig JD: Am J Public Health 85(49):494, 1995.)

in the newborns or karyotypic abnormalities in the spontaneous abortuses of women who conceived while using spermicides.

BARRIER TECHNIQUES

Diaphragm

A diaphragm must be carefully fitted by the health care provider. The largest size that does not cause discomfort or undue pressure on the vaginal mucosa should be used. After the fitting, the woman should remove the diaphragm and reinsert it herself. She should then be examined to make sure the diaphragm is covering the cervix. The diaphragm should be used with a spermicide and be left in place for at least 8 hours after the last coital act. If repeated intercourse takes place or coitus occurs more than 8 hours after insertion of the diaphragm, additional spermicide should be used. Although advisable, it may not be necessary to use a spermicide with the diaphragm, since it has not been conclusively demonstrated that pregnancy rates are lower when a spermicide is used with a diaphragm than when the diaphragm is used alone. The number of urinary tract infections in women who use diaphragms is significantly higher than in nonusers, probably because of the mechanical obstruction of the outflow of urine by the diaphragm. Diaphragm users should also be cautioned not to leave the device in place for more than 24 hours, as ulceration of the vaginal epithelium may occur with prolonged usage. One report, however, indicated that among a group of women who left the diaphragm in place without using spermicide, removing it only once daily to wash it before immediately reinserting it, as well as removing it during menses, the 12-month failure rate was only 2.8%. This rate was lower than the failure rate of 9.8% among a group of women who inserted the diaphragm with a spermicide in the usual manner only when having sexual intercourse and then leaving it in for 8 hours thereafter.

Data from the Oxford/Family Planning Association Contraceptive Study indicate that the diaphragm is an effective method of contraception in married, motivated women and that failure rates decline with increasing age and increasing duration of use. Analyses of data from two large clinical trials comparing use of the diaphragm with that of the cervical cap or sponge indicate that the failure rate during the first year of use for the diaphragm ranged from 12.5% to 17.1% among all users and was reduced to 4.3% to 5.3% with perfect use.

Cervical Cap

The cervical cap, a cup-shaped plastic or rubber device that fits around the cervix, has been used as a barrier contraceptive for decades, mainly in Britain and other parts of Europe.

There has been a recent resurgence of interest in the use of this older method, since the cervical cap can be left in place longer than the diaphragm and is more comfortable. The various types of caps are manufactured in different sizes and should be fitted to the cervix by a clinician. The cervical cap should not be left in place for more than 48 hours because of the possibility of ulceration, unpleasant odor, and infection.

The Prentif cavity-rim cervical cap was approved for general use in the United States in 1988. The product labeling stipulates that the cap should be left on the cervix for no more than 48 hours and that a spermicide should always be placed inside the cap before use. The cap is manufactured in four sizes and requires more training than the diaphragm, both for the provider to fit it and for the user to place it correctly.

Failure rates with the cervical cap are similar to those observed with the diaphragm. In a large, randomized clinical trial of the cap and diaphragm, 1-year pregnancy rates were 17.4% for the cap and 16.7% for the diaphragm. Of the pregnancies with the cap, one third were method failures and two thirds were user-related failures. In other studies, pregnancy rates at 1 and 2 years with the use of the cervical cap ranged from 8% to 17% and 14% to 38%, respectively, with good continuation rates. Because of concern about a possible adverse effect of the cap on cervical tissue, the cervical cap should be used only by women with normal cervical cytology, and it is recommended that users have another cervical cytologic examination 3 months after starting to use this method.

Male Condom

Use of the male condom by individuals with multiple sex partners should be encouraged. The male condom is the most effective method of contraception to prevent transmission of sexually transmitted diseases. The male condom should not be applied tightly. The tip should extend beyond the end of the penis by about half an inch to collect the ejaculate. Care must be taken upon withdrawal not to spill the ejaculate. When used by strongly motivated couples, the male condom is highly effective.

Barrier techniques are effective methods of contraception in women 30 years of age or older. In a U.S. study, the first-year failure rates for male condom use among women wishing no more pregnancies ranged between 3% and 6% when the woman was over age 30 but between 8% and 10% when the woman was under age 25.

Female Condom

A female condom was approved for marketing in the United States in 1994. It consists of a soft, loose-fitting sheath and two flexible polyurethane rings. One ring lies inside the vagina at the closed end of the sheath and serves as an insertion mechanism and internal anchor. The outer ring forms the external edge of the device and remains outside the vagina after insertion, thus providing protection to the labia and the base of the penis during intercourse. The condom is prelubricated and is intended for one-time use only. Fitting by a health professional is not required.

Compared with the male condom, the female condom has the advantage of being able to be inserted prior to beginning sexual activity and to be left in place for a longer time after ejaculation has occurred. Because the female condom also covers the external genitalia, it should offer greater protection against the transfer of certain sexually transmitted organisms, particularly genital herpes. Because polyurethane is stronger than the latex used in male condoms, the female condom is less likely to rupture. In a multicenter clinical trial the cumulative pregnancy rates in U.S. centers at 6 months was 12.4%. The 6-month pregnancy rate with perfect use was 2.6%, indicating that the probable 1-year pregnancy rate with perfect use would be slightly more than 5%. At the end of 6 months in the U.S. study about one third of the women had discontinued use of this method.

Because clinical trials with the female condom have not compared its use with other barrier techniques, an exact comparison with other contraceptive methods cannot be made. Trussell et al., using the data of other studies, concluded that with perfect use efficacy rates of the female condom would be similar to that of the diaphragm and cervical cap but with typical use the failure rates of the female condom would be higher than that of the diaphragm. Because of the lack of prospective clinical trials with the male condom, no statistical comparison of the effectiveness of the two types of condoms can be made. No data exist in which the effectiveness of the female condom for reducing sexual disease transmission is analyzed. Because polyurethane does not allow virus transmission it should reduce the risk of a woman acquiring HIV infection.

Barrier Techniques and Sexually Transmitted Diseases

Barrier methods have the advantage of reducing the rate of transmission of sexually transmitted diseases. Several studies have shown that spermicides reduce the frequency of clinical infection with sexually transmitted diseases, both bacterial and viral. Several in vitro studies have demonstrated that condoms prevent the transmission of viruses, specifically the herpesvirus and the human immunodeficiency virus, as well as *Chlamydia trachomatis* bacteria, which is a frequent cause of salpingitis. Serial epidemiologic studies, both case-control and cohort, indicate that the use of the condom or diaphragm protects both men and women from clinically apparent gonorrheal infection.

An epidemiologic study of women with infertility caused by tubal obstruction found that the past use of barrier techniques protected women against tubal damage. The greatest protection occurred with the use of diaphragms or condoms in conjunction with spermicides. The incidence of cervical neoplasia was also markedly diminished among the female members of couples using condoms or diaphragms, probably because of the decreased transmission of human papillomavirus (HPV). This antiviral action may be the reason that women who use spermicides are only one third as likely to have cervical cancer as are members of a control group. Certain strains of this virus have been causally linked to the later development of cervical neoplasia. Unfortunately, the pregnancy failure rates of diaphragm or condom users are highest for persons younger than 25 years, those most likely to become infected with sexually transmitted diseases. Therefore, to prevent the transmission of these diseases as well as prevent unwanted pregnancy in this age group, the use of a barrier technique, together with one of the four most effective reversible methods of contraception, is advisable.

PERIODIC ABSTINENCE

The avoidance of sexual intercourse during the days of the menstrual cycle when the ovum can be fertilized is used by many highly motivated couples as a means of preventing pregnancy. Wilcox et al. reported that conception can only occur if coitus takes place during the 5 days preceding ovulation or the day of ovulation. Thus, if couples would only avoid coitus on these 6 days each month, conception would not occur. Because a woman cannot precisely determine when she will ovulate, four techniques of periodic abstinence have been utilized. The oldest of these is the calendar rhythm method. With this method, the period of abstinence is determined solely by calculating the length of the individual woman's previous menstrual cycle. The rationale for the rhythm method is based on three assumptions: (1) the human ovum is capable of being fertilized for only about 24 hours after ovulation, (2) spermatozoa retain their fertilizing ability for only about 48 hours after coitus, and (3) ovulation usually occurs 12 to 16 days (14 ± 2 days) before the onset of the subsequent menses. According to these assumptions, after the woman records the length of her cycles for several months, she establishes her fertile period by subtracting 18 days from the length of her previous shortest cycle and 11 days from her previous longest cycle. Then, in each subsequent cycle, the couple abstains from coitus during this calculated fertile period.

This method requires abstinence by the majority of women with regular menstrual cycles for nearly half the days of each cycle and cannot be used by women with irregular menstrual cycles. Although calendar rhythm is the most widely used technique of periodic abstinence, pregnancy rates are high, ranging from 14.4 to 47 per 100 woman-years, mainly because most couples fail to abstain for the relatively long periods required. The use of the calendar rhythm method by itself is currently not advocated or taught to couples who are interested in practicing periodic abstinence.

In the past two decades, new techniques have been developed whereby women rely on physiologic change during each cycle to determine the fertile period. The term *natural family planning* has been used instead of *rhythm* to describe these new techniques. They include the temperature method, the cervical mucus method, and the symptothermal method. Each of these techniques requires a great amount of motivation and training. In most reports of use of these methods pregnancy rates are relatively high and continuation rates are low.

The temperature method relies on measuring basal body temperature daily. The woman is required to abstain from intercourse from the onset of the menses until the third consecutive day of elevated basal temperature. Because abstinence is required for the entire preovulatory period in ovulatory cycles and for the entire cycle in anovulatory cycles, the temperature method alone is no longer commonly used.

The cervical mucus method requires that the woman be taught to recognize and interpret cyclic changes in the presence and consistency of cervical mucus; these changes occur in response to changing estrogen and progesterone levels. Abstinence is required during the menses and every other day after the menses ends, because of the possibility of confusing semen with ovulatory mucus, until the first day that copious, slippery mucus is observed to be present. Abstinence is required every day thereafter until 4 days after the last day when the characteristic mucus is present, called the "peak mucus day." In two well-designed, randomized clinical trials, the pregnancy rates for new users of this method in the first year after they completed a 3- to 5-month training period were 20% and 24%, with the discontinuation rates between 72% and 74%. In a 5-country study of 725 highly motivated couples sponsored by the World Health Organization, the use failure rate during the first year after the completion of 3 cycles of training was 19.6%, with a method failure rate of 3.5%. Three fourths of these pregnancies resulted from conscious deviation from the rules of the method. The mean length of the fertile period in this study was 9.6 days, and abstinence was therefore required for about 17 days of each cycle. In this study the continuation rate after 1 year was high, 64.4%.

The symptothermal method, rather than relying on a single physiologic index, uses several indexes to determine the fertile period—most commonly calendar calculations and changes in the cervical mucus to estimate the onset of the fertile period and changes in mucus or basal temperature to estimate its end. Because several indexes need to be monitored, this method is more difficult to learn than the single-index methods, but it is more effective than the cervical mucus method alone. In two large, randomized studies comparing these methods, the pregnancy rates at the end of 1 year of use, after the training phase, were 10.9% and 19.8% with the symptothermal method, compared with 20% and 24% for the cervical mucus method. In addition, the continuation rate among the women who used the sympothermal method in these studies was higher after 1 year, about 50% in each study, than that among the women who used the cervical mucus method (26% and 40%).

The major reason for the lack of acceptance of natural family planning, as well as the relatively high pregnancy rates among users of these methods, is the need to avoid having sexual intercourse for a large number of days during each menstrual cycle. To overcome this problem, many women use barrier methods or spermicides during the fertile period. In a study of women who used the symptothermal method with barrier contraceptives or withdrawal during the fertile period, the failure rate during the first year was 9.9%, and the discontinuation rate was 33%.

Because the use of any method of contraception other than abstinence is unacceptable to many couples, simple, self-administered tests to detect hormonal changes have been developed to reduce the number of days of abstinence required in each cycle to a maximum of seven. Enzyme immunoassays for urinary estrogen and pregnanediol glucuronide have been developed. These assays can easily be used at home at minimal cost, and they require minimal time to perform. Such tests have to be performed by the woman for about 12 days each month, but they should reduce the number of days of abstinence required. It remains to be determined to what extent this aid to natural family planning will be used when it becomes generally available.

ORAL STEROID CONTRACEPTIVES

Oral steroid contraceptives (OCs) were initially marketed in the United States in 1960. Because of their extremely high rate of effectiveness and ease of administration, within a few years of their introduction they became the most widely used method of reversible contraception among both married and unmarried women. The major effect of the synthetic progestin component is to inhibit ovulation and produce other contraceptive actions such as thickening of the cervical mucus. The major effect of the synthetic estrogen is to maintain the endometrium and prevent unscheduled bleeding as well as inhibit follicular development. Most OC formulations contain a combination of a synthetic progestin and a synthetic estrogen in a single tablet. The initially marketed formulations of OCs contained 150 µg of the estrogen component mestranol and 9.85 mg of the progestin component norethynodrel. With the high doses of steroids in the original formulations, minor side effects such as nausea, breast tenderness, and weight gain were common and frequently were of such magnitude as to cause discontinuation of use. During the past 41 years, many other formulations have been developed and marketed with steadily decreasing dosages of both the estrogen and progestin components. All the formulations initially marketed after 1975 contain less than 50 μg of ethinyl estradiol and 1 mg or less of several progestins. Use of these lower steroid dose formulations is associated with very low pregnancy rates, similar to those for formulations with higher doses of steroid, and a significantly lower incidence of severe adverse cardiovascular effects and minor adverse symptoms.

Because contraceptive steroid formulations with more than 50 μg of estrogen were associated with a greater incidence of adverse effects without greater efficacy, they are no longer marketed for contraceptive use in the United States, Canada, and Great Britain. Indications for prescribing formulations with 50 μg of estrogen are very uncommon. OC formulations currently marketed in the United States, excluding generic brands, are listed in Table 13-3.

Pharmacology

There are three major types of OC formulations: fixed-dose combination, combination phasic, and daily progestin. The combination formulations are the most widely used and most effective. They consist of tablets containing both an estrogen and progestin given continuously for 3 weeks. No steroids are given for the next 7 days, except for one formulation in which a low dose of estrogen is given for 5 additional days, after which time the active combination is given for an additional 3 weeks. Uterine bleeding usually occurs in the week when no steroid is ingested. Without estrogenic stimulation the endometrium usually begins to slough 1 to 3 days after stopping steroid ingestion. Withdrawal bleeding usually lasts 3 to 4 days, and uterine blood loss averages about 25 ml, less than the mean of about 35 ml that occurs during menses in a normal ovulatory cycle.

The combination phasic formulations currently marketed contain two or three different amounts of the same estrogen and progestin. Each of the tablets containing one of these various dosages is given for intervals varying from 5 to 11 days during the 21-day medication period. These formulations have been described as biphasic or triphasic and are generally referred to as *multiphasic*. The rationale given for use of this type of formulation is that a lower total dose of steroid is administered without increasing the incidence of unscheduled uterine bleeding. However, there have been no published reports of comparative clinical trials in which multiphasic combinations have been shown to have significantly fewer adverse effects than fixed-dose combination formulations. The third type of contraceptive formulation, consisting of tablets containing a progestin without any estrogen, are ingested once every day without a steroid-free interval.

All currently marketed formulations are made from synthetic steroids and contain no natural estrogens or progestins. There are two major types of synthetic progestins: derivatives of 19-nortestosterone and derivatives of 17α-acetoxyprogesterone. The latter group are C21 progestins, called *pregnanes*, and are structurally related to progesterone. Medroxyprogesterone acetate and megestrol acetate are C21 progestins marketed as tablets for noncontraceptive usage. In contrast to the 19-nortestosterone derivatives, when high dosages of the C21 progestins were given to female beagle dogs (an animal previously used for OC toxicology testing), the animals developed an increased incidence of mammary cancer. Because of this carcinogenic effect, oral contraceptives containing these progestins are no longer marketed despite the fact that the beagle, unlike the human, metabolizes C21 progestins to estrogen that then stimulates mammary nodules, which can become carcinogenic in this animal. An injectable contraceptive containing a C21 progestin, medroxyprogesterone acetate, is currently marketed in the United States and other countries.

The steroid structure of the 19-nortestosterone progestins more closely resembles testosterone than the C21 acetoxy progestins. Therefore, all progestational agents currently used in OCs have some degree of androgenic activity. The 19-nortestosterone progestins used in OCs are of two major types, called *estranes* and *gonanes*. Although the original estrane norethynodrel is no longer used in currently marketed OCs, other estranes, norethindrone and its derivatives with one or two acetates, norethindrone acetate and ethynodiol diacetate, are used in several marketed formulations (Figure 13-2). Gonanes have greater progestational activity per unit weight than do estranes, and thus a smaller amount of the gonane type of progestin is used in OC formulations (Figure 13-3). The parent compound of the gonanes is *dl*-norgestrel, which consists of two isomers, dextro and levo. Only the levo form is biologically active. Both *dl*-norgestrel and its active isomer levonorgestrel are present in several OC formulations. Three less androgenic derivatives of levonorgestrel, namely desogestrel, norgestimate, and gestodene, have also been synthesized. Formulations with each of these latter three progestins have been marketed in Europe for many years, and formulations with desogestrel and norgestimate, but not gestodene, have been marketed in the United States since 1992.

Except for two daily progestin-only formulations, the progestins are combined with varying dosages of two estrogens, ethinyl estradiol and ethinyl estradiol 3-methyl ether, also known as mestranol (Figure 13-4). All the older higher-dosage OC formulations contained mestranol, and this steroid is still present in some 50-μg formulations. All formulations with less than 50 μg of estrogen contain only the parent compound ethinyl estradiol. In common usage formulations with 50 μg or more of estrogen (ethinyl estradiol or mestranol) have been termed *first-generation* OCs. Those with less than 50 μg

TABLE 13-3
OC Formulations Marketed in the United States, Excluding Generic Brands

Manufacturer/Product	Type*	Progestin Component	Estrogen Component (Ethinyl Estradiol Unless Noted)
Berlex			
Lerlite	Comb.	0.1 mg levonorgestrel	20 μg
Levlen	Comb.	0.15 mg levonorgestrel	30 μg
Tri-Levlen 6/	Comb., triphasic	0.05 mg levonorgestrel	30 μg
5/		0.075 mg levonorgestrel	40 μg
10/		0.125 mg levonorgestrel	30 μg
Warner Chilcott			
Ovcon 35	Comb.	0.4 mg norethindrone	35 μg
Ovcon 50	Comb.	1.0 mg norethindrone	50 μg
Organon			
Desogen	Comb.	0.15 mg desogestrel	35 μg
Mircette	Comb.	0.15 mg desogestrel	20 μg
		none	10 μg
Ortho-MacNeil Pharmaceutical			
Micronor	Prog.	0.35 mg norethindrone	
Modicon	Comb.	0.5 mg norethindrone	35 μg
Ortho-Cept	Comb.	0.15 mg desogestrel	30 μg
Ortho-Cyclen	Comb.	0.25 mg norgestimate	35 μg
Ortho-Novum 1/35	Comb.	1.0 mg norethindrone	35 μg
Ortho-Novum 1/50	Comb.	1.0 mg norethindrone	50 μg†
Ortho-Novum 7/	Comb., triphasic	0.5 mg norethindrone	35 μg
7/		0.75 mg norethindrone	35 μg
7/		1.0 mg norethindrone	35 μg
Ortho-Novum 10/11	Comb., biphasic	0.5 mg norethindrone	35 μg
10/11		1.0 mg norethindrone	35 μg
Ortho-Tricyclin	Comb., triphasic	0.18 mg norgestimate	35 μg
		0.215 mg norgestimate	35 μg
		0.25 mg norgestimate	35 μg
Pfizer			
Estro-step	Comb., Triphasic	1 mg norethindrone acetate	20 μg
		1 mg norethindrone acetate	30 μg
		1 mg norethindrone acetate	35 μg
Loestrin 1/20	Comb.	1.0 mg norethindrone acetate	20 μg
Loestrin 1.5/30	Comb.	1.5 mg norethindrone acetate	30 μg
Norlestrin 1/50	Comb.	1.0 mg norethindrone acetate	50 μg†
Norlestrin 2.5/50	Comb.	2.5 mg norethindrone acetate	50 μg†
Pharmacia			
Brevicon	Comb.	0.5 mg norethindrone	35 μg
Demulen 1/35	Comb.	1.0 mg ethynodiol diacetate	35 μg
Demulen 1/50	Comb.	1.0 mg/ethynodiol diacetate	50 μg
Demulen 1/35	Comb.	1.0 mg ethynodiol diacetate	35 μg
Demulen 1/50	Comb.	1.0 mg/ethynodiol diacetate	50 μg
Norinyl 1 + 35	Comb.	1.0 mg norethindrone	35 μg
Norinyl 1 + 50	Comb.	1.0 mg norethindrone	50 μg
Nor-Q.D.	Prog.	0.35 mg norethindrone	
Tri-Norinyl 7/	Comb., triphasic	0.5 mg norethindrone	35 μg
9/		1 mg norethindrone	35 μg
5/		0.5 mg norethindrone	35 μg
Wyeth-Ayerst			
Allesse	Comb.	0.1 mg levonorgestrel	20 μg
Lo/Ovral	Comb.	0.3 mg norgestrel	30 μg
Nordette	Comb.	0.15 mg levonorgestrel	30 μg
Ovral	Comb.	0.5 mg norgestrel	50 μg
Ovrette	Prog.	75 mg norgestrel	30 μg
Triphasil 6/	Comb., triphasic	50 mg levonorgestrel	40 μg
5/		75 mg levonorgestrel	40 μg
10/		125 mg levonorgestrel	30 μg

*Comb., Combination; Prog., Progestin only.   †Mestranol.

of estrogen, 20 to 35 μg of ethinyl estradiol, are called *second-generation* products if they contain any progestin except the three newest levonorgestrel derivatives. Those formulations with desogestrel, norgestimate, and gestodene are called *third-generation* formulations. All the synthetic estrogens and progestins in OCs have an ethinyl group at position 17. The presence of this ethinyl group enhances the oral activity of these agents, because their essential functional groups are not as rapidly metabolized as they pass through the intestinal mucosa and liver via the portal system, in contrast to what occurs when natural sex steroids are ingested orally. The synthetic steroids thus have greater oral potency per unit of weight than do the natural steroids. It has been estimated that ethinyl estradiol has about 100 times the potency of an equivalent weight of conjugated equine estrogen or estrone sulfate for stimulating synthesis of various hepatic globulins.

The various modifications in chemical structure of the different synthetic progestins and estrogens also affect their biologic activity. Thus one cannot define the pharmacologic activity of the progestin or estrogen in a particular contraceptive steroid formulation based only on the amount of steroid present. The biologic activity of each steroid also has to be considered. Using established tests for progestational activity in animals, it has been found that a given weight of norgestrel is several times more potent than the same weight of norethindrone. Studies in humans, using delay of menses or endometrial histologic alterations such as subnuclear vacuolization as end points, also determined that norgestrel is about 10 times more potent than the same weight of norethindrone. Norethindrone acetate and ethynodiol diacetate are metabolized in the body to norethindrone and have equivalent potency per unit weight to the parent compound, norethindrone, whereas levonorgestrel is 10 to 20 times as potent. Each of the three most recently developed levonorgestrel derivatives has been shown in animal, but not human, studies to have similar or greater progestogenic potency than an equivalent weight of levonorgestrel, with less androgenic

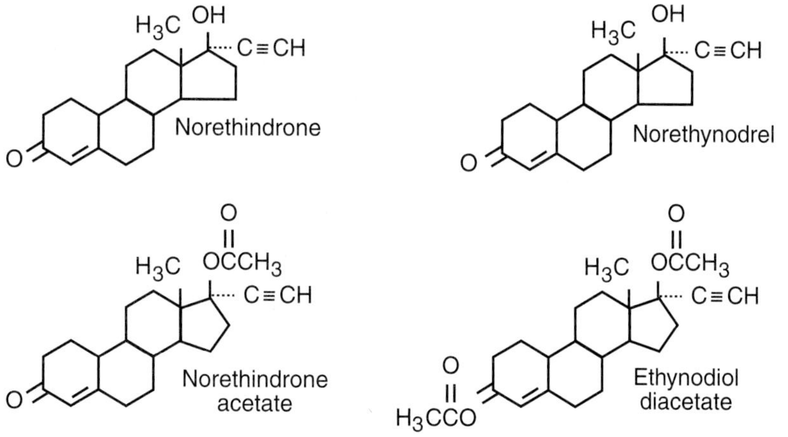

FIGURE 13-2 Chemical structures of the estrane progestins used in oral contraceptives.

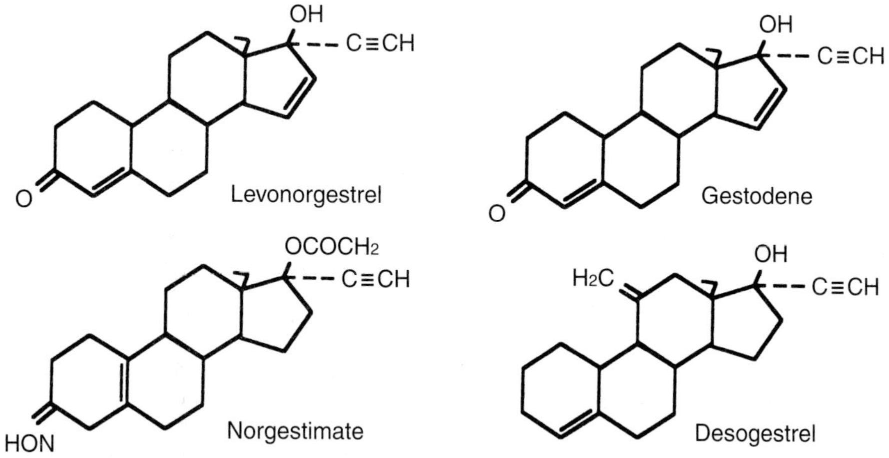

FIGURE 13-3 Chemical structure of the gonane progestins used in oral contraceptives.

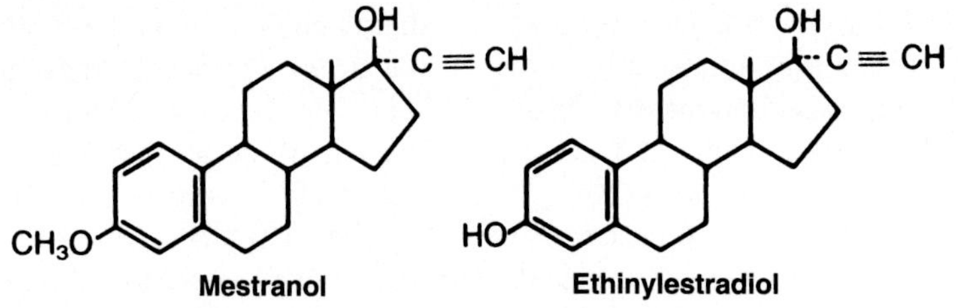

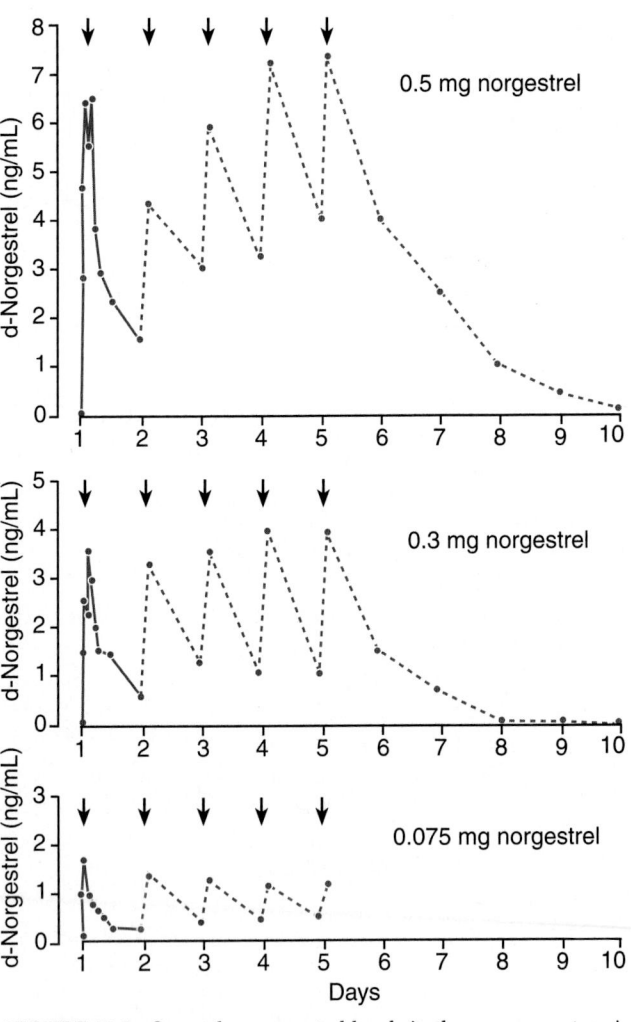

FIGURE 13-4   Structures of the two estrogens used in combination oral contraceptives.

activity. The magnitude of difference in androgenic and progestational effects produced by each progestin is called *selectivity.*

The two estrogenic compounds used in OCs, ethinyl estradiol and its 3-methyl ether mestranol, also have different biologic activity in women. To become biologically effective, mestranol must be demethylated to ethinyl estradiol, because mestranol does not bind to the estrogen cytosol receptor. The degree of conversion of mestranol to ethinyl estradiol varies among individuals; some are able to convert it completely, whereas others convert only a portion of it. Thus, in some women, a given weight of mestranol is as potent as the same weight of ethinyl estradiol, and in other women it is only about half as potent. Overall, it has been estimated, using human endometrial response and effect on liver corticosteroid-binding globulin (CBG) production as end points, that ethinyl estradiol is about 1.7 times as potent as the same weight of mestranol. The biologic activity, as well as the quantity of both steroid components, need to be evaluated when comparing potency of the various formulations.

Radioimmunoassay methods have been developed to measure blood levels of these synthetic estrogens and progestins. Peak plasma levels of ethinyl estradiol are lower and occur later, about 2 to 4 hours, after ingestion of mestranol than after ingestion of ethinyl estradiol. The delay is due to the time necessary for mestranol to be demethylated to ethinyl estradiol in the liver.

When different doses of *dl*-norgestrel were administered to women, we found that the serum levels of levonorgestrel were related to the dosage. Peak serum levels were found 0.5 to 3 hours after oral administration, followed by a rapid, sharp decline (Figure 13-5). However, 24 hours after ingestion, 20% to 25% of the peak level of levonorgestrel was still present in the serum. After 5 days of norgestrel administration, measurable amounts of levonorgestrel were present for at least the following 5 days.

Brenner et al. measured serum levels of levonorgestrel, follicle-stimulating hormone (FSH), luteinizing hormone (LH), estradiol, and progesterone 3 hours after ingestion of a combination OC containing 0.5 μg of *dl*-norgestrel and 50 mg of ethinyl estradiol in three women during two consecutive cycles, as well as during the intervening pill-free interval. Daily levels of levonorgestrel rose during the first few days of ingestion, plateaued thereafter, and

declined after ingestion of the last pill. Nevertheless, substantial amounts of levonorgestrel remained in the serum for at least the first 3 to 4 days after the last pill was ingested. These steroid levels were sufficient to suppress gonadotrophin release during the 1-week interval when no steroid was administered. Thus, follicle maturation, as

FIGURE 13-5   Serum levonorgestrel levels in three women at various times after ingestion of 0.5, 0.3, and 0.075 mg of *dl*-norgestrel once a day for 5 days. Arrows indicate days drug was ingested. (From Mishell DR Jr, Stanczyk F, Hiroi M, et al: Steroid contraception. In Crosignani PG and Mishell DR Jr, editors: Ovulation in the human, London, 1976, Academic Press.)

evidenced by rising estradiol levels, did not occur during the week when no steroid was being ingested. When lower doses of steroids are administered, follicular growth but not ovulation may occur because of initiation of growth of the dominant follicle during the time that no steroid is being ingested.

From these data it seems reasonable to conclude that accidental pregnancies during OC use probably do not occur because of failure to ingest one to two pills more than a few days after a treatment cycle is initiated but rather because initiation of the next cycle of medication is delayed for a few days. Therefore, it is important that the pill-free interval is not extended more than 7 days. This is best accomplished by ingesting either a placebo or iron tablet daily during the steroid-free interval (the so-called 28-day package). If a 3-week pill package is used, treatment is best started on the first Sunday after menses begins instead of the first or fifth day of the cycle. It is easier to remember to start the new package on a Sunday. Women should be advised that the most important pill to remember to take is the first one of each cycle.

Physiology

Mechanism of Action

The estrogen-progestin combination is the most effective type of OC formulation, because these preparations consistently inhibit the midcycle gonadotrophin surge and thus prevent ovulation. The progestin-only formulations have a lower dose of progestin than do the combined agents and do not consistently inhibit ovulation. Both types of formulations also act on other aspects of the reproductive process. They alter the cervical mucus, making it thick, viscid, and scanty, which retards sperm penetration. They also alter motility of the uterus and oviduct, thus impairing transport of both ova and sperm. Furthermore, they alter the endometrium so that its glandular production of glycogen is diminished and less energy is available for the blastocyst to survive in the uterine cavity. Finally, they may alter ovarian responsiveness to gonadotrophin stimulation. With both types of formulations, neither gonadotrophin production nor ovarian steroidogenesis is completely abolished. Levels of endogenous estradiol in the peripheral blood during ingestion of high-dose combination OCs are similar to those found in the early follicular phase of the normal cycle.

Contraceptive steroids prevent ovulation mainly by interfering with release of gonadotrophin-releasing hormone (GnRH) from the hypothalamus. In rats and in a few studies in humans, this inhibitory action of the contraceptive steroids could be overcome by the administration of GnRH. However, in the majority of other human studies, most women who had been ingesting combination OCs had suppression of the release of LH and FSH after infusion of GnRH, indicating that the steroids had a direct inhibitory effect on the pituitary and the hypothalamus.

It is possible that when hypothalamic inhibition is prolonged, the mechanism for synthesis and release of gonadotrophins may become refractory to the normal amount of GnRH stimulation. However, in studies of a few OC users, after serial daily administration of GnRH, there was still a refractory response to a GnRH infusion. Thus the combination contraceptive steroids probably do have a direct inhibitory effect on the gonadotrophin-producing cells of the pituitary, in addition to affecting the hypothalamus. Direct pituitary inhibition occurs in about 80% of women ingesting high-dose combination OCs. Pituitary suppression is unrelated to the age of the woman or the duration of steroid use but is related to the potency of the formulation. The effect is more pronounced with formulations containing a more potent progestin and with those containing 50 μg or more of estrogen than with 30- to 35-μg estrogen-containing formulations. It has not been demonstrated that the amount of pituitary suppression is related to the occurrence of amenorrhea after stopping OC use, but if there is a relationship, the lower-dose formulations should be associated with a lower frequency of this entity. There are data showing that the mean time to conception after discontinuation of OC use is shorter in women ingesting preparations with less than 50 μg of estrogen (4.01 cycles) than in those ingesting formulations with 50 μg of estrogen or more (4.79 cycles).

The daily progestin-only preparations do not consistently inhibit ovulation. They exert their contraceptive action via the other mechanisms listed above, but because of the inconsistent ovulation inhibition, their effectiveness is significantly less than that of the combination types of OCs. Because a lower dose of progestin is used in these formulations than in the combination tablets, it is important that these preparations be consistently taken at the same time of day to ensure that blood levels do not fall below the effective contraceptive level.

No significant difference in clinical effectiveness has been demonstrated among the various combination formulations currently available in the United States (see Table 13-3). As long as no tablets are omitted (perfect use), the pregnancy rate is less than 0.2% at the end of 1 year with all marketed combination formulations.

Metabolic Effects

The synthetic steroids in OC formulations have many metabolic effects in addition to their contraceptive actions (Table 13-4). These metabolic effects can produce both the more common, less serious side effects, as well as the rare, potentially serious complications. The magnitude of these effects is directly related to the dosage and potency of the steroids in the formulations. Fortunately, in most instances the more common adverse effects are relatively mild.

TABLE 13-4
Metabolic Effects of Contraceptive Steroids

	Effects	
	Chemical	Clinical
Estrogen-Ethinyl Estradiol		
*Proteins**		
Albumin	↓	None
Amino Acids	↓	None
Globulins	↑	
Angiotensinogen		↑Blood pressure
Clotting Factors		Hypercoagulability
Carrier proteins (CBG, TBG, SHBG, transferrin, ceroloplasmin)		None
Carbohydrate		
Plasma insulin	None	None
Glucose tolerance	None	None
Lipids†		
Cholesterol	↑	None
Triglyceride	↑	None
HDL cholesterol	↑	? ↓ cardiovascular disease
LDL cholesterol	↓	? ↓ cardiovascular disease
Electrolytes		
Sodium excretion	↓	Fluid retention
		Edema
Vitamins		
B complex	↓	None
Ascorbic acid	↓	None
Vitamin A	↑	None
Other		
Breast	↑	Breast tenderness
Endometrial steroid receptors	↑	Hyperplasia
Skin	↓	Sebum production
		Facial pigmentation
Progestins—19-Nortestosterone Derivatives		
Proteins	↓ SHBG	None
Carbohydrate		
Plasma insulin	↑	None
Glucose tolerance	↓	None
Lipids		
Cholesterol	↓	None
Triglyceride	↓	None
HDL cholesterol	↓	? ↓ Cardiovascular disease
LDL cholesterol	↑	? ↓ Cardiovascular disease
Other		
Nitrogen retention	↑	↑ Body weight
Skin-sebum production	↑	↑ Acne
CNS effects	↑	Nervousness, fatigue, depression
Endometrial steroid receptors	↓	No withdrawal bleeding

*CBG, Corticosteroid-binding globulin; TBG, thyroxine-binding globulin.

†HDL, High-density lipoprotein; LDL, low-density lipoprotein.

The most frequent symptoms produced by the estrogen component include nausea (a central nervous system effect), breast tenderness, and fluid retention (which usually does not exceed 3 to 4 pounds of body weight) caused by decreased sodium excretion. Minor, clinically insignificant changes in circulating vitamin levels also occurred after ingestion of the higher-dosage OCs. These changes included a decrease in levels of the B complex vitamins and ascorbic acid and increases in levels of vitamin A. Even with use of the high-steroid–dose agents, dietary vitamin supplementation was not necessary, as the changes in circulating vitamin levels were small and clinically insignificant. Estrogen can also cause melasma, pigmentation of the malar eminences, to develop. Melasma is accentuated by sunlight and usually takes a long time to disappear after OCs are discontinued. The incidence of all these estrogenic side effects is much less with use of lower-estrogen–dose formulations than that which occurred with use of high-estrogen–dose formulations. With high doses of estrogen OC usage was found to accelerate the development of the symptoms of gallbladder disease in young women but did not increase the overall incidence of cholelithiasis. The results of the large British Family Planning Association Study and a recent case-control study indicate that the use of high-dose OCs does not increase the incidence of gallbladder disease in women. When the data were stratified among women of different body weight or age, no increased risk of gallbladder disease was found in any subgroup. These results indicate that development of gallbladder disease is not a risk factor associated with OC use, even if these agents contain high doses of steroids and are used for more than 8 years.

It was previously postulated that high dosages of the synthetic estrogens could also produce changes in mood and depression brought about by diversion of tryptophan metabolism from its minor pathway in the brain to its major pathway in the liver. The end product of tryptophan metabolism, serotonin, is thus decreased in the central nervous system, and it was postulated that the resultant lowering of serotonin could produce depression in some women and sleepiness and mood changes in others. Analysis of the data from the Royal College of General Practitioners (RCGP) cohort study indicated that OC use was positively correlated with the incidence of depression, which in turn was directly related to the dose of estrogen in the formulation. In this study an increased incidence of depression was not found to occur among users of OCs containing less than 50 μg of estrogen. Data from postmenopausal women receiving estrogen therapy alone, as well as from estrogen-progestin sequential therapy, indicate that administration of physiologic doses of estrogen alone, which is less potent than the pharmacologic dose used in OCs, improves the mood of women, whereas the addition of a progestin increases the amount of depression, irritability, tension, and fatigue. These studies indicate that the progestin component of the agents may be the major cause of the adverse mood changes and tiredness observed in some women after ingestion of OCs, but it has not been definitely established which of the steroid components is the major factor in producing adverse mood changes. Possibly both are involved.

The progestins, because they are structurally related to testosterone, also produce certain adverse androgenic effects. These include weight gain, acne, and a symptom perceived by some women as nervousness. Some women gain a considerable amount of weight when they take OCs, and this weight gain is believed to be produced by the anabolic effect of the progestin component. Although estrogens decrease sebum production, progestins increase it and can cause acne to develop or worsen. Thus women who have acne should be given a formulation with a low progestin-estrogen ratio. One formulation, containing estrogen and a nonandrogenic progestin, norgestimate, has been shown in a randomized controlled trial to reduce acne to a greater extent than placebo. The treatment of acne is now an approved indication for use of this agent. The final symptom produced by the progestin component is failure of withdrawal bleeding or amenorrhea. Because the progestins decrease the synthesis of estrogen receptors in the endometrium, endometrial growth is decreased, and some women have failure of withdrawal bleeding. This symptom is not important medically, but since bleeding serves as a signal that the woman is not pregnant, it is desirable to have some amount of periodic withdrawal bleeding during the days she is not taking these steroids. The two steroid components can act together to produce irregular bleeding.

Unscheduled (breakthrough) bleeding (which is usually produced by insufficient estrogen, too much progestin, or a combination of both), as well as failure of withdrawal bleeding, can be alleviated by increasing the amount of estrogen in the formulation or by switching to a more estrogenic formulation. Many women taking OCs complain of an increased frequency of headaches. It has not been determined what is the exact relation, if any, between each of the steroids in OCs and the occurrence of headaches.

Protein

The synthetic estrogens used in OCs cause an increase in the hepatic production of several globulins. Progesterone and androgenic progestins do not affect the synthesis of globulins except that of sex hormone binding globulin (SHBG). Synthesis of SHBG is reduced by androgens, including the androgenic progestins. Some of the globulins that are increased by ethinyl estradiol ingestion, such as Factor V, VIII, X, and fibrinogen, enhance thrombosis, while another globulin, angiotensinogen, may be converted to angiotensin and increase blood pressure in some users. The circulating levels of each of these globulins are directly correlated with the amount of estrogen in the OC formulation (Table 13-5). Epidemiologic studies have shown that the incidence of both venous and arterial thrombosis is also directly related to the dose of estrogen.

TABLE 13-5
Mean Factor VII and Fibrinogen Levels* in Relation to Oral Contraceptive Use and Estrogen Dose

	OC Estrogen Dose		
	Not Taking OCs	30 µg	50 µg
No. of patients	243	15	65
Factor VII (%)	83.08	96.6	121.1
Fibrinogen (g/L)	2.52	2.84	2.89

From Meade TW: Am J Obstet Gynecol 142:758, 1982.

*Age-adjusted values.

Although angiotensinogen levels are lower in women who ingest formulations with 30 to 35 µg of ethinyl estradiol than in those who ingest higher-estrogen–dosage formulations, a slight but significant increase in mean blood pressure still occurs in women who ingest the lower-dosage formulations and about 1 in 200 women will develop clinical hypertension. Thus blood pressure should be monitored in all users of OCs. There is some indirect evidence that the progestin component may also raise blood pressure. However, women who receive progestins without estrogen do not have an increase in blood pressure over time, indicating that the estrogen component is the major cause of elevated blood pressure in a few users of OCs.

Another globulin, sex hormone binding globulin (SHBG), binds circulating levels of estrogens and androgens. Progesterone is bound to corticosteroid-binding globulin but since the progestins used in oral contraceptives are 19-nortestosterone compounds, they are bound to SHBG. Estrogens increase SHBG levels while androgens, including 19-nortestosterone derivatives, decrease SHBG levels. Thus measurement of SHBG is one way to determine the relative estrogenic/androgenic balance of different OC formulations. Van der Vange et al. measured SHBG levels before and 6 months following ingestion of several OC formulations containing about the same amount of ethinyl estradiol. The greatest increase occurred with formulations containing cyproterone acetate, (not used in OC formulations in the United States), desogestrel, and gestodene. SHBG increases of lesser magnitude occurred following ingestion of formulations containing low doses of norethindrone and levonorgestrel. Since SHBG binds endogenous testosterone and prevents it acting on the target tissue, formulations causing the greatest increase in SHBG should be associated with the least amount of androgenic effects. These formulations are particularly useful for treating women with symptoms of hyperandrogenism such as polycystic ovarian syndrome.

Carbohydrate

The effect of OCs on glucose metabolism is mainly related to the dose, potency, and chemical structure of the progestin. Conflicting data exist as to whether the estrogen component affects carbohydrate metabolism. The estrogen may act synergistically with the progestin to impair glucose tolerance. In general the higher the dose and potency of the progestin, the greater the magnitude of impaired glucose metabolism. The amount of alteration appears to be greater with gonanes than with estranes. Several studies have shown that formulations with a low dose of progestin, including one containing levonorgestrel, do not significantly alter levels of glucose, insulin, or glucagon after a glucose load in healthy women or in those with a history of gestational diabetes. However, other studies indicate that the multiphasic formulations with norgestrel, but not those with norethindrone, produce some deterioration of glucose tolerance in normal women, as well as in those with a history of gestational diabetes. Some studies have shown increased levels of both glucose and insulin when glucose tolerance tests were administered to women ingesting desogestrel containing OCs.

Data from 20 years of experience using mainly high-dose formulations in the large Royal College of General Practitioners (RCGP) cohort study indicated that there was no increased risk of diabetes mellitus developing among current OC users (relative risk [RR], 0.80) or former OC users (RR, 0.82) even among women who had used OCs for 10 years or more. More than 1 million person-years of follow-up of OC users in the large Nurses Health Study cohort, which was initiated in 1976, were analyzed in 1992. Although type 2 diabetes mellitus developed in more than 2000 women, the risk was not increased among current OC users (RR, 0.71) and only marginally increased in past OC users (RR, 1.11) and occurred only among women who had used high-dose formulations many years previously, not for those who had used lower-dose formulations. Kjos et al. followed a group of women with a history of gestational diabetes mellitus for several years after the end of the pregnancy. Three years after delivery women ingesting low-dose norethindrone combination and low-dose levonorgestrel combination containing OCs had no greater risk of developing diabetes mellitus than the control group not taking OCs. When prescribing oral contraceptives for women with a history of glucose intolerance, it is probably preferable to use formulations with a low dose of a norethindrone-type progestin than a levonorgestrel type and to monitor glucose tolerance periodically.

Lipids

The estrogen component of OCs cause an increase in high-density lipoprotein (HDL) cholesterol, a decrease in low-density lipoprotein (LDL) levels, and an increase in total cholesterol and triglyceride levels. The progestin component causes a decrease in HDL and an increase in LDL levels while causing a decrease in both total cholesterol and triglyceride levels.

The older formulations with high doses of progestin had adverse effects upon the lipid profile although they also contained high doses of the synthetic estrogen. These progestin-dominant formulations produced a decrease in HDL cholesterol levels and an increase in LDL cholesterol levels. They also caused an increase in serum triglyceride because the estrogen has a greater effect on triglyceride synthesis than does the progestin. Short-term longitudinal studies of several phasic formulations containing levonorgestrel and norethindrone found that a significant increase in triglyceride levels still occurred but there was little change in either HDL cholesterol or LDL cholesterol levels, as well as total cholesterol levels, because the effects of each steroid on lipid synthesis were offset by the other.

In a cross-sectional study in which lipid levels were measured in a large number of women ingesting several OC formulations and compared with non-OC users, Godsland et al. reported that there were insignificant differences in HDL and LDL cholesterol levels compared with non-OC users when low-dose monophasic and triphasic levonorgestrel and norethindrone formulations were ingested. The women ingesting formulations with only 0.5 mg of norethindrone or 150 μg of desogestrel had a significant increase in HDL cholesterol levels and a significant decrease in LDL cholesterol levels (Figure 13-6). The three most recently developed progestins have less androgenic activity than do the older progestins and, as such, when combined with an estrogen would be expected to have less adverse effect on lipid metabolism than on the older formulations. Speroff et al. in 1993 reviewed data from the published studies in which lipid levels were measured in women ingesting formulations with the three less androgenic progestins. They reported that with use of these formulations there was a significant increase in HDL cholesterol levels, a significant decrease in LDL cholesterol levels, little change in total cholesterol levels, and a substantial increase in triglyceride levels (Table 13-6). The long-term effect, if any, of these changes in lipid parameters remains to be determined.

Coagulation Parameters

The estrogen component of oral contraceptives increases the synthesis of several coagulation factors, including fibrinogen, which enhance thrombosis, in a dose-dependent manner. The effect of OCs on parameters that inhibit coagulation, such as protein C, protein S, and antithrombin III, is less clear because of the diversity of techniques used to measure these parameters in different laboratories (Figure 13-7). A similar lack of consistency occurs when parameters that enhance fibrinolysis, such as plasminogen, or inhibit fibrinolysis, such as plasminogen activator inhibitor-1, are measured in OC users. Changes in most of these coagula-

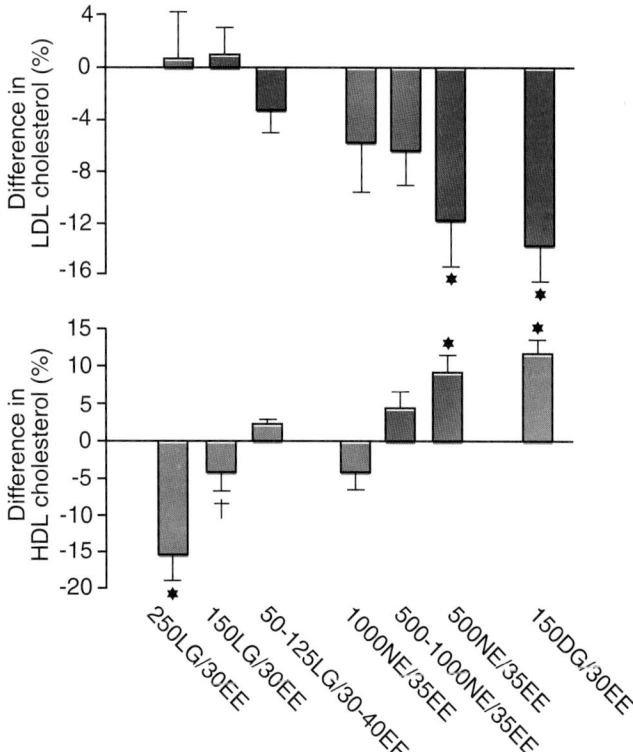

FIGURE 13-6 Percent differences in HDL and LDL cholesterol levels and in the incremental area for insulin in response to the OGTT between women taking one of seven combination oral contraceptives and those not taking oral contraceptives. The T bars indicate 1 SD. The asterisk (p < 0.001) and dagger (p < 0.01) indicate significant differences between users and nonusers in the mean values for the principal metabolic variables. (Modified from Godsland IF, Crook D, Simpson R, et al: N Engl J Med 323:1375, 1990.)

tion parameters in OC users are very small, if they occur at all, and there is no evidence that these minor alterations in levels of coagulation parameters measured in the laboratory have any effect upon the clinical risk of developing venous or arterial thrombosis. Nevertheless, if the woman has an inherited coagulation disorder that increases her risk of developing thrombosis, such as protein C, protein S, or antithrombin III deficiency or the more common activated protein C resistance, her risk of developing thrombosis is increased severalfold if she ingests estrogen-containing oral contraception. Vandenbroucke et al. reported that the relative risk of developing deep venous thrombosis (DVT) among women with activated protein C resistance and OC use was increased thirtyfold compared with non-OC users without the mutation. They estimated that the annual incidence of DVT in a woman of reproductive age with this genetic mutation was about 6 per 10,000 women if she did not take OCs and about 30 per 10,000 women if she took them. Currently, it is not recommended that screening for these coagulation deficiencies be undertaken before starting OC use unless the woman has a personal or family history of thrombotic events.

TABLE 13-6
Lipid Changes with Oral Contraceptives Containing New Progestins

Progestin	N	% Change from Baseline					
		TG	C	LDL-C	HDL-C	Apo B	Apo A-1
Desogestrel	608	29.3	2.8	−2.1	12.9	10.5	11.3
Gestodene	296	38.3	3.8	−2.5	8.1	16.0	7.1
Norgestimate	>2550	14.8	4.3	−0.2	9.9	5.3	7.3

From Speroff L, DeCherney A, and the advisory board for the new progestins: Obstet Gynecol 81:1034, 1993.

TG, triglyceride; C, total cholesterol; LDL-C, low-density lipoprotein cholesterol; HDL-C, high-density lipoprotein cholesterol; apo, apoprotein.

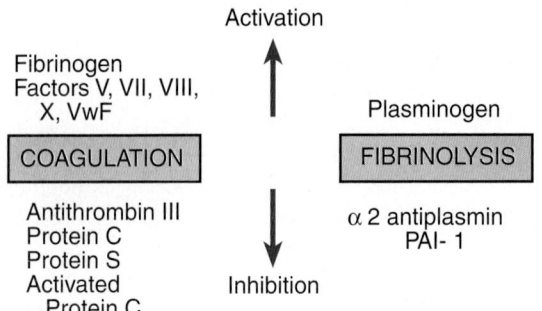

FIGURE 13-7 Factors involved in coagulation and fibrinolysis.

Cardiovascular Effects

The cause of the increased incidence of both venous and arterial cardiovascular disease, including myocardial infarction, in users of OCs appears to be thrombosis and not atherosclerosis.

Venous Thromboembolism

Gerstman et al. analyzed the effect of OCs with different doses of estrogen on the incidence of venous thromboembolism (VTE) in a historical cohort study of more than 230,000 women aged 15 to 44 in Michigan between 1980 and 1986. Among users of OC formulations with less than 50 μg of estrogen, the rate of VTE per 10,000 woman-years was 4.2; among users of formulations with 50 μg of estrogen, the rate was 7.0; and among users of formulations with greater than 50 μg of estrogen, the rate increased to 10.0 per 10,000 woman-years (Table 13-7). These data confirm earlier findings that indicate that the risk of VTE is directly related to the dose of estrogen in the formulation. The background rate of VTE in women of reproductive age is about 0.8 per 10,000 woman-years. An observational study by Farmer and Preston from nearly 700,000 women aged 14 to 45 years assessed the incidence of venous thromboembolic events associated with pregnancy and exposure to combined OCs containing more

than 20, but less than 50, μg of estrogen. The incidence of venous thromboembolic events among OC users was 3 per 10,000 woman-years, which was about 4 times the background rate but half the rate of 6 per 10,000 woman-years associated with pregnancy.

Several observational studies have been performed to determine the risk of VTE in users of OCs containing mainly less than 50 μg estrogen. These studies were consistent and showed that the risk of deep-vein thrombosis was increased approximately fourfold among women using OCs compared with women not using OCs.

Thus use of OCs containing less than 50 μg of estrogen is associated with about a threefold to fourfold increased risk of VTE compared with a nonpregnant population not taking OCs but about a 50% reduction in risk of VTE compared with a pregnant or recently postpartum population. The increased risk of VTE is similar in women ingesting the same dose of progestin with 20 μg of estrogen or 30 μg of estrogen. Thus, as stated in a WHO report, among users of combined oral contraceptive preparations containing less than 50 μg of ethinyl estradiol, the risk of venous thromboembolism is not related to the dose of estrogen.

In late 1995 and early 1996 results of four observational studies reported that the risk of VTE among women ingesting low-estrogen–dose formulations containing desogestrel or gestodene was increased about 1.5 to 2.5 times that of women ingesting formulations containing less than 50 μg of estrogen and levonorgestrel. Because none of these studies were prospective clinical trials, controversy exists as to whether the increased risk of VTE was causally related to formulations containing these progestins or whether the increased risk was due to certain types of bias. Selection bias, diagnostic bias, and referral bias could have accounted for the differences, but a causal relation cannot be disproved. Little data has been published to date regarding the risk of VTE with norgestimate-containing compounds, so it remains uncertain whether formulations containing this progestin are also associated with an increased risk of VTE compared with use of low-estrogen–dose levonorgestrel compounds.

TABLE 13-7
Rates of Deep Venous Thromboembolic Disease in Oral Contraceptive Estrogen Dose-Refined Cohorts

Estrogen-defined cohorts (μg)	No. of cases	Person-years (× 10,000)	Rates/ 10,000 person-years
<50	53	12.7	4.2
50	69	9.8	7.0
>50	20	2.0	10.0
All	142	24.5	5.8

From Gerstman BB, Piper JM, Tomita DK, et al: Am J Epidemiol 133:32, 1991.

Myocardial Infarction (MI)

Neither epidemiologic studies of humans nor experimental studies with subhuman primates have observed an acceleration of atherosclerosis with the ingestion of OCs. Nearly all the published epidemiologic studies indicate that there is no increased risk of myocardial infarction among former users of OCs. The incidence of cardiovascular disease is also not correlated with the duration of oral contraceptive use. Further data, which indicate that the increased risk of MI in OC users is due to thrombosis, not atherosclerosis, is provided by an angiographic study performed in 1982 by Engel et al. of young women who had an MI. In this study only 36% of users of OCs containing 50 μg ethinyl estradiol had evidence of coronary atherosclerosis compared with 79% of nonusers. A study with cynomolgus macaque monkeys found that the ingestion of an oral contraceptive containing high doses of norgestrel and ethinyl estradiol lowered HDL cholesterol levels significantly. However, after 2 years of ingesting this formulation and being fed an atherogenic diet, these animals had a significantly smaller area of coronary-artery atherosclerosis than did a control group of female monkeys not ingesting OCs but fed the same diet. Another group of monkeys, who received levonorgestrel without estrogen, also had lowered HDL cholesterol levels. In this group, the extent of coronary atherosclerosis was significantly increased compared with that of the controls. The results of this study have since been confirmed in a larger study with two high-dose estrogen-progestin formulations. Both of these compounds lowered the HDL cholesterol levels by half and tripled the cholesterol/HDL cholesterol ratio. In this study, the mean extent of coronary-artery plaque formation in the high-risk control group of female animals was more than 3 times greater than that found in animals ingesting a high-dose norgestrel compound and more than 10 times greater than that found in animals ingesting a high-dose ethynodiol diacetate compound with that of controls (Figure 13-8).

These studies suggest that the estrogen component of OCs has a direct protective effect on the coronary arteries, reducing the extent of atherosclerosis that would otherwise be accelerated by decreased levels of HDL cholesterol.

The epidemiologic studies that reported an increased incidence of MI in older users of OCs were published in the late 1970s and thus used as data base women who only ingested formulations with 50 μg or more of estrogen. In these case-control and cohort studies, a significantly increased incidence of MI was found mainly among older users who had risk factors that caused arterial narrowing, such as preexisting hypercholesterolemia, hypertension, diabetes mellitus, or smoking more than 15 cigarettes a day.

Data accumulated during the first 10 years of the RCGP study (1968 to 1978), in which the majority of users ingested formulations with more than 50 μg of estrogen and high doses of progestin, showed that a significantly increased relative risk of death from circulatory disease occurred only among women over 35 years of age who also smoked. A more recent analysis of data obtained during the first 20 years of this study (1968 to 1988) revealed that there was no significant increased relative risk of acute MI among current or former users of oral contraceptives who did not smoke any cigarettes (Table 13-8). Women who smoked and did not use OCs had a greater risk of MI than did nonsmokers whether or not they used OCs. Even though most of the women in this study used high-dose formulations, a significantly increased risk of MI with OC use compared with smokers

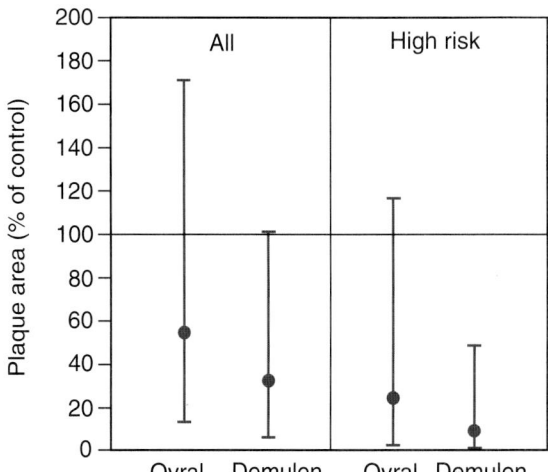

FIGURE 13-8 The 95% confidence intervals of the ratio of coronary artery atherosclerosis extent (measured as cross-sectional plaque area in mm²) of the OC treatment groups versus the control group, for all of the animals in the study and for the high-risk subset. (Estimates are based on sample sizes of 23, 23, and 25 for all monkeys in the control, Ovral, and Demulen groups, respectively; and 11, 9, and 12 for the high-risk monkeys in the control, Ovral, and Demulen groups, respectively. (From Clarkson TB, Shively CA, Morgan TM, et al: Obstet Gynecol 75:217, 1990.)

TABLE 13-8
Relative Risk of Myocardial Infarction in Relation to Smoking and Oral Contraceptive Use (RCGP Study, 1968–1987) ($N = 158$)

Smoking	Oral Contraceptive Use		
	Never (CL)	Previously (CL)	Current (CL)
Never	1.0	1.1 (0.6–2.2)	0.9 (0.3–2.7)
<15 cig./day	2.0 (1.0–3.9)	1.3 (0.6–2.8)	3.5 (1.3–9.5)
≥15 cig./day	3.3 (1.6–6.7)	4.3 (2.3–8.0)	20.8 (5.2–83.1)

Modified from Croft P and Hannaford PC: Br Med J 298:165, 1989.
CL, Confidence limits.

not using OCs occurred only among both mild (less than 15 cigarettes per day) and heavy cigarette smokers; OC users who were heavy smokers had a greater relative risk than mild smokers. A case-control study analyzed the relation between OC use and the risk of MI among women admitted to a group of New England hospitals between 1985 and 1988. The relative risk of MI among current OC users was not significantly increased, RR 1.1 (confidence interval [CI], 0.4 to 3.1). Among women who smoked at least 25 cigarettes a day, current OC use increased the risk of MI thirtyfold. Smoking alone, without use of OCs, increased the risk of myocardial infarction about ninefold. Thorogood et al. performed a case-control study between 1986 and 1988 to investigate the association between fatal MI and low-dose OCs. The overall risk associated with current use of OCs was estimated to be 1.1 (CI, 0.7 to 4.9). With formulations containing 50 µg of estrogen, the estimated risk increased to 4.2 (CI, 0.5 to 39.2). Cigarette smoking without the use of OCs was associated with a relative risk factor of MI of approximately 19. The data indicate that cigarette smoking is an independent risk factor for MI, but the use of high-dose OCs by cigarette smokers significantly enhances their risk of experiencing an MI, the two factors acting synergistically. Current or prior OC use is not associated with an increased risk of MI in nonsmokers.

The mechanism whereby cigarette smoking increases the risk of arterial thrombosis in OC users appears to be due to the effect of nicotine on the coagulation process. Although OCs increase the concentration of factors involved in producing blood coagulation, they also affect the activity of factors inhibiting coagulation. Notelovitz et al. found that smokers who ingested low-dose OCs had a significantly greater decrease in levels of endogenous coagulation inhibitors, mainly antithrombin III, than did OC users who did not smoke. Dynamic tests of coagulation and fibrinolysis by these investigators showed an altered procoagulant activity only among the OC users who also smoked. Mileikowsky et al. reported that platelet aggregation was increased only among OC users who also smoked and not among women who smoked and did not use OCs. This thrombotic effect was probably related to prostacyclin inhibition, as prostacyclin formation was reduced only among the women in the study who smoked and used OCs. The usual balance of prostacyclin and thromboxane is thus altered when OC users smoked, producing a relative excess of thromboxane. The results of this study therefore suggest that the synergistic effect of OCs and smoking on the effects of arterial thrombosis, such as MI and cerebral thrombosis, are produced by activation of the thromboxane A2-mediated mechanism of platelet aggregation brought about by reduction of prostacyclin only during nicotine intake. Thus former cigarette smokers do not have a risk of enhanced thrombosis, and nicotine administered in any form can increase the risk. Both the Royal College and WHO study reported that the risk of myocardial infarction in OC users was several-fold greater if they had hypertension than if they did not. Two recent large case-control studies in the United States have shown no significantly increased risk of MI in OC users. For many years in the United States OCs were not prescribed to women with uncontrolled hypertension or those older than age 35 who smoked cigarettes. A recent WHO Technical Report stated that women who do not smoke, who have their blood pressure checked, and who do not have hypertension or diabetes are at no increased risk of myocardial infarction if they use combined oral contraceptives regardless of their age.

Stroke

Although epidemiologic data from studies performed in the 1970s indicated that there was possibly a causal relation between ingestion of high-dose OC formulations and stroke, the data was conflicting, with some studies showing a significantly increased risk of ischemic stroke, others an increased risk of hemorrhagic stroke, and still others no significantly increased risk of either entity. Furthermore, as occurred with MI, the studies that did show a significantly increased risk of stroke in OC users indicated that the increased risk was mainly limited to older women who also smoked and/or were hypertensive. The monkey study performed by Clarkson et al. revealed that the animals ingesting high-dose OCs, which lowered HDL cholesterol, had no greater extent of carotid artery atherosclerosis than did the control group of female animals. Epidemiologic studies consistently report that there is no increased risk of either ischemic or hemorrhagic stroke in past users of OCs compared to never users.

Data from the epidemiologic studies of OC use and cardiovascular disease performed in the 1960s and 1970s are not relevant to their current use, as the dose of both steroid components in the formulations now being marketed is markedly less, and women with cardiovascular risk factors such as uncontrolled hypertension are no longer receiving these agents. Furthermore, it is strongly recommended not to prescribe OCs to women over age 35 who also smoke.

A nested case-control analysis by Hannaford et al. examined the data obtained between 1968 and 1990 during the Royal College of General Practitioners' (RCGP) Oral Contraception Study to determine the relationship between OC use and the risk of first-ever stroke, including the diagnosis of subarachnoid hemorrhage, cerebral hemorrhage, or ischemic stroke. Women using OCs containing a high estrogen dose (more than 50 μg) had nearly a six-fold increase in the risk of stroke, while women ingesting OC formulations containing 30 to 35 μg estrogen did not have an increased risk. Similar data were reported from a WHO study. The risk of ischemic stroke among women ingesting OCs with 50 μg or more of estrogen was 5.3 compared with nonusers but only 1.5 (insignificant) in women ingesting OCs with less than 50 μg of estrogen. An analysis of strokes occurring in a large health maintenance organization in California from 1991 to 1994 by Pettiti et al. indicated that the users had no significant increase of either ischemic or hemorrhagic stroke with OC use. In this study the relative risk of ischemic stroke and hemorrhagic stroke for OC users was 1.18 and 1.13, respectively, compared with never users and past users. Another case study by Schwartz et al. analyzed this data as well as data from the state of Washington. The relative risk of ischemic and hemorrhagic stroke in OC users compared to nonusers was 1.4 and 1.3. Neither of these figures was statistically significant.

The results of these recent epidemiologic studies indicate that use of low estrogen-progestin–dose OC formulation by nonsmoking women without risk factors for cardiovascular disease is not associated with an increased incidence of either myocardial infarction or ischemic or hemorrhagic stroke. Smoking is a risk factor for arterial but not venous thrombosis. Combination OCs should not be prescribed to women over the age of 35 who smoke cigarettes or use alternative forms of nicotine.

Reproductive Effects

In an attempt to determine whether the reproductive endocrine system recovers normally after cessation of OC therapy, Klein and Mishell measured serum levels of FSH, LH, estradiol, progesterone, and prolactin in six women every day for 2 months after they discontinued use of high-dose OCs. Except for a variable prolongation of the follicular phase of the first postcontraceptive cycle, the patterns and levels of all of these hormones were indistinguishable from those found in normal ovulating subjects. In these six women, the initial LH peak occurred from 21 to 28 days after ingestion of the last tablet. These results indicate that after a variable, but usually short, interval after the cessation of oral steroids, their suppressive effect on the hypothalamic-pituitary-ovarian axis disappears.

After the initial recovery, completely normal endocrine function occurs.

As previously mentioned the delay in the return of fertility is greater for women discontinuing use of OCs with 50 μg of estrogen or more than with those containing lower doses of estrogen. However, use of the low-dose formulations still causes a significant reduction in time to conception rates, with a mean of 5.88 cycles for OC users, compared with 3.18 cycles for women discontinuing other contraceptive methods. Among women stopping use of OCs in order to conceive, the reduced probability of conception compared with women stopping use of other methods is greatest in the first month after stopping their use and decreases steadily thereafter (Figure 13-9). There is little, if any, effect of duration of OC use on the length of delay of subsequent conception but the magnitude of the delay to return of conception after OC use is greater among older primiparous women than among others.

Thus, for about 2 years after the discontinuation of contraceptives in order to conceive, the rate of return of fertility is lower for users of OCs than for women who have used barrier methods, but eventually the percentage of women who conceive after ceasing to use each of these contraceptive methods becomes the same. Thus the use of OCs does not cause permanent infertility.

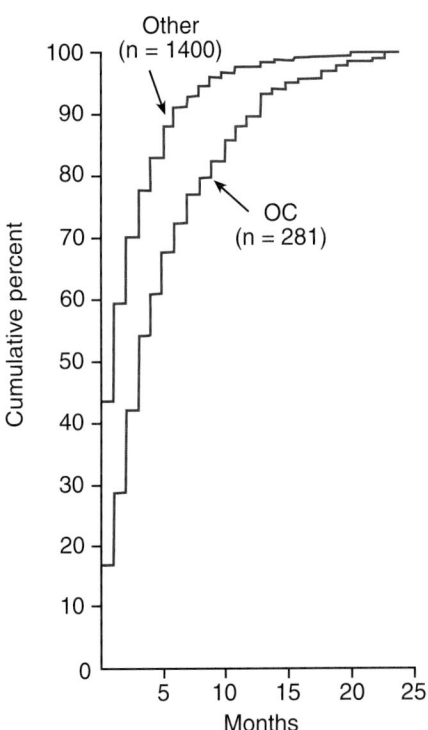

FIGURE 13-9 Cumulative conception rates for former oral contraceptive and other contraceptive users, Yale-New Haven Hospital 1980 to 1982. (From Bracken MB, Hellenbrand KG, and Holford TR: Fertil Steril 53:21, 1990.)

Because the resumption of ovulation is delayed for variable periods after OCs are stopped, it is difficult to estimate the expected date of delivery if conception takes place before spontaneous menses return. For this reason, when women stop OCs in order to conceive, it is probably best that they use barrier methods for about 1 to 2 months, until regular cycles resume. If conception occurs before resumption of spontaneous menses, gestational age should be estimated by serial sonography. Neither the rate of spontaneous abortion nor the incidence of chromosomal abnormalities in abortuses is increased in women who conceive in the first or subsequent months after ceasing to use OCs.

Several cohort and case-control studies of large numbers of babies born to women who stopped using OCs have been undertaken. These studies indicate that these infants have no greater chance of being born with any type of birth defect than do infants born to women in the general population, even if conception occurred in the first month after the medication was discontinued. If OCs are accidentally ingested during the first few months of pregnancy, a large cohort study reported that there is no significantly increased risk of congenital malformations among the offspring of users overall or among those of nonsmoking users. Smokers who used OCs after conception had a threefold higher risk of delivering infants with anomalies than did the entire study group. Smoking by itself has been shown to have an adverse effect on reproductive outcome, increasing the risk of abortion. Although an increased risk of certain anomalies was reported in some case-control studies of women ingesting OCs after conception, the results could have been influenced by both recall bias and the confounding effect of smoking. A statement warning of a possible teratogenic effect of ingestion of OCs during pregnancy has been deleted from current product labeling for OCs.

Neoplastic Effects

OCs have been extensively used for more than 35 years, and numerous epidemiologic studies of both cohort and case-control design have been performed to determine the relation between use of these agents and the development of various types of neoplasms. Because as yet no elderly women have used OCs during their early reproductive years, the studies thus far published usually restrict the analysis to women under 60 years of age. The most comprehensive of these studies is an analysis of a large number of U.S. women from several geographic areas aged 20 to 54 with cancer initially diagnosed between 1980 and 1983 and an appropriate control group. This study, the Cancer and Steroid Hormone (CASH) study, was performed by the U.S. Centers for Disease Control. Because hormones are mainly considered to be promoters, not initiators, of cancers, any adverse oncologic effects of these steroids should show a dose response, as demonstrated by

an increased risk occurring with increased duration of use. In 1995 Schlesselman addressed this issue by performing a meta-analysis of the epidemiologic studies reported between 1980 and 1994 that analyzed the effect of OCs according to their duration of use on cancer of the breast, organs of the female reproductive tract, and liver.

Breast Cancer

Schlesselman in 1995 performed a meta-analysis of 25 studies that analyzed the risk of breast cancer diagnosis associated with different durations of OC use in women between the ages of 45 and 60. In this analysis of nearly 20,000 women with breast cancer, of whom nearly half used OCs, he found there was a nonsignificant trend of slightly increasing breast cancer risk with increasing duration of use (Figure 13-10). The RR for 4, 8, and 12 years of OC use was 1.06, 1.068, and 1.072, respectively. Since each of these risk estimates are not significantly increased, the data support the conclusion that there is no adverse effect of OC use on the risk of diagnosis of breast cancer between the ages of 45 and 60. The CASH data and these findings are compatible with the hypothesis that OC use, like early first-term pregnancy, increases the risk of breast cancer diagnosis at a young age, with no appreciable effect on lifetime risk of breast cancer and possibly a decreased risk during the perimenopausal years when the disease becomes most common. No data regarding the effect of OC use on the risk of breast cancer in women older than age 55 has been published to date.

In 1996 a large, international collaborative group reanalyzed the entire worldwide epidemiologic data that had investigated the relation between risk of breast cancer and use of OCs. Analysis was performed on data from 54 studies performed in 25 countries, involving more than 53,000 women with breast cancer and more than 100,000 controls. The analysis indicated that while women took OCs

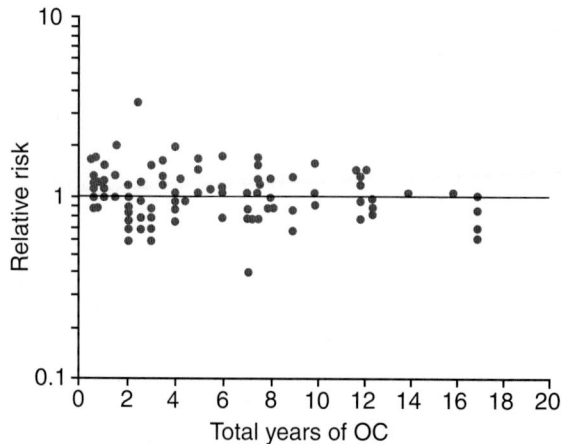

FIGURE 13-10   Relative risk of breast cancer by total years of oral contraceptive use. (From Schlesselman JJ: Obstet Gynecol 85:793, 1995.)

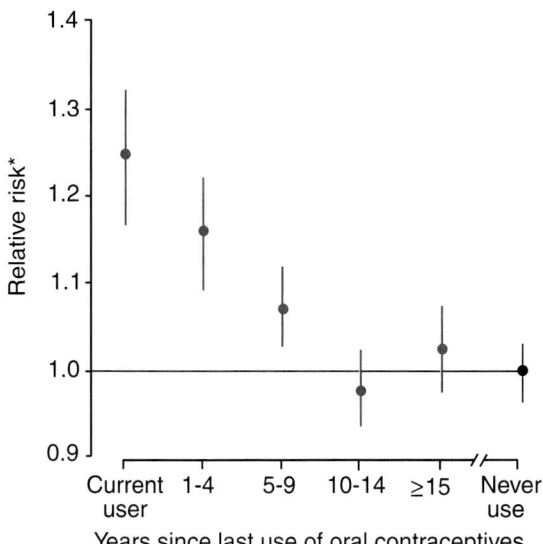

FIGURE 13-11 Relative risk of breast cancer by time since last use of combined oral contraceptives. (From Collaborative Group on Hormonal Factors in Breast Cancer: Lancet 347:1713, 1996.)

*Relative risk (given with 95% CI) relative to never-users, stratified by study, age at diagnosis, parity, age at first birth, and age at which risk of conception ceased.

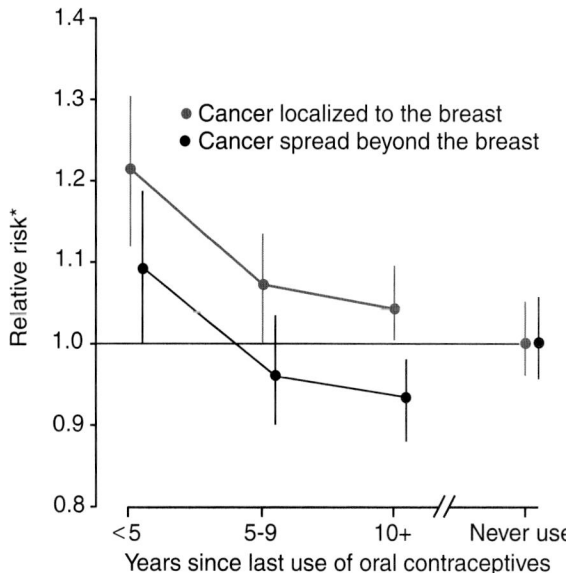

FIGURE 13-12 Relative risk of breast cancer by time since last use of combined oral contraceptives, according to the extent of tumor spread. (From Collaborative Group on Hormonal Factors in Breast Cancer: Contraception 54:1S, 1996.)

*Relative risk (given with 95% CI) relative to never use, stratified by study, age at diagnosis, parity, age at first birth, and age at which risk of conception ceased.

they had a slightly increased risk of having breast cancer diagnosed (RR, 1.24 [CI, 1.15 to 1.30]). The magnitude of risk of having breast cancer diagnosed declined steadily after stopping OCs so there was no longer a significantly increased risk 10 or more years after stopping their use (RR, 1.01 [CI, 0.96 to 1.05]) (Figure 13-11). It is of interest that the cancers diagnosed in women taking OCs were less advanced clinically than occurred in the nonusers. The risk of having breast cancer that had spread beyond the breast compared with a localized tumor was significantly reduced (RR, 0.88 [CI, 0.81 to 0.95]) in OC users compared with nonusers. The group concluded that these results could be explained by the fact that breast cancer is diagnosed earlier in OC users than in nonusers or could be due to biologic effects of the oral contraceptives. It was also found that women who had stopped using OCs more than 10 years earlier and developed breast cancer were significantly less likely to have nonlocalized disease than were women of similar age who had never used OCs (Figure 13-12).

The clinical meaning of this vast amount of epidemiologic data with small changes in relative risk is difficult to interpret. It appears that the dose or type of either steroid, as well as duration of OC use, is not related to breast cancer risk. Because there is no relation between dose or duration of use of estrogen, it is unlikely that OCs initiate breast cancer. Furthermore, the collaborative analysis found there was no significant increase in risk of breast cancer with OC use at very young ages, use before a first birth, or use by women with a family history of breast cancer. Two findings are important. One is that with current OC use or use within 5 years, the risk of breast cancer

diagnosis is increased by about 25%. The second is that the increased risk of breast cancer in current OC users is limited to localized disease, and OC users have a significantly reduced incidence of disease that has spread beyond the breast. A decreased risk of advanced disease is also found in older women. Since the increased risk of breast cancer with OC use is confined to current and recent users, if there is an excess in incidence the magnitude of increased incidence is small because breast cancer is uncommon under age 45. Furthermore, the contraceptive steroids probably act to promote the growth or increase the chance of diagnosis of existing cancers as breast cancer has been thought to usually take many years to become clinically evident after the cancer is initiated. Overall the large body of data regarding OC use and breast cancer risk is very reassuring.

Cervical Cancer

The epidemiologic data regarding the risk of invasive cervical cancer, as well as cervical intraepithelial neoplasia, and OC use is conflicting. Confounding factors, such as the woman's age at first sexual intercourse, the number of sexual partners, exposure to human papillomavirus (possibly greater among OC users), cytologic screening (probably more frequent among OC users), and the use of barrier contraceptives or spermicides (primarily by women in the control group), as well as cigarette smoking (an independent risk factor for this disease), could account for the

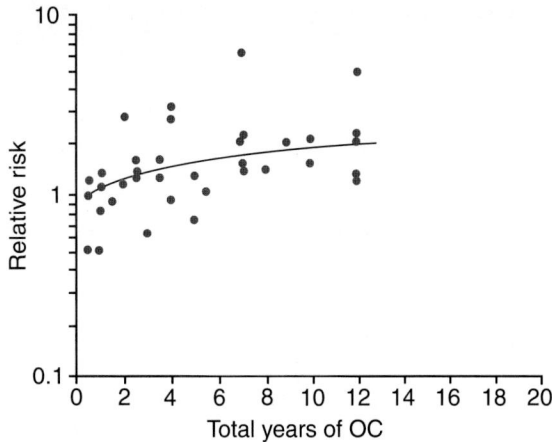

FIGURE 13-13   Relative risk of cervical cancer by total years of oral contraceptive use. (From Schlesselman JJ: Obstet Gynecol 85:793, 1995.)

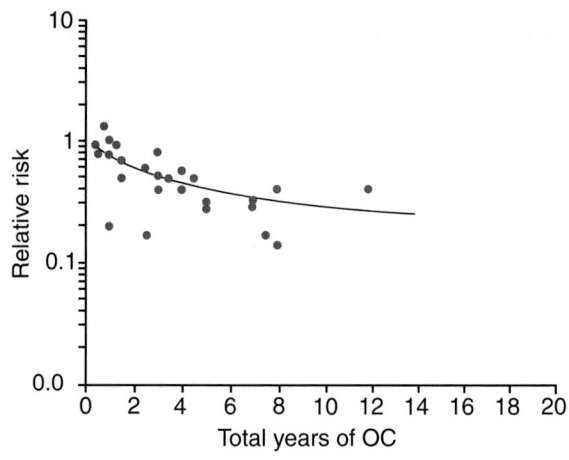

FIGURE 13-14   Relative risks of endometrial cancer by total years of oral contraceptive use. (From Schlesselman JJ: Obstet Gynecol 85:793, 1995.)

different results in different studies. In most of these studies statistical corrections were made for these confounding factors, and in many of them the control group did not use barrier methods of contraception.

As reported by Schlesselman's review of 14 studies of more than 3800 women with invasive cervical cancer, there is a significant trend of increased risk of this disease with increased duration of OC use (Figure 13-13). The relative risk of disease with 4, 8, and 12 years of OC use increased from 1.37 to 1.60 to 1.77, respectively.

Two prospective studies and two of three recent case-control studies also reported that the risk of invasive cervical cancer was significantly increased with long-term OC use, with an RR between 1.5 to 2.5. Three recent case-control studies have reported that the risk of adenocarcinoma of the cervix was significantly increased, about twofold, among OC users compared with nonusers. In two of these studies, the risk of developing this type of tumor increased with increasing duration of use and in one study reached a fourfold increased risk with more than 12 years of OC use. Adenocarcinoma of the cervix is uncommon under age 55, with an incidence of about 1 per 1000 women. In contrast to these findings the majority of well-controlled studies indicate that there is no change in risk of cervical intraepithelial neoplasia with OC use. Since invasive epithelial cervical cancer is usually preceded by dysplasia, the relation between OC use and increased risk of epithelial cervical cancer is unlikely to be causal. However, it is possible that a causal relation exists between OC use and an increased risk of cervical adenocarcinoma.

Although it is uncertain whether OCs themselves increase the risk of cervical cancer, act as a cocarcinogen, or have no effect, users of OCs as a group are at high risk for cervical neoplasia and require at least annual screening of cervical cytology, especially if they have used OCs for more than 5 years.

Endometrial Cancer

Twelve case-control studies and three cohort studies have examined the relation between OCs and endometrial cancer, and all but two of these studies have indicated that the use of these agents has a protective effect against endometrial cancer, the third most common cancer among U.S. women. Women who use OCs for at least 1 year have an age-adjusted relative risk of 0.5 for development of endometrial cancer between ages 40 and 55 compared with nonusers. This protective effect is related to duration of use, increasing from a 20% reduction in risk with 1 year of use to a 40% reduction with 2 years of use to about a 60% reduction with 4 years of use. In Schlesselman's review of 10 studies of more than 1200 women with endometrial cancer, the risk of developing endometrial cancer was decreased by 54% with 4 years' use, 66% with 8 years' use, and 72% with 12 years' use (Figure 13-14). This protective effect appears within 10 years of initial use and persists for at least 15 years after stopping use of OCs. In the study by Jick et al. of 142 cases of endometrial cancer among women 50 to 64 years of age the risk of endometrial cancer was decreased by 50% among former OC users compared with never users (RR, 0.48 [CI, 0.26 to 0.84]). The greatest protective effect is in nulliparous women (RR, 0.2) or women of low parity, who are at greater risk of acquiring this disease. Voight et al. reported the protective effect of OCs on endometrial cancer occurred with use of combination formulations with both high and low doses of progestin.

Ovarian Cancer

As summarized by Hankinson et al. in 1994 there were 20 published reports examining the use of OCs with subsequent development of ovarian cancer, and 18 of these found a reduction in risk specifically of the most common

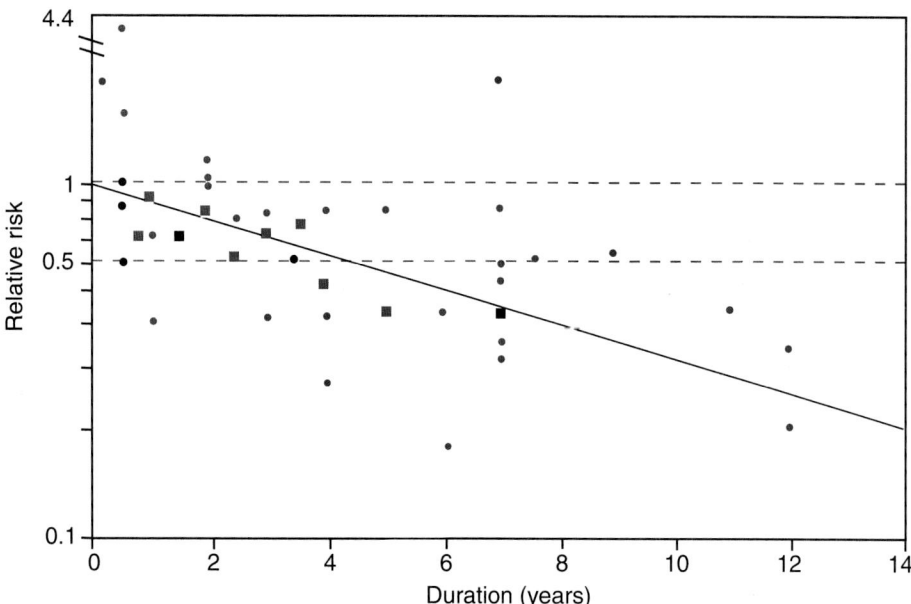

FIGURE 13-15 Relative risk of ovarian cancer associated with different durations of oral contraceptive use; findings of 15 studies. Study categories, indicating category weights ranging from smallest (weight in bottom 25% of range) to largest (weight in top 25% of range): blue circles = 1 (smallest); blue squares = 2; black circles = 3; black squares = 4 (largest). (From Hankinson SE, Colditz GA, Hunter DJ, and Rosner B: Obstet Gynecol 80:708, 1992.)

type—epithelial ovarian cancers (Figure 13-15). The summary relative risk of development of ovarian cancer among ever users of OCs was 0.64, a 36% reduction. OCs reduce the risk of the four main histologic types of epithelial ovarian cancer—serous, mucinous, endometrioid, and clear-cell—and the risk of both invasive ovarian cancers, as well as those with low malignant potential, is reduced. The magnitude of the decrease in risk is directly related to the duration of OC use, increasing from about a 40% reduction with 4 years of use, to a 53% reduction with 8 years of use, and a 60% reduction with 12 years of use. Beyond 1 year there is about an 11% reduction in ovarian cancer risk for each of the first 5 years of use. The protective effect begins within 10 years of first use and continues for at least 20 years after the use of OCs ends. A recent study by Rosenberg et al. found a similar level of protection with low-dose monophasic formulations, as well as higher-dose agents. Insufficient data on ovarian cancer risk with use of phasic formulations is currently available. As with endometrial cancer, the protective effect occurs only in women of low parity (≤4), who are at greatest risk for this type of cancer.

Liver Adenoma and Cancer

The development of a benign hepatocellular adenoma is a rare occurrence in long-term users of OCs, and the increased risk of this tumor was associated with prolonged use of high-dose formulations, particularly those containing mestranol. Although two British studies reported an increased risk of liver cancer among users of OCs, the number of patients was small and the results could have been influenced by confounding factors. The rate of death from the disease has remained unchanged in the United States over the past 25 years, a period when millions of women have used these agents. Data from a large, multi-center epidemiologic study coordinated by the World Health Organization found no increased risk of liver cancer associated with OC users in countries with a high prevalence rate of this neoplasm. This study found no change in risk with increasing duration of use or time since first or last use.

Pituitary Adenoma

OCs mask the predominant symptoms produced by prolactinoma—amenorrhea and galactorrhea. When OC use is discontinued, these symptoms occur, suggesting a causal relation. However, data from three studies indicate that the incidence of pituitary adenoma among users of OCs is not higher than that among matched controls.

Malignant Melanoma

Several epidemiologic studies have been undertaken to assess the relation of OC use and the development of malignant melanoma. The results are ambiguous, since an increased risk, a decreased risk, and no effect have all been reported. In a review by Prentice and Thomas in 1987, the summary relative risk for eight case-control studies was

1.0 and for three cohort studies 1.4—an insignificant increase. A more recent analysis of the 2 large British cohort studies involving more than 40,000 women, which were initiated in 1968, reported that the adjusted RR of incidence developing in OC users was 0.92 and 0.85. The results of these large studies of long duration indicate that OC use does not increase the risk of development of malignant melanoma.

Oral Contraceptive Use and Overall Mortality

In 1989 Vessey et al. reported the causes of mortality (through 1987) among OC users and nonusers enrolled in the Oxford Family Planning Association Cohort Study between 1968 and 1974. During this 20-year follow-up of 17,032 women, there were 238 deaths. The overall risk of death among the OC users was 0.9 (CI, 0.7 to 1.2) compared with the women of similar age and socioeconomic status who used a diaphragm or condom for contraception. The risk of death from breast cancer in OC users compared with nonusers was 0.9 (CI, 0.4 to 1.4), from cervical cancer 3.3 (CI, 0.9 to 17.9), and from ovarian cancer 0.4 (CI, 0.1 to 1.2). These cancer mortality rates are consistent with the other epidemiologic data reported earlier in this chapter. The death rate for circulatory disease was 1.5 (CI, 0.7 to 3.0), and nearly all these deaths in OC users occurred in women who were also smokers. In 1994 Colditz et al. reported mortality rates among the 166,755 women enrolled in the Nurses Health Study in 1976 that were followed through 1980. A total of 2879 deaths occurred in this group of women, and the relative risk of death among ever users of OCs compared with never users was 0.93. There was no change in risk of death with long-term use. Among women who had used OCs for 10 or more years the relative risk of mortality was 1.06 compared with nonusers. There was no change in risk of deaths caused by cardiovascular disease or cancer. The risk of death from ovarian cancer was 0.79, from endometrial cancer 0.33, and from breast cancer 1.07. None of these differences were statistically significant. In 1999 Beral et al. reported mortality in the 25-year follow-up of the 46,000 women enrolled in the RCGP study. There were 1599 deaths reported. For current and recent (within 10 years) users, the risk of death from ovarian cancer was 0.2, cervical cancer 2.5, and cerebrovascular disease 1.9. Ten or more years after stopping OCs, mortality rates for all causes, as well as most specific causes, were similar in women who had and those who had not used OCs. The mortality rate for breast cancer was nearly identical in OC users and nonusers. It thus appears that high-dose OC use has no appreciable risk on overall mortality. With exclusive use of low-dose formulations given to women without cardiovascular risk factors who have frequent cervical cytologic screening, an overall beneficial effect on mortality with OC use may be expected.

Contraindications to Oral Contraceptive Use

OCs can be prescribed for the majority of women of reproductive age, because these women are young and generally healthy. However, there are certain absolute contraindications; these include a history of vascular disease, including thromboembolism, thrombophlebitis, atherosclerosis, and stroke; and systemic disease that may affect the vascular system, such as lupus erythematosus or diabetes with retinopathy or nephropathy. Cigarette smoking by OC users over age 35 and uncontrolled hypertension are also contraindications. One of the contraindications listed in the product labeling is cancer of the breast or endometrium, although there are no data indicating that OCs are harmful to women with these diseases.

Pregnant women should not ingest OCs, because it has been theorized that there is a masculinizing effect of the 19 nonprogestins on the external genitalia of female fetuses. As mentioned earlier, concerns that OCs might produce other deleterious fetal effects, such as limb reduction and heart defects, have not proved valid. These concerns were raised by articles linking ingestion of any progestational agent in pregnancy to an increased incidence of congenital abnormalities. However, the major use of progestins in pregnancy had previously been for treatment of threatened abortion. Bleeding in pregnancy is itself associated with an increased incidence of anomalies. The incidence of birth defects has not decreased since the use of progestins for threatened abortion has been discontinued.

Women with functional heart diseases should not use OCs, because the fluid retention they produce could result in congestive heart failure. There is no evidence, however, that individuals with asymptomatic mitral valve prolapse should not use OCs. Women with active liver disease should not take OCs. However, women who have recovered from liver disease, such as viral hepatitis, and whose liver function tests have returned to normal, can safely take OCs.

Relative contraindications to OC use include heavy cigarette smoking under age 35, migraine headaches, undiagnosed causes of amenorrhea, and depression. About 20% of women have migraine headaches, and their frequency and severity can be worsened by OC use. There is no evidence that the risk of stroke is significantly increased in women with migraine headaches who use OCs compared with non-OC users. Unless the women have peripheral neurologic symptoms with the migraine headaches, OCs can be used. If fainting, temporary loss of vision or speech, or paresthesias develop in an OC user, the use of OCs should be stopped because of their hypercoaguable effect.

Since OC use may mask the symptoms produced by a prolactin-secreting adenoma—amenorrhea and galactorrhea—amenorrheic women should not receive OCs until the diagnosis for this symptom is established. If galactorrhea develops during OC use, OCs should be discontinued, and after 2 weeks a serum prolactin level should be measured. If elevated, further diagnostic evaluations are indicated. The presence of a prolactin-secreting macroadenoma, but not a microadenoma, is a contraindication for OC use. Use of OCs does not cause enlargement of prolactin-secreting pituitary microadenomas or worsen functional prolactinoma as was previously believed. Women with gestational diabetes can take low-dose OC formulations, because these agents do not affect glucose tolerance or accelerate the development of diabetes mellitus. Insulin-dependent diabetes without vascular disease is also not a contraindication for low-dose OC use.

Beginning Oral Contraceptives

Adolescents

In deciding whether a sexually active pubertal girl should use OCs for contraception, the clinician should be more concerned about compliance with the regimen than about possible physiologic harm. As long as she has demonstrated maturity of the hypothalamic-pituitary-ovarian axis with at least three regular, presumably ovulatory, menstrual cycles, it is safe to prescribe OCs without concern that their use will permanently alter future reproductive endocrinologic function. It is not necessary to be concerned about accelerating epiphyseal closure in the postmenarcheal female. Endogenous estrogens have already initiated the process a few years before menarche, and use of contraceptive steroids will not hasten it.

After Pregnancy

There is a difference in the relationship of the return of ovulation and bleeding between the postabortal woman and one who has had a term delivery. The first episode of menstrual bleeding in the postabortal woman is usually preceded by ovulation. After a term delivery, the first episode of bleeding is usually, but not always, anovulatory. Ovulation occurs sooner after an abortion, usually between 2 and 4 weeks, than after a term delivery, when ovulation is usually delayed beyond 6 weeks but may occur as early as 4 weeks in a woman who is not breast-feeding.

Thus, after spontaneous or induced abortion of a fetus of less than 12 weeks' gestation, OCs should be started immediately to prevent conception after the first ovulation. For women who deliver after 28 weeks and are not nursing, the combination pills should be initiated 2 to 3 weeks after delivery. If the termination of pregnancy occurs between 21 and 28 weeks, contraceptive steroids should be started 1 week later. The reason for delay in the latter instances is that the normally increased risk of thromboembolism occurring postpartum may be further enhanced by the hypercoagulable effects of combination OCs. Because the first ovulation is delayed for at least 4 weeks after a term delivery, there is no need to expose the woman to this increased risk.

Estrogen inhibits the action of prolactin in breast tissue receptors; therefore, the use of combination OCs (those containing both estrogen and progestin) diminishes the amount of milk produced by OC users who breast-feed their babies. Although the diminution of milk production is directly related to the amount of estrogen in the contraceptive formulation, only one study has been published in which the amount of breast milk was measured by breast pump in women using formulations with less than 50 μg of estrogen. In this study the use of this low dose of estrogen reduced the amount of breast milk. Thus, it is probably best for women who are nursing not to use combination OCs unless supplemental feeding is given to the infant.

Women who are breast-feeding every 4 hours, including during the night, will not ovulate until at least 10 weeks after delivery and thus do not need contraception before that time. Because only a small percentage of breast-feeding women will ovulate as long as they continue full nursing and remain amenorrheic, either a barrier method or a progestin-only OC can be used until menses resume. Progestins do not diminish the amount of breast milk, and progesin-only OCs are effective in this group of women. Once supplemental feeding is introduced, ovulation can resume promptly and effective contraception is then needed. Combination OCs should be used once supplemental feeding is initiated.

Cycling Women

At the initial visit, after a history and physical examination have determined that there are no medical contraindications for OCs, the woman should be informed about the benefits and risks. For medicolegal reasons it is best to note on the patient's medical record that the benefits and risks have been explained to her.

Type of Formulation

In determining which formulation to use, it is best initially to prescribe a formulation with less than 50 μg of ethinyl estradiol, as these agents are associated with less cardiovascular risk as well as with fewer estrogenic side effects than formulations with 50 μg of estrogen. It would also appear reasonable to use formulations with the lowest androgenic potency of progestin, as there would be less androgenic metabolic and clinical adverse effects associated with their use. The development of multiphasic formulations has allowed the total dose of progestin to be reduced compared with some monophasic formulations, without increasing the incidence of breakthrough bleeding. However, several monophasic formulations have a lower total dose of progestin per cycle than the multiphasic formulations and the incidence of follicular enlargement is more frequent with multiphasic than with monophasic formulations.

The FDA has stated that the product prescribed should be one that contains the least amount of estrogen and progestin that is compatible with a low failure rate and the needs of the individual woman. Because few randomized studies have been performed comparing the different marketed formulations, until large-scale comparative studies are performed, the clinician must decide on the formulation to use based on which has the least adverse effects among women in his or her practice. If estrogenic or progestogenic side effects occur with one formulation, a different agent with less estrogenic or progestogenic activity can be given.

The contraceptive formulations containing progestins and no estrogen have a lower incidence of adverse metabolic effects than do the combination formulations. Because the factors that predispose to thromboembolism are caused by the estrogen component, the incidence of thromboembolism in women ingesting these compounds is probably not increased. Furthermore, blood pressure is not affected, nausea and breast tenderness are eliminated, and milk production and quality are unchanged. Despite these advantages, these agents have the disadvantages of a high frequency of intermenstrual and other abnormal bleeding patterns (including amenorrhea) and a lower rate of effectiveness than the combined formulations. The failure rate of these preparations is higher than with the combined formulations, and a relatively high percentage of the pregnancies that do occur are ectopic. Since nursing mothers have reduced fertility and are amenorrheic, the major disadvantages of these preparations are minimized for these individuals. Furthermore, since milk production and quality are unaffected in contrast to the changes produced by combination pills, the formulations with only a progestin may be offered to these women while they are nursing. However, a small portion of these synthetic steroids have been detected in breast milk. The long-term effects (if any) of these progestins on the infant are not known, but none have been detected to date. A long-term follow-up study of breast-fed children whose mothers ingested 50 mg of estrogen in combined OCs while they were lactating revealed no difference in mean body weight or height up to 8 years of age compared with breast-fed children whose mothers did not ingest OCs. There was also no difference of occurrence of disease or in intellectual or psychologic behavior between the two groups.

Follow-up

If a healthy woman has no contraindications to OC use, it is unnecessary to perform any laboratory tests, including cervical cytology, unless these are necessary for routine health maintenance. At the end of 3 months, the woman should be seen again; at this time a nondirected history should be obtained and the blood pressure measured. After this visit the woman should be seen annually, at which time a nondirected history should again be taken, blood pressure and body weight measured, and a physical examination (including breast, abdominal, and pelvic examination with cervical cytology) performed. It is important to perform annual cervical cytologic screening on OC users, as they are a relatively high-risk group for development of cervical neoplasia. The routine use of other laboratory tests is not indicated unless the woman has a family history of diabetes or vascular disease at a younger age. Routine use of these tests in women is not indicated, because the incidence of positive results is extremely low. However, if the woman has a family history of vascular disease, such as myocardial infarction occurring in family members under the age of 50, it would be advisable to obtain a lipid panel before OC use is started, as hypertriglyceridemia may be present and OC use will further raise triglycerides. Because the low-dose formulations do not adversely alter the lipid profile except for triglycerides it is not necessary to measure lipids, other than the routine cholesterol screening every 5 years, in women with no cardiovascular risk factors, even if they are over age 35. If the woman has a family history of diabetes or evidence of diabetes during pregnancy, a 2-hour postprandial blood glucose test should be performed before OCs are started, and if blood glucose is elevated, a glucose-tolerance test should be performed. If the woman has a history of liver disease, a liver panel should be obtained to make certain that liver function is normal before OCs are started.

Drug Interactions

Although synthetic sex steroids can retard the biotransformation of certain drugs (e.g., phenazone and meperidone) as a result of substrate competition, such interference is not important clinically. OC use has not been shown to inhibit the action of other drugs. However, some drugs can interfere clinically with the action of OCs by inducing liver enzymes that convert the steroids to more polar and less biologically active metabolites. Certain drugs have been shown to accelerate the biotransformation of steroids in humans. These include barbiturates, sulfonamides, cyclophosphamide, and rifampin. Several investigators have reported a relatively high incidence of OC failure in women ingesting rifampin, and these two agents should not be given concurrently. The clinical data concerning OC failure in users of other antibiotics (e.g., penicillin, ampicillin, and sulfonamides), analgesics (e.g., phenytoin), and barbiturates are less clear. A few anecdotal studies have appeared in the literature, but reliable evidence for a clinical inhibitory effect of these drugs on OC effectiveness, such as occurs with rifampin, is not available. One study by Murphy et al. showed that when 2 g of tetracycline were given daily in divided doses the levels of both ethinyl estradiol and norethindrone in OC users were similar to those before antibiotic use. Women with epilepsy requiring medication probably should be treated with formulations containing 50 μg of estrogen, because a higher incidence of abnormal bleeding has been reported in these women with the use of lower-dose–estrogen formulations due to lower circulating levels of ethinyl estradiol brought about by the action of most antiepileptic medications.

Noncontraceptive Health Benefits

In addition to being the most effective method of contraception, OCs provide many other health benefits. Some are due to the fact that the combination OCs contain a potent, orally active progestin, as well as an orally active estrogen, and there is no time when the estrogenic target tissues are stimulated by estrogens without a progestin (unopposed estrogen).

Both natural progesterone and the synthetic progestins inhibit the proliferative effect of estrogen, the so-called antiestrogenic effect. Estrogens increase the synthesis of both estrogen and progesterone receptors, whereas progesterone decreases their synthesis. Thus one mechanism whereby progesterone exerts its antiestrogenic effects is by decreasing the synthesis of estrogen receptors. Relatively little progestin is needed to exert this action, and the amount present in OCs is sufficient. Another way progesterone produces its antiestrogenic action is by stimulating the activity of the enzyme estradiol-17 β-dehydrogenase within the endometrial cell. This enzyme converts the more potent estradiol to the less potent estrone, reducing estrogenic action within the cell.

Benefits from Antiestrogenic Action of Progestins

As a result of the antiestrogenic action of the progestins in OCs, the height of the endometrium is less than in an ovulatory cycle, and there is less proliferation of the endometrial glands. These changes produce several substantial benefits for the OC user. One is a reduction in the amount of blood loss at the time of endometrial shedding. In an ovulatory cycle the mean blood loss during menstruation is about 35 ml, compared with 20 ml for women ingesting OCs. This decreased blood loss makes the development of iron deficiency anemia less likely for OC users than for nonusers. Data from the RCGP study showed that OC users were about half as likely to develop iron deficiency anemia as were controls. Moreover, the beneficial effect persisted to a similar degree in women who had previously used OCs and then stopped using them, probably because of an increase in the iron stores that remained for several years after the drug was discontinued.

Because OCs produce regular withdrawal bleeding, it would be expected that OC users would have fewer menstrual disorders than controls. The results of the RCGP study confirmed the fact that OC users were significantly less likely to have menorrhagia, irregular menstruation, or intermenstrual bleeding develop. Because these disorders are frequently treated by curettage and/or hysterectomy,

OC users require these procedures less frequently than do nonusers.

Because progestins inhibit the proliferative effect of estrogens on the endometrium, as mentioned earlier, adenocarcinoma of the endometrium is significantly less likely to develop in women who use OCs.

Estrogen exerts a proliferative effect on breast tissue, which also contains estrogen receptors. Progestins may also inhibit the synthesis of estrogen receptors in this organ. Several studies have shown that OCs reduce the incidence of benign breast disease, and two prospective studies have indicated that this reduction is directly related to the amount of progestin in the compounds.

Data from the Oxford study indicate that current users of OCs have an 85% reduction in the incidence of fibroadenomas and 50% reductions in chronic cystic disease and nonbiopsied breast lumps, compared with controls using intrauterine contraceptive devices (IUDs) or diaphragms. The risk of development of these three diseases decreased with increased duration of OC use and persisted for about 1 year after discontinuation of OCs, after which no reduction in risk was observed. Rohn and Miller reported results of a large cohort study which showed that long-term use of OCs was associated with a significant reduction in the diagnosis of benign breast disease of the proliferative type.

Benefits from Inhibition of Ovulation

Other noncontraceptive medical benefits of OCs result from their main action—inhibition of ovulation. Some disorders, such as dysmenorrhea and premenstrual tension, occur much more frequently in ovulatory than in anovulatory cycles. In fact, inhibition of ovulation by exogenous steroids has been used for decades as therapy for severe dysmenorrhea. The RCGP study showed that OC users had 63% less dysmenorrhea and 29% less premenstrual tension than did controls. Another study indicated that OC users were less likely to have variation in the degree of feeling of well-being throughout the cycle than non-OC users.

Another potentially serious adverse effect of ovulatory menstrual cycles is the development of functional ovarian cysts—specifically, follicular and luteal cysts—that frequently require surgical management because of enlargement, rupture, or hemorrhage. When ovulation is inhibited, functional cysts do not usually develop. In a survey performed by the Boston Collaborative Drug Surveillance Program, less than 2% of women with a discharge diagnosis of functional ovarian cysts were taking OCs, in contrast to 20% of controls. However, 20% of women with nonfunctional cysts were taking OCs, an incidence similar to that observed in the controls. Although authors of one small case series postulated that the formation of functional ovarian cysts may be increased in users of multiphasic OCs, the rate of hospitalization for ovarian cysts in the United States has remained unchanged after the widespread use of multiphasic formulations.

TABLE 13-9

Rate Ratio Estimates for Functional Ovarian Cysts Comparing Each Oral Contraceptive Category with No Oral Contraception

	Rate Ratio*	95% Confidence Interval
No prescription	1.00	Reference category
Active prescription:		
Multiphasic	0.91	0.30–2.31
≤35 µg estrogen	0.52	0.17–1.33
>35 µg estrogen	0.24	0.01–1.34

From Lanes AF, Birmann B, Walter AM, and Singer S: Am J Obstet Gynecol 166:956, 1992.

*Rate ratios standardized to age distribution of index (i.e., "exposed") category.

Lanes et al. studied the rate of functional cysts more than 2 cm in diameter by ultrasound, which required either hospitalization or outpatient surgery. They found that low-dose monophasic formulations resulted in about a 50% reduction in functional cysts, lower than the 75% reduction with high-dose formulations, while use of multiphasic formulations had only a slight reduction of ovarian cyst development (Table 13-9).

Another disorder linked to incessant ovulation is ovarian cancer. As mentioned earlier, the development of ovarian cancer is significantly reduced in OC users, with a duration-dependent decrease in risk.

Other Benefits

Several European studies, including the RCGP study, showed that the risk of development of rheumatoid arthritis in OC users was only about half that in controls. Another benefit is protection against salpingitis, commonly referred to as pelvic inflammatory disease (PID). At least 11 published epidemiologic studies have estimated the relative risk of PID developing among OC users. Seven of these studies compared OC use with nonuse of any other contraception. The relative risk of PID developing among OC users in most of these studies was about 0.5, a 50% reduction. It has been estimated that between 15% and 20% of women with cervical gonorrheal infection will develop salpingitis. In a Swedish study, all women with culture-proven cervical gonococcal infection had a diagnostic laparoscopy 1 day after hospital admission to determine whether salpingitis was present. Of those who used contraception other than the IUD and oral steroids, salpingitis developed in 15%; salpingitis developed in only about half as many, 8.8%, of those who used OCs. The results of this study indicate that OCs reduce the clinical development of salpingitis in women infected with gonorrhea. Although the incidence of cervical infection with *Chlamydia tra-*

chomatis is increased in OC users compared with controls, Wølner-Hanssen et al. reported that the incidence of chlamydial salpingitis in OC users was only half that of controls. This protection may be related to the decreased duration of menstrual flow, which permits a small number of organisms to ascend to the upper genital tract and allows the body's defenses to eliminate them more easily. One sequela of PID is ectopic pregnancy, an entity that has tripled in incidence in the past decade. OCs reduce the risk of ectopic pregnancy by more than 90% in current users and may reduce the incidence in former users by decreasing their chance of developing salpingitis.

Since the lower-dose agents contain a progestin that inhibits estrogenic mitotic activity and also inhibits ovulation, the scope and magnitude of beneficial effects should be similar with all combination formulations currently marketed. It is unfortunate that the infrequent adverse effects of OCs have received widespread publicity, while the more common noncontraceptive health benefits have attracted little attention. In a study of women attending a Yale Health Center, about 80% of these well-educated women were unaware of these noncontraceptive health benefits. A nationwide survey sponsored by the American College of Obstetricians and Gynecologists also found that there was limited awareness of the noncontraceptive benefits of OCs by U.S. women, with less than half the women interviewed being aware of any benefit other than contraception.

There is also epidemiologic data that indicate that OCs reduce bone loss particularly in perimenopausal women with oligomenorrhea. Michaelsson recently reported that OC use by women after the age of 40 decreased the risk of subsequent hip fracture. There are noncontraceptive health benefits associated with continuing OC use beyond age 40 into the perimenopausal years. There are limited data regarding metabolic risks of OC use by women over age 40, but Godsland et al. reported that there were no changes in cardiovascular risk markers with long-term OC use. Because the estrogen given for hormone replacement is not as thrombophillic as is the estrogen dose currently used in OCs, it is best to switch from OCs to estrogen replacement about age 50. To avoid discontinuing OC use when the woman is still ovulating, measurement of the FSH and E_2 levels on the last day of the pill-free interval provides information about ovarian follicular activity. If the FSH level is elevated and the E_2 level low, OCs may be discontinued and estrogen hormonal replacement begun.

LONG-ACTING CONTRACEPTIVE STEROIDS

To avoid contraceptive failure associated with the need to remember to take oral contraceptives daily, methods of administering contraceptive steroid formulations at infrequent intervals have been developed. To date, two types of long-acting steroids—injectable suspensions and subdermal implant formulations—have been developed and are being used by women in the United States and elsewhere. Clinical trials with a contraceptive skin patch and intravaginal ring have also been performed, and these long-acting methods of contraception should soon be available. Because most of the long-acting steroid formulations contain only a progestin, without an estrogen, endometrial integrity is not maintained and uterine bleeding occurs at irregular and unpredictable intervals. Therefore women wishing to use these methods need to be counseled beforehand about the development of irregular bleeding to enhance continuity of use.

Injectable Suspensions

Three types of injectable steroid formulations are currently in use for contraception throughout the world. These include depo-medroxyprogesterone acetate (DMPA), given in a dose of 150 mg every 3 months; norethindrone enanthate, given in a dose of 200 mg every 2 months; and several once-a-month injections of combinations of different progestins and estrogens. Only the first of these three types is currently available in the United States. Injectable contraceptives are a popular method of contraception worldwide. In the United States they are used by about 3% of women of reproductive age.

Medroxyprogesterone acetate (MPA) is a 17-acetoxy progesterone compound and is the only progestin used for contraception that is not a 19-nortestosterone derivative. In all currently marketed oral contraceptives, the progestins are all 19-nortestosterone compounds, either estranes or gonanes, and as such have varying degrees of androgenic activity.

The 17-acetoxy progestins, which do not have androgenic activity and are structurally related to progesterone instead of testosterone, were used in oral contraceptive formulations about 30 years ago. Although approved for contraception in many Western countries in the 1960s, regulatory approval for these agents in the United States was stopped when tests on beagle dogs showed that ingestion of oral contraceptives with 17-acetoxy progestins was associated with an increased risk of mammary cancer. It was discovered later that unlike humans and other animals the beagle uniquely metabolizes 17-acetoxy progestins to estrogen, which causes mammary hyperplasia. Thus, when MPA is ingested by the beagle, it behaves differently than it does in the human, where it is not metabolized to estrogen. After epidemiologic studies showed that DMPA does not increase the risk of breast cancer in humans, regulatory approval for marketing this agent as a contraceptive was obtained in the United States in 1992.

Depot Formulation of MPA

MPA is a 17-acetoxy-6-methyl progestin that has progestogenic activity in the human (Figure 13-16). Since MPA is not metabolized as rapidly as the parent compound progesterone, it can be given in smaller amounts than

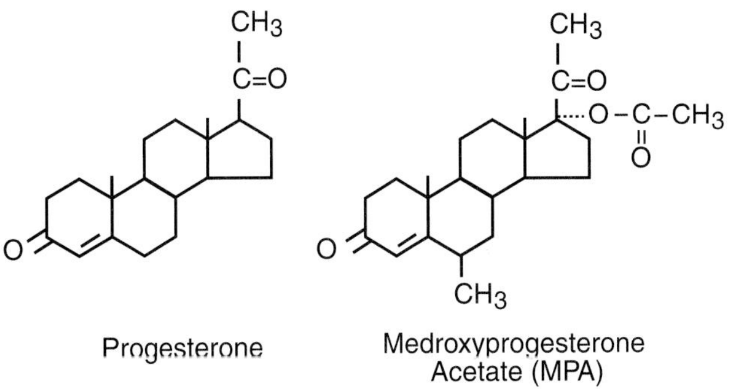

FIGURE 13-16 Comparative structures of progesterone and MPA.

progesterone, with an equivalent amount of progestational activity. Depo-medroxyprogesterone acetate (DMPA), the long-acting injectable formulation of MPA, consists of a crystalline suspension of this progestational hormone. The effective contraceptive dosage is 150 mg DMPA, which is given by injection deep into the gluteal or deltoid muscle, after which the progestin is released slowly into the systemic circulation. The area should not be massaged, so that the drug is released slowly into the circulation and maintains its contraceptive effectiveness for at least 4 months.

DMPA is an extremely effective contraceptive. In a large World Health Organization clinical trial studying use of DMPA, the pregnancy rate at 1 year was only 0.1%, and at 2 years the cumulative rate was 0.4%. Three mechanisms of action are involved. The major effect is inhibition of ovulation. Second, the endometrium becomes thin and does not secrete sufficient glycogen to provide nutrition for a blastocyst entering the endometrial cavity. Third, DMPA keeps the cervical mucus thick and viscous, so sperm are unlikely to reach the oviduct and fertilize an egg. With these multiple mechanisms of action, DMPA is one of the most effective reversible methods of contraception currently available.

PHARMACOKINETICS. MPA can be detected in the systemic circulation within 30 minutes after its intramuscular injection. Although serum MPA levels vary among individuals, they rise steadily to contraceptively effective blood levels (> 0.5 ng/ml) within 24 hours after the injection.

The pattern of MPA clearance from the circulation varies among different studies according to the type of assay used. After DMPA was administered to three subjects, Ortiz et al. assayed blood MPA levels daily for 2 weeks, then 3 times a week for the next 3 months, and then weekly until MPA was undetectable. In 2 subjects MPA levels initially plateaued at 1.0 to 1.5 ng/ml for about 3 months, after which they declined slowly to about 0.2 ng/ml during the fifth month (Figure 13-17). In a third subject, the blood levels were higher during the first month, then ranged between 1.0 and 1.5 ng/ml for the next 2 months, after which there was a further decline. MPA levels remained detectable in the circulation, > 0.2 ng/ml, for 7 to 9 months in all 3 subjects, after which it was not detectable. Estradiol levels were found to be in the early to midfollicular phase range, but consistently below 100 pg/ml during the first 4 months after injection. After 4 to 6 months, when MPA levels decreased to < 0.5 ng/ml, estradiol concentrations rose to preovulatory levels, indicating follicular activity, but ovulation did not occur, as evidenced by persistently low progesterone levels. Return of follicular activity preceded the return of luteal activity by 2 to 3 months. This delay in resumption of luteal activity is probably due to the fact that the circulating MPA levels inhibit the positive feedback effect of the rise of estradiol on the hypothalamic-pituitary axis, which in the absence of MPA would stimulate the midcycle release of luteinizing hormone (LH). The return of luteal activity in this study, indicated by a rise in serum progesterone levels, did not occur until 7 to 9 months after the injection, when the MPA levels were < 0.1 ng/ml.

In another study, performed by Kirton and Cornette using a different assay, MPA levels were much higher, although the pattern was similar to that found in the study by Ortiz et al., and luteal activity also did not occur until about 7 months after the injection.

A third study of DMPA pharmacokinetics was reported by Fotherby et al. and showed an entirely different pattern of MPA clearance after the injection. In this study the MPA levels fell more rapidly than in the other 2 studies, and the progesterone levels initially rose about 3.5 months after the injection. Based on this study the product labeling states that if the time interval after the last injection is more than 13 weeks the provider should determine that the woman is not pregnant before administering the drug. Additional studies are needed to determine more precisely the pharmacodynamics of MPA clearance and time of initial resumption of ovulation because of the differences observed in previous studies.

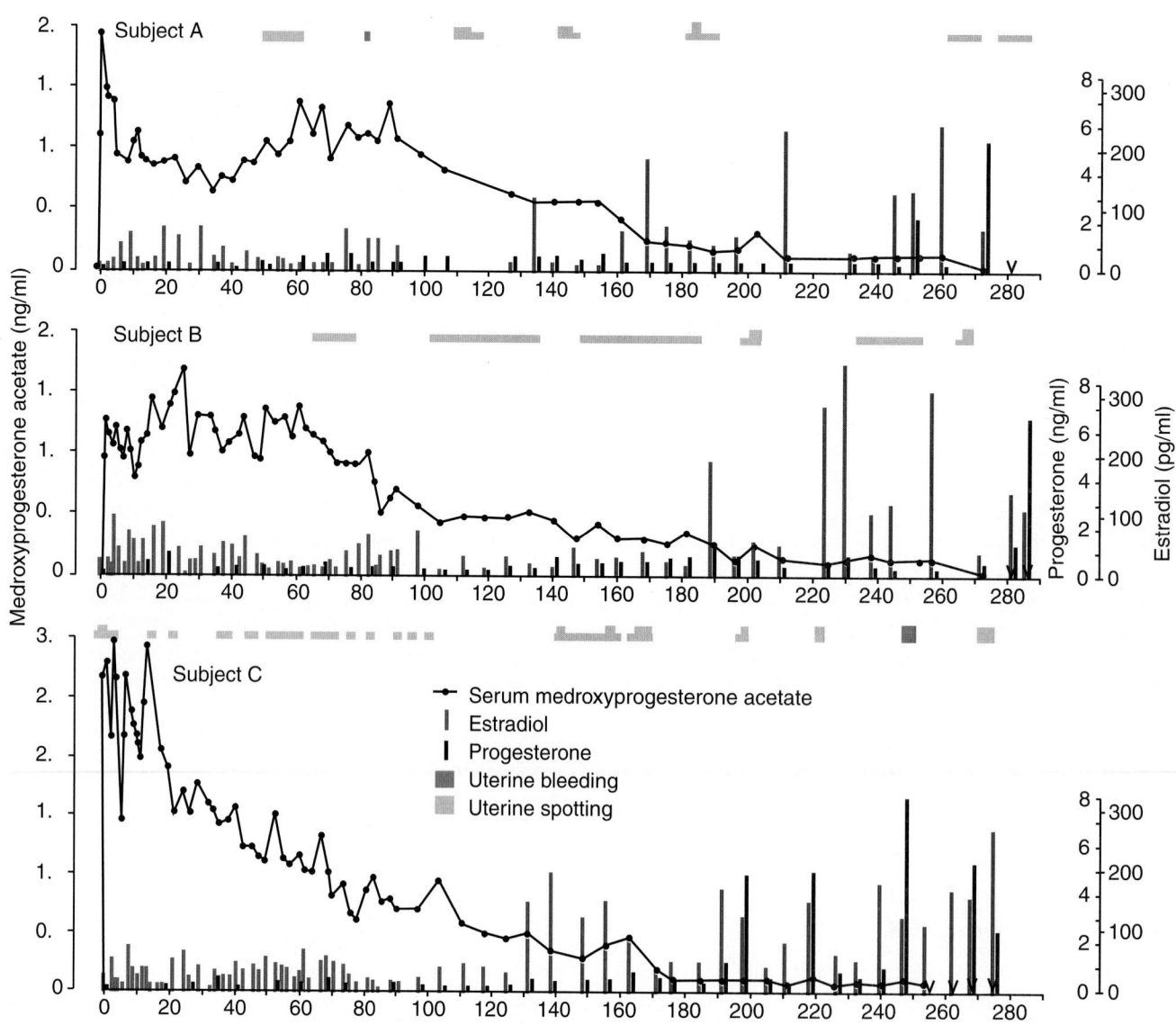

FIGURE 13-17   Serum MPA concentrations in 3 subjects during the first 24 hours after intramuscular injection of 150 mg of MPA. (From Ortiz A, Hiroi M, Stanczyk FZ, et al: J Clin Endocrinol Metab 44:32, 1977.)

OVULATORY SUPRESSION. To determine the effect of DMPA on the hypothalamic-pituitary axis, Mishell et al. measured serum LH and follicle stimulating hormone (FSH) levels daily during a control cycle and then for 2 months after a single injection was given. Although the midcycle LH peak was suppressed after the injection, LH was still being secreted in a pulsatile manner, and tonic serum levels were about the same as those found in the follicular phase of the control cycle (Figure 13-18). The normally occurring peak level of FSH at midcycle was also suppressed after the injection, but tonic FSH levels were in the range of those found in the luteal phase of the control cycle, indicating a lack of complete suppression of the hypothalamic-pituitary axis.

Goldzieher et al. measured FSH and LH levels in single blood samples from women who received injections of DMPA every 3 months for up to 2 years. In this cross-sectional study, the investigators found that both FSH and LH levels remained in the mean range of those in a control menstrual cycle. Therefore long-term use of DMPA also does not cause complete suppression of the hypothalamic-pituitary axis.

Mishell et al. reported that daily progesterone levels were consistently in the follicular phase range during the first 2 months after the initial injection of DMPA (see Figure 13-18). To obtain suppression of ovulation in the initial injection cycle, DMPA has to be administered within several days after the onset of menses. Siriwongse et al. reported that when the drug was initially given on days 5 or 7 of the cycle none of the women ovulated but when it was given on day 9, 2 of 13 subjects had presumptive evidence of ovulation. The results of this study indicated that DMPA should be given no later than 7 days after the onset of menses to be effective in the first ovulatory cycle. The product labeling states that to ensure the woman is not pregnant at the time of the first injection, it must be given during the first 5 days of the cycle.

Mishell et al. reported that circulating estradiol levels during the first 2 months after the initial 150-mg injection of DMPA were similar to the levels found in the follicular

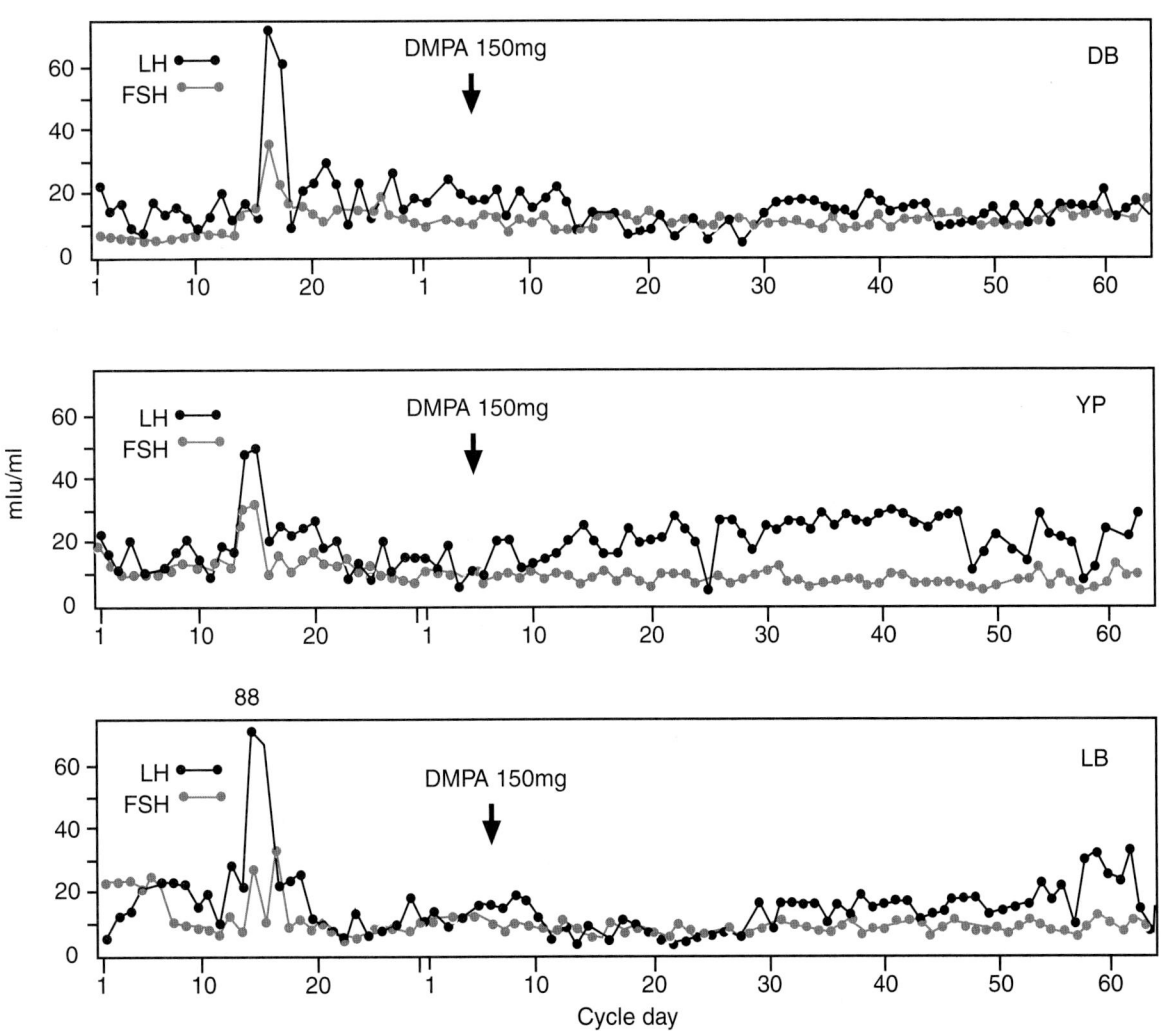

FIGURE 13-18 Daily serum LH and FSH levels in 3 women for 1 control cycle and 2 months after receiving an injection of 150 mg of DMPA. (From Mishell DR Jr, Kharma KM, and Thorneycroft IH: Am J Obstet Gynecol 113:372, 1972.)

phase of the control cycle (see Figure 13-19). Therefore there is incomplete suppression of follicular activity in the first two cycles after an injection of DMPA.

A cross-sectional study was performed by Mishell et al. on 121 women who received 150 mg of DMPA every 3 months for more than 1 year. An assay performed on a serum sample obtained on the day of the next scheduled injection showed marked differences in the estradiol levels, which varied from approximately 15 pg/ml to nearly 100 pg/ml (mean approximately 42 pg/ml) (Figure 13-20). A similar range and mean value were also found among women who had been receiving DMPA for 1 to 2 years and those who had used it for 4 to 5 years. All these women had moist, well-rugated vaginas, and none stated that her breast size had decreased. None of the women complained of hot flushes. This use of contraceptive doses of DMPA does not decrease endogenous estradiol levels to the postmenopausal range and does not cause symptoms of estrogen deficiency.

RETURN OF FERTILITY.   Because of the lag time in clearing DMPA from the circulation, resumption of ovulation is delayed for a variable period of time, which may last as long as 1 year after the last injection. Women who wish to become pregnant and stop using DMPA should be informed that there will be a delay in the resumption of fertility until the drug is cleared from the circulation. After this initial delay, fecundability resumes at a rate

similar to that found after discontinuing a barrier contraceptive (Figure 13-21). Thus use of DMPA does not prevent return of fertility; it only delays the time at which conception will occur. Because of its long and unpredictable duration of release from the injection site, the time until resumption of fertility may be delayed for 1 year or more after the last injection. Information about the possibility of a very long duration DMPA action needs to be given to women who are considering this method of contraception.

Because the half-life of the drug is constant, the return of fertility is not related to the number of injections that a woman receives. Schwallie and Assenzo reported that the median time to conception varied between 9 and 12 months after the last injection but did not differ according to the number of injections. With 10 or more injections, the median delay to the onset of fertility is similar to that in a woman who received only a few injections.

These investigators did find that the median time to conception after DMPA was discontinued varied according to body weight. As body weight increased, there was a similar concomitant increase in the median time to resumption of conception, most likely because the drug had been absorbed into adipose tissue and not cleared as rapidly.

ENDOMETRIAL CHANGES.   The histology of the endometrium at various intervals after starting DMPA was

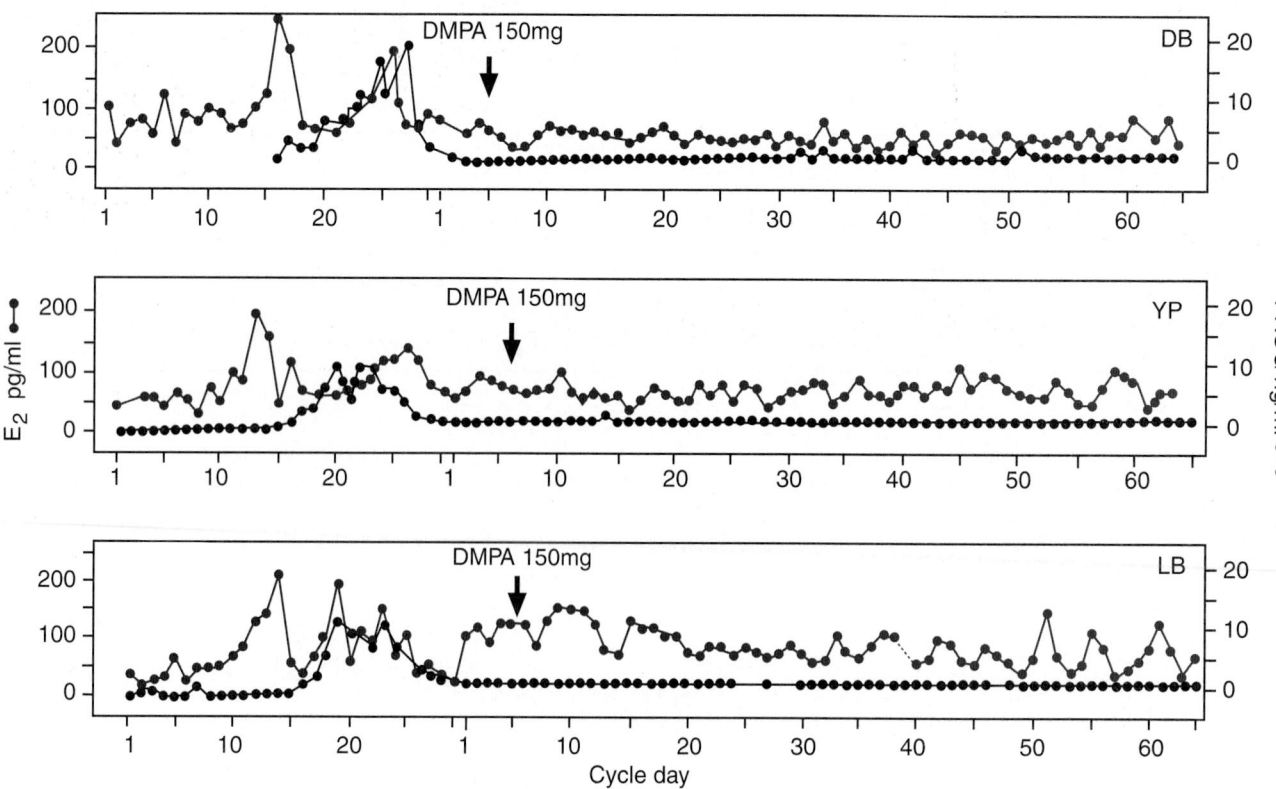

FIGURE 13-19   Daily serum estradiol and progesterone levels in 3 women for 1 control cycle and 2 months after receiving an injection of 150 mg of DMPA. (From Mishell DR Jr, Kharma KM, and Thorneycroft IH: Am J Obstet Gynecol 113:372, 1972.)

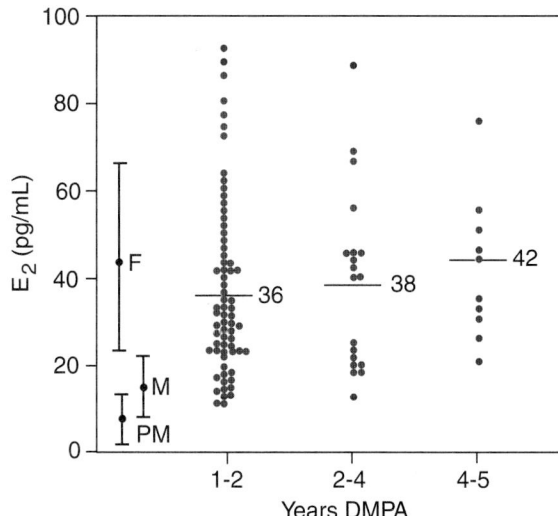

FIGURE 13-20 Serum estradiol (E₂) levels in 121 women who had used DMPA for contraception for more than 1 year. The horizontal bar in each time period represents the mean value. Vertical bars represent mean (●) ± SD of serum estradiol levels in cycling women in the early follicular phase (F), normal males (M), and postmenopausal women (PM). (From Mishell DR Jr, Kharma KM, and Thorneycroft IH: Am J Obstet Gynecol 113:372, 1972.)

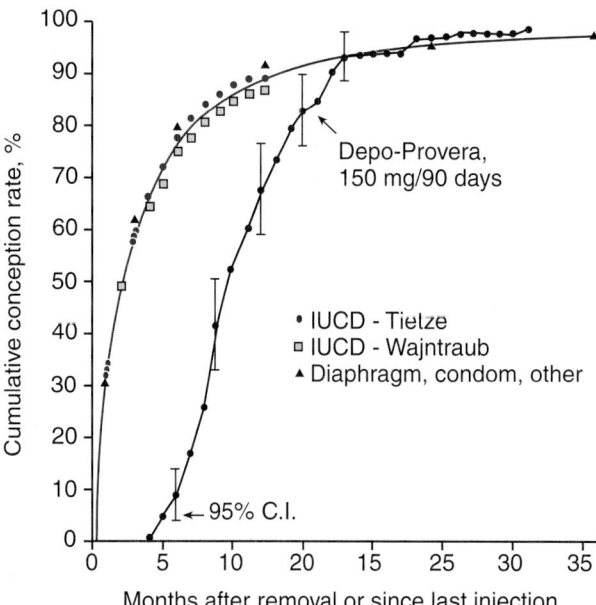

FIGURE 13-21 Cumulative conception rates of women who discontinued a contraceptive method to become pregnant. (From Schwallie PC and Assenzo JR: Contraception 10(2):181, 1974.)

examined by Mishell et al. Histologic examination of endometrial biopsies revealed three types of patterns: proliferative, quiescent, and atrophic. Secretory endometrium was not seen. Most of the women had a quiescent pattern, characterized by narrow, widely spaced glands and decidualization of the stroma.

Endometrial biopsies were performed at intervals of 1.5, 3, 6, 9, and 12 months after the first DMPA injection in a group of women receiving DMPA every 3 months. About half the biopsies showed that proliferative endometrium was present 6 weeks after the first injection. The percentage of women with proliferative endometrium then steadily declined, and after the second injection, less than 10% of the biopsies were proliferative. The majority of the biopsy specimens showed a quiescent type of endometrium, but after 1 year of DMPA, about 40% of the specimens were characterized as atrophic.

ADVERSE EFFECTS

Clinical. The major side effect of DMPA is complete disruption of the menstrual cycle. In the first 3 months after the first injection, about 30% of women are amenorrheic and another 30% have irregular bleeding and spotting occurring more than 11 days per month. The bleeding is usually light in amount and does not cause anemia to occur. As duration of therapy increases, the incidence of frequent bleeding steadily declines and the incidence of amenorrhea steadily increases, so that at the end of 2 years about 70% of the women treated with DMPA are amenorrheic (Figure 13-22). Women who use this method of contraception should be counseled that

with time the irregular bleeding episodes will cease and amenorrhea will most likely occur.

After treatment with DMPA is discontinued, about half of the women resume a regular cyclic menstrual pattern within 6 months and about three fourths have regular menses within 1 year. When bleeding does resume after the effect of the last injection is dissipated, it is initially regular in about half the women and irregular in the remainder. In a study involving 36 women who stopped using DMPA, Gardner and Mishell reported that in the first 3 months, 27 women were amenorrheic, and 9 had irregular menses, which was usually characterized as spotting. During the next 3 months, about half the women began regular menses. The incidence of regular menses steadily increased, and 2 years after the last injection all the women were having regular menses or were pregnant. In this group of women, amenorrhea did not persist for more than 6 months after the last injection.

Weight changes. In five cross-sectional studies, users of DMPA weighed more than a comparison group not using hormonal contraceptives. Several longitudinal studies have indicated that DMPA users gain between 1.5 to 4 kg in their first year of use and continue to gain weight thereafter. None of these studies included a control group so the weight could be due to factors other than DMPA use. In one retrospective, comparative, longitudinal study Moore et al. found no significant change in mean weight of DMPA, progestin implant, and oral contraceptive users. Thus the effect among DMPA on body weight remains unclear. If DMPA users gain weight they should

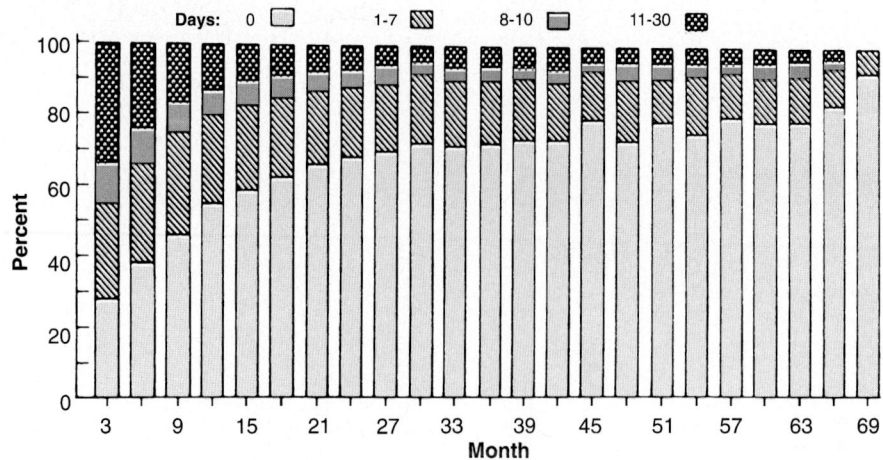

FIGURE 13-22 Percentage of patients with bleeding or spotting on spotting days 0, 1 to 7, 8 to 10, or 11 to 30 per 30-day cycle while receiving injectable DMPA, 150 mg, every 3 months. (From Schwallie PC and Assenzo JR: Fertil Steril 24:331, 1973.)

be counseled to decrease caloric intake and increase their expenditure of energy.

Mood changes. The product labeling lists depression and mood changes as side effects of DMPA. Several studies, however, indicate that the incidence of depression and mood change in women using this method of contraception is less than 5%. No clinical trials with a comparison group not using DMPA have been performed to determine whether a causal relation between use of DMPA and development of depression exists.

Headache. Although development of headaches is the most frequent medical event reported by DMPA users and a common reason for discontinuation of its use, there are no comparative studies to indicate that use of DMPA increases the incidence or severity of tension or migraine headaches. Therefore the presence of migraine headaches is not an absolute contraindication for use of DMPA. However, women should be counseled that if the frequency or severity of headaches increases after the injection is given it may be several months before the drug is cleared from the circulation. For this reason the presence of migraine headaches may be considered to be a relative contraindication for use of DMPA.

Metabolic effects.

Protein. Because DMPA does not increase liver globulin production as does the estrogen component of oral contraceptives (ethinyl estradiol), no alteration in blood-clotting factors or angiotensinogen levels is associated with its use. Thus, unlike OCs, DMPA has not been associated with an increased incidence of hypertension or thromboembolism. A WHO study reported that mean blood pressure measurements were unchanged in DMPA users after 2 years of injections.

Carbohydrate. There have been two studies in which oral glucose tolerance tests have been performed on long-term DMPA users and matched controls not using hormonal contraceptives. The mean glucose levels were slightly greater among the DMPA users than among the controls in one, but not the other, study. Mean insulin levels were also higher. The slight deterioration in glucose tolerance among DMPA users is probably not clinically significant and returns to normal after stopping use of DMPA.

Lipids. Westhoff reviewed the findings of 11 studies that evaluated plasma lipids among groups of women using DMPA. Most of the studies were cross-sectional and compared lipid levels among DMPA users with women not using hormonal methods of contraception. There was little or no change in mean triglyceride and total cholesterol levels, but in all seven studies in which mean HDL cholesterol levels were measured, the levels were lower among the DMPA users. Of the five studies in which LDL cholesterol was measured, three noted an increase among the DMPA users. There are no studies in which the incidence of cardiovascular events among current or former long-term DMPA users was compared with the incidence among controls. Therefore, although the lipid changes with DMPA use are not beneficial, there is no evidence to date that they are associated with an acceleration of atherosclerosis.

Bone loss. Several observational studies performed in several different countries with women of different ethnic groups indicate that the use of DMPA is associated with some degree of bone loss. The amount and location of the bone loss varied in the different studies, as well as the age groups most likely to experience this problem when using DMPA. Although there are scant data, the bone loss appears reversible after stopping use of DMPA. There are also no reports of an increased risk of fractures in DMPA users. It would appear useful to encourage calcium intake of 1500 mg/day in adolescent DMPA users and to consider performing a bone scan in women who have used DMPA for 5 or more years to determine whether they have a decreased amount of bone mineral density.

NEOPLASTIC EFFECTS. Approval of DMPA for contraceptive use in the United States was delayed for many years because of concern about a causal relation between use of this agent and an increased risk of cervical, breast, and endometrial cancer. These concerns were raised because of studies showing an increased risk of abnormal cervical cytology in women using DMPA and studies reporting an increased risk of breast cancer in beagle dogs treated with DMPA and endometrial cancer in monkeys receiving long-term DMPA. These neoplastic concerns were found to be unwarranted as a result of several large epidemiologic studies, the majority of which were undertaken by the World Health Organization. In the WHO studies the risk of neoplasia development among a large group of DMPA users in three countries—Kenya, Thailand and Mexico—was investigated.

Breast cancer. Two large case-control studies, the WHO study and a New Zealand study, indicated that the relative risk of developing breast cancer among all DMPA users was not significantly increased (RR of 1.2 [CI, 0.96 to 1.15] and 1.0 [CI, 0.8 to 1.3], respectively). When the data from these studies were pooled, the overall breast cancer risk among DMPA users was 1.1 (CI, 0.97 to 1.4). In long-term users, that is, in those who had used the drug more than 5 years and those who had started use more than 14 years earlier, the risk of developing breast cancer was also not increased (RR of 1.0 [CI, 0.70 to 1.5] and 0.89 [CI, 0.6 to 1.3], respectively). However, among those women who had started use within the past 5 years and were mainly under age 35 there was a significant increased risk of developing breast cancer (RR 2.0 [CI, 1.5 to 2.8]), similar to that found with use of oral contraceptives and women with first-term pregnancy at an early age. Thus DMPA, like other contraceptive steroids, does not appear to change the overall incidence of developing breast cancer and women should be counseled accordingly.

Endometrial cancer. A WHO case-control study found the risk of developing endometrial cancer to be significantly reduced among DMPA users (RR, 0.21 [CI, 0.06 to 0.79]). This reduction in risk persisted for at least 8 years after stopping use and was similar in magnitude to the protective effect observed with combination oral contraceptives.

Ovarian cancer. In a WHO case-control study the risk of developing ovarian cancer among DMPA users was unchanged (RR, 1.07 [CI, 0.6 to 1.8]). These findings do not demonstrate a protective effect similar to that observed with oral contraceptives despite inhibition of ovulation with both agents. The lack of a protective effect observed with DMPA was probably due to the fact that in the countries studied DMPA was given only to multiparous women, women at low risk of developing epithelial ovarian cancer, who differ from the higher-risk women taking oral contraceptives.

Noncontraceptive Health Benefits of Contraceptive Use of DMPA

Definite
Salpingitis
Endometrial cancer
Iron deficiency anemia
Sickle cell problems

Probable
Ovarian cysts
Dysmenorrhea
Endometriosis
Epileptic seizure
Vaginal candidiasis

Cervical cancer. In a large WHO case-control study the risk of developing invasive cancer of the cervix was not increased (RR, 1.1 [CI, 0.96 to 1.29]), similar to findings observed in a large case-control study in Costa Rica. Long-term use and long time since first use were also not associated with a significant increase in risk of cervical cancer in these studies. The risk of developing cancer in situ was slightly increased in the WHO study (RR, 1.4 [CI, 1.2 to 1.7]), but not in the Costa Rica study (RR, 1.0 [0.6 to 1.8]) or two New Zealand studies investigating the risk of cancer dysplasia. Thus the reports in which the neoplastic effects of DMPA on breast and reproductive tract neoplasia have been investigated are very reassuring.

NONCONTRACEPTIVE HEALTH BENEFITS. In a recent summarization by Cullins, there is good epidemiologic evidence that use of DMPA reduces the risk of developing iron deficiency anemia, pelvic inflammatory disease, and endometrial cancer. It has a beneficial effect on hematologic parameters in women with sickle cell disease and reduces their incidence of clinical problems (see box on this page). DMPA also reduces seizure frequency in women with epilepsy and probably should reduce the incidence of primary dysmenorrhea, ovulation pain, and functional ovarian cyst because it inhibits ovulation. DMPA also reduces the symptoms of endometriosis and in two small studies it reduced the incidence of vaginal candidiasis.

CLINICAL RECOMMENDATIONS. Women should be thoroughly counseled about the occurrence of abnormal bleeding and development of amenorrhea with use of DMPA prior to receiving the first injection. It has been shown that pretreatment counseling improves continuation rates. In addition, women should be counseled that the duration of action may last as long as 1 year following the last injection if they decide to discontinue use in order to become pregnant or because of side effects.

In cycling women the initial injection should be given no later than day 5 of the cycle to be certain to inhibit ovulation in the initial treatment cycle. Because of an absence of thrombogenic effects, the first injection should be given within 5 days postpartum in nonlactating women but for women who exclusively breast-feed their infants the product labeling states that the first injection should not be given until at least 6 weeks postpartum. DMPA does not affect the quantity or quality of breast milk or the health of children who breast-feed during its use. If a woman with lactational amenorrhea wishes to commence DMPA use and if a qualitative test for hCG is negative, it is unlikely she is pregnant and therefore can receive the injection at that time. If concern about pregnancy exists, use of a barrier contraceptive should be advised for 2 additional weeks, at which time the assay for hCG should be repeated. If it is still negative, the injection can be given. A similar protocol can be utilized for the woman who has previously received DMPA but is delayed beyond 13 weeks in returning for her next injection and is still amenorrheic. If accidental pregnancy does occur in a woman receiving DMPA, there is no evidence that the agent is teratogenic or adversely affects the outcome of the pregnancy.

Norethindrone Enanthate

Norethindrone enanthate (NET-EN) is another injectable progestagen that has been approved for contraceptive use in more than 40 countries but not in the United States. It is administered in an oily suspension and thus has pharmacodynamics different from those of DMPA. Because of a shorter duration of action, it is recommended that NET-EN be given every 60 days for at least the first 6 months and no less often than every 12 weeks thereafter. The WHO recommends that the drug be given at intervals no shorter than 46 days and no longer than 74 days.

Progestin-Estrogen (Once Monthly) Injectable Formulations

Because the major reason for discontinuance of all progestin injectable contraceptives is menstrual irregularity, several combined progestin-estrogen injectables designed for once-a-month administration and production of regular withdrawal bleeding have been developed. They consist of a low dose of a long-acting progestin plus a small amount of an estradiol ester. Although many different formulations have been developed, currently four of them are most widely used. An injectable formulation containing 17α-hydroxyprogesterone caproate 250 mg and estradiol valerate, 5 mg estimated to be used by at least 1% of all contraceptive users in China. A combination of dihydroxyprogesterone acetophenide, 150 mg plus estradiol oenanthate, 10 mg is widely used in Mexico and other Latin American countries and is marketed under different brand names. The WHO has developed two new formulations that are being used by several national family-planning programs. A combination of medroxyprogesterone acetate, 25 mg and estradiol cypi-

onate, 5 mg is marketed as Cyclofem and also called Cyclo-provera. This agent may soon be approved for marketing in the United States with the name Lunelle. The last compound is a combination of norethisterone enanthate, 50 mg and estradiol valerate, 5 mg called Mesigyna. Lunelle is formulated as a microcrystalline suspension given in 0.5 ml of an aqueous solution, while Mesigyna is formulated in 1 ml of an oily solution of castor oil and benzyl benzoate, 60:40. Both of these formulations are administered as deep intramuscular injections into the deltoid anterior thigh or gluteal muscle every 23 to 33 days (28 ± 5 days) with the first injection being given between 1 to 5 days after the onset of menses. The estradiol levels peak at 250 pg/ml 2 to 7 days after the injection and gradually decline thereafter reaching half the peak at 8 days at which time uterine bleeding usually occurs. Estradiol levels fall to baseline about 2 weeks after the injection. Medroxyprogesterone acetate levels peak about 3 days after injection at 1.25 ng/ml. Levels decline slowly with a half-life of 14.7 days. Nondetectable levels are reached between 63 to 84 days. Steady-state conditions are reached after the first injection. Ovulation is inhibited for 63 to 112 days after the injection after which there is a prompt return of fertility.

Newton et al. summarized the results of clinical trials with these compounds. The combined preparations offered better cycle control and less intermenstrual spotting than did the progestagen-only preparations of medroxyprogesterone acetate and norethisterone enanthate. Amenorrhea rates were also lower with the combination injections, and about 85% of all cycles were regular following the first early bleed about 15 days after the first injection.

The results of five clinical trials with Mesigyna and Lunelle demonstrated a high level of effectiveness, with 12-month pregnancy rates of 0.4% or less for Mesigyna and 0.2% or less for Lunelle. Rates of discontinuation for amenorrhea varied between 0.8% and 4.2% for Mesigyna and 2.1% and 5.2% for Lunelle. Those for bleeding-related reasons were 5.4% to 12.0% with Mesigyna and 6.3% to 12.7% with Lunelle. The main bleeding disturbances were heavy, prolonged, and irregular bleeding.

Results of a 1-year nonrandomized U.S. study of Lunelle and a combination OC were reported by Kaunitz et al. No pregnancies occurred in the 782 women accumulating 8008 women-cycle of use with Lunelle. After 3 months regular menses occur in women treated with both the injection and OC, but bleeding irregularities were more common with the injection. Also women receiving the injection had more days of bleeding and spotting than those receiving the OCs as well as greater variability of cycle length. The WHO Task Force that studied Lunelle found no significant changes in the hemostatic parameters, lipid levels, or carbohydrate metabolism with Lunelle and in clinical studies involving more than 12,000 women no venous or arterial cardiovascular events were recorded. Indications and contraindications for Lunelle are similar to oral contraceptives.

Subdermal Implants

Subdermal implants of capsules made of polydimethyl-siloxane (Silastic) containing levonorgestrel for use as contraceptives have been developed and patented by The Population Council as Norplant. Clinical trials of this long-acting, effective, reversible method of contraception were initiated in 1975. It was approved by the FDA in 1990, and marketing in this country began in 1991. As with all steroid-containing Silastic devices, the rate of steroid delivery is directly proportional to the surface area of the capsules, whereas duration of action depends on the amount of steroid within the capsules. To produce effective blood levels of norgestrel, it was found necessary to use six capsules filled with crystalline levonorgestrel. The cylindric capsules are 3.4 cm long and 2.4 mm in outer diameter, with the ends sealed with Silastic medical adhesive. Each capsule contains 36 mg of crystalline levonorgestrel for a total amount of 215 mg in each 6-capsule set.

Insertion is performed in an outpatient setting, and the entire procedure takes about 5 minutes. After infiltration of the skin with local anesthesia, a 3-mm incision is made with a scalpel, usually in the upper arm, although the lower arm, the inguinal, scapular, and gluteal regions have also been used. When the capsules are inserted in any area of subcutaneous tissue, the steroid diffuses into the circulation at a relatively constant rate. The capsules are implanted into the subcutaneous tissue in a radial pattern through a 10- to 12-gauge trocar, and the incision is closed with adhesive. Sutures are not necessary. Because polydimethysiloxane is not biodegradable, the capsules have to be removed through another incision when desired by the user or at the end of 5 years, which is the duration of maximal contraceptive effectiveness.

After insertion, blood levels of levonorgestrel rise rapidly to reach levels between 1000 and 2000 pg/ml in 24 hours. These levels fall markedly in the first week and then gradually in the first month and then remain relatively constant during the first year of use, with mean levels ranging between 250 to 600 pg/ml, which is usually sufficient to inhibit ovulation (Figure 13-23). At the end of 5 years, mean levonorgestrel levels range between 170 and 350 pg/ml. Blood levels vary considerably among women, mainly because of differences in body weight. Heavier women have lower circulating levonorgestrel levels than do thin women. When the amount of steroid was measured in capsules removed from women after various times, it was found that the rate of release was fairly constant during the first year of use, averaging about 50 μg of levonorgestrel per day from the 6-capsule set. From about the end of the first year of use until 8 years of use, daily release rates declined to about 30 μg per day but remained constant during each day.

With this low level of levonorgestrel, gonadotrophin levels are not completely suppressed, and ovarian follicular activity results in periodic peaks of estradiol. Since the level of circulating levonorgestrel is usually sufficient to inhibit the positive feedback effect of these estradiol peaks on LH release, LH levels are lower than normal, even in Norplant users with regular cycles, and ovulation during the first 2 years of use occurs infrequently.

It is difficult to determine the exact incidence of ovulatory cycles in Norplant users because different investigators have used different minimum levels of serum progesterone as a definition of presumptive ovulation and serum samples have been obtained at various time intervals in different studies. When serum progesterone levels above 3 ng/ml with twice-weekly blood sampling are used as a

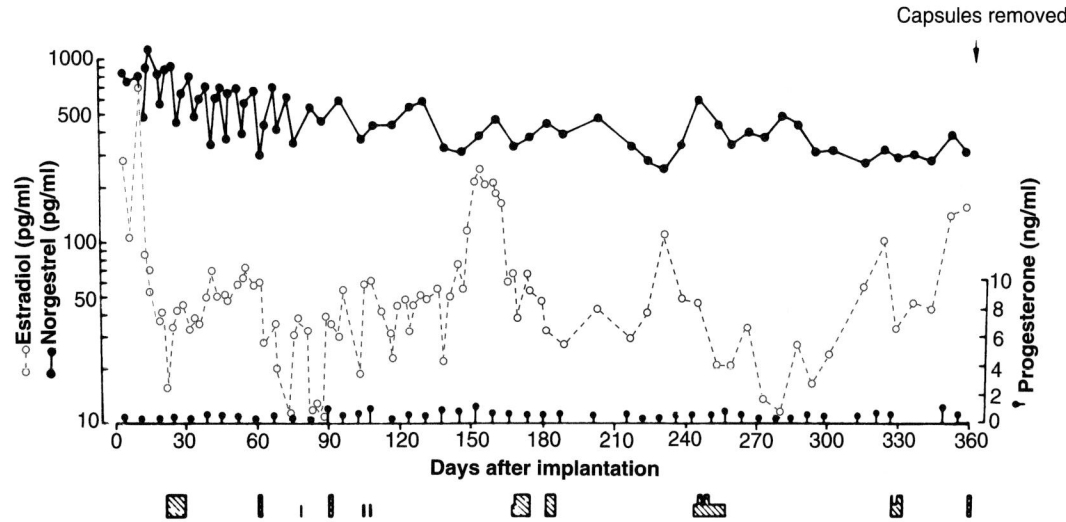

FIGURE 13-23 Serum levels of estradiol, progesterone, and *d*-norgestrel in a subject with six polysiloxanne capsules, each containing 33.9 mg of *d*-norgestrel, implanted on day 0. Hatched bars represent uterine bleeding. (From Moore DE, Roy S, Stanczyk FZ, et al: Contraception 17:315, 1978.)

definition of presumptive ovulation, Brache et al. reported that about one third of the cycles of Norplant users are ovulatory, with the incidence of luteal activity increasing beyond the second year of use. However, this incidence of ovulation is an overestimate, as the mean peak progesterone level, duration of elevated progesterone levels, and thus total luteal amount of progesterone is significantly less in Norplant users than in control cycles, indicating a high incidence of luteal deficiency and/or anovulatory, luteinized follicles. Daily ultrasonographic scanning of ovaries of Norplant users with regular cycles and elevated luteal-phase progesterone levels revealed that only about one third of these cycles had ovarian morphologic changes consistent with a normal ovulatory pattern. Since only about half the cycles of Norplant users have a fairly regular pattern, probably less than 20% of the cycles are ovulatory and a high percentage of these have deficient progesterone production.

Thus inhibition of ovulation is one of the major mechanisms of action of this method of contraception. The consistently elevated circulating levels of norgestrel also prevent the normal midcycle thinning of the cervical mucus from occurring. The cervical mucus remains scanty and viscid, and normal sperm penetration does not take place, as demonstrated by both in vivo and in vitro studies. These two mechanisms of action result in a very high level of contraceptive effectiveness for 5 years duration of use. In the initial studies, the Norplant capsules were made of a denser type of tubing than is now being used, and serum levels of norgestrel were slightly lower than occurred with the currently used less dense tubing.

Thus, with the less dense tubing, annual pregnancy rates for the first 5 years of use are about 0.2 per 100 women of all body weights, yielding a cumulative 5-year pregnancy rate of 1.1%. A recent analysis by Sivin of 7-year experience with the less dense tubing found the cumulative pregnancy rate to be 1.1 per 100 women at 5 years and 1.9 at 7 years (Table 13-10). However all the pregnancies that occurred between 5 and 7 years were in women weighing more than 70 kg at the time of insertion. Thus for women weighing less than 70 kg, the implants remain effective for 7 years of use, 2 more years than stated in the product labeling. Thus the Norplant implants are one of the most effective methods of reversible contraception available. As with all progestin-only methods of contraception, when pregnancies occur with Norplant, a high percentage, about 20%, are ectopic. However, because of its high rate of effectiveness, the overall rate of ectopic pregnancies in Norplant users, 0.28 per 1000 woman-years of use, is reduced compared with ectopic pregnancy rates in the entire U.S. population of women of reproductive age, 1.5 per 1000 women annually.

TABLE 13-10
Annual and Cumulative Life Table Pregnancy Rates by Weight Group

Year	Weight Group (kg)				
	<50	50-59	60-69	70-79	≥80
Annual rates per 100 and standard errors					
1	0	0	0	0	0
2	0	0	0	0	0
3	0	0.3 ± 0.3	0	0	2.2 ± 2.2
4	0	0	0	0	0
5	0	0	0.6 ± 0.6	2.9 ± 2.0	6.1 ± 4.3
6	0	0.7 ± 0.6	0	2.0 ± 2.0	0
7	0	0	0	0	5.6 ± 5.4
Cumulative rates per 100 and standard errors					
1	0	0	0	0	0
2	0	0	0	0	0
3	0	0.3 ± 0.3	0	0	2.2 ± 2.2
4	0	0.3 ± 0.3	0	0	2.2 ± 2.2
5	0	0.3 ± 0.3	0.6 ± 0.6	2.9 ± 2.0	8.1 ± 4.5
6	0	1.0 ± 0.7	0.6 ± 0.6	4.8 ± 2.8	8.1 ± 4.5
7	0	1.0 ± 0.7	0.6 ± 0.6	4.8 ± 2.8	13.2 ± 6.6
Number					
At admission	179	492	344	129	66
Completed 5 years	78	198	150	55	28
Entered month 84	53	119	86	37	14
Completed 7 years	46	103	77	34	14
Pregnancies	0	2	1	3	4

From: Sivin I, Mishell DR, Jr, Diaz S, Biswas A, et al: Prolonged effectiveness of Norplant capsule implants: a 7-year study, Contraception 61:187, 2000.

Mean estradiol levels in Norplant users, whether they are ovulatory or anovulatory, are about the same as in women with regular ovulatory cycles who used IUDs, and three patterns of estradiol activity have been observed. About half of Norplant users have periodic, irregular peaks of estradiol within the normal range (up to 400 pg/ml), 30% have fluctuating estradiol levels with high broad peaks above 400 pg/ml, and about 10% have consistently low estradiol levels below 75 pg/ml. After a fall in estradiol, endometrial sloughing and uterine bleeding or spotting usually occur. Because the peaks and declines in estradiol levels occur at irregular intervals, uterine bleeding also occurs at irregular intervals in the majority of Norplant users.

The major side effect of Norplant use is the irregular pattern of uterine bleeding. Other alterations in uterine blood flow involve changes in duration and volume, with most bleeding episodes being scanty in amount. About half the bleeding episodes can be characterized as fairly regular, with the interval between bleeding episodes ranging between 21 and 35 days; about 40% as irregular, with intervals outside this range; and about 10% as amenorrheic, with no bleeding for more than a 13-month interval. Because of the high incidence of bleeding irregularities, potential Norplant users must be thoroughly counseled about this problem prior to insertion. Bleeding episodes tend to be more prolonged and irregular during the first year of use, after which there is greater frequency of a more regular pattern. Shoupe et al. reported that during the first year of use about 25% of the cycles were regular, 66% were irregular, and 7% were amenorrheic (Figure 13-24). By the fifth year about two thirds of the cycles were regular, one third were irregular, and none were amenorrheic. The mean number of days of bleeding also declined steadily with time from 54.3 days in the first year to 44.1 days in the fifth year. Mean total blood loss in Norplant users is about 25 ml per month, slightly less than the average monthly blood loss of normally cycling women. Several clinical studies have shown that the mean hemoglobin concentration in the first 3 years of Norplant use tends to rise slightly. Even women who stop using the method because of bleeding problems have been found to have an increase in mean hemoglobin levels. When pregnancies occur in Norplant users, they almost always occur in women with a recent history of regular cyclic uterine bleeding. Thus women who are amenorrheic or have infrequent episodes of uterine bleeding do not need to be monitored by periodic assays for hCG.

Other problems associated with this method of contraception include infection, local irritation, or painful reaction at the insertion site. Occasionally, expulsion of a capsule occurs, usually in association with infection. The incidence of insertion-site infection is less than 1%. Headache is the single most frequent medical problem causing removal of the implants, accounting for about 30% of the medical reasons for removal. Weight gain was a common reason for

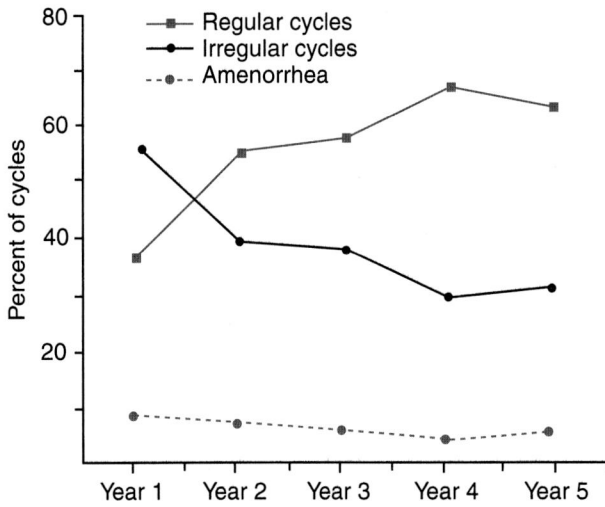

FIGURE 13-24 Bleeding patterns calculated on a monthly basis in implant users during 5 years of use. (From Shoupe D, Mishell DR Jr, Bopp BL, and Fielding M: Obstet Gynecol 77:256, 1991.)

medical removal in U.S. studies, whereas weight loss was more common in the Dominican Republic. Other medical problems among Norplant users include acne, mastalgia, and mood changes, including anxiety, depression, and nervousness. Because ovarian follicular development without subsequent ovulation is common among Norplant users, adnexal enlargement caused by persistent unruptured follicles has been noted during routine bimanual pelvic examination in many Norplant users. These enlarged follicles, which may reach 5 to 7 cm in diameter, usually spontaneously regress in 1 to 2 months without therapy.

A great number of metabolic studies have been performed among Norplant users in various population groups. Studies of carbohydrate metabolism, serum chemistries, liver function, serum cortisol levels, thyroid function, and blood coagulation have revealed only minimal changes, which remain within the normal range. Several studies have been performed in different countries in which lipoproteins were measured before and after Norplant insertion. In most of these studies, levels of triglycerides, total cholesterol, and LDL cholesterol declined, whereas HDL cholesterol declined slightly or increased. There was little change in the cholesterol/high density lipoprotein cholesterol ratio, indicating that Norplant should not enhance the development of atherosclerosis.

The removal process is, like the insertion procedure, performed in the clinic area, using local anesthesia and a small skin incision. Removal of Norplant is a more difficult process than insertion, because fibrous tissue develops around the capsule and must be cut prior to removing the capsules. It is important to insert the capsules superficially to enhance the ease of removal; deeply implanted capsules are more difficult to remove.

After removal the incision is closed without sutures, and a pressure dressing is applied for about 24 hours. If the woman wishes to continue use, another set can be inserted through the same incision or in the opposite arm. If another set of Norplant is not inserted after removal, the steroid is rapidly cleared from the circulation and serum levels of norgestrel fall rapidly, reaching nearly undetectable levels in 96 hours. If pregnancy is desired, return to ovulation is prompt and is similar to that in women discontinuing other nonhormonal methods of reversible contraception, reaching 50% at 3 months and 86% at 1 year.

Continuation rates with the Norplant method of contraception are very high, ranging from 76% to 99% at 1 year in different countries and from 33% to 78% at 5 years. These high continuation rates are similar to those observed with IUDs and are due in large part to the fact that to discontinue use of these methods the user is required to return to the clinic. This requirement is the main reason why Norplant implants and the IUD have the highest continuation rates of any methods of contraception in use today.

Manufacture of the capsules is complicated, and placing or removing six capsules creates some difficulties; therefore, norgestrel has been fabricated into solid rods that are a homologous mixture of Silastic and crystalline levonorgestrel covered with Silastic tubing. The rods are easier to manufacture, insert, and remove than the capsules. Because of different properties of diffusion, higher blood levels of norgestrel are achieved with a smaller total surface area of the rods. Thus, with two 4-cm covered rods with the same diameter as the capsules, the same release rate for norgestrel, about 50 µg per day, can be achieved as with placement of six 3-cm capsules. During a 5-year clinical study comparing rods and capsules, the serum norgestrel levels, bleeding patterns, and incidence of elevated progesterone levels were similar. A multicenter clinical study has confirmed these findings, and use of the two covered rods has been approved by the U.S. FDA for clinical use for 3 years. Nevertheless the manufacturer has to date not decided to market the 2-rod system, which is named Jadelle. Single implants with other progestins have been manufactured and studied in clinical trials. These implants have a probable duration of action of 3 years, are extremely effective, and are much easier to insert and remove than the multiple levonorgestrel-releasing implants. A single ethylene vinyl acetate 4-cm implant containing etonogestrel (3-keto desogestrel) is only 2 mm in diameter and can be inserted through a needle without making a skin incision. Clinic trials with this implant reported no pregnancies and an acceptable bleeding pattern.

EMERGENCY CONTRACEPTION

Morris and Van Wagenen suggested in 1966 that high doses of estrogen administered in the early postovulatory period will accelerate tubal transport of the morula so it arrives in the endometrial cavity prior to the time when adequate glycogen is present for continued growth. Various estrogenic compounds have been used for emergency contraception or what is commonly referred to as the "morning-after pill." The estrogen compounds that have been used for this purpose include diethylstilbestrol (DES), 25 to 50 mg per day; ethinyl estradiol, 5 mg per day; and conjugated estrogen, 30 mg per day. Treatment is continued for 5 days. If it is begun within 72 hours after an isolated midcycle act of coitus, its effectiveness is very good. If more than one episode of coitus has occurred, or if treatment is initiated later than 72 hours after coitus, the method is less effective.

Pregnancy rates among the women treated with ethinyl estradiol were 0.6%; with DES 0.7%; and with conjugated estrogen 1.6%. None of the trials included a control group, but it has been estimated that the clinical pregnancy rate after a single act of midcycle coitus without use of a contraceptive is about 7%. Thus high-dose estrogen is an effective method of emergency contraception.

Side effects associated with this high-dose estrogen therapy are common and severe. They include nausea, vomiting, breast soreness, and menstrual irregularities, which tend to reduce compliance.

Because the side effects of high-dose estrogens cause many women to fail to complete the 5-day treatment course, a regimen of four tablets of ethinyl estradiol, 0.05 mg, and *dl*-norgestrel, 0.5 mg, combination oral contraceptive (Ovral), given in doses of two tablets 12 hours apart, was initially tested in Canada by Yuzpe. This regimen was found to have a similar degree of effectiveness with a shorter duration of adverse symptoms than with 5 days of estrogen.

Trussell et al. pooled the data from studies that were published between 1977 and 1993 involving 5226 women treated with this regimen. They calculated that the failure rate was 1.5% and that use of this regimen prevented about 75% of the expected pregnancies. The United States Food and Drug Administration has approved a product containing 4 tablets of these contraceptive steroids (Preven) for emergency contraception. Nevertheless combinations of other products that provide an equivalent dose of ethinyl estradiol and norgestrel can also be used. In one large Canadian study 30% of the subjects treated with this regimen reported having nausea without vomiting and another 20% had nausea with vomiting. These investigators included an antiemetic, a 50-mg tablet of dimenhydrinate, in the package and instructed the women to take it together with the second dose of contraceptive steroid if they experienced nausea after the first dose. They also reported that the time to onset of the subsequent menses was slightly shortened in the users of this regimen.

Thus the effectiveness of this method appears to be slightly less than that of higher dosages of estrogen alone. However, there is also a lower incidence of abnormal bleeding and delayed menses, as well as gastrointestinal side effects, with this regimen than with the high-dose estrogen. In addition, because of the 1-day treatment regimen, patient compliance is greater with this technique. Thus this method is more widely used than the high-dose estrogens. Nevertheless, as reported by Grossman et al., this method is very underutilized in the United States as there is a lack of public awareness of emergency contraception.

Ho and Kwan reported results of a randomized trial comparing the use of 4 tablets of ethinyl estradiol and levonorgestrel taken in divided doses 12 hours apart with a single tablet of 0.75 mg levonorgestrel taken initially and another one 12 hours later. Both regimens were ingested within 48 hours of unprotected intercourse. Failure rates of both regimens, about 2%, were similar, but there was significantly less nausea and vomiting with the progestin alone than with the one combined with estrogen. Subsequently the WHO performed a randomized trial of the 2 regimens in about 2000 women in 21 centers. Levonorgestrel alone was more effective and had fewer side effects than the estrogen-levonorgestrel combined oral contraceptive, which had a 3.2% pregnancy rate when given within 72 hours after a single act of unprotected sexual intercourse. The authors calculated that levonorgestrel prevented 85% of pregnancies compared with 57% for the combined OC. There was also less nausea and vomiting with the levonorgestrel compound. Furthermore, in contrast to an earlier summary of results of studies of emergency contraception, effectiveness was greater when the agents were given within 24 hours of sexual intercourse than when they were given in the subsequent 48 hours. A strip of 4 tablets of 0.75 mg levonorgestrel is marketed in several countries including the United States under a variety of brand names. In the United States it is called Plan B.

Another method of emergency contraception, the administration of danazol, 400 to 600 mg in 2 doses separated by 12 hours, has been tried by 2 groups of investigators. A total of 998 women were treated in these trials, and the pregnancy rate of 2.0% was similar to that of the 2 doses of combined oral contraceptives. However, the incidence of side effects, particularly nausea, was less with danazol, and thus acceptability was high. If the woman has a continuing need for contraception after the cycle in which either of these techniques is used, one of the conventional methods should be prescribed.

Several authors have advocated that intrauterine insertion of a copper IUD within 5 to 10 days of midcycle coitus is an effective method to prevent continuation of the pregnancy. Fasoli et al. summarized the results of 4 published studies in 9 countries involving 875 women. Cost and concern about introducing pathogens into the upper genital tract with IUD insertion limit its widespread use.

Glasier et al. have shown that mifepristone is extremely effective when used as a postcoital contraceptive and is given as a single 600-mg dosage. Side effects were fewer and efficacy was similar to that with the use of 2 tablets of oral contraceptives taken 12 hours apart.

INTRAUTERINE DEVICES

The main benefits of IUDs are: (1) a high level of effectiveness, (2) a lack of associated systemic metabolic effects, and (3) the need for only a single act of motivation for long-term use. Despite these advantages less than 1% of married women of reproductive age use the IUD for contraception in the United States, compared with 15% to 30% in most European countries and Canada. In contrast to other types of contraception, there is no need for frequent motivation to ingest a pill daily or to use a coitus-related method consistently. These characteristics, as well as the necessity for a visit to a health care facility to discontinue the method, account for the fact that IUDs have the highest continuation rate of all currently available reversible methods of contraception.

Unlike other contraceptives, such as the barrier methods, which rely on frequent use by the individual to be effective and therefore have higher typical-failure rates than perfect-failure rates, the IUD has similar rates of failure for typical or perfect use. First-rate failure rates with the copper T 380A IUD are less than 1% and with the progesterone-releasing IUD are 2%. Pregnancy rates are related to the skill of the clinician inserting the device. With experience, correct high-fundal insertion occurs more frequently, and there is a lower incidence of partial or complete expulsion, with resultant lower pregnancy rates. Furthermore, the annual incidence of accidental pregnancy decreases steadily after the first year of IUD use. The cumulative pregnancy rate after 12 years use of the copper T 380A IUD is only 1.7%. The incidence of all major adverse events with IUDs, including pregnancy, expulsion, or removal for bleeding and/or pain, steadily decrease with increasing age. Thus the IUD is especially suited for older parous women who wish to prevent further pregnancies (Table 13-11).

TABLE 13-11
Cumulative Discontinuation Rate for Copper T 380A IUD

Event	Years Since Insertion		
	3	**5**	**7**
Pregnancies	1.0	1.4	1.6
Expulsions	7.0	8.2	8.6
Medical removals	14.6	20.8	25.8
Nonmedical removals	13.8	25.6	34.4
Loss to follow-up	10.2	15.5	22.1
All discontinuations	32.2	46.7	56.3
Woman-months	38,571	56,010	67,885

Modified from World Health Organization (WHO): Contraception 42:141, 1990.

Types of IUDs

In the past 35 years, many types of IUDs have been designed and used clinically. The devices developed and initially used in the 1960s were made of a plastic, polyethylene, impregnated with barium sulfate to make them radiographic. In the 1970s, in order to diminish the frequency of the side effects of increased uterine bleeding and pain, smaller plastic devices covered with copper were developed and widely utilized. In the 1980s devices bearing a larger amount of copper, including sleeves on the horizontal arm, such as the copper T 380A and the copper T 220C, were developed, as well as the Multiload CU 250 and CU 375. These devices have a longer duration of high effectiveness and thus need to be reinserted at less frequent intervals than do the devices bearing a smaller amount of copper. The copper T 380A IUD is the only copper-bearing IUD currently marketed in the United States, but the Multiload CU 375 is widely used in Europe (Figure 13-25).

Because of the constant dissolution of copper, which amounts daily to less than that ingested in the normal diet, all copper IUDs have to be replaced periodically. The copper T 380A is currently approved for use in the United States for 10 years and maintains its effectiveness for at least 12 years. At the scheduled time, the device can be removed and another inserted during the same office visit.

Adding a reservoir of progesterone to the vertical arm also increases the effectiveness of the T-shaped devices. The currently marketed progesterone-releasing IUD allows 65 mg of progesterone to diffuse into the endometrial cavity each day. This amount is sufficient to prevent pregnancy by local action within the endometrial cavity but is not enough to cause a measurable increase in peripheral serum progesterone levels. Because of the progestational effect on the endometrium, the amount of uterine bleeding is reduced with use of this device and it has been used therapeutically to treat menorrhagia. The currently approved progesterone-releasing IUD needs to be replaced annually, because the reservoir of progesterone becomes depleted after about 18 months of use and the surface area of plastic in this small device is insufficient to produce a sufficiently large leukocytic response to yield a high level of contraceptive effectiveness without progesterone.

A T-shaped device containing a reservoir of levonorgestrel on the vertical arm has been developed and undergone extensive clinical testing. A large comparative trial of the copper T 380A and the levonorgestrel-releasing IUD found that the effectiveness and continuation rates of both devices were similar. A T-shaped device containing a reservoir of levonorgestrel on the vertical arm has been marketed in Europe for many years and will soon be available for use in the United States. About 20 µg levonorgestrel is released each 24 hours. This device is extremely effective with a 5-year pregnancy rate of 0.7 per 100 women. Because levonorgestrel is released more slowly than progesterone, the levonorgestrel-releasing IUD has a high level of effectiveness for at least 5 years. This IUD also reduces menstrual blood loss and has been used therapeutically to treat abnormal uterine bleeding.

Mechanisms of Action

The main mechanism of contraceptive action of copper-bearing IUDs in the human is as a spermicide. This effect is caused by a local, sterile, inflammatory reaction produced by the presence of the foreign body in the uterine cavity. There is an approximate 1000% increase in the number of leukocytes in washings of the human endometrial cavity 18 weeks after the insertion of an IUD compared with washings obtained before insertion. In addition to causing phagocytosis of spermatozoa, tissue breakdown products of these leukocytes are toxic to all cells, including spermatozoa and the blastocyst. The amount of inflammatory reaction, and thus contraceptive effectiveness, is directly related to the size of the intrauterine foreign body. Copper markedly increases the extent of the inflammatory reaction, so this metal has been added to the small-sized frame of T-shaped devices. In addition, copper impedes sperm transport and viability in the cervical mucus. Since the copper T 380 has about twice as much copper surface area as the formerly marketed copper 7 IUD, the former IUD has a lower failure rate than the latter. Sperm transport from the cervix to the oviduct in the first 24 hours after coitus is markedly impaired in women wearing IUDs. Because of the spermicidal action of IUDs, very few, if any, sperm reach the oviducts, and the ovum usually does not become fertilized.

Further evidence for this spermicidal action of IUDs was reported by a group of investigators who performed oviductal flushing in 56 women wearing IUDs and 45 using no method of contraception who were sterilized by salpingectomy soon after ovulation. These women had unprotected sexual intercourse shortly before ovulation.

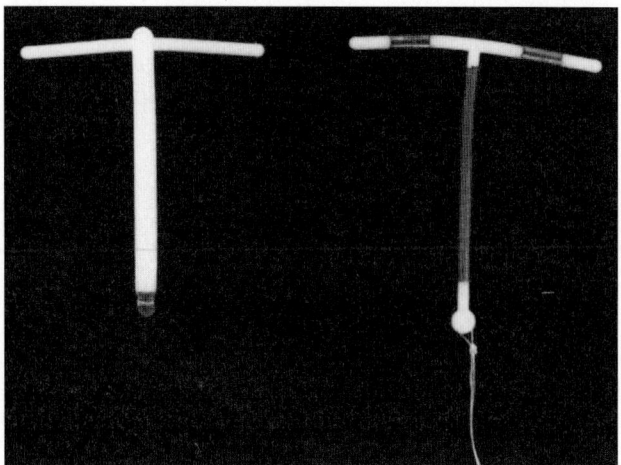

FIGURE 13-25 Intrauterine devices currently being marketed in the United States. *Left,* Progesterone-releasing IUD; *right,* copper T 380A.

Normally cleaving, fertilized ova were found in the tubal flushings of about half of the women not wearing IUDs, whereas no eggs that had the microscopic appearance of a normally developing embryo were found in the oviducts of the women wearing IUDs.

A long-term study of women wearing the copper T 380A IUD revealed that while the intrauterine pregnancy rate gradually increased with duration of IUD use, the ectopic pregnancy rate remained low and constant after the first year of use. If fertilization occurred frequently with IUD use and its main mechanism of action was to prevent uterine implantation of the blastocyst, the ectopic pregnancy rate would be expected to increase at a rate more rapidly than the intrauterine pregnancy rate, and this outcome did not occur. Thus the principal mechanism of action of the copper T 380A IUD is as a spermicide, preventing fertilization of the ovum. The progesterone-releasing IUD has a much higher ectopic pregnancy rate than does the copper IUD and probably acts mainly by slowing tubal transport of the embryo, as well as by preventing implantation of the blastocyst because of the presence of a high level of progesterone in the uterine cavity. The levonorgestrel-releasing IUD, like the copper device, has a very low ectopic pregnancy rate. Therefore fertilization does not occur and its main mechanism of action is also spermicidal.

Upon removal of the IUD, the inflammatory reaction rapidly disappears. Resumption of fertility following IUD removal is prompt and occurs at the same rate as resumption of fertility following discontinuation of the barrier methods of contraception. The incidence of term deliveries, spontaneous abortion, and ectopic pregnancies in conceptions occurring after IUD removal is the same as in the general noncontracepting population.

Time of Insertion

Although it is widely believed that the optimal time for insertion of an IUD is during the menses, there are data indicating that the IUD can be safely inserted on any day of the cycle provided the woman is not pregnant. An analysis was made of 2-month event rates of about 10,000 women who had copper T 200s inserted on various days of the cycle. Differences in event rates with insertion occurring on different days of the cycle were small and of little clinical relevance. Therefore the IUD can be inserted on any day of the cycle. Since bacteria are introduced into the endometrial cavity at the time of IUD insertion, it may be preferable to insert the IUD after the menses cease to avoid providing a good environment for bacterial growth.

It has also been recommended that IUDs not be inserted until more than 2 to 3 months have elapsed after completing a term pregnancy. However, in 1982 we analyzed event rates in our clinic among women who had copper T IUDs inserted between 4 and 98 weeks postpartum and more than 8 weeks postpartum. The 1- and 2-year event rates for all causes were similar for the two groups, indicating that copper T IUDs can be safely inserted at the time of the routine postpartum visit. No uterine perforations occurred in this series, in which the withdrawal technique of insertion was used. Although one report suggested that the uterine perforation rate was increased if the IUD is inserted when a woman is lactating, this finding has not been confirmed in several other studies.

The effect of breast-feeding on performance of the copper T 380A IUDs was evaluated from data obtained from a large, multicenter, clinical trial in which the device was inserted into 559 breast-feeding women and 590 non-breast-feeding women, all of whom were at least 6 weeks postpartum. There were significantly fewer problems with pain and bleeding at the time of insertion in the group that was breast-feeding. The expulsion rate, which was low, and the continuation rate, which was high, were similar in the breast-feeding and nonbreast-feeding groups 6 months after insertion. Therefore insertion of the IUD can be performed in postpartum women who are breast-feeding their infants, as well as in those who are not nursing at the time of the routine postpartum visit.

Adverse Effects

Incidence

In general, in the first year of use, copper IUDs have less than a 1% pregnancy rate, a 10% expulsion rate, and a 15% rate of removal for medical reasons, mainly bleeding and pain. The incidence of each of these events, especially expulsion, diminishes steadily in subsequent years.

In an ongoing World Health Organization study of the copper T 380A, termination rates for adverse effects continued to decline annually following the first year after insertion for each of the 12 years in which sufficient data had been accumulated. In this study, the cumulative percentage discontinuation rate for pregnancy, bleeding and pain, and expulsion at the end of 7 years was 1.6, 22.7, and 8.6, respectively and at the end of 12 years they were 1.7, 35.2, and 12.5 (Table 13-12).

Uterine Bleeding

The majority of women discontinuing this method of contraception do so for medical reasons. Nearly all the medical reasons accounting for removal of copper-bearing or inert IUDs involve one or more types of abnormal bleeding: heavy and/or prolonged menses or intermenstrual bleeding. The heavy bleeding may be produced by a premature and increased rate of local release of prostaglandins brought about by the presence of the intrauterine foreign body. The stimulation of uterine contractions by excessive levels of prostaglandins may prolong the duration of the menstrual flow, which is significantly longer in women wearing IUDs than in normally cycling women.

TABLE 13-12

Selected Cumulative Net Probabilities of Discontinuation (Standard Errors) per 100 Women Using Copper T 380A at 8, 10, and 12 Years of Use– WHO Study Excluding Chinese Centers

	8 years	10 years	12 years
Total pregnancies	1.7 (0.6)	1.7 (0.6)	1.7 (0.6)
Total medical removals	30.9 (1.8)	37.5 (2.2)	40.1 (2.4)
Total nonmedical removals	49.1 (2.0)	57.2 (2.1)	64.9 (2.2)
Continuation rate	19.3 (1.1)	12.6 (1.0)	7.9 (0.8)
Number of insertions	1195		
Number of women completing the interval	230	151	94
Woman-years experience	4947	5313	5537

Adapted from United Nations Development Programme/United Nations Population Fund/World Health Organization/World Bank, Special Programme of Research, Development and Research Training in Human Reproduction: Long-Term Reversible Contraception: Twelve years of experience with the TCU 380A, Contraception 56:341, 1997.

The amount of blood lost in each menstrual cycle is significantly greater in women using inert, as well as copper-bearing IUDs than in nonusers. The copper T 380A IUD is associated with about a 55% increase in menstrual blood loss (MBL). In contrast, with the progesterone-releasing IUD, the amount of blood loss is significantly reduced to about 25 ml/cycle. There is also reduced blood loss with the levonorgestrel-releasing IUD.

In a study of Swedish women in whom the copper T 380 was inserted, there was no significant change in mean measurements of several hematologic parameters, including hemoglobin, hematocrit, and erythrocyte count at 3, 6, and 12 months after IUD insertion compared with mean values before insertion.

A sensitive indicator of tissue iron stores is the serum ferritin level. In a study of women wearing the copper T 380A IUD there was no significant change in mean serum ferritin levels at 3, 6, and 12 months after IUD insertion. None of the women with low ferritin levels had a decrease in hemoglobin levels. They probably had an increase in intestinal iron absorption to compensate for the increased MBL as none of these women developed anemia. There is a significant reduction of MBL, about 60%, during the use of the levonorgestrel IUD. This reduction is seen as early as 3 months after insertion and persists for the duration of use of the device. The reduction of MBL results in an improvement of blood hemoglobin levels. Thus the levonorgestrel-releasing IUD is useful in the prevention and the treatment of iron deficiency anemia and the depletion of iron stores by heavy menstrual blood loss.

Excessive bleeding in the first few months following IUD insertion should be treated with reassurance and supplemental oral iron, as well as systemic administration of one of the prostaglandin synthetase inhibitors during menses. The bleeding usually diminishes with time, as the uterus adjusts to the presence of the foreign body.

Mefenamic acid ingested in a dosage of 500 mg three times a day during the days of menstruation has been shown to reduce MBL significantly in IUD users. If excessive bleeding continues despite this treatment, the device should be removed. After a 1-month interval, another type of device may be inserted if the woman still wishes to use an IUD for contraception. Consideration should be given to using a progestin-releasing IUD, because this device is associated with less blood loss than the copper-bearing IUDs.

Perforation

Although uncommon, one of the potentially serious complications associated with use of the IUD is perforation of the uterine fundus. Perforation always occurs at the time of insertion. Sometimes only the distal portion of the IUD penetrates the uterine muscle at insertion. Then uterine contractions over the next few months force the IUD into the peritoneal cavity. IUDs correctly inserted entirely within the endometrial cavity do not wander through the uterine muscle into the peritoneal cavity. The incidence of perforation is generally related to the shape of the device and/or amount of force used during its insertion, as well as the experience of the clinician performing the insertion. Perforation of the uterus is best prevented by straightening the uterine axis with a tenaculum and then probing the cavity with a uterine sound before IUD insertion.

Perforation rates for the copper T 380A are only about 1 in 3000 insertions. Since the perforations occurring at the time of insertion are nearly always asymptomatic, the clinician should always suspect that perforation has occurred if the user cannot feel the appendage but did not observe that the device was expelled. One should not assume that an unnoticed expulsion has occurred when the appendage is not visualized. Sometimes the IUD is still in its correct position in the uterine cavity, but the appendage has been withdrawn into the cavity as the position of the IUD has changed. In this situation, after pelvic examination has been performed and the possibility of pregnancy excluded, the uterine cavity should be probed.

If the device cannot be felt with a uterine sound or biopsy instrument, a pelvic sonogram or x-ray should be obtained. If the device is not visualized with pelvic ultrasonography, an x-ray visualizing the entire abdominal cavity should be performed because IUDs that have been pushed thorough the uterus may be located anywhere in the peritoneal cavity, even in the subdiaphragmatic area.

Any type of IUD found to be outside the uterus, even if asymptomatic, should be removed from the peritoneal cavity because complications such as severe adhesions and bowel obstruction have been reported with intraperitoneal

IUDs. Therefore it is best to remove intraperitoneal IUDs shortly after the diagnosis of perforation is made. Unless severe adhesions have developed, most intraperitoneal IUDs can be removed by means of laparoscopy.

Perforation of the cervix has also been reported with devices having a straight vertical arm, such as the copper T. A plastic ball has been added to the distal vertical arm of the copper T 380A to reduce the rate of cervical perforation. When follow-up examinations are performed after IUD insertion, the cervix should be carefully inspected and palpated, because often perforations do not extend completely through the ectocervical epithelium. Cervical perforation is not a major problem, but devices that have perforated downward should be removed through the endocervical canal with uterine packing forceps. Their downward displacement is associated with reduced contraceptive effectiveness.

Complications Related to Pregnancy

Congenital Anomalies

When pregnancy occurs with an IUD in place, implantation takes place away from the device itself, so the device is always extraamniotic. Although there is a paucity of published data, so far there is no evidence of an increased incidence of congenital anomalies in infants born with a plastic, copper-bearing, or progesterone-releasing IUD in utero.

Data from 2 studies of more than 300 babies conceived with a copper IUD in utero suggest that its presence does not exert a deleterious effect on fetal development or increase the risk of birth defects. Although relatively few infants have been born following gestation in a uterus containing a progesterone-releasing IUD, examination of these infants has revealed no evidence of cardiac or other anomalies.

Spontaneous Abortion

In all reported series of pregnancies with any type of IUD in situ, the incidence of fetal death was not significantly increased; however, a significant increase in spontaneous abortion has been consistently observed. If a woman conceives while wearing an IUD that is not subsequently removed, the incidence of spontaneous abortion is about 55%, approximately 3 times greater than would occur in pregnancies without an intrauterine IUD.

After conception, if the IUD is spontaneously expelled, or if the appendage is visible and the IUD is removed by traction, the incidence of spontaneous abortion is significantly reduced. In one study of women who conceived with copper T devices in place, the incidence of spontaneous abortion was only 20% if the device was removed or spontaneously expelled. This figure is similar to the normal incidence of spontaneous abortion and signifi-cantly less than the 54% incidence of abortion reported in the same study among women retaining the devices in utero. Thus, if a woman conceives with an IUD in place and wishes to continue the pregnancy, the IUD should be removed if the appendage is visible, to significantly reduce the chance of spontaneous abortion. If the appendage is not visible, blind probing of the uterine cavity may increase the chance of abortion, as well as sepsis. However, several recent reports indicate that with sonographic guidance it is possible during early gestation to remove intrauterine IUDs in the lower uterine cavity without a visible appendage and not adversely affect the outcome of the pregnancy.

Septic Abortion

If the IUD cannot be removed from the uterine cavity during early gestation, some evidence suggests that the risk of septic abortion may be increased if the IUD remains in place. Most of the evidence was based on data from women who conceived while wearing the shield type of IUD. This device, with its multifilament tail, was extensively used in the United States during the 1970s. The structure of the shield's appendage allowed vaginal bacteria to steadily enter the spaces between the filaments of the tail beneath the surrounding sheath. This action differs from the inability of bacteria to enter the monofilament tails or migrate along their surface through the cervical mucus barrier. During pregnancy, when the shield was drawn upward into the uterine cavity as gestation advanced, the bacteria in the tail string could exit into the uterine cavity and cause a severe and sometimes fatal uterine and systemic infection. This infection usually became manifest during the second trimester of pregnancy.

Although there is an increased risk of septic abortion if a patient conceived with a shield IUD in place, because of the structure of the shield's appendage, there is no conclusive evidence that IUDs with monofilament tail strings cause sepsis during pregnancy. In a British study, there was no significant difference in the incidence of septic abortion among women who conceived with an IUD in place and those who conceived while using other methods. In another study of 918 women who conceived with the copper T in situ, there were only two instances of septic abortion, both occurring in the first trimester. These data indicate that there is no increase in sepsis in pregnancy caused by the presence of an IUD except for the shield device. However, about 2% of all spontaneous abortions are septic, and the continued presence of an intrauterine IUD is associated with about a 50% risk of having a spontaneous abortion. Therefore the overall incidence of septic abortion may be increased with any IUD in place because the incidence of spontaneous abortion is increased, not because the presence of the IUD increases the risk of sepsis by itself.

Ectopic Pregnancy

Because copper-bearing IUDs principally act by preventing fertilization through a cytotoxic effect on spermatozoa, the incidence of both ectopic pregnancy and intrauterine pregnancy are decreased with their use. The risk of the pregnancy being ectopic is increased about threefold from 1.4% to 6% if a woman becomes pregnant with a copper IUD in place than if she continues using no contraception method. However, because the copper T 380A IUD so effectively prevents all pregnancies, the estimated ectopic pregnancy rate is only 0.2 to 0.4 per 1000 woman-years. This rate is one tenth the rate in women using no contraception, 3 per 1000 woman-years (Table 13-13). If a woman uses a copper T 380A IUD, her risk of having an ectopic pregnancy is reduced by 90% compared with use of no contraception.

In the 7-year WHO study of the copper T 380A IUD, the cumulative ectopic pregnancy rate at the end of 7 years was only 0.1 per 100 women. These data confirm that the copper T 380A reduces the risk of having both intrauterine and ectopic gestations.

Because fertilization of the egg probably occurs more frequently with the small, plastic progesterone-releasing IUD than with the copper-bearing devices, one would expect the ectopic pregnancy rate with the progesterone-releasing IUD to be higher also. Clinical data with this device confirms this belief. The progesterone-releasing IUD has a pregnancy rate of about 30 per 1000 woman-years and an ectopic pregnancy rate of 6.8 per 1000 woman-years. Thus about 1 in 4 pregnancies occurring in women using the device will be ectopic. The rate of ectopic pregnancies of 6.8 per 1000 woman-years in women using this device is higher than the 3.25 to 4.5 rate of ectopic pregnancy per 1000 noncontracepting women per year.

With this IUD the action of progesterone on oviductal motility increases the relative risk of having an ectopic pregnancy 1.5 to 1.8 times compared with women using no method of contraception. Thus the two types of IUDs currently marketed in the United States have differing effects on the risk of ectopic pregnancy. The copper T 380 IUD lowers the risk, and the progesterone IUD increases the risk compared with use of no contraception. Because a woman who becomes pregnant with either IUD in place has a greater risk of the pregnancy being ectopic compared with the overall population of pregnant women, appropriate diagnostic studies should take place early in gestation to establish the diagnosis before tubal rupture occurs. The levonorgestrel-releasing IUD has a very low rate of both intrauterine and ectopic pregnancies. The 5-year ectopic pregnancy rate with this device is 0.1, similar to the copper 380A IUD.

The increased risk of ectopic pregnancy for a woman who conceives while wearing an IUD is temporary and does not persist after removal of the IUD. In two large European studies women wishing to conceive after they had an ectopic pregnancy had a much greater chance of having a subsequent intrauterine pregnancy if they were using an IUD at the time of their ectopic pregnancy than were those who had an ectopic pregnancy and were not using an IUD.

Prematurity

In the previously cited study of conceptions occurring in the presence of copper T devices, the rate of prematurity among live births was 4 times greater when the copper T was left in place than when it was removed.

If a pregnant woman has an IUD in place and the device cannot be removed but she wishes to continue her gestation, she should be warned of the increased risk of prematurity, as well as that of spontaneous abortion and ectopic pregnancy. She should also be informed of the possible increased risk of septic abortion and advised to report promptly the first signs of pelvic pain or fever. There is no evidence that pregnancies with IUDs in utero are associated with an increased incidence of other obstetric complications. There is also no evidence that prior use of an IUD results in a greater incidence of complications in pregnancies occurring after its removal.

TABLE 13-13

Intrauterine and Ectopic Pregnancy Rates for IUDs and Controls per 1000 Woman-Years

	Total Pregnancy Rate	Ectopic Pregnancy Ratio per 1000 Pregnancies	Ectopic Pregnancy Rate	Relative Risk Ectopic Pregnancy
No contraception	400–500	14	3.25–4.5	1.0
CuT 380	3.4	59	0.2	0.1
Progesterone-releasing IUD	29.4	231	6.8	1.5

Modified from Sivin I: Obstet Gynecol 78:291, 1991.

Infection in the Nonpregnant IUD User

In the 1960s, despite great concern among clinicians that use of the IUD would markedly increase the incidence of salpingitis, or pelvic inflammatory disease (PID), there was little evidence that such an increase did occur. During that decade the IUD was inserted mainly into parous women, and the incidence of sexually transmitted disease was not as high as occurred subsequently. In 1966 a study was performed in which aerobic and anaerobic cultures were made of homogenates of endometrial tissue obtained transfundally from uteri removed by vaginal hysterectomy at various intervals after insertion of the loop IUD. During the first 24 hours after IUD insertion, the normally sterile endometrial cavity was consistently infected with bacteria. Nevertheless, in 80% of uteri removed during the following 24 hours, the women's natural defenses had destroyed these bacteria and the endometrial cavities were sterile. In this study, when transfundal cultures were obtained more than 30 days after IUD insertion, the endometrial cavity, the IUD, and the portion of the thread within the cavity were always found to be sterile (Figure 13-26). These findings indicate that development of PID more than a month after insertion of the IUD is due to infection with a sexually transmitted pathogen and is unrelated to the presence of the device.

Results of a large multicenter clinical study coordinated by the WHO confirmed these findings. In this study of 22,908 women inserted with IUDs, the PID rate was highest in the first 3 weeks after insertion but remained lower and constant during the 8 years thereafter at 0.5 per 1000 woman-years (Figure 13-27). An IUD should not be inserted into a woman who may have been recently infected with gonococci or *Chlamydia.* Insertion of the device will transport these pathogens from the cervix into the upper genital tract, where the large number of organisms may overcome the host defense and cause salpingitis. If there is clinical suspicion of infectious endocervicitis, cultures should be obtained and the IUD insertion delayed until the results reveal no pathogenic organisms are present. It does not appear to be cost-effective to administer systemic antibiotics routinely with every IUD insertion, but the insertion procedure should be as aseptic as possible.

A randomized trial comparing use of azithromycin ingested just prior to IUD insertion with a placebo control reported no significant difference in the subsequent rate of pelvic inflammation. The rate was 0.1% in both study arms. In a study of the copper T 380A IUD, the rate of removal because of infection during the first year of use was only 0.3%. In a study of the copper T 380A IUD, the rate of removal for infection in the first year of use was only 0.3% (Table 13-14).

Other epidemiologic studies have shown that the presence of an IUD with monofilament tail strings does not increase the incidence of PID after the insertion interval. One study determined the incidence of tubal infertility among former IUD users. It was reported that nulliparous women with a single sexual partner who had previously used an IUD had no increased risk of tubal infertility, whereas women with multiple sexual partners who used an IUD did have an increased risk of tubal infertility.

Analysis of this large amount of data indicates that PID occurring more than a month following insertion of IUDs with monofilament tail strings is due to a sexually transmitted pathogen and not related to the presence of the IUD.

The increased risk of impairment of future fertility from PID developing in the first month after IUD insertion, as well as the possibility of ectopic pregnancy in the event of contraceptive failure, must be considered when deciding whether to use an IUD in a nulliparous woman, especially if she has multiple sexual partners. Contraceptive steroids reduce the risk of developing salpingitis in

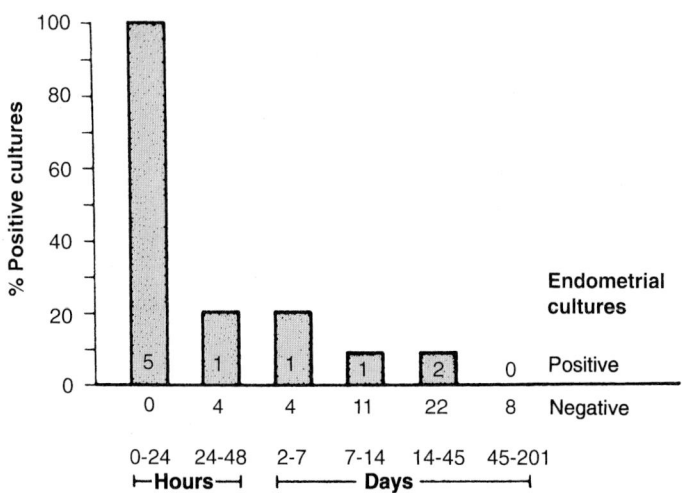

FIGURE 13-26 Relationship between incidence of positive endometrial cultures and duration of IUD use beyond hysterectomy. (From Mishell DR Jr, Bell JH, Good RG, et al: Am J Obstet Gynecol 96:119, 1966.)

women infected with gonorrhea and should be offered to such women. However, for women with medical reasons for not using contraceptive steroids, the IUD is the only other effective reversible method of contraceptive and can be used. The use of condoms should be advised to reduce the risk of transmission of pathogens.

Symptomatic PID can usually be successfully treated with antibiotics without removing the IUD until the woman becomes symptom-free. For women with clinical evidence of a tuboovarian abscess, the IUD should be removed only after a therapeutic serum level of appropriate parenteral antibiotics has been reached, preferably after a clinical response has been observed. An alternative method of contraception should be substituted in women who develop PID with an IUD in place.

There is evidence that IUD users may have an increased risk for colonizing actinomycosis organisms in the upper genital tract. The relationship of actinomycosis to PID is

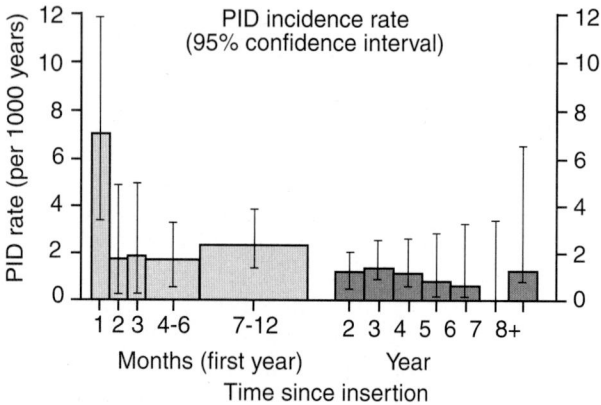

FIGURE 13-27 PID incidence by time since insertion. Incidence rate was estimated by the number of PID cases and years of exposure in each time interval. 95% confidence intervals were calculated from the Poisson distribution. (From Farley TM, Rosenberg MJ, Rowe PJ, et al: Lancet 339:785, 1992.)

TABLE 13-14
First-Year Event Rates per 100 Women
for Copper T 380A

Event	1 Year Parous
Pregnancy	0.5
Expulsion	2.3
Bleeding/pain	3.4
Infection	0.3
Other medical	0.5
Planning pregnancy	0.6
Other personal	0.7

From Rosenberg MJ, Foldesy R, Mishell DR Jr, et al: Contraception 53:197, 1996.

unclear, as many women without IUDs have actinomycosis in their vagina and are asymptomatic. If actinomycosis organisms are identified on the routine examination of cervical cytology and the woman is asymptomatic, she may be treated with appropriate antimicrobial therapy to eradicate the organisms or followed without therapy. The IUD should not be removed from an asymptomatic woman who is colonized but not infected with actinomycosis. If pelvic infection is present, the woman should be treated with antibiotics and the IUD removed.

Contraindications

It is logical and consistent with good medical practice that IUDs not be inserted into women with the following seven conditions, which are listed as contraindications to IUD insertion in the United States: (1) pregnancy or suspicion of pregnancy, (2) acute pelvic inflammatory disease, (3) postpartum endometritis or infected abortion in the past 3 months, (4) known or suspected uterine or cervical malignancy, (5) genital bleeding of unknown etiology, (6) untreated acute cervicitis, and (7) a previously inserted IUD that has not been removed. However, little data are available to indicate that the complications of Wilson's disease, allergy to copper, and genital actinomycosis are true contraindications for insertion of copper-bearing IUDs and, because of the infrequency of these conditions, it is unlikely that data will ever become available.

The remaining contraindications for IUD use listed in the product labeling—abnormalities of the uterus resulting in distortion of the uterine cavity; history of pelvic inflammatory disease; vaginitis, including bacterial vaginosis, until infection is controlled; patient or her partner has multiple sexual partners; and conditions associated with increased susceptibility to infections with microorganisms—remain questionable because of the lack of clinical studies of copper IUD use in women with these conditions.

The reason why the IUD is stated to be contraindicated in women who have multiple sexual partners or whose partner has multiple sexual partners is unclear. Such women should be counseled to have their partners use condoms to protect against transmission of diseases and to use the IUD to effectively prevent pregnancy if they so desire.

Conditions previously believed to preclude IUD use, but are no longer considered to be contraindications, include diabetes mellitus, valvular heart disease (including mitral valve prolapse), past history of ectopic pregnancy (except progesterone-containing IUD), nulliparity, treated cervical dysplasia, irregular menses due to anovulation, breast-feeding, corticosteroid use, and age less than 25.

Overall Safety

Several long-term studies have indicated that the IUD is not associated with an increased incidence of endometrial or cervical carcinoma and may actually be associated with a reduction in risk of developing these neoplasms during and following its use. The IUD is a particularly useful method of contraception for women who have completed their families and do not wish permanent sterilization and have contraindications to, or do not wish to use, other effective methods of reversible contraception. A recent analysis reported that after 5 years of use the IUD was the most cost-effective method of all methods of contraception, including sterilization (see Figure 13-1). Women in the United States who use an IUD have a higher level of satisfaction with their method of contraception than women using any of the other methods of reversible contraception.

STERILIZATION

In 1995 in the United States, sterilization of one member of a couple was the most widely used method of preventing pregnancy. The popularity of sterilization was greatest if (1) the wife was over age 30, (2) the couple had been married more than 10 years, and (3) the couple desired no additional children. In contrast to the other methods of contraception, which are reversible or temporary, sterilization should be considered permanent. Although reanastomosis after vasectomy or tubal ligation is possible, the reconstructive operation is much more difficult than the original sterilizing procedure and the results are variable. Pregnancy rates after reanastomosis of the vas range from 45% to 60%, whereas those after oviduct reanastomosis range from 50% to 80%, depending on the amount of tissue damage associated with the original procedure, as well as technical competency.

Voluntary sterilization is legal in all 50 states, and the decision to be sterilized should be made solely by the individual in consultation with the provider. Because all currently available sterilization procedures require surgical techniques, individuals who request sterilization should be counseled regarding both the risks and the irreversibility of the procedures. It is advisable to inform the individual fully, and the spouse if possible, of the benefits and risks of these surgical procedures. In addition, it has been useful to have more than one counselor when sterilization is requested by a woman younger than age 25, as well as all women without children.

The rationale for such careful scrutiny of younger candidates for sterilization is that they tend to change their minds more often, their attitudes may be less fixed, and they face a longer period of reproductive life during which divorce, remarriage, or death among their children can occur. About 1% of sterilized women subsequently request reversal. In the United States approximately 7000 women request reversal each year.

The most effective, least destructive method of tubal occlusion is the most desirable in younger women, since ovarian dysfunction and adhesion formation are diminished, while the incidence of successful reversal procedures is increased. The effective laparoscopic band techniques or the modified Pomeroy technique (also called partial salpingectomy) (Figure 13-28) should be used in women younger than age 25. Reversal after this method of sterilization is followed by pregnancy in approximately 75% of women, a rate that is higher than that reported after most laparoscopic fulgurations, where more tube is destroyed.

Male Sterilization

Sterilization in the male is performed by vasectomy, an outpatient procedure that takes about 20 minutes and requires only local anesthesia. The vas deferens is isolated and cut. The ends of the vas are closed, either by ligation or by fulguration; they are then replaced in the scrotal sac, and the incision is closed. Complications of vasectomy include hematoma (in up to 5% of the subjects), sperm granulomas (inflammatory responses to sperm leakage), and spontaneous reanastomosis. When the latter occurs, it usually does so within a short time after the procedure. Usually about 14 to 20 ejaculations are required after the operation before the man is sterile. Although in the United States reversal requests range from 5% to 7% of men who had a vasectomy, vas reanastomosis is a difficult and meticulous procedure that has an optimal success rate of about 50%.

Female Sterilization

Sterilization of the female is more complicated, requiring a transperitoneal incision and usually general anesthesia. Postpartum sterilization is performed by making a small infraumbilical incision and performing either a Pomeroy or modified Irving type of tubal ligation. These simple and rapid procedures can be performed either in the delivery room immediately after delivery or in the operating room the following day without prolonging the hospital stay. The same operative techniques can be used for female sterilization at times other than the puerperium, but additional techniques are also used for what has been termed *interval sterilization*. Ligation of the oviducts by the Pomeroy technique can be easily and rapidly performed through a small abdominal incision termed *minilaparotomy*. On occasion a colpotomy incision may also be used, but this incision is associated with a higher incidence of postoperative infection.

The development of fiberoptic light sources has made laparoscopy a popular gynecologic operative technique. By using various accessories in addition to the laparoscope, the operator can fulgurate and cut the oviducts without making an intraperitoneal incision other than one or two small punctures. Most gynecologists find the two-puncture technique for laparoscopy sterilization easier to learn and perform than the single-puncture technique. General anesthesia is usually employed for laparoscopic sterilization, but overnight hospitalization is unnecessary. Because the pregnancy rate after fulguration and transection is

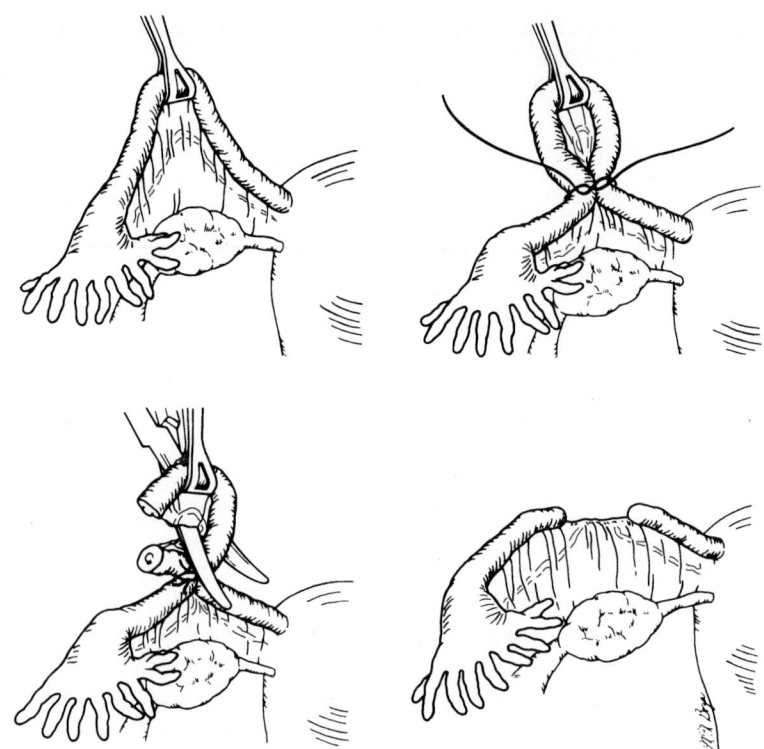

FIGURE 13-28   Modified Pomeroy technique of female sterilization. (From Sciarra JJ: Surgical procedures for tubal sterilization. In Sciarra JJ, Zatuchni GI, and Daly MJ: Gynecology and obstetrics, vol 6, Philadelphia, 1984, Harper & Row, Publishers.)

similar to that after fulguration alone, it is now recommended that the oviducts not be cut after fulguration. The incidence of complications after laparoscopic fulguration ranges from 1% to 6%; major complications (hemorrhage, puncture, or cautery of bowel) occur in about 0.6% of patients.

In an attempt to eliminate the problem of bowel injury, bipolar forceps were developed to replace the unipolar apparatus, which has a grounding plate attached to the patient through which the current passes. In the bipolar system the current passes from one prong of the forceps, through the tissue, to the other prong, producing a limited area of coagulation with destruction of a small segment of the oviduct. After coagulation, if division is to be performed, scissors are introduced to cut the oviduct. If division is not to be performed, some operators perform a coagulation of two or three contiguous burns on each oviduct to ensure adequate obliteration of the lumen. When the unipolar apparatus is used, a single 1-cm burn on each oviduct is sufficient. However, even with this small amount of coagulation, local tissue damage after unipolar coagulation is extensive, and attempts at reanastomosis have a very low rate of success. Because bipolar coagulation not only is safer but also is associated with a higher success rate after a reanastomosis procedure, this technique is now preferred.

Because of the problems of electrocoagulation, efforts have been made to develop safer methods that destroy less

tissue. Nonelectrical tubal occlusion techniques that may be performed through the laparoscope are those using spring-loaded clips and the Silastic band (falope ring). All these techniques require a modification of the conventional laparoscope, as well as specialized training in their use.

Female sterilization by surgical removal of a portion of the oviduct or mechanically occluding a portion of the lumen by clips, bands, or electrocoagulation was previously believed to be the most effective form of pregnancy prevention. This belief was based on studies that reported that failure rates during the first year of use of any type of reversible contraceptive were higher than the first-year failure rate of female sterilization. The results of a long-term study by Peterson et al. indicate that pregnancies continue to occur for many years after the sterilization procedure. The failure rate increased from 0.55 per 100 women at 1 year to 1.31 at 5 years, and 1.85 10 years after the operation for all methods of tubal interruption, being higher for bipolar coagulation and spring clips and lower for partial salpingectomy. For women 18 to 27 years of age, 2.8% became pregnant 5 to 10 years after bipolar coagulation of the oviduct. There are several reversible methods of contraception, with failure rates similar to those of tubal sterilization. Cumulative 5-year failure rates with Norplant are 1.1 per 100 women; with the copper T 380 IUD, 1.2 per 100 women; and with female sterilization, 1.3 per 100 women. Furthermore, among women who become pregnant after female sterilization, about one third have ectopic pregnancies compared with one fourth with Norplant and 5% with the copper T 380 IUD. Because the copper T 380 IUD has an effective life span of 10 years, with a failure rate comparable to that of female sterilization and a lower ectopic pregnancy rate, as well as being less expensive and more convenient to use, it should be considered as an alternative to tubal sterilization.

INDUCED ABORTION

Induced abortion is one of the most common gynecologic operations performed in the United States and in many other countries. As determined by the landmark *Roe v. Wade* Supreme Court decision, the state may not interfere with the practice of abortion in the first trimester. In the second trimester, states may regulate abortion services in the interest of preserving the health of the woman. However, restrictions limiting the performance of second-trimester abortions to hospitals have been declared unconstitutional.

From 1973 through 1980, the number of induced abortions performed annually in the United States steadily increased from 750,000 to about 1,600,000. The annual number of abortions stabilized at this figure from 1980 until 1990. Since 1990 there has been a gradual decline in the annual number of abortions performed in the United States, reaching 1,360,000 in 1996. In 1996 the abortion ratio (number of abortions per 100 pregnancies) was 26, whereas the abortion rate (number of abortions per 1000 women aged 15 to 44) was 23. In the United States the abortion rates have declined gradually since 1980 but are higher than in all Western European countries and about 1 in 4 pregnancies in the United States are terminated by elective abortion. Approximately one third of abortions are performed in women under age 20, another third in women ages 20 to 24, and the remaining third among women age 25 and older. Only one fourth of abortions are obtained by married women. Ninety percent of abortions are performed within the first 12 weeks of pregnancy, and about 50% of abortions are performed during the first 8 weeks of pregnancy. In the United States nearly all abortions are performed by various surgical techniques, while in Europe and a few U.S. centers many abortions are terminated with the use of drugs.

Methods

Three principal methods are used for elective abortion: transcervical evacuation, induction of labor, and major operations. Suction curettage is the predominant method of performing abortion in the United States, accounting for approximately 75% of all abortion procedures; the remainder are performed by dilation and evacuation (curettage techniques in the second trimester), labor induction, and major operations.

Curettage Methods

Curettage by vacuum aspiration is the predominant method of performing abortion in the first trimester. Very early in pregnancy, *endometrial aspiration*, also termed *menstrual extraction*, can be done with a small, flexible, plastic cannula without dilation or anesthesia. Abortions performed to terminate pregnancies with a gestational age of 8 weeks or more generally require dilation of the cervix and some type of anesthesia, either local or general.

Dilation of the cervix can be facilitated by use of osmotic dilators. These are usually placed in the cervical canal for several hours or overnight to produce gradual dilation. Most commonly *Laminaria japonica*, made of seaweed sticks, are utilized. Synthetic osmotic dilators include a polyvinyl alcohol sponge impregnated with magnesium sulfate and a hygroscope plastic polymer. Use of such osmotic dilators in nulliparous women substantially reduces the risk of uterine trauma, such as perforation and cervical injury.

Dilation and evacuation (D&E) is the predominant method of abortion used beyond the first trimester. Because a greater amount of cervical dilation is usually needed, osmotic dilators are usually inserted for several hours or several days before the procedure. Although recent data are lacking, earlier studies indicated that D&E was substantially safer than induction of labor or major operations for abortions of 13 to 16 weeks' gestation. For later abortions, D&E and induction of labor appear to have comparable risks of morbidity and mortality, although the range of complications varies by technique. Disadvantages of D&E include the requirement of technical expertise, the emotional burden for participating physicians and medical personnel, and possible long-term deleterious effects upon the cervix. Advantages include less emotional stress for the woman, avoidance of the need for hospitalization, greater convenience, and lower cost than induction of uterine contractions.

Induction of Uterine Contractions

Second-trimester abortion is also performed by induction of uterine contractions. One technique uses instillation of hypertonic solution into the amniotic cavity. The solution most frequently used was hypertonic saline (2000 ml of 20% saline), although hypertonic glucose and urea were also employed. Uterine contractions usually began within 12 to 24 hours, and abortion occurred within a few hours thereafter. Use of an ancillary agent such as *Laminaria* or oxytocin facilitates the process. Uterine instillation of hypertonic solution is currently performed infrequently.

The most common method now used for medical termination in the second trimester is administration of prostaglandins. Prostaglandin E_2, administered as a vaginal suppository; a prostaglandin E_2 methyl analogue, misoprostol; APGE, given as tablets orally or vaginally; and 15-methyl prostaglandin $E_{2\alpha}$, administered as an intramuscular injection, have all been used. These techniques have the advantage of easy administration. Each compound is given at 2- to 6-hour intervals until evacuation of the gestational material is achieved. Disadvantages include gastrointestinal side effects and, with the prostaglandin E_2 suppositories, hyperpyrexia. Jain and Mishell reported that the intravaginal placement of 2 100-μg tablets of misoprostol every 12 hours was as successful as prostaglandin E_2, with fewer side effects and less cost. The success rate after 48 hours of treatment was nearly 90%.

Major Operations

Hysterotomy and hysterectomy are infrequently used for performing abortion in the United States. Both procedures have a much higher risk of morbidity and mortality than do alternative methods. Hysterectomy should be reserved for those instances in which preexisting gynecologic pathology, such as carcinoma in situ of the cervix or large leiomyomata, also exist.

Pharmacologic Agents

PROGESTERONE ANTAGONISTS. A few years ago Healy et al. synthesized a progestogenic steroid compound that had weak progestational activity but marked affinity for progesterone receptors in the endometrium. This compound, called RU 486, or mifepristone (Figure 13-29), because of its high receptor affinity prevents progesterone from binding to its receptors and thus inhibits the action of circulating progesterone on its target tissue. In clinical trials it was found that if a single 600-mg dose of RU 486 were administered orally in early pregnancy, prior to 7 weeks after the onset of the last menses, that about 85% of the pregnancies spontaneously terminated. When this treatment was combined with administration of a prostaglandin 36 to 48 hours later, the efficacy increased to 96%. However, side effects include nausea, vomiting, and abdominal pain. Two prostaglandin analogues, intramuscular sulprostone and vaginal gemeprost, were the agents initially used after mifepristone. Sulprostone is no longer marketed for this purpose, as three women who received this agent with mifepristone suffered a myocardial infarction. Gemeprost is much more expensive than misoprostol, a prostaglandin analogue widely used to prevent peptic ulcer disease. Therefore oral administration of misoprostol is now being used more extensively than gemeprost after mifepristone.

The results of a randomized trial with misoprostol given vaginally or orally suggest that when misoprostol is given vaginally instead of orally it is more effective and has fewer side effects. A large, multicenter, clinical trial with mifepristone followed by oral misoprostol was recently performed in the United States. Therefore, when this drug combination does become available for use in this country, the oral administration of misoprostol will most likely be recommended, even though vaginal administration probably is preferable. The main disadvantage of this medical abortifacient is prolonged and sometimes heavy uterine bleeding that on occasion can cause anemia, necessitating a blood transfusion and possibly curettage. The mean duration of bleeding after administration of this drug is about 12 days when administered alone and 9 days when used with a prostaglandin. Currently, distribution of mifepristone is limited to a few European countries and China, but compounds with similar activity or steroid enzymatic inhibitors that prevent progesterone synthesis are also being studied.

Since mifepristone is unavailable in most countries, including the United States, other pharmacologic agents have been used to terminate early gestation. Studies with 800 μg of misoprostol tablets placed in the vagina and moistened with saline for 1, 2, or 3 applications 24 hours apart report about a 90% effectiveness when given to women less than 8 weeks' gestational age. Side effects such as vomiting and diarrhea are frequent and can be lessened with use of prophylactic medications. Several investigators have administered methotrexate intramuscularly in a dosage of 50 mg/m² followed 3 to 7 days later by vaginal administration of 800 mg of misoprostol to groups of women with pregnancies less than 8 weeks' gestational age and found that about 90% of the pregnancies aborted. However, with this regimen only about two thirds of the women aborted within 1 day after receiving the misoprostol. The mean time to abortion in the remainder was about 3 weeks. The mean length of time during which uterine bleeding occurred in the entire study group was more than 2 weeks. Because of these problems, as well as the need to determine the true incidence of side effects, this treatment regimen should still be considered to be experimental and only used after an investigative protocol has been approved and the woman has signed an informed consent.

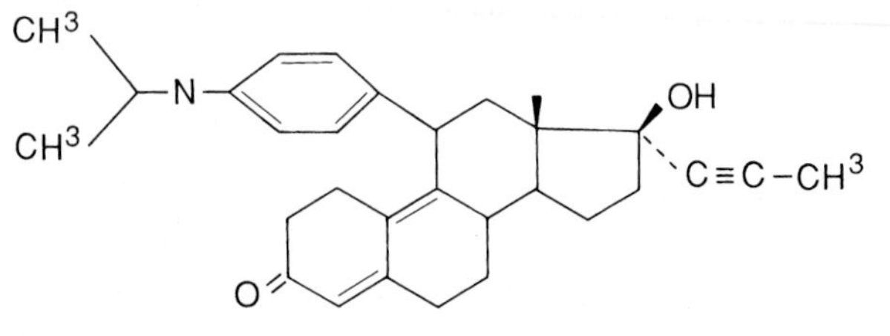

FIGURE 13-29 Molecular structure of RU 486. Molecular weight is 430, and empirical formula is $C_{29}H_{35}NO_2$. (From Healy DL, Baulieu EE, and Hodgen GD: Fertil Steril 40:253, 1983.)

Ancillary Techniques

A qualitative assay for hCG should always be performed before an abortion is undertaken unless there is sonographic evidence of pregnancy. Performing a qualitative pregnancy test 2 weeks after the procedure will ensure that the pregnancy has been successfully aborted. In the first trimester, sonography should be done to determine gestational age when a substantial discrepancy occurs between the menstrual history and clinical examination; when uterine abnormalities, such as leiomyomata, are present; or when the presence of an ectopic gestation is suspected. Sonography should always be performed before initiating second-trimester abortions and has avoided the problem of misestimation of gestational age, which is an important cause of complications. Performing ultrasonography during a D&E may facilitate the procedure.

Complications

Elective abortion in the United States is a very safe operation. Complications are infrequent, and the overall mortality is less than 1 per 100,000 procedures. Two important determinants of complications are the gestational age and method of abortion chosen. When abortion is performed in pregnancies of 6 weeks or less gestational age there are slightly higher complication rates than when the gestational age is between 7 to 10 weeks. Beyond 10 weeks, abortion complication rates increase progressively with gestational age. Suction curettage is the safest surgical method of abortion, followed by D&E, induction of labor, and major operations.

The most common complication is infection, and the routine use of preoperative antibiotic prophylaxis has been shown to reduce this risk. Other complications include hemorrhage, the consequences of uterine perforation, and anesthetic hazards.

KEY POINTS

- In 1994, of the 58 million women in the United States aged 15 to 44 years, approximately one third were not exposed to pregnancy and 64%, 39 million, were using a method of contraception. About 5% of women of reproductive age were sexually active and not using any contraceptive.

- In 1994 there were about 6 million pregnancies in the United States. There were 3.9 million births and about 1.4 million elective abortions. About 25% of all pregnancies were electively terminated. Half of all pregnancies were unwanted.

- Of women using contraceptives in the United States in 1995, male and female sterilization were used by 40%, oral contraceptives by 27%, male condom by 20%, the progestin injection by 3%, and the implant and IUD by less than 1%.

- Typical- and perfect-use failure rates in the first year of use range between 5% to 27% for coitus-related methods and between 0.1% to 3% for oral contraceptives (OCs). The IUD, injection, and implants have failure rates less than 1%.

- Contraceptive failure rates are increased in inverse relation to the user's age, level of education, and socioeconomic class.

- Pregnancy results from failure of spermicide use are not associated with an increased risk of fetal malformations.

- The active ingredient in spermicides is a surfactant, usually nonoxynol 9, which immobilizes or kills sperm on contact.

- Barrier techniques reduce the rate of transmission of sexually transmitted diseases, both bacterial and viral.

- Pregnancy (failure rates) with the cervical cap are similar to those with the diaphragm.

- The most effective type of periodic abstinence is the symptothermal method.

- OC formulations in the United States consist of varying dosages of one of the following estranes: norethindrone, norethindrone acetate, ethynodiol diacetate, or gonanes: norgestrel (or its active isomere, levonorgestrel), desogestrol, norgestimate, and either of two estrogens, ethinyl estradiol or ethinyl estradiol-3-methyl ether, also called *mestranol*.

- A given weight of norgestrel or the other gonanes has 5 to 10 times more progestational activity than the equivalent weight of norethindrone, whereas norethindrone acetate and ethinyodiol deacetate are similar in potency to norethindrone.

- Metabolic effects of the estrogen component of OCs include an increase in serum globulins and altering of the lipid profile to increase triglycerides and HDL cholesterol and lower LDL cholesterol.

- Metabolic effects of the progestin component of OCs include peripheral insulin resistance and lowering HDL cholesterol and raising LDL cholesterol.

- Ethinyl estradiol is approximately 1.7 times as potent as an equivalent weight of mestranol.

- No significantly increased risk of breast cancer occurs among ever users of OC or in various high-risk subgroups of OC users. While using OCs young women have a slightly increased risk of having nonmetastatic breast cancer diagnosed but have a decreased risk of having metastatic breast cancer diagnosed compared with non-OC users.

- The risk of breast cancer developing 10 years after stopping OCs is similar to that of nonusers.

- OC users have an increased risk of developing invasive cervical cancer, particularly adenocarcinoma, compared with users of no contraception, but a causal relation has not been established.

- The rate of return of fertility after stopping OCs is delayed, but eventually the percentage of women who conceive after stopping all methods of contraception, including OCs, is the same.

- Babies born to women who discontinue OCs or who conceive while ingesting OCs have no greater incidence of any type of birth defect.

- All OC formulations with less than 50 µg of estrogen increase the risk of venous thrombosis and embolism three- to four-fold.

- A significantly increased risk of developing myocardial infarction occurs only in current OC users over age 35 who smoke.

- Users of low-dose OCs do not have a significantly increased risk of developing ischemic or hemorrhagic stroke if they do not smoke or have hypertension.

- The cause of myocardial infarction in older OC users who smoke is arterial thrombosis.

- Adverse effects produced by the estrogenic component of OCs include nausea, breast tenderness, fluid retention, temporary increase in blood pressure, thrombosis, changes in mood, and chloasma. Progestins produce certain androgenic adverse effects, including weight gain, nervousness, depression, tiredness, and acne, as well as failure of withdrawal bleeding or amenorrhea.

- In an ovulatory cycle the mean blood loss during menstruation is approximately 35 ml, compared with 20 ml for women ingesting OCs.

- OC users are about half as likely to develop iron deficiency anemia as are control subjects.

- OC users are significantly less likely to develop menorrhagia, irregular menstruation, or intermenstrual bleeding than nonusers.

- The risk of developing endometrial cancer, as well as ovarian cancer, in OC users and former users is only half that in control subjects. OC users also have a 50% reduction in the incidence of benign breast disease.

- OC users have approximately 50% less dysmenorrhea and 39% less premenstrual tension than do control subjects.

- Functional ovarian cysts occur less frequently in OC users than in nonusers if they use monophasic, but not multiphasic, formulations.

- Prior use of OCs does not affect mortality rates in women.

- OCs reduce the clinical development of salpingitis (pelvic inflammatory disease [PID]) in women infected with gonorrhea or *Chlamydia* by 50%, and the overall incidence of PID in OC users is reduced by 50%.

- OCs reduce the risk of ectopic pregnancy by more than 90% in women currently using them.

- There are three types of injectable contraception: depo-medroxyprogesterone acetate (DMPA), norethindrone enanthate, and several progestin-estrogen combinations. All are very effective.

- Women using injectable DMPA (150 mg every 3 months) have a first-year pregnancy rate of 0.1%.

- Injectable DMPA is associated with loss of bone density that appears to recover after DMPA is stopped.

- Women treated with injectable progestins for contraception have complete disruption of the normal menstrual cycle and a totally irregular bleeding pattern that is usually followed by amenorrhea.

- The monthly estrogen-progestin combination injection produces regular bleeding and is extremely effective, with first-year pregnancy rates less than 0.5%.

- Norplant releases sufficient amounts of levonorgestrel daily to maintain blood levels of 300 to 400 pg/ml for 5 years. The annual pregnancy rate with this method is approximately 0.2%, and its major side effect is abnormal bleeding.

- The most effective method of emergency contraception is ingestion of two tablets of 750 µg of levonorgestrel taken 12 hours apart with a failure rate about 1%. The most widely used is four tablets of 50 µg ethinyl estradiol and 0.5 mg norgestrel taken in doses of two tablets 12 hours apart. The latter, called the Yuzpe regimen, has a failure rate of about 2% to 3%.

- The cumulative incidence of accidental pregnancy with the copper T 380A IUD is 1.6% after 7 years of use and 1.7% after 12 years of use. This IUD is approved for 10 years' use.

- The incidence of adverse events with IUDs steadily decreases with increasing age of the woman.

- The main mechanism of contraceptive action of the copper IUD is production of a local sterile inflammatory reaction of leukocytes, which destroys sperm and prevents fertilization.

- Resumption of fertility after IUD removal is not delayed and occurs at the same rate as resumption after discontinuation of use of mechanical contraceptive methods.

- A copper or progesterone-releasing IUD can be removed and a new one reinserted immediately afterward. The IUD can be safely inserted on any day of the cycle.

- In the first year of use, the copper T 380 IUD has approximately a 0.5% pregnancy rate, a 10% expulsion rate, and a 15% rate of removal for medical reasons, and the incidence of each of these events diminishes steadily in subsequent years.

- In women wearing a copper T IUD, 50 to 60 ml of blood is lost per cycle; with the progesterone-releasing IUD, the amount of blood loss is 25 ml per cycle.

- Mefenamic acid, 500 mg twice daily during menses, significantly reduces menstrual blood loss in IUD users.

- The fundal perforation rate with the copper T 380 IUD is about 1 per 3000 insertions.

- The incidence of congenital anomalies is not increased in infants born with any type of IUD in utero.

- If a woman conceives with an IUD in place and the IUD is not removed, the incidence of spontaneous abortion is about 55%, approximately 3 times greater than would occur without an IUD. If, after conception, the IUD is removed, the incidence of spontaneous abortion is reduced to about 20%.

- If a woman conceives with a copper IUD in place, her chances of having an ectopic pregnancy is about 5%, approximately 10 times greater than occurs in conceptions without an IUD.

- Women using a copper T 380 IUD have approximately a 90% lower overall risk of having an ectopic pregnancy than women using no method of contraception.

- The rate of prematurity among live births occurring with an IUD in utero is increased about 2 to 4 times.

- The overall risk of PID in users of IUDs with a monofilament tail string is increased only during the first 3 weeks after insertion.

- Pregnancy rates after reanastomosis of the vas range from 45% to 60%, whereas those after oviduct reanastomosis range from 50% to 80%.

- About 1% of sterilized women request reversal. In the United States approximately 7000 women request reversal each year.

- Usually about 15 to 20 ejaculations are required after vasectomy before a man is sterile.

- After vasectomy, two aspermic ejaculates are required before the male is considered sterile.

- After sterilization by tubal interruption, the 1-year failure rate is 0.55 per 100 women, the 5-year failure rate is 1.31 per 100 women, and the 10-year failure rate is 1.85 per 100 women. About one third of the pregnancies are ectopic.

- Complication rates are 3 to 4 times higher for second-trimester abortions than for first-trimester abortions.

- The most effective medical means to terminate pregnancies less than 8 weeks' gestation is the combination of mifepristone followed by misoprostol, with a failure rate less than 5%. The combination of methotrexate followed by misoprostol and misoprostol alone are slightly less effective.

BIBLIOGRAPHY

Adams MR, Clarkson TB, Kortinik DR, et al: Contraceptive steroids and coronary artery atherosclerosis in cynomolgus macaques, Fertil Steril 47:1010, 1987.

Alvarez F, Gujiloff E, Brache V, et al: New insights on the mode of action of intrauterine contraceptive devices in women, Fertil Steril 49:768, 1988.

Anderson ABM, Haynes PJ, Guillebaud J, et al: Reduction of menstrual blood loss by prostaglandin synthetase inhibitors, Lancet 1:774, 1976.

Austin H, Louv WC, and Alexander WJ: A case-control study of spermicides and gonorrhea, JAMA 251:2822, 1984.

Back DJ, Breckenridge AM, Crawford FE, et al: The effects of rifampicin on the pharmacokinetics of ethinylestradiol in women, Contraception 21:135, 1980.

Bahamondes L, Lavin P, Ojeda G, et al: Return of fertility after discontinuation of the once-a-month injectable contraceptive Cyclofem, Contraception 55:307, 1997.

Beral V, Hermon C, Kay C, et al: Mortality associated with oral contraceptive use: 25 year follow up of cohort of 46000 women from Royal College of General Practitioners' Oral Contraception Study, BMJ 318:96, 1999.

Bloemenkamp KWM, Rosendaal FR, Helmerhorst FM, et al: Enhancement of Factor V Leiden mutation of risk of deep-vein thrombosis associated with oral contraceptives containing a third-generation progestagen, Lancet 346:1593, 1995.

Bokarewa MI, Falk G, Sten-Linder M, et al: Thrombotic risk factors and oral contraception, J Lab Clin Med 126:294, 1995.

Brache V, Alvarez-Sanchez F, Faundes A, et al: Ovarian endocrine function through five years of continuous treatment with Norplant® subdermal contraceptive implants, Contraception 41:169, 1990.

Brache V, Faundes A, Johansson E, et al: Anovulation, inadequate luteal phase and poor sperm penetration in cervical mucus during prolonged use of Norplant® implants, Contraception 31:261, 1985.

Bracken MB, Hellenbrand KG, and Holford TR: Conception delay after oral contraceptive use: the effect of estrogen dose, Fertil Steril 53:21, 1990.

Bracken MB and Vita K: Frequency of non-hormonal contraception around conception and association with congenital malformations in offspring, Am J Epidemiol 117:281, 1983.

Brenner PF, Goebelsmann U, Stanczyk FZ, and Mishell DR Jr: Serum levels of ethinylestradiol following its ingestion alone or in oral contraceptive formulations, Contraception 22:85, 1980.

Brenner PF, Mishell DR Jr, Stanczyk FZ, et al: Serum levels of d-norgestrel, luteinizing hormone, follicle-stimulating hormone, estradiol, and progesterone in women during and following ingestion of combination oral contraceptives containing dl-norgestrel, Am J Obstet Gynecol 129:133, 1977.

Brinton LA, Reeves WC, Brenes MM, et al: Oral contraceptive use and risk of invasive cervical cancer, Int J Epidemiol, 19:4, 1990.

Brinton LA, Vessy MP, Flavell R, et al: Risk factors for benign breast disease, Am J Epidemiol 113:203, 1981.

Brown JB, Blackwell LF, Billings JJ, et al: Natural family planning, Am J Obstet Gynecol 157:1082, 1987.

Castracane VD, Gimpel T, and Goldzieher JW: When is it safe to switch from oral contraceptives to hormonal replacement therapy? Contraception 52:371, 1995.

Celentano DD, Klassen AC, Weisman CS, and Rosenshein NB: The role of contraceptive use in cervical cancer: the Maryland cervical cancer case-control study, Am J Epidemiol 126:592, 1987.

Centers for Disease Control: Combination oral contraceptives use and risk of endometrial cancer, JAMA 257:976, 1987.

Chasan-Taber L, Colditz GA, Willett WC, et al: A prospective study of oral contraceptives and NIDDM among U.S. women, Diabetes Care 20:330, 1997.

Chasan-Taber L, Willett WC, Manson JE, et al: Prospective study of oral contraceptives and hypertension among women in the United States, Circulation 94:483, 1996.

Chi IC, Potts M, Wilkens LR, et al: Performance of the copper T-380A intrauterine device in breast feeding women, Contraception 39:603, 1989.

Chow WH, Daling JR, Weiss NS, et al: IUD use and subsequent tubal pregnancy, Am J Public Health 66:131, 1986.

Clarkson TB, Shively CA, Morgan TM, et al: Oral contraceptives and coronary artery atherosclerosis of cynomolgus monkeys, Obstet Gynecol 75:217, 1990.

Coenen CMH, Thomas CMH, Borm GF, et al: Changes in androgens during treatment with four low-dose contraceptives, Contraception 53:171, 1996.

Coker AL, McCann MF, Hulka BS, and Walter LA: Oral contraceptive use and cervical intraepithelial neoplasia, J Clin Epidemiol 45:1111, 1992.

Colditz GA for The Nurses' Health Study Research Group: Oral contraceptive use and mortality during 12 years follow-up: the Nurses' Health Study, Ann Intern Med 120:821, 1994.

Collaborative Group on Hormonal Factors in Breast Cancer: Breast cancer and hormonal contraceptives: collaborative reanalysis of individual data on 53,297 women with breast cancer and 100,239 women without breast cancer from 54 epidemiological studies, Lancet 347:1713, 1996.

Collaborative Group on Hormonal Factors in Breast Cancer: Breast cancer and hormonal contraceptives: further results, Contraception 54:1S, 1996.

Conant M, Hardy D, Sernatinger J, et al: Condoms prevent transmission of AIDS-associated retrovirus, JAMA 255:1706, 1986.

Conant MA, Spicer DW, and Smith CD: Herpes simplex virus transmission: condom studies, Sex Transm Dis 11:94, 1984.

Craig S and Hepburn S: The effectiveness of barrier methods of contraception with and without spermicide, Contraception 26:347, 1982.

Croft P and Hannaford PC: Risk factors for acute myocardial infarction in women, Br Med J 298:165, 1989.

Cromer BA, Blair JM, Mahan JD, et al: A prospective comparison of bone density in adolescent girls receiving depot medroxyprogesterone acetate (Depo-Provera), levonorgestrel (Norplant), or oral contraceptives, J Pediatr 129:671, 1996.

Cullins VE: Noncontraceptive benefits and therapeutic uses of depot medroxyprogesterone acetate, J Reprod Med 41(9):428, 1996.

Cundy T, Cornish J, Evans MC, et al: Recovery of bone density in women who stop using medroxyprogesterone acetate, Br Med J 308:247, 1994.

Cundy T, Evans M, Roberts H, et al: Bone density in women receiving depot medroxyprogesterone acetate for contraception, Br Med J 303:13, 1991.

Diaz S, Pavez M, Miranda P, et al: Long-term follow-up of women treated with Norplant® implants, Contraception 33:551, 1987.

Dong W, Colhoun HM, and Poutler NR: Blood pressure in women using oral contraceptives: Results from the Health Survey for England 1994, J Hypertens 15:1063, 1997.

Dorflinger L: Relative potency of progestins used in oral contraceptives, Contraception 557:31, 1985.

El-Rafaey H, Rajasekar D, Abdalla M, et al: Induction of abortion with mifepristone (RU 486) and oral or vaginal misoprostol, N Engl J Med 332:983, 1995.

Engel HJ, Engel E, and Lichtlen PR: Coronary atherosclerosis and myocardial infarction in young women: role of oral contraceptives, Eur Heart J 4:1, 1983.

Farley TM, Rosenberg MJ, Rowe PJ, et al: Intrauterine devices and pelvic inflammatory disease: an international perspective, Lancet 339:785, 1992.

Farmer RDT and Preston NTD: The risk of venous thrombosis associated with low oestrogen oral contraceptives, J Obstet Gynecol 15:195, 1995.

Farr G, Gabelnlick H, Sturgen K, and Dorflinger L: Contraceptive efficacy and acceptability of the female condom, Am J Public Health 84:1960, 1994.

Ferreira AE, Araujo MJ, Regina CH, et al: Effectivnesss of the diaphragm, used continuously, without spermicide, Contraception 48:29, 1993.

Fihn SD, Latham RH, Roberts P, et al: Association between diaphragm use and urinary tract infection, JAMA 254:240, 1986.

Forman D, Vincent TJ, and Doll R: Cancer of the liver and the use of oral contraceptives, Br Med J 292:1357, 1986.

Gambacciani M, Spinetti A, Toponeco F, et al: Longitudinal evaluation of perimenopausal vertebral bone loss: effects of a low-dose oral contraceptive preparation on bone mineral density and metabolism, Obstet Gynecol 83:392, 1993.

Gerstman BB, Piper JM, Tomita DK, et al: Oral contraceptive estrogen dose and the risk of deep venous thromboembolic disease, Am J Epidemiol 133:32, 1991.

Glasier A, Thong KJ, Dewar M, et al: Mifepristone (RU486) compared with high-dose estrogen and progestogen for emergency postcoital contraception, N Engl J Med 327:1041, 1992.

Godsland IF, Crook D, Simpson R, et al: The effects of different formulations of oral contraceptive agents on lipid and carbohydrate metabolism, N Engl J Med 323:1375, 1990.

Godsland IF, Crook D, Worthington M, et al: Effects of a low-estrogen, desogestrel-containing oral contraceptive on lipid and carbohydrate metabolism, Contraception 48:217, 1993.

Godsland IF, Crook D, and Wynn V: Clinical and metabolic considerations of long-term oral contraceptive use, Am J Obstet Gynecol 166:1955, 1992.

Gray RH and Pardthaisong T: In utero exposure to steroid contraceptives and survival during infancy, Am J Epidemiol 134:804, 1991.

Grossman RA and Grossman BD: How frequently is emergency contraception prescribed? Fam Plann Perspect 26:270-271, 1994.

Guillebaud J: Copper IUDs and pregnancy (letter), Br J Fam Plan 7:88, 1981.

Hall P, Bahamondes L, Diaz J, et al: Introductory study of the once-a-month, injectable contraceptive Cyclofem in Brazil, Chile, Colombia, and Peru, Contraception 56:353, 1997.

Hankinson SE, Colditz GA, Hunter DJ, et al: A quantitative assessment of oral contraceptive use and risk of ovarian cancer, Obstet Gynecol 80:708, 1992.

Hannaford PC, Croft PR, and Kay CR: Oral contraception and stroke: evidence from the Royal College of General Practitioners' Oral Contraception Study, Stroke 25:935, 1993.

Hannaford PC and Kay CR: Oral contraceptives and diabetes mellitus, Br Med J 299:315, 1989.

Hannaford PC, Villard-Mackintosh L, Vessey MP, and Kay CR: Oral contraceptives and malignant melanoma, Br J Cancer 63:430, 1991.

Harlap S, Shiono PH, and Ramcharan S: Congenital abnormalities in the offspring of women who used oral and other contraceptives around the time of conception, Int J Fertil 30:39, 1985.

Helms SE, Bredle DL, Zajic J, et al: Oral contraceptive failure rates and oral antibiotics, J Am Acad Dermatol 36:705, 1997.

Henshaw SK: Unintended pregnancy in the United States, Fam Plann Perspect 30:24, 1998.

Henshaw SK and Von Vort J: Abortion services in the United States, 1991 and 1992, Fam Plann Perspect 26:100, 1994.

Hicks DR, Martin LS, Getchell JP, et al: Inactivation of HTLV-III/LAV-infected cultures of normal human lymphocytes by nonoxynol-9 in vitro, Lancet 2:1422, 1985.

Ho PC and Kwan MSW: A prospective randomized comparison of levonorgestrel with the Yuzpe regimen in post-coital contraception, Hum Reprod 8:389, 1993.

Jain JK and Mishell DR Jr: A comparison of misoprostol with and without laminaria tents for induction of second-trimester abortion, Am J Obstet Gynecol 175:173, 1996.

Janerich DT, Piper JM, and Glebatis DM: Oral contraceptives and birth defects, Am J Epidemiol 112:73, 1980.

Jick H, Hanna MT, Stergachis A, et al: Vaginal spermicides and gonorrhea, JAMA 248:1619, 1982.

Jick SS, Walker AM, and Jick H: Oral contraceptives and endometrial cancer, Obstet Gynecol 82:931, 1993.

Kimmerle R, Weiss R, Berger M, and Kurz KH: Effectiveness, safety, and acceptability of a copper intrauterine device (CU Safe 300) in type 1 diabetic women, Diabetes Care 16:1227, 1993.

Kirton KT and Cornette JC: Return of ovulatory cyclicity following an intramuscular injection of medroxyprogesterone acetate (Provera®), Contraception 10:39, 1974.

Kjaer SK, Engholm G, Dahl C, et al: Case-control study of risk factors for cervical squamous-cell neoplasia in Denmark. III. Role of oral contraceptive use. Cancer Causes Control 4:513, 1993.

Kjos SL, Ballagh SA, LaCour M, et al: The copper T380A intrauterine device in women with type II diabetes mellitus, Obstet Gynecol 84:1006, 1994.

Kjos SL, Shoupe D, Douhan S, et al: Effect of low-dose oral contraceptives on carbohydrate and lipid metabolism in women with recurrent gestational diabetes: results of a controlled randomized prospective study, Am J Obstet Gynecol 163:1822, 1990.

Klaus H: Natural family planning: a review, Obstet Gynecol Surv 37:128, 1982.

Lanes AF, Birmann B, Walter AM, and Singer S: Oral contraceptive type and functional ovarian cysts, Am J Obstet Gynecol 166:956, 1992.

La Vecchcia C, Negri E, D'Avanzo B, et al: Oral contraceptives and noncontraceptive oestrogens in the risk of gallstone disease requiring surgery, J Epidemiol Community Health 46:234, 1992.

Lee NC and Rubin GL: The intrauterine device and pelvic inflammatory disease revisited: new results from the women's health study, Obstet Gynecol 72:1, 1988.

Lidegaard O and Milsom I: Oral contraceptives and thrombotic diseases: impact of new epidemiological studies, Contraception 53:135, 1996.

Lieu DFM, Ng CSA, Yong YM, et al: Long-term effects of depo-provera on carbohydrate and lipid metabolism, Contraception 31:51, 1985.

Linn S, Schoenbaum SC, Monson RR, et al: Lack of association between contraceptive usage and congenital malformations in offspring, Am J Obstet Gynecol 147:923, 1983.

Louik C, Mitchell AA, Werler MM, et al: Maternal exposure to spermicides in relation to certain birth defects, N Engl J Med 317:474, 1987.

Luyckx AS, Gaspard UJ, Romus MA, et al: Carbohydrate metabolism in women who used oral contraceptives containing levonorgestrel or desogestrel: a 6-month prospective study, Fertil Steril 45:635, 1986.

Mattson RH, Cramer JA, Caldwell BVD, et al: Treatment of seizures with medroxyprogesterone acetate: preliminary report, Neurology 34:1255, 1984.

Mattson RH and Rebar RW: Contraceptive methods for women with neurologic disorders, Am J Obstet Gynecol 168:2027, 1993.

Meade TW: Oral contraceptives, clotting factors, and thrombosis, Am J Obstet Gynecol 142:758, 1982.

Meade TW, Greenberg G, and Thompson SG: Progestogens and cardiovascular reactions associated with oral contraceptives and a comparison of the safety of 50- and 30-μg oestrogen preparations, Br Med J 280:1157, 1980.

Michaelsson K, Baron JA, Farahmand BY, et al: Oral-contraceptive use and risk of hip fracture: a case-control study, Lancet 353:1481, 1999.

Mileikowsky GN, Nadler JL, Huey F, et al: Evidence that smoking alters prostacyclin formation and platelet aggregation in women who use oral contraceptives, Am J Obstet Gynecol 159:1547, 1988.

Milson I, Anderson K, Jonasson K, et al: The influence of the Gyne-T 380A IUD on menstrual blood loss and iron status, Contraception 52:175, 1995.

Mishell DR Jr: Noncontraceptive benefits of oral contraceptives. J Reprod Med 1993; 38: 1021-9.

Mishell DR Jr, Ballagh S, and Kjos SL: Determining contraindications to IUDs. In Bardin WC and Mishell DR Jr, editors: Proceedings from the Fourth International Conference on IUDs, Boston, Mass, 1994, Butterworth-Heinemann, p 239.

Mishell DR Jr: Bell JH, Good RG, et al: The intrauterine device: a bacteriologic study of the endometrial cavity, Am J Obstet Gynecol 96:119, 1966.

Mishell Dr Jr, Keltzky OA, Brenner PF, et al: The effect of contraceptive steroids on hypothalamic-pituitary function, Am J Obstet Gynecol 130:817, 1978.

Mishell DR Jr, Kharma KM, Thorneycroft IH, et al: Estrogenic activity in women receiving an injectable progestogen for contraception, Am J Obstet Gynecol 113:372, 1972.

Mishell DR Jr and Roy S: Copper intrauterine contraceptive device event rates following insertion 4 to 8 weeks postpartum, Am J Obstet Gynecol 143:29, 1981.

Moore DE, Roy S, Stanczyk FZ, et al: Bleeding and serum d-norgestrel, estradiol, and progesterone patterns in women using d-norgestrel subdermal polysiloxane capsules for contraception, Contraception 17:315, 1978.

Moore LL, Valuck R, McDougall C, et al: A comparative study of one-year weight gain among users of medroxyprogesterone acetate, levonorgestrel implants, and oral contraceptives, Contraception 52:215, 1995.

Murphy AA., Zacur HA, Charache P, and Burkmand RT: The effect of tetracycline on levels of oral contraceptives, Am J Obstet Gynecol 164:28, 1991.

Naessen T, Olsson SE, and Gudmundson J: Differential effects on bone density of progestogen-only methods for contraception in premenopausal women, Contraception 52:35, 1995.

Newton JR, d'Arcangues C, and Hall PE: Once-a-month combined injectable contraceptives, J Obstet Gynecol 14(suppl 1):S1, 1994.

The New Zealand Contraception and Health Study Group: Risk of cervical dysplasia in users of oral contraceptives, intrauterine devices or depot medroxyprogesterone acetate, Contraception 50:431, 1994.

Ortiz A, Hiroi M, Stanczyk FZ, et al: Serum medroxyprogesterone acetate (MPA) concentrations and ovarian function following intramuscular injection of depo-MPA, J Clin Endocrinol Metab 44:32, 1977.

Pabinger I and Schneider B: Thrombotic risk of women with hereditary antithrombin III-protein C- and protein S-deficiency taking oral contraceptive medication: the GTH Study Group on Natural Inhibitors, Thromb Haemost 71:548, 1994.

Parazzini F, La Vecchia C, Negri E, and Maggi R: Oral contraceptive use and invasive cervical cancer, Int J Epidemiol 19:259, 1990.

Peipert JF and Gutmann J: Oral contraceptive risk assessment: a survey of 247 educated women, Obstet Gynecol 82:112, 1993.

Persson E, Holmberg K, Dahlgren S, et al: *Actinomyces israelii* in genital tract of women with and without intrauterine contraceptive devices, Acta Obstet Gynecol Scand 62:563, 1983.

Petersen KR, Skouby SO, and Pedersen RG: Desogestrel and gestodene in oral contraceptives: 12 months' assessment of carbohydrate and lipoprotein metabolism, Obstet Gynecol 78:666, 1991.

Peterson HB, for the US Collaborative Review of Sterilization Working Group (National Center for Chronic Disease Prevention and Health Promotion, Atlanta GA): The risk of pregnancy after tubal sterilization: findings from the U.S. Collaborative Review of Sterilization, Am J Obstet Gynecol 174:1161, 1996.

Peterson HB, Xia Z, Hughes JM, et al: The risk of pregnancy after tubal sterilization: findings from the U.S. Collaborative Review of Sterilization, Am J Obstet Gynecol 174:1161, 1996.

Petitti DB, Sidney S, Bernstein A, et al: Stroke in users of low-dose oral contraceptives, N Engl J Med 335:8, 1996.

Piccinino LJ and Mosher WD: Trends in contraceptive use in the United States: 1982-1995, Fam Plann Perspect 30(1):4-10 and 46, 1998.

Pituitary Adenoma Study Group: Pituitary adenomas and oral contraceptives: a multicenter case-control study, Fertil Steril 39:753, 1983.

Poulter NR, for the World Health Organization Collaborative Study of Cardiovascular Disease and Steroid Hormone Contraception: Venous thromboembolic disease and combined oral contraceptives: results of international multicentre case-control study, Lancet 346:1571, 1995.

Powell LMG, Mears BJ, Deber RB, and Ferguson D: Contraception with the cervical cap: effectiveness, safety, continuity of use, and user satisfaction, Contraception 33:215, 1986.

Rosenberg L, Palmer JR, Lesko SM, et al: Oral contraceptive use and the risk of myocardial infarction, Am J Epidemiol 131:1009, 1990.

Rosenberg L, Palmer JR, and Zauber AG: A case-control study of oral contraceptive use and invasive epithelial ovarian cancer, Am J Epidemiol 139:654, 1994.

Rosenberg MJ, Waugh MS, and Stevens CM: Smoking and cycle control among oral contraceptive users, Am J Obstet Gynecol 174:628, 1996.

Rothman KJ and Louik C: Oral contraceptives and birth defects, N Engl J Med 299:522, 1978.

Rowe PJ, for United Nations Development Programme/United Nations Population Fund/World Health Organization: Long-term reversible contraception: Twelve years of experience with the Tcu380A and Tcu220C. Contraception 56:341, 1997.

Ryden G, Fahraeus L, Molin L, et al: Do contraceptives influence the incidence of acute pelvic inflammatory disease in women with gonorrhea? Contraception 20:149, 1979.

Sandvei R, Ulstein M, and Woolen AL: Fertility following ectopic pregnancy with special reference to previous use of an intrauterine contraceptive device (IUCD), Acta Obstet Gynecol Scand 66:131, 1987.

Schlesselman JJ: Net effect of oral contraceptive use on the risk of cancer in women in the United States, Obstet Gynecol 85:793, 1995.

Schwartz SM, Petitti DB, Siscovick DS, et al: Stroke and use of low-dose oral contraceptives in young women: a pooled analysis of two US studies, Stroke 29:2277, 1998.

Schwallie PC and Assenzo JR: Contraceptive use: efficacy study utilizing medroxyprogesterone acetate administered as an intramuscular injection once every 90 days, Fertil Steril 24:331, 1973.

Schwallie PC and Assenzo JR: The effect of depo medroxyprogesterone acetate on pituitary and ovarian function, and the return of fertility following its discontinuation: a review, Contraception 10(2):181, 1974.

Senanayake P and Kramer DG: Contraception and the etiology of pelvic inflammatory disease: new perspectives, Am J Obstet Gynecol 138:852, 1980.

Shalev E, Edelstein S, Engelhard J, et al: Ultrasonically controlled retrieval of an intrauterine contraceptive device (IUCD) in early pregnancy, J Clin Ultrasound 15:525, 1987.

Shoupe D, Mishell DR Jr, Bopp BL, and Fielding M: The significance of bleeding patterns in Norplant implant users, Obstet Gynecol 77:256, 1991.

Sidney S, Petitti DB, Quesenberry CP Jr, et al: Myocardial infarction in users of low-dose oral contraceptives, Obstet Gynecol 88:939, 1996.

Sivin I: Dose- and age-dependent ectopic pregnancy risks with intrauterine contraception, Obstet Gynecol 78:291, 1991.

Sivin I: Contraception with Norplant® implants, Hum Reprod 9:1818, 1994.

Sivin I, Stern J, Diaz J, et al: Two years of intrauterine contraception with levonorgestrel and with copper: a randomized comparison of the TCU 380A and levonorgestrel 20 μg/day devices, Contraception 35:245, 1987.

Skegg DC, Noonan EA, Paul C, et al: Depot medroxyprogesterone acetate and breast cancer: a pooled analysis of the World Health Organization and New Zealand studies, JAMA 273:799, 1995.

Skouby SO and Milsted-Pedersen L: Consequences of intrauterine contraception in diabetic women, Fertil Steril 42:468, 1984

Spector TD, Romas E, and Silman AJ: The pill, parity, and rheumatoid arthritis, Arthritis Rheum 33:782, 1990.

Speroff L, DeCherney A, and the Advisory Board for the New Progestins: Evaluation of a new generation of oral contraceptives, Obstet Gynecol 81:1034, 1993.

Spitzer WO, Lewis MA, Heinemann LAJ, et al: Third generation oral contraceptives and risk of venous thromboembolic disorders: an international case-control study, Br Med J 312:83, 1996.

Tatum HJ, Schmidt FH, and Jain AK: Management and outcome of pregnancies associated with the Copper T intrauterine contraceptive device, Am J Obstet Gynecol 126:869, 1976.

Tredway DR, Uymezaki CU, Mishell DR Jr, et al: Effect of intrauterine devices on sperm transport in the human being: preliminary report, Am J Obstet Gynecol 123:734, 1975.

Trussell J: Contraceptive efficacy. In Contraceptive technology, ed 17, Hatcher RA, Trussell J, Stewart F, Cates W Jr, Stewart GK, Guest F, Kowal D, editors: Ardent Media Inc, New York, 1998, p. 779.

Trussell J, Ellertson C, and Stewart F: The effectiveness of the Yuzpe regimen of emergency contraception, Fam Plann Prospect 28:58, 1996.

Trussell J, Hatcher RA, Cates W Jr, Stewart FH, Kost K: Contraceptive failure in the United States: an update. Studies in Family Planning 21(1):51, 1990.

Trussell J, Kost K: Contraceptive failure in the United States: a critical review of the literature. Studies in Family Planning 18(5):237, 1987.

Trussell J, Leveque JA, Koenig JD, et al: The economic value of contraception: a comparison of 15 methods, Am J Public Health 85:494, 1995.

Trussell J, Strickler J, and Vaughan B: Contraceptive efficacy of the diaphragm, the sponge and the cervical cap, Fam Plann Perspect, 25:100 and 135, 1993.

Trussell J, Sturgen K, Strickler J, and Dominik R: Comparative contraceptive efficacy of the female condom and other barrier methods, Fam Plann Perspect 26:66, 1994.

United Nations Development Programme/United Nations Population Fund/World Health Organization/World Bank, Special Programme of Research, Development and Research Training in Human Reproduction: Long-Term Reversible Contraception: Twelve years of experience with the TCU 380A, Contraception 56:341, 1997.

Ursin G, Peters RK, Henderson BE, et al: Oral contraceptive use and adenocarcinoma of cervix, Lancet 344:1390, 1994.

Vandenbroucke JP, Koster T, Briet E, et al: Increased risk of venous thrombosis in oral-contraceptive users who are carriers of Factor V Leiden Mutation, Lancet 344:1453, 1994.

Van der Vange N, Blankenstein MA, Kloosterboer HJ, et al: Effects of seven low-dose combined oral contraceptives on sex hormone binding globulin, corticosteroid binding globulin, total and free testosterone, Contraception 41:345, 1990.

Van der Vange N, Kloosterboer HG, and Haspels AA: Effect of seven low-dose combined oral contraceptive preparations on carbohydrate metabolism, Am J Obstet Gynecol 156:918, 1987.

Vessey MP, Lawless M, McPherson K, et al: Fertility after stopping use of intrauterine contraceptive device, Br Med J 286:106, 1983.

Vessey M and Painter R: Oral contraceptive use and benign gallbladder disease revisited, Contraception 50:167, 1994.

Vessey MP, Villard-Mackintosh L, McPherson K, et al: Mortality among oral contraceptive users: 20 year follow up of women in a cohort study, Br Med J 299:1487, 1989.

Virutamasen P, Wongsrichanalai C, Tangkeo P, et al: Metabolic effects of depot medroxyprogesterone acetate in long-term users: a cross-sectional study, Int J Gynaecol Obstet 24:291, 1986.

Von Hertzen H, for the Task Force on Postovulatory Methods of Fertility Regulation (World Health Organization, Geneva): Randomised controlled trial of levonorgestrel versus the Yuzpe regimen of combined oral contraceptives for emergency contraception, Lancet 352:428, 1998.

Walsh T, for the IUD Study Group. Randomised controlled trial of prophylactic antibiotics before insertion of intrauterine devices, Lancet 351:1005, 1998.

Warner P and Bancroft J: Mood, sexuality, oral contraceptives and the menstrual cycle, J Psychosom Res 32:417, 1988.

Westhoff C: Depot medroxyprogesterone acetate contraception: metabolic parameters and mood changes, J Reprod Med 41(suppl 5): 401, 1996.

White MK, Ory HW, Rooks JB, et al: Intrauterine device termination rates and the menstrual cycle day of insertion, Obstet Gynecol 55:220, 1980.

Wilcox AJ, Weinberg CR, and Baird DD: Timing of sexual intercourse in relation to ovulation: effects on the probability of conception, survival of the pregnancy, and sex of the baby, New Engl J Med 333:1517, 1995.

Williams P, Johnson B, and Vessey M: Septic abortion in women using intrauterine devices, Br Med J 4:253, 1975.

Wilson JG and Brent RL: Are female sex hormones teratogenic? Am J Obstet Gynecol 141:567, 1981.

Wølner-Hanssen P, Svensson L, Mrdh PA, et al: Laparoscopic findings and contraceptive use in women with signs and symptoms suggestive of acute salpingitis, Obstet Gynecol 66:233, 1985.

World Health Organization: A prospective multicentre trial of the ovulation method of natural family planning. II. The effectiveness phase. Fertil Steril 36:591, 1981.

World Health Organization Expanded Programme of Research, Development and Research Training in Human Reproduction Task Force on Long-Acting Systemic Agents for the Regulation of Fertility: Multinational comparative clinical evaluation of two long-acting injectable contraceptive steroids: norethisterone enanthate and medroxyprogesterone acetate. Final report, Contraception 18:1, 1983.

World Health Organization: Combined oral contraceptives and liver cancer, Int J Cancer 43:254, 1989.

World Health Organization (WHO): The TCu220C, multiload 250 and Nova T IUDs at 3.5 and 7 years of use: results from three randomized multicentre trials, Contraception 42:141, 1990.

WHO Collaborative Study of Neoplasia and Steroid Contraceptives: Depot medroxyprogesterone acetate (DMPA) and risk of endometrial cancer, Int J Cancer 49:186, 1991.

WHO Collaborative Study of Neoplasia and Steroid Contraceptives: Depot medroxyprogesterone acetate (DMPA) and risk of epithelial ovarian cancer, Int J Cancer 49:191, 1991.

WHO Collaborative Study of Neoplasia and Steroid Contraceptives: Depot medroxyprogesterone acetate (DMPA) and risk of squamous cell cervical cancer, Contraception 45:299, 1992.

World Health Organization Collaborative Study of Cardiovascular Disease and Steroid Hormone Contraception. Venous thromboembolic disease and combined oral contraceptives: results of international multicenter case-control study, Lancet 346:1575, 1995.

World Health Organization Collaborative Study of Cardiovascular Disease and Steroid Hormone Contraception. Effect of different progestagens in low-oestrogen oral contraceptives on venous thromboembolic disease, Lancet 346:1582, 1995.

Wright NH, Vessey MP, Kenward B, et al: Neoplasia and dysplasia of the cervix uteri and contraception: a possible protective effect of the diaphragm, Br J Cancer 38:273, 1978.

Breast Diseases
Diagnosis and Treatment of Benign and Malignant Disease

KEY TERMS AND DEFINITIONS

Axillary Tail of Spence. A lateral projection of glandular tissue that extends from the upper, outer portion of the breast toward the axilla.

Cluster. A mammographic finding of five or more calcifications within a volume of a cubic centimeter.

Cooper's Ligaments. Fibrous septa that extend from the skin through the breast to the underlying pectoralis fascia.

Cystosarcoma Phyllodes. Fibroepithelial breast tumors that are rare and may arise from fibroadenomas.

Digital Radiography. The technique by which x-ray photons are detected after passing through the breast tissue and the radiographic image is recorded electronically in a digital format and stored in a computer.

Fibroadenomas. Firm, freely mobile, solitary, solid, benign breast masses.

Fibrocystic Changes. This is a general descriptive term that includes any change in contour of breast tissue. There is a wide spectrum and variation in clinical symptoms and palpable findings. Similarly, this term refers to a broad spectrum of benign histopathologic changes in the breast.

Intraductal Papilloma. Benign breast mass that is usually microscopic but may grow to 2 to 3 mm in diameter. The predominant symptom of an intraductal papilloma is spontaneous discharge from one nipple.

Lumpectomy. Conservative surgical procedure for breast carcinoma that involves removal of a wide margin of normal breast tissue surrounding a breast carcinoma less than 4 cm in diameter.

Modified Radical Mastectomy. An operation that includes removal of the breast and only the fascia over the pectoralis major muscle.

Montgomery glands. Accessory glands located around the periphery of the areola. They represent an intermediate gland in between sebaceous glands and true mammary glands and as such can secrete milk.

Myoepithelial Cells. Specialized cells in the lactiferous ducts that are peripheral to epithelial cells, thus forming a double cellular layer in the ductal system. These cells are believed to be involved in the milk letdown phenomenon.

Paget's Disease. Rare breast carcinoma that has an innocent appearance and looks like eczema or dermatitis of the nipple.

Polymastia. More than two breasts.

Polythelia. More than two nipples.

Radical Mastectomy. An operation that includes en bloc removal of the breast, as well as underlying pectoralis major and pectoralis minor muscles.

Simple Mastectomy. An operation that includes removal of the breast without underlying muscle or fascial tissue.

Thermography. Potential technique to diagnose breast disease by directly measuring either cutaneous temperatures of the breast or infrared radiation from the breast by electronic detectors.

Virginal Hypertrophy of the Breasts. Rare condition in which there is massive hypertrophy of the breasts at puberty.

The importance of early detection and diagnosis of breast carcinoma cannot be overemphasized. Breast carcinoma is the most common malignancy of women and is one of the two leading causes of all cancer deaths in women. It is the number one cause of death in women in their 40s. One in 8 women (12.5% of American women) develops carcinoma of the breast if she lives beyond age 90. Presently, the incidence of breast cancer in the United States is relatively stable. There has been an important reduction in breast cancer mortality in recent years. Since 1989, death rates from breast cancer have decreased an average of 1.8% per year. An increase in public awareness combined with recent improvements in mammography and newer imaging techniques has facilitated earlier detection of breast carcinoma. Combined with improvements in breast cancer therapy, improved survival rates are being reported. With the advent of chemoprevention of the high-risk woman, there is an opportunity to alter the natural course of the disease. The majority of women in whom breast cancer is diagnosed will not die of the disease.

The prognosis for and survival of a woman with breast carcinoma are improved by early discovery. Thus every gynecologist has an obligation to educate patients concerning self-examination of the breast and to develop a routine for carefully screening patients for breast disease. Detailed physical examination of the breast must be an integral step in evaluating every female patient.

Our culture attaches great significance to the female breast. An individual patient may react to the tremendous anxiety of suspected breast disease with behavior that varies from frequent visits to the physician for breast pain to denial of the presence of an obvious mass. The patient's description of her problem and her reactions to diagnoses and treatment must never be taken out of the context of this anxiety.

The major emphasis of this chapter is the epidemiology, detection, and diagnosis of breast carcinoma. Also, the chapter covers the chemoprevention of breast cancer as well as a discussion of benign breast diseases. Galactorrhea is presented in Chapter 39.

ANATOMY

The breasts are large, modified sebaceous glands contained within the superficial fascia of the anterior chest wall. A lateral projection of glandular tissue extends from the upper, outer portion of the breast toward the axilla and is called the *axillary tail of Spence.* The average weight of the adult breast is 200 to 300 g during the menstruating years. The mature breast consists of approximately 20% glandular tissue and 80% fat and connective tissue. The periphery of breast tissue is predominantly fat, while the central area contains more glandular tissue.

The breast is composed of 12 to 20 lobes arranged in radial fashion from the nipple. Each lobe is triangular and has one central excretory duct that opens to the exterior at the nipple. Milk originates in the secretory cells of the alveoli. It is subsequently transported by the branching collecting ducts of the lobules into the lactiferous sinuses and terminally into the excretory ducts of each respective lobe of

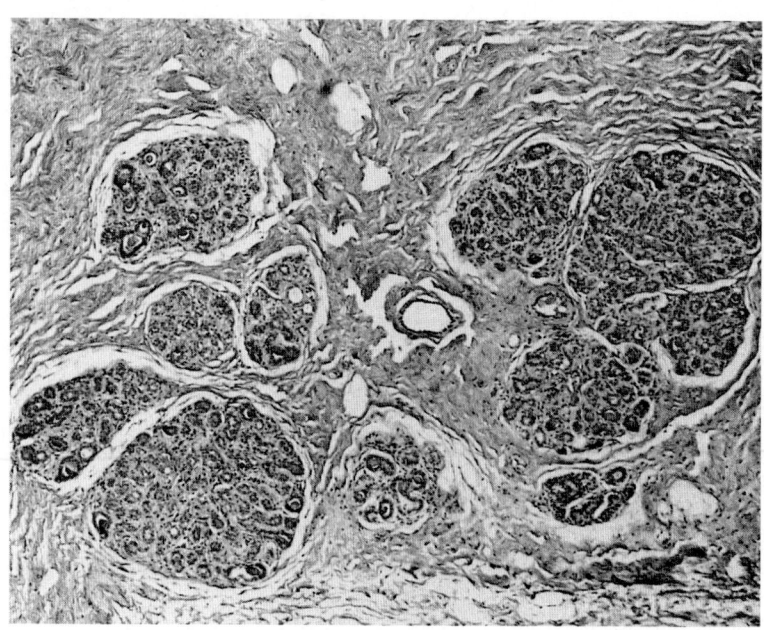

FIGURE 14-1 This low-power photomicrograph of a lobule illustrates the centrally located terminal duct and the peripherally arranged clusters of small glandular structures grouped within a loose fibrovascular stroma. The stroma exterior to the lobule and the terminal duct is composed of collagen-rich connective tissue. (From Powell DE: The normal breast: structure, function, and epidemiology. In Powell DE and Stelling CB, editors: The diagnosis and detection of breast disease, St. Louis, 1994, Mosby–Year Book, Inc.)

the breast. There is a wide range in number of lobules, between 10 and 100, in each lobe of the breast (Figure 14-1). *Montgomery glands* are accessory glands located around the periphery of the areola. Because they are structurally intermediate between true mammary and sebaceous glands, they can secrete milk. Fibrous septa, *Cooper's ligaments,* extend from the skin to the underlying pectoralis fascia (Figure 14-2). They are believed to offer support to the breast. Invasion of these ligaments by malignant cells produces skin retraction, which is a sign of advanced breast carcinoma.

The lymphatic distribution of the breast is complex. Approximately 75% of the lymphatic drainage goes to regional nodes in the axilla. The axilla contains a varying number of nodes, usually between 30 and 60. Other metastatic routes include lymphatics adjacent to the internal mammary vessels. After direct spread into the mediastinum, lymphatic drainage may go to the intercostal glands, which are located posteriorly along the vertebral column, and to subpectoral and subdiaphragmatic areas (Figure 14-3). Lymph drainage usually flows toward the most adjacent group of nodes. This concept represents the basis for sentinel node mapping in breast cancer. In most instances breast cancer spreads in an orderly fashion within the axillary lymph node basin based on the anatomic relationship between the primary tumor and its associated regional (sentinel) nodes. However, lymphatic

metastases from one specific area of the breast may be found in any or all of the groups of regional nodes. Krag et al. reported a large multicenter study to validate the use of sentinel node biopsy in women with breast cancer. All of the women studied had positive nodes. However, in just 3% of these women was the only positive node outside of the axilla. Metastases from one breast across the midline to the other breast or chest wall occur occasionally.

Breast tissue is sensitive to the cyclic changes in hormonal levels. The epithelium of the breast responds to fluctuating levels of estrogen and progesterone similar to other hormonally sensitive tissue. The stroma of the breasts and the myoepithelial cells of the breasts also respond to estrogen and progesterone. Women often experience breast tenderness and fullness during the luteal phase of the cycle. The average increase in volume of the premenstrual breasts is 25 to 30 ml, as measured by water displacement techniques. Premenstrual breast symptoms are produced by an increase in blood flow, vascular engorgement, and water retention. There is a corresponding enlargement in the lumina of ducts and an increase in ductal and acinar cellular secretory activity. During the follicular phase, there is parenchymal proliferation of the ducts. During the luteal phase, there is dilation of the ductal system and differentiation of the alveolar cells into secretory cells. The alveolar elements respond to both

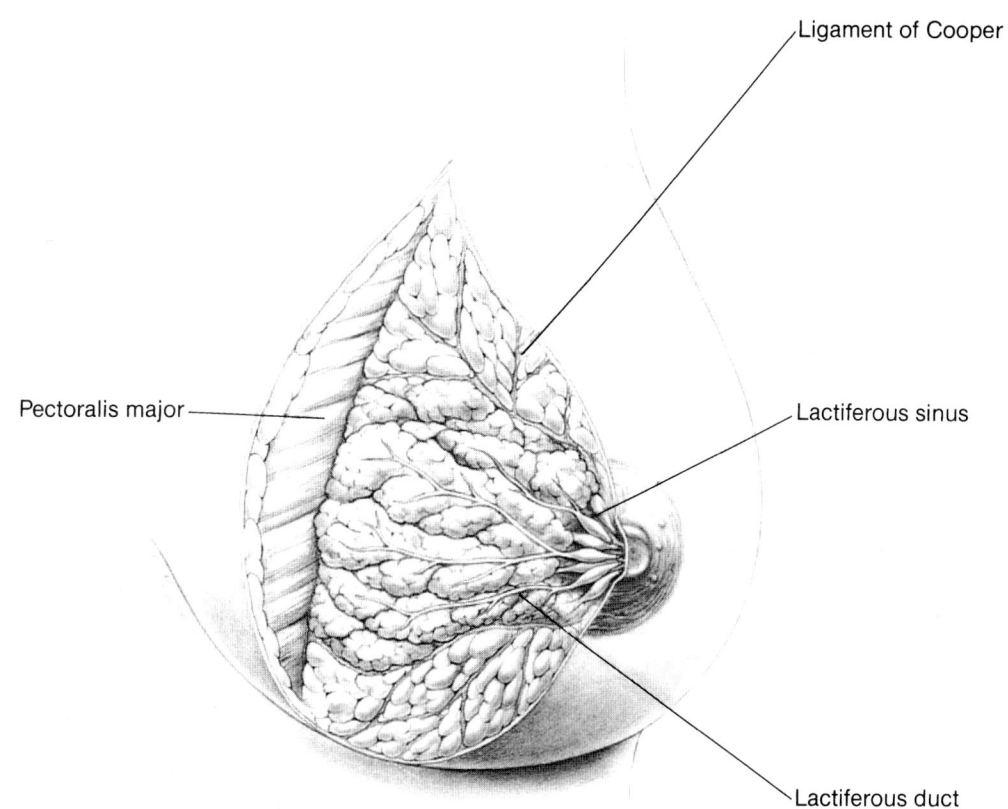

FIGURE 14-2 Anatomy of breast. (From Rehman I: Embryology and anatomy of the breast. In Gallager HS, Leis HP, Synderman RK, et al, editors: The breast, St. Louis, 1978, Mosby–Year Book, Inc, p 6.)

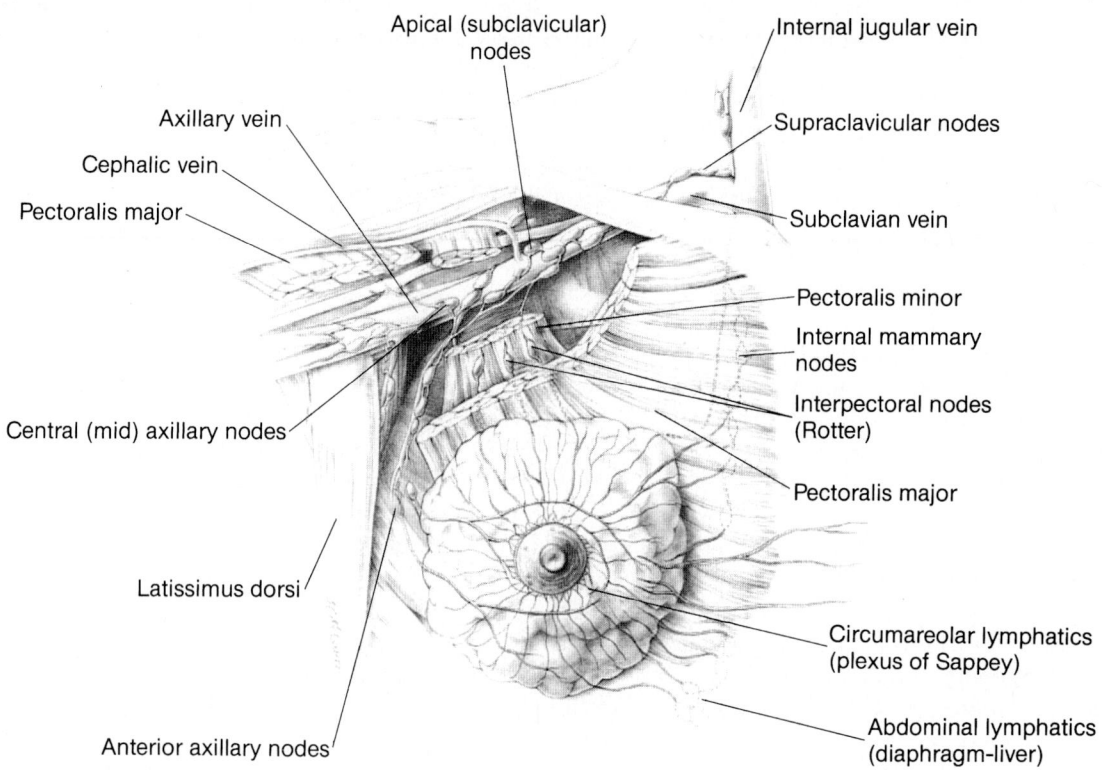

FIGURE 14-3 Lymphatics of breast. (From Rehman I: Embryology and anatomy of the breast. In Gallager HS, Leis HP, Synderman RK, et al, editors: The breast, St. Louis, 1978, Mosby–Year Book, Inc, p 17.)

estrogen and progesterone. When menstruation begins, there is a regression of cellular activity in the alveoli and the ducts become smaller.

Accessory breasts or nipples can occur along the breast lines, which run from the axilla to the groin. Supernumerary nipples (polythelia) or breasts (polymastia) are common anomalies (Figure 14-4), which may be well developed and functional or rudimentary. They occur in approximately 1% to 2% of Caucasian women and 5% to 6% of Asian women. Underdevelopment of one breast in relationship to the other is a common anomaly. In a recent study of 8408 mammograms, 3% were notable for asymmetric volume reduction relative to the contralateral breast. This asymmetry represented a benign, normal variation unless an associated palpable abnormality was present. Massive hypertrophy of the breasts at puberty (virginal hypertrophy) is a rare occurrence that has a deeply disturbing effect on a teenager's self-image (Figure 14-5). This condition is best managed by skillful cosmetic surgery.

BENIGN BREAST DISEASE

The classifications and terminologies of benign breast disease are confusing. Nevertheless, an understanding of these conditions is important. The symptomatology and physical findings of benign disease cause anxiety and fear in the patient, who often thinks the symptoms may be related to breast cancer. The common symptoms of breast disease—pain and tenderness—and the signs—a mass or nipple discharge—may result from either a benign or a malignant process. However, breast pain is a comparatively late symptom in women with breast carcinoma and is the sole presenting symptom in less than 10% of these women. During the second half of the menstrual cycle, the breasts increase in size, density, and nodularity. These three changes are often associated with increased sensitivity or pain.

Numerous epidemiologic studies have found an increased risk of developing breast carcinoma in women with benign breast disease with associated atypical epithelial hyperplasia. This risk varies from twofold to fivefold, depending on the degree of epithelial hyperplasia. The pathophysiology of the association between cellular atypia and subsequent carcinoma is straightforward and similar in concept to endometrial disease.

Dupont and Page performed the classic study on the relationship between benign breast disease and subsequent development of carcinoma. They followed more than 3000 women for at least 15 years after benign breast biopsy. The study population was divided into three groups of women according to histology of the original biopsy. The first group consisted of 70% of the women. Their biopsies

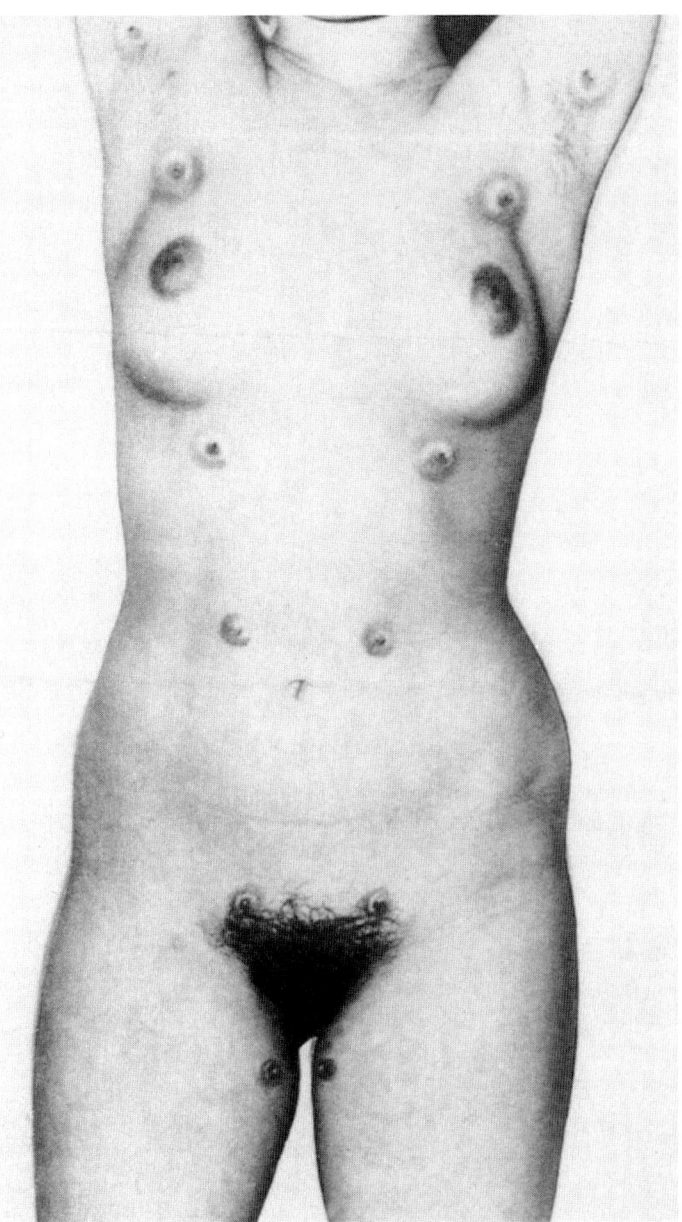

FIGURE 14-4 Extensive polythelia along milk line. (From Degrell I: Atlas of diseases of the mammary gland, Basel, Switzerland, 1976, S Karger AG, p 41.)

revealed no proliferative changes, and their diagnoses included adenosis, apocrine metaplasia, duct ectasia, and mild epithelial hyperplasia. During the 15 years of follow-up, only 2% of these women developed breast carcinoma. The second group of women, 26%, had breast biopsies that demonstrated varying degrees of epithelial hyperplasia but without atypia. Of these women, 4% developed breast carcinoma during the 15 years; their relative risk was increased 1.6-fold. The last group consisted of the 4% of women with histology that demonstrated atypical ductal or lobular hyperplasia. Their relative risk was 4 to 5 times greater for developing malignancy; 8% developed carcinoma during the 15-year follow-up.

Fibrocystic Changes

Fibrocystic changes are the most common of all benign breast conditions. Often, clinicians use the nonspecific term *fibrocystic changes* to describe multiple irregularities in contour and cyclically painful breasts. The term *fibrocystic disease* is a misnomer and probably should not be used. This condition has a prolific terminology that includes over 35 different names, with mammary dysplasia and chronic cystic mastitis being the two most common. The exact incidence of fibrocystic changes is difficult to establish. Frantz et al. found histologic evidence of fibrocystic changes in 53% of "normal breasts" examined

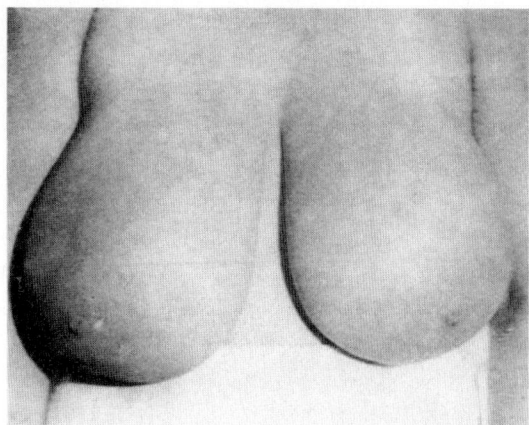

FIGURE 14-5 Virginal hypertrophy, age 13. (From Degrell I: Atlas of diseases of the mammary gland, Basel, Switzerland, 1976, S Karger AG, p 46.)

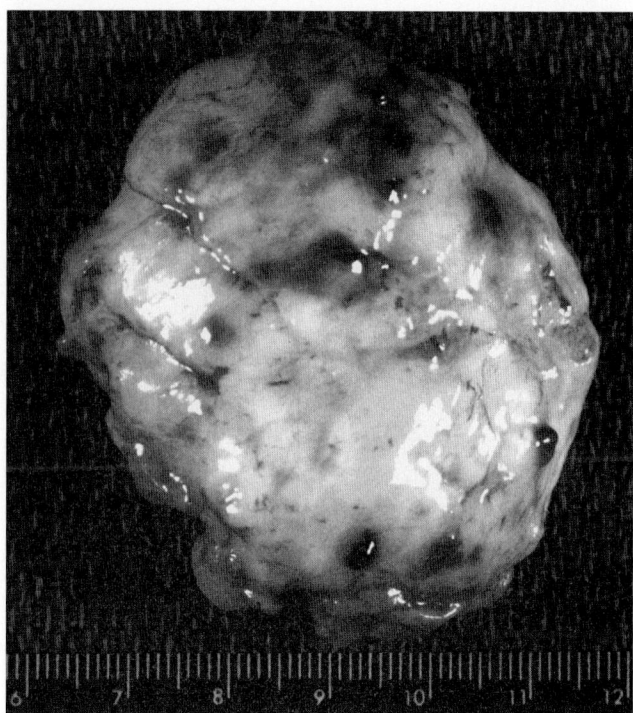

FIGURE 14-6 Breast biopsy from a 38-year-old woman demonstrating characteristic gross appearance of fibrocystic changes. Note multiple cysts interspersed between the dense fibrous connective tissue. (Courtesy Fidel Valea.)

in a series of 225 autopsies. Clinical evidence of fibrocystic changes is discovered in breast examinations of approximately one in two premenopausal women.

Fibrocystic changes are believed to be an exaggeration of the normal physiologic response of breast tissue to the cyclic levels of ovarian hormones. However, no consistent abnormality of circulating hormone levels has been proven. The condition is most common in women between the ages of 20 and 50 and unusual after the menopause unless associated with exogenous hormone use. Some postulate the etiology to be a subtle imbalance of the ratio of estrogen to progesterone. However, others have postulated that fibrocystic changes are secondary to increased daily prolactin production. Women with fibrocystic changes have enhanced prolactin production in response to thyroid-releasing hormone.

The classic symptom of fibrocystic changes is cyclic bilateral breast pain. The signs of fibrocystic change include increased engorgement and density of the breasts, excessive nodularity, rapid change and fluctuation in the size of cystic areas, increased tenderness, and occasionally spontaneous nipple discharge. Both signs and symptoms are more prevalent during the premenstrual phase of the cycle. The breast pain is bilateral, and it is often difficult for the patient to localize. The pain is most frequently located in the upper, outer quadrants of the breasts. Often the pain radiates to the shoulders and upper arms. Severe localized pain may occur when a simple cyst undergoes rapid expansion. The pathophysiology that produces these symptoms and signs includes cyst formation, epithelial and fibrous proliferation, and varying degrees of fluid retention. The differential diagnosis of breast pain includes referred pain from a dorsal radiculitis or inflammation of the costal chondral junction (Tietze's syndrome). The latter two conditions have symptoms that are not cyclic and are unrelated to the menstrual cycle.

On physical examination the findings of excessive

nodularity of fibrocystic changes have been described as similar to palpating the surface of a plateful of peas. Multiple solid areas are described as ill-defined thicknesses or areas of "palpable lumpiness" that are rubbery in consistency and may seem more two dimensional than the three-dimensional mass usually associated with a carcinoma (Figure 14-6). During palpation the larger cysts have a consistency similar to a balloon filled with water.

There are three indistinct clinical stages, with each stage having predominant histologic findings. Clinically these stages have considerable overlap. The stages are described to allow understanding of the condition's natural history.

The first stage occurs in women in their 20s and is termed *mazoplasia* (mastoplasia). Breast pain is noted primarily in the upper, outer quadrants of the breast. The indurated axillary tail is in the most tender area of the breast. During this phase there is intense proliferation of the stroma.

The second clinical stage of *adenosis* occurs generally in women in their 30s. The breast pain and tenderness are premenstrual but less severe. Multiple small breast nodules vary from 2 to 10 mm in diameter. The histologic picture of adenosis demonstrates marked proliferation and hyperplasia of ducts, ductules, and alveolar cells.

The last stage is termed the *cystic* phase and usually

occurs in women in their 40s. There is no severe breast pain unless a cyst increases rapidly in size. In this situation a woman experiences a sudden pain with point tenderness and discovers a lump. Cysts are tender to palpation and vary from microscopic to 5 cm in diameter. The cysts in fibrocystic changes often regress in size. The fluid aspirated from a large cyst is straw colored, dark brown, or green, depending on the chronicity of the cyst.

Women with a clinical diagnosis of fibrocystic changes have a wide variety of histopathologic findings. The histology of fibrocystic changes is characterized by proliferation and hyperplasia of the lobular, ductal, and acinar epithelium. Usually proliferation of fibrous tissue occurs and accompanies epithelial hyperplasia. Many histologic variants of fibrocystic change have been described, including cysts (from microscopic to large, blue, domed cysts), adenosis (florid and sclerosing), fibrosis (periductal and stromal), duct ectasia, apocrine metaplasia, intraductal epithelial hyperplasia, and papillomatosis. Ductal epithelial hyperplasia and atypia and apocrine metaplasia with atypia are the most prominent histologic findings directly associated with the subsequent development of breast carcinoma. If these two conditions are discovered on breast biopsy, the chance of breast carcinoma in the future is approximately fivefold greater than in controls.

The proper management of women with fibrocystic changes, depending on their age, includes appropriate imaging techniques, fine-needle aspiration cytology, as well as histologic evaluation with either a core needle or excision biopsy when indicated. If there is a persistent dominant mass or any uncertainty in the examination, a biopsy of the area should be performed to rule out a malignancy. There is a wide range of options for treating this condition. The treatment of fibrocystic change depends on the severity of symptoms and varies from mechanical support of the breast to extremely rare instances of surgical therapy for intractable pain. The vast majority of symptoms can be controlled by medical therapy. Initial therapy of fibrocystic changes consists of the patient wearing a "support" bra, which provides adequate support for the breasts both night and day. Diuretics during the premenstrual phase occasionally relieve breast discomfort. Minton has advocated advising patients to reduce their consumption of methylxanthines and tobacco. Methylxanthines are commonly found in coffee, tea, cola drinks, chocolate, and many nonprescription medications. Minton studied 106 women with clinical fibrocystic changes and found that in 68% the condition resolved and in another 24% the clinical symptoms improved by decreasing consumption of methylxanthines and nicotine. However, four recent case-control studies have found no association between caffeine or methylxanthine consumption and benign breast disease.

Oral contraceptives or supplemental progestins during the secretory phase of the cycle have both been used to treat fibrocystic change. Approximately 40% of women will have a recurrence of their symptomatology following discontinuation of oral contraceptives.

The drug of choice for severe symptoms is danazol. It is the only drug approved by the Food and Drug Administration for the treatment of mastalgia. Dosages of 100, 200, and 400 mg daily continuously for 4 to 6 months have been employed. Therapy should not continue more than 6 months because side effects are common and the dosage should be tapered as described by Harrison in one report and Sutton in another. Danazol relieves breast symptoms and decreases nodularity of the breast in approximately 90% of patients. This effect lasts for several months after discontinuation of danazol. Patients who do not respond to danazol should receive a trial of bromocriptine or tamoxifen. Bromocriptine, an inhibitor of prolactin, is given continuously in a dosage of 5 mg daily. Tamoxifen is a synthetic antiestrogen commonly used as a chemotherapeutic agent for breast carcinoma. Tamoxifen competes with estradiol for estrogen receptors in the breast. Small clinical studies have documented a 70% relief of breast symptoms when tamoxifen is prescribed for fibrocystic changes. Women with cyclic breast pain seem to respond better than those with chronic mastalgia.

Severe cyclical mastalgia has been associated with abnormal levels of certain essential fatty acids. Gateley reports a 58% response rate with cyclical mastalgia and 38% response rate with noncyclical mastalgia using dietary supplementation of gamma-linoleic acid with evening primrose oil. A dose of 3 g/day is well tolerated with few side effects.

On rare occasions a woman with severe fibrocystic changes is treated medically with GnRH agonists or surgically by total mastectomy. Subcutaneous mastectomy produces a better cosmetic result. However, it does not remove all the breast tissue. Thus, if the surgery is being performed prophylactically, the risk of breast cancer remains. Indications for surgery include intractable pain not relieved by medical therapy or biopsy evidence of a precancerous lesion.

Fibroadenomas

Fibroadenomas are firm, rubbery, freely mobile, solid, usually solitary breast masses. They are the second most common type of benign breast disease. Fibroadenomas most frequently present in adolescents and women in their 20s. Typically the young woman discovers the painless mass accidentally while bathing. Growth of the mass is usually extremely slow but may be quite rapid. Fibroadenomas do not change in size with the menstrual cycle, and they do not produce breast pain or tenderness. Approximately 30% of fibroadenomas will disappear and 10% to 12% become smaller when followed for many years. Pathophysiologically, fibroadenomas should be considered as an abnormality of normal development rather than true neoplasm. However, the long-term risk of invasive breast cancer is approximately 2 times higher than control patients. Women with fibroadenomas should be made aware of this risk and encouraged to maintain annual mammographic screening commencing at age 40.

The average fibroadenoma is 2.5 cm in diameter. Multiple fibroadenomas are discovered in 15% to 20% of patients. After surgical removal, fibroadenomas recur in approximately 20% of women.

Sometimes it is difficult to distinguish a fibroadenoma from a cyst. Mammography is rarely indicated in a woman under age 35. However, ultrasound is helpful in differentiating a solid from a cystic mass. If the etiology of the mass cannot be established by fine-needle aspiration, surgical removal is indicated. Regardless of age, any mass that rapidly increases in size should be removed as should any solid mass in a woman over age 35. Fibroadenomas can be removed without difficulty under local anesthesia. They are rubbery in consistency, well circumscribed, and easily delineated from surrounding breast tissue (Figure 14-7). Nonoperative management is appropriate for small fibroadenomas discovered in women under the age of 35 if three separate clinical parameters support the diagnosis of fibroadenoma. The three parameters are clinical exam, imaging evaluation (either mammogram or ultrasound), and fine-needle aspiration cytology. The characteristic features of a fibroadenoma are found in approximately 95% of all fibroadenomas. Thus conservative management can be considered with follow-up every 6 months. The only way to distinguish a fibroadenoma from a malignancy is

with either a histologic or cytologic evaluation. Despite the option of conservative management of a fibroadenoma, most women usually prefer to have the lesion excised.

Cystosarcoma Phyllodes

Cystosarcoma phyllodes are fibroepithelial breast tumors. However, microscopically, it is the hypercellularity of the connective tissue that is the distinctive characteristic of the tumor. Cystosarcoma phyllodes are rare in that they represent only 2.5% of fibroepithelial tumors and 1% of breast malignancies. They are the most frequent breast sarcoma. These rapidly growing tumors are most common in the fifth decade of life. In large series, the mean diameter of the tumor at time of diagnosis was approximately 5 cm. One in four of these tumors is malignant, yet only one out of ten metastasizes. If metastatic disease is discovered, it is the stromal tissue that predominates. Differentiation of benign from malignant tumors by strict histologic criteria has resulted in poor correlation in some series. Recent studies using flow cytometry have improved on the predictive value in differentiating the biologic nature of the neoplasia. The treatment of a benign cystosarcoma phyllode is excision of the mass, including a wide margin of normal tissue. Presence of microscopic tumor at the margins of the excised specimen is the major factor in predicting whether there will be a local recurrence of the tumor.

Intraductal Papilloma

The classical symptom of an intraductal papilloma is spontaneous bloody discharge from one nipple. This symptom usually appears in a woman in the perimenopausal age group. The discharge from the nipple is *spontaneous* and intermittent. The consistency of the discharge associated with an intraductal papilloma can be watery, serous, or serosanguineous. The amount of discharge varies from a few drops to several milliliters of fluid. Approximately 75% of intraductal papillomas are located beneath the areola. Often these tumors are difficult to palpate because they are small and soft. During examination of the breast, it is important to circumferentially put radial pressure on different areas of the areola. This technique helps to identify whether the discharge emanates from a single duct or multiple openings. When the discharge comes from a single duct, the differential diagnosis involves both intraductal papilloma and carcinoma. If multiple ducts are involved, the diagnosis of carcinoma is more likely. Radiologically, the involved duct may be identified by injecting contrast material into the duct with a small catheter (galactography). Intraductal papillomas are usually microscopic but may grow to 2 to 3 mm in diameter, extending radially from the alveolar margin. Treatment of an intraductal papilloma is excisional biopsy of the involved duct and a small amount of surrounding tissue. Although these tumors tend to regress in postmenopausal women and

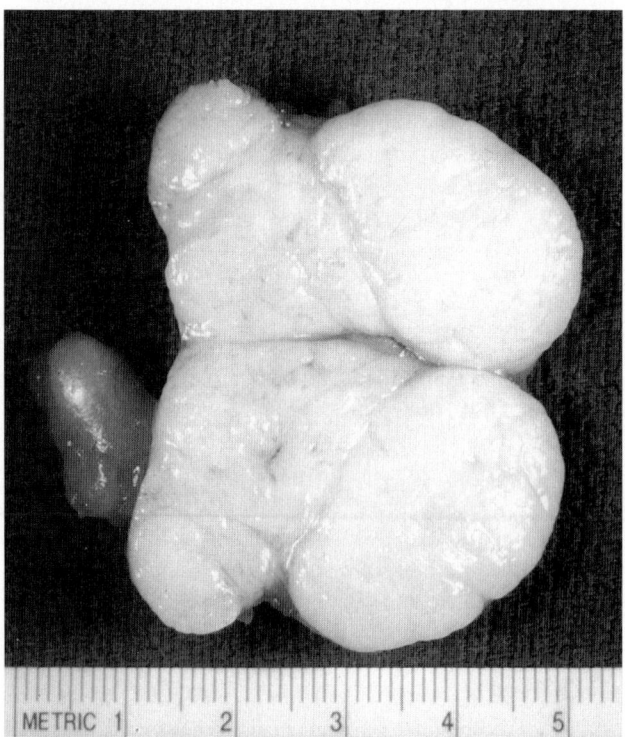

FIGURE 14-7   Classic fibroadenoma of the breast. (Courtesy Fidel Valea.)

occasionally diminish in size in premenopausal women, they should be excised. In Carter's series, women with a solitary papilloma showed an approximately twofold increased risk of subsequent development of carcinoma.

Nipple Discharge

Nipple discharge may be a complaint of women with either benign or malignant breast disease. Nipple discharge is a complaint of 10% to 15% of women with benign breast disease. However, nipple discharge is present in less than 3% of women with breast carcinoma. Leis reported a series of 7588 women with breast operations; 85% had a mass, and 7% had a chief complaint of discharge from the nipple. Of the 560 patients operated on for nipple discharge, 493 findings were benign and 67 malignant. If the nipple discharge is from a single duct, the chances of carcinoma are much less (Table 14-1).

To be medically significant, discharge from the breast should be spontaneous and persistent in a nonlactating woman. Many normal women can express a few drops of sticky gray, green, or black viscous fluid. The importance of diagnosing the etiology of *spontaneous* nonmilky discharge from the nipple is to rule out carcinoma. The color of the discharge does not differentiate a benign from a malignant process. Malignancies have been associated with clear, serous, serosanguineous or bloody nipple discharges. Importantly, bloody discharge from the nipple, gross or microscopic, should be considered to be related to carcinoma until this diagnosis has been ruled out. Cytology of the discharge is important but often not diagnostic. Most series document a false-negative rate of approximately 20%. Therefore a negative cytology should not deter surgical biopsy.

Before excisional biopsy a patient with a persistent discharge of any type should have mammography. In a young woman with a suspected intraductal papilloma, the involved duct, which is usually blue, and a small area of surrounding breast tissue can be removed. Table 14-2 documents that intraductal papillomas and fibrocystic changes are the two most common etiologies of spontaneous nonmilky nipple discharge. In this series, 50 of 432 patients had a carcinoma diagnosed by breast biopsy.

Fat Necrosis

Fat necrosis is rare but important because it is often confused with carcinoma. The patient presents with a firm, tender, indurated, ill-defined mass that may have an area of surrounding ecchymosis. Sometimes the area of fat necrosis liquefies and becomes cystic in consistency. Mammography may demonstrate fine, stippled calcification and stellate contractions. Occasionally there is skin retraction, which further confuses the prebiopsy diagnosis. The usual etiology of fat necrosis is trauma. However, the majority of women do not remember the event that injured the breast. Treatment of fat necrosis is excisional biopsy. There is no relationship between fat necrosis and subsequent breast carcinoma.

TABLE 14-1
Causes of Single Duct Nipple Discharge in 170 Patients (Nottingham 1988)

Diagnosis	Number (%)
Duct papilloma	77 (45)
Benign disease (for example, duct ectasia)	80 (47)
Cancer in situ	2 (7)
No abnormality	1 (0.6)

From Chetty U: Nipple discharge. In Smallwood JA and Taylor I, editors: Benign breast disease, Baltimore, 1990, Urban & Schwarzenberger.

TABLE 14-2
Relation Between Nipple Discharge and Diagnosis in 432 Operations from New York Medical College, 1960–1975

Discharge	Galactorrhea	Duct Ectasia	Infection	Intraductal Papilloma	Fibrocystic Disease	Cancer
Milky	2	0	0	0	0	0
Multicolored and sticky	0	46	0	0	0	0
Purulent	0	0	14	0	0	0
Watery	0	0	0	3	1	5
Serous	0	5	0	79	52	11
Serosanguineous	0	8	0	59	34	14
Sanguineous	0	6	0	45	28	20
TOTAL	2	65	14	186	115	50

Reprinted with permission from Pilnik S: J Reprod Med 22:286, 1979.

BREAST CARCINOMA

Epidemiology

The etiology of breast carcinoma is poorly understood despite extensive investigation. Epidemiologists have documented some risk factors that provide clues in understanding the pathophysiology of the disease's development in certain high-risk groups of women (Table 14-3). The risk factors can be divided into several categories: heredity, age, hormones, nutrition, demography, radiation, and previous breast disease. Generalizations concerning etiology follow similar categories: genetic predisposition, environmental carcinogens, viral agents, and radiation exposure.

Three problems obscure a clear understanding of the risk factors of breast cancer. One is the long latent period before the development of clinically recognizable carcinoma. Second, is the consideration both of the duration and the intensity of factors that may induce or promote cancer. For example, the peak incidence of breast carcinoma in Japanese women after the bombing of Hiroshima and Nagasaki occurred in women who were in the premenarcheal age group at the time of the atomic explosions. Subsequently these teenagers developed breast carcinoma in their mid-30s after the characteristic prolonged latent period. Korenman's estrogen window hypothesis suggests that the radiation (cancer inducer) acted with the background of the unopposed estrogen of adolescence (cancer

TABLE 14-3
Established and Probable Risk Factors for Breast Cancer

Risk Factor	Comparison Category	Risk Category	Typical Relative Risk
Family history of breast cancer	No first-degree relatives affected	Mother affected before the age of 60	2.0
		Mother affected after the age of 60	1.4
		Two first-degree relatives affected	4–6
Age at menarche	16 yr	11 yr	1.3
		12 yr	1.3
		13 yr	1.3
		14 yr	1.3
		15 yr	1.1
Age at birth of 1st child	Before 20 yr	20–24 yr	1.3
		25–29 yr	1.6
		≥30 yr	1.9
		Nulliparous	1.9
Age at menopause	45–54 yr	After 55 yr	1.5
		Before 45 yr	0.7
		Oophorectomy before 35 yr	0.4
Benign breast disease	No biopsy or aspiration	Any benign disease	1.5
		Proliferation only	2.0
		Atypical hyperplasia	4.0
Radiation	No special exposure	Atomic bomb (100 rad)	3.0
		Repeated fluoroscopy	1.5–2.0
Obesity	10th percentile	90th percentile:	
		Age, 30–49 yr	0.8
		Age, ≥50 yr	1.2
Height	10th percentile	90th percentile:	
		Age, 30–49 yr	1.3
		Age, ≥50 yr	1.4
Oral contraceptive use	Never used	Current use*	1.5
		Past use*	1.0
Postmenopausal estrogen-replacement therapy	Never used	Current use all ages	1.4
		Age, <55 yr	1.2
		Age, 50–59 yr	1.5
		Age, ≥60 yr	2.1
		Past use	1.0
Alcohol use	Nondrinker	3 drinks/day	2.0

Modified from Harris JR et al: N Engl J Med 327:319, 1992.

*Relative risks may be higher for women given a diagnosis of breast cancer before the age of 40.

promoter). Third, observational studies concentrating on a single risk factor often reach contrary conclusions.

Although there are limits in the clinical applicability of risk factors, selected women at increased risk may benefit from screening at more frequent intervals or consider some risk reduction measures. Pharmacologic or surgical prophylaxis has been proven to significantly decrease the risk of developing breast cancer. Many risk factors are additive. Risk factors are estimates developed by epidemiologists that allow patients and physicians to consider the probability of developing the disease. They have been widely publicized in the lay press. The fact that has not been emphasized is that risk factors identify *only* 25% of women who will eventually develop breast carcinoma.

The United States has one of the highest rates of breast carcinoma in the world. Incidence rates increased gradually from 1940 to 1990. Subsequently, they appear to have remained stable. The stabilization of rates probably results from the increase in detection and screening that occurred in the 1980s. The American Cancer Society estimates approximately 184,200 new cases of invasive breast cancer are anticipated in the year 2000 with approximately 41,200 deaths. The specific risk to an American woman of developing a breast carcinoma is 1 in 8 (12.5%) during her entire lifetime. The lifetime risk for an American woman without a single risk factor is 1 in 17 (6%). Therefore the message concerning risk should be that every woman in the United States is at risk for breast carcinoma.

Berg has made an interesting comparison contrasting breast cancer with another common gynecologic neoplasm, carcinoma of the cervix. In women ages 35 to 39, the rate of breast carcinoma is 55:100,000 women per year. This rate is 3 times greater than the rate for cervical carcinoma in the same age group. The risk of breast carcinoma during a woman's lifetime is similar to the risk of lung cancer in a heavy smoker.

Approximately 5% to 10% of breast cancers have a familial or genetic link. Genetic predisposition to develop breast carcinoma has been recognized in some families. In these families breast cancer tends to occur at a younger age and there is a higher prevalence of bilateral disease. Recently, mutations in BRCA family of genes have been identified that confer a lifetime risk of breast cancer that approaches 85%. BRCA1 and BRCA2 genes are involved in the majority of inheritable cases of breast cancer. These genes function as tumor suppressor genes and several mutations have been described on each of these genes. BRCA1 was mapped to chromosome 17, and in 1994 the DNA sequence of the gene was determined by Miki et al. Although the lifetime risk of breast cancer is approximately 85%, the risk of ovarian cancer is variable depending on the location of the mutation. The average lifetime risk of ovarian cancer is approximately 40% to 50%. The BRCA2 gene was mapped to chromosome 13, and the DNA sequence was determined by Schutte et al. in 1995. A woman with a BRCA2 gene mutation has an 85% lifetime

risk of breast cancer and a 15% to 20% lifetime risk of ovarian cancer. This mutation is also associated with male breast cancer, conferring a 5% to 10% lifetime risk for a male with the mutation. BRCA3 gene has been recently mapped to chromosome 8, but the details of the clinical syndrome have not yet been described. Because of multiple mutations of each gene and the possibility of differing penetrance of the mutations, the most appropriate clinical use of this genetic information continues to be a matter of intense debate. Presently, management recommendations vary from earlier and increased interval screening tests to prophylactic measures such as chemoprevention with tamoxifen, mastectomy, and oophorectomy. A task force convened by the Cancer Genetics Studies Consortium in 1997 recommended breast self-examination beginning by age 20, annual or semiannual clinical examination beginning at age 25 to 35 years, and annual mammograms beginning at age 25 to 35 years. They made no recommendation for or against prophylactic surgery in these patients. Hartmann recently presented the Mayo Clinic experience with 28 patients who had a BRCA gene mutation and underwent prophylactic bilateral mastectomy. In this series, the risk reduction was estimated at 91%.

The frequency of breast carcinoma increases directly with the patient's age (see box below and Figure 14-8). Breast carcinoma is almost nonexistent before puberty; the incidence gradually increases during the reproductive years. Eighty-five percent of breast carcinoma occurs after age 40. After menopause the incidence of breast carcinoma increases directly with a woman's age.

The relationship between endogenous ovarian hormones and breast carcinoma has been studied extensively. Several clinical observations support the hypothesis that the risk of breast carcinoma is related to the intensity and duration of exposure to unopposed endogenous estrogen.

Risk By Age: A Woman's Risk of Developing Breast Cancer

By age 25	1 in 19,608
30	1 in 2525
35	1 in 622
40	1 in 217
45	1 in 93
50	1 in 50
55	1 in 33
60	1 in 24
65	1 in 17
70	1 in 14
75	1 in 11
80	1 in 10
85	1 in 9
Ever	1 in 8

Data from National Cancer Institute. Painter K: Factoring in cost of mammograms, USA Today, p 11D, Dec. 5, 1996.

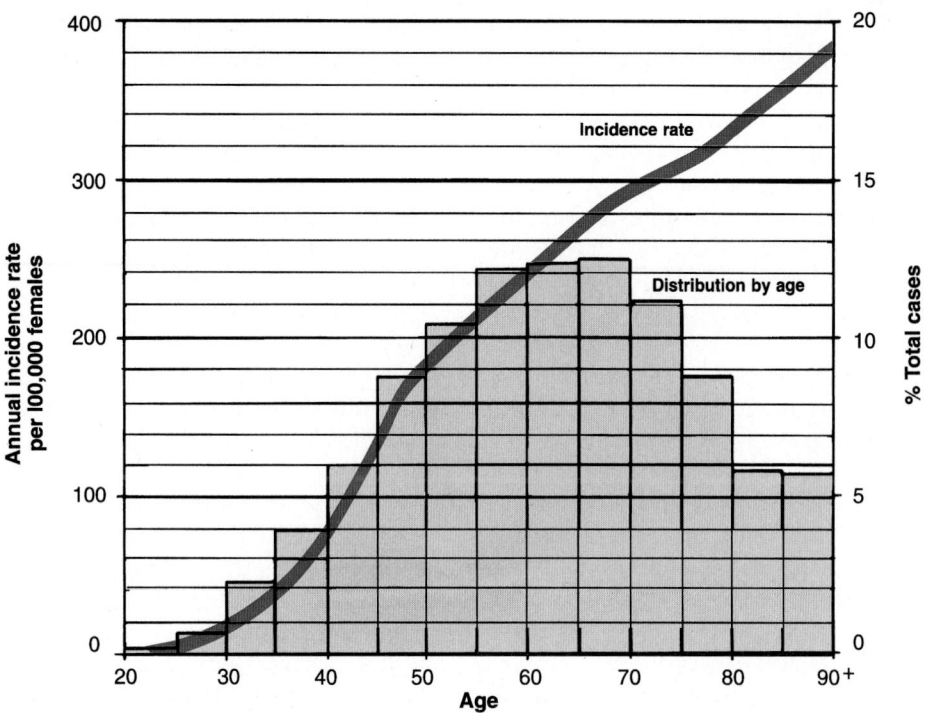

FIGURE 14-8 Incidence in the United States, by age, of female breast cancer. (From Seidman H and Mushinski MH: Breast cancer incidence, mortality, survival, and prognosis. In Feig SA and McLelland R, editors: Breast carcinoma: current diagnosis and treatment, New York, 1983, Masson Publishing USA, Inc. Copyright by American College of Radiology.)

Breast cancer is most unusual in the prepubertal female. Bilateral oophorectomy before age 35, without hormonal replacement, reduces the risk of breast carcinoma by 70%. Women have an incidence of breast carcinoma 100 times greater than that of men.

Obese women are at a higher risk for developing breast carcinoma during the postmenopausal years. The pathophysiology of this tendency is believed to be an increased amount of peripheral conversion of androstenedione to estrone and decreased levels of sex hormone–binding globulin. Marchant et al. described the increased risk associated with prolonged menstrual function. Women with spontaneous menopause before age 45 experience half the risk of developing breast carcinoma as do women who are still menstruating at age 54. A similar study documented a twofold increased risk for women who menstruated for 40 years or longer contrasted with that for women who menstruated for 30 years or less.

Demographic data describe significant variations in the incidence of breast carcinoma from country to country. In a descriptive review of the epidemiology of breast carcinoma, De Waard points out that women living in the United States have a much higher rate of breast carcinoma than women living in Africa, Asia, or the Middle East. The age-specific incidence of breast carcinoma in American women is 6 times greater than among women in Japan. Interestingly, studies of Japanese families who moved to the United States demonstrate that their rate of breast car-

cinoma becomes similar to that of American women after two generations. The demographic data were initially believed to be due to differences in total dietary fat and obesity. Epidemiologic studies performed within the same culture have demonstrated differences in incidences of breast cancer directly related to the amount of fat in the diet. However, recent epidemiologic studies, such as the Nurses' Health Study, failed to show any association between dietary fat and the risk of breast cancer. It is interesting to note that high consumption of olive oil modestly reduces breast cancer risk. Recently, the differences in breast cancer rates among the various groups is speculated to be due to caloric restriction in childhood. Dietary or lifestyle modification that shows the biggest reduction in risk is avoidance of weight gain in adulthood. Alcohol consumption has also been associated with breast cancer risk. Several studies have reported a 40% to 50% increase in the risk of developing breast cancer related to alcohol consumption. Longnecker showed that the risk of breast cancer was strongly related to the amount of alcohol consumed and that even light drinking was associated with a 10% increase in risk. Zhang reported that light consumption of alcohol was not associated with an increased risk of breast cancer. At the present time the effects of light consumption of alcohol on breast cancer risk is uncertain.

Ionizing radiation is a definite risk factor because of the long-accepted relationship between radiation and malignant transformation. The experience of Japanese women who survived the atomic bomb has been discussed. There are small groups of women who received multiple radiation treatments for postpartum mastitis, irradiation of the thymus in infancy, or multiple fluoroscopic examinations during treatment for tuberculosis who have subsequently developed breast carcinoma at an increased rate. The data concerning relative risk of developing breast carcinoma are most consistent with a linear dose-response relationship.

Previous history of breast disease is an important risk factor. Although the risk varies between premenopausal and postmenopausal women with breast cancer, once the patient has developed carcinoma of one breast, her risk is approximately 1% per year of developing cancer in the other breast. As emphasized previously, the extent of epithelial hyperplasia and atypia in women with benign breast disease determines the magnitude of risk for developing carcinoma. Women with ovarian, endometrial, or colon carcinoma have a twofold to fourfold greater risk of also developing breast carcinoma.

The age at which a woman delivers her first child is more important as a risk factor than parity. If a woman's first term birth occurs before age 20, she has 50% less risk than a nulliparous woman. If the first term pregnancy occurs after age 35, the risk is 1.5 times greater than for women who have their first baby before age 26. For many years it was believed that nursing an infant offered a protective effect for the future development of breast neoplasia. Subsequent studies have documented that this finding may be confounded by parity, timing of first pregnancy, and the relative length of anovulation. Newcomb et al. reported that after adjusting for parity, age at first delivery, and other confounding factors lactation was associated with a slight reduction in the risk of breast cancer among premenopausal women compared with those who had never lactated (relative risk, 0.78 [95% CI, 0.6 to 0.91]). Reserpine, which elevates prolactin levels, has been shown not to be a risk factor. Rosenberg et al. could find no relationship between cigarette smoking and the incidence of breast cancer.

There is no consensus on the association of exogenous estrogen administration, either as hormone replacement or in the form of oral contraceptives, and the risk of breast cancer. Numerous epidemiologic studies have failed to consistently demonstrate a detrimental impact of exogenous estrogen administration and breast cancer risk. Although some studies demonstrate a slight increased risk in the exogenous estrogen group, this risk is less than that associated with postmenopausal obesity or daily alcohol consumption. Recently, Schairer et al. concluded that current and recent users of an estrogen-progestin regimen had a higher increased risk of breast cancer than a patient using estrogen alone with relative risks of 1.4 (1.1 = 1.8) and 1.2 (1.0 = 1.4). This increase in relative risk was significant only in lean women. Estrogens are considered tumor promoters in respect to the pathophysiology of breast carci-

noma rather than inducers or initiators of carcinoma. Thus any adverse effect should increase with duration of use, and a dose-response curve should be recognized. Some recently reported epidemiologic studies have found an elevated risk for subsets of women under age 45. However, no consistent evidence showed an increase in breast cancer risk through middle age, even in long-term oral contraceptive users or in women with a family history of breast carcinoma (Chapters 13 and 42). If there is an increased risk, it appears to be small compared to other risk factors. The decision to use postmenopausal hormone replacement in patients with risk factors should be individualized, and the patient should be informed of the risks and benefits so she can make an informed decision.

Prevention

Breast cancer risk reduction should be considered throughout a woman's life. Although there is no proven benefit for women with low to normal risk, lifestyle modifications such as weight control, avoidance of smoking, decreased alcohol consumption, and exercise are associated with good general health. Most importantly, women with a high risk of breast cancer have proven options that can decrease their risk of breast cancer. In the National Surgical Adjuvant Breast and Bowel Project (NSABP) B-14 trial, tamoxifen users had a significant decrease in the incidence of contralateral breast cancers compared to placebo. As a result, the Breast Cancer Prevention Trial (BCPT) was designed to assess whether tamoxifen would decrease the incidence of breast cancer in a high-risk population as determined by the Gail model for breast cancer risk assessment. The trial enrolled 13,388 women in a double-blinded, randomized, placebo-controlled trial to evaluate the effects of tamoxifen on risk reduction. The trial was closed prematurely because of a large discordance between the two groups. Tamoxifen significantly reduced the incidence of breast cancer in this population of patients by 49% compared to controls ($p < 0.00001$). It did not reduce the incidence of estrogen receptor negative cancers.

Two other trials, the Royal Marsden Hospital trial and the Italian tamoxifen prevention study, failed to confirm this reduction in risk with prophylactic tamoxifen use. However, both studies were smaller and enrolled a lower risk population than the BCPT. Raloxifene, another selective estrogen receptor modulator, also reduces the relative risk. In a trial designed to test the efficacy of raloxifene on the prevention of bone fractures, 7705 postmenopausal women were treated with either raloxifene or a placebo. There was a 76% reduction in the incidence of breast cancer in the raloxifene group after 40 months of follow-up. As a result, the Study of Tamoxifen and Raloxifene (STAR) trial was designed and is currently enrolling women to determine which of the two drugs is superior in risk reduction. Until the results of the STAR trial are known, tamoxifen should be considered for breast cancer risk reduction in the high-risk patient according to the Gail model of breast cancer risk assessment. There is still no conclusive data on the use of tamoxifen in a population of patients with a BRCA gene mutation.

Surgical prophylaxis is another option for the woman who desires risk reduction. In a recent retrospective cohort of 639 patients, Hartmann was able to demonstrate a 90% risk reduction for the patient with a high risk of breast cancer after prophylactic bilateral mastectomy. In a follow-up study Hartmann was also able to demonstrate a similar risk reduction in a population of women with BRCA gene mutations. Although prophylactic bilateral mastectomy provides the greatest risk reduction it is usually reserved for the very high-risk patient because of the associated physiologic and complicated psychologic consequences. While most women who have undergone prophylactic bilateral mastectomy do not regret having undergone the procedure, approximately 5% to 20% report dissatisfaction according to Chlebowski.

Detection and Diagnosis

Detection of breast carcinoma is defined as the use of screening tests in asymptomatic women at periodic intervals to discover breast malignancies. The advantage of screening tests that facilitate early detection and diagnosis is reduced mortality because of smaller-sized cancers, more localized lesions, and a lower percentage of positive nodes. Established methods of detection include self-examination of the breasts, periodic examination by physicians, and mammography.

Physical examination and mammography are complementary procedures that must be considered together. Breast self-examination (BSE) has the major advantages of no cost to the patient and convenience. Diagnosis can be established only by biopsy or, sometimes, by fine-needle aspiration. Most importantly, a negative mammogram does not rule out breast carcinoma.

The kinetics of growth in breast carcinoma are important for understanding screening and detection. The average breast mass doubles in volume every 100 days and doubles in diameter every 300 days. A breast carcinoma grows for 6 to 8 years before reaching a diameter of 1 cm. In slightly less than another year the carcinoma will reach 2 cm in diameter. The mean diameter of a breast mass discovered by women who perform BSE at monthly intervals is 2 cm.

Greenwald et al. studied the results of BSE and of physician examination on the stage of breast carcinoma at initial diagnosis. Of 293 women with breast carcinoma, cancer was detected in clinical stage I in 54% when the detection method was routine physical examination, in 38% when the detection method was BSE, and in only 27% when the detection of the mass was accidental. In this study, only 50% of women who performed BSE did so on a monthly basis. These authors estimated that the breast cancer mortality might be reduced 19% by BSE and 24% by annual examination of the breasts by physicians.

In another study, Foster and Costanza determined the relationship between BSE and survival of breast cancer patients. Their study group included 1004 newly diagnosed invasive breast carcinoma in Vermont from July 1975 to December 1982. During this time, there was not widespread use of screening mammography in their state. The survival rate at 5 years was 75% for women who examined their own breasts versus 57% for women who did not examine their breasts. The authors concluded that in their population, BSE was responsible for earlier detection, improved survival, smaller tumor size, and fewer axillary node metastases. Their findings persisted after controlling the analysis for the potential bias of confounding variables, such as age, length-biased sampling, and lead-time bias.

In summary, present methods of screening for breast carcinoma are not ideal. Nevertheless, screening tests result in a reduction in mortality rate from breast cancer of approximately 25% to 30%.

Self-Examination of the Breasts

The majority of breast masses are initially discovered by the patient, either accidentally or during BSE. In a group of women having annual mammography and physical examinations by physicians, one of three carcinomas was discovered by the patients in the interval between professional detection methods. Even with widespread national publicity, approximately 50% of women do not perform monthly BSE. However, over 90% of women who regularly practice BSE were instructed in the techniques by their physicians. In Foster and Costanza's study of newly diagnosed carcinomas, 424 women performed BSE and 411 did not. The average size of the breast mass in women who performed BSE monthly was 2.1 cm. For those who performed BSE less than monthly, it was 2.4 cm; for the nonexaminers, 3.2 cm.

Although BSE has long been advocated, based on the studies cited here, its efficacy has been questioned because of the potential for bias. Several other studies have failed to show a benefit to BSE. In a recent case-controlled study within the Canadian National Breast Screening Study, Harvey demonstrated an odds ratio of 2.2 (95% CI 1.30 to 3.71) for cancer mortality or distant metastatic disease for women who omitted any part of the BSE. Although not conclusive, proficient BSE may reduce the risk of death from breast cancer.

The most effective teaching of BSE occurs in a one-to-one relationship. It is ideal to test the patient's ability to palpate masses in manufactured breast models. These models should contain masses with diameters as small as 0.3 to 0.5 cm.

Instructions for the patient concerning the techniques of breast self-palpation should emphasize timing, inspection, and palpation. The few days immediately after a menstrual period are the best time to detect changes in normal lumps or texture of the breasts. Postmenopausal women or women who have had a hysterectomy should be instructed to perform BSE on the same calendar days each month.

Women should be instructed that bilateral soft thickening and nodularity are normal physical findings. Palpation should begin in the shower, since many women have increased tactile sensitivity by using a "wet" technique. After the shower the woman should lie down, initially with one arm at her side and subsequently with the same arm underneath her head. She should be instructed to use the pads of her second, third, and fourth fingers to palpate the contralateral breast. Using the pads of her fingers, in a massaging motion with firm pressure, she should examine the entire breast and surrounding chest wall in a systematic fashion. One of the easier techniques to follow is to palpate the breasts in a clockwise fashion beginning at the nipple and gradually circumscribing larger circles. It is pragmatic not to include specific instructions for the woman to try to express secretions from her nipples.

Physical Examination

The ability to detect breast lumps varies widely from physician to physician. Fletcher et al. tested the physical examination techniques of 80 different physicians using manufactured breast models. The simulated breasts of the mannequins had a volume of 250 ml and the consistency of the breast tissue of a 50-year-old woman. The ability to detect the mass was directly related to the size of the mass; 87% of 1 cm, 33% of 0.5 cm, and 14% of 0.3 cm masses were discovered. The most disturbing finding was the wide range of detection rates among physicians, from 17% to 83%. In general, physicians with higher discovery rates spent more time performing the examination. The number of masses detected by a physician increased in those who used a consistent geometric pattern of examination with variable pressure exerted by the fingertips.

Although there has been widespread acceptance of physical exam as part of the screening for breast cancer, for ethical reasons there have not been randomized trials comparing physical exam to no screening. Several studies included the physical exam in addition to mammography, but only the HIP study demonstrated a significant reduction in breast cancer. Because 67% of the cancers in the HIP study group were detectable by physical exam, it was postulated that physical exam alone could have contributed to the reduction in breast cancer mortality. One randomized trial that compared physical exam with physical exam plus mammography for women over the age of 50 was the Canadian National Breast Screening Study II. Although there was no difference in mortality between the two groups it generated interest in screening by physical exam. In a recent meta-analysis of clinical breast exam by Barton, there was indirect evidence of the effectiveness of the clinical exam. Clinical breast exam discovered approximately 15% to 20% of breast cancers that were missed by mammography.

A thorough breast examination by the physician should take 3 to 5 minutes to complete. This time is also an ideal opportunity to instruct the patient in the technique of BSE. A complete breast examination involves inspecting and palpating the breasts with the patient in the sitting as well as the supine position.

Initially, with a woman sitting on the examining table, the physician inspects the contour, symmetry, and vascular pattern of the breasts and the skin for irritation, retraction, or edema. It is important to have the patient place her arms above her head and subsequently place her hands on her hips. This sequence will contract the pectoralis muscles, which may allow the physician to visualize an abnormality. The patient in the sitting position is in the optimal position for the physician to determine the presence of adenopathy in the axilla (Figure 14-9).

The woman's breasts should be subsequently examined with the woman in the supine position. It is important to examine both nipples for retraction, skin irritation, or a discharge. The areola should be compressed to identify any discharge. The normal breast has a small depression directly below the nipple. The skin of the breast is again carefully inspected for unusual vascular patterns, edema, erythema, or retraction.

Palpation is performed with both the woman's arms at her side and raised above her head and should not be limited to the breast tissue alone. A small pillow placed under the shoulder of the breast being examined often improves the examination. The examiner should palpate the axilla, the supraclavicular areas, and the adjacent chest wall. Palpation should use the pads of the first three fingers placed together, exerting firm but gentle pressure. Each physician

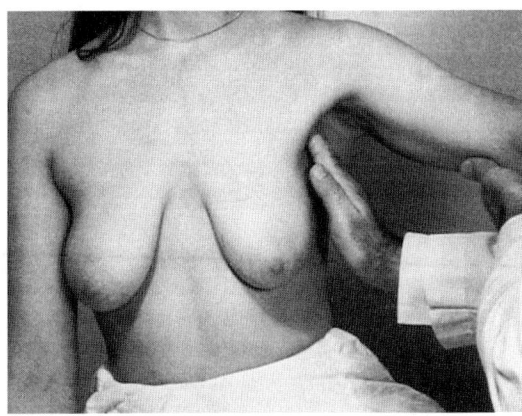

FIGURE 14-9 Examination of axilla in sitting position during breast examination. (From Marchant DJ: Clin Obstet Gynecol 25:361, 1982.)

determines his or her own systematic approach to examining all quadrants of the breast, the majority preferring concentric circles. It is very important that the physician draw a descriptive picture of any positive finding. This picture should include notations concerning the site, shape, size, consistency, and mobility of the mass. Special notation should be made as to whether the mass is tender and whether it is attached to skin or deep structures (Figure 14-10). Physical examination is excellent as a screening procedure, but extremely poor in predicting the histopathology of the lesion. Studies have demonstrated that 30% to 40% of breast masses suspected by palpation to be malignant were found after biopsy to be benign. Conversely, 15% to 20% of benign-appearing masses during a physical examination subsequently are discovered to be carcinoma by histopathology.

Mammography

Mammography currently is the most practical method of detecting breast carcinoma at an early and highly curable stage, ideally discovering an occult cancer (less than 5 mm in diameter). The clinical advantages of discovering breast carcinoma during its earliest stage include higher percentage of localized disease, lower incidence of positive regional nodes, and reduced mortality. The 5-year survival of women whose breast cancer is believed to be localized to the breast with negative axillary nodes is approximately 85%. In contrast, the 5-year survival is only 53% when axillary nodes are positive. Ten-year survival statistics in women with negative nodes are approximately 74%, and 39% in women with positive nodes. Mammography is also the most accurate conventional method of detecting

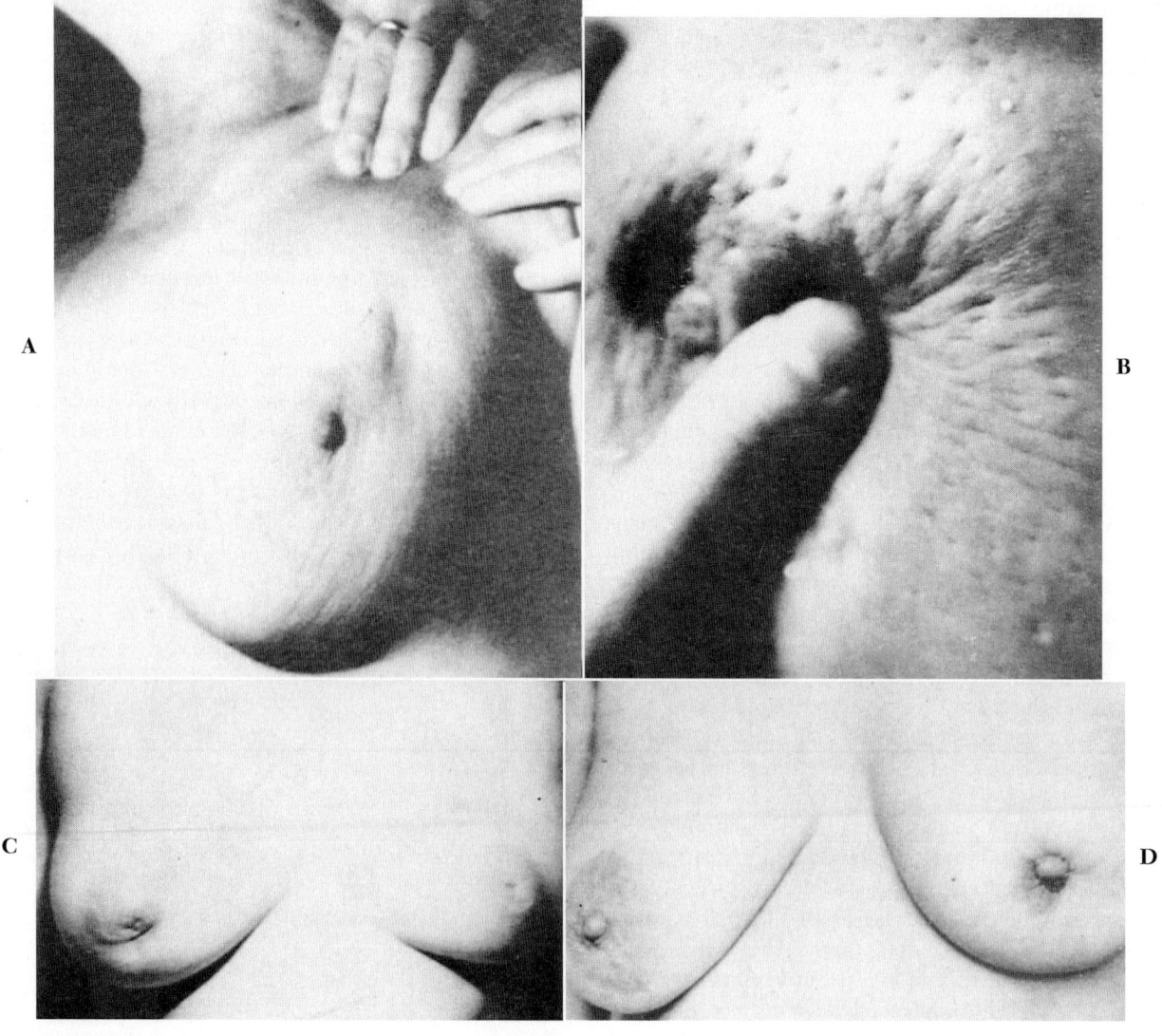

FIGURE 14-10   Signs of breast carcinoma. **A,** Retraction found during physical examination. **B,** Peau d'orange from underlying carcinoma. **C,** Retraction of right nipple. **D,** Retraction of left nipple from carcinoma. (From Degrell I: Atlas of diseases of the mammary gland, Basel, Switzerland, 1976, S Karger AG, p 20.)

nonpalpable breast carcinoma. Therefore, with increasing emphasis on conservative surgery for early carcinomas, mammography will not only save lives but also conserve breasts. The number of women receiving screening mammography has increased dramatically over the past 10 years. Mammography is not as precise in younger women or in women with dense breasts secondary to fibroglandular tissue. Mammography is most sensitive in older women in which the majority of the breast is composed of fatty tissue.

Most physicians are able to consistently palpate breast masses when they are 1 cm in diameter or greater. Mammography may discover fine calcifications in breast neoplasms months to years before the carcinoma enlarges to a size that may be palpated on physical examination. Studying the kinetics of growth of breast cancer helps the clinician to appreciate why breast carcinoma is so often a systemic disease. Breast carcinoma must develop neovascularization to grow beyond 1 to 2 mm in diameter. Neovascularization provides the breast carcinoma the capability of metastasizing via the vascular system. It has been demonstrated that the development of angiogenesis as measured by microvessel density in histopathologic sections is the strongest independent predictor of relapse-free survival in women with node-negative breast cancer. The average breast carcinoma grows for 3 years, to enlarge from 1 mm to 1 cm.

Image quality in mammography has undergone major improvements since the 1980s. New equipment has decreased the radiation exposure associated with mammography approximately tenfold. The vast majority of screening mammography in the mid-1990s is performed by dedicated mammographic equipment. Recently, there has been an increase in the routine use of grids and automatic exposure control. New film/screen combinations and improved film processing have facilitated superior images and sometimes reduced radiation dose. Conservative estimates are that 50 million American women should be screened by mammography each year. This challenge to radiologists has been summarized by McLelland. He believes there are two definite restraints on the optimal use of mammography to identify early breast carcinoma: a lack of properly trained and committed radiologists and the cost of the test. McLelland emphasizes that mammography is a technically demanding procedure that requires an experienced and meticulous interpretation of the films, as well as correlation of the images with a thorough clinical examination. Recently, Elmore et al. reported the diagnostic consistency between pairs of radiologists in interpretation of mammograms. This consistency was moderate, with a median weight for percent of agreement at 78%. The frequency of the radiologists' recommendations for an immediate workup ranged from 74% to 96% in the woman with cancer and from 11% to 67% in the woman without cancer.

Historically, two landmark studies laid the foundation for the scientific credibility of mammography as a screening procedure. The first large, randomized control study was undertaken in the early 1960s by the Health Insurance Plan of New York (HIP). The HIP investigation involved yearly screening by both mammography and physical examination for 5 years. The women were followed for 10 to 14 years, and the study demonstrated a 30% reduction in mortality from breast carcinoma in the women who had annual mammography compared with the control group.

The second pivotal study was performed in 29 centers throughout the United States during the late 1970s. This immense undertaking was sponsored by the National Institutes of Health and was named the Breast Cancer Detection Demonstration Project (BCDDP). The BCDDP involved screening 275,000 women, and during the 5 years of the project, 3557 breast carcinomas were found, 42% discovered only by mammography.

The definite improvements in mammographic diagnosis over the 12-year interval between the two studies is documented by comparing their results. Cancer detection was approximately two times more frequent in the BCDDP study. In women ages 40 to 49, mammography found 39% of carcinomas in the HIP investigation, compared with 85% identified in the BCDDP project. Most important, in the detection of carcinoma less than 1 cm, the results were 36% in the BCDDP versus 8% in the HIP.

Present studies demonstrate that screening mammography reduces breast cancer mortality by approximately 33% in women 50 to 70 years of age. Even though screening mammography does not show a similar benefit for women 40 to 49 years of age, the most recent international randomized trials show about a 17% reduction in breast cancer mortality for women screened in this age group. Obviously, the sensitivity and specificity of a screening test are key factors in the success of the early detection of cancer.

Hormone replacement may alter the effectiveness of mammographic screening. Lundström et al. demonstrated that an increase in mammographic density was much more common in women receiving continuous combination hormone replacement (52%) than women using cyclic (13%) and estrogen only (18%) treatment. This was further substantiated by Greendale et al., who noted an increase in mammographic density for patients on hormone replacement. However, almost all the changes occurred within the first year of use. Laya et al. demonstrated that the specificity of mammography was significantly lower in current users of estrogen replacement therapy (82%), than in women who had never had estrogen replacement therapy (85%). Similarly, sensitivity also was significantly lower in current users (69%) versus 94% for never users. Thurfjell et al. did not detect any decrease in sensitivity of screening mammography in women currently using hormone replacement therapy, but there was some marginal decrease in specificity varying with the regimen and duration of treatment.

Present recommendations to detect breast cancer include encouraging all adult women to perform BSE monthly. The American Cancer Society recommends a clinical breast exam every 3 years for women under 40 and yearly for women over 40 years of age. Because one third of breast carcinomas occur before age 50, increasing emphasis is being placed on early discovery in young women. After many years of debate there is consensus among the American Cancer Society, the American College of Radiology, and the American College of Obstetricians and Gynecologists that annual screening mammography should be offered to all women starting at the age of 40. There is a benefit to screening, although the reduction in mortality may not be as great for women age 40 to 49 years. In the United States more than 10,000 deaths occur each year in women who initially developed breast carcinoma between the ages of 40 and 49. Sickles and Kopans have reported that a meta-analysis of recent studies shows a 21% mortality reduction in women who have had mammographic screening compared with those in control groups. They further conclude that screening is at least as beneficial for women who are ages 40 to 49 as it is for those ages 50 to 64 years.

Obviously, many other nonscientific factors affect an individual physician and an individual woman's decision. Among the more prominent of these are the cost of the test and the patient's anxiety regarding breast cancer. In addition, the anxiety related to false-positive mammograms can be an obstacle to screening. Elmore et al. performed a 10-year retrospective cohort study of breast cancer screening and discovered that over 10 years, one third of the women screened had additional evaluations because of abnormal screening tests. Multiple studies document that the primary barrier to mammographic screening is the lack of a strong recommendation from the woman's primary care physician. More frequent physical examinations and mammograms may be indicated, depending on individual risk factors and the finding of precursors of breast carcinoma.

Mammography is established as part of the diagnostic workup of women with breast symptoms. Often significant occult disease is identified in another quadrant of the same breast or in the contralateral breast. All patients with breast masses or persistent spontaneous nipple discharge should have mammograms of both breasts before biopsy. Mammography is also indicated in evaluating a breast mass the patient has found but that the physician cannot confirm by palpation. This technique is helpful in difficult clinical problems, such as the evaluation of large breasts or following augmentation mammoplasty. It is important to stress once again that mammography and physical examination are complementary procedures. One procedure does not replace the necessity of carefully performing the other.

Optimal identification of early breast carcinoma by mammography depends on a competent technician obtaining excellent images and the radiologist searching for subtle changes. For screening mammography, two views of each breast are performed: the mediolateral oblique (MLO) and the craniocaudal (CC). The MLO is the most effective single view because it includes the greatest amount of breast tissue and is the only view that includes all of the upper-outer quadrant and axillary tail. Sickles emphasized the importance of firm breast compression of the breast during mammography for the following reasons (Figure 14-11). First, it holds the breast still to prevent motion artifact. It brings the objects closer into view reducing the amount of blur. It also serves to separate overlapping tissues that can obscure an underlying lesion. Finally, it decreases the amount of radiation exposure by making the breast thinner and easier to penetrate with less radiation. Sickles further advocated the importance of side-by-side comparison of both breasts and evaluating current films with previous ones. This facilitates identification of the less classic, indirect signs of breast carcinoma, such as a single dilated duct with intraductal carcinoma, asymptomatic architectural distortion in dense breasts, and a developing density.

Breast cancer may be detected by visualizing clusters of fine calcifications, spiculations, or poorly defined multinodular masses with irregular contours, all characteristic of malignancy. Isolated clusters of tiny calcifications are the most common and important diagnostic sign of an early carcinoma. Calcifications are often smaller than 0.5 mm in diameter and thus must be identified by a magnifying lens. The presence of five or more calcifications within a volume of 1 cm^3 is termed a *cluster*. Subsequent breast biopsies will find 25% of clusters associated with cancer and 75% with benign disease. Conversely, approximately 68% of occult breast carcinomas and 34% of palpable breast cancers demonstrate calcifications on mammographic examination.

Standardized terminology should be used to describe mammographic findings. As a result, the American College of Radiology Breast Imaging Reporting and Data System (BIRADS) was devised to standardize mammographic terminology, reduce confusing interpretations, and facilitate the monitoring of outcomes. The report includes an overall assessment of the likelihood that the finding represents a malignancy. There are six assessment categories, each associated with a specific risk of cancer. In the conclusion of every mammogram report, the final assessment is provided to prevent confusion and to guide the referring health care professional as to a recommended plan of action.

Computer-aided diagnosis has been an area of active investigation in recent years. Delineation by computer program of microcalcifications and masses gives the radiologist a second opinion of the mammographic films. It has been long established that double-reading of a mam-

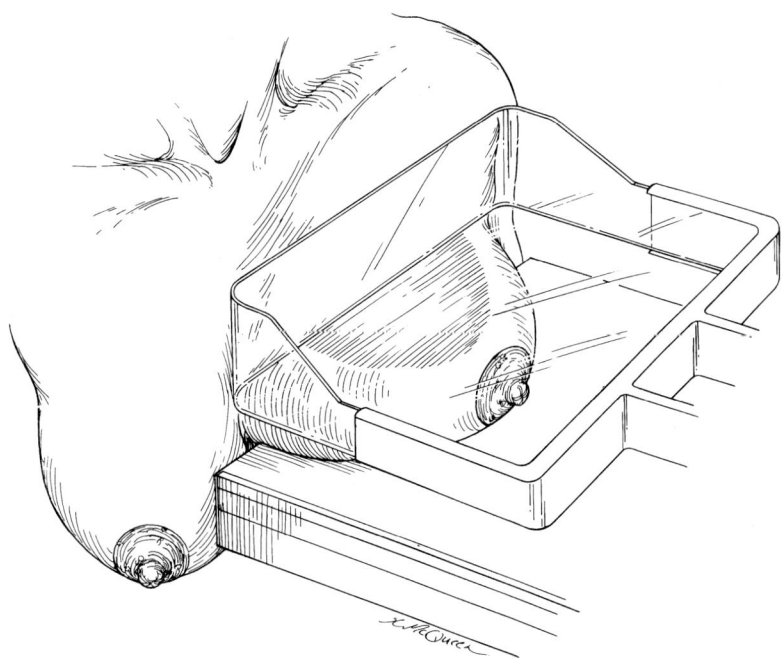

FIGURE 14-11 Mammography being performed with appropriate compression applied. (Redrawn from Wilson OL: Mammographic technique. In Parsons CA, editor: Diagnosis of breast disease: imaging, clinical features, and pathology, London. Copyright 1983, Chapman & Hall Ltd, p 67.)

mographic study by two independent observers improves the breast cancer detection rate by approximately 10%. Obviously, it also increases the cost of screening. Computer-aided diagnosis shows promise of potentially detecting lesions that would not be identified by double-reading.

The relationship between high levels of radiation and increased risk for breast carcinoma raises questions concerning the relative risk of the carcinogenic effect of mammography. The measured radiation dose to the breast by state-of-the-art mammography equipment is approximately 0.1 rad (0.001 Gy) for a two-view examination. Mettler et al. have summarized the recent literature regarding the benefits versus the risks from screening mammography. Their findings are that for a woman beginning annual screening at age 50 and continuing until age 75 the benefit exceeds the risk secondary to radiation by a factor of almost 100. For a high-risk woman who begins annual screening at age 35 the benefit/risk in reduced mortality is more than twenty-fivefold (Table 14-4). Thus the benefits of screening far outweigh any possible radiation risk.

The incidence of breast carcinoma in the United States is 1000 cases per million women per year for women in their early 40s. In summary, the risk of radiation from mammography is negligible compared with the benefits of the discovery of early and potentially curable breast carcinoma.

Diagnostic mammography is a comprehensive radio-logic examination that usually involves multiple individualized and specialized equipment and views. The extra views and magnification increase the sensitivity and specificity of the procedure. Often mammography is used to locate a breast lesion prior to open biopsy or to obtain stereotactic core biopsy during mammographic imaging. Although the primary role of mammography is to screen women with no symptoms or signs of breast cancer, mammography is also used diagnostically. The diagnostic follow-up to an abnormal screening mammogram is individualized depending on a woman's risk factors, physical examination, and age. The BIRADS classification of screening mammograms can be helpful in assessing risk and devising a management plan (Figure 14-12). Obviously, it is ideal to use nonsurgical methods to manage low-risk women and try to perform stereotactic or open biopsy depending on relative risk.

Ultrasound

Ultrasound has a definite role as a complementary procedure to other imaging techniques in the diagnosis of breast disease, particularly in differentiating cystic from solid masses. It should not be used as a "screening test" except for women with very dense breasts who cannot be adequately screened with mammography. Ultrasound screening increased the detection of otherwise occult cancers by 37% in a recent study involving 3626 women aged 42 to 67, with dense breasts and no visi-

TABLE 14-4
Breast Cancer Benefit/Risk Ratio for a Woman Having Annual Mammography Beginning at Age 35

Age	Annual Baseline Breast Cancer Incidence per 100,000	Fatal Radiation-Induced Cases	Fatal Cases Prevented by Mammography	Benefit/Risk Ratio
35	66	0	1.3	
36	66	0	1.3	
37	66	0	1.3	
38	66	0	1.3	
39	66	0	1.3	
40	129	0	12.9	>400
41	129	0	12.9	
42	129	0	12.9	
43	129	0	12.9	
44	129	0	12.9	
45	187	<0.1	18.7	352
46	187	<0.1	18.7	181
47	187	0.2	18.7	120
48	187	0.2	18.7	91
49	187	0.3	18.7	73
50	220	0.3	22	66
51	220	0.4	22	61
52	220	0.4	22	57
53	220	0.4	22	53
54	220	0.4	22	50
55	268	0.6	26.08	47
56	268	0.6	26.8	44
57	268	0.6	26.8	43
58	268	0.7	26.8	41
59	268	0.7	26.8	39
60	339	0.9	33.9	38
61	339	0.9	33.9	37
62	339	0.9	33.9	36
63	339	1	33.9	35
64	339	1	33.9	34
65	391	1.2	39.1	33
66	391	1.2	39.1	33
67	391	1.2	39.1	32
68	391	1.3	39.1	31
69	391	1.3	39.1	30
70	421	1.4	42.1	30
71	421	1.4	42.1	29
72	421	1.5	42.1	29
73	421	1.5	42.1	28
74	421	1.5	42.1	28
75	421	1.5	42.1	27

From Mettler FA et al: Cancer 77:903, 1996.

Tables assume reduction in mortality from breast cancer as a result of screening as follows: age 35–39, 5%; 40–49, 15%; and 50–75, 25%.

ble abnormalities on mammography. In the general population the effectiveness of ultrasound "screening" is more limited. Sickles et al. reported a comparison study using state-of-the-art equipment. Mammography detected 62 of 64 (97%) carcinomas, whereas ultrasound diagnosed only 37 of 64 (58%). Only 8% of carcinomas smaller than 1 cm in diameter were discovered by ultrasound. The conclusion of this study was that the majority of breast carcinomas visualized by ultrasound can be pal-

pated clinically and there was little use for the ultrasound as a screening tool. The primary advantage of ultrasound is the ability to produce images of breast tissue on multiple occasions without harmful effects. It is most useful in evaluating solitary masses greater than 1 cm in diameter. The greatest limitation of ultrasonography of the breast is the limited spatial resolution. Microcalcifications are not visualized because resolution of less than 2 mm is difficult with ultrasound. Whether it can distinguish benign from

BI-RAD class	Description	Probability of malignancy (%)	Follow-up
0	Needs additional evaluation	1	Diagnostic mammogram, ultrasound
1	Normal mammogram	0	Yearly screening
2	Benign lesion	0	Yearly screening
3	Probably benign lesion	<2	Short interval follow-up
4	Suspicious for malignancy	20	Biopsy
5	Highly suspicious malignancy	90	Biopsy

BI-RAD = Breast Imaging Reporting and Data Systems

FIGURE 14-12 BI-RAD classification of mammographic lesions. (From Pazdur R, Coia LR, Hoskins WJ, and Wagman LD, editors, Cancer management: a multidisciplinary approach, ed. 4, Melville, NY, PRR, p. 143.)

malignant lesions has been a topic of great debate. In one series, Stavros et al. described the sonographic evaluation of 750 solid breast nodules (palpable and nonpalpable) all of which had subsequent histologic confirmation. The negative predictive value of sonography was 99.5%. This is a higher negative predictive value than a BIRAD 3 mammogram for which a 6-month follow-up is recommended. It can be used to evaluate mammographically detected lesions. A low-risk lesion according to strict sonographic criteria can either be aspirated or safely observed. When the lesion is believed to be intermediate risk it should undergo histologic evaluation because 10% to 15% will be malignant.

Ultrasonography of the breast is usually performed by a handheld, real-time, high-frequency probe. It is a highly operator- and reader-dependent test with a great deal of variation among different centers. Breast cancer is usually hypoechoic, and early cancers are difficult to distinguish from surrounding normal hypoechoic breast tissue. The most important use of ultrasound is to differentiate a cystic breast mass from a solid mass. The accuracy rate of ultrasound to diagnose a cystic mass is 96% to 100% and exceeds the combined accuracy of mammography and physical examination. Ultrasound may be used as a guide for needle aspiration, needle core biopsy, and in localization procedures. It has also been used to localize tumors intraoperatively without a guide wire with excellent success rates. In one series, pathologically negative margins were achieved in 97% of the cases by using sonography alone to localize the lesion intraoperatively. This imaging technique also may be useful in women with augmentation mammoplasty, in the differential diagnosis of masses

in the dense breast tissue of younger women, evaluating a breast abscess, and possibly determining lymph node status in a woman with carcinoma. Although it can be used to evaluate the integrity of a silicone breast implant, most believe that MRI is better at detecting implant ruptures.

Duplex Doppler ultrasonography is a new technique; however, preliminary results do not demonstrate a high sensitivity or specificity.

In summary, ultrasound should not be used as a sole imaging technique for breast disease. Because of its lack of sensitivity and specificity for early breast carcinoma, it should not be used in an attempt to detect subclinical disease in the general population at this time.

Digital Radiography

Digital radiography is the technique by which x-ray photons are detected after passing through the breast tissue and the radiographic image is recorded electronically in a digital format and stored in a computer. Digital technology has multiple advantages compared with conventional mammography. Image acquisition, display, and storage are much faster, and image manipulation through adjustments in contrast, brightness, and electronic magnification of selected regions enables radiologists to obtain superior views. This technology makes it possible to subtract various layers of computerized imagery in order to examine suspicious areas and improve the ability to detect and diagnose breast carcinoma. Digital mammography is particularly helpful in screening women with very dense breasts and breast implants. With the ability to manipulate the images, digital mammography will reduce the number of women recalled for more images. Computer-aided diagnosis is also possible with this technique as well as the ability to transmit the image electronically. Because of low background "noise" and superior contrast capabilities, the final image is superior to conventional mammography.

The disadvantages of digital mammography include the high cost of the equipment, the limited image storage capacity, and the reduced spatial resolution due in part to inadequate resolution of current monitors. Although not yet FDA approved, there are several clinical trials underway designed to evaluate its utility as a screening test. The Department of Defense Digital Mammography Screening Trial is recruiting approximately 15,000 women to compare both conventional and digital mammography. The interim results revealed no difference in the number of cancers missed by either group. However, digital mammography is associated with a significantly lower recall rate (11.5% vs. 14.1%) and a higher rate of positive findings at the time of biopsy (43.3% vs. 23.7%). Although promising, for the near future the high cost per test will make it financially impractical to implement widespread digital radiography for screening purposes. This imaging technique will be the screening modality of the future, as it also requires less radiation exposure than modern mammographic equipment because of the increased quantum efficiency of the digital equipment.

Computed Tomography

Computed tomography (CT) has limited value when compared with mammography because of higher radiation dose and longer study times. The thickness of cross-sectional slices with CT miss the majority of areas of microcalcification. CT scans have demonstrated some preclinical cancers after injection with radiocontrast media. This imaging technique is excellent for studying the most medial and lateral aspects of the breast. It is sometimes used for preoperative wire location of a mass that is difficult to localize by mammography. However, the increased expense and radiation exposure virtually eliminate CT scans for screening programs.

Magnetic Resonance Imaging

Preliminary research studies using magnetic resonance imaging (MRI) in the workup of women suspected of having breast carcinoma are promising. Because of higher costs, this imaging technique will not be used in screening but as a diagnostic test. The ability of MRI to differentiate benign from malignant tissue may help to reduce the frequency of breast biopsy, especially in women with dense, fibroglandular breasts. MRI has been proven effective in detecting new tumors in patients with previous lumpectomy because it can accurately distinguish between scar tissue and cancerous lesions. This is best accomplished by the gadolinium-enhanced MRI. Other potential uses or indications for MRI are to improve imaging of structures close to the chest wall, to improve imaging of women with breast prosthesis, and to evaluate for prosthesis rupture. It is useful in the patient who presents with axillary adenopathy and no apparent mass in the breast. Because the average examination takes about 45 minutes to an hour, MRI will not be used in mass screening programs. MRI cannot identify microcalcifications. Another limitation of MRI is the loss of image quality with respiratory movements. Its role in the screening of very high-risk women is being evaluated.

Thermography

Thermography is unreliable as a screening technique for breast carcinoma or as a technique to determine women at increased risk for subsequent breast neoplasia. Lawson first described the elevation of skin temperature associated with breast carcinoma in 1956. Although thermography has been used clinically since that time, it has extremely high false-positive and false-negative rates.

Thermography is ineffective in detection of occult or preclinical cancers. This technique was initially included in the national multicenter breast cancer detection demonstration program. However, the detection rate with thermography was 42% as compared to 92% for mammography. The major fault of a normal thermography examination is the false sense of security engendered in the symptom-free woman. The addition of thermography to other established diagnostic methods increases costs without providing useful clinical information.

Transillumination

Transillumination, or dynamic optical breast imaging (DOBI), is a radiation-free technique that measures the light transmitted through breast tissue. The breast acts as a filter for the light; the hypothesis is that malignant tissue absorbs more infrared light than does benign tissue. Although this technique is inexpensive it is still experimental and unproven. To date, results of research studies using transillumination do not compare with results obtained with mammography.

Mammoscintigraphy (Scintimammography)

Mammoscintigraphy is a radionuclide imaging test for the detection of breast cancer. Technetium-99m sestamibi is a radiotracer with reported high sensitivity and high negative predictive value for breast cancer. It has a high diagnostic accuracy for the detection of breast cancer in all women, including women who may be unsuitable for conventional mammography. In a study designed to describe the diagnostic utility of mammoscintigraphy in women with a breast mass, Howarth et al. studied 115 patients and noted an overall sensitivity for the detection of breast cancer of 84% for scintimammography and 66% for conventional mammography. The specificity of scintimammography was also significantly better than conventional mammography, 84% and 67%, respectively. The high negative predictive value of this test for breast cancer potentially makes it an important adjunct to mammography by potentially reducing the number of biopsies performed for benign findings. Mammoscintigraphy is useful for locating tumors in the lateral areas of dense breasts as well as detecting metastatic disease in the lymph nodes of the axilla. Additional studies are needed before this test is widely accepted and its utility proven.

Other Imaging Techniques

There are several other imaging techniques that are currently being evaluated. Diffraction enhanced imaging (DEI) is one such technique. With this technique an analyzing crystal is placed in the x-ray beam between the breast and an image-creating medium such as film or digital detector. The crystal diffracts the x-ray beam and produces two separate images, one based on standard x-ray and the other based on refraction. The result is an excellent quality image with superior tumor visibility. Digital thermal imaging is another new technique that uses the principles of thermography as well as digital technology to create an image base determined by temperature differences between the cancer and the normal breast. Microwave radiography is a portable, noninvasive adjuvant diagnostic approach that involves passive measurement of microwave emissions from breast tissue. All these techniques must undergo further appropriate testing to determine their safety and efficacy in the management of breast cancer.

Fine-Needle Aspiration

Fine-needle aspiration (FNA) of a breast mass is a well-established diagnostic test. It is a simple office-based procedure that is well accepted by women because it is sometimes less painful than a venipuncture. Most physicians do not use anesthesia, although some prefer to use a small amount of local anesthetic (1 cc of 1% lidocaine). The skin over the breast is the most sensitive area as the breast tissue itself has few pain fibers. The anesthetic procedure has more disadvantages than advantages. The major disadvantage is that if excessive amounts of anesthetic are injected into the skin, or if a hematoma develops, the mass may be obscured and the accuracy of the FNA is decreased. However, an injection of local anesthesia into a small area of the skin will help to reduce the patient's anxiety. The skin is usually prepared for an FNA with either an alcohol or iodine solution. The slides for the aspirate should be properly labeled or preferably a cytotechnologist should be available to process the slides and assess the adequacy of the specimen. The breast mass is secured with one hand and the other hand introduces a 20- or 22-gauge needle attached to a 10- or 20-ml syringe into the mass. If the mass is a cyst, one feels a "give" or reduced resistance after puncturing the cyst wall. It may be technically easier to manipulate the smaller needles without the syringe attached. Complete aspiration of all the fluid from the cyst is facilitated by negative pressure from the syringe and firm pressure on the cyst wall (Figure 14-13). With withdrawal of the fluid the cyst wall collapses, and usually a residual mass cannot be palpated. After withdrawal of the needle, firm pressure is applied for 5 to 10 minutes to reduce the possibility of hematoma formation. Complications of needle aspiration are minimal, with hematoma formation being the only substantial one. Infection is very

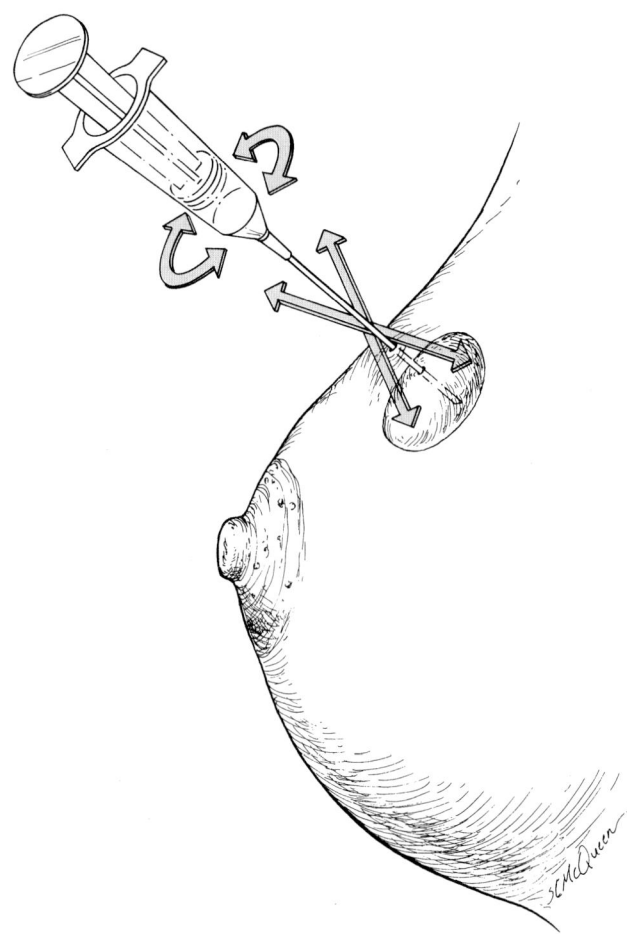

FIGURE 14-13 Needle biopsy and aspiration with negative pressure. Needle is rotated, moved back and forth, and slightly in and out to aspirate representative specimen. (From Vorherr H: Am J Obstet Gynecol 148:128, 1984.)

rare. The theoretic risk of spreading cancer along the needle track has not been substantiated. The relief of a patient's anxiety produced by successfully aspirating a newly discovered breast mass is most gratifying.

The color of the fluid obtained via aspiration varies from clear to grossly bloody. It is not uncommon to find yellow, brown, and even green fluid in a cyst. If the aspirated fluid is clear, it is not necessary to submit it for cytologic evaluation. One study in the literature documents no breast cancers discovered from almost 7000 consecutive nonbloody cyst aspirates. If the aspirated fluid is turbid or bloody, it should be placed on a cover slip and sent for cytologic interpretation and the mass should be further evaluated with a biopsy. Although bloody fluid is usually from a traumatic tap one must consider the possibility of a carcinoma.

No further workup is necessary if the aspirated fluid is clear and no residual mass is palpated immediately after the procedure and again 1 month later. However, if the mass remains after aspiration, a biopsy should be performed even if the cytologic analysis of the fluid was negative. Cysts that recur within 2 weeks or necessitate more than one repeat aspiration should be biopsied. Slightly less than 20% of cysts recur after a single aspiration and less than 10% recur after two aspirations. The percentage of false-positive, fine-needle aspirations is very rare, usually less than 2%.

In the event that no fluid is obtained, the breast mass is probably solid and several passes are made through the mass with continuous suction from the syringe. Moving the needle within a single tract will give a satisfactory cellular yield in the majority of cases. The cellular specimen within the needle should be placed on a slide and fixed for analysis. Definitive diagnosis by open biopsy or core needle biopsy should be considered if there is any suspicion from the aspirate, the mammogram, or on physical exam. This triple test has been advocated by many as a reliable alternative to biopsy. According to the National Cancer Institute's committee opinion on fine-needle aspirate, if the physical exam, imaging findings, and cytologic evaluation of the mass all confirm the same benign process, the mass can be safely followed. However, if there is any suspicion from any of these assessments, the mass should be biopsied. The false-negative rate of triple test diagnosis approaches that of surgical biopsy, and the false-positive rate is comparable to that of frozen section. Although optimal performance of FNA is operator dependent, the results of the triple test for palpable masses have proven quite reliable. The sensitivity of FNA for palpable masses is approximately 90% with a false-negative rate that varies from 0.7% to 22%. In experienced hands, the false-negative rate of FNA is approximately 3% to 10%. The major drawbacks of FNA are that it cannot distinguish invasive from noninvasive breast carcinoma and it is unable to confirm in histologic terms a definitive benign diagnosis.

Biopsy

The definitive diagnosis and ultimate foundation for treatment of breast carcinoma depends on histologic diagnosis of the biopsy material. Breast biopsy is one of the most common surgical procedures performed, but with the increasing acceptance of mammography and the development of less invasive procedures there has been a shift from the traditional open biopsy to the less invasive and more popular core-needle biopsy. The common indications for tissue biopsy include bloody discharge from the nipple, a persistent three-dimensional mass, and/or suspicious mammography. Nipple retraction or elevation and skin changes, such as erythema, induration, or edema, are also indications for breast biopsy. Obviously, the suspicious area must be sampled appropriately. This can be accomplished several ways.

Nonpalpable breast lesions are most commonly discovered through screening mammography, and they represent a large proportion of the suspicious areas investigated by biopsy. Although these lesions are relatively easy to identify, intraoperative localization and subsequent adequate excision can be very challenging. Until recently, the best available method was to perform a mammographically guided wire localized excisional biopsy. With this method a wire is placed percutaneously in the vicinity of the abnormality by the radiologist using mammogram guidance. Subsequently, the woman is taken to the operating suite where the surgeon uses the wire as a guide to excise the abnormal area. The specimen is removed with the wire in place and it is radiographed to confirm the removal of the abnormal area. More recently a needle is placed over the wire to help localize the lesion.

Mammographically guided wire localized excisional biopsy is more invasive than the more widely accepted stereotactic core-needle biopsy. This latter procedure has changed dramatically how mammographically detected lesions are managed. The woman is placed prone on the stereotactic biopsy table with the breast in a dependent position. The breast is imaged and the lesion is localized using computer-assisted positioning and targeting devices. A small nick is made in the skin and the core biopsy needle is advanced into the lesion. The lesion is sampled and the "cores" of tissue are sent to pathology for histologic evaluation. Although this technique is very accurate, the finding of atypical hyperplasia or carcinoma in situ requires open wire localized excisional biopsy to rule out an underlying invasive cancer. The false-negative rate for this procedure is less than 2%.

Palpable lesions can be evaluated by several techniques. The type of technique used is dependent on many factors including the location and size of the lesion as well as patient and physician preference. Options include incisional or excisional biopsy, as well as core-needle biopsy. A small incisional biopsy may be appropriate for a large mass. However, it is important to obtain a large wedge of breast tissue so as not to miss an occult carcinoma identified by mammography. The intent of excisional biopsy is to remove the mass with a surrounding margin of normal tissue.

Today the majority of open breast biopsies are performed under local anesthesia on an outpatient basis. Twenty-five years ago, it was common practice to perform a biopsy, frozen section, and definitive surgery during the same operation. The modern two-step approach significantly decreases anxiety for the patient. The 1- to 2-week interval between biopsy and therapy gives the woman a chance to contemplate alternative choices in therapy. Cosmetic results are important, and the majority of biopsies can be performed with curvilinear incisions, often in the circumareolar area. An open biopsy should be performed using a cold knife rather than electrocautery. The use of electrocautery on the biopsy material may blur the margin of normal tissue around the tumor and cause abnormally low receptor levels. It is important to send the laboratory a small sample (1 g of suspicious tissue) to determine the presence or absence of estrogen and progesterone receptors. These receptors are heat labile, and therefore the tissue must be frozen within 30 minutes. The incidence of carcinoma in biopsies corresponds directly with the patient's age. Approximately 20% of breast biopsies in women aged 50 are positive, and this figure increases to 33% in women aged 70 or older.

Classification

Breast cancer is usually asymptomatic before the development of advanced disease. Breast pain is experienced by only 10% of women with early breast carcinoma. The classic sign of a breast carcinoma is a solitary, solid, three-dimensional, dominant breast mass. The borders of the mass are usually indistinct, which makes it difficult to define precisely the size of the mass. Often the mass is not freely mobile. Far-advanced local disease produces changes in the skin and nipples of the breast, including retraction, dimpling, induration, edema (peau d'orange), ulceration, and signs of inflammation.

The prognosis and treatment of breast carcinoma are primarily related to the stage of the disease and extent of spread to regional nodes (Figure 14-14). Variations in histologic types and degree of cellular atypia of breast cancer are of secondary importance. There have been numerous classifications of breast carcinoma that contain mixtures of both clinical and pathologic subgroups. The neoplasm is classified based on the predominate histologic cells; however, several cellular patterns may be found in any one tumor. A condensed classification is presented in Table 14-5. Most carcinomas originate in the epithelium of the collecting ducts or terminal lobular ducts. Both in situ and invasive carcinoma have been described, often in the same quadrant of the breast. Bilateral breast carcinoma occurs in approximately 1% of all newly diagnosed cases. The prevalence of bilateral breast cancer is twofold greater in lobular neoplasia.

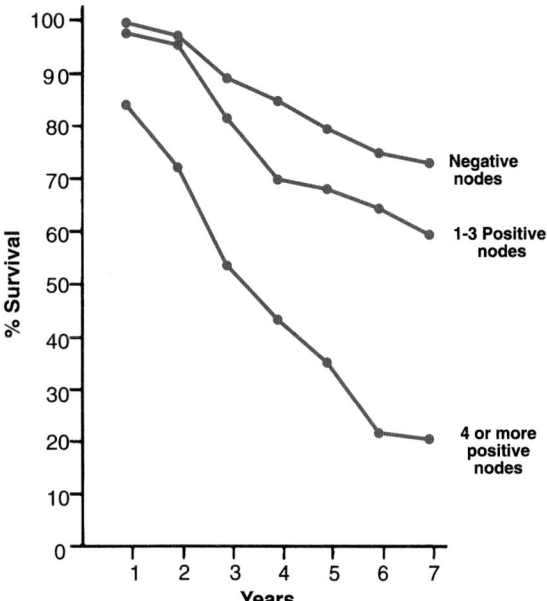

FIGURE 14-14 Survival with breast carcinoma in relation to positive nodes. (From Gambrell RD: Am J Obstet Gynecol 150:122, 1984.)

TABLE 14-5
Simplified Classification of Breast Carcinoma

Type of Carcinoma	Percentage of All Cases Diagnosed
Ductal carcinoma	
In situ	5%
Infiltrating	80%
Lobular carcinoma	
In situ	3%
Infiltrating	9%
Inflammatory carcinoma	2%
Paget's disease	1%

Intraductal carcinoma in situ is a disease in which the cellular abnormalities are limited to the ductal epithelium and have not penetrated the base membrane. It is most commonly discovered in perimenopausal and postmenopausal women. Intraductal carcinoma in situ is not usually detected by palpation because the disease does not produce a definitive mass. Mammography sometimes demonstrates the fine stippling of microcalcifications. The histologic diagnosis of intraductal carcinoma in situ includes a heterogeneous group of tumors with varying malignant potential. Reviews by Betsill et al. and Page et al. document carcinoma developing in approximately 35% of women with this disease within 10 years of initial diagnosis usually in the same quadrant of the breast as the original biopsy. If the primary treatment is simple mastectomy, 5% to 10% of women will have a simultaneous invasive carcinoma in the same breast.

Lobular carcinoma in situ should not be treated as a cancer or as a precursor of breast cancer. It is considered to be a marker for an increased breast cancer risk. It does not have the same malignant potential as intraductal carcinoma in situ. However, it has a much greater tendency to be bilateral and to present as multifocal disease. Three of four patients are in the premenopausal age group. Lobular carcinoma in situ is not detected by palpation, and mammography shows no characteristic pattern. However, it should be considered as a major risk factor for the subsequent development of breast carcinoma. The latent period is longer than with intraductal carcinoma in situ; often over 20 years will elapse before infiltrating carcinoma develops. Approximately 20% of women with this disease will develop invasive breast carcinoma during the remainder of their life. Interestingly, most of the subsequent carcinomas are ductal, not lobular (Table 14-6).

Infiltrating ductal carcinoma is the most common breast malignancy. Histologically, nonuniform malignant epithelial cells of varying sizes and shapes infiltrate the surrounding tissue. The degree of fibrous response to the invading epithelial cells determines the firmness to palpation and texture during biopsy. Often the stromal reaction may be extensive, thus the outdated term *cirrhosis carcinoma.* Approximately 10% of infiltrating ductal carcino-

mas are of a uniform histologic picture and are classified as medullary, colloid, comedo, tubular, or papillary carcinomas. In general the specialized forms are grossly softer, mobile, and well delineated. They are usually smaller and have a more optimistic prognosis than the more common nonhomogeneous variety. Medullary carcinomas are soft, with extensive stromal infiltration by lymphocytes and plasma cells. Colloid carcinomas have a similar soft consistency, with extensive deposition of extracellular mucin.

Infiltrating lobular carcinomas are characterized by the uniformity of the small, round neoplastic cells. Often the malignant epithelial cells infiltrate the stroma in a single-file fashion. This neoplasia tends to have a multicentric origin in the same breast and tends to involve both breasts more often than infiltrating ductal carcinoma. Histologic subdivisions of infiltrating lobular carcinoma include small cell, round cell, and signet cell carcinomas.

Inflammatory carcinomas comprise approximately 2% of breast cancers. This type is recognized clinically as a rapidly growing, highly malignant carcinoma. Infiltration of malignant cells into the lymphatics of the skin produces a clinical picture that simulates a skin infection. There is not a specific histologic cell type.

Paget's disease of the breast is rare, comprising slightly less than 1% of breast carcinomas (Figure 14-15). This lesion has an innocent appearance and looks like eczema or a dermatitis of the nipple. The clinical picture is produced by an infiltrating ductal carcinoma that invades the epidermis. Paget's disease has an excellent prognosis.

Treatment

The treatment of breast carcinoma is complex, with many variables to consider. The most appropriate treatment varies from woman to woman. The four most important variables for treatment selection are the tumor's size; its inherent aggressiveness, as determined by the histology of the initial lesion; the presence of positive nodes; and the receptor status of the tumor. A widely recognized staging system based on both clinical and pathologic criteria, the TNM system, represents the extent of the tumor, the lymph node involvement, and the presence of metastasis (Table 14-7). When generalizations are offered concerning the preferred method of therapy, it is important to remember that breast carcinoma is a heterogeneous group of neoplasms. Unfortunately, neither clinical nor pathologic staging of the disease is nearly as precise as one would postulate in a carcinoma involving an external organ. Axillary nodes will be negative for metastatic disease at initial surgery in approximately 60% of women. However, approximately 25% of these women will develop recurrent carcinoma. Microscopic metastatic disease occurs early via both hematogenous and lymphatic routes. For example, 30% to 40% of women without gross adenopathy in the axilla will have positive nodes discovered during histo-

---

TABLE 14-6
Salient Characteristics of In Situ Ductal (DCIS) and Lobular (LCIS) Carcinoma of the Breast

	LCIS	DCIS
Age (years)	44–47	54–58
Incidence*	2%–5%	5%–10%
Clinical signs	None	Mass, pain, nipple discharge
Mammographic signs	None	Microcalcifications
Premenopausal	2/3	1/3
Incidence synchronous invasive carcinoma	5%	2%–46%
Multicentricity	60%–90%	40%–80%
Bilaterality	50%–70%	10%–20%
Axillary metastasis	1%	1%–2%
Subsequent carcinomas:		
Incidence	25%–35%	25%–70%
Laterality	Bilateral	Ipsilateral
Interval to diagnosis	15–20 years	5–10 years
Histology	Ductal	Ductal

From Frykberg ER, Ames FC, and Bland KI: Current concepts for management of early (in situ and occult invasive) breast carcinoma. In Bland KI and Copeland EM, editors: The breast, Philadelphia, 1991, WB Saunders, p 736.

*Among biopsies of mammographically detected breast lesions.

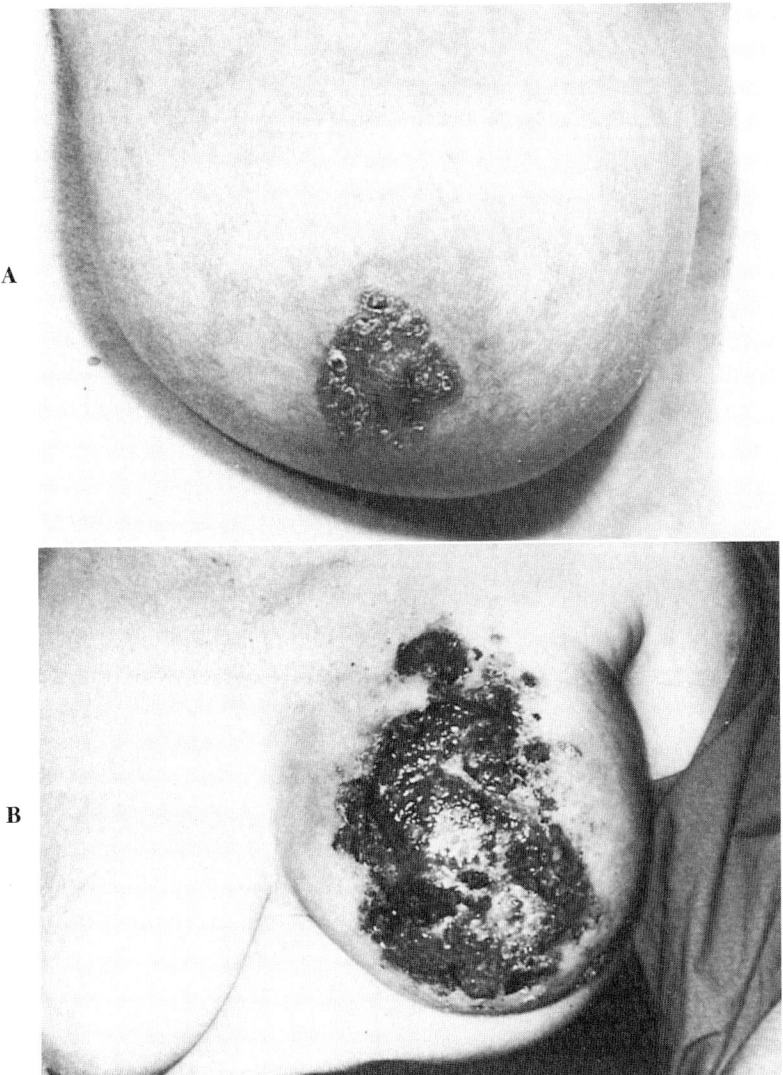

FIGURE 14-15 A, Paget's disease of left nipple. **B,** Extensive Paget's disease involving skin of breast. (From McKinna JA: Clinical features of breast disease. In Parsons CA, editor: Diagnosis of breast disease: imaging, clinical features, and pathology, London. Copyright 1983, Chapman & Hall Ltd, p 38.)

logic examination. With the additional assessment tools of immunohistochemical staining for the presence of cytokeratin and serial sectioning of axillary nodes, 10% to 30% of women considered to have negative nodes by standard histologic analysis are found to be node-positive. Approximately two thirds of all women with breast carcinoma eventually develop distant metastatic disease regardless of the type of initial therapy.

It is important to understand the natural history of untreated breast carcinoma. In series of women refusing therapy, 20% will be alive at 5 years and 5% will be alive at 10 years. Breast carcinoma is a systemic disease that may recur many years, sometimes decades, after initial diagnosis. However, women with negative nodes have a 10-year survival rate of 75% (Table 14-8).

The major changes in management of breast carci-

noma over the past two decades have resulted from changing concepts regarding the biology of the disease, with the understanding that many women with breast carcinoma have systemic disease at the time the diagnosis is initially established. The natural history of the majority of developing breast carcinomas results in years of growth of the neoplasm before discovery. Because occult vascular dissemination is likely to occur prior to diagnosis, treatment of breast carcinoma involves both local and systemic therapy. It is beyond the scope of this book to present the details of treatment of breast carcinoma. Thorough clinical and surgical staging is the cornerstone of any treatment plan. In the TNM classification, the tumor size and characteristics are described (T), regional lymph node involvement is documented (N), and distant metastases are noted (M).

TABLE 14-7
TNM Staging of Breast Cancer

Primary tumor (T)

TX	Primary tumor cannot be assessed
T0	No evidence of primary tumor
Tis*	Carcinoma in situ. Intraductal carcinoma, lobular carcinoma in situ, or Paget's disease of the nipple with no tumor
T1	Tumor is 2.0 cm or less in greater dimension
T1a	Tumor is 0.5 cm or less in greatest dimension
T1b	Tumor is more than 0.5 cm but not more than 1.0 cm in greatest dimension
T1c	Tumor is more than 1.0 cm but not more than 2.0 cm in greatest dimension
T2	Tumor is more than 2.0 cm but not more than 5.0 cm in greatest dimension
T3	Tumor is more than 5.0 cm in greatest dimension
T4	Tumor of any size with direct extension to chest wall or skin
T4a	Extension to chest wall
T4b	Edema (including peau d'orange) or ulceration of the skin of the breast or satellite skin nodules confined to the same breast
T4c	Both T4a and T4b above
T4d	Inflammatory carcinoma

Regional lymph node involvement (N) (Clinical)

NX	Regional lymph nodes cannot be assessed (e.g., previously removed)
N0	No regional lymph node metastasis
N1	Metastasis to movable ipsilateral axillary lymph node(s)
N2	Metastasis to ipsilateral axillary lymph node(s) fixed to one another or the other structures
N3	Metastasis to ipsilateral mammary lymph node(s)

Distant metastasis (M)

MX	Presence of distant metastasis cannot be assessed
M0	No distant metastasis
M1	Distant metastasis (includes metastasis to ipsilateral supraclavicular lymph node[s])

Stage grouping

Stage 0	Tis	N0	M0
Stage I	T1	N0	M0
Stage IIa	T0	N1	M0
	T1	N1*	M0
	T2	N0	M0
Stage IIb	T2	N1	M0
	T3	N0	M0
Stage IIIa	T0	N2	M0
	T1	N2	M0
	T2	N2	M0
	T3	N1, N2	M0
Stage IIIb	T4	Any N	M0
	Any T	N3	M0
Stage IV	Any T	Any N	M1

From Eberlein TJ: Ann Surg 220:121, 1994.

Paget's disease associated with a tumor is classified according to the size of the tumor. Chest wall includes ribs, intercostal muscles, and serratus anterior muscle but not pectoral muscle.

*The prognosis of patients with pN1a is similar to that of patients with pN0.

Veronesi et al. have listed the three major objectives of treating breast carcinoma: control of local disease, treatment of distant metastasis, and improved quality of life for women treated for the disease. There are several methods for controlling local disease. However, no difference in long-term survival rates has been documented, regardless of the extent of surgical therapy or aggressiveness of local radiotherapy. During the past 15 years, revolutionary changes have involved multiple therapeutic options in both local and systemic therapy for breast carcinoma. Women are assuming an increasingly active role in deciding their own treatment regimen. Breast conservation is a frequent choice for the control of local disease. Sentinel node resection is becoming standard practice in the treatment of early stage breast cancer. Chemotherapy is used not only

TABLE 14-8
Stages and Survival of Women with Breast Cancer

Clinical Staging (American Joint Committee)	Crude 5-Year Survival (%)	Range of Survival (%)
Stage 1 Tumor <2 cm in diameter Nodes, if present, not felt to contain metastases Without distant metastases	85	82–94
Stage II Tumor <5 cm in diameter Nodes, if palpable, not fixed Without distant metastases	66	47–74
Stage III Tumor >5 cm or, Tumor of any size with invasion of skin or attached to chest wall Nodes in supraclavicular area Without distant metastases	41	7–80
Stage IV With distant metastases	10	—

Histologic Staging (NSABP*)	Crude Survival (%)		5-Year Disease-Free Survival (%)
	5-Year	10-Year	
All patients	63.5	45.9	60.3
Negative axillary lymph nodes	78.1	64.9	82.3
Positive axillary lymph nodes	46.5	24.9	34.9
1–3 positive axillary lymph nodes	62.2	37.5	50.0
>4 positive axillary lymph nodes	32.0	13.4	21.1

From Henderson IC and Canellos GP: N Engl J Med 302:18, 1980. Reprinted by permission of The New England Journal of Medicine.

*National Surgical Adjuvant Breast Project.

TABLE 14-9
Ten-Year Disease-Free Survival Rates
of Women with Breast Cancer

	Conservation Surgery and Radiation	Radical or Modified Radical Mastectomy Alone
Minimal breast cancer	92%	95%
Stage I	78%	80%
Stage II	73%	65%

Reprinted with permission from Montague ED: Cancer 53:702, 1984.

for patients with proved metastatic disease but also for women at high risk for the development of primary or recurrent disease. Recent emphasis on conservative surgery plus radiation therapy to control multifocal cancer in the same breast and on reconstructive surgery after mastectomy has improved the quality of life of women with breast carcinoma (Table 14-9).

Surgical Therapy

The decision concerning appropriate therapy and extent of the surgical operation to treat breast carcinoma should be made by the woman in consultation with the surgeon, radiotherapist, and medical oncologist who will treat her. As emphasized, the size of the tumor, the initial extent of disease, virulence of the neoplasms, and presence of estrogen and progesterone receptors are the key medical factors in the decision. The initial size of the breast carcinoma is the single best predictor of the likelihood of positive axillary nodes. The presence and number of axillary node metastasis is the single best predictor of survival. Intensive discussions concerning breast reconstruction or external prostheses are important to help the woman contemplate the effects of surgery on body image. Morris et al. have studied the psychologic and social adjustments to mastectomy in 160 women. They were followed at intervals of 3, 12, and 24 months after surgery. One in four women was still having problems with depression and associated marital and sexual problems 2 years after initial therapy.

Until approximately 25 years ago, radical mastectomy

was the standard operation for carcinoma of the breast. Radical mastectomy was designed to control local disease by an extensive en bloc removal of the breast and underlying pectoralis major and pectoralis minor muscles and complete axillary dissection. It is a cosmetically disfiguring operation, leaving a major deformity of the chest wall. With an increased understanding that cancer of the breast is often a systemic disease, the therapeutic emphasis has changed to less radical surgery and increased use of radiotherapy and chemotherapy. It has also been recognized that often patients are not cured even with extensive local therapy. Thus protocols have been designed for more conservative approaches to local disease, and less radical operations have grown in popularity. The modified radical mastectomy removes the breast and only the fascia over the pectoralis major muscle. The pectoralis minor muscle may be removed to facilitate the axillary dissection. Simple mastectomy includes removal of the breast without underlying muscle tissue.

The primary therapy for the vast majority of women with stages I and II breast cancer is conservative surgery, which preserves the breast, followed by radiation therapy. Lazovic et al. reported that 60% of women with stage I and 39% of women with stage II breast carcinoma were treated with conservative surgery in a review of 9 recent population-based cancer registries. Resection of a wider area of the breast than lumpectomy is referred to as *quadrantectomy*. The latter operation is more effective in preventing local recurrences. However, the cosmetic result is not as satisfactory. In trials with either lumpectomy or quadrantectomy without irradiation the rate of recurrence in the treated breast was approximately 40% compared with 10% when irradiation was given. Thus almost all women with conservative surgical therapy for invasive breast carcinoma receive radiotherapy. Interestingly, there was no definite difference in overall survival at 10 years. Radiotherapy may not be necessary in some selected instances in women over age 55.

Veronesi et al. published a controlled study of 701 women with carcinomas measuring less than 2 cm in diameter without palpable axillary lymph nodes. The women were randomized preoperatively into two treatment groups. One group of 349 patients had radical mastectomy. The other group included 352 women who had excision of a quadrant of the breast to control the primary lesion, axillary dissection, and radiotherapy involving both external and interstitial sources. Five-year survival rates were virtually identical—90% in both groups. Five-year disease-free survival rates were similar, 83% and 84%. Fisher et al., in the National Surgical Adjuvant Breast Project, have reported similar findings with breast carcinomas less than 4 cm, if the surgical margins were free of tumor. Three additional randomized prospective studies found no difference in therapeutic results contrasting conservative surgery and postoperative irradiation versus radical surgery for stage I or II breast carcinoma. These studies

found local recurrence rates of 5% at 5 years and approximately 10% at 10 years. Radiotherapy was begun 1 to 2 weeks postoperatively and given for approximately 5 weeks. The radiotherapeutic dosage was 180 to 200 cGy per day for a total dose of approximately 5000 cGy.

Another conservative approach to the treatment of breast cancer involves the use of sentinel lymph node mapping as an alternative to axillary dissection. Although the presence of axillary node metastasis is an important prognostic factor for patients with breast cancer, there is a high incidence of chronic complications associated with axillary dissection. By injecting the primary tumor with radioactive colloid tracers and dyes, the surgeon can identify the first set of regional lymph nodes that receive lymphatic drainage from the tumor. These are termed *sentinel lymph nodes*. Subsequently, these nodes can be removed and the axillary dissection can be deleted if they are negative. In a large multi-institutional trial, Krag et al. were able to identify the sentinel nodes in 93% of the cases. The accuracy of sentinel node mapping in this series for predicting the status of axillary nodes was 97%. The positive predictive value was 100% and the negative predictive value was 96%. Although sentinel lymph node mapping can accurately predict the status of the axillary nodes, the procedure can be technically challenging and the success rates vary according to the surgeon's expertise with the procedure.

It is important to offer every woman alternatives in treatment for stages I and II breast carcinoma. The cosmetic result obtained by lumpectomy and radiation therapy depends on the size and shape of the breast and the size of the initial tumor. For some women, mastectomy followed by reconstructive surgery may give a superior cosmetic result. Also, the management of the axillary nodes should be considered and the woman should be informed concerning all of her options.

Medical Therapy

Adjuvant systemic chemotherapy decreases the odds of dying from breast cancer during the first 10 years following diagnosis by approximately 25%. The two major factors in predicting the likelihood of systemic disease in breast carcinoma are the diameter of the primary tumor and the number of positive axillary nodes. Women whose initial tumor is less than 1 cm in diameter and who have negative axillary nodes have excellent disease-free survival, with a 10-year relapse rate of less than 10%. Multiple other determinations have been used as prognostic factors in clinical trials, including the presence of estrogen and progesterone receptors, the DNA content, mitotic index, growth rate measured by flow cytometry, epidermal growth factor receptor, overgrowth of the oncogene erbB-2 (HER2 or neu) and the expression of various proteins such as heat/shock proteins, collagenase type IV, and many others. The majority of breast carcinomas are adenocarcinomas. Nevertheless, they represent microscopically a heterogenous group of tumors. It is not established whether the response to chemotherapy of specific histologic subtypes differs because women in various chemotherapeutic studies have not been randomized according to histologic type.

The presence and concentration of receptors should be obtained at the initial diagnostic surgery, as receptor status may change after radiotherapy or chemotherapy. In general, receptor-positive tumors are usually more well differentiated and exhibit a less aggressive clinical behavior, including a lower risk of recurrence and lower capacity to proliferate. When estrogen receptors are positive, approximately 60% of breast cancers will respond to hormonal therapy; an 80% response is noted when both estrogen and progesterone receptors are present. If estrogen receptors are negative, less than 10% of tumors respond to hormonal manipulation.

Hormonal therapy may include ablative surgery but is usually accomplished by drugs that change endocrine function by blocking receptor sites or blocking synthesis of hormones. In the past the most commonly used ablative surgery was bilateral oophorectomy in a premenopausal woman with breast carcinoma. Hormonal therapy is effective in producing a response in advanced metastatic carcinoma for approximately 1 year. Metastatic disease in soft tissue and bone is the most sensitive to hormonal manipulation. Tamoxifen, an oral antiestrogen, is an alternative to surgical castration and presently is the most frequently prescribed hormonal agent for breast carcinoma. Adrenalectomy or hypophysectomy has largely been replaced by medical adrenalectomy using aminoglutethimide in select cases. Depot-medroxyprogesterone, androgens, danazol, and gonadotrophin hormone-releasing hormone (GH-RH)

agonists have also been used to treat breast carcinoma. Two endocrine agents used simultaneously do not produce better results than a single agent.

Adjuvant chemotherapy has produced positive responses and an increase in disease-free survival in many clinical studies. Initially, chemotherapy was selected to treat women with positive axillary nodes or remote disease. Chemotherapy has proved effective in shrinking measurable metastatic disease in both premenopausal and postmenopausal women.

The role for adjuvant therapy in the management of breast cancer continues to expand. Adjuvant chemotherapy has been shown to improve disease-free and overall survival in all patients with operable breast cancer with the exception of select node-negative patients with small (less than 1 cm.) tumors that have no high-risk features. A recent update of the NSABP B-20 trial indicated a significant advantage in the estrogen receptor-positive, node-negative patient who received chemotherapy in addition to tamoxifen. Even women in the postmenopausal age group with estrogen receptor-positive, node-negative breast cancers that traditionally would be treated with tamoxifen alone have been shown to benefit from the combination of chemotherapy and tamoxifen. There is only limited data from randomized trials regarding women over the age of 70. In the absence of other comorbidities chemotherapy can be considered in this population of older women. The indications for adjuvant chemotherapy are summarized in Table 14-10. It is important to note that improvements in disease-free survival have not always been followed by similar improvements in overall survival.

It is firmly established that combinations of cytotoxic drugs are superior to a single agent. In the past, combina-

TABLE 14-10

Indications for Adjuvant Systemic Therapy After Surgery in Women with Operable Breast Cancer

Type of Disease	Adjuvant Therapy Indicated*
Breast cancer without evidence of invasion	
Noninvasive breast cancer (ductal or lobular carcinoma in situ)	None
Breast cancer with evidence of invasion, but negative axillary lymph nodes	
Microinvasive breast cancer (<1 mm in largest diameter)	None
Invasive ductal or lobular carcinoma <1 cm in largest diameter	None
Invasive carcinoma <3 cm in largest diameter with favorable histologic findings (pure tubular, mucinous, or papillary)	None
Invasive ductal or lobular carcinoma ≥1 cm in largest diameter	Chemotherapy, hormonal therapy, or both
Invasive carcinoma ≥3 cm in largest diameter with favorable histologic findings (pure tubular, mucinous, or papillary)	Chemotherapy, hormonal therapy, or both
Invasive breast cancer with positive axillary lymph nodes	
All tumors, regardless of size or histologic findings	Chemotherapy, hormonal therapy, or both

*Chemotherapy consists of fluorouracil, doxorubicin, and cyclophosphamide (FAC); doxorubicin and cyclophosphamide (AC); or cyclophosphamide, methotrexate, and fluorouracil (CMF). Hormonal therapy consists of tamoxifen or ovarian ablation (either surgical or chemical).

From Hortobagyi GN: N Engl J Med, 339:977, 1998.

tions included drugs such as cyclophosphamide, methotrexate, adriamycin, 5-fluorouracil, and vinblastine. Presently, it is believed that anthracycline-containing combinations are more effective than regimens that do not contain anthracyclines. Recently, paclitaxel has also become available for the treatment of breast cancer with very promising results. Preliminary results from a Cancer and Leukemia Group B (CALGB) study indicated that the addition of four cycles of paclitaxel to four cycles of the adriamycin and cyclophosphamide regimen improved disease-free and overall survival in patients with node-positive breast cancer. Other drugs currently under investigation for the treatment of breast cancer include anthrapyrazoles, liposomal anthracyclines, and gemcitabine. The average total response rate to combined chemotherapy is 55%. Approximately 10% to 20% of women treated with combination chemotherapy experience a complete remission for about 18 months. The major short-term toxic effects of chemotherapy are alopecia and fatigue. Some women develop premature ovarian failure.

Tamoxifen has the greatest effect in postmenopausal women. As one would expect, tamoxifen is of greater benefit in women with tumors that have estrogen receptors than in tumors that are negative for estrogen receptors. There is no significant improvement in survival in patients with estrogen receptor-negative tumors. However, even in receptor-negative patients, 5 years of tamoxifen use will decrease the risk of a second primary or contralateral breast cancer by as much as 45%. Extending tamoxifen therapy beyond 5 years is not associated with further reduction in risk. Chronic tamoxifen therapy increases the prevalence of intrauterine polyps and endometrial hyperplasia and carcinoma. Recent clinical trials have investigated the use of extremely intensive chemotherapeutic regimens followed by transplantation of autologous bone marrow in women with advanced or recurrent disease. Obviously, this therapy is expensive, requires prolonged hospitalization, and has a mortality rate of approximately 15%. Some women have experienced complete remission for longer than 1 year, but to date there is no convincing evidence that high-dose chemotherapy is superior to conventional treatment. Its use should be limited to clinical trials until sufficient data support its efficacy.

KEY POINTS

- One out of 8 women (12.5% of American females) develops carcinoma of the breast if she lives beyond age 90.

- The breast consists of approximately 20% glandular tissue and 80% fat and connective tissue.

- Lymph drainage of the breast usually flows toward the most adjacent group of nodes. This concept represents the basis for sentinel node mapping in breast cancer. In most instances, breast cancer spreads in an orderly fashion within the axillary lymph node basin based on the anatomic relationship between the primary tumor and its associated regional (sentinel) nodes.

- Numerous epidemiologic studies have found an increased risk of developing breast carcinoma in women with benign breast disease only if there is associated atypical epithelial hyperplasia. This risk varies from twofold to fivefold, depending on the degree of epithelial hyperplasia.

- Clinical evidence of fibrocystic changes is discovered in breast examination of approximately one in two premenopausal women.

- The classic symptom of fibrocystic changes is cyclic bilateral breast pain. The signs of fibrocystic changes include increased engorgement and density of the breasts, excessive nodularity, rapid change and fluctuation in the size of cystic areas, increased tenderness, and occasionally spontaneous nipple discharge.

- Fibroadenomas most frequently present in adolescents and women in their 20s.

- Approximately 30% of fibroadenomas will disappear and 10% to 12% become smaller when followed for many years.

- Approximately 75% of intraductal papillomas are located beneath the areola. Often these tumors are difficult to palpate because they are small and soft.

- Nipple discharge is a complaint of 10% to 15% of women with benign breast disease. However, nipple discharge is present in less than 3% of women with breast carcinoma.

- The importance of diagnosing the etiology of *spontaneous* discharge from the nipple is to rule out carcinoma. The color of the nonmilky discharge does not differentiate a benign from a malignant process.

- Bloody discharge from the nipple, gross or microscopic, should be considered to be related to carcinoma until this diagnosis has been ruled out.

- Intraductal papilloma and fibrocystic changes are the two most common etiologies of spontaneous nonmilky nipple discharge.

- Fat necrosis caused by trauma may present as a firm, indurated, poorly defined mass that has a mammographic appearance of stippled calcifications.

- Risk factors identify only 25% of women who will eventually develop breast carcinoma.

- Approximately 5% to 10% of breast cancers have a familial or genetic link. Genetic predisposition to develop breast carcinoma has been recognized in some families. In these families breast cancer tends to occur at a younger age and there is a higher prevalence of bilateral disease.

- Mutations in BRCA family of genes have been identified that confer a lifetime risk of breast cancer that approaches 85%. BRCA1 and BRCA2 genes are involved in the majority of inheritable cases of breast cancer. These genes function as tumor suppressor genes and several mutations have been described on each of these genes.

- The frequency of breast carcinoma increases directly with the patient's age; 85% occur after 40 years of age.

- Once a woman has developed carcinoma of one breast, her risk is approximately 1% per year of developing cancer in the other breast.

- Women with a high risk of breast cancer have proven options that can decrease their risk of breast cancer. Both tamoxifen and raloxifene significantly decrease the relative risk of developing breast carcinoma.

- Present methods of screening for breast carcinoma are not ideal. Nevertheless, screening tests result in a reduction of mortality from breast cancer of approximately 25% to 30%.

- Physical examination is excellent as a screening procedure but extremely poor in predicting the histopathology of the lesion. Studies have demonstrated 30% to 40% of breast masses suspected by palpation to be malignant were found after biopsy to be benign. Conversely, 15% to 20% of benign-appearing masses during a physical examination subsequently are discovered to be carcinoma by histopathology.

- The 5-year survival of a woman whose breast carcinoma is believed to be localized to the breast with negative axillary nodes is 85%. In contrast, the 5-year survival is only 53% when axillary nodes are positive.

- The number of women receiving screening mammography has increased dramatically over the past 10 years. Mammography is not as precise in younger women or in women with dense breasts secondary to fibroglandular tissue. Mammography is most sensitive in older women in which the majority of the breast is composed of fatty tissue.

- Present studies demonstrate that screening mammography reduces breast cancer mortality by approximately 33% in women 50 to 70 years of age.

- For screening mammography, two views of each breast are performed: the mediolateral oblique (MLO) and the craniocaudal (CC). The MLO is the most effective single view because it includes the greatest amount of breast tissue and is the only view that includes all of the upper-outer quadrant and axillary tail.

- Mammographic signs of carcinoma include isolated clusters of fine, irregular calcifications or poorly defined masses with irregular contours.

- Double-reading of a mammographic study by two independent observers improves the breast cancer detection rate by approximately 10%. Obviously, it also increased the cost of screening. Computer-aided diagnosis shows promise of potentially detecting lesions that would not be identified by double-reading.

- The radiation dose to the breast by state-of-the-art mammography equipment is 0.1 rad (0.001 Gy) for a two-view examination.

- The most important use of ultrasound is to differentiate a cystic breast mass from a solid mass.

- Ultrasound should not be used as a sole imaging technique for breast disease. Because of its lack of sensitivity and specificity for early breast carcinoma, it should not be used in an attempt to detect subclinical disease.

- Digital technology has multiple advantages compared with conventional mammography. Image acquisition, display, and storage are much faster, and image manipulation through adjustments in contrast, brightness, and electronic magnification of selected regions enables radiologists to obtain superior views.

- Digital technology makes it possible to subtract various layers of computerized imagery in order to examine suspicious areas and improve the ability to detect and diagnose breast carcinoma. Digital mammography is particularly helpful in screening women with very dense breasts and breast implants. With the ability to manipulate the images, digital mammography will reduce the number of women recalled for more images.

- The ability of MRI to differentiate benign from malignant tissue may help to reduce the frequency of breast biopsy, especially in women with dense, fibroglandular breasts. MRI has been proven effective in detecting new tumors in women with previous lumpectomy because it can accurately distinguish between scar tissue and cancerous lesions.

- If the aspirated fluid from a breast cyst is clear and no residual mass is palpated immediately after the procedure and again 1 month later, no further workup is necessary.

- Palpable lesions can be evaluated by several techniques. The type of technique used is dependent on many factors including the location and size of the lesion as well as patient and physician preference. Options include incisional or excisional biopsy, as well as core-needle biopsy.

- The incidence of carcinoma in biopsies corresponds directly with the patient's age. Approximately 20% of breast biopsies in women age 50 are positive, and this figure increases to 33% in women age 70 or older.

- Breast cancer is usually asymptomatic before the development of advanced disease. Breast pain is experienced by only 10% of women with early breast carcinoma.

- The classic sign of a breast carcinoma is a solitary, solid, three-dimensional, dominant breast mass. The borders of the mass are usually indistinct.

- Bilateral breast carcinoma occurs in approximately 1% of all newly diagnosed cases. The prevalence of bilateral breast cancer is twofold greater in lobular neoplasia.

- Infiltrating ductal carcinoma is the most common breast malignancy.

- Microscopic metastatic disease occurs early via both hematogenous and lymphatic routes. For example, 30% to 40% of women without gross adenopathy in the axilla will have positive nodes discovered during histologic examination. With the additional assessment tools of immunohistochemical staining for the presence of cytokeratin and serial sectioning of axillary nodes, 10% to 30% of patients considered to have negative nodes by standard histologic analysis are found to be node positive.

- Approximately two thirds of all women with breast carcinoma eventually develop distant metastatic disease regardless of the type of initial therapy.

- Three major objectives of treating breast carcinoma are control of local disease, treatment of distant metastasis, and improved quality of life for women treated for the disease.

- Breast conservation is a frequent choice for the control of local disease. Sentinel node resection is becoming standard practice in the treatment of early stage breast cancer. Chemotherapy is used not only for patients with proved metastatic disease, but also for women at high risk for the development of primary or recurrent disease.

- Recent emphasis on conservative surgery plus radiation therapy to control multifocal cancer in the same breast and on reconstructive surgery after mastectomy has improved the quality of life of women with breast carcinoma.

- The initial size of the breast carcinoma is the single best predictor of the likelihood of positive axillary nodes. The presence and number of axillary node metastasis is the single best predictor of survival.

- The primary therapy for the vast majority of women with stages I and II breast cancer is conservative surgery, which preserves the breast, followed by radiation therapy.

- Another conservative approach to the treatment of breast cancer involves the use of sentinel lymph node mapping as an alternative to axillary dissection.

- Adjuvant systemic chemotherapy decreases the odds of dying from breast cancer during the first 10 years following diagnosis by approximately 25%.

- When estrogen receptors are positive, approximately 60% of breast cancers will respond to hormonal therapy. If estrogen receptors are negative, less than 10% of tumors respond to a hormonal manipulation.

- Adjuvant chemotherapy has been shown to improve disease-free and overall survival in all patients with operable breast cancer with the exception of select node-negative patients with small (less than 1 cm) tumors that have no high-risk features.

- Approximately 10% to 20% of women treated with combination chemotherapy experience a complete remission for about 18 months.

- The major effect of multiagent systemic therapy has been on the disease-free interval rather than the effect on overall survival. In general, multiple-agent chemotherapy has greater effect than single-agent chemotherapy, especially in the premenopausal woman. Tamoxifen has the greatest effect in postmenopausal women.

- Recent clinical trials have investigated the use of extremely intensive chemotherapeutic regimens followed by transplantation of autologous bone marrow in women with advanced breast cancer or recurrent disease. Obviously, this therapy is expensive, requires prolonged hospitalization, and has a mortality rate of approximately 15%.

BIBLIOGRAPHY

American Cancer Society: Cancer Facts & Figures—2000.

Baines CJ: Breast self-examination, Cancer 69:1942, 1992.

Barton MB, Harris R, and Fletcher SW: Does this patient have breast cancer? The screening clinical breast examination: should it be done? How? JAMA 282:1270, 1999.

Bassett LW and Gambhir S: Breast imaging in the 1990s, Semin Oncol 18:80, 1991.

Bassett LW, Giuliano AE, and Gold RH: Staging for breast carcinoma, Am J Surg 157:250, 1989.

Berg JW: Clinical implications of risk factors for breast cancer, Cancer 53:589, 1984.

Berkel H, Birdsell DC, and Jenkins H: Breast augmentation: a risk factor for breast cancer? N Engl J Med 326:1649, 1992.

Betsill WL, Rosen PP, Lieberman PH, et al: Intraductal carcinoma: long-term follow-up after treatment by biopsy alone, JAMA 239:1863, 1978.

Biro FM, Lucky AW, Huster GA, et al: Hormonal studies and physical maturation in adolescent gynecomastia, J Pediatr 116:450, 1990.

Black WC and Fletcher SW: Effects of estrogen on screening mammography: another complexity, J Natl Cancer Inst 88:62, 1996.

Bland KI and Copeland EM III: Breast. In Schwartz SI, Shires GT, and Spencer FE, editors: Principles of surgery, ed 6, New York, 1994, McGraw Hill, p 562.

Boothroyd A and Carty H: Breast masses in childhood and adolescence: a presentation of 17 cases and a review of the literature, Pediatr Radiol 24:81, 1994.

Bottels K, Chan JS, and Holly EA: Cytologic criteria for fibroadenoma: a step wise logistic regression analysis, Am J Clin Pathol 89:707, 1988.

Brenner RJ, Bein ME, Sarti DA, and Vinstein AL: Spontaneous regression of interval benign cysts of the breast, Radiology 193:365, 1994.

Burke W, Daly M, Garber J, et al: Recommendations for follow-up care of individuals with an inherited predisposition to cancer, JAMA 277:997, 1997.

Buzdar AU and Hortobagyi GN: Recent advances in adjuvant therapy of breast cancer, Semin Oncol 26 (suppl 12):21, 1999.

Cant PJ, Madden MV, Coleman MG, and Dent DM: Nonoperative management of breast mass diagnosed as fibroadenoma, Br J Surg 82:792, 1995.

Carter D: Intraductal papillary tumors of the breast: a study of 78 cases, Cancer 39:1689, 1977.

Chlebowski RT: Reducing the risk of breast cancer, N Eng J Med 343:191, 2000.

Chua CL, Thomas A, and Ng BK: Cystosarcoma phyllodes: a review of surgical options, Surgery 105:141, 1989.

Colditz GA, Stampher MS, Willett WC, et al: Prospective study of estrogen replacement therapy and risk of breast cancer in postmenopausal women, JAMA 264:2648, 1990.

Colditz GA, Stampher MS, Willett WC, et al: Type of postmenopausal hormone use and risk of breast cancer: 12-year follow-up from the Nurses' Health Study, Cancer Causes Control 3:433, 1992.

Corley D, Rowe J, Curtis MT, et al: Postmenopausal bleeding from unusual endometrial polyps in women on chronic tamoxifen therapy, Obstet Gynecol 79:111, 1992.

Cummings SR, Eckert S, Krueger KA, et al: The effect of raloxifene on risk of breast cancer in postmenopausal women: results from the MORE randomized trial, JAMA 281:2189, 1999.

Davis PL, Staiger MJ, Harris KB, et al: Breast cancer measurements with magnetic resonance imaging, ultrasonography, and mammography, Breast Cancer Res Treat 37:1, 1996.

Dershaw DD and Chaglassian TA: Mammography after prosthesis placement for augmentation or reconstruction mammoplasty, Radiology 170:69, 1989.

De Waard F: Epidemiology of breast cancer: a review, Eur J Cancer Clin Oncol 19:1671, 1983.

Dupont WD and Page DL: Risk factors for breast cancer in women with proliferative breast disease, N Engl J Med 312:136, 1985.

Dupont WD, Page DL, Parl FF, et al: Long-term risk of breast cancer in women with fibroadenoma, N Engl J Med 331:10, 1994.

Early Breast Cancer Trialists' Collaborative Group: Effects of adjuvant tamoxifen and of cytotoxic therapy on mortality in early breast cancer, N Engl J Med 319:1681, 1988.

Early Breast Cancer Trialists' Collaborative Group: Effects of radiotherapy and surgery in early breast cancer: an overview of the randomized trials, N Engl J Med 333:1444, 1995.

Eberlein TJ: Current management of carcinoma of the breast, Ann Surg 220:121, 1994.

Eklund GW, Cardenosa G, and Parsons W: Assessing adequacy of mammographic image quality, Radiology 190:297, 1994.

Elmore JG, Barton MB, Moceri VM, et al: Ten-year risk of false positive screening mammograms and clinical breast examinations, N Engl J Med 338:1089, 1998.

Elmore JG, Wells CK, Lee CH, et al: Variability in radiologists' interpretations of mammograms, N Engl J Med 331:1493, 1994.

Feig SA: Age-related accuracy of screening mammography: how should it be measured? Radiology 214:633, 2000.

Feig SA and Ehrlich SM: Estimation of radiation risk from screening mammography: recent trends and comparison with expected benefits, Radiology 174:638, 1990.

Fisher B, Costantino J, Redmond C, et al: Lumpectomy compared with lumpectomy and radiation therapy for the treatment of intraductal breast cancer, N Engl J Med 328:1581, 1993.

Fisher B, Bauer M, Margolese R, et al: Five-year results of a randomized clinical trial comparing total mastectomy and segmental mastectomy with or without radiation in the treatment of breast cancer, N Engl J Med 312:665, 1985.

Fisher B, Costantino J, Redmond C, et al: A randomized clinical trial evaluating tamoxifen in the treatment of patients with node-negative breast cancer who have estrogen-receptor-positive tumors, N Engl J Med 320:479, 1989.

Fisher B, Costantino JP, Wickerham DL, et al: Tamoxifen for the prevention of breast cancer: report of the National Surgical Adjuvant Breast and Bowel Project P-1 study, J Natl Cancer Inst 90:1371, 1998.

Fisher B, Redmond C, Dimitrov NV, et al: A randomized clinical trial evaluating sequential methotrexate and fluorouracil in the treatment of patients with node-negative breast cancer who have estrogen-receptor-negative tumors, N Engl J Med 320:473, 1989.

Fletcher SW, O'Malley MS, and Bunce LA: Physicians' abilities to detect lumps in silicone breast models, JAMA 253:2224, 1985.

Folkman J: Angiogenesis and breast cancer, J Clin Oncol 12:441, 1994.

Foster RS and Costanza MC: Breast self-examination practices and breast cancer survival, Cancer 53:999, 1984.

Fowler PA, Casey CE, and Cameron GG: Cyclic changes in composition and volume of the breast during the menstrual cycle, measured by magnetic resonance imaging, Br J Obstet Gynaecol 97:595, 1990.

Frantz VK, Pickren JW, Melcher GW, et al: Incidence of chronic cystic disease in so-called "normal breasts," Cancer 4:762, 1951.

Gail MH, Brinton LA, Byar DP, et al: Projecting individualized probabilities of developing breast cancer for white females who are being examined annually, J Natl Cancer Inst 81:1879, 1989.

Gasparini G and Harris AL: Clinical importance of the determination of tumor angiogenesis in breast carcinoma: much more than a new prognostic tool, J Clin Oncol 13:765, 1995.

Gateley CA, Miers M, Mansel RE, and Hughes LE: Drug treatments for mastalgia: 17 year experience in the Cardiff mastalgia clinic, J R Soc Med 85(1):12, 1992.

Goldhirsch A, Gelber RD, Price KN, et al: Effect of systemic adjuvant treatment on first sites of breast cancer relapse, Lancet 343:377, 1994.

Greendale GA, Reboussin BA, Sie A, et al: Effects of estrogen and estrogen-progestin on mammographic parenchymal density, Ann Inter Med 130:262, 1999.

Greenlee RT, Murray T, Bolden S, and Wingo PA: Cancer Statistics, 2000, CA Cancer J Clin 50:7, 2000.

Greenwald P, Nasca PC, Lawrence CE, et al: Estimated effect of breast self-examination and routine physician examinations on breast-cancer mortality, N Engl J Med 299:271, 1978.

Gusberg SB: The treatment of breast cancer: should we play a role? Gynecol Oncol 49:277, 1993.

Harris JR, Lippman ME, Morrow M, and Hellman S, editors: Diseases of the breast, Philadelphia, 1996, Lippincott-Raven.

Harris JR, Lippman ME, Veronesi U, and Willett W: Breast cancer: first of three parts, N Engl J Med 327:319, 1992.

Harris JR, Lippman ME, Veronesi U, and Willett W: Breast cancer: second of three parts, N Engl J Med 327:319, 1992.

Harris JR, Lippman ME, Veronesi U, and Willett W: Breast cancer: third of three parts, N Engl J Med 327:319, 1992.

Harris R and Leininger L: Clinical strategies for breast cancer screening: weighing and using the evidence, Ann Intern Med 122:539, 1995.

Harrison BJ, Maddox PR, and Mansel RE: Maintenance therapy of cyclical mastalgia using low-dose danazol, J R Coll Surg Edinb 34:79, 1989.

Hartmann LC, Schaid DJ, Sellers T, et al: Bilateral prophylactic mastectomy (PM) in BRCA1/2 mutation carriers, Proc Am Assoc Cancer Res 41:222, 2000. Abstract.

Hartmann LC, Schaid DJ, Woods JE, et al: Efficacy of prophylactic mastectomy in women with a family history of breast cancer, N Eng J Med 340:77, 1999.

Harvey BJ, Miller AB, Baines CJ, and Corey PN: Effect of breast self-examination techniques on the risk of death from breast cancer, Can Med Assoc J 157:1205, 1997.

Henderson IC, Hayes DF, Parker LM, et al: Adjuvant systemic therapy for patients with node-negative tumors, Cancer 65:2132, 1990.

Hildreth NG, Shore RE, Dvoretsky PM, et al: The risk of breast cancer after irradiation of the thymus in infancy, N Engl J Med 321:1281, 1989.

Hindle WH: Breast disease for gynecologists, Norwalk, Conn, 1990, Appleton & Lange.

Hindle WH and Alonzo LJ: Conservative management of breast fibroadenomas, 164:1647, 1991.

Hindle WH, Payne PA, and Pan EY: The use of fine-needle aspiration in the evaluation of persistent palpable dominant breast masses, Am J Obstet Gynecol 168:1814, 1993.

Hortobagyi GN: Treatment of breast cancer, N Engl J Med 339:974, 1998.

Hoskins KF, Stopfer JE, Calzone KA, et al: Assessment and counseling for women with a family history of breast cancer: a guide for clinicians, JAMA 273:577, 1995.

Howarth D, Sillar R, Lan L, et al: Scintimammography: an adjunct test for the detection of breast cancer, MJA 170:588, 1999.

Huang Z, Hankinson SE, Colditz GA, et al: Dual effects of weight and weight gain on breast cancer risk, JAMA 278:1407, 1997.

Hughes LE: Benign breast disorders: the clinician's view, Ca Detec Preven 16:1, 1992.

Jensen RA, Page DL, DuPont WD, et al: Invasive breast cancer risk in women with sclerosing adenosis, Cancer 64:1977, 1989.

Kerlikowske K, Grady D, Rubin SM, et al: Efficacy of screening mammography: a meta-analysis, JAMA 273:149, 1995.

Kopans DB, Swann CA, White G, et al: Asymmetric breast tissue, Radiology 171:639, 1989.

Korenman SG: Estrogen window hypothesis of the etiology of breast cancer, Lancet 1:700, 1980.

Korenman SG: The endocrinology of breast cancer, Cancer 46:874, 1980.

Kornguth PJ, Rimer BK, Conaway MR, et al: Impact of patient-controlled compression on the mammography experience, Radiology 186:99, 1993.

Krag D, Weaver D, Ashikaga T, et al: The sentinel node in breast cancer, N Eng J Med 339:941, 1998.

Lancaster JM, Wiseman RW, and Berchuck A: An inevitable dilemma: prenatal testing for mutations in the BRCA1 breast-ovarian cancer susceptibility gene, Obstet Gynecol 87:306, 1996.

Land CE: Studies of cancer and radiation dose among atomic bomb survivors, JAMA 274:402, 1995.

Laya MB, Larson EB, Taplin SH, and White E: Effect of estrogen replacement therapy on the specificity and sensitivity of screening mammography, J Natl Cancer Inst 88:643, 1996.

Layde PM, Webster LA, Baughman AL, et al: The independent associations of parity, age at first full-term pregnancy, and duration of breastfeeding with the risk of breast cancer, J Clin Epidemiol 42:963, 1989.

Lazovich D, Solomon CC, Thomas DB, et al: Breast conservation therapy in the United States following the 1990 National Institutes of Health Consensus Development Conference on the treatment of patients with early stage invasive breast carcinoma, Cancer 86:628, 1999.

Leis HP and Kwon CS: Fibrocystic disease of the breast, J Reprod Med 22:291, 1979.

Leis HP Jr: The significance of nipple discharge. In Schwartz GF and Marchant D, editors: Breast disease, diagnosis and treatment, New York, 1980, Symposia Specialists, p 111.

Liljegren G, Holmberg L, Bergh J, et al: 10-year results after sector resection with or without postoperative radiotherapy for stage I breast cancer: a randomized trial, J Clin Oncol 17:2326, 1999.

Longnecker MP: Alcoholic beverage consumption in relation to risk of breast cancer: meta-analysis and review, Cancer Causes Control 5:73, 1994.

Love RR, Mazess RB, Barden HS, et al: Effects of tamoxifen on bone mineral density in postmenopausal women with breast cancer, N Engl J Med 326:852, 1992.

Love SM, Gelman RS, and Silen W: Fibrocystic "disease" of the breast—non-disease? N Engl J Med 307:1010, 1982.

Ludwig Breast Study Group: Prolonged disease-free survival after one course of perioperative adjuvant chemotherapy for node-negative breast cancer, N Engl J Med 320:491, 1989.

Lundström E, Wilczek B, von Palffy Z, et al: Mammographic breast density during hormone replacement therapy: differences according to treatment, Am J Obstet Gynecol 181:348, 1999.

Mansour EG, Gray R, Shatila AH, et al: Efficacy of adjuvant chemotherapy in high-risk, node-negative breast cancer: an intergroup study, N Engl J Med 320:485, 1989.

Marchant DJ, Kase NG, and Berkowitz RL, editors: Breast disease, New York, 1986, Churchill Livingstone, Inc, pp 6-7.

McGuckin MA, Cummings MC, Walsh MD, et al: Occult axillary node metastases in breast cancer: their detection and prognostic significance, Br J Cancer 73:88, 1996.

McLelland R: Mammography 1984: challenge to radiology, AJR 143:1, 1984.

Mettler FA, Upton AC, Kelsey CA, et al: Benefits versus risks from mammography: a critical reassessment, Cancer 77:903, 1996.

Meyer JE, Eberlein TJ, Stomper PC, et al: Biopsy of occult breast lesions: analysis of 1261 abnormalities, JAMA 263:2341, 1990.

Meyer JE, Frenna TH, Polger M, et al: Enlarging occult fibroadenomas, Radiology 183:639, 1992.

Miki Y, Swensen J, Shattuck-Eidens D, et al: A strong candidate for the breast and ovarian cancer susceptibility gene BRCA1, Science 266:66, 1994.

Miller AB, Baines CJ, To T, and Wall C: Canadian National Breast Screening Study II: breast cancer detection and death rates among women aged 50–59 years, Can Med Assoc J 147:1477, 1992.

Miller AB, Howe GR, Sherman GJ, et al: Mortality from breast cancer after irradiation during fluoroscopic examinations in patients being treated for tuberculosis, N Engl J Med 321:1285, 1989.

Minton JP: Methylxanthines in breast disease. In Schwartz GF and Marchant D, editors: Breast disease, diagnosis and treatment, New York, 1980, Symposia Specialists, p 143.

Moffat CJC, Pinder SE, Dixon AR, et al: Phyllodes tumors of the breast: a clinicopathological review of thirty-two cases, Histopathology 27:205, 1995.

Monsonego J, Destable MD, Florent GDS, et al: Fibrocystic disease of the breast in premenopausal women: histohormonal correlation and response to luteinizing hormone releasing hormone analog treatment, Am J Obstet Gynecol 161:1181, 1991.

Morris T, Greer HS, and White P: Psychological and social adjustments to mastectomy, Cancer 40:2381, 1977.

Morrow M, Schmidt RA, Cregger B, et al: Preoperative evaluation of abnormal mammographic findings to avoid unnecessary breast biopsies, Arch Surg 129:1091, 1994.

Murad TM, Hines JR, Beal J, et al: Histopathological and clinical correlations of cystosarcoma phyllodes, Arch Pathol Lab Med 112:752, 1988.

National Cancer Institute Conference: The uniform approach to breast fine-needle aspiration biopsy, Am J Surg 174:371, 1997.

NCI Breast Cancer Screening Consortium: Screening mammography: a missed clinical opportunity? JAMA 264:54, 1990.

Newcomb PA, Storer BE, Longnecker MP, et al: Lactation and a reduced risk of premenopausal breast cancer, N Engl J Med 330:81, 1994.

NIH Consensus Conference: Treatment of early-stage breast cancer, JAMA 265:391, 1991.

Olivotto IA, Bajdik CD, Plenderleith IH, et al: Adjuvant systemic therapy and survival after breast cancer, N Engl J Med 330:805, 1994.

O'Malley MS and Fletcher SW: Screening for breast cancer with breast self-examination: a critical review, JAMA 257:2197, 1987.

Page DL, Dupont WD, Rogers LW, et al: Intraductal carcinoma of the breast: follow-up after biopsy only, Cancer 49:751, 1982.

Painter K: Factoring in cost of mammograms, USA Today p 11D, Dec. 5, 1996.

Palmer MD, DeRisi DC, Pelikan A, et al: Treatment options and recurrence potential for cystosarcoma phyllodes, Surg Obstet Gynecol 170:193, 1990.

Pisano E: Current status of full-field digital mammography, Radiology 214:26, 2000.

Powell DE and Stelling CB, editors: The diagnosis and detection of breast disease, St. Louis, 1994, Mosby–Year Book, Inc.

Powles T, Eeles R, Ashley S, et al: Interim analysis of the incidence of breast cancer in the Royal Marsden Hospital tamoxifen randomized chemoprevention trial, Lancet 352:98, 1998.

Recht A and Houlihan MJ: Axillary lymph nodes and breast cancer: a review, Cancer 76:1491, 1995.

Sacks MPM and Baum M: Primary management of carcinoma of the breast, Lancet 342:1402, 1993.

Schairer C, Lubin J, Triosi R, et al: Menopausal estrogen and estrogen-progestin replacement therapy and breast cancer risk, JAMA 283:485, 2000.

Schnitt SJ, Silen W, Sadowsky NL, et al: Ductal carcinoma in situ (intraductal carcinoma) of the breast, N Engl J Med 318:898, 1988.

Schutte M, Rozenblum E, Moskaluk CA, et al: An integrated high-resolution physical map of the DPC/BRCA2 region at chromosome 13q12, Cancer Res 55:4570, 1995.

Seitz S, Rohde K, Bender E, et al: Strong indication for a breast cancer susceptibility gene on chromosome 8p12-p22: linkage analysis in German breast cancer families, Oncogene 14:741, 1997.

Shah AK, Girishkumar HT, Parithivel VS, et al: Stereotactic needle breast biopsy: a review of current status and practice, Prim Care Update Ob/Gyns 6:147, 1999.

Shapiro S: The call for change in breast cancer screening guidelines, Am J Public Health 84:10, 1994.

Shattuck-Eidens D, McClure M, Simard J, et al: A collaborative survey of 80 mutations in the BRCA1 breast and ovarian cancer susceptibility gene: implications for presymptomatic testing and screening, JAMA 273:535, 1995.

Shimizu Y, Schull WJ, and Kato H: Cancer risk among atomic bomb survivors: the RERF life span study, JAMA 264:601, 1990.

Sickles EA: Breast masses: mammographic evaluation, Radiology 173:297, 1989.

Sickles EA, Filly RA, and Callen PW: Breast cancer detection with sonography and mammography: comparison using state-of-the-art equipment, AJR 140:843, 1983.

Sickles EA and Kopans DB: Mammographic screening for women aged 40 to 49 years: the primary care practitioner's dilemma, Ann Intern Med 122:534, 1995.

Sigurdsson H, Baldetorp B, Borg A, et al: Indicators of prognosis in node-negative breast cancer, N Engl J Med 322:1045, 1990.

Speroff L: Postmenopausal hormone therapy and breast cancer, Obstet Gynecol 87:44S, 1996.

Stavros AT, Thickman D, Rapp CL, et al: Solid breast nodules: use of sonography to distinguish between benign and malignant lesions, Radiology 196:123, 1995.

Strawbridge HTG, Bassett AA, and Foldes I: Role of cytology in management of lesions of the breast, Surg Gynecol Obstet 152:1, 1981.

Sutherland HJ, Lockwood GA, and Boyd NF: Ratings of the importance of quality of life variables: therapeutic implications for patients with metastatic breast cancer, J Clin Epidemiol 43:661, 1990.

Sutton GLJ and O'Malley UP: Treatment of cyclical mastalgia with low dose short-term danazol, Br J Clin Pract 40:68, 1986.

Thurfjell EL, Holmberg LH, and Persson IR: Screening mammography: sensitivity and specificity in relation to hormone replacement therapy, Radiology 203:339, 1997.

Veronesi U, Luini A, Del Vechio M, et al: Radiotherapy after breast-preserving surgery in women with localized cancer of the breast, N Engl J Med 328:1587, 1993.

Veronesi U, Maisonneuve P, Costa A, et al: Prevention of breast cancer with tamoxifen: preliminary findings from the Italian randomized trial among hysterectomized women, Lancet 352:93, 1998.

Veronesi V, Sacozzi R, Del Vecchio M, et al: Comparing radical mastectomy with quadrantectomy, axillary dissection, and radiotherapy in patients with small cancers of the breast, N Engl J Med 305:6, 1981.

Vorherr H: Breast aspiration biopsy, Am J Obstet Gynecol 148:127, 1984.

Walker MJ, Osborne MD, Young DC, et al: The natural history of breast cancer with more than 10 positive nodes, Am J Surg 169:575, 1995.

Weber BL: Genetic testing for breast cancer, Sci Am Sci Med Jan/Feb:12, 1996.

Weidner N: Prognostic factors in breast carcinoma, Curr Opin Obstet Gynecol 7:4, 1995.

Wolf DM and Jordan C: Gynecologic complications associated with long-term adjuvant tamoxifen therapy for breast cancer, Gynecol Oncol 45:118, 1992.

Zhang Y, Kreger BE, Dorgan JF, et al: Alcohol consumption and risk of breast cancer: the Framingham study revisited, Am J Epidemiol 149:93, 1999.

Adult Sequelae of Fetal Exposure to Diethylstilbestrol (DES)

Diagnosis, Monitoring, Fertility Management, Health Outcomes

Abnormal Transformation Zone. Area in the vagina or on the cervix that may contain columnar epithelium and squamous metaplasia and that often contains intraepithelial neoplasia that has an abnormal colposcopic pattern.

Adenosis. The presence of glandular (columnar) epithelium in the vagina. The tuboendometrial type is associated in some cases with the development of clear cell adenocarcinoma.

Cervicovaginal Ridge. A structural change in the cervix or upper vagina of DES-exposed females (hood, cockscomb, pseudopolyp, collar). In many cases it spontaneously disappears.

Clear Cell Adenocarcinoma of the Vagina and Cervix. Rare genital tract malignancy that occurs with increased frequency in DES females.

Diethylstilbestrol (DES). An orally active synthetic nonsteroidal estrogen.

Ectropion. The presence of glandular (columnar) epithelium on the ectocervix (portio of the cervix).

Müllerian Ducts. Paired structures in the embryo that in part lead to the formation of the female reproductive tract, primarily the upper vagina, cervix, uterus, and fallopian tubes.

Normal Transformation Zone. Area of columnar epithelium and squamous metaplasia in the vagina or on the cervix that has normal colposcopic patterns.

Squamous Metaplasia. Physiologic process by which squamous epithelium replaces the columnar epithelium of adenosis and ectropion.

Uterine Constriction Ring and T-Shaped Uterus. Types of abnormal shapes of the endometrial cavity diagnosed by hysterosalpingogram in DES females.

Diethylstilbestrol (DES) was initially synthesized in 1938 and was the first commercially available, orally active estrogen. It is derived from the stilbene molecule and biologically acts in a fashion similar to steroidal estrogens such as estradiol (Figure 15-1). Because it was relatively inexpensive and is orally active, its use for human therapy became widespread. In the late 1940s, DES treatment was used during pregnancy to prevent complications such as threatened abortion and prematurity. Many initial studies reported beneficial effects for DES pregnancy therapy, but some investigations in the early 1950s did not confirm these initial claims. The popularity of the drug for pregnancy support subsequently waned but continued into the 1960s. Finally, in 1971 it was noted that young women whose mothers took DES during pregnancy were at increased risk to develop a rare malignancy, clear cell adenocarcinoma of the vagina, and the use of estrogens for treatment of pregnancy complications in the United States was proscribed by the Food and Drug Administration.

In the United States it is estimated there have been approximately 3 million pregnant women treated with nonsteroidal synthetic estrogens, primarily DES. After the

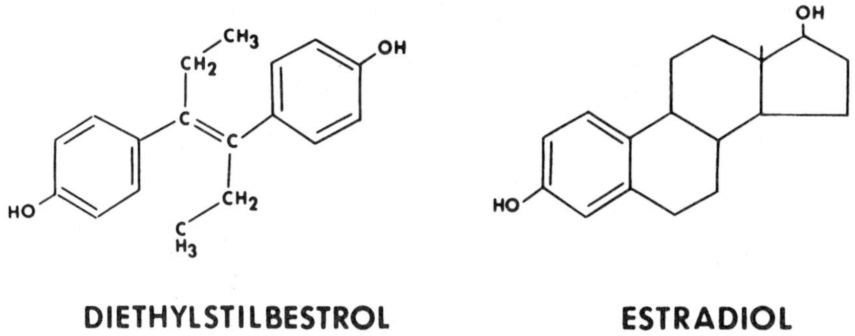

DIETHYLSTILBESTROL   **ESTRADIOL**

FIGURE 15-1   Structures of diethylstilbestrol and estradiol.

initial association with clear cell adenocarcinoma of the vagina and cervix, a number of nonmalignant epithelial structural abnormalities of the female genital tract have also been discovered in this population.

This chapter reviews the various genital tract changes in DES-exposed females, including those that have been observed in their reproductive functions. The histogenesis of DES-associated genital changes is reviewed. In addition, a brief summary is provided of the current health status of DES-exposed males and mothers. The management of clear cell adenocarcinoma of the vagina is discussed in Chapter 33.

LOWER GENITAL TRACT (VAGINA AND CERVIX) ABNORMALITIES

Several nonneoplastic abnormalities of the cervix and vagina are found frequently in the genital tract of females exposed to DES in utero. These changes include vaginal adenosis, cervical ectropion, structural abnormalities of the cervix and upper vagina, and alterations in the shape of the endometrial cavity.

Vaginal adenosis (Figure 15-2) consists of glandular (columnar) epithelium or its mucinous products in the vagina; cervical ectropion refers to similar changes on

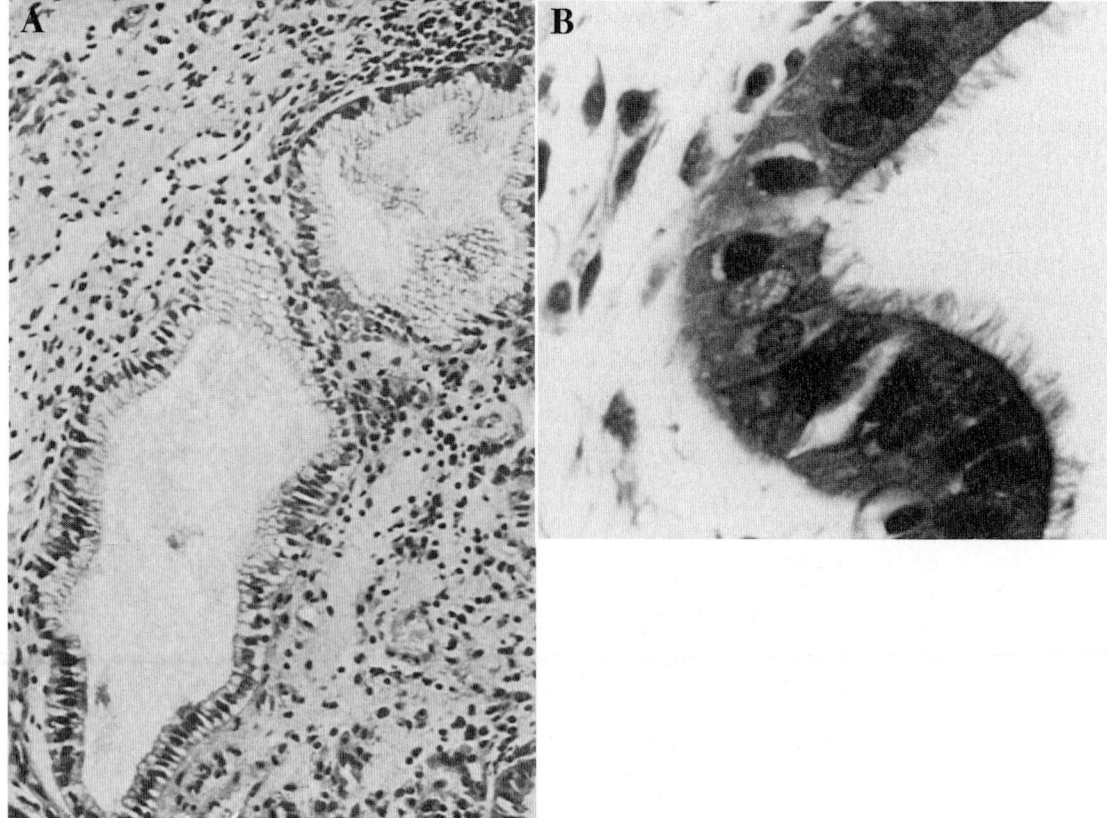

FIGURE 15-2   Vaginal adenosis. **A,** Glands are lined by endocervical-type epithelium (×200). **B,** Glands are lined by ciliated tuboendometrial cells (×890). (**A** from Herbst AL and Scully RE: Cancer 25:745, 1970. **B** from Herbst AL, ed: Intrauterine exposure to diethylstilbestrol in the human, Washington, DC, 1978, American College of Obstetricians and Gynecologists.)

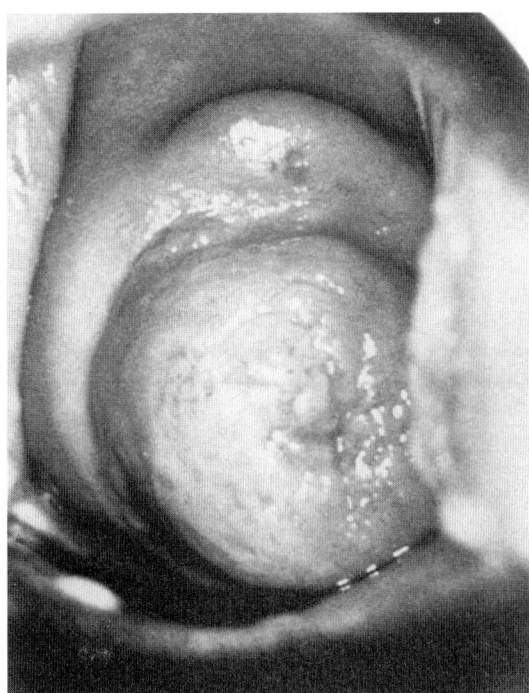

FIGURE 15-3 Vaginal hood. (From Robboy SJ, Scully RE, and Herbst AL: J Reprod Med 15:13, 1975.)

the ectocervix. The columnar epithelium of vaginal adenosis usually contains various cell types. One resembles the epithelium of the endocervix (Figure 15-2, *A*), and the other contains cells similar to the epithelium of the endometrium and fallopian tubes (so-called tuboendometrial cells) (Figure 15-2, *B*). It appears that the clear cell adenocarcinomas arise from the tuboendometrial cells. Intestinal metaplasia in DES-associated vaginal adenosis

has been described, raising the theoretic possibility of enteric-type neoplasms developing in the future.

Squamous metaplasia is frequently seen with adenosis and ectropion and is the physiologic process by which columnar epithelium is replaced by squamous epithelium. This process occurs normally in both DES-exposed and unexposed females.

Structural malformations of the lower genital tract, including transverse ridges, cervical collars, hoods, cockscombs, hypoplasia of the cervix, and pseudopolyps, have been described (Figure 15-3). Upper genital tract abnormalities (changes in the shape of the endometrial cavity) have also been identified on hysterosalpingogram examinations (Figure 15-4).

Frequency

Adenosis has been reported to occur in 30% to 90% of DES-exposed subjects. However, data from case-control studies that are not influenced by the potential bias of self-selection or physician referral suggest the overall prevalence is 30% to 40%. The term *vaginal epithelial changes* (VECs) has been used by some investigators to indicate the changes of vaginal adenosis and squamous metaplasia in the vagina.

The highest rate of adenosis occurs among those whose mothers began taking DES in early pregnancy, and changes are rarely observed in subjects whose mothers started treatment after the eighteenth week. A larger dosage of the drug also leads to a greater frequency of adenosis. As subjects grow older, the columnar epithelium is replaced in many instances by squamous metaplasia. Over years the healing process appears to proceed in most cases to complete healing.

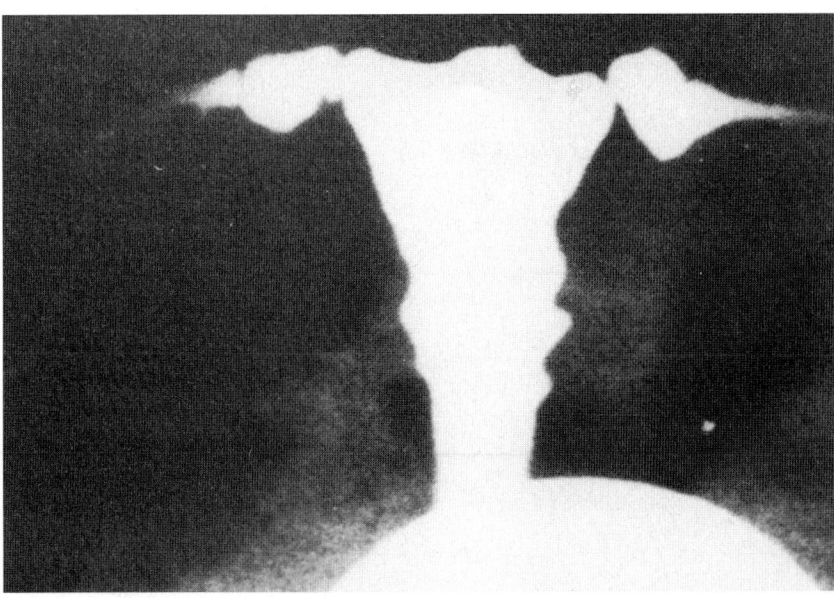

FIGURE 15-4 Hysterosalpingogram. Constrictions are noted in proximal portion of hornlike extension from uterine cavity. Uterine cavity is somewhat irregular. (From Kaufman RH, Adam H, Binder GL, et al: Am J Obstet Gynecol 137:299, 1980.)

The factors that promote the changes of squamous metaplasia are not clearly identified, although some have theorized that a more acid pH of the vagina may accelerate the process. Cervicovaginal structural abnormalities (ridges, hoods, collars, etc.) occur in approximately 25% of DES-exposed subjects. These structural changes are also more common with higher dosages of maternal medication and initiation of DES treatment early in pregnancy. These structural abnormalities also recede over a period of years and in some subjects disappear entirely.

Examination of the DES-Exposed Female

The initial examination of the DES-exposed female is conducted much like a thorough gynecologic pelvic examination (Chapter 6). One difference is that careful inspection and palpation of the entire vaginal mucosa and cervix are performed first. Surgical lubricants should not be used, since they interfere with the interpretation of cytologic specimens (Pap smear). After thorough palpation is completed, an appropriately sized speculum is inserted into the vagina. The speculum is gently rotated to allow full visualization of the entire vagina and cervix, with care taken not to obscure any small lesion of the anterior or posterior vaginal wall.

Cytologic samples are obtained from the vagina, including the fornices, as well as from the ectocervix and the endocervical canal (cytobrush [Medscand] or similar instrument—see Chapter 28). These three samples are submitted separately to identify the location of abnormal cells, if any, seen on the smears. Colposcopy (Chapter 28) is usually performed to allow detailed assessment of the cervicovaginal epithelium (transformation zone) but is not mandatory unless squamous cell abnormalities are being evaluated.

The colposcopic appearance of vaginal adenosis is often similar to the "grapelike" appearance of columnar epithelium on the cervix. Squamous metaplasia may give rise to an atypical-appearing transformation with areas of "mosaicism" and "punctation," findings that often suggest the presence of intraepithelial neoplasia in the unexposed female. However, in DES-exposed offspring such changes often indicate the presence of active squamous metaplasia (Figure 15-5) rather than a dysplastic process. Colposcopy allows for the careful evaluation of the transformation zone and provides a guide for biopsy sites in individuals whose Pap smears indicate squamous intraepithelial neoplasia. However, colposcopy is of little value in the detection of clear cell adenocarcinomas, which have no unique colposcopic vascular pattern, unlike squamous cell carcinomas. Biopsies should be performed on any suspicious nodular areas or from the most abnormal parts of the transformation zone if there is an atypical Pap smear. A careful bimanual vaginal and rectal examination completes the evaluation.

The intervals for follow-up examinations depend on the findings, as well as the completeness, of the initial examination. Yearly intervals are adequate for most individuals.

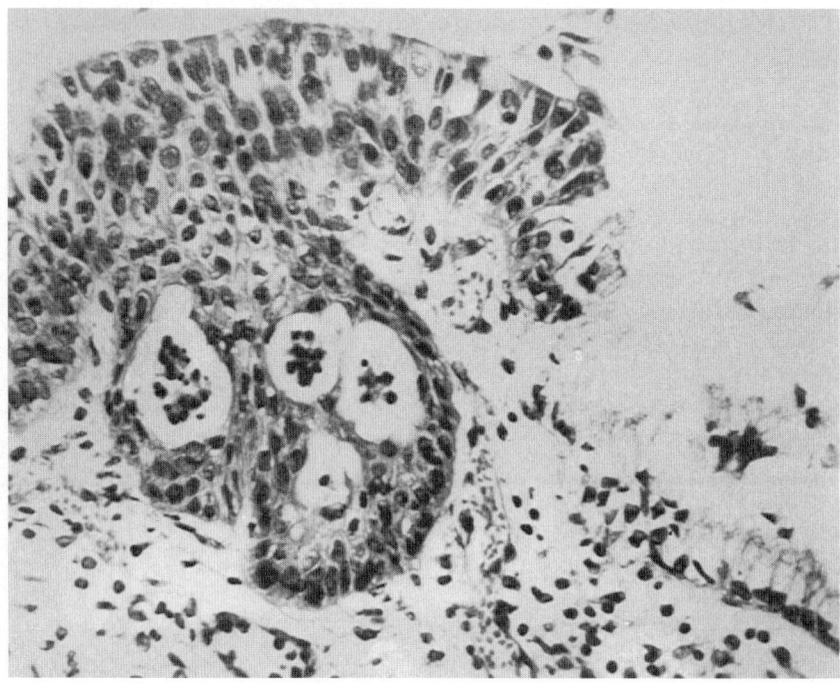

FIGURE 15-5   Squamous metaplasia of surface epithelium and underlying gland (×310). (From Herbst AL, Scully RE, and Robboy SJ: Hosp Pract 10:51, 1975.)

Semiannual examinations are often done for those who have large areas of vaginal adenosis, while the findings of cellular atypia in the vagina or cervical epithelium also necessitate more frequent follow-up.

Management

The tuboendometrial glands of vaginal adenosis are believed capable of providing the origin of clear cell adenocarcinoma. However, the risk of these tumors developing in an area of adenosis is extremely small. Therefore, unless atypia of the columnar epithelium is determined on biopsy or suggested cytologically, therapy for adenosis is not needed.

Because the extensive transformation zone in the DES-exposed female often extends far into the vagina, it has been hypothesized that a higher incidence of dysplasia or intraepithelial neoplasia may occur (Chapter 28). This larger transformation zone would theoretically provide a greater surface area of immature metaplastic epithelium that could be influenced by potential carcinogens. As noted by Bornstein et al. other factors, including increased rates of herpes simplex virus and human *Papillomavirus* infections, were observed among the DES exposed in that study, and a clear-cut association was not established. A new multi-institutional National Cancer Institute–sponsored follow-up by Hatch, Herbst, Hoover, et al. has shown approximately a 2-fold increase in occurrence of cervical dysplasia in DES-exposed. This study also suggests that moderate and severe dysplasia were more likely in those women whose mothers started DES prior to the eighth week of pregnancy. Exposed women also had a higher frequency of genital infections. Thus far follow-up studies have not demonstrated an increased risk of invasive cervical squamous carcinoma.

Although abnormal colposcopic findings (white epithelium, punctation, and mosaicism) are found frequently in DES-exposed women, it has been demonstrated that these abnormal colposcopic areas often contain active squamous metaplasia rather than a neoplastic process. It is important that therapy be based on an accurate histologic diagnosis and not be influenced by the history of DES exposure.

The therapy of intraepithelial neoplasia (dysplasia and carcinoma in situ) of the vagina and cervix in the DES-exposed female involves the same considerations as in those not exposed and is considered in detail in Chapters 28 and 32. Local destruction of the entire area of intraepithelial neoplasia is important. In the vagina this can be accomplished by local surgical excision or laser vaporization. In the cervix, laser treatment can also be utilized and occasionally local surgical therapy in the form of conization or a loop electroexcision procedure (LEEP) is indicated. Although cryotherapy (freezing) has been used successfully to treat intraepithelial neoplasia of the cervix in the unexposed woman, it has been reported to be followed by cervical stenosis and infertility in DES-exposed

females. For that reason this modality of therapy should be avoided, and therapy should be limited to those abnormal areas that require treatment.

Contraceptive Advice

No data indicate that any contraceptive method, including oral contraceptives, is contraindicated in the DES-exposed female. There has been concern regarding the potential increased risk of endocrine-related tumors, such as endometrial or breast carcinomas, in those offspring who have already been exposed in utero to high doses of exogenous estrogens. Concern involves potential future risks of increasing the lifetime exposure to any estrogen. However, ovarian preservation in patients treated for clear cell adenocarcinoma does not worsen the prognosis, and as noted subsequent oral contraceptive use does not increase the risk of clear cell adenocarcinoma of the vagina.

Barrier contraceptives and jellies have been frequently prescribed and appear to have the same risks and benefits for the DES-exposed female as for the unexposed population. The intrauterine device has also been used, although there is concern about prescribing it for use by the DES-exposed female because of the abnormal contours of the endometrial cavity that have been demonstrated on hysterosalpingograms in many subjects.

The diaphragm offers an effective method (Chapter 13) without major risk of side effects. Oral contraceptives provide a very effective and convenient form of contraception, and no data exist to indicate an increase in adverse risk factors in DES-exposed women who use this method of contraception.

DEVELOPMENT OF KIDNEYS AND URETERS

A number of studies have been done comparing the results of x-ray examinations of the kidneys and ureters (intravenous pyelograms) to evaluate the frequency of anatomic changes, such as duplication of a ureter or absence of a kidney. It appears that such changes have been observed in about 5% of the DES-exposed subjects studied, and this is the frequency anticipated in the general population. Thus DES exposure does not appear to cause anatomic abnormalities of the urinary tract.

IMMUNE FUNCTION

There has been some concern based on animal studies that DES-exposed offspring may have an altered immune state and may be subject to an increased frequency of autoimmune diseases. Noller et al. studied 1171 DES-exposed females and 922 controls. There was a trend of an increase of autoimmune diseases among the DES-exposed females

(49 in 1162) compared with controls (15 in 922), with a relative prevalence of 1.8, but the 95% confidence limits overlapped 1.0 (0.99 to 3.1). While not establishing a definitive clinical association, these data raise concern of a possibility of altered immune function in DES-exposed females, and this is currently the subject of a collaborative NIH study. A recent study of 13 DES-exposed women by Burke et al. demonstrated altered function in vitro of T-cell function in response to mitogens.

REPRODUCTION

Hysterosalpingogram Studies

Various abnormalities in the shape of the endometrial cavity have been identified on hysterosalpingograms (HSGs) performed on DES-exposed females (see Figure 15-4). Irregularities in the shape and size of the endometrial cavity have been observed, characterized by a T-shaped uterus; constriction rings near the entrance of the fallopian tubes into the uterus, as well as irregular contours of the surface; and a smaller than normal

endometrial cavity. HSG abnormalities occur in more than half of DES-exposed subjects. It appears that those who have cervicovaginal structural abnormalities or vaginal epithelial changes also are at greater risk for HSG abnormalities. These associations are related to the increased risk for uterine changes in individuals whose mothers began DES treatment in early pregnancy. Garbin et al. reported reduced pregnancy loss in 23 DES-exposed females who underwent hysteroscopic metroplasty and recommend the technique for those experiencing recurrent loss or prolonged severe infertility with a malformed uterus.

Menstrual Patterns

There are conflicting reports regarding menstrual function in the DES-exposed female. In general, it has been reported that menarche in the DES exposed is comparable to that of the general population—about 12 years of age. A prospective case control study by Hornsby et al. indicates that DES-exposed daughters have shorter duration of menstrual bleeding and less flow than comparable unexposed controls (Figure 15-6).

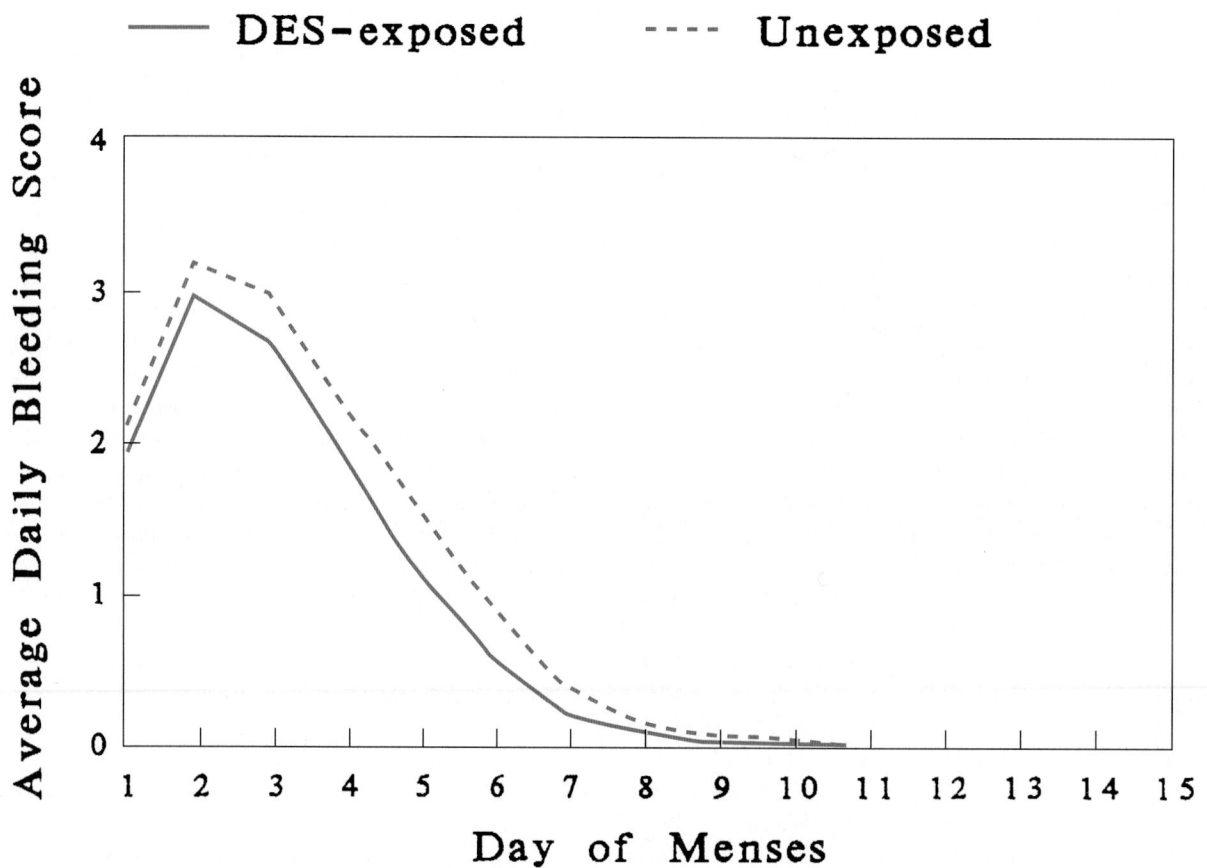

FIGURE 15-6 Composite menstrual period for DES-exposed and unexposed women. For each day, the average bleeding score was computed on the basis of all women. (From Hornsby PP, Wilcox AJ, Weinberg CR, and Herbst AL: Am J Obstet Gynecol 170:709, 1994.)

Moreover, Wilcox et al. showed no difference in onset of menstruation between DES-exposed granddaughters and unexposed controls, suggesting that the "third" generation has not been affected, and this is also being evaluated in a current NIH study. There are no case-control data at present to indicate alterations in cessation of ovarian activity such as a heightened risk of premature ovarian menopause in these women.

Fertility

Some studies have suggested decreased fertility among DES-exposed women. Table 15-1 summarizes the findings in four case-control studies that evaluated fertility in this group and adds a recent large NIH-sponsored collaborative trial. Two studies found no differences, while in the other two studies the differences were significant. The follow-up study of Senekjian et al. evaluated the causes of primary infertility and, not surprisingly, noted abnormal HSGs in approximately half the exposed subjects and in none of the controls. While there is no evidence the abnormal HSGs contributed to the primary infertility, the study demonstrated that a "tubal factor" was significantly more likely to occur in the DES-exposed subjects. The recent study of Palmer et al. confirmed a higher risk of infertility in DES-exposed females, associated with uterine or tubal problems. The tubal factor appears to be primarily related to adhesions secondary to pelvic inflammatory disease (PID) in the exposed subjects. It has not been established that DES-exposed women are more susceptible to PID, but they should be vigorously treated with appropriate intravenous antibiotics if PID is thought to exist (Chapter 23), since it is known that delayed care of PID is a risk factor for infertility as shown in the CDC-Collaborative Study by Hillis et al.

TABLE 15-1
Fertility in DES Exposed and Unexposed Females

Study	Conception Rate	
	Exposed	Unexposed
Herbst et al. (1980)	67%	86%
Barnes et al. (1980)	47%	50%
Cousins et al. (1980)	46%	41%
Senekjian et al. (1988)*	82%	95%
Palmer (2000)	72%	84%

*Follow-up of Herbst et al. (1980). Rates of at least one pregnancy.

TABLE 15-2
First Pregnancy Outcome in DES Exposed and Unexposed Females

Evaluable Pregnancy Outcome	Exposed (N = 158)		Unexposed (N = 157)	
Term birth	85	(54%)	130	(83%)
Premature*	32	(20%)	8	(5%)
Second-trimester loss (weeks 14 to 26)	4 ⎱	(19%)	1 ⎱	(12%)
Spontaneous abortion (≤13 weeks)	26 ⎰		18 ⎰	
Ectopic pregnancy	11	(7%)	0	

Adapted from Herbst AL, Senekjian EK, and Frey KW: Semin Reprod Endocrinol 7:124, 1989.

*Births were scored as premature if the duration of pregnancy was 26 weeks or more and birth weight was less than 2500 g.

All but one premature baby in each group survived.

Pregnancy Outcome

Unfavorable pregnancy outcomes, including premature live birth, ectopic pregnancy, and nonviable birth, have been reported more commonly among DES-exposed females. The most reliable source of data to evaluate these outcomes derives from case-control studies that have calculated the outcome of first pregnancies. Table 15-2 summarizes the results of one such study among DES-exposed females and unexposed controls. Seven percent of exposed women experienced ectopic pregnancy ($P < 0.01$) in their initial pregnancy. It also appears that unfavorable outcome may be more frequent among those noted to have cervicovaginal ridges on pelvic examination. However, these ridges are not stable and can disappear with time; their relation to adverse pregnancy outcome is not certain. Herbst et al. (1989) also noted that 12 of 30 exposed women who had cervical therapy with cautery or cryosurgery experienced at least one subsequent pregnancy loss compared with only 2 of 17 controls ($P < 0.05$), again suggesting that these modalities should be avoided. Although reproductive performance has been associated with an increased proportion of unfavorable outcomes, more than 80% of DES-exposed females who desire pregnancy have delivered at least one live-born infant. Thorp et al. reported DES gravidas were at increased risk for cesarean section, manual removal of the placenta, and postpartum hemorrhage.

Management

Although there may be an increased risk for unfavorable outcome in DES-exposed females with an abnormal hysterosalpingogram, the results of this examination have not been correlated with any individual or specific adverse pregnancy outcome. Therefore routine hysterographic evaluation of DES-exposed females is not warranted. The indications for obtaining HSGs in these individuals are similar to those for unexposed women who are undergoing infertility evaluation.

Careful prenatal care is required for the DES-exposed woman. An early vaginal ultrasound should be performed to confirm intrauterine pregnancy and detect any early ectopic pregnancy. Careful surveillance in the second and third trimesters is needed to treat preterm dilation of the cervix. Michaels et al. studied DES-exposed and unexposed women during pregnancy to monitor for cervical dilation (Figure 15-7). Cervical cerclage was placed when indicated by their ultrasound findings. Five of 21 DES-exposed patients required cerclage for cervical incompetence. The results were comparable, except control subjects delivered on the average 8 days later. There were no pregnancy losses among the exposed or unexposed patients because of cervical incompetence, and the technique appears safe and effective. Levine and Berkowitz found similar pregnancy outcomes among those DES-exposed women with or without genital tract anatomic deformities. They observed most losses in the first trimester and confirmed routine cerclage is not indi-

cated. If cerclage is needed for those with a hypoplastic cervix, Ludmir et al. used ultrasound and achieved transvaginal cerclage placement.

CLEAR CELL ADENOCARCINOMA OF THE VAGINA AND CERVIX

A special registry exists to centralize data on the clinical outcome, histopathology, and epidemiology of clear cell adenocarcinomas of the vagina and cervix that occur in women born after 1948. All such cancers are studied, regardless of a history of maternal hormone ingestion. As of early 2000 more than 715 cases of these rare carcinomas had been added. Approximately 60% of the cases reported are associated with a positive maternal history, whereas about one quarter show no history of DES-type treatment. The remainder of the cases had therapy for high-risk pregnancy either with unidentified or with non–DES-type drugs. It is likely that some of the so-called negative cases may be due to faulty memory or incomplete medical records, but some are undoubtedly negative, insofar as these cancers were also known to occur in young women in the pre-DES era. The fact that these tumors can occur in

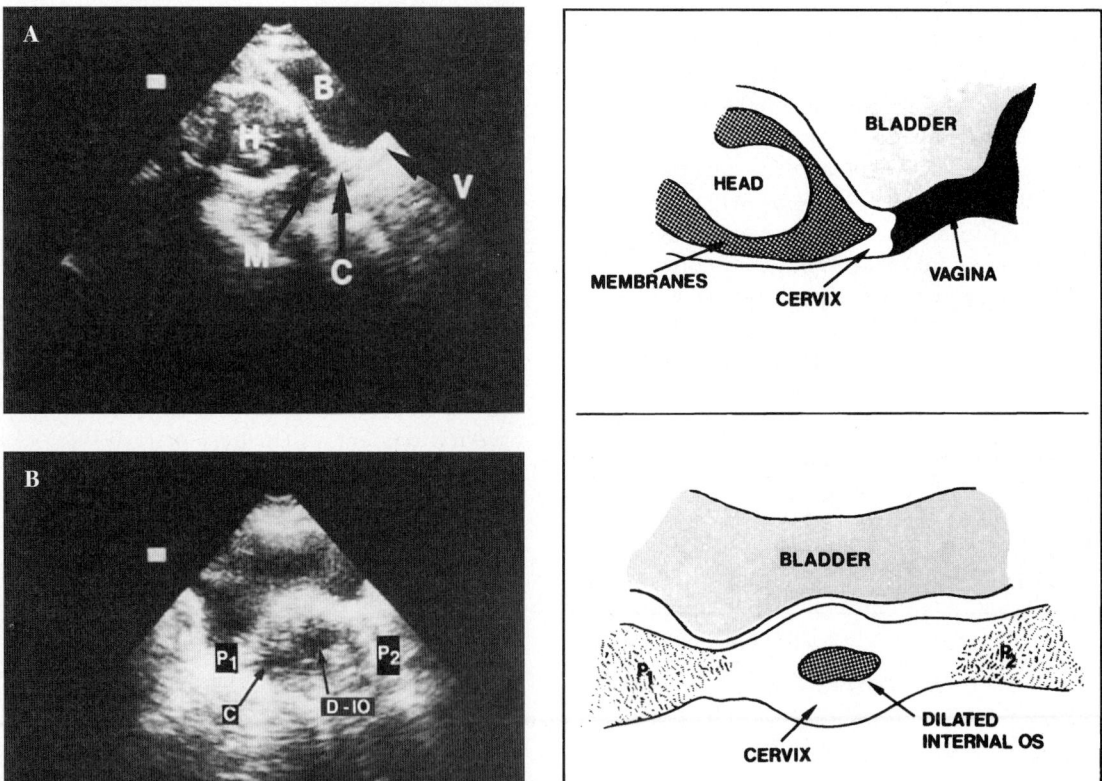

FIGURE 15-7   DES-exposed patient, 21.1 weeks pregnant, with membrane herniation. Internal os dilated to 20 mm, and cervix to 10 mm. **A,** Longitudinal view. **B,** Transverse view. *H,* Head; *M,* membrane herniation; *B,* bladder; *C,* cervix; *V,* vagina; *P1,* right parametrium; *P2,* left parametrium; *D-IO,* dilated internal os. (Reprinted with permission from Michaels WH, Thompson HO, Schreiber FR, et al: Obstet Gynecol 73:230, 1989.)

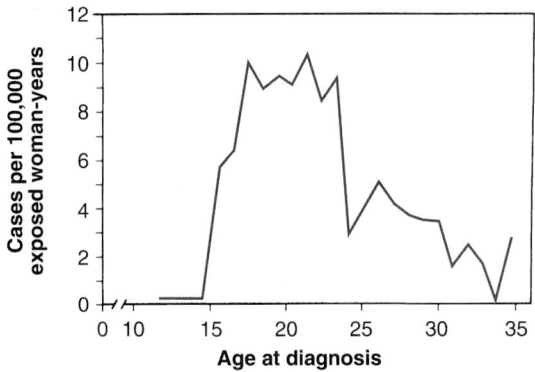

FIGURE 15-8   Incidence rates of clear cell adenocarcinoma, according to age, among white female residents of the United States who were prenatally exposed to diethylstilbestrol. (Reprinted with permission from Melnick S, Cole P, Anderson D, et al: N Engl J Med 316:514, 1987.)

the absence of DES exposure was recently confirmed by Kjorstad et al., who found three vaginal and seven cervical clear cell cases in Norway in women under age 40, yet DES was not used for pregnancy support in that country.

The age of DES patients diagnosed with clear cell adenocarcinoma has varied from 7 to 48 years. Figure 15-8 shows an age-incidence curve for these individuals up to age 35. It can be seen that the tumors are extraordinarily rare before age 14. Then the age-incidence curve rises rapidly, plateauing at about age 19, after which it drops through the 20s and 30s. Similar results for DES history and age distribution were reported by Hanselaar et al. on 55 patients from the Netherlands.

These tumors are uncommon, even among DES-exposed females, and the risk of cancer occurring in this population is estimated to be less than 1 cancer per 1000 exposed women. It does appear, however, that the risk of clear cell adenocarcinoma is increased among those females whose mothers began DES treatment in early pregnancy. However, recent studies have shown that DES-associated clear cell adenocarcinomas (CCA) have a better prognosis than those developing in unexposed females. This is similar to an improved outlook that has been reported in other estrogen-associated tumors including carcinomas of the endometrium and breast.

As noted previously, vaginal adenosis is also more frequent among those whose mothers started taking DES early in pregnancy. In addition a maternal history of miscarriage and premature birth also appear to be factors contributing to the development of clear cell adenocarcinoma. A recent analysis by Palmer et al. showed that neither subsequent pregnancy nor oral contraceptive use increased the risk of CCA. However, DES is a primary factor. In addition, a recent study indicates that maternal vaginal bleeding during the index pregnancy *reduces* the risk of clear cell adenocarcinoma and vaginal adenosis, providing further evidence that DES, rather than a problem preg-

nancy, is the primary factor in the development of these lesions. Insofar as clear cell adenocarcinomas have developed in DES-exposed females through their 20s and early 30s, these cancers will continue to be diagnosed for a number of years, since DES pregnancy usage is known to have continued, albeit on a limited basis, until 1971. An additional potential problem is raised by Merchant and Gale, who reported intestinal (mucinous) metaplasia in DES-associated vaginal adenosis, as well as by the report of DeMars et al. of mucinous-type vaginal adenocarcinoma developing in DES-exposed women. The therapeutic results of treatment of these tumors are considered in Chapter 33.

HISTOGENESIS OF DES-ASSOCIATED ABNORMALITIES

Although there are various interpretations, the development of the human vagina is believed to evolve primarily from the müllerian ducts and the urogenital sinus. The paired müllerian (paramesonephric) ducts arise as invaginations of the celomic epithelium near the urogenital ridge, extend caudally, and then fuse at the urogenital sinus. The müllerian-derived columnar epithelium is then replaced by a solid core of squamous epithelium that arises from the vaginal plate (Figure 15-9). The vaginal plate grows cephalad from the urogenital sinus, and the solid core of squamous epithelium ultimately canalizes to form the permanent lining of the vagina, which consists primarily of squamous epithelium.

The laboratory mouse has been used frequently to study the effects of hormones on the developing genital tract. In the newborn mouse the vagina is immature, and the reproductive tract continues to develop neonatally, similar to the changes that occur in humans during the latter part of intrauterine life. By administering estrogens, such as estradiol or DES, to neonatal mice, it has been found that the squamous transformation of columnar epithelium is arrested, resulting in the persistence of müllerian-type columnar epithelium in the upper vagina and cervix.

In utero exposure to DES in humans may have a similar effect, that is, a DES-induced persistence of glandular epithelium in the vagina leading to adenosis. The increased risk of clear cell adenocarcinoma in subjects whose mothers began DES treatment in early pregnancy may in part be due to the larger area of ectopic glandular epithelium in the vagina of these patients. Insofar as clear cell adenocarcinomas are related to the tuboendometrial cell of adenosis, increased areas of tuboendometrial-type epithelium in patients exposed to DES in early gestation may provide a greater area for interaction with an unidentified carcinogen. Endogenous estrogens could act as such a promoter insofar as the adenocarcinomas primarily occur after the onset of menstruation. However, not all the factors that lead to the appearance of these tumors are understood at present.

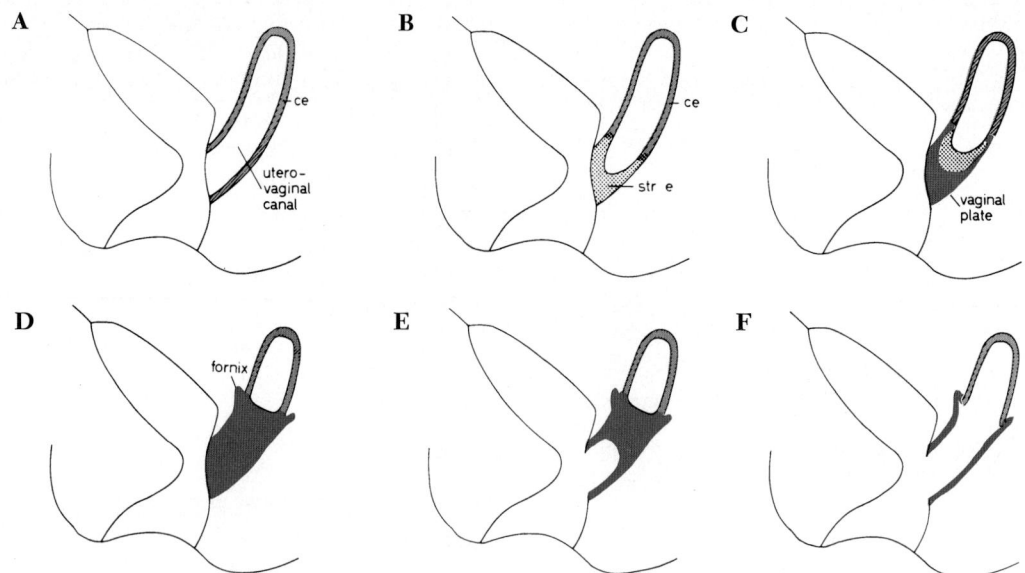

FIGURE 15-9 Diagrams of successive stages in development of human vagina. **A,** Uterovaginal canal is lined with columnar epithelium *(ce)*, which later, **B,** undergoes transformation into stratified squamous type *(str e)*. Transition between these two epithelial types is indefinite. At same time as transformation takes place, uterovaginal canal is changed into solid structure in same region, **B. C,** Vaginal plate has appeared between dorsal wall of urogenital sinus and region with stratified epithelium in uterovaginal anlage. Vaginal plate grows cranially, stratified epithelium is resorbed, and plate finally is in contact with columnar epithelium, **D.** Lumen formation in solid vaginal plate begins caudally, **E,** and progresses cranially, **F.** (From Forsberg JG and Kalland T: Embryology of the genital tract in humans and in rodents. In Herbst AL and Bern HA, eds: Developmental effects of diethylstilbestrol [DES] in pregnancy, New York, 1981, Thieme-Stratton, Inc.)

The structural abnormalities of the uterus and cervicovaginal areas may also be associated with anomalous development of the müllerian ducts. Although the mechanism is not clear, some unfavorable pregnancy outcomes observed in DES-exposed women appear to be related to the configuration of the endometrial cavity or to anomalies of the cervix. A defect in the development of the myometrium or in cervical-uterine connective tissue may also contribute. Recently it has been shown experimentally that the stroma of different parts of the embryonic female genital tract can have inductive effects that determine the histology of the overlying epithelium (Figure 15-10). For example, combining cervical stroma with uterine epithelium leads to cervical differentiation, while combining vaginal stroma with cervical epithelium leads to vaginal epithelial development. These observations suggest a primarily stromal action of DES that could account for both the epithelial and the connective tissue abnormalities often observed. Presumably, DES ingested by the mother crosses the uteroplacental barrier and enters the fetal circulation. It is known that estrogen receptors develop in the fetal genital tract in early intrauterine life. Insofar as DES is a nonsteroidal estrogen, it appears that it may not be metabolized in the fetal tissues in the same manner as steroidal estrogens. This would allow it to have the developmental effects noted in exposed offspring.

The genital abnormalities associated with DES in humans pertain to the ingestion of any stilbene-type estrogen (see Figure 15-1). Ingestion of steroidal estrogens during pregnancy has not been reported to be associated with such changes.

DES-EXPOSED MALES

Abnormalities have been described in DES-exposed males, including cryptorchidism, hypoplasia of the testis, more frequent epididymal cysts, and abnormalities in semen analyses. It should be remembered that the effect of DES on the female genital tract appears to occur primarily on the müllerian ducts. In the male genital tract the müllerian remnants are found in the epididymis of the testis and the utricle of the prostate. An increased risk in development of malignancy in DES-exposed males has not been demonstrated. The testicular and semen changes observed with increased frequency among DES-exposed males in some studies have not been verified in others. Studies in the 1980s suggested possible infertility problems in DES-exposed males. However, follow-up studies by Wilcox et al. indicate that intrauterine DES exposure did not impair fertility or sexual function in adult men.

DES-EXPOSED MOTHERS

Because of the high doses of estrogen taken during pregnancy by DES mothers, there have been concerns of an increased risk of estrogen-sensitive tumors in this group.

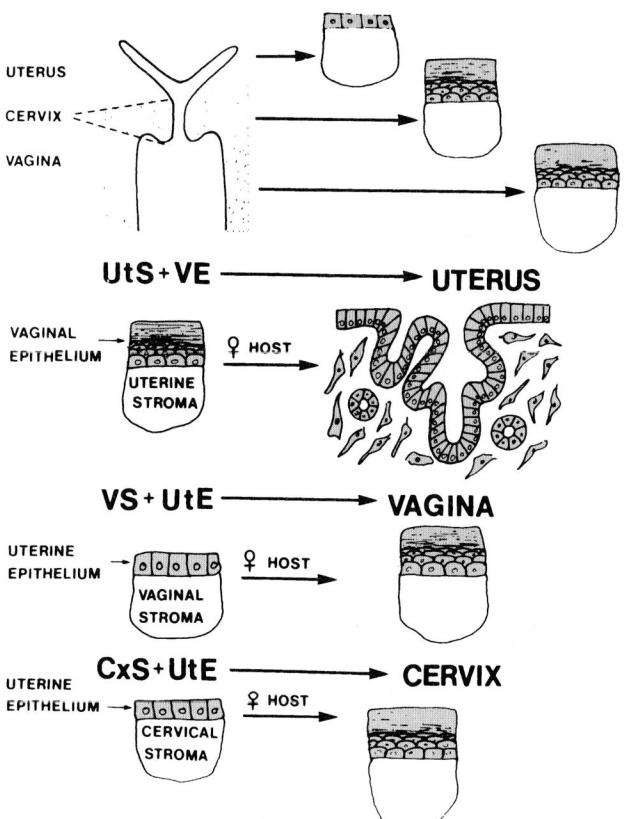

FIGURE 15-10 Summary of recombination experiments between epithelium and stroma from uterus, cervix, and vagina from neonatal mice (1 to 5 days old). Upper portion of figure depicts morphologic organization of epithelium in these organs: uterine epithelium is a simple columnar glandular epithelium, whereas vaginal and cervical epithelium is stratified squamous. Uterine stroma *(UtS)* induces uterine morphogenesis and cytodifferentiation from vaginal epithelium *(VE)*. In reciprocal recombination composed of vaginal stroma *(VS)* plus uterine epithelium *(UtE),* simple columnar epithelium normally is induced to differentiate as vaginal epithelium. Similarly, cervical stroma *(CxS)* induces development of stratified epithelium from *UtE.* (From Cunha GR and Fujii H: Stromal parenchymal interactions in normal and abnormal development of the genital tract. In Herbst AL and Bern HA, eds: Developmental effects of diethylstilbestrol [DES] in pregnancy, New York, 1981, Thieme-Stratton, Inc.)

TABLE 15-3
Breast Cancer Occurrence

	DES-Exposed	Unexposed	Relative Risk	95% Confidence Intervals
Bibbo, 1978	32/693	21/668	1.5	
Herbst, 1981*	35/655	28/645	1.2	
Greenberg, 1984	118/3033	80/3033	1.4	1.1 to 1.0
Hadjimichael, 1984	38/1531	24/1405	1.5	
Herbst, 1990*	50/692	45/666	1.1	
Colton, 1993	185/3029	140/3029†	1.35	1.05 to 1.74

*Follow-up study of Bibbo, 1978.

†Follow-up of Greenberg, 1984. No increased risk with time.

In particular, breast cancer and endometrial cancer, as well as other genital tract cancers, have been evaluated in case-control studies. Table 15-3 summarizes the occurrence of breast cancer incidence, citing studies that have evaluated this in DES-exposed women. Calle et al. evaluated mortality statistics from 501,556 females who participated in a breast cancer prevention study. Approximately a 30% excess of mortality from breast cancer was noted among the exposed. These data taken with the recent incidence study of Titus-Ernstoff et al. indicate a slight increase in risk for breast cancer in DES mothers. It is important that these patients follow regular breast cancer screening guidelines (Chapter 14). Furthermore, all studies show no increased risk with prolonged follow-up, as is shown in Table 15-3.

KEY POINTS

- Vaginal adenosis occurs in about one third of DES-exposed females.

- Cervicovaginal ridges occur in about one fourth of DES-exposed females.

- Vaginal adenosis is more frequent among those whose mothers took DES in early pregnancy, in those whose mothers took DES at a higher dose, and in exposed females who are younger at the time of examination.

- Adenosis and ectropion usually heal by the physiologic process of squamous metaplasia.

- Adenosis, ectropion, and cervicovaginal ridges heal spontaneously in many but not all DES-exposed females.

- Unfavorable pregnancy outcomes, particularly premature birth, midtrimester loss, and ectopic pregnancy, occur in about half of DES-exposed females.

- DES-exposed females have an approximately 2-fold increase in risk for moderate and severe cervical dysplasia. This risk is greatest for those whose mothers started therapy prior to the eighth week of gestation.

- DES females appear to be at increased risk for the development of genital infection.

- More than 80% of DES daughters have a live-born child.

- Routine hysterosalpingogram studies are not indicated for DES-exposed females.

- Primary infertility is more frequent in DES females, and tubal factors appear to be a contributory cause. An increased frequency of endometriosis has not been demonstrated. Adverse effects on male fertility have not been demonstrated.

- The risk of development of clear cell adenocarcinoma of the vagina and cervix is increased in DES-exposed females, but these tumors occur in less than 1 per 1000 exposed females and have been noted in those 7 to 48 years of age.

- Abnormal development of the müllerian ducts in utero results in reproductive tract alterations in the DES-exposed female.

- Factors that appear to increase the risk of development of clear cell adenocarcinoma, in addition to uterine DES exposure, include history of miscarriage in the mother and the daughter's prematurity. Oral contraceptive use does not alter the risk.

- DES females have menstrual periods of shorter duration and diminished flow compared with unexposed controls.

- Preliminary studies thus far have not shown any "third" generation effects.

- DES mothers have a slightly elevated risk for breast cancer. This risk has not thus far been demonstrated in DES daughters.

BIBLIOGRAPHY

Bibbo M, Gill WB, Azizi F, et al: Follow-up study of male and female offspring of DES-exposed mothers, Obstet Gynecol 49:1, 1977.

Bornstein J, Adam E, Adler-Storthz K, et al: Development of cervical and vaginal squamous cell neoplasia as a late consequence of in utero exposure to diethylstilbestrol, Obstet Gynecol Surv 43:15, 1988.

Burke L, Seagall-Blank M, Lorenzo C, et al: Altered immune responsivity in adult women exposed to diethylstilbestrol in utero. Am J Obstet Gynecol, in press.

Calle EE, Mervis CA, Thus MJ, et al: Diethylstilbestrol and risk of fatal breast cancer in a prospective cohort of US women. Am J Epidemiol 144:645, 1996.

Cousins L, Karp W, Lacey C, et al: Reproductive outcome of women exposed to diethylstilbestrol in utero, Obstet Gynecol 56:70, 1980.

Cunha G and Fujii H: Stromal-parenchymal interactions in normal and abnormal development of the genital tract. In Herbst AL and Bern HA, eds: Developmental effects of diethylstilbestrol (DES) in pregnancy, New York, 1981, Thieme-Stratton, Inc.

DeCherney AH, Cholst I, and Naftolin A: Structure and function of the fallopian tubes following exposure to diethylstilbestrol (DES) during gestation, Fertil Steril 36:741, 1981.

DeMars LR, Van Le L, Huang I, and Fowler WC: Case report: primary non-clear cell adenocarcinomas of the vagina in older DES-exposed women, Gynecol Oncol 58:389, 1995.

Dieckmann WE, Davis ME, Rynkiewicz SM, et al: Does the administration of diethylstilbestrol during pregnancy have therapeutic value? Am J Obstet Gynecol 66:1062, 1953.

Dodds EC, Goldberg L, Larson W, et al: Oestrogenic activity of certain synthetic compounds, Nature 141:247, 1938.

Fishman DA, Williams S, Small W Jr, et al: Late recurrences of vaginal clear cell adenocarcinoma, Gynecol Oncol 62:128, 1996.

Forsberg MD and Kalland T: Embryology of the genital tract in humans and in rodents. In Herbst AL and Bern HA, eds: Developmental effects of diethylstilbestrol (DES) in pregnancy, New York, 1981, Thieme-Stratton, Inc.

Fu Y, Robboy SJ, and Prat J: Nuclear DNA study of vaginal and cervical squamous cell abnormalities in DES-exposed progeny, Obstet Gynecol 52:129, 1978.

Garbin O, Ohl J, Bettahar-Lebugle K, et al: Hysteroscopic metroplasty in diethylstilbestrol-exposed and hypoplastic uterus: a report of 24 cases. Hum Reprod 13:2751, 1998.

Greenberg ER, Barnes AB, Resseguie L, et al: Follow-up study of mothers exposed to diethylstilbestrol in pregnancy, N Engl J Med 311:1393, 1984.

Hadjimichael OC, Meigs JW, Falcier FW, et al: Cancer risk among women exposed to exogenous estrogens during pregnancy, JNCI 73:831, 1984.

Hanselaar AGJM, Van Leusen NDM, DeWilde PCM, and Vooijs GP: Clear cell adenocarcinoma of the vagina and cervix: a report of the Central Netherlands Registry with emphasis on early detection and prognosis, Cancer 67:1971, 1991.

Hatch EE, Herbst AL, Hoover R, et al: Incidence of cervical dysplasia in DES-exposed daughters: Update and long-term follow-up of the NCI DES Follow-up study cohorts. Submitted.

Hatch EE, Palmer JR, Titus-Ernstoff L, et al: Cancer risk in women exposed to diethylstilbestrol in utero. JAMA 280:630, 1998.

Herbst AL: Behavior of estrogen-associated female genital tract cancer and its relation to neoplasia following intrauterine exposure to diethylstilbestrol (DES). Gynecol Oncol 76:147, 2000.

Herbst AL and Anderson D: Recent advances in clear cell adenocarcinoma of the vagina and cervix secondary to intrauterine exposure to DES, Semin Surg Oncol 6:343, 1990.

Herbst AL, Anderson S, Hubby M, et al: Risk factors for the development of DES-associated clear cell adenocarcinoma: a case control study, Am J Obstet Gynecol 154:814, 1986.

Herbst AL and Bern HA, eds: Developmental effects of diethylstilbestrol (DES) in pregnancy, New York, 1981, Thieme-Stratton, Inc.

Herbst AL, Cole P, Colton T, et al: Age-incidence and risk of diethylstilbestrol-related clear cell adenocarcinoma of the vagina and cervix, Am J Obstet Gynecol 128:43, 1977.

Herbst AL, Hubby MM, Azizi F, et al: Reproductive and gynecologic surgical experience in diethylstilbestrol-exposed daughters, Am J Obstet Gynecol 141:1019, 1981.

Herbst AL, Hubby MM, Blough RR, et al: A comparison of pregnancy experience in DES-exposed and DES-unexposed daughters, J Reprod Med 24:62, 1980.

Herbst AL and Scully RE: Adenocarcinoma of the vagina in adolescence: a report of 7 cases including 6 clear cell carcinomas (so-called mesonephromas), Cancer 25:745, 1970.

Herbst AL, Scully RE, and Robboy SJ: Effects of maternal DES ingestion on the female genital tract, Hosp Pract 10:51, 1975.

Herbst AL, Senekjian EK, and Frey KW: Abortion and pregnancy loss among diethylstilbestrol-exposed women, Semin Reprod Endocrinol 7:124, 1989.

Herbst AL, Ulfelder H, and Poskanzer DC: Adenocarcinoma of the vagina: association of maternal stilbestrol therapy with tumor appearance in young women, N Engl J Med 284:878, 1971.

Hillis SD, Riduan J, Marchbanks PA, et al: Delayed care of pelvic inflammatory disease as a risk factor for impaired fertility, Am J Obstet Gynecol 168:1503, 1993.

Hornsby PP, Wilcox AJ, Weinberg CR, and Herbst AL: Effects on the menstrual cycle of in utero exposure to diethylstilbestrol, Am J Obstet Gynecol 170:709, 1994.

Jeffries JA, Robboy SJ, O'Brien PC, et al: Structural anomalies of the cervix and vagina in women enrolled in the Diethylstilbestrol Adenosis (DESAD) Project, Am J Obstet Gynecol 148:59, 1984.

Kaufman RH, Adam H, Binder GL, et al: Upper genital tract changes and pregnancy outcome in offspring exposed in utero to diethylstilbestrol, Am J Obstet Gynecol 137:299, 1980.

Kaufman RH, Noller KL, Adam E, et al: Upper genital tract abnormalities and pregnancy outcome in diethylstilbestrol-exposed progeny, Am J Obstet Gynecol 148:973, 1984.

Kjorstad KE, Bergstrom J, and Abeler V: Clear cell adeno-carcinoma of the uterus and vagina in young women in Norway, J Norwegian Med Assoc 109:1634, 1989.

Levine RU and Berkowitz KM: Conservative management and pregnancy outcome in diethylstibestrol-exposed women with and without gross genital tract abnormalities, Am J Obstet Gynecol 169:1125, 1993.

Ludmir J, Jackson GM, and Samuels P: Transvaginal cerclage under ultrasound guidance in cases of severe cervical hypoplasia, Obstet Gynecol 78:1067, 1991.

Melnick S, Cole P, Anderson D, et al: Rates and risks of diethylstilbestrol-related clear cell adenocarcinoma of the vagina and cervix: an update, N Engl J Med 316:514, 1987.

Merchant WJ and Gale J: Intestinal metaplasia in stilboestrol-induced vaginal adenosis, Histopathology 23:373, 1993.

Michaels WH, Thompson HO, Schreiber FR, et al: Ultrasound surveillance of the cervix during pregnancy in diethylstilbestrol-exposed offspring, Obstet Gynecol 73:230, 1989.

Mittendorf R and Herbst AL: Diethylstilbestrol: an update, Cancer Prevention, 1–12, August, 1992.

Noller KL, Blair PB, O'Brien PC, et al: Increased occurrence of autoimmune disease among women exposed in utero to diethylstilbestrol, Fertil Steril 49:1080, 1988.

Noller KL, Townsend DE, Kaufman RH, et al: Maturation of vaginal and cervical epithelium in women exposed in utero to diethylstilbestrol (DESAD Project), Am J Obstet Gynecol 146:279, 1983.

Palmer JR, Anderson D, Helmrich SP, et al: Risk factors for diethylstilbestrol-associated clear cell adenocarcinoma. Obstet Gynecol, 95:814, 2000.

Palmer J, Hatch E, Hoover R, Herbst A, Kaufman R, Noller K, and Titus L: Infertility among women exposed prenatally to diethylstilbestrol. Am J Obstet Gynecol (submitted).

Robboy SJ, Noller KL, O'Brien P, et al: Increased incidence of cervical and vaginal dysplasia in 3980 DES-exposed young women, JAMA 252:2979, 1984.

Robboy SJ, Scully RE, and Herbst AL: Pathology of vaginal and cervical abnormalities associated with prenatal exposure to diethylstilbestrol (DES), J Reprod Med 15:5, 1975.

Senekjian EK, Potkul RK, Frey K, et al: Infertility among daughters either exposed or not exposed to diethylstilbestrol, Am J Obstet Gynecol 158:493, 1988.

Sharp GB and Cole P: Vaginal bleeding and diethylstilbestrol exposure during pregnancy: relationship to genital tract clear cell adenocarcinoma and vaginal adenosis in daughters, Am J Obstet Gynecol 162:994, 1990.

Thorp JM, Fowler WC, Donehoo R, et al: Antepartum and intrapartum events in women exposed in utero to diethylstilbestrol, Obstet Gynecol 76:828, 1990.

Titus-Ernstoff L, Hatch EE, Hoover RN, et al: Long-term cancer risk in women given diethylstilbestrol (DES) during pregnancy, Br. J. Cancer (in press).

Trimble EL, Rubinstein LV, Menck HR, et al: Vaginal clear cell adenocarcinoma in the United States, Gynecol Oncol 61:113, 1996.

Waggoner SE, Mittendorf RL, Biney N, et al: Influence of in utero diethylstilbestrol exposure on the prognosis and biologic behavior of vaginal clear cell adenocarcinoma. Gynecol Oncol 55:238, 1994.

Wilcox AJ, Baird DD, Weinberg CR, et al: Fertility in men exposed prenatally to diethylstilbestrol, N Engl J Med 332:1411, 1995.

Wilcox AJ, Umbach DM, Hornsby PP, and Herbst AL: Age at menarche among diethylstilbestrol granddaughters, Am J Obstet Gynecol 173:835, 1995.

Spontaneous and Recurrent Abortion
Etiology, Diagnosis, Treatment

KEY TERMS AND DEFINITIONS

Anembryonic Gestation (Blighted Ovum). Ultrasonic visualization of a gestational sac more than 17 mm in diameter without an embryo present. Sonographically, an embryo should be visualized in the uterine cavity beyond 43 days' gestational age.

Abortion. Termination of pregnancy before 20 weeks' gestation calculated from date of onset of last menses. An alternative definition is delivery of a fetus with a weight of less than 500 g. If abortion occurs before 12 weeks' gestation, it is called *early;* from 12 to 20 weeks it is called *late.*

Aneuploid Abortus. An abortus with the number of chromosomes less than or greater than the normal 46.

Anticardiolipin Antibody. An antiphospholipid antibody that is present in 5% to 15% of women with recurrent spontaneous abortion but in less than 2% of women with normal pregnancies.

Cerclage. A circular ligature used to treat the incompetent cervix. The suture is placed beneath the epithelium of the cervix at the level of the internal cervical os.

Complete Abortion. Spontaneous expulsion of all fetal and placental tissue from the uterine cavity before 20 weeks' gestation.

Conceptional Age. The duration of gestation from the date of conception.

Embryonic Death. Sonographic visualization of an embryo between 4 and 15 mm in length without cardiac activity.

Embryo. The human conceptus during the period of 35 to 70 days' gestational age.

Euploid Abortus. An abortus in which the chromosome complement is normal, 46,XX or 46,XY.

Fetus. The human conceptus during the period beyond 70 days' gestational age until delivery.

Gestational Sac. Fluid-filled structure in endometrial cavity. Earliest sonographic indicator of presence of intrauterine gestation.

Gestational Age. The duration of gestation from the date of onset of the last menstrual period before conception, usually considered to be 14 days longer than the conceptional age.

Incompetent Cervix (Cervical Incompetence). Condition whereby the internal cervical canal dilates at 16 weeks of gestation or later, resulting in recurrent premature pregnancy loss.

Incomplete Abortion. Passage of some but not all fetal or placental tissue from the uterine cavity through the cervical canal before 20 weeks' gestation.

Induced Abortion. Intentional medical or surgical termination of pregnancy before 20 weeks' gestation. Also called *elective pregnancy termination* if performed for the woman's desires or *therapeutic abortion* if performed to maintain the mother's health.

Inevitable Abortion. Uterine bleeding from a gestation of less than 20 weeks accompanied by cervical dilation but without expulsion of any placental or fetal tissue through the cervix.

Intrauterine Fetal Death. Sonographic visualization of fetus more than 15 mm long, crown-rump length, without fetal heart activity.

Lupus Anticoagulant. An antibody directed against the negatively charged phospholipids of the prothrombin activator complex. This antibody prolongs the phospholipid-dependent coagulation tests in vitro. The presence of this antibody is associated with recurrent pregnancy loss.

Metroplasty. A surgical procedure to unify the endometrial cavity of a bicornuate uterus or remove the septum of a septate uterus.

Missed Abortion. Fetal death before 20 weeks' gestation without expulsion of any fetal or maternal tissue for at least 8 weeks thereafter.

Recurrent Spontaneous Abortion. The loss of three or more pregnancies before 20 weeks' gestation. In practice it is advisable to perform a diagnostic evaluation for recurrent spontaneous abortion after two first-trimester pregnancy losses or one second-trimester loss.

Septic Abortion. Any type of abortion that is accompanied by uterine infection.

Subchorionic Hematoma. Sonographically visible hematoma elevating the membranes surrounding the amniotic sac.

Threatened Abortion. Uterine bleeding from a gestation of less than 20 weeks without any cervical dilation or effacement.

Uterine Adhesions. Tissue within the uterine cavity that obliterates part or all of the endometrium. Also called uterine synechia.

About 15% to 20% of all known human pregnancies terminate in clinically recognized abortion. However, the incidence of total human embryonic loss is estimated to be much higher. Wilcox et al. measured hCG in daily urine samples of a group of 221 healthy women attempting to conceive. Of the 198 pregnancies that occurred, 22% ended before the pregnancy was clinically recognized and the total pregnancy loss, including clinically recognized abortions, was 31%. Because some fertilized ova do not implant and thus do not secrete detectable hCG and other abnormal pregnancies do not secrete sufficient intact hCG to be detectable by immunoassay, the rate of human pregnancy loss is probably much higher; it has been estimated by Léridon to be as high as 70% (Table 16-1). Therefore the process of human reproduction is inefficient. However, because most early pregnancy losses are the result of chromosomal or genetic abnormalities, the high frequency of abortion, as stated by Austin, is "an important and valuable provision of Nature . . . and . . . is in the best interests of the race," because "disadvantageous features from gene mutation are prevented from being incorporated into the overall hereditary pattern."

Obtaining accurate data to determine the true incidence of clinical spontaneous abortion overall, as well as in particular subgroups of women, is difficult because of possible sources of bias produced by the selection process. Probably the most accurate data come from a study by Regan et al. In this study 630 women who were contemplating pregnancy were interviewed before conception and examined by ultrasonography as soon as pregnancy was suspected and then serially throughout the first trimester. The overall incidence of spontaneous abortion was 12%, and half had occurred before 8 weeks' gestation. The abortion rate in primigravidas was only 5%, whereas it was 14% in multigravidas (Table 16-2).

Women whose last pregnancy was successful also had a low abortion rate (5%), whereas women whose last pregnancy aborted had about a 20% abortion rate. The highest rate of abortion (24%) occurred in that group of women who had been pregnant in the past but in whom all the prior pregnancies had terminated in abortion. This study indicates that reproductive history is the most relevant predictive factor for pregnancy, outcome in a subsequent pregnancy, and the risk of abortion in primigravidas is less than previously believed.

TABLE 16-1

Life Table for Intrauterine Mortality in the Human (Per 100 Ova Exposed to Risk of Fertilization)

Week After Ovulation	Death (Expulsion of Dead Embryos)	Survivors
—	16 (not fertilized)	100
0	15 (failed to cleave)	84 (fertile)
1	27	69 (implanted)
2	5.0	42
6	2.9	37
10	1.7	34.1
14	0.5	32.4
18	0.3	31.9
22	0.1	31.6
26	0.1	31.5
30	0.1	31.4
34	0.1	31.3
38	0.2	31.32
Live births (including birth defects)		31
Natural wastage		69

From Léridon H: Intrauterine mortality. In Léridon H, editor: Human fertility, Chicago, 1977, The University of Chicago Press.

Warburton and Fraser studied the incidence of abortion over a 10-year period in a group of more than 2000 women who had at least one pregnancy of at least 20 weeks' gestation. The overall incidence of clinical abortion was 14.7%, and the risk of a pregnancy terminating in spontaneous abortion increased with increasing parity, maternal age, and paternal age (Table 16-3). Each of these parameters was an independent risk factor for abortion, and this information has been confirmed in other studies. These investigators also found that in this group of women who had previously delivered at least one live-born infant, the incidence of clinical abortion was 12.3% if they had no prior abortion. After having one or more abortions, there was a 24% to 32% risk of abortion in successive pregnancies that did not vary greatly with the number of abortions. They also reported that a woman with multiple abortions has a tendency to abort at about the same gestational length.

Knudsen et al. reviewed the data for all patients admitted to hospitals in Denmark between 1980 and 1984. There were 33,900 spontaneous abortions during this 5-year period. The overall incidence of spontaneous abortion was 11.3%, which increased in women over age 35. The abortion risk in women 35 to 40 was 21% and for women over 40 it was 42% (Table 16-4). The rate of spontaneous abortion also increased steadily with the number of prior abortions. The risk of abortion in women with no live births with one prior abortion was 13%. With two prior abortions it was 25%, with three it was 45% and with four prior abortions the risk of abortion increased to 54% (Table 16-5). Several other studies have reported the chance of having a subsequent abortion after three prior abortions is about 50%. These figures obtained from clinical studies are much lower than the theoretic value of 84% for a similar population reported by Malpas using mathematic assumptions.

About 80% of clinical abortions occur in the first trimester, with the incidence decreasing with increasing gestational age. Harlap et al. reported that the incidence of *clinical* abortion is relatively stable during each week of gestation before 12 weeks and declines steadily thereafter (Figure 16-1). Goldstein followed a group of women with serial sonograms in early pregnancy. He reported that once an intrauterine gestational sac was visualized sonographically the rate of pregnancy loss between 4.5 and 8.5 weeks' gestational age was 11.5%. If the pregnancy was viable at 8.5 weeks' gestation, then no pregnancy loss occurred until beyond 15.5 weeks' gestation, when an additional 2.4% fetal deaths occurred. Thus the majority of pregnancy failure occurs in the embryonic period, and about two thirds of these are due to chromosomal abnormalities.

Several other studies also reported that when embryonic heart activity is present between 8 and 12 weeks' gestational age, the incidence of subsequent pregnancy loss is between 2% and 3%. However, when sonography is performed earlier in gestation, beginning between 5.5 and 6 weeks, the subsequent spontaneous abortion rate after embryonic heart activity is seen has been reported to vary between 6% and 8%. There is an inverse relation between increasing length of gestational age between 5 and 8 weeks, in which embryonic heart activity is seen, and the risk of subsequent abortion. The later in early gestation that heart activity is seen, the lower the rate of subsequent abortion. Although spontaneous expulsion of the products of conception, clinical abortion, usually occurs between 8 and 12 weeks gestational age, nearly all embryonic deaths take place several days or weeks prior to the initiation of uterine bleeding and cramping.

TABLE 16-2
Effect of Mother's Reproductive History on Risk of Spontaneous Abortion (*N* = 407)

History	No. of Patients	No. of Patients Aborting	Percentage
Last pregnancy aborted	214	40	19
Only abortions in the past	98	24	24
Only pregnancy aborted	59	12	20
Last pregnancy successful	95	5	5
All pregnancies successful	73	3	4
Only pregnancy successful	62	3	5
Previous termination of pregnancy	32	2	6
Primigravida	87	4	5
TOTAL	407		

From Regan L et al: Br Med J 299:541, 1989.

TABLE 16-3
Relation of Abortion Frequency to Maternal and Paternal Age at Conception

Maternal Age	% Abortion Frequency	Paternal Age	% Abortion Frequency
<20	12.2	<20	12.0
20–24	14.3	20–24	11.8
25–29	13.7	25–29	15.7
30–34	15.5	30–34	13.1
35–39	18.7	35–39	15.8
40–44	25.5	40–44	19.5
		44 +	23.1
MEAN	14.7	MEAN	14.7

From Warburton D and Fraser FC: Am J Hum Genet 16:1, 1964.

TABLE 16-4
Overall Risk of Abortion, According
to Age of Mother*

Age of Mother	Number of Pregnancies	Spontaneous Abortions (%)
–19	1105	10.8 (9.0–12.7)
20–29	13,173	9.7 (9.2–12.7)
30–34	3900	11.5 (10.6–12.6)
35–39	1299	21.4 (19.2–23.7)
40+	260	42.2 (35.1–47.4)
Overall	19,737	11.3 (10.9–11.8)

From Knudsen UB, Hansen V, Juul S, and Secher NJ: Eur J Obstet Gynecol Reprod Biol 39:31, 1991.

*The table is calculated from a 6.6% sample of the study pregnancies. Figures in brackets: 95% confidence limits. X^2 (trend) = 244; df = 1; p < 0.0001.

TABLE 16-5
Risk of Subsequent Pregnancy Ending
in a Spontaneous Abortion*

No. of Previous Abortions	No. of Pregnancies Studied	Abortion Risk (%)
0	18,164	10.7 (10.3–11.2)
1	21,054	15.9 (15.4–16.4)
2	2231	25.1 (23.4–27.0)
3	353	45.0 (39.8–50.4)
4	94	54.3 (43.7–64.4)
Overall	19,737	11.3 (10.9–11.8)

From Knudsen UB, Hansen V, Juul S, and Secher NJ: Eur J Obstet Gynecol Reprod Biol 39:31, 1991.

*The table is calculated from a 6.6% sample of the study pregnancies. Figures in brackets: 95% confidence limits. X^2 (trend) = 728; df = 1:p < 0.001.

The loss rate after visualization of embryonic heart activity, according to Siddiqi et al., increases about 2 to 3 times when maternal age is over 34 compared with younger women. If uterine bleeding occurs when embryonic heart activity is present in the first trimester, the risk of abortion increases about threefold to about 15%, compared with pregnancies without uterine bleeding. Women with uterine bleeding and a viable embryo are more likely to abort if the serum CA-125 is elevated. In one study of a group of women with first-trimester threatened abortion and a viable embryo, 15 of 16 aborted if the CA-125 was above 120 IU/ml and the hCG was less than 45,000 mIU/ml. The presence of a subchorionic hematoma, visualized sonographically with a viable embryo, does not increase the risk of subsequent pregnancy loss.

ETIOLOGY

Genetic

The causes of spontaneous abortion can be divided into two major categories: fetal and maternal, also called *genetic* and *environmental*. By far the major causes of abortion are genetic. There have been several large cytogenetic studies of the tissue expelled from the uterus at the time of abortion. Cytogenic studies of this material following tissue culture indicated that the incidence of chromosomal anomalies is about 50%.

Several investigators have subsequently performed cytogenic studies by direct analysis of chorionic villi of first-trimester embryonic deaths or anembryonic gestations. Samples of chorionic villi were obtained by uterine sampling or by tissue removed by curettage after nonviability was found sonographically. Cytogenic analyses of this tissue revealed that between 70% and 85% of the chorionic villi had chromosomal abnormalities. The higher incidence of aneuploidy found in these recent studies may be caused by several factors. First, a rapid direct cytogenic technique was used instead of long-term tissue culture. Second, the tissue was obtained from the uterine cavity instead of after spontaneous expulsion. Furthermore, most of the direct analyses were performed from tissue obtained earlier in gestation than when the cell culture technique was performed. Finally, cytogenic analysis was performed on chorionic villi, not directly on embryonic tissue. The incidence of chromosomal abnormalities in chorionic villi is higher than in fetal tissue. The very high incidence of aneuploidy found with both techniques should assist when counseling parents regarding the cause of the spontaneous abortion when it occurs in the first trimester.

The vast majority of the abnormal karyotypes in the gestational tissue are numeric abnormalities as a result of errors occurring during gametogenesis (chromosomal nondisjunction during meiosis), fertilization (triploidy as a result of digyny or dispermy), or the first division of the fertilized ovum (tetraploidy or mosaicism). Only about 5% of the abnormal karyotypes of the gestations are abnormalities in the structure of individual chromosomes, such as translocation.

In most surveys of chromosomal anomalies of abortuses the relative frequency of the different types of anomalies is similar. The most common type of anomaly is autosomal trisomy, which accounts for about half the abnormal karyotypes when cell cultures were used and about two thirds of the abnormal karyotypes when chorionic villi analysis was performed directly (Table 16-6).

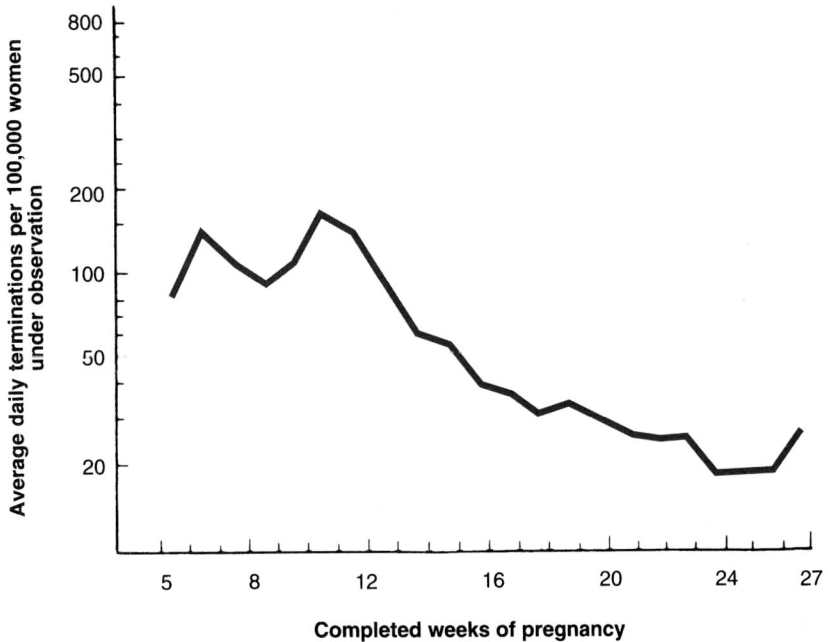

FIGURE 16-1 Spontaneous abortion by week of pregnancy. (From Harlap S, Shiono PH, and Ramcharan S: A life table of spontaneous abortions and the effects of age, parity, and other variables. In Porter IH and Hook EB, editors: Human embryonic and fetal death, New York, 1980, Academic Press.)

Trisomies of all autosomes except for autosome 1 have been reported after karyotyping of abortions, with trisomy 16 being the most common. About one third of all autosomal trisomies in abortuses are trisomy 16, with trisomy 22 the next most frequent. Many trisomies occurring in abortions have not been reported in live births, probably because the genotype is incompatible with fetal development.

The second most common chorionic abnormality is polyploidy, most frequently triploidy, and less commonly tetraploidy. Polyploidy occurs in about 10% of the aneuploid abortions, and monosomy 45,X occurs in about 7% of the abnormal karyotypes in tissue examined by direct analysis. The survival rate of 45,X gestations is about 1 in 300. To summarize, autosomal trisomy is the most common abnormal karyotype (50% to 65%), followed in decreasing frequency by monosomy 45,X (7% to 15%), triploidy (15%), tetraploidy (10%), and structural abnormalities (5%). The most common single chromosomal abnormality is monosomy 45,X. Karyotypes of abortuses of women who have had more than one abortion tend to be similar if the first abortus had either a normal karyotype or an autosomal trisomy. Except for monosomy, it is possible to determine the parental origin of the chromosomal abnormality. Jacobs and Hassold reported that 26% of all fetal loss is caused by errors of maternal gametogenesis, 5% by errors of paternal gametogenesis, 4% by errors of fertilization, and 4% by errors of zygote division.

TABLE 16-6
Chromosome Results of 447 Abortuses

	Karyotyped (Banded)	% of All Known Karyotype
Chromosomally normal		
46,XY	111	24.8
46,XX	95	21.3
TOTAL	206	46.1
Chromosomally abnormal		
45,X	44	9.8
Primary autosomal trisomy	138	30.9
Double trisomy	7	1.7
Triple trisomy	1	0.4
Triploidy	29	6.5
Tetraploidy	8	1.8
Mosaicism	1	0.4
Structural rearrangement	11	2.5
Others (XXY, Monosomy 21)	2	0.8
TOTAL	241	53.9

From Kajii T and Ferrier A: Hum Genet 55:87, 1980.

The various surveys have revealed no seasonal variability in the incidence of any type of chromosomal abnormality in abortions. There is also no effect of paternal age. Maternal age, however, is directly related to the incidence of trisomies, mainly those in the D and G group. Maternal age has no effect on the incidence of the other chromosomal anomalies in abortions, although there is evidence that monosomy 45,X is associated with a younger maternal age than other aneuploid or euploid abortions. Chromosomal abnormalities in the parents are an uncommon cause of abortions—more than 95% of couples who have two or more spontaneous abortions are chromosomally normal.

In most studies the rate of chromosomal abnormalities is highest when abortion occurs between 8 and 15 weeks' gestational age. Kajii et al. reported that the greatest prevalence of chromosomally abnormal abortions (74%) occurred when clinical abortion occurred at 9 weeks' gestational age and gradually decreased thereafter. The lower prevalence of abnormal karyotypes occurring in gestations terminating at less than 9 weeks may be artifactual, because the success of karyotyping by culture is less likely if an embryo is not present, and the frequency of anembryonic gestation is greatest in abortions of 8 weeks or less.

Abortion of chromosomally normal conceptuses is found to occur later in gestation than abortion of chromosomally abnormal ones. The peak incidence of euploid abortion is about 12 to 13 weeks of gestation. The incidence of chromosomally normal abortions increases markedly after maternal age 35, rising to more than 30% of clinically recognized conceptions after age 40 (Figure 16-2). Whether this increase in risk of abortion of euploid conceptions is the result of an increase in genetic abnormalities or abnormalities in the maternal environment or both has not been determined, but there is an increased incidence of both first- and second-trimester abortions after age 35, and uterine abnormalities generally are a cause of second-trimester abortion.

Tharapel et al. reviewed the cytogenic results of the 79 published surveys of couples with 2 or more pregnancy losses, comprising a total of 8208 women and 7834 men. The composite prevalence of major chromosomal abnormalities in either parent was about 3%, 5 to 6 times higher than the general population. Since this review several large studies, including the one by De Braekeleer and Dao, indicate that the prevalence of chromosomal abnormalities in one member of the couple may be as high as 5%. Abnormalities occur in the female parent about twice as frequently as in the male. About half of all chromosomal abnormalities are balanced reciprocal translocations, and one fourth are Robertsonian translocations. About 12% are sex chromosomal mosaicism in the female, and the rest are inversions and other sporadic abnormalities. Thus karyotypes of both members of couples with two or more spontaneous abortions should be performed. If translocation is found in one parent, about 80% of the couple's subsequent pregnancies will abort. If abortion does not occur in a subsequent pregnancy, fetal cytogenic studies are indicated, because there is about a 3% to 5% incidence of unbalanced fetal karyotype in these gestations. Therefore, if an abnormal karyotype is found in one of the members of the couple with recurrent abortion, genetic counseling is indicated. Use of donor gametes should be considered in subsequent pregnancy attempts.

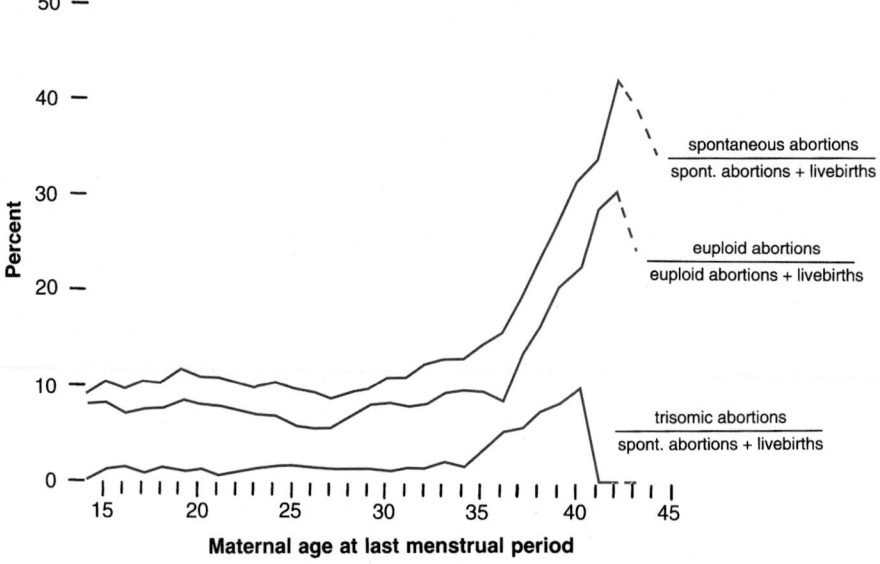

FIGURE 16-2 Estimated rates (%) of spontaneous abortion, euploid abortion, and trisomic abortion by maternal age for private and public patients combined. *Broken line,* denominator less than 25. (From Stein Z, Kline J, Susser E, et al: Maternal age and spontaneous abortion. In Porter IH and Hook EB, editors: Human embryonic and fetal death, New York, 1980, Academic Press.)

There are many possible causes for abortion of chromosomally normal conceptions. Simpson has postulated that a common, but yet unproved, cause is a genetic abnormality, most probably a mutation, or polygenic factors. He based this assumption on the fact that about 2% of live births have a disorder involving a single gene mutation or polygenic inheritance, whereas only 0.5% of live births have a chromosomal abnormality. Thus, in humans, genetic abnormalities are more common than are chromosomal abnormalities. These genetic disorders could produce abortion by interfering with fetal metabolism or embryonic structural differentiation.

Several investigators have reported an increased incidence of histocompatibility locus antigen (HLA) sharing at the A, B, and DR locus among couples with recurrent abortion than among controls and have postulated that the abortion occurs because of the absence of a maternal immunologic blocking factor normally produced in response to paternal antigens. Because the majority of women with repeated abortions have a normal maternal lymphocytic immune response to stimulation by paternal lymphocytes, it is more likely that the cause of the recurrent abortions in couples with HLA sharing is genetic, not immunologic. Homozygosity for recessive major histocompatibility complex genes could be the responsible factor for the abortion. In several animal species, genes contributing to spontaneous abortion are located in the region of the chromosome that controls the major histocompatibility complex. In humans the histocompatibility complex is found in the HLA locus on chromosome 6. The sharing of the HLA antigens could be just the detectable marker for the segment of the chromosome that carries recessive genes that are potentially lethal.

Weitkamp and Schacter reported that chromosomally normal couples who experience recurrent abortion, in addition to having increased sharing of HLA-A alleles, also have an increased incidence of the transferrin C3 allele and a decreased frequency of the most common transferrin allele, C1. These transferrin alleles are located on chromosome 3. Although transferrin genes have been associated with abortion in several animal species, the effect of transferrin on spontaneous abortion may not be necessarily direct but, as with HLA antigens, could be an effect of genes closely located to the transferrin locus. Jin et al. used a new shared allele test to compare the frequency of shared alleles among couples with recurring spontaneous abortion. They reported that there was an excess of HLA-DR sharing, but not HLA-A or HLA-B, among couples with recurrent spontaneous abortion. They also found there was excessive sharing of other HLA alleles in couples with unexplained infertility and various immunologic, metabolic, neoplastic, and developmental diseases. They therefore postulated that these problems are due to the presence of recessive genes located on different parts of the HLA allele.

These reports support the concept that the presence of certain recessive genes located on chromosomes 3 and 6 can interfere with normal fetal development and increase the possibility of spontaneous abortion of an euploid embryo. Further evidence for a genetic mechanism is the fact that in the gestation after a spontaneous abortion in a primigravida, there is an increased frequency of congenital malformations and perinatal deaths.

Environmental

In contrast to the frequent genetic causes of abortion, maternal or environmental causes are less common. Uterine abnormalities, either congenital or acquired, may not provide the optimal environment for nourishment and survival of the embryo and thus may cause abortion of a genetically normal embryo. Congenital uterine abnormalities can be divided into those brought about by abnormal uterine fusion, those produced by maternal diethylstilbestrol (DES) ingestion, and those caused by abnormal cervical function. The latter condition, the incompetent cervix, can also be acquired after mechanical cervical dilation.

Congenital Uterine Anomalies

ANOMALIES OF UTERINE DEVELOPMENT. Anomalies of uterine development are relatively common, with the incidence reported in the literature ranging from about 1:200 to 1:600 women. Overall, about 20% to 25% of women with anomalies of uterine fusion have problems with reproduction, recurrent abortion being the most serious. Although it has been stated that the bicornuate and septate uteri are the anomalies most frequently associated with abortion, this belief has arisen from the fact that these anomalies can be corrected surgically and thus are more frequently reported as a cause of abortion before surgical correction. In a study of all 182 women with uterine anomalies detected during an 18-year period at a large Finnish hospital, Heinonen et al. reported that the least common uterine anomaly, the unicornuate uterus, was associated with the greatest incidence of spontaneous abortion, about 50%. This incidence was higher than the 25% to 30% incidence of abortion that occurred in women with either a septate or bicornuate uterus.

Surgical correction of bicornuate and septate uteri is possible by using one of the transfundal metroplasty techniques originally described by Strassmann, Jones, or Tompkins, or by transcervical hysteroscopic resection of the uterine septum or cerclage of the cervix. The Strassmann technique of metroplasty was used for a bicornuate uterus, and the Jones and Tompkins techniques were used for resection of a uterine septum. In the series of Heinonen et al., about one fifth of the women with bicornuate and septate uteri had a metroplasty performed, and the abortion rate declined from 84% to 12%. In other series the live birth rate increased from 7% to 76% after metroplastic unification of the uterine cavity. The treatment of uterine anomalies associated with recent pregnancy loss by these major surgical procedures has now been replaced by treatment with minor operations. Hysteroscopic resection of the uterine septum is now used to treat this anomaly, and cervical cerclage is used to treat recurrent pregnancy loss associated with a bicornuate uterus.

March and Israel reported that it was possible to incise the septum, even those thicker than 1 cm, of all 82 women with recurrent abortion, using flexible scissors placed transcervically through the hysteroscope. After this treatment the abortion rate declined from 95% to 13%. Similar results have been reported by others, and now hysteroscopic incision is the treatment of choice for women with a septate uterus and a history of pregnancy loss. Two groups in Israel, Golan et al. and Bider et al., have reported that when cervical cerclage was used to treat women with a bicornuate uterus and recurrent pregnancy loss the incidence of viable pregnancies markedly increased. In one series of 41 women with bicornuate uteri and recurrent abortion, 85% had a successful pregnancy outcome after cervical cerclage and in the other all 18 women had a term delivery following this minor operative procedure.

UTERINE ANOMALIES AFTER DIETHYLSTILBESTROL (DES). Comparative studies have shown that women exposed to DES during their fetal life have a significantly greater incidence of spontaneous abortion than do controls. Kaufman et al. reported that the percentage of first or all pregnancies in women exposed to DES that ended in spontaneous abortion was similar whether or not their hysterosalpingogram revealed abnormalities in the shape of the uterine cavity or intrauterine defects. Haney et al. reported that the endometrial cavity of women exposed to DES in utero had a significantly smaller surface area than normal, which could perhaps contribute to the increased spontaneous abortion rate in women exposed to DES in utero. No therapy, including cerclage, has been shown to significantly lower the abortion rate in women exposed to DES who have abnormalities of the uterine cavity and recurrent abortion unless they also have cervical incompetence. Because the length of gestation tends to increase with subsequent pregnancies among women who had fetal DES exposure, most of these women ultimately have a viable pregnancy.

CERVICAL INCOMPETENCE. Cervical incompetence is characterized by an asymptomatic dilation of the internal cervical os, leading to dilation of the cervical canal and external os during the second trimester of pregnancy. The consequent lack of support of the fetal membranes leads to their spontaneous rupture, which is usually followed by expulsion of the fetus and placenta. The incidence of this problem was previously estimated to vary from 1 in 57 to 1 in 1730 pregnancies. Although excessive mechanical cervical dilation at the time of dilation and curettage was formerly the most common cause of this problem, since recognition of this syndrome, the use of excessive

mechanical cervical dilation is now uncommon. Consequently, now the most common cause of cervical incompetence is believed to be a congenital defect in the cervical tissue, and the incidence of this disorder as a cause of recurrent abortion is infrequent. In a recent series of 500 consecutive unselected women with recurrent abortion reported by Clifford et al., none of the 176 women with late abortions had a history of cervical incompetence. There is no satisfactory test available for the diagnosis of cervical incompetence. Therefore the diagnosis is usually made by obtaining a history of second-trimester pregnancy loss accompanied by spontaneous rupture of the fetal membranes without preceding uterine contractions. Cervical incompetence is associated with the presence of uterine anomalies, particularly uterus didelphys, as well as with anomalies produced by fetal DES exposure.

The best treatment of cervical incompetence is placement of a concentric nonabsorbable silk or Mersilene suture at the level of the internal os (cerclage), using the technique described by McDonald (Figure 16-3). If strict criteria are used to diagnose cervical incompetence, fetal survival rates after cerclage have been reported to increase from 20% to 80%. However, if the criteria for diagnosis are less certain, in several randomized clinical trials, there is only a slight increase in the incidence of term deliveries after cerclage is performed. It is recommended that the suture be placed electively between 10 to 14 weeks of gestation after major embryogenesis has been completed and the incidence of spontaneous abortion caused by genetic abnormalities has markedly lessened. An ultrasound examination should be performed before the cerclage is placed to document that a normal gestation is present. Occasionally, if there is a markedly shortened cervix or placement of the McDonald cerclage has failed to maintain the pregnancy, a transabdominal cerclage should be performed. If the suture is placed externally, it is usually removed at 38 weeks' gestation, and vaginal delivery is permitted to occur. However, because of cervical scarring, cesarean section is required in about 15% of pregnancies after the cerclage is removed.

Acquired Uterine Defects

LEIOMYOMAS. Leiomyomas are common benign uterine tumors that are present in about one fourth of women of reproductive age. Uterine leiomyomas, especially if they are submucosal, can be associated with repetitive abortion. Although a causal relationship is difficult to establish, in a review of the literature, Buttram and Reiter reported that when myomectomy was performed for recurrent abortion in a total of 1941 women, the rate of spontaneous abortion was reduced from 41% to 19%. These data indicate that, on occasion, uterine leiomyomas are a cause of abortion.

INTRAUTERINE ADHESIONS. Adhesions in the uterine cavity can cause partial or complete obliteration of the endometrium leading to menstrual abnormalities and amenorrhea, as well as being a cause of abortion. The lat-

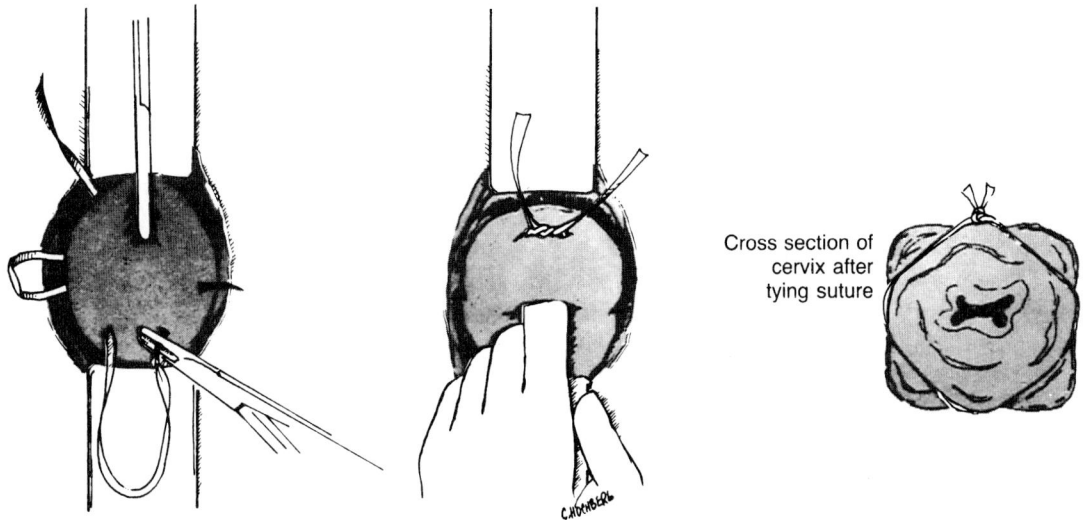

FIGURE 16-3 Steps in performing McDonald cerclage using Mersilene suture. Index finger is used to ensure closure of internal os. (From March CM: Recurrent abortion. In Mishell DR Jr and Davajan V, editors: Infertility, contraception, and reproductive endocrinology, ed 3, Oradell, NJ, 1991, Medical Economics Books. Reproduced with permission. All rights reserved.)

ter is thought to be the result of insufficient endometrium to support adequate fetal growth. The major cause of adhesions is curettage of the endometrial cavity in association with a pregnancy or in the early puerperium (Table 16-7). In the series of March and Israel the most common antecedent factor was curettage for incomplete abortion. Curettage after a missed abortion or after postpartum hemorrhage is associated with a high incidence of subsequent intrauterine adhesion (IUA) formation. On occasion IUAs develop after a diagnostic curettage, as well as in women with genital tuberculosis. The diagnosis of IUA is usually made by the finding of filling defects seen at the time of hysterosalpingogram. The defects are typically irregular, with sharp contours and homogeneous opacity that persist in a series of films (Figure 16-4). The diagnosis is best confirmed by hysteroscopy.

The recommended treatment for IUA is lysis of the adhesions by miniature scissors during hysteroscopy. After adhesion lysis, either an IUD or small Foley catheter is usually placed in the cavity, and high-dose estrogen (conjugated equine estrogen 2.5 mg bid) is administered for 60 days. Medroxyprogesterone acetate 10 mg per day is added for the last 5 to 10 days, and then the foreign body is removed. March and Israel reported that the abortion rate decreased from 83% to 13% after hysterographic lysis of adhesions. To minimize the chances of development of IUA, curettage of the pregnant or recently pregnant uterus should be gentle and superficial and not extend deep into the muscle. After curettage for missed abortion or postpartum hemorrhage, consideration should be given to prophylactic high-dose estrogen treatment orally for 1 to 2 months to enhance endometrial growth.

Endocrine Causes

Progesterone Deficiency

Maintenance of the endometrium for the first 7 weeks of gestation depends on progesterone produced by the corpus luteum. After this time the corpus luteum regresses, and progesterone synthesized by the trophoblast maintains the decidual tissue. Luteal progesterone synthesis is dependent upon hCG produced by the trophoblast. When progesterone secretion from the corpus luteum is lower than normal or the endometrium has an inadequate response to normal circulating levels of progesterone, endometrial development may be inadequate to support the implanted blastocyst and may lead to spontaneous abortion. Several investigators have reported that in conception cycles, midluteal peak progesterone levels in the circulation are always greater than 9 ng/ml. Horta et al. measured daily plasma progesterone levels during the luteal phase of a group of normal fertile women, as well as in a group of women whose previous three gestations terminated in spontaneous abortion. In the former group the lowest midluteal peak progesterone level was 9 ng/ml, whereas in the latter group mean progesterone levels reached a peak of 6 ng/ml, significantly lower than the normal fertile group. Therefore, if midluteal serum progesterone levels are consistently less than 10 ng/ml in several cycles, the diagnosis of luteal insufficiency can be made.

Diagnosis of luteal insufficiency has also been made by performing histologic examination of the endometrium and finding a discrepancy of 3 days or more between the expected and actual endometrial dating pattern in at least two menstrual cycles. Several investigators using this method of diagnosis have reported luteal deficiency to

TABLE 16-7
Definite Causes of IUA in 1856 Cases

	No. of Cases	Percent
Trauma associated with pregnancy		
Curettage after abortion	1237	66.7
Spontaneous	544	
Induced	557	
Unknown	136	
Postpartum curettage	400	21.5
Cesarean section	38	2.0
Evacuation of hydatidiform mole	11	0.6
Trauma without pregnancy		
Myomectomy	24	1.3
Diagnostic curettage	22	1.2
Cervical manipulation (biopsy, polypectomy, etc.)	10	0.5
Curettage because of menometrorrhagia	8	0.4
Insertion of IUD	3	
Insertion of radium	1	0.3
Without known trauma		
Postpartum; after abortion; others	28	1.5
Genital tuberculosis	74	4.0
TOTAL	1856	100.00

From Schenker JG and Margalioth EJ: Fertil Steril 37:593, 1982. Reproduced with permission of the publisher, The American Fertility Society.

occur in as many as one third of women with recurrent abortion, whereas others have reported it to be an uncommon cause of abortion. This discrepancy may have occurred because the precision of endometrial dating by histologic examination varies among different observers and different criteria are used for determining the day of ovulation.

Several investigators have treated women with recurrent abortion and evidence of luteal deficiency with progesterone vaginal suppositories 25 mg twice daily or with intramuscular progesterone 12.5 mg/day beginning 3 days after ovulation and continuing throughout the first trimester. With this treatment, term pregnancy rates have been reported to range from 80% to 90%. However, no randomized clinical trials with a placebo control group have been undertaken to verify whether progesterone significantly reduces the incidence of abortion in women who have documented luteal insufficiency. Goldstein et al. performed a meta-analysis of randomized control trials of the use of progestational agents given to women in early pregnancy who had a history of two or more abortions without a specific diagnosis of luteal deficiency. There was no significant reduction in the rate of abortion with the use of progestational agents. It is therefore unsettled whether luteal insufficiency is a cause of recurrent sponta-

neous abortion and/or whether administration of progesterone in the luteal phase of the cycle in which conception occurs, as well as during early pregnancy, is beneficial.

There is no evidence that administration of synthetic progestins, which themselves may be luteolytic, are of benefit in reducing the incidence of abortion. There is also no benefit to be derived by initiating progesterone therapy or administering exogenous hCG after the expected menstrual period is missed, especially if the woman develops symptoms of threatened abortion. Low progesterone levels at this gestational age are a result, not the cause, of the abortion.

Thyroid Disease

Although older studies suggested that hypothyroidism may be a cause of abortion, a study by Montoro et al. reported that no abortions occurred in 11 pregnancies of 9 markedly hypothyroid women. In three recent studies of large numbers of women with recurrent abortion, only a few women in one of the studies were found to have abnormal thyroid function. Thus there is no definitive evidence that hypothyroidism is a cause of spontaneous abortion. There are, however, several studies that indicate that the presence of antithyroid antibodies are risk markers for spontaneous abortion.

Stagnaro-Green et al. measured thyroglobulin and thyroid peroxidase antibodies in 552 unselected women in the first trimester of pregnancy. An antithyroid antibody was found in 20% of these women. Among the group of women in whom thyroid antibodies were detected, the spontaneous abortion rate was twice as high, 17% rather than the 8.4% incidence in the group of women without antibodies. Lejeune et al. measured these 2 antithyroid antibodies in 730 euthyroid women in early pregnancy and reported that 1 of these antibodies was present in 24% of women who had a first-trimester abortion but in only 5% of those with viable pregnancies and in 1 of 8 women with a second-trimester abortion.

Pratt et al. measured these antibodies prior to conception in a group of euthyroid women with a history of recurrent first-trimester abortion. Antibodies were detected in one third of the women. In the next pregnancy one third of the entire group had an early abortion and two thirds of the women who aborted their pregnancies had an antithyroid antibody. When an antibody was present, 62% of the women had an abortion in the next pregnancy and when it was absent only 14% had an early abortion. Bussen and Steck also found that one third of euthyroid women with recurrent abortion had one of the two antithyroid antibodies present compared with 5% in a group of controls. Wilson et al. studied a group of women with recurrent abortion all of whom had thyroid antibodies present. In a subsequent pregnancy there was a direct correlation between the level of thyroid antibody titer and occurrence of abortion. The findings of these studies indicate that the presence of

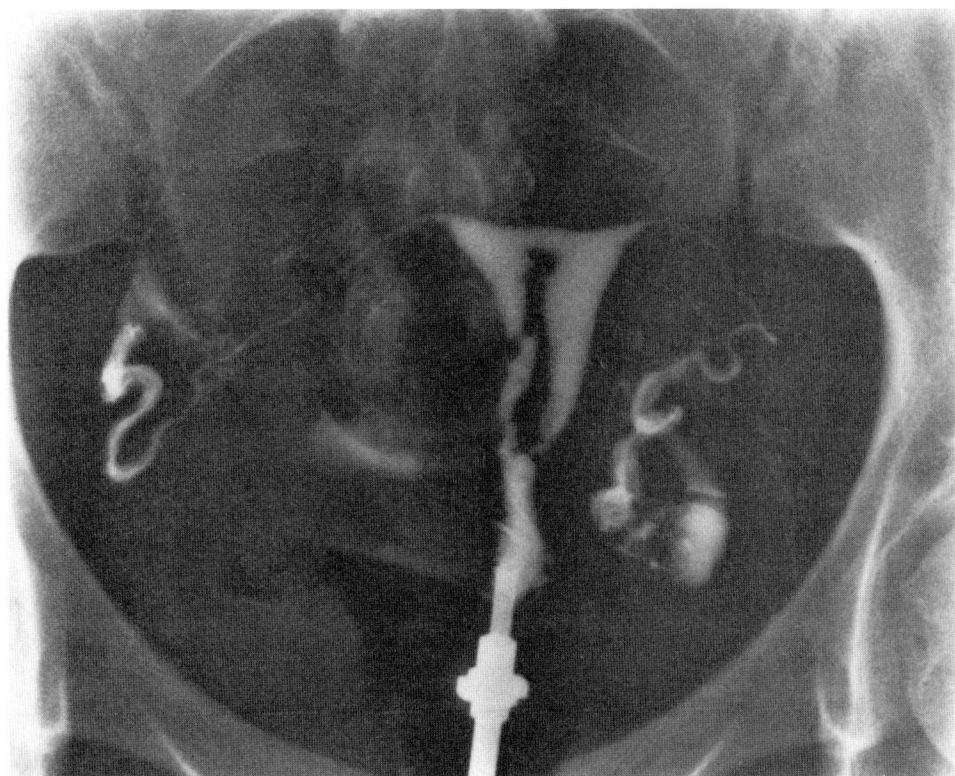

FIGURE 16-4 Endometrial adhesions. The patient was a 23-year-old gravida 5, para 0, spontaneous abortus 4, ectopic 1 (G5 PO SAB4 ECT), with previous left linear salpingostomy, being evaluated for recurrent abortion. Irregular, linear filling defect represents adhesions between anterior and posterior walls of endometrial cavity, extending from internal os to level near fundus. (From Richmond JA: Hysterosalpingography. In Mishell DR Jr and Davajan V, editors: Infertility, contraception, and reproductive endocrinology, ed 3, Oradell, NJ, 1991, Medical Economics Books. Reprinted with permission. All rights reserved.)

thyroid antibodies is a risk marker for abortion. Since the antibodies are found in euthyroid women it is likely that they are a marker for some type of immunologic-mediated cause of abortion that is likely to reoccur in subsequent pregnancies. Kiprov et al. treated a group of women with recurrent abortion and antithyroid and other autoimmune antibodies with intrauterine gamma globulin infusions throughout pregnancy. There was an 80% rate of viable pregnancies. Randomized trials are needed to determine whether this high rate of successful pregnancies was causally related to the gamma globulin infusion.

Diabetes Mellitus

Although uncontrolled diabetes mellitus has been associated with an increased abortion rate, Crane and Wahl found the incidence of spontaneous abortion was similar in a group of women with either gestational diabetes (12.3%) or frank diabetes (12.2%) and matched control groups (10.9% and 14.5%). In this study the diabetes was controlled with insulin. They also reported that the number of women with multiple spontaneous abortions was similar in the diabetic and control groups. Mills et al. performed a prospective study of insulin-dependent diabetic

and nondiabetic women enrolled within 3 weeks of conception. The spontaneous abortion rate in both groups was 16%. However, a small group of diabetic women who were not well controlled and had elevated blood glucose and glycosylated hemoglobulin levels had a significantly increased risk of spontaneous abortion. Thus it appears that diabetes, when controlled by diet or insulin, is not a cause of abortion. However, diabetes without good metabolic control is associated with an increased risk of early pregnancy loss, and a direct correlation exists between the level of hemoglobin A_1 and the rate of abortion.

Hypersecretion of LH

Homburg et al. reported that about one third of women with polycystic ovarian syndrome who conceive after undergoing ovulation induction have a spontaneous abortion, more than twice the incidence of spontaneous abortion of women with hypogonadotropic hypogonadism who conceive after ovulation induction. The incidence of spontaneous abortion was only increased in those women with polycystic ovarian syndrome who had elevations of follicular phase plasma LH levels, not those in whom the LH levels were in the normal range. Regan et al. prospectively measured follicular phase LH levels in a group of

193 women with regular menstrual cycles who were planning to become pregnant, the majority of whom had a history of one or more previous spontaneous abortions. Within 18 months 88% of women with normal LH levels (less than 10 IU/l) conceived, compared with 67% of women whose LH levels were elevated. These investigators found that of the women who conceived with elevated LH levels, 65% of the pregnancies ended in abortion while only 12% of the pregnancies in women with normal LH levels aborted. Thus, if the LH levels were elevated on day 8 of the cycle, there was a significantly greater risk of the pregnancy ending in abortion, as well as a greater risk of infertility. These investigators concluded that hypersecretion of LH among women with and without polycystic ovarian syndrome is a cause of spontaneous abortion. The exact mechanism whereby elevated LH levels cause abortion has not been determined but may be due to a direct effect on the ovaries, causing premature aging of the oocyte, or a direct effect on the endometrium, adversely affecting implantation. Clifford et al. studied a group of 500 consecutive women with recurrent spontaneous abortion who were referred to a special clinic to study this problem. Sonographic findings of polycystic ovaries were found in 56% of these women, but only 12% of them had elevated follicular phase serum LH levels. However, it was found that nearly 60% of the women with polycystic ovaries had elevated urinary LH levels. Urinary LH may be a more sensitive marker of LH hypersecretion than of serum LH since LH is secreted in a pulsatile manner. Clifford et al. performed a randomized controlled trial of women with recurrent abortion and elevated LH levels, comparing therapy of GnRH analogs with no therapy. The viable birth rate was similar in the 2 groups indicating that LH suppression with a GnRH analog is not beneficial for improving live birth rates.

Immunologic Factors

As mentioned, the foreign antigens produced by the fetus should cause it to be rejected by the mother's immune system. Although some protection from this immunologic effect is offered by progesterone, it has been hypothesized that a maternal blocking factor, an IgG antibody, coats the foreign fetal antigens and prevents the fetus from being rejected. It has also been suggested that some women with recurrent abortion lack this blocking factor and as a result, abortions occur in each pregnancy.

It has also been postulated that if there is sharing of major histocompatability locus antigens (HLA) between the male and the female in the couple with recurrent abortion, then natural blocking factors would be less likely to develop and abortion would be more likely to occur. Numerous studies have investigated the degree of HLA sharing at several loci in groups of couples with recurrent abortion in whom no etiology for the problem could be detected. Bellingard et al., in addition to performing their own study, summarized the results of 23 previously published studies that investigated the degree of HLA sharing between spouses of couples with recurrent abortion. The findings were divided among the studies. HLA-A sharing was reported to be present in 11 and absent in 12 of the 23 studies, and HLA-B sharing was present in 10 but absent in 13 of the 23 studies. In the 17 studies in which HLA-DR sharing was investigated, 11 found sharing of this allele to be more frequent among couples with recurrent abortion of undetected etiology than controls. In their own study of women with three successive spontaneous abortions, Bellingard et al. found that the number of couples with HLA sharing in each of the three alleles was not significantly different among women with a known etiology for their recurrent abortion and those with unexplained recurrent abortion, as well as a control group of parous women without spontaneous abortion.

Sargent et al. performed a prospective study of couples with recurrent abortion before and after conception and found no difference in the incidence of HLA sharing among the couples who subsequently had a successful pregnancy and those whose pregnancies aborted. Furthermore, they could not confirm that after pregnancy occurred in these women, as well as in normal controls, there was an increase in production of maternal immunologic factors to fetal (paternal) HLA antigens. Thus HLA sharing does not appear to cause abortion by an immunologic mechanism. Since HLA alleles are probably the location for potentially lethal recessive genes as previously mentioned, it is more likely that sharing of these alleles increases the risk of abortion by a genetic mechanism. However, in 1985 Mowbray et al. performed a randomized treatment trial in a group of women with recurrent abortion and no detectable antibody against paternal lymphocytes. In this study women injected with paternal white cells had a significantly greater chance of a subsequent successful pregnancy (78%) than did those injected with their own white cells (37%). The investigators concluded that infusion of the foreign leukocytes increased maternal production of the blocking factors that would prevent rejection of the fetal tissues. However, in two subsequent studies performed by Cowchock and Smith, as well as by Hwang et al., after paternal leukocytes were given to the female the outcome of the subsequent pregnancy was not related to the development of either maternal antipaternal antibodies or blocking factors. After paternal white cell immunotherapy was performed, neither the formation of antipaternal antibodies nor blocking factors was associated with a decrease in the spontaneous abortion rate or an increase in term pregnancy rate compared with pregnancies after immunotherapy in which these factors did not substantially increase (Table 16-8).

Following the study of Mowbray et al. there have been several other prospective clinical trials involving the use of

TABLE 16-8
Pregnancy Outcome with Respect to Development of Lymphocytotoxic Antibody and/or Mixed Lymphocyte Reaction Blocking Factors After Immunization.

| Pregnancy Outcome | Lymphocytotoxic Acetate | | | | Mixed Lymphocyte Reaction Blocking Factors | | | |
| | Neg → Pos | | Neg → Neg | | Neg → Pos | | Neg → Neg | |
	Number	Percentage	Number	Percentage	Number	Percentage	Number	Percentage
Aborted	20/27	74	7/27	26	9/25	36	16/25	64
Delivered	10/21	48	11/21	52	6/18	33	12/18	67

From Smith JB and Cowchock FS: J Reprod Immunol 14:99, 1988.

paternal leukocyte infusion to treat recurrent spontaneous abortion. In 1995 Jeng et al. performed a meta-analysis of the results of 4 published and 4 unpublished clinical trials, as well as a meta-analysis of pooling original patient data from 15 completed or ongoing trials. The relative risk (RR) of having a live birth was significantly greater after the leukocyte infusion only when the data from four of the published clinical trials were analyzed, RR = 1.29 (CI 1.03 to 2.60). However, when all the individual patient data from these trials (RR = 1.17) or the data from individual patients in four unpublished trials (RR = 1.01) were analyzed, there was no longer a significantly increased relative risk of having a live birth after immunotherapy (Figure 16-5). Jeng concluded that the effect of immunotherapy to treat women with recurrent spontaneous abortion remains inconclusive.

Thus the data regarding an immunologic cause of abortion are conflicting, with the majority of the evidence failing to confirm an immunologic etiology. There are potential risks associated with leukocytic immunotherapy, including the possibility of virus transmission and the development of autoimmune disease. For these reasons, at present it is not cost effective or necessary to perform the expensive HLA typing of each member of the couple with a history of recurrent abortion. Infusion of paternal leukocytes should only be performed under experimental protocols with informed consent, because the procedure has not been proven to be beneficial and has serious potential health risks. Since 1994 several groups of investigators have given intravenous immunoglobulin (IVIG) to women with unexplained recurrent abortion in an attempt to suppress immunologic factors that could cause abortion. The time of initiation of therapy, intervals of therapy, and amount of IVIG given differ in the various trials. Nevertheless the majority of randomized controlled trials indicate that IVIG therapy is not associated with a significantly higher viable birth rate than placebo. Therefore use of this expensive therapy should currently be considered experimental and should be performed only under a research protocol.

The Lupus Anticoagulant

The presence of either the lupus anticoagulant or the anticardiolipin antibody but not other antiphospholipid antibodies has been found to be associated with an increased rate of spontaneous abortion and intrauterine fetal death. These antiphospholipid antibodies are immunoglobulins of the IgG or IgM class. Although in vitro these immunoglobulins have anticoagulant activity by interfering with activation of the prothrombin activator complex and thus prolonging the partial thromboplastin time, clinically the presence of these antibodies is associated with thrombosis. Although the exact mechanism for the increased incidence of thrombosis is not known, some investigators have shown that when either antibody is present, it inhibits prostacyclin production from endothelial tissues, leading to a relative excess of thromboxane, which could enhance thrombosis. The presence of lupus anticoagulant activity is usually documented by performing one of the phospholipid-dependent coagulation tests. These include the activated partial thromboplastin time, the Kaolin clotting time, or the dilute Russell Viper venom time. The latter test has been reported to be the most sensitive for detection of the lupus anticoagulant. If the coagulation test is prolonged, an equal amount of normal plasma is added to the woman's plasma and the test is repeated. If it is still prolonged, the presence of lupus anticoagulant is likely and can be confirmed by correcting the coagulation test with the addition of phospholipid. The presence of the anticardiolipin antibody can be determined by specific solid-phase or enzyme-linked immunoassays. Rai et al. reported that if tests for either of these antibodies are positive, when repeat testing is done after an interval of 2 months or more only two thirds of those women originally found to have lupus anticoagulant and one third of these with anticardiolipins remained positive. Deleze et al. reported that about 80% of women with systemic lupus erythematosus (SLE) and recurrent fetal loss had antiphospholipid antibodies, whereas they were present in

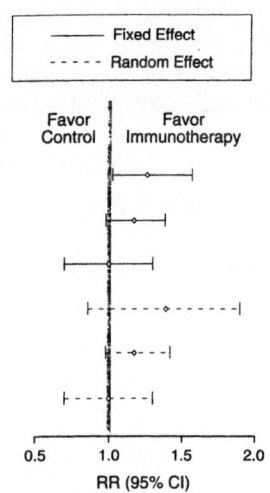

FIGURE 16-5   Publication bias: comparisons of published trials (original and updated) and unpublished trials. Number of trials, number of patients, relative live-term ratios (Rs), and 95% confidence intervals (CIs) are displayed. (From Jeng GT, Scott JR, and Burmesiter LF: JAMA 274:830, 1995.)

only 15% of women with SLE without fetal loss. These antibodies are also found in women (1) with other immunologic diseases, (2) with subclinical autoimmune disease, and (3) with recurrent abortion, thrombosis, or thrombocytopenia. Several groups, including the large unselected series of women with recurrent abortion reported by Rai et al., have reported that lupus anticoagulant is found in about 10% of women with recurrent spontaneous abortion of undetermined etiology. Anticardiolipin antibody has been reported to occur in 6% to 40% of such individuals, with the lower incidence being found in the large unselected series of 500 women. Thus about 15% of women with recurrent spontaneous abortion of undetermined etiology will have one of these antiphospholipid antibodies present. The prevalence of either lupus anticoagulant or anticardiolipin antibodies in a normal obstetric population is only 1% for each antibody. Therefore tests to detect the presence of both lupus anticoagulant and anticardiolipin antibody should be performed in individuals with recurrent abortion, since a causal relation apparently exists. Since a transient positive test is common, it is necessary to demonstrate that the antibody is present on at least two occasions more than 2 months apart.

Retrospective studies of women with recurrent abortion who have antiphospholipid antibodies report that abortion occurs in as many as 90% of their pregnancies. Rai et al. in a prospective study found that if one of these antibodies was present in women with recurrent abortion and no treatment was given, spontaneous abortion occurred in 90% of their next pregnancies. In a group of women with recurrent abortion without these antibodies present, abortion occurred in only 34% of the subsequent pregnancies. In this study 94% of the abortions in women with the antibodies occurred in the first trimester, and

fetal heart activity was present in 86% of these pregnancies. Thus first-trimester loss of embryonic, not anembryonic, pregnancies are the most common feature of abortion in association with antiphospholipid antibodies.

Currently there is no general agreement about therapy for individuals with recurrent abortion and the presence of lupus anticoagulant or anticardiolipin antibodies. Different investigators have used corticosteroids, aspirin, heparin, intravenous gamma globulin, or various combinations of these agents. Corticosteroids suppress the levels of antiphospholipid antibodies, aspirin inhibits platelet aggregation, and heparin prevents thrombosis. Previously the most widely used therapeutic regimen was daily ingestion of 20 to 60 mg of prednisone with 75 to 80 mg of aspirin. The overall live birth rate with this therapy was about 80%.

Since serious maternal and fetal complications have been reported to occur when high-dose corticosteroid therapy is given throughout pregnancy, a randomized multicenter trial comparing corticosteroid plus aspirin with heparin plus aspirin for the therapy of recurrent abortion was undertaken. In this small series of 23 women, live birth rates of 75% occurred in both treatment groups. However, the incidence of preterm birth and maternal morbidity were significantly higher in the group treated with corticosteroids and aspirin than heparin and aspirin. The results of two randomized trials by Rai, Cohen, Dave, et al. comparing the use of heparin plus aspirin with aspirin alone reported viable pregnancy rates with heparin plus aspirin to range between 70% and 80%, significantly better than the 42% to 44% rate with the use of aspirin alone. Therefore it is now suggested that the treatment of women with a history of recurrent abortion and the presence of either of these antibodies should be 80 mg of aspirin daily beginning when hCG is first detected throughout pregnancy and heparin 5,000 units every 12 hours daily, administered subcutaneously as soon as fetal heart activity is demonstrated sonographically. The heparin dose is adjusted downward until the activated partial thromboplastin time is within the normal range. Individuals with antiphospholipid antibodies, even when treated with aspirin and heparin, have a rate of pregnancy complications and need close monitoring during their gestation.

Activated Protein C Resistance

There is evidence from several studies that the incidence of activated protein C resistance (Factor V Leiden) is increased in women with unexplained recurrent abortion. Therefore, tests should be performed to determine if this abnormality is present. If present, treatment with aspirin and heparin can be given. However, no randomized trials have demonstrated an improved viable birth rate in women with activated protein C resistance treated with aspirin and heparin.

Hyperhomocystenemia

A few studies suggest that hyperhomocystenemia may be a cause of recurrent miscarriage because the incidence of abortions is higher in women with hyperhomocystenemia than controls. If this abnormality is present, therapy with folic acid and pyridoxine has been shown to normalize homocystene levels and results in viable births in a high rate of small case series. The dosage of these agents and their efficacy in achieving a viable pregnancy remains to be determined in randomized trials.

Infections

Numerous infectious agents present in the cervix, uterine cavity, or seminal fluid have been postulated to be etiologic factors for abortion. Although there is evidence that clinical endometritis caused by any infectious agent can produce an abortion, the evidence is unclear as to whether subclinical infections with certain microorganisms or viruses are a cause of spontaneous abortion. The parasite *Toxoplasma gondii* may infect the embryo and cause an abortion. However, it is difficult to document the presence of this organism before abortion occurs because there is a lack of correlation between serologic immunoassays for this organism and its detection in the endometrium by immunofluorescence. Furthermore, Kimball et al. reported that there was a similar incidence of positive immunologic screening tests for this organism in women with a history of none, one, or more than one abortion.

Although *Listeria monocytogenes* produces abortion in several animal species, there is no evidence that it is an abortifacient in women. Rabau and David found no bacteriologic or serologic evidence of *Listeria* infection in 554 women who had aborted, including 74 with recurrent abortions, and Stray-Pedersen et al. were unable to isolate this organism from a group of 48 women with recurrent abortion. *Chlamydia trachomatis* is a common sexually transmitted pathogen, but there is no evidence that it causes abortion in asymptomatic women.

Infection with herpes simplex virus in the genital tract has been reported to cause abortion. Nahmias et al. reported that if genital herpes initially occurred in the first half of pregnancy, the abortion rate was about 34%. Naib et al. reported that if pregnancy occurred within 18 months after initial detection of herpes infection, the abortion rate was 55%. Both these rates were significantly higher than the 11.5% abortion rate in the control population.

Several authors have suggested that T strain mycoplasma, both *Ureaplasma urealyticum* and *Mycoplasma hominis,* can cause abortion. Data indicating that the first organism is a cause of abortion are stronger than for the latter. Stray-Pedersen et al. found that although the incidence of cervical colonization of *U. urealyticum* was similar in a group of women with recurrent abortion and controls, the incidence of endometrial colonization was significantly more common (28%) in the group with recurrent abortions than in the control group (7%). In this study the cultures were obtained at least 6 months after the last abortion, and there were no clinical or laboratory signs of infection in any of the women. These investigators could not correlate the presence of *M. hominis* in the uterus with an increased frequency of abortion.

Stray-Pedersen and Stray-Pedersen reported that eradication of *U. urealyticum* in the endometrium by tetracyline treatment for 10 days resulted in a significantly lower subsequent abortion rate (19%). However, there are no randomized placebo-controlled clinical trials to prove that these organisms cause abortion and that treatment is effective.

Environmental Factors

Smoking

In a retrospective study Kline et al. reported that women who smoked during pregnancy had a significantly greater chance of having a spontaneous abortion than did a control group (Table 16-9). For women who smoked more than 14 cigarettes per day the risk of having an abortion was 1.7 times greater than for women who did not smoke, but smoking less than this amount did not result in a significantly greater incidence of abortion. These investigators found that heavy smokers had an increased risk of aborting chromosomally normal embryos only. There was no increased risk of an aneuploid abortion in smokers. These data indicate that smoking acts as a toxic agent to destroy chromosomally normal fetuses.

TABLE 16-9

Frequency (%) of Smoking Among Women Experiencing Spontaneous Abortions (Cases) and Women Delivering at 28 Weeks' Gestation or Later (Controls)

No. of Cigarettes Per Day	% Distribution		Adjusted Odds Ratio	95% Confidence Interval
	Cases	Controls		
None	62.0	69.8	1.00	—
1–13	20.5 ⎫	20.5 ⎫	1.07 ⎫	.80–1.42
14–80	17.4 ⎭ 37.9	10.2 ⎭ 30.2	1.73 ⎭ 1.28	1.23–2.43
TOTAL	648	645		

From Kline J, Stein Z, Susser M, et al: Environmental influences on early reproductive loss in a current New York City study. In Porter IH and Hook EB, editors: Human embryonic and fetal death, New York, 1980, Academic Press.

TABLE 16-10

Frequency (%) of Alcohol Consumption Among Women Experiencing Spontaneous Abortions (Cases) and Women Delivering at 28 Weeks' Gestation or Later (Controls)

Frequency of Alcohol Consumption During Pregnancy	% Distribution		Adjusted Odds Ratio	95% Confidence Interval
	Cases	Controls		
Never	42.6	43.7	1.00	
Twice a month and less	28.9	38.0	.77	.59–.99
Less than twice a month	10.8	10.4	1.04	.71–1.52
2 to 6 days a week	13.3 ⎫	6.5 ⎫	1.96 ⎫	1.30–2.95
Daily	4.5 ⎭ 17.9	1.4 ⎭ 7.9	3.00 ⎭ 2.36	1.39–6.49
TOTAL	648	645		

From Kline J, Stein Z, Susser M, et al: Environmental influences on early reproductive loss in a current New York City study. In Porter IH and Hook EB, editors: Human embryonic and fetal death, New York, 1980, Academic Press

Alcohol

Kline et al. also reported that drinking alcohol, acting independently from smoking, was a risk factor for abortion (Table 16-10). Women who drank alcohol at least 2 days a week had about a twofold greater risk of having an abortion than women who did not drink during pregnancy, with the risk increasing to threefold with daily ingestion of alcohol. As with smoking, an increased risk of abortion was confined to chromosomally normal embryos, indicating that drinking alcohol, like smoking, can act as a toxic agent on the normal embryo to cause its death. Harlap and Shiono found that even moderate drinking of alcohol increased the risk of second, but not first, trimester pregnancy loss, confirming the toxic effect of alcohol on the embryo.

Coffee, Caffeine, and Cocaine

There are some epidemiologic data suggesting that each of these substances may be an independent risk factor for abortion, but the data are inconsistent. Because there may be a causal relation between these agents and abortion, women who become pregnant should avoid their use.

Irradiation

Animal studies have shown that ionizing radiation can produce congenital malformation, growth retardation, and embryonic death. These effects are dose related, and there is a threshold dose below which an adverse effect does not occur. Although there is evidence in the human that high-energy radiation exposure is associated with teratogenic effects and growth retardation, there is no conclusive evi-

TABLE 16-11

Estimation of Abortigenic Hazards of X-Irradiation to Human Embryo from Animal Experiments

Stage of Human Gestation (Days)	Lethal Dose/50 (Rads)	MLD (Rads)
1	70–100	10
14	140	25
18	150	25
28	220	50
50	260	50
Late fetus to term	300–400	50

From Brent RL: Radiation-induced embryonic and fetal loss from conception to birth. In Porter IH and Hook EB, editors: Human embryonic and fetal death, New York, 1980, Academic Press.

dence that similar exposure increases the risk of spontaneous abortion.

Extrapolation from animal data indicates that the embryo is most sensitive to the lethal effect of irradiation during the day of implantation and a few days later (Table 16-11). The sensitivity decreases during the period of early embryogenesis, after which the minimum lethal dose (MLD) remains constant to term gestation. Brent reported that the MLD of irradiation to rats is 5 rads on the day of implantation. These data thus indicate that there is little likelihood that irradiation of less than 5 rads (severalfold greater than the amount used in nearly all diagnostic procedures) will cause an abortion in the human, even if it is administered during the time of implantation.

Environmental Toxins

Little valid information exists concerning the effect of environmental toxins on human abortion. Although some studies have shown an increased risk of abortion among female anesthesiologists, other studies have not found such an effect. Most studies reporting such a relation are retrospective questionnaire studies of marginal validity. A well-done case-control study by Axelsson and Rylander indicated that the incidence of abortion in women exposed to anesthetic gases was not significantly increased.

Information concerning a possible abortifacient effect after increased exposure to other environmental toxins is even less clear. Vianna and Polan reported that the entire population of women exposed to toxic chemical wastes in the Love Canal area had no significant excess of spontaneous abortions, although groups of women living in certain areas with a higher exposure may have had an increased risk of abortion.

DIAGNOSIS

Threatened Abortion

It has been estimated that bleeding occurs during the first 20 weeks of pregnancy in about 30% to 40% of human gestations, with about half of these pregnancies ending in spontaneous abortion. The risk of abortion is greater among those women who bleed for 3 or more days (24%) than among those who bleed only 1 or 2 days (7%). There is no evidence that women with gestational bleeding who do not abort have an increased incidence of complications of pregnancy, but they may have a slightly increased incidence of fetal anomalies and preterm birth. To determine the prognosis of the pregnancy in a woman with threatened abortion, ultrasonography, endocrinologic studies, and a combination of both techniques have been used.

The refinement of sonographic technology and the development of the vaginal probe have made it possible for a high-frequency transducer crystal in the probe to be placed in close proximity to the uterus. The images produced by this technique have much greater resolution than do those obtained by the transabdominal transducer. With use of the vaginal probe, it is now possible to always detect a gestational sac in a normal intrauterine pregnancy when the hCG level is between 1000 and 1500 mIU/ml, by at least 33 days' gestational age. The diameter of the gestational sac should be more than 3 mm at this stage of gestation. Between 34 to 38 days of gestation, when the gestational sac is more than 10 mm in diameter, the yolk sac should be visualized sonographically. Between 39 to 43 days' gestation, when the hCG concentration is more than 13,000 mIU/ml, the gestational sac should be more than 18 mm in diameter and an embryo with embryonic heart activity should be visualized in a normal gestation. If the gestational sac is more than 18 mm in diameter and no embryo is seen, an anembryonic gestation is present.

There are several sonographic parameters found in an early gestation that are predicators of a viable birth. As previously mentioned, if embryonic heart activity is seen at 6 weeks' gestational age, the chance of spontaneous abortion is about 7%. If heart activity is still present after 8 weeks' gestation, the chance of spontaneous abortion falls to about 2%.

Schats et al. and Achiron et al. reported that if the embryonic heart rate is much slower or faster than the normal rate of 100 to 120 beats per minute in early gestation, the risk of spontaneous abortion is elevated. Nazari et al. reported that if the diameter of the gestational sac and embryonic crown-rump length at 8 weeks' gestation were more than 1.5 standard diameters less than the mean lengths in normal gestations, the risk of spontaneous abortion was also very high. It has also been reported by Bromley et al. and Dickey et al. that if the difference between the diameter of the gestational sac and crown-rump length was less than 5 mm, the risk of spontaneous abortion was 80% or more. Thus early oligohydramnios is a very poor prognostic sign. These sonographic predictors of viable birth have less prognostic value among couples with recurrent spontaneous abortion because the pregnancy loss in those instances is more likely due to maternal disorders instead of problems with the gestation. Opsahl and Pettit and Stern and Coulam have reported that in contrast to the 7% abortion rate found after embryonic heart activity in all gestations when embryonic heart activity was seen in early gestation, among women with recurrent abortion the subsequent abortion rate was between 22% and 30%. Opsahl and Pettit also reported that if the difference in diameter between the gestational sac and crown-rump length was more than 8 mm in normal gestations, the spontaneous abortion rate was only 5%, but among women with recurrent abortion, the spontaneous abortion rate was 20%.

In addition to facilitating visualization of gestational structures much sooner after conception, use of vaginal sonography has also enabled the etiology and prognosis of the symptom of threatened abortion to be established with greater accuracy than had previously been possible with transabdominal ultrasonography. The diagnosis of intrauterine death or anembryonic gestation can be easily established and the contents of the uterus promptly evacuated, avoiding the occurrence of missed abortion. There have been several reports of ultrasonographic studies of groups of women with threatened abortion by Joupilla, Mantoni, and Cashner. In about two thirds of such pregnancies a live fetus is present, and about 85% of these fetuses subsequently are delivered and survive. The incidence of low birth weight or preterm birth in such pregnancies was increased in one series and not in another. The remaining 15% of the pregnancies abort, usually in the second trimester. Of the one third of women with a threatened abortion who do not have a live fetus present, about half have an anembryonic gestation, with the remainder being about equally divided between embryonic death and incomplete abortion, with an occasional molar gestation. Siddiqi reported that if embryonic heart activity is visualized early in gestation, the risk of the pregnancy ending in spontaneous abortion was increased about threefold if uterine bleeding occurred, from 5% without bleeding to 16% with bleeding.

Inevitable, Incomplete, and Complete Abortions

In a patient bleeding during the first half of pregnancy the diagnosis of inevitable abortion is strengthened if the bleeding is profuse and associated with uterine cramping pains. Women with threatened abortion who do not abort usually do not have cramps. When bleeding or pain in the first half of pregnancy is severe enough to require hospitalization, the most likely diagnosis is inevitable or incomplete abortion, occurring in more than 60% of women

who are hospitalized for vaginal bleeding in the first half of pregnancy (Table 16-12). The diagnosis can be confirmed by examination of the cervical os. If cervical dilation has occurred with or without rupture of membranes, the abortion is inevitable. If only a portion of the products of conception have been expelled and the cervix remains dilated, a diagnosis of incomplete abortion is made. However, if all fetal and placental tissue has been expelled, the cervix is closed, bleeding from the canal is minimal or decreasing, and uterine cramps have ceased, a diagnosis of complete abortion can be made. A complete abortion usually occurs *before* 6 weeks' and *after* 14 weeks' gestation. Abortions occurring *between* 6 weeks' and 14 weeks' gestation are usually incomplete and may be accompanied by profuse uterine bleeding.

Missed Abortion

The diagnosis of missed abortion is suspected clinically when the uterus fails to continue to enlarge with or without uterine bleeding or spotting. Typically after an episode of bleeding subsides, a continuous brown vaginal discharge is noted. When a dead fetus is retained in the uterus beyond 5 weeks after fetal death, consumptive coagulability with resultant hypofibrogenemia may occur. The incidence of this condition is correlated with both the length of gestation and the duration of fetal death: it is uncommon in gestations of less than 14 weeks' duration or duration of fetal death less than 6 weeks. With the use of ultrasonography the term *missed abortion* is no longer relevant because the diagnosis of anembryonic gestation or fetal death can be easily determined without delay. The uterus can then be promptly evacuated, avoiding the possibility of the adverse consequences associated with prolonged retention of necrotic fetal tissue.

TABLE 16-12
Causes of Vaginal Bleeding Before
Twentieth Week of Pregnancy

Final Diagnosis	No. of Patients	Percentage
Threatened abortion	211	13.6
Inevitable and incomplete abortion	951	61.4
Complete abortion	203	13.1
Septic abortion	67	4.3
Missed abortion	27	1.7
Benign hydatidiform mole	12	0.8
Tubal pregnancy	78	5.1
TOTAL	1549	

From Cavanagh D, Fleisher A, and Ferguson JH: Am J Obstet Gynecol 90:216, 1964.

Septic Abortion

Infection occurs in about 1% to 2% of all spontaneous abortions, with the incidence increasing if the abortion has been induced by a nonsterilized instrument. All women with uterine bleeding or spotting during the first half of pregnancy accompanied by clinical signs of infection must be considered to have a septic abortion if no obvious source of infection outside the genital tract is evident.

Septic abortions can be threatened, inevitable, or incomplete. The infection frequently spreads from the endometrium through the myometrium to the parametrium and sometimes to the peritoneum. Thus, in addition to endometritis, parametritis and peritonitis frequently occur in women with septic abortions. In addition to an elevated temperature and leukocytosis, lower abdominal tenderness, cervical motion tenderness, and a foul uterine discharge are signs of septic abortion. The cause of the infection is usually polymicrobial, with *Escherichia coli* and other aerobic gram-negative rods frequently involved. Group B beta-hemolytic streptococci, anaerobic streptococci, *Bacteroides* species, and on occasion *Clostridium perfringens* are other organisms that can cause septic abortion. Because endotoxins can be released from the gram-negative bacilli, endotoxic shock may accompany septic abortion, particularly if it is caused by insertion of nonsterile agents into the uterine cavity.

TREATMENT

Threatened Abortion

Although some physicians recommend that women with threatened abortion restrict their physical activities or stay at bed rest, there is no evidence that these measures or any active medical therapy improves the prognosis of threatened abortion. Treatment with natural progesterone, synthetic progestins, or hCG was previously advocated, but there is no evidence that such therapy improves the prognosis. Because such treatment may increase the probability of having a missed abortion, the use of this or any type of hormonal therapy is contraindicated. Nevertheless, staying at home with restriction of physical activities and avoidance of coitus is usually advised until the bleeding ceases. If bleeding increases, especially if it is accompanied by uterine cramps, it is likely that the abortion is becoming inevitable and the woman should be examined in a medical facility. Serial hCG measurements and uterine sonography aid in predicting the outcome. If ultrasonography reveals the presence of an anembryonic gestation or intrauterine fetal death, it is best to evacuate the uterine contents medically with an oxytocic agent or prostaglandin or surgically with curettage, depending on the stage of gestation. A recent study by Zalanyi et al. reported that vaginal administration of 200 μg misoprostol every 4 hours for up to 4 doses was an effective method to evacuate the uterine contents of women with a nonviable fetus in early gestation without the need to perform surgical evacuation.

Inevitable and Incomplete Abortion

Most abortions that occur between 8 and 14 weeks of pregnancy are incomplete and require surgical evacuation. This procedure can usually be accomplished on an outpatient basis in a hospital or surgical outpatient facility, since bleeding may be profuse and it may be necessary to administer a blood transfusion. Women with an incomplete abortion who do not develop sepsis or hypotension can usually be treated in the emergency room. After measurement of vital signs and placement of an intravenous line with an 18-gauge needle, blood is drawn for a complete blood count, as well as typing and cross matching for possible transfusion. An infusion of 10 to 30 units of oxytocin in 1000 ml of 5% Ringer's lactate should be initiated, and an intramuscular analgesic (meperidine [Demerol] 75 mg and diazepam [Valium] 5 mg) given, followed by placement of a paracervical block at 3 and 9 o'clock with 10 ml of 1% lidocaine (Xylocaine). Approximately 5 to 10 minutes later the uterine contents should be evacuated with sponge forceps and the cavity curetted gently with a sharp curette. Deep curettage should be avoided to prevent the subsequent development of uterine adhesions. After the procedure the vital signs and amount of vaginal bleeding should be monitored for 4 to 8 hours, after which the woman may be discharged home to remain at bed rest for 24 hours and avoid intercourse for 2 weeks. Oral ergonovine maleate 0.2 mg should be administered every 4 to 6 hours for 1 to 2 days. In addition, iron sulfate 200 mg should be administered orally three times a day until hemoglobin levels return to normal and tissue iron stores are replenished. If the mother is Rh negative and the father Rh positive, 50 μg anti-D gamma globulin should be administered intramuscularly. Numerous investigations, including the large series reported by Decenzo and Cavanagh, have shown this management approach to have good results.

Women with a complete abortion, usually before 8 weeks' gestation, need not be hospitalized but can be treated as outpatients with administration of ergonovine maleate. However, if the woman is already in the hospital and is believed to have spontaneously passed all the products of conception, sonography should be performed to confirm this fact prior to hospital discharge. If gestational tissue is still present in the uterine cavity, it should be surgically evacuated. Several studies including that of Chung et al. have shown that evacuation of retained products of conceptus after an incomplete abortion can be accomplished with the use of misoprostol, a prostaglandin E_2 analog. Thus curettage or vacuum aspiration is not needed.

Septic Abortion

Septic abortion is a potentially fatal condition, with an estimated fatality rate of 0.4 to 0.6 per 100,000 spontaneous abortions. All women with the diagnosis of septic abortion should have a complete blood count, urinalysis, chemistry, and electrolyte panel obtained. In addition, a specimen of the uterine discharge should be sent to the laboratory for culture and sensitivity. A Gram stain of the discharge should be performed in the admitting area. If the woman is seriously ill, blood cultures, a chest x-ray examination, and tests of blood coagulability should be obtained. Antibiotics should be administered intravenously, and the uterine contents evacuated. It is best to use combination antibiotic therapy, including an agent that will be effective against anaerobic bacteria. After adequate blood levels of antibiotics are obtained, usually within 2 hours, the uterus should be evacuated as described previously.

If the uterus is larger than 14 weeks' gestation and the cervix is closed (threatened septic abortion), management is more difficult. The uterine cavity needs to be evacuated to provide drainage of the infected material. This can be performed either by curettage, dilation and evacuation, oxytocics, or prostaglandins. Sometimes it is necessary to perform a hysterectomy if the sepsis is severe and the uterus cannot be evacuated through the cervical canal. All women with septic abortions need to have close monitoring of vital signs and urinary output. If signs of septic shock should develop, a central venous pressure catheter should be placed and additional intravenous fluids administered. Additional therapeutic agents, such as nasal oxygen, vasopressor agents, digitalis, and corticosteroids, may also be used.

Recurrent Abortion

The calculated probability of a woman's having three consecutive spontaneous abortions is about 0.3% to 0.4%, but the actual incidence is reported to range from 0.4% to 0.8%, indicating that there is a specific cause for recurrent pregnancy loss in some women.

The abortuses of women who have three or more abortions are more likely to be chromosomally normal (80% to 90%) than those of women with a single spontaneous abortion. Women with recurrent abortions also have a tendency to abort later in gestation, with two thirds of such abortions occurring beyond 12 weeks' gestation, indicating that maternal or environmental factors are a more likely cause of repeated pregnancy loss. Recurrent abortion is also called *habitual abortion*, but this term implies that every subsequent pregnancy in these women will end in an abortion. Clifford et al. reported the pregnancy outcome of 201 women with a history of unexplained recurrent abortion who received no pharmacologic therapy for the subsequent pregnancy. The abortion rate in the subsequent pregnancy was 29% and 27% for those with 3 or 4 prior abortions and 44% and 53% for those with 5 or 6 or more prior abortions, respectively. Overall nearly 70% of the women had a viable birth in their subsequent pregnancy without treatment. Thus the term *habitual abortion* should not be used and all studies of potential therapeutic agents should have a placebo control arm to determine true efficacy.

Couples with recurrent abortion require careful, sympathetic management by the practitioner, because an abortion is an emotionally traumatic experience that can result in as much grief as intrauterine fetal death in late pregnancy or a neonatal death. With recurrent abortion this emotional trauma is magnified, and the practitioner needs to express sympathy and understanding as counseling is performed and a diagnostic regimen is outlined.

Because the etiology of a second-trimester loss is more likely to be uterine in origin and thus more likely to be able to be diagnosed, a diagnostic evaluation should be performed after a woman has had only one second-trimester spontaneous abortion. There is no need to wait for a woman to have three first-trimester abortions with their accompanying emotional trauma before beginning a diagnostic evaluation. Because one early abortion is relatively common, it is recommended that diagnostic evaluation be initiated after a woman has had two first-trimester abortions.

After a history and physical examination are performed with pertinent questions regarding cervical incompetence, a complete blood count, a serum TSH, a midfollicular serum LH level, a midluteal serum progesterone measurement, as well as measurement of homocysteine levels and tests for antithyroid antibodies, should be obtained. Tests to detect lupus anticoagulant and anticardiolipin antibodies as well as activated protein C resistance should also be performed. If all these tests are normal a hysterogram, hydrosonography, or hysteroscopy should be performed to rule out congenital uterine anomalies, submucous leiomyomas, and intrauterine adhesions. Keltz et al. reported that hydrosonography, or sonohysterography is a very sensitive, specific, and accurate screening method to assess abnormalities in the uterine cavity of women with recurrent miscarriage. This technique avoids the need of radiation exposure. If no abnormalities are found, a karyotype of the husband and wife should be performed to determine if a chromosomal anomaly exists. It is not necessary to obtain endometrial bacteriologic cultures or perform HLA typing of the husband and wife.

If any of these tests reveals an abnormality that can be corrected with appropriate surgical or medical therapy as described, such therapy should be initiated. If a chromosomal abnormality is found, genetic counseling is indicated. There have been three series of large numbers of couples with recurrent abortion who have undergone a comprehensive diagnostic evaluation. Although different criteria for abnormal diagnostic tests were used by each group of investigators, no specific etiologic factor for the recurrent abortion (all tests normal) was found in 35% to 44% of the couples studied.

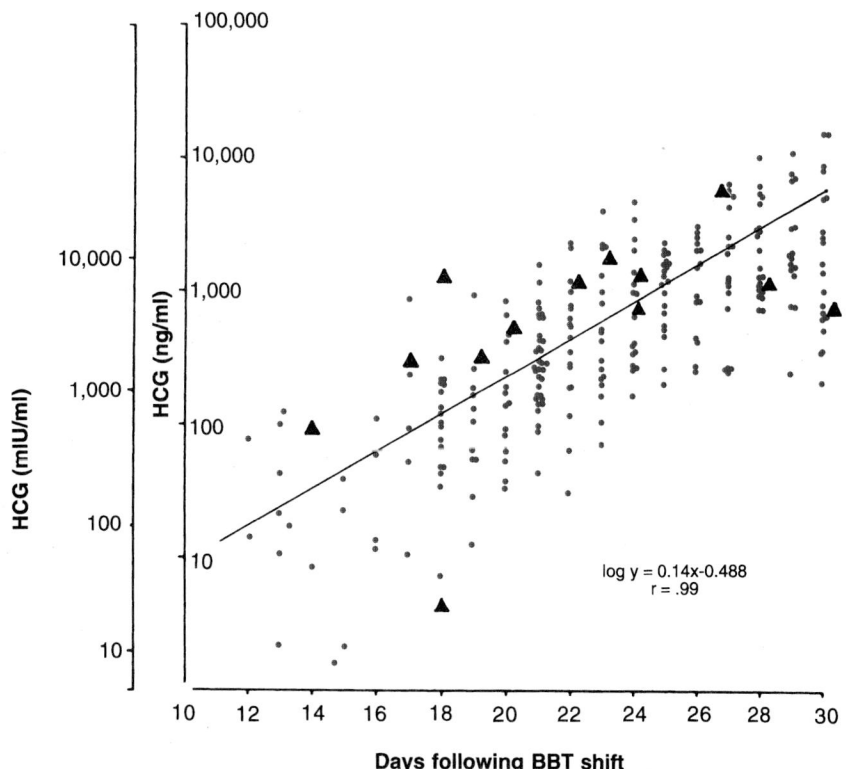

FIGURE 16-6 β-hCG RIA values during first 30 days of successful pregnancies. Each point represents concentration of hCG on specific day from 189 successful pregnancies. ▲, twin gestation. Line represents linear regression of means of data taken by days (5.7 mIU; 1 ng). (From Batzer FR, Schlaff S, Goldfarb AF, et al: Fertil Steril 35:307, 1981. Reproduced with permission of the publisher, The American Fertility Society.)

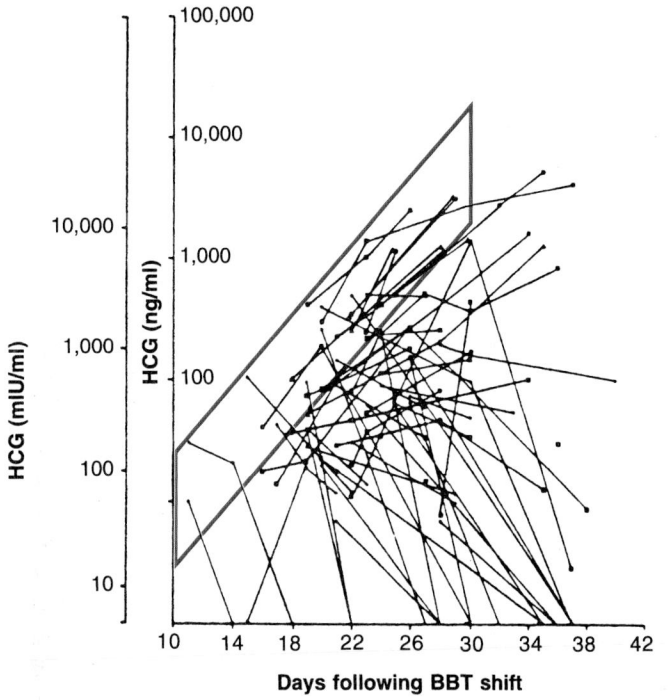

FIGURE 16-7 Serial β-hCG RIA values in 53 patients who aborted spontaneously. Twenty-six patients had a negative slope. Five patients with a normal slope aborted in second trimester. Blue line encloses 95% confidence limits in successful pregnancies. (From Batzer FR, Schlaff S, Goldfarb AF, et al: Fertil Steril 35:307, 1981. Reproduced with permission of the publisher, The American Fertility Society.)

If no diagnosis is obtained, the couple should be counseled regarding the probability of abortion in a subsequent pregnancy as described earlier. After conception, measurement of hCG levels twice weekly will provide information early in gestation regarding the prognosis of the outcome of the pregnancy. In normal gestations the levels of hCG double about every 2 days, and the rate of increase in a particular woman can be compared with the expected normal rate of increase (Figure 16-6). In most individuals with an early abortion, levels of hCG will rise at a slower rate than normal, plateau, and then decline (Figure 16-7). Batzer et al. found that when β-hCG doubling time in the first month of gestation was normal, it predicted a good outcome 88% of the time, and when abnormal, predicted a poor outcome 76% of the time. Pelvic sonography should be performed initially after hCG levels reach 1500 mIU/ml, at which time a gestational sac should be visualized. The sonogram should be repeated 2 weeks later, when an embryo with normal cardiac activity should be seen. These findings are reassuring, both to the woman and to the clinician but are of less prognostic value to couples with recurrent abortion than to the rest of the population.

Some individuals recommend that prophylactic antibiotic treatment be given to the husband and wife in the conception cycle or that progesterone supplementation be given to all women with recurrent abortion in the first trimester of pregnancy. Neither of these modalities has been demonstrated to improve the outcome of the pregnancy. However, three studies have demonstrated that extensive counseling and emotional support throughout early gestation results in significantly greater live birth rates than when only routine care is given. Stray-Pederson and Stray-Pederson reported that when a group of women with a history of unexplained recurrent abortion were given extensive antenatal counseling and psychologic support the live birth rate was 86%. Liddell et al. also reported that when a program of focused emotional support and close supervision was given to a group of 42 women with unexplained recurrent abortion the live birth rate was 86%. Clifford et al. reported that women with unexplained recurrent miscarriage given supportive care early in pregnancy had a 74% viable birth rate without other therapy. When only routine antenatal care was given to a similar group of women, the live birth rate in these three reports was between 33% and 51%, significantly less. Thus, intensive psychological support during early pregnancy appears to be very beneficial for improving the prognosis of couples with recurrent abortion whose etiology remains undetermined.

KEY POINTS

- About 15% to 20% of all human pregnancies terminate in clinically recognized abortion.

- In the human the total embryonic loss before 12 weeks' gestation is about 30%.

- About 80% of abortions occur in the first trimester, with the incidence decreasing with increasing gestational age.

- If embryonic cardiac activity is seen sonographically at 6 weeks' gestation, then the subsequent abortion rate is about 6% to 8%. If the embryo is viable at 8 weeks, then the subsequent abortion rate is only about 2% to 3%.

- The risk of a pregnancy terminating in spontaneous abortion increases independently with increasing parity, maternal age, and paternal age.

- The risk of abortion occurring when embryonic heart activity is seen early in pregnancy is increased if uterine bleeding is present, when the maternal age is over 35, and when serum CA-125 levels are elevated. Women with multiple abortions have a tendency to abort at about the same gestational age.

- For a woman with a reproductive history of three pregnancies terminating in abortion with no live births, her chance of having an abortion in a subsequent pregnancy is about 50%; if she has had at least one live birth and three spontaneous abortions, the chance that her next pregnancy will terminate in abortion is only about 30%.

- The major cause of abortion is genetic. The incidence of chromosomal anomalies in abortuses is about 50% when tissue culture is performed but is as high as 85% with direct cytogenetic analysis of chorionic villus tissue.

- Only about 5% of the abnormal karyotypes of abortuses are structural abnormalities of the chromosomes, such as translocation.

- Autosomal trisomy is the most common abnormal karyotype (50%), followed in decreasing frequency by monosomy 45,X (20%), triploidy (15%), tetraploidy (10%), and structural abnormalities (5%).

- The most common single chromosomal abnormality is monosomy 45,X.

- It is not cost effective or necessary to perform HLA typing of each member of the couple that has recurrent abortion.

- Lupus anticoagulant is found in about 10% of women with recurrent spontaneous abortion of undetermined etiology and anticardiolipin antibody is found in about 5% of these women.

- Karyotypes of abortuses of women who have had more than one abortion tend to be similar if the first abortus had either a normal karyotype or an autosomal trisomy.

- Maternal age is directly related to the incidence of trisomic abortions.

- Monosomy 45,X abortion is associated with a younger maternal age than other aneuploid or euploid abortions.

- Abortion of chromosomally normal conceptuses is found to occur later in gestation than abortion of chromosomally abnormal conceptuses does, with the peak incidence of euploid abortion being about 12 to 13 weeks of gestation; the peak incidence of aneuploid abortions is about 11 weeks.

- The incidence of chromosomally normal abortions increases markedly after a maternal age of 35, rising to more than 30% of clinically recognized conceptions after age 40.

- About 20% to 25% of women with anomalies of uterine fusion have severe problems with reproduction, with recurrent abortion being the most serious.

- The least common uterine anomaly, the unicornuate uterus, is associated with the greatest incidence of spontaneous abortion, about 50%.

- Women with either a septate or bicornuate uterus have a 25% to 30% incidence of spontaneous abortion.

- Women with recurrent abortion as a result of bicornuate and septate uteri have a decline in the abortion rate from about 88% to 15% after surgical correction.

- Women exposed to DES who subsequently conceive have a significantly greater incidence of spontaneous abortion than controls do.

- In women with an incompetent cervix the rate of fetal survival increases from about 20% to 80% after cerclage.

- Spontaneous and induced abortions cause about two thirds of intrauterine adhesions.

- Diabetes, if controlled by diet or insulin, is not a cause of abortion, whereas if uncontrolled, it is a cause.

- In women who smoke more than 14 cigarettes per day the risk of having an abortion is 1.7 times greater than in women who do not smoke.

- Smoking and drinking alcohol introduce toxic agents that can destroy chromosomally normal fetuses.

- Women who drink alcohol at least 2 days a week have about a twofold greater risk of having an abortion.

- Irradiation of less than 5 rads will not cause an abortion in the human.

- Threatened abortion occurs in about 30% to 40% of human gestations, with only about half of these pregnancies ending in spontaneous abortion.

- The prevalence of major chromosomal abnormalities present in either partner of a couple with two or more pregnancy losses is about 3% to 5%, 5 to 6 times higher than in the general population. Abnormalities occur in the female parent about twice as frequently as the male, with balanced reciprocal translocations occurring in half of these individuals.

- The most widely used therapeutic regimen to treat women with recurrent abortion and the presence of lupus anticoagulant or anticardiolipin antibody is 75 to 80 mg of aspirin per day together with 10,000 μg heparin daily.

- Complete abortion usually occurs *before* 6 weeks' and *after* 14 weeks' gestation. Abortions occurring *between* 6 weeks' and 14 weeks' gestation are usually incomplete.

- When a dead fetus is retained in the uterus beyond 5 weeks after fetal death, consumptive coagulability with resultant hypofibrogenemia may occur.

- About 1% to 2% of all spontaneous abortions become infected.

- The expected probability of a woman's having three consecutive abortions is about 0.3% to 0.4%, but the actual incidence is reported to range from 0.4% to 0.8%.

- The abortuses of women who have had three or more abortions are more likely to be chromosomally normal (80% to 90%) than those of women with a single spontaneous abortion.

- Women with recurrent abortions also have a tendency to abort later in gestation, with two thirds of such abortions occurring beyond 12 weeks' gestation, indicating that maternal or environmental factors are a more likely cause of repeated pregnancy loss.

- A diagnostic evaluation should be performed after a woman has had only one second-trimester spontaneous abortion or two first-trimester abortions.

- In most individuals with an early abortion, levels of hCG will rise at a slower rate than normal, plateau, and then decline.

- Sharing of histocompatability locus antigens at the H and B locus probably does not occur more frequently in women with recurrent abortion, but sharing at the DR locus probably does occur more frequently. The cause of abortion in couples with this finding is more likely due to a recessive gene, not an immunologic cause.

- Maternal immunization with paternal white cells has not been proven to increase the incidence of live births. This therapy has risks and should be considered to be experimental.

- Hypothyroidism has not been shown to be a cause of abortion, but women who have an abortion are more likely to have antithyroid antibodies indicative of a possible immunologic problem.

- Women with elevated follicular phase LH levels, with and without polycystic ovaries, are more likely to have an abortion than are women with normal LH levels.

- With use of the vaginal probe a gestational sac should always be seen when hCG levels reach 1500 mIU/ml. When embryonic size is 4 mm or more, cardiac activity should be observed.

- About two thirds of pregnancies in women with threatened abortion have a live embryo or fetus present, and about 85% of these will survive. Of the one third without a live fetus, half will have an anembryonic gestation, the remainder being divided equally between embryonic death and incomplete abortion.

- Intravenous immunoglobulin infusions have been used to treat unexplained recurrent abortions as well as women with abortion and antithyroid antibodies. The majority of randomized trials indicate that this therapy is not associated with a significantly higher viable birth rate than placebo.

- Three studies have shown that intensive supportive care in early pregnancy of women with recurrent spontaneous abortion yields viable pregnancy rates of 70% to 80%, significantly higher than occurs with routine prenatal care.

BIBLIOGRAPHY

Achiron R, Tadmor O, and Mashiach S: Heart rate as a predictor of first-trimester spontaneous abortion after ultrasound-proven viability, Obstet Gynecol 78:330, 1991.

Al-Sebai MAH, Kingsland CR, Diver M, et al: The role of a single progesterone measurement in the diagnosis of early pregnancy failure and the prognosis of fetal viability, Br J Obstet Gynaecol 102:364, 1995.

Axelsson G and Rylander R: Exposure to anaesthetic gases and spontaneous abortion: response bias in a postal questionnaire study, Int J Epidemiol 11:250, 1982.

Backos M, Rai R, Baxter N, et al: Pregnancy complications in women with recurrent miscarriage associated with antiphospholipid antibodies treated with low dose aspirin and heparin, Br J Obstet Gynaecol 106:102, 1999.

Balasch J, Font J, Lopez-Soto A, et al: Antiphospholipid antibodies in unselected patients with repeated abortion, Hum Reprod 5:43, 1990.

Ballen AH, Tan SL, Jacobs HS: Hypersecretion of luteinising hormone: a significant cause of infertility and miscarriage, Br J Obstet Gynaecol 100:1082, 1993.

Barnes AB, Colton T, Gundersen J, et al: Fertility and outcome of pregnancy in women exposed in utero to diethylstilbestrol, N Engl J Med 302:609, 1980.

Batzer FR, Schlaff S, Goldfarb AF, et al: Serial β-subunit human chorionic gonadotropin doubling time as a prognosticator of pregnancy outcome in an infertile population, Fertil Steril 35:307, 1981.

Bellingard V, Hedon B, Eliaou JF, et al: Immunogenetic study of couples with recurrent spontaneous abortions, Eur J Obstet Gynecol Reprod Endocrinol 60:53, 1995.

Berry CW, Brambati B, Eskes TKAB, et al: The Euro-Team early pregnancy (ETEP) protocol for recurrent miscarriage, Hum Reprod 10:1516, 1995.

Bider D, Kokia AE, Seidman DS, et al: Cervical cerclage for anomalous uteri, J Reprod Med 37:138, 1992.

Boué J, Boué A, and Lazar P: Retrospective and prospective epidemiological studies of 1500 karyotyped spontaneous human abortions, Teratology 12:11, 1975.

Brent RL: Radiation-induced embryonic and fetal loss from conception to birth. In Porter IH and Hook EB, editors: Human embryonic and fetal death, New York, 1980, Academic Press.

Bromley B, Harlow BL, Laaboda LA, and Benacerraf BR: Small sac size in the first trimester: a predictor of poor fetal outcome, Radiology 178:375, 1991.

Bussen S and Steck T: Thyroid autoantibodies in euthyroid non-pregnant women with recurrent spontaneous abortions, Hum Reprod 10:2938, 1995.

Buttram VC and Gibbons WE: Müllerian anomalies: a proposed classification (an analysis of 144 cases), Fertil Steril 32:40, 1979.

Buttram VC Jr and Reiter RC: Uterine leiomyomata: etiology, symptomatology, and management, Fertil Steril 36:433, 1981.

Cacciatore B, Tiitinen A, Stenman UH, and Ylostalo P: Normal early pregnancy: serum HCG levels and vaginal ultrasonographic findings, Br J Obstet Gynaecol 97:899, 1990.

Cashner KA, Christopher CR, and Dysert GA: Spontaneous fetal loss after demonstration of a live fetus in the first trimester, Obstet Gynecol 70:827, 1987.

Chipchase J, and James DE: Randomised trial of expectant versus surgical management of spontaneous miscarriage, Br J Obstet Gynecol 104:840, 1997.

Christiansen OB, Mathiesen O, Husth M, et al: Prognostic significance of maternal DR histocompatibility types in Danish women with recurrent miscarriages, Hum Reprod 8:1843, 1993.

Christiansen OB, Mathiesen O, Husth M, et al: Placebo-controlled trial of active immunization with third party leukocytes in recurrent miscarriage, Acta Obstet Gynecol Scand 73:261, 1994.

Chung T, Leung P, Cheung LP, et al: A medical approach to management of spontaneous abortion using misoprostol: Extending misoprostol treatment to a maximum of 48 hours can further improve evacuation of retained products of conception in spontaneous abortion, Acta Obstet Gynecol Scand 76:248, 1997.

Chung TKH, Lee DTS, Cheung LP, et al: Spontaneous abortion: a randomized, controlled trial comparing surgical evacuation with conservative management using misoprostol, Fertil Steril 71:1054, 1999.

Clifford K, Rai R, and Regan L: Future pregnancy outcome in unexplained recurrent first trimester miscarriage, Hum Reprod 12:387, 1997.

Clifford K, Rai R, Watson H, and Regan L: An informative protocol for the investigation of recurrent miscarriage: preliminary experience of 500 consecutive cases, Hum Reprod 9:1328, 1994.

Clifford K, Rai R, Watson H, et al: Does suppressing luteinising hormone secretion reduce the miscarriage rate? Results of a randomised controlled trial, BMJ 312:1508, 1995.

Copumans ABC, Huijgens PC, Jakobs C, et al: Haemostatic and metabolic abnormalities in women with unexplained recurrent abortion, Human Reprod 14:21, 1999.

Coulam CB: Immunologic tests in the evaluation of reproductive disorders: a critical review, Am J Obstet Gynecol 167:1844, 1995.

Coulam CB, Krysa L, Stern JJ, and Bustillo M: Intravenous immunoglobulin for treatment of recurrent pregnancy loss, Am J Reprod Immunol 34:333, 1995.

Cowchock FS, Reece EA, Balaban D, et al: Repeated fetal losses associated with antiphospholipid antibodies: a collaborative randomized trial comparing prednisone with low-dose heparin treatment, Am J Obstet Gynecol 166:1318, 1992.

Cowchock FS and Smith JB: Fertility among women with recurrent spontaneous abortions: the effect of paternal cell immunization treatment, Am J Reprod Immunol 33:176, 1995.

Crane JP and Wahl N: The role of maternal diabetes in repetitive spontaneous abortion, Fertil Steril 36:477, 1981.

Daya S and Gunby J: The recurrent miscarriage immunotherapy trialists group: the effectiveness of allogeneic leukocyte immunization in unexplained primary recurrent spontaneous abortion, Am J Reprod Immunol 32:294, 1994.

Daya S, Gunby J, and Clark DA: Intravenous immunoglobulin therapy for recurrent spontaneous abortion: a meta-analysis, Am J Reprod Immunol 39:69, 1998.

De Braekeleer M and Dao TN: Cytogenetic studies in couples experiencing repeated pregnancy losses, Hum Reprod 5:519, 1990.

Deleze M, Alarcon-Segovia D, Valdes-Macho E, et al: Relationship between antiphospholipid antibodies and recurrent fetal loss in patients with systemic lupus erythematosus and apparently healthy women, J Rheumatol 16:768, 1989.

Dickey RP, Olar TT, Taylor SN, et al: Relationship of small gestational sac-crown-rump length differences to abortion and abortus karyotypes, Obstet Gynecol 79:554, 1992.

Dickey RP, Gasser RF, Olar TT, et al: The relationship of initial embryo crown-rump length to pregnancy outcome and abortus karyotype based on new growth curves for the 2-31 mm embryo, Hum Reprod 9:366, 1994.

Fraser EJ, Grimes DA, and Schulz KF: Immunization as therapy for recurrent spontaneous abortion: a review and meta-analysis, Obstet Gynecol 82:854, 1993.

Goldstein P, Berrier J, Rosen S, et al: A meta-analysis of randomized control trials of progestational agents in pregnancy, Br J Obstet Gynaecol 96:265, 1989.

Goldstein SR: Embryonic ultrasonographic measurements: crown-rump length revisisted, Am J Obstet Gynecol 165:497, 1991.

Goldstein SR: Significance of cardiac activity on endovaginal ultrasound in very early embryos, Obstet Gynecol 80:670, 1992.

Goldstein SR: Embryonic death in early pregnancy: a new look at the first trimester, Obstet Gynecol 84:294, 1994.

Goldstein SR and Wolfson R: Endovaginal ultrasonographic measurement of early embryonic size as a means of assessing gestational age, J Ultrasound Med 13:27, 1994.

Harlap S and Shiono PH: Alcohol, smoking, and incidence of spontaneous abortions in the first and second trimester, Lancet 2:173, 1980.

Heinonen PK, Saarikoski S, and Pystynen P: Reproductive performance of women with uterine anomalies, Acta Obstet Gynecol Scand 61:157, 1982.

Hill LM, Guzick D, Fries J, and Hixson J: Fetal loss rate after ultrasonically documented cardiac activity between 6 and 14 weeks, menstrual age, J Clin Ultrasound 19:221, 1991.

Horta JLH, Fernandez JG, Soto de Leon B, et al: Direct evidence of luteal insufficiency in women with habitual abortion, Obstet Gynecol 49:705, 1977.

Hwang JL, Hsieh CY, Ho HN, et al: The role of blocking factors and antipaternal lymphocytotoxic antibodies in the success of pregnancy in patients with recurrent spontaneous abortion, Fertil Steril 58:691, 1992.

Illeni MT, Marelli G, Parazzini F, et al: Immunotherapy and recurrent abortion: a randomized clinical trial, Hum Reprod 9:1247, 1994.

Jablonowska B, Selbing A, Palfi M, et al: Prevention of recurrent spontaneous abortion by intravenous immunoglobulin: a double-blind placebo-controlled study, Hum Reprod 14:838, 1999.

Jeng GT, Scott JR, and Burmiester LF: A comparison of meta-analytic results using literature vs individual patient data, JAMA 274:830, 1995.

Jin K, Ho H-N, Speed TP, and Gill TJ III: Reproductive failure and the major histocompatibility complex, Am J Hum Genet 56:1456, 1995.

Kajii T, Ferrier A, Niikawa N, et al: Anatomic and chromosomal anomalies in 639 spontaneous abortuses, Hum Genet 55:87, 1980.

Kaufman RH, Noller K, Adam E, et al: Upper genital tract abnormalities and pregnancy outcome in diethylstilbestrol-exposed progeny, Am J Obstet Gynecol 148:973, 1984.

Keltz MD, Olive DL, Kim AH, et al: Sonohysterography for screening in recurrent pregnancy loss, Fertil Steril 67:670, 1997.

Kilpatrick DC and Liston WA: Influence of histocompatibility antigens in recurrent spontaneous abortion and its relevance to leukocyte immunotherapy, Hum Reprod 8:1645, 1993.

Kimball AC, Kean BH, and Fuchs F: The role of toxoplasmosis in abortion, Am J Obstet Gynecol 111:219, 1971.

Kiprov DD, Nachtigall RD, Weaver RC, et al: The use of intra-venous immunoglobulin in recurrent pregnancy loss associated with combined alloimmune and autoimmune abnormalities, Am J Reprod Immunol 36:228, 1996.

Kline J, Shrout P, Stein ZA, et al: Drinking during pregnancy and spontaneous abortion, Lancet 2:176, 1980.

Kline J, Stein ZA, Susser M, et al: Smoking: a risk factor for spontaneous abortion, N Engl J Med 297:793, 1977.

Knudsen UB, Hansen V, Juul S, and Secher NJ: Prognosis of a new pregnancy following previous spontaneous abortions, Eur J Obstet Gynaecol 39:31, 1991.

Laboda LA, Estroff JA, and Benacerraf BR: First trimester brady-cardia: a sign of impending fetal loss, J Ultrasound Med 8:561, 1989.

Lejeune B, Grun JP, DeNayer P, et al: Antithyroid antibodies underlying thyroid abnormalities and miscarriage or pregnancy induced hypertension, Br J Obstet Gynaecol 100:669, 1993.

Li TC, Spring PG, Bygrave C, et al: The value of biochemical and ultrasound measurements of predicting pregnancy outcome in women with a history of recurrent miscarriage, Hum Reprod 13:3525, 1998.

Liddell HS, Pattison NA, and Zanderigo A: Recurrent miscarriage: outcome after supportive care in early pregnancy, Aust N Z J Obstet Gynaecol 31:320, 1991.

March CM and Israel R: Gestational outcome following hysteroscopic lysis of adhesions, Fertil Steril 36:455, 1981.

March CM and Israel R: Hysteroscopic management of recurrent abortion secondary to septate uterus, Am J Obstet Gynecol 156:834, 1987.

Marzuseh K, Dietl J, Klein R, et al: Recurrent first trimester spontaneous abortion associated with antiphospholipid antibodies: a pilot study of treatment with intravenous immunoglobulin, Acta Obstet Gynecol Scand 74:922, 1996.

Mills JL, Simpson JL, Driscoll SG, et al: Incidence of spontaneous abortion among normal women and insulin-dependent diabetic women whose pregnancies were identified within 21 days of conception, N Engl J Med 319:1618, 1988.

Montoro M, Collea JV, Frasier D, et al: Successful outcome of pregnancy in women with hypothyroidism, Ann Intern Med 94:31, 1981.

Mowbray JF, Gibbings C, Liddell H, et al: Controlled trial of treatment of recurrent spontaneous abortion by immunisation with paternal cells, Lancet 1:941, 1985.

MRC/RCOG Working Party on Cervical Cerclage: Final report of the Medical Research Council/Royal College of Obstetricians and Gynaecologists multicentre randomised trial of cervical cerclage, Br J Obstet Gynaecol 100:516, 1993.

Nahmias AJ, Josey WE, Naib ZM, et al: Perinatal risk associated with maternal genital herpes simplex virus infection, Am J Obstet Gynecol 110:825, 1971.

Naib ZM, Nahmias AJ, Josey WE, et al: Association of maternal genital herpetic infection with spontaneous abortion, Obstet Gynecol 35:260, 1970.

Naylor AF and Warburton D: Sequential analysis of spontaneous abortion. II. Collaborative study data show that gravidity determines a very substantial rise in risk, Fertil Steril 31:282, 1979.

Nazari A, Check JH, Epstein RH, et al: Relationship of small-for-dates sac size to crown-rump length and spontaneous abortion in patients with a known date of ovulation, Obstet Gynecol 78:369, 1991

Ness RB, Grisso JA, Hirschinger N, et al: Cocaine and tobacco use and the risk of spontaneous abortion, N Engl J Med 340:333, 1999.

Ogasawara M, Aoyama T, Kajiura S, et al: Are serum progesterone levels predictive of recurrent miscarriage in future pregnancies? Fertil Steril 68:806, 1997.

Ohno M, Maeda T, and Matsunobu A: A cytogenetic study of spontaneous abortions with direct analysis of chorionic villi, Obstet Gynecol 77:394, 1991.

Opsahl MS and Pettit DC: First trimester sonographic characteristics of patients with recurrent spontaneous abortion, J Ultrasound Med 12:507, 1993.

Out HJ, Bruinse HW, and Derksen RHWM: Antiphospholipid antibodies and pregnancy loss, Hum Reprod 6:889, 1991.

Parazzini F, Chatenoud L, DiCintio E, et al: Coffee consumption and risk of hospitalized miscarriage before 12 weeks of gestation, Hum Reprod 13:2286, 1998.

Pattison NS, Chamley LW, McKay EJ, et al: Antiphospholipid antibodies in pregnancy: prevalence and clinical associations, Br J Obstet Gynaecol 100:909, 1993.

Pedersen JF and Mantoni M: Prevalence and significance of subchorionic hemorrhage in threatened abortion: a sonographic study, Am J Roentgenol 154:535, 1990.

Perino A, Vassiliadis A, Vucetich A, et al: Short-term therapy for recurrent abortion using intravenous immunoglobulins: results of a double-blind placebo-controlled Italian study, Hum Reprod 12:2388, 1997.

Poland BJ, Miller JR, Jones DC, et al: Reproductive counseling in patients who have had a spontaneous abortion, Am J Obstet Gynecol 127:685, 1977.

Portnoi MF, Joye N, Van Den Akker J, et al: Karyotypes of 1142 couples with recurrent abortion, Obstet Gynecol 72:31, 1988.

Pratt DE, Karande V, Kaberlein G, et al: The association of antithyroid antibodies in euthyroid nonpregnant women with recurrent first trimester abortions in the next pregnancy, Fertil Steril 60:1001, 1993.

Quere I, Bellet H, Hoffet M, et al: A woman with five consecutive fetal deaths: case report and retrospective analysis of hyperhomocystenemia prevalence in 100 consecutive women with recurrent miscarriages, Fertil Steril 69:152, 1998.

Rabau E and David A: *Listeria monocytogenes* in abortion, J Obstet Gynaecol Br Comm 70:481, 1963.

Rai R, Clifford K, and Regan L: The modern preventative treatment of recurrent miscarriage, Br J Obstet Gynaecol 103:106, 1996.

Rai R, Cohen H, Dave M, et al: Randomised controlled trial of aspirin and aspirin plus heparin in pregnant women with recurrent miscarriage associated with phospholipid antibodies (or antiphospholipid antibodies), BMJ 314:253, 1997.

Rai R, Regan L, Hadley E, et al: Second-trimester pregnancy loss is associated with activated protein C resistance, Br J Haematol 92:489, 1996.

Rai RS, Clifford K, Cohen H, and Regan L: High prospective fetal loss rate in untreated pregnancies of women with recurrent miscarriage and antiphospholipid antibodies, Hum Reprod 10:3301, 1995.

Rai RS, Regan L, Clifford K, et al: Antiphospholipid antibodies and β_2-glycoprotein-I in 500 women with recurrent miscarriage: results of a comprehensive screening approach, Hum Reprod 10:2001, 1995.

Regan L, Braude PR, and Trembath PL: Influence of past reproductive performance on risk of spontaneous abortion, Br Med J 299:541, 1989.

Regan L, Owen EJ, and Jacobs HS: Hypersecretion of luteinising hormone, infertility, and miscarriage, Lancet 336:1141, 1990.

Reznikoff-Etievant MF, Cayol V, Zou GM, et al: Habitual abortions in 1678 healthy patients: investigation and prevention, Human Reprod 14:2106, 1999.

Ridker PM, Miletich JP, Buring JE, et al: Factor V Leiden mutation as a risk factor for recurrent pregnancy loss, Ann Intern Med 128:1000, 1998.

Roberts JM and Laros RK: Hemorrhagic and endotoxic shock: a pathophysiologic approach to diagnosis and management, Am J Obstet Gynecol 110:1041, 1971.

Sachs ES, Jahoda MGJ, Van Hemel JO, et al: Chromosome studies of 500 couples with two or more abortions, Obstet Gynecol 65:375, 1985.

Sargent IL, Wilkins T, Redman CWG: Maternal immune responses to the fetus in early pregnancy and recurrent miscarriage, Lancet 2:1099, 1988.

Sbracia M, Mastrone M, Scarpellini F, and Grasso JA: Influence of histocompatibility antigens in recurrent spontaneous abortion couples and on their reproductive performances, Am J Reprod Immunol 35:85, 1996.

Scarpellini F, Mastrone M, Sbracia M, and Scarpellini L: Serum CA 125 and first trimester abortion, Int J Gynaecol Obstet 49:259, 1995.

Schats R, Jansen CAM, and Wladimiroff JW: Embryonic heart activity: appearance and development in early human pregnancy, Br J Obstet Gynaecol 97:989, 1990.

Siddiqi TA, Caligaris JT, Miodovnik M, et al: Rate of spontaneous abortion after first trimester sonographic demonstration of fetal cardiac activity, Am J Perinatol 5:1, 1988.

Silver RK, MacGregor SN, Sholl JS, et al: Comparative trial of prednisone plus aspirin versus aspirin alone in the treatment of anticardiolipin antibody-positive obstetric patients, Am J Obstet Gynecol 169:1411, 1993.

Simpson JL: Genes, chromosomes, and reproductive failure, Fertil Steril 33:107, 1980.

Smith A and Gaha TJ: Data on families of chromosome translocation carriers ascertained because of habitual spontaneous abortion, Aust N Z J Obstet Gynaecol 30:57, 1990.

Smith JB and Cowchock FS: Immunological studies in recurrent spontaneous abortion: effects of immunization of women with paternal mononuclear cells on lymphocytotoxic and mixed lymphocyte reaction blocking antibodies and correlation with sharing of HLA and pregnancy outcome, J Reprod Immunol 14:99, 1988.

Stagnaro-Green A, Roman SH, Cobin RH, et al: Detection of at-risk pregnancy by means of highly sensitive assays for thyroid autoantibodies, JAMA 264:1422, 1990.

Stein Z, Kline J, Susser E, et al: Maternal age and spontaneous abortion. In Porter IH and Hook EB, editors: Human embryonic and fetal death, New York, 1980, Academic Press.

Stern JJ and Coulam CB: Mechanism of recurrent spontaneous abortion. I. Ultrasonographic findings. Am J Obstet Gynecol 166:1844, 1992.

Stray-Pedersen B and Stray-Pedersen S: Etiologic factors and subsequent reproductive performance in 195 couples with a prior history of habitual abortion, Am J Obstet Gynecol 148:140, 1984.

Stray-Pedersen B, Eng J, and Reikvam TM: Uterine T-mycoplasma colonization in reproductive failure, Am J Obstet Gynecol 130:307, 1978.

Strobino BA and Pantel-Silverman J: First-trimester vaginal bleeding and the loss of chromosomally normal and abnormal conceptions, Am J Obstet Gynecol 157:1150, 1987.

Tadmor OP, Achiron R, Rabinowiz R, et al: Predicting first-trimester spontaneous abortion: ratio of mean sac diameter to crown-rump length compared to embryonic heart rate, J Reprod Med 39:459, 1994.

Tharapel AT, Tharapel SA, and Bannerman RM: Recurrent pregnancy losses and parental chromosome abnormalities: a review, Br J Obstet Gynaecol 92:899, 1985.

The German RSA/IVIG Group: Intravenous immunoglobulin in the prevention of recurrent miscarriage, Br J Obstet Gynaecol 101:1072, 1994.

The Recurrent Miscarriage Immunotherapy Trialists Group L worldwide collaborative observational study and meta-analysis on allogenic leukocyte immunotherapy for recurrent spontaneous abortion, Am J Reprod Immunol 32:55, 1994.

Tho PT, Byrd TR, and McDonough PG: Etiologies and subsequent reproductive performance of 100 couples with recurrent abortion, Fertil Steril 32:389, 1979.

Tulppala M, Palosuo T, Ramsay T, et al: A prospective study of 63 couples with a history of recurrent spontaneous abortion: contributing factors and outcome of subsequent pregnancies, Hum Reprod 8:764, 1993.

Vianna NJ and Polan AK: Incidence of low birth weight among Love Canal residents, Science 226:1217, 1984.

Warburton D and Fraser FC: Spontaneous abortion risks in man: data from reproductive histories collected in a medical genetics unit, Am J Hum Genet 16:1, 1964.

Watson H, Kiddy DS, Hamilton-Fairley D, et al: Hypersecretion of luteinizing hormone and ovarian steroids in women with recurrent early miscarriage, Hum Reprod 8:829, 1993.

Wilcox AJ, Weinberg CR, O'Connor JF, et al: Incidence of early loss of pregnancy, N Engl J Med 319:189, 1988.

Wilson R, Ling lH, MacLean MA, et al: Thyroid antibody titer and avidity in patients with recurrent miscarriage, Fertil Steril 71:558, 1999.

Wong KS, Ngai CSW, Yeo ELK, et al: A comparison of two regimens of intravaginal misoprostol for termination of second trimester pregnancy: a randomized comparative trial, Hum Reprod 15:709, 2000.

World Health Organisation Task Force on Post-ovulatory Methods of Fertility Regulation. Special Programme of Research, Development and Research Training, World Health Organisation, Geneva: Comparison of two doses of mifepristone in combination with misoprostol for early medical abortion: a randomised trial. Br J Obstet Gynaecol 107:524, 2000.

Yamada H, Kishida T, Kobayashi N, et al: Massive immunoglobulin treatment in women with four or more recurrent spontaneous primary abortions of unexplained aetiology, Hum Reprod 13:2620, 1998.

Zalanyi S: Vaginal misoprostol alone is effective in the treatment of missed abortion, Br J Obstet Gynaecol 105:1026, 1998.

Ectopic Pregnancy
Etiology, Pathology, Diagnosis, Management, Fertility Prognosis

KEY TERMS AND DEFINITIONS

Abdominal Pregnancy. Pregnancy that develops in any portion of the peritoneal cavity. It usually occurs after a secondary implantation of the trophoblast after tubal abortion (secondary abdominal pregnancy). A primary abdominal pregnancy is one that implants directly into the peritoneal cavity.

Arias-Stella Reaction. Hypersecretory appearance of endometrial glands. The cells demonstrate hyperchromatism, pleomorphism, increased mitotic activity, and hypertrophy.

Cervical Pregnancy. Pregnancy developing in the cervical canal below the level of the internal os.

Chronic Ectopic Pregnancy. Ectopic gestational tissue in the peritoneal cavity after tubal abortion or rupture. It produces chronic symptoms of lower abdominal pain and usually forms adhesions to bowel and peritoneum.

Cornual Pregnancy. Pregnancy developing in one horn of a bicornuate uterus.

Culdocentesis. Aspiration of fluid in cul-de-sac (pouch) of Douglas via a needle placed through the vagina.

Decidual Cast. Sloughing of nearly all of the decidua lining the endometrial cavity.

Ectopic Pregnancy. Pregnancy that develops after implantation of the blastocyst anywhere other than the endometrium lining the uterine cavity.

Hemoperitoneum. Blood in the peritoneal cavity. The blood from a ruptured ectopic pregnancy initially clots and then lyses so that hemoperitoneum is a combination of blood clots and hemorrhagic fluid that will not clot.

Heterotopic Pregnancy. Combined intrauterine and extrauterine pregnancy.

Interstitial Pregnancy. Pregnancy developing in the interstitial portion of the oviduct.

Ovarian Pregnancy. Pregnancy developing in the ovary. For the diagnosis to be made, the following four characteristics must be fulfilled. (1) the tube on the affected side should be intact, (2) the gestational site must occupy the normal position of the ovary, (3) the gestational site must be connected to the uterus by the ovarian ligament, and (4) histologically identified ovarian tissue must be present in the sac wall.

Persistent Ectopic Pregnancy. Continued growth of viable trophoblastic tissue after conservative treatment of an unruptured ectopic pregnancy; manifestations include hCG titers that do not decline and/or pelvic pain.

Ruptured Ectopic Pregnancy. Ectopic pregnancy that has eroded through the tissue in which it has implanted, producing hemorrhage from exposed vessels.

Salpingitis Isthmica Nodosa (Tubal Diverticulum). Direct invasion of the tubal muscularis by the tubal epithelium for varying distances between the lumen and the serosa.

Salpingostomy. Surgical incision of the oviduct, which is followed by removal of a tubal pregnancy for the purpose of retaining the oviduct. After hemostasis is achieved, the incision is left open.

Salpingotomy. Surgical incision of the oviduct, followed by removal of a tubal pregnancy and closure of the incision.

Tubal Abortion. Tubal pregnancy that has extruded out of the fimbrial end of the oviduct.

Tubal Pregnancy. Pregnancy occurring in the oviduct in either the ampulla, fimbria, or isthmus. Pregnancy in the oviduct is the most common site of ectopic pregnancy.

Unruptured Tubal Gestation. Tubal pregnancy that has not yet eroded through the wall of the oviduct.

ctopic pregnancy was probably first described in AD 963 by Albucasis, an Arab writer. In 1876, before the initiation of surgical therapy, the mortality from ectopic pregnancy was estimated to be 60%. The first successful operative treatment of ectopic pregnancy was performed in 1883 by Lawson Tait in England. In 1887 he reported that he had performed salpingectomy on four women with ectopic pregnancy and that they all survived.

EPIDEMIOLOGY

The incidence of ectopic pregnancy is expressed in different ways in the literature. The most common denominator used is the number of recognized conceptions, with the incidence expressed as the number of ectopic pregnancies per 1000 conceptions. Other denominators include the number of women of reproductive age, expressed as the number of ectopic pregnancies per 10,000 women aged 14 to 44, and the number of total births expressed as the number of ectopic pregnancies per 1000 births.

It would be best to be able to calculate the incidence of ectopic pregnancies per 1000 total conceptions; however, since most spontaneous abortions and many elective abortions are not reported, the denominator is always smaller than the actual number, yielding a spuriously increased incidence. Nevertheless, since an unknown number of ectopic pregnancies remain asymptomatic and thus are not reported, the numerator is also lower. Thus the true incidence of ectopic pregnancies per 1000 total conceptions can never be accurately calculated. The incidences reported in the literature, however, are good approximations and, since the same methodology is used, can be validly compared.

The incidence of ectopic pregnancy varies among different countries, with rates as high as 1 in 28 and 1 in 40 deliveries reported in Jamaica and Vietnam. In the United States in 1989 the annual ectopic pregnancy rate per 10,000 women aged 15 to 44 was 15.5, similar to that in Finland but higher than the rate in France.

During the past 40 years the incidence of ectopic pregnancy has been steadily increasing in the United States, as well as in most European countries. In the United States, between 1970 and 1989 there was a fivefold increase in the annual number of women hospitalized for ectopic pregnancies (from 17,800 to 88,400), and there was a tripling of the rate per 1000 pregnancies (from 4.5 to 16.0). Since 1987 there has been an increasing trend toward treating ectopic pregnancy on an ambulatory basis without overnight hospitalization. With earlier detection of ectopic pregnancy a steadily increasing percentage of women with this problem are now being treated before tubal rupture occurs by outpatient laparoscopic procedures or by medical treatment with methotrexate. An analysis of both hospital discharge data, as well as an ambulatory medical care survey, revealed that the estimated number of hospitalizations for ectopic pregnancy in the United States declined from nearly 90,000 in 1989 to about 45,000 in 1994. However, in 1992 about half of all women with ectopic pregnancy in the United States were treated as outpatients, and the estimated number of total ectopic pregnancies in this year was 108,000, for a rate of 19.7 per 1000 reported pregnancies (Figure 17-1). Thus in the United States in 1992 about 2 of every 100 women who were known to conceive had an ectopic gestation. This increased incidence of ectopic pregnancy is thought to be due to two factors: (1) the increased incidence of salpingitis, due to increased infection with *Chlamydia trachomatis* or other sexually transmitted pathogens, and (2) improved diagnostic techniques, which

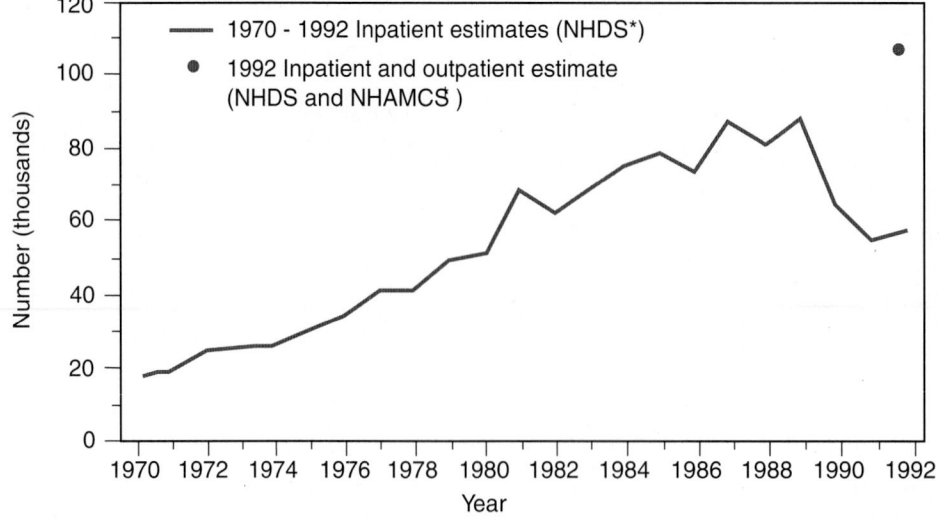

FIGURE 17-1 Number of ectopic pregnancies, United States, 1970-1992. (From Ectopic Pregnancy—United States, 1990-1992, MMWR 44[suppl 3]:47, 1996.)

*NHDS, National Hospital Discharge Survey. †NHAMCS, National Hospital Ambulatory Medical Care Survey.

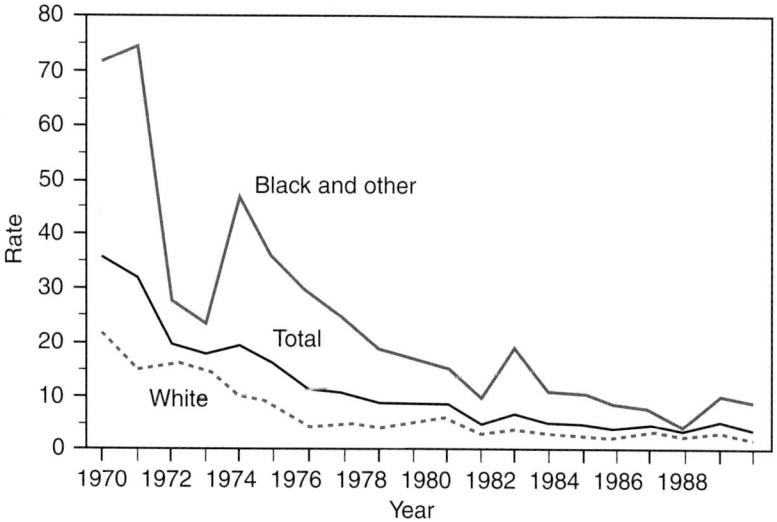

FIGURE 17-2 Ectopic pregnancy death rates, by race, United States, 1970-1989. (From Ectopic pregnancy, United States, 1988-1989, MMWR 41[suppl 32]:591, 1992.)

enable diagnosis of unruptured ectopic pregnancy to be made with more precision and earlier in gestation before asymptomatic resolution of the pregnancy could occur.

There is a marked increase in the rate of ectopic pregnancy with increasing age when calculated as incidence per 1000 reported conceptions. In the United States the rate increased from 6.6 in women aged 15 to 24 years to 21.5 in those aged 35 to 44 years. However, when the number was calculated per 10,000 women aged 15 to 44, the rate of ectopic pregnancy was lowest in the older group, reflecting the lower total number of pregnancies in this age group. These data indicate that the incidence rate of ectopic pregnancy should be calculated using total pregnancies as the denominator to determine the actual risk for a woman exposed to pregnancy. Because of the lower pregnancy rate in older women, overall only about 11% of ectopic pregnancies in the United States occur in women aged 35 to 44, whereas more than half, 58%, occur in women aged 25 to 34.

Most ectopic pregnancies occur in multigravid women. Only 10% to 15% of ectopic pregnancies occur in nulligravid women, whereas more than half occur in women who have been pregnant three or more times.

In the United States the rates of ectopic pregnancy are similar in each section of the country, but the rates are higher for nonwhite than white women. About 3% of all reported pregnancies in nonwhite women aged 35 to 44 in the United States were ectopic.

MORTALITY

Even with the increased use of surgery and blood transfusions and earlier diagnosis, ectopic pregnancy remains a major cause of maternal death in the United States today.

In 1988 there were 44, and in 1989 there were 34 deaths from complications related to ectopic pregnancy in the United States. Ectopic pregnancy is the most common cause of maternal death in the first half of pregnancy. Although the percentage of all maternal deaths in the United States that are the result of ectopic pregnancy increased from 8% in 1970 to 13% in 1989, the percentage of ectopic pregnancies that become fatal has decreased. The overall death-to-case rate of ectopic pregnancy has decreased tenfold, from 35 per 10,000 women with ectopic pregnancy in 1970 to 3.8 in 1989 (Figure 17-2). The death-to-case rate is similar in all age groups but is 4 times higher in blacks and other nonwhites than in white women. Because the incidence of ectopic pregnancy is also higher in blacks in the United States, a pregnant black woman is about 5 times more likely to die of ectopic pregnancy than a white woman. Ectopic pregnancy is the most common single cause of all maternal deaths among black women, causing about one fifth of such deaths. Unmarried women of all races have a 1.7 times greater chance of dying of ectopic pregnancy than married women do. Overall risk of death from ectopic pregnancy is about 10 times greater than the risk of childbirth and more than 50 times greater than the risk of legal abortion.

Atrash et al. studied the clinical aspects of deaths resulting from ectopic pregnancy in the United States from 1979 to 1982. They found that blood loss was the major cause of death (88%), with infection (3%) and anesthesia complications (2%) much less common. Dorfman et al. reported that about 80% of these gestations were in the oviduct itself and the other 20% were interstitial or abdominal gestations. Because the overall incidence of ectopic pregnancy occurring in these latter locations is slightly less than 4%, interstitial and abdominal ectopic pregnancies have about a 5 times greater risk of being fatal than those pregnancies located in the portion of the tube distal to the uterus. About three fourths of the women with fatal ectopic pregnancies initially developed symptoms and died in the first 12 weeks of gestation. Of the remaining one fourth who developed symptoms and died after the first trimester, 70% had interstitial or abdominal pregnancies. Patient delay in consulting a physician after development of symptoms accounted for one third of the deaths, whereas treatment delay resulting from misdiagnosis contributed to the death in half. More than half of the women died of hemorrhage without emergency surgery. The most common misdiagnoses were intestinal disorders and intrauterine pregnancy.

ETIOLOGY

The major cause of ectopic pregnancy is acute salpingitis. Its morphologic sequelae account for about half of the initial episodes of ectopic pregnancy. Although other morphologic factors have been identified as a cause of ectopic pregnancy, in the majority of the remaining first episodes no such factor can be identified. Thus in about 40% of instances the cause cannot be determined and is presumed to be a physiologic disorder that results in delay of passage of the embryo into the uterine cavity so it remains in the oviduct at the gestational age (7 days) when implantation occurs. Ovulation from the contralateral ovary has been implicated as a cause of delay of blastocyst transport, and Breen reported contralateral ovulation to occur in about one third of tubal gestations treated by laparotomy. However, Saito et al. observed that the portion of the tube where implantation occurred in women with ectopic pregnancies was similar whether the corpus luteum was ipsilateral or contralateral to the pregnancy. If transmigration was a factor, they hypothesized that there would be a greater incidence of distal tubal pregnancies with ovulation in the contralateral ovary. Furthermore, women who have an ipsilateral oophorectomy together with salpingectomy for ectopic pregnancy have a repeat ectopic pregnancy rate similar to the rate in those who do not have the ovary removed. For these reasons it is unlikely that transmigration of the ovum from the opposite ovary is a common cause of ectopic pregnancy.

A more likely physiologic cause is hormonal imbalance, as elevated circulating levels of either estrogen or progesterone can alter normal tubal contractility. An increased rate of ectopic pregnancies has been reported in women who conceive with physiologically and pharmacologically elevated levels of progestins. The latter condition can be produced locally with a progesterone-releasing IUD, as well as systemically with progestin-only oral contraceptives. Iatrogenic, physiologically increased levels of estrogen and progesterone occur after ovulation induction with either clomiphene citrate or human menopausal gonadotrophins, and an increased rate of ectopic pregnancies has

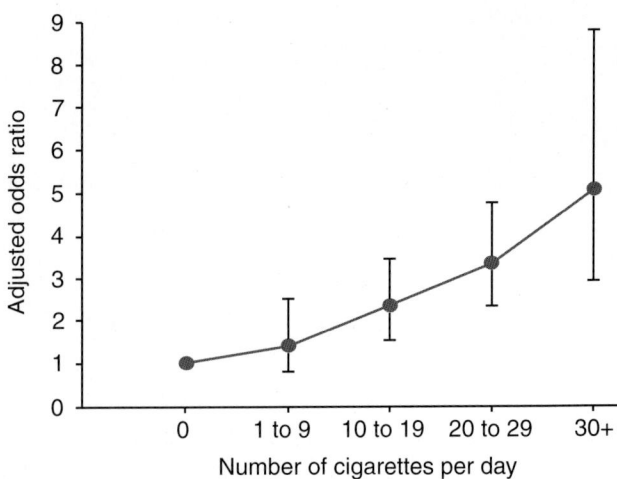

FIGURE 17-3   Dose response curve for smoking and ectopic pregnancy among women with no prior spontaneous abortion, adjusted for maternal age and race. (From Handler A, Davis F, Ferre C, and Yeko T: Am J Public Health 79:1239, 1989.)

been reported in women conceiving after each of these treatment modalities.

Another probable etiology is an abnormality of embryonic development. Stratford examined 44 human conceptuses from ectopic gestations by microdissection and histologic sections and found that about two thirds were abnormal and half had gross structural abnormalities. These types of abnormalities could interfere with normal tubal transport. Elias et al., using cell culture technique, reported that the chromosomal complement of ectopic gestations was similar to that of intrauterine gestations of comparable gestational age. However, Karikoski et al., using DNA flow cytometry, found aneuploidy to be present in one third of tubal gestations. These investigators suggested that this high incidence of chromosomal abnormalities could be a factor causing ectopic implantation. Inherited genetic abnormalities are most probably not a cause of ectopic pregnancy, because there is no increased incidence among first-degree relatives. Several epidemiologic studies indicate that cigarette smoking is associated with about a twofold increased risk of ectopic pregnancy, even when the data were controlled for the presence of other risk factors. The risk of ectopic pregnancy was directly related to the number of cigarettes smoked per day, with a fourfold increased risk noted among women who smoked 30 or more cigarettes per day (Figure 17-3).

The major causes of ectopic pregnancy will now be discussed in more detail.

Tubal Pathology

The permanent agglutination of the plicae (folds) of the endosalpinx produced by salpingitis can allow normal passage of the smaller sperm while preventing normal transport of the larger morula. The morula can be trapped in blind pockets formed by adhesions of the endosalpinx. In their 20-year longitudinal study, Weström et al. found that nearly half (45.3%) of the women with ectopic pregnancy had a clinical history or histologic findings of a prior episode of acute salpingitis. This figure is in close agreement with the 40% incidence of histologic evidence of prior salpingitis found by several groups of investigators in the pathologic review of oviducts removed from women with ectopic pregnancy (Figure 17-4).

Weström et al. prospectively followed 900 women age 15 to 34 who had laparoscopically confirmed diagnosis of acute salpingitis and found that the subsequent ectopic pregnancy rate was 68.8 per 1000 conceptions, yielding a sixfold increase in the risk of ectopic pregnancy after acute salpingitis compared with a control group of women without prior clinical evidence of salpingitis. The risk that the first pregnancy after acute salpingitis would be ectopic increased both with the number of episodes of infection and with increasing age of the women at the time of infection.

In two histopathologic studies of oviducts removed from women with ectopic pregnancy, Majmudar et al. and Green and Kott found that about half contained lesions of salpingitis isthmica nodosa (SIN) when numerous sections of the tube were examined. In their control groups only 5% of oviducts had SIN. SIN was defined as the microscopic presence of tubal epithelium within the myosalpinx or beneath the tubal serosa (Figure 17-5). With serial sectioning it has been determined that SIN is actually a diverticulum or intrauterine extension of the tubal lumen (Figure 17-6). Associated histologic evidence of chronic salpingitis was seen in only 6% of the oviducts in the first series, indicating that SIN was not necessarily the result of infection. These findings are in agreement with those of Persaud, who observed tubal diverticula (histologically similar to SIN) in the isthmus and proximal ampulla of half of the oviducts removed for tubal pregnancy. In both these series the tubal pregnancy usually implanted in a portion of the tube distal to the SIN, indicating that mechanical entrapment of the morula is not the mechanism whereby SIN causes tubal gestation. These investigators postulated that SIN itself or associated tubal anomalies may be responsible for dysfunction of the tubal transport mechanism without anatomic obstruction.

It is likely that adhesions between the tubal serosa and bowel or peritoneum may interfere with normal tubal motility and cause ectopic pregnancy because, as reported in two series respectively, 17% to 27% of women with ectopic pregnancy have had previous abdominal surgical procedures not involving the oviduct. On the other hand, neither endometriosis nor congenital anomalies of the tube have been associated with an increased incidence of ectopic pregnancy.

An operative procedure on the oviduct itself is a cause of ectopic pregnancy whether the oviduct is morphologically normal, as occurs with sterilization procedures, or abnormal, as occurs with postsalpingitis reconstructive surgery. The incidence of ectopic pregnancy occurring

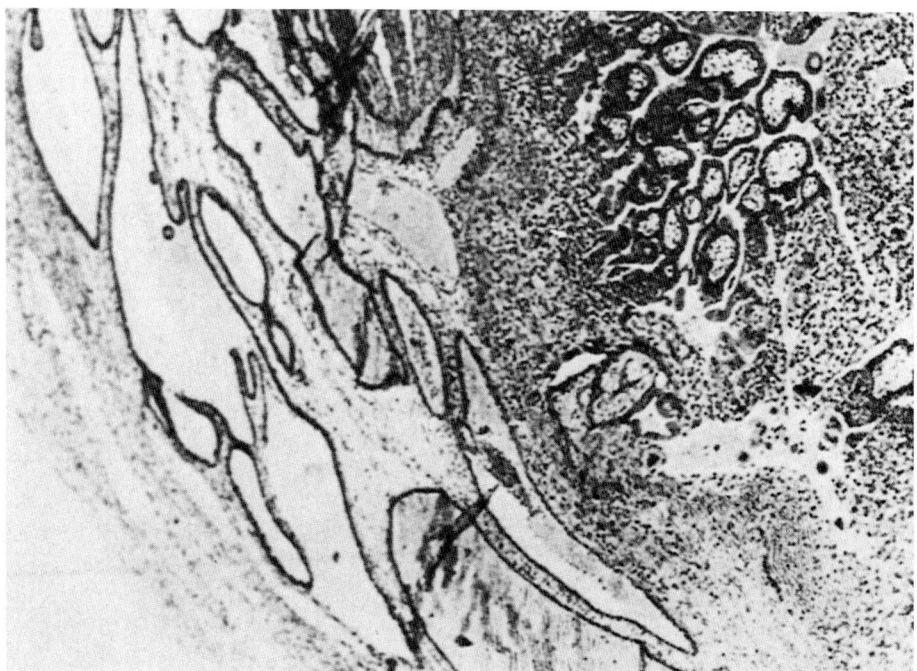

FIGURE 17-4 Tubal pregnancy with placental villi and trophoblastic cells to the right and wall of the tube to the left showing marked degree of follicular salpingitis. (Original magnification, ×70.) (From Bone NL and Greene RR: Am J Obstet Gynecol 82:1166, 1961.)

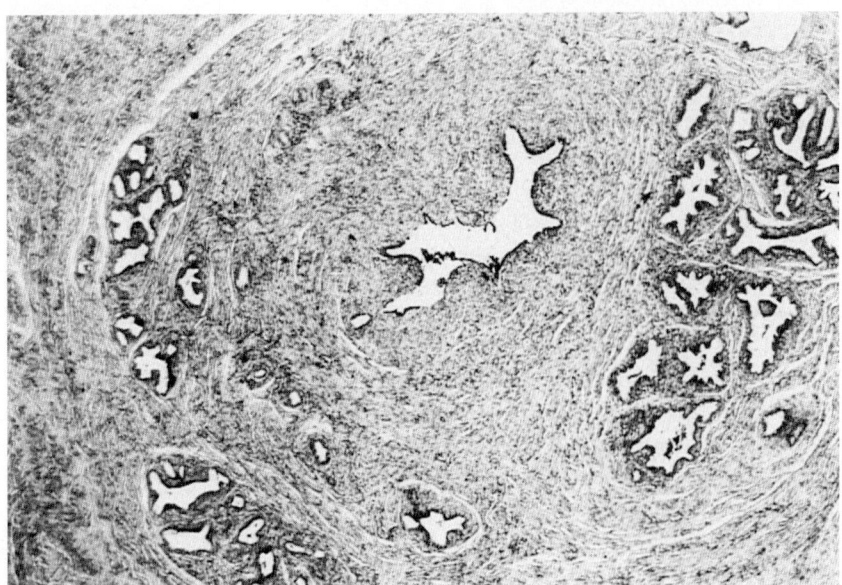

FIGURE 17-5 Microscopic section of fallopian tube showing typical lesion of salpingitis isthmica nodosa. Multiple glandular inclusions of tubal mucosa are seen in myosalpinx without continuity with luminal epithelium. (H&E, ×12.) (From Majmudar B, Henderson PH III, and Semple E: Obstet Gynecol 62:73, 1983. Reprinted with permission from The American College of Obstetricians and Gynecologists.)

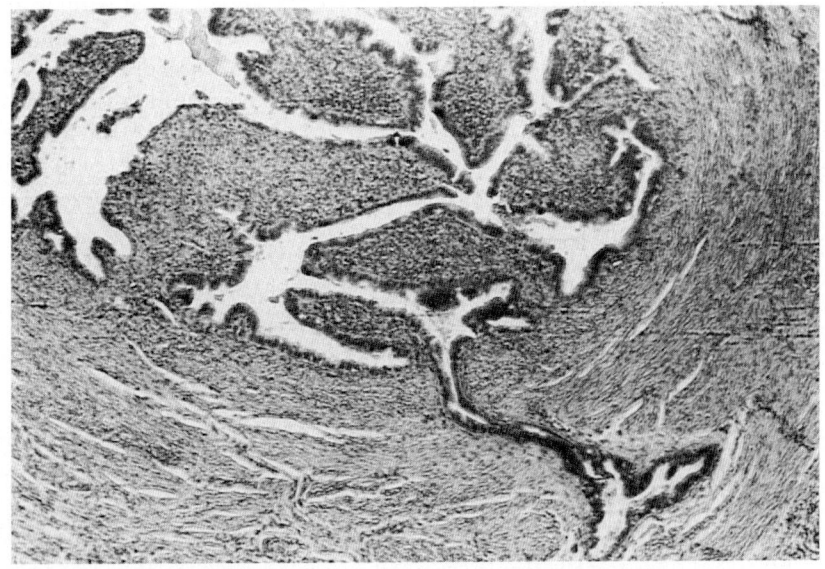

FIGURE 17-6 Tubal mucosa showing its actual extension into myosalpinx. (H&E, ×12.) (From Majmudar B, Henderson PH III, and Semple E: Obstet Gynecol 62:73, 1983. Reprinted with permission from The American College of Obstetricians and Gynecologists.)

after salpingoplasty or salpingostomy procedures to treat distal tubal disease ranges from 15% to 25%, probably because the damage to the endosalpinx remains. The rate of ectopic pregnancy after reversal of sterilization procedures is lower, about 4%, because the tubes have not been damaged by infection.

Women who have had a prior ectopic pregnancy, even if treated by unilateral salpingectomy, are at increased risk for having a subsequent ectopic pregnancy. Of women who conceive after having one ectopic pregnancy, about 25% of subsequent pregnancies are ectopic. In two large series of women with ectopic pregnancy, 7% had a history of a prior ectopic pregnancy.

Herbst et al., as well as others, have shown that the incidence of ectopic gestation is significantly greater (4 to 5 times) in women who have been exposed to diethylstilbestrol (DES) in utero than in a control group. In various series the rate of ectopic pregnancy in such women is about 4% to 5%. Kaufman et al. reported that among women exposed to DES whose hysterosalpingograms demonstrated abnormalities in the uterine cavity, the ectopic pregnancy rate was 13%.

Contraception Failure

For several decades sterilization has been the most popular method of contraception used by couples in the United States. Since the development of laparoscopic surgery, female tubal sterilization is performed about twice as frequently as vasectomy. In a recent analysis of the long-term risk of pregnancy after tubal sterilization reported by Peterson et al., it was found that within 10 years after the procedure the cumulative life-table probability of pregnancy was 1.85%. The 10-year failure rate after bipolar coagulation of the oviducts was 2.48%, which rose to 5.43% if the sterilization procedure was performed when the woman was less than 28 years of age. These investigators reported that for all 143 pregnancies occurring after tubal sterilization, 43, or 32.9%, were ectopic pregnancies.

Several investigators have reported that if pregnancy occurred after tubal sterilization by laparoscopic fulguration without concomitant transection, the ectopic pregnancy rate was about 50%. McCausland hypothesized that with the extensive tissue destruction caused by electrocoagulation, a uteroperitoneal fistula could develop that would allow sperm to pass into the distal segment of the oviduct and fertilize the egg (Figure 17-7). Such fistulas were demonstrated radiographically by Shah et al. in 11% of 150 women after laparoscopic electrocoagulation and demonstrated histologically by McCausland, who called the process endosalpingosis or endosalpingoblastosis. McCann and Kessel also reported a 50% ectopic pregnancy rate after failure of laparoscopic electrocoagulation after failure of sterilization with metal clips or silicone rings. Peterson et al. reported that within 10 years after the sterilization procedure twice as many women sterilized by bipolar coagulation had ectopic pregnancies than those sterilized with metal clips or silicone bands. The ectopic pregnancy rate after bipolar coagulation sterilization was 1.7%.

With the marked increase in use of female sterilization techniques, failure of sterilization is becoming a more common cause of ectopic pregnancy. In contrast to a large series of ectopic pregnancies in the United States in the 1950s and 1960s in which only 0.6% of women with ectopic pregnancy had a prior tubal sterilization, Brenner et al. reported that 3% of 300 ectopic pregnancies occurring in 1976 to 1977 were the result of tubal sterilization failure. The incidence is probably even greater at present because tubal sterilization failure occurs throughout a woman's reproductive life. Peterson et al. reported that among women sterilized under age 28, 2.8% became pregnant between 5 to 10 years after the procedure. Because about one third of pregnancies that occur after tubal sterilization are ectopic, women should be counseled that if they do not experience the expected menses at any time following tubal sterilization before menopause, a test to detect hCG should be performed rapidly, and if they are pregnant a diagnostic evaluation to exclude the presence of ectopic pregnancy is necessary.

As summarized by Tatum and Schmidt, pregnancies occurring as a result of failure of certain contraceptive methods have a greater chance of being ectopic than among women becoming pregnant who were not using contraception. Although women who become pregnant while using diaphragms or combination oral contraceptives do not have an increased chance of having an ectopic pregnancy, women who become pregnant while using a Copper T380 IUD or progestin-only oral contraceptives have about a 5% chance of having an ectopic pregnancy. The incidence of ectopic pregnancy in women who become pregnant with the progesterone-releasing IUD is even higher, about 23%. Women using these methods of contraception who elect to have their pregnancies terminated should have a histologic examination of the tissue removed from the uterine cavity to be certain the pregnancy was intrauterine. If no chorionic villi are observed, a diagnostic evaluation to detect ectopic pregnancy should be performed.

Women using any type of contraception have a significantly decreased chance of having an ectopic pregnancy compared with sexually active, noncontraceptive users. Thus women using any of the most effective reversible contraceptive methods are about 90% less likely to have an ectopic pregnancy than if they are sexually active and use no method of contraception. However, because the progesterone-releasing IUD inhibits tubal contractions and has a higher failure rate than the copper IUD, women using this method of contraception have about twice the risk of ectopic pregnancy (7.5 per 1000 woman-years) than women using no method of contraception (3.5 per 1000 woman-years).

Hormonal Alterations

As occurs with exogenous progesterone administration, if increased levels of exogenous or endogenous estrogens are present shortly after the time of ovulation, the incidence of ectopic pregnancy is increased. Morris and Van Wagenen reported that 3 of 30 pregnancies were ectopic in women receiving postovulatory high-dose estrogen to prevent pregnancy. Several investigators have reported

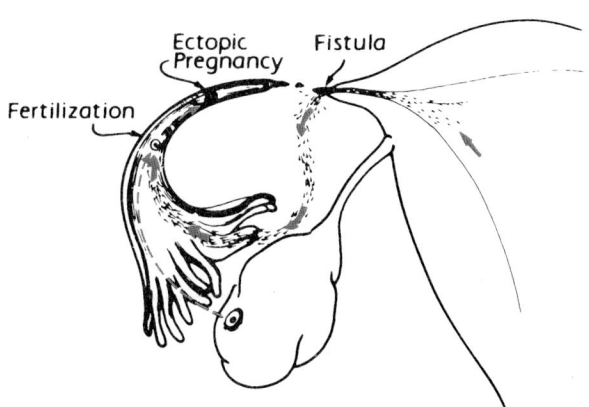

FIGURE 17-7 Mechanism of ectopic pregnancy after sterilization. (From Corson SL and Batzer FR: J Reprod Med 31:78, 1986.)

that the ectopic pregnancy rate is about 1.5% for conceptions occurring after ovulation has been induced with clomiphene citrate. The ectopic rate in pregnancies occurring after ovulation is induced with human menopausal gonadotrophin (hMG) has been reported to range between 3% and 4%. McBain et al. reported that if the urinary estrogen excretion during human menopausal gonadotrophin therapy exceeded 200 µg per day and conception occurred the ectopic pregnancy rate was 12.5%. Fernandez et al. in a case-control study found the risk of ectopic pregnancy was increased about fourfold among ovulatory women treated with controlled ovarian hyperstimulation, either clomiphene citrate, hMG, or a combination of both, for the treatment of unexplained infertility. These reports indicate that increased levels of estrogen, as well as of progesterone, interfere with tubal motility and increase the chance of ectopic gestation. Ectopic gestations occur in about 5% of pregnancies that develop after in vitro fertilization and embryonic transfer. The etiology for this increased incidence is likely due to one or more of several factors: increased sex steroid hormone levels, presence of proximal tubal disease, flushing an embryo directly into the oviduct, and increased probability of early diagnosis before an asymptomatic tubal abortion could occur.

Previous Abortion

Although some studies have suggested that a prior induced abortion increases the risk of ectopic pregnancy, Levin et al. showed that when statistical techniques were used to control the effects of other risk factors, the history of one prior induced abortion did not significantly increase the risk of ectopic pregnancy (Table 17-1). In this study, the risk for ectopic pregnancy doubled if a woman had had two or more prior induced abortions,

which (although not significant) indicates a possible association between multiple induced abortions and subsequent ectopic gestation, probably related to postabortal infection. A more recent study by Holt et al., using a different type of control group, reported no significantly increased incidence of ectopic pregnancy in women having one prior abortion (RR = 0.9) or two or more prior abortions (RR = 1.2).

PATHOLOGY

Most ectopic pregnancies occur in the oviduct. In Breen's series 97.7% of the ectopic pregnancies were tubal, 1.4% were abdominal, and less than 1% were ovarian or cervical (Figure 17-8). The majority of tubal gestations, 81%, were located in the ampullary portion of the oviduct, being about equally divided between the distal and middle third of the tube. About 12% of tubal gestations occur in the isthmus and 5% in the fimbrial region. Although Breen considered pregnancies located in the cornual area of the uterus to be uterine in origin, they are in fact pregnancies implanted in the interstitial portion of the oviduct. About 2% of all ectopic pregnancies are interstitial and are frequently associated with severe morbidity, because they become symptomatic later in gestation than do other tubal pregnancies, are difficult to diagnose, and frequently produce massive hemorrhage when they rupture (Figure 17-9). A true cornual pregnancy is one located in the rudimentary horn of a bicornuate uterus, and this occurrence is quite rare. In a review of 240 true cornual pregnancies reported by O'Leary and O'Leary, about 90% of them ruptured with massive hemorrhage.

About 1 in 200 ectopic pregnancies are true ovarian pregnancies that fulfill the four criteria originally described by Spiegelberg. Many women with ovarian pregnancies are believed clinically to have a ruptured corpus luteum cyst. In Hallatt's series of 25 primary ovarian pregnancies, the correct diagnosis was made during the surgical procedure in only 28%. In his series the hemorrhagic mass was always located adjacent to the corpus luteum, never within it. Ovarian pregnancy is also associated with profuse hemorrhage, with 81% of Hallatt's cases having a hemoperitoneum greater than 500 ml. Nevertheless, most can be successfully treated by ovarian resection and not oophorectomy.

Most abdominal pregnancies occur secondary to tubal abortion with secondary implantation in the peritoneal cavity (Figure 17-10). On rare occasions a primary abdominal pregnancy may occur. For the latter diagnosis to be made the following three criteria originally set forth by Studdiford must be present: (1) the tubes and ovaries must be normal, with no evidence of recent or past injury; (2) there must be no evidence of a uteroplacental fistula; and (3) the pregnancy must be related only to the peritoneal surface and early enough in gestation to eliminate

---

TABLE 17-1
Standardized* Relative Risks of Ectopic Pregnancy and 95% Confidence Intervals According to Selected Characteristics

History Characteristic	Relative Risk	95% Confidence Interval
One induced abortion	1.3	0.6–2.7
Two or more induced abortions	2.6	0.9–7.4
Ectopic pregnancy	7.7	1.9–31.5
Pelvic infection	7.5	3.5–16.0
Pelvic operation	2.6	1.4–4.6

From Levin AA, Schoenbaum SC, Stubbfield PG, et al: Am J Public Health 72:253, 1982.

*Standardized using the multiple logistic regression model.

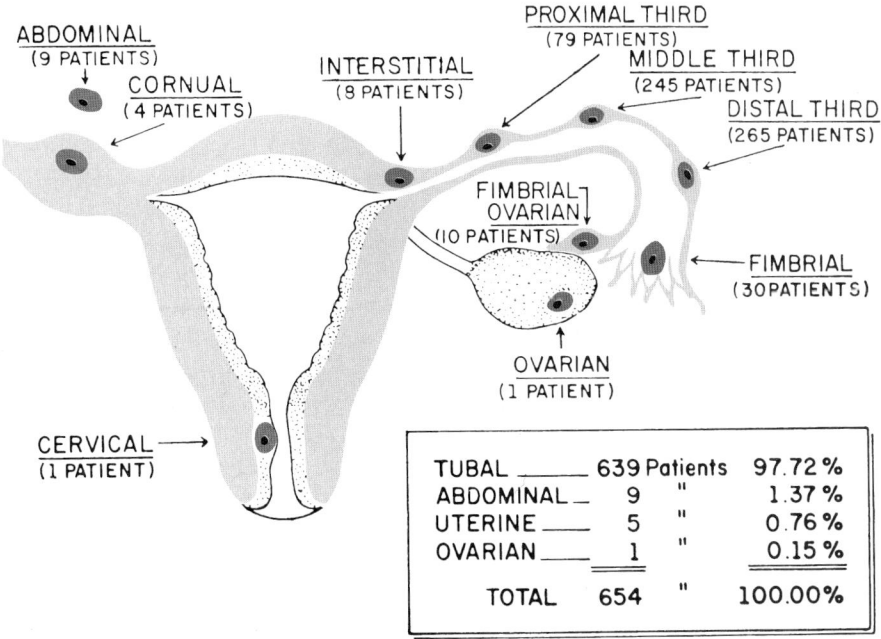

FIGURE 17-8 Anatomic site of ectopic pregnancy. (From Breen JL: Am J Obstet Gynecol 106:1004, 1970.)

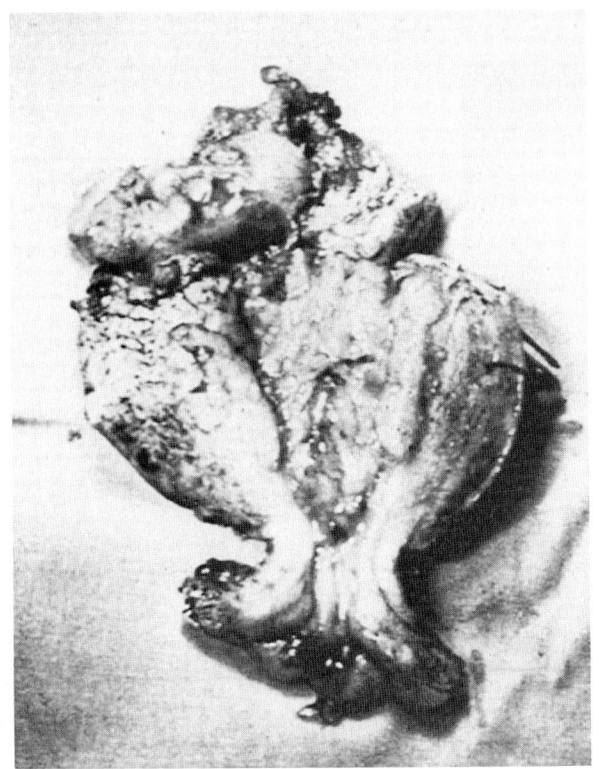

FIGURE 17-9 Anterior view of uterus that has been opened with an anterior **Y** incision, showing conceptus replaced in site it had formerly occupied in cornual bed. (From Kalchman GG and Meltzer RM: Am J Obstet Gynecol 96:1139, 1966.)

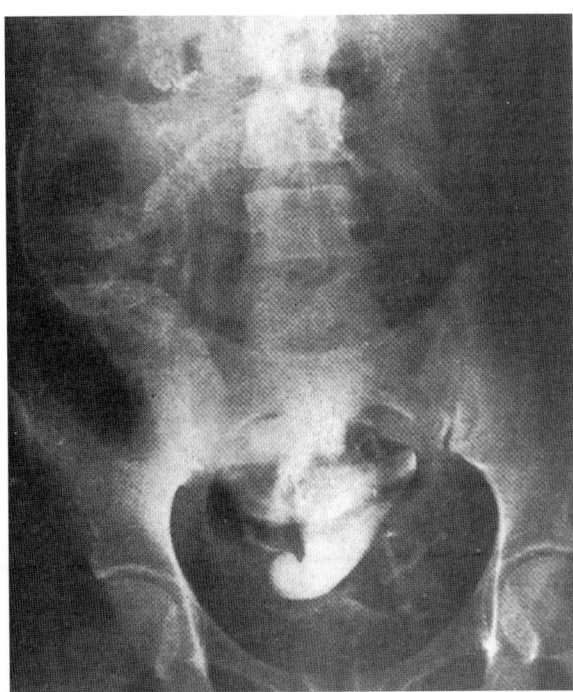

FIGURE 17-10 Hysterosalpingography demonstrating size of uterus and fetus, which is located outside of uterus. (From Clark JF and Guy RS: Am J Obstet Gynecol 96:511, 1966.)

the possibility of secondary implantation after primary tubal nidation. An unusual type of primary abdominal pregnancy may implant in the spleen or liver and produce massive intraperitoneal hemorrhage.

The prognosis for fetal survival in abdominal pregnancy is poor, found to be 11% by Clark and Guy. Diagnosis is difficult but has become easier with the use of ultrasonography. Once the diagnosis is established, a laparotomy with removal of the fetus should be performed immediately to prevent a possible fatal hemorrhage. On occasion, when the placenta is tightly adherent to bowel and blood vessels, it should be left in the abdominal cavity. In such instances the placental tissue usually resorbs, but symptoms of abdominal pain and intermittent fever may persist for many months as a result of partial bowel obstruction and abscess formation. Thus, when it is surgically feasible, the placenta should be entirely removed. Partial removal may result in massive hemorrhage.

The four pathologic criteria for the diagnosis of cervical pregnancy as reported by Rubin et al. are (1) cervical glands must be present opposite the placental attachment, (2) the attachment of the placenta to the cervix must be intimate, (3) the placenta must be below the entrance of the uterine vessels or below the peritoneal reflection of the anteroposterior surface of the uterus, and (4) fetal elements must not be present in the corpus uteri (Figure 17-11).

The clinical criteria for the diagnosis of cervical pregnancy described by Paalman and McElin are (1) uterine bleeding after amenorrhea without cramping pain, (2) a softened cervix that is disproportionately enlarged to a size equal to or larger than the corpus, (3) complete confinement and firm attachment of the products of conception to the endocervix, and (4) a snug internal os.

Most cervical pregnancies occur after a previous sharp uterine curettage. The differential diagnosis is difficult and includes incomplete abortion, placenta previa, carcinoma of the cervix, and degenerative leiomyoma. Although this entity was previously associated with a high mortality because of massive hemorrhage, currently, with better methods of diagnosis and modern techniques of treatment, death is rare. More than half of the women with cervical pregnancy require a hysterectomy for treatment, and it is nearly always necessary if the pregnancy has advanced more than 18 weeks' gestational age. Even if a hysterectomy is not performed, the prognosis for future fertility is poor.

There have been several case reports in which cervical pregnancy was successfully treated by systemic methotrexate. Other case reports have shown that after angiographic uterine artery embolization evacuation of the pregnancy can be easily performed transcervically with minimal blood loss. Frates et al. reported that transvaginal ultrasound-guided injections of potassium chloride directly into the embryonic gestational sac of six cervical pregnancies successfully terminated the pregnancies. Local injection of methotrexate, with or without uterine artery

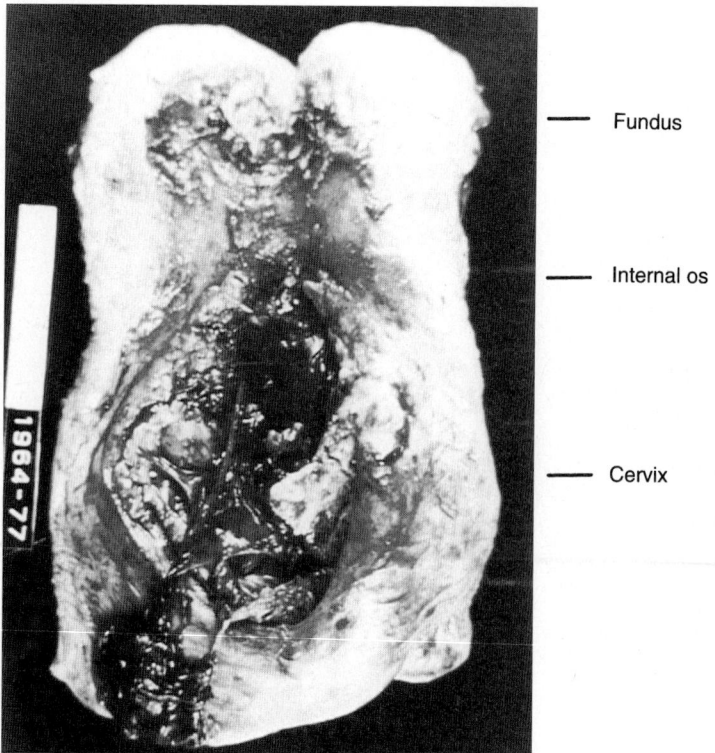

Fundus

Internal os

Cervix

FIGURE 17-11 Cervical pregnancy, 10 weeks' gestation. (From Parente JT, Ou CS, and Levy J: Obstet Gynecol 62:79, 1983. Reprinted with permission from The American College of Obstetricians and Gynecologists.)

embolization, has also been used to successfully treat cervical ectopic pregnancy.

Another uncommon form of ectopic gestation is combined intrauterine and extrauterine pregnancy (94% tubal and 6% ovarian). With the use of mathematic calculation the incidence of this entity has previously been estimated to be either 1 in 16,000 or 1 in 30,000 pregnancies. However, a review of the recent experience at one institution by Reece et al. revealed that 1 of 8000 pregnancies was combined intrauterine and extrauterine and 1 of 70 ectopic pregnancies was associated with an intrauterine pregnancy. Bello et al. estimated that the incidence of heterotopic pregnancy may be as high as 1 of 4000 pregnancies. Combined intrauterine and extrauterine pregnancy may be more common after pharmacologic ovulation induction with the subsequent increase in multiple ovulation. With the increased use of ovulation-inducing agents, as well as an increased incidence of salpingitis, combined intrauterine and extrauterine pregnancy now occurs more frequently than previously estimated. In several large series, the incidence of heterotopic pregnancy ranges from 1% to 3% of all pregnancies occurring after in vitro fertilization. The incidence was higher when tubal damage was present and/or four or more embryos were transferred. Heterotopic pregnancy should be suspected when any of the following clinical criteria are present: (1) a fundus compatible with gestational age estimated by date of onset of last menses in a woman believed to have an ectopic gestation; (2) two corpora lutea seen at the time of laparotomy or laparoscopy and an enlarged, soft, and globular uterus; (3) the absence of withdrawal bleeding and the presence of pregnancy symptoms after excision of an ectopic pregnancy; (4) hemoperitoneum after the termination of an intrauterine pregnancy; and (5) the combination of abdominal pain, adnexal mass with pain and tenderness, peritoneal irritation, and a uterus enlarged more than 8 weeks' gestational age.

A chronic ectopic pregnancy occurs when the intraperitoneal hemorrhage associated with tubal abortion or rupture is relatively minor and ceases spontaneously but the ectopic gestation neither resolves completely nor implants and continues to develop as an abdominal pregnancy. The trophoblast continues to secrete human chorionic gonadotrophin (hCG) in small amounts, with the circulating levels less than 1000 mIU/ml in 50% and less than 100 mIU/ml in 20%. In the series of Cole and Corlett about 6% of all surgically treated ectopic pregnancies in one institution were classified as chronic. The most common (72%) gross pathologic finding was dense adhesions produced by the inflammatory response to the trophoblast. These adhesions attach omentum and bowel to the site of the ectopic pregnancy. In one third of the cases a collection of clotted blood or old hematoma was present. Cole and Corlett reported that because of the extensive disease it was necessary to perform a hysterectomy in 25% and an

oophorectomy in 60% of women with a chronic ovarian ectopic pregnancy.

HISTOPATHOLOGY

When the morula implants in the oviduct, it does not grow mainly in the tubal lumen as has been assumed for many years. In a review of the pathology of tubal gestation, Budowick et al. found that after implanting on the mucosa of the endosalpinx, the trophoblast invades the lamina propria and then the muscularis of the oviduct and grows mainly between the lumen of the tube and its peritoneal covering (Figure 17-12). Growth occurs both parallel to the long axis of the oviduct and circumferentially around it. As the trophoblast invades vessels, retroperitoneal tubal hemorrhage occurs that is mainly extraluminal but may extrude from the fimbriated end and create a hemoperitoneum before tubal rupture (Figure 17-13).

The stretching of the peritoneum covered by this hemorrhage results in episodic pain before the final perforation into the peritoneal cavity. Rupture occurs when the serosa is maximally stretched, producing necrosis secondary to an inadequate blood supply.

Hemoperitoneum is nearly always found in advanced ruptured ectopic pregnancy other than that which is cervical in origin. Usually there is a combination of clotted and unclotted blood in the peritoneal cavity. The unclotted blood does not clot upon removal from the peritoneal cavity because it originates from lysis of blood that has previously coagulated, similar to what occurs during menstrual bleeding. The hematocrit value of this nonclotting blood is nearly always greater than 15%, such a finding being reported in 98% of specimens obtained by culdocentesis in the series of ectopic pregnancies reported by Brenner et al. At the time of laparotomy for a ruptured ectopic pregnancy, about half of the women have less than 500 ml of hemoperitoneum, one quarter between 500 and 1000 ml, and one fifth more than 1000 ml.

When the oviduct is removed and examined histologically, inflammatory cells are nearly always seen. These include plasma cells, lymphocytes, and histiocytes. The presence of chorionic villi, which are frequently degenerated or hyalinized, as well as nucleated red cells, establish the diagnosis of ectopic pregnancy. Decidual reaction in the tube is uncommon.

Because of limited space or inadequate nourishment, the trophoblastic tissue of most ectopic pregnancies does not grow as rapidly as that of pregnancies within the uterine cavity. As a result, hCG production does not increase as rapidly as in a normal pregnancy, and although steroid production of the corpus luteum is initiated, elevated progesterone levels cannot be maintained. Thus initially the endometrium becomes decidualized because of continued progesterone production by the corpus luteum. Sometimes the secretory cells of

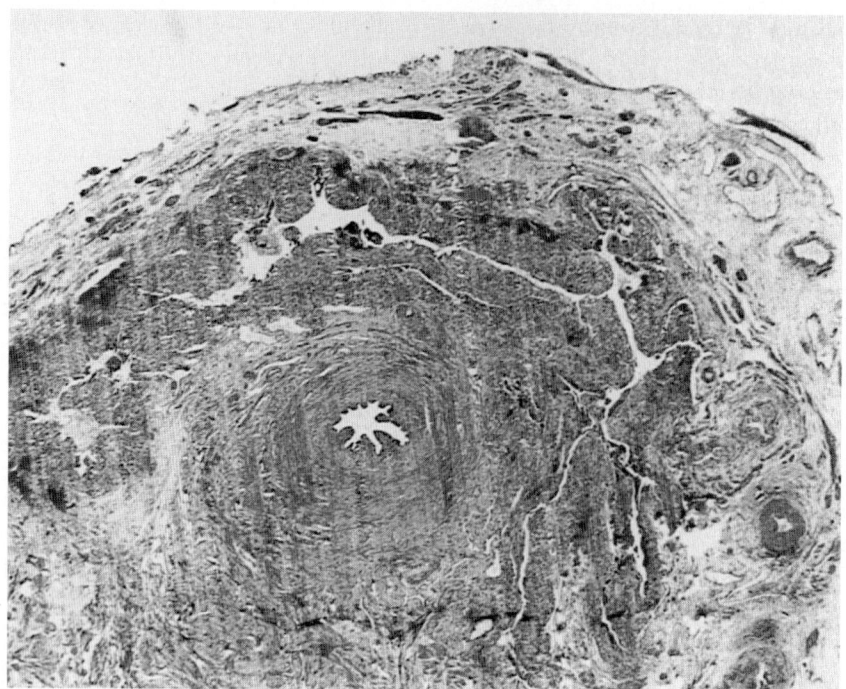

FIGURE 17-12 Low-power photograph showing tube almost completely surrounded by cleftlike space. Closer inspection revealed that cleft was produced by trophoblast that had implanted elsewhere, perforated wall of tube, and was dissecting along broad ligament between tube and peritoneum. (From Budowick M, Johnson TRB, Genadry R, et al: Fertil Steril 34:169, 1980. Reproduced with permission of the publisher, The American Fertility Society.)

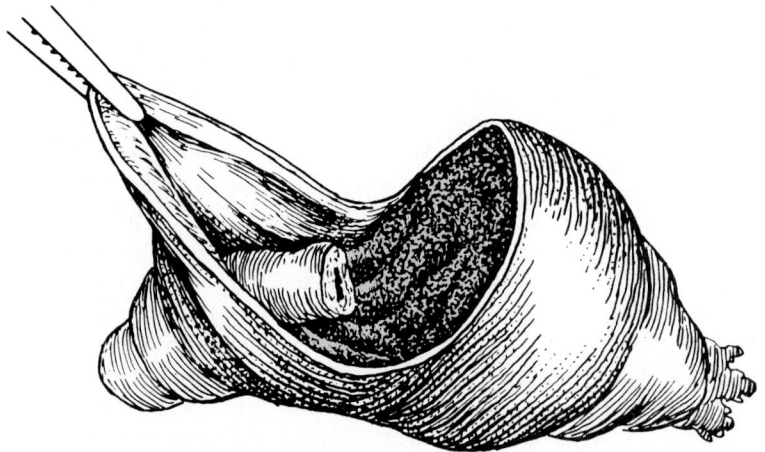

FIGURE 17-13 Artist's rendition of dissected ampullary ectopic pregnancy showing space between tube and peritoneum, revealed when blood clots and placenta were removed. Toward fimbriated end, no dissection was performed and external appearance is that of dilated tube. (From Budowick M, Johnson TRB, Genadry R, et al: Fertil Steril 34:169, 1980. Reproduced with permission of the publisher, The American Fertility Society.)

the endometrial glands become hypertrophied with hyperchromatism, pleomorphism, and increased mitotic activity, as originally described by Arias-Stella (Figure 17-14). The Arias-Stella reaction can be confused with neoplasia, but it is not unique for ectopic pregnancy, because it can occur with intrauterine pregnancy, as well as after ovarian stimulation with clomiphene citrate. In a histologic study of the endometrium in 84 women

with ectopic pregnancies, Ollendorff and Felgin found that about 40% had secretory endometrium, with the remainder being about equally divided among proliferative endometrium, decidual reaction, and Arias-Stella reaction. When progesterone levels fall as a result of insufficient daily increase of hCG, endometrial integrity is no longer maintained, and it sloughs, producing uterine bleeding. Sometimes nearly all the decidua is passed

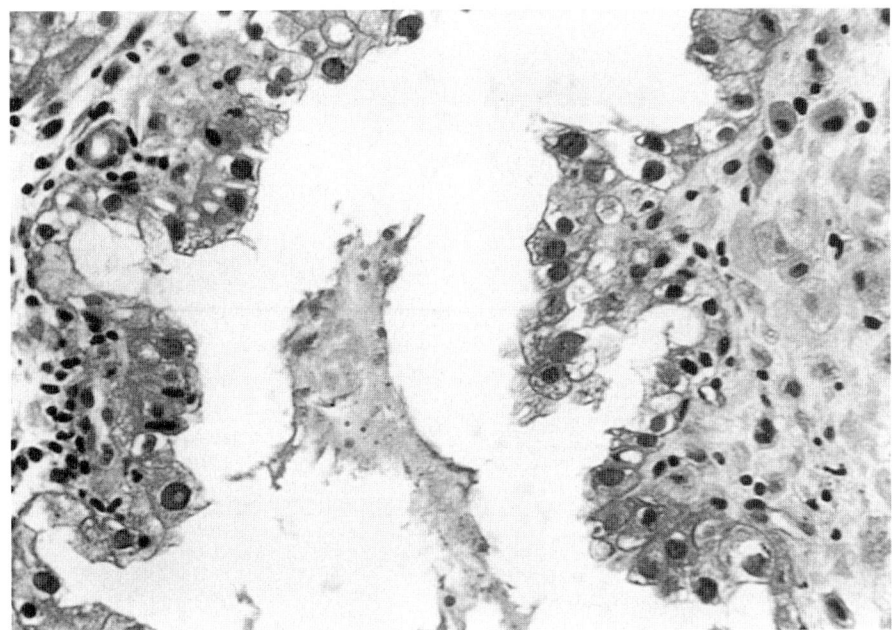

FIGURE 17-14 Arias-Stella reaction. (From DeCherney AH and Maheux R: Curr Probl Obstet Gynecol 6:2, 1983. Reproduced with permission.)

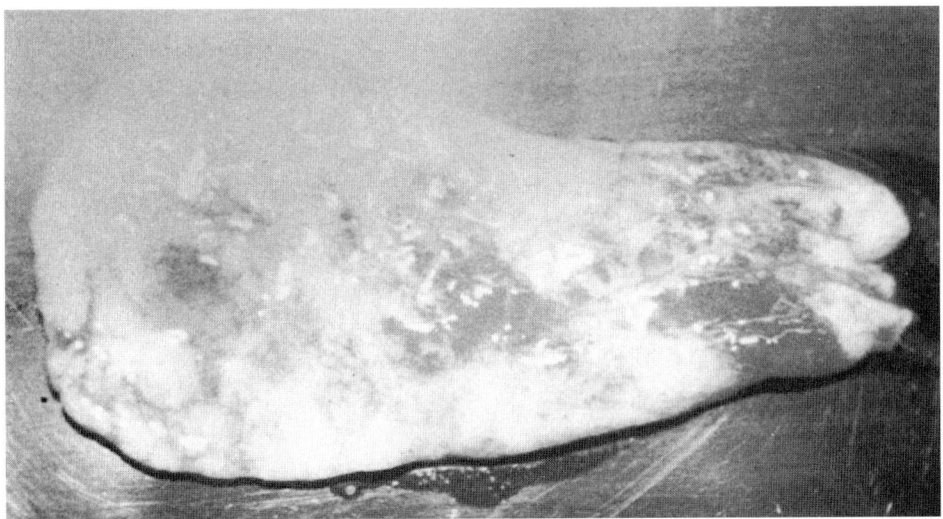

FIGURE 17-15 Decidual cast. (From DeCherney AH and Maheux R: Curr Probl Obstet Gynecol 6:2, 1983. Reproduced with permission.)

through the cervix intact, producing a decidual cast that may be clinically confused with a spontaneous abortion (Figure 17-15).

SYMPTOMS

Among women with risk factors for ectopic pregnancy, with the use of early hormonal testing and vaginal sonography, it is now frequently possible to establish the diagnosis of ectopic pregnancy before symptoms develop. However, when the gestational age increases and intra-peritoneal bleeding occurs from extrusion of blood through the fimbrial end of the oviduct or from tubal rupture, symptoms develop. It is important to be aware of the symptoms of ectopic gestation because this potentially fatal condition can occur in any sexually active woman of reproductive age whether or not she is using contraceptives or has undergone tubal sterilization.

The most common symptoms of ectopic pregnancy are abdominal pain, absence of menses, and irregular vaginal bleeding (Table 17-2). Abdominal pain is nearly a universal symptom of intraperitoneal bleeding but its characteristics are similar with different causes of bleeding. Before

TABLE 17-2
Symptoms of Ectopic Pregnancy

Symptoms	% Patients with Symptom
Abdominal pain	90–100
Amenorrhea	75–95
Vaginal bleeding	50–80
Dizziness, fainting	20–35
Urge to defecate	5–15
Pregnancy symptoms	10–25
Passage of tissue	5–10

From Weckstein LN: Obstet Gynecol Surv 40:259, 1985.

TABLE 17-3
Signs of Ectopic Pregnancy

Sign	% Patients with Sign
Adnexal tenderness	75–90
Abdominal tenderness	80–95
Adnexal mass*	50
Uterine enlargement	20–30
Orthostatic changes	10–15
Fever	5–10

From Weckstein LN: Obstet Gynecol Surv 40:259, 1985.

*20% present on the side opposite the ectopic pregnancy.

rupture occurs, the pain may be characterized as only a vague soreness or colicky in nature. Its location may be generalized, unilateral, or bilateral. Shoulder pain occurs in about one fourth of women with ruptured ectopic pregnancy as a result of diaphragmatic irritation from the hemoperitoneum. During rupture of the oviduct the pain usually becomes intense. Syncope occurs in about one third of women with tubal rupture. Other symptoms that occur following tubal rupture include dizziness and an urge to defecate.

The majority of women with ectopic pregnancy fail to have menses at the expected time but have one or more episodes of irregular vaginal bleeding when the decidual endometrial tissue is sloughed. The interval of amenorrhea is usually 6 weeks or more. The bleeding is usually characterized as spotting but may simulate menstrual bleeding. It is rarely as heavy as that which occurs in spontaneous abortion. About 5% to 10% of women with an advanced ectopic pregnancy will note passage of a decidual cast.

SIGNS

The most common presenting sign in a woman with symptomatic ectopic pregnancy is abdominal tenderness, which, together with adnexal tenderness elicited at the time of the bimanual pelvic examination, is present in nearly all women with an advanced or ruptured ectopic pregnancy (Table 17-3). It is possible to palpate an adnexal mass in half of the women, and about one third have some degree of uterine enlargement that is nearly always smaller than a normal 8-week intrauterine gestation except when an interstitial gestation is present. Tachycardia and hypotension can occur after rupture if blood loss is profuse, but temperature elevation is an uncommon finding, being present in only about 5% to 10% of women with tubal rupture, and is rarely greater than 38° C.

DIAGNOSIS

Laboratory Tests

A hematocrit of less than 30% is found in about one fourth of women with ruptured ectopic pregnancy at the time of rupture. About half have a normal leukocyte count, with a mild elevation of 10,000 to 15,000/mm³ in one third and a greater elevation in one fifth.

HCG is present in the circulation of nearly every woman with an ectopic gestation, but the levels are lower than 3000 mIU/ml in about half. The incidence of positive qualitative pregnancy tests depends on the sensitivity of the assay. With use of the sensitive enzyme-linked immunosorbent assays (ELISA), more than 90% of women with an ectopic pregnancy will have a positive pregnancy test. This incidence increases to nearly 100% if a radioimmunoassay for hCG is used.

Differential Diagnosis of Symptomatic Ectopic Pregnancy

The diagnosis is usually obvious for women with the classic symptoms of ruptured ectopic pregnancy: a history of irregular bleeding followed by sudden onset of pain and syncope accompanied by signs of peritoneal irritation. However, before rupture the symptoms and signs are nonspecific and may also occur with other gynecologic disorders. Entities frequently confused with ectopic pregnancy include salpingitis, threatened or incomplete abortion, ruptured corpus luteum, appendicitis, dysfunctional uterine bleeding, adnexal torsion, degenerative uterine leiomyoma, and endometriosis.

In the series of Brenner et al., about 50% of the women with ruptured ectopic pregnancy had at least one consultation with a physician without the condition being correctly diagnosed before admission to a health care facility, where the correct diagnosis was made. About 33% of the women were seen once, 11% twice, and the remainder 3 to 5 times before the diagnosis was made. Other studies have confirmed that there is a high frequency of misdiagnosis and physician delay in determining that an ectopic pregnancy is present. Because of the possibility of a fatal outcome from undiagnosed ruptured ectopic pregnancy, it is essential that the diagnosis of ectopic pregnancy be considered in any woman of childbearing age with abdominal pain and irregular uterine bleeding even if she has had a previous tubal sterilization procedure or is using an effective method of reversible contraception.

Ectopic pregnancy should be suspected in any woman who develops the symptoms listed earlier, particularly if she has previously had a pelvic operation, especially tubal surgery, either a tubal reconstructive procedure or a sterilization procedure. Other risk factors include one or more episodes of salpingitis, a previous ectopic gestation, current use of a progesterone-releasing IUD, use of a progestin-only oral contraceptive, use of pharmacologic methods of ovulation induction, and a history of infertility. In any woman with the symptoms of ectopic gestation the diagnosis is facilitated by a quantitative assay for hCG and pelvic ultrasonography and can be established by laparoscopy or laparotomy. Culdocentesis and measurement of serum progesterone levels may also be of assistance.

Procedures Used to Aid the Diagnosis of Severely Symptomatic Ectopic Pregnancy

Culdocentesis

Prior to the development of pelvic sonography with a vaginal transducer, the finding of nonclotting blood at the time of culdocentesis, especially if the hematocrit was above 15%, was of great assistance in establishing the diagnosis of ruptured ectopic pregnancy. With the use of pelvic sonography, if available, the presence of intraperitoneal fluid can be easily visualized and it is unnecessary to perform a culdocentesis. In the literature review of Cartwright et al. of nearly 5000 ectopic pregnancies, most series reported that nonclotting blood was obtained by culdocentesis in more than 90% of women with symptomatic ectopic pregnancies. If nonclotting blood is obtained by culdocentesis it indicates that hemoperitoneum is present. The hemoperitoneum may be caused by other pathologic conditions, most frequently a hemorrhagic corpus luteum, or upper abdominal pathology. However, about 85% of women with hemoperitoneum suspected of having an ectopic pregnancy do have one. The finding of nonclotting blood at the time of culdocentesis does not always indicate that rupture of the oviduct has occurred, as tubal abortion can also cause intraperitoneal bleeding. Mild degrees of hemoperitoneum can occur without causing symptoms or signs of peritoneal irritation.

Laparoscopy

A definitive diagnosis of ectopic pregnancy can nearly always be made by direct visualization of the pelvis with laparoscopy. However, sometimes because of hemoperitoneum, adhesions, or obesity, it is difficult to visualize the pelvic organs. In a study by Samuellson and Sjovall, 4 of 166 ectopic pregnancies were not visualized by the laparoscopist, and 6 of 120 women with an intrauterine pregnancy were thought to have ectopic pregnancies. Thus there is a 2% to 5% chance of a false-positive or false-negative diagnosis with laparoscopy. If sufficient hemoperitoneum is present to prevent adequate laparoscopic visualization of the pelvic organs, an exploratory laparotomy should be performed.

Procedures Used for the Diagnostic Evaluation of the Asymtomatic or Mildly Symptomatic Woman with Suspected Ectopic Pregnancy

Human Chorionic Gonadotrophin

Although a negative qualitative urine test for hCG does not rule out ectopic pregnancy, if a sensitive serum immunoassay is negative, the diagnosis is unlikely. If β-hCG is not detected with use of radioimmunoassay of serum, the diagnosis of ectopic pregnancy can, with a rare exception, be ruled out. Although about 85% of women with ectopic pregnancy have serum hCG levels lower than those seen in normal pregnancy at a similar gestational age, a single quantitative hCG assay cannot be used to diagnose ectopic pregnancy because the actual dates of ovulation and conception are not known for most women. Even if the date of ovulation is known, 2.5% of women with normal gestations will have hCG levels lower than the normal 95% confidence limits. Furthermore, low hCG levels are also found in women with various stages of spontaneous abortion, conditions that must be considered in the differential diagnosis. Intact hCG and free β-hCG levels were measured in a large group of women in early pregnancy who presented with symptoms of ectopic pregnancy. Although mean levels of intact hCG and free β-hCG were significantly lower in the group of women with ectopic pregnancy and those who aborted than in those with viable intrauterine pregnancies, the individual hCG levels among the three conditions overlapped too much to devise a cut-off level for diagnostic purposes (Figure 17-16).

In normal pregnancies in early gestation the levels of circulating hCG double about every 2 days. Levels should double in two thirds of women with normal pregnancies in 2 days and in all women in 3 days (Table 17-4). In abnormal pregnancies, ectopic gestations and those destined to abort, hCG levels usually do not increase at the same rate. Kadar et al. reported that if the percentage increase in hCG during a 2-day period is less than 66%, the chance that the woman has an abnormal pregnancy is high.

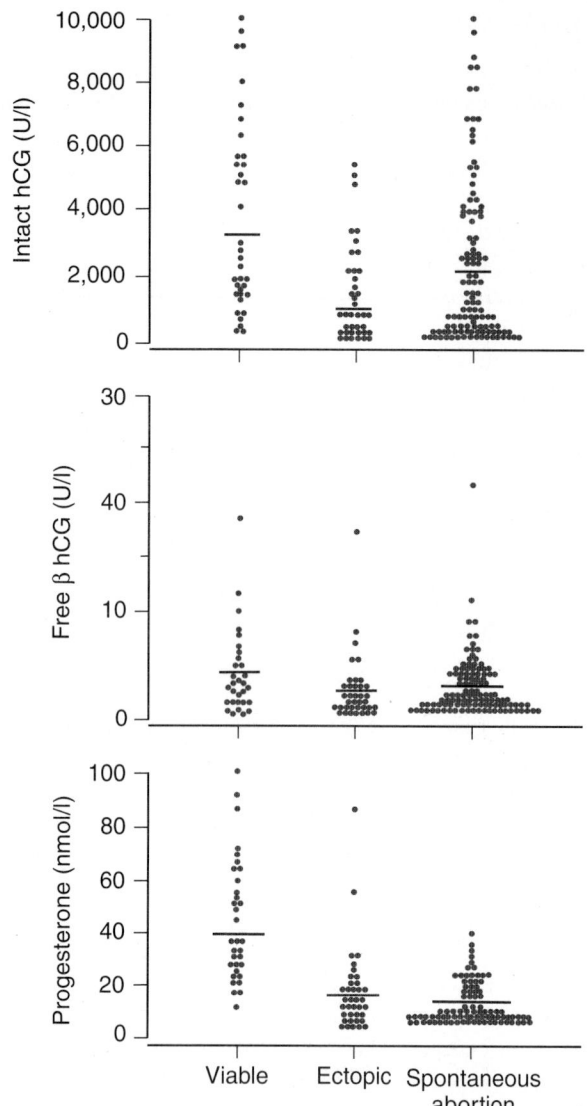

FIGURE 17-16 The distribution of serum concentrations of progesterone, intact human chorionic gonadotrophin (hCG) and free β-hCG in viable and ectopic pregnancies and spontaneous abortions. Means are indicated by horizontal bars (———). (From Ledger WL, Sweeting VM, and Chatterjee S: Hum Reprod 9:157, 1994.)

TABLE 17-4
Lower Normal Limits of Percentage Increase of Serum hCG during Early Pregnancy

Sampling Interval (Days)	Increase in hCG (%)
1	29
2	66
3	114
4	175
5	255

From Kadar N, Caldwell BV, and Romero R: Obstet Gynecol 58:162, 1981. Reprinted with permission from The American College of Obstetricians and Gynecologists.

In their series only 15% of normal pregnancies failed to have this amount of increase while only 13% of ectopic pregnancies had this normal rate of increase.

Cartwright and DiPietro reported that when serial hCG measurements were performed before surgical excision of an ectopic pregnancy in 25 women 20 had a plateau or decrease in hCG levels during a 2-day or longer duration before surgical excision (Figure 17-17).

Romero et al. reported that 90% of women with ectopic pregnancies had one of two main patterns of serial hCG values. About half had falling hCG levels, and the other half had a subnormal rate of increase with a slope of less than 0.11 (corresponding to a 66% increase in 48 hours and a 114% increase in 3 days). Thus the sensitivity of measuring serial hCG levels to diagnose ectopic pregnancy compared with a normal intrauterine pregnancy is 90%. However, the false-positive rate of intrauterine pregnancies with a subnormal slope was 12.5%. Kratzer and Taylor reported similar results when comparing the rates of hCG increase in ectopic and intrauterine pregnancies. Lindblom et al. refined this technique by plotting the slope of the rise of serial β-hCG levels against the initial level and reported that the positive predictive value for the diagnosis of ectopic pregnancy was 95% compared with intrauterine pregnancy. Gronlund and Marushak measured 2 serum hCG levels at intervals of more than 2 days in 21 women with ectopic pregnancy and compared the median slope with that of 39 women with normal intrauterine pregnancies of less than 8 weeks' gestational age. The median slopes of increase were significantly different, with very little overlap. An increase of 1000 mIU/ml of hCG in 2 days was able to differentiate between an ectopic and a normal pregnancy, with a predictive value of 90%, sensitivity of 86%, and specificity of 93% (Figure 17-18). These studies indicate that serial measurements of hCG are of great assistance in the early diagnosis of unruptured ectopic pregnancy. However, a differentiation between ectopic pregnancies and impending spontaneous abortion cannot be made with this technique because the rate of increase of hCG in women with an ectopic pregnancy is similar to that found in women with an impending intrauterine abortion.

Progesterone

Since a single hCG determination does not provide sufficient information to diagnose ectopic pregnancy because of the inability to determine gestational age with precision, and serial determinations require a 2- to 3-day delay, a single serum progesterone measurement in early gestation has been found by several groups to be of great use in differentiating an ectopic from an intrauterine gestation. Several investigators have shown that when an ectopic pregnancy is present the corpus luteum does not secrete as much progesterone as occurs in normal pregnancies with similar levels of hCG. Stern et al. prospectively measured

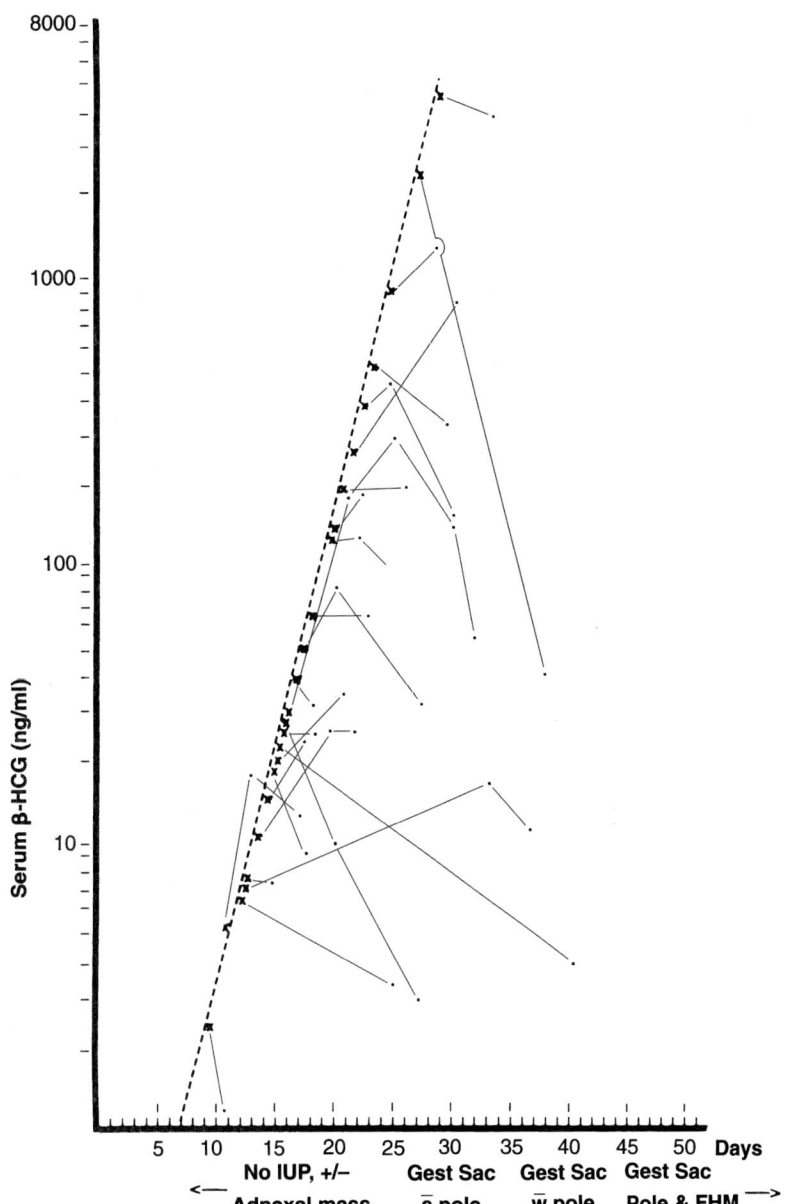

FIGURE 17-17 Serial quantitated serum β-hCG levels for 25 patients with ectopic pregnancy. Broken line represents average hCG progression for first 30 days of normal pregnancy, with corresponding sonographic findings below. Each patient's first determined value is arbitrarily placed on standard line. (From Cartwright PS and DiPietro DL: Obstet Gynecol 63:76, 1984. Reprinted with permission from The American College of Obstetricians and Gynecologists.)

progesterone, as well as hCG, in serum samples at 4, 5, and 6 weeks of known gestational age from a group of women with infertility or a history of recurrent abortion who conceived. They found that in the women with ectopic pregnancies, mean serum progesterone levels were significantly lower at each of these gestational ages than in the women with intrauterine gestations whether or not these gestations subsequently aborted or continued to viability (Table 17-5). They also reported that at 4 weeks' gestation a threshold progesterone level of 5 ng/ml was able to differentiate ectopic from intrauterine gestations, with a sensi-

tivity of 100% and a specificity of 97%. At 5 weeks' gestation the threshold level of progesterone increased to 10 ng/ml and at 6 weeks to 20 ng/ml, but the sensitivity and specificity of the use of serum progesterone measurement to differentiate ectopic from intrauterine gestations decreased as the gestational age increased.

Ledger et al. also found a significant difference in mean progesterone levels between women in early pregnancy with a viable intrauterine gestation and those with an ectopic gestation or those who had a spontaneous abortion (see Figure 17-16). Hahlin et al. found that in a group of

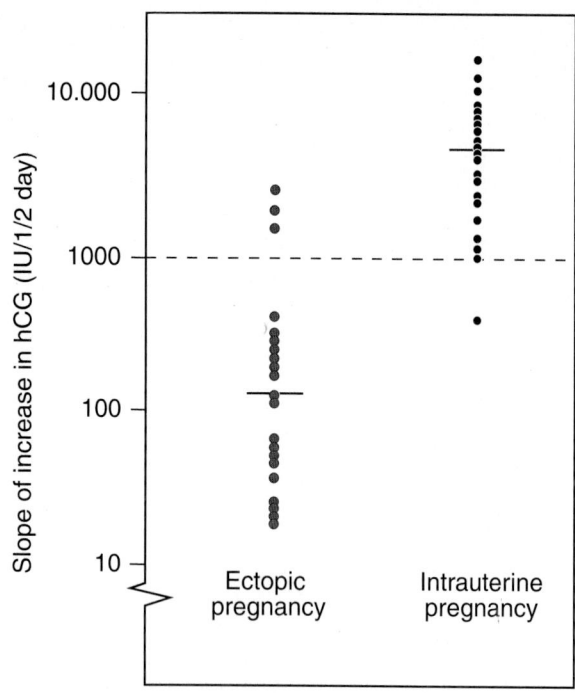

FIGURE 17-18 The slope of hCG rise in patients with ectopic (*N* = 2) and intrauterine pregnancy (*N* = 29). Solid lines are median slopes. Dotted line at 980 IU/1/2 days. (From Gronlund B and Marushak A: Aust N Z J Obstet Gynaecol 33:312, 1993.)

women presenting with symptoms of ectopic pregnancy no woman with a viable intrauterine pregnancy had progesterone levels less than 30 nM/L (10 ng/ml), whereas 88% of ectopic pregnancies and 83% of spontaneous abortions had progesterone values less than this amount.

Stovall et al. measured both hCG and serum progesterone levels in more than 1000 women in the first trimester of pregnancy. They found that all those women with a serum progesterone level less than 5 ng/ml had either an ectopic gestation or a nonviable intrauterine ges-

tation, while 97% of women with a serum progesterone level above 25 ng/ml had a viable intrauterine gestation. They calculated that a single progesterone level of less than 15 ng/ml was as sensitive and more specific than lack of a rise of 66% of two hCG levels measured 48 hours apart for the detection of an abnormal pregnancy. This same group showed that the probability of an ectopic or abnormal intrauterine pregnancy decreased with rising progesterone levels, with less than a 10% likelihood of an abnormal pregnancy occurring with the progesterone level above 17.6 mg/µl (Figure 17-19). O'Leary et al. reported that a combination of hCG less than 3000 IU/L and a progesterone less than 13 ng/ml predicted an abnormal gestation, either ectopic pregnancy or nonviable intrauterine gestation, in 97% of women.

Sauer et al. reported that measurement of pregnanediol glucuronide in a single random urine specimen by a rapid enzyme immunoassay was also very useful to differentiate ectopic from intrauterine pregnancy when a level of 9 µg/ml was used to discriminate the two entities. In their study, this single rapid assay was as effective as measurement of serum progesterone in distinguishing ectopic from intrauterine pregnancies between 5 and 8 weeks from the onset of the last menses.

Ultrasonography

With the use of abdominal ultrasonography, Kadar et al. reported in 1981 that if the hCG level was greater than 6500 mIU/ml and no gestational sac was seen in the uterus, nearly all the women had an ectopic pregnancy. However, this technique was not clinically useful, because about 90% of women with ectopic pregnancies had hCG levels below this threshold.

Development of the transvaginal transducer probes with 5.0 to 7.0 MHz scanning frequency has enabled more precise imaging of the pelvic organs in early pregnancy than is possible with transabdominal ultrasonography. With these probes it is usually possible to identify an

TABLE 17-5

Mean Progesterone Concentrations Obtained at Weeks 4, 5, and 6 of Gestation from Women Whose Pregnancies Subsequently Terminated in Live Births, Spontaneous Abortions, or Ectopic Pregnancies

Pregnancy Outcome	*n*	Progesterone Concentrations at Different Gestational Ages (Weeks) (Mean ± SEM, ng/ml)			
		4	5	6	Mean All Gestations
Live birth	242	35.5 ± 6.2	31.0 ± 6.0	27.5 ± 5.3	31.2 ± 5.9
Spontaneous abortion	81	32.9 ± 4.62	23.9 ± 2.8	23.3 ± 2.6	26.7 ± 3.0
Ectopic	15	*1.9 ± 0.9	*11.9 ± 1.4	*7.0 ± 3.3	*7.0 ± 2.9

From Stern JJ, Voss, F, and Coulam, CB: Hum Reprod 8(5):775, 1993.

*Significantly lower than other values in same column (*P* = 0.0005).

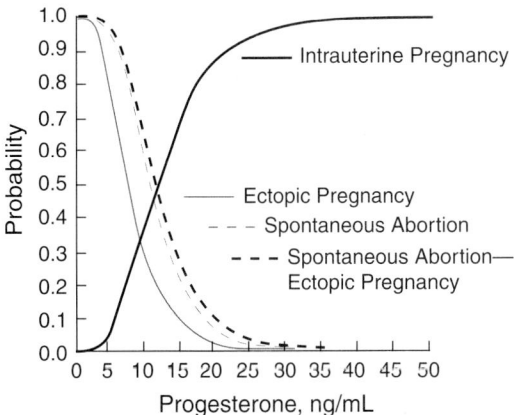

FIGURE 17-19 Predicted pregnancy outcome versus P concentrations. The probability of EP and SAB decreases with rising P, forming a negative-sloping signoid-shaped curve, a mirror image of the IUP curve, with its slope decreasing sharply at approximately 5 ng/ml (15.9 nmol/l) and increasing sharply at approximately 17 ng/ml (54.1 nmol/l). (From McCord ML, Arheart KL, Muram D, et al: Fertil Steril 66:513, 1996.)

intrauterine gestational sac when the hCG level reaches 1500 mIU/ml and always possible to identify a gestational sac in the uterus when the hCG level exceeds 2000 mIU/ml (1st International Reference Preparation [1st IRP], now called the Third International Standard), about 5 to 6 weeks after the last menses. Kadar et al. reported that in both singleton and multiple gestations a gestational sac should always be seen sonographically beyond 24 days after conception, 38 days gestational age. Because combined extrauterine and intrauterine pregnancy is a rare event, the finding of an intrauterine gestational sac should nearly always exclude the presence of an ectopic pregnancy. When a gestational sac is not present and the hCG level is more than 1500 mIU/ml, a pathologic pregnancy, either an ectopic or a nonviable intrauterine gestation, is most likely present and should be suspected. Usually an adnexal mass and/or a gestational sac-like structure can be identified in the oviduct when an ectopic pregnancy is present that produces levels of hCG above 2500 mIU/ml (Figure 17-20).

Thus diagnostic criteria for the ultrasonographic diagnosis of ectopic pregnancy with the use of a vaginal probe include the detection of a complex or cystic adnexal mass or visualization of an embryo in the adnexa, and/or the absence of an intrauterine gestational sac when the gestational age is known to be more than 38 days, and/or the hCG level is above a certain threshold, usually between 1500 and 2500 mIU/ml.

About two thirds of women presenting with symptoms of ectopic pregnancy have hCG levels above 2500 mIU/ml, and when this occurs, the diagnosis of ectopic pregnancy can usually be made sonographically. For the other one third with lower hCG levels, unless a gestational sac is evident on ultrasonography, other diagnostic techniques, such as measurement of a serum progesterone level and serial hCG determination, should be performed. Repeat ultrasonographic examinations at 3- to 5-day intervals are often helpful in establishing a correct diagnosis.

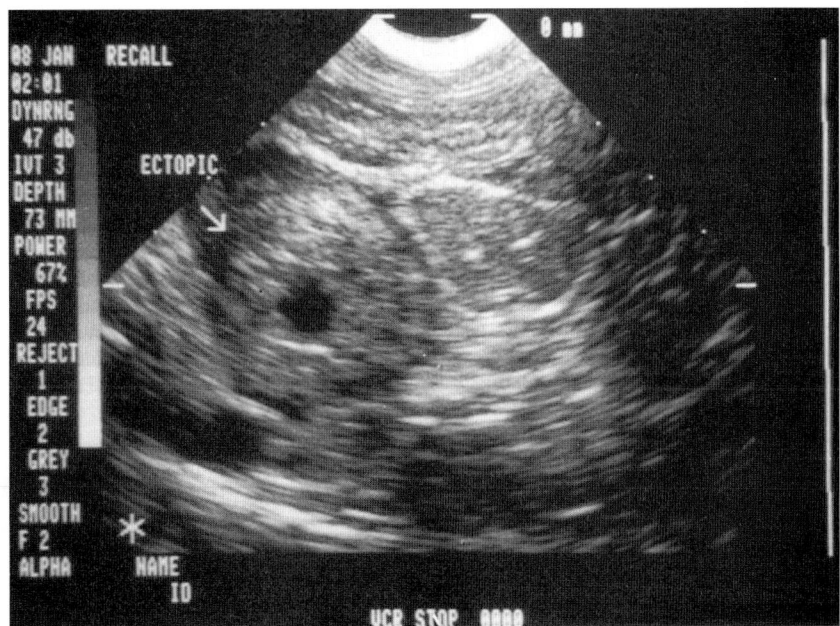

FIGURE 17-20 Ultrasound of etopic pregnancy. (Photo courtesy of Advanced Technology Laboratories, Bothell, Washington, 1991.)

Several investigators have shown that with the use of endovaginal color Doppler flow imaging it is possible to establish the diagnosis of ectopic pregnancy with greater sensitivity and specificity than with ordinary endovaginal sonography. With endovaginal color flow imaging of the pelvic structures in the presence of an ectopic pregnancy about a 20% difference in the degree of tubal blood flow between the adnexae has been found compared with less than an 8% difference with intrauterine gestations. Use of endovaginal color flow compared with routine transvaginal sonography increased the sensitivity of the diagnosis of ectopic pregnancy from 71% to 95%, with a specificity of 96% to 100% in various studies. Unfortunately, the restricted availability of these expensive color flow sonography units limits their availability for routine diagnostic use.

Dilation and Curettage

When serum hCG levels are more than 1500 mIU/ml, the gestational age exceeds 38 days, or the serum progesterone level is less than 5 ng/ml and no intrauterine gestational sac is seen with vaginal ultrasonography, a curettage of the endometrial cavity with histologic examination of the tissue removed, by frozen section if desired, can be undertaken to determine if any gestational tissue is present. Spandorfer et al. reported that frozen section was 93% accurate in identifying chorionic villi. If no chorionic villi are visualized in the removed tissue, a presumptive diagnosis of ectopic pregnancy can be made and treatment undertaken.

Diagnostic Evaluation of Women with Suspected Ectopic Pregnancy

Flow sheets have been developed by several authors to aid the clinician in establishing the diagnosis of an asymptomatic or mildly symptomatic ectopic pregnancy. They involve the use of vaginal probe pelvic ultrasonography, measurement of serial quantitative hCG and single serum progesterone levels, and uterine curettage (Figure 17-21). These diagnostic aids are of particular use when following an asymptomatic woman with risk factors for ectopic pregnancy, beginning shortly after conception. Performing a quantitative hCG assay twice weekly and calculating the rate of increase, measuring serum progesterone levels at 4, 5, and 6 weeks' gestational age; and performing serial ultrasonography beginning 3 weeks after ovulation will help to establish the diagnosis of ectopic pregnancy before tubal rupture. The combination of these two techniques is particularly applicable for stable women treated in institutions with adequate facilities for ultrasound and rapid serial quantitative β-hCG assays. If a woman with or without risk factors for ectopic pregnancy develops mild symptoms consistent with an ectopic gestation and is hemodynamically stable, vaginal sonography, measurement of serum progesterone and serial hCG levels, as well as uterine curettage, if indicated, will aid in establishing the diagnosis. The use of a quantitative serum hCG assay and transvaginal sonography enables the diagnosis of ectopic gestation of hemodynamically stable women to be made with a sensitivity of 97% to 100% and a specificity of 95% to 99% (Figure 17-22).

If a woman develops symptoms of a ruptured ectopic pregnancy that are of sufficient hemodynamic severity to require emergency care, a sensitive qualitative pregnancy test and vaginal sonography are usually all the diagnostic aids necessary to establish the diagnosis. If vaginal sonography is not immediately available culdocentesis may be performed. If hCG is present and peritoneal fluid is seen sonographically, it is most likely that an ectopic pregnancy is present, and laparoscopy or laparotomy, or both, should be performed, depending on the findings of the physical examination. If peritoneal fluid is observed sonographically or nonclotting blood is obtained by culdocentesis, and a qualitative hCG assay is negative, the diagnosis of ruptured corpus luteum is likely and either a laparoscopy or laparotomy should be performed.

MANAGEMENT

Surgical Therapy

The treatment of ectopic gestations in uncommon locations other than the oviduct was discussed earlier in the chapter (see "Pathology"). An interstitial pregnancy, because it usually becomes symptomatic at a late gestational age, is usually large and may require hysterectomy. Otherwise a resection of the cornual region of the uterus may be sufficient. Nearly all ruptured ectopic pregnancies require surgical treatment, which can be either a radical or a conservative procedure. Radical operation consists of salpingectomy with or without accompanying oophorectomy or hysterectomy, while a conservative procedure, salpingostomy or segmental resection, does not remove the entire oviduct. If the rupture has produced extensive damage to the oviduct or if no further pregnancies are desired, a radical procedure is usually performed; otherwise a conservative procedure is usually done. It was previously advocated that an elective ipsilateral oophorectomy be performed in a woman wishing future fertility. The theoretic reason for this recommendation was to increase the chance of conception and reduce the chance of another ectopic pregnancy by having ovulation occur each month from the ovary proximal to the remaining tube. Results from various studies yield conflicting data. Some studies report similar conception rates in women treated with salpingectomy and salpingo-oophorectomy, whereas others report both

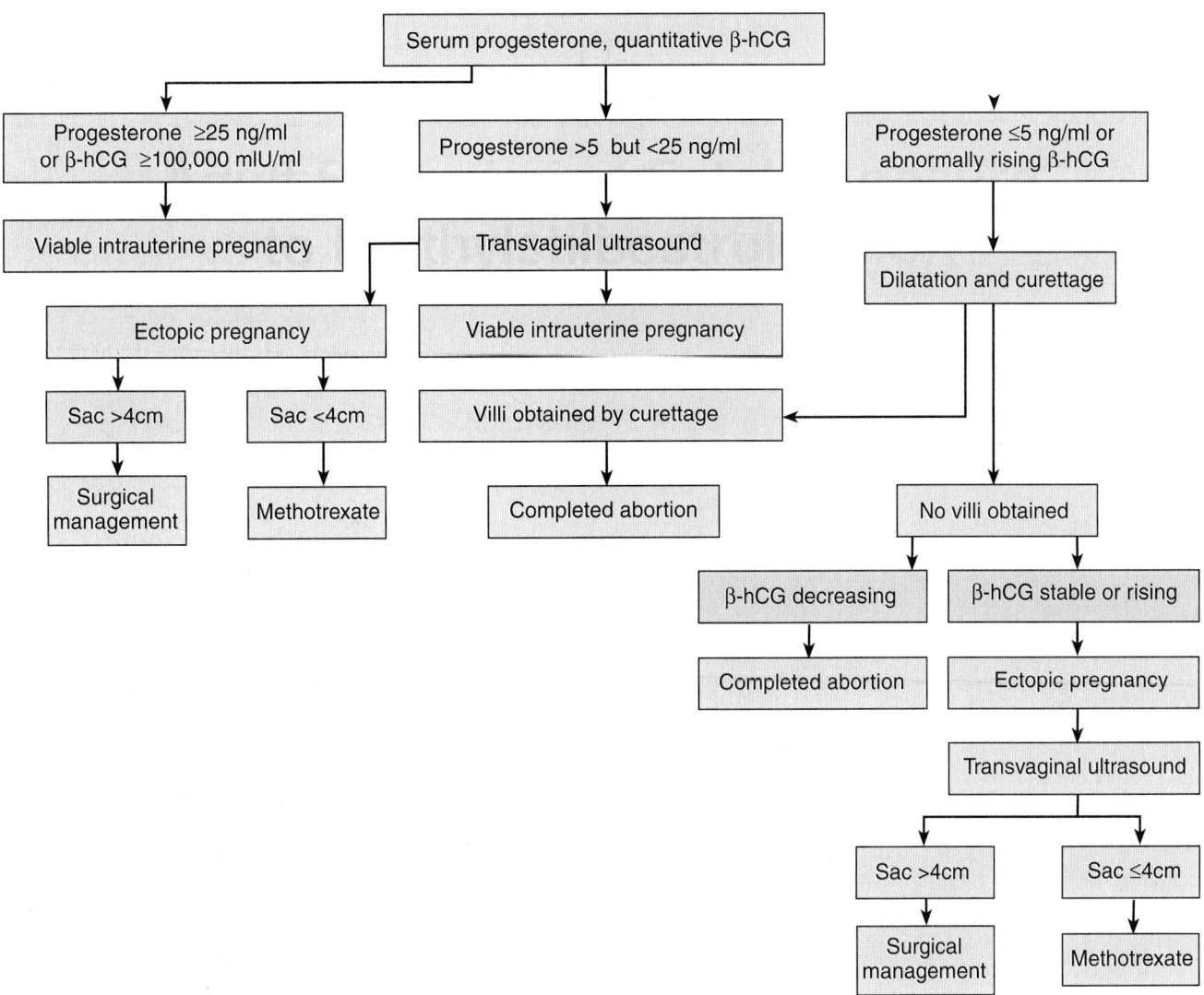

FIGURE 17-21 Algorithm for the diagnosis of unruptured ectopic pregnancy without laparoscopy. Progesterone measurements increase the sensitivity of the algorithm by screening large numbers of patients inexpensively during the first trimester of pregnancy. Definitive diagnosis is made by transvaginal ultrasound or uterine curettage and does not depend on the serum progesterone concentrations obtained during screening, β-hCG, β-human chorionic gonadotrophin. (From Buster JE and Carson SA: Curr Opin Obstet Gynecol 7:168, 1995.)

higher and lower pregnancy rates in women having the ovary removed. Because the subsequent ectopic pregnancy rate in these studies was not decreased when oophorectomy was performed and because the number of oocytes available for in vitro fertilization is greater with two ovaries, it is best not to remove the ipsilateral ovary unless its involvement in the pathologic process necessitates its removal for technical reasons.

Removal of the uterus may sometimes be indicated if another disease, such as leiomyoma, is present. On occasion a hysterectomy can be performed if the woman has undergone a prior tubal sterilization and develops a tubal pregnancy. However, because of the increased operating time and morbidity associated with hysterectomy, as well

as the need for extensive preoperative counseling, elective hysterectomy should usually not be performed at the time of laparotomy for ectopic pregnancy. If a woman develops an ectopic pregnancy after tubal sterilization, it is usually advisable to perform a bilateral salpingectomy to prevent the development of a subsequent ectopic pregnancy in the contralateral oviduct.

Resection of the distal portion of the interstitial oviduct, commonly called a cornual resection, is frequently performed at the time of salpingectomy, but the procedure is unnecessary because it does not prevent a subsequent interstitial pregnancy. Of the 75 cases of interstitial pregnancy after homolateral salpingectomy reported by Kalchman and Meltzer, 20% had been preceded by a cornual

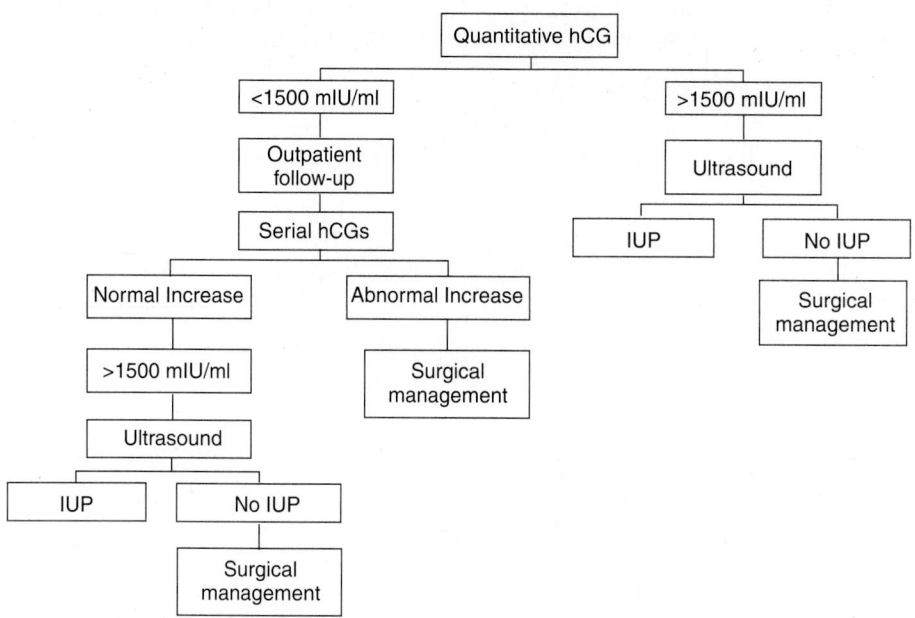

FIGURE 17-22 Algorithm for the diagnosis of ectopic pregnancy in patients presenting to an emergency department without evidence of shock. Human chorionic gonadotropin values are according to the First International Reference Preparation. IUP, intrauterine pregnancy. (From Barnhart K, Mennuti MT, Benjamin I, et al: Obstet Gynecol 84:1010, 1994.)

resection. In Hallatt's series of repeat ectopic pregnancies, 8 of 10 ruptured homolateral interstitial pregnancies were preceded by deep cornual resection. Thus cornual resection does not prevent a subsequent interstitial pregnancy, and if it is performed, it should only be a superficial excision.

Although a colpotomy incision has been used to perform salpingectomy when an unruptured tubal pregnancy exists, as well as to aid in establishing the diagnosis, because of the extensive use of laparoscopy for diagnosis, this incision is used infrequently.

Conservative treatment (not removing the oviduct) for an unruptured ectopic pregnancy is being used with increasing frequency for women who desire future fertility. No randomized trials have compared future fertility or the incidence of ectopic or intrauterine pregnancies after salpingostomy or salpingectomy. However observational studies suggest that when conservative surgery is correctly performed for an unruptured ectopic pregnancy, the repeat ectopic pregnancy rate is not increased compared with that of salpingectomy, whereas the subsequent live birth rate is increased. In the large review by Yao and Tulandi of women with an ectopic pregnancy attempting to conceive after salpingostomy, 60% had a intrauterine pregnancy and 15% an ectopic pregnancy. After salpingectomy 38% had an intrauterine pregnancy and 10% an ectopic pregnancy. Therefore for hemodynamically stable women who wish to preserve fertility and have an unruptured tubal pregnancy, laparoscopic salpingostomy should be performed. The conservative

surgical techniques used include salpingotomy, salpingostomy, fimbrial evacuation, and partial salpingectomy, also called segmental resection of the portion of the oviduct containing the ectopic pregnancy. Fimbrial evacuation of the gestational products by digital expression or blunt curettage traumatizes the endosalpinx and is associated with a high rate of recurrent ectopic pregnancy (24%), about twice as high as the rate after salpingectomy. In addition, this procedure may not remove the entire tubal gestation, and another operative procedure may be required a few days later. The best results of conservative operation occur after salpingotomy or salpingostomy. The latter technique is used more frequently in the United States (Figure 17-23). Tulandi and Guralnick reported that the 2-year cumulative rates of intrauterine pregnancy after salpingotomy and salpingostomy were similar, about 45%, but the 1-year rates were twice as great when salpingostomy was performed (45% versus 21%), indicating that there is a more rapid return of normal tubal function when the incision heals by secondary intention than when it is sutured (Figure 17-24).

These techniques can be used to treat the vast majority of unruptured tubal pregnancies not located in the isthmic portion of the oviduct. It is best to use microsurgical principles when performing salpingostomy. When the unruptured pregnancy is small (less than 5 cm), it is usually possible to perform the salpingostomy with a laparoscopic procedure. Vermesh et al. performed a prospective randomized trial of use of either laparoscopy or laparo-

Ectopic Pregnancy **465**

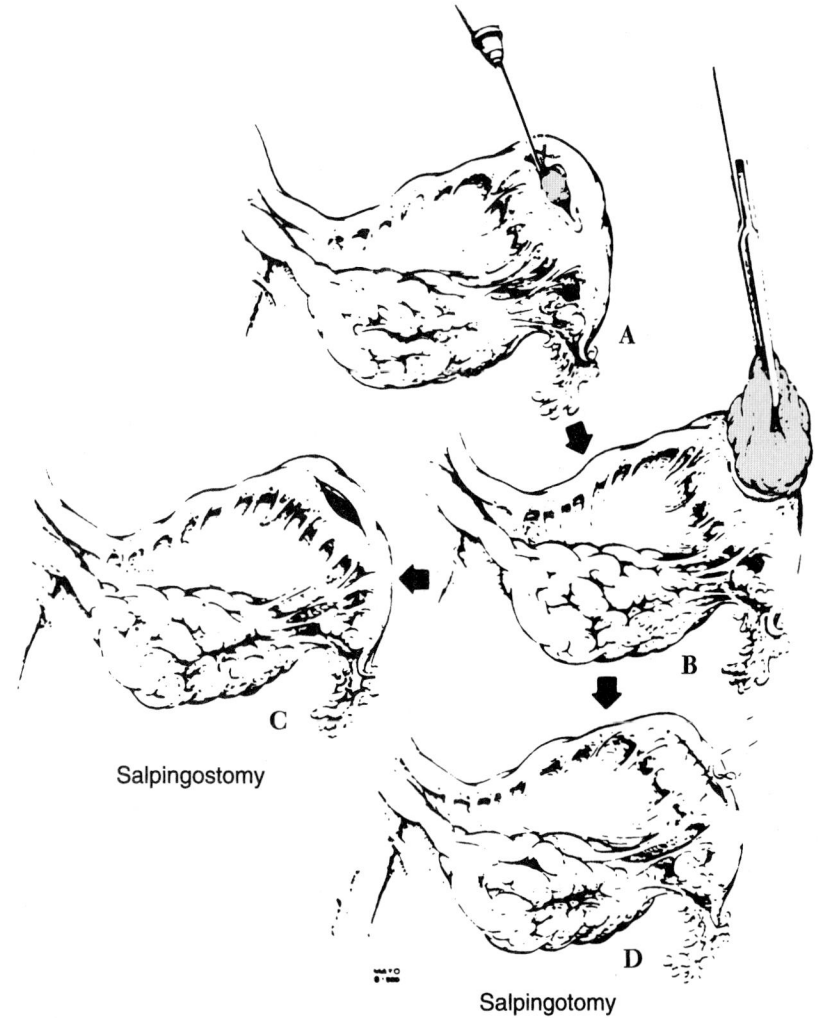

FIGURE 17-23 **A,** Incision is made into the antimesenteric border of the fallopian tube. **B,** Ectopic pregnancy is gently removed from within the fallopian tube. **C,** Salpingostomy site is allowed to heal by secondary intention. **D,** Salpingotomy is completed by primary closure. (From Leach RE and Ory SJ: J Reprod Med 34:325, 1989.)

tomy for the treatment of unruptured ectopic gestation by linear salpingostomy. They found both techniques to be safe and effective, but the estimated blood loss and length of hospital stay and cost were all significantly less in the group treated by laparoscopy and recovery was faster. It was found following a randomized trial of these two techniques by Lundorff et al. that there was significantly more subsequent pelvic adhesion formation when ectopic pregnancies were treated by laparotomy than by laparoscopy. However, the risk of persistent ectopic pregnancy (PEP) in several series has been found to be significantly greater if the salpingostomy is performed laparoscopically rather than by laparotomy. Seifer et al. reported that the incidence of PEP was 16% following laparoscopic salpingostomy but only 2% when a laparotomy was performed, an eightfold increase with the former technique. If hemostasis cannot be maintained after a salpingostomy, which frequently occurs for those unrup-

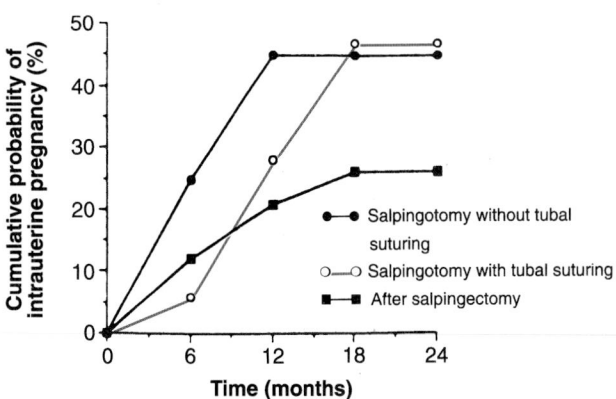

FIGURE 17-24 Cumulative probability of IUP after conservative surgical treatment of tubal EP by salpingotomy without tubal suturing; salpingotomy with tubal suturing; and after salpingectomy. (From Tulandi T and Guralnick M: Fertil Steril 55:53, 1991.)

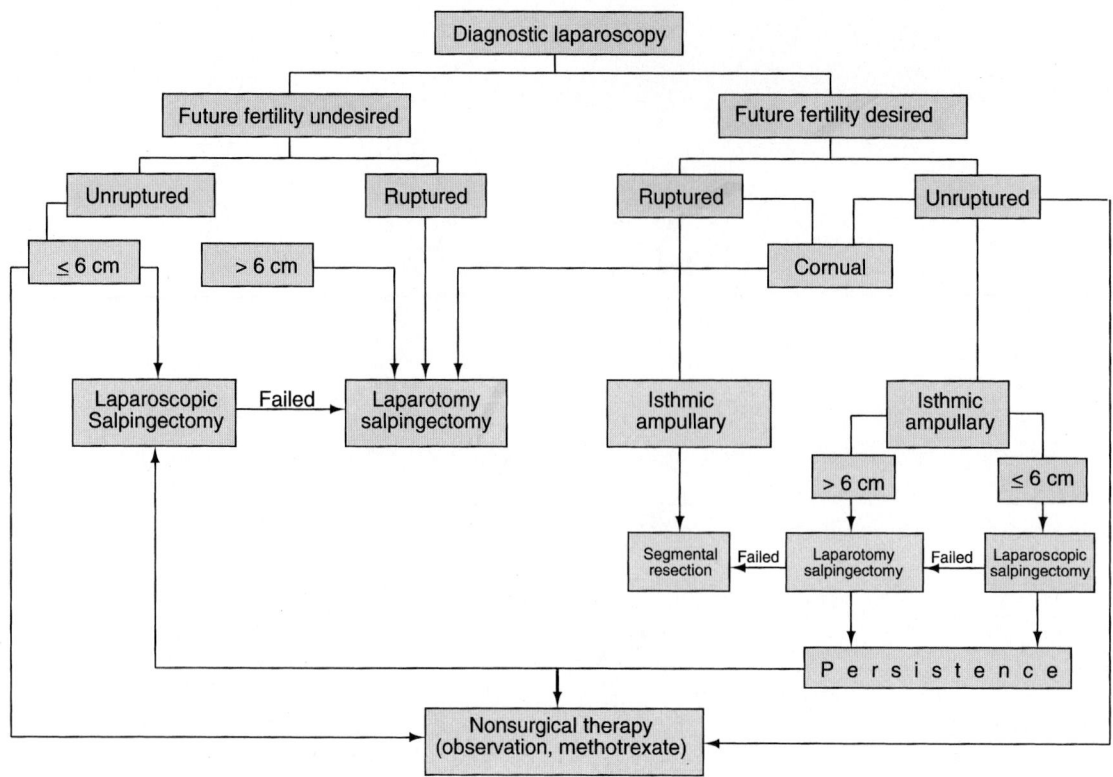

FIGURE 17-25 Conservative management of ectopic gestation. (From Vermesh M: Fertil Steril 51:559, 1989.)

tured pregnancies located in the isthmus, a segmental resection of the oviduct can be performed and a reanastomosis done a few months later. Timonen and Nieminen reported that women who had a segmental resection had a lower subsequent term pregnancy rate (17%) than did women who had salpingectomy (29%). Therefore it is recommended that a partial salpingectomy be performed only if it is not technically possible to do a salpingostomy and the contralateral oviduct is absent or irrevocably damaged.

In his review of the conservative management of ectopic gestation, Vermesh presented a useful flow sheet developed to guide the clinician (Figure 17-25).

Persistent Ectopic Pregnancy

With increasing use of conservative surgical treatment instead of salpingectomy for the treatment of ectopic pregnancy, the entity of persistent ectopic pregnancy (PEP) is becoming more common. Manifestations of PEP include either acute abdominal symptoms and/or persistent or rising hCG levels after conservative treatment of an unruptured ectopic gestation. The overall mean incidence of PEP after linear salpingostomy is about 5%, being higher when the procedure is performed laparoscopically and lower when performed by laparotomy. After

fimbrial expression or tubal abortion the incidence of persistence ranges from 12% to 15%.

Stock reviewed the histologic findings of five women with persistent ectopic gestation treated by subsequent salpingectomy. He observed that in all five instances the implantation sites in the oviduct were medial to the original salpingostomy incision site. The original incision was made over the maximally dilated area of the tube, which contained blood clots and some gestational tissue, but some gestational tissue remained medial to the incision.

Persistent ectopic pregnancy is uncommon when the preoperative hCG level is below 3000 mIU/ml. When preoperative hCG levels are greater than 3000 mIU/ml, the incidence of PEP has been reported to range from about 22% to 42%. If the hCG level is above 1000 mIU/ml 7 days after surgery or is more than 15% of the original level at this time, PEP is nearly always present. If the day 7 hCG level is under 1000 mIU/ml or less than 15% of the initial value, PEP is very unlikely. Vermesh et al. measured both hCG and progesterone levels preoperatively and every 3 days after conservative tubal surgery for an unruptured ectopic gestation in a group of 114 women. Of these 114, 6 (5.3%) had PEP. All six had an initial sharp drop in hCG levels to 25% of the pretreatment levels 6 days after surgery, similar to the remainder of the group who did not have PEP. After 6 days, titers of the former group plateaued or rose slightly

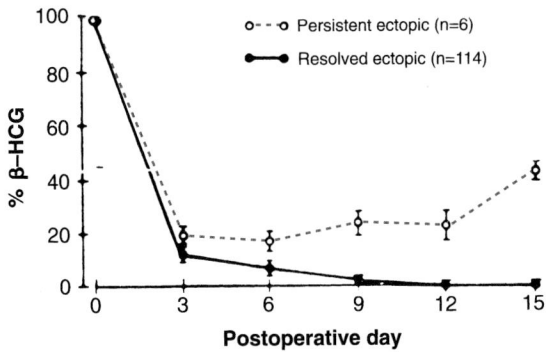

FIGURE 17-26 Serum β-hCG patterns in persistent and resolved ectopic gestations after conservative surgery. (From Vermesh M, Silva PD, Rosen GF, et al: Fertil Steril 50:584, 1988.)

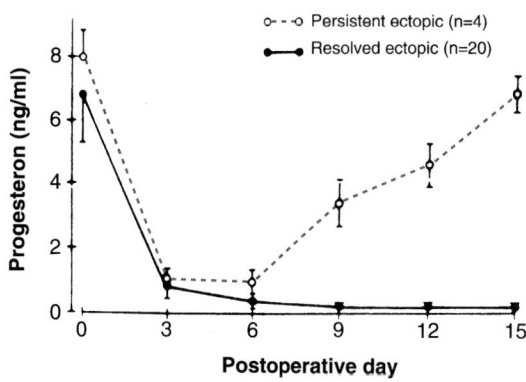

FIGURE 17-27 Serum progesterone patterns in persistent and resolved ectopic gestations after conservative surgery. (From Vermesh M, Silva PD, Rosen GF, et al: Fertil Steril 50:584, 1988.)

(Figure 17-26). Progesterone levels showed the same type of pattern (Figure 17-27).

Based on these data, PEP is presumed to be present if a day 9 serum hCG level is more than 10% of the initial level and/or a day 9 serum progesterone level is higher than 1.5 ng/ml. It is now recommended that after linear salpingostomy either hCG or progesterone levels be measured initially on day 6 postoperatively and at 3-day intervals thereafter. Increasing levels of either of these hormones beyond day 6 or a day-6 level of hCG more than 1000 mIU/ml or more than 15% of the original value are all indicators of persistent ectopic gestation. Because tubal rupture is likely to occur with PEP, it is best to treat the entity before this emergency situation occurs.

Methods used to treat PEP include salpingectomy, salpingostomy, methotrexate, or expectant management. Expectant management is usually reserved for the asymptomatic woman whose hCG titers plateau but do not rise. Surgical management, either by laparoscopy or laparotomy, should be utilized for those women who develop symptoms of persistent lower abdominal pain. The remaining women with PEP are best treated with methotrexate. A single dose of 50 mg/m² of methotrexate is usually sufficient to cause resolution of PEP. Hoppe et al. used this therapy in 19 consecutive women with PEP, and all had resolution of the PEP. Graczykowski and Mishell performed a randomized trial in which a single dose of methotrexate or placebo was given within 24 hours after salpingostomy. The use of methotrexate reduced the risk of developing PEP by nearly 90%. The prophylactic use of a single dose of methotrexate may be considered in women unable or unwilling to have serial hCG measurements made after salpingostomy.

Medical Therapy

In 1982 Tanaka et al. reported the successful use of methotrexate for the sole treatment of an unruptured interstitial pregnancy, and in the following year Miyazaki et al. reported the first series of women with small, unruptured ectopic pregnancies that were successfully treated with systemic methotrexate.

Initially methotrexate was administered at a dose of 1 mg/kg on alternate days for four to five doses, with administration of citrovorum factor (reduced folate) on the intervening days. About 20% of women so treated developed side effects such as stomatitis or abnormal liver function tests. Stovall et al. suggested stopping the methotrexate when the hCG levels fell more than 15% in 48 hours or when four doses of the drug had been given. With this regimen only 29% of women received four doses of the drug and only 8% experienced side effects. By 1995, as reviewed by Buster and Carson, 11 series involving 262 women treated with this regimen had been published and there was a cumulative 94% success rate, with subsequent evidence of tubal patency in 82% and fertility in 66% (Table 17-6). These rates are similar to those reported with treatment of unruptured tubal pregnancy by salpingostomy. Criteria believed necessary for methotrexate treatment of asymptomatic or mildly symptomatic unruptured ectopic pregnancy include diameter of the gestational mass, as measured sonographically, to be less than 4 cm, and no clinical evidence of active bleeding or tubal rupture. It has been estimated that with monitoring early in gestation at least one third of women with ectopic pregnancies will satisfy these criteria and can be treated medically instead of surgically. In addition there should not be sonographic evidence of intraperitoneal fluid outside the pelvic cavity and no evidence of hepatic, hematologic, or renal disease.

Other regimens have subsequently been utilized for administration of methotrexate both locally and systemically. In 1993 Stovall and Ling reported their experience with use of a single dose of systemic methotrexate 50 mg/m² without the use of citrovorum. In 4 series of 228 women treated with this regimen 90% resolved without surgery. Of this group 10% required a second dose of methotrexate because hCG levels did not fall suf-

TABLE 17-6

Outcome of Various Methods Used to Treat Unruptured Ectopic Pregnancy Since 1980

Therapy	Reports	n	Success (%)	Tubal Patency (%)	Total Fertility (%)	Intrauterine Pregnancy (%)	Ectopic Pregnancy
Laparoscopic salpingostomy	23	1218	95	81	74	61	13
Variable dose methotrexate	12	262	94	82	63	59	7
Single dose methotrexate	4	228	90	81	69	61	8
Direct tubal injection of methotrexate	11	295	83	88	82	78	4
Expectant management	11	216	61	100	NA	NA	NA

Adapted from Carson SA and Buster JE: N Engl J Med 329:1174, 1993.

ficiently. About 85% of patients treated with methotrexate have a transient rise in hCG level between 1 and 4 days after treatment. Between 4 and 7 days after methotrexate is administered the hCG levels should fall at least 15%. If this amount of decrease does not occur or there is less than a 15% decrease in hCG levels in each subsequent week, an additional dose of methotrexate should be given for a maximum of 3 doses. If after 3 doses of methotrexate hCG levels do not decline by 15% weekly, a surgical procedure should be performed. Saraj et al. reported that serum progesterone levels fall more rapidly than hCG levels after methotrexate, and a progesterone level of less than 1.5 ng/ml was an excellent predictor of resolution of the ectopic pregnancy. The rates of tubal patency and subsequent fertility with the single-dose regimen were similar to those with the multiple-dose regimen. Because of the need for surgical treatment in a higher percentage of the women treated with a single dose rather than with multiple doses of methotrexate, some investigators still advocate that use of the intermittent regimen is preferable. To reduce the incidence of tubal rupture with systemic methotrexate it is advisable to perform only a single bimanual pelvic examination before and after initiating treatment. Between 3 to 7 days after initiating therapy severe pelvic pain lasting up to 12 hours frequently occurs. This symptom, probably caused by tubal abortion, needs to be differentiated from the symptoms of tubal rupture. Serial monitoring of vital signs and measurement of hematocrit levels are helpful. If the woman remains hemodynamically stable and the pain disappears, a tubal abortion has probably taken place and no further therapy is necessary. Lipson et al. analyzed predictors of success in 350 women treated with methotrexate. A total of 30 women, 9%, were treatment failures. There were no significant differences between women treated successfully and failures regarding age, parity, volume of the ectopic mass, or presence or absence of free peritoneal fluid. The mean hCG and progesterone level as well as frequency of cardiac activity were

TABLE 17-7

Success Rates of Methotrexate Treatment in Women with Ectopic Pregnancies as a Function of Their Initial Serum Chorionic Gonadotropin Concentrations

Serum Chorionic Gonadotropin Concentrations (mIU/ml)	Success No.	Failure No.	Success Rate (95% CI)* Percent
<1000	118	2	98 (69–100)
1000–1999	40	3	93 (85–100)
2000–4999	90	8	92 (86–97)
5000–9999	39	6	87 (79–98)
10,000–14,999	18	4	82 (65–98)
≥15,000	15	7	68 (49–88)

*CI denotes confidence interval. Treatment was successful in 320 women and failed in 30.

lower in the successfully treated group than the failures. If the initial hCG titer was less than 5000 mIU/ml the success rate was more than 90%; if it was more than 15,000 mIU/ml the success rate was only 68% (Table 17-7).

There have been two randomized trials comparing the results of systemic methotrexate with laparoscopic salpingostomy for the treatment of unruptured ectopic pregnancy. In a Dutch study, a similar degree of success was achieved with each treatment methodology. In the group treated medically, 14% required surgical intervention; in the group treated surgically, 20% required methotrexate treatment for persistent ectopic pregnancy.

In another study by Saraj et al., 2 of 38 women treated with methotrexate required subsequent surgery and 3 of

37 treated by salpingostomy required medical treatment for persistent ectopic pregnancy. Resolution following salpingostomy was more rapid than after methotrexate. The mean time to disappearance occurred about 20 days after salpingostomy and 27 days after methotrexate.

To avoid the toxicity of systemic methotrexate administration, a smaller dose of the drug has been administered directly into the oviduct with either laparoscopic or sonographic visualization. In the summary of Buster and Carson, of 11 series involving 295 women treated with tubal injection of methotrexate, only 83% had successful resolution of the ectopic pregnancy but subsequent tubal patency rates were 88% and fertility rates were 82% (Table 17-6).

Because of the lower success rate and need for direct needle placement with local injection, most clinicians are now using systemic methotrexate. There have also been several reports of direct intratubal injection of other substances, including potassium chloride, hypertonic glucose, and prostaglandins, but use of these agents is generally less successful than methotrexate.

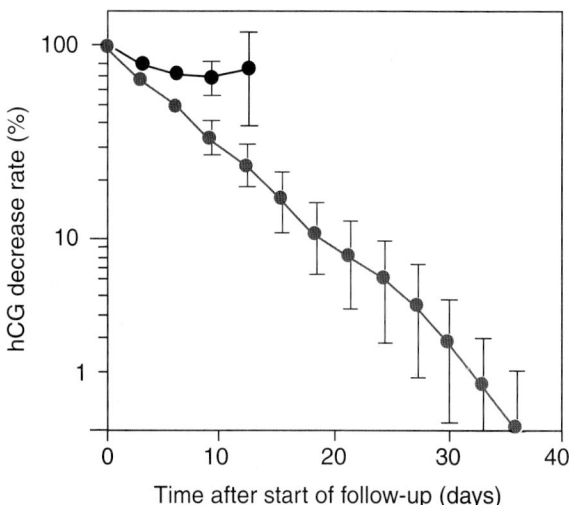

FIGURE 17-28 Mean value and 95% confidence limits for ratio of serum hCG concentrations to starting value 9% during expectant management in patients with a spontaneous resolution and in those later treated by laparoscopy. ● Spontaneous resolution; ●, Laparoscopy. (From Korhonen J, Stenman UH, Ylöstalo P: Fertil Steril 61:632, 1994.)

Expectant Management

In 1955 Lund reported a series of 119 women with unruptured tubal pregnancy treated expectantly with only bed rest and frequent observation while hospitalized. Of these 119, 68 (57%) were eventually discharged without the need for a surgical procedure, but about 60% of them required hospitalization for more than 1 month. The remainder had a tubal rupture or required operative intervention for other reasons. The subsequent fertility rates were similar in the group treated surgically and those treated expectantly. In 1982 Mashiach et al. reported that if at the time of the initial laparoscopy a small unruptured tubal pregnancy was found and that if serial hCG levels subsequently fell, it was possible to avoid surgical therapy, although they performed a repeat laparoscopy before discharge.

Other investigators subsequently reported similar results. In published reports of 347 women with ectopic pregnancy treated expectantly, since 1980 the success rate was 69%, with a high subsequent tubal patency rate (Table 17-6). At present, if it is necessary to perform a laparoscopy for diagnostic purposes, it is best to excise the unruptured ectopic pregnancy to avoid the additional expense of hospitalization, serial hCG assays, and possibly a second laparoscopic procedure. Nevertheless, in an asymptomatic woman, expectant management can be undertaken if certain criteria are present and the presumptive diagnosis of unruptured ectopic pregnancy has been made without a laparoscopy. These criteria include sonographic diameter of the tubal mass less than 3 cm, an initial hCG level less than 1000 mIU/ml, and no rise in hCG levels during a 2-day period. If the woman remains asymptomatic and hCG levels subsequently fall, no other therapy is needed.

Trio et al. with multivariate analysis reported that an initial hCG titer of less than 1000 mIU/ml and a decrease in hCG levels between the initial serum sample and one obtained a few days later were each independent predictors of successful spontaneous resolution while sonographic visualization of an ectopic gestational sac was not an independent predictor of failure. In their series of 49 women managed expectantly, 88% of those with an initial hCG level less than 1000 mIU/ml had successful resolution.

Korhonen et al. measured serial hCG levels before and during outpatient expectant management of a group of 118 women with ectopic pregnancies. This group comprised one fourth of all the women with the diagnosis of ectopic pregnancy seen at their institution during 3 years. Initially their median gestational age was 44 days, and the median hCG level was 374 mIU/ml. Spontaneous resolution occurred in two thirds of the 118 women (16% of the entire group of women with ectopic pregnancies). If the initial hCG level was less than 200 mIU/ml, the rate of successful spontaneous resolution was 88%. When the initial hCG level was more than 2000 mIU/ml, the rate of spontaneous resolution was only 25%. When spontaneous resolution occurred, hCG levels declined to undetectable levels in 4 to 67 days, with a mean of 20 days. A distinct difference in the rate of decline of hCG levels in those who did and did not require surgery was not observed until 7 days after the initial examination (Figure 17-28). If hCG levels had not fallen more than two thirds of the initial level in 7 days, two thirds of this group of women needed surgical treatment for either rising hCG levels, clinical symptoms, or sonographic findings of intraperitoneal bleeding. Atri et al. reported that when serial sonography is performed some of the tubal pregnancies can increase in size and become more vascular as they resolve.

Rh Factor

It is recommended that all Rh-negative, unsensitized women with ectopic pregnancies receive Rh immunoglobulin at a dosage of 50 μg if the gestation is of less than 12 weeks' duration and 300 μg if it is beyond 12 weeks. However, Grimes et al. have reported that because most of their hospitalizations were unscheduled and not preceded by Rh screening, the majority of women with ectopic pregnancies in the United States who are Rh negative do not receive Rh(D) immunoglobulin. The magnitude of the risk of sensitization is unknown but is estimated to vary from nil at 1 month to about 9% at 3 months' gestation. Because of the potential benefits and lack of risk, this treatment should be utilized in all Rh-negative, unsensitized women with ectopic pregnancy.

PROGNOSIS FOR SUBSEQUENT FERTILITY

If a woman wishes to conceive after having an ectopic pregnancy, three possibilities exist. She may remain infertile. She may conceive and have an intrauterine gestation (with a viable birth or spontaneous abortion), or she may conceive and have an ectopic gestation. Overall the subsequent conception rate in women following all ectopic pregnancies is about 60%, with the other 40% remaining infertile. About one third of the pregnancies occurring after the initial ectopic pregnancy are another ectopic pregnancy and one sixth are spontaneous abortions. Therefore, only about half the pregnancies are viable and only one third of all women with an ectopic pregnancy have a subsequent live birth. However, these overall figures are modified by several factors, particularly age, parity, history of infertility, evidence of contralateral tubal disease, whether the ectopic pregnancy is ruptured or intact, and use of an IUD at the time of the ectopic gestation. The subsequent fertility rate is significantly higher in parous women under the age of 30. However, if the ectopic pregnancy occurs in a woman's first pregnancy, her overall subsequent conception rate is only about 35%, being lower with a history of infertility and higher with no such history. On the other hand, women with high parity (more than three births) who develop an ectopic pregnancy have a relatively high rate, about 80%, of subsequent conception. The subsequent conception rate is lower in women who have a history of salpingitis, as well as those who have visual evidence of pathologic changes in the opposite oviduct as a result of previous salpingitis. Several studies have reported that women who were using an IUD at the time of ectopic

pregnancy have normal rates of subsequent fertility and no increased risk of a subsequent ectopic pregnancy. Future fertility is significantly higher in women who have an unruptured tubal pregnancy than in those with tubal rupture so that early diagnosis is desirable. In the report of Sherman et al., only 65% of women with a ruptured ectopic pregnancy subsequently conceived, while the conception rate in women with an unruptured tubal pregnancy was 82%.

In two large groups of women with unruptured ectopic pregnancy treated by conservative surgery, Langer et al. and Pouly et al. reported a high incidence of subsequent fertility (80% to 86%) and a low incidence of subsequent ectopic pregnancy (11% to 22%). The intrauterine pregnancy rates were 64% to 70%. In both series the intrauterine pregnancy rates were highest (82% to 86%) in women with no history of infertility or gross evidence of prior salpingitis. The intrauterine pregnancy rates were significantly lower (41% to 56%) in women with these problems. Sherman et al. and Tuomivaara and Kauppila reported that among women with a normal contralateral tube and no history of infertility, pregnancy rates were similar whether salpingectomy or salpingostomy was performed. However, in the group of women with evidence of prior tubal infection and/or a history of infertility, subsequent intrauterine conception rates were higher when they were treated with salpingostomy (73% to 76%) than with salpingectomy (43% to 44%). Most studies in the literature indicate that the overall subsequent ectopic pregnancy rate is similar among women treated radically or conservatively, and these two studies indicate that conservative surgery is most beneficial for women with evidence of contralateral tubal damage or peritubal adhesions, and/or history of infertility.

Vermesh and Presser analyzed the reproductive outcome for 3 years in a group of 60 women with unruptured tubal pregnancy treated by salpingostomy who were randomized to have the procedure performed by laparoscopy or laparotomy. At the end of 3 years 74% and 86%, respectively, had conceived after each procedure. The women treated by laparoscopy conceived sooner than those treated by laparotomy, and there were more ectopic pregnancies in the latter group. Overall, 68% and 71% of women in the two groups, respectively, had an intrauterine pregnancy, and 5% and 19% had an ectopic pregnancy.

Pouly et al. attempted to provide criteria for women with an unruptured ectopic pregnancy to determine whether a salpingostomy or salpingectomy should be performed to enhance the rate of subsequent pregnancy and decrease the rate of subsequent ectopic pregnancy. In this study the future fertility rate was lower in nulliparous than in parous women only if the former had a history of infertility. Future fertility or chance of subsequent ectopic pregnancy was unaffected by the size of the ectopic gestation or its location. A history of prior abdomino-pelvic surgery or use of an IUD also did not affect the risk of future fertility or subsequent ectopic pregnancy. Although the presence of

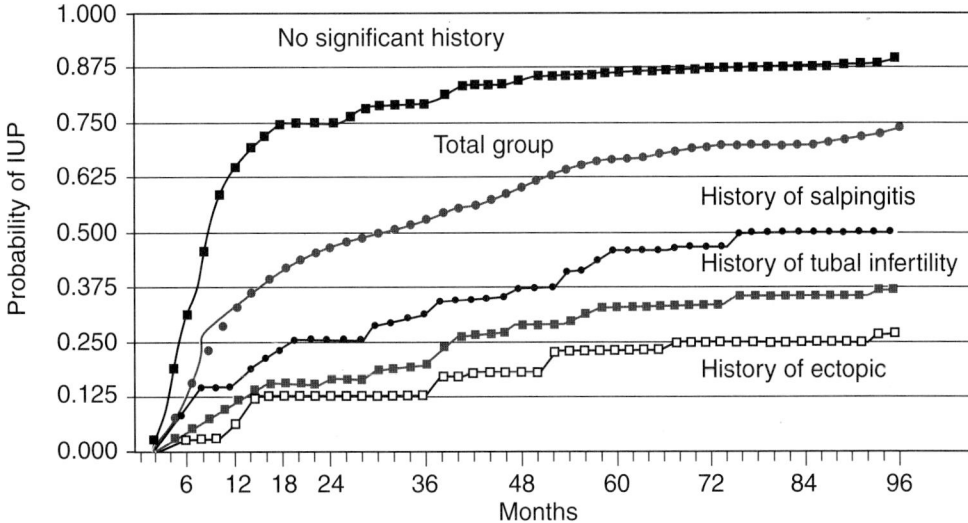

FIGURE 17-29   Cumulative PR according to the patients' history.

adnexal adhesions increased the rate of infertility, it did not affect the risk of recurrence of ectopic pregnancy.

However, a history of infertility (particularly resulting from tubal disease), previous salpingitis, a prior ectopic pregnancy, or the presence of only one oviduct were each independent factors that decreased the rate of subsequent fertility and also increased the risk of subsequent ectopic pregnancy (Figure 17-29). These authors suggested that if more than one of these factors were present it was preferable to perform a salpingectomy than salpingostomy since 80% of the recurrent ectopic pregnancies occurred in the same tube as the initial ectopic pregnancy.

The rate of repeat ectopic pregnancies after a single ectopic pregnancy ranges from 8% to 27%, with a mean of about 20%. Since the overall pregnancy rate is in the 60% to 80% range, about one of three to four conceptions after an ectopic pregnancy is a repeat ectopic pregnancy. Women with an ectopic pregnancy who become pregnant again should be monitored by sonography early in pregnancy because of the high incidence of another ectopic pregnancy as well as spontaneous abortion. Only about one of three nulliparous women who have had an ectopic pregnancy ever conceives again (35%), and about one third of these conceptions are an ectopic pregnancy, for an overall rate of 13%. Skeldestad et al. followed up on 697 women with an ectopic pregnancy if they conceived again. The reported ectopic pregnancy rate was 21%, the viable birth rate was about 55%, and the spontaneous abortion rate was about 25%. Risk factors for a repeat ectopic pregnancy were ectopic pregnancy as first pregnancy, age less than 25, evidence of tubal infection, and history of infertility (Table 17-8). With two ectopic pregnancies the subsequent fertility rate is decreased even further. If a woman has two consecutive ectopic pregnancies treated by salpingostomy, about half will

TABLE 17-8
Odds of Repeat Ectopic Pregnancy in Subsequent Pregnancies

	Adjusted OR	95% CI
Pregnancy order		
1st subsequent	11.8	2.0, 68.0
2nd subsequent	3.0	0.5, 21.1
3rd or more subsequent	1.0	Reference
Repeat ectopic pregnancy		
1 repeat (2nd) ectopic pregnancy	9.5	2.5, 36.6
No repeat (1st) ectopic pregnancy	1.0	Reference
Status at index ectopic pregnancy		
Age (yr)		
≤24	3.1	1.1, 8.9
≥25	1.0	Reference
Infectious pathology*		
Yes	2.7	1.5, 5.0
No	1.0	Reference
Have started infertility work-up		
Yes	2.3	1.0, 5.1
No	1.0	Reference
Conceived with intrauterine device in situ at index pregnancy		
Yes	0.4	0.1, 0.9
No	1.0	Reference

*Defined as either adhesions or macroscopic damage to the contralateral tube or both.

OR, odds ratio; CI, confidence interval.

Reprinted with permission from American College of Obstetricians and Gynecologists, Obstet Gynecol 91(1):129–135, 1997.

subsequently conceive, but as reported by Vermesh and Presser the majority of them will be a repeat ectopic pregnancy. Therefore it is probably better to perform in vitro fertilization if a woman has two consecutive ectopic pregnancies in order to enhance the possibility of a viable pregnancy and reduce the risk of having a third ectopic pregnancy.

There have been several reports of the use of conservative surgery, either salpingostomy or salpingotomy, in women with an unruptured tubal pregnancy in the only remaining oviduct. In the great majority of the subjects the other oviduct had been removed for another ectopic gestation. Of 90 women so treated in six different centers, the conception rate was 81%, with an intrauterine pregnancy rate of 57% (Table 17-9). About one fourth of the women who conceived had a subsequent ectopic gestation, similar to the rate among all ectopic pregnancies. Thus conservative surgery or medical therapy may be performed when an unruptured ectopic pregnancy occurs in the only remaining oviduct.

TABLE 17-9

Results of Conservative Surgery for Tubal Pregnancy in Women with a Solitary Tube

Author	Year	No. of Patients Desiring Pregnancy	IUP	EUP
Henri-Suchet et al.	1979	14	8	2
DeCherney et al.	1982	12	6	2
Langer et al.	1982	8	5	2
Valle and Lifchez	1983	11	11	0
Oelsner et al.	1986	21	10	9
Pouly et al.	1986	24	11	7
TOTAL		90	51 (57%)	22 (24%)

From Vermesh M: Fertil Steril 51:559, 1989.

KEY POINTS

- The annual ectopic pregnancy rates in the United States are about 1.5 per 1000 women aged 15 to 44.

- In the United States in 1992 about 2 of every 100 women who were known to conceive had an ectopic gestation.

- In the United States the rate of ectopic pregnancy increased from 6.6 per 1000 conceptions in women aged 15 to 24 to 21.5 per 1000 conceptions in those aged 25 to 34.

- Only 10% to 15% of ectopic pregnancies occur in nulligravid women, and more than half of the ectopic pregnancies occur in women who have been pregnant three or more times.

- Nonclotting blood is obtained by culdocentesis in more than 90% of ruptured ectopic pregnancies.

- About 85% of women with an ectopic pregnancy have serum hCG levels lower than those seen in normal pregnancy at a similar gestational age.

- In women with an ectopic gestation, about 90% have an abnormal pattern of serial hCG levels. Half of these have falling levels and half have a subnormal increase.

- Laparoscopy has a 2% to 5% misdiagnosis rate (false-positive or false-negative) for ectopic pregnancy.

- Ultrasonography with a vaginal probe allows visualization of an intrauterine gestation when the hCG level is between 1500 and 2500 mIU/ml depending on the transducer.

- Criteria for the ultrasonographic diagnosis of ectopic pregnancy with use of currently available vaginal transducers include the finding of an adnexal mass and/or the absence of a gestational sac when the hCG level is above a certain threshold, about 1500 to 2500 mIU/ml.

- About two thirds of women with symptomatic ectopic pregnancy have hCG levels above 2500 mIU/ml and thus can be reliably diagnosed by ultrasonography.

- Similar subsequent conception rates and ectopic pregnancy rates occur in women with an ectopic pregnancy treated with salpingectomy or salpingo-oophorectomy.

- Cornual resection does not prevent a subsequent interstitial pregnancy.

- If the ectopic pregnancy has produced rupture of the oviduct or has involved the entire oviduct or if no further pregnancies are desired, salpingectomy is the treatment of choice.

- When an unruptured ectopic pregnancy is present, the repeat ectopic pregnancy rate with salpingostomy is not increased compared with salpingectomy, whereas the subsequent live birth rate is increased if the other tube is grossly abnormal or if there is a history of infertility.

- Fimbrial evacuation of the gestational products by digital expression has about twice the rate of recurrent ectopic pregnancy as treatment by salpingectomy.

- It is recommended that all Rh-negative unsensitized women with ectopic pregnancies receive Rh immunoglobulin.

- Overall the subsequent conception rate in women with an ectopic pregnancy is about 60%. A little less than half of these pregnancies terminate in another ectopic pregnancy or spontaneous abortion, so only about one third of women with an ectopic pregnancy have a subsequent live birth.

- If the ectopic pregnancy occurs in a woman's first pregnancy, her chance of subsequent conception is only about 35%.

- The subsequent conception rate following an ectopic pregnancy is lower in women who have a history of salpingitis, as well as in those who have gross evidence of damage in the opposite oviduct caused by previous salpingitis.

- Future fertility is significantly higher among women who have an unruptured tubal pregnancy than in those with a ruptured ectopic pregnancy.

- Conservative tubal surgery is most beneficial in women with evidence of contralateral tubal damage or peritubal adhesions or a history of infertility.

- About one of four conceptions after an ectopic pregnancy is a repeat ectopic pregnancy.

- About one third of nulliparous women with an ectopic pregnancy have a subsequent ectopic pregnancy.

- In women with one remaining oviduct when an unruptured ectopic pregnancy is treated by salpingostomy, the conception rate is 81%, with an intrauterine pregnancy rate of 56% and a subsequent ectopic gestation rate of 24%.

- The overall risk of ectopic pregnancy after tubal sterilization failure is about 30%, reaching 50% if the sterilization technique was bilateral tubal fulguration.

- The incidence of heterotopic ectopic pregnancy is about 1% of all pregnancies occurring after in vitro fertilization.

- If the hCG level is less than 3000 mIU/ml and the progesterone level is less than 12 ng/ml, the likelihood of ectopic pregnancy or nonviable intrauterine gestation is 97%.

- If the serum progesterone level is less than 5 ng/ml, the pregnancy is nonviable, whether in an ectopic or intrauterine location.

- All women with a serum progesterone level more than 25 ng/ml have a viable intrauterine gestation.

- With a gestational age more than 38 days and/or a serum hCG level more than 2500 mIU/ml, if an intrauterine gestation is present it should be visualized sonographically.

- The diagnosis of an asymptomatic ectopic pregnancy can usually be made with the use of vaginal probe pelvic sonography, serial hCG levels, and/or a serum progesterone measurement.

- The overall incidence of persistent ectopic pregnancy after conservative tubal surgery is about 5%, being higher when the procedure is performed laparoscopically than by laparotomy.

- The incidence of persistent ectopic pregnancy increases when the preoperative serum hCG is more than 3000 mIU/ml and can be diagnosed by a finding of an hCG level above 1000 mIU/ml or a decrease of hCG above 15% of the preoperative level 7 days after the salpingostomy.

- Asymptomatic persistent ectopic pregnancy can be treated expectantly or with methotrexate.

- The best medical treatment of unruptured ectopic pregnancy is to give methotrexate in a single intramuscular dose of 50 mg/m^2 without citrovorum factor.

- With monitoring in early gestation, at least one third of women with ectopic pregnancies can be treated medically.

- Expectant management of unruptured ectopic pregnancy can be used if the size of the tubal mass is less than 3 cm and the initial hCG level is less than 1000 mIU/ml without a rise in levels in 2 days.

- The hCG level should fall at least 15% between days 4 and 7 after the methotrexate injection and at least 15% weekly thereafter.

- The best predictor of successful treatment of ectopic pregnancy with methotrexate is the initial hCG level. If the level is less than 5000 mIU/ml the success rate is 90%.

- Factors that increase the risk of ectopic pregnancy after consecutive tubal surgery include a history of infertility, previous salpingectomy or a prior ectopic pregnancy, and the presence of only one oviduct.

BIBLIOGRAPHY

Atrash HK, Friede A, Hogue CJ: Ectopic pregnancy mortality in the United States, 1970-1983, Obstet Gynecol 70:817, 1987.

Aleem FA, DeFazio M, and Gintautas J: Endovaginal sonography for the early diagnosis of intrauterine and ectopic pregnancies, Hum Reprod 5:755, 1990.

Ankum WM, Van der Veen F, Hamerlynck JVThH, and Lammes FB: Laparoscopy: a dispensable tool in the diagnosis of ectopic pregnancy, Hum Reprod 8:1301, 1993.

Ankum WM, Van der Veen F, Hamerlynck JVThH, and Lammes FB: Transvaginal sonography and human chorionic gonadotrophin measurements in suspected ectopic pregnancy: a detailed analysis of a diagnostic approach, Hum Reprod 8:1307, 1993.

Atri M, Bret PM, and Tulandi T: Spontaneous resolution of ectopic pregnancy: initial appearance and evolution at transvaginal US, Radiology 186:83, 1993.

Atri M, Bret PM, Tulandi T, and Senterman MK: Ectopic pregnancy: evolution after treatment with transvaginal methotrexate, Radiology 185:749, 1992.

Barnhart K, Mennuti MT, Benjamin I, et al: Prompt diagnosis of ectopic pregnancy in an emergency department setting, Obstet Gynecol 84:1010, 1994.

Bengtsson G, Brytman I, Thorburn J, and Lindblom B: Low-dose oral methotrexate as second-line therapy for persistent trophoblast after conservative treatment of ectopic pregnancy, Obstet Gynecol 79:589, 1992.

Breen JL: A 21-year survey of 654 ectopic pregnancies, Am J Obstet Gynecol 106:1004, 1970.

Brenner PF, Roy S, and Mishell DR Jr: Ectopic pregnancy: a study of 300 consecutive surgically treated cases, JAMA 243:673, 1980.

Budowick M, Johnson TRB, Genadry R, et al: The histopathology of the developing tubal ectopic pregnancy, Fertil Steril 34:169, 1980.

Buster JE and Carson SA: Ectopic pregnancy: new advances in diagnosis and treatment, Curr Opin Obstet Gynecol 7:168, 1995.

Cacciatore B, Korhnone J, Stenman UH, and Ylöstalo P: Transvaginal sonography and serum HCG in monitoring of presumed ectopic pregnancies selected for expectant management, Ultrasound Obstet Gynecol 5:297, 1995.

Cacciatore B, Stenman UH, Ylöstalo P, et al: Diagnosis of ectopic pregnancy by vaginal ultrasonography in combination with a discriminatory serum HCG level of 1000 IU/1 (IRP), Br J Obstet Gynaecol 97(10):904, 1990.

Carson SA and Buster JE: Ectopic pregnancy, N Engl J Med 329:1174, 1993.

Cartwright PS and DiPietro DL: Ectopic pregnancy: changes in serum human chorionic gonadotropin concentration, Obstet Gynecol 63:76, 1984.

Cartwright PS, Vaughn B, and Tuttle D: Culdocentesis and ectopic pregnancy, J Reprod Med 29:88, 1984.

Clark JF and Guy RS: Abdominal pregnancy, Am J Obstet Gynecol 96:511, 1966.

Clausen I: Conservative versus radical surgery for tubal pregnancy: a review, Acta Obstet Gynecol Scand 75:8, 1996.

Cole T and Corlett R Jr: Chronic ectopic pregnancy, Obstet Gynecol 59:63, 1982.

Corson SL and Batzer FR: Ectopic pregnancy: a review of the etiologic factors, J Reprod Med 31:78, 1986.

Cosin JA, Bean M, Grow D, et al: The use of methotrexate and arterial embolization to avoid surgery in a case of cervical pregnancy, Fertil Steril 67:1169, 1997.

DeCherney AH and Kase N: The conservative surgical management of unruptured ectopic pregnancy, Obstet Gynecol 54:451, 1979.

DeCherney AH and Maheux R: Modern management of tubal pregnancy, Curr Probl Obstet Gynecol 6:1, 1983.

DeCherney AH, Romero R, and Naftolin F: Surgical management of unruptured ectopic pregnancy, Fertil Steril 35:21, 1981.

Delke I, Veridiano NP, and Tancer ML: Abdominal pregnancy: review of current management and addition of 10 cases, Obstet Gynecol 60:200, 1982.

Di Marchi JM, Kosasa TS, Kobara TY, and Hale RW: Persistent ectopic pregnancy, Obstet Gynecol 70:555, 1987.

Dimitry ES, Margara R, Subak-Sharpe R, et al: Nine cases of heterotopic pregnancies in 4 years of in vitro fertilization, Fertil Steril 53:107, 1990.

Dorfman SF, Grimes DA, Cates W Jr, et al: Ectopic pregnancy mortality—United States, 1979 to 1980: clinical aspects, Obstet Gynecol 64:386, 1984.

Elias S, LeBeau M, Simpson JL, et al: Chromosome analysis of ectopic human conceptuses, Am J Obstet Gynecol 141:698, 1981.

Emerson DS, Cartier MS, Altieri LA, et al: Diagnostic efficacy of endovaginal color Doppler flow imaging in an ectopic pregnancy screening program, Radiology 183:413, 1992.

Fernandez H, Baton C, Benifla JL, et al: Methotrexate treatment of ectopic pregnancy: 100 cases treated by primary transvaginal injection under sonographic control, Fertil Steril 59:773, 1993.

Fernandez H, Coste J, and Job-Spira N: Controlled ovarian hyperstimulation as a risk factor for ectopic pregnancy, Obstet Gynecol 78:656, 1991.

Fernandez H, Lellaidier C, Thouvenez V, and Frydman R: The

use of a pretherapeutic, predictive score to determine inclusion criteria for the non-surgical treatment of ectopic pregnancy, Hum Reprod 6:995, 1991.

Fernandez H, Olivenes F, Pauthier S, et al: Ultrasound-guided injection of methotrexate versus laparoscopic salpingotomy in ectopic pregnancy, Fertil Steril 63:25, 1995.

Frates MC, Benson CB, Doubilet PM, et al: Cervical ectopic pregnancy: results of conservative treatment, Radiology 191:773, 1994.

Gaetano V and Henno D: Combined pregnancy: the Mount Sinai experience, Obstet Gynecol Surv 41:603, 1986.

Glock JL, Johnson JV, and Brumsted JR: Efficacy and safety of single-dose systemic methotrexate in the treatment of ectopic pregnancy, Fertil Steril 62:715, 1994.

Goldner TE, Lawson HW, Xia Z, and Atrash HK: Surveillance for ectopic pregnancy—United States, 1970-1989, MMWR 42(suppl 6):73, 1993.

Graczykowski JW, Mishell DR Jr: Methotrexate prophylaxis for persistent ectopic pregnancy after conservative treatment by salpingostomy, Obstet Gynecol 89: 118, 1997.

Green LK and Kott ML: Histopathologic findings in ectopic tubal pregnancy, Int J Gynecol Pathol 8:255, 1989.

Grimes DA, Geary FH Jr, and Hatcher RA: Rh immunoglobulin utilization after ectopic pregnancy, Am J Obstet Gynecol 140:246, 1981.

Gronlund B and Marushak A: Serial human chorionic gonadotrophin determination in the diagnosis of ectopic pregnancy, Aust N Z J Obstet Gynaecol 33:312, 1993.

Gruft L, Bertola E, Luchini L, et al: Determinants of reproductive prognosis after ectopic pregnancy, Hum Reprod 9:1333, 1994.

Hagstrom HG, Hahlin M, Bennegard-Eden B, et al: Prediction of persistent ectopic pregnancy after laparoscopic salpingostomy, Obstet Gynecol 84:798, 1994.

Hahlin M, Wallin A, Sjoblom P, and Lindblom B: Single progesterone assay for early recognition of abnormal pregnancy, Hum Reprod 5:662, 1990.

Hajenius PJ, Mol BWJ, Ankum WM, et al: Clearance curves of serum human chorionic gonadotrophin for the diagnosis of persistent trophoblast, Hum Reprod 10:683, 1995.

Hallatt JG: Primary ovarian pregnancy: a report of twenty-five cases, Am J Obstet Gynecol 143:55, 1982.

Handler A, Davis F, Ferre C, and Yeko T: The relationship of smoking and ectopic pregnancy, Am J Public Health 79:1239, 1989.

Hay DL, de Crespigny LC, and McKenna M: Monitoring early pregnancy with transvaginal ultrasound and choriogonadotrophin levels, Aust N Z J Obstet Gynaecol 29:165, 1989.

Herbst AL, Hubby MM, Azizi F, et al: Reproductive and gynecologic surgical experience in diethylstilbestrol-exposed daughters, Am J Obstet Gynecol 141:1019, 1981.

Holt VL, Daling JR, Voigt LF, et al: Induced abortion and the risk of subsequent ectopic pregnancy, Am J Public Health 70:1234, 1989.

Hoppe DE, Bekkar BE, and Nager MD: Single-dose systemic methotrexate for the treatment of persistent ectopic pregnancy after conservative surgery, Obstet Gynecol 83:51, 1994.

Ichinoe K, Wake H, Shinkai N, et al: Nonsurgical therapy to preserve oviduct function in patients with tubal pregnancies, Am J Obstet Gynecol 156:484, 1987.

Job-Spira N, Bouyer J, Pouly JL, et al: Fertility after ectopic pregnancy: first results of a population-based cohort study in France, Hum Reprod 11:99, 1996.

Johnson MR, Riddle AF, Irvine R, et al: Corpus luteum failure in ectopic pregnancy, Hum Reprod 8:1491, 1993.

Kadar N, Bohrer M, Kemmann E, and Shelden R: The discriminatory human chorionic gonadotropin zone for endovaginal sonography: a prospective, randomized study, Fertil Steril 61:1016, 1994.

Kadar N, Caldwell BV, and Romero R: A method of screening for ectopic pregnancy and its indications, Obstet Gynecol 58:162, 1981.

Kalchman GG and Meltzer RM: Interstitial pregnancy following homolateral salpingectomy, Am J Obstet Gynecol 196:1139, 1966.

Karikoski R, Aine R, and Heinonen PK: Abnormal embryogenesis in the etiology of ectopic pregnancy, Gynecol Obstet Invest 36:158, 1993.

Kaufman RH, Noller K, Adam E, et al: Upper genital tract abnormalities and pregnancy outcome in diethylstilbestrol-exposed progeny, Am J Obstet Gynecol 148:973, 1984.

Kirchler HC, Seebacher S, Alge AA, et al: Early diagnosis of tubal pregnancy: changes in tubal blood flow evaluated by endovaginal color Doppler sonography, Obstet Gynecol 82:561, 1993.

Korhonen J, Stenman UH, and Ylöstalo P: Serum human chorionic gonadotropin dynamics during spontaneous resolution of ectopic pregnancy, Fertil Steril 61:632, 1994.

Kratzer PG and Taylor RN: Corpus luteum function in early pregnancies is primarily determined by the rate of change of human chorionic gonadotropin levels, Am J Obstet Gynecol 163:1497, 1990.

Langer R, Raszier A, Ron-El R, et al: Reproductive outcome after conservative surgery for unruptured tubal pregnancy: a 15-year experience, Fertil Steril 53:227, 1990.

Ledger WL, Sweeting VM, and Chatterjee SP: Rapid diagnosis of early ectopic pregnancy in an emergency gynaecology service: are measurements of progesterone, intact and free β human chorionic gonadotrophin helpful? Hum Reprod 9:157, 1994.

Levin AA, Schoenbaum SC, Stubblefield PG, et al: Ectopic pregnancy and prior induced abortion, Am J Public Health 72:253, 1982.

Lindblom B, Hahlin M, Lundorff P, and Thorburn J: Treatment of tubal pregnancy by laparoscopy-guided injection of prostaglandin Fa$_2$, Fertil Steril 54:404, 1990.

Lindblom B, Hahlin M, Sjöblom P: Serial human chorionic gonadotropin determinations by fluoroimmunoassay for differentiation between intrauterine and ectopic gestation, Am J Obstet Gynecol 161:397, 1989.

Lipscomb GH, Bran D, McCord ML, et al: Analysis of three hundred fifteen ectopic pregnancies treated with single-dose methotrexate, Am J Obstet Gynecol 178:1354, 1998.

Lobel SM, Meyerovitz MF, Benson CC, et al: Preoperative angiographic uterine artery embolization in the management of cervical pregnancy, Obstet Gynecol 766:938, 1990.

Luc Pouly J, Canis M, Chapron C, et al: Multifactorial analysis of fertility after conservative laparoscopic treatment of ectopic pregnancy in a series of 223 patients, Fertil Steril 56:543, 1991.

Lund J: Early ectopic pregnancy, J Obstet Gynaecol Br Emp 62:70, 1955.

Lundorff P, Hahlin M, Sjöblom P, and Lindblom B: Persistent trophoblast after conservative treatment of tubal pregnancy: prediction and detection, Obstet Gynecol 77:129, 1991.

Lundorff P, Thorburn J, Hahlin M, et al: Adhesion formation after laparoscopic surgery in tubal pregnancy: a randomized trial versus laparotomy, Fertil Steril 55:911, 1991.

Majmudar B, Henderson PH III, and Semple E: Salpingitis isthmica nodosa: a high-risk factor for tubal pregnancy, Obstet Gynecol 62:73, 1983.

Makinen JI, Salmi TA, Nikkanen VPJ, and Koskineew EYJ: Encouraging rates of fertility after ectopic pregnancy, Int J Fertil 34:46, 1989.

Marchbanks PA and Annegers JF: Risk factors for ectopic pregnancy: population based study, JAMA 259:1823, 1988.

Mashiach S, Carp HA, and Serr DM: Nonoperative management of etopic pregnancy: a preliminary report, J Reprod Med 1:127, 1982.

Matthews CP, Coulson P, and Wild RA: Serum progesterone levels as an aid in the diagnosis of ectopic pregnancy, Obstet Gynecol 68:390, 1986.

McBain JC, Evans JH, Pepperell RJ, et al: An unexpectedly high rate of ectopic pregnancy following the induction of ovulation with human pituitary and chorionic gonadotrophin, Br J Obstet Gynaecol 87:5, 1980.

McCann MF and Kessel E: International experience with laparoscopic sterilization: follow-up of 8500 women, Adv Planned Parent 12.199, 1978.

McCausland A: Endosalpingosis ("endosalpingoblastosis") following laparoscopic tubal coagulation as an etiologic factor of ectopic pregnancy, Am J Obstet Gynecol 143:12, 1982.

McCord ML, Arheart KL, Muram D, et al: Single serum progesterone as a screen for ectopic pregnancy: exchanging specificity and sensitivity to obtain optimal test performance, Fertil Steril 66:513, 1996.

Mitra AG, Harris-Owens, M: Conservative medical management of advanced cervical ectopic pregnancies. Obstetrical and Gynecological Survey 55(6):385, 2000.

Miyazaki Y, Shrina Y, Wake N, et al: Studies on nonsurgical therapy of tubal pregnancy, Acta Obstet Gynaecol Jpn 35:489, 1983.

MMWR, Ectopic pregnancy—United States, 1988-1989, 41(suppl 32): 591, 1992.

MMWR, Ectopic pregnancy—United States, 1990-1992, 44(suppl 3):47, 1996.

Molloy D, Hynes J, Deambrosis W, et al: Multiple-sited (heterotopic) pregnancy after in vitro fertilization and gamete intrafallopian transfer, Fertil Steril 53:1068, 1990

Morris JM and Van Wagenen G: Interception: the use of postovulatory estrogens to prevent implantation, Am J Obstet Gynecol 115:101, 1973.

Nakajima ST, Nason FG, Badger GJ, and Gibson M: Progesterone production in early pregnancy, Fertil Steril 55:516, 1991.

Niles JH and Clark JJ: Pathogenesis of tubal pregnancy, Am J Obstet Gynecol 105:1230, 1969.

O'Leary JL and O'Leary JA: Rudimentary horn pregnancy, Obstet Gynecol 22:371, 1963.

O'Leary P, Nicols C, Feddema P, et al: Serum progesterone and human chorionic gonadotrophin measurements in the evaluation of ectopic pregnancy, Aust NS J Obstet Gynaecol 36:319, 1996.

Ollendorff BA and Felgin MD: The value of curettage in the diagnosis of ectopic pregnancy, Am J Obstet Gynecol 157:71, 1987.

Ory SJ: New options for diagnosis and treatment of ectopic pregnancy, JAMA 267(4):534, 1992.

Paalman RJ and McElin TW: Cervical pregnancy, Am J Obstet Gynecol 77:1261, 1959.

Pansky M, Golan A, Bukovsky I, and Caspi E: Nonsurgical management of tubal pregnancy, Am J Obstet Gynecol 164:888, 1991.

Parente JT, Ou CS, and Levy J: Cervical pregnancy analysis: a review and report of five cases, Obstet Gynecol 62:79, 1983.

Parker J and Bisits A: Laparoscopic surgical treatment of ectopic pregnancy: salpingectomy or salpingostomy? Aust NZ J Obstet Gynaecol 37:115, 1997.

Parker J, Permezel M, and Thompson D: Review of the management of ectopic pregnancy in a major teaching hospital: laparoscopic surgical treatment and persistent ectopic pregnancy, Aust N Z J Obstet Gynaecol 34:575, 1994.

Pellerito JS, Taylor KJ, Quedens-Case C, et al: Ectopic pregnancy: evaluation with endovaginal color flow imaging, Radiology 183:407, 1992.

Persaud V: Etiology of tubal ectopic pregnancy, Obstet Gynecol 36:257, 1970.

Peterson HB: Extratubal ectopic pregnancies, J Reprod Med 31:108, 1986.

Peterson HB, Xia Z, Hughes JM, et al. for the U.S. Collaborative Review of Sterilization Working Group: The risk of pregnancy after tubal sterilization: findings from the U.S. Collaborative Review of Sterilization, Am J Obstet Gynecol 174:1161, 1996.

Peterson HB, for the US Collaborative Review of Sterilization Working Group: The risk of ectopic pregnancy after tubal sterilization, N Engl J Med 336:762, 1997.

Pouly JL, Canis M, Chapron C, et al: Multifactorial analysis of fertility after conservative laparoscopic treatment of ectopic pregnancy in a series of 223 patients, Fertil Steril 56:453, 1991.

Pouly JL, Mahnes H, Mage G, et al: Conservative laparoscopic treatment of 321 ectopic pregnancies, Fertil Steril 46:1093, 1986.

Ransom MX, Garcia AJ, Bohrer M, et al: Serum progesterone as a predictor of methotrexate success in the treatment of ectopic pregnancy, Obstet Gynecol 83:1033, 1994.

Reece EA, Petrie RH, Sirmans MF, et al: Combined intrauterine and extrauterine gestations: a review, Am J Obstet Gynecol 146:323, 1983.

Risquez F, Reidy J, Forman R, et al: Transcervical cannulation of the fallopian tube for the management of ectopic pregnancy: prospective multicenter study, Fertil Steril 58:1131, 1992.

Romero R, Kadar H, Castro D, et al: The value of serial human chorionic gonadotropin testing as a diagnostic tool in ectopic pregnancy, Am J Obstet Gynecol 155:392, 1986.

Rose PG and Cohen SM: Methotrexate therapy for persistent ectopic pregnancy after conservative laparoscopic management, Obstet Gynecol 76:947, 1990.

Rubin GL, Peterson HB, Dorfman SF, et al: Ectopic pregnancy in the United States 1970 through 1978, JAMA 249:1725, 1983.

Saito M, Koyama T, Yaoi Y, et al: Site of ovulation and ectopic pregnancy, Acta Obstet Gynecol Scand 54:227, 1975.

Samuellson S and Sjovall A: Laparoscopy in suspected ectopic pregnancy, Acta Obstet Gynecol Scand 51:31, 1972.

Saraj AJ, Wilcox JG, Najmabadi S, et al: Resolution of hormonal markers of ectopic gestation: a randomized trial comparing single-dose intramuscular methotrexate with salpingostomy, Obstet Gynecol 92:989, 1998.

Sauer MV, Vermesh M, Anderson R, et al: Rapid measurement

of urinary pregnanediol glucuronide to diagnose ectopic pregnancy, Am J Obstet Gynecol 159:1531, 1988.

Seifer DB, Gutmann JN, Grant WD, et al: Comparison of persistent ectopic pregnancy after laparoscopic salpingostomy versus salpingostomy at laparotomy for ectopic pregnancy, Obstet Gynecol 81:378, 1993.

Shah A, Courney NG, Cunanan RG: Pregnancy following laparoscopic tubal electrocoagulation and division, Am J Obstet Gynecol 1129:459, 1977.

Shalev E, Romano S, Peleg D, et al: Spontaneous resolution of ectopic tubal pregnancy: natural history, Fertil Steril 63:15, 1995.

Sherman D, Langer R, Sadovsky G, et al: Improved fertility following ectopic pregnancy, Fertil Steril 37:497, 1982.

Sivin I: Copper T IUD use and ectopic pregnancy rates in the United States, Contraception 19:151, 1979.

Skeldestad FE, Hadgu A, and Eriksson N: Epidemiology of repeat ectopic pregnancy: a population-based prospective cohort study, Obstet Gynecol 91:129, 1998.

Spandorfer SD, Menzin AW, Barnhart KT, et al: Efficacy of frozen-section evaluation of uterine curettings in the diagnosis of ectopic pregnancy, Am J Obstet Gynecol 175:603, 1996.

Spandorfer SD, Sawin SW, Benjamin I, and Barnhart KT: Postoperative day 1 serum human chorionic gonadotropin level as a predictor of persistent ectopic pregnancy after conservative surgical management, Fertil Steril 68:430, 1997.

Stern JJ, Voss F, and Coulam CB: Early diagnosis of ectopic pregnancy using receiver-operator characteristic curves of serum progesterone concentrations, Hum Reprod 8:775, 1993.

Stock RJ: Persistent tubal pregnancy, Obstet Gynecol 77:267, 1991.

Stovall TG and Ling FW: Single-dose methotrexate: an expanded clinical trial, Am J Obstet Gynecol 168:1759, 1993.

Stovall TG, Ling FW, Anderson RN, and Buster JE: Improved sensitivity and specificity of a single measurement of serum progesterone over serial quantitative beta-human chorionic gonadotrophin in screening for ectopic pregnancy, Hum Reprod 7:723, 1992.

Stovall TG, Ling FW, Carson SA, and Buster JE: Serum progesterone and uterine curettage in differential diagnosis of ectopic pregnancy, Fertil Steril 67:456, 1992.

Stovall TG, Ling FW, Cope BJ, and Buster JE: Preventing ruptured ectopic pregnancy with a single serum progesterone, Am J Obstet Gynecol 160:1425, 1989.

Stovall TG, Ling FW, Gray LA, et al: Methotrexate treatment of unruptured ectopic pregnancy: a report of 100 cases, Obstet Gynecol 77:749, 1991.

Stovall TG, Ling F, Kellerman AL, and Buster JE: Outpatient chemotherapy of unruptured ectopic pregnancy, Fertil Steril 51:435, 1989.

Stratford B: Abnormalities of early human development, Am J Obstet Gynecol 107:1223, 1970.

Tanaka T, Hayashi H, Kutsuzawa T, et al: Treatment of interstitial ectopic pregnancy with methotrexate: report of a successful case, Fertil Steril 37:851, 1982.

Tatum HJ and Schmidt FH: Contraceptive and sterilization practices and extrauterine pregnancy: a realistic perspective, Fertil Steril 28:407, 1977.

Timonen S and Nieminen U: Tubal pregnancy, choice of operative method of treatment, Acta Obstet Gynecol Scand 46:327, 1967.

Trio D, Lapinski RH, Strobelt N, et al: Prognostic factors for successful expectant management of ectopic pregnancy, Fertil Steril 63:469, 1995.

Tulandi T, Falcone T, Atri M, et al: Transvaginal intratubal methotrexate treatment of ectopic pregnancy, Fertil Steril 58:98, 1992.

Tulandi T and Guralnick M: Treatment of tubal ectopic pregnancy by salpingotomy with or without tubal suturing and salpingectomy, Fertil Steril 55:53, 1991.

Tummon IS, Nisker JA, Whitmore NA, et al: Transferring more embryos increases risk of heterotopic pregnancy, Fertil Steril 61:1065, 1994.

Tuomivaara L and Kauppila A: Radical or conservative surgery for ectopic pregnancy? A follow-up study of fertility of 323 patients, Fertil Steril 50:580, 1988.

Vermesh M: Conservative management of ectopic gestation, Fertil Steril 51:559, 1989.

Vermesh M and Presser SC: Reproductive outcome after linear salpingostomy for ectopic gestation: a prospective 3-year follow-up, Fertil Steril 57:682, 1992.

Vermesh M, Silva PD, Rosen GF, et al: Management of unruptured ectopic gestation by linear salpingostomy: a prospective, randomized clinical trial of laparoscopy versus laparotomy, Obstet Gynecol 73:400, 1989.

Vermesh M, Silva PD, Rosen GF, et al: Persistent tubal ectopic gestation: patterns of circulation β-human chorionic gonadotropin and progesterone and management options, Fertil Steril 50:584, 1988.

Weckstein LN: Current perspective on ectopic pregnancy, Obstet Gynecol Surv 40:259, 1985.

Weckstein LN, Boucher AR, Tucker H, et al: Accurate diagnosis of early ectopic pregnancy, Obstet Gynecol 65:393, 1985.

Weström L, Bengtsson LPH, and Mårdh PA: Incidence, trends and risks of ectopic pregnancy in a population of women, Br Med J 282:15, 1981.

Wong YH, Liang EY, and Lau, KY: A cervical ectopic pregnancy managed by medical treatment and angiographic embolization. Aust NZ J Obstet Gynecol 39(4):493, 1999.

Yao M, Tulandi T: Current status of surgical and nonsurgical management of ectopic pregnancy, Fertil Steril 67:421, 1997.

Yeko TR, Gorrill MJ, Hughes LH, et al: Timely diagnosis of early ectopic pregnancy using a single blood progesterone measurement, Fertil Steril 48:10, 1987.

Ylöstalo P, Cacciatore B, Sjoberg J, et al: Expectant management of ectopic pregnancy, Obstet Gynecol 80:345, 1992.

CHAPTER
18

Benign Gynecologic Lesions
Vulva, Vagina, Cervix,
Uterus, Oviduct, Ovary

KEY TERMS AND DEFINITIONS

Brenner Tumor. A small, smooth, solid fibroepithelial tumor of the ovary. It may be benign or malignant.

Degeneration of a Myoma. The process by which a myoma outgrows its blood supply and begins to necrose centrally. Forms of degeneration include hyaline, myxomatous, calcific, cystic, fat, and red degeneration.

Dermoid (Benign Cystic Teratoma). A benign germ cell tumor that contains well-differentiated derivatives of all three germ cell layers.

Dysontogenetic Cysts. Thin-walled cysts of embryonic origin.

Endometrial Polyp. A localized outgrowth of endometrial glands and stroma projecting beyond the surface of the endometrium and including a vascular stalk.

Follicular Hematoma. Follicular cysts filled with blood, usually from hemorrhage in the vascular theca zone.

Gartner's Duct Cysts. Cysts primarily of mesonephric origin found laterally in the vagina.

Hematometra. A uterus distended with blood, secondary to partial or complete obstruction of any portion of the lower genital tract.

Hidradenitis Suppurativa. A chronic infection involving skin, subcutaneous tissue, and apocrine glands.

Hidradenoma. A rare, small, benign vulvar tumor originating from apocrine sweat glands.

Hydatid Cysts of Morgagni. Pedunculated paratubal cysts found near the fimbria of the oviduct.

Hydrometra. A collection of clear fluid in the uterine cavity.

Hyperreactio Luteinalis. Multiple theca lutein cysts causing bilateral ovarian enlargement during pregnancy.

Intravenous Leiomyomatosis. An extremely rare condition in which benign smooth muscle fibers invade and slowly grow into the venous channels of the pelvis.

Itch-Scratch Cycles. Repetitive cycles of itching leading to scratching. The scratching leads to excoriation, irritation, and healing, with subsequent irritation and itching.

Leiomyoma (Myoma or Fibroid). A benign tumor of muscle cell origin found in any tissue that contains smooth muscle.

Leiomyomatosis Peritonealis Disseminata. A benign disease with multiple small nodules over the surface of the pelvis and abdominal peritoneum, grossly mimicking disseminated carcinoma or sarcoma.

Lichenification. Changes in the skin from chronic irritation, characterized by whiteness, thickening, and leathery appearance.

Luteoma of Pregnancy. A rare, specific, benign, hyperplastic reaction of ovarian theca lutein cells during pregnancy.

Meigs' Syndrome. The constellation of symptoms of ascites and hydrothorax associated with a benign ovarian fibroma, resolving after the removal of the tumor.

Nabothian Cysts. Cervical retention cysts lined by endocervical-type columnar cells.

Parasitic Myoma. A myoma that outgrows its uterine blood supply and obtains a secondary blood supply from another organ, such as the omentum.

Prominence or Tubercle of Rokitansky. The protrusion of solid elements of a dermoid into the cyst cavity.

479

Pruritus. A symptom of intense itching with an associated desire to scratch.

Pyometra. A collection of pus in the uterine cavity.

Struma Ovarii. A specialized ovarian teratoma that consists of thyroid tissue as a major or exclusive component. Rarely, it may produce sufficient thyroid hormone to induce hyperthyroidism.

Submucosal Myoma. A myoma located immediately below the endometrial lining.

Subserosal Myoma. A myoma found just beneath the serosa of the uterus.

Syringoma. A benign tumor of the eccrine sweat glands.

Vulvodynia. A term describing chronic vulvar discomfort.

This book is divided primarily into chapters dealing with benign diseases and chapters dealing with malignant ones. For the clinician, however, the difference is not always clear. As in many areas of medicine, gynecologic problems do not fall into definitive categories, and those that include malignant disease often overlap with those that include benign disease. When the diagnosis from the history, physical examination, and laboratory tests is clear, management is usually self-evident. When a specific diagnosis is unclear, tissue biopsy is appropriate. This chapter deals primarily with benign lesions; however, the symptoms and differential diagnoses of these lesions have definite overlap with those of malignant disease.

The discussions in this chapter are arranged anatomically, beginning with the vulva and subsequently covering the vagina, cervix, uterus, oviducts, and ovaries. This chapter does not attempt to be encyclopedic; rather, lesions have been selected based on their clinical importance and prevalence. Therefore, extremely rare lesions such as glomus tumors of the vulva or papillomas of the cervix have been omitted. Because several nonneoplastic abnormalities and lesions present in ways similar to those of benign tumors, this chapter also discusses entities that are not specifically abnormal growths. Clinical problems such as torsion of the ovary, lacerations of the vagina, and hematomas of the vulva are examples of common conditions included in this chapter.

The successful clinician must use both deductive and inductive reasoning in solving a problem. To have mastered both these techniques, he or she not only must be adept at history taking and physical examination but also must be able to form a complete list of possible lesions that may be involved in the patient's complaint. An understanding of the entities of this chapter will be helpful toward that goal.

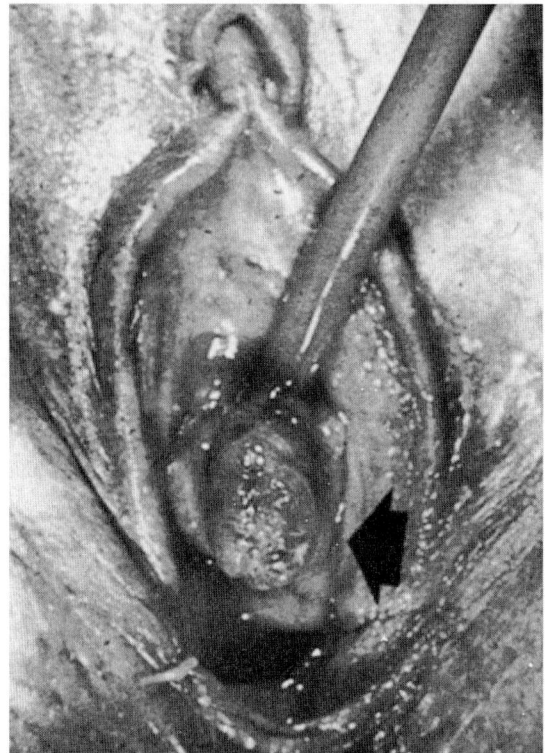

FIGURE 18-1 Large benign urethral caruncle, thought clinically to be urethral carcinoma because of its size *(arrow)*. (From Marshall FC, Uson AC, and Melicow MM: Surg Gynecol Obstet 110:724, 1960. By permission of Surgery, Gynecology & Obstetrics.)

VULVA

Urethral Caruncle

A urethral caruncle is a small, fleshy outgrowth of the distal edge of the urethra. The tissue of the caruncle is soft, smooth, friable, and bright red and initially appears as an eversion of the urethra (Figure 18-1). Urethral caruncles are generally small, single, and sessile but may be pedunculated and grow to be 1 to 2 cm in diameter. They occur most frequently in postmenopausal women and must be differentiated from urethral carcinomas. Urethral caruncles are believed to arise from an ectropion of the posterior urethral wall associated with retraction and atrophy of the postmenopausal vagina. The growth of the caruncle is secondary to chronic irritation or infection. Histologically the caruncle is composed of transitional and stratified squamous epithelium with a loose connective tissue (Figure 18-2). Often the submucosal layer contains relatively large dilated veins. Caruncles are

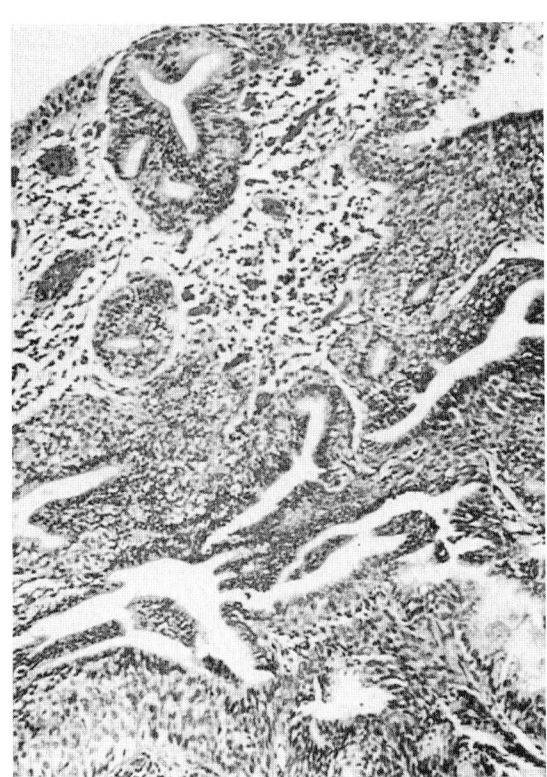

FIGURE 18-2 Urethral caruncle. Hyperemia, inflammation, and some infolding of transitional epithelium. (H&E stain.) From Kaufman RH: Solid tumors. In Kaufman RH and Faro S, editors: Benign diseases of the vulva and vagina, ed 4, St. Louis, 1994, Mosby–Year Book.)

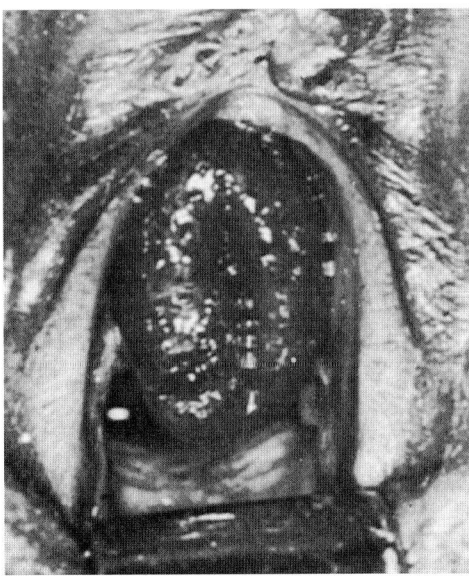

FIGURE 18-3 Prolapse of urethral mucosa in 7-year-old child. Edematous red collar of tissue surrounds urethral meatus. (From Kaufman RH: Solid tumors. In Kaufman RH and Faro S, editors: Benign diseases of the vulva and vagina, ed 4, St. Louis, 1994, Mosby–Year Book.)

frequently subdivided by their histologic appearance into papillomatous, granulomatous, and angiomatous varieties. They are often secondarily infected, producing ulceration and bleeding. If the diagnosis of a urethral caruncle is entertained in a child, most likely the correct diagnosis is urethral prolapse.

The symptoms associated with urethral caruncles are variable. Many women are asymptomatic, whereas others experience dysuria, frequency, and urgency. Sometimes the caruncle produces point tenderness after contact with undergarments or during intercourse. Ulcerative lesions usually produce spotting on contact more commonly than hematuria.

The differential diagnosis of urethral caruncles includes primary carcinoma of the urethra and prolapse of the urethral mucosa. Although urethral caruncles are not a precursor for urethral carcinoma, grossly the two are often confused. Marshall et al. reported a series of 394 urethral tumors. A clinical diagnosis of urethral caruncle was made in 376 of these women. Histologic examination of biopsy material demonstrated urethral carcinoma in nine patients in their series. Approximately 1 in 40 women with a clinical diagnosis of urethral caruncle has a malignant urethral neoplasm. Urethral carcinoma is pri-

marily a disease of elderly women. The majority of urethral carcinomas are of squamous cell origin. Most of these rare carcinomas arise from the distal urethra. The symptoms of a urethral carcinoma include bleeding, urinary frequency, and dysuria, and the signs include a mass protruding from the urethra, with associated tenderness and induration of the urethra.

The diagnosis of a urethral caruncle is established by biopsy under local anesthesia. Initial therapy is oral or topical estrogen and avoidance of irritation. If the caruncle does not regress or is symptomatic, it may be destroyed by cryosurgery, laser therapy, fulguration, or operative excision. Following operative destruction, a Foley catheter should be left in place for 48 to 72 hours. Follow-up is necessary to ensure that the patient does not develop urethral stenosis. Often the caruncle may recur. Small, asymptomatic urethral caruncles do not need treatment.

Urethral prolapse is predominantly a disease of the premenarchal female (Figure 18-3), although it does occur in postmenopausal women. Patients may have dysuria; however, the majority are asymptomatic. The annular rosette of friable, edematous, prolapsed mucosa does not have the bright-red color of a caruncle and is not as circumscribed in gross configuration. It may be ulcerated with necrosis or grossly edematous. Therapy of a prolapsed urethra is hot sitz baths and antibiotics to reduce inflammation and infection. Topical estrogen cream is sometimes an effective treatment. In rare cases it may be necessary to excise the redundant mucosa.

Cysts

The most common large cyst of the vulva is a cystic dilation of an obstructed Bartholin's duct. Approximately 2% of new gynecologic patients present with an asymptomatic Bartholin's duct cyst. Treatment is not necessary in women younger than 40 unless the cyst becomes infected or enlarges enough to produce symptoms. A more complete discussion of Bartholin's duct cysts and abscesses is included in Chapter 22. Occasionally the ducts of mucous glands of the vestibule are occluded. The resulting cysts may be clear, yellow, or blue. Similar small mucous cysts occur in the periurethral region. Wolffian duct cysts or mesonephric cysts are rare, but when they do occur, they are found near the clitoris and lateral to the hymeneal ring. These cysts have thin walls and contain clear serous fluid.

The most common small vulvar cysts are epidermal inclusion cysts or sebaceous cysts. Because these cysts cannot be differentiated grossly and since a continuing controversy exists with respect to their histogenesis, these two cysts are discussed together in this chapter. However, numerically, many more epithelial cysts are discovered, sebaceous cysts of the vulva being a rarity. These cysts are located immediately beneath the epidermis. Most commonly they are discovered on the anterior half of the labia majora. These cysts are usually multiple, freely movable, round, slow growing, and nontender. They are firm to shotty in consistency, and their contents are usually under pressure. Grossly, they are white or yellow, and the contents are caseous, like a thick cheese. Local scarring of the adjacent skin sometimes occurs when rupture of the contents of the cyst produces an inflammatory reaction in the subcutaneous tissue.

An inclusion cyst may develop following trauma when an infolding of squamous epithelium has occurred beneath the epidermis in the site of an episiotomy or obstetric laceration. Most inclusion cysts of the vagina are directly related to previous trauma, while most inclusion cysts of the vulva are not related to trauma. Alternative theories of histogenesis include embryonic remnants and occlusion of pilosebaceous ducts of sweat glands. The histology of these cysts is characterized by an epithelial lining of keratinized, stratified squamous epithelium with a center of cellular debris that grossly resembles sebaceous material. Most vulvar epidermal cysts do not have sebaceous cells or sebaceous material identified on microscopic examination. Usually there are multiple cysts, with the vast majority being less than 1 cm in diameter. These cysts are asymptomatic unless they are secondarily infected. Large epidermal cysts may be confused with fibromas, lipomas, and hidradenomas.

Most of these cysts require no treatment. If the cyst becomes infected, treatment consists of heat applied locally and incision and drainage. Cysts that become recurrently infected or produce pain should be excised when the acute inflammation has subsided.

Nevus

A nevus, commonly referred to as a *mole*, is a localized nest or cluster of melanocytes. These undifferentiated cells arise from the embryonic neural crest and are present from birth. Many nevi are not recognized until they become pigmented at the time of puberty. Vulvar nevi are one of the most common benign neoplasms in females. As with nevi in other parts of the body, they exhibit a wide range in depth of color, from blue to dark brown to black, and some may be amelanotic. The diameter of most nevi ranges from a few millimeters to 2 cm. Grossly, a benign nevus may be flat, elevated, or pedunculated. Other pigmented lesions in the differential diagnosis include hemangiomas, endometriosis, malignant melanoma, vulvar intraepithelial neoplasia, and seborrheic keratosis.

Vulvar nevi are generally asymptomatic. Most women do not closely inspect their vulvar skin and are unaware of biologic changes in gross appearance of these lesions. Histologically the lesions are subdivided into three major groups: junctional, compound (Figure 18-4), and intradermal nevi.

Although the vulvar area contains approximately 1% of the skin surface of the body, 5% to 10% of all malignant melanomas in women arise from this region. The biologic reasons for this discrepancy are unknown. Speculation includes the hypothesis that junctional activity is common in vulvar nevi, and the many irritants to which vulvar skin is exposed may lead to malignancy. It is estimated that 50% of malignant melanomas arise from a preexisting nevus. The majority of women who develop melanomas are in their 50s.

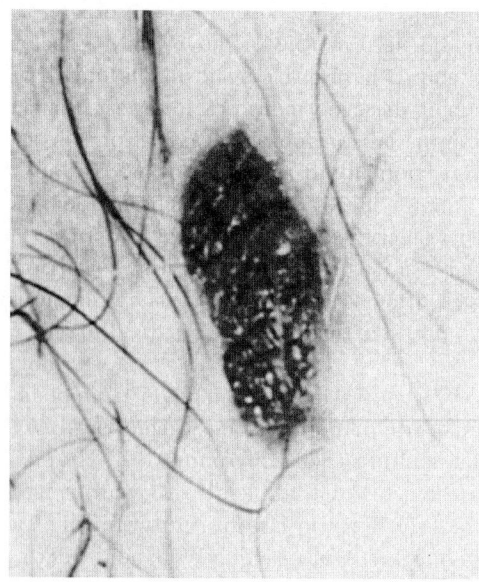

FIGURE 18-4 Compound nevus, usually a slightly elevated pigmented lesion. (From Kaufman RH: Solid tumors. In Kaufman RH and Faro S, editors: Benign diseases of the vulva and vagina, ed 4, St. Louis, 1994, Mosby–Year Book.)

Ideally, all flat vulvar nevi should be excised and examined histologically. Special emphasis should be directed toward the flat junctional nevus and the dysplastic nevus for they have the greatest potential for malignant transformation. The lifetime risk of a woman developing melanoma from a congenital junctional nevus that measures greater than 2 cm in diameter is estimated to be approximately 10%. The dysplastic nevus is characterized by being more than 5 mm in diameter, with irregular borders and patches of variegated pigment. Removal may be accomplished with local anesthesia or coincidentally with obstetric delivery or gynecologic surgery. Proper excisional biopsy should be three dimensional and adequate in width and depth. Approximately 5 to 10 mm of normal skin surrounding the nevus should be included, and the biopsy should include the underlying dermis as well. Some patients are reluctant to have a "normal"-appearing nevus removed. Nevi that are raised or contain hair rarely undergo malignant change. However, if they are frequently irritated or bleed spontaneously, they should be removed. Recent changes in growth or color, ulceration, bleeding, pain, or the development of satellite lesions mandate biopsy. Friedman et al. (1985) listed the characteristic clinical features of an early malignant melanoma, which may be remembered by thinking ABCD: *asymmetry*, *border* irregularity, *color* variegation, and a *diameter* usually greater than 6 mm.

Hemangioma

Hemangiomas are rare malformations of blood vessels rather than true neoplasms. Vulvar hemangiomas frequently are discovered initially during childhood. They are usually single, 1 to 2 cm in diameter, flat, and soft, and they range in color from brown to red or purple. Histologically the multiple channels of hemangiomas are predominantly thin-walled capillaries arranged randomly and separated by thin connective tissue septa. These tumors change in size with compression and are not encapsulated. Most hemangiomas are asymptomatic; occasionally they may become ulcerated and bleed.

There are at least five different types of vulvar hemangiomas. The strawberry and cavernous hemangiomas are congenital defects discovered in young children. The strawberry hemangioma is usually bright red to dark red, is elevated, and rarely increases in size after age 2. Approximately 60% of vulvar hemangiomas discovered during the first years of life spontaneously regress in size by the time the child goes to school. Cavernous hemangiomas are usually purple in color and vary in size, with the larger lesions extending deeply into the subcutaneous tissue. These hemangiomas initially appear during the first few months of life and may increase in size until age 2. Similar to strawberry hemangiomas, spontaneous resolution generally occurs before age 6. Senile or cherry angiomas are common small lesions that arise on the labia majora, usually in postmenopausal women. They are most often less than 3 mm in diameter, multiple, and red-brown to dark blue. Angiokeratomas are approximately twice the size of cherry angiomas, are purple or dark red, and occur in women between the ages of 30 and 50. They are noted for their rapid growth and tendency to bleed during strenuous exercise. In the differential diagnosis of an angiokeratoma is Kaposi's sarcoma and angiosarcoma. Pyogenic granulomas are an overgrowth of inflamed granulation tissue. These lesions grow under the hormonal influence of pregnancy, with similarities to lesions in the oral cavity. Pyogenic granulomas are usually approximately 1 cm in diameter and may be mistaken clinically for malignant melanomas, basal cell carcinomas, vulvar condylomas, or nevi. Treatment of pyogenic granulomas involves wide and deep excision to prevent recurrence.

The diagnosis is usually established by gross inspection of the vascular lesion. Asymptomatic hemangiomas and hemangiomas in children rarely require therapy. In adults, initial treatment of large symptomatic hemangiomas that are bleeding or infected may require subtotal resection. When the differential diagnosis is questionable, excisional biopsy should be performed. A hemangioma that is associated with troublesome bleeding may be destroyed by cryosurgery or use of an argon laser. Cryosurgical treatment usually involves a single freeze/thaw cycle repeated three times at monthly intervals. Obviously, if the histologic diagnosis is questionable, any bleeding vulvar mass should be treated by excisional biopsy so that the definitive pathologic diagnosis can be established. Surgical removal of a large, cavernous hemangioma may be technically quite difficult. Lymphangiomas of the vulva do exist but are extremely rare.

Fibroma

Fibromas are the most common benign solid tumors of the vulva. They are more frequent than lipomas, the other common benign tumors of mesenchymal origin. Fibromas occur in all age groups and most commonly are found in the labia majora (Figure 18-5). However, they actually arise from deeper connective tissue. Thus they should be considered as dermatofibromas. They grow slowly and vary from a few centimeters to one gigantic vulvar fibroma reported to weigh more than 250 pounds. The majority are between 1 and 10 cm in diameter. The smaller fibromas are discovered as subcutaneous nodules. As they increase in size and weight, they become pedunculated. Smaller fibromas are firm; however, larger tumors often become cystic after undergoing myxomatous degeneration. Sometimes the vulvar skin over a fibroma is compromised by pressure and ulcerates.

Fibromas have a smooth surface and a distinct contour. On cut surface the tissue is gray-white. Fat or muscle cells microscopically may be associated with the interlacing fibroblasts. Fibromas have a low-grade potential for

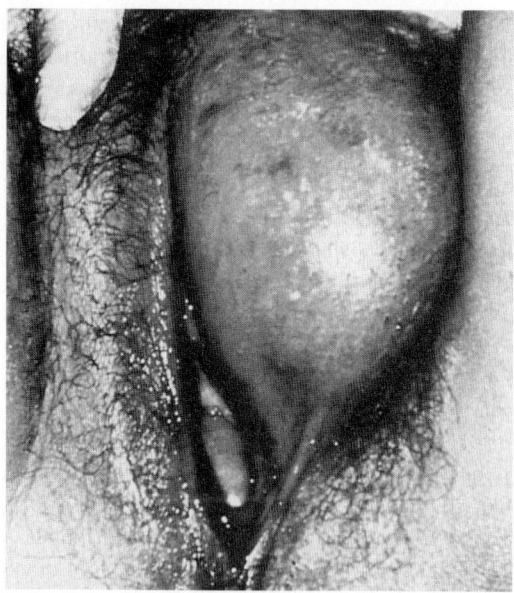

FIGURE 18-5 Vulvar fibroma, which is the most common benign solid tumor of the vulva. (From Friedrich EG, editor: Vulvar disease, ed 2, Philadelphia, 1983, WB Saunders Co, p 283.)

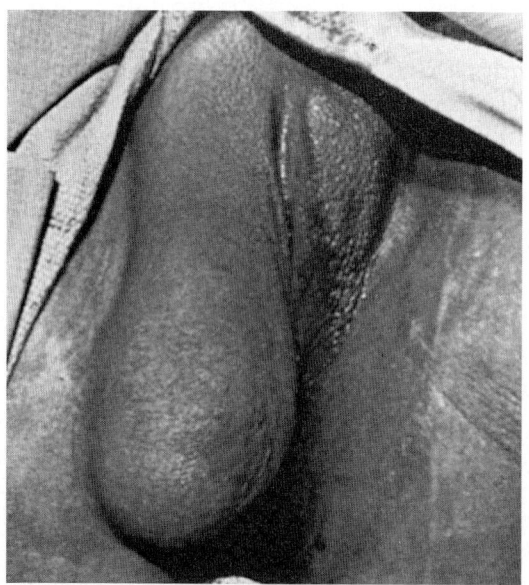

FIGURE 18-6 Lipoma. (From Friedrich EG, editor: Vulvar disease, ed 2, Philadelphia, 1983, WB Saunders Co, p 233.)

becoming malignant. Smaller fibromas are asymptomatic; larger tumors may produce chronic pressure symptoms or acute pain when they degenerate. Treatment is operative removal if the fibromas are symptomatic and/or continue to grow. Occasionally they are removed for cosmetic reasons.

Lipoma

Lipomas are benign, slow-growing, circumscribed tumors of fat cells arising from the subcutaneous tissue of the vulva (Figure 18-6). Lipomas of the vulva are similar to lipomas of other parts of the body. When discovered they are softer and usually larger than fibromas. The majority of lipomas in the vulvar region are smaller than 3 cm in diameter. The largest vulvar lipoma reported in the literature weighed 44 pounds. Lipomas are the second most frequent benign vulvar mesenchymal tumor. Because of the fat distribution of the vulva, most lipomas are discovered in the labia majora and are superficial in location. They are slow growing, and their malignant potential is extremely low.

When a lipoma is cut, the substance is soft, yellow, and lobulated. Histologically, lipomas are usually more homogeneous than fibromas. Prominent areas of connective tissue occasionally are associated with the mature adipose cells of a true lipoma. Unless extremely large, lipomas do not produce symptoms. Excision is usually performed to establish the diagnosis, although smaller tumors may be followed conservatively.

Hidradenoma

The hidradenoma is a rare, small, benign vulvar tumor that originates from apocrine sweat glands of the inner surface of the labia majora and nearby perineum. Occasionally, they may originate from eccrine sweat glands. For unknown reasons, they are discovered exclusively in white women between the ages of 30 and 70, most commonly in the fourth decade of life. These tumors have not been reported prior to puberty. Hidradenomas may be cystic or solid. In a review by Woodworth et al., 55% were cystic. While 38% originated from the labia majora, 26% arose from the labia minora. Approximately 50% of hidradenomas are less than 1 cm in diameter.

These tumors are well defined and usually sessile, pinkish-gray nodules not larger than 2 cm in diameter. In most cases the surface epithelium is white, but occasionally necrosis of a central indented area occurs, with a protrusion of reddish-brown granulation tissue. These latter lesions may be confused with pyogenic granulomas.

These tumors have well-defined capsules. These papillary tumors arise deep in the dermis. Histologically, because of its hyperplastic, adenomatous pattern, a hidradenoma may be mistaken at first glance for an adenocarcinoma. On close inspection, however, although there is glandular hyperplasia with numerous tubular ducts, there is a paucity of mitotic figures and a lack of significant cellular and nuclear pleomorphism (Figure 18-7). Hidradenomas are generally asymptomatic. However, they may cause pruritus or bleeding if the tumor undergoes necrosis. Excisional biopsy is the treatment of choice.

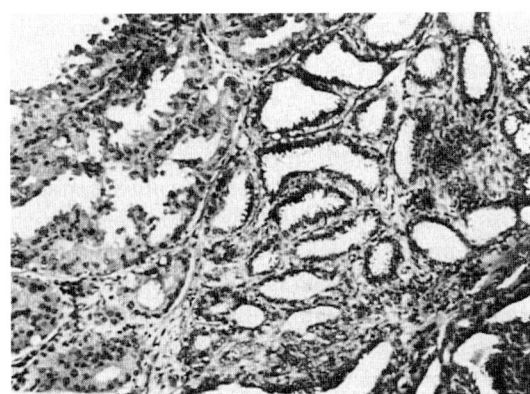

FIGURE 18-7 Hidradenoma. Numerous acini. Distinct apocrine gland-type epithelium is present on left. (H&E stain.) (From Kaufman RH: Cystic tumors. In Kaufman RH and Faro S, editors: Benign diseases of the vulva and vagina, ed 4, St. Louis, 1994, Mosby–Year Book.)

Syringoma

The syringoma is a very rare, cystic, asymptomatic, benign tumor that is an adenoma of the eccrine sweat glands. It appears as small subcutaneous papules, less than 5 mm in diameter, that are either skin colored or yellow and that may coalesce to form cords of firm tissue. In the vulvar area, these asymptomatic papules are usually located in the labia majora. Identical tumors are often found in the eccrine glands of the eyelids. This tumor is usually treated by excisional biopsy or cryosurgery. The most common differential diagnosis is Fox-Fordyce disease, a condition of multiple retention cysts of apocrine glands accompanied by inflammation of the skin. The latter disease often produces intense pruritus, while syringoma is generally asymptomatic. Fox-Fordyce disease is treated by oral or topical estrogens and topical retinoic acid.

Endometriosis

Endometriosis of the vulva is rare. Only 1 in 500 women with endometriosis will present with vulvar lesions. The firm, small nodule or nodules may be cystic or solid and vary from a few millimeters to several centimeters in diameter. The subcutaneous lesions are blue, red, or purple, depending on their size, activity, and closeness to the surface of the skin. The gross and microscopic pathologic picture of vulvar endometriosis is similar to endometriosis of the pelvis (Chapter 19). Vulvar adenosis may appear similar to endometriosis. The former condition occurs following laser therapy of condyloma acuminata.

Endometriosis of the vulva is usually found at the site of an old, healed obstetric laceration, episiotomy site, an area of operative removal of a Bartholin's duct cyst, or along the canal of Nuck. The pathophysiology of develop-

ment of vulvar endometriosis may be secondary to metaplasia, retrograde lymphatic spread, or potential implantation of endometrial tissue during operation. Paull and Tedeschi documented 15 cases of vulvar endometriosis they believed were associated with prophylactic postpartum curettage of the uterus to prevent postpartum bleeding. In their series there was not a single case of vulvar endometriosis in 13,800 deliveries without curettage, but 15 cases of vulvar endometriosis were associated with 2028 deliveries with prophylactic curettage. In general, symptoms do not appear for many months following implantation.

The most common symptoms of endometriosis of the vulva are pain and introital dyspareunia. The classic history is cyclic discomfort and an enlargement of the mass associated with menstrual periods. Treatment of vulvar endometriosis is by wide excision or laser vaporization depending on the size of the mass. Recurrences are common following inadequate operative removal of all the involved area.

Granular Cell Myoblastoma

Granular cell myoblastoma is a rare, slow-growing, solid vulvar tumor. The tumor originates from neural sheath (Schwann) cells and is sometimes called a *schwannoma*. These tumors are found in connective tissues throughout the body, most commonly in the tongue, and occur in any age group. Approximately 7% of solitary granular cell myoblastomas are found in the subcutaneous tissue of the vulva. Twenty percent of multiple granular cell myoblastomas are located in the vulva. The tumors are usually located in the labia majora, but occasionally involve the clitoris.

These tumors are subcutaneous nodules, usually 1 to 5 cm in diameter. They are benign but characteristically infiltrate the surrounding local tissue. The tumors are slow growing, but as they grow, they may cause ulcerations in the skin. The overlying skin often has hyperplastic changes that may look similar to invasive squamous cell carcinoma. Grossly, these tumors are not encapsulated. The cut surface of the tumor is yellow. Histologically, there are irregularly arranged bundles of large, round cells with indistinct borders and pink-staining cytoplasm. Initially the cell of origin was believed to be striated muscle; however, electron microscopic studies have demonstrated that this tumor is from cells of the neural sheath.

The tumor nodules are painless. Treatment involves wide excision to remove the filamentous projections into the surrounding tissue. If the initial excisional biopsy is not adequate and aggressive enough, these benign tumors tend to recur. Recurrence occurs in approximately one in five of these vulvar tumors. The appropriate therapy is a second operation with wider margins, since these tumors are not radiosensitive.

von Recklinghausen's Disease

The vulva is sometimes involved with the benign neural sheath tumors of von Recklinghausen's disease (generalized neurofibromatous and café-au-lait spots). The vulvar lesions of this disease are fleshy, brownish red, polypoid tumors. Approximately 18% of women with von Recklinghausen's disease have vulvar involvement. Excision is the treatment of choice for symptomatic tumors.

Other Abnormal Tissue

Other examples of diseases or aberrant tissue presenting as vulvar masses include leiomyomas, myomas, squamous papillomas, sebaceous adenomas, dermoids, accessory breast tissue and müllerian or wolffian duct remnants, epidermal inclusion cysts, sebaceous cysts, mucous cysts, and skin diseases such as seborrheic keratosis, condyloma acuminata, and molluscum contagiosum. Some of these diseases are discussed in this chapter, others in Chapter 22.

Hematomas

Hematomas of the vulva are usually secondary to blunt trauma such as a straddle injury from a fall, an automobile accident, or a physical assault. Traumatic injuries producing vulvar hematomas have been reported secondary to a wide range of recreational activities, including bicycle, motorcycle, and go-cart riding; sledding; water skiing; cross-country skiing; and amusement park rides (Figure 18-8). Spontaneous hematomas are rare and usually occur from rupture of a varicose vein during pregnancy or the postpartum period.

The management of nonobstetrical vulvar hematomas is usually conservative unless the hematoma is greater than 10 cm in diameter or is rapidly expanding. The bleeding that produces a vulvar hematoma is usually venous in origin. Therefore it may be controlled by direct pressure. Compression and application of an ice pack to the area are appropriate therapy. If the hematoma continues to expand, operative therapy is indicated in an attempt to identify and ligate the damaged vessel. Often identification of the "key responsible vein" is a futile operative procedure. However, obvious bleeding vessels are ligated, and a pack is placed to promote hemostasis. During the operation careful inspection and, if needed, endoscopy is performed to rule out injury to the urinary bladder and rectosigmoid.

The majority of small hematomas regress with time. However, Reid et al. have emphasized the problems associated with a chronic expanding hematoma. The most familiar clinical example of this problem is the chronic subdural hematoma, but a similar situation may accompany vulvar hematomas. The underlying pathophysiology is the repetitive episodes of bleeding from capillaries in the granulation tissue of the hematoma, which result in a chronic,

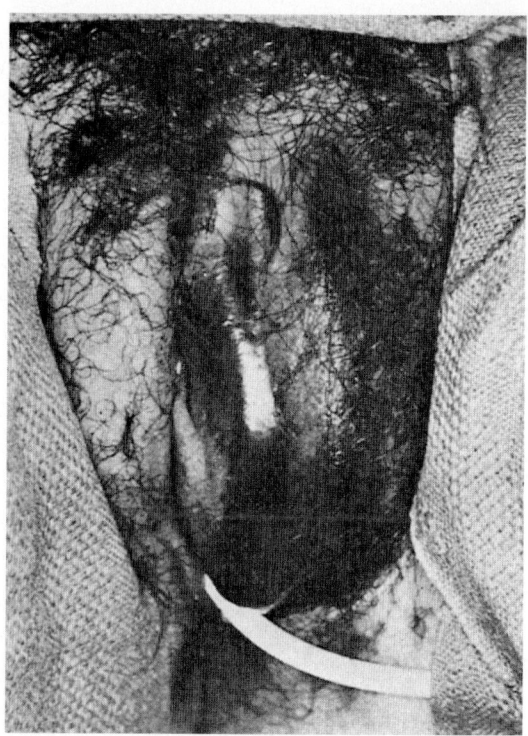

FIGURE 18-8   Vulva hematoma from straddle injury that produced urethral obstruction. (From Naumann RO and Droegemueller W: Am J Obstet Gynecol 142:358, 1982.)

slowly expanding vulvar mass. Treatment of a chronic expanding hematoma is drainage and debridement.

DERMATOLOGIC DISEASES

The skin of the vulva is similar to the skin over any surface of the body and is therefore susceptible to any generalized skin disease or involvement by systemic disease. The most common skin diseases involving the vulva include contact dermatitis, neurodermatitis, psoriasis, seborrheic dermatitis, cutaneous candidiasis, and lichen planus. The majority of vulvar skin problems are red, scalelike rashes, and the woman's primary complaint is of pruritus. The diagnosis and treatment of these lesions are often obscured or modified by the environment of the vulva. The combination of moisture and heat of the intertriginous areas may produce irritation, maceration, and a wet, weeping surface. Therefore it is important that the gynecologist examine the skin of the entire body, because the patient may have more classic lesions of the dermatologic disease in another location. The skin of the vulva is susceptible to acute infections produced by streptococcus or staphylococcus, such as folliculitis, furunculitis, impetigo, and a special chronic infection, hidradenitis suppurativa.

The nonspecific symptom complex of vulvar pruritus

and burning is presented next as an introduction to the discussion of dermatologic diseases of the vulva.

Pruritus and Vulvodynia

Pruritus is a symptom of intense itching with an associated desire to scratch and rub the affected area. In some women pruritus becomes an almost unrelenting symptom, with the development of repetitive "itch-scratch" cycles. The itch-scratch cycle is a complex of itching leading to scratching, producing excoriation and then healing. The healing skin itches, leading to further scratching. *Vulvodynia* is a term developed to describe chronic vulvar discomfort, including burning, stinging, and "rawness." Patients with persistent vulvodynia in which a physical cause has not been identified are often grouped under the semantic term *burning vulvar syndrome.* Pruritus and vulvodynia are nonspecific symptoms, and they are not interrelated. Their differential diagnosis includes a wide range of vulvar diseases, including skin infections, sexually transmitted diseases, specific dermatosis, vulvar dystrophies, lichen sclerosus, premalignant and malignant disease, contact dermatitis, neurodermatitis, atrophy, diabetes, drug allergies, vitamin deficiencies, pediculosis, scabies, psychologic causes, and systemic diseases such as leukemia and uremia. The differential diagnosis of vulvodynia also includes neurologic diseases, especially of the nerve roots; herpes simplex infection; vulvar vestibulitis; contact dermatitis; and psychogenic causes.

The management of pruritus or vulvodynia involves establishing a diagnosis, treating the offending cause, and improving local hygiene. Importantly, women with vulvodynia have greater psychologic distress than women who have other vulvar problems. These psychologic concerns must be addressed as part of the therapeutic management. For successful treatment the itch-scratch cycle must be interrupted before the condition becomes chronic, resulting in *lichenification* of the skin. During the latter process the skin becomes white, thickened, and "leathery." The resulting dry, scaly skin frequently cracks, forms fissures, and becomes secondarily infected, thus complicating the treatment. Chapter 32 discusses vulvar dystrophies.

Vulvar Vestibulitis

Vulvar vestibulitis, also known as *vestibular adenitis,* is a rare syndrome of unknown etiology. Patients experience severe introital dyspareunia, vulvar burning and pain at the introitus, particularly the area of the vulvar vestibule. Signs of this syndrome include focal ulceration and inflammation of the mucosa of the vestibule. Grossly, there are small areas of erythematous epithelium that are punctate and 3 to 10 mm in diameter, and sometimes there are associated small ulcerations. The woman is able to identify these small foci of pain when tested by repetitively touching the area with a cotton-tipped applicator.

Classically, most patients have 1 to 10 lesions, with 75% being located in the skin between the two Bartholin's glands. Vulvar vestibulitis is similar to interstitial cystitis, another condition in which tissue that arose from the urogenital sinus produces a chronic pain syndrome without a recognized etiology. The pathophysiology of the condition is believed to be secondary to local neural hyperplasia and/or sympathetically maintained pain loops. Vulvar vestibulitis has a spontaneous remission in approximately one of three patients. It may be treated medically with topical anesthetics such as viscous Xylocaine or amitriptyline hydrochloride (Elavil). However, refractory cases are treated by surgical removal of the involved skin.

Contact Dermatitis

The vulvar skin, especially the intertriginous areas, is a frequent site of contact dermatitis. The vulvar skin is more reactive to exposure by irritants than other skin areas such as the extremities. Contact dermatitis may be one of two basic pathophysiologic processes: a primary irritant (nonimmunologic) or a definite allergic (immunologic) etiology. Substances that are irritants produce immediate symptoms such as a stinging and burning sensation when applied to the vulvar skin. The symptoms and signs secondary to an irritant disappear within 12 hours of discontinuing the offending substance. In contrast, allergic contact dermatitis requires 36 to 48 hours to manifest its symptoms and signs. Often the signs of allergic contact dermatitis persist for several days despite removal of the allergen. Commonly, biologic fluids such as urine and feces cause irritation of the vulvar skin. Rarely, some women will be allergic to latex or semen. The majority of chemicals that produce hypersensitivity of the vulvar skin are cosmetic or therapeutic agents, including vaginal contraceptives, lubricants, sprays, perfumes, douches, fabric dyes, fabric softeners, synthetic fibers, bleaches, soaps, chlorine, dyes in toilet tissues, and local anesthetic creams. External chemicals that trigger the disease process must be avoided. Some of the most severe cases of contact dermatitis involve lesions of the vulvar skin secondary to poison ivy or poison oak.

Acute contact dermatitis results in a red, edematous, inflamed skin. The skin may become weeping and eczematoid. The most severe skin reactions form vesicles, and any stage may become secondarily infected. The common symptoms of contact dermatitis include superficial vulvar tenderness, burning, and pruritus.

The foundation of treatment of contact dermatitis is to withdraw the offending substance. Sometimes the distribution of the vulvar erythema helps to delineate the irritant. For example, localized erythema of the introitus often results from vaginal medication, while generalized erythema of the vulva is secondary to an allergen in clothing. It is possible to use a vulvar chemical innocuously for many months or years before the topical vulvar "allergy" develops.

Initial treatment of severe lesions is with wet compresses of Burow's solution (diluted 1 to 20) for 30 minutes several times a day. This is followed by drying the vulva with cool air from a hair dryer. The vulvar skin should be kept clean and dry. Use of a lubricating agent such as petroleum jelly or Eucerin cream will reduce the pruritus by rehydrating the skin. Cotton undergarments that allow the vulvar skin to aerate should be worn, and constrictive, occlusive, or tight-fitting clothing such as pantyhose should be avoided. Vulvar dryness may be facilitated by using a nonmedicated cornstarch baby powder. Hydrocortisone (0.5% to 1%) and fluorinated corticosteroids (Valisone, 0.1%, or Synalar, 0.01%) as lotions or creams may be rubbed into the skin two to three times a day for a few days to control symptoms. Synthetic systemic corticosteroids (prednisone, 50 mg a day for 7 to 10 days) are sometimes necessary for treatment of poison ivy and poison oak. Antipruritic medications, such as antihistamines, are not of great therapeutic benefit except as soporific agents.

Psoriasis

Psoriasis is a common, generalized skin disease of unknown etiology. Generally, women develop psoriasis during their teenage years, with approximately 3% of adult women being affected. Approximately 20% of these have involvement of vulvar skin. The disease is chronic and relapsing, with an extremely variable and unpredictable course marked by spontaneous remissions and exacerbations. Twenty-five percent of women have a family history of the disease. Genetic susceptibility to develop psoriasis is believed to be multifactorial. Common areas of involvement are the scalp and fingernails. When psoriasis involves the vulvar skin, it produces both anxiety and embarrassment. Similar to candidiasis, psoriasis may be the first clinical manifestation of HIV infection.

Vulvar psoriasis usually affects intertriginous areas and is manifested by red to red-yellow papules. These papules tend to enlarge, becoming well-circumscribed, dull-red plaques. The classic silver scales and bleeding on gentle scraping of the plaque help to establish the diagnosis. In the vulvar region the amount of scales is extremely variable and they are often absent. Under the influence of the moisture and heat of the vulva, vulvar psoriasis may resemble candidiasis. Sometimes dermatologists treat refractory cases of psoriasis with oral retinoids. The margins of psoriasis are more well defined than the common skin conditions in the differential diagnosis including candidiasis, seborrheic dermatitis, and eczema. Initial treatment is 1% hydrocortisone cream. If the patient has pain secondary to chronic fissures, a 4-week course of fluorinated corticosteroid cream should be given. If this treatment is not successful, a dermatologist should be consulted. Systemic steroids often produce a rebound flare-up of the disease.

Seborrheic Dermatitis

Seborrheic dermatitis is a common chronic skin disease of unknown etiology that classically affects the face, scalp, sternum, and the area behind the ears. Rarely, the mons pubis and vulvar areas may be involved. Vulvar lesions are pale to yellow-red, erythematous, and edematous, and they are covered by a fine, nonadherent scale that is usually oily. Excessive sweating and emotional tension precipitate attacks. The etiology of the condition is most likely a yeast, *Pityrosporum ovale.* Approximately 2% to 4% of women have some form of the disease. The pruritus associated with seborrheic dermatitis varies from mild to severe. Treatment is similar to that for contact dermatitis, with hydrocortisone cream being the most effective medication. Refractory cases sometimes respond to topical ketoconazole cream. The differential diagnosis of seborrheic dermatitis includes psoriasis, cutaneous candidiasis, and contact dermatitis. Often it is difficult to differentiate between the cutaneous manifestations of psoriasis and seborrheic dermatitis. Clinically and pragmatically, the exact diagnosis is only of academic interest because the treatment is similar.

Lichen Planus

Lichen planus is a unique, chronic eruption of shiny, violaceous papules. These tiny flat papules appear in women over 30 years of age on flexor surfaces, mucous membranes, and vulvar skin. Most lesions are located on the inner aspects of the vulva, especially the labia minora and vestibule. Both the vulvar and vaginal lesions are painful. Papules often develop in linear scratch marks. The lesions are intensely pruritic and sometimes painful. The initial onset usually follows a time of intense emotional stress. The etiology of this disease is believed to be related to a local autoimmune cell-mediated response. This chronic disease tends to have spontaneous remissions and exacerbations that last for weeks to months. Some women also develop an erosive desquamative vaginitis even though they have normal circulating levels of estrogen. This ulcerative vaginitis may be mistakenly treated as atrophic vaginitis. Correct diagnosis is confirmed by a small punch biopsy of the vagina or vulva. Treatment of local lesions is by use of a potent topical steroid cream such as clobetasone. If the patient is intensely symptomatic, oral steroids may be necessary. Dapsone, 50 mg daily for several months, is sometimes effective in chronic resistant cases. Women with this condition should be monitored at periodic intervals because of an associated increased risk to develop vulvar carcinoma.

Hidradenitis Suppurativa

Hidradenitis suppurativa is a chronic, unrelenting, refractory infection of the skin and subcutaneous tissue. Initially it develops from one or more subcutaneous nodules.

Subsequently, deep scars and pits are formed. The patient undergoes great emotional distress as this condition is both painful and associated with a foul-smelling discharge. The disease is primarily found in reproductive-aged women. The lesions involve the mons pubis, the genitocrural folds, and the buttocks. If treatment is unsuccessful with long-term antibiotic therapy and topical steroids, other medical therapies of the early stages of the disease include antiandrogens, isotretinoin, and cyclosporin. The early phase of the disease is infection of the follicular epithelium. Gradually a deep-seated chronic infection of apocrine glands develops, with occlusion of dilated ducts with inspissated keratin material. In the advanced stages, hidradenitis suppurativa progresses to multiple draining abscesses and sinuses. The diagnosis should be confirmed by biopsy. The treatment of refractory cases is aggressive, wide operative excision of the infected skin. The differential diagnosis of hidradenitis suppurativa includes simple folliculitis, Crohn's disease of the vulva, and granulomatous sexually transmitted diseases.

Edema

Edema of the vulva may be a symptom of either local or generalized disease. Two of the most common causes of edema of the vulva are secondary reactions to inflammation or to lymphatic blockage. Vulvar edema is often recognized before edema in other areas of the female body is noted. The loose connective tissue of the vulva and its dependent position predispose to early development of pitting edema. Systemic causes of vulvar edema include circulatory and renal failure, ascites, and cirrhosis. Vulvar edema also may occur after intraperitoneal fluid is instilled to prevent adhesions or for dialysis. Local causes of vulvar edema include allergy, neurodermatitis, inflammation, trauma, and lymphatic obstruction caused by carcinoma or infection. Infectious diseases that are associated with vulvar edema include necrotizing fasciitis, tuberculosis, syphilis, filariasis, and lymphogranuloma venereum.

VAGINA

Urethral Diverticulum

A urethral diverticulum is a permanent, epithelialized, saclike projection that arises from the posterior urethra. Often they present as a mass of the anterior vaginal wall. It is a common problem, being discovered in approximately 1% to 3% of women. Most urogynecologists have noted a decline in the prevalence of this condition during the past two decades. The majority of cases are initially diagnosed in reproductive-age females, with the peak incidence in the fourth decade of life. The symptoms of a urethral diverticulum are nonspecific and are identical to the symptoms of a lower urinary tract infection. To diagnose this elusive condition, one should suspect urethral diverticulum in any woman with chronic or recurrent lower urinary tract symptoms. The urologic aspects of this condition are discussed in Chapter 21. Histologically the diverticulum is lined by epithelium; however, there is a lack of muscle in the saclike pocket.

Urethral diverticula may be congenital or acquired. Few urethral diverticula present in children; therefore it is assumed that most diverticula are not congenital. Huffman made the analogy that anatomically the urethra is similar to a tree with many stunted branches that represent the periurethral ducts and glands. It is assumed that the majority of urethral diverticula result from repetitive or chronic infections of the periurethral glands. The suburethral infection may cause obstruction of the ducts and glands, with subsequent production of cystic enlargement and retention cysts. These cysts may rupture into the urethral lumen and produce a suburethral diverticulum. Occasionally a suburethral diverticulum has associated stone formation in the dilated retention cyst. Urethral diverticula are small, from 3 mm to 3 cm in diameter. The majority of urethral diverticula open into the midportion of the urethra (Table 18-1). Occasionally, multiple suburethral diverticula occur in the same woman.

Classically, the symptoms associated with the urethral diverticulum are extremely chronic in nature and they have not resolved with multiple courses of oral antibiotic therapy. The most common symptoms associated with urethral diverticula are urinary urgency, frequency, and dysuria. Ginsburg and Genadry discovered that 90% of their patients had symptoms of chronic lower urinary tract infection as the presenting complaint. Approximately 15% of women with urethral diverticula experience hematuria. Other authors have stressed the three Ds associated with a diverticulum: *dysuria, dyspareunia,* and *dribbling* of the urine. Although for years postvoiding dribbling has been termed a classic symptom of urethral diverticulum, it is reported by fewer than 10% of women with this condition. In Lee's series a palpable, tender mass was discovered in 56 of 108 patients. Ginsburg and Genadry found a palpable

---

TABLE 18-1

Location of the Ostium in 108 Female Patients with Diverticulum of the Urethra

Site	No. of Patients
Distal (external) third of the urethra	11
Middle third of the urethra	55
Proximal (inner) third of the urethra (including vesical neck)	18
Multiple sites	18
Unknown	6

From Lee RA: Clin Obstet Gynecol 27:491, 1984.

mass in 46 of 70 women with a urethral diverticulum. It is interesting that in most large series, approximately 20% of the women are asymptomatic. A classic sign of a suburethral diverticulum is the expression of purulent material from the urethra after compressing the suburethral area during a pelvic examination.

The foundation of diagnosing urethral diverticulum is the physician's awareness of the possibility of this defect occurring in women with chronic symptoms of lower urinary tract infection. Subsequently it is important to appreciate that a single diagnostic procedure may not identify the diverticulum. The two most common methods of diagnosing urethral diverticulum are voiding cystourethrography and cystourethroscopy. Approximately 70% of urethral diverticula will be filled by contrast material on a postvoiding x-ray film with a lateral view. Cystourethroscopy will demonstrate the urethral opening of the urethral diverticulum in approximately 6 of 10 cases. Other diagnostic tests used to identify urethral diverticula include urethral pressure profile recordings, vaginal ultrasound, magnetic resonance imaging, and positive-pressure urethrography. The latter test is done with a special double-balloon urethral catheter (Davis catheter) (Figure 18-9). Classically, the recordings of the pressure profile of the urethra demonstrate a biphasic curve in a woman with a urethral diverticulum. If a woman has a urethral diverticulum and urinary incontinence, performing a stress urethral pressure profile will help to differentiate the etiology. The differential diagnosis includes Gartner's duct cyst, an ectopic ureter that empties into the urethra, and Skene's glands cysts.

Several different operations can correct urethral diverticula. Excisional surgery should be scheduled when the diverticulum is not acutely infected. Operative tech-

niques can be divided into transurethral and transvaginal approaches, with most gynecologists preferring the transvaginal approach as described by Lee. The vast majority of diverticula enter into the posterior aspect of the urethra. Diverticula of the distal one third may be treated by simple marsupialization. Following operations, approximately 80% of patients obtain complete relief from symptoms. Some diverticula have multiple openings into the urethra. Complete excision of this network of fistulous connections is important. The recurrence rate varies between 10% and 20%, and many failures are due to incomplete surgical resection. The most serious consequences of surgical repair of urethral diverticula are urinary incontinence and urethrovaginal fistula. Postoperative incontinence usually follows operative repairs of large diverticula that are near the bladder neck. This incontinence may be secondary to damage to the urethral sphincter. The incidence of each of these complications is approximately 1% to 2%.

Inclusion Cysts

Inclusion cysts are the most common cystic structures of the vagina. In Deppisch's series of 64 women with cystic masses of the vagina, 34 had inclusion cysts. The cysts are usually discovered in the posterior or lateral walls of the lower third of the vagina. Inclusion cysts vary from 1 mm to 3 cm in diameter. Deppisch reported a mean diameter of 1.6 cm. Similar to inclusion cysts of the vulva, inclusion cysts of the vagina are more common in parous women. Inclusion cysts usually result from birth trauma or gynecologic surgery. Often they are discovered in the site of a previous episiotomy or at the apex of the vagina following hysterectomy.

Histologically, inclusion cysts are lined by stratified squamous epithelium. These cysts contain a thick, pale-yellow substance that is oily and formed by degenerating epithelial cells. Often these cysts are erroneously called sebaceous cysts in the misbelief that the central material is sebaceous. Similar to vulvar inclusion cysts, the etiology is either a small tag of vaginal epithelium buried beneath the surface following a gynecologic or obstetric procedure or a misplaced island of embryonic remnant that was destined to form epithelium.

The majority of inclusion cysts are asymptomatic. If the cyst produces dyspareunia or pain, the treatment is excisional biopsy.

Dysontogenetic Cysts

Dysontogenetic cysts of the vagina are thin-walled, soft cysts of embryonic origin. Whether the cysts arise from the mesonephros (Gartner's duct cyst), the perimesonephrium (müllerian cyst), or the urogenital sinus (vestibular cyst) is predominantly of academic rather than clinical importance. The cysts may be differentiated histologically by the epithelial lining. Most mesonephric cysts

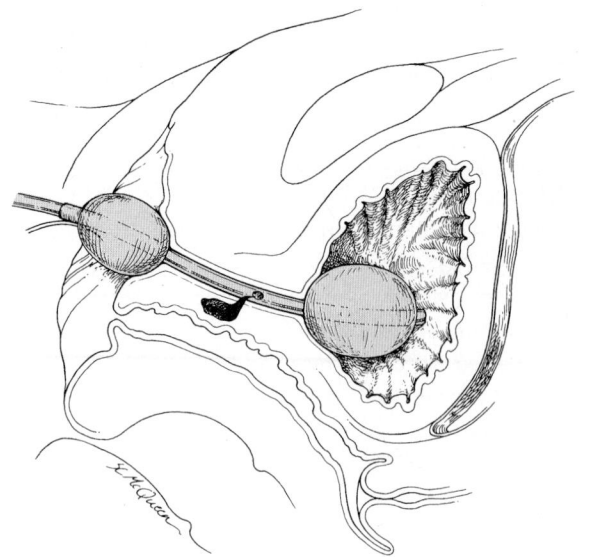

FIGURE 18-9 Double-balloon catheter in use for positive-pressure urethrography.

have cuboidal, nonciliated epithelium. Most perimesonephric cysts have columnar, endocervical-like epithelium. Occasionally pressure produced by the cystic fluid produces flattening of the epithelium, which makes histologic diagnosis less reliable. Although most commonly single, dysontogenetic cysts may be multiple. The cysts are usually 1 to 5 cm in diameter and are usually discovered in the upper half of the vagina. Sometimes multiple small cysts may present like a string of large, soft beads. A large cyst presenting at the introitus may be mistaken for a cystocele, anterior enterocele, or obstructed aberrant ureter. Approximately 1 in 200 females develop these cysts.

Embryonic cysts of the vagina, especially those discovered on the anterior lateral wall, are usually Gartner's duct cysts. In the embryo the distal portion of the mesonephric duct runs parallel with the vagina. It is assumed that a segment of this embryonic structure fails to regress, and the obstructed vestigial remnant becomes cystic. These cysts are most commonly found in the lower one third of the vagina.

Most of these benign cysts are asymptomatic, sausage-shaped tumors that are discovered only incidentally during pelvic examination. Small asymptomatic Gartner's duct cysts may be followed conservatively. Deppisch, in a series of 25 women undergoing operations for symptomatic dysontogenetic cysts, reported a wide range of symptoms, including dyspareunia, vaginal pain, urinary symptoms, and a palpable mass. Sometimes large cysts interfere with the use of tampons.

Operative excision is indicated for chronic symptoms. Rarely, one of these cysts becomes infected, and if operated on during the acute phase, marsupialization of the cyst is preferred. Excision of the vaginal cyst may be a much more formidable operation than anticipated. The cystic structure may extend up into the broad ligament and anatomically be in proximity to the distal course of the ureter.

Tampon Problems

The vaginal tampon has achieved immense popularity and ubiquitous use by women. It is not surprising that there are rare associated risks with tampon usage: vaginal ulcers, the "forgotten" tampon, and toxic shock syndrome. The latter, related to toxins elaborated by *Staphylococcus aureus*, is discussed in Chapter 22.

Wearing tampons for a few days has been associated with microscopic epithelial changes. The majority of women develop epithelial dehydration and epithelial layering, and some will develop microscopic ulcers. These minor changes take between 48 hours to 7 days to heal. Friedrich, in a study of colposcopic changes related to the tampon, found serial changes of epithelial drying, peeling, layering, and ultimately microulceration. In his study, 15% of women wearing tampons only during the time of normal menstruation developed microulcerations. No clin-

ical symptoms were associated with these microscopic changes. Theoretically, these microulcerations are a potential portal of entry for the HIV virus.

Barrett et al. were the first to describe large macroscopic ulcers of the vaginal fornix in four women who were tampon "abusers." Each of these young women wore vaginal tampons for prolonged lengths of time for persistent vaginal discharge or spotting, changing the individual tampon several times per day. The ulcers had a base of clean granulation tissue with smooth, rolled edges. Jimmerson and Becker found birefractal foreign body fragments in biopsy specimens (fibers from tampons) in the vaginal ulcers of 4 of 10 women. The pathophysiology of the ulcer is believed to be secondary to drying and pressure necrosis induced by the tampon. Obviously, many of these young women use tampons for the identical symptoms that are associated with a vaginal ulcer, that is, spotting and vaginal discharge. Often the intermenstrual spotting is believed to be breakthrough bleeding from oral contraceptives, and the possibility of a vaginal ulcer from chronic tampon usage is overlooked.

Vaginal ulcers are not uncommon secondary to several types of foreign objects, including diaphragms, pessaries, and medicated silicon rings. Management is conservative, because the ulcers heal spontaneously when the foreign object is removed. Any persistent ulcer should be biopsied to establish the etiology.

A woman with a "lost" or "forgotten" tampon presents with a classic foul vaginal discharge and occasionally spotting. The tampon is usually found high in the vagina. The odor from a forgotten tampon is overwhelming. The woman should be treated with an antibiotic vaginal cream for the next 5 to 7 days.

Local Trauma

The most frequent etiology of trauma to the lower genital tract of adult females is coitus. Approximately 80% of vaginal lacerations occur secondary to sexual intercourse. Other causes of vaginal trauma are straddle injuries, penetration injuries by foreign objects, sexual assault, vaginismus, and water skiing accidents. The management of vulvar and vaginal trauma in children is discussed in Chapter 12.

The predisposing factors believed to be related to coital injury include virginity, the postpartum and postmenopausal vaginal epithelium, pregnancy, intercourse after a prolonged period of abstinence, hysterectomy, and inebriation. Smith et al. reviewed 19 injuries from normal coitus; 12 of the women in his series were between the ages of 16 and 25 and 5 were over age 45. The most common injury is a transverse tear of the posterior fornix. Similar linear lacerations often occur in the right or left vaginal fornices. The location of the coital injury is believed to be related to the poor support of the upper vagina, which is supported only by a thin layer of connective tissue. The most prominent symptom of a coital vaginal laceration is profuse or prolonged vaginal bleeding. Many women experienced sharp pain during intercourse, and 25% noted persistent abdominal pain. The most troublesome but extremely rare complication of vaginal laceration is vaginal evisceration.

Often the history of the coital injury is not obtained, and, for personal reasons, the woman may even give misleading information. However, coital injury to the vagina should be considered in any woman with profuse or prolonged abnormal vaginal bleeding.

Management of coital lacerations involves prompt suturing under adequate anesthesia. Secondary injury to the urinary and gastrointestinal tracts should be ruled out.

CERVIX

Endocervical and Cervical Polyps

Endocervical and cervical polyps are the most common benign neoplastic growths of the cervix. In an extensive series Farrar and Nedoss reported an incidence of endocervical polyps in 4% of gynecologic patients. Endocervical polyps are most common in multiparous women in their 40s and 50s. Cervical polyps usually present as a single polyp, but multiple polyps do occur occasionally. The majority are smooth, soft, reddish-purple to cherry red, and fragile. They readily bleed when touched. Endocervical polyps may be single or multiple and are a few millimeters to 4 cm in diameter. The stalk of the polyp is of variable length and width (Figure 18-10). Polyps may arise from either the endocervical canal (endocervical polyp) or ectocervix (cervical polyp). Endocervical polyps are more common than are cervical polyps. Often the terms *endocervical* and *cervical* polyps are used to describe the same abnormality. Polyps whose base is in the endocervix usually have a narrow, long pedicle and occur during the reproductive years, while polyps that arise from the ectocervix have a short, broad base and usually occur in postmenopausal women.

The hypothesis of the origin of endocervical polyps is that they are usually secondary to inflammation or abnormal focal responsiveness to hormonal stimulation. Focal hyperplasia and localized proliferation are the response of the cervix to local inflammation. The color of the polyp depends in part on its origin, with most endocervical polyps being cherry red and most cervical polyps grayish-white.

The classic symptom of an endocervical polyp is intermenstrual bleeding, especially following contact such as coitus or a pelvic examination. Sometimes an associated leukorrhea emanates from the infected cervix. Many endocervical polyps are asymptomatic and recognized for the first time during a routine speculum examination. Often the polyp seen on inspection is difficult to palpate because of its soft consistency.

Histologically the surface epithelium of the polyp is columnar or squamous epithelium, depending on the site of origin and the degree of squamous metaplasia (Figure 18-11). The stalk is composed of an edematous, inflamed, loose, and richly vascular connective tissue. Six different histologic subtypes have been described: adenomatous, cystic, fibrous, vascular, inflammatory, and fibromyomatous. Greater than 80% are of the adenomatous type. During pregnancy, focal areas of decidual changes may develop in the stroma. Often there is ulceration of the stalk's most dependent portion, which explains the symptom of contact bleeding. Malignant degeneration of an endocervical polyp is extremely rare. The reported incidence is less than 1 in 200. Considerations in the differential diagnosis include endometrial polyps, small prolapsed myomas, retained products of conception, squamous papilloma, sarcoma, and cervical malignancy. Microglandular endocervical hyperplasia sometimes presents as a 1- to 2-cm polyp. This is an exaggerated histologic response, usually to oral contraceptives.

Most endocervical polyps may be managed in the office by grasping the base of the polyp with an appropriately sized clamp. The polyp is avulsed with a twisting motion and sent to the pathology laboratory for microscopic evaluation. The polyp is usually friable. If the base is broad or bleeding ensues, the base may be treated with chemical cautery, electrocautery, or cryocautery. After the polyp is removed, endometrial sampling should be performed to diagnose a coexisting endometrial hyperplasia or carcinoma in both symptomatic and asymptomatic women. Pradhan et al. discovered significant endometrial pathology in approximately 5% of asymptomatic women with endocervical polyps. It is rare for a polyp to recur following removal.

Nabothian Cysts

Nabothian cysts are retention cysts of endocervical columnar cells occurring where a tunnel or cleft has been covered by squamous metaplasia. These cysts are so common that they are considered a normal feature of the adult cervix. Many women have multiple cysts. Grossly, these cysts may be translucent or opaque whitish or yellow in color. Nabothian cysts vary from microscopic to macroscopic size, with the majority between 3 mm and 3 cm in diameter. Rarely, a woman with several large nabothian cysts may develop gross enlargement of the cervix. These mucous retention cysts are produced by the spontaneous healing process of the cervix. The area of the transformation zone of the cervix is in an almost constant process of repair, and squamous metaplasia and inflammation may block the cleft of a gland orifice. The endocervical columnar cells continue to secrete, and thus a mucous retention cyst is formed. Nabothian cysts are asymptomatic, and no treatment is necessary.

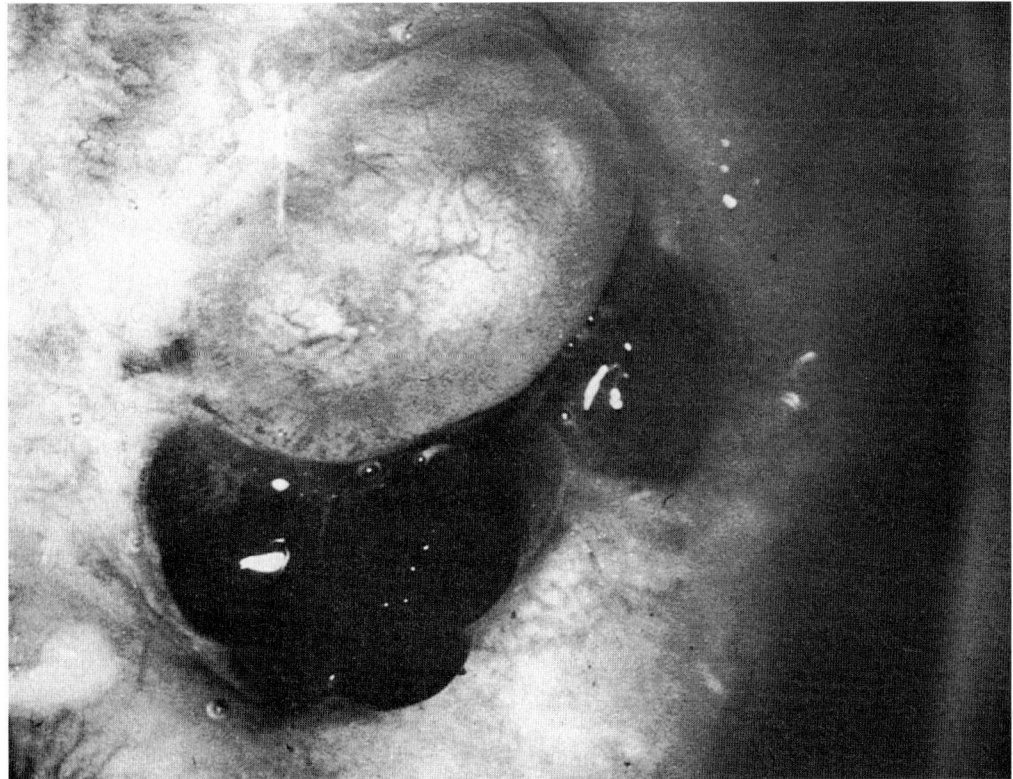

FIGURE 18-10 Endocervical polyp: clinical appearance. (From Gompel C and Silverberg SG, editors: Pathology in gynecology and obstetrics, ed 2, Philadelphia, 1977, JB Lippincott Co, p 74.)

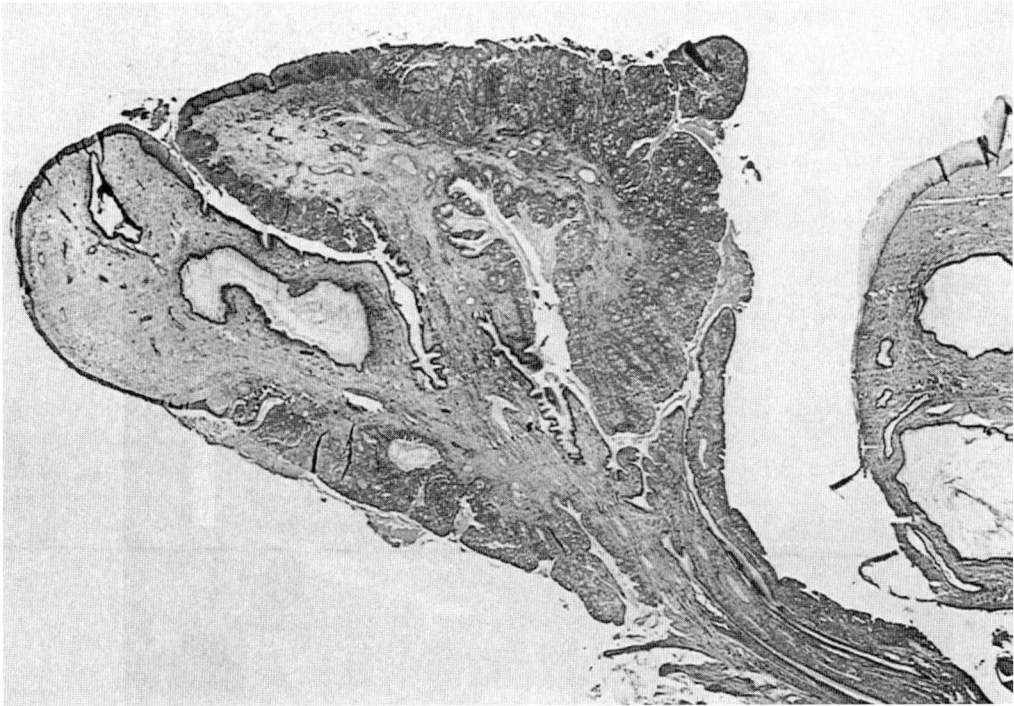

FIGURE 18-11 Endocervical polyp with zones of squamous metaplasia. (From Gompel C and Silverberg SG, editors: Pathology in gynecology and obstetrics, ed 2, Philadelphia, 1977, JB Lippincott Co, p 74.)

Lacerations

Cervical lacerations frequently occur with both normal and abnormal deliveries. Lacerations may occur in non-pregnant women with mechanical dilation of the cervix. Obstetric lacerations vary from minor superficial tears to extensive full-thickness lacerations at 3 and 9 o'clock, respectively, which may extend into the broad ligament. In gynecology the atrophic cervix of the postmenopausal woman predisposes to the complication of cervical laceration when the cervix is mechanically dilated for a diagnostic dilation and curettage.

Acute cervical lacerations bleed and should be sutured. Cervical lacerations that are not repaired may give the external os of the cervix a fish-mouthed appearance; however, they are usually asymptomatic. The use of laminaria tents to slowly soften and dilate the cervix before mechanical instrumentation of the endometrial cavity has reduced the magnitude of iatrogenic cervical lacerations. Furthermore, the practice of routine inspection of the cervix, stabilized with one or more ring forceps, following every second- or third-trimester delivery has enabled physicians to discover and repair extensive cervical lacerations. Lacerations should be palpated to determine the extent of cephalad extension of the tear. Extensive cervical lacerations especially those involving the endocervical stroma may lead to incompetence of the cervix during a subsequent pregnancy.

Cervical Myomas

Cervical myomas are smooth, firm masses that are similar to myomas of the fundus (Figures 18-12 and 18-13). A cervical myoma is usually a solitary growth in contrast to uterine myomas, which in general, are multiple. Depending on the series, 3% to 8% of myomas are categorized as cervical myomas. Because of the relative paucity of smooth muscle fibers in the cervical stroma, the majority of myomas that appear to be cervical actually arise from the isthmus of the uterus.

Most cervical myomas are small and asymptomatic. When symptoms do occur, they are dependent on the direction in which the enlarging myoma expands. The expanding myoma produces symptoms secondary to mechanical pressure on adjacent organs. Cervical myomas may produce dysuria, urgency, urethral or ureteral obstruction, dyspareunia, or obstruction of the cervix. Occasionally a cervical myoma may become pedunculated and protrude through the external os of the cervix. These prolapsed myomas are often ulcerated and infected. A very large cervical myoma may produce distortion of the cervical canal and upper vagina. Rarely, a cervical myoma causes dystocia during childbirth.

The diagnosis of a cervical myoma is by inspection and palpation. Grossly and histologically, cervical myomas are identical to and indistinguishable from myomas of the

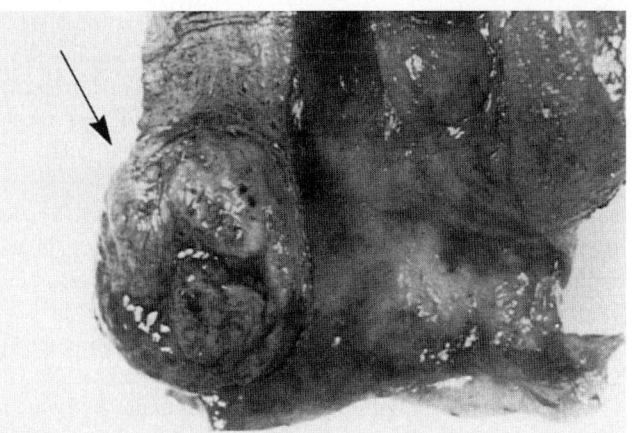

FIGURE 18-12 Leiomyoma, originating in cervix and dilating endocervical canal. It is soft, showing degenerative changes. (From Janovski NA, editor: Color atlas of gross gynecologic and obstetric pathology, New York, 1969, McGraw-Hill Book Co, p 71.)

corpus of the uterus. Occasionally the histologic picture of cervical myomas will demonstrate many hyalinized, thick-walled blood vessels that are postulated to be the source of the neoplastic smooth muscle tumor. This latter subtype of cervical myoma is termed a *vascular leiomyoma*. Management is similar to that of uterine myomas in that asymptomatic, small myomas may be observed for rate of growth. The occurrence and persistence of symptoms from a cervical myoma are an indication for medical therapy with gonadotrophin-releasing hormone (GnRH) agonists and/or myomectomy or hysterectomy, depending on the patient's age and future reproductive plans. Treatment of cervical myomas that grow laterally may become a challenge if myomectomy is the operation of choice, because of both a complex blood supply and involvement with the distal course of the ureter. Recently, some centers are treating cervical myomas by radiologic catheter embolization. Prolapsed uterine myomas are discussed later in this chapter.

Cervical Stenosis

Cervical stenosis most often occurs in the region of the internal os. Cervical stenosis may be divided into congenital or acquired types. The causes of acquired cervical stenosis are operative, radiation, infection, neoplasia, or atrophic changes. Cone biopsy and cautery of the cervix, either electrocautery or cryocoagulation, are the operations that most commonly cause cervical stenosis. According to recent reports, cervical stenosis has occurred following LEEP procedures in women with low circulating estrogen levels such as secondary to periodic injections of depot-medroxyprogesterone.

The symptoms of cervical stenosis depend on whether the patient is premenopausal or postmenopausal and

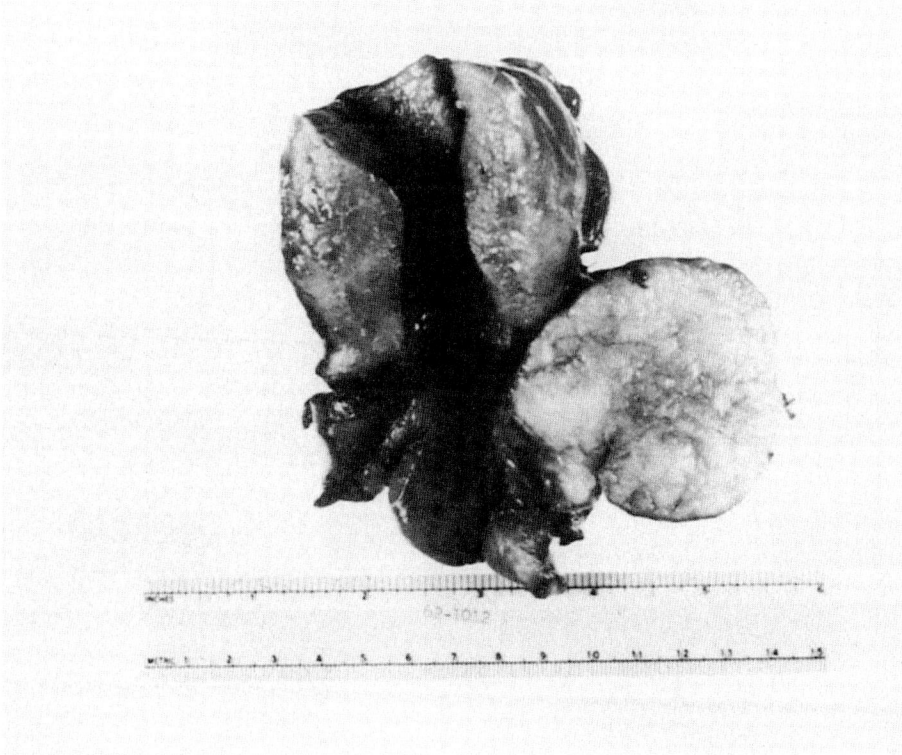

FIGURE 18-13   Leiomyoma of cervix most likely developing from lateral endocervix and protruding into broad ligament. Tumor is whitish, firm, and poorly encapsulated. (From Janovski NA, editor: Color atlas of gross gynecologic and obstetric pathology, New York, 1969, McGraw-Hill Book Co, p 69.)

whether the obstruction is complete or partial. Common symptoms in premenopausal women include dysmenorrhea, pelvic pain, abnormal bleeding, amenorrhea, and infertility. The infertility is usually associated with endometriosis, which is commonly found in reproductive-aged women with cervical stenosis. Postmenopausal women are usually asymptomatic for a long time. Slowly they develop a hematometra (blood), hydrometra (clear fluid), or pyometra (exudate).

The diagnosis is established by inability to introduce a 1 to 2 mm dilator into the uterine cavity. If the obstruction is complete, a soft, slightly tender, enlarged uterus is appreciated as a midline mass. Management of cervical stenosis is dilation of the cervix with dilators under ultrasound guidance. If stenosis recurs, monthly laminaria tents may be used. Similarly, office follow-up and sounding of the cervix of women who have had a cone biopsy or cautery of the cervix is important to establish patency of the endocervical canal. Postmenopausal women with pyometra usually do not need antibiotics. After the acute infection has subsided, endometrial carcinoma and endocervical carcinoma should be ruled out by appropriate diagnostic biopsies. After cervical dilation it is often useful to leave a T tube or latex nasopharyngeal airway as a stent in the cervical canal for a few days to maintain patency. Two small series from Birmingham,

England, and Syracuse, New York, reported the use of the CO_2 laser for treatment of cervical stenosis. In these series approximately 70% of patients were relieved of their cervical stenosis. The success of treatment depends on the proper use of the laser and the quality and quantity of residual columnar epithelium remaining in the endocervix.

UTERUS

Endometrial Polyps

Endometrial polyps are localized overgrowths of endometrial glands and stroma that project beyond the surface of the endometrium. They are soft, pliable, and may be single or multiple. Most polyps arise from the fundus of the uterus. *Polypoid hyperplasia* is a benign condition in which numerous small polyps are discovered throughout the endometrial cavity. Endometrial polyps vary from a few millimeters to several centimeters in diameter, and it is possible for a single large polyp to fill the endometrial cavity. Endometrial polyps may have a broad base (sessile) or be attached by a slender pedicle (pedunculated). In Novak and Woodruff's review of 1100 women with polyps, the growths were discovered in all age groups, with a peak incidence between the ages of 40 and 49. The prevalence of endometrial polyps in reproductive-aged women is 20% to 25%. Endometrial polyps are noted in approximately 10% of women when the uterus is examined at autopsy. The etiology of endometrial polyps is unknown. Because polyps are often associated with endometrial hyperplasia, unopposed estrogen may be the cause.

The majority of endometrial polyps are asymptomatic. Those that are symptomatic are associated with a wide range of abnormal bleeding patterns. No single abnormal bleeding pattern is diagnostic for polyps; however, menorrhagia, premenstrual and postmenstrual staining, and scanty postmenstrual spotting are the most common. Occasionally a pedunculated endometrial polyp with a long pedicle may protrude from the external cervical os. Sometimes large endometrial polyps may contribute to infertility.

Polyps are succulent and velvety, with a large central vascular core. The color is usually gray or tan but may occasionally be red or brown. Histologically an endometrial polyp has three components: endometrial glands, endometrial stroma, and central vascular channels (Figures 18-14 and 18-15). Epithelium must be identified on three sides, like a peninsula. Approximately two of three polyps consist of immature endometrium that does not respond to cyclic changes in circulating progesterone. This immature endometrium differs from surrounding endometrium and often appears as a "Swiss cheese" cystic hyperplasia during all phases of the menstrual cycle. The other one third of endometrial polyps consist of functional endometrium that will undergo cyclic histologic changes. The tip of a prolapsed polyp often undergoes squamous metaplasia, infection, or ulceration. The clinician cannot distinguish whether the abnormal bleeding originates from the polyp or is secondary to the frequently coexisting endometrial hyperplasia. Approximately one in four reproductive-aged women with abnormal bleeding will have endometrial polyps discovered in their uterine cavity.

Malignant transformation in an endometrial polyp has been estimated to be as high as 0.5%. However, an epidemiologic, population-based, case-control study from Sweden by Pettersson et al. estimates that the increased risk of subsequent endometrial carcinoma in women with endometrial polyps is only twofold. This study provides a more realistic appraisal of the risk. Malignant change, when found in an endometrial polyp, is usually curable, and the endometrial carcinoma is most often of a low stage and grade. It is interesting that benign polyps have been found in approximately 20% of uteri removed for endometrial carcinoma. Recently, unusual polyps have been described in association with chronic administration of the nonsteroidal anti-estrogen tamoxifen. The incidence of endometrial abnormalities associated with chronic tamoxifen therapy is polyps 20% to 35%, endometrial hyperplasia 2% to 4%, and endometrial carcinoma 1% to 2%.

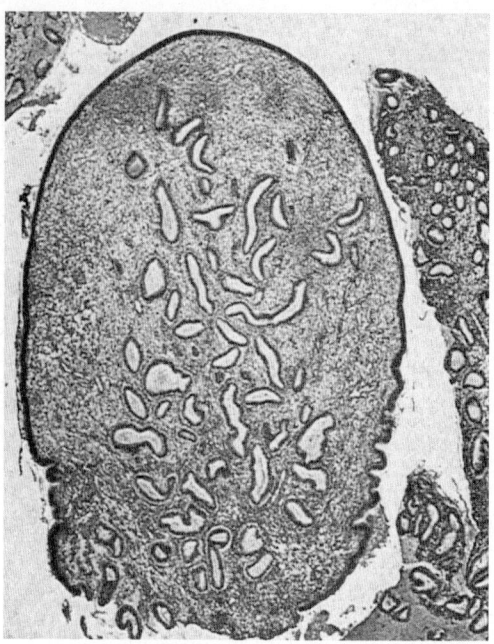

FIGURE 18-14 Typical small endometrial polyp. (From Novak ER and Woodruff JD, editors: Novak's gynecologic and obstetric pathology, ed 6, Philadelphia, 1967, WB Saunders Co, p 206.)

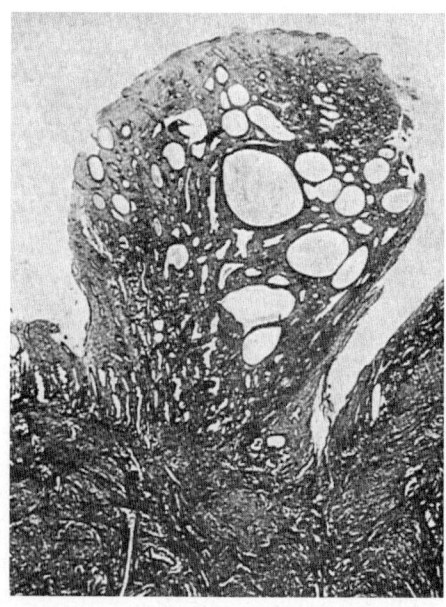

FIGURE 18-15 Endometrial polyp showing hyperplastic, nonfunctioning structure. This is much more common than the functioning type. (From Novak ER and Woodruff JD, editors: Novak's gynecologic and obstetric pathology, ed 6, Philadelphia, 1967, WB Saunders Co, p 207.)

Because most endometrial polyps are asymptomatic, the diagnosis is not usually established until the uterus is opened following hysterectomy for other reasons. Endometrial polyps are often discovered by vaginal hydrosonography, hysteroscopy, and/or hysterosalpingography during the diagnostic workup of a woman with a refractory case of abnormal uterine bleeding. A well-defined, uniformly hyperechoic mass that is less than 2 cm in diameter, identified by vaginal ultrasound within the endometrial cavity, is usually a benign endometrial polyp.

The management of endometrial polyps is removal by curettage or via the hysteroscope. Because of the frequent association of endometrial polyps and other endometrial pathology, it is important to examine histologically both the polyp and the associated endometrial lining. Polyps, because of their mobility, often tend to elude the curette. Postcurettage hysteroscopic studies have demonstrated that routine use of a long, narrow polyp forceps at the time of curettage at best results in discovery and removal of only approximately one in four endometrial polyps. The differential diagnosis of endometrial polyps includes submucous leiomyomas, adenomyomas, retained products of conception, endometrial hyperplasia, carcinoma, and uterine sarcomas.

Hematometra

A hematometra is a uterus distended with blood and is secondary to gynatresia, which is partial or complete obstruction of any portion of the lower genital tract. Obstruction of the isthmus of the uterus, cervix, or vagina may be congenital or acquired. The two most common congenital causes of hematometra are an imperforate hymen and a transverse vaginal septum. Among the leading causes of acquired lower tract stenosis are senile atrophy of the endocervical canal and endometrium, scarring of the isthmus by synechiae, cervical stenosis associated with surgery, radiation therapy, cryocautery or electrocautery, malignant disease of the endocervical canal, and cervical obstruction by tissue following suction curettage.

The symptoms of hematometra depend on the age of the patient, her menstrual history and the rapidity of the accumulation of blood in the uterine cavity, and the possibility of secondary infection producing pyometra. Thus common symptoms of hematometra include primary or secondary amenorrhea and possibly cyclic lower abdominal pain. During the early teenage years the combination of primary amenorrhea and cyclic, episodic cramping lower abdominal pains suggests the possibility of a developing hematometra. Occasionally the obstruction is incomplete, and there is associated spotting of dark-brown blood. Hematometra in postmenopausal women may be entirely asymptomatic. On pelvic examination a mildly tender, globular uterus is usually palpated.

The diagnosis of hematometra is generally suspected by the history of amenorrhea and cyclic abdominal pain. The diagnosis is usually confirmed by vaginal ultrasound or probing the cervix with a narrow metal dilator, with release of dark brownish-black blood from the endocervical canal. Sometimes the blood retained inside the uterus becomes secondarily infected and has a foul odor.

Management of hematometra is dependent on operative relief of the lower tract obstruction. Treatment of congenital obstruction is discussed in Chapter 11. Appropriate biopsy specimens of the endocervical canal and endometrium should be obtained to rule out malignancy when the cause of hematometra is not obvious. If the uterus is significantly enlarged or if there is any suspicion that the retained fluid is infected, drainage should be accomplished first. Biopsy should be postponed for approximately 1 month to diminish the chances of infection or uterine perforation. Hematometra following operations or cryocautery usually resolves with cervical dilation. Hematometra following a first-trimester abortion is treated by repeat suction aspiration of the products of conception that are blocking the internal os.

Leiomyomas

Leiomyomas, also called *myomas,* are benign tumors of muscle cell origin. These tumors are often referred to by their popular names, *fibroids* or *fibromyomas,* but both terms are semantic misnomers if one is referring to the cell of origin. Most leiomyomas contain varying amounts of fibrous tissue, which is believed to be secondary to degeneration of some of the smooth muscle cells.

Leiomyomas are the most frequent pelvic tumors, with the highest prevalence occurring during the fifth decade of a woman's life. Although leiomyomas arise throughout the body in any structure containing smooth muscle, in the pelvis the majority are found in the corpus of the uterus. Occasionally, leiomyomas may be found in the fallopian tube or the round ligament, and approximately 5% of uterine myomas originate from the cervix. Myomas may be single but most often are multiple. Myomas are discovered in one of four white women and one of two black women. They vary greatly in size from microscopic to multinodular uterine tumors that may weigh more than 50 pounds and literally fill the patient's abdomen. Myomas are more prone to grow and become symptomatic in nulliparous women. The question as to why some women develop myomas while others do not is unanswered. However, genetic determinants definitely contribute to their development. Symptomatic uterine leiomyomas are the primary indication for approximately 30% of all hysterectomies.

Initially most myomas develop from the myometrium, beginning as intramural myomas. As they grow, they remain attached to the myometrium with a pedicle of varying width and thickness. Myomas are classed into subgroups by their relative anatomic relationship and position to the layers of the uterus (Figure 18-16). The three most common types of myomas are intramural, subserous, and submucous, with special nomenclature for broad ligament and parasitic myomas (Figures 18-17 and 18-18). Continued growth in one direction determines which myomas will be located just below the endometrium (submucosal) and which will be found just beneath the serosa (subserosal) (Figure 18-19). Although only 5% to 10% of myomas become submucosal, they usually are the most troublesome clinically. These submucosal tumors may be associated with abnormal vaginal bleeding or distortion of the uterine cavity that may produce infertility or abortion. Rarely, a submucosal myoma enlarges and becomes pedunculated. The uterus will try to expel it, and the prolapsed myoma may protrude through the external cervical os. Subserosal myomas give the uterus its knobby contour during pelvic examination.

Further growth of a subserosal myoma may lead to a pedunculated myoma wandering into the peritoneal cavity. This myoma may outgrow its uterine blood supply and obtain a secondary blood supply from another organ, such as the omentum, and become a parasitic myoma.

Growth of a myoma in a lateral direction from the uterus may result in a broad ligament myoma (Figure 18-20). The clinical significance of broad ligament myomas is that they are difficult to differentiate on pelvic examination from a solid ovarian tumor. Large, broad ligament myomas may produce a hydroureter as they enlarge.

Small myomas are round, firm, solid tumors. With continued growth the myometrium at the edge of the tumor is compressed and forms a pseudocapsule. Although myomas do not have a true capsule, this pseudocapsule is a valuable surgical plane during a myomectomy.

The etiology of uterine leiomyomas is incompletely understood. It is known that each tumor results from an original single muscle cell. Each individual uterine myoma is monoclonal. All the cells are derived from one progenitor myocyte. Cytogenetic analysis has demonstrated multiple chromosomal abnormalities. Approximately 60% of myomas have normal karyotypes and 40% have abnormal karyotypes with a significantly lower DNA content. The current hypothesis is that cytogenetic semantic mutation in uterine myomas are often associated with change in the dependency on steroid hormones which alter the growth potential of the myomas.

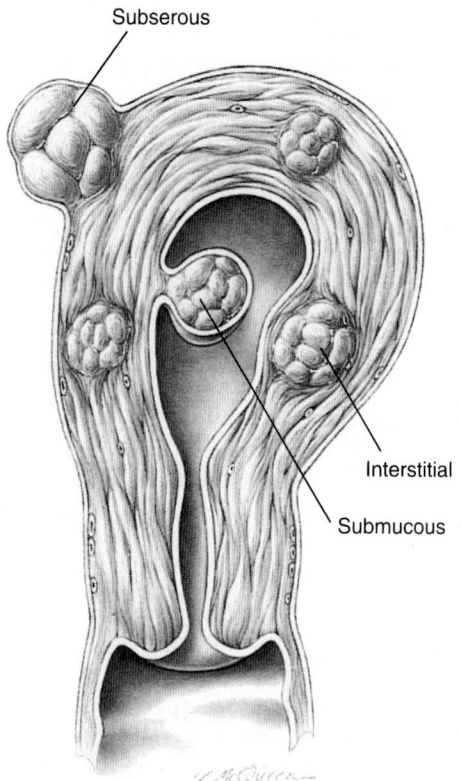

FIGURE 18-16 Drawing of cut surface of uterus showing characteristic whorl-like appearance and varying locations of leiomyomas. (From Novak ER and Woodruff JD, editors: Novak's gynecologic and obstetric pathology, ed 6, Philadelphia, 1967, WB Saunders Co, p 215.)

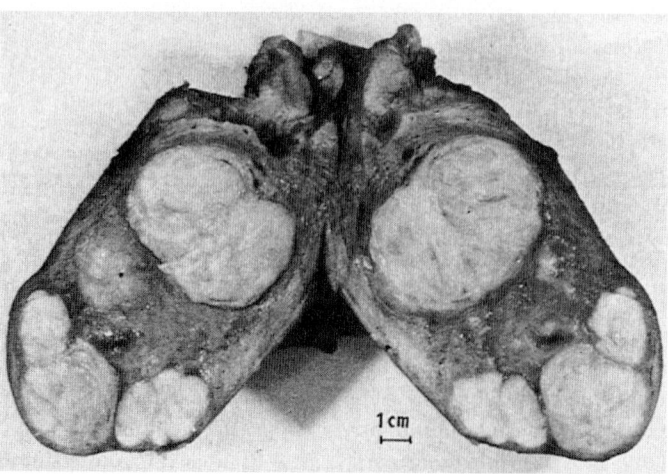

FIGURE 18-17 Intramural leiomyomata. (From Gompel C and Silverberg SG, editors: Pathology in gynecology and obstetrics, ed 2, Philadelphia, 1977, JB Lippincott Co, p 186.)

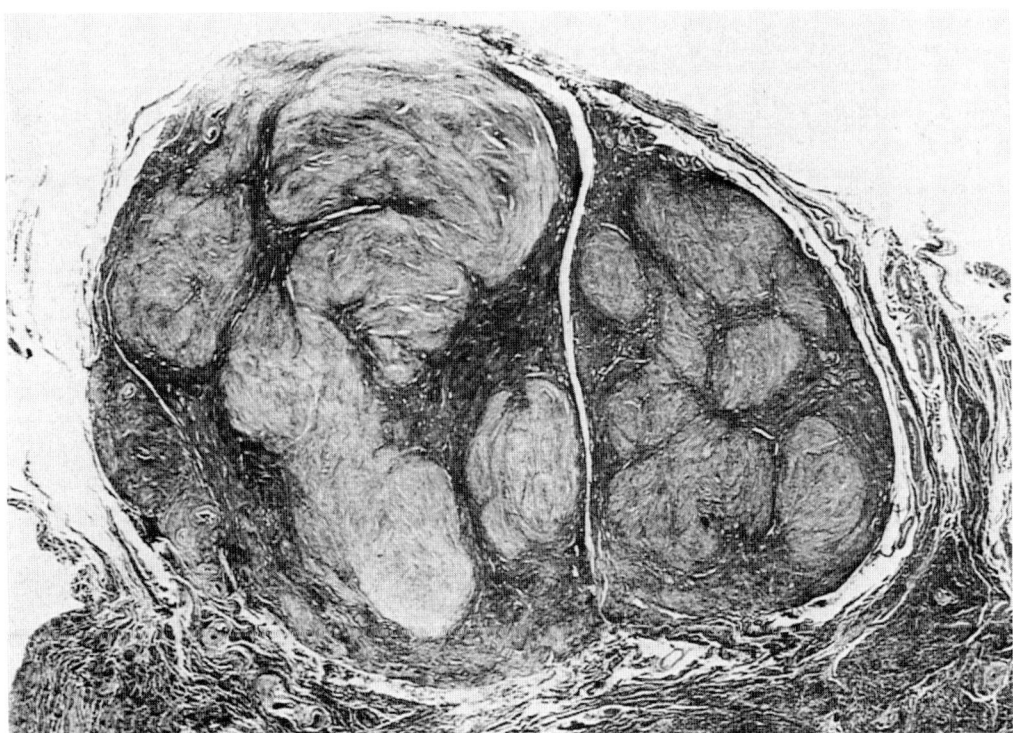

FIGURE 18-18   Intramural leiomyoma. (From Gompel C and Silverberg SG, editors: Pathology in gynecology and obstetrics, ed 2, Philadelphia, 1977, JB Lippincott Co, p 187.)

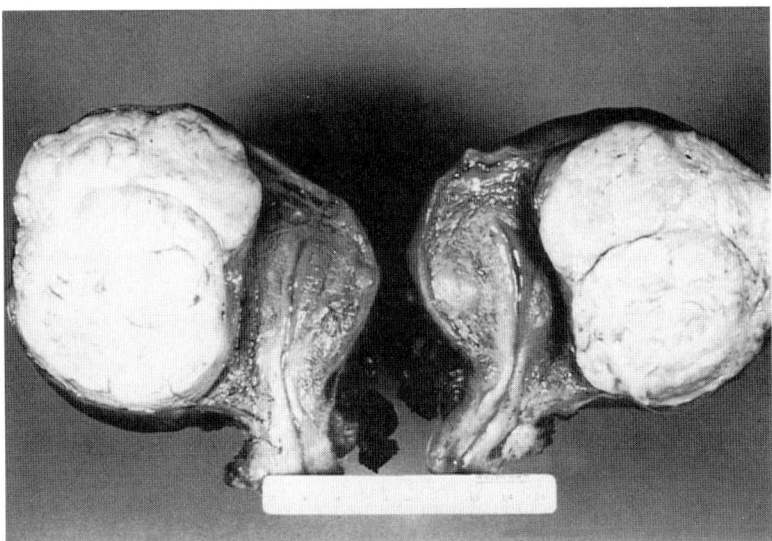

FIGURE 18-19   Large subserosal myoma. (Courtesy William Droegemueller and Vern L. Katz.)

The present thoughts regarding the pathogenesis of uterine myomas is that neoplastic transformation is probably a somatic mutation of normal myometrium to leiomyoma influenced by estrogen and progesterone and local growth factors such as epidermal growth factor, insulin-like growth factor 1, and platelet-derived growth factor (Figure 18-21). Both estrogen and progesterone receptors are found in uterine myomas. The exact stimulus for growth of myomas is also unclear; however, the growth may be influenced by relative levels of estrogen and/or progesterone. Myomas are rare before menarche, and most myomas diminish in size following menopause with the reduction of a significant amount of circulating estrogen. Myomas often enlarge during pregnancy and occasionally enlarge secondary to oral contraceptive therapy. Medically induced hypoestrogenic states produce reductions in the

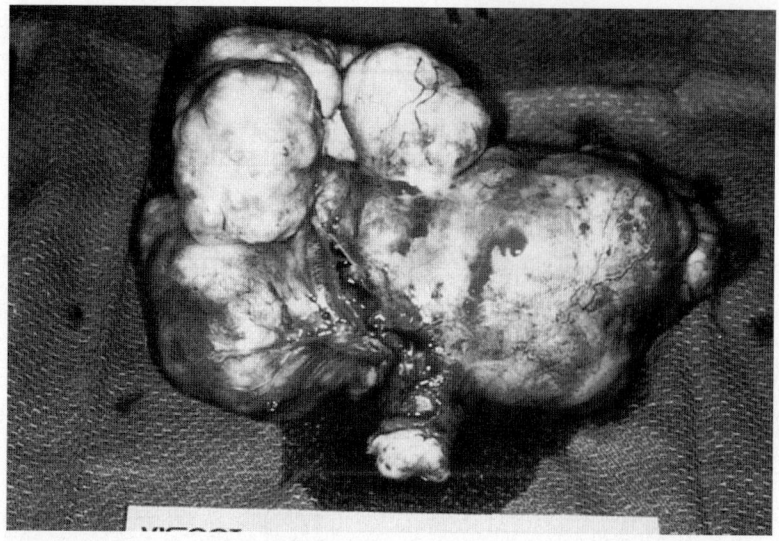

FIGURE 18-20 Hysterectomy specimen of myomatous uterus. (Courtesy Vern L. Katz and William Droegemueller.)

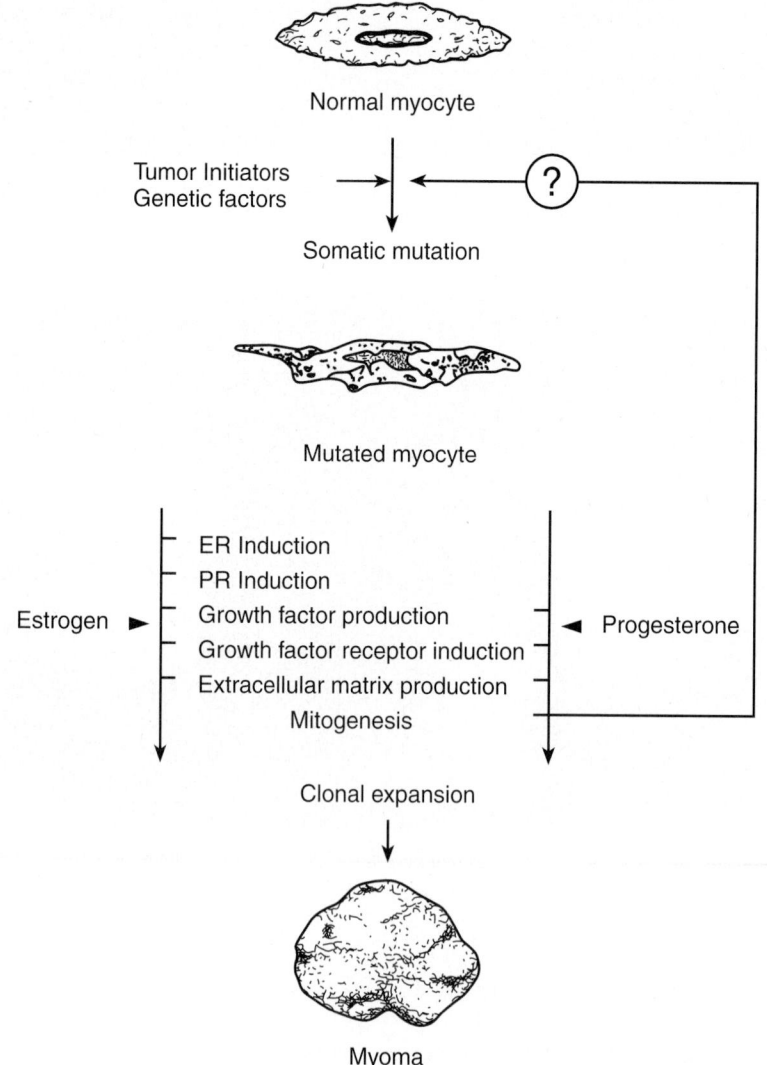

Normal myocyte

Tumor Initiators
Genetic factors

?

Somatic mutation

Mutated myocyte

Estrogen ►

ER Induction
PR Induction
Growth factor production
Growth factor receptor induction
Extracellular matrix production
Mitogenesis

◄ Progesterone

Clonal expansion

Myoma

FIGURE 18-21 The initiation and growth of myomas likely involves a multistep cascade of separate tumor initiators and promoters. The initial neoplastic transformation of the normal myocyte involves somatic mutations. Although the initiators of the somatic mutations remain unclear, the mitogenic effect of progesterone may enhance the propagation of somatic mutations. Myoma proliferation is the result of clonal expansion and likely involves the complex interactions of estrogen, progesterone, and local growth factors. Estrogen and progesterone appear equally important as promoters of myoma growth. *ER,* Estrogen receptor; *PR,* progesterone receptor. (Modified from Rein MS, Barbieri RL, and Friedman AJ: Am J Obstet Gynecol 172:14, 1995).

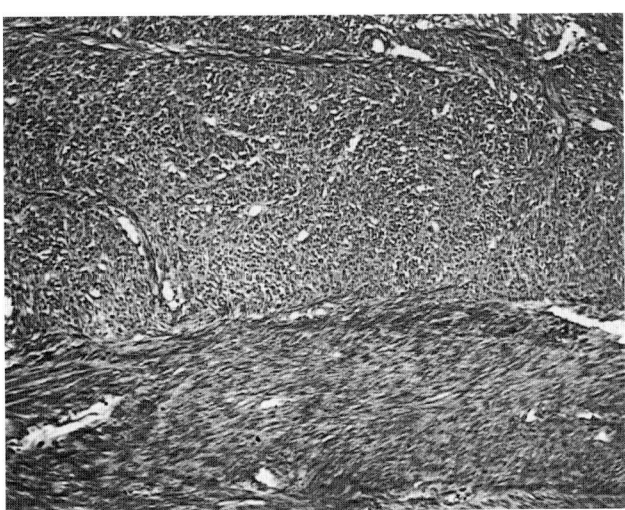

FIGURE 18-22 Histologic section of leiomyoma. (Courtesy Daniel R. Mishell, Jr., M.D.)

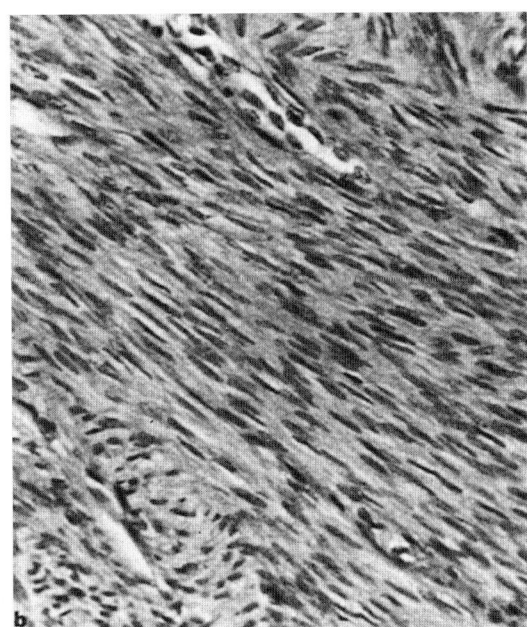

FIGURE 18-23 Leiomyoma showing interlacing bundles of smooth muscles with spindle nuclei without degeneration. (From Demopoulos RI: Benign lesions of the myometrium. In Blaustein A, editor: Pathology of the female genital tract, New York, 1977, Springer-Verlag New York, Inc, p 302.)

size of myomas. Estrogen and progesterone receptors are found in higher concentrations in myomas than in the surrounding myometrium. Women who smoke cigarettes and are thus relatively estrogen deficient have a lower incidence of myomas. Many women, though, have small myomas that do not grow under the influence of high circulating estrogen levels. Thus the relationship between estrogen and progesterone levels and myoma growth is complex. Cramer et al. are studying the growth potential of uterine leiomyomas in vitro and have found heterogeneity in hormonal responsiveness.

Grossly, a myoma has a lighter color than the normal myometrium. On cut surface the tumor has a glistening, pearl-white appearance, with the smooth muscle arranged in a trabeculated or whorled configuration. Histologically there is a proliferation of mature smooth muscle cells. The nonstriated muscle fibers are arranged in interlacing bundles. Between bundles of smooth muscle cells are variable amounts of fibrous connective tissue, especially toward the center of any large tumor (Figures 18-22 to 18-24). The amount of fibrous tissue is proportional to the extent of atrophy and degeneration that has occurred over time.

The eventual fate of some myomas is determined by their relatively poor vascular supply. This supply is found in one or two major arteries at the base or pedicle of the myoma. The arterial supply of myomas is significantly less than that of a similar-sized area of normal myometrium. Thus, with continued growth, degeneration occurs because the tumor outgrows its blood supply. The severity of the discrepancy between the myoma's growth and its blood supply determines the extent of degeneration: hyaline, myxomatous, calcific, cystic, fatty, or red degeneration and necrosis. The mildest form of degeneration of a myoma is hyaline degeneration. Grossly, in this condition

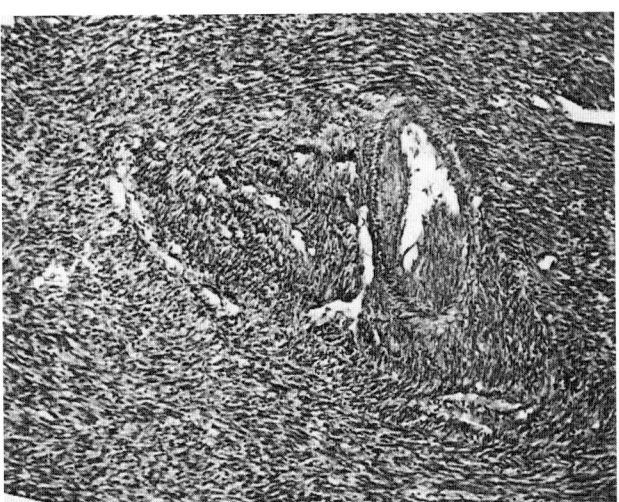

FIGURE 18-24 Leiomyoma histologic section of a cellular myoma. (Courtesy Daniel R. Mishell, Jr., M.D.)

the surface of the myoma is homogeneous with loss of the whorled pattern. Histologically, with hyaline degeneration, cellular detail is lost as the smooth muscle cells are replaced by fibrous connective tissue. A recent interesting study by Huang et al. using transvaginal color Doppler ultrasound documented that the intratumoral blood flow correlated with reduced tumor size and tumor volume, but did not correlate with angiogenesis or cell proliferation.

The most acute form of degeneration is red, or carneous, infarction. This acute muscular infarction causes severe pain and localized peritoneal irritation. This form of degeneration occurs during pregnancy in approximately 5% to 10% of gravid women with myomas. The ultrasound appearance of painful myomas is one of mixed echodense and echolucent areas. Serial ultrasound examinations have also demonstrated that most (80%) myomas do not change size during pregnancy; if a change in size does occur, it is usually not associated with painful symptomatology. During pregnancy this complication should be treated medically, for attempts at operative removal may result in profuse blood loss. If the patient is not pregnant, acute degeneration is not a contraindication to myomectomy. Obviously the more advanced forms of degenerating myomas may become secondarily infected, especially when large necrotic areas exist. The histologic changes of degeneration are found more commonly in larger myomas. However, two thirds of all myomas show some degree of degeneration, with the three most common types being hyaline degeneration (65%), myxomatous degeneration (15%), and calcific degeneration (10%).

The literature emphasizes that the incidence of malignant degeneration is estimated to be between 0.3% and 0.7%. The term *malignant degeneration* is ambiguous and may be incorrect. It is unknown as to whether myomas degenerate into sarcomas or if sarcomas arise spontaneously in myomatous uteri. In a series of 1429 hysterectomies in patients with a preoperative diagnosis of symptoms related to myomas, leiomyosarcomas were found histologically in 0.49%. The incidence increases in each advancing decade of life. The possibility of a uterine tumor being a leiomyoma sarcoma is 10 times greater in a woman in her 60s than in a woman in her 40s.

The most common symptoms related to myomas are pressure from an enlarging pelvic mass, pain including dysmenorrhea, and abnormal uterine bleeding. The severity of symptoms is usually related to the number, location, and size of the myomas. However, the majority of women with uterine myomas are asymptomatic.

One of three women with myomas experiences pelvic pain. Acquired dysmenorrhea is the most frequent complaint, with a study by Iosif and Akerlund from Sweden documenting an associated increase in myometrial activity. Various forms of vascular compromise, either acute degeneration or torsion of the pedicle, produce severe pelvic pain. Milder pelvic discomfort is described as pelvic heaviness or a dull, aching sensation that may be secondary to edematous swelling in the myoma.

An enlarged myoma or myomas often produce pressure symptoms similar to those of an enlarging pregnant uterus. Sometimes a woman will notice that her abdominal girth is increasing without appreciable change in weight. Alternately, an anterior myoma pressing on the bladder may produce urinary frequency and urgency. In general, urinary symptoms are more common than rectal symptoms. Extremely large myomas and broad ligament myomas may produce a unilateral or bilateral hydroureter. Abnormal bleeding is experienced by 30% of women with myomas. The most common symptom is menorrhagia, but intermenstrual spotting and disruption of a normal pattern are other frequent complaints. The exact cause-and-effect relationship between myomas and abnormal bleeding is difficult to determine and is poorly understood. The explanation is straightforward when there are areas of ulceration over submucous myomas. However, ulceration is a rare finding. The most popular theory is that myomas result in an abnormal microvascular growth pattern and function of the vessels in the adjacent endometrium. The theory that the amount of menorrhagia is directly related to an increase of endometrial surface area has been disproved. One of three women with abnormal bleeding and submucous myomas also has endometrial hyperplasia, which may be the cause of the symptom.

Occasionally, myomas are the only identifiable abnormality after a detailed infertility investigation. Because the data relating myomas to infertility are weak, myomectomy is indicated only in long-standing infertility and recurrent abortion after all other potential factors have been investigated and treated. Successful term pregnancy rates of 40% to 50% have been reported following a myomectomy. The success of an operation is most dependent on the age of the patient, the size of the myomas, and the number of compounding factors that affect the couple's fertility.

Rapid growth of a uterine myoma after menopause is a disturbing symptom. This is the classic symptom of a leiomyosarcoma, and thus the patient should have a total abdominal hysterectomy so that the tissue may be examined histologically.

Rarely, a secondary polycythemia is noted in women with uterine myomas. This syndrome is related to elevated levels of erythropoietin. The polycythemia diminishes following removal of the uterus.

The diagnosis of uterine myomas is usually confirmed by palpating an enlarged, firm, irregular uterus during pelvic examination. The three conditions that commonly enter into the differential diagnosis include pregnancy, adenomyosis, and an ovarian neoplasm. The discrimination between large ovarian tumors and myomatous uteri may be difficult. Extension of myomas laterally may make palpation of normal ovaries impossible during the pelvic examination. Degeneration of myomas may cause a change of consistency from firm to soft, and some may become cystic. Often, if pregnancy has been excluded, placing a metal sound in the uterine cavity will help to establish the clinical diagnosis. The uterine cavity is generally enlarged and often irregular with myomas, while an ovarian tumor is usually associated with a normal-sized uterus. The mobility of the pelvic mass and whether the mass moves independently or as part of the uterus may be helpful diagnostically. Submucosal myomas may be diagnosed by vaginal ultrasound, hysteroscopy, or occasionally as a filling defect on hysterosalpingography.

Although the majority of uterine myomas may be diagnosed by pelvic examination, difficult cases will benefit from ultrasound examination or a search for concentric calcifications on an abdominal x-ray film. There are several recent reports of computed tomography (CT) and magnetic resonance imaging (MRI) studies of uterine myomas. However, these imaging techniques are more expensive than ultrasound. Until CT and MRI can distinguish between benign and malignant myomas, they will rarely be ordered in routine clinical management of myomas. MRI is helpful in differentiating adenomyosis or an adenomyoma from a single, solitary myoma especially in a woman desiring preservation of her fertility. Serial ultrasound examinations have been used to evaluate progression in size of myomas or response to therapy. However, in a recent study Cantuaria et al. compared bimanual pelvic exam and ultrasound imaging prior to hysterectomy for uterine myomas. They found a strong correlation in determining the size of myoma between bimanual and ultrasound exams.

The management of a woman with small, asymptomatic myomas is judicious observation. When the tumor is first discovered, it is appropriate to perform a pelvic examination at 6-month intervals to determine the rate of growth. The majority of women will not need an operation, especially those women in the perimenopausal period, where the condition usually improves with diminishing levels of circulating estrogens.

Women with abnormal bleeding and leiomyomas should be investigated thoroughly for concurrent problems such as endometrial hyperplasia. If their symptoms do not improve with conservative management, operative therapy may be considered. The choice between a myomectomy and hysterectomy is usually determined by the patient's age, parity, and most important, future reproductive plans. In comparison studies the relative morbidity of abdominal hysterectomy and myomectomy is similar when one controls for uterine size.

Classic indications for a myomectomy include a rapidly expanding pelvic mass, persistent abnormal bleeding, pain or pressure, or enlargement of an asymptomatic myoma to more than 8 cm in a woman who has not completed childbearing. The causal relationship of myomas and adverse reproductive outcomes is poorly understood. Long-standing infertility or repetitive abortion directly related to myomas is rare. Contraindications to a myomectomy include pregnancy, advanced adnexal disease, malignancy, and the situation in which enucleation of the myoma would result in a severe reduction of endometrial surface so that the uterus would not be functional. The choice between the two operations is not always an easy one. To quote Richard TeLinde, "All indications and contraindications in medicine are relative, a fact that is especially true when one considers hysterectomy versus myomectomy."

Within 20 years of the myomectomy operation, one in four women subsequently has a hysterectomy performed, the majority for recurrent leiomyomas. In recent years myomectomy has been performed in selected women using innovative laparoscopic techniques. Some centers excise uterine myomas vaginally using an anterior or posterior colpotomy. They believe that vaginal myomectomy is an alternative surgical plan even in women with moderately enlarged tumors. Submucous myomas may be resected via the cervical canal using the hysteroscope. Although preliminary studies using laser surgery have been reported, most investigators advocate using an operative resectoscope. Three out of four women have long-term relief of their menorrhagia secondary to uterine myomas following hysteroscopic resection of the myomas.

The indications for hysterectomy for myomas are similar to indications for myomectomy, with a few additions. Some gynecologists selectively perform a hysterectomy for asymptomatic myomas when the uterus has reached the size of a 14- to 16-week gestation. The hypothesis is that most myomas of this size will eventually produce symptoms. However, it is impossible to predict which individual woman will most likely develop symptoms. A previously mentioned indication for hysterectomy is rapid growth of a myoma after the menopause. Prolapse of a myoma through the cervix is optimally treated by vaginal removal and ligation of the base of the myoma, with antibiotic coverage. Hysteroscopic resection has greatly aided transvaginal removal of a prolapsed myoma.

It is possible to treat leiomyomas medically by reducing the circulating level of estrogen and progesterone. GnRH agonists, medroxyprogesterone acetate (Depo-Provera), danazol, and the antiprogesterone RU 486 have undergone clinical trials. Recent studies in the past 10 years have emphasized the use of GnRH agonists, sometimes with add-back hormonal therapy, to treat myomas. Reduction in mean uterine volume and myoma size by 40% to 50% has been documented. However, individual response varies greatly, from no response to an 80% reduction in uterine size. The vast majority of the reduction in size occurs within the first 3 months. After cessation of therapy, myomas gradually resume their pretreatment size. By 6 months after treatment, most myomas will have returned to their original size. During treatment, Doppler flow studies have demonstrated increased resistance in the uterine arteries and in the smaller arteries feeding the myoma. Also during treatment, the proliferative activity of the myoma and binding of epidermal growth factor is reduced. Several investigators have advocated preoperative treatment of myomas with GnRH agonists. Reduction in blood loss at the time of hysterectomy or myomectomy is anticipated in selected cases. The advantages and disadvantages of preoperative GnRH agonist therapy are listed in the box on page 504. Most important, medical therapy is useful perimenopausally to avoid hysterectomy.

**Advantages and Disadvantages
of Preoperative GnRH Agonist Treatment**

Advantages Gained by Uterine-Fibroid Shrinkage
May allow vaginal hysterectomy
May decrease intraoperative blood loss
May allow Pfannenstiel incision
May facilitate endoscopic myomectomy

Advantages Gained by Induction of Amenorrhea
May correct hypermenorrhea-menorrhagia-associated anemia
May improve ability to donate blood
May decrease need for nonautologous blood transfusion
May atrophy endometrium, facilitating hysteroscopic resection of submucosal tumors

Disadvantages
Delay to final tissue diagnosis
Degeneration of some leiomyomas, necessitating piecemeal enucleation at myomectomy
Hypoestrogenic side effects (e.g., trabecular bone loss, vasomotor flushes)
Cost
Need to self-administer or receive injections in many cases
Vaginal hemorrhage in approximately 2% of patients

From Friedman AJ: Clin Obstet Gynecol 36:650, 1993.

The newest modality to manage uterine myomas is transcatheter uterine artery embolization as an ambulatory nonsurgical technique. Multiple embolic materials have been used including gelatin sponge (Gelfoam) silicone spheres, metal coils, and polyvinyl alcohol (PVA) particles of various diameters. Postprocedural abdominal and pelvic pain is common for the first 24 hours. Success rates in regard to decreasing menorrhagia and reduction in uterine size are promising. However, a recent national conference reported 4 deaths among the first 4000 women receiving this therapy. Obviously, a large-scale, randomized clinical trail is desperately needed.

Two associated but rare diseases should be noted: intravenous leiomyomatosis and leiomyomatosis peritonealis disseminata. *Intravenous leiomyomatosis* is a rare condition in which benign smooth muscle fibers invade and slowly grow into the venous channels of the pelvis. The tumor grows by direct extension and grossly appears like a "spaghetti" tumor. Only 25% of tumors extend beyond the broad ligament; however, case reports exist of tumor growth into the vena cava and right heart.

Leiomyomatosis peritonealis disseminata (LPD) is a benign disease with multiple small nodules over the surface of the pelvis and abdominal peritoneum. Grossly, LPD mimics disseminated carcinoma (Figure 18-25). However, histologic examination demonstrates benign-appearing myomas. This disorder is usually associated with a recent pregnancy.

OVIDUCT

Leiomyomas

Both benign and malignant tumors of the oviduct are uncommon compared with other gynecologic neoplasms. Although these tumors are underreported, fewer than 100 women with myomas or leiomyomas of the oviduct are described in the literature. Tubal leiomyomas may be single or multiple and usually are discovered in the interstitial portion of the tubes. They usually coexist with the more common uterine leiomyomas. Myomas may originate from muscle cells in the walls of the tube or blood vessels or from smooth muscle in the broad ligament.

Leiomyomas of the tube present as smooth, firm, mobile, usually nontender masses that may be palpated

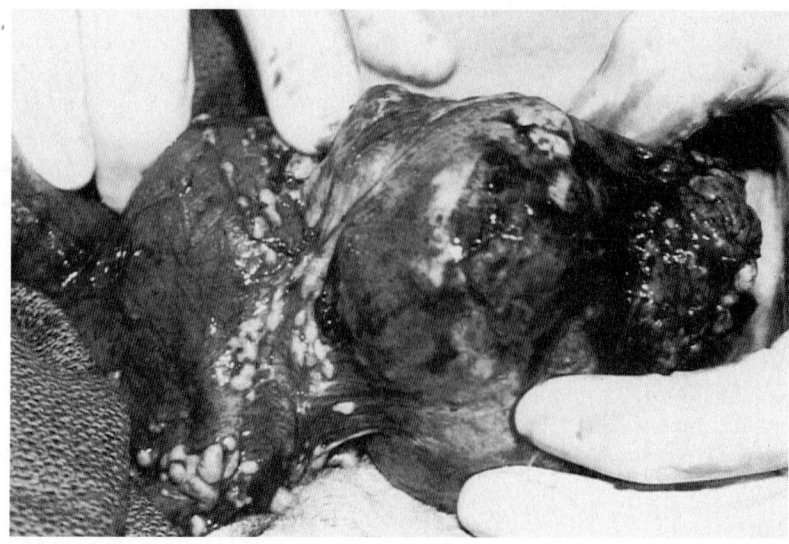

FIGURE 18-25   Photograph of leiomyomatosis peritonealis disseminata. (Courtesy William Droegemueller and Vern L. Katz.)

during the bimanual examination. Similar to uterine myomas, they may be subserosal, interstitial, or submucosal. During laparoscopy the myomas appear as a spherical mass that protrudes from beneath the peritoneal surface. They vary from a few millimeters to 15 cm in diameter. Histologically they are identical to uterine leiomyomas.

The majority of the myomas of the oviduct are asymptomatic. Rarely, they may undergo acute degeneration or be associated with unilateral tubal obstruction or torsion. Treatment of a symptomatic tubal leiomyoma is excision.

Adenomatoid Tumors

The most prevalent benign tumor of the oviduct is the *angiomyoma* or *adenomatoid tumor*. They are small, gray-white, circumscribed nodules, 1 to 2 cm in diameter. These tumors are usually unilateral and present as small nodules just under the tubal serosa. These small nodules do not produce pelvic symptoms or signs. These benign tumors also are found below the serosa of the fundus of the uterus and the broad ligament. Microscopically they are composed of small tubules lined by a low cuboidal or flat epithelium. Histologic studies have established that the thin-walled channels that comprise these tumors are of mesothelial origin. These tumors do not become malignant; however, they may be mistaken for a low-grade neoplasm when initially viewed during a frozen-section evaluation.

Paratubal Cysts

Paratubal cysts are frequently incidental discoveries during gynecologic operations for other abnormalities. They are often multiple and may vary from 0.5 cm to more than 20 cm in diameter. The majority of cysts are small, asymptomatic, and slow growing and are discovered during the third and fourth decades of life. When paratubal cysts are pedunculated and near the fimbrial end of the oviduct, they are called *hydatid cysts of Morgagni* (Figure 18-26). Cysts near the oviduct may be of mesonephric, mesothelial, or paramesonephric origin. Sometimes the histologic differentiation is difficult because of mechanically produced changes in the cells that line the cyst. These cysts are translucent and contain a clear or pale yellow fluid.

The histogenesis of the majority of paratubal cysts had been believed to be from the mesonephric duct, with the cysts arising from the main duct or accessory tubules. These latter cysts often develop between the leaves of the broad ligament in the mesosalpinx, with the ovary being separate. However, a histologic study of 79 paratubal cysts by Samaha and Woodruff has documented that 60 of the cysts were of tubal origin. Thus the majority of grossly identified "paratubal cysts" are in reality accessory lumina of the fallopian tubes. The remaining 19 cysts in Samaha and Woodruff's series were of mesothelial origin. Paratubal cysts are thin walled and smooth and contain clear

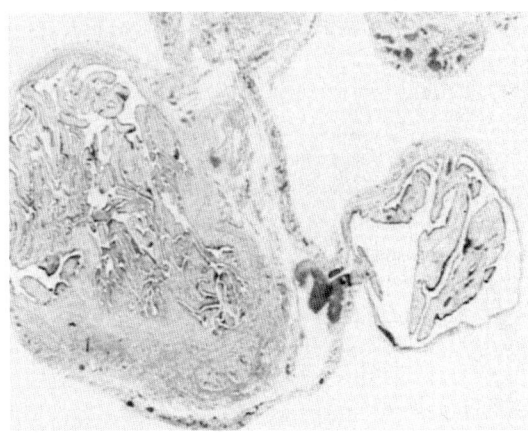

FIGURE 18-26 Normal tube on left, with pedunculated hydatid cyst of Morgagni to right (accessory lumen with papillary fronds, really mucosal folds of tube). (From Samaha M and Woodruff JD: Obstet Gynecol 65:692, 1985. Reprinted with permission from The American College of Obstetricians and Gynecologists.)

fluid. Often there are multiple small cysts. These cysts are thin walled and are filled with clear fluid. Occasionally there is a papillomatous proliferation on the internal wall of these cysts. Inflammatory cysts of the peritoneum may be found anywhere in the pelvis.

The majority of paratubal cysts are asymptomatic and are usually discovered incidentally during gynecologic operations. When paratubal cysts are symptomatic, they generally produce a dull pain. During a pelvic examination it is difficult to distinguish a paratubal cyst from an ovarian mass. At operation the oviduct is often found stretched over a large paratubal cyst. The oviduct should not be removed in these cases, because it will return to normal size after the paratubal cyst is excised. Stein et al. recently reported a retrospective 10-year review of 168 women with parovarian tumors. Three low-grade malignant neoplasms were found in this series. These malignancies were in women of reproductive age who had cysts greater than 5 cm in diameter with internal papillary projections. The authors cautioned that the differentiation between benign and malignant parovarian masses cannot be made by external examination of the cyst. Therefore they expressed concern about the practice of aspirating cysts via the laparoscope because of the potential hazard of missing or disseminating a malignant disease.

Paratubal cysts may grow rapidly during pregnancy, and most of the cases of torsion of these cysts have been reported during pregnancy or the puerperium. Treatment is simple excision.

Torsion

Acute torsion of the oviduct is a rare event; however, it has been reported with both normal and pathologic fallopian tubes. Pregnancy predisposes to this problem. Tubal torsion usually accompanies torsion of the ovary, as they have a common vascular pedicle. (See discussion of ovarian torsion later in this chapter.) Torsion of the fallopian tube is secondary to an ovarian mass in approximately 50% to 60% of patients. The right tube is involved more frequently than is the left (Figure 18-27). The degree of tubal torsion varies from less than one turn to four complete rotations. Torsion of the oviduct is usually seen in women of reproductive age. However, it occurs also in preadolescent children, especially when part of the tube is enclosed in the sac of a femoral or inguinal hernia.

Youssef et al. have subdivided the pathophysiology and etiology of tubal torsion into intrinsic and extrinsic causes. Prominent intrinsic causes include congenital abnormalities, such as increased tortuosity caused by excessive length of the tube, and pathologic processes, such as hydrosalpinx, hematosalpinx, tubal neoplasms, and previous operation, especially tubal ligation. Torsion of the fallopian tube following tubal ligation is usually of the distal end. Extrinsic causes of tubal torsion are ovarian and peritubal tumors, adhesions, trauma, and pregnancy.

The most important symptom of tubal torsion is acute lower abdominal and pelvic pain. The onset of this pain may be gradual or sudden, and the pain is usually located in the iliac fossa, with radiation to the thigh and flank. The duration of pain is generally less than 48 hours, and it is associated with nausea and vomiting in two thirds of the cases. Usually, the pelvic pain, secondary to hypoxia, is so intense that it is difficult to perform an adequate pelvic exam. Unless there is associated torsion of the ovary, a specific mass is usually not palpable on pelvic examination.

The preoperative diagnosis of tubal torsion is made in less than 20% of reported cases. However, the number of cases diagnosed preoperatively has increased dramatically with the use of vaginal ultrasonography. Because of the severity of the pain, a wide differential diagnosis of abdominal and pelvic pathology must be considered. The differential diagnosis includes acute appendicitis, ectopic pregnancy, pelvic inflammatory disease, and rupture or torsion of an ovarian cyst.

Exploratory operation determines the extent of hypoxia and the choice of operative techniques. With tubal torsion, usually the tubes are gangrenous and must be excised. The twisted tube is usually filled with a bloody or serous fluid. Occasionally, with a minor degree of torsion, it is possible to restore normal circulation to the tube and salvage it. The tube is usually sutured into a secure position to prevent recurrence.

OVARY

Functional Cysts

Follicular Cysts

Follicular cysts are by far the most frequent cystic structures in normal ovaries. The cysts are frequently multiple and may vary from a few millimeters to as large as 15 cm in diameter. However, a normal follicle may physiologically become cystic, and therefore it is important to have a minimal diameter for a follicular cyst. This diameter is generally considered to be between 2.5 and 3 cm. Follicular cysts are not neoplastic and are believed to be dependent on gonadotrophins for growth. They arise from a temporary variation of a normal physiologic process. Clinically they may present with the signs and symptoms of ovarian enlargement and therefore must be differentiated from a true ovarian neoplasm. Functional cysts may be solitary or multiple. These cysts are found most commonly in young, menstruating women. Solitary cysts may occur during the fetal and neonatal periods and rarely during childhood, but there is an increase in frequency during the perimenarchal period. Wolf et al. studied 149 postmenopausal women and found simple cysts ranging in size from 0.4 to 4.7 cm in 15% of them. Large solitary follicular cysts in which the lining is luteinized are occasionally discovered during pregnancy and the puerperium. Multiple follicular cysts in which the lining is luteinized are associated with either intrinsic or extrinsic elevated levels of gonadotrophins. Interestingly, reproductive-aged women with cystic fibrosis appear to have an increased propensity to develop individual follicular cysts.

Follicular cysts are translucent, thin walled, and are filled with a watery, clear to straw-colored fluid. If a small opening in the capsule of the cyst suddenly develops, the cyst fluid under pressure will squirt out. These cysts are situated in the ovarian cortex, and sometimes they appear as translucent domes on the surface of the ovary. Histologically the lining of the cyst is usually

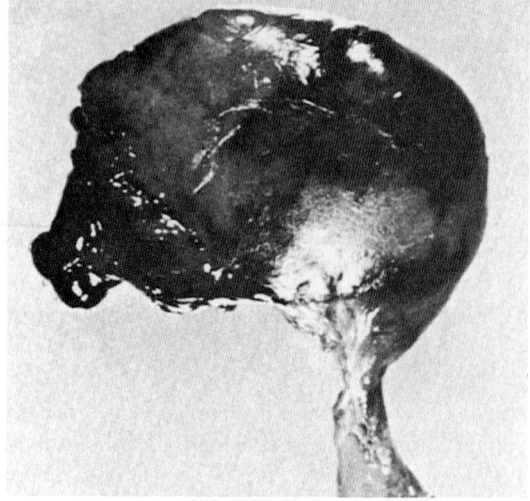

FIGURE 18-27 Right fallopian tube showing hemorrhage, edema, and infarction secondary to torsion. (From Chambers JT, Thiagarajah S, and Kitchin JD: Obstet Gynecol 54:488, 1979. Reprinted with permission from The American College of Obstetricians and Gynecologists.)

composed of a closely packed layer of round, plump granulosa cells, with the spindle-shaped cells of the theca interna deeper in the stroma. In many cysts the lining of granulosa cells is difficult to distinguish, having undergone pressure atrophy. All that remains is a hyalinized connective tissue lining.

The temporary disturbance in follicular function that produces the clinical picture of a follicular cyst is poorly understood. Follicular cysts may result from either the dominant mature follicle's failing to rupture (persistent follicle) or an immature follicle's failing to undergo the normal process of atresia. In the latter circumstance the incompletely developed follicle fails to reabsorb follicular fluid. Some follicular cysts lose their ability to produce estrogen, while in others the granulosa cells remain productive, with prolonged secretion of estrogens. Occasionally, follicular cysts are better termed *follicular hematomas*, because blood from the vascular theca zone fills the cavity of the cyst.

The majority of follicular cysts are asymptomatic and are discovered during ultrasound imaging of the pelvis or a routine pelvic examination. Because of their thin walls, these cysts may rupture during examination. The patient may experience a transient tenderness or no pain whatsoever. Rarely is significant intraperitoneal bleeding associated with the rupture of a follicular cyst. However, women who are chronically anticoagulated may bleed, not infrequently, from either a follicular or corpus luteum cyst. Occasionally, menstrual irregularities and abnormal uterine bleeding may be associated with follicular cysts, which produce elevated blood estrogen levels. The syndrome associated with such follicular cysts consists of a regular cycle with a prolonged intermenstrual interval, followed by episodes of menorrhagia. Some women with larger follicular cysts notice a vague, dull sensation or a heaviness in the pelvis.

The initial management of a suspected follicular cyst is conservative observation. The majority of follicular cysts disappear spontaneously by either reabsorption of the cyst fluid or silent rupture within 4 to 8 weeks of initial diagnosis. However, a persistent ovarian mass necessitates operative intervention to differentiate a physiologic cyst from a true neoplasm of the ovary. There is no way to make the differentiation on the basis of signs, symptoms, or the initial growth pattern during early development of either process. Endovaginal ultrasound examination may help to differentiate simple from complex cysts and also may help during conservative management by providing dimensions to determine if the cyst is increasing in size. When the diameter of the cyst remains stable for greater than 10 weeks or enlarges, a neoplasia should be ruled out. Spanos suggested prescribing oral contraceptives for 4 to 6 weeks for young women with adnexal masses. This therapy removes any influence that pituitary gonadotrophins may have on the persistence of the ovarian cyst. It also allows for several weeks of observation. In Spanos's series,

80% of cystic masses 4 to 6 cm in size disappeared during the time the patient was taking oral contraceptives. Steinkampf et al. performed a randomized prospective study of the effect of oral contraceptives on functional ovarian masses in women of reproductive age. Their study group consisted of women with infertility who had recently been treated by ovulation induction. In their series there was no difference in the rate of disappearance of functional ovarian cysts between the group that received oral contraceptives and the control group.

Operative management is cystectomy, not oophorectomy. Many clinicians will manage simple cysts with the laparoscope. Since this procedure has an accompanying risk of spilling malignant cells into the peritoneal cavity if the cyst is an early carcinoma, strict preoperative criteria should be fulfilled before laparoscopy is attempted. These include the woman's age, size of the mass, and ultrasonic characteristics, such as nonadherent smooth and thin-walled cysts, without papillae or internal echoes. The use of color Doppler for examination of vascularity and vascular resistance may also be helpful in the preoperative assessment of simple cysts. DeWilde et al., in a series of follicular cysts averaging 6 cm in diameter, found that the recurrence rate following laparoscopic fenestration was approximately 2%. Higher rates of recurrence, up to 40%, have been reported for simple drainage of multiple types of benign cysts. When cysts are drained, it is essential to remember that cytologic examination of cyst fluid has poor predictive value and poor sensitivity in differentiating benign from malignant cysts. One recent report of fine-needle aspiration of ovarian cysts found sensitivity of 25%, specificity of 90%, false-positive rate of 73%, and false-negative rate of 12%. In a preliminary study of chemical analysis of adnexal cystic fluid, lactic dehydrogenase (LDH) levels were the most promising marker to differentiate benign from malignant disease. Thus, if there is any suspicion of malignancy, a tissue sample for histopathology should be obtained.

Corpus Luteum Cysts

Corpus luteum cysts are less common than follicular cysts, but clinically they are more important. This discussion collectively combines corpus luteum cysts and persistently functioning mature corpora lutea (Figure 18-28). Pathologists are sometimes able to make a distinction between a hemorrhagic cystic corpus luteum and a corpus luteum cyst, but at other times this difference cannot be established. All corpora lutea are cystic with gradual reabsorption of a limited amount of hemorrhage, which may form a cavity. Clinically, corpora lutea are not termed *corpus luteum cysts* unless they are a minimum of 3 cm in diameter. Corpus luteum cysts may be associated with either normal endocrine function or prolonged secretion of progesterone. The associated menstrual pattern may be normal, delayed menstruation, or amenorrhea.

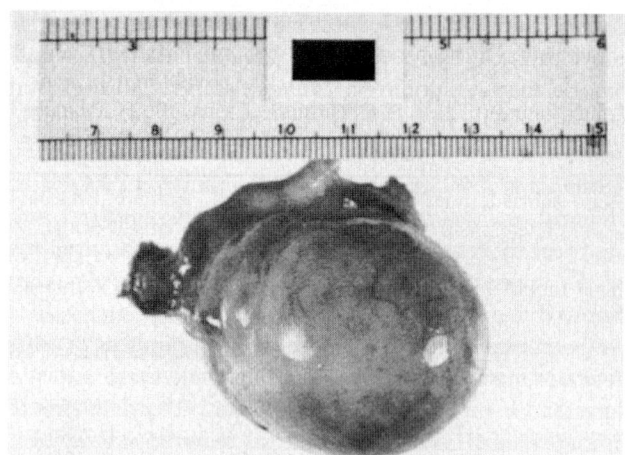

FIGURE 18-28   Corpus luteum cyst, 3 to 4 cm in diameter, externally smooth. (From Janovski NA, editor: Color atlas of gross gynecologic and obstetric pathology, New York, 1969, McGraw-Hill Book Co, p 155.)

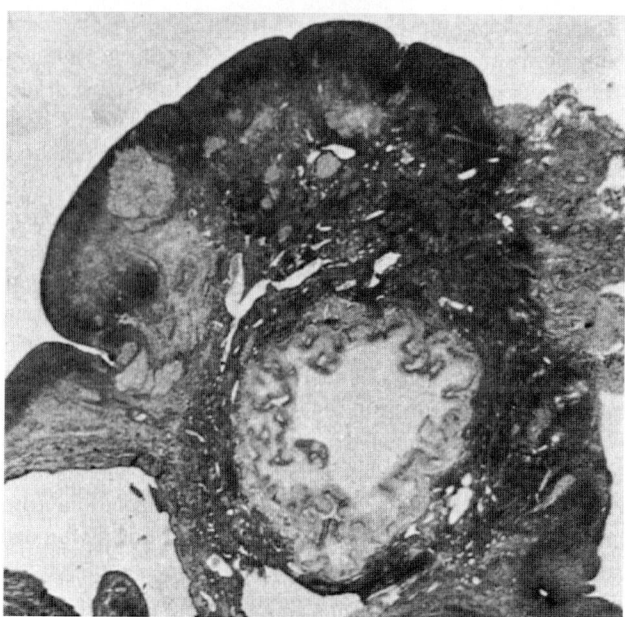

FIGURE 18-29   Corpus albicans cyst. Lining of cyst is composed of hyalinized connective tissue. (From Blaustein A: Nonneoplastic cysts of the ovary. In Blaustein A, editor: Pathology of the female genital tract, New York, 1977, Springer-Verlag New York, Inc, p 396.)

Corpora lutea develop from mature graafian follicles. Intrafollicular bleeding does not occur during ovulation. However, 2 to 4 days later, during the stage of vascularization, thin-walled capillaries invade the granulosa cells from the theca interna. Spontaneous but limited bleeding fills the central cavity of the maturing corpus luteum with blood. Subsequently this blood is absorbed, forming a small cystic space. When the hemorrhage is excessive, the cystic space enlarges. If the hemorrhage into the central cavity is brisk, intracystic pressure increases and rupture of the corpus luteum is a possibility. If rupture does not occur, the size of the resulting corpus luteum cyst usually varies between 3 and 10 cm. Occasionally a cyst may be 11 to 15 cm in diameter. If a cystic central cavity persists, blood is replaced by clear fluid, and the result is a hormonally inactive corpus albicans cyst (Figure 18-29). A corpus luteum of pregnancy is normally 3 to 5 cm in diameter with a central cystic structure, occupying at least 50% of the ovarian mass.

Most corpus luteum cysts are small, the average diameter being 4 cm. Grossly, they have a smooth surface and, depending on whether the cyst represents acute or chronic hemorrhage, are purplish red to brown (Figure 18-30). When a corpus luteum is cut, the convoluted lining is yellowish-orange, and the center contains an organizing blood clot. Both the granulosa and the theca cells undergo luteinization. In chronic corpus luteum cysts the wall becomes gray-white, and the polygonal luteinized cells usually undergo pressure atrophy. Hallatt et al. reviewed 173 ruptured corpora lutea with hemoperitoneum. In their institution the frequency of serious bleeding from a corpus luteum cyst compared with ectopic pregnancy was one in four.

Corpus luteum cysts vary from being asymptomatic masses to those causing catastrophic and massive intra-

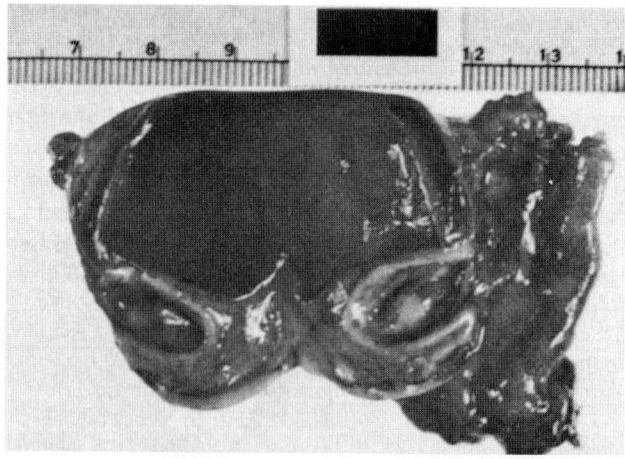

FIGURE 18-30   Corpus luteum cyst with thickened cyst wall and definite lutein cell lining recognized by its color. Cyst is filled with hemorrhagic gelatinous material. (From Janovski NA, editor: Color atlas of gross gynecologic and obstetric pathology, New York, 1969, McGraw-Hill Book Co, p 157.)

peritoneal bleeding associated with rupture. Many corpus luteum cysts produce dull, unilateral, lower abdominal and pelvic pain. The enlarged ovary is moderately tender on pelvic examination. Depending on the amount of progesterone secretion associated with cysts, the menstrual bleeding may be normal or delayed several days to weeks with subsequent menorrhagia. Halban in 1915 described a syndrome of a persistently functioning corpus luteum cyst that has clinical features similar to an unruptured ectopic pregnancy. Halban's classic triad was a delay in a normal period followed by spotting, unilateral pelvic pain, and a small, tender adnexal mass. This triad of symptomatology is similar to the triad of an anomalous period or delay in a normal period, spotting, and unilateral pelvic pain that is exhibited by the classic ectopic pregnancy. The differential diagnosis between these two conditions without a sensitive pregnancy test is difficult.

Corpus luteum cysts may cause intraperitoneal bleeding. The amount of bleeding varies from slight to clinically significant hemorrhage, necessitating blood transfusion. Internal bleeding often follows coitus, exercise, trauma, or a pelvic examination. However, episodes of bleeding usually do not recur, which differs from an ectopic pregnancy. Women with a bleeding diathesis or undergoing chronic warfarin (Coumadin) therapy are especially prone to develop ovarian hemorrhage from a corpus luteum cyst. Bleeding occurs usually between days 20 to 26 of their cycle, and these women have a 31% chance for subsequent hemorrhage from a recurrent corpus luteum cyst. Oral contraceptives are sometimes used to suppress ovulation and avoid recurrent hemorrhage.

Hallatt et al. reported that sudden, severe, lower abdominal pain was a prominent symptom in women with hemoperitoneum caused by a ruptured corpus luteum cyst (Table 18-2). One of three women also noted unilateral cramping and lower abdominal pain for 1 to 2 weeks before overt rupture. The right ovary was the source of hemorrhage in 66% of their series. Tang et al. have also reported a right-sided predominance in the incidence of

hemorrhage from corpus luteum cysts. They postulated that the difference is related to a higher intraluminal pressure on the right side because of the differences in ovarian vein architecture. Most ruptures occur between days 20 and 26 of the cycle, although in the series of Hallatt et al. 28% of the women had a delay in menses not explained by pregnancy (Table 18-3).

The differential diagnosis of a woman with acute pain and suspected ruptured corpus luteum cyst includes ectopic pregnancy, a ruptured endometrioma, and adnexal torsion. A sensitive serum or urinary assay for human chorionic gonadotrophin (hCG) will help to differentiate a bleeding corpus luteum from ectopic pregnancy (Chapter 17). Vaginal ultrasound is useful in establishing a preoperative diagnosis. Occasionally, culdocentesis is helpful in establishing the severity of the hemorrhage. If the hematocrit of the fluid obtained from the posterior cul-de-sac is greater than 15%, operative therapy becomes a necessity. Cystectomy is the operative treatment of choice, with preservation of the remaining portion of the ovary. In the series of DeWilde et al. of persistent corpus luteum cysts treated by fenestration via the laparoscope, 6 of 44 (14%) recurred. Obviously, it was impossible for the authors to distinguish between a recurrent corpus luteum cyst and the development of a new corpus luteum. Unruptured corpus luteum cysts may be followed conservatively. Raziel et al. reported on a series of 70 women with ruptured corpora lutea. Ultrasonic evidence of large amounts of peritoneal fluid and severe pain were indications for operative intervention. In 12 of 70 patients with small amounts of intraperitoneal fluid and mild to moderate pain, observation alone was associated with resolution of symptoms.

TABLE 18-2
Symptoms of 173 Women with Ruptured Corpus Luteum

	Number	Percent
Location		
Right ovary	114	66
Left ovary	56	32
Unknown	3	2
Abdominal pain	173	100
Onset with intercourse	29	17
Right ovary	21	72
Left ovary	8	28
Duration		
Less than 24 hours	94	54
1 to 7 days	40	23
Over 7 days	14	8
Unknown	25	15
Nausea or vomiting or diarrhea	60	35

From Hallatt JG, Steele CH, and Snyder M: Am J Obstet Gynecol 149:6, 1984.

TABLE 18-3
Menstrual History in 173 Women with Ruptured Corpus Luteum

Last menstrual period to operation	
Under 14 days	5
14 to 31 days (pregnant = 2)	77
31 to 60 days (pregnant = 15)	56
Over 60 days (pregnant = 10)	18
No menstrual period	14
Hysterectomy	5
Amenorrhea after oral contraceptives	5
Secondary amenorrhea	2
Menarche	1
Menopause	1
History of irregular menses	14
Unknown	3

From Hallatt JG, Steele CH, and Snyder M: Am J Obstet Gynecol 149:6, 1984.

Theca Lutein Cysts

Theca lutein cysts are by far the least common of the three types of physiologic ovarian cysts (Figure 18-31). Unlike corpus luteum cysts, theca lutein cysts are almost always bilateral and produce moderate to massive enlargement of the ovaries. The individual cysts vary in size from 1 cm to 10 cm or more in diameter. These cysts arise from either prolonged or excessive stimulation of the ovaries by endogenous or exogenous gonadotrophins or increased ovarian sensitivity to gonadotrophins. The condition of ovarian enlargement secondary to the development of multiple luteinized follicular cysts is termed *hyperreactio luteinalis*. Approximately 50% of molar pregnancies and 10% of choriocarcinomas have associated bilateral theca lutein cysts (Chapter 31). In these patients the hCG from the trophoblast produces luteinization of the cells in immature, mature, and atretic follicles. The cysts are also discovered in the latter months of pregnancies often with conditions that produce a large placenta, such as twins, diabetes, and Rh sensitization. It is not uncommon to iatrogenically produce theca lutein cysts in women receiving drugs to induce ovulation. Theca lutein cysts are occasionally discovered in association with normal pregnancy, as well as in newborn infants secondary to transplacental effects of maternal gonadotrophins. Rarely, these cysts are found in young girls with juvenile hypothyroidism. Bakri et al. reported a case of theca lutein cysts in normal pregnancy that may have been associated with the patient's hypothyroidism. The authors speculated that similarities in the alpha subunit of TSH, hCG, and FSH may have led to the ovarian enlargement.

Grossly the total ovarian size may be voluminous, 20 to 30 cm in diameter, with multiple theca lutein cysts. Bilateral ovarian enlargement is produced by multiple gray to bluish-tinged cysts. The bilateral enlargement is secondary to hundreds of thin-walled locules or cysts producing a honeycombed appearance. Grossly the external surface of the ovary appears lobulated. The small cysts contain a clear to straw-colored or hemorrhagic fluid. Histologically the lining of the cyst is composed of theca lutein cells (paralutein cells), believed to originate from ovarian connective tissue. Occasionally there is also luteinization of granulosa cells. These voluminous and congested ovaries are slow growing. The vast majority of women with smaller cysts are asymptomatic. Generally only the larger cysts produce vague symptoms, such as a sense of pressure in the pelvis. Ascites and increasing abdominal girth have been reported with hyperstimulation from exogenous gonadotrophins. Rarely, associated adnexal torsion may occur. Montz et al., in reviewing the natural history of 102 women with theca lutein cysts, found that approximately 1% of patients experienced acute complications of either torsion or intraperitoneal bleeding. They also discovered that theca lutein cysts persisted in some women for weeks after hCG levels were nondetectable.

The presence of theca lutein cysts is established by palpation and often confirmed by ultrasound examination. Treatment is conservative because these cysts gradually regress. If these cysts are discovered incidentally at cesarean delivery, they should be handled delicately. No attempt should be made to drain or puncture the multiple cysts because of the possibility of hemorrhage. Bleeding is difficult to control in these cases because of the thin walls that comprise the cysts.

A condition related to theca lutein cysts is the *luteoma* of pregnancy. The condition is rare and not a true neoplasm but rather a specific, benign, hyperplastic reaction of ovarian theca lutein cells (Figure 18-32). These nodules do not arise from the corpus luteum of pregnancy. Fifty percent of luteomas are multiple, and approximately 30% of those reported

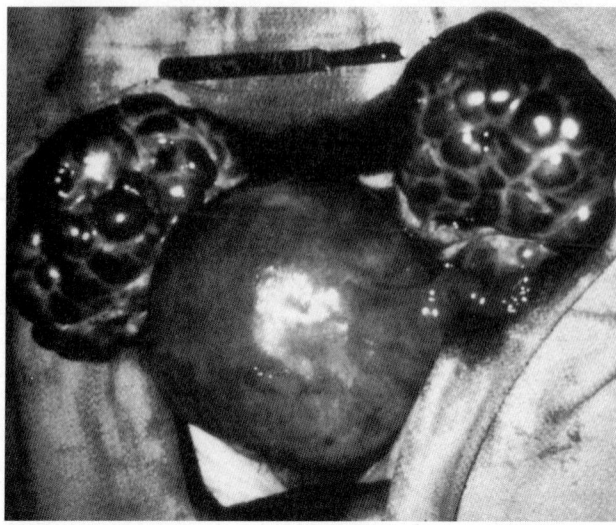

FIGURE 18-31 Bilateral theca lutein cysts. (Courtesy Daniel R. Mishell, Jr., M.D.)

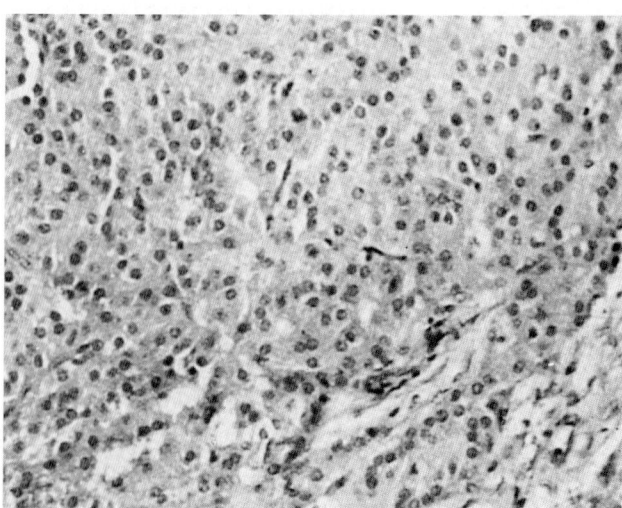

FIGURE 18-32 Luteoma. Solid mass of uniform polygonal "luteinized" cells with spherical nuclei. (H&E stain; ×220.) (From Dische FE and Ritchie JM: J Pathol 100:77, Plate XXXVI, 1970.)

have bilateral nodules. In appearance they are discrete and brown to reddish brown and may be solid or cystic.

The majority of patients with luteomas are asymptomatic. The solid, fleshy, often hemorrhagic, nodules are discovered incidentally at cesarean delivery or postpartum tubal ligation. Most reported cases are in multiparous black women. Masculinization of the mother occurs in 30% of cases, and masculinization of the external genitalia of the female fetus may sometimes occur. These tumors regress spontaneously following completion of the pregnancy.

Benign Neoplasms of the Ovary

Benign Cystic Teratoma (Dermoid Cyst, Mature Teratoma)

Benign ovarian teratomas are usually cystic structures that on histologic examination contain elements from all three germ cell layers. The word *teratoma* was first advanced by Virchow and translated literally means "monstrous growth." Teratomas of the ovary may be benign or malignant. Although *dermoid* is a misnomer, it is the most common term used to describe the benign cystic tumor, composed of mature cells, whereas the malignant variety is composed of immature cells (immature teratoma). *Dermoid* is a descriptive term in that it emphasizes the preponderance of ectodermal tissue with some mesodermal and rare endodermal derivatives. Malignant teratomas that are immature are usually solid with some cystic areas and histologically contain immature or embryonic-appearing tissue. (See Chapter 31 for further discussion of malignant teratomas.) Benign teratomas may undergo malignant transformation. This occurs in approximately 1% to 2% of dermoids, usually in women over age 40. The malignant component is generally a squamous carcinoma. Nonovarian teratomas may arise in any midline structure of the body where the germ cell has resided during embryonic life.

Benign teratomas are among the most common ovarian neoplasms. They account for over 90% of germ cell tumors of the ovary. These slow-growing tumors occur from infancy to the postmenopausal years. Depending on the series, dermoids represent 20% to 25% of all ovarian neoplasms and approximately 33% of all benign tumors, if follicular and corpus luteum cysts are excluded. Dermoids are the most common ovarian neoplasm in prepubertal females and are also common in teenagers. However, more than 50% of benign teratomas are discovered in women between the ages of 25 and 50 years. In the series of Lakkis et al. of 118 women with dermoids, 86% of the women were less than 40 years of age, and 3.4% had recurrences (Figure 18-33). Similarly, in the series by Comerci et al. of 573 tumors in 517 women the mean age was 32 years and 86% were less than 43 years of age. In most large series of benign tumors in postmenopausal women, dermoids account for approximately 20% of the neoplasms.

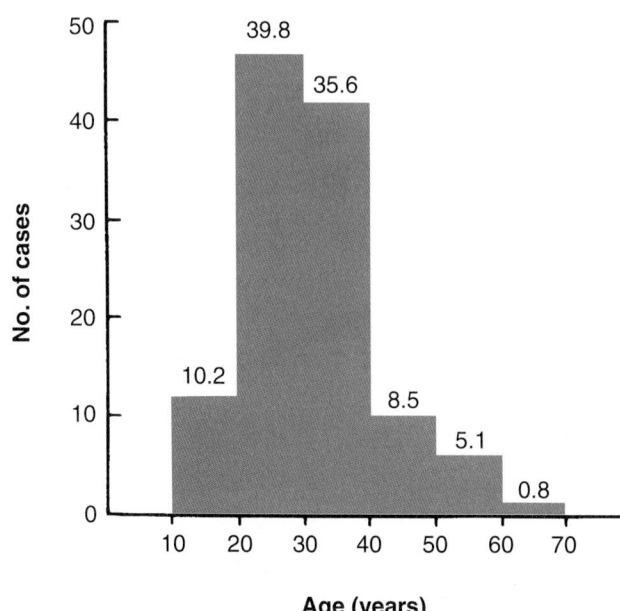

FIGURE 18-33 Age distribution of cystic teratomas. (From Lakkis WG, Martin MC, and Gelfand MM: Originally published in Canadian Journal of Surgery 28:444, 1985.)

Dermoids vary from a few millimeters to 25 cm in diameter. Comerci et al. reported a large tumor weighing 7657 g in a woman who was asymptomatic. However, 80% are less than 10 cm. These tumors may be single or multiple, with as many as nine individual dermoids having been reported in the same ovary. Benign teratomas occur bilaterally 10% to 15% of the time. Often, dermoid cysts are pedunculated. These cysts make the ovary heavier than normal, and thus they are usually discovered either in the cul-de-sac or anterior to the broad ligament. On palpation these tumors, which have both cystic and solid components, have a doughy consistency (Figure 18-34).

The cysts are usually unilocular. The walls of the cyst are a smooth, shiny, opaque white color. When they are opened, thick sebaceous fluid pours from the cyst, often with tangled masses of hair and firm areas of cartilage and teeth (Figure 18-35). The sebaceous material is a thick fluid at body temperature but solidifies when it cools in room air.

Benign teratomas are believed to arise from a single germ cell after the first meiotic division. Therefore they develop from totipotential stem cells, and they are neoplastic sequelae from a transformed germ cell. Dermoids have a chromosomal makeup of 46,XX. Linder et al., in a series of experiments using chromosome banding techniques and electrophoretic variance, discovered that the chromosomes of dermoids were different from the chromosomes of the host. They postulated that dermoids began by parthenogenesis from secondary oocytes. An alternative hypothesis was that the dermoid resulted from fusion of the second polar body with the oocyte. The studies by Linder et al. ruled out the possibility that dermoids arise from somatic cells or from an oogonium before the first stage of meiosis. The first meiotic division occurs at approximately 13 weeks of gestation. Thus dermoids begin in fetal life sometime after the first trimester.

Histologically, benign teratomas are composed of mature cells, usually from all three germ layers (Figure 18-36). A combination of skin and skin appendages, including sebaceous glands, sweat glands, hair follicles, muscle fibers, cartilage, bone, teeth, glial cells, and epithelium of the respiratory and gastrointestinal tracts, may be

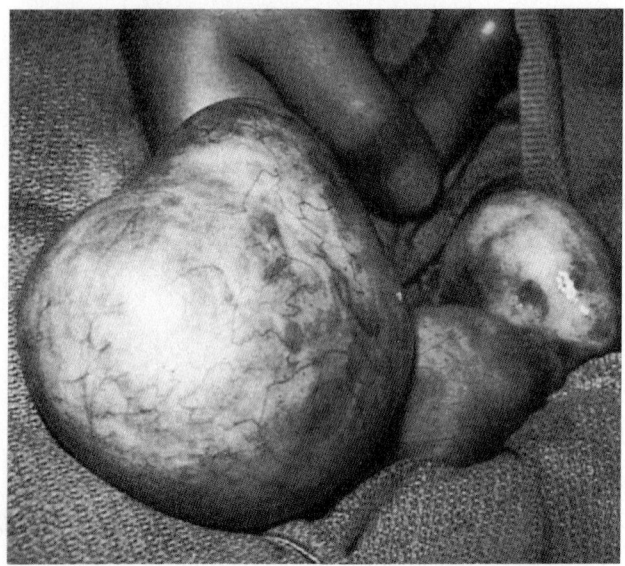

FIGURE 18-34   Gross appearance of bilateral dermoid cysts of the ovary. (Courtesy Daniel R. Mishell, Jr., M.D.)

visualized. Teeth are predominantly premolar and molar forms. The fluid in dermoid cysts is usually sebaceous. Most solid elements arise and are contained in a protrusion or nipple (mamilla) in the cyst wall termed the *prominence* or *tubercle of Rokitansky*. This prominence may be visualized by ultrasound as an echodense region, thus aiding in the sonographic diagnosis. The wall of the cyst will often contain granulation tissue, giant cells, and pseudoxanthoma cells.

From 50% to 60% of dermoids are asymptomatic and are discovered during a routine pelvic examination, coincidentally visualized by an abdominal x-ray or ultrasound examination, or found incidentally at laparotomy. Presenting symptoms of dermoids include pain, and the sensation of pelvic pressure. Specific complications of dermoid cysts include torsion, rupture, infection, hemorrhage, and malignant degeneration. Three medical diseases also may be associated with dermoid cysts: thyrotoxicosis, carcinoid syndrome, and autoimmune hemolytic anemia. Torsion of a dermoid is the most frequent complication, occurring in 11% of the series by Pantoja et al. and 3.5% of the time in Comerci's series. Because of its weight, the benign teratoma is often pedunculated, which may predispose to torsion. Torsion is more common in younger women (Figure 18-37). Small dermoid cysts, less than 6 cm in diameter, grow slowly at an approximate rate of 2 mm per year.

Rupture or perforation of the contents of a dermoid into the peritoneal cavity or an adjacent organ is a most serious complication. The incidence varies between 0.7% and 4.6%. However, most series report less than 1%. Rupture is more common in pregnancy. Rupture may occur either catastrophically, which produces an acute abdomen, or by a slow leak of the sebaceous material. The latter is clinically more common, with the sebaceous

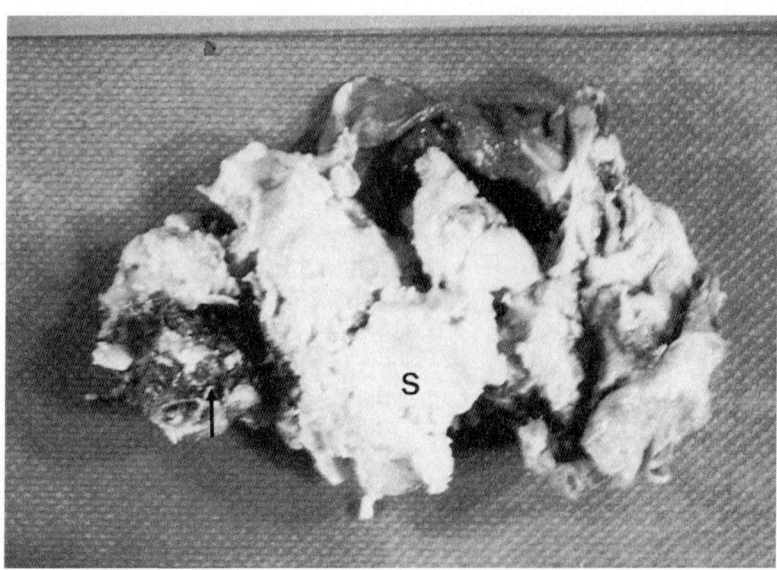

FIGURE 18-35   Benign cystic teratoma. This section from the tumor demonstrates areas of hair *(dark arrows)* and solid sebaceous material *(S)*. (Courtesy Deborah Jean Dotters, M.D.)

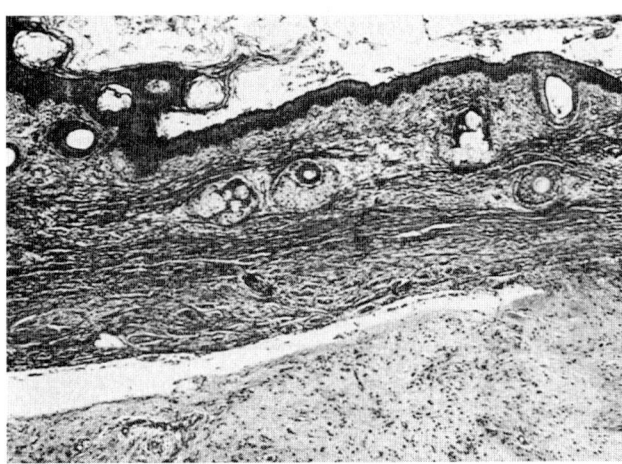

FIGURE 18-36 Mature cystic teratoma. Lining of cyst is composed of skin with its appendages. Mature neural tissue is seen beneath the cutaneous structures. (H&E stain; ×61.) (Reprinted by permission from Talerman A: Germ cell tumors of the ovary. In Blaustein A, editor: Pathology of the female genital tract, New York, 1977, Springer-Verlag New York, Inc, p 559.)

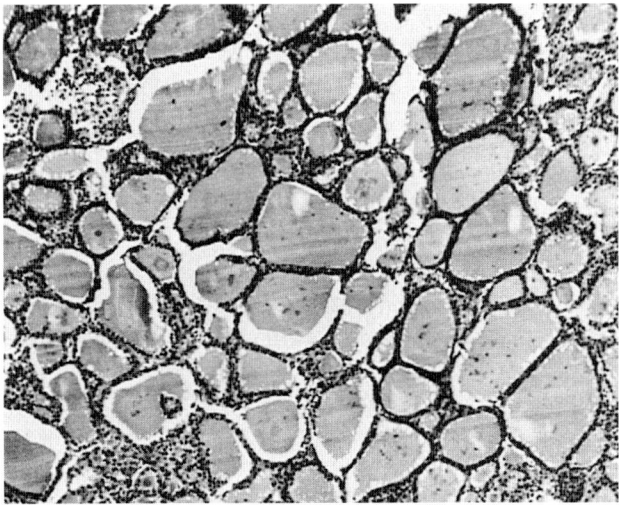

FIGURE 18-38 Struma ovarii. Tumor is composed of normal thyroid tissue. (H&E stain; ×76.) (Reprinted by permission from Talerman A: Germ cell tumors of the ovary. In Blaustein A, editor: Pathology of the female genital tract, New York, 1977, Springer-Verlag New York, Inc, p 563.)

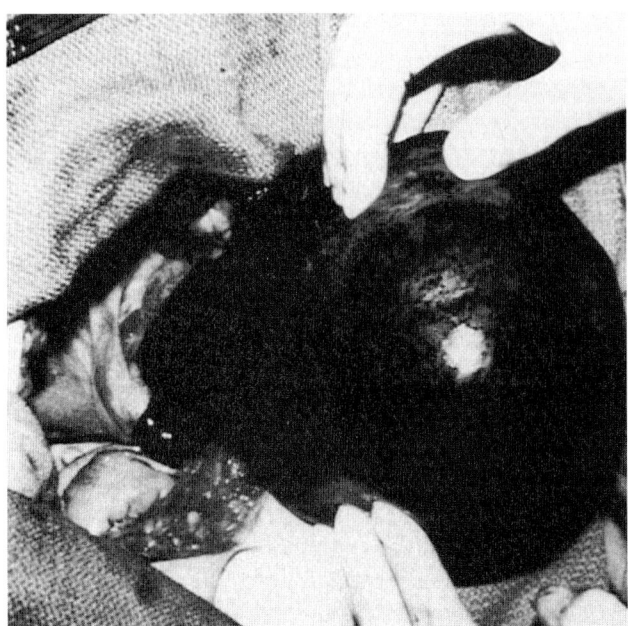

FIGURE 18-37 Torsion of the ovary. (Courtesy Daniel R. Mishell, Jr., M.D.)

material producing a severe chemical granulomatous peritonitis. Waxman and Boyce warn that this possibility should be considered and a frozen section obtained so that the true diagnosis is established. Thus a young woman will not be mistakenly treated for suspected ovarian carcinoma with metastasis because of the identical gross appearance of a slow-leaking dermoid cyst. Infection, hemorrhage, and malignant degeneration are

all unusual complications of dermoids, occurring in less than 1% of patients.

Adult thyroid tissue is discovered microscopically in approximately 12% of benign teratomas. *Struma ovarii* is a teratoma in which the thyroid tissue has overgrown other elements and is the predominant tissue (Figure 18-38). Strumae ovarii comprise 2% to 3% of ovarian teratomas. These tumors are usually unilateral and measure less than 10 cm in diameter. Less than 5% of women with struma ovarii develop thyrotoxicosis, which may be secondary to the production of increased thyroid hormone by either the ovarian or the thyroid gland.

Another rare finding with dermoids is the presence of a primary carcinoid tumor from the gastrointestinal or respiratory tract epithelium contained in the dermoid. One of three of these tumors is associated with the typical carcinoid syndrome even without metastatic spread. If the carcinoid is functioning, it may be diagnosed by measuring serum serotonin levels or urinary levels of 5-hydroxyindoleacetic acid. The autoimmune hemolytic anemia associated with dermoids is the rarest of the three medical complications.

The diagnosis of a dermoid cyst is often established when a semisolid mass is palpated anterior to the broad ligament. Approximately 50% of dermoids have pelvic calcifications on x-ray examination. Often an ovarian teratoma is an incidental finding during radiologic investigation of the genitourinary or gastrointestinal tract. Many, but not all, dermoids have a characteristic ultrasound picture. These characteristics include a dense echogenic area within a larger cystic area, a cyst filled with bands of mixed echoes, and an echoic dense cyst. Laing et al. have found that only one of three dermoids have this "typical picture." In their series of 45 patients with 51 biopsy-proven dermoid cysts, 24% of the dermoid cysts were predominantly solid, 20% were almost entirely cystic, and 24% were not visible. Operative treatment of benign cystic teratomas is cystectomy with preservation of as much normal ovarian tissue as possible.

Endometriomas

Endometriosis of the ovary is usually associated with endometriosis in other areas of the pelvic cavity. Approximately two out of three women with endometriosis have ovarian involvement. Interestingly, only 5% of these women have enlargement of the ovaries that is detectable by pelvic examination. However, because of the prevalence of the disease, endometriosis is one of the most common causes of enlargement of the ovary. Because most authors do not classify endometriosis as a neoplastic disease, the diagnosis of endometriosis may not be given due consideration in the differential diagnosis of an adnexal mass. Ovarian endometriosis is similar to endometriosis elsewhere and is described in greater detail in Chapter 19.

The size of ovarian endometriomas varies from small, superficial, blue-black implants that are 1 to 5 mm in diameter to large, multiloculated, hemorrhagic cysts that may be 5 to 10 cm in diameter (Figure 18-39). Clinically, large ovarian endometriomas, greater than 20 cm in diameter, are extremely rare. Areas of ovarian endometriosis that become cystic are termed *endometriomas*. Rarely, large chocolate cysts of the ovary may reach 15 to 20 cm (Figure 18-40). Larger cysts are frequently bilateral. The surface of an ovary with endometriosis is often irregular, puckered, and scarred. Depending on their size, endometriomas replace a portion of the normal ovarian tissue.

Although most women with endometriomas are asymptomatic, the most common symptoms associated with ovarian endometriosis are pelvic pain, dyspareunia, and infertility. Approximately 10% of the operations for endometriosis are for acute symptoms, usually related to a ruptured ovarian endometrioma that was previously asymptomatic. Smaller cysts generally have thin walls, and perforation occurs commonly secondary to cyclic hemorrhage into the cystic cavity.

On pelvic examination the ovaries are often tender and immobile, secondary to associated inflammation and adhesions. Most commonly the ovaries are densely adherent to surrounding structures, including the peritoneum of the pelvic sidewall, the oviduct, the broad ligament, and sometimes the small or large bowel. Endometrial glands, endometrial stroma, and large phagocytic cells containing hemosiderin may be identified histologically (Figure 18-41). Pressure atrophy may lead to the loss of architecture of the endometrial glands.

The choice between medical and operative management depends on several factors, including the patient's age, future reproductive plans, and severity of symptoms. Medical therapy is rarely successful in treating ovarian endometriosis if the disease has produced ovarian enlargement. Often surgical therapy is complicated by formation of de novo and recurrent adhesions.

On pathologic examination, it is important to distinguish endometriosis from benign endometrial tumors, which are usually adenofibromas. The latter tumor is a true neoplasm, and there is a malignant counterpart.

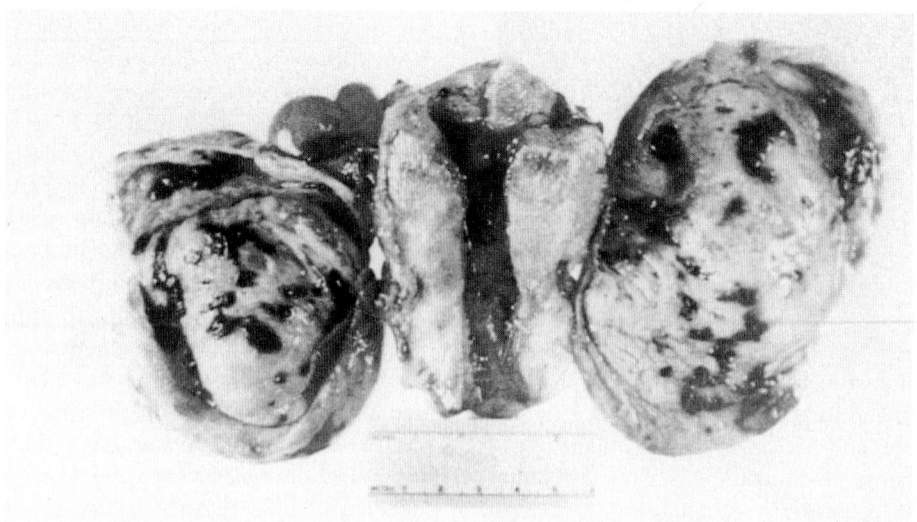

FIGURE 18-39 Endometriosis of ovaries. Wall of endometriotic cyst is thickened and fibrotic. Inner surface shows areas of dark brown discoloration. (From Janovski NA, editor: Color atlas of gross gynecologic and obstetric pathology, New York, 1969, McGraw-Hill Book Co, p 159.)

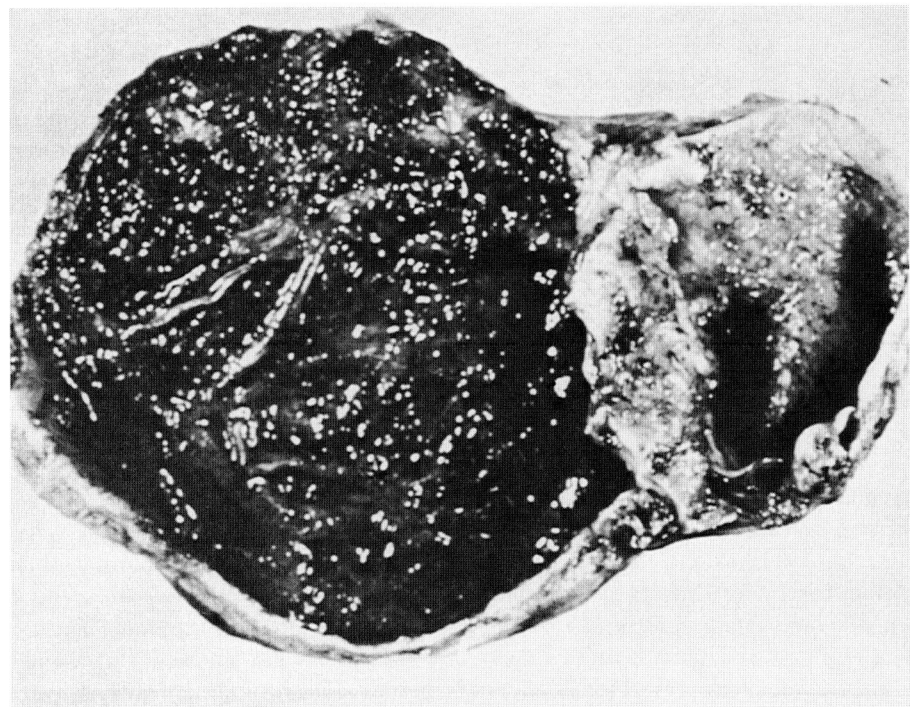

FIGURE 18-40 Opened endometrioma showing large cyst lined by hemorrhagic tissue. (From Czernobilsky B: Primary epithelial tumors of the ovary. In Blaustein A, editor: Pathology of the female genital tract, New York, 1977, Springer-Verlag New York, Inc, p 476.)

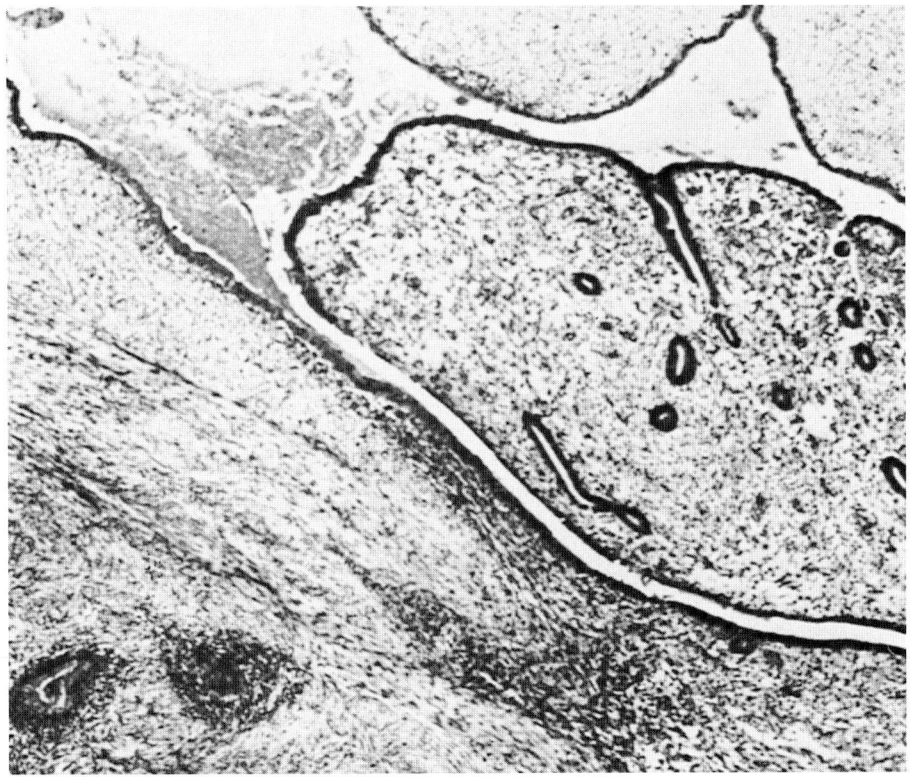

FIGURE 18-41 Wall of endometrioma lined by endometrial-type epithelium with underlying endometrial stroma. Note polypoid projections of endometrial tissue projecting into cyst lumen. (H&E stain; ×40.) (From Czernobilsky B: Primary epithelial tumors of the ovary. In Blaustein A, editor: Pathology of the female genital tract, New York, 1977, Springer-Verlag New York, Inc, p 476.)

Fibroma

Fibromas are the most common benign, solid neoplasms of the ovary. Their malignant potential is low, less than 1%. These tumors comprise approximately 5% of benign ovarian neoplasms and approximately 20% of all solid tumors of the ovary.

Fibromas vary in size from small nodules to huge pelvic tumors weighing 50 pounds. One of the predominant characteristics of fibromas is that they are extremely slow-growing tumors. The average diameter of a fibroma is approximately 6 cm; however, some tumors have reached 30 cm in diameter. In most series, less than 5% of fibromas are greater than 20 cm in diameter. The diameter of a fibroma is important clinically, because the incidence of associated ascites is directly proportional to the size of the tumor. Many ovarian fibromas are misdiagnosed and are believed to be leiomyomas prior to operation. Ninety percent of fibromas are unilateral; however, multiple fibromas are found in the same ovary in 10% to 15% of cases. The average age of a woman with an ovarian fibroma is 48. Thus this tumor often presents in a postmenopausal woman. The tumor arises from the undifferentiated fibrous stroma of the ovary. Bilateral ovarian fibromas are commonly found in women with the rare genetic transmitted basal cell nevus syndrome.

The pelvic symptoms that develop with growth of fibromas include pressure and abdominal enlargement, which may be secondary to both the size of the tumor and ascites. Smaller tumors are asymptomatic because these tumors do not elaborate hormones. Thus there is no change in the pattern of menstrual flow. Fibromas may be pedunculated and therefore easily palpable during one examination yet difficult to palpate during a subsequent pelvic examination. Sometimes on pelvic examination the fibromas appear to be softer than a solid ovarian tumor because of the edema and/or occasional cystic degeneration.

Meigs' syndrome is the association of an ovarian fibroma, ascites, and hydrothorax. Both the ascites and the hydrothorax resolve after removal of the ovarian tumor. The ascites is caused by transudation of fluid from the ovarian fibroma. Samanth and Black reported that the incidence of ascites was directly related to the size of the fibroma. Fifty percent of patients have ascites if the tumor is greater than 6 cm. However, true Meigs' syndrome is rare, occurring in less than 2% of ovarian fibromas. The hydrothorax develops secondary to a flow of ascitic fluid into the pleural space via the lymphatics of the diaphragm. Statistically the right pleural space is involved in 75% of reported cases, the left in 10%, and both sides in 15%. The clinical features of Meigs' syndrome are not unique to fibromas, and a similar clinical picture is found with many other ovarian tumors.

Grossly, fibromas are heavy, solid, well encapsulated, and grayish-white. The cut surface usually demonstrates a

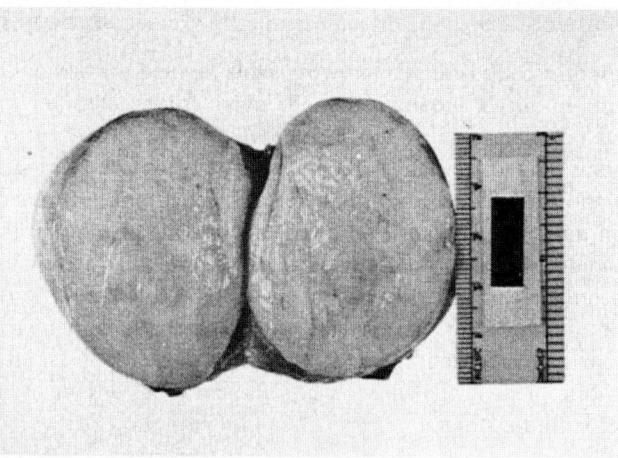

FIGURE 18-42 Fibroma of ovary. Cut surface shows somewhat edematous, interlacing bundles of connective tissue. (From Janovski NA, editor: Color atlas of gross gynecologic and obstetric pathology, New York, 1969, McGraw-Hill Book Co, p 163.)

homogeneous white or yellowish-white solid tissue with a trabeculated or whorled appearance similar to that of myomas. The vast majority of fibromas are grossly edematous (Figure 18-42). Less than 10% of fibromas have calcifications or small areas of hyaline or cystic degeneration. Histologically, fibromas are composed of connective tissue, stromal cells, and varying amounts of collagen interposed between the cells. The connective tissue cells are spindle-shaped, mature fibroblasts. They are arranged in an imperfect pattern. A few smooth muscle fibers may be occasionally identified. It is sometimes difficult to distinguish fibromas from nonneoplastic thecomas. Histologically the pathologist must differentiate fibromas from stromal hyperplasia, fibrosarcomas, and also look for epithelial elements of an associated Brenner tumor.

The management of fibromas is straightforward because any woman with a solid ovarian neoplasm should have an exploratory operation soon after the tumor is discovered. Simple excision of the tumor is all that is necessary. Following excision of the tumor, there is resolution of all symptoms, including ascites. Because these tumors are frequently discovered in postmenopausal women, often a bilateral salpingo-oophorectomy and total abdominal hysterectomy are performed. Conversely, it is important to note that most women who preoperatively have the combination of a solid ovarian tumor and ascites are found to have ovarian carcinoma.

Transitional Cell Tumors—Brenner Tumors

Brenner tumors are rare, small, smooth, solid, fibroepithelial ovarian tumors that are generally asymptomatic. The semantic classification of neoplasms changes and the current preferred term for benign Brenner tumor is *transitional cell tumor*. The benign, proliferative (low malignant potential), and malignant forms together comprise approximately 2% of ovarian tumors. These tumors usually occur in women aged 40 to 60 years. Approximately 30% of transitional cell tumors are discovered as small, solid tumors in association with a concurrent serous cystic neoplasia, such as serous or mucinous cystadenomas of the ipsilateral ovary. Some are microscopic, with the entire tumor contained in a single low-powered microscopic field, and others may reach a diameter of 20 cm; the majority are less than 5 cm in diameter. The tumor is unilateral 85% to 95% of the time.

The Brenner tumor was first described in 1898. Robert Meyer in 1932 postulated that it was a distinct, independent neoplasm from granulosa cell tumors. Since that time there has been a controversy in the gynecologic pathology literature as to the histogenesis of the neoplasm. Presently, most authorities accept the theory that most of these tumors result from metaplasia of coelomic epithelium into uroepithelium. Detailed three-dimensional histologic studies have demonstrated a downward growth in a cordlike fashion of epithelium from the surface of the ovary to deeper areas in the ovarian cortex. Others have postulated that sometimes the solid nests of epithelial cells of the tumor originate from the rete ovarii or Walthard rests. Shevchuk et al., in an electron microscopy study, confirmed the histologic and ultrastructural similarity between epithelium in Brenner tumors and transitional epithelium. These authors argue that because of the histogenesis from coelomic inclusion cysts and also the mixture of müllerian-type epithelium in 30% of

Brenner tumors, it might be appropriate to classify Brenner tumors in the epithelial group of ovarian neoplasms.

Approximately 90% of these small neoplasms are discovered incidentally during a gynecologic operation, although large tumors may produce unilateral pelvic discomfort. Postmenopausal bleeding is sometimes associated with Brenner tumors, as endometrial hyperplasia is a coexisting abnormality in 10% to 16% of cases. It is postulated that luteinization of the stroma produces estrogen with resulting hyperplasia. Recent reports by Moon et al. and Outwater et al. describe the CT and MR imaging characteristics of Brenner tumors of the ovary. The extensive fibrous content of these tumors results in lower signal intensity in T2-weighted images. During CT scanning, Brenner tumors characteristically demonstrate a finding of extensive amorphous calcification within the solid components of the ovarian mass.

Grossly, Brenner tumors are smooth, firm, gray-white, solid tumors that grossly resemble fibromas. Similar to fibromas, transitional cell tumors are slow growing. Upon sectioning, the tumor usually appears gray; however, occasionally there is a yellowish tinge with small cystic spaces (Figure 18-43). Approximately 1% to 2% of these tumors undergo malignant change (Chapter 31). Histologically, Brenner tumors have two principal components: solid masses or nests of epithelial cells and a surrounding fibrous stroma. The epithelial cells are uniform and do not appear anaplastic (Figure 18-44). The histology and ultrastructure of the epithelial cells of a Brenner tumor are similar to transitional epithelium of the urinary bladder.

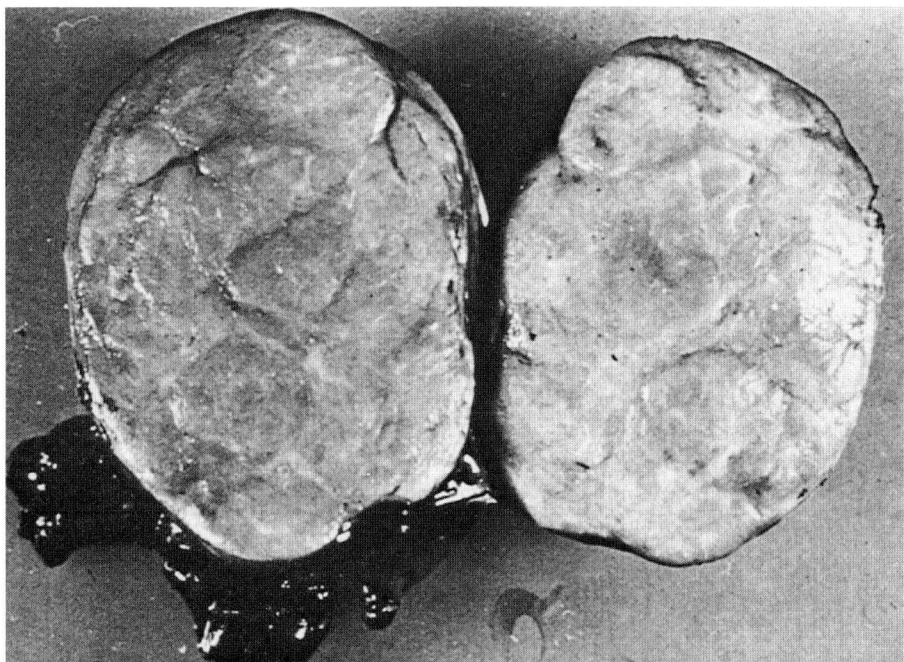

FIGURE 18-43   Cut section of solid, nodular Brenner tumor. (From Czernobilsky B: Primary epithelial tumors of the ovary. In Blaustein A, editor: Pathology of the female genital tract, New York, 1977, Springer-Verlag New York, Inc, p 489.)

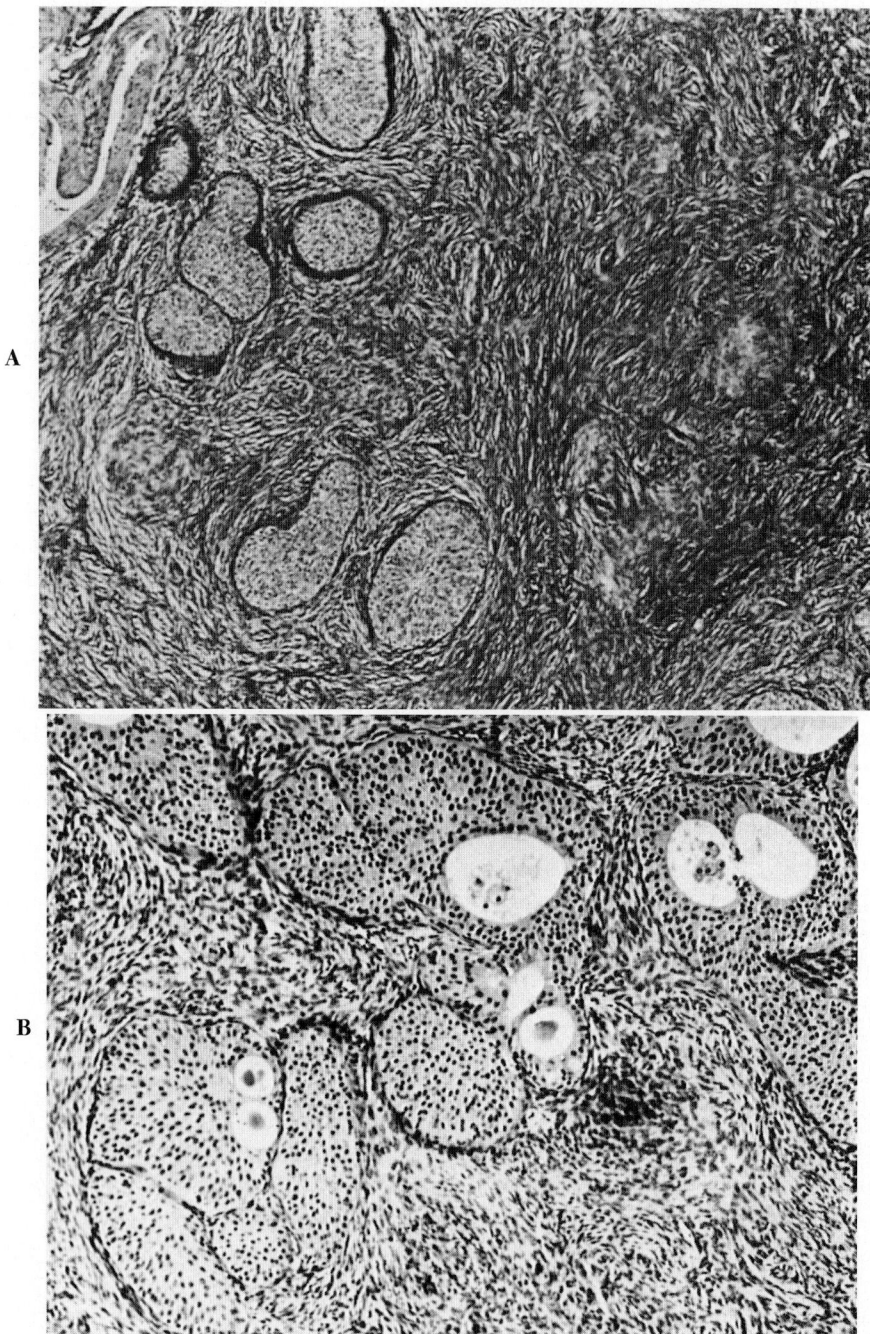

FIGURE 18-44   A, Brenner tumor of ovary that measured 3 mm in diameter; shows characteristic nests of epithelium in dense fibrous stroma. Tumor was an incidental microscopic finding. (H&E stain; ×25.) **B,** Brenner tumor showing solid and partly cystic epithelial nest in dense fibrous stroma. (H&E stain; ×113.) (**A** from Balasa RW, Adcock LL, Prem KA, et al: Obstet Gynecol 50:121, 1977; **B** from Czernobilsky B: Primary epithelial tumors of the ovary. In Blaustein A, editor: Pathology of the female genital tract, New York, 1977, Springer-Verlag New York, Inc, p 490.)

The pale epithelial cells have a "coffee bean"–appearing nucleus, which is also described as a longitudinal groove in the cell's nucleus. Electron microscopy has demonstrated that the longitudinal groove during routine microscopy is produced by prominent indentation of the nuclear membrane. An additional ovarian neoplasm is frequently found associated with Brenner tumors. Balasa et al., in a review of 302 tumors, reported 100 other concurrent neoplasms, with the majority being serous and mucinous cystadenomas or teratomas.

Management of Brenner tumors is operative, with simple excision being the procedure of choice. However, as with ovarian fibromas, the patient's age often is the principal factor in deciding the extent of the operation.

Adenofibroma and Cystadenofibroma

Adenofibromas and cystadenofibromas are closely related. Both of these benign firm tumors consist of fibrous and epithelial components. The epithelial element is most commonly serous, but histologically may be mucinous and endometrioid or clear cell. They differ from benign epithelial cystadenomas in that there is a preponderance of connective tissue. Most pathologists emphasize that at least 25% of the tumor consists of fibrous connective tissue. Obviously, cystadenofibromas have microscopic or occasional macroscopic areas that are cystic. The varying degree of fibrous stroma and epithelial elements produces a spectrum of tumors, which have resulted in a confusing nomenclature with terms such as *papillomas, fibropapillomas,* and *fibroadenomas.*

Adenofibromas are usually small fibrous tumors that arise from the surface of the ovary. They are bilateral in 20% to 25% of women. They usually occur in postmenopausal women and are 1 to 15 cm in diameter. Grossly, they are gray or white tumors, and it is difficult to distinguish them from fibromas. Papillary adenofibromas, which project from the surface of the ovary, at first glance may appear to be external excrescences of a malignant tumor. Histologically, small precursors of adenofibromas are identified in many normal ovaries. Under the microscope, true cystic gland spaces lined by cuboidal epithelium are characteristic. However, differing from serous cystadenomas, the fibrous connective tissue surrounding the cystic spaces is abundant and is the predominant tissue of the tumor.

Smaller tumors are asymptomatic and are only discovered incidentally during abdominal or pelvic operations. Large tumors may cause pressure symptoms or, rarely, undergo adnexal torsion. Recently a small series of the MR features of these tumors has been reported. Similar to Brenner tumors, the fibrous component produces a very low signal intensity on T2-weighted images. This interest in imaging results from an attempt to distinguish, prior to operation, whether a predominately solid ovarian mass is benign or malignant. Because adenofibromas are usually discovered in postmenopausal women, the treatment of choice is bilateral salpingo-oophorectomy and total abdominal hysterectomy. Because these tumors are benign and because malignant transformation is rare, simple excision of the tumor and inspection of the contralateral ovary is appropriate in younger women.

Torsion

Torsion of the ovary or both the oviduct and the ovary (adnexal torsion) is uncommon but an important cause of acute lower abdominal and pelvic pain. Torsion of the ovary may occur separately from torsion of the fallopian tube, but most commonly the two adnexal structures are affected together. In Hibbard's review of 128 cases of adnexal torsion, this syndrome accounted for approximately 3% of gynecologic operative emergencies at the University of Southern California Medical Center.

Adnexal torsion occurs most commonly during the reproductive years, with the average patient being in her mid-20s. Adnexal torsion is also a complication of benign ovarian tumors in the postmenopausal woman. Pregnancy appears to predispose women to adnexal torsion, with approximately one in five women being pregnant when the condition is diagnosed. Most susceptible are ovaries that are enlarged secondary to ovulation induction during early pregnancy. One series reported 4 cases of adnexal torsion in 648 pregnancies resulting from ovulation induction. The most common etiology of adnexal torsion is ovarian enlargement by an 8- to 12-cm benign mass of the ovary. However, smaller ovaries may also undergo torsion. Ovarian tumors are discovered in 50% to 60% of women with adnexal torsion. Torsion of a normal ovary or adnexum is also possible and occurs more frequently in children. Hibbard reports that because of their relative prevalence, dermoids are the tumor most frequently reported in a series of women with adnexal torsion. However, the relative risk of adnexal torsion is higher with parovarian cysts, solid benign tumors, and serous cysts of the ovary. The right ovary has a greater tendency to twist (3 to 2) than does the left ovary. Torsion of a malignant ovarian tumor is comparatively rare.

Patients with adnexal torsion present with acute, severe, unilateral, lower abdominal and pelvic pain. Often the patient relates the onset of the severe pain to an abrupt change of position. A unilateral, extremely tender adnexal mass is found in more than 90% of patients. Approximately two thirds of patients have associated nausea and vomiting. These associated gastrointestinal symptoms sometimes lead to a preoperative diagnosis of acute appendicitis or small intestinal obstruction. Many patients have noted intermittent previous episodes of similar pain for several days to several weeks. The hypothesis is that previous episodes of pain were secondary to partial torsion, with spontaneous reversal without significant vascular compromise. With progressive torsion, initially venous and lymphatic obstruction occurs. This produces a cyanotic, edematous ovary, which on pelvic examination presents as a unilateral, extremely tender adnexal mass. Further progression of the torsion interrupts the major arterial supply to the ovary, resulting in hypoxia, adnexal necrosis, and a concomitant low-grade fever and leukocytosis. Fever is more common in women who have developed necrosis of the adnexa. Approximately 10% of women with adnexal torsion have a repetitive episode affecting the contralateral adnexum.

Most patients with adnexal torsion present with symptoms and signs severe enough to demand operative intervention. Some authors have reported the successful use of Doppler ultrasound to evaluate ovarian arterial blood flow to help diagnose torsion. Abnormal color Doppler flow is highly predictive of torsion of the ovary. However, approximately 50% of women with surgically confirmed adnexal torsion will have a normal Doppler flow study. Increasingly, women with ovarian torsion are being treated via laparoscopic surgery. The most common gynecologic conditions that may be confused with adnexal torsion are a ruptured corpus luteum or an adnexal abscess. In recent series emphasizing the early diagnosis of adnexal torsion, conservative operative management has been possible in 75% of cases.

Because the majority of cases of adnexal torsion occur in young women, a conservative operation is ideal. The clinician should maintain a high index of suspicion for adnexal torsion so that early and conservative surgery is possible. Although salpingo-oophorectomy has been the routine treatment for ovarian torsion, many authors have reported large series of conservative management. Conservative surgery either through the laparoscope or via laparotomy entails gentle untwisting of the pedicle, possibly cystectomy, and stabilization of the ovary with sutures. McHutchison et al. have suggested the use of intravenous fluorescein intraoperatively with subsequent inspection of the untwisted ovary with an ultraviolet light to document vascular integrity. A recent review of the literature documented the risk of pulmonary embolus with adnexal torsion as approximately 0.2%. The risk was similar regardless of whether the condition was managed by conservative surgery with untwisting or adnexal removal without untwisting. With severe vascular compromise, the appropriate operation is unilateral salpingo-oophorectomy. The vascular pedicle should be clamped with care so as not to injure the ureter, which may be tented up by the torsion.

Ovarian Remnant Syndrome

Chronic pelvic pain secondary to a small area of functioning ovarian tissue following intended total removal of both ovaries is termed *ovarian remnant syndrome*. Most of the women who develop this condition had endometriosis or chronic pelvic inflammatory disease and extensive pelvic adhesions discovered during previous surgical procedures.

The chronic pelvic pain is usually cyclic and exacerbated following coitus. The masses are small, approximately 3 cm in diameter, and located in the retroperitoneal space immediately adjacent to either ureter. Histologically, the mass contains both ovarian follicles and stroma. If the mass cannot be palpated during pelvic examination, imaging studies such as vaginal ultrasound or MRI are often helpful. Premenopausal levels of FSH and/or estradiol help to establish the diagnosis in a woman who has a history of a bilateral salpingo-oophorectomy. However, sometimes a small area of ovarian tissue does not produce enough circulating estrogen to suppress gonadotrophins. Difficult cases have been diagnosed by challenging and stimulating the suspected ovarian remnant with either clomiphene citrate or a GnRH agonist.

Once the diagnosis is suspected, the most effective treatment is surgical removal of the ovarian remnant. The tissue should be removed by laparoscopy or laparotomy with wide excision of the mass using meticulous techniques so as to protect the integrity of the ureter. The recurrence rate is approximately 10%.

KEY POINTS

- Some urethral caruncles are asymptomatic; others cause dysuria, frequency, and urgency. In elderly women they must be differentiated from urethral carcinoma by biopsy. Treatment of urethral caruncles is topical or oral estrogen therapy.

- The majority of urethral carcinomas are of squamous cell origin. Most of these rare carcinomas arise from the distal urethra.

- Urethral prolapse is predominantly a disease of the premenarchal female, although it does occur in postmenopausal women.

- The most common large cyst of the vulva is a cystic dilation of an obstructed Bartholin's duct. The most common small vulvar cysts are epidermal inclusion cysts or sebaceous cysts.

- The vulva contains 1% of the skin surface of the body, but 5% to 10% of all malignant melanomas in women arise from this region.

- Ideally, all vulvar nevi should be excised and examined histologically. Special emphasis should be directed toward the flat junctional nevus and the dysplastic nevus for they have the greatest potential for malignant transformation. The dysplastic nevus is characterized by being more than 5 mm in diameter, with irregular borders and patches of variegated pigment.

- Symptoms of an early malignant melanoma include *asymmetry, border* irregularity, *color* variegation, and a *diameter* usually greater than 6 mm (ABCD).

- Vulvar hemangiomas frequently are discovered initially during childhood. Approximately 60% of vulvar hemangiomas discovered during the first years of life spontaneously regress in size by the time the child goes to school.

- Fibromas are the most common benign solid tumors of the vulva. Lipomas are the second most frequent benign vulvar mesenchymal tumor.

- Hidradenomas are rare, small, benign, asymptomatic vulvar tumors originating from apocrine glands and are found in white women between 30 and 70 years of age.

- Endometriosis of the vulva is rare, with only 1 in 500 women with endometriosis having vulvar involvement.

- The most common symptoms of endometriosis of the vulva are pain and introital dyspareunia. The classic history is cyclic discomfort and an enlargement of the mass associated with menstrual periods.

- The management of nonobstetrical vulvar hematomas is usually conservative unless the hematoma is greater than 10 cm in diameter or rapidly increasing.

- The majority of vulvar skin problems are red, scalelike rashes, and the woman's primary complaint is of pruritus.

- Substances that are irritants produce immediate symptoms such as a stinging and burning sensation when applied to the vulvar skin. The symptoms and signs secondary to an irritant disappear within 12 hours of discontinuing the offending substance. In contrast, allergic contact dermatitis requires 36 to 48 hours to manifest its symptoms and signs. Often the signs of allergic contact dermatitis persist for several days despite removal of the allergen.

- The most common causes of vulvar contact dermatitis are cosmetic and local therapeutic agents. External chemicals that trigger the disease process must be avoided.

- Women usually develop psoriasis during their teenage years, with approximately 3% of adult women being affected. Approximately 20% of these have involvement of the vulvar skin.

- The margins of psoriasis are more well defined than the common skin conditions in the differential diagnosis including candidiasis, seborrheic dermatitis, and eczema.

- Hidradenitis suppurativa is a chronic, unrelenting, refractory infection of the skin and subcutaneous tissue. The diagnosis should be confirmed by biopsy.

- Urethral diverticula occur in approximately 1% to 3% of women.

- Classically, the symptoms associated with the urethral diverticulum are extremely chronic in nature and they have not resolved with multiple courses of oral antibiotic therapy.

- The two most common methods of diagnosing urethral diverticula are voiding cystourethrography and cysto-urethroscopy. Other diagnostic tests used to identify urethral diverticula include urethral pressure profile recordings, vaginal ultrasound, positive-pressure urethrography, and magnetic resonance imaging.

- Embryonic cysts of the vagina, especially those on the anterior lateral wall, are usually Gartner's duct cysts. These cysts are most commonly found in the lower one third of the vagina.

- Prolonged tampon use may be associated with ulcerations of the vagina, discharge, and bleeding.

- Endocervical polyps are smooth, soft, red, fragile masses. They are found most commonly in multiparous women in their 40s and 50s.

- After the endocervical polyp is removed, endometrial sampling should be performed to diagnose a coexisting endometrial hyperplasia or carcinoma.

- Depending on the series, 3% to 8% of myomas are categorized as cervical myomas. Because of the relative paucity of smooth muscle fibers in the cervical stroma, the majority of myomas that appear to be cervical actually arise from the isthmus of the uterus.

- The causes of acquired cervical stenosis are operative, radiation, infection, neoplasia, or atrophic changes. Cone biopsy and cautery of the cervix, either electrocautery or cryocoagulation, are the operations that most commonly cause cervical stenosis.

- Endometrial polyps are noted in approximately 10% of women when the uterus is examined at autopsy. Approximately one in four women with abnormal bleeding will have an endometrial polyp.

- Malignant transformation of endometrial polyps has been estimated to occur in 0.5% of cases and is most often an endometrial carcinoma of low grade and stage.

- Hematometra in postmenopausal women is often asymptomatic. Appropriate biopsy specimens of the endocervical canal and endometrium should be obtained to rule out malignancy when the cause of hematometra is not obvious.

- Leiomyomas are the most frequent pelvic tumors, with the highest prevalence occurring during the fifth decade of a woman's life.

- Symptomatic uterine leiomyomas are the primary indication for approximately 30% of all hysterectomies.

- Five to ten percent of myomas are submucosal, often presenting with symptoms of abnormal vaginal bleeding.

- The etiology of uterine leiomyomas is incompletely understood. It is known that each tumor results from an original single muscle cell. Each individual uterine myoma is monoclonal. All the cells are derived from one progenitor myocyte.

- Acute muscular infarction, as is seen with red degeneration of a myoma, causes severe pain and localized peritoneal irritation.

- The majority of women with uterine myomas are asymptomatic, but one of three will experience pelvic pain, with dysmenorrhea being the most frequent complaint.

- Abnormal bleeding is experienced by 30% of women with myomas, with the most common symptom being menorrhagia, but intermenstrual spotting and disruption of the normal pattern are other frequent complaints.

- The management of women with small, asymptomatic myomas is conservative, and the majority of women will not need operations.

- Women with abnormal bleeding and leiomyomas should be investigated thoroughly for concurrent problems, such as endometrial hyperplasia.

- In comparison studies, the relative morbidity of abdominal hysterectomy and myomectomy is similar when one controls for uterine size.

- Classic indications for myomectomy include rapidly expanding pelvic mass, persistent abnormal bleeding, pain or pressure, or enlargement of an asymptomatic myoma to more than 8 cm in a woman who has not completed childbearing.

- Prolapse of a myoma through the cervix is optimally treated by vaginal removal and ligation of the base of the myoma.

- It is possible to treat leiomyomas medically by reducing the circulating level of estrogen and progesterone. Gonadotrophin-releasing hormone (GnRH) agonists will reduce the mean uterine volume and myoma size by 40% to 50%. However, individual response varies greatly, from no response to an 80% reduction in uterine size. The vast majority of the reduction in size occurs within the first 3 months.

- The newest modality to manage uterine myomas is transcatheter uterine artery embolization as an ambulatory nonsurgical technique. Postprocedural abdominal and pelvic pain is common for the first 24 hours. Success rates in regard to decreasing menorrhagia and reduction in uterine size are promising.

- The most prevalent benign tumor of the oviduct is the *angiomyoma* or *adenomatoid tumor*. They are small, gray-white, circumscribed nodules, 1 to 2 cm in diameter.

- The main symptom of torsion of the tube is pain, usually located in the iliac fossa, with radiation to the thigh and flank. In two thirds of cases the pain is associated with nausea and vomiting.

- Follicular cysts are the most common cystic structures in normal ovaries. The cysts are frequently multiple and may vary from a few millimeters to as large as 15 cm in diameter.

- The initial management of a suspected follicular cyst is conservative observation. The majority of follicular cysts disappear spontaneously by either reabsorption of the cyst fluid or silent rupture within 4 to 8 weeks of initial diagnosis.

- Corpus luteum cysts may be associated with either normal endocrine function or prolonged secretion of progesterone. The associated menstrual pattern may be normal, delayed menstruation, or amenorrhea.

- Women with a bleeding diathesis or taking warfarin (Coumadin) are especially prone to develop hemorrhage from rupture of a corpus luteum cyst. Bleeding occurs usually between days 20 to 26 of their cycle.

- The differential diagnosis of a woman with acute pain and a suspected ruptured corpus luteum cyst includes ectopic pregnancy, a ruptured endometrioma, and adnexal torsion.

- The treatment of unruptured corpus luteum cysts is conservative. However, if the cyst persists or intraperitoneal bleeding occurs, necessitating operation, the treatment is cystectomy.

- Theca lutein cysts arise from either prolonged or excessive stimulation of the ovaries by endogenous or exogenous gonadotrophins or increased ovarian sensitivity to gonadotrophins. The condition of ovarian enlargement secondary to the development of multiple luteinized follicular cysts is termed *hyperreactio luteinalis*. Approximately 50% of molar pregnancies and 10% of choriocarcinomas have associated bilateral theca lutein cysts.

- Benign ovarian teratomas vary from a few millimeters to 25 cm, may be single or multiple, and are bilateral 10% to 15% of the time.

- Dermoids are believed to arise during fetal life from a single germ cell. They are 46,XX in karyotype.

- Histologically, benign teratomas are composed of mature cells, usually from all three germ layers. Most solid elements arise and are contained in a protrusion or nipple (mamilla) in the cyst wall termed the *prominence* or *tubercle of Rokitansky*. This prominence may be visualized by ultrasound as an echodense region, thus aiding in the sonographic diagnosis.

- Although most dermoids are asymptomatic, torsion and rupture are two important complications.

- Operative treatment of benign cystic teratomas is cystectomy with preservation of as much normal ovarian tissue as possible.

- The most common symptoms associated with of ovarian endometriosis are pelvic pain, dyspareunia, and infertility.

- Medical therapy is rarely successful in treating ovarian endometriosis if the disease has produced ovarian enlargement. Often, surgical therapy is complicated by formation of de novo and recurrent adhesions.

- Fibromas are the most common, benign, solid neoplasms of the ovary. They have a low malignant potential.

- Many ovarian fibromas are misdiagnosed and are believed to be leiomyomas prior to operation.

- Fibromas vary in size from small nodules to huge pelvic tumors weighing as much as 50 pounds. Ninety percent of fibromas are unilateral and have an average diameter of 6 cm.

- Fifty percent of patients with an ovarian fibroma will have ascites if the tumor is greater than 6 cm. The incidence of associated ascites is directly proportional to the size of the tumor.

- Transitional cell tumors (Brenner tumors) are small, smooth, solid, fibroepithelial tumors of the ovary. They usually occur in women between the ages of 40 and 60 and are predominantly unilateral.

- Adnexal torsion occurs most commonly in the reproductive years, with the average age of patients being in the mid-20s. Pregnancy predisposes to adnexal torsion.

- Ovarian tumors are discovered in 50% to 60% of women with adnexal torsion.

- Abnormal color Doppler flow is highly predictive of torsion of the ovary. However, approximately 50% of women with surgically confirmed adnexal torsion will have a normal Doppler flow study.

- A recent review of the literature documented the risk of pulmonary embolus with adnexal torsion as approximately 0.2%. The risk was similar regardless of whether the condition was managed by conservative surgery with untwisting or adnexal removal without untwisting.

- Chronic pelvic pain secondary to a small area of functioning ovarian tissue following intended total removal of both ovaries is termed *ovarian remnant syndrome*.

BIBLIOGRAPHY

Abulafia O and Sherer DM: Transcatheter uterine artery embolization for the management of symptomatic uterine leiomyomas, Obstet Gynecol Surv 54:745, 1999.

Aghajanian A, Bernstein L, and Grimes DA: Bartholin's duct abscess and cyst: a case-control study, SMJ 87:26, 1994.

Ahnaimugan S and Asuen MI: Coital laceration of the vagina, Aust N Z J Obstet Gynaecol 20:180, 1980.

Al-Took S, Murray C, and Tulandi T: Effects of pirfenidone and dermoid cyst fluid on adhesion formation, Fertil Steril 69:341, 1998.

Andersen PG, Christensen S, Detlefsen GU, and Kern-Hansen P: Treatment of Bartholin's abscess: marsupialization versus incision, curettage and suture under antibiotic cover. A randomized study with 6 months' follow-up, Acta Obstet Gynecol Scand 71:59, 1992.

Axe S, Parmley T, Woodruff JD, et al: Adenomas in minor vestibular glands, Obstet Gynecol 68:16, 1986.

Bakour SH, Khan KS, and Gupta JK: The risk of premalignant and malignant pathology in endometrial polyps, Acta Obstet Gynecol Scand 79:317, 2000.

Bakri YN, Bakhashwain M, and Hugosson C: Massive theca-lutein cysts, virilization, and hypothyroidism associated with normal pregnancy, Acta Obstet Gynecol Scand 73:153, 1994.

Balasa RW, Adcock LL, Prem KA, et al: The Brenner tumor, Obstet Gynecol 50:120, 1977.

Baldauf JJ, Dreyfus M, Ritter J, et al: Risk of cervical stenosis after large loop excision or laser conization, Obstet Gynecol 88:933, 1996.

Barbieri RL: Ambulatory management of uterine leiomyomata, Clin Obstet Gynecol 42:196, 1999.

Barbieri RL, Dilena M, Chumas J, et al: Leuprolide acetate depot decreases the number of nucleolar organizer regions in uterine leiomyomata, Fertil Steril 60:569, 1993.

Baron JA, LaVecchia C, and Levi F: The antiestrogenic effect of cigarette smoking in women, Am J Obstet Gynecol 162:502, 1990.

Barrett KF, Bledsoe S, Greer BE, et al: Tampon-induced vaginal or cervical ulceration, Am J Obstet Gynecol 127:332, 1977.

Bayer AI and Wiskind AK: Adnexal torsion: can the adnexa be saved? Am J Obstet Gynecol 171:1506, 1994.

Bazot M, Cortez A, Sananes S, et al: Imaging of dermoid cysts with foci of immature tissue, J Comput Assist Tomogr 23:703, 1999.

Belardi MG, Maglione MA, Vighi S, and di Paola GR: Syringoma of the vulva: a case report, J Reprod Med 39:957, 1994.

Bernardus RE, Van Der Slikke JW, Roex AJM, et al: Torsion of the fallopian tube: some considerations on its etiology, Obstet Gynecol 64:675, 1984.

Bider D, Maschiach S, Dulitzky M, et al: Clinical, surgical and pathologic findings of adnexal torsion in pregnant and non-pregnant women, Surg Gynecol Obstet 173:363, 1991.

Birch HW and Sondag DR: Granular-cell myoblastoma of the vulva, Obstet Gynecol 18:443, 1961.

Blickstein I, Feldberg E, Dgani R, et al: Dysplastic vulvar nevi, Obstet Gynecol 78:968, 1991.

Bornstein J, Zarfati D, Goldik Z, and Abramovici H: Vulvar vestibulitis: physical or psychosexual problem? Obstet Gynecol 93:876, 1999.

Bradham DD, Stovall TG, and Thompson CD: Use of GnRH agonist before hysterectomy: a cost simulation, Obstet Gynecol 85:401, 1995.

Brosens I, Deprest J, Dal Cin P, and Van Den Berghe H: Clinical significance of cytogenetic abnormalities in uterine myomas, Fertil Steril 69:232, 1998.

Brosens I, Johannison E, Dal Cin P, et al: Analysis of the karyotype and desoxyribonucleic acid content of uterine myomas in premenopausal, menopausal, and gonadotropin-releasing hormone agonist-treated females, Fertil Steril 66:376, 1996.

Burton CA, Grimes DA, and March CM: Surgical management of leiomyomata during pregnancy, Obstet Gynecol 74:707, 1989.

Candiani GB, Fedele L, Parazzini F, and Villa L: Risk of recurrence after myomectomy, Br J Obstet Gynaecol 98:385, 1991.

Canis M, Mage G, Pouly JL, et al: Laparoscopic diagnosis of adnexal cystic masses: a 12-year experience with long-term follow-up, Obstet Gynecol 83:707, 1994.

Canis M, Mage G, Wattiez A, et al: Second-look laparoscopy after laparoscopic cystectomy of large ovarian endometriomas, Fertil Steril 58:617, 1992.

Cantuaria GHC, Angioli R, Frost L, et al: Comparison of bimanual examination with ultrasound examination before hysterectomy for uterine leiomyoma, Obstet Gynecol 92:109, 1998.

Carlson KJ, Nichols DH, and Schiff I: Indications for hysterectomy, N Engl J Med 328:856, 1993.

Carneiro SJC, Gardner HL, and Knox JM: Syringoma: three cases with vulvar involvement, Obstet Gynecol 39:95, 1972.

Carr BR, Marshburn PB, Weatherall PT, et al: An evaluation of the effect of gonadotropin-releasing hormone analogs and medroxyprogesterone acetate on uterine leiomyomata volume by magnetic resonance imaging: a prospective, randomized, double-blind, placebo-controlled, crossover trial, J Clin Endocrinol Metab 76:1217, 1993.

Caspi B, Appleman Z, Rabinerson D, et al: The growth pattern of ovarian dermoid cysts: a prospective study in premenopausal and postmenopausal women, Fertil Steril 68:501, 1997.

Chambers JT, Thiagarajah S, and Kitchin JD: Torsion of the normal fallopian tube in pregnancy, Obstet Gynecol 54:487, 1979.

Cin PD, Vanni R, Marras S, et al: Four cytogenetic subgroups can be identified in endometrial polyps, Cancer Res 55:1565, 1995.

Coates JB and Hales JS: Granular cell myoblastoma of the vulva, Obstet Gynecol 41:796, 1973.

Cohen LS and Valle RF: Role of vaginal sonography and hysterosonography in the endoscopic treatment of uterine myomas, Fertil Steril 73:197, 2000.

Cohen Z, Shinhar D, Kopernik G, and Mares AJ: The laparoscopic approach to uterine adnexal torsion in childhood, J Pediatr Surg 31:1557, 1006.

Comerci JT Jr, Licciardi F, Bergh PA, et al: Mature cystic teratoma: a clinicopathologic evaluation of 517 cases and review of the literature, Obstet Gynecol 84:22, 1994.

Corley D, Rowe J, Curtis MT, et al: Postmenopausal bleeding from unusual endometrial polyps in women on chronic tamoxifen therapy, Obstet Gynecol 79:111, 1992.

Cramer SF, Robertson AL, Ziats NP, et al: Growth potential of human uterine leiomyomas: some in vitro observations and their implications, Obstet Gynecol 66:36, 1985.

Danikas D, Goudas VT, Rao CV, and Brief DK: Luteinizing hormone receptor expression in leiomyomatosis peritonealis disseminata, Obstet Gynecol 95:1009, 2000.

Davies A, Hart R, and Magos AL: The excision of uterine fibroids by vaginal myomectomy: a prospective study, Fertil Steril 71:961, 1999.

DeCrespigny LC, Robinson HP, Davoren RAM, et al: The 'simple' ovarian cyst: aspirate or operate? Br J Obstet Gynaecol 96:1035, 1989.

Deppisch LM: Cysts of the vagina, Obstet Gynecol 45:623, 1975.

DeWilde R, Bordt J, Hesseling M, et al: Ovarian cystostomy, Acta Obstet Gynecol Scand 68:363, 1989.

Dische FE and Ritche JM: Luteoma of pregnancy, J Pathol 100:77, 1970.

Dmochowski RR, Ganabathi K, Zimmern PE, and Leach GE: Benign female periurethral masses, J Urol 152:1943, 1994.

Dottino PR, Levine DA, Ripley DL, and Cohen CJ: Laparoscopic management of adnexal masses in premenopausal and postmenopausal women, Obstet Gynecol 93:223, 1999.

Dreyer L, Simson IW, Sevenster CBO, et al: Leiomyomatosis peritonealis disseminata: a report of two cases and a review of the literature, Br J Obstet Gynaecol 92:856, 1985.

Dubuisson JB, Lecuru F, Foulot H, et al: Myomectomy by laparoscopy: a preliminary report of 43 cases, Fertil Steril 56:827, 1991.

Duckman S, Suarez JR, and Sese LQ: Giant cervical polyp, Am J Obstet Gynecol 159:852, 1988.

Dunnihoo DR and Wolff J: Bilateral torsion of the adnexa: a case report and a review of the world literature, Obstet Gynecol 64:55S, 1984.

Dunton CJ, Kautzky M, and Hanau C: Malignant melanoma of the vulva: a review, Obstet Gynecol Surv 50:739, 1995.

Emanuel MH, Vamsteker K, Hart AAM, et al: Long-term results of hysteroscopic myomectomy for abnormal uterine bleeding, Obstet Gynecol 93:743, 1999.

Evans AT, Symmonds RE, and Gaffey TA: Recurrent pelvic intravenous leiomyomatosis, Obstet Gynecol 57:260, 1981.

Farber EM and Nall L: Genital psoriasis, Cutis 50:263, 1992.

Farrar HK and Nedoss BR: Benign tumors of the uterine cervix, Am J Obstet Gynecol 81:124, 1961.

Fedele L, Bianchi S, Dorta M, et al: Transvaginal ultrasonography in the diagnosis of diffuse adenomyosis, Fertil Steril 58:94, 1992.

Fedele L, Vercellini P, Bianchi S, et al: Treatment with GnRH agonists before myomectomy and the risk of short-term myoma recurrence, Br J Obstet Gynaecol 97:393, 1990.

Fischer G: The commonest causes of symptomatic vulvar disease: a dermatologist's perspective, Austl J Dermatol 57:12, 1996.

Fischer G, Spurrett B, and Fischer A: The chronically symptomatic vulva: aetiology and management, Br J Obstet Gynaecol 102:773, 1995.

Friedel W and Kaiser IH: Vaginal evisceration, Obstet Gynecol 45:315, 1975.

Friedman AJ: Use of gonadotropin-releasing hormone agonists before myomectomy, Clin Obstet Gynecol 36:650, 1993.

Friedman AJ, Daly M, Juneau-Norcross M, and Rein MS: Predictors of uterine volume reduction in women with myomas treated with a gonadotropin-releasing hormone agonist, Fertil Steril 58:413, 1992.

Friedman AJ and Haas ST: Should uterine size be an indication for surgical intervention in women with myomas? Am J Obstet Gynecol 168:751, 1993.

Friedman AJ, Hoffman DI, Comite F, et al: Treatment of leiomyomata uteri with leuprolide acetate depot: a double-blind, placebo-controlled, multicenter study, Obstet Gynecol 77:720, 1991.

Friedman RJ, Rigel DS, and Kopf AW: Early detection of malignant melanoma: the role of physician examination and self-examination of the skin, CA 35:130, 1985.

Friedrich EG: Tampon effects on vaginal health, Clin Obstet Gynecol 24:395, 1981.

Friedrich EG and Wilkinson EJ: Vulvar surgery for neurofibromatosis, Obstet Gynecol 65:135, 1985.

Gerber GS and Schoenberg HW: Female urinary tract fistulas, J Urol 149:229, 1993.

Ginsburg D and Genadry R: Suburethral diverticulum: classification and therapeutic considerations, Obstet Gynecol 61:685, 1983.

Goldenberg M, Sivan E, Sharabi Z, et al: Outcome of hysteroscopic resection of submucous myomas for infertility, Fertil Steril 64:714, 1995.

Goodwin SC, McLucas B, Lee M, et al: Uterine artery embolization for the treatment of uterine leiomyomata midterm results, JVIR 10:1159, 1999.

Gordon JD, Hopkins KL, Jeffrey RB, and Giudice LC: Adnexal torsion: color Doppler diagnosis and laparoscopic treatment, Fertil Steril 61:383, 1994.

Grimes DA and Hughs JM: Use of multiphasic oral contraceptives and hospitalizations of women with functional ovarian cysts in the United States, Obstet Gynecol 73:1037, 1989.

Haefner HK, Andersen F, and Johnson MP: Vaginal laceration following a jet-ski accident, Obstet Gynecol 78:986, 1991.

Hallatt JG, Steele CH, and Snyder M: Ruptured corpus luteum with hemoperitoneum: a study of 173 surgical cases, Am J Obstet Gynecol 149:5, 1984.

Hart WR: Paramesonephric mucinous cysts of the vulva, Am J Obstet Gynecol 107:1079, 1980.

Herndon JH: Itching: the pathophysiology of pruritus, Int J Dermatol 14:465, 1975.

Hibbard LT: Adnexal torsion, Am J Obstet Gynecol 152:456, 1985.

Higgins RV, Matkins JF, and Marroum MC: Comparison of fine-needle aspiration cytologic findings of ovarian cysts with ovarian histologic findings, Am J Obstet Gynecol 180:550, 1999.

Hillis SD, Marchbanks PA, and Peterson HB: Uterine size and risk of complications among women undergoing abdominal hysterectomy for leiomyomas, Obstet Gynecol 87:539, 1996.

Huang SC, Yu CH, Huang RT, et al: Intratumoral blood flow in uterine myoma correlated with a lower tumor size and volume, but not correlated with cell proliferation or angiogenesis, Obstet Gynecol 87:1019, 1996.

Huddock JJ, Dupayne N, and McGeary JA: Traumatic vulvar hematomas, Am J Obstet Gynecol 70:1064, 1955.

Huffman JW: The detailed anatomy of the paraurethral ducts in the adult human female, Am J Obstet Gynecol 55:86, 1948.

Iosif CS and Akerlund M: Fibromyomas and uterine activity, Acta Obstet Gynecol Scand 62:165, 1983.

Israel SL: The clinical similarity of corpus luteum cyst and ectopic pregnancy, Am J Obstet Gynecol 44:22, 1942.

Iverson RE Jr, Chelmow D, Strohbehn K, et al: Relative morbidity of abdominal hysterectomy and myomectomy for management of uterine leiomyomas, Obstet Gynecol 88:415, 1996.

Iverson RE Jr, Chelmow D, Strohbehn K, et al: Myomectomy fever: testing the dogma, Fertil Steril 72:104, 1999.

Jimmerson SD and Becker JD: Vaginal ulcers associated with tampon usage, Obstet Gynecol 56:97, 1980.

Joura EA, Zeisler H, Bancher-Todesca D, et al: Short-term effects of topical testosterone in vulvar lichen sclerosus, Obstet Gynecol 89:297, 1997.

Kampraath S, Possover M, and Schneider A: Description of a laparoscopic technique for treating patients with ovarian remnant syndrome, Fertil Steril 68:663, 1997.

Katz VL, Dotters DJ, and Droegemueller W: Complications of uterine leiomyomas in pregnancy, Obstet Gynecol 73:593, 1989.

Kaufman RH, Faro S, Friedrich EG Jr, and Gardner HL: Benign diseases of the vulva and vagina, ed 4, St. Louis, 1994, Mosby.

Kemmann E, Ghazi DM, and Corsan GH: Adnexal torsion in menotropin-induced pregnancies, Obstet Gynecol 76:403, 1990.

Klein HZ and Smith RL: Fibromyoma of the uterine tube, Obstet Gynecol 26:515, 1965.

Koonings PP and Grimes DA: Adnexal torsion in postmenopausal women, Obstet Gynecol 73:11, 1989.

Kruger E and Heller DS: Adnexal torsion: a clinicopathologic review of 31 cases, J Reprod Med 44:71, 1999.

Kupfer MC, Schiller VL, Hansen GC, and Tessler FN: Transvaginal sonographic evaluation of endometrial polyps, J Ultrasound Med 13:535, 1994.

Kurjak A, Schulman H, Sosic A, et al: Transvaginal ultrasound, color flow, and Doppler waveform of the postmenopausal adnexal mass, Obstet Gynecol 80:917, 1992.

Kurman RJ, editor: Blaustein's pathology of the female genital tract, ed 4, New York, 1994, Springer-Verlag New York, Inc.

Lafferty HW, Angiioli R, Rudolph J, and Penalver MA: Ovarian remnant syndrome: experience at Jackson Memorial Hospital, University of Miami, 1985 through 1993, Am J Obstet Gynecol 174:641, 1996.

Lahiti E, Vuopala S, Kauppila A, et al: Maturation of vaginal and endometrial epithelium in postmenopausal breast cancer patients receiving long-term tamoxifen, Gynecol Oncol 55:410, 1994.

Laing FC, Van Dalsem VF, Marks WM, et al: Dermoid cysts of the ovary: their ultrasonographic appearances, Obstet Gynecol 57:99, 1981.

Lakkis WG, Martin MC, and Gelfand MM: Benign cystic teratoma of the ovary: a 6-year review, Can J Surg 28:444, 1985.

Lambert B and De Brux J: Theca lutein cysts of pregnancy without mole or chorioepithelioma, Obstet Gynecol 22:643, 1963.

LaMorte AI, Lalwani S, and Diamond MP: Morbidity associated with abdominal myomectomy, Obstet Gynecol 82:897, 1993.

Lee RA: Diverticulum of the female urethra: postoperative complications and results, Obstet Gynecol 61:52, 1983.

Lee RA: Diverticulum of the urethra: clinical presentation, diagnosis, and management, Clin Obstet Gynecol 27:490, 1984.

Leibsohn S, d'Ablaing G, Mishell DR Jr, et al: Leiomyosarcoma in a series of hysterectomies performed for presumed uterine leiomyomas, Am J Obstet Gynecol 162:968, 1990.

LevGur M and Levie MD: The myomatous erythrocytosis syndrome: a review, Obstet Gynecol 86:1026, 1995.

Lewis FM: Vulvar lichen planus, Br J Dermatol 138:569, 1998.

Linder D, McCau BK, and Hecht F: Parthenogenic origin of benign ovarian teratomas, N Engl J Med 292:63, 1975.

Lipitz S, Seidman DS, Menczer J, et al: Recurrence rate after fluid aspiration from sonographically benign-appearing ovarian cysts, J Reprod Med 37:845, 1992.

Loffer FD: Removal of large symptomatic intrauterine growths by the hysteroscopic resectoscope, Obstet Gynecol 76:836, 1990.

Luxman D, Bergman A, Sagi J, and David MP: The postmenopausal adnexal mass: correlation between ultrasonic and pathologic findings, Obstet Gynecol 77:726, 1991.

Maiman M, Seltzer V, and Boyce J: Laparoscopic excision of ovarian neoplasms subsequently found to be malignant, Obstet Gynecol 77:563, 1991.

Mais V, Guerriero S, Ajossa S, et al: Transvaginal ultrasonography in the diagnosis of cystic teratoma, Obstet Gynecol 85:48, 1995.

Mann MS and Kaufman RH: Erosive lichen planus of the vulva, Clin Obstet Gynecol 34:605, 1991.

Marshall LM, Spiegelman D, Barbieri RL, et al: Variation in the incidence of uterine leiomyoma among premenopausal women by age and race, Obstet Gynecol 90:967, 1997.

Marshall FC, Uson AC, and Melicow MM: Neoplasms and caruncles of the female urethra, Surg Gynecol Obstet 110:723, 1960.

Matta WHM, Shaw RW, and Nye M: Long-term follow-up of patients with uterine fibroids after treatment with the LHRH agonist buserelin, Br J Obstet Gynaecol 96:200, 1989.

McGovern PG, Noah R, Koenigsberg R, and Little AB: Adnexal torsion and pulmonary embolism: case report and review of the literature, Obstet Gynecol Surv 54:601, 1999.

McHutchison LLB, Koonings PP, Ballard CA, and d'Ablaing G III: Preservation of ovarian tissue in adnexal torsion with fluorescein, Am J Obstet Gynecol 168:1386, 1993.

McKay M: Vulvodynia versus pruritus vulvae, Clin Obstet Gynecol 28:123, 1985.

McKay M: Vulvar dermatoses, Clin Obstet Gynecol 34:614, 1991.

McLennan MT and Bent AE: Suburethral abscess: a complication of periurethral collagen injection therapy, Obstet Gynecol 92:650, 1998.

Meigs JV, Armstrong SH, and Hamilton HH: A further contribution to the syndrome of fibroma of the ovary with fluid in the abdomen and chest, Meigs' syndrome, Am J Obstet Gynecol 46:19, 1943.

Meloni AM, Surti U, Contento AM, et al: Uterine leiomyomas: cytogenetic and histologic profile, Obstet Gynecol 80:209, 1992.

Minke T, DePond W, Winkelmann T, and Blythe J: Ovarian remnant syndrome: study in laboratory rats, Am J Obstet Gynecol 171:1440, 1994.

Montz FJ, Schlaerth JB, and Morrow CP: The natural history of theca lutein cysts, Obstet Gynecol 72:247, 1988.

Moon WJ, Koh BH, Kim SK, et al: Brenner tumor of the ovary: CT and MR findings, J Comput Assist Tomogr 24:72, 2000.

Moran O, Menczer J, Ben-Baruch G, et al: Cytologic examination of ovarian cyst fluid for the distinction between benign and malignant tumors, Obstet Gynecol 82:444, 1993.

Mulvaney NJ, Slavin JL, Östör AG, and Fortune DW: Intravenous leiomyomatosis of the uterus: a clinicopathologic study of 22 cases, Int J Gynecol Pathol 13:1, 1994.

Murphy AA, Morales AJ, Kettel LM, and Yen SSC: Regression of uterine leiomyomata to the antiprogesterone RU 486: dose-response effect, Fertil Steril 64:187, 1995.

Mutter GL: Teratoma genetics and stem cells: a review, Obstet Gynecol Surv 42:661, 1987.

Nanda VS: Common dermatoses, Am J Obstet Gynecol 173:488, 1995.

Naumann RO and Droegemueller W: Unusual etiology of vulvar hematomas, Am J Obstet Gynecol 142:357, 1982.

Neuwirth RS: Urethral prolapse—a cause of vaginal bleeding in young girls, Obstet Gynecol 22:290, 1963.

Ngadiman S and Yang GCH: Adenomyomatous, lower uterine segment and endocervical polyps in cervicovaginal smears, Acta Cytol 39:643, 1995.

Nichols DH and Julian PJ: Torsion of the adnexa, Clin Obstet Gynecol 28:375, 1985.

NIH Consensus Development Panel on Early Melanoma: Diagnosis and treatment of early melanoma, JAMA 268:1314, 1992.

Niv J, Lessing JB, Hartuv J, and Peyser MR: Vaginal injury resulting from sliding down a water chute, Am J Obstet Gynecol 166:930, 1992.

Novak ER and Woodruff JD, editors: Novak's gynecologic and obstetric pathology with clinical and endocrine relations, ed 8, Philadelphia, 1979, WB Saunders Co.

Nucci MR, Young RH, and Fletcher CDM: Cellular pseudosarcomatous fibroepithelial stromal polyps of the lower female genital tract: an underrecognized lesion often misdiagnosed as sarcoma, Am J Surg Pathol 24:231, 2000.

Oelsner G, Bider D, Goldenberg M, et al: Long-term follow-up of the twisted ischemic adnexa managed by detorsion, Fertil Steril 60:976, 1993.

Outwater EK, Siegelman ES, Kim B, et al: Ovarian Brenner tumors: MR imaging characteristics, Magn Reson Imaging 16:1147, 1998.

Outwater EK, Siegelman ES, Talerman A, and Dunton C: Ovarian fibromas and cystadenofibromas: MRI features of the fibrous component, J Magn Reson Imaging 7:465, 1997.

Paavonen J: Diagnosis and treatment of vulvodynia, Ann Med 27:175, 1995.

Paavonen J: Vulvodynia—a complex syndrome of vulvar pain, Acta Obstet Gynecol Scand 74:243, 1995.

Pantoja E, Rodriguez-Ibanez I, Axtmayer RW, et al: Complications of dermoid tumors of the ovary, Obstet Gynecol 45:89, 1975.

Parker MF, Conslato SS, Chang AS, et al: Chemical analysis of adnexal cyst fluid, Gynecol Oncol 73:16, 1999.

Parker WH and Berek JS: Management of selected cystic adnexal masses in postmenopausal women by operative laparoscopy: a pilot study, Am J Obstet Gynecol 163:1574, 1990.

Parker WH, Fu YS, and Berek JS: Uterine sarcoma in patients operated on for presumed leiomyoma and rapidly growing leiomyoma, Obstet Gynecol 83:414, 1994.

Patrizi A, Neri I, Marzaduri S, et al: Syringoma: a review of twenty-nine cases, Acta Derm Venereol 78:460, 1998.

Paull T and Tedeschi LG: Perineal endometriosis at the site of episiotomy scar, Obstet Gynecol 40:28, 1972.

Peckham EM, Maki DG, Patterson JJ, et al: Focal vulvitis: a characteristic syndrome and cause of dyspareunia, Am J Obstet Gynecol 154:855, 1986.

Peña JE, Ufberg D, Cooney N, and Denis AL: Usefulness of Doppler sonography in the diagnosis of ovarian torsion, Fertil Steril 73:1047, 2000.

Peters WA, Thiagarajah S, and Thornton WN: Ovarian hemorrhage in patients receiving anticoagulant therapy, J Reprod Med 22:82, 1979.

Peterson WF and Novak ER: Endometrial polyps, Obstet Gynecol 8:40, 1956.

Pettersson B, Adami HO, Lindgren A, et al: Endometrial polyps and hyperplasia as risk factors for endometrial carcinoma, Acta Obstet Gynecol Scand 64:653, 1985.

Platt LD, Agarwal SK, and Greene N: The use of chorionic villus biopsy catheters for saline infusion sonohysterography, Ultrasound Obstet Gynecol 15:83, 2000.

Popp LW, Schwiedessen JP, and Gaetje R: Myometrial biopsy in the diagnosis of adenomyosis uteri, Am J Obstet Gynecol 169:546, 1993.

Pradhan S, Chenoy R, and O'Brien PMS: Dilatation and curettage in patients with cervical polyps: a retrospective analysis, Br J Obstet Gynaecol 102:415, 1995.

Price FV, Edwards R, and Buchsbaum HJ: Ovarian remnant syndrome: difficulties in diagnosis and management, Obstet Gynecol Surv 45:151, 1990.

Rafla N: Vaginismus and vaginal tears, Am J Obstet Gynecol 158:1043, 1988.

Ravina JH, Vigneron NC, Aymard A, et al: Pregnancy after embolization of uterine myoma: report of 12 cases, Fertil Steril 73:1241, 2000.

Raziel A, Ron-El R, Pansky M, et al: Current management of ruptured corpus luteum, Eur J Obstet Gynecol Reprod Biol 50:77, 1993.

Reid JD, Kommareddi S, Lankerani M, et al: Chronic expanding hematomas, JAMA 244:2441, 1980.

Rein MS, Barbieri RL, and Friedman AJ: Progesterone: a critical role in the pathogenesis of uterine myomas, Am J Obstet Gynecol 172:14, 1995.

Rein MS, Friedman AJ, Stuart JM, et al: Fibroid and myometrial steroid receptors in women treated with gonadotropin-releasing hormone agonist leuprolide acetate, Fertil Steril 53:1018, 1990.

Reiter RC, Wagner PL, and Gambone JC: Routine hysterectomy for large asymptomatic uterine leiomyomata: a reappraisal, Obstet Gynecol 79:481, 1992.

Ribeiro SC, Reich H, Rosenberg J, et al: Laparoscopic myomectomy and pregnancy outcome in infertile patients, Fertil Steril 71:571, 1999.

Richardson DA, Hajj SN, and Herbst AL: Medical treatment of urethral prolapse in children, Obstet Gynecol 59:69, 1982.

Ridgeway LE: Puerperal emergency: vaginal and vulvar hematomas, Obstet Gynecol Clin North Am 22:275, 1995.

Ridley CM and Neill SM, editors: The vulva, ed 2, Malden, Mass., 1999, Blackwell Science Ltd.

Robboy SJ, Ross JS, Prat J, et al: Urogenital sinus origin of mucinous and ciliated cysts of the vulva, Obstet Gynecol 51:347, 1978.

Roberts DB: Necrotizing fasciitis of the vulva, Am J Obstet Gynecol 157:568, 1987.

Robson S and Kerin JF: Acute adnexal torsion before oocyte retrieval in an in vitro fertilization cycle, Fertil Steril 73:650, 2000.

Roehrborn CG: Long-term follow-up study of the marsupialization technique for urethral diverticula in women, Surg Gynecol Obstet 167:191, 1988.

Rulin MC and Preston AL: Adnexal masses in postmenopausal women, Obstet Gynecol 70:578, 1987.

Samaha M and Woodruff JD: Paratubal cysts: frequency, histogenesis, and associated clinical features, Obstet Gynecol 65:691, 1985.

Samanth KK and Black WC: Benign ovarian stromal tumors associated with free peritoneal fluid, Am J Obstet Gynecol 107:538, 1970.

Scialli AR and Jestila KJ: Sustained benefits of leuprolide acetate with or without subsequent medroxyprogesterone acetate in the nonsurgical management of leiomyomata uteri, Fertil Steril 64:313, 1995.

Scott RT, Beatse SN, Illinois EH, and Snyder RR: Use of the GnRH agonist stimulation test in the diagnosis of ovarian remnant syndrome: a report of three cases, J Reprod Med 40:143, 1995.

Seoud M, Shamseddine A, Khalil A, et al: Tamoxifen and endometrial pathologies: a prospective study, Gynecol Oncol 75:15, 1999.

Shalev E and Peleg D: Laparoscopic treatment of adnexal torsion, Surg Gynecol Obstet 176:448, 1993.

Shevchuk MM, Fenoglio CM, and Richart RM: Histogenesis of Brenner tumors. I. Histology and structure, Cancer 46:2607, 1980.

Siddall-Allum J, Rae T, Rogers V, et al: Chronic pelvic pain caused by residual ovaries and ovarian remnants, Br J Obstet Gynaecol 101:979, 1994.

Siegelman ES, Banner MP, Ramchandani P, and Schnall MD: Multicoil MR imaging of symptomatic female urethral and periurethral disease, Radiographics 17:349, 1997.

Sims JA, Brzyski R, Hansen, and Coddington CC III: Use of a gonadotropin releasing hormone agonist before vaginal surgery for cervical leiomyomas: a report of two cases, J Reprod Med 39:660, 1994.

Smith NC, Van Coeverden de Groot HA, and Gunston KD: Coital injuries of the vagina in nonvirginal patients, S Afr Med J 64:746, 1983.

Soper DE, Patterson JW, Hurt WG, et al: Lichen planus of the vulva, Obstet Gynecol 72:74, 1988.

Spanos WJ: Preoperative hormonal therapy of cystic adnexal masses, Am J Obstet Gynecol 116:551, 1973.

Steege JF: Ovarian remnant syndrome, Obstet Gynecol 70:64, 1987.

Stein AL, Koonings PP, Schlaerth JB, et al: Relative frequency of malignant parovarian tumors: should parovarian tumors be aspirated? Obstet Gynecol 75:1029, 1990.

Steinkampf MP, Hammond KR, and Blackwell RE: Hormonal treatment of functional ovarian cysts: a randomized prospective study, Fertil Steril 54:775, 1990.

Stewart DE, Reicher AE, Gerulath AH, and Boydell KM: Vulvodynia and psychological distress, Obstet Gynecol 84:587, 1994.

Stovall TG, Muneyyirci-Delale O, Summit RL, et al: GnRH agonist and iron versus placebo and iron in the anemic patient before surgery for leiomyomas: a randomized controlled trial, Obstet Gynecol 86:65, 1995.

Summitt RL Jr and Stovall TG: Urethral diverticula: evaluation by urethral pressure profilometry, cystourethroscopy, and the voiding cystourethrogram, Obstet Gynecol 80:695, 1992.

Tang LCH, Cho HKM, Chan SYW, et al: Dextropreponderance of corpus luteum rupture, J Reprod Med 30:764, 1985.

Tepper R, Zalel Y, Markov S, et al: Ovarian volume in postmenopausal women—suggestions to an ovarian size nomogram for menopause age, Acta Obstet Gynecol Scand 74:208, 1995.

Thomas R, Barnhill D, Bibro M, et al: Hidradenitis suppurativa: a case presentation and review of the literature, Obstet Gynecol 66:592, 1985.

Thorp JM Jr, Wells SR, and Droegemueller W: Ovarian suspension in massive ovarian edema, Obstet Gynecol 76:912, 1990.

Valente PT: Leiomyomatosis peritonealis disseminata, Arch Pathol Lab Med 108:669, 1984.

Van Bogaert LJ: Clinicopathologic findings in endometrial polyps, Obstet Gynecol 71:771, 1988.

van der Putte SCJ: Mammary-like glands of the vulva and their disorders, Int J Gynecol Pathol 13:150, 1994.

Van Voorhis BJ, Schwaiger J, Syrop CH, and Chapler FK: Early diagnosis of ovarian torsion by color Doppler ultrasonography, Fertil Steril 58:215, 1992.

Van Winter JT and Stanhope CR: Giant ovarian leiomyoma associated with ascites and polymyositis, Obstet Gynecol 80:560, 1992.

Varasteh NN, Neuwirth RS, Levin B, and Keltz MD: Pregnancy rates after hysteroscopic polypectomy and myomectomy in infertile women, Obstet Gynecol 94:168, 1999.

Vercellini P, Crosignani PG, Mangioni C, et al: Treatment with a gonadotropin releasing hormone agonist before hysterectomy for leiomyomas: results of a multicentre, randomised controlled trial, Br J Obstet Gynaecol 105:1148, 1998.

Vercellini P, Ragni G, Trespidi L, et al: Adenomyosis: a déjà vu? Obstet Gynecol Surv 48:789, 1993.

Vercellini P, Zàina B, Yaylayan L, et al: Hysteroscopic myomectomy: long-term effects on menstrual pattern and fertility, Obstet Gynecol 94:341, 1999.

Verkauf BS: Changing trends in treatment of leiomyomata uteri, Curr Opin Obstet Gynecol 5:301, 1993.

Visco A and Del Priore G: Postmenopausal Bartholin gland enlargement: a hospital-based cancer risk assessment, Obstet Gynecol 87:286, 1996.

Vollenhoven BJ, Shekleton P, McDonald J, et al: Clinical predictors for buserelin acetate treatment of uterine fibroids: a prospective study of 40 women, Fertil Steril 54:1032, 1990.

Waxman M and Boyce JG: Intraperitoneal rupture of benign cystic ovarian teratoma, Obstet Gynecol 48:95, 1976.

Weissberg SM and Dodson MG: Recurrent vaginal and cervical ulcers associated with tampon use, JAMA 250:1430, 1983.

Weissman A, Barash A, Manor M, et al: Acute changes in endometrial thickness after aspiration of functional ovarian cysts, Fertil Steril 69:1142, 1998.

Wenström LV and Willén R: Vestibular nerve fiber proliferation in vulvar vestibulitis syndrome, Obstet Gynecol 91:572, 1998.

Wertheim I, Fleischhacker D, McLachlin CM, et al: Pseudomyxoma peritonei: a review of 23 cases, Obstet Gynecol 84:17, 1994.

Whittman LR and McGibbon DH: The management of psoriasis, Int J Clin Pract 52:487, 1998.

Wolf SI, Gosnik BB, Feldesman MR, et al: Prevalence of simple adnexal cysts in postmenopausal women, Radiol 180: 65, 1991.

Wood C, Maher P, and Hill D: Biopsy diagnosis and conservative surgical treatment of adenomyosis, Aust N Z J Obstet Gynaecol 33:319, 1993.

Woodworth H, Dockerty MB, Wilson RB, et al: Papillary hidradenoma of the vulva: a clinicopathologic study of 69 cases, Am J Obstet Gynecol 110:501, 1971.

Young SB, Rose PG, and Reuter KL: Vaginal fibromyomata: two cases with preoperative assessment, resection, and reconstruction, Obstet Gynecol 78:972, 1991.

Youssef AF, Fayad MM, and Shafeek MA: Torsion of the fallopian tube, Acta Obstet Gynecol Scand 41:291, 1962.

Zellis S and Pincus SH: Treatment of vulvar dermatoses, Semin Dermatol 15:71, 1996.

Zweizig S, Perron J, Grubb D, and Mishell DR Jr: Conservative management of adnexal torsion, Am J Obstet Gynecol 168:1791, 1993.

Endometriosis and Adenomyosis
Etiology, Pathology, Diagnosis, Management

Adenomyoma. An isolated area of endometrial glands and stroma in the uterine musculature that can be identified grossly.

Adenomyosis. The growth of endometrial glands and stroma into the uterine myometrium to a depth of at least 2.5 mm from the basalis layer of the endometrium.

Chocolate Cyst. A cystic area of endometriosis in the ovary.

Coelomic Metaplasia. The potential ability of coelomic epithelium to develop into several different histologic cell types.

Danazol. A synthetic steroid, an attenuated androgen, that is active when taken orally.

Dyschezia. Difficult or painful evacuation of feces from the rectum.

Endometrioma. A small area of endometriosis that can be identified macroscopically.

Endometriosis. The presence and growth of glands and stroma identical to the lining of the uterus in an aberrant location.

GnRH Agonists. A group of synthetic hormones that suppresses gonadotrophin secretion, causing secondary diminution of ovarian steroidogenesis.

Retrograde Menstruation. The flow of menstrual blood, endometrial cells, and debris via the fallopian tubes into the peritoneal cavity.

ENDOMETRIOSIS

Endometriosis is a benign, but in many women, a progressive disease. The wide spectrum of clinical problems that occur with endometriosis has frustrated gynecologists, fascinated pathologists, and burdened patients for years. The classic studies of Sampson in the 1920s were the first to emphasize the clinical and pathologic correlations of endometriosis. Even today, many aspects of the disease remain enigmatic.

By definition, endometriosis is the presence and growth of the glands and stroma of the lining of the uterus in an aberrant or heterotopic location. Adenomyosis is the growth of endometrial glands and stroma into the uterine myometrium to a depth of at least 2.5 mm from the basalis layer of the endometrium. Adenomyosis is sometimes termed *internal endometriosis;* however, this is a semantic misnomer because most likely they are separate diseases.

It is usually stated that the incidence of endometriosis has been increasing over the past 30 years. This "opinion" is secondary to an enlightened awareness of mild endometriosis as diagnosed by the increasing use of laparoscopy. During the past 10 years diagnostic delay, the average time to the first diagnosis of the disease, has decreased dramatically. Evers has advanced a provocative hypothesis that endometrial implants in the peritoneal cavity are a physiologic finding secondary to retrograde menstruation and their presence does not confirm a disease process. The age-specific incidence or prevalence of endometriosis is unknown. Any statements concerning the incidence or prevalence of endometriosis are approximations. Many patients are diagnosed incidentally during laparoscopy or exploratory celiotomy performed for a variety of other indications. Conservative estimates find that endometriosis is present in 5% to 15% of celiotomies performed on reproductive-age females. The prevalence of active endometriosis is approximately 33% of women with chronic pelvic pain. The incidence of endometriosis is 30% to 45% in women with infertility. It must be emphasized that all studies of the prevalence of endometriosis are subject to selection bias and are dependent on the definition of "active disease."

The etiology of endometriosis is uncertain and may involve retrograde menstruation, vascular dissemination, metaplasia, genetic predisposition, immunologic changes, and hormonal influences. Visualization in the vast majority of endometriosis cases necessitates either laparoscopy or celiotomy. Clinically, it is most difficult to predict the natural course of endometriosis in any one individual. For example, the clinician is uncertain as to which woman with mild disease in her 20s will progress to severe disease at a later age.

The typical patient with endometriosis is in her mid-30s, is nulliparous and involuntarily infertile, and has symptoms of secondary dysmenorrhea and pelvic pain. The classic symptom of endometriosis is pelvic pain. However, in clinical practice the majority of cases are not "classic." The diagnosis and treatment of infertility associated with endometriosis is discussed in Chapter 41. Aberrant endometrial tissue grows under the cyclic influence of ovarian hormones; therefore the disease is most commonly found during the reproductive years. Approximately 5% of women with endometriosis are diagnosed following menopause. Postmenopausal endometriosis is usually stimulated by exogenous estrogen. Teenagers with endometriosis should be investigated for obstructive reproductive tract abnormalities that increase the amount of retrograde menstruation.

Endometriosis is a disease not only of great individual variability but also of contrasting pathophysiologic processes (Table 19-1). It is a benign disease, yet it has the characteristics of a malignancy—locally infiltrative, invasive, and widely disseminating. Although the growth of ectopic endometrium is stimulated by physiologic levels of estrogen and progesterone, both low ("pseudomenopause") and high ("pseudopregnancy") levels of these hormones are usually therapeutic. Another contrast often noted is the inverse relationship between the extent of pelvic endometriosis and the severity of pelvic pain. Women with extensive endometriosis may be asymptomatic, whereas other patients with minimal implants may have incapacitating chronic pelvic pain. However, as would be expected, women with deep infiltrating endometriosis, especially in retroperitoneal spaces, often experience severe episodes of pain. Finally, there is speculation as to

TABLE 19-1
Endometriosis: A Disease of Clinical Contrasts

Characteristics	Contrasts
Benign disease	Locally invasive Widespread disseminated foci Proliferates in pelvic lymph nodes
Minimal disease	Severe pain
Many large endometriomas	Asymptomatic patient
Cyclic hormones cause growth	Continuous hormones reverse the growth pattern

the underlying pathophysiology that produces infertility in women with endometriosis.

Until the natural history of endometriosis is understood, the clinician will have more questions than answers concerning this benign, usually progressive, and sometimes recurrent disease. These questions are a stimulating challenge to future investigators.

Etiology

There are several theories to explain the histogenesis of endometriosis. However, no single theory adequately explains the protean manifestations of the disease. Most important, there is only speculation as to why some women develop endometriosis, while others do not. Some postulate that there is a complex interplay between a dose-response curve of the amount of retrograde menstruation and an individual woman's immunologic response.

Retrograde Menstruation

The most popular theory is that endometriosis results from retrograde menstruation. Sampson suggested that pelvic endometriosis was secondary to implantation of endometrial cells shed during menstruation. These cells attach to the pelvic peritoneum and under hormonal influence grow as homologous grafts. Endometriosis is discovered most frequently in areas immediately adjacent to the tubal ostia or in the dependent areas of the pelvis.

A number of experiments in monkeys and clinical observations in humans support this hypothesis. Monkeys developed classic endometriosis when the cervix was sutured to prevent the normal egress of menstrual blood. In these experiments the development of endometriosis was dependent on repetitive "seeding" of the peritoneal cavity. Retrograde menstruation is the rule rather than the exception in all women. This fact has been noted at laparoscopy during the first days of menstrual flow. Studies by Blumenkrantz et al. observed bloody dialysate fluid 24 to 48 hours before menstruation in the majority of women being treated with peritoneal dialysis. This bloody peritoneal fluid contained viable endometrial cells. Endometriosis is frequently found in women with outflow obstruction of the genital tract.

Metaplasia

In contrast to the theory of seeding from retrograde menstruation is the theory that endometriosis arises from metaplasia of the coelomic (celomic) epithelium or proliferation of embryonic rests. The müllerian ducts and nearby mesenchymal tissue form the majority of the female reproductive tract. The müllerian duct is derived from the coelomic epithelium during fetal development. The metaplasia hypothesis postulates that the coelomic epithelium retains the ability for multipotential development. The decidual reaction of isolated areas of peritoneum during pregnancy is an example of this process. It is well known that the surface epithelium of the ovary can differentiate into several different histologic cell types. Endometriosis has been discovered in prepubertal girls, women with congenital absence of the uterus, and very rarely in men. These examples support the coelomic metaplasia theory.

Metaplasia occurs after an "induction phenomenon" has stimulated the multipotential cell. The induction substance may be a combination of menstrual debris and the influence of estrogen and progesterone. Batt and Smith have hypothesized that the histogenesis of endometriosis in peritoneal pockets of the posterior pelvis results from a congenital anomaly involving rudimentary duplication of the müllerian system. The peritoneal pockets that they describe are found in the posterior pelvis, the posterior aspects of the broad ligament, and the cul-de-sac of Douglas. Similarly, Nisolle and Donnez postulate that metaplasia of the celomic epithelium that invaginates into the ovarian cortex is the pathogenesis for the development of ovarian endometriosis.

Lymphatic and Vascular Metastasis

The theory of endometrium being transplanted via lymphatic channels and the vascular system helps to explain rare and remote sites of endometriosis, such as the spinal column and nose. Endometriosis has been observed in the pelvic lymph nodes of approximately 30% of women with the disease. Hematogenous dissemination of endometrium is the best theory to explain endometriosis of the forearm and thigh, as well as multiple lesions in the lung.

Iatrogenic Dissemination

Endometriosis of the anterior abdominal wall is sometimes discovered in women after a cesarean delivery. The hypothesis is that endometrial glands and stroma are implanted during the procedure. The aberrant tissue is found subcutaneously at the abdominal incision. Rarely, iatrogenic endometriosis may be discovered in an episiotomy scar.

Immunologic Changes

One of the most perplexing, unanswered questions concerning the pathophysiology of endometriosis is that some women with retrograde menstruation develop endometriosis while the majority do not. Multiple investigations have suggested that changes in the immune system, especially altered function of immune-related cells, are directly related to the pathogenesis of endometriosis. Whether endometriosis is an autoimmune disease has been intensely debated during the past 15 years. Studies have demonstrated abnormalities in cell-mediated and humoral components of the immune system in both peripheral blood and peritoneal fluid. In the past 15 years approximately 400 articles have been published on the basic science of endometriosis.

Most likely the primary immunologic change involves an alteration in the function of the peritoneal macrophages so prevalent in the peritoneal fluid of patients with endometriosis. Halme et al. hypothesize that women who do not develop endometriosis have monocytic-type macrophages in their peritoneal fluid that have a short life span and limited function. Conversely, women who develop endometriosis have more peritoneal macrophages that are larger. These hyperactive cells secrete multiple growth factors and cytokines that enhance the development of endometriosis. The attraction of leukocytes to specific areas is controlled by chemokines, which are chemotactic cytokines (Figure 19-1). Changes in the expression of integrins also may be an important local factor. Recent literature has focused attention on elevated levels of vascular endothelial growth factor and interleukin-6. They are postulated to promote angiogenesis, which facilitates the growth of endometriosis. Recently, Tsudo et al. have reported increased levels of tumor necrosis factor-α, altered gene expression, and protein secretion of interleukin-6 in women with endometriosis. Poetically, he commented, "the peritoneal fluid contains a rich cocktail of cytokines" (Figure 19-2). To further complicate our understanding, cytokines and growth factors also may be produced by the ectopic endometrium or stroma. Other immunologic abnormalities that may be important in the pathophysiology of endometriosis include changes in the secretory products of T-lymphocytes and decreased activity of natural killer cells. Lastly, intrinsic biochemical differences do exist in the eutopic endometrium of women with endometriosis, which may explain why these cells are able to implant on the peritoneal surface. In summary, the basic science of the pathophysiology of endometriosis is rapidly expanding and, hopefully, all the pieces of the puzzle will be in place sometime during the next few years.

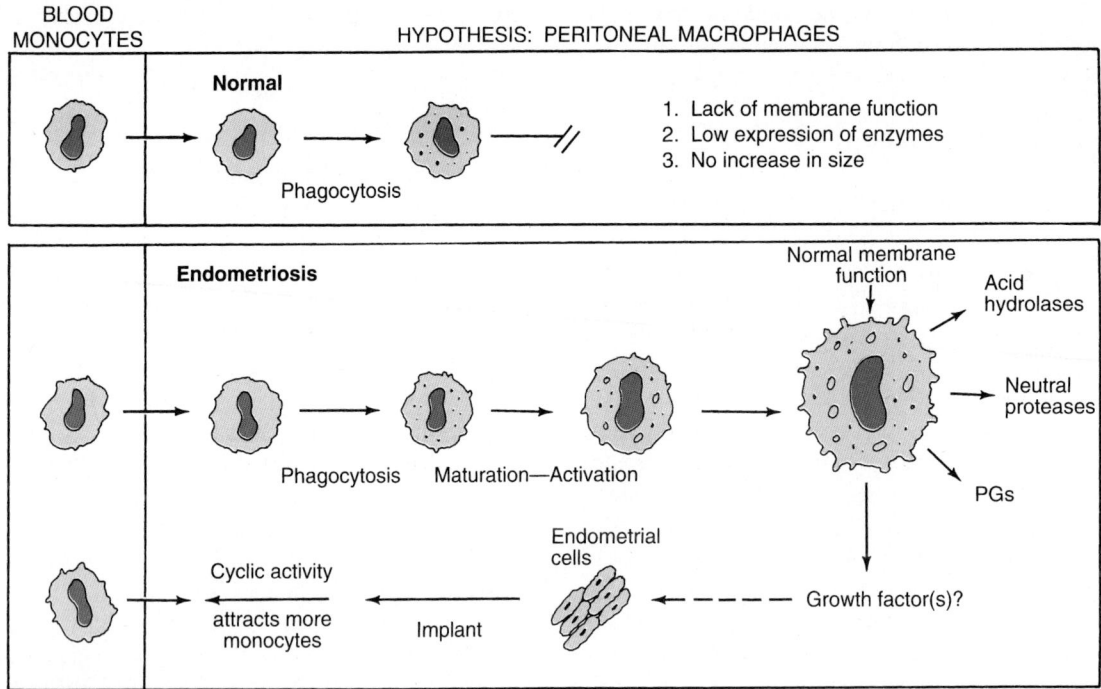

FIGURE 19-1 Hypothesis regarding pathophysiologic characteristics of human peritoneal macrophages in endometriosis. The presence of higher numbers and larger, more mature macrophages in endometriosis may lead to secretion of putative growth factors facilitating implantation and growth of endometrial cells. (Redrawn from Halme J et al: Am J Obstet Gynecol 156:787, 1987.)

Genetic Predisposition

Several studies have documented a familial predisposition to endometriosis with grouping of cases of endometriosis in mothers and their daughters. An investigation by Simpson et al. demonstrated a sevenfold increase in the incidence of endometriosis in relatives of women with the disease compared with controls. One of 10 women with severe endometriosis will have a sister or mother with clinical manifestations of the disease. Women who have a family history of endometriosis are likely to develop the disease earlier in life and to have more advanced disease than women whose first-degree relatives are free of the disease. Recent studies have identified deletions of genes, most specifically increased heterogenicity of chromosome 17 and aneuploidy, in women with endometriosis compared to controls. The expression of this genetic liability most likely depends on an interaction with environmental factors. Preliminary data suggest some bilateral ovarian endometrial cysts may arise independently from different clones.

In summary, most authorities believe that several factors are involved in the etiology of endometriosis, including retrograde transport of endometrium, potentially coelomic metaplasia, an immunologic change, and a genetic predisposition. Each factor may contribute to the development of this enigmatic disease, and their relative importance varies among individuals (see box at right).

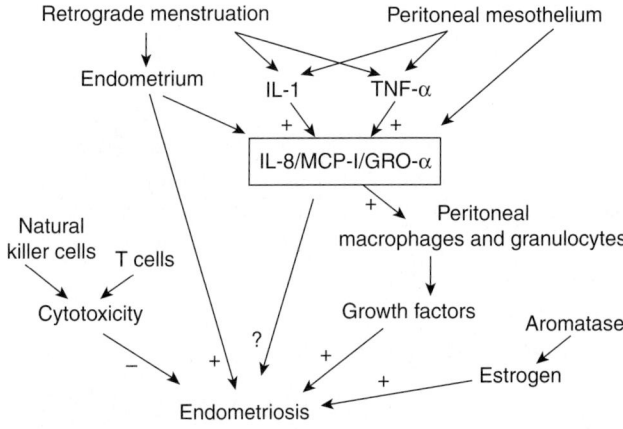

FIGURE 19-2 The role of different chemokines in the pathogenesis of endometriosis. (From Garcia-Velasco JA and Arici A: Chemokines and human reproduction, Fertil Steril 71:983, 1999.)

Etiology of Endometriosis

Retrograde menstruation
Coelomic metaplasia
Activation of embryonic rests
Lymphatic and vascular metastases
Immunologic changes
Genetic predisposition
Iatrogenic dissemination

Pathology

The majority of endometrial implants are located in the dependent portions of the female pelvis (Figure 19-3). The ovaries are the most common site, being involved in two of three women with endometriosis. In most of these women the involvement is bilateral. The pelvic peritoneum over the uterus, the anterior and posterior cul-de-sac, and the uterosacral, round, and broad ligaments are also common sites where endometriosis develops. Pelvic lymph nodes are involved in 30% of cases (Figure 19-4). The cervix, vagina, and vulva are other possible pelvic locations. Recently Brosens et al. have emphasized the importance of distinguishing between superficial and deep lesions of endometriosis. Deep lesions, penetrations of greater than 5 mm, represent a more progressive form of the disease.

Approximately 10% to 15% of women with advanced disease have lesions involving the rectosigmoid. Depending on the amount of associated scarring, endometriosis of the bowel may be difficult to differentiate grossly from a primary neoplasm of the large intestine.

Rare sites of endometriosis include the umbilicus, areas of previous surgical incisions of the anterior abdominal wall or perineum, the bladder, ureter, kidney, lung, arms, legs, and even the male urinary tract (Table 19-2).

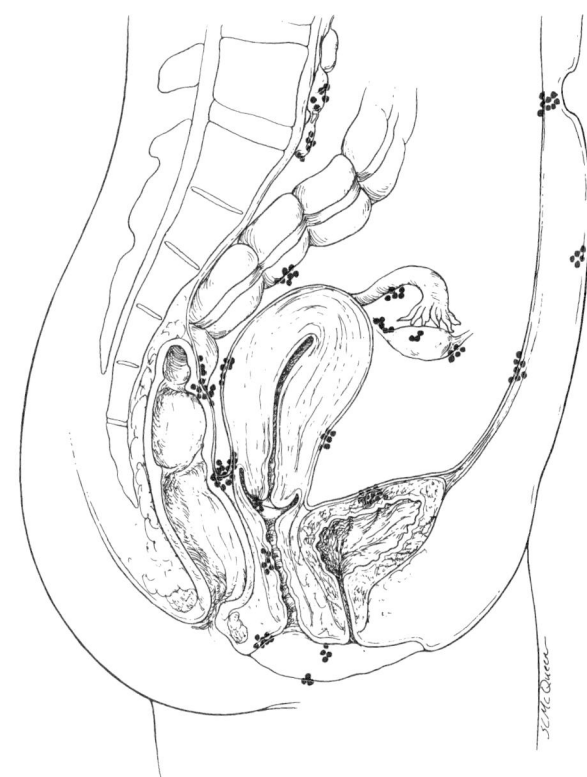

FIGURE 19-3 Common pelvic sites of endometriosis.

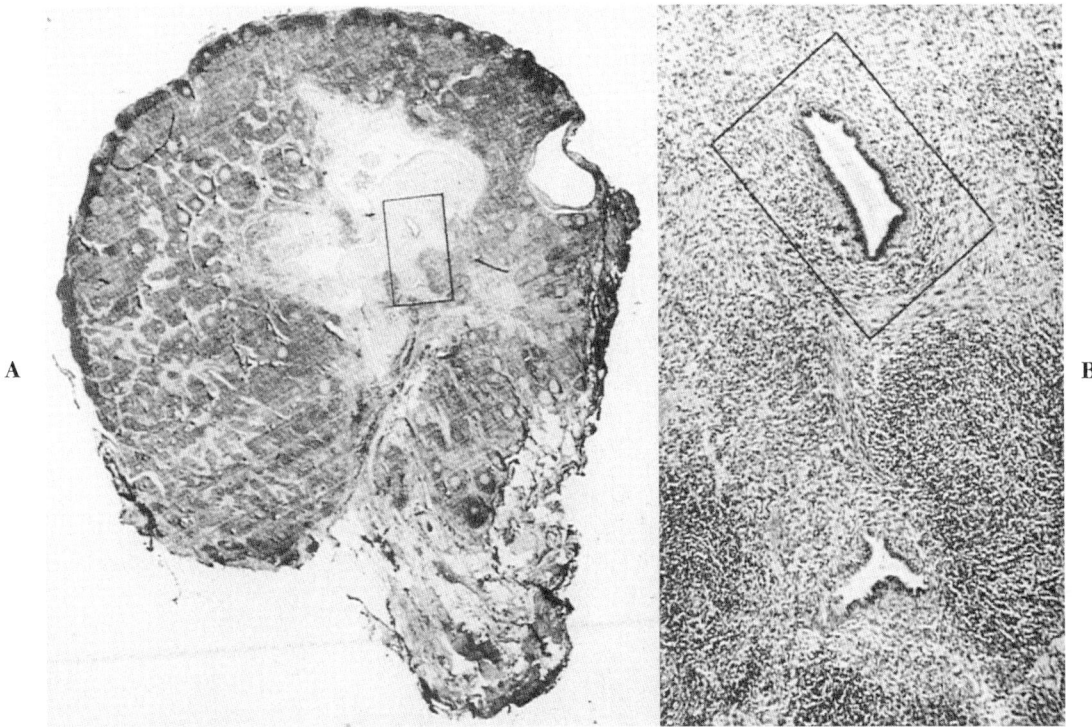

FIGURE 19-4 Endometriosis in right ureteral lymph node. **A,** Low-power view. **B,** Higher-power view showing two glands and surrounding stroma. (From Javert CT: Cancer 2:403, 1949.)

TABLE 19-2
Anatomic Distribution of Endometriosis

Common Sites	Rare Sites
Ovaries	Umbilicus
Pelvic peritoneum	Episiotomy scar
Ligaments of the uterus	Bladder
Sigmoid colon	Kidney
Appendix	Lungs
Pelvic lymph nodes	Arms
Cervix	Legs
Vagina	Nasal mucosa
Fallopian tubes	Spinal column

TABLE 19-3
Terminology Used to Describe Peritoneal
Endometriosis

Powder-burn, puckered black lesions
Vascularized glandular papules
Vesicular lesions
    Serous, surrounded by marked vascularization
    Red hemorrhagic
Red, flamelike
Petechial peritoneum
Hypervascularized area
Discolored area
    Yellow-brown
    Blue
    White
White scarring
Peritoneal defects
Cribriform peritoneal
Subovarian adhesions

From Brosens IA: Endometriosis: a disease because it is characterized by bleeding, Am J Obstet Gynecol 176:265, 1997.

Gross pathologic changes of endometriosis exhibit wide variability in color, shape, size, and associated inflammatory and fibrotic changes. The visual manifestations of endometriosis in the female pelvis are protean and have many appearances. Increased awareness and anticipation have focused on the subtle lesions of endometriosis. Recently, clinicians closely inspect the pelvic peritoneum to identify abnormal areas and small, nonhemorrhagic lesions. More emphasis has been placed on biopsy confirmation of endometriosis because of increasing awareness of subtle lesions. The gross appearance of the implant depends on the site, activity, relationship to day of menstrual cycle, and chronicity of the area involved. The color of the lesion varies widely and may be red, brown, black, white, or yellow or a pink, clear, or red vesicle. The predominant color depends on the blood supply and the amount of hemorrhage and fibrosis. The color also appears related to the size of the lesion, degree of edema, and the amount of inspissated material (Table 19-3). Other peritoneal lesions that grossly appear similar to endometriosis, but on histologic examination are not, include necrotic areas of an ectopic pregnancy, fibrotic reactions to suture, hemangiomas, adrenal rest, Walthard's rest, breast cancer, ovarian cancer, epithelial inclusions, residual carbon from laser surgery, peritoneal inflammation, psammoma bodies, peritoneal reactions to oil-based hysterosalpingogram dye, and splenosis.

New lesions are small, bleb-like implants that are less than 1 cm in diameter. Initially these areas are raised above the surrounding tissues. Red, blood-filled lesions have been shown, by histologic and biochemical studies, to be the most active phase of the disease. With time the areas of endometriosis become larger and assume a light or dark brown color, and they may be described as "powder burn" areas or "chocolate cysts." The older lesions have more intense scarring and are usually puckered or retracted from the surrounding tissue.

The pattern of ovarian endometriosis is also variable

(Figure 19-5). Individual areas range from 1 mm to large chocolate cysts greater than 8 cm in diameter. The associated adhesions may be filmy or dense. Larger cysts are usually densely adherent to the surrounding pelvic sidewalls or broad ligament.

The three cardinal histologic features of endometriosis are ectopic endometrial glands, ectopic endometrial stroma, and hemorrhage into the adjacent tissue (Figures 19-6 and 19-7). Previous hemorrhage can be discovered by identifying large macrophages filled with hemosiderin near the periphery of the lesion. In the majority of cases the aberrant endometrial glands and stroma respond in cyclic fashion to estrogen and progesterone. These changes may or may not be in synchrony with the endometrial lining of the uterus. The ectopic endometrial stroma will undergo classic decidual changes similar to pregnancy when exposed to high physiologic or pharmacologic levels of progesterone.

In approximately 25% of the cases of endometriosis, viable endometrial glands and stroma cannot be identified. Repetitive episodes of hemorrhage may lead to severe inflammatory changes and result in the glands and stroma undergoing necrobiosis secondary to pressure atrophy or lack of blood supply. In these cases a presumptive diagnosis of endometriosis is made by visualizing the intense inflammatory reaction and the large macrophages filled with blood pigment.

The natural history of endometriosis is a subject of intense speculation. Spontaneous regression or disappear-

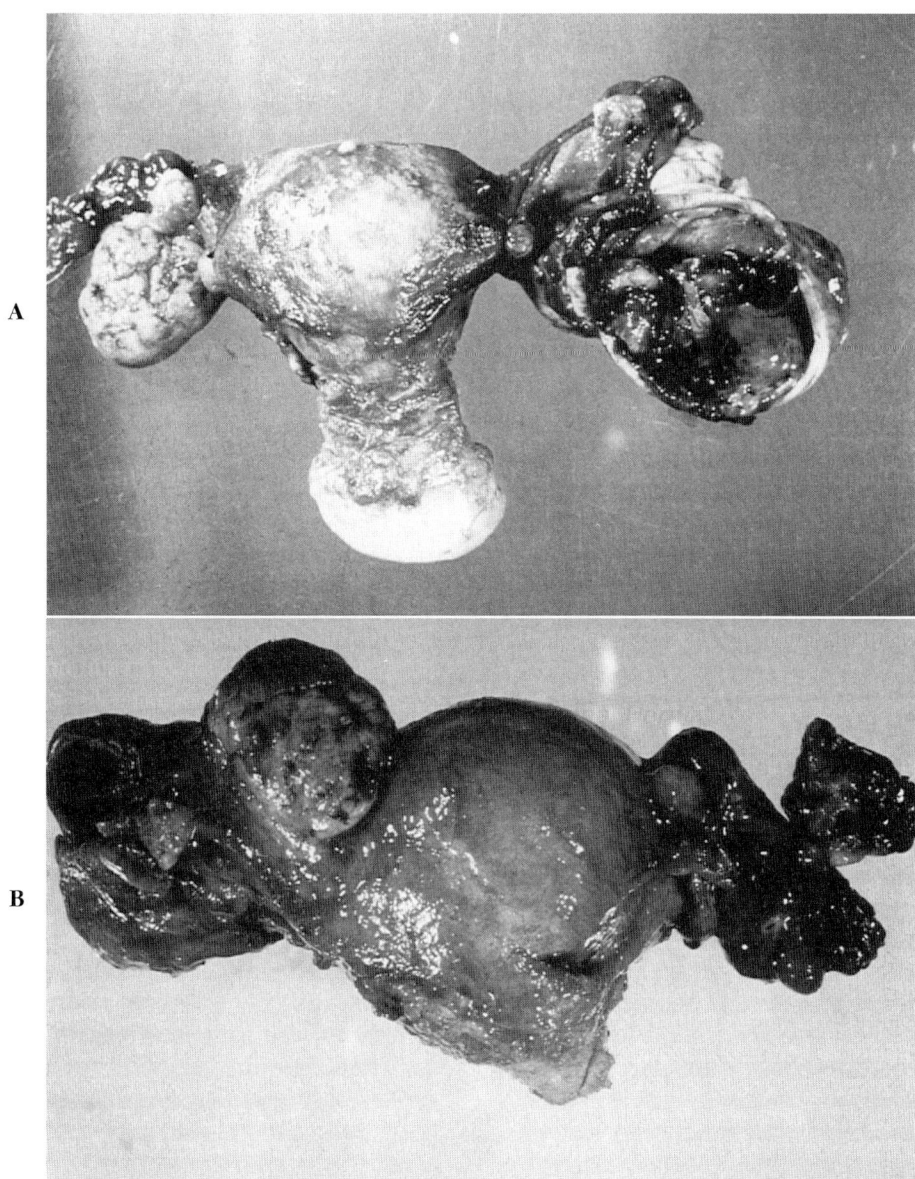

FIGURE 19-5 A, Total hysterectomy specimen from woman with endometriosis. Right ovary was partially destroyed by endometrioma. **B,** Anterior view of same specimen. Note small endometrial implants on surface of right ovary. (Courtesy Fred Askin, M.D.)

ance of active disease is common. The pathophysiology of progression from subtle endometriosis to severe disease is presently unknown.

Clinical Diagnosis

Symptoms

It is important to reemphasize that endometriosis has many different clinical presentations, with one in three women being asymptomatic. Most importantly, the disease has an extremely unpredictable course. The classic symptoms of endometriosis are cyclic pelvic pain and infertility. The chronic pelvic pain usually presents as sec-

ondary dysmenorrhea and/or dyspareunia. Secondary dysmenorrhea usually begins 36 to 48 hours prior to the onset of menses. However, approximately one third of patients with endometriosis are asymptomatic, with the disease being discovered incidentally during an abdominal operation or visualized at laparoscopy for an unrelated problem. Conversely, endometriosis is discovered in approximately one of three women whose primary symptom is chronic pelvic pain.

Clinicians have appreciated the paradox that the extent of pelvic pain is often inversely related to the amount of endometriosis in the female pelvis. Women with large, fixed adnexal masses sometimes have minor symptoms, while other patients with only a few small foci with deep

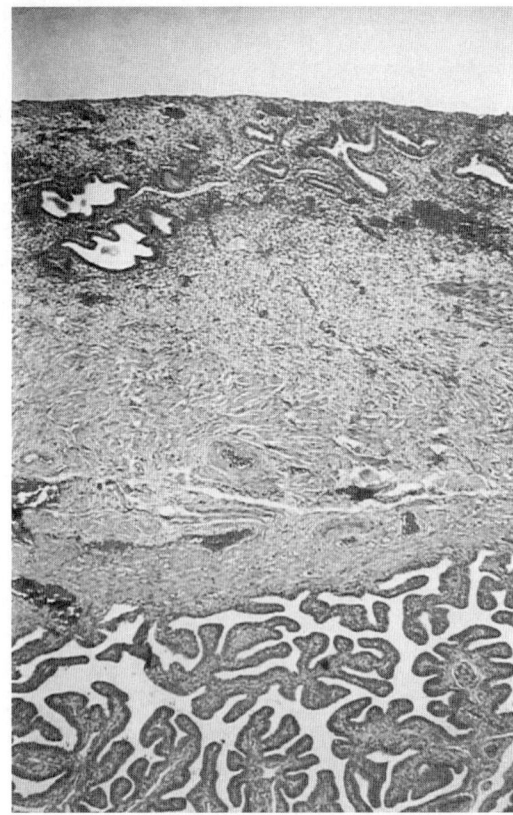

FIGURE 19-6 Endometriosis on fallopian tube. Serosa of tube is being invaded by glands and stroma. (Courtesy Fred Askin, M.D.)

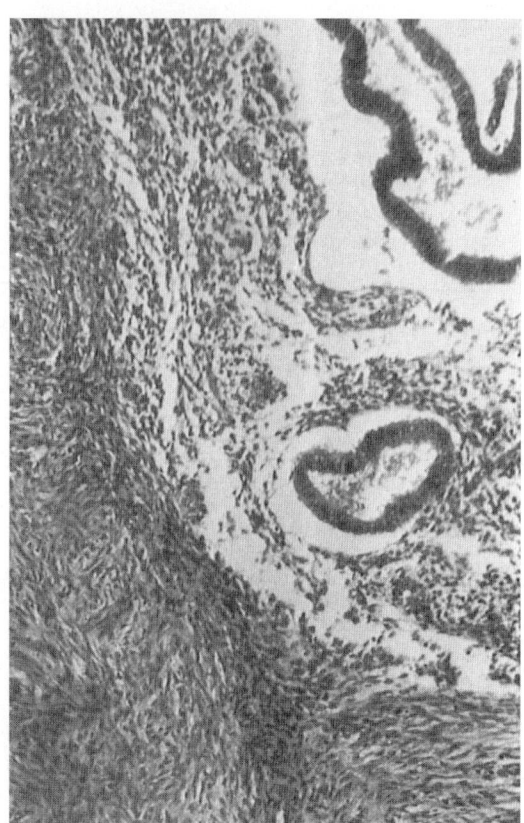

FIGURE 19-7 High-power view of endometrial glands in ovarian stroma. (Courtesy Fred Askin, M.D.)

infiltration may experience moderate to severe chronic pain. Fedele et al. could find no correlation between the anatomic stage of the disease and the patient's perception of severity of pelvic pain. In their study, 124 women were staged according to the revised scoring system of the American Society of Reproductive Medicine. No relationship was found between stage of the disease and frequency or severity of pain symptoms.

The cyclic pelvic pain is related to the sequential swelling and the extravasation of blood and menstrual debris into the surrounding tissue. The chemical mediators of this intense sterile inflammation and pain are believed to be prostaglandins and cytokines. Infiltrative endometriosis, which involves extensive areas of the retroperitoneal space, often is associated with moderate to severe pelvic pain. Recently, studies of pain mapping by laparoscopy under minimal sedation have found that the pelvic pain arises from areas of normal peritoneum adjacent to areas of endometriosis.

The secondary dysmenorrhea is constant pain. It varies from a dull ache to severe pelvic pain. It may be unilateral or bilateral and may radiate to the lower back, legs, and groin. Patients often complain of pelvic heaviness or a perception of their internal organs being swollen. Unlike primary dysmenorrhea, the pain may last for many days, including several days before and after the menstrual flow.

The dyspareunia associated with endometriosis is described as pain deep in the pelvis. The etiology of this symptom seems to be immobility of the pelvic organs during coital activity or direct pressure on areas of endometriosis in the uterosacral ligaments or the cul-de-sac of Douglas. Sometimes patients describe areas of point tenderness. The acute pain, experienced during deep penetration, may continue for several hours following intercourse.

Abnormal bleeding is a symptom noted by 15% to 20% of women with endometriosis. The most frequent complaints are premenstrual spotting and menorrhagia. Usually this abnormal bleeding is not associated with an anovulatory pattern. On the other hand, patients with endometriosis frequently have ovulatory dysfunction. Approximately 15% of women with endometriosis have coincidental anovulation.

An increased incidence of first-trimester abortion in women with untreated endometriosis has been reported. However, recent epidemiologic studies question a true increased incidence and, if there is, raise serious doubt as to a cause-and-effect relationship.

Less common yet troublesome are the symptoms resulting from endometriosis influencing the gastrointestinal and urinary tracts. Cyclic abdominal pain, intermittent constipation, diarrhea, dyschezia, urinary frequency, dysuria, and

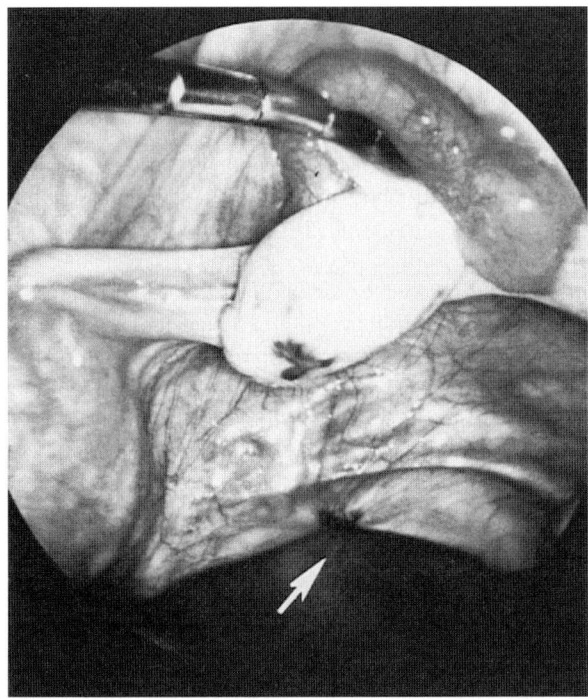

FIGURE 19-8 Laparoscopic view of ovarian and pelvic endometriosis. Tube is being elevated by a probe. Note retracted area of broad ligament around endometriosis *(arrow)*. (Courtesy Jaroslav Hulka, M.D.)

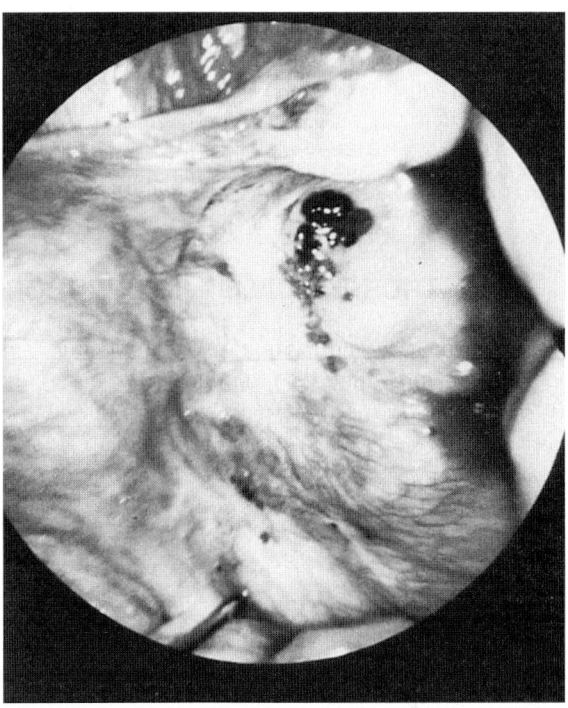

FIGURE 19-9 Laparoscopic view of endometriosis on posterior leaf of broad ligament and cul-de-sac. Note the many adhesions. (Courtesy Jaroslav Hulka, M.D.)

hematuria are all possible symptoms. Bowel obstruction and hydronephrosis may occur. One rare clinical manifestation of endometriosis is catamenial hemothorax, bloody pleural fluid occurring during menses. Massive ascites is a rare symptom of endometriosis, but it is important because the disease process initially masquerades as ovarian carcinoma.

Signs

The classic pelvic finding of endometriosis is a fixed retroverted uterus, with scarring and tenderness posterior to the uterus. The characteristic nodularity of the uterosacral ligaments and cul-de-sac of Douglas may be palpated on rectovaginal examination in approximately one third of women with the disease. Advanced cases have extensive scarring and narrowing of the posterior vaginal fornix. The ovaries may be enlarged and tender and are often fixed to the broad ligament or lateral pelvic sidewall. The adnexal enlargement is rarely symmetric, as one might expect in some benign pelvic conditions. In one study of 561 women with ovarian endometriomas, bilateral cysts were observed in 158. In women with unilateral endometriomas, 63% were found in the left ovary.

Endometriosis is a disease that produces tenderness of the pelvic structures and scarring that restricts movement of the pelvic organs. Occasionally the physician discovers endometriosis in an old surgical incision or a site of a previous amniocentesis. Speculum examination may demonstrate small areas of endometriosis on the cervix or upper vagina.

Lateral displacement or deviation of the cervix is visualized or palpated by digital exam of the vagina and cervix in approximately 15% of women with moderate or severe endometriosis. The diagnosis is straightforward if a patient presents with secondary dysmenorrhea, deep dyspareunia, and infertility and if during a pelvic examination the physician discovers a fixed posterior uterus, bilateral adnexal tenderness, and beading of the uterosacral ligaments. An experienced clinician may instruct the patient to return for a pelvic examination during the first or second day of her menstrual flow when the diagnosis of endometriosis is in doubt. This is the time of maximum swelling and tenderness in the areas of endometriosis. The diagnosis can be confirmed in most cases by direct laparoscopic visualization of endometriosis with its associated scarring and adhesion formation. In many patients it is discovered for the first time during an infertility investigation. Biopsy of selected implants gives confirmation of the diagnosis. However, sometimes the pathologist may be unable to find glandular elements and endometrial stroma in the biopsy specimens.

When laparoscopy is undertaken to establish the diagnosis of endometriosis, it is important to describe systematically the extent of the pathology (Figures 19-8 and 19-9). In 1993 a committee of the American Society for Reproductive Medicine developed a detailed form to help the clinician document and assign numeric values illustrating the operative appearance of the disease including the most important features of endometriosis and pelvic pain (Figure 19-10). The key elements of this form

MANAGEMENT OF ENDOMETRIOSIS IN THE PRESENCE OF PELVIC PAIN
A Clinical Instrument to Document the Extent of Endometriosis and Pelvic Pain[1]

Patient's Name _____ Age _____ Date _____

PRE-OPERATIVE ASSESSMENT OF PELVIC PAIN

Complaints _____

_____

Describe the patient's symptoms of pain quality and position, and any limitation caused by these symptoms. Abbreviate quality of pain as **A = mild, B = discomforting, C = distressing, D = horrible, E = excruciating.** On the anatomic drawings below, draw a **SOLID LINE** around the area(s) of pain described by the patient, and mark the most intense area(s) with an **X.**

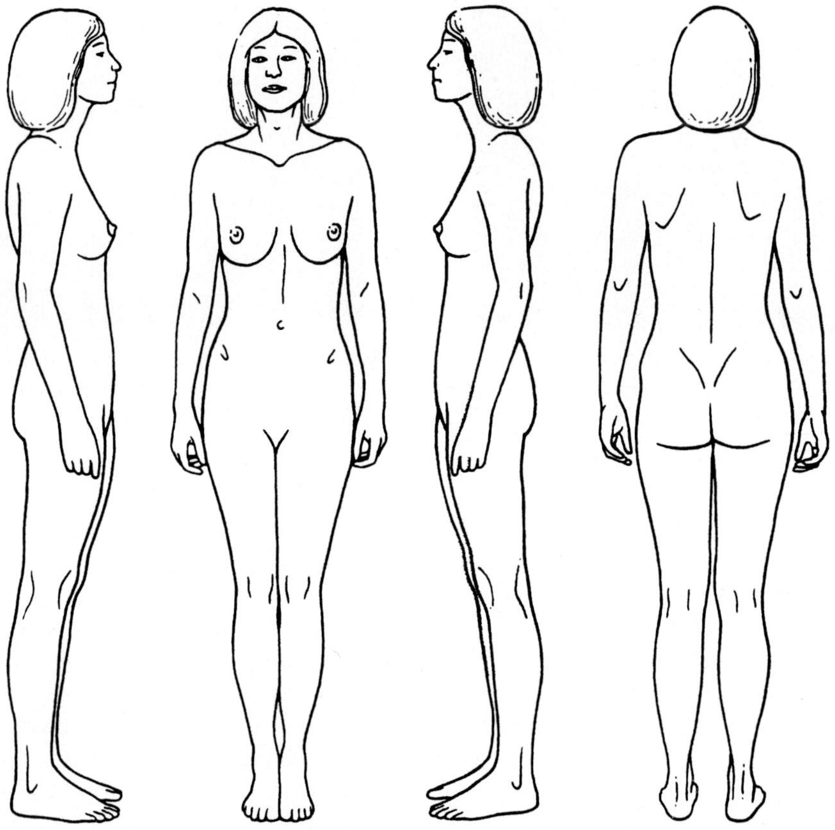

Physical findings _____

_____

Identify the quality and site of tenderness caused by palpation, extent of nodularity, diffuse or focal distribution, and/or fixation of uterus/adnexa. On the anatomic drawings above, draw a **BROKEN LINE** around the area(s) of tenderness found on examination.

Adjuncts: [ ] IVP?   [ ] BE?   [ ] Sigmoidoscopy?   [ ] Other? _____

_____

_____

[1] The association of pelvic pain and endometriosis remains enigmatic because the extent of disease by the previous AFS classifications does not dependably relate to the severity of pelvic pain or tenderness. This form was designed by the AFS Committee on Classification of Endometriosis to carefully document the location and intensity of pelvic pain and tenderness in addition to distribution of endometriosis and pelvic adhesions. Constant recording of this data will permit consistent management of the patient with endometriosis and pelvic pain, and facilitate clinical research.

FIGURE 19-10   Form for the management of endometriosis in the presence of pelvic pain. (From The American Fertility Society: Fertil Steril 60:953, 1993.)

Procedure _____

_____

OPERATIVE DESCRIPTION OF PELVIC ADHESIONS

Describe the location, points of attachment and characteristics of adhesions. Abbreviate characteristics as **A = avascular/thin, T = thick/dense, B = band/string-like, S = sheet-like.** Draw a picture of these adhesions at the appropriate location in each quadrant.

IIa (Left lateral)

I (Anterior)

IIb (Right lateral)

IV (Other sites)

III (Posterior)

OPERATIVE APPEARANCE OF THE DISTRIBUTION OF ENDOMETRIOSIS

After mobilizing the pelvic viscera, measure the size (mean diameter in millimeters) and depth of each visible lesion. Use a calibrated endoscopic probe, if necessary. Record the location, dimension, visual appearance and histologic confirmation of these lesions. Abbreviate the visual appearance as **C = clear, V = vesicles/blebs, P = pink, R = red/flame-like, B = black/blue, Y = yellow/brown, W = white, F = peritoneal fibrosis.** Document the site of each lesion by positioning the index number (No. on the table below) at the appropriate location in each quadrant.

IIa (Left lateral)

I (Anterior)

IIb (Right lateral)

IVa (Other intra-abdominal sites)

IVb (Outside peritoneal cavity)

III (Posterior)

No.	Size in mm	Depth	Appearance	Histology	Location	No.	Size in mm	Depth	Appearance	Histology	Location
i.e.	*8 m*	*2 mm*	*F*	*Glands & stroma*	*III*						
1						11					
2						12					
3						13					
4						14					
5						15					
6						16					
7						17					
8						18					
9						19					
10						20					

Histology _____

Results _____

FIGURE 19-10, cont'd   For legend see opposite page.

and point scoring system include a complete description of the location, width, and depth of the implants, and the presence and severity of adhesive disease by location thickness and points of attachment. An updated scoring system developed in 1996 by the American Society for Reproductive Medicine was designed primarily to record the progress of the disease in fertility patients. It is easy to combine this form with a numeric pain scale to periodically document specific pain symptoms and the physical findings of tenderness during pelvic exam (Figure 19-11).

Unfortunately, ultrasound examination shows no specific pattern to screen for pelvic endometriosis. Ultrasound may be helpful in differentiating solid from cystic lesions and may help distinguish an endometrioma from other adnexal abnormalities. Therefore, pelvic ultrasound or magnetic resonance imaging (MR) may give additional and confirmatory information but cannot be used for primary screening.

Although a benign disease, endometriosis exhibits characteristics of both malignancy and sterile inflammation. Therefore the common considerations in the differential diagnosis include chronic pelvic inflammatory disease, ovarian malignancy, degeneration of myomas, hemorrhage or torsion of ovarian cysts, adenomyosis, primary dysmenorrhea, and functional bowel disease.

Occasionally a large endometrioma of the ovary may rupture into the peritoneal cavity. This results in an acute surgical abdomen and brings into the differential diagnosis conditions such as ectopic pregnancy, appendicitis, diverticulitis, and a bleeding corpus luteum cyst. Studies have not demonstrated any temporal relationship between the timing of an endometrioma's acute rupture and the day of the menstrual cycle.

Natural History

Endometriosis is a chronic and sometimes progressive disease. The disease is usually first diagnosed in a woman during her mid to late 20s. The rate of progression of the disease varies widely from one patient to another. Serial pelvic examinations are a poor indicator of progression of the disease. Therefore the natural history of the disease is largely speculation. In some centers, second-look or reassessment laparoscopy is performed routinely. These limited studies have given insight into the success of therapy. During the past few years interest has centered on measuring serum levels of cancer antigen-125 (CA-125) as a chemical marker and noninvasive test for endometriosis. CA-125 levels are elevated in most patients with endometriosis and increase incrementally with advanced stages. However, assays for serum levels of CA-125 have a low specificity because they also increase with other pelvic conditions such as myomas, acute pelvic inflammatory disease, and the first trimester of pregnancy. Similarly, serum CA-125 levels have a low sensitivity for the diag-

nosis of early or minimal endometriosis. Therefore it is unlikely that this assay will become a screening or diagnostic test. Serial CA-125 levels are of limited utility in following the course of the disease or results of medical therapy.

It would be optimal to identify women who are going to develop endometriosis. Clinicians should note the genetic factors in endometriosis and identify family members at risk. The optimal preventive therapy for a young teenager not desirous of pregnancy until her late 20s is unknown. Clinical options include no treatment, continuous use of oral contraceptives, or cyclic oral contraceptive therapy. Controlled prospective studies are needed to answer the difficult clinical question of the best method to inhibit progression of the disease.

Approximately 10% of teenagers who develop endometriosis have associated congenital outflow obstruction. Therefore teenagers with pelvic pain should be examined for this possibility.

At one time there was a general belief that pregnancy improved endometriosis. A careful study by McArthur and Ulfelder of external endometriosis, which could be observed throughout the pregnancy, discovered that this generalization was not invariably true. In some cases endometriomas rapidly increase in size during the first few weeks of pregnancy. In general, during the third trimester, symptoms are less severe and the size of the external lesions decreases.

Endometriosis is dependent on ovarian hormones to stimulate growth. With a natural menopause, there is a gradual relief of symptoms. Following surgical menopause, areas of endometriosis rapidly disappear. However, it is important to note that 5% of symptomatic cases of endometriosis present after menopause. The vast majority of the cases in women in their late 50s or early 60s are related to the use of exogenous estrogen.

Management

The two primary short-term goals in treating endometriosis are the relief of pain and promotion of fertility. The latter is discussed in Chapter 41. The primary long-term goal in the management of a woman with endometriosis is attempting to prevent progression or recurrence of the disease process. Presently, there is a paucity of definitive, evidence-based literature upon which to select the most appropriate method of treatment. The appropriate treatment for endometriosis varies widely because of the vast differences in the spectrum of clinical symptoms and in the extent of the disease from one woman to another. Therefore the treatment plan must be individualized. Choice of therapy, for women whose primary symptom is pelvic pain, depends on multiple variables, including the patient's age, her future reproductive plans, the location and extent of her disease, the severity of her symptoms, and associated pelvic pathology.

Patient's Name _____ Date _____

Stage I   (Minimal) - 1-5
Stage II (Mild)   - 6-15
Stage III (Moderate) - 16-40
Stage IV (Severe)   - > 40

Laparoscopy _____ Laparotomy _____ Photography _____

Recommended Treatment _____

_____

Total _____

Prognosis _____

	ENDOMETRIOSIS	< 1cm	1- 3cm	> 3cm
PERITONEUM	Superficial	1	2	4
	Deep	2	4	6
OVARY	R Superficial	1	2	4
	Deep	4	16	20
	L Superficial	1	2	4
	Deep	4	16	20

	POSTERIOR CULDESAC OBLITERATION	Partial		Complete	
		4		40	

	ADHESIONS	< 1/3 Enclosure	1/3-2/3 Enclosure	> 2/3 Enclosure
OVARY	R Filmy	1	2	4
	Dense	4	8	16
	L Filmy	1	2	4
	Dense	4	8	16
TUBE	R Filmy	1	2	4
	Dense	4*	8*	16
	L Filmy	1	2	4
	Dense	4*	8*	16

*If the fimbriated end of the fallopian tube is completely enclosed, change the point assignment to 16.
Denote appearance of superficial implant types as red [(R), red, red-pink, flamelike, vesicular blobs, clear vesicles], white [(W), opacifications, peritoneal defects, yellow-brown], or black [(B) black, hemosiderm deposits, blue]. Denote percent of total described as R ____%, W ____ % and B ____ %. Total should equal 100%.

Additional Endometriosis: _____

_____

_____

_____

Associated Pathology: _____

_____

_____

_____

To Be Used with Normal
Tubes and Ovaries

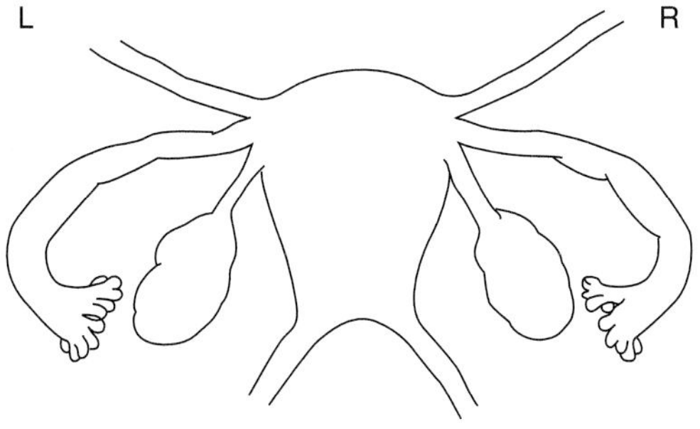

L   R

To Be Used with Abnormal
Tubes and/or Ovaries

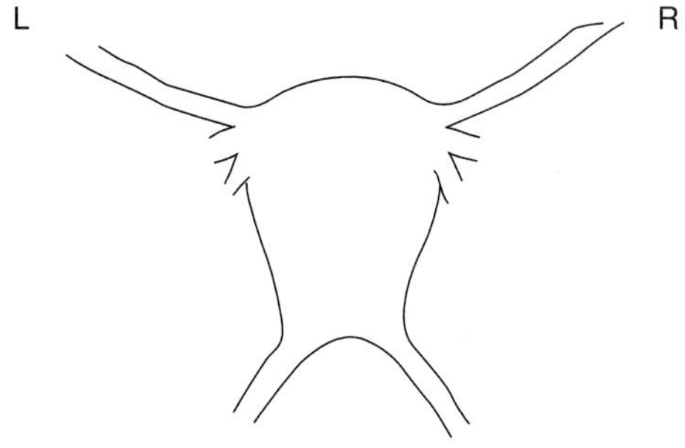

L   R

FIGURE 19-11 Updated scoring system to record the progress of endometriosis in fertility patients. (From American Society for Reproductive Medicine: Fertil Steril 67:817, 1997.)

Most patients should undergo a diagnostic laparoscopy to establish the nature and extent of endometriosis before therapy. However, if other gynecologic conditions such as chronic pelvic inflammatory disease or neoplasia have been ruled out, empiric medical therapy for 3 months with a GnRH agonist is a reasonable choice.

Treatment of endometriosis can be medical, surgical, or a combination of both. Most of the sex steroids, alone or in combination, have been tried in clinical studies to suppress the growth of endometriosis. Optimal regression secondary to medical treatment is observed in small endometriomas that are less than 1 to 2 cm in diameter. Response in larger areas of endometriosis may be minimal with medical therapy. A poor therapeutic result may be governed by the reduction of blood supply to the mass caused by surrounding scar tissue.

Surgical therapy is divided into conservative and definitive operations. Conservative surgery involves the resection or destruction of endometrial implants, lysis of adhesions, and attempts to restore normal pelvic anatomy. Definitive surgery involves the removal of both ovaries, the uterus, and all visible ectopic foci of endometriosis.

Medical Therapy

The primary goal of the hormonal treatment of endometriosis is induction of amenorrhea. Recurrent bleeding in the ectopic implants is one of the most important pathophysiologic processes to interrupt. Brosens has advanced the hypothesis that endometriosis is a physiologic process unless recurrent bleeding in the ectopic implants produces progressive disease and symptoms. Therefore, he postulates that effective medical therapy can be established by amenorrhea without the induction of hypoestrogenism. Recent clinical studies confirm that effective medical treatment can be achieved without the induction of severe hypoestrogenism. It is hoped that hormonal treatment will create an environment that will inhibit growth and promote regression of the disease. Medical therapy is very effective in relieving pain while the patient is taking medication. However, symptoms often recur several months after discontinuing therapy. Both clinical symptomatology and findings on second-look laparoscopy have demonstrated that clinical improvement directly correlates with establishment of amenorrhea. The choice of medical therapy for the individual patient depends on the clinician's evaluation of adverse effects, side effects, cost of therapy, and expected patient compliance. The clinical effectiveness, as measured by relief of symptoms and recurrence rates of current medical therapies, are similar. The recurrence rate following medical therapy is 5% to 15% in the first year and increases to 40% to 50% in 5 years. Obviously the chance of recurrence is directly related to the extent of initial disease. In summary, medical therapy usually suppresses symptomatology and prevents progression of endometriosis, but it does not provide a long-lasting cure of the disease. The recurrence rate in women who initially had minimal disease is approximately 35% while in those women whose initial disease was severe the rate is approximately 75%.

DANAZOL. Danazol was approved by the Food and Drug Administration in the mid-1970s for the treatment of endometriosis. In recent years, clinicians most frequently select GnRH agonists, medroxyprogesterone, or oral contraceptives as their drug of choice for medical therapy of endometriosis. Danazol also may be prescribed for women with benign cystic mastitis, menorrhagia, and hereditary angioneurotic edema. Danazol is an attenuated androgen that is active when given orally. Chemically it is a synthetic steroid that is the isoxazole derivative of ethisterone (17-alpha-ethinyltestosterone) (Figure 19-12). Danazol produces a hypoestrogenic and hyperandrogenic effect on steroid-sensitive end organs. The drug is mildly androgenic and anabolic. Many of danazol's side effects are directly related to these two properties. The androgenic effects of testosterone are approximately 200 times greater than those of danazol.

Danazol was initially prescribed for its "pseudomenopausal effect." The drug significantly decreases follicle-stimulating hormone (FSH) and luteinizing hormone (LH) levels in castrated females. However, in premenopausal women, basal levels of gonadotrophins are not influenced.

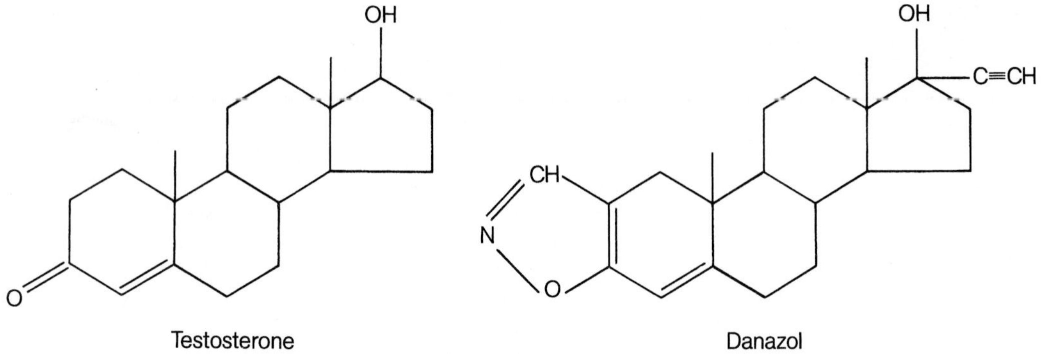

Testosterone   Danazol

FIGURE 19-12 Chemical structures of danazol and testosterone.

The midcycle surge of FSH and LH is eliminated by a dose of 800 mg a day. The term *pseudomenopause* is a misnomer because during the physiologic menopause, gonadotrophins are elevated.

Danazol binds to androgen and progesterone receptors and also binds to sex hormone–binding globulin. The latter effect results in a threefold increase in endogenous free testosterone levels. Danazol directly inhibits several steroidogenic enzymes in both the ovary and the adrenal gland, thus reducing circulating steroid levels. In vitro and in vivo studies have shown that danazol may also modulate immunologic functions through an effect on macrophages and/or T lymphocytes.

The explanations of the exact mechanism of action and underlying pharmacologic properties of danazol are controversial and speculative. Dosages of 800 mg daily produce amenorrhea and inhibition of ovulation within 4 to 6 weeks after the onset of therapy. Plasma levels of estrogen and progesterone remain in the early follicular range. Danazol induces atrophic changes in the endometrium of the uterus and similar changes in endometrial implants (Figure 19-13). An endometrial biopsy performed after several weeks of therapy shows endometrial atrophy with few glands and an inactive stroma. It would be difficult to differentiate the biopsy of a young woman taking danazol from the biopsy of a postmenopausal woman.

The standard prescribed dosage of danazol is 400 to 800 mg a day for approximately 6 months. The half-life of this oral drug is between 4 and 5 hours. Therefore, for the 800-mg dosage regimen, it is best to recommend one tablet four times a day rather than two tablets in the morning and two at night. Prescribing danazol 200 mg every 6 hours results in mean serum estradiol concentrations that are 40% lower than with the alternative regimen, 400 mg twice a day. Traditionally the drug is started on the fifth day after the onset of menses. The length of therapy of oral danazol should be individualized, depending partly on the stage of endometriosis. Women should use mechanical contraceptives for the first month, as danazol has produced female pseudohermaphroditism in a developing fetus. If one is certain the patient is not pregnant, danazol is begun on the first day of the menstrual bleeding. By starting the hormone earlier in the cycle, the patient will experience less breakthrough bleeding during the first 4 to 6 weeks.

Many investigators have reduced the total daily dosage of the drug comparing 600, 400, 200, and even 100 mg of danazol daily. The relief of the symptoms of endometriosis was directly related to the incidence of amenorrhea. The lower dosages of danazol are not as effective at producing amenorrhea and anovulation. The clinical success rates using lower dosages are slightly less with advanced disease than when 400 to 800 mg daily is used. Women with atrophic endometrium may experience breakthrough bleeding.

Side effects of the hormonal changes are encountered by 80% of patients taking danazol. Approximately 10% to 20% of women discontinue the drug because of the side

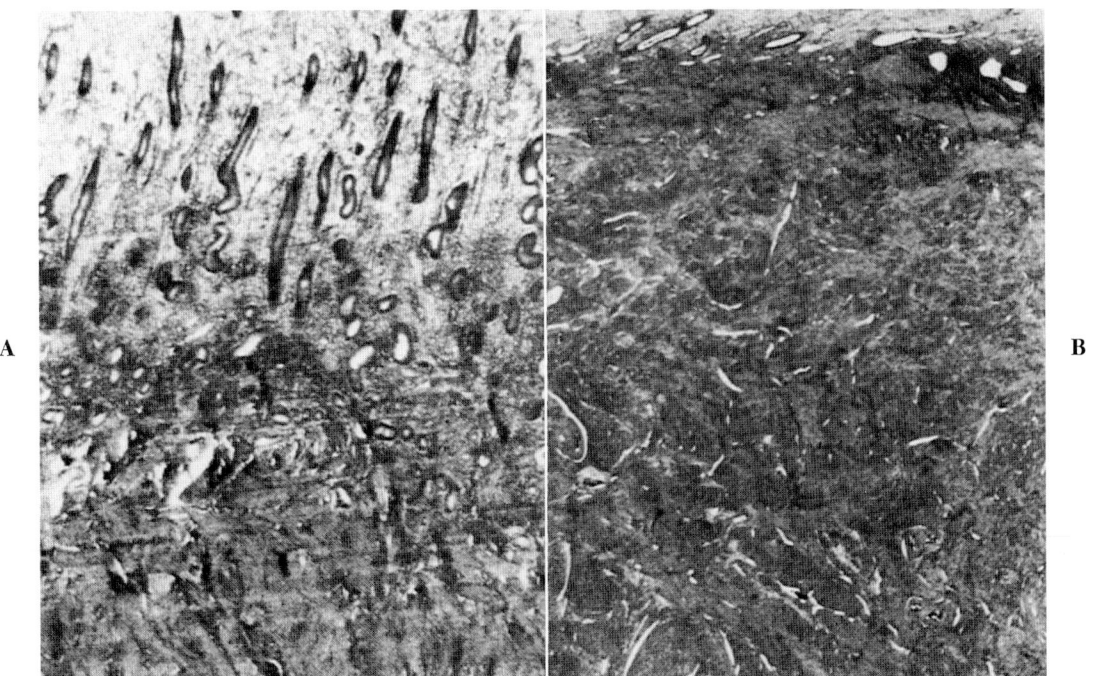

FIGURE 19-13   A, Untreated endometrium. **B,** Endometrium after 4 months of treatment with danazol. (From Greenblatt RP, Dmowski WP, Mahesh VB, and Scholer HFL: Fertil Steril 22:108, 1971. Reproduced with permission of the publisher, American Fertility Society.)

effects. Virtually all of the symptoms disappear on cessation of drug therapy. However, there are scattered reports of deepening of the voice that did not resolve after discontinuing the drug. Symptoms that have been related to danazol therapy include menopausal hot flushes, atrophic vaginitis, emotional lability, weight gain averaging 8 to 10 pounds, fluid retention, migraine headaches, dizziness, fatigue, depression, oily skin, facial hair, and deepening of the voice (Table 19-4). Studies have demonstrated that danazol decreases high-density lipoprotein (HDL) levels and elevates low-density lipoprotein (LDL) levels. However, the clinical impact of these changes occurring for a few months in young women is not known.

Danazol is metabolized in the liver with cleavage of the isoxazole ring. Mild elevation in serum liver enzyme levels has been reported in women treated for endometriosis. Clinicians should be alert to these changes, and women who take danazol for longer than 6 months should have serum liver enzyme determinations.

The standard length of treatment with danazol is 6 to 9 months. Approximately three of four patients note significant improvement in their symptoms, and about 90% have objective improvement discovered at second-look laparoscopy. The uncorrected fertility rate following danazol therapy is approximately 40%. Unfortunately, 15% to 30% of women will have recurrence of symptoms within 2 years following therapy.

TABLE 19-4
Adverse Reactions to Danazol (800 mg/day)

Androgenic action

Acne	17%
Edema	6%
Weight gain	5%
Hirsutism	6%
Voice changes	3%

Antiestrogenic action

Flushes and sweats	15%
Uterine spotting	10%
Decrease in breast size	5%
Change in libido	3% to 5%
Atrophic vaginitis	3%

Idiopathic drug reactions

GI disturbances	8%
Weakness, dizziness	8%
Muscle cramps	4%
Skin rashes	3%
Headaches	2%
Sleep disturbances	Uncommon

From Luciano AA: Contemp OB/GYN 19:228, 1982. Modified from Greenblatt R, editor: Recent advances in endometriosis: proceedings of a symposium, Augusta, Ga, March 5–6, 1975. Excerpta Medica, 1976, p 368.

Several randomized, double-blind clinical studies have compared the therapeutic effectiveness of danazol with gonadotrophin-releasing hormone (GnRH) agonists. The results do not show significant differences between the efficacies of these two drugs.

GnRH AGONISTS. In 1971 Schally and Guellemin first characterized and sequenced the structure of the native decapeptide, gonadotrophin-releasing hormone (GnRH). This discovery led to their winning the Nobel prize and also to the development of GnRH analogue-agonists, which are 10 to 200 times more potent and have much longer half-lives than the natural hormone. With chronic administration of GnRH agonists, specific suppression of gonadotrophin secretion occurs, with secondary diminution of ovarian steroidogenesis. The GnRH agonists bind with receptors for a prolonged time and induce protracted periods of downward regulation.

Multiple GnRH agonists have been developed. These agonists may be administered by intravenous, intramuscular, subcutaneous, intravaginal, or intranasal routes. The oral route is not practical because the hormone is inactivated by enzymes in the gastrointestinal tract. Representative agonists are leuprolide acetate (Lupron, injectable), nafarelin acetate (Synarel, intranasal), and goserelin acetate (Zoladex, subcutaneous implant). The usual dose of leuprolide acetate is 3.75 mg intramuscularly once per month or 11.25 mg depot injection every 3 months. Nafarelin acetate nasal spray is given in a dose of one spray (200 g) in one nostril in the morning and one spray (200 g) in the other nostril in the evening up to a maximum of 800 μg daily. Goserelin acetate is given in a dosage of 3.6 mg every 28 days in a biodegradable subcutaneous implant.

Studies have determined the dose-response curve of the GnRH agonists, establishing the optimal dose to produce sufficient down regulation and desensitization of the pituitary to produce extremely low levels of circulating estrogen and amenorrhea. Chronic use of GnRH agonists produces a "medical oophorectomy." A dramatic reduction occurs in serum estrone, estradiol, testosterone, and androstenedione levels similar to the hormonal levels in castrated women (Figure 19-14). The total serum estrone and estradiol levels and the free serum estradiol concentration are 25% to 50% of those measured in women taking danazol chronically for endometriosis.

GnRH agonists have no effect on sex hormone–binding globulin. Thus the androgenic side effects from danazol caused by the increase in free serum testosterone are not observed. Similarly, no significant changes occur in total serum cholesterol, HDL, or LDL levels during therapeutic periods of as long as 6 months. Endometrial samples obtained after several months of chronic agonist therapy demonstrated either atrophic or early proliferative endometrium.

GnRH AGONISTS IN ENDOMETRIOSIS

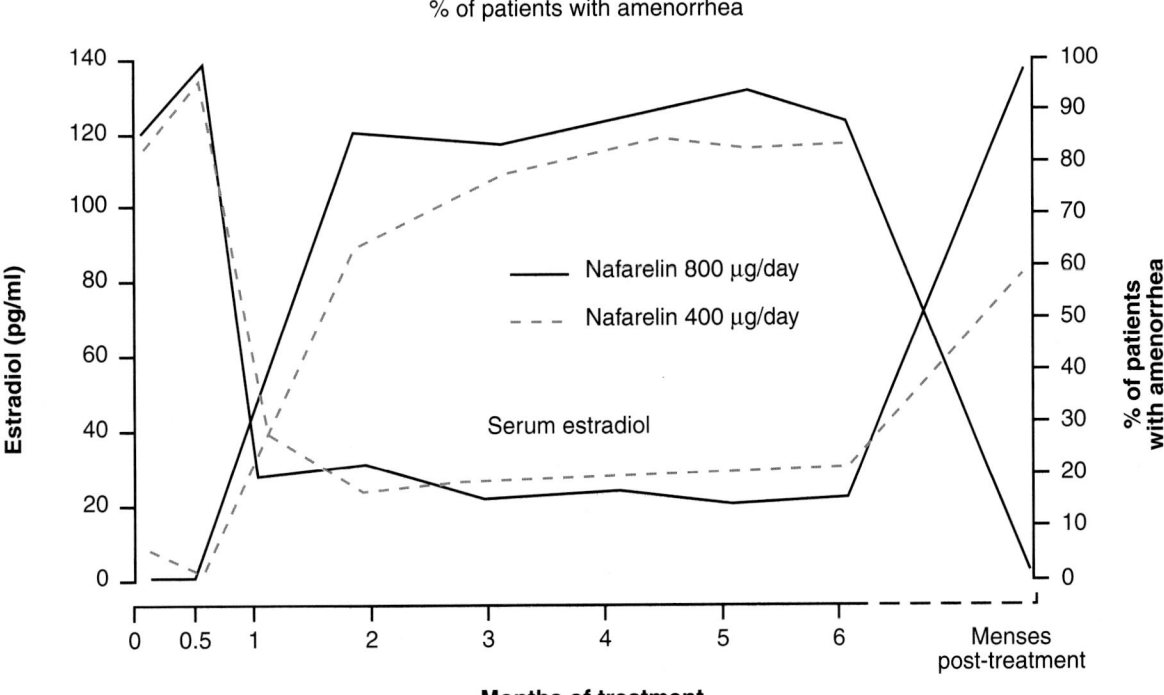

FIGURE 19-14 Decrease in serum estradiol levels and the development of amenorrhea in patients receiving nafarelin. (Redrawn from Henzl MR: Clin Obstet Gynecol 31:847, 1989.)

The side effects associated with GnRH agonist therapy are primarily those associated with estrogen deprivation, similar to menopause. The three most common symptoms are hot flushes, vaginal dryness, and insomnia. A decrease in bone mineral content has been demonstrated in the trabecular bone of the lumbar spine by quantitative computer tomography. This decrease in bone density is not seen in the compact bone of the distal radius. There is a decrease in measured bone mass of 2% to 7% during a 6-month course of agonist therapy. However, it has been established that the decrease in bone density associated with 6 months of therapy with GnRH agonist completely recovers between 12 and 24 months after discontinuing therapy.

The clinical response to agonist therapy depends on when the therapy is initiated in regard to the menstrual cycle. If agonist therapy is begun during the follicular phase, an initial rapid rise in FSH and E_2 levels occurs for approximately 3 weeks. FSH levels fall to basal levels by the third to fourth week of therapy. E_2 levels rapidly decline after 21 days of therapy. The expected LH surge does not occur, and serum progesterone levels do not become elevated. Amenorrhea is induced within 6 to 8 weeks. In contrast, beginning agonist therapy during the luteal phase diminishes the length of the initial hormonal response. LH levels are elevated for approximately 1 week, and serum estradiol levels are suppressed to those of a castrated female

within 2 weeks. Amenorrhea is induced in 4 to 5 weeks. It is important to ensure that the patient is not pregnant when beginning GnRH agonist therapy during the luteal phase.

GnRH agonist therapy results in amelioration of symptomatology in 75% to 90% of patients with endometriosis, depending on the extent of the disease in the study group. Growth of endometriosis is either arrested, diminished, or eliminated. The greatest therapeutic effects are seen in patients whose areas of endometriosis are less than 1 cm in diameter. In comparison studies, the results of GnRH agonist therapy are directly comparable with those obtained with danazol.

Henzl et al. performed a multicenter, double-blind, double-placebo randomized study of GnRH agonist and danazol therapy in which neither physicians nor patients were aware of their group's status. The 235 patients had laparoscopy both before and after 6 months of treatment and were assigned to three different protocols. One group received 400 g of intranasal nafarelin acetate per day; the second, 800 g of intranasal nafarelin per day; and the third, 800 mg of oral danazol per day. This investigation demonstrated that the therapeutic response to the two drugs was similar. More than 80% of patients had a reduction in the extent of endometriosis, according to the American Society for Reproductive Medicine classification. Before therapy, 46% had stage III or IV disease; after therapy, 26% had stage III or IV disease. Endometriosis was progressive in 4% to 8% of patients throughout the study. Interestingly, basic research has demonstrated that approximately 5% of implants of endometriosis do not contain estrogen or progesterone receptors.

Ovarian function will return to normal in 6 to 12 weeks after 6 months of GnRH agonist therapy. Large ovarian endometriomas and severe adhesive disease have not responded to hormonal therapy. The primary advantage of GnRH agonists over danazol is better patient compliance. Most patients find the side effects of GnRH agonists more tolerable.

Currently many clinicians "add-back" hormone replacement therapy with dosages similar to menopausal therapy in combination with chronic GnRH agonist regimens. The daily "add-back" therapy is begun simultaneously with the initial dose of the agonist. The clinical hypothesis is that the "add-back" medication will reduce or eliminate the vasomotor symptoms, vaginal atrophy, and also diminish or overcome the demineralization of bone. Barbieri has suggested that there is a therapeutic window that he estimates is a circulating level of approximately 30 pg per ml of estradiol. He postulates that this level of estradiol is enough to protect the body from substantial bone loss and is not a high enough level to interfere with the inhibition of growth of endometriosis (Figures 19-15 and 19-16). Multiple randomized series have demonstrated that "add-back" therapy does not interfere in the effectiveness of agonists to relieve the pelvic pain from endometriosis. The majority of studies have also demonstrated no diminished therapeutic efficacy when "add-back" therapy is initiated simultaneously with the GnRH agonist. Some clinicians additionally give organic bisphosphonates and calcium with the low-dose progestins and estrogen. Add-back regimens not only reduce or eliminate adverse clinical and metabolic side effects associated with hypoestrogenism, but also facilitate safe and effective prolongation of GnRH agonist therapy for up to 12 months (Figure 19-17).

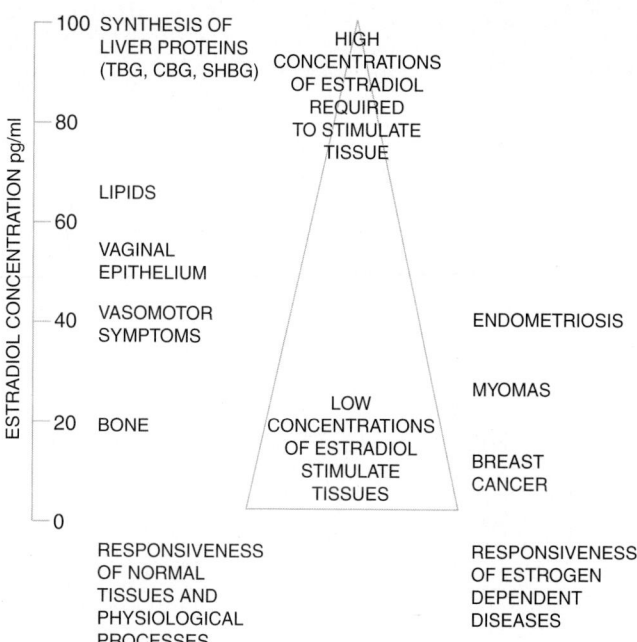

FIGURE 19-15 Estrogen dose-response hierarchy. Normal tissues vary in their sensitivity to estradiol stimulation. Menopause is associated with an estradiol concentration in the range of 5-20 pg/ml. Vasomotor symptoms are significantly suppressed by estradiol in the range of 30 pg/ml. Bone metabolism begins to respond to estrogen stimulation at low concentrations of estradiol (30-60 mg/ml). Stimulation of the synthesis of liver proteins, such as thyroxine-binding globulins, may require estradiol concentrations >80 pg/ml. Estrogen-dependent disease processes also vary in their sensitivity to estradiol. Breast cancer cells may be stimulated to grow at an estradiol concentration in the range of 10-20 pg/ml. Endometriosis lesions may require estradiol concentrations >20-40 pg/ml to grow. (From Barbieri RL: Endometriosis and the estrogen threshold theory: relation to surgical and medical treatment, J Reprod Med 43:287, 1998.)

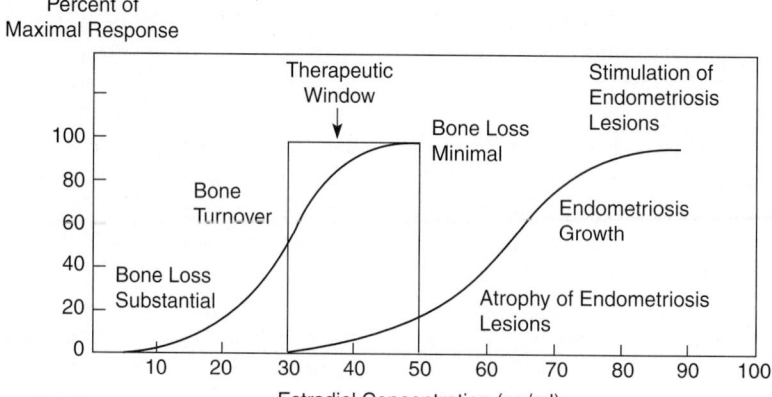

FIGURE 19-16 Estradiol therapeutic window. The concentration of estradiol required to cause growth of endometriosis lesions may be greater than the concentration required to stabilize bone mineral density. (From Barbieri RL: Hormone treatment of endometriosis: the estrogen threshold hypothesis, Am J Obstet Gynecol 166:740, 1992.)

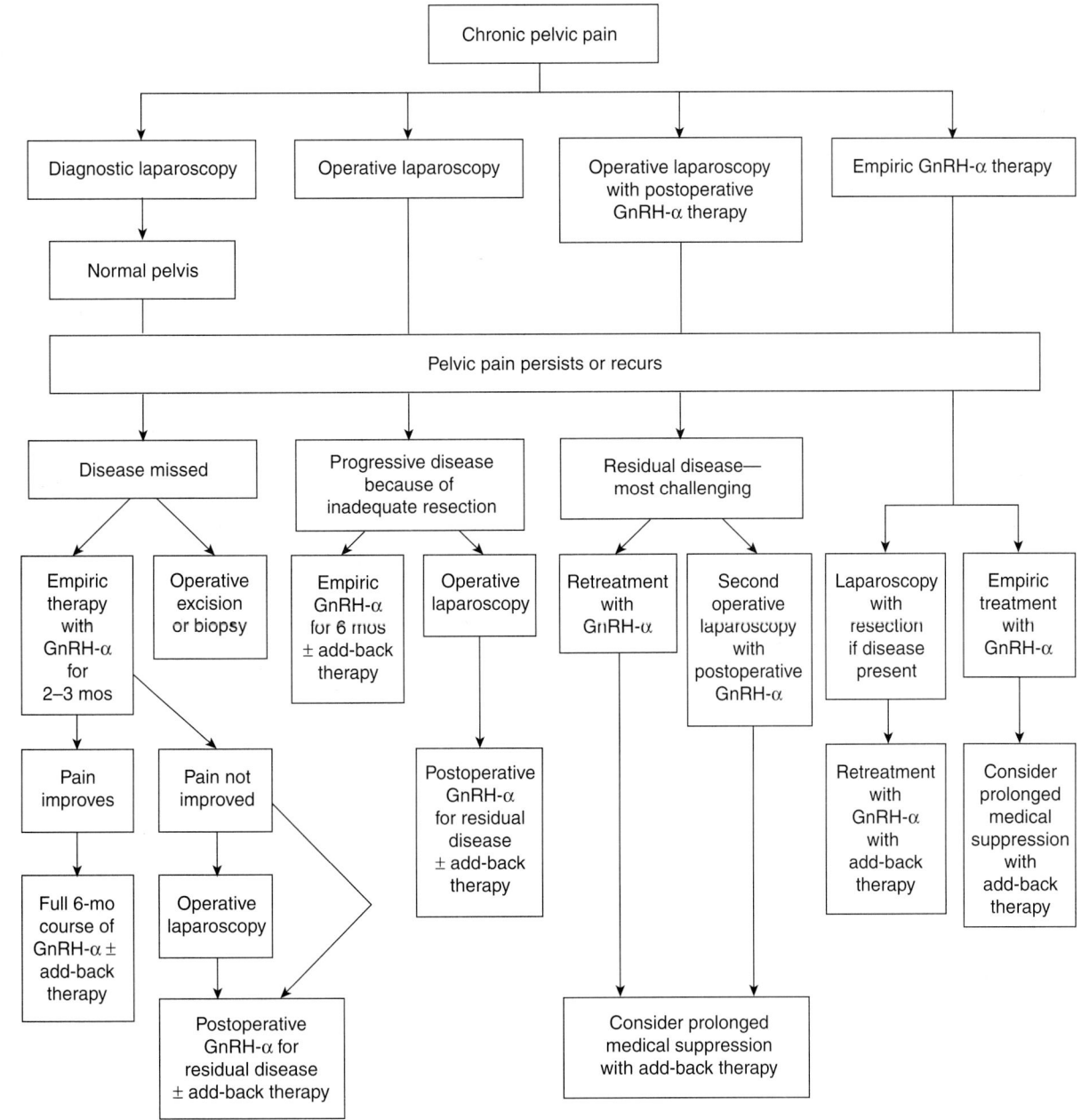

FIGURE 19-17 Algorithm for treatment of women with endometriosis with chronic pelvic pain who presently do not desire fertility yet are reluctant to have a hysterectomy and/or bilateral oophorectomy. (From Lindheim SR: Treatment options for recurrent endometriosis, Contemp OB/GYN 43:34, 1998.)

In summary, when comparing Danazol and GnRH agonists, the greatest advantage of GnRH agonists is their production of a pseudomenopause or medical castration without the androgenic side effects of danazol on other steroid-sensitive organs.

ORAL CONTRACEPTIVES. Kistner was the first to popularize the continuous use of high-dosage, combination oral contraceptives for endometriosis. In the late 1950s up to 40 mg of norethynodrel with mestranol (Enovid) daily were given to produce amenorrhea and a "pseudopregnancy." Most of the published studies involved the first-generation, high-estrogen-content oral contraceptives.

However, more recent reports have established that the present low-estrogen monophasic combination pills, specifically the ones with a relatively high progestin potency, are equally effective when used in a continuous fashion. Over the past 30 years, the most economical regimen for the treatment of women with mild or moderate symptoms of endometriosis has been continuous daily oral contraceptives for 6 to 12 months.

The regimen is started by a single daily monophasic oral contraceptive tablet beginning on the third day of the patient's period. The pills are taken continuously until breakthrough bleeding occurs, and then the daily dosage is doubled to relieve breakthrough bleeding. After 5 days of a double dose, the majority of patients can return to one to two pills a day, thereby maintaining their amenorrhea on a comparatively low dosage of steroids. As in other hormonal regimens for endometriosis, amenorrhea is the desired endpoint. The optimal regimen is the lowest daily dose of steroids that will produce amenorrhea in the individual patient. Most patients are able to maintain the amenorrhea for 6 to 9 months, using at most three to four contraceptive tablets a day. It is necessary to emphasize to the patient the importance of continuous rather than intermittent oral contraceptive therapy.

The initial histologic response is similar to that of normal pregnancy, with an increase in vascularity and edema in the endometrial implants. This transient growth phase may cause an acute exacerbation of the clinical symptoms. Occasionally, large ovarian endometriomas rupture, resulting in an acute surgical abdomen during the first 6 weeks of oral contraceptive therapy. During prolonged therapy the endometrial glands atrophy and the stroma undergoes a marked decidual reaction. Subsequently, in most smaller endometriomas that are less than 1 to 2 cm, there is necrobiosis and absorption.

The most common side effects of inducing amenorrhea with oral contraceptives include weight gain and breast tenderness. Approximately one of three women discontinue this therapy because of side effects.

The results of continuous oral contraceptive therapy include a decrease in symptomatology in approximately 80% of patients during therapy.

OTHER HORMONAL TREATMENTS. For women who cannot tolerate the high dosage of estrogen in the pseudopregnancy regimen or who have a contraindication to estrogen therapy, treatment with progestins only has been successful. Medroxyprogesterone (Provera), 30 mg orally per day or depomedroxyprogesterone (Depo-Provera) in a dosage of 150 mg intramuscularly every 3 months to a maximum of 200 mg every month, will produce a prolonged amenorrhea. The medication is most appropriate for the older woman who has completed childbearing. The time of resumption of ovulation following discontinuation of injectable medroxyprogesterone is prolonged and extremely variable. Some women will not ovulate for more than a year after their last injection. Therefore this form of therapy should not be prescribed for a young woman who is contemplating pregnancy in the near future. Oral medroxyprogesterone in a dosage of 30 mg a day is an alternative mode of therapy.

The most prominent side effects while taking medroxyprogesterone are breakthrough spotting or bleeding. Approximately 40% of patients develop abnormal bleeding associated with high-dose progestin therapy. If there is no contraindication to estrogen, this symptom can be alleviated by small doses of oral estrogen. Many women find unacceptable the changes in mood, depression, and irritability produced by high-dose progestins. Gestrinone is a progestin originally developed as a once-a-week oral contraceptive. Recently, this drug has undergone clinical trials for endometriosis with dosages ranging from 2.5 to 7.5 mg per week. Gestrinone acts as an agonist-antagonist of progesterone receptors and an agonist of androgen receptors and also binds weakly to estrogen receptors. At completion of therapy in a randomized trial, a tendency for prolonged pain relief was observed for gestrinone when compared to GnRH agonist.

Clinical results with progestin-only therapy are similar to those with continuous oral contraceptives. Some pathologists postulate that suppression of growth of endometriosis by progestins equals the suppression by oral contraceptives, but there is less necrobiosis and absorption.

There have been successful limited trials of using the antiprogestin mifepristone RU 486 to produce amenorrhea and to treat endometriosis. A daily dose of 50 mg per day improved symptoms and caused regression of endometriosis. In the future, one of the newer antiprogestins may be more effective for the treatment of endometriosis. No large-scale trial or comparison study has been published.

Surgical Therapy

The choice between medical treatment to suppress endometriosis and surgical therapy to remove it depends on the patient's age, symptomatology, and reproductive desires. Surgical therapy often occurs concurrently during the laparoscopy to establish the diagnosis of the disease. Obviously, surgical therapy is the only option for failed medical therapy. Because endometriosis is a puzzling disease, with great individual variation in its natural course, many therapeutic regimens exist. Thus the time-honored admonition that each patient must have individualized treatment still holds (Table 19-5).

Surgery has been the foundation of treatment for women with moderate or severe endometriosis especially those with adhesions and when the disease involves organs other than the pelvic genital tract. A surgical approach is mandatory in cases involving acute rupture of large endometriomas, ureteral obstruction, compromise in the large bowel's function, ovarian endometriomas greater than 2 cm, or adnexal enlargements with a diameter of 8 cm or larger. During the past 20 years, clinicians have increasingly emphasized laparoscopic treatment of endometriosis.

Wheeler and Malinak use the term "manage" rather than "treat" endometriosis. Their rationale is that the diagnosed recurrence rate of endometriosis is approximately one in three patients after 5 years, and since many patients do not have second-look laparoscopy, the actual recurrence rate is probably higher. This recurrence rate reflects both persistence and proliferation of microscopic disease. The recurrence rate is directly related to the initial stage of the disease and is as high as 75% in women who initially had severe disease.

TABLE 19-5
Endometriosis Treatment Algorithm

| Chief Complaint | Desires Childbearing | | Childbearing Complete |
	Infertility	Pelvic Pain	Pelvic Pain
Stages I and II	1. Expectant Rx 2. Laparoscopic Rx 2. Medical Rx 3. CSEL ± PSN 3. IVF/ET	1. Laparoscopic Rx 2. Medical Rx 3. CSEL + PSN	1. Laparoscopic Rx 2. Medical Rx 3. TAH ± BSO 3. CSEL ± PSN
Stage III	1. Laparoscopic Rx 1. CSEL ± PSN 2. Medical Rx 3. IVF/ET	1. Laparoscopic Rx 2. CSEL + PSN 3. Medical Rx	1. Laparoscopic Rx 2. Medical Rx 3. TAH ± BSO 3. CSEL + PSN
Stage IV	1. CSEL + perioperative medical Rx 2. CSEL alone 3. Laparoscopic Rx + post- operative medical Rx 4. IVF/ET	1. CSEL + PSN + perioperative medical Rx 2. Medical Rx 3. Laparoscopic Rx + medical Rx	1. TAH ± BSO 1. CSEL + PSN + medical Rx 2. Laparoscopic Rx + medical Rx

From Wheeler JM and Malinak LR: Obstet Gynecol Clin North Am 31:150, 1989.

Rx, Treatment; *CSEL,* Conservative surgery for endometriosis at laparotomy; *PSN,* Presacral neurectomy; *TAH,* Total abdominal hysterectomy; *BSO,* Bilateral salpingo-oophorectomy; *IVF/ET,* In vitro fertilization/embryo transfer; ±, Indicates adjunctive treatment option based on individual patient findings.

Laparoscopy is employed frequently for both diagnostic and therapeutic reasons. The major advantage of treating endometriosis with the laparoscope, using either surgical instruments, the laser, or electrocautery, is that patients may be treated at the time of diagnosis. Depending on the operative technique chosen, endometriosis is coagulated, vaporized, and/or resected. The vast majority of surgical treatment for endometriosis occurs via laparoscopy rather than laparotomy because of a shorter recovery period and reduction in the extent of subsequent adhesions.

Adhesions in the pelvis have varying characteristics. They may be minimal or extensive, filmy or dense, and avascular or vascular. If the laser is used, the surgeon must adjust spot size, power setting (watts), and time of application to control depth of penetration. The laser is preferable to electrocautery when endometriosis is adjacent to the ureter, bladder, or bowel because the depth of penetration can be controlled. Follow-up studies have documented pain improvement in 70% to 80% of patients treated via the laparoscope.

The surgical difficulties in treating invasive carcinoma and endometriosis are similar. The infiltrative nature of both disease processes and the associated scarring from endometriosis result in a loss of cleavage planes and tedious, difficult dissections. Technically it is easier to palpate rather than visualize the extent of the infiltrative process of endometriosis. Special care must be taken not to injure the bladder or bowel during excision of areas impinging on these structures.

Conservative surgery has as its goal the removal of all macroscopic, visible areas of endometriosis with preservation of ovarian function and restoration of normal pelvic anatomy. Conservative operations include removal or destruction of implants, removal of endometriomas, lysis of adhesions, appendectomy, and sometimes presacral neurectomy. Throughout these procedures the surgeon observes the principles of microsurgery and plastic surgery, including minimal and gentle handling of tissues, avoiding hypoxia of the peritoneum, and attempting to restore the pelvic anatomy to normal. Approximately one in four women will have a second operation for a recurrence of endometriosis. Laparoscopy has been proven to be equally as effective and reliable as laparotomy in the treatment of ovarian endometriomas. The rate of recurrence is directly dependent on the duration of follow-up and is highest in women with stage 4 disease and a history of previous surgery for endometriosis. Recent studies have documented that excision of an ovarian endometrioma is associated with a lower reoperation rate than using a fenestration technique. Transabdominal or transvaginal aspiration of ovarian endometriomas has been technically successful using a 20 gauge spinal needle under ultrasound guidance. However, clinically, this procedure is rarely utilized because of its high recurrence rate.

If the patient has midline pain, such as dysmenorrhea or dyspareunia, occasionally a presacral neurectomy or resection of the uterosacral ligaments may be performed. When ablation of the utero-sacral nerves is performed via the laparoscope, the operation is referred to by the acronym LUNA procedure. A successful presacral neurectomy relieves only midline pain and does not diminish pain in other areas of the pelvis.

Somewhere between conservative and definitive surgery for endometriosis there is a place for total abdominal hysterectomy with ovarian preservation of one or both ovaries. This operation is selected for women who have completed childbearing and are in their late 20s or 30s. It is interesting that without repetitive episodes of retrograde menstruation, the endometriosis remains quiescent in the majority of these women. Approximately one out of three women develop recurrent symptoms and they subsequently have a second operation involving oophorectomy.

Definitive surgical treatment is reserved for patients with far-advanced disease and for whom future fertility is not a consideration. Patients with pain that continues after medical and conservative surgery are treated by definitive surgery. Definitive surgery involves total abdominal hysterectomy, bilateral salpingo-oophorectomy, and the removal of all visible endometriosis. If the surgeon believes that it is not possible to surgically remove all the areas of endometriosis, it is best to treat a premenopausal woman with medroxyprogesterone or continuous oral contraceptive therapy for approximately 6 to 12 months before beginning cyclic hormonal therapy. Malignant transformation of endometriosis is a rare phenomenon. Approximately 75% of reported cases are found associated with ovarian endometriosis. Based on an unproven hypothesis, some clinicians invariably prescribe a progestin with estrogen replacement in hopes of reducing the potential of developing adenocarcinoma in residual endometriosis.

Medical therapy and surgical therapy are often performed in combination for advanced stages of the disease. Clinicians debate the advantages of either preoperative or postoperative medical therapy. Presently the majority favor preoperative medical treatment followed by surgery. It is postulated that preoperative therapy facilitates the subsequent operative procedure.

Photodynamic therapy for endometriosis is undergoing preliminary trials. This procedure involves intravenous injection of a special dye that is concentrated in areas of endometriosis. A laser light produces a photochemical reaction to destroy the areas.

If a patient has recurrent symptoms following definitive surgery for endometriosis and has not been taking exogenous estrogen, it is possible that she has a remnant of residual ovary, which can be diagnosed by measuring serum gonadotrophin levels. If the FSH and LH levels are not in menopausal range, some viable ovarian tissue remains, usually in the retroperitoneal space. Operative management is the preferred method of treatment for persistent pelvic pain secondary to retroperitoneal remnants of active ovarian tissue. In rare instances, when recurrent operative procedures fail to relieve the symptoms of recurrent endometriosis, it is appropriate to ablate the remnants using external radiotherapy with a total dose of 10 to 20 Gy.

Most surgeons routinely remove the appendix when performing surgery for endometriosis not related to infertility. In a series of more than 100 consecutive patients with endometriosis, 13% had histologic evidence of endometriosis in the appendix. This involvement could be discovered by gross examination in only 60% of patients.

The efficacy of medical therapy immediately before or following surgery for endometriosis is unresolved in clinical practice. Those who advocate hormones before surgery believe that it makes the dissection easier, but it does not result in changes in prevalence of pain relief or rate of recurrence. Oral contraceptives carry the additional hazard of producing a hypercoagulable state during the perioperative period. Postoperatively, medical therapy may help diminish microscopic endometriosis.

Gastrointestinal Tract Endometriosis

The frequency of gastrointestinal tract involvement in series of women with histologically proven endometriosis varies from 3% to 34%. Most large series document a frequency of approximately 5%. Implants that involve the gastrointestinal tract are the most common site of extrapelvic endometriosis. The severity and extent of involvement of the bowel by ectopic endometrium varies from the incidental finding of a spot on the serosa of the bowel to obstruction of the rectosigmoid. In most cases the implants do not produce clinical symptoms. In the majority of cases, endometriosis of the gastrointestinal tract involves the sigmoid colon and the anterior wall of the rectum (Figure 19-18). An important clinical marker is the finding that women with endometriosis of the ovaries have an increased frequency of extensive, invasive disease of the large intestine.

Endometriosis of the appendix is fairly common. The incidence in patients with pelvic endometriosis is reported between 1% and 13% (Figure 19-19). Endometriosis of the appendix is usually an incidental pathologic finding. It is not clinically important because pathophysiologically the aberrant endometrium in the appendix wall does not produce symptoms.

Endometriosis of the small bowel is rare. Approximately 200 cases of endometriosis of the ileum have been reported in the literature. This is a troublesome process because of the high incidence of associated small bowel obstruction.

Classic symptoms of endometriosis of the large bowel include cyclic pelvic cramping and lower abdominal pain and rectal pain with defecation, especially during the menstrual period. Associated with the abdominal and pelvic pain is a change in bowel function, diarrhea and/or constipation (see Table 19-6). Mathias et al. have demonstrated a consistent and distinct dysfunction of the enteric nervous system, which they believe is the primary etiology of the abnormalities of bowel function in women with endometriosis. It is difficult to differentiate the symptoms associ-

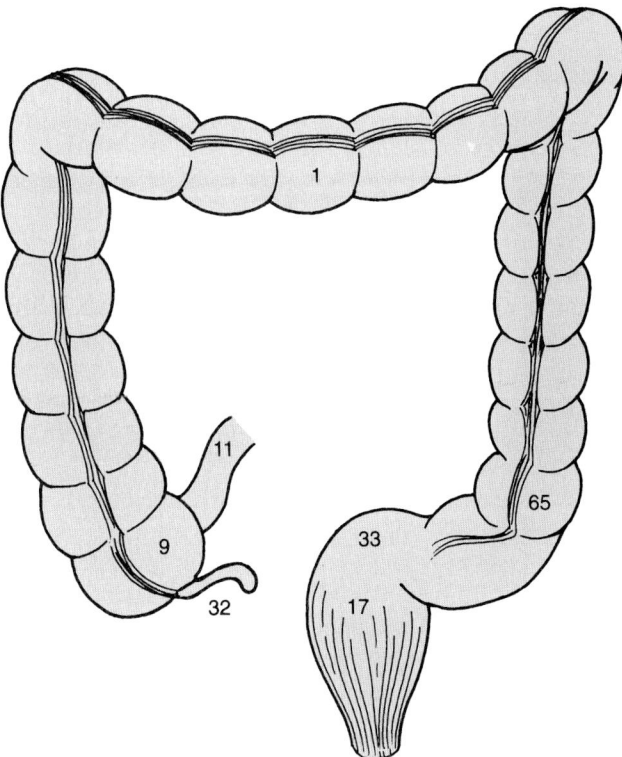

FIGURE 19-18 Locations of 168 bowel lesions found in 163 patients with endometriosis of the bowel. (Redrawn from Weed JC and Ray JE: Obstet Gynecol 69:727, 1987.)

ated with endometriosis from the constellation of symptoms associated with inflammatory disease of the colon or malignancy. Women with a gastrointestinal malignancy usually experience intermittent rather than cyclic intestinal bleeding. Early diagnosis of gastrointestinal endometriosis demands a high index of suspicion by the physician. The initial clue to the diagnosis of the patient with multiple symptoms is the cyclic nature of these symptoms. Bowel resection is indicated for obstruction of the bowel or with extensive lesions in which malignancy may not be ruled out. On pathologic examination the aberrant endometrial glands and stroma penetrate the serosa of the bowel and muscularis. It is unusual for endometriosis to involve the submucosa of the bowel. However, studies have demonstrated that 25% to 35% of women with advanced endometriosis of the large bowel experience episodic rectal bleeding from endometriosis extending into the submucosa.

Diagnosis of endometriosis invading the rectosigmoid is usually suspected by palpation of a pelvic mass or "rectal shelf" on rectovaginal examination. Sigmoidoscopy usually demonstrates absence of a mucosal lesion in addition to fixation and immobility of the anterior rectal wall. Donnez et al. speculate that endometriosis of the rectovaginal septum is a disease process more closely related to foci of adenomyosis than endometriosis.

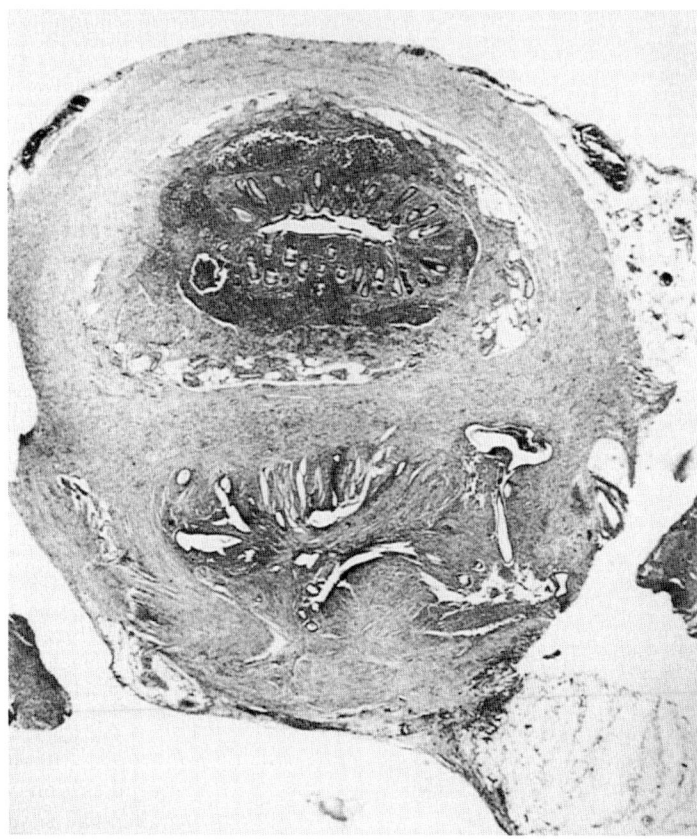

FIGURE 19-19   Cross section of appendix showing lumen of bowel and island of endometriosis. (From Dougherty CM: Surgical pathology of gynecologic disease, New York, 1968, Harper & Row, Publishers, Inc, p 636.)

TABLE 19-6
Preoperative Symptoms in 130 Patients
Undergoing Colorectal Resection
for Endometriosis

Symptom	No. of Patients	(%)
Pelvic pain	111	(85)
Rectal pain	68	(52)
Cyclic rectal bleeding	24	(18)
Diarrhea	55	(42)
Constipation	53	(41)
Diarrhea and constipation	18	(14)
Dyspareunia	83	(64)

From Bailey HR, Ott MT, and Hartendorp P: Dis Colon Rectum 37:747, 1994,
p 748.

They postulate that the nodules originate from müllerian rests in the rectovaginal space. Colonoscopy and an air-contrast barium enema are important steps in suspected cases, since they help to establish the differential diagnosis and the degree of obstruction. There is no specific radiologic appearance for endometriosis. However, a filling defect and absence of a mucosal lesion with the presence of extramucosal involvement are usually demonstrated. The definitive diagnosis and differentiation of endometriosis from carcinoma of the bowel may be delayed until a frozen section is obtained during exploratory surgery.

The treatment of endometriosis of the gastrointestinal tract is dependent on the extent and severity of symptoms. Endocrine therapy is not recommended for advanced cases. The importance of preoperative preparation of the bowel should not be forgotten. Surgical procedures vary from superficial excision of the endometriosis to bowel resection with anastomosis.

Urinary Tract Endometriosis

Endometriosis in the female pelvis occasionally produces dysfunction in adjacent pelvic organs. Approximately 10% of women with endometriosis have involvement of the urinary tract by implants of endometriosis and associated retroperitoneal fibrosis. In most cases an incidental finding of aberrant endometrial glands and stroma is discovered on the bladder peritoneum and anterior cul-de-sac. The most serious consequence of urinary tract involvement is ureteral obstruction, which occurs in about 1% of women with moderate or severe pelvic endometriosis. The pathogenesis of endometriosis of the bladder is controversial. Interestingly, approximately 50% of women with endometriosis of the urinary tract have a history of previous

pelvic surgery. The lesions may develop from implanted endometrium during cesarean delivery or may be an extension from adenomyosis of the anterior uterine wall.

Patients with endometriosis involving the urinary tract have nonspecific clinical presentations. Hematuria and flank pain are experienced by less than 25% of women. One of three women with documented complete ureteral obstruction secondary to endometriosis has no pelvic symptoms whatsoever. The clinical challenge is to diagnose minimal ureteral obstruction at an early stage, before loss of renal function. The obstruction is almost always in the distal one third of the course of the ureter. The importance of an imaging study to diagnose ureteral compromise in all women with retroperitoneal endometriosis cannot be overemphasized.

Endometriosis of the bladder is discovered most often in the region of the trigone or the anterior wall of the bladder. Bladder endometriosis produces midline, lower abdominal, and suprapubic pain, dysuria, and, occasionally, cyclic hematuria. Treatment of endometriosis of the peritoneum over the bladder can be accomplished by medical or surgical means. Ureteral obstruction may be intrinsic, from active endometriosis, or extrinsic, from longstanding fibrotic reactions to retroperitoneal inflammation. Extrinsic endometriosis is 3 to 5 times more common than the intrinsic form. There are few reports of endometriosis of the ureter responding to danazol or GnRH agonists. However, long-term follow-up with serial ultrasound imaging or intravenous pyelograms must be undertaken to ensure that the disease process does not recur.

Surgical therapy is preferred for ureteral obstruction secondary to endometriosis. The operations are rare and should be individualized. However, operative removal of the uterus and both ovaries and the relief of urinary obstruction by ureterolysis or by ureteroneocystostomy are the most common choices. If ureterolysis is the operation chosen, peristalsis in the involved segment of the ureter should be observed, along with adequate resection of the endometriosis and surrounding inflammation in the retroperitoneal space. Ureteroneocystostomy has the advantage of bypassing the urinary obstruction and making it technically easier to resect the area of endometriosis and associated retroperitoneal fibrosis.

ADENOMYOSIS

Adenomyosis is frequently referred to as *endometriosis interna*. This term is misleading because endometriosis and adenomyosis are discovered in the same patient in less than 20% of women. More important, endometriosis and adenomyosis are most likely clinically different diseases. The only common feature is the presence of ectopic endometrial glands and stroma. Adenomyosis is derived from aberrant glands of the basalis layer of the endometrium. Therefore these glands do not usually undergo the traditional proliferative and secretory changes that are associated with cyclic ovarian hormone production. Leyondecker believes that endometriosis is a disease with extreme pleomorphism. He postulates that adenomyosis is an early manifestation and the primary lesion of endometriosis with other sites of pelvic endometriosis being merely a sequelae. Whether endometriosis and adenomyosis are one or two different diseases has been debated for the past 80 years.

Adenomyosis is usually diagnosed incidentally by the pathologist examining histologic sections of surgical specimens. The frequency of the histologic diagnosis is directly related to how meticulously the pathologist searches for the disease. If multiple serial sections of the uterus are obtained, the incidence may exceed 60% in women 40 to 50 years of age. Adenomyosis is also a common incidental finding during autopsy. Serial histologic slides confirm the continuity of benign downward growth of the basalis layer of the endometrium. Thus the histogenesis of adenomyosis is direct extension from the endometrial lining.

The pathogenesis of adenomyosis remains unknown. For an unknown reason the barrier between the endometrium and myometrium is broken. Initially the stroma and subsequently the glands begin to invade the myometrium along the path of least resistance. In most instances this growth is adjacent to lymphatic and vascular channels.

Pathology

There are two distinctly different pathologic presentations of adenomyosis. Most common is a diffuse involvement of both anterior and posterior walls of the uterus. The poste-rior wall is usually involved more than the anterior wall. The individual areas of adenomyosis are not encapsulated. The second presentation is a focal area or adenomyoma. This results in an asymmetric uterus, and this special area of adenomyosis may have a pseudocapsule. Diffuse adenomyosis is found in approximately two thirds of cases, and focal adenomyosis is found in one third.

In the more common, diffuse type of adenomyosis the uterus is uniformly enlarged, usually 2 to 3 times normal size. Sometimes it is difficult to distinguish grossly from uterine leiomyomas. When the myometrium is transected by a knife, the cut surface protrudes convexly and has a spongy appearance. The cut surface of a uterus with adenomyosis is darker than the white surface of a myoma. Sometimes there are discrete areas of adenomyosis that are not densely encapsulated and contain small, dark cystic spaces. There is not a distinct cleavage plane around focal adenomyomas as there is with uterine myomas.

Benign endometrial glands and stroma are seen within the myometrium. These glands rarely undergo the same cyclic changes as the normal uterine endometrium. Studies have demonstrated both estrogen and progesterone receptors in tissue samples from adenomyosis.

The standard criterion used in diagnosis of adenomyosis is the finding of endometrial glands and stroma more than one low-powered field (2.5 mm) from the basalis layer of the endometrium (Figure 19-20). The small areas of adenomyosis have the same general appearance as the basalis layers of the endometrium. Histologically the glands exhibit an inactive or proliferative pattern. Rarely, one sees cystic hyperplasia or a pseudodecidual pattern. In general there is

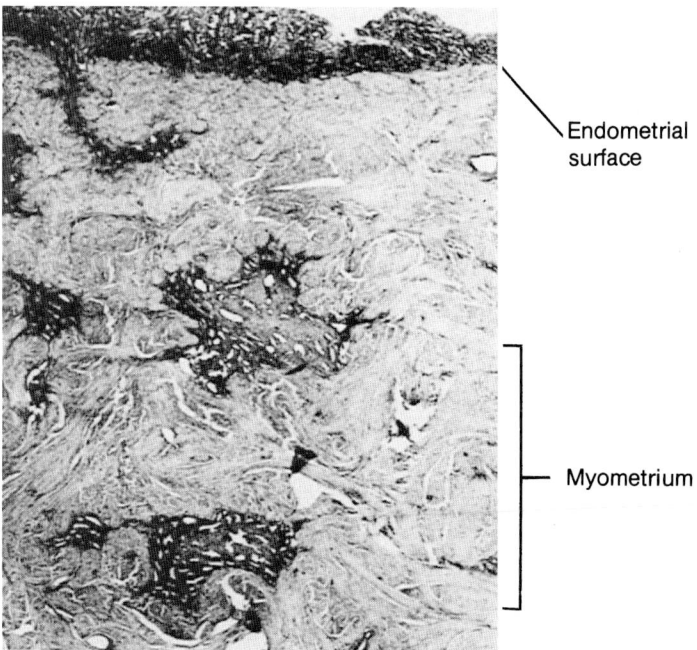

FIGURE 19-20 Adenomyosis. Note islands of endometrial tissue deep within myometrium. (From Janovski NA and Dubrauszky V: Atlas of gynecologic and obstetric diagnostic histopathology, New York, 1967, McGraw-Hill Book Co, p 217.)

a lack of inflammatory cells surrounding the fossae of adenomyosis. Although the areas do not undergo full menstrual-type changes, bleeding may occur in these ectopic areas, as evidenced by both gross and microscopic findings. It is not unusual to see histologic variability in several different areas deep in the walls of the myometrium from the same uterus. Some fossae of adenomyosis undergo decidual changes either during pregnancy or during estrogen-progestin therapy for endometriosis. The reaction of the myometrium to the ectopic endometrium is hyperplasia and hypertrophy of individual muscle fibers (Figure 19-21). Surrounding most foci of glands and stroma are localized areas of hyperplasia of the smooth muscle of the uterus. This change in the myometrium produces the globular enlargement of the uterus.

Clinical Diagnosis

The majority of women with adenomyosis are asymptomatic or have minor symptoms that do not annoy them enough to seek medical care. They attribute the increase in dysmenorrhea or menstrual bleeding to the aging process and tolerate the symptoms. Symptomatic adenomyosis usually presents in women between the ages of 35 and 50. The majority of women with symptomatic adenomyosis are parous. The severity of pelvic symptoms increases proportionally to the depth of penetration and the total volume of disease in the myometrium.

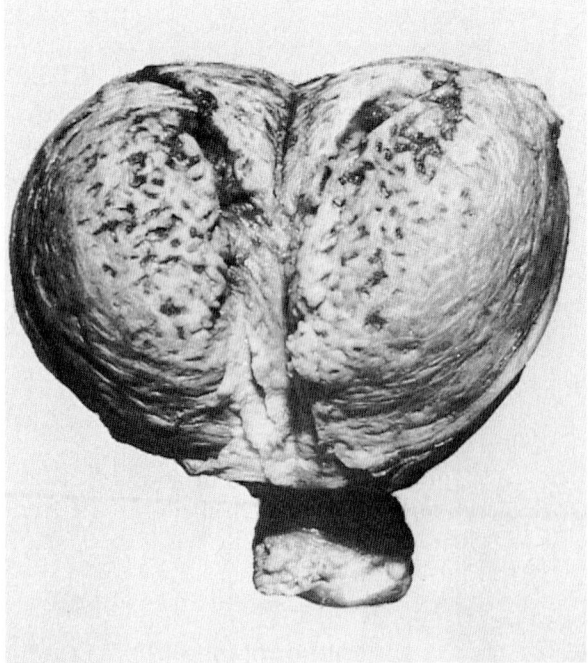

FIGURE 19-21 Adenomyosis. This hysterectomy specimen from a 32-year-old woman has been bisected to demonstrate the hypertrophied myometrium. (From Jeffcoate TNA: Principles of gynaecology, ed 4, London, 1975, Butterworths, p 353.)

The classic symptoms of adenomyosis are secondary dysmenorrhea and menorrhagia. The acquired dysmenorrhea becomes increasingly more severe as the disease progresses. Occasionally the patient complains of dyspareunia, which is midline in location and deep in the pelvis. On pelvic examination the uterus is diffusely enlarged, usually 2 to 3 times normal size. It is most unusual for the uterine enlargement associated with adenomyosis to be greater than a 14-week–size gestation unless the patient also has uterine myomas. The uterus is globular and tender immediately before and during menstruation (Figure 19-22).

The diagnosis of adenomyosis is usually confirmed following histologic examination of the hysterectomy specimen. Frequently the clinical diagnosis is inaccurately assigned to the patient who has chronic pelvic pain. Traditionally the patient will have endometrial sampling to rule out other organic causes of abnormal bleeding. Many times adenomyosis is diagnosed retrospectively following a hysterectomy for other indications. Attempts have been made to establish the diagnosis preoperatively by transcervical needle biopsy of the myometrium. However, even with multiple needle biopsies, the sensitivity of the test is too low to be of practical clinical value. Adenomyosis may coexist with both endometrial hyperplasia and endometrial carcinoma. Approximately two of three women with adenomyosis have coexistent pelvic pathology, most commonly myomas but also endometriosis, endometrial hyperplasia, and salpingitis isthmica nodosa. Emge speculated that unopposed estrogen is a potential cause of adenomyosis. The two most common conditions in the differential diagnosis of adenomyosis are small uterine myomas and dysfunctional uterine bleeding in the slightly enlarged uterus of a multiparous woman. Ultrasound and magnetic resonance imaging are useful to help differentiate between adenomyosis and uterine myomas in a young woman desiring future childbearing. Diagnosing adenomyosis by transvaginal ultrasonography has a reported sensitivity between 53% and 89% and a specificity of 50% to 89%. In some series, magnetic resonance imaging is more sensitive, ranging between 88% and 93%, and has a higher specificity of 66% to 91% than ultrasonography in the diagnosis of adenomyosis. In summary, magnetic resonance imaging is clinically useful in differentiating adenomyosis from uterine leiomyoma, especially preoperatively in women who desire future fertility.

Management

There is no satisfactory proven medical treatment for adenomyosis. Occasionally, patients with adenomyosis are treated with GnRH agonists, cyclic hormones, or prostaglandin synthetase inhibitors for their abnormal bleeding and pain. A preliminary report observed a decrease in uterine size and marked relief from menorrha-

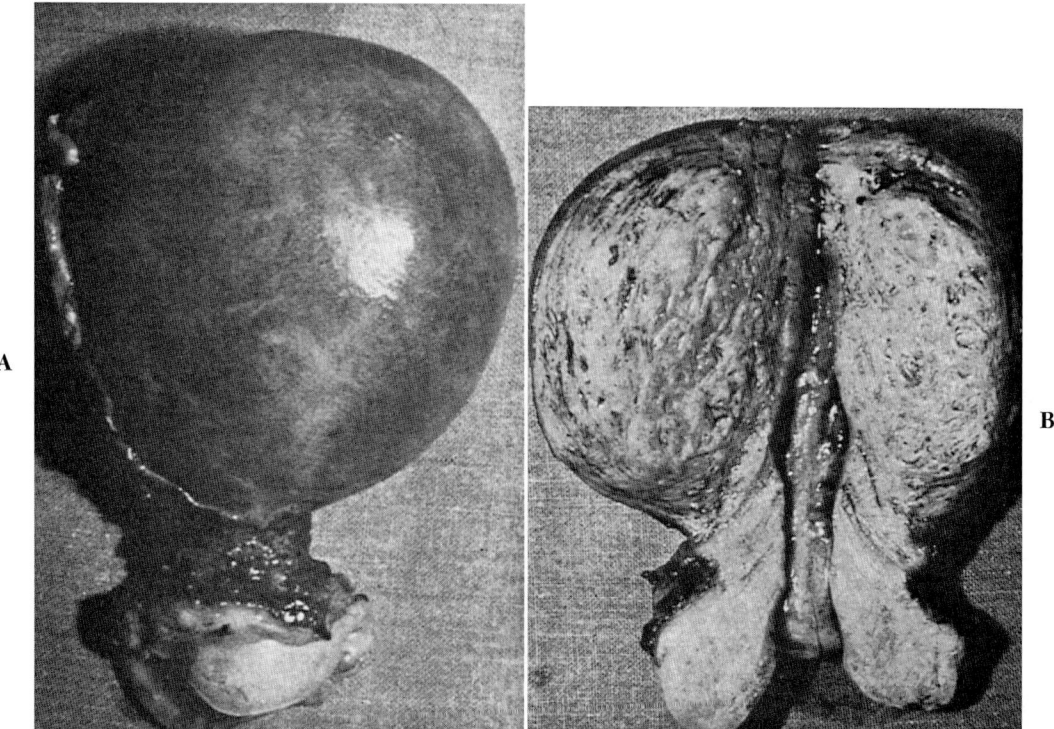

FIGURE 19-22 **A,** Hysterectomy specimen from 37-year-old woman showing adenomyosis. Note globular appearance of uterus. **B,** Bisection of posterior wall of uterus. (From Emge LA: Am J Obstet Gynecol 83:1551, 1962.)

gia in women using a progestin-releasing intrauterine device. Hysterectomy is the definitive treatment if this therapy is appropriate for the woman's age, parity, and plans for future reproduction. Size of the uterus, degree of prolapse, and presence of associated pelvic pathology determine the choice of abdominal or vaginal route for the hysterectomy. For the woman in her late 40s, the ovaries are often removed as a prophylactic measure against ovarian carcinoma, regardless of whether the woman has an abdominal or vaginal hysterectomy.

KEY POINTS

- Endometriosis is a benign, usually progressive, and sometimes recurrent disease that invades locally and disseminates widely.

- Endometriosis is present in 5% to 15% of celiotomies performed on women of reproductive age.

- The incidence of endometriosis is 30% to 45% in women with infertility.

- Approximately 5% of women with endometriosis are diagnosed following menopause. Postmenopausal endometriosis is usually secondary to the use of exogenous estrogen.

- Possible etiologic factors of endometriosis include retrograde menstruation, coelomic metaplasia, vascular metastasis, immunologic changes, iatrogenic dissemination, and a genetic predisposition.

- Some postulate that there is a complex interplay between a dose-response curve of the amount of retrograde menstruation and an individual woman's immunologic response.

- One of 10 women with severe endometriosis will have a sister or mother with clinical manifestations of endometriosis.

- The ovaries are the most common site, being involved in two of three women with endometriosis. The pelvic peritoneum over the uterus, the anterior and posterior cul-de-sac, and the uterosacral, round, and broad ligaments are also common sites where endometriosis develops. Pelvic lymph nodes are involved in 30% of cases.

- Grossly, endometriosis appears in many forms, including red, brown, black, white, yellow, pink, or clear vesicles and lesions. Biopsy is important to establish the diagnosis.

- Red, blood-filled lesions have been shown, by histologic and biochemical studies, to be the most active phase of endometriosis.

- Three cardinal features of microscopic endometriosis are ectopic endometrial glands, ectopic endometrial stroma, and hemorrhage into the adjacent tissue.

- Viable endometrial glands and stroma cannot be identified on pathologic examination in approximately 25% of cases of endometriosis.

- Classic symptoms of endometriosis are cyclic pelvic pain and infertility. However, approximately one third of patients with endometriosis are asymptomatic.

- Endometriosis is discovered in approximately one of three women whose primary symptom is chronic pelvic pain.

- Secondary dysmenorrhea usually begins 36 to 48 hours prior to the onset of menses. Unlike primary dysmenorrhea, the pain may last for many days, including several days before and after the menstrual flow.

- The most prominent pelvic sign of endometriosis is a fixed, retroverted uterus with scarring and tenderness posterior to the uterus. The characteristic nodularity of the uterosacral ligaments and cul-de-sac of Douglas may be palpated on rectovaginal examination.

- Serum CA-125 levels have a low sensitivity for the diagnosis of early or minimal endometriosis.

- Approximately 10% of teenagers who develop endometriosis have associated congenital outflow obstruction.

- The two primary short-term goals in treating endometriosis are the relief of pain and promotion of fertility. The primary long-term goal in the management of a woman with endometriosis is attempting to prevent progression or recurrence of the disease process.

- Recurrent bleeding in the ectopic implants is one of the most important pathophysiologic processes to interrupt.

- Optimal regression secondary to medical treatment is observed in small endometriomas that are less than 1 to 2 cm in diameter.

- The choice of medical therapy for the individual patient depends on the clinician's evaluation of adverse effects, side effects, cost of therapy, and expected patient compliance. The recurrence rate following medical therapy is 5% to 15% in the first year and increases to 40% to 50% in 5 years.

- The side effects of danazol are related to its androgenic and anabolic properties, as well as to the "pseudomenopause" produced by the drug.

- Approximately three of four women note significant improvement in symptoms following danazol therapy. Unfortunately, 15% to 30% of women will have a recurrence of symptoms within 2 years following completion of medical therapy.

- With chronic administration of GnRH agonists, specific suppression of gonadotrophin secretion occurs, with secondary diminution of ovarian steroidogenesis. The GnRH agonists bind with receptors for a prolonged time and induce protracted periods of downward regulation.

- GnRH agonists produce a "medical oophorectomy" without the side effects of danazol on steroid-sensitive target organs.

- The side effects associated with GnRH agonist therapy are primarily those associated with estrogen deprivation, similar to menopause. The three most common symptoms are hot flushes, vaginal dryness, and insomnia. A decrease in bone mineral content of trabecular bone has been demonstrated in the cortical bone on the lumbar spine by quantitative computer tomography.

- It has been established that the decrease in bone density associated with 6 months of therapy with GnRH agonist completely recovers between 12 and 24 months after discontinuing therapy.

- Initial clinical response to GnRH agonist therapy depends on when the therapy is begun in relation to the menstrual cycle.

- Many clinicians "add-back" very low doses of estrogen, low doses of progestins, or both in combination with chronic GnRH agonist therapy.

- Laparoscopy is employed frequently for both diagnostic and therapeutic reasons. The major advantage of treating endometriosis with the laparoscope, using either surgical instruments, laser, or electrocautery, is that patients may be treated at the time of diagnosis.

- The goals of conservative surgery for endometriosis include removal of macroscopic endometriosis, lysis of adhesions, and restoration of normal anatomy.

- Classic symptoms of endometriosis of the large bowel include cyclic pelvic cramping and lower abdominal pain and rectal pain with defecation, especially during the menstrual period.

- The pathogenesis of endometriosis of the bladder is controversial. Interestingly, approximately 50% of women with endometriosis of the urinary tract have a history of previous pelvic surgery.

- Endometriosis of the bladder is discovered most often in the region of the trigone or the anterior wall of the bladder. Bladder endometriosis produces midline, lower abdominal, and suprapubic pain, dysuria, and, occasionally, cyclic hematuria.

- Surgical therapy is preferred for ureteral obstruction secondary to endometriosis.

- Adenomyosis is frequently asymptomatic. If multiple serial sections of the uterus are obtained, the incidence may exceed 60% in women 40 to 50 years of age.

- Symptomatic adenomyosis primarily occurs in parous women over age 35. The classic symptoms are secondary dysmenorrhea and menorrhagia. The most common physical sign is a diffusely enlarged uterus, usually 2 to 3 times normal size.

- The severity of pelvic symptoms associated with adenomyosis increases proportionally to the depth of penetration and the total volume of disease in the myometrium.

- Adenomyosis rarely causes uterine enlargement greater than a size at 14 weeks' gestation unless there is concomitant uterine pathology.

BIBLIOGRAPHY

Adamson GD: Diagnosis and clinical presentation of endometriosis, Am J Obstet Gynecol 162:568, 1990.

American Fertility Society: Management of endometriosis in the presence of pelvic pain, Fertil Steril 60:952, 1993.

American Society for Reproductive Medicine: Revised American Society for Reproductive Medicine classification of endometriosis: 1996, Fertil Steril 67:817, 1997.

Arnold LL, Ascher SM, and Simon JA: Familial adenomyosis: a case report, Fertil Steril 61:1165, 1994.

Ascher SM, Arnold LL, Patt RH, et al: Adenomyosis: prospective comparison of MR imaging and transvaginal sonography, Radiology 190:803, 1994.

Bailey HR, Ott MT, and Hartendorp P: Aggressive surgical management for advanced colorectal endometriosis, Dis Colon Rectum 37:747, 1994.

Barbieri RL: Gonadotropin-releasing hormone agonists: treatment of endometriosis, Clin Obstet Gynecol 36:636, 1993.

Barbieri RL: Hormone treatment of endometriosis: the estrogen threshold hypothesis, Am J Obstet Gynecol 166:740, 1992.

Barbieri RL and Gordon AC: Hormonal therapy of endometriosis: the estradiol target, Fertil Steril 56:820, 1991.

Barlow D: Today's treatments: how do you choose? Int J Gynaecol Obstet 64:S15, 1999.

Bateman BG, Kolp LA, and Mills S: Endoscopic versus laparo-

tomy management of endometriomas, Fertil Steril 62:690, 1994.

Batt RE and Smith RA: Embryologic theory of histogenesis of endometriosis in peritoneal pockets, Obstet Gynecol Clin North Am 16:15, 1989.

Berga SL: A skeleton in the closet? Bone health and therapy for endometriosis revisited, Fertil Steril 65:702, 1996.

Bergqvist A: Different types of extragenital endometriosis: a review, Gynecol Endocrinol 7:207, 1993.

Bergqvist A: Extragenital endometriosis: a review, Eur J Surg 158:7, 1992.

Bird CC, McElin TW, and Manalo-Estrella P: The elusive adenomyosis of the uterus-revisited, Am J Obstet Gynecol 112:583, 1972.

Blumenkrantz MJ, Gallagher N, Bashore RA, et al: Retrograde menstruation in women undergoing chronic peritoneal dialysis, Obstet Gynecol 57:667, 1981.

Bozdech JM: Endoscopic diagnosis of colonic endometriosis, Gastrointest Endosc 38:568, 1992.

Brosens IA: New principles in the management of endometriosis, Acta Obstet Gynecol Scand 159:S18, 1994.

Brosens IA: Endometriosis—a disease because it is characterized by bleeding, Am J Obstet Gynecol 176:263, 1997.

Brosens IA and Brosens JJ: Redefining endometriosis: is deep endometriosis a progressive disease? Hum Reprod 15:1, 2000.

Brosens JJ and Barker FG: The role of myometrial needle biopsies in the diagnosis of adenomyosis, Fertil Steril 63:1347, 1995.

Busacca M, Marana R, Caruana P, et al: Recurrence of ovarian endometrioma after laparoscopic excision, Am J Obstet Gynecol 180:519, 1999.

Byun JY, Kim SE, Choi BG, et al: Diffuse and focal adenomyosis: MR imaging findings, Radiographics 19:S161, 1999.

Candiani GB, Fedele L, Vercellini P, et al: Presacral neurectomy for the treatment of pelvic pain associated with endometriosis: a controlled study, Am J Obstet Gynecol 167:100, 1992.

Candiani GB, Fedele L, Vercellini P, et al: Repetitive conservative surgery for recurrence of endometriosis, Obstet Gynecol 77: 421, 1991.

Cedars MI, Lu JKH, Meldrum DR, et al: Treatment of endometriosis with a long-acting gonadotropin-releasing hormone agonist plus medroxyprogesterone acetate, Obstet Gynecol 75:641, 1990.

Cornillie FJ, Oosterlynck D, Lauweryns JM, et al: Deeply infiltrating pelvic endometriosis: histology and clinical significance, Fertil Steril 53:978, 1990.

Coronado C, Franklin RR, Lotze EC, et al: Surgical treatment of symptomatic colorectal endometriosis, Fertil Steril 53:411, 1990.

Crosignani PG and Vercellini P: New clinical guidelines are needed for the treatment of endometriosis, Hum Reprod 9:2205, 1994.

Darrow SL, Selman S, Batt RE, et al: Sexual activity, contraception, and reproductive factors in predicting endometriosis, Am J Epidemiol 140:500, 1994.

Dawood MY: Impact of medical treatment of endometriosis on bone mass, Am J Obstet Gynecol 168:674, 1993.

Dawood MY, Lewis V, and Ramos J: Cortical and trabecular bone mineral content in women with endometriosis: effect of gonadotropin-releasing hormone agonist and danazol, Fertil Steril 52:21, 1989.

Dawood MY, Obasiolu CW, Ramos J, and Khan-Dawood FS: Clinical, endocrine, and metabolic effects of two doses of gestrinone in treatment of pelvic endometriosis, Am J Obstet Gynecol 176:387, 1997.

Dawood MY, Ramos J, and Khan-Dawood FS: Depot leuprolide acetate versus danazol for treatment of pelvic endometriosis: changes in vertebral bone mass and serum estradiol and calcitonin, Fertil Steril 63:1177, 1995.

Dickinson CJ: Could tight garments cause endometriosis? B J Obstet Gynaecol 106:1003, 1999.

D'Hooghe TM, Bambra CS, Raeymaekers BM, and Koninokx PR: Serial laparoscopies over 30 months show that endometriosis in captive baboons (*Papio anubis, Papio cynocephalus*) is a progressive disease, Fertil Steril 65:645, 1996.

diZerega GS: Contemporary adhesion prevention, Fertil Steril 61:219, 1994.

Dlugi AM, Miller JD, Knittle J, et al: Lupron depot (leuprolide acetate for depot suspension) in the treatment of endometriosis: a randomized, placebo-controlled, double-blind study, Fertil Steril 54:419, 1990.

Dmowski WP: Danazol-induced pseudomenopause in the management of endometriosis, Clin Obstet Gynecol 31:829, 1989.

Dmowski WP, Gebel HM, and Braun DP: The role of cell-mediated immunity in pathogenesis of endometriosis, Acta Obstet Gynecol Scand 159:7, 1994.

Dochi T, Lees B, Sidhu M, and Stevenson JC: Bone density and endometriosis, Fertil Steril 61:175, 1994.

Dodin S, Lemay A, Maheux R, et al: Bone mass in endometriosis patients treated with GnRH agonist implant or danazol, Obstet Gynecol 77:410, 1991.

Donnez J: Today's treatments: medical, surgical and in partnership, Int J Gynaecol Obstet 64:S5, 1999.

Donnez J, Nisolle M, Gillerot S, et al: Rectovaginal septum adenomyotic nodules: a series of 500 cases, Br J Obstet Gynaecol 104:1014, 1997.

Evers JLH: Endometriosis does not exist; all women have endometriosis, Hum Reprod 9:2206, 1994.

Farquhar C and Sutton C: The evidence for the management of endometriosis, Curr Opin Obstet Gynecol 10:321, 1998.

Fedele L, Arcaini L, Vercellini P, et al: Serum CA-125 measurements in the diagnosis of endometriosis recurrence, Obstet Gynecol 72:19, 1988.

Fedele L, Bianchi S, Bocciolone L, et al: Pain symptoms associated with endometriosis, Obstet Gynecol 79:767, 1992.

Fedele L, Bianchi S, Raffaelli R, et al: Treatment of adenomyosis-associated menorrhagia with a levonorgestrel-releasing intrauterine device, Fertil Steril 68:426, 1997.

Fedele L, Bianchi S, Viezzoli T, et al: Gestrinone versus danazol in the treatment of endometriosis, Fertil Steril 51:781, 1989.

Fedele L, Marchini M, Bianchi S, et al: Endometrial patterns during danazol and buserelin therapy for endometriosis: comparative structural and ultrastructural study, Obstet Gynecol 76:79, 1990.

Fedele L, Parazzini F, Bianchi S, et al: Stage and localization of pelvic endometriosis and pain, Fertil Steril 53:155, 1990.

Fedele L, Piazzola E, Raffaelli R, and Bianchi S: Bladder endometriosis: deep infiltrating endometriosis or adenomyosis? Fertil Steril 69:972, 1998.

Fong YF and Singh K: Medical treatment of a grossly enlarged adenomyotic uterus with the levonorgestrel-releasing intrauterine system, Contraception 60:173, 1999.

Friedman AJ and Hornstein MD: Gonadotropin-releasing hormone agonist plus estrogen-progestin "add-back" therapy for endometriosis-related pelvic pain, Fertil Steril 60:236, 1993.

Friedman AJ, Juneau-Norcross M, and Rein MS: Adverse effects of leuprolide acetate depot treatment, Fertil Steril 59:448, 1993.

Fujii S: Secondary müllerian system and endometriosis, Am J Obstet Gynecol 165:219, 1991.

Gannon MJ and Brown SB: Photodynamic therapy and its applications in gynaecology, Br J Obstet Gynecol, 106:1246, 1999.

García-Velasco JA and Arici A: Chemokines and human reproduction, Fertil Steril 71:983, 1999.

Gehr TWB and Sica DA: Case report and review of the literature: ureteral endometriosis, Am J Med Sci 294:346, 1987.

Gestrinone Italian Study Group: Gestrinone versus a gonadotropin-releasing hormone agonist for the treatment of pelvic pain associated with endometriosis: a multicenter, randomized, double-blind study, Fertil Steril 66:911, 1996.

Graham B and Mazier WP: Diagnosis and management of endometriosis of the colon and rectum, Dis Colon Rectum 31:952, 1988.

Guerrieros S, Mais V, Ajossa S, et al: Transvaginal ultrasonography combined with CA-125 plasma levels in the diagnosis of endometrioma, Fertil Steril 65:293, 1996.

Guilbeault H, Wilson SR, and Lickrish GM: Massive uterine enlargement with necrosis: an unusual manifestation of adenomyosis, J Ultrasound Med 13:326,1994.

Halme J, Becker S, and Haskill S: Altered maturation and function of peritoneal macrophages: possible role in pathogenesis of endometriosis, Am J Obstet Gynecol 156:783, 1987.

Halme J, White C, Kauma S, et al: Peritoneal macrophages from patients with endometriosis release growth factor activity in vitro, J Clin Endocrinol Metab 66:1044, 1988.

Han AC, Hovenden S, Rosenblum NG, and Salazar H: Adenocarcinoma arising in extragonadal endometriosis: an immunohistochemical study, Cancer 83:1163, 1998.

Henzl MR: Gonadotropin-releasing hormone and its analogues: from laboratory to bedside, Clin Obstet Gynecol 36:617, 1993.

Henzl MR, Corson SL, Moghissi K, et al: Administration of nasal nafarelin as compared with oral danazol for endometriosis: a multicenter double-blind comparative clinical trial, N Engl J Med 318:485, 1988.

Hirata JD, Moghissi KS, and Ginsburg KA: Pregnancy after medical therapy of adenomyosis with a gonadotropin-releasing hormone agonist, Fertil Steril 59:444, 1993.

Hornstein MD, Gleason RE, and Barbieri RL: A randomized double-blind prospective trial of two doses of gestrinone in the treatment of endometriosis, Fertil Steril 53:237, 1990.

Hornstein MD, Hemmings R, Yuzpe AA, and Henrichs WL: Use of nafarelin versus placebo after reductive laparoscopic surgery for endometriosis, Fertil Steril 68:860, 1997.

Hornstein MD, Thomas PP, Gleason RE, and Barbieri RL: Menstrual cyclicity of CA-125 in patients with endometriosis, Fertil Steril 58:279, 1992.

Hornstein MD, Surrey ES, Weisberg GW, et al: Leuprolide acetate depot and hormonal add-back in endometriosis: a 12-month study, Obstet Gynecol 91:16, 1998.

Hoshiai H, Ishikawa M, Sawatari Y, et al: Laparoscopic evaluation of the onset and progression of endometriosis, Am J Obstet Gynecol 169:714, 1993.

Ishimaru T and Masuzaki H: Peritoneal endometriosis: endometrial tissue implantation as its primary etiologic mechanism, Am J Obstet Gynecol 165:210, 1991.

Israel R: Pelvic endometriosis. In Mishell DR, Davajan V, and Lobo RA, editors: Infertility, contraception and reproductive endocrinology, ed 3, Oradell, NJ, 1990, Medical Economics Books.

Jain S and Dalton ME: Chocolate cysts from ovarian follicles, Fertil Steril 72:852, 1999.

Javert CT: Pathogenesis of endometriosis based on endometrial homeoplasia, direct extension exfoliation and implantation, lymphatic and hematogenous metastasism, Cancer 2:399, 1949.

Jimbo H, Hitomi Y, Yoshikawa H, et al: Clonality analysis of bilateral ovarian endometrial cysts, Fertil Steril 72:1142, 1999.

Joseph J and Sahn SA: Thoracic endometriosis syndrome: new observations from an analysis of 110 cases, Am J Med 100:164, 1996.

Kane C and Drouin P: Obstructive uropathy associated with endometriosis, Am J Obstet Gynecol 151:207, 1985.

Kauma S, Clark MR, White C, et al: Production of fibronectin by peritoneal macrophages and concentrations of fibronectin in peritoneal fluid from patients with or without endometriosis, Obstet Gynecol 72:13, 1988.

Kauppila A: Changing concepts of medical treatment of endometriosis, Acta Obstet Gynecol Scand 72:324, 1993.

Kennedy SH, Williams IA, Brodribb J, et al: A comparison of nafarelin acetate and danazol in the treatment of endometriosis, Fertil Steril 53:998, 1990.

Kettel LM, Murphy AA, Morales AJ, et al: Treatment of endometriosis with the antiprogesterone mifepristone (RU 486), Fertil Steril 65:23, 1996.

Kettel LM, Murphy AA, Mortola JF, et al: Endocrine responses to long-term administration of the antiprogesterone RU 486 in patients with pelvic endometriosis, Fertil Steril 56:402, 1991.

Kinkel K, Chapron C, Balleyguier C, et al: Magnetic resonance imaging characteristics of deep endometriosis, Human Reprod 14:1080, 1999.

Kitawaki J, Kusuki I, Koshiba H, et al: Detection of aromatase cytochrome P-450 in endometrial biopsy specimens as a diagnostic test for endometriosis, Fertil Steril 72:1100, 1999.

Klein RS and Cattolica EV: Ureteral endometriosis, Urology 13:477, 1979.

Knapp VJ: How old is endometriosis? Late 17th- and 18th-century European descriptions of the disease, Fertil Steril 72:10, 1999.

Koninckx PR: Is mild endometriosis a disease? Is mild endometriosis a condition occurring intermittently in all women? Hum Reprod 9:2202, 1994.

Kosugi Y, Elias S, Malinak LR, et al: Increased heterogeneity of chromosome 17 aneuploidy in endometriosis, Am J Obstet Gynecol 180:792, 1999.

Koutsilieris M, Akoum A, Lazure C, et al: N–terminal truncated forms of insulin-like growth factor binding protein-3 in the peritoneal fluid of women without laparoscopic evidence of endometriosis, Fertil Steril 63:314, 1995.

Langlois NEI, Park KGM, and Keenan RA: Mucosal changes in the large bowel with endometriosis: a possible cause of misdiagnosis of colitis? Hum Pathol 25:1030, 1994.

Letterie GS, Stevenson D, and Shah A: Recurrent anaphylaxis to a depot form of GnRH analogue, Obstet Gynecol 78:943, 1991.

Leyendecker G: Endometriosis is an entity with extreme pleomorphism, Hum Reprod 15:4, 2000.

Lim YT and Schenken RS: Interleukin-6 in experimental endometriosis, Fertil Steril 59:912, 1993.

Ling FW and Pelvic Pain Study Group: Randomized controlled trial of depot leuprolide in patients with chronic pelvic pain and clinically suspected endometriosis, Obstet Gynecol 93:51, 1999.

Low WY, Edelmann RJ, and Sutton C: Short term psychological outcome of surgical intervention for endometriosis, Br J Obstet Gynaecol 100:191, 1993.

Luciano AA, Turksoy RN, and Carleo J: Evaluation of oral medroxyprogesterone acetate in the treatment of endometriosis, Obstet Gynecol 72:323, 1988.

Luster AD: Chemokines-chemotactic cytokines that mediate inflammation, N Engl J Med 338:436, 1998.

MacDonald SR, Klock SC, and Milad MP: Long-term outcome of nonconservative surgery (hysterectomy) for endometriosis-associated pain in women <30 years old, Am J Obstet Gynecol 180:1360, 1999.

Mahmood TA, Templeton AA, Thomson L, and Fraser C: Menstrual symptoms in women with pelvic endometriosis, Br J Obstet Gynaecol 98:558, 1991.

Mahnke JL, Dawood MY, and Huang JC: Vascular endothelial growth factor and interleukin-6 in peritoneal fluid of women with endometriosis, Fertil Steril 73:166, 2000.

Mathias JR, Franklin R, Quast DC, et al: Relation of endometriosis and the neuromuscular disease of the gastrointestinal tract: new insights, Fertil Steril 70:81, 1998.

McArthur JW and Ulfelder H: The effect of pregnancy upon endometriosis, Obstet Gynecol Surv 20:709, 1965.

McCausland AM: Hysteroscopic myometrial biopsy: its use in diagnosing adenomyosis and its clinical application, Am J Obstet Gynecol 166:1619, 1992.

Meek SC, Hodge DD, and Musich JR: Autoimmunity in infertile patients with endometriosis, Am J Obstet Gynecol 158:1365, 1988.

Miller JD, Shaw RW, and Casper RFJ: Historical prospective cohort study of the recurrence of pain after discontinuation of treatment with danazol or a gonadotropin-releasing hormone agonist, Fertil Steril 70:283, 1998.

Moen MH and Magnus P: The familial risk of endometriosis, Acta Obstet Gynecol Scand 72:560, 1993.

Moghissi KS: Gonadotropin-releasing hormones: clinical applications in gynecology, J Reprod Med 35:1097, 1990.

Moghissi KS: Treatment of endometriosis with estrogen-progestin combination and progestogens alone, Clin Obstet Gynecol 31:823, 1989.

Moghissi KS, Schlaff WD, Olive DL, et al: Goserelin acetate (Zoladex) with or without hormone replacement therapy for the treatment of endometriosis, Fertil Steril 69:1056, 1998.

Mol BWJ, Bayram N, Lijmer JG, et al: The performance of CA-125 measurement in the detection of endometriosis: a meta-analysis, Fertil Steril 70:1101, 1998.

Myers WC, Kelvin FM, and Jones RS: Diagnosis and surgical treatment of colonic endometriosis, Arch Surg 114:169, 1979.

Nafarelin European Endometriosis Trial Group: Nafarelin for endometriosis: a large-scale, danazol-controlled trial of efficacy and safety, with 1-year follow-up, Fertil Steril 57:514, 1992.

Namnoum AB, Hickman TN, Goodman SB, et al: Incidence of symptom recurrence after hysterectomy for endometriosis, Fertil Steril 64:898, 1995.

Nelson JR and Corson SL: Long-term management of adenomyosis with a gonadotropin-releasing hormone agonist: a case report, Fertil Steril 59:441, 1993.

Nishida M: Relationship between the onset of dysmenorrhea and histologic findings in adenomyosis, Am J Obstet Gynecol 165:229, 1991.

Nisolle M and Donnez J: Peritoneal endometriosis, ovarian endometriosis, and adenomyotic nodules of the rectovaginal septum are three different entities, Fertil Steril 68:585, 1997.

Olive DL and Henderson DY: Endometriosis and müllerian anomalies, Obstet Gynecol 69:412, 1987.

Oosterlynck DJ, Meuleman C, Sobis H, et al: Angiogenic activity of peritoneal fluid from women with endometriosis, Fertil Steril 59:778, 1993.

Oosterlynck DJ, Meuleman C, Waer M, et al: Transforming growth factor- activity is increased in peritoneal fluid from women with endometriosis, Obstet Gynecol 83:287, 1994.

Outwater EK, Siegleman ES, and Van Deerlin V: Adenomyosis: current concepts and imaging considerations, AJR 170:437, 1998.

Parazzini F, Fedele L, Busacca M, et al: Postsurgical medical treatment of advanced endometriosis: results of a randomized clinical trial, Am J Obstet Gynecol 171:1205, 1994.

Patel A, Thorpe P, Ramsay JWA, et al: Endometriosis of the ureter, Br J Urol 69:495, 1992.

Popp LW, Schwiedessen JP, and Gaetje R: Myometrial biopsy in the diagnosis of adenomyosis uteri, Am J Obstet Gynecol 169:546, 1993.

Propst AM, Storti K, and Barbieri RL: Lateral cervical displacement is associated with endometriosis, Fertil Steril 70:568, 1998.

Prystowsky JB, Stryker SJ, Ujiki GT, et al: Gastrointestinal endometriosis, Arch Surg 123:855, 1988.

Ramey JW and Archer DF: Peritoneal fluid: its relevance to the development of endometriosis, Fertil Steril 60:1, 1993.

Redwine DB: Is "microscopic" peritoneal endometriosis invisible? Fertil Steril 50:665, 1988.

Redwine DB: Ovarian endometriosis: a marker for more extensive pelvic and intestinal disease, Fertil Steril 72:310, 1999.

Reimnitz C, Brand E, Nieberg RK, et al: Malignancy arising in endometriosis associated with unopposed estrogen replacement, Obstet Gynecol 71:444, 1988.

Reinhold C, Atri M, Mehio A, et al: Diffuse uterine adenomyosis: morphologic criteria and diagnostic accuracy of endovaginal sonograph, Radiology 197: 609, 1995.

Reinhold C, Tafazoli F, Mehio A, et al: Uterine adenomyosis: endovaginal US and MR imaging features with histopathologic correlation, Radiographics 19:S147, 1999.

Rivlin ME, Krueger RP, and Wiser WL: Danazol in the management of ureteral obstruction secondary to endometriosis, Fertil Steril 44:274, 1985.

Rivlin ME, Miller JD, Krueger RP, et al: Leuprolide acetate in the management of ureteral obstruction caused by endometriosis, Obstet Gynecol 75:532, 1990.

Rock JA: Endometriosis and pelvic pain, Fertil Steril 60:950, 1993.

Rock JA, Truglia JA, Caplan RJ, and Zoladex Endometriosis Study Group: Zoladex (goserelin acetate implant) in the treatment of endometriosis: a randomized comparison with danazol, Obstet Gynecol 82:198, 1993.

Rock JA and Zoladex Endometriosis Study Group: The revised American Fertility Society classification of endometriosis: reproducibility of scoring, Fertil Steril 63:1108, 1995.

Rolland R and van der Heijden PFM: Nafarelin versus danazol in the treatment of endometriosis, Am J Obstet Gynecol 162:586, 1990.

Rose PG, Alvarez B, and MacLennan GT: Exacerbation of endometriosis as a result of premenopausal tamoxifen exposure, Am J Obstet Gynecol 183:507, 2000.

Rovati V, Faleschini E, Vercellini P, et al: Endometrioma of the liver, Am J Obstet Gynecol 163:1490, 1990.

Ryan IP and Taylor RN: Endometriosis and infertility: new concepts, Obstet Gynecol Surv 52:365, 1997.

Saleh A and Tulandi T: Reoperation after laparoscopic treatment of ovarian endometriomas by excision and fenestration, Fertil Steril 72:322, 1999.

Sampson JA: Peritoneal endometriosis due to menstrual dissemination of endometrial tissue into peritoneal cavity, Am J Obstet Gynecol 14:422, 1927.

Schenken RS: Gonadotropin-releasing hormone analogs in the treatment of endometriosis, Am J Obstet Gynecol 162:579, 1990.

Schenken RS and Guzick DS: Revised endometriosis classification: 1996, Fertil Steril 67:815, 1997.

Seltzer VL and Benjamin F: Treatment of pulmonary endometriosis with a long-acting GnRH agonist, Obstet Gynecol 76:929, 1990.

Shah M, Tager D, and Feller E: Intestinal endometriosis masquerading as common digestive disorders, Arch Intern Med 155:977, 1995.

Shaw RW: A risk benefit assessment of drugs used in the treatment of endometriosis, Drug Saf 11:104, 1994.

Shaw RW and Zoladex Endometriosis Study Team: An open randomized comparative study of the effect of goserelin depot and danazol in the treatment of endometriosis, Fertil Steril 58:265, 1992.

Siegler AM and Camilien L: Adenomyosis, J Reprod Med 39:841, 1994.

Simpson JL, Elias S, Malinak LR, et al: Heritable aspects of endometriosis, Am J Obstet Gynecol 137:327, 1980.

Spitzer M and Benjamin F: Ascites due to endometriosis, Obstet Gynecol Survey 50:628, 1995.

Stahl C and Grimes EM: Endometriosis of the small bowel: case reports and review of the literature, Obstet Gynecol Surv 42:131, 1987.

Stripling MC, Martin DC, Chatman DL, et al: Subtle appearance of pelvic endometriosis, Fertil Steril 49:427, 1988.

Suginami H: A reappraisal of the coelomic metaplasia theory by reviewing endometriosis occurring in unusual sites and instances, Am J Obstet Gynecol 165:214, 1991.

Surrey ES and the Add-Back Consensus Working Group: Add-back therapy and gonadotropin-releasing hormone agonists in the treatment of patients with endometriosis: can a consensus be reached? Fertil Steril 71:420, 1999.

Surrey ES, Gambone JC, Lu JKH, et al: The effects of combining norethindrone with a gonadotropin-releasing hormone agonist in the treatment of symptomatic endometriosis, Fertil Steril 53:620, 1990.

Surrey ES, Voigt B, Fournet N, and Judd HL: Prolonged gonadotropin-releasing hormone agonist treatment of symptomatic endometriosis: the role of cyclic sodium etidronate and low-dose norethindrone "add-back" therapy, Fertil Steril 63:747, 1995.

Sutton C: Laser treatment of endometriosis, Practitioner 237:601, 1993.

Tahara M, Matsuoka T, Yokoi T, et al: Treatment of endometriosis with a decreasing dosage of a gonadotropin-releasing hormone agonist (nafarelin): a pilot study with low-dose agonist therapy ("draw-back" therapy), Fertil Steril 73:799, 2000.

Takahashi K, Okada S, Okada M, et al: Magnetic resonance imaging and serum Ca-125 in evaluating patients with endometriomas prior to medical therapy, Fertil Steril 65:288, 1996.

Takayama K, Zeitoun K, Gunby RT, et al: Treatment of severe postmenopausal endometriosis with an aromatase inhibitor, Fertil Steril 69:709, 1998.

Thomas EJ: Endometriosis, 1995—confusion or sense? Int J Gynecol Obstet 48:149, 1995.

Thomas WW, Hughes LL, and Rock J: Palliation of recurrent endometriosis with radiotherapeutic ablation of ovarian remnants, Fertil Steril 68:938, 1997.

Torkelson SJ, Lee RA, and Hidahl DB: Endometriosis of the sciatic nerve: a report of two cases and a review of the literature, Obstet Gynecol 71:473, 1988.

Treloar SA, O'Connor DT, O'Connor VM, and Martin NG: Genetic influences on endometriosis in an Australian twin sample, Fertil Steril 71:701, 1999.

Troiano RN and Taylor KJW: Sonography guided therapeutic aspiration of benign-appearing ovarian cysts and endometriomas, AJR 171:1601, 1998.

Tsudo T, Harada T, Iwabe T, et al: Altered gene expression and secretion of interleukin-6 in stromal cells derived from endometriotic tissues, Fertil Steril 73:205, 2000.

Urbach DR, Reedijk M, Richard CS, et al: Bowel resection for intestinal endometriosis, Dis Colon Rectum 41:1158, 1998.

Vercellini P, Aimi G, De Giorgi O, et al: Is cystic ovarian endometriosis an asymmetric disease? Br J Obstet Gynaecol 105:1018, 1998.

Vercellini P, Aimi G, Panazza S, et al: A levonorgestrel-releasing intrauterine system for the treatment of dysmenorrhea associated with endometriosis: a pilot study, Fertil Steril 72:505, 1999.

Vercellini P, Cortesi I, and Crosignani PG: Progestins for symptomatic endometriosis: a critical analysis of the evidence, Fertil Steril 68:393, 1997.

Vessey MP, Villard-Mackintosh L, and Painter R: Epidemiology of endometriosis in women attending family planning clinics, Br Med J 306:182, 1993.

Waller KG and Shaw RW: Gonadotropin-releasing hormone analogues for the treatment of endometriosis: long-term follow-up, Fertil Steril 59:511, 1993.

Weed JC and Ray JE: Endometriosis of the bowel, Obstet Gynecol 69:727, 1987.

Wheeler JM and Malinak LR: Recurrent endometriosis: incidence, management, and prognosis, Am J Obstet Gynecol 146:247, 1983.

Wheeler JM and Malinak LR: The surgical management of endometriosis, Obstet Gynecol Clin North Am 16:147, 1989.

Wild RA, Hirisave V, Bianco A, et al: Endometrial antibodies versus CA-125 for the detection of endometriosis, Fertil Steril 55:90, 1991.

Wolf GC and Singh KB: Cesarean scar endometriosis: a review, Obstet Gynecol Surv 44:89, 1989.

Worthington M, Irvine LM, Crook D, et al: A randomized comparative study of the metabolic effects of two regimens of gestrinone in the treatment of endometriosis, Fertil Steril 59:522, 1993.

Yu J and Grimes DA: Ascites and pleural effusions associated with endometriosis, Obstet Gynecol 78:533, 1991.

Anatomic Defects of the Abdominal Wall and Pelvic Floor

Abdominal and Inguinal Hernias, Cystocele, Urethrocele, Enterocele, Rectocele, Uterine and Vaginal Prolapse, and Rectal Incontinence: Diagnosis and Management

KEY TERMS AND DEFINITIONS

Abdominal Wall Hernia. An outpouching of peritoneum, with or without intraabdominal contents, through weak areas of the abdominal wall.

Anal Incontinence. Fecal incontinence due to damage to the anal sphincter at the time of vaginal delivery with or without neuronal injury.

Anal Manometry. A commonly used test that objectively assesses the resistance to spontaneous defecation provided by the anorectal sphincter mechanism and the sensory capabilities of the rectum to provide a feeling of imminent defecation.

Cystocele. Protrusion of the bladder into the vagina, signifying the relaxation of fascial supports of the bladder.

Descensus of Cervix and Uterus (Prolapse, Procidentia). Protrusion of the cervix and uterus into the barrel of the vagina.
First Degree. Prolapse into the upper vagina.
Second Degree. Prolapse to or near the introitus.

Third Degree (Complete). Prolapse through the introitus.

Dovetail Sign. Loss of anterior perianal folds indicating a defect in the external anal sphincter (EAS) or chronic third degree laceration.

Electromygraphy (EMG). Evaluates the bioelectrical action potentials that are generated by depolarization of skeletal striated muscle. EMG evaluation consists of systematic examination of spontaneous activity, recruitment patterns, and the waveform of the motor unit action potentials (MUAP).

Enterocele. Herniation of the pouch of Douglas (cul-de-sac) between the uterosacral ligaments into the rectovaginal septum; usually contains small bowel.

Fecal Incontinence. The inability to defer the elimination of stool or gas until there is a socially acceptable time and place to do so.

Femoral Hernia. A hernia that occurs through the femoral triangle. The hernia sac passes beneath the inguinal ligament through Hesselbach's triangle (an area bounded laterally by the inferior epigastric artery, inferiorly by the inguinal ligament, and medially by the lateral margin of the rectus sheath).

Incarcerated Hernia. A hernia whose contents cannot be reduced readily.

Incisional Hernia. A hernia that occurs in a surgical incision.

Inguinal Hernia. A hernia that occurs through the inguinal canal.

Pessary. A prosthesis inserted into the vagina to help support pelvic structures.

Pudendal Nerve Terminal Motor Latencies (PNTML). Nerve conduction studies that measure the time from stimulation of a nerve to a response in the muscle it innervates.

Rectoanal Inhibitory Reflex (RAIR). A reflex response to increased pressure in the rectum from gas or stool. Normally, the IAS relaxes to allow a sampling of the rectal contents by the anal canal to determine if the contents are gas or stool and whether it is an appropriate time to defecate or pass flatus.

Rectocele. Protrusion of the rectum into the vagina, signifying a relaxation of rectal supports.

Reducible Hernia. A hernia whose contents can be reduced from the sac.

Sliding Hernia. A hernia in which the organ protruding makes up a portion of the wall of the hernia sac.

Spigelian Hernia. A rare hernia at a point where the vertical linea semilunaris joins the lateral border of the rectus muscle.

Strangulated Hernia. A hernia whose contents are incarcerated and whose blood supply to the content's structures is compromised.

Umbilical Hernia. A hernia protruding through the umbilicus.

Urethrocele. Protrusion of the urethra into the vagina, signifying loss of fascial supports of the urethra.

The structural supports of the abdomen and pelvis are susceptible to a number of stresses. In the female these supports are affected by congenital anatomic weaknesses, the stresses of childbearing, injury, surgical damage, and straining. In addition, a combination of chronic stresses, such as lifting heavy objects, chronic cough, straining at stool, or activities that require frequent stretching, plus the aging process, may make older women more susceptible to such abnormalities. This chapter considers hernias of the abdominal wall and pelvic region, as well as conditions that are a result of the loss of pelvic supports. In addition it considers the etiology, diagnosis, and treatment of rectal incontinence.

ABDOMINAL WALL HERNIAS

The abdominal wall is made up of the following structures beginning externally: skin; subcutaneous connective tissue; external oblique, internal oblique, and transversus abdominis muscles with their investing fascia; and parietal peritoneum. The rectus abdominis muscles run longitudinally in the midline from the xiphoid to the pubic symphysis. The investing fasciae of the external oblique, internal oblique, and transversus abdominis muscles completely encase the rectus abdominis muscles cephalic to the semilunar line. Caudally from the semilunar line the muscle is completely behind the aponeurosis of the fasciae of these muscles and lies directly on the peritoneum (Figure 20-1).

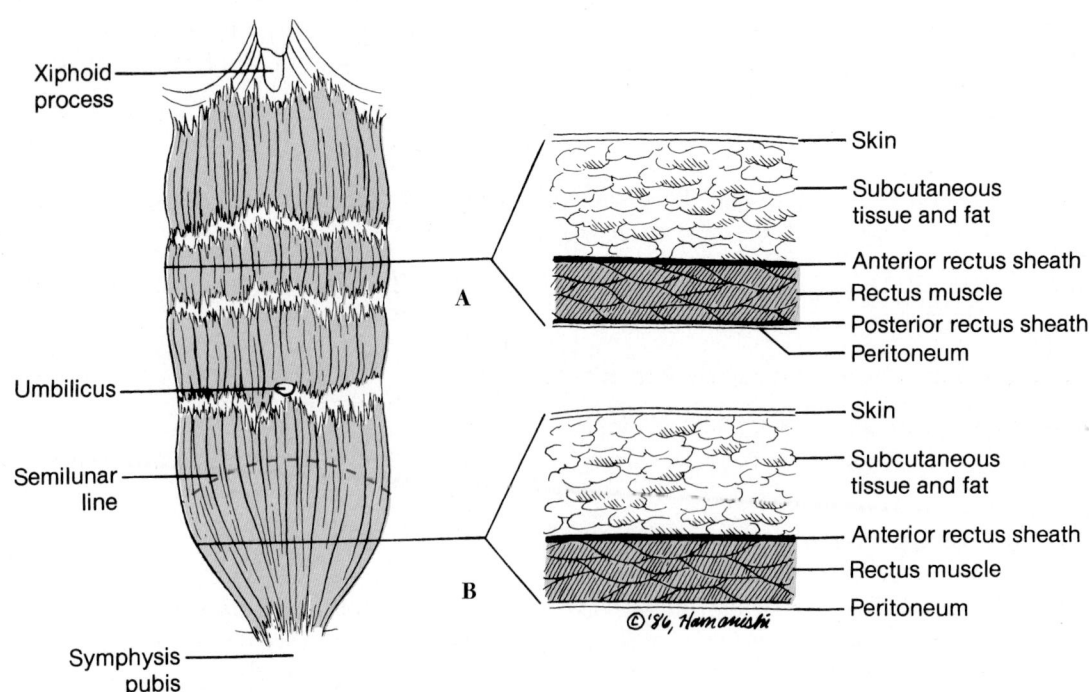

FIGURE 20-1 Graphic representation of layers of the abdominal wall. **A,** Above semilunar line. **B,** Below semilunar line.

Normally the investing fasciae join in the midline after surrounding the rectus abdominis muscles.

In the male the descent of the testes from their original retroperitoneal site to the scrotum necessitates passing through the abdominal wall to the inguinal region. At the level of the transversalis fascia where the descent begins, the internal inguinal ring is formed. The medial margin of this ring is defined by the inferior epigastric artery as it courses from the external iliac artery medially and superiorly into the rectus sheath. The inguinal canal runs from the internal inguinal ring obliquely downward, emerging through the external inguinal ring and opening in the external oblique aponeurosis just above the pubic spine and then continuing into the scrotum. This allows for passage of the testes and for the presence of part of the spermatic cord.

In the female the round ligament courses in the same direction but ends short of the labia. An inguinal hernia, that is, a bulge of peritoneum through the internal inguinal ring and into the inguinal canal, is less common in the female than in the male and is frequently identified after stretching of the abdominal wall during or after pregnancy. It may be related to a congenital weakness of this area. Occasionally a femoral-type groin hernia may develop. In this case the defect in the transversalis fascia occurs in Hesselbach's triangle, which is an area bounded laterally by the inferior epigastric artery, inferiorly by the inguinal ligament, and medially by the lateral margin of the rectus sheath (Figure 20-2). The hernia sac passes under the inguinal ligament into the femoral triangle rather than coursing through the inguinal canal. Femoral hernias are more common in females than in males.

The hernia is said to be *reducible* if the contents can be returned to the abdominal cavity. If the contents cannot be reduced, the hernia is said to be incarcerated. An incarcerated hernia may be acute, accompanied by pain, or may be longstanding and asymptomatic. If the blood supply to the incarcerated structure is compromised, the hernia is said to be *strangulated*. Because the hernia sac is primarily prolapsed peritoneum, the hernia itself is not strangulated but only its contents.

On rare occasions a portion of the wall of the hernia sac is composed of an organ such as the sigmoid colon or the cecum. In these instances the hernia is called a *sliding hernia.*

A ventral hernia occurs in the abdominal wall away from the groin. Examples include umbilical hernias, which are caused by congenital relaxation of the umbilical ring, and incisional hernias, which are herniations through separation of fascial planes after operative incision. Two special ventral hernias include the epigastric hernia, which occurs in a defect of the linea alba above the umbilicus, and the rare spigelian hernia, which is a herniation at a point where the vertical linea semilunaris joins the lateral border of the rectus muscle.

Incisional hernias generally involve the separation of the fascia of the abdominal wall with the hernia sac palpated beneath the skin and subcutaneous tissue. The sac wall is composed of peritoneum.

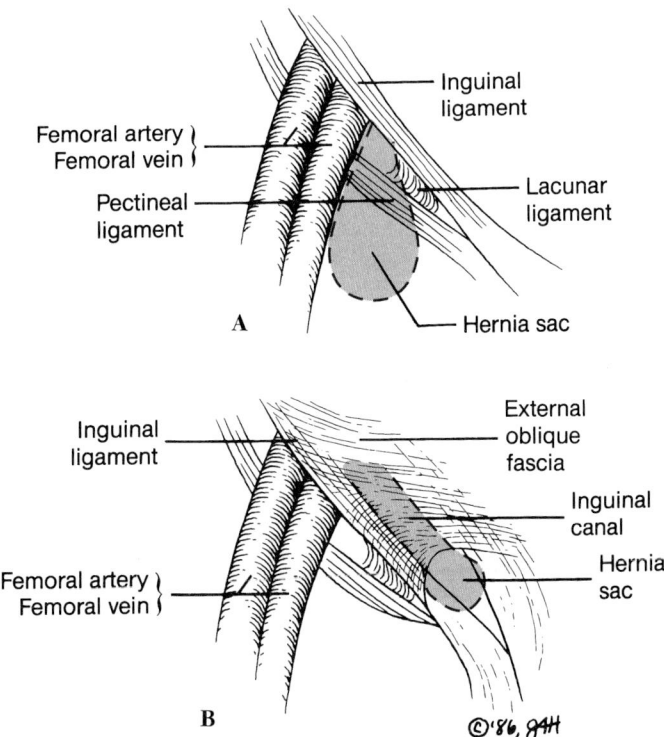

FIGURE 20-2   Graphic representation of right femoral (**A**) and right inguinal (**B**) hernias in the female.

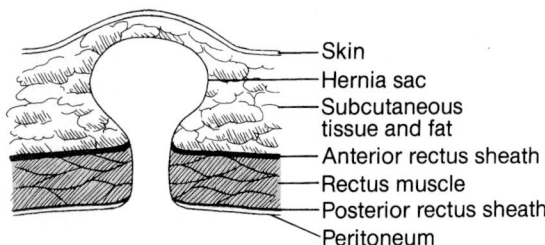

- Skin
- Hernia sac
- Subcutaneous tissue and fat
- Anterior rectus sheath
- Rectus muscle
- Posterior rectus sheath
- Peritoneum

FIGURE 20-3   Graphic representation of umbilical hernia.

Because the umbilicus consists of a fusion of skin, fascia, and peritoneum, an umbilical hernia generally occurs because the fascial ring is grossly separated, allowing the hernia sac to protrude. This occurs most frequently in obese women. The hernia sac itself is made up of peritoneum and subcutaneous tissue beneath the skin (Figure 20-3).

Etiology

Hernias may be the result of a congenital malformation. The umbilical hernia is the best example. Before 10 weeks' gestation the abdominal contents are partially herniated through the umbilicus into the extra embryonic coelomic cavity. However, after 10 weeks the viscera normally return to the abdominal cavity, and the defect in the abdominal wall closes during subsequent fetal growth. Generally at birth only the space occupied by the umbilical cord remains patent. Following the cutting of the cord the area heals so that the skin in the area of the umbilicus fuses above the closed fascial layer. Some infants at birth will show a small umbilical hernia, but in most instances the fascial defect closes during the first 3 years of life. If it does not close, an umbilical hernia will form. In rare cases the abdominal wall closure process is less complete, leading to an omphalocele, which is a hernia sac at the umbilicus covered only by peritoneum and including bowel and other abdominal contents. Omphaloceles are usually seen in infants with other malformations and possibly chromosome anomalies, such as trisomy 13.

Black infants have umbilical hernias more often than do white infants. Occasionally, umbilical hernias occur in adults after the distention of the abdominal cavity with pregnancy or with ascites.

Inguinal hernias are more common in males than in females. Femoral hernias occur primarily in females. Hernias that occur in adults are often associated with trauma or injury. In many instances the hernia bulge develops slowly after years of heavy labor. It is likely that a congenital anatomic defect was always present but became exaggerated over time, leading to the development of a hernia. Zimmerman and Anson thought that such lesions resulted from inadequate muscle support at the lower area of the inguinal canal, primarily caused by a defect in the internal oblique muscle. Stretching of this area in pregnancy may

initiate a hernia, but other factors, such as chronic cough caused by smoking or chronic respiratory disease, may be responsible.

Incisional hernias generally occur because of poor healing of the fascia. This may be secondary to poor nutrition, infection, or necrosis of the fascia secondary to suturing. It may also occur because absorbable suture loses its tensile strength before healing is complete. Stress and strain secondary to chronic cough or retching in the postoperative period may contribute to the process.

Symptoms and Signs

Bulges in the abdominal wall lead to the discovery of most ventral or groin hernias in women, either by a physician at the time of physical examination or by the patient. These hernias are generally symptom free. Occasionally, excessive straining or trauma will be implicated, and the patient may experience a feeling of tearing of tissue. Frequently the bulges are noted during an increase in intraabdominal pressure, such as with pregnancy or ascites. Most hernias are asymptomatic, but in some cases, particularly with larger ones, there may be aching or discomfort. Should intraabdominal organs move into the sac, the patient may experience some discomfort. Organs that strangulate within the sac cause acute pain and discomfort. Incarcerated organs may give nonspecific visceral pain, which is most likely the result of mesenteric stretching.

In cases where a hernia exists but no contents are within the sac, physical examination reveals a weakening at the site of the hernia. It is often possible to feel the "ring" of the hernia as one palpates the defect through the skin and subcutaneous tissue. The patient's straining will generally accentuate the hernia, making it more palpable and visible. In the case of inguinal and femoral hernias it may be necessary for the patient to be standing for one to palpate the hernia.

When there are intraabdominal contents within the hernia sac, the hernia is more easily palpated. The physician should then decide, based on his or her attempts to gently milk the contents from the sac back through the defect ring, whether the contents are reducible. For a hernia that does not reduce easily but in which there is no evidence of vascular compromise it is sometimes useful to apply ice packs to the abdomen in the area of the incarcerated hernia before additional attempts are made to reduce it. In cases of strangulated hernia, evidence of devitalization of an organ, such as fever, leukocytosis, and evidence for an acute abdomen, may be noted.

Management

Nonoperative management of hernias of the ventral wall and groin in women is often feasible. Umbilical hernias in little girls will generally close by age 3 or 4 years and rarely become incarcerated. An incisional hernia, if not too large, can frequently be managed by a corset, which prevents it from becoming incarcerated. Unincarcerated groin hernias are often small and become uncomfortable only with an increase in intraabdominal pressure, such as occurs with pregnancy. Many authors advocate repair, however, because the small neck of these hernias may make incarceration more likely. With pregnancy the opportunity for incarceration is reduced because the increasing size of the uterus pushes bowel contents away from the area of the herniation. Trusses and other supports are generally difficult to fit and are of little value in women.

Larger hernias, hernias that continuously contain intraabdominal contents, hernias that cause continuing discomfort, and those that have been incarcerated should be repaired. Some general principles of operative repair can be stated. The first principle involves the anatomy of the hernia. The hernia almost always consists of a sac of peritoneum with a narrow neck and a fascial defect of some sort. In rare instances, if a peritoneal sac is broad based, it may be possible to simply reduce the sac through the fascial defect without opening it and then to repair the fascial defect. However, if a narrow-necked sac exists, it must be dissected free of the fascial defect, emptied of its contents, and then excised and sutured at the neck (base). The fascial defect is then mobilized completely to remove stress and scarring, and it is closed with permanent suture. In rare cases the fascial defect may be large and the degree of mobilization that is required may be impossible. In such instances, patching with inert material, such as Mersilene mesh, may be necessary. This is rarely required in women except in the presence of large incisional hernias.

The second principle involves management of the contents of the hernia sac. Usually the hernia sac reduces with ease, but if intraabdominal contents are fixed to the sac wall by adhesions, the sac must be opened and the adhesions carefully separated. Care must be taken not to damage the organs or their blood supply. When these organs are reduced from the sac, the sac may be handled in the usual fashion. When incarceration has occurred, the organs must be inspected for viability before replacement.

Umbilical Hernia

A curved incision is made at the inferior margin of the umbilicus (Figure 20-4). The umbilicus is dissected free of the sac and reflected upward. The sac is then dissected free of the fascial defect and either reduced or excised, depending on the circumstances. The fascial edges are freshened and either closed by direct approximation anterior to posterior using nonabsorbable sutures or mobilized and closed in a "vest over pants" manner, suturing the anterior edge to the posterior edge in an overlapping fashion. Studies have not shown that either of these closures is superior to the other, and the approach taken generally is the one that best fits the circumstances. The umbilicus is then tacked to the fascial defect and the skin margin approximated.

Incisional Hernia

Repair of an incisional hernia can be accomplished by incising the skin through the old scar or via a parallel incision and dissecting through the subcutaneous tissue to identify both margins of the separated fascial defect. The peritoneum of the hernia sac is then isolated, dissected free of the margins, and reduced in the most appropriate fashion, with the surgeon exercising care not to damage any organs that may be fixed in the sac by adhesions. The fascial edges are then mobilized completely and closed side to side with interrupted nonabsorbable suture. Rarely the defect is so large that a patch has to be sutured over the defect. With care, however, it is generally possible to mobilize the fascia so that this is not necessary.

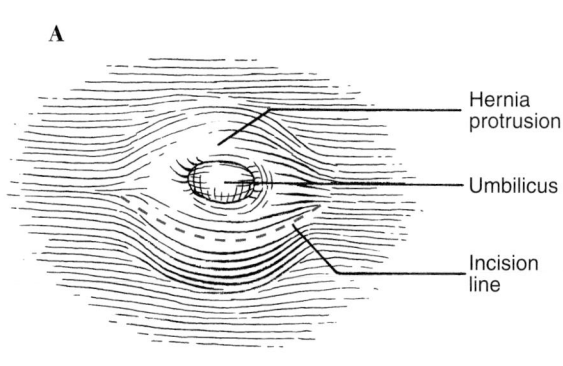

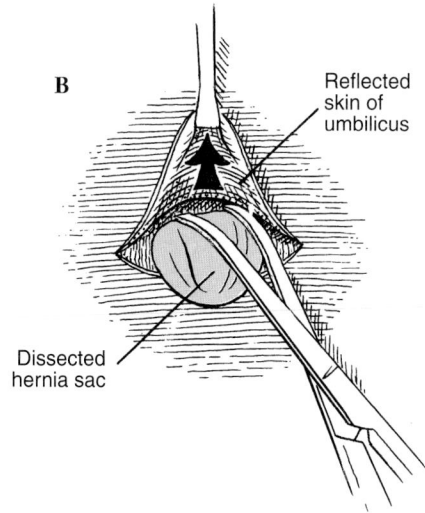

FIGURE 20-4 Repair of umbilical hernia. **A,** Site of incision. **B,** Umbilicus dissected free of sac and reflected upward.

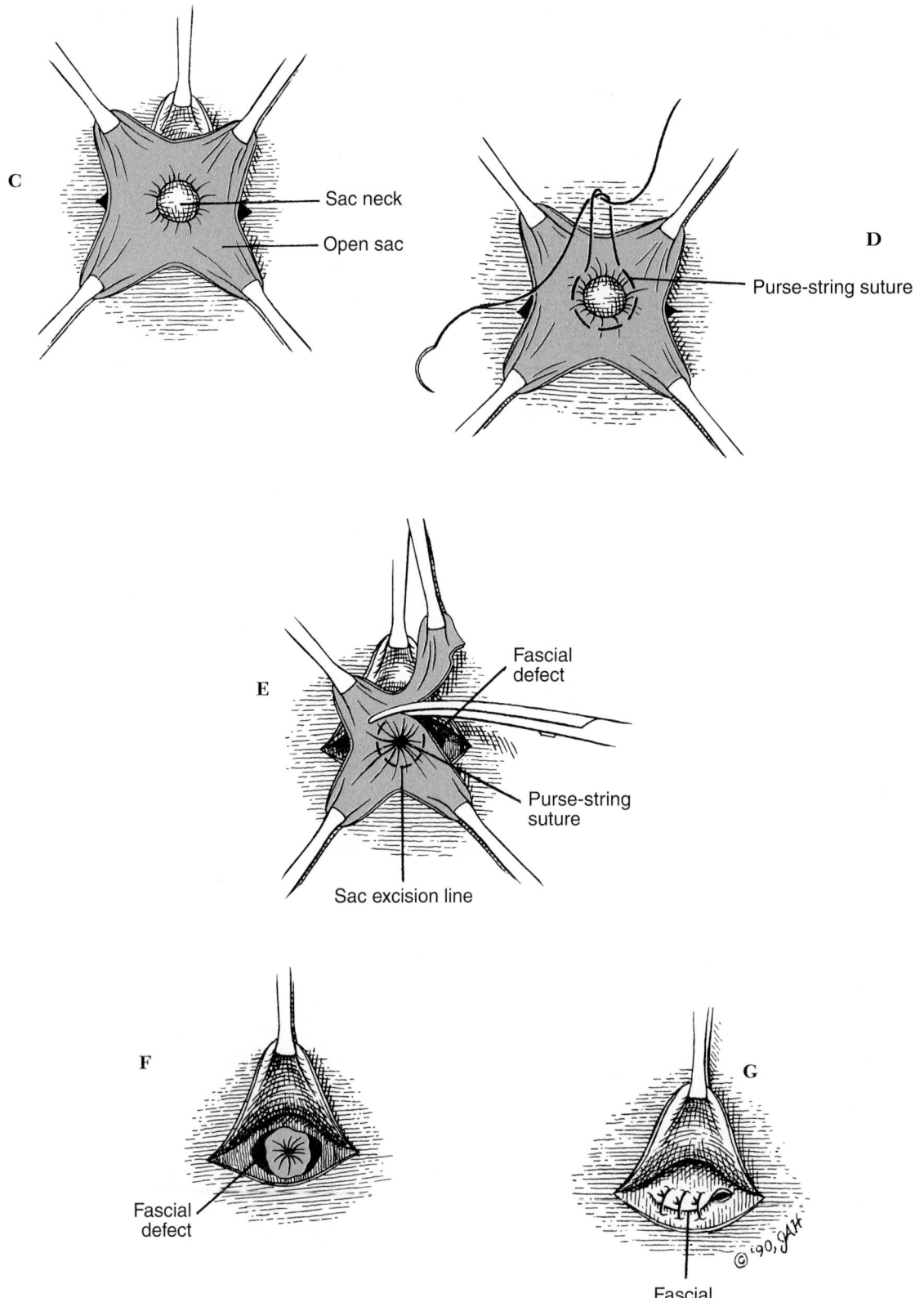

FIGURE 20-4, cont'd.   **C,** Appearance of sac that is cut open. **D,** Placement of purse-string suture at neck of sac. **E,** Sac dissected free of fascial defect after suture is tied. **F,** Appearance of fascial defect after sac excised. **G,** Fascial defect closed; umbilicus will be tacked to it.

Groin Hernia

To repair an inguinal or femoral hernia, an incision is made above the inguinal ligament, usually parallel to its medial portion. Subcutaneous tissue is separated, and the aponeurosis of the external oblique muscle is exposed. The external oblique is then incised from above down through the external inguinal ring, with the surgeon taking care to avoid the ilioinguinal nerve, which is frequently adherent to the external ring. The sac is identified and by careful dissection excised down to its emergence through the transversalis fascia. The sac is opened, and the intraperitoneal contents are reduced. The surgeon should place his or her finger through the sac neck into the peritoneal cavity and palpate the structures immediately within to be sure that there are no other hernia sacs protruding, particularly into the femoral canal. The sac neck is then ligated and transfixed away from the ring, often to Cooper's ligament. The transversalis fascia is approximated with nonabsorbable suture. The external oblique aponeurosis is then closed with nonabsorbable suture, and the skin and subcutaneous tissue are closed. Occasionally on opening the external oblique aponeurosis, only a mass of fat is found. In such instances the diagnosis of a hernia was made in error and no sac is present. Often, however, there is both fat and a sac, and the surgeon must be careful to determine the contents of the inguinal canal.

Femoral Hernia

When the sac is protruding beneath the inguinal ligament and through the femoral canal, an attempt may be made to reduce it from above. Frequently it is necessary to incise the inguinal ligament to free up the sac neck. In either case the sac should be ligated at its base, with the surgeon making sure that its contents are not damaged and that they are reduced. The sac, as in all cases, is generally handled by excising excess peritoneum and placing a purse-string suture of absorbable material about the base. Although it is probably not necessary to repair the inguinal ligament, most surgeons will do so. To prevent recurrent hernia in the transversalis fascia, the sac neck is sutured to Cooper's ligament beneath the inguinal ligament. To support the transversalis fascia repair, the external oblique aponeurosis is sutured over the transversalis fascia for extra support, all with interrupted, nonabsorbable suture material.

Recently, many groin hernias have been repaired laparoscopically. This may be carried out both in the preperitoneal space and intraperitoneally. In most instances a mesh patch is placed across the defect and fixed with either staples or sutures. Although many different materials may be utilized, Mersilene mesh seems to be popular and safe. Intraperitoneal exploration by laparoscopy often makes it possible to see a small hernia developing on the opposite side, which can also be fixed. In a study by Panton and Panton, of 79 patients undergoing a repair of inguinal hernia, 25% were found to have a hernia on the contralat-

eral side. Operative complications occur in 5% to 10% of patients and include lateral thigh parathesia, inferior epigastric artery injury, enterotomy from adhesiolysis, bowel obstruction secondary to herniation through trocar sites, and bladder injury. Recurrence rates are reported as 1% to 2% in most studies.

DISORDERS OF PELVIC SUPPORT

Pelvic support structures are often weakened by childbirth, other pelvic trauma, stress and strain, and the aging process. Abnormalities that result from these relaxation problems include urethrocele, cystocele, rectocele, enterocele, and uterine prolapse (descensus of the cervix and uterus). If a hysterectomy has been performed, prolapse of the vagina may also be a problem. It is unusual to have only one of these conditions. In most cases the relaxation affects all the support structures of the pelvis. Frequently, relaxation of the urethra, the bladder neck, and the bladder (urethrocele, cystocele) is associated with urinary incontinence, which is discussed in Chapter 21.

Urethrocele and Cystocele

Attenuation or rupture of the pubovesicle cervical fascia for any reason may allow the descent of the urethra (urethrocele), bladder neck, or bladder (cystocele) into the vaginal canal. Often only a cystocele is present (Figure 20-5), and generally in these cases the patient is continent. When a urethrocele is present as well, the woman usually suffers from stress incontinence. Urethroceles seem to be more common in women with wide subpubic arches (gynecoid type), which allow the full force of the fetal head against this area during descent in labor. Narrower arches, such as those associated with the android or anthropoid pelvic types, seem to protect this region from the descent of the fetal head.

Symptoms and Signs

Symptoms and signs of urethrocele and cystocele consist of a sensation of fullness or pressure and at times a feeling that organs are falling out, stress incontinence, occasional urgency, and often a feeling of incomplete emptying with voiding. The patient and the physician note a soft, bulging mass of the anterior vaginal wall. In some patients this mass must be replaced manually before the patient can void. Strain or cough accentuates the bulge. The mass may descend to or beyond the introitus. Although urethroceles and cystoceles almost always occur in parous women, they have been noted in nulliparous women who have poor structural supports. This is particularly true in women who have congenital malformations or weaknesses of the endopelvic connective tissue and musculature of the pelvic floor. Most parous women demonstrate some degree of cystocele, and when asymptomatic, they do not require therapy.

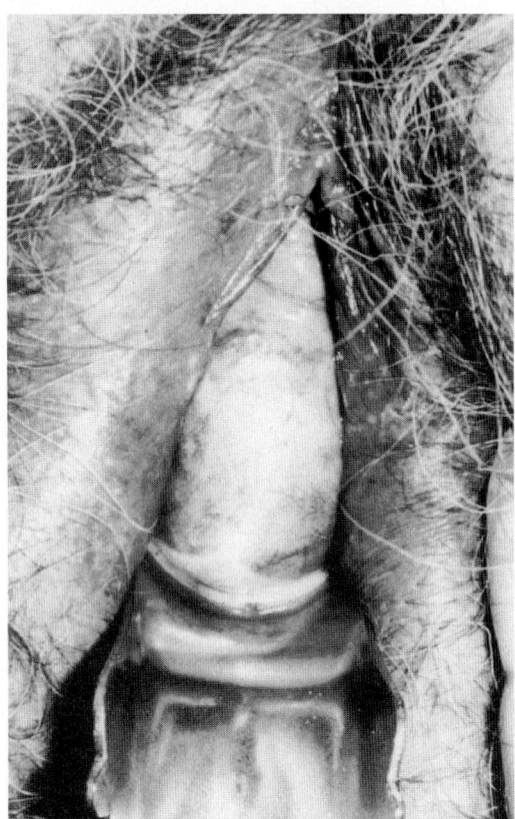

FIGURE 20-5 Cystocele.

Diagnosis

The urethrocele and the cystocele are best demonstrated with a patient in the lithotomy position. A retractor or posterior wall blade of a Graves speculum is used to depress the posterior wall. The patient is then asked to strain, and the degree of the cystocele or urethrocele is noted. The physician should palpate the bladder neck and note whether it is well supported. Generally, if the supports of the bladder neck are adequate, the urethra is adequately supported. If a cystocele and a urethrocele are present, it invariably follows that the bladder neck is not supported. The examination for cystocele and urethrocele is best performed with the bladder at least partially filled (100 to 250 ml).

Urethroceles must be differentiated from inflamed and enlarged Skene's glands and urethral diverticula. Cystoceles must be differentiated from bladder tumors and bladder diverticula, both of which are rare but may occur. Urethroceles and cystoceles are generally soft, pliable, and nontender. Although diverticula may be reducible, a sensation of a mass is usually present. Inflamed Skene's glands are generally tender, and it may be possible to express pus from the urethra when they are palpated. Pus may be expressed also in the presence of a diverticulum of the urethra. In such cases gonococcal and chlamydial infections should be considered.

Management

Treatment of urethroceles and cystoceles may be nonoperative or operative. Nonoperative treatment consists of supporting the herniation of the bladder into the vagina with the use of the Smith-Hodge or inflatable pessary (see Figure 20-12) or even with the intermittent use of a large tampon. Kegel exercises (see Chapter 21) help to strengthen the pelvic floor musculature and thereby may relieve some of the pressure symptoms produced by the cystocele. In an older woman the use of estrogen systemically or in a vaginal cream may improve both the tone of the pelvic support structures and the vascular supply of these tissues.

A younger woman with a large cystocele should be encouraged to avoid operative repair until she has completed her family. Occasionally the abnormality is so uncomfortable that repair must be performed before childbearing is complete. If this is the case, cesarean delivery should be considered for subsequent pregnancies.

Operative repair of a cystocele is generally performed in conjunction with the repair of a rectocele. It is unusual for anterior supports of the vagina to relax without an accompanying relaxation of the posterior wall. Repair therefore usually consists of an anterior and posterior colporrhaphy. If uterine descensus is noted, this must also be treated. Frequently an enterocele accompanies a cystocele and rectocele and where present must be excised and repaired. These problems are discussed later in this chapter.

Anterior wall repair (colporrhaphy) is performed by incising the vaginal epithelium transversally just above the anterior lip of the cervix in the region of the bladder reflection (Figure 20-6). If the woman has undergone a hysterectomy in the past, the incision may be made approximately 1 to 1.5 cm anterior to the vaginal scar. The vagina is then incised longitudinally from the transverse incision to the level of the bladder neck. If no urethrocele is present, this incision is sufficient. If a urethrocele is present, the incision must be continued under the urethra as well. The longitudinal incision is made by separating the vaginal wall from the underlying tissue progressively, using Metzenbaum scissors. When the longitudinal incision is complete, the cut edge of the vagina is held under tension and the pubocervical fascia that is attached is separated from it by blunt and sharp dissection. This is repeated on each side. At this point the bladder is free of the pubocervical fascia, which is itself free of the vaginal wall. The surgeon then places a suture over the bladder neck (Kelly stitch), bringing together the pubocervical fasciae on either side. The stitch should be placed in such a fashion that the pubocervical fascia is sutured as far away from the cut edge as possible and parallel to the previous incision. A similar stitch is taken on the opposite side, and the suture tied. Most appropriate for this closure is 0 or 2-0 polyglycol suture. With the bladder neck well identified and supported, the pubocervical fascia is then closed with progressive similar stitches to completely imbricate the fascia over the bladder. If the urethrocele is present, similar sutures are also placed over the urethra. (In Chapter 21 the replacement of the bladder neck behind the pubic symphysis to correct incontinence is described. The reader may wish to review these steps.) After the imbrication of the pubocervical fascia is completed, the vaginal edges are trimmed and the vagina closed with a row of interrupted 2-0 polyglycol or catgut sutures.

Postoperatively the bladder should be drained for about 3 to 5 days. There are several ways to accomplish this. The first is to leave a No. 16 Foley catheter in place for 2 to 5 days, remove the catheter on the second to fifth day, and allow the patient to try to void. After voiding of at least 200 ml the patient should be catheterized for the presence of residual urine. If residual urine is found in a quantity of more than 150 ml on two successive voidings or if the amount voided is less than 200 ml, the physician should

consider replacing the catheter for 24 to 48 hours. If residual urine amounts are less than 150 ml on two consecutive voidings, no further steps are necessary. Occasionally, after an anterior repair, voiding does not occur after 5 days of bladder drainage. At that point the patient may require catheterization for 24 to 48 hours longer, or she may be treated with a Foley catheter in place for continuous drainage for a week, to be rechecked for voiding and residual urine as an outpatient in 1 week. It is rarely necessary to treat the patient with antibiotics during this period; however, lower urinary tract infections are common and should be treated as they occur. In some patients who have had chronic urinary tract infections, prophylactic antibiotics, such as a sulfa preparation or nitrofurantoin (Furadantin), can be administered.

Alternatives to the above regimen include suprapubic catheter drainage or placing an infant feeding tube (No. 5) through the urethra and attaching it with a labial suture. In both methods the drainage tube can be clamped,

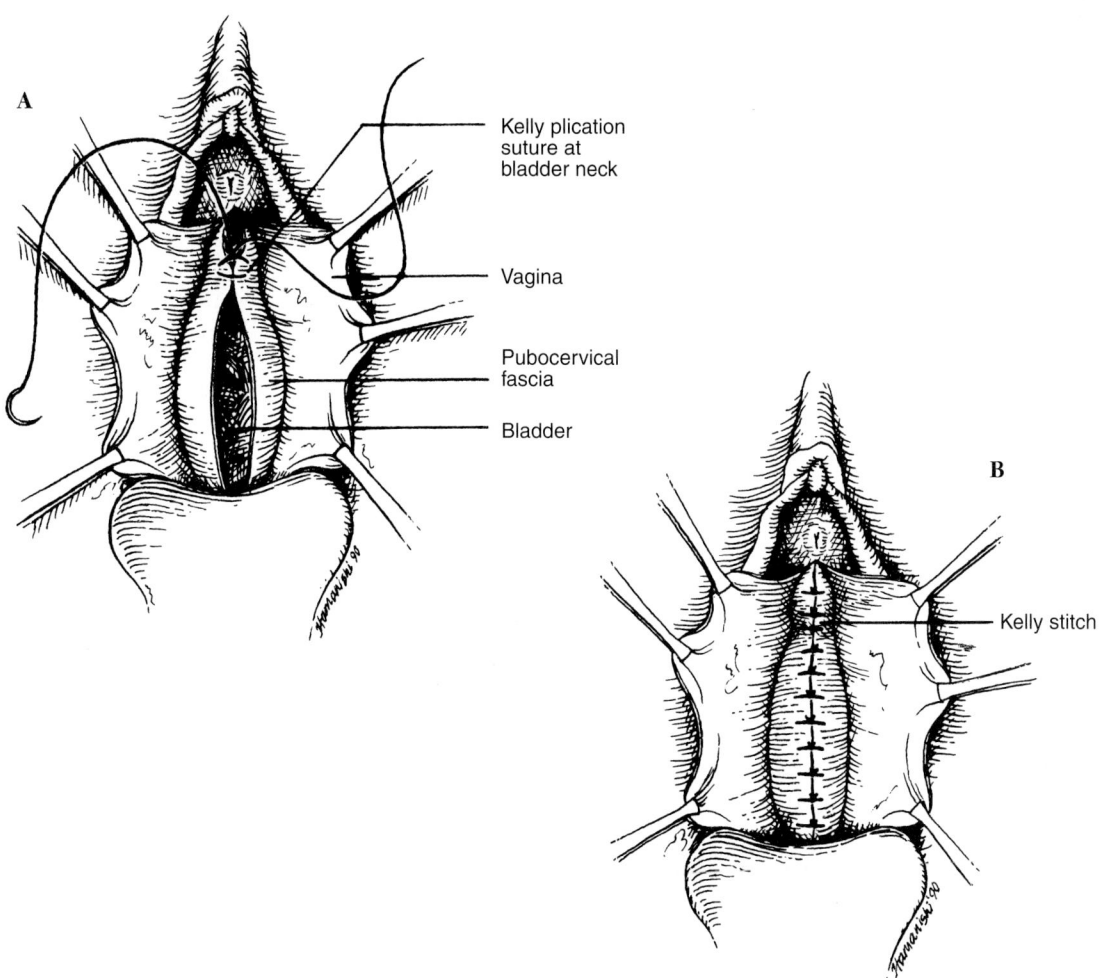

FIGURE 20-6 Cystourethrocele repair. **A,** The placement of Kelly stitch in the pubocervical fascia at the junction of the urethra with the bladder neck. **B,** The repair of the cystocele as the pubocervical fascia is sutured. Thus the cystocele is plicated. (Redrawn from Symmonds RE: Relaxation of pelvic supports. In Benson RC, editor: Current obstetric and gynecologic diagnosis and treatment, ed 5, Los Altos, Calif, 1984, Lange Medical Publications.)

allowing the patient to void when she can and allowing residual urine measurements to be taken. The suprapubic technique is simple to use and seems to have a lower incidence of infection than does transurethral catheterization, but patients may complain of extravasation of urine around the site and occasionally of hematoma formation. The surgeon should decide which method is best suited to the needs of his or her institution and develop a system that the surgeon and nursing team understand and can follow.

Postoperatively it is important to emphasize to the patient that heavy lifting, straining, or prolonged periods of standing should be avoided for 3 months. The healing process is slow, and the tissue is generally weak initially. Complete healing should be ensured before the tissue is stressed by normal activities.

Kohli et al. studied the recurrence rate of cystocele in 27 patients who underwent anterior colporrhaphy for symptomatic cystocele and 40 patients who underwent anterior colporrhaphy and needle suspension for cystocele and genuine stress incontinence. Recurrence of the cystocele occurred in 2 of the 27 cystocele patients and 13 of the 40 cystoceles with genuine stress incontinent patients in an average of 13 months. They speculated that the increased recurrency rate was due to the retropubic dissection necessary for the needle suspension. It is possible that the incontinent patients in the latter group suffered from a different pathologic problem such as nerve damage, collagen defect, and so on, and that this may have been responsible for the poorer outcome.

Rectocele

Symptoms and Signs

The patient with a rectocele often complains of a heavy or "falling out" feeling in the vagina. She may complain of constipation and occasionally may need to splint the vagina with her fingers to effect a bowel movement. She may also have a feeling of incomplete emptying of the rectum at the time of the bowel movement.

Diagnosis

A rectocele may be identified by retracting the anterior vaginal wall upward and again having the patient strain. The rectum will bulge into the vagina, and this bulge may protrude through the introitus (Figure 20-7). The physician should then place one finger in the rectum and one in the vagina and palpate the hernia. Often the rectovaginal septum is paper thin, and the rectocele can be palpated to its upper margin. If an enterocele is present, it may be possible to differentiate it from the rectocele by having the patient strain. Frequently, however, the diagnosis of a small enterocele is established only at the time of operation.

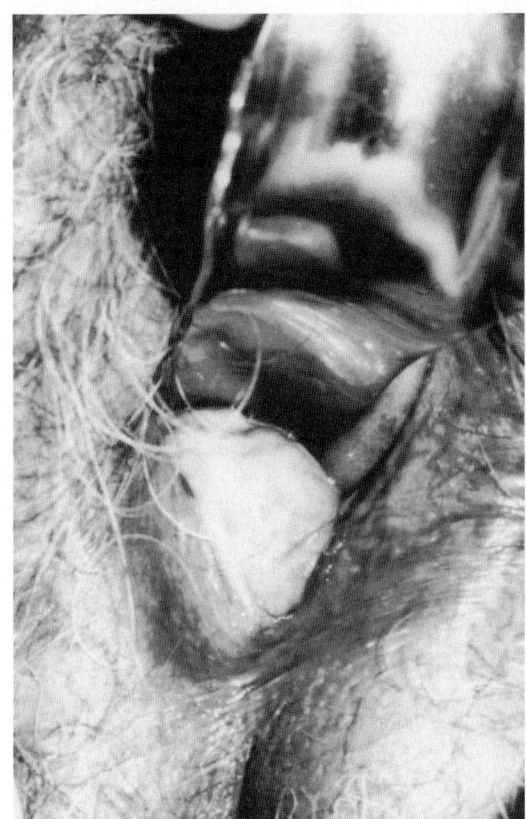

FIGURE 20-7 Rectocele.

Management

Nonoperative management of a rectocele is similar to that mentioned for a cystocele. Pessaries, Kegel exercises, and estrogen may be useful in the appropriate situations.

Operative management of a rectocele (posterior colporrhaphy) is generally performed at the time of an anterior colporrhaphy with or without enterocele repair or operation for descensus. Most women with rectoceles also have gaping vaginas and weakness in their perineal body. Therefore as part of a rectocele repair a perineorrhaphy is performed as well. The surgeon should estimate at the time of starting the posterior repair what degree of perineorrhaphy he or she wishes to perform. The margins of the perineum to be narrowed are generally marked by placing Allis clamps at their extreme at the introital opening (Figure 20-8). The tissue of the introitus is then incised between these clamps, and the vaginal wall is separated from the underlying tissue and rectum in a progressive manner longitudinally in the midline, beginning at the introital incision and being carried forward to the apex of the vagina above the limit of the rectocele. This is done by progressive separation and incision using the Metzenbaum scissors in a fashion similar to that described for cystocele repair.

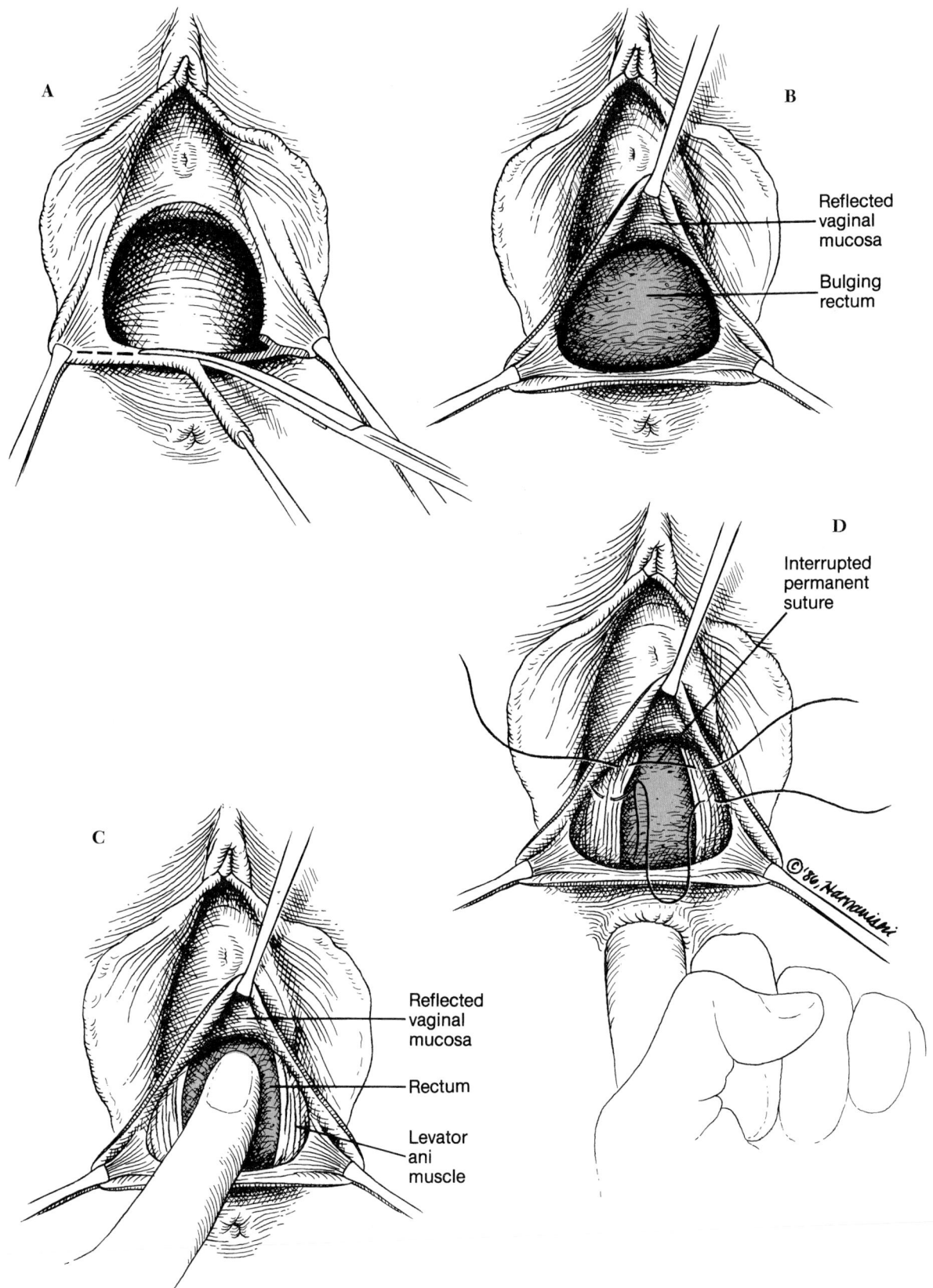

FIGURE 20-8 Repair of rectocele. **A,** Placement of Allis clamps at margins of perineal incision; perineal incision is being made. **B,** Reflected vaginal mucosa with rectum bulging. **C,** Depression of rectum identifying margins of levator ani muscle. **D,** Placement of sutures in perirectal tissue and levator ani bundles.

When the vaginal wall is completely incised, the edges are grasped and placed under tension, and the perirectal connective tissue is separated from the vaginal mucosa by blunt and sharp (if necessary) dissection. This is carried out bilaterally until it is possible for the operator to palpate the perirectal space on each side. The operator then places a finger of his or her nondominant hand into the rectum using a double-glove technique while an assistant picks up perirectal tissue on either side. The operator then places an 0 nonabsorbable suture (silk or dermalon) into the perirectal tissue on either side. Approximately three to five of these stitches are placed, and these are held without tying. The operator should use his or her finger in the rectum to ensure that no suture is placed into the rectum. The perirectal tissue usually includes portions of the levator ani muscles. When the sutures are tied, these tissues are interposed between rectum and vagina, thereby reducing the rectocele. These sutures also serve to tack the vagina to the levator ani area, thereby, it is hoped, avoiding future vaginal prolapse if a hysterectomy has also been performed. The vaginal edges are then trimmed and the vagina closed with a row of either continuous or interrupted catgut suture.

Attention is then turned to the perineorrhaphy, which is closed in the following fashion. Polyglycol sutures are placed in the lateral margins of the transverse incision, essentially bringing bulbocavernosal muscles together from either side to the midline. The operator should be sure that the bulbocavernosal muscle insertions are included in the sutures by pulling on the suture and noting whether the tension identifies the muscle bundles. The remainder of the perineal incision is then closed with a row of 2-0 polyglycol sutures to the deep tissue, and the skin of the perineum is closed with either interrupted or continuous subcuticular suture of 3-0 chromic catgut or polyglycol.

Enterocele

Enteroceles frequently occur after an abdominal or vaginal hysterectomy and generally are the result of a weakened support for the pouch of Douglas. In the prevention of enteroceles, the uterosacral and cardinal ligaments are the most important support structures and should be incorporated into the vault repair at the time of a hysterectomy and the ligaments from each side joined together.

Diagnosis

An enterocele is not always easy to diagnose. It is a true hernia of the peritoneal cavity emanating from the pouch of Douglas between the uterosacral ligaments and into the rectovaginal septum (Figure 20-9). It may be noticed as a separate bulge above the rectocele, and at times it may be large enough to prolapse through the vagina (Figure 20-10). If such is the case, it may be possible to make the

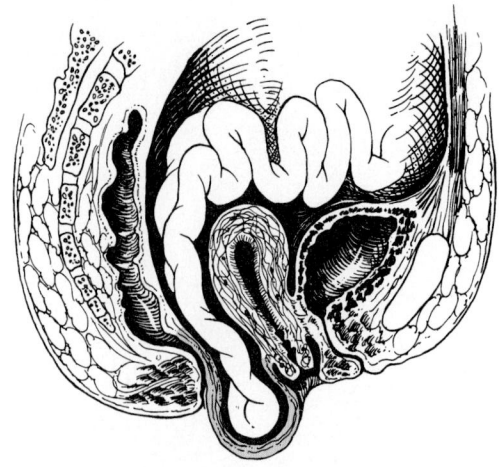

FIGURE 20-9 Enterocele and uterine prolapse. (Reproduced with permission from Symmonds RE: Relaxation of pelvic supports. In Benson RC, editor: Current obstetric and gynecologic diagnosis and treatment, ed 5, Los Altos, Calif, 1984, Lange Medical Publications.)

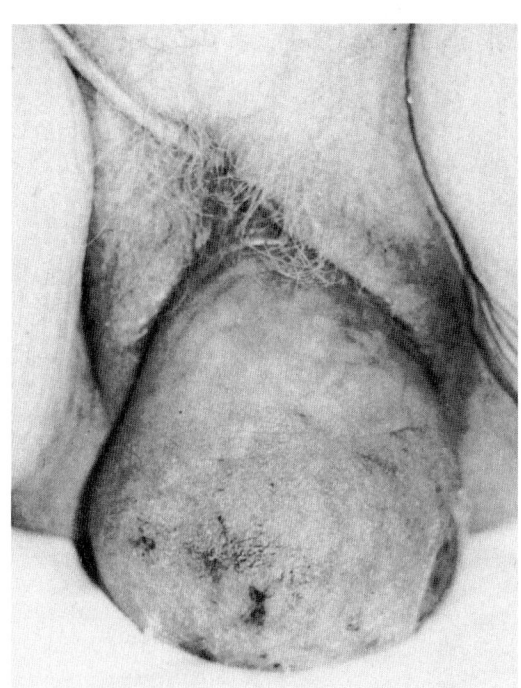

FIGURE 20-10 Elderly patient with vaginal prolapse who proved to have large enterocele with ulcers on the vagina.

specific diagnosis of enterocele by transilluminating the bulge and seeing small bowel shadows within the sac. It may also be possible to differentiate the enterocele from a rectocele by rectovaginal examination. The contents of an enterocele are always small bowel and may also include omentum. The contents may be easily reducible or may be fixed to the peritoneum of the sac by adhesions.

Management

Enteroceles may be reduced transabdominally as a primary procedure or at the time of other abdominal procedures. In the primary procedure the sac should be reduced upward if possible, and if the uterosacral ligaments are present, these may be brought together in the midline. If the uterosacral ligaments cannot be identified, as with large enteroceles after previously performed hysterectomy, the cul-de-sac may be obliterated by concentric purse-string sutures in the endopelvic fascia. Care must be taken to avoid damaging the ureters, rectum, and sigmoid colon. It is best to perform this procedure with permanent suture. The enterocele has probably occurred because of weakening of pelvic floor structures. Therefore, for optimum results, repair of the lower pelvis using a vaginal approach is probably indicated, even though the enterocele is obliterated abdominally.

Repair of the enterocele can be carried out at the time of the posterior colporrhaphy. The sac will be visualized as the vagina is separated from the rectum. The sac must then be dissected free of underlying tissue and isolated at its neck. It should be opened to ensure that all contents are replaced. The neck of the hernia is then sutured with a purse-string 0-chromic or polyglycol suture ligature and the sac excised (Figure 20-11).

It is important to support the neck of the enterocele sac as much as possible. If uterosacral ligaments can be identified or if they are present when a vaginal hysterectomy has been performed in association with an enterocele repair, they should be used in the repair. This can be accomplished by fixing the uterosacral ligaments to the peritoneum of the sac and the vaginal vault using a suture of 0 polyglycol, beginning on one side of the vagina and continuing through the uterosacral ligament of that side, the peritoneum of the sac, and the uterosacral ligament and vagina of the opposite side. Multiple sutures can be placed if space allows. This technique was described by McCall and is often called the *McCall stitch*. It effectively shortens the cul-de-sac and supports the enterocele neck. If uterosacral ligaments cannot be identified, as is often the case if the uterus has been previously removed, the rectocele repair should be continued to the area of the enterocele sac neck to reinforce this area and support the cul-de-sac as high as possible. This usually involves the joining of the levator ani muscles up to the area of the enterocele sac.

Correctly repaired enteroceles usually will not recur. Enteroceles repaired without proper attention to ligation of the neck of the sac and without appropriate rectocele repair may recur. In such cases a subsequent operation with special attention to these surgical principles is indicated. Often when an enterocele recurs, it is appropriate not only to repair the enterocele, either from above or below, but also to obliterate the cul-de-sac with imbricating suture through an abdominal incision.

Uterine Prolapse (Descensus, Procidentia)

Descensus of the uterus and cervix into or through the barrel of the vagina is associated with injuries of the endopelvic fascia, including the cardinal and uterosacral ligaments, as well as injury to or relaxation of the pelvic floor muscles, particularly the levator ani muscles. Occasionally, prolapse is the result of increased intraabdominal pressure, such as with ascites or large pelvic or intraabdominal tumors superimposed on poor pelvic supports. In some instances, sacral nerve disorders, especially injuries to S_1 to S_4, or diabetic neuropathy may be responsible. Using computed tomography, Sze et al. demonstrated that women with advanced genital prolapse had larger transverse inlet diameters, but not anterior-posterior diameters than do women without prolapse, suggesting an anatomic predisposition. Associated factors that increase tension on pelvic floor musculature, such as chronic respiratory disease including chronic bronchitis, asthma, and bronchiectasis, or severe obesity, may be associated. Congenitally damaged or relaxed pelvic floor supports may cause prolapse in young, nulliparous women. Most of the time, however, the patients are multiparous, with the prolapse being at least in part a result of childbirth trauma. Descensus is almost always associated with rectocele and cystocele and, at times, enterocele, supporting the concept of overall relaxation of the pelvic support structures.

A prolapse into the upper barrel of the vagina is called *first degree*. If the prolapse is through the vaginal barrel to the region of the introitus, it is *second degree*. If the cervix and uterus prolapse out through the introitus, it is called *third degree* or *total*. In total prolapse the vagina is everted around the uterus and cervix and completely exteriorized. When this occurs, the patient is in danger of developing dryness, thickening, and chronic inflammation of the vaginal epithelium. Stasis ulcers may result as edema and interference with blood supply to the vaginal wall occur. These ulcers rarely become cancerous, but biopsies should always be taken to ensure that they are not. In almost every case of acquired prolapse, the perineal supports are poor and the perineal body is damaged.

In 1996 a standardized terminology for the description of female pelvic organ prolapse and pelvic floor dysfunction was adapted by the International Continence Society, the American Urogynecologic Society, and the Society of Gynecologic Surgeons. This is an objective, site-specific system for describing, quantitating, and staging pelvic support and was developed to enhance both clinical and academic communication with respect to individual patients and populations of patients. The terminology replaces such terms as *cystocle, rectocele, enterocele*, and *urethrovesical junctions* with precise descriptions relating to specific anatomic landmarks. The first points are on the anterior vaginal wall and categorize anterior vaginal wall prolapse accordingly.

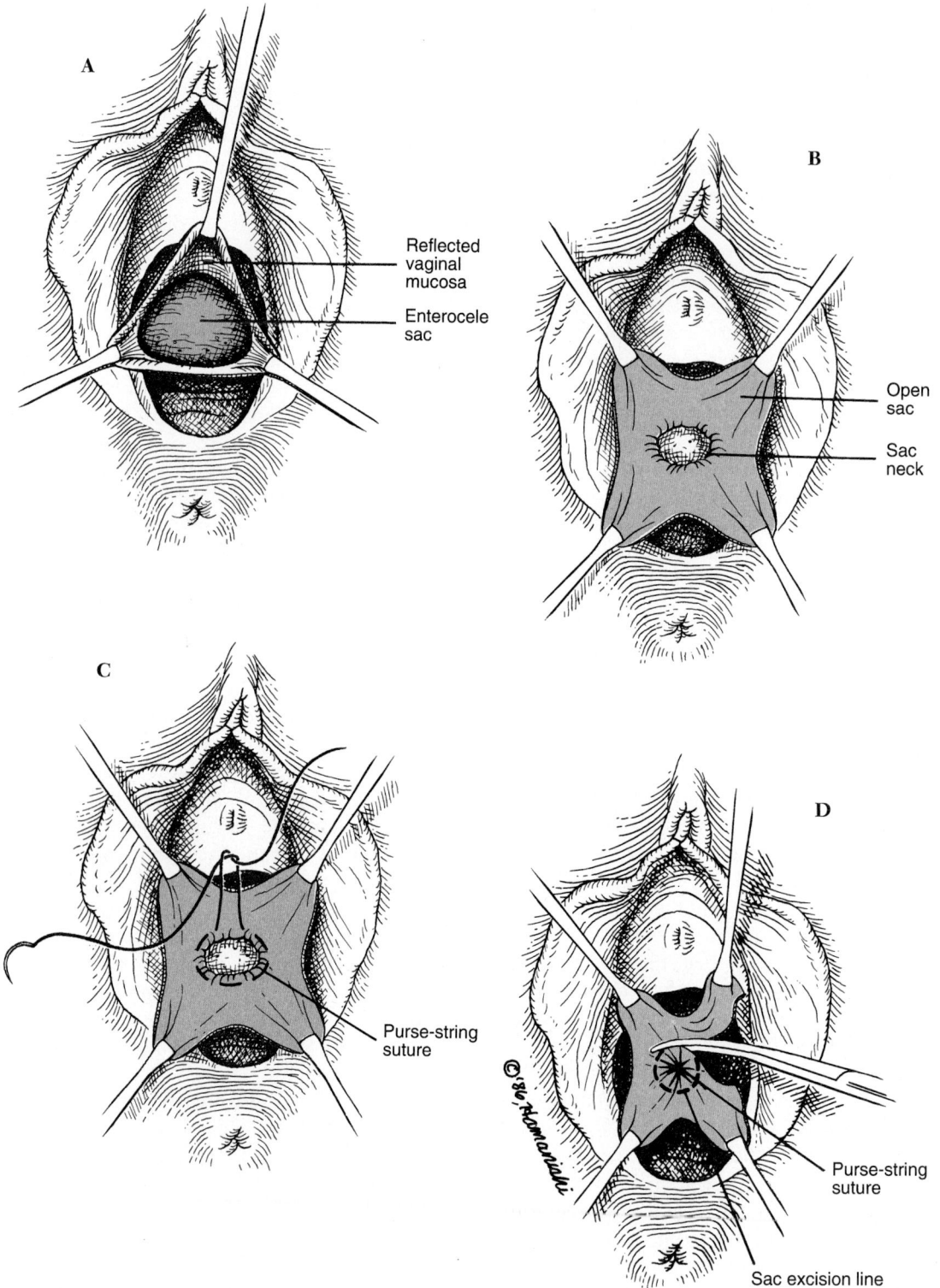

FIGURE 20-11 Repair of enterocele. **A,** Appearance of enterocele sac with vaginal wall reflected. **B,** Appearance of open enterocele sac with sac neck identified. **C,** Placing of purse-string suture at the neck of the enterocele sac. **D,** Excision of enterocele sac.

TABLE 20-1
Staging of Pelvic Floor Prolapse Using
International Continence Society Terminology

Stage 0   No prolapse is demonstrated. Points Aa, Ap, Ba, and Bp are all at –3 cm and either point C or D is between total vaginal length –2 cm.

Stage I   Criteria for stage 0 are not met, but the most distal portion of the prolapse is >1 cm above the level of the hymen.

Stage II   The most distal portion of the prolapse is less or equal to 1 cm proximal or distal to the plane of the hymen.

Stage III   The most distal portion of the prolapse is >1 cm below the plane of the hymen, but protrudes no further than 2 cm less than the total vaginal length in centimeters.

Stage IV   Essentially complete eversion of the total length of the lower genital tract.

Point Aa is a point located in the midline of the anterior wall 3 cm proximal to the urethral meatus and is roughly the location of the urethrovesicle crease. Point Ba represents the most distal position of any part of the anterior vaginal wall. Point C represents either the most distal edge of the cervix or the leading edge of the vagina if a hysterectomy has been performed. Point D represents the location of the posterior fornix (pouch of Douglas) in a woman with a cervix. Point Bp is a point most distal of any part of the upper posterior vaginal wall and Point Ap is a point located in the midline of the posterior vaginal wall 3 cm proximal to the hymen. To record measurements, these points should be expressed in cm above or below the hymen. It is important for the examining individual to express the position and other circumstances of the examination (i.e., straining or not, patient flat on table or in examining chair, etc.).

When the examination is recorded according to the anatomic points just cited, staging may be performed (listed in Table 20-1). These organizations hope that by using this system, a clearer understanding of a patient's prolapse will be achieved, and the transmittal of this information to others will be made more accurate. They also expect that this system will make it possible to standardize research information.

Symptoms and Signs

Major symptoms noted by patients with descensus are a feeling of heaviness, fullness, or "falling out" in the perineal area. In cases where the cervix and uterus are low in the vaginal canal, the cervix may be seen protruding from the introitus, giving the patient the impression that a tumor is bulging out of her vagina. Where total descensus has occurred, the patient is aware that a mass has actually prolapsed out of the introitus. Because prolapse almost always is related to anterior and posterior vaginal wall relaxation, symptoms that were reported earlier for cystocele and rectocele may be present as well.

It is not uncommon for the cervix or vaginal epithelium to become damaged or ulcerated, in which case the patient may report pain or vaginal bleeding. There is often discharge from the cervix and vagina when secondary infection occurs.

Management

Minimum prolapse does not require therapy unless the patient is very uncomfortable. Degrees of prolapse that place the cervix at or through the introitus probably cause greater discomfort and are usually more bother-some to the patient. Medical management of such conditions involves the use of a pessary, usually of the Smith-Hodge, donut, cube, or inflatable variety (Figure 20-12). These

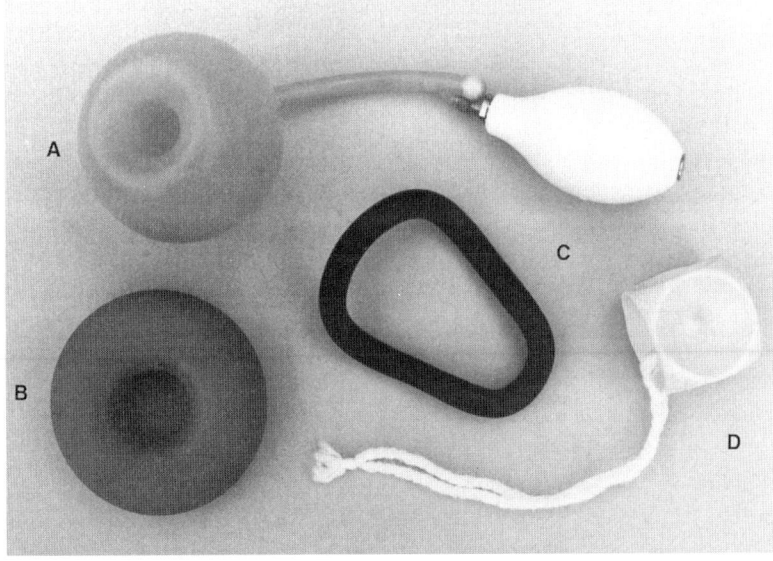

FIGURE 20-12   Examples of pessaries. **A,** Inflatable; **B,** donut; **C,** Smith-Hodge; **D,** cube type.

require the replacement of the uterus and cervix to their usual position in the pelvis and then the institution of support using one of these devices. Pessaries are available in varying sizes and should be properly fitted to the patient. In general the perineum must be capable of holding the pessary in place, or the pessary will frequently fall out. If the patient is a young woman and pregnant, it is important to replace the uterus before it enlarges and becomes trapped in the lower pelvis or vagina. If this happens, edema may cause incarceration and even loss of blood supply to the uterus. In a postmenopausal woman, estrogen replacement for at least 30 days in the form of systemic estrogen or vaginal estrogen cream may help improve the vitality of the vaginal epithelium, the cervix, and the vasculature of these organs, making the operative procedure and the healing process more efficient. The patient should not undergo operation until all ulcers of the vagina and cervix are healed, because to do otherwise is to risk infection and breakdown of the repair.

Operative repair for prolapse of the uterus and cervix generally involves a vaginal hysterectomy with anterior and posterior colporrhaphy. The hysterectomy is performed carefully, isolating the uterosacral and cardinal ligaments so that they may be used in the support of the vaginal vault. The uterosacral ligaments should be sutured together so that the cul-de-sac is shortened or obliterated and the risk of a subsequent enterocele is lessened.

In some cases a vaginal hysterectomy is not advisable. These circumstances include previous intraabdominal operation for an inflammatory process, such as endometriosis or pelvic inflammatory disease. Where such is the case an abdominal hysterectomy may be performed, followed by a vaginal anterior and posterior colporrhaphy. Under these circumstances the cardinal and uterosacral ligaments should be treated as noted earlier. As an alternative, a laparoscopically assisted vaginal hysterectomy may be performed in such situations.

In some women the cervix is hypertrophied and elongated to the area of the introitus, but the supports of the uterus itself are good. A cystocele and rectocele may be present, and operative repair can consist of a Manchester-Fothergill operation. This operation combines an anterior and posterior colporrhaphy with the amputation of the cervix and the use of the cardinal ligaments to support the anterior vaginal wall and bladder. Although it was suggested for repair in young women who wish to maintain their reproductive abilities, the loss of the cervix may interfere with fertility or lead to incompetence of the internal cervical os. The operation has value in older women who have an elongated cervix and well-supported uterus because it is technically easier and has a shorter operative time than the vaginal hysterectomy in such cases, and the entering of the peritoneal cavity is avoided.

Recently, Thomas et al., in a retrospective chart analysis, compared the data on 88 consecutive Manchester procedures to 105 randomly selected vaginal hysterectomy patients. All operations were performed at Mt. Sinai Hospital in New York between 1984 and 1988. Patients undergoing a Manchester procedure tended to be older and postmenopausal but were less likely to have significant medical illnesses than were patients who underwent vaginal hysterectomy. Operative time was shorter and blood loss less in patients undergoing a Manchester procedure, and long-term operative outcomes were similar for the two groups.

In older women who are no longer sexually active a simple procedure for reducing prolapse is a partial colpocleisis. The classic procedure was described by Le Fort (Figure 20-13) and involves the removal of a strip of anterior and posterior vaginal wall, with closure of the margins of the anterior and posterior wall to each other. This procedure may be performed with or without the presence of a uterus and cervix, and when it is completed, a small vaginal canal exists on either side of the septum, which is produced by the suturing of the lateral margins of the excision. The line of dissection of the vaginal wall is carried to the level of the bladder neck anteriorly and to the reflection of bladder onto cervix at the upper margin of the vagina. Posteriorly the dissection is carried from just inside the introitus to a position just posterior to the cervix. If a hysterectomy has been previously performed, the dissection may begin approximately 1 cm on either side of the vaginal scar. When the procedure is completed, the bladder neck is spared from any scarring, and urinary incontinence is generally avoided. Bladder neck plication may be carried out if the patient is incontinent. After healing of the plication a small introital area is noted; this has cosmetic benefits in older women. In addition, narrow canals are noted on each lateral vaginal wall. If the cervix and uterus are still present and intrauterine pathology occurs, bleeding along these canals could take place, alerting the physician to a potential problem.

The Goodall-Power modification of the Le Fort operation (Figure 20-14) allows for the removal of a triangular piece of vaginal wall beginning at the cervical reflection or 1 cm above the vaginal scar at the base of the triangle, with the apex of the triangle just beneath the bladder neck anteriorly and just at the introitus posteriorly. The cut edge of vaginal wall making up the base of the triangle anteriorly is sutured to the similar wall posteriorly, and the vaginal incision is then closed with a row of interrupted sutures beginning beneath the bladder neck and carried side to side to the area of the introitus. This procedure works well for relatively small prolapses, whereas the Le Fort is best for larger ones.

When a colpocleisis is performed, if an enterocele is found when the vaginal wall is stripped away, the sac must be identified, its neck ligated, and the peritoneum of the sac excised to prevent recurrence of the enterocele behind the colpocleisis.

In most cases a perineorrhaphy is performed with a colpocleisis to reinforce the introitus.

Prognosis for a colpocleisis procedure to reduce the prolapse and prevent recurrence is generally excellent. Ridley

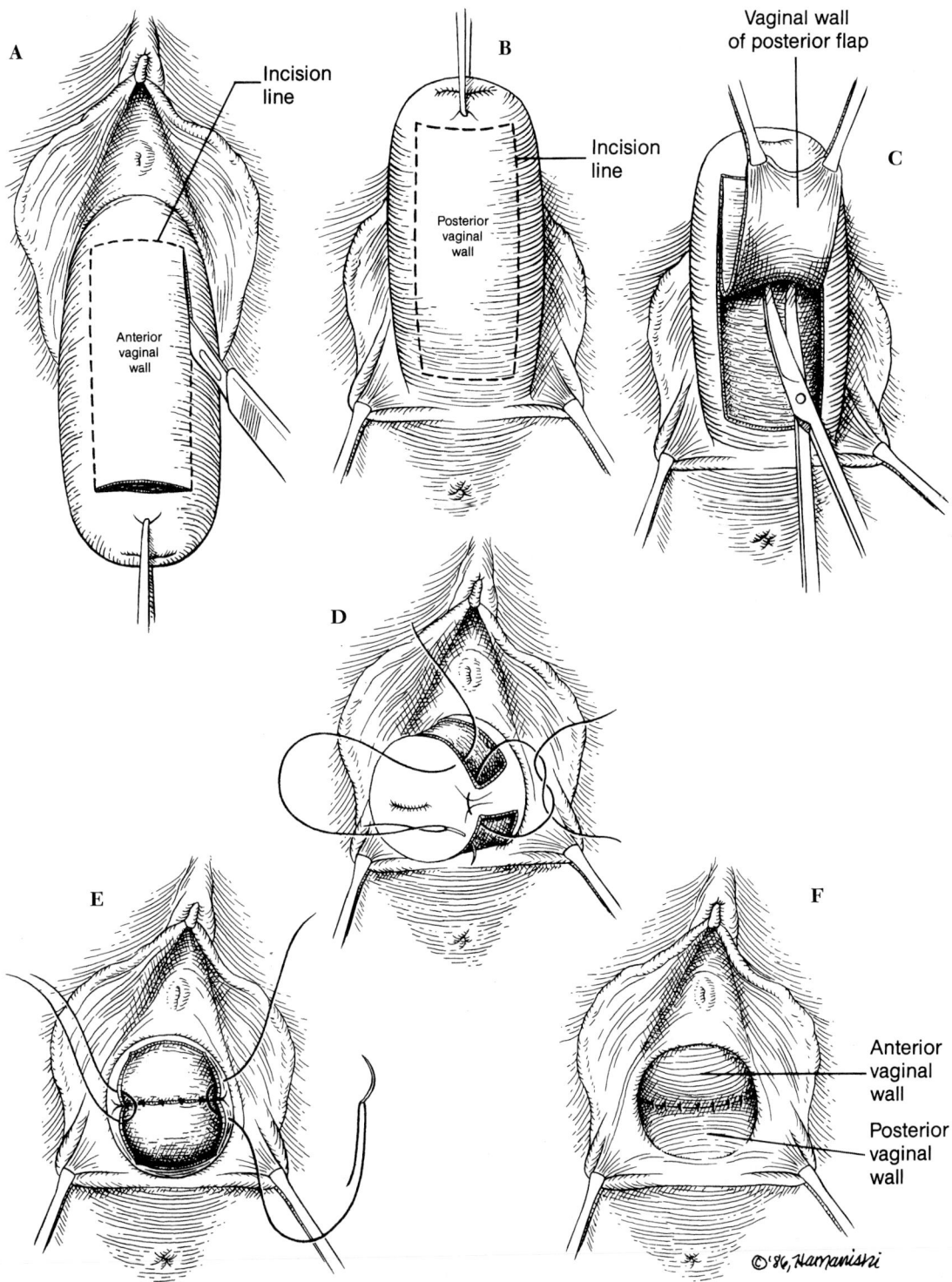

FIGURE 20-13   Le Fort procedure. **A,** Incision of anterior vaginal wall strip. **B,** Incision of posterior wall strip. **C,** Removal of vaginal strip. **D** and **E,** Placement of sutures. **F,** Appearance of vagina after procedure is completed but before perineorrhaphy is performed.

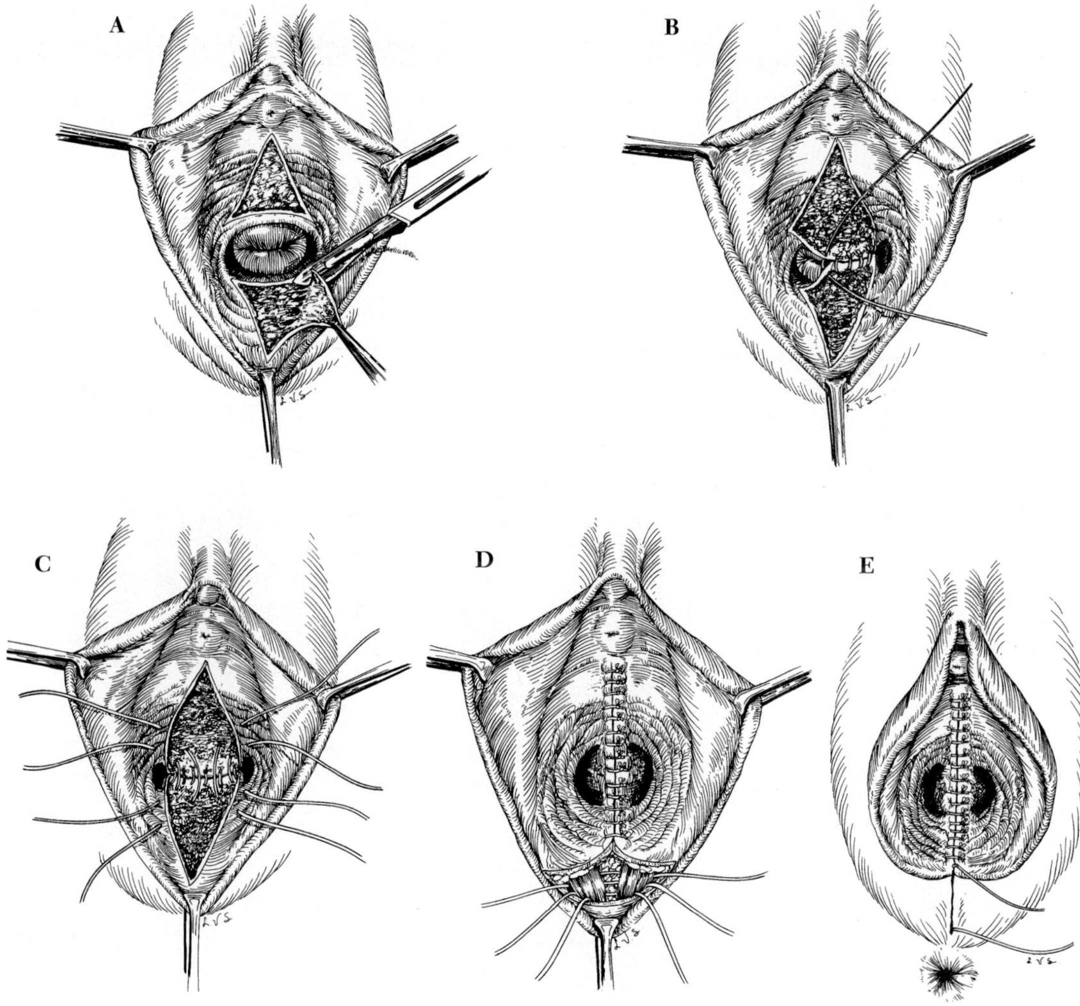

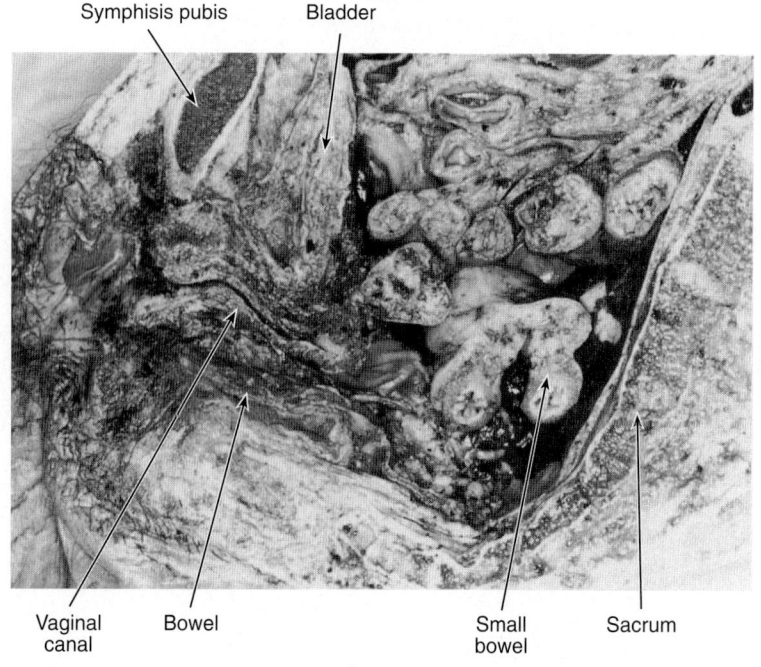

FIGURE 20-14 Goodall-Power modification of Le Fort operation. **A,** Representation of vaginal incision on anterior and posterior wall. **B,** Early placement of sutures. **C,** Later placement of sutures. **D,** Vaginal incision completely closed; perineorrhaphy being performed. **E,** Appearance at completion of procedure. (Reprinted with permission from Symmonds RE: Relaxation of pelvic supports. In Benson RC, editor: Current obstetric and gynecologic diagnosis and treatment, ed 5, Los Altos, Calif, 1984, Lange Medical Publications.)

Symphisis pubis   Bladder

Vaginal   Bowel   Small   Sacrum
canal   bowel

FIGURE 20-15 Pelvis of a dissected cadaver in supine position demonstrating vaginal canal orientation in the pelvis. (Courtesy Richard Hebertson, M.D.)

reports no prolapse recurrences in 58 patients unless an incomplete procedure was performed in an attempt to salvage vaginal depth and function. Three patients developed stress incontinence where none was present preoperatively.

Denehy et al. compared 25 elderly women (average age 82 years) in poor health and with a uterovaginal prolapse treated by colpocleisis with 42 women who also had a similar prolapse but were treated with vaginal hysterectomy, anterior colporrhaphy, and posterior colporrhaphy. Members of the vaginal hysterectomy group were considerably younger, with an average age of 66 (range 39 to 80). Average operating time for the Le Fort procedure was 75 minutes compared with 150 minutes for the vaginal hysterectomy. There was one postoperative death in the Le Fort group, but 19 of the 20 remaining Le Fort patients had excellent results for a follow-up of an average of 25 months (range 4 to 40 months). These authors performed Kelly urethral plication and posterior colpoperineoplasty in all patients as suggested earlier.

A special circumstance involves the treatment of women who wish to maintain their fertility despite the fact that they have a total uterine prolapse. Kovac and Cruikshank have demonstrated that uterosacral ligaments bilaterally could be sutured to the sacrospinus ligaments, thereby reversing the prolapse. In 19 such patients treated, 5 delivered a total of 6 babies (1 delivered twice).

Vaginal Stump Prolapse

Prolapse of the vaginal stump at some time remote to the performance of either abdominal or vaginal hysterectomy has been reported as occurring in 0.1% to 18.2% of patients. The prolapse may be total and may be accompanied by a cystocele, a rectocele, an enterocele, or some combination thereof. Occasionally the prolapse involves only one of those entities and not the entire vaginal stump. In a study in Munich, Richter reported that of 97 vaginal stump prolapses, 6.2% were cystocele only, 5.1% rectocele only, 9.3% primarily an enterocele type, and 72.2% of mixed type. Specific classification was not given for 7.2%.

Vaginal stump prolapse is probably the result of continuing pelvic support weakness and failure of the vaginal support structures, namely, the cardinal and uterosacral ligaments, to maintain their tone or attachment to the vagina.

Symptoms and Signs

Symptoms and signs of vaginal stump prolapse are similar to those delineated for descensus of the uterus. They include pelvic heaviness, backache, and a mass protruding through the introitus. At times, stress incontinence, urgency, frequency, dribbling, vaginal bleeding or discharge (if there is an ulcer), and, depending on the size of the mass, difficulty with sitting or walking may occur.

Diagnosis

Examination may help determine the contents of the herniation depending on where the vaginal scar is located in relation to the protruding mass and the extent to which the supports of the pelvis are lost. Rectovaginal examination is often helpful in delineating an enterocele from a rectocele.

Management

Although the management of descensus with the uterus present is uniformly agreed to be vaginal hysterectomy with anterior and posterior colporrhaphy, there is much controversy over the appropriate procedure for vaginal stump prolapse. Nevertheless, certain principles and facts are important. The first is that the normal position of the vagina in the standing position is against the rectum and no more than 30 degrees from the horizontal (Figure 20-15). The second principle is that pelvic relaxation is a part of the problem and dictates that an existing cystocele, rectocele, or enterocele must be repaired as part of the procedure. The third principle acknowledges that the perineal body is almost always severely weakened in such patients and must therefore be reconstructed as well. Nonsurgical management, such as the use of pessaries, estrogen, and the healing of ulcers, should be used as appropriate. Pessaries, however, are rarely retained in such patients, and attempts to treat these patients nonsurgically are generally met with frustration.

The choices of operative procedures are many. These include those that use the abdominal route, the vaginal route, or some combination thereof. For the abdominal approach a variety of procedures have been tried. These include fixation of the vaginal vault to the anterior abdominal wall, to the lumbar spine, to the sacral promontory, to various tendonous lines in the musculature of the true pelvis, and to the sacrospinous ligament. The anterior abdominal wall fixation increases the diameters of the pouch of Douglas and frequently adds to the risk of subsequent enterocele development, often creating a recurrence in short order. Fixation to the lumbar spine or the sacral promontory is often difficult to achieve directly and frequently requires the interposition of a different material. In the past, ox fascia lata, fascial aponeurosis from the patient, or inert materials such as Mersilene have been used. In such procedures it is important to cover the stent with peritoneum, thereby rendering it retroperitoneal to avoid troublesome adhesions and internal hernias at a future date. After such procedures the pouch of Douglas may still be large enough to allow an enterocele to develop. Fixation to various aspects of the pelvic wall or to the sacrospinous ligament has had encouraging degrees of success, the latter being the most successful. Using the sacrospinous ligament can frequently be accomplished vaginally. Randall and Nichols report excellent success with both abdominal and vaginal approaches. In 18 patients treated with fixation of the vaginal vault to the sacrospinous ligament via the vaginal route, all had successful outcomes.

Morley and DeLancey reported the results of 100 patients treated at the University of Michigan for vaginal vault prolapse or posthysterectomy enterocele with sacrospinous ligament suspension of the vaginal vault. Of 71 patients who were followed for 1 year or more, 64 (90%) had complete symptomatic relief, 10 had some asymptomatic relaxation of the vaginal walls, and 9 had either vaginal stenosis or stress incontinence. In addition, four patients developed cystoceles, and three had recurrent prolapse of the vagina. Other authors have reported equally encouraging results using this procedure.

Sze and Karram reviewed the literature on transvaginal vault prolapse repair in 1997. They compared the cumulative results for sacrospinus ligament fixation (*n* = 1062) and endopelvic fascia vault fixation (*n* = 322). Of the sacrosciatic ligament fixation group, 193 (18%) developed recurrent relaxation including 32 vault eversions, 81 anterior wall and 24 posterior wall prolapses, and 56 other or multiple defects. Of the endopelvic fascia fixation groups, 34 (11%) developed recurrent relaxation including 9 vault prolapses, 2 anterior and 11 posterior wall prolapses, and 12 other defects. Follow-up was from 1 to 12 years, and these authors concluded that the true efficacy of these procedures remains inconclusive.

Figure 20-16 depicts the fixation of the vaginal vault to the sacrospinous ligament and the direction of the vagina after the procedure. Miyazaki reports the use of an instrument, the Miya hook ligature carrier, to lessen the difficulty of placing a suture into the sacrospinous ligament. This is depicted in Figure 20-17. Some surgeons favor the use of this instrument in the performance of this procedure. Sharp has reported equally good results using an orthopedic instrument, the Shutt Suture Punch System, as an alternative to the Miya hook ligature carrier. Several special ligature carriers and auto-suturing devices have also been found useful. It is likely that other instruments will be developed for this purpose.

A variety of vaginal procedures have been designed. The best success, however, occurs in procedures in which adequate vaginal length is maintained and the vagina is positioned against the rectum nearly parallel to the horizontal. Thornton and Peters reported on 41 women who underwent repair of vaginal stumps, in which the vaginal approach was used with good, lasting success. Of these patients, 20 required a repair of an enterocele and a posterior repair, which especially detailed the attachment of the posterior wall of the vagina to the perirectal fascia and levator ani muscles. In addition, 21 patients underwent a repair of an enterocele with both an anterior and a posterior repair because a cystocele was believed to be a major part of their prolapse problem. Long-term follow-ups were effected, and the success rate was said to be excellent.

Richter and Albrich combined the repair of cystocele, rectocele, and enterocele where necessary with a unilateral or bilateral vaginal sacrospinal fixation procedure. They

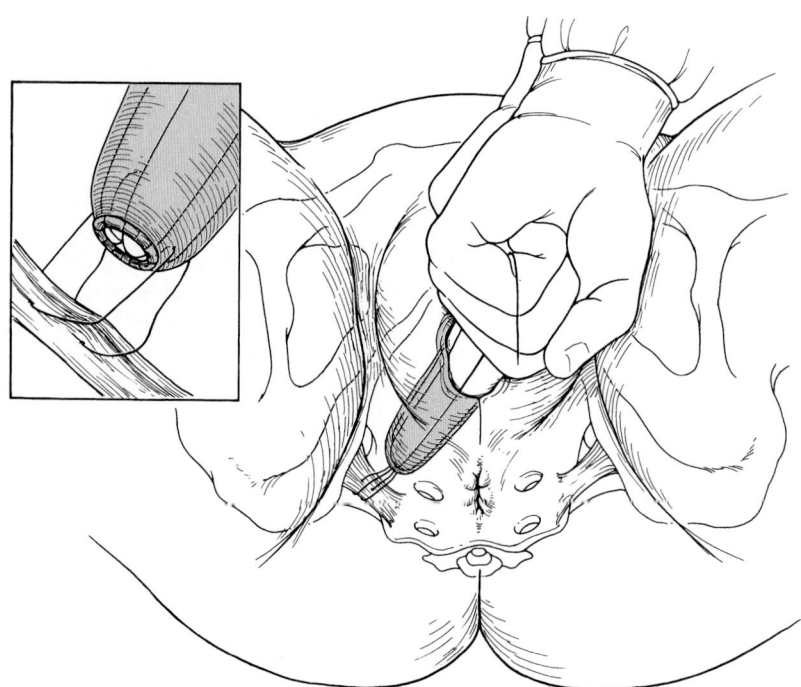

FIGURE 20-16 Sutures tied to bring the new vaginal apex into contact with the ligament and overlying muscle. Vaginal wall is advanced toward the sacrospinous ligament while tying sutures. A "suture bridge" is to be avoided. (Redrawn from Morley GW and DeLancey JO: Am J Obstet Gynecol 158:872, 1988.)

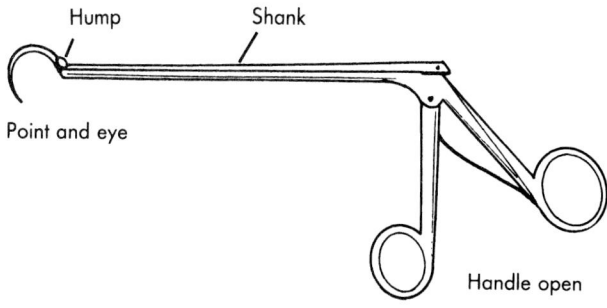

FIGURE 20-17 The Miya hook ligature carrier. (From Miyazaki FS: Obstet Gynecol 70:286, 1987.)

also stressed the importance of suturing the vagina in its physiologic position to the perirectal support tissue. The success in their group of 97 patients was also excellent, in that 61.7% of the patients had what were considered ideal results in long-term follow-up. There was a recurrence of cystocele in 14.8%, rectocele in 8.6%, and enterocele in 3.7%. Stress incontinence was reported in 3.7% of their patients and urgency incontinence in 2.5% with long-term follow-up. For operative procedures that fix the vaginal vault to an anterior structure (i.e., the anterior abdominal wall) an obliteration of the cul-de-sac must be carried out as part of the operative procedure to prevent enteroceles from forming.

An equally good technique for suspending the vaginal vault is the fixation of the vault to the sacrum. This generally requires the use of a stent, which can be a fascial strip taken from the patient or an inert mesh such as Mersilene. The stent is sutured to the upper vaginal vault and the opposite end to the ligamentum flavum of the sacral promintory or the anterior longitudinal ligament of the sacrum. Care must be taken to avoid the middle sacral artery and the plexus of veins in its vicinity. The stent should be made retroperitoneal by bringing the peritoneum in front of it. The procedure should also include an obliteration of the cul-de-sac. Snyder and Krantz reported on 147 patients undergoing abdominal sacral colpoplexy using a Dacron graft and reported good long-term results. Four patients experienced a graft erosion and one patient a recurrent prolapse. Other authors have reported similarly good outcomes.

Few studies have been performed to attempt to compare the efficacy of vaginal versus abdominal repair of vault prolapse. Benson et al. performed a randomized trial of bilateral sacrospinous vault suspensions and paravaginal repair (*n* = 48) and colposacral suspension and paravaginal repair (*n* = 40). Surgical effectiveness as judged by recurrent prolapse was optimal in 29% of the vaginal and 58% of the abdominal group and was unsatisfactory leading to reoperation in 33% of the vaginal and 16% of the abdominal group.

In older women who are no longer sexually active, and

particularly in those who have medical reasons to avoid a longer procedure, a Le Fort–type colpocleisis operation may be performed with excellent results.

Vaginal colpocleisis procedures for women who are elderly and are no longer sexually active are appropriate. It is extremely important to identify and repair enteroceles in such women, but this can readily be done as part of the procedure. Perineorrhaphy should always be performed as part of any procedure to repair a vaginal stump prolapse.

The question of continuing sexual activity after vaginal vault repairs is obviously an important one. With an adequate vaginal operation (with the exception of colpocleisis), intercourse is achievable in most patients who wish to maintain this activity.

Weber at al. studied sexual function in 81 women who were sexually active before undergoing surgery for either pelvic prolapse or urinary incontinence, or both. All remained sexually active after surgery, but dyspareunia was likely to occur if a combination of the Burch procedure and posterior colporrhaphy was performed.

FECAL INCONTINENCE

Fecal incontinence is one of the most devastating of all physical disabilities. Yet, because of the social embarrassment and psychologic impact, most patients fail to report their symptoms and many physicians do not ask. Therefore, the exact prevalence of this condition is unknown. Estimates range from 2% to 11% of community dwelling women older than 64 years of age. Over 30% of women reporting urinary incontinence also report fecal incontinence, known as dual incontinence.

Fecal incontinence is the inability to defer the elimination of stool or gas until there is a socially acceptable time and place to do so. Because maintaining continence is a complex physiologic process that requires a person's ability to perceive the type of fecal bolus, store or retain when necessary, and to excrete when desirable, the loss of that ability is equally as complex.

In the evaluation of fecal incontinence, it is important for the physician to understand the patient's symptoms, type of loss (i.e., flatus or stool), frequency of incontinence, and impact on the quality of the patient's life. Fecal incontinence affects each patient's life in a different manner. What may be acceptable for one patient may be intolerable to another. Evaluation and treatment should be directed by the severity of the patient's symptoms and the expected goals of therapy.

Physiology of Fecal Continence

Fecal continence requires normal stool consistency and volume, normal colonic transit time, a compliant rectum, innervation of the pelvic floor and anal sphincter, and the interplay between the puborectalis muscle, rectum, and anal sphincters. Loss of one or more of these abilities can lead to fecal incontinence.

As a bolus of stool or gas passes from the sigmoid colon to the rectal canal, receptors within the wall of the puborectalis sense the distention of the rectum. As long as the pressure in the anal canal is maintained at a higher level than the rectal pressure, continence is maintained. Anal canal pressure is dependent on a functional internal anal sphincter (IAS) and external anal sphincter (EAS). The IAS is a thickened continuation of the circular muscle of the colon and provides 75% to 85% of the resting tone of the anal canal. The IAS, under autonomic control, maintains the high pressure zone or continence zone and along with the EAS keeps the anal canal closed. The shape of the combined IAS and EAS is nearly cylindrical as it encircles the anal canal. The sphincter complex averages 18.3 mm in thickness and 2.8 cm in length in the midline anteriorly. Fifty-four percent of the anterior thickness is attributable to the IAS and the remainder to the EAS. The EAS provides the voluntary squeeze pressure that prevents incontinence with increasing rectal or abdominal pressure. The EAS is innervated by the hemorrhoidal branch of the pudendal nerve from the S_2-S_4 nerve roots. Contraction of the EAS, either voluntarily or through a spinal reflex, doubles the anal canal pressure.

The third muscular component of the sphincter complex is the puborectalis muscle (Figure 20-18). The puborectalis, part of the levator ani muscle complex, originates from the pubic bone on either side of the midline, passes beside the vagina and rectum, and fuses posteriorly behind the anorectal junction to form the U-shaped sling that cradles the rectum while also sending some fibers onto the walls of the anal canal. Unlike most other striated muscles, the puborectalis, like the EAS, maintains a constant muscle tone that is directly proportional to the volume of the rectal content and pressure, and relaxes at the time of defecation. Both the puborectalis and EAS contain a majority of type I or slow twitch muscle fibers, which are ideally suited to maintaining a constant contraction or tone. Each muscle group also contains a small proportion of type II or fast twitch fibers that allow for quick responses to rapid increases in intraabdominal pressure. The puborectalis is innervated by direct branches from S_3 and S_4 and, to a lesser degree, from the pudendal nerve. The constant contraction of the puborectalis creates a 90° angle between the rectum and anal canal. This angle, known as the anorectal angle, has been the source of much discussion and evaluation in determining its role in the maintenance of continence. Parks postulated that this angle creates a flap-valve effect that presses the anterior rectal wall down onto the upper anal canal and thereby prevents rectal contents from entering the anal canal when intraabdominal pressure is applied. The anterior rectal wall therefore acts as a plug. However, Bartolo found that when the anal sphincter was maximally stressed and the rectum was visualized radiographically, there was no contact between the rectal wall and anal canal. In addition,

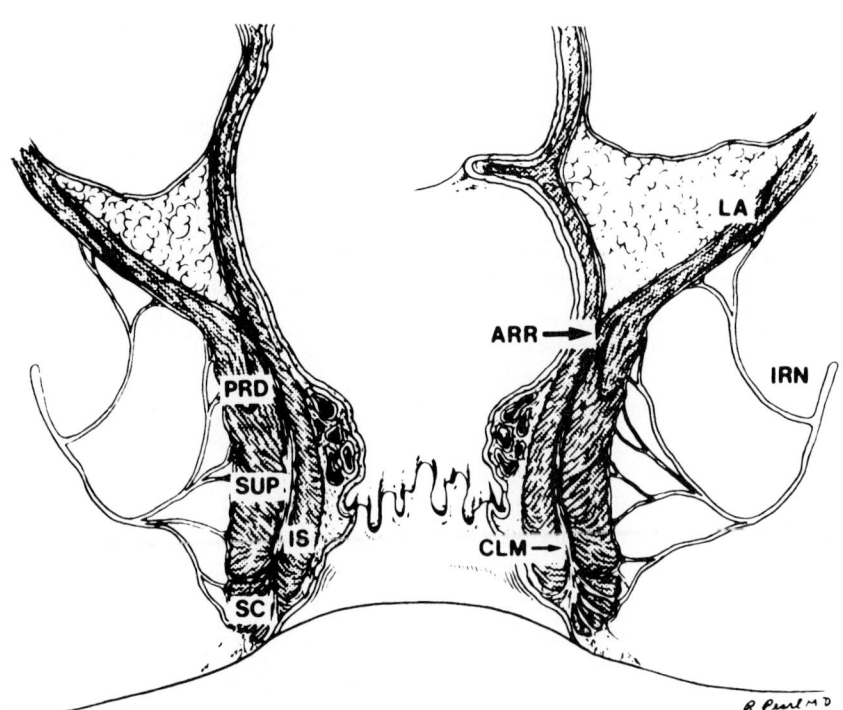

FIGURE 20-18 Coronal section of the anal canal and lower rectum. LA = levator ani muscles; ARR = level of anorectal ring; PRD = puborectalis/deep external sphincter complex; SC = subcutaneous external sphincter; CLM = conjoined longitudinal muscle; IRN = inferior rectal nerve. (From Pearl RK: Practical guide to anorectal testing, Smith L, editor, New York, 1995, Igula-Shoin.)

TABLE 20-2
Anal Incontinence: An Underrecognized, Undertreated Problem

Component	Function	Symptoms of Deficit
External anal sphincter	Provides emergency control for liquid stool and flatus	Fecal urgency; urge-related incontinence of liquid stool and flatus
Puborectalis	Maintains continence of solid stool	Incontinence of solid stool
Internal anal sphincter	Keeps anal canal closed at rest; allows sampling of stool content and enhances continence of liquid stool and flatus	Fecal soiling Incontinence of liquid stool and flatus
Anal sensation	Allows discrimination of gas, liquid, and solid stool Provides warning of pending incontinence	Fecal soiling Fecal leakage that is promptly halted by voluntary contraction or conscious detection
Colonic motility	Controls stool volume, consistency, and delivery rate to the rectum	Incontinence of liquid/loose stools during prolonged or severe diarrheal states
Rectal reservoir	Maintains adequate reservoir under low pressure	Incontinence of solid stool associated with sudden rectal distension Fecal urgency and urge-related incontinence

From Toglia M: Anal incontinence: An underrecognized, undertreated problem, The Female Patient 21:27, 1996.

surgeries that try to recreate this angle in hopes of restoring continence have not proven effective.

When a bolus of stool or gas is sensed in the rectum, the IAS has a reflex relaxation that allows for colonic contents to be sampled by the anal canal to distinguish solid, liquid, and gas forms of fecal material. After the sampling, the IAS contracts and the fecal material is pushed back into the rectum. The reflex, known as the rectoanal inhibitory reflex, or RAIR, is absent in patients with Hirschprung's disease. This reflex can also be inhibited by chronic dilation of the anus with fecal impaction leading to incontinence. If the impaction is cured, the reflex and anal tone can return to normal.

If the rectum has normal compliance and the person chooses to defer defecation, the IAS, EAS sphincters, and puborectalis remain contracted until the appropriate time to eliminate. As seen in Table 20-2, loss of any of these important components can lead to incontinence of flatus, liquid, or solid stool.

Etiology and Pathophysiology

There are many etiologies of fecal incontinence as seen in Table 20-3. One way to categorize the causes of fecal incontinence is to separate the initial etiology into those that start outside the pelvis with a normal pelvic floor from those causes that start with an abnormal pelvic floor. Etiologies that start outside the pelvis include all of the pathologies that cause diarrhea or increased intestinal motility, overflow incontinence from fecal impaction, and rectal neoplasms. Known or diagnosable neurologic conditions such as multiple sclerosis, diabetic neuropathy,

TABLE 20-3
Common Causes of Fecal Incontinence

Obstetric Injury
  Disruption of internal anal sphincter
  Disruption of external anal sphincter
  Pelvic floor denervation

Trauma
  Pelvic fracture
  Accidental injury
  Anorectal surgery
  Rectovaginal fistula

Diarrheal States
  Irritable bowel
  Infectious diarrhea
  Inflammatory bowel disease
  Short-gut syndrome
  Laxative abuse
  Radiation enteritis

Rectal Neoplasia

Rectal Prolapse

Rectocele

Overflow
  Impaction
  Encopresis

Neurologic Disease
  Congenital anomalies (i.e., myelomeningocele)
  Multiple sclerosis
  Diabetic neuropathy
  Neoplasms or injury of brain, spinal cord, cauda equina
  Pudendal neuropathy (childbirth, chronic straining, perineal descent)

Congenital Anomalies of Anorectum/Pelvis

trauma, or neoplasms in the spinal cord or cauda equina initially begin as pathologies outside of the pelvis and the pelvic floor is presumed normal. As these neuropathies progress, there is damage to the pelvic floor musculature or in rectal sensation, resulting in fecal incontinence.

Fecal incontinence secondary to an abnormal pelvic floor is due to congenital anorectal malformations, surgery, obstetric injury, aging, or pelvic floor denervation without a known neurologic disease. Historically, incontinence secondary to denervation has been designated as idiopathic and represents 80% of patients with fecal incontinence. Pelvic floor denervation has been studied extensively in the last 10 years in women with urinary and fecal incontinence as well as pelvic organ prolapse. Denervation may be secondary to vaginal delivery, chronic straining with constipation, rectal prolapse, or descending perineal syndrome. Histologic studies of the EAS and puborectalis show fibrosis, scarring, and fiber-type grouping consistent with nerve damage and reinervation in women with idiopathic fecal incontinence. Electromyographic studies (EMG) have demonstrated reinnervation of the pelvic floor with increased fiber density and prolongation of nerve conduction on pudendal terminal motor latency studies.

In women, a common cause of fecal incontinence is damage to the anal sphincters at the time of vaginal delivery with or without neuronal injury. This type of incontinence is often referred to as anal incontinence. Damage can occur by mechanical disruption or separation of the internal anal sphincter (IAS) and/or external anal sphincter (EAS) or by damage to the muscle innervation by stretching or crushing the pudendal and pelvic nerves. Sultan showed that 13% of primiparas and 23% of multiparas developed fecal incontinence or fecal urgency 6 weeks postpartum. By anal ultrasound, all but one of the women had evidence of anal sphincter disruption. The incidence of occult external anal sphincter disruption after vaginal delivery determined by endoanal ultrasound ranges from 11% to 35%. The chance of muscular injury is increased with midline episiotomy, instrumented delivery, and vaginal delivery of larger infants. Other risk factors include increasing maternal age, prolonged second stage (greater than 2 hours), and clinically diagnosed sphincter laceration at the time of delivery. The first vaginal delivery appears to have the greatest impact on pelvic floor function and risk of EAS disruption, but subsequent deliveries can increase the risk of permanent damage, especially in women with transient symptoms of fecal incontinence after their first delivery. Not all risk factors are known and not all women are susceptible to pelvic floor and sphincter damage with vaginal delivery.

Detection of Fecal Incontinence

For fecal incontinence, even more than urinary incontinence, if the physician does not ask, the patient will not volunteer the information. Ideally, a question such as,

"How often do you leak gas, liquid, or solid stool?" should be placed on the standard office intake questionnaire. Several reports have shown that twice as many patients complain of fecal or flatual incontinence when given written questionnaires rather than answering verbal questioning.

Since approximately one in ten women will develop some fecal incontinence or fecal urgency after one vaginal delivery, it is especially important to incorporate open-ended questions concerning flatal or fecal incontinence as part of the 6-week postpartum visit. In addition, as women age, the chances of developing fecal incontinence increase, so it is also important to target older women for questioning.

Evaluation

Assessment of the patient with fecal incontinence must include a thorough history because the etiology of the problem may be the single most important criterion of therapy.

The history should include onset, duration, severity of the condition, impact on the patient's daily activities, pad use, frequency of bowel movements, consistency of bowel movements, use of laxatives, fiber intake, and dietary habits. Specific questions concerning diarrhea, amount of flatus, the average number of stools per day, passage of mucus, and bloating should be asked. Physicians and patients define normal bowel function differently. Diarrhea may mean frequent bowel movements to one person but loose and watery bowel movements to another. It is best to have the patient quantitate the number of bowel movements and incontinent episodes and describe the stool consistency. A diary of bowel habits and incontinent episodes can be useful, and several standardized classification systems are used. Table 20-4 gives a frequently used scoring system developed by Jorge and Wexner. The patient circles the appropriate number on each line of the scale. The numbers are then added. A perfect score or 0 indicates no incontinence and a score of 20 indicates complete incontinence. The value of this scale is that it can be utilized before and after treatment to determine efficacy of the intervention. A standardized questionnaire should be used whenever possible to direct diagnosis and treatment and to assess treatment success.

The history should also identify specific complaints such as feelings of incomplete emptying, straining with bowel movements, fecal urgency, pain with defecation, and insensible loss of stool. It is important to determine if the patient senses the need to have a bowel movement or if she is unaware that she needs to defecate, but finds stool in her undergarments. A sensory impairment or hygiene problem is implied when stool leakage occurs without warning. If the patient is aware of impending incontinence, but cannot prevent the passage of stool, a motor impairment is suggested. Patients may have pseudoincon-

TABLE 20-4
Continence Grading Scale

Type of Incontinence	Frequency				
	Never	Rarely	Some-times	Usually	Always
Solid	0	1	2	3	4
Liquid	0	1	2	3	4
Gas	0	1	2	3	4
Wears pad	0	1	2	3	4
Lifestyle alteration	0	1	2	3	4

From Jorge JM, Wexmer SD: Etiology and management of fecal incontinence, Dis Colon Rectum 36:77, 1993.

0 = perfect.
20 = complete incontinence.
Never = 0 (never).
Rarely = <1/month.
Sometimes = <1/week, ≥1/month.
Usually = <1/day, ≥1/week.
Always = ≥1/day.

The continence score is determined by adding points from the above table, which takes into account the type and frequency of incontinence and the extent to which it alters the patient's life.

tinence secondary to soiling from prolapsing hemorrhoids or rectovaginal or anovaginal fistulas.

The review of systems should include abdominal pain or cramping, lower back or pelvic pain, any changes in pelvic or lower extremity sensation, or changes in sexual response. Changes in the neurologic function of the pelvis or lower extremities or a history of an acute onset of fecal incontinence should direct the physician to rule out a neurologic disease such as multiple sclerosis or a neoplasm of the brain or lumbar/sacral spinal cord.

Past medical history should include detailed history of vaginal deliveries, including birth weights, length of second stage, episiotomies or lacerations, and use of forceps. Any breakdown or complications of episiotomy healing should be noted. Past history of abdominal and pelvic surgeries or trauma to the back or pelvis should be reviewed. Details and operative reports of any anal dilatations, anal sphincterotomy, hemorrhoidectomy, rectovaginal fistula repairs, or posterior colporrhaphy should be obtained. Patients should also be questioned about previous evaluations and results of flexible sigmoidoscopy, colonoscopy, and/or barium enemas. Any family history of colon cancer, inflammatory bowel disease, or familial polyposis should be elicited.

Many medications also affect bowel function. The patient should not only be asked about laxatives and bowel stimulants, but a complete list of all prescription and over-the-counter medications should be reviewed. Many medications, including anticholinergics, antidepres-

sants, iron, narcotics, nonsteroidals, and pseudoephedrine, can cause chronic constipation that may contribute to overflow incontinence or pelvic floor neuropathy secondary to straining.

Physical Examination

Undergarments or pads should be inspected for stool, mucus, blood, or pus. If material is found, the patient should be asked if this is her normal leakage. Physical examination begins with inspection of the perineum and anal region. Pruritus ani, or discoloration and irritation of the perianal skin, is commonly seen with fecal incontinence of liquid stool and chronic diarrhea. Perianal skin creases or folds should completely encircle the anus. Note the presence of protruding tissue around or from the anus and determine if there are external hemorrhoids or mucosal or full-thickness rectal wall prolapse. The dovetail sign or loss of anterior perineal folds indicates a defect in the external anal sphincter (EAS) or chronic third-degree laceration (Figure 20-19). Previous episiotomy, laceration, or surgical scars should be noted. The size of the genital hiatus and the presence of genital prolapse should be assessed as an indicator of pelvic floor neuromuscular function. The innervation of the EAS can be grossly tested by eliciting the clitoral-anal or bulbocavernosis reflex. Using a cotton swab, a gentle, quick touch beside the clitoris or over the bulbocavernosis muscle should elicit a contraction of the EAS. If intact, the reflex implies that the pudendal nerve afferents and the rectal or external hemorrhoidal branch of the pudendal efferent nerves are functional. Unlike males, who should always exhibit this reflex, about 10% of women lack this reflex naturally. However, if absent, and in the presence of fecal incontinence, further neurologic testing is indicated. Sensation in the S_2-S_4 dermatomes should be screened by dull and pinprick discrimination when touching the perineum. Loss of sensation should direct the clinician to further neurologic or radiologic assessment of the nervous system.

Next, the patient should be asked to squeeze as if trying to not pass gas. Inspection of the perianal folds should be evaluated for a concentric contraction and some upward movement of the perineal body as she contracts the EAS and levator ani. Substitution with contraction of the buttocks, upper thighs, or abdomen should be noted. The patient should then be asked to bear down as if trying to have a bowel movement. She should be reassured that it is expected she may pass flatus during this part of the examination. The degree of perineal descent and any prolapse of the vagina, pelvic viscera, or rectum should be noted. If there appears to be any pelvic organ prolapse, the examination should be performed in the standing position or after straining on a commode to maximize the prolapse.

Rectal examination is used to assess both resting and squeeze tone of the anal canal. The resting tone of the anal

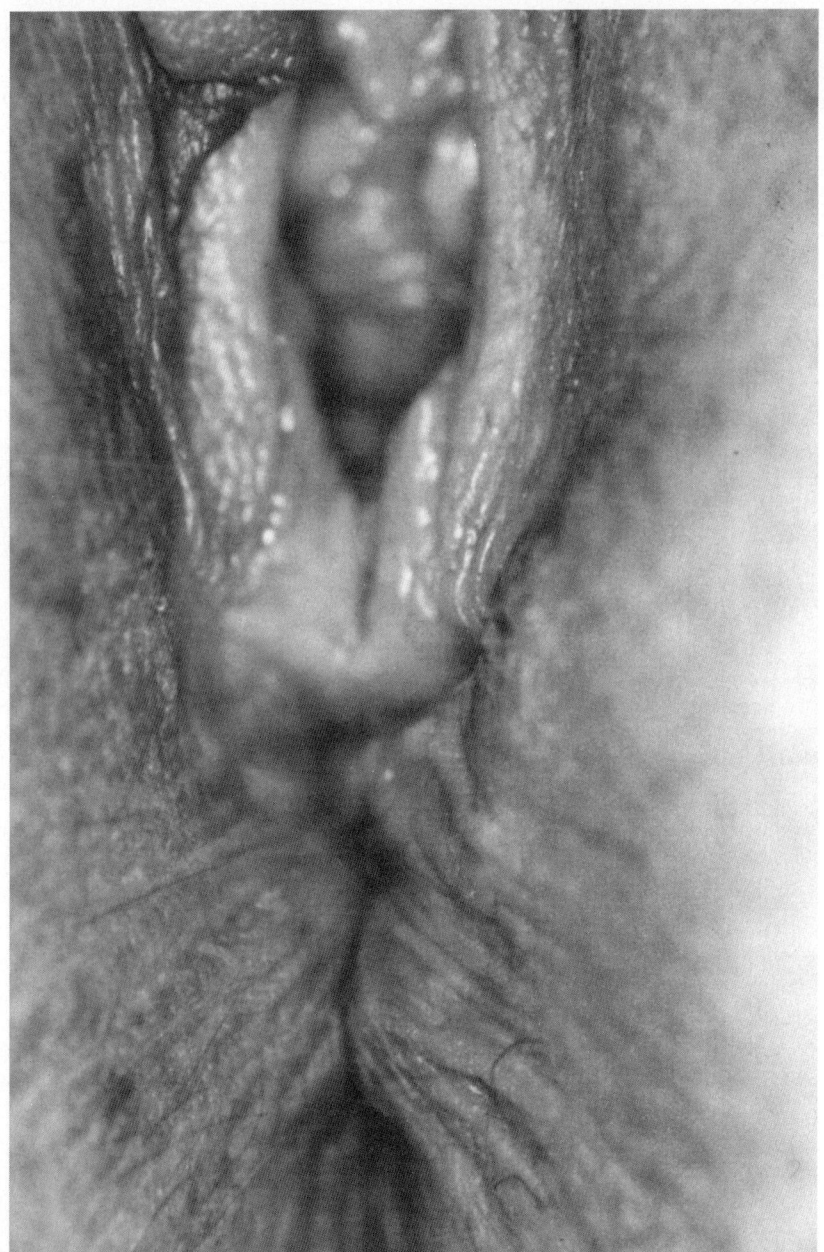

FIGURE 20-19 Perineum with chronic laceration of external anal sphincter (EAS). Inspection of the perineum shows the classic "dovetail" sign with loss of the anal skin creases anteriorly due to a chronic third-degree laceration of the EAS. Normally, with an intact sphincter, the skin creases are arranged radially around the anus. (From Atlas of clinical gynecology, Stenchever MA and Benson JT, editors, New York, 2000, McGraw-Hill.)

canal is an indicator of internal anal sphincter (IAS) function. When asked to squeeze, a circumferential contraction and tightening should be felt. An upward movement of the rectum and posterior compartment of the pelvis should be seen as the levator ani muscles contract. As these muscles also play an important role in anal continence, palpation of the levators for strength and symmetry should be performed by palpating the muscles on each side of the vagina at the introitus.

In addition to assessing rectal tone, the anal canal and rectum should be palpated for masses and a dilated rectum or the presence of stool in the rectal vault. A chronically distended rectum, either with stool, a tumor, or an intussusepting bowel, will disrupt the normal rectoanal inhibitory reflex that allows the highly sensitive anal canal to sample the stool contents by relaxing the IAS while at the same time contracting the EAS to prevent incontinence. If this reflex is suppressed, the anal canal remains dilated, the EAS fatigues, and incontinence will occur.

While doing the rectal examination, the patient is also asked to strain to diagnose the presence of a rectocele, enterocele, rectal prolapse, or bowel intussusception. With a finger in the rectum the integrity of the rectovaginal septum, posterior vaginal wall, and perineal body can be assessed by palpating through the vagina via bimanual examination.

Testing

Clinical diagnosis based on physical examination and history alone will be accurate in a majority of patients. However, further evaluation, including radiologic and physiologic tests, have been shown in a prospective study at a tertiary colorectal referral clinic to alter the final diagnosis of the cause of fecal incontinence in 19% of cases. Which tests to consider should be based on history and physical examination, prior treatment, and proposed therapy. The algorithm outlined in Figure 20-20 recommends further evaluation based on history and the rectal tone. Normal rectal tone directs the clinician away from anal incontinence and toward a metabolic or colonic etiology. Metabolic tests including thyroid stimulating hormone and glucose should be checked.

Poor resting tone on rectal examination directs the clinician to a neuromuscular etiology. A normal resting tone, with an anterior sphincter defect, indicates a chronic third-degree laceration of the EAS.

Evaluation or further testing is not only performed for diagnostic purposes, but also to determine which nonsurgical and surgical therapies are most likely to benefit the patient. In addition, certain tests, such as anal manometry or a sphincter ultrasound, can be used for baseline assessment for which post-treatment assessment or function can be compared. Whenever the patient's history does not match her physical examination, further testing should be considered. In addition, if the patient has had prior surgery, or has other pelvic floor dysfunction, testing before treatment, especially surgical, may help direct care. It is important to remember that the patient may have more than one etiology or pathology contributing to her fecal incontinence such as pudendal neuropathy and an anal sphincter defect or irritable bowel in combination with a weakened pelvic floor (Table 20-5).

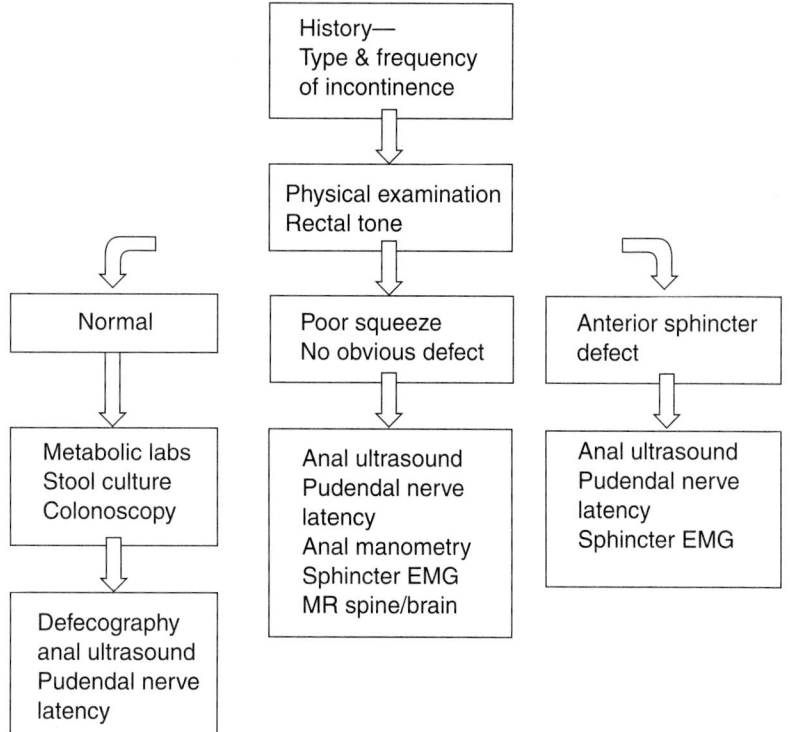

FIGURE 20-20 Evaluation of fecal incontinence. A detailed history differentiates incontinence of gas, liquid, or solid stool, along with frequency, onset, and effect on the patient's quality of life. The history should assess the possibility of Crohn's disease, ulcerative colitis, irritable bowel syndrome, radiation to the pelvis, neurologic diseases such as multiple sclerosis, and prior anorectal surgeries. A detailed obstetric history should include type of delivery, weight of largest infant, length of second stage, episiotomy or lacerations, and use of forceps or vacuum extraction. Rectal examination should assess resting and squeeze tone, presence of a rectocele or rectal mass, and fecal impaction. Inspection of the rectum and vagina should evaluate for a rectovaginal fistula, prolapsing hemorrhoids, or rectal prolapse. Further evaluation, including radiologic and physiologic tests, have been shown in a prospective study at a tertiary colorectal referral clinic to alter the final diagnosis of the cause of fecal incontinence in 19% of the cases. EMG, electromyography; MRI, magnetic resonance imaging. Modified from Atlas of clinical gynecology, Stenchever MA and Benson JT, editors, New York, 2000, McGraw-Hill.

TABLE 20-5
Tests of Anorectal Function for Patients with Fecal Incontinence

Test	Measures	Indication
Anal Manometry	Resting anal pressures Maximum squeeze pressure Rectoanal inhibitory reflex Rectal sensation	Low resting and squeeze pressure on rectal exam Prior radiation Fecal urgency Fecal impaction
Single Fiber EMG	Fiber density Muscle activity	Deinnervation Reinnervation injury Map EAS defect
Pudendal Nerve Motor Latency	Speed of signal along pudendal nerve	Pudendal nerve damage from childbirth or straining Perineal descent
Endoscopic Ultrasound	IAS and EAS defect	Obstetric or traumatic sphincter injuries
Defecating Proctogram	Movement of pelvic floor Pelvic floor defects	Perineal descent Posterior compartment deficits

Diagnostic Procedures

Colonoscopy

A colonoscopy is indicated for any patient with chronic diarrhea to evaluate for inflammatory bowel disease and infectious diarrhea.

Transanal Ultrasound

Transanal ultrasound has significantly enhanced the ability to delineate defects of both the internal (IAS) and external (EAS) sphincters. The integrity, thickness, and length of the IAS and EAS can be determined. The internal sphincter is visible as a hypoechoic circle, and the EAS is seen as a hyperechoic circle (Figure 20-21). Transanal ultrasound is most useful in evaluation of patients for chronic third-degree lacerations or occult sphincter tears. Knowing the boundaries of the sphincter defect and if both the EAS and IAS are disrupted can direct the surgeon at time of anal sphincteroplasty. Similar information can be obtained from electromyography of the EAS when used to map the sphincter defect. In general, transanal ultrasound is less painful and better tolerated by the patient.

Anal Manometry

Anal manometry is a commonly used test that objectively assesses the resistance to spontaneous defecation provided by the anorectal sphincter mechanism and the sensory capabilities of the rectum to provide a feeling of imminent defecation. Anal manometry is helpful for patients who have had prior surgery to the anorectal canal or radiation therapy that could have altered the rectal storage function. In patients who, by history, report a normal sensation to defecate, anal manometry has been largely replaced by transanal ultrasound and pudendal nerve terminal motor latencies or sphincter EMG alone. Although these studies do not give information on rectal function, they are more accurate in assessing the neuromuscular function of the anal sphincters.

Anal manometry uses a rectal balloon to assess rectal sensation, rectal compliance, the rectoanal inhibitory reflex (RAIR), and maximal tolerable rectal volume (Figure 20-22). The RAIR is a reflex response to increased pressure in the rectum from gas or stool. Normally, the IAS relaxes to allow a sampling of the rectal contents by the anal canal to determine if the contents are gas or stool and whether it is an appropriate time to defecate or pass flatus. At the same time, the EAS squeezes to prevent incontinence.

In addition to rectal function, resting and squeeze pressures in the anal canal are obtained by pulling a perfusion catheter with radial ports (4 or 8) through the anal canal. The IAS contributes 80% of the resting pressure. Voluntary contraction of the EAS should double the resting pressure (Figure 20-23). While objective documentation is useful for diagnosis or preoperative baseline, normal resting and squeeze pressures can be accurately assessed on rectal examination by most experienced clinicians.

Electromyography

Electromyography (EMG) is used for mapping of the EAS defect and for determining the presence and degree of neuropathy and denervation and reinvation. EMG evaluates the bioelectrical action potentials that are generated by depolarization of skeletal striated muscle. EMG evaluation consists of systematic examination of spontaneous activity, recruitment patterns, and the waveform of the motor unit action potentials (MUAP).

Performance and interpretation of EAS electromyography requires special training and experience. A needle electrode is inserted into the skeletal muscle of the EAS.

A
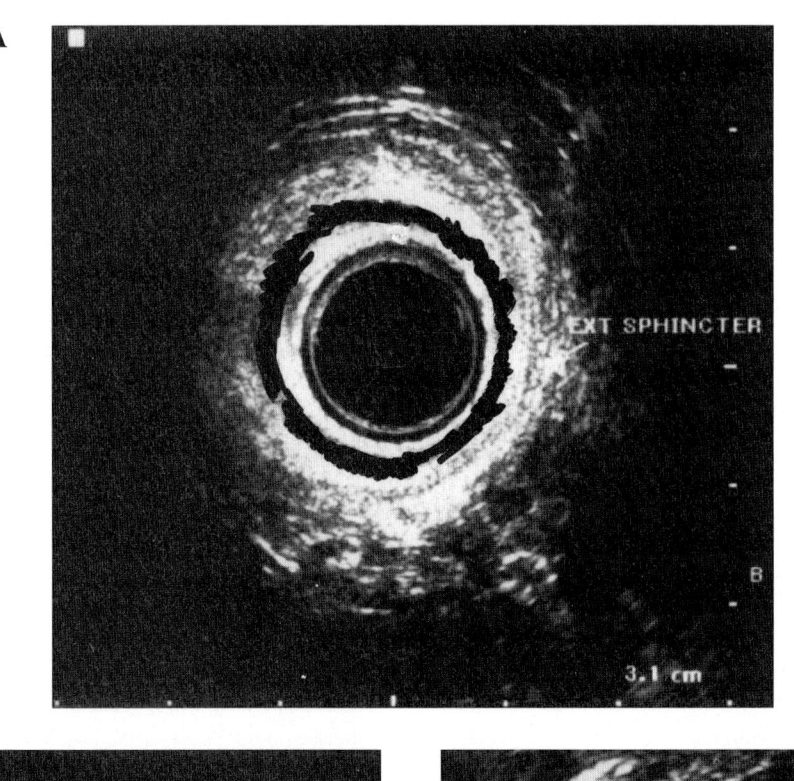

B
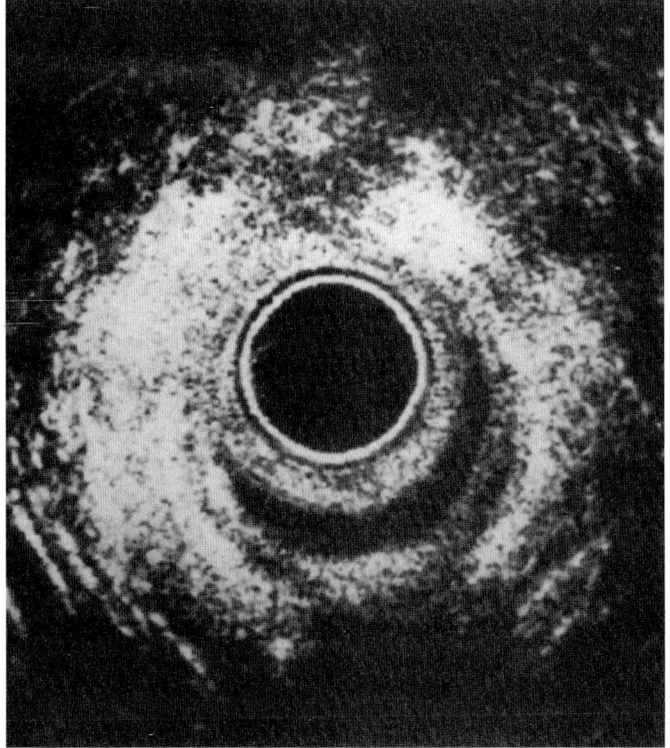

C
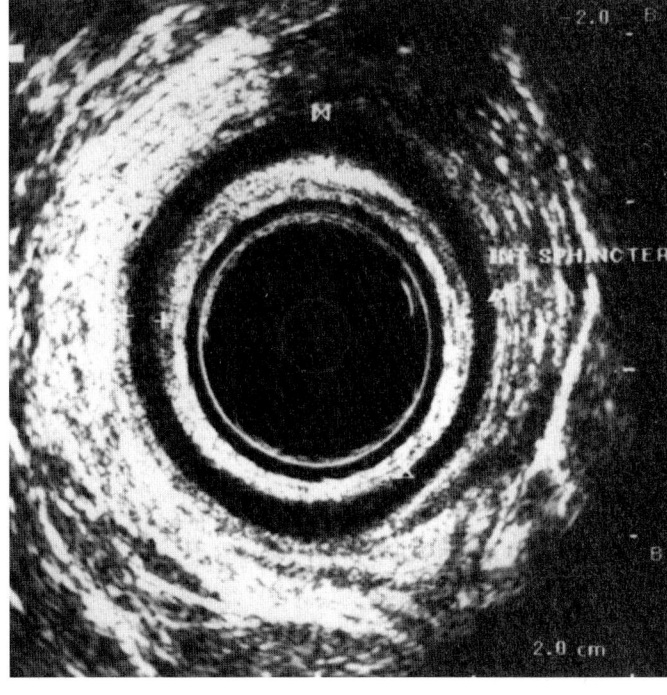

FIGURE 20-21   Anal ultrasound. **A.** Anal ultrasound has significantly enhanced the ability to delineate defects of the internal and external anal sphincters. The internal anal sphincter (IAS) is visible as a hypoechoic circle, and the external anal sphincter (EAS) is seen as a hyperechoic circle. Scarred areas have a homogeneous, gray appearance. Both IAS and EAS are intact. **B.** With the patient supine, a defect in the AIS from 3 o'clock to 9 o'clock and a defect at 12 o'clock in the EAS is shown. **C.** Again, with the vagina at the 12 o'clock position, there is an intact IAS and defect in the EAS. (From Atlas of clinical gynecology, Stenchever MA and Benson JT, editors, New York, 2000, McGraw-Hill.)

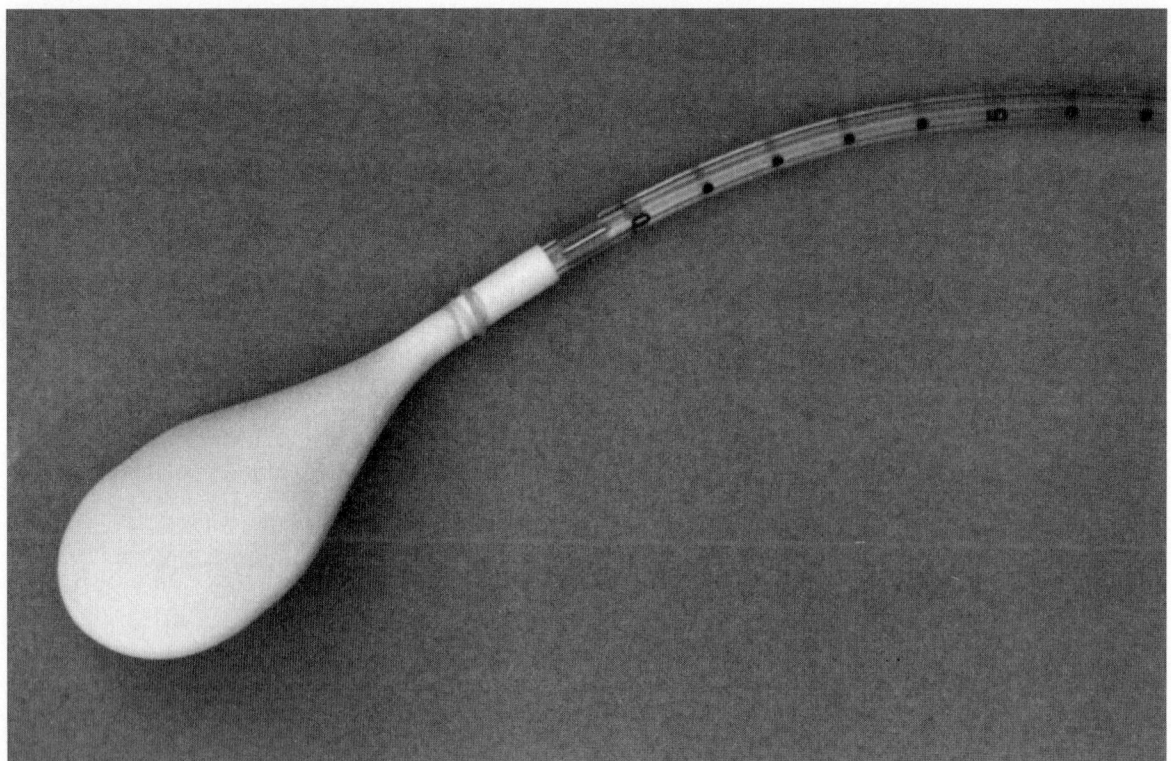

FIGURE 20-22 Anal manometer, a four-channel perfusion catheter with balloon tip. There are many different types and methods for performing anal manometry. A balloon or probe is inserted into the rectum and a pressure transducer relays information to a recorder or computer. Important manometric parameters include sphincter length, resting and squeeze pressures, rectal sensation, and the presence of the anorectal inhibitory reflex (RAIR). The balloon is placed in the rectum and inflated by 10 cc increments to determine rectal sensation and compliance. The presence of the RAIR is determined with balloon inflation and seeing the IAS relax and the EAS contract to allow for the "sampling" of rectal contents. The four radical ports are perfused with sterile water, and resting and squeeze pressures around the anal canal are measured at centimeter intervals along the anal canal. The catheter can be pulled at a constant rate to determine the length of the sphincter and "high pressure" or incontinence zone.

First, spontaneous activity is heard and seen. Next, the patient voluntarily squeezes her pelvic floor and recruitment activity is recorded. Straining should decrease activity and coughing should increase recruitment. The final step in analysis is evaluation of the MUAP waveform. Following nerve damage, as seen with a vaginal delivery, reinveration of the muscle fibers leads to a single motor unit innervating multiple muscle fibers. On single-fiber EMG the MUAPs have larger amplitudes, longer duration, and more phases or crossings of the baseline.

Pudendal Nerve Terminal Motor Latencies (PNTML)

Nerve conduction studies measure the time from stimulation of a nerve to a response in the muscle it innervates The PNTML is determined by using a glove-mounted electrode known as a St. Mark's pudendal electrode, connected to a pulsed stimulus generator and, with the examiner's index finger in the vagina or anus, the pudendal nerve is stimulated at the ischial spine.

The latent period between the pudendal nerve stimula-

tion and the electromechanical response of the muscle is measured. Normal PNTML is 2.0 + 0.2 ms. A normal PNTML is the measurement of the fastest response of the pudendal nerve and does not necessarily mean the entire nerve is normal (Figure 20-24). Prolonged PNTMLs have been found in patients with idiopathic fecal incontinence and in patients with rectal prolapse and may be predictive of continence following surgical repair.

PNTML measurement is particularly important in suspected neurogenic incontinence and prior to sphincter repair. PNTML has been found to be the most sensitive predictor of functional outcome of overlapping EAS repairs (Table 20-6). Gilland and Wexner found in reviewing 100 patients at a median of 24 months after surgery that pudendal neuropathy was the only significant predictor of surgical success. Neither patient age, parity, prior sphincteroplasty, cause or duration of incontinence, extent of electromyographic damage, size of the endoanal ultrasound defect, or pressures on anal manometry successfully predicted postoperative continence. However, 62% of 59 patients with bilaterally normal pudendal nerve terminal latencies had a successful outcome compared with 1 of 12 patients with unilateral or bilateral prolonged pudendal

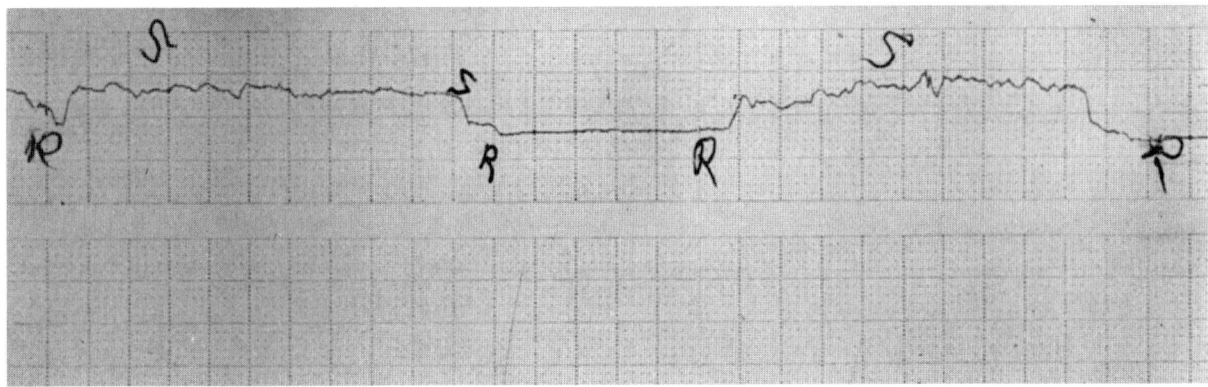

FIGURE 20-23 A single-channel recording of the resting pressure of the anal canal (R) and the squeeze pressure (S). The IAS contributes 80% of the resting pressure. Voluntary contraction or squeezing of the EAS should double the resting pressure.

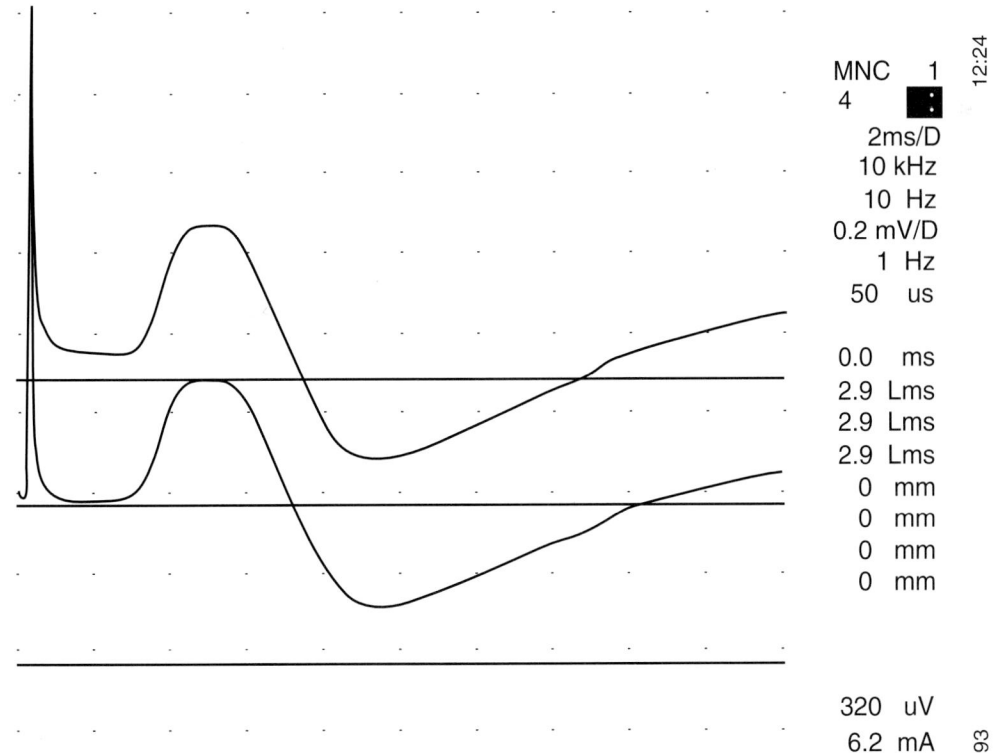

MNC 1
4
2ms/D
10 kHz
10 Hz
0.2 mV/D
1 Hz
50 us

0.0 ms
2.9 Lms
2.9 Lms
2.9 Lms
0 mm
0 mm
0 mm
0 mm

320 uV
6.2 mA

FIGURE 20-24 Pudendal nerve terminal motor latencies (PNTML). Normal bilateral PNTML have been shown to be 2.0 + 0.2 ms. The latency response is measured from the onset of the stimulus to the onset of the response in the external anal sphincter. A normal PNTML is the measurement of the fastest response of the pudendal nerve and does not necessarily mean the entire nerve is normal. Neither does an abnormal latency indicate abnormal muscle function. A damaged nerve can heal and reinnervate the muscle, and although the PNTML may be slightly prolonged, the muscle functions normally. (From Atlas of clinical gynecology, Stenchever MA and Benson JT, editors, New York, 2000, McGraw-Hill.)

nerve terminal motor latencies (<0.01). The high failure rate seen with prolonged PNTML may occur for several reasons. First, prolongation of the PNTMLs is associated with increased mean fiber density of the EAS, resulting in a less efficient sphincter. Second, as the pudendal nerves also convey sensory nerve fibers from the levator muscles, the sensation of rectal distention may be diminished. Loss of rectal sensation leads to rectal distention and decreased anal resting tone leading to incontinence.

Defecography

Dynamic cystoproctography or defecography is an imaging technique that has been widely used in the evaluation of anorectal function and anatomy, dating back to the mid-1960s. Defecography may be used as an adjunct to physical examination in patients with chronic constipation and pelvic floor defects or hernias that may be contributing to their fecal incontinence. Intussusception or rectal prolapse

TABLE 20-6
Influence of Pudendal Neuropathy on Outcome After Sphincteroplasty

| | | | % Success | | |
Author	Institution	No. of Patients	Patients with Neuropathy	Patients without Neuropathy	P Value
Laurberg et al., 1988	St. Marks	19	80	11	<0.05
Wexner et al., 1991	Cleveland Clinic, Florida	16	92	50	ns
Engel et al., 1994	St. Marks	55	not recorded	not recorded	ns
Simmang et al., 1994	Washington University	14	100	67	ns
Londono-Schimmer et al., 1994	St. Marks	94	55	30	<0.001
Sitzler and Thompson, 1996	St. Marks	31	67	63	ns
Felt-Bersma et al., 1996	Vrije University	18	not recorded	not recorded	ns
Sangwan et al., 1996	Lahey Clinic	15	100	14	<0.005
Gilliland et al., 1998	Cleveland Clinic, Florida	100	63	10	<0.01

From Gilliland R, Altomare DF, Moviera H, et al: Pudendal neuropathy is predictive of failure following anterior overlapping sphincteroplasty, Dis Colon Rectum 41:1516, 1998.

can be seen on defecography along with rectoceles that do not empty at the time of defecation. Stool retained in the rectocele can cause chronic distention of the rectum and loss of rectal sensation. The loss of rectal sensation leads to chronic constipation or impaction, causing further neuromuscular damage to the pelvic floor and ultimately fecal incontinence. Perineal descent and the anorectal angle can be objectively measured using defecography.

Magnetic Resonance Imaging of the Anal Sphincters

Magnetic resonance imaging (MRI) of the anal sphincters has the ability to evaluate both muscular and connective tissue supports of the pelvis. Recent advances in MRI technologies using the endoanal cil, rapid sequencing, and cinematic display have replaced defecography in evaluation of the pelvic floor and defecation disorders in a few centers. Muscular defects along with pelvic organ prolapse and perineal descent can be assessed. Specialized dynamic MRI may replace defecography and transanal ultrasound in the future.

Transit Study

A transit study is used to evaluate colonic motility and is most often used in the evaluation of chronic constipation. For patients where fecal impaction or overflow incontinence is high on the differential, a transit study may be indicated. There are numerous variations of the study. The patient ingests a Sitzmark capsule containing 20 or 25 radio-opaque rings. She does not take any laxatives or bowel stimulants. Five days after taking the capsule, an abdominal flat plate is obtained. Normally, 80% of the capsules should have been passed. Diffuse or global colon dys-

function is indicated if the rings are dispersed throughout the colon or segmental abnormalities can be seen if the rings are clustered in one area or trapped in a rectocele.

Treatment

Treatment of fecal incontinence includes medications, biofeedback, electrical stimulation, and surgery. Obstructive devices, including transanal plugs, have been marketed but are not widely used.

Fecal incontinence should, obviously, be treated based on diagnosis as in medications or surgery for inflammatory bowel disease or surgery for a neoplasm of the cauda equina. For patients with fecal incontinence associated with liquid or watery stools, dietary modifications and medications are the first line of therapy. Increasing dietary fiber with diet changes or bulking agents or fiber supplements such as methyl cellulose or psyllium helps to increase stool size. A larger more formed stool may improve rectal sensation and emptying. To slow intestinal transit and allow for increased water absorption, several medications (Table 20-7) are available. For some patients, a daily cleansing of the rectum with an enema allows for several hours of freedom from their incontinence.

Biofeedback

For fecal incontinence, like urinary incontinence, biofeedback requires a motivated patient, a feedback device, and a planned exercise program. Although the patient may not perceive normal sensation or be able to contract her pelvic floor voluntarily, she must be neurologically intact in order to benefit from biofeedback. No correlation has been seen with premanometry testing as long as some neuro-

TABLE 20-7
Medications for Treatment of Diarrhea

Drug	Dosage	Mechanism of Action
Loperamide	2 mg TID or 4 mg followed by 2 mg after loose BM Max 16 mg/day	Inhibits circular and longitudinal muscle contraction
Diphenoxylate with atropine	10 mg QID	Direct action of circular smooth muscle to decrease peristalis
Hyoscyamind sulfate	375 mg	Anticholinergic
Alosetron	1 mg BID	5 HT$_3$ receptor antagonist
Cholestyramine	4 mg pack qd or BID	Binds bile acids after cholecystectomy

muscular function is present. About 60% to 70% of patients with fecal incontinence secondary to an abnormal pelvic floor will have a 90% reduction in incontinence.

Biofeedback of any type is founded on the patient hearing, seeing, or sensing a response from a planned exercise. A measuring device, either electrode or pressure transducer, is used transvaginally or transanally to record and give feedback to the patient on how she is squeezing the pelvic floor. She then uses this feedback to increase or lengthen the pelvic floor contraction. If the patient has incontinence secondary to a sensory deficit in the rectum, rectal balloons can be used to "retrain" the patient to perceive rectal distention while, at the same time, squeezing her external sphincter in response to rectal distention. The patient can be taught by a physical therapist who not only provides encouragement but also instructs on proper technique. Although initially labor intensive, biofeedback has no side effects or morbidity and can be used in conjunction with other treatment modalities, including surgery. In addition, for patients with urinary and fecal incontinence, a single therapy may improve both conditions.

Electrical Stimulation Therapy

Functional electrical stimulation therapy has been shown to improve fecal incontinence in patients with a weakened pelvic floor and who are unable to contract their EAS or puborectalis on command. Because of the expense, electrical stimulation is generally reserved for patients who are unable to respond to traditional biofeedback protocols. Both transvaginal and transrectal probes are available. Most protocols recommend high-frequency stimulation at a maximum tolerable stimulation of 50 mHz for 15 to 20 minutes twice a day. Response to therapy is usually seen in 6 weeks with maximum improvement by 12 weeks.

Preliminary reports indicate that using sacral nerve stimulation with implantable electrodes may provide an additional treatment modality for patients with fecal incontinence.

Surgery

Surgical management of fecal incontinence includes repair of rectal prolapse, anal sphincteroplasty, anal sphincter neomuscular flaps, and the implantation of artificial sphincters. Unfortunately, postanal repair or posterior levatorplasty has not been shown to be effective in the treatment of fecal incontinence in most patients and will not be discussed.

Repair of rectal prolapse, either transrectally or transabdominally, restores continence in 50% of patients. Success is dependent on the neuromuscular function of the pelvic floor.

Overlapping anterior anal sphincterplasty provides symptomatic control of incontinence in 60% to 80% of patients (Table 20-8). Patients who have both an anal sphincter defect and prolonged PNTML should be counseled that their chance of continence following surgery may be decreased. But unless there is absolutely no nerve function, surgical repair should be considered. Repair of an anal sphincter laceration includes not only repair of the EAS, but identification and repair of any IAS defects. Since the IAS maintains the resting tone of the anus, it is important to restore sphincter integrity, especially for control of flatus.

The surgery is performed through a transperineal incision from 11 o'clock to 2 o'clock over the EAS defect. With a gloved hand in the rectum, the internal sphincter is identified and plicated in the midline with 3-0 prolonged absorbable suture. Next, the ends of the EAS are identified. The use of a nerve stimulator can facilitate identification of the sphincter ends. The fibrous scar tissue at the ends of the sphincter is kept for added strength. The sphincter ends are dissected free to allow overlap in the midline without tension. The sphincter is then closed with 2 or 3-0 prolonged absorbable sutures by overlapping the sphincter ends (Figure 20-25). The advantage of the overlapping sphincteroplasty over the traditional end-to-end repair is decreased tension to prevent separation of the suture line once anesthesia no longer prevents sphincter contraction.

Neosphincters

There are basically two types of neosphincters, one using the patient's own skeletal muscle, usually the gracilis, and the other using an artificial silastic cuff connected to a fluid reservoir to occlude the anal canal. The gracilis muscle wrap has been shown to have inconsistent results. Initially described by Pickrell in 1952, the entire muscle is mobilized and its distal portion is wrapped snugly around the anus and anchored to the contralateral ischial tuberosity. Recently, the addition of chronic, low-frequency electrical stimulation of the nerve or muscle has been used to

TABLE 20-8
Outcome After Sphincteroplasty

Author	Institution	No. of Pts.	F/U Period (mean [range]; months)	Success (%)	Improved (%)
Fang et al., 1984	Minnesota	76	35 (2–62)	82	89
Browning and Motson, 1988	St. Marks	83	39.2 (4–116)	78	91
Ctercteko et al., 1988	Cleveland Clinic, Ohio	44	50	75	
Laurberg et al., 1988	St. Marks	19	18 (median: 9–36)	47	79
Yoshioka and Keighley, 1989	Birmingham	27	48 (median: 16–108)		74.1
Wexner et al., 1991	Cleveland Clinic, Florida	16	10 (3–16)	76	87.5
Fleshman et al., 1991	Washington University	55	0 (12–24)	72	87
Simmang et al., 1994	Washington University	14	0 (6–12)	71	93
Engel et al., 1994	St. Marks	55	15 (6–36)	60.4	
Engel et al., 1994	Amsterdam	28	46 (median: 15–116)	75	
Londono-Schimmer et al., 1994	St. Marks	94	58.5 (median: 12–98)	50	75
Sitzler and Thompson, 1996	St. Marks	31	0 (1–36)	74	
Felt-Bersma et al., 1996	Vrije University	18	14 (3–39)		72
Oliveira et al., 1996	Cleveland Clinic, Florida	55	29 (3–61)	70.1	80
Nikiteas et al., 1996	Birmingham	42	38 (median: 12–66)	60	
Gilliland et al., 1998	Cleveland Clinic, Florida	100	24 (median: 2–96)	55	69

From Gilliand R, Altomare DF, Moviera H, et al: Pudendal neuropathy is predictive of failure following anterior overlapping sphincteroplasty, Dis Colon Rectum 41:1516, 1998.

convert fatigue-prone type II muscle fibers to fatigue-resistant type I fibers. Once converted, the muscle may be continuously stimulated, resulting in prolonged closure of the anal canal. A report by the Dynamic Graciloplasty Therapy Study Group reported on 123 adults treated at 20 institutions with dynamic graciloplasty and found 90% of patients reported a 50% or greater improvement in incontinent events 1 year after surgery. Another 11% noted some improvement and 26% reported not improved or worse. There was one surgery-related death and 74% of patients experienced an adverse event related to the treatment with 40% of patients requiring an additional surgery. Despite these frequent complications, most patients showed a significant improvement in quality of life following the surgery.

Artificial sphincters are indicated in patients with anal incontinence caused by neuromuscular disease or trauma. Complications include infection and mechanical breakdown. Seventy-five percent success rates and 33% complication rates, similar to the muscle transpositions, have been reported.

RECTOVAGINAL FISTULAS

Although not a true source of fecal incontinence by definition, rectovaginal fistulas (RVF) are common enough complications of vaginal birth and gynecologic surgeries to be addressed under this heading. Any time a patient presents complaining of fecal or flatal incontinence, a rectovaginal fistula should be included in the differential diagnosis.

The etiology of rectovaginal fistulas, as seen in Table 20-9, include operative, inflammatory, and neoplastic sources, but obstetric injuries are, by far, the most common etiology. It is estimated that 0.1% of vaginal births will result in a RVF.

A fistula occurring caudad or adjacent to the EAS is termed an anovaginal fistula and is managed differently from a rectovaginal fistula. Fistulas that occur more than 3 cm above the anal verge are true rectovaginal fistulas.

Most rectovaginal fistulas secondary to obstetric injury occur in the lower third of the vagina and may be associated with a sphincter defect in the EAS. It is important to evaluate the EAS as outlined earlier with either a transanal ultrasound or EMG to map any defects prior to surgical treatment.

Fistulas secondary to surgical trauma, malignancy, or inflammatory process may occur anywhere along the vaginal wall, including the apex. If a fistula develops after a difficult surgery, such as following pelvic inflammatory disease, or after radiation, it is important to check for more than one fistula prior to repair. If the patient has a history of malignancy, examination with biopsies should be performed to rule out cancer as the cause of the fistula.

Depending on the size and location of the fistula, the patient may be nearly asymptomatic or complain of a small amount of flatus passing into her vagina with a low, small fistula. With a large fistula, she may have formed stool coming through the vagina with every bowel movement, causing significant distress and hygiene problems.

Evaluation of a patient includes history and physical examination to determine etiology. If there is suspicion of

A

C

B

D

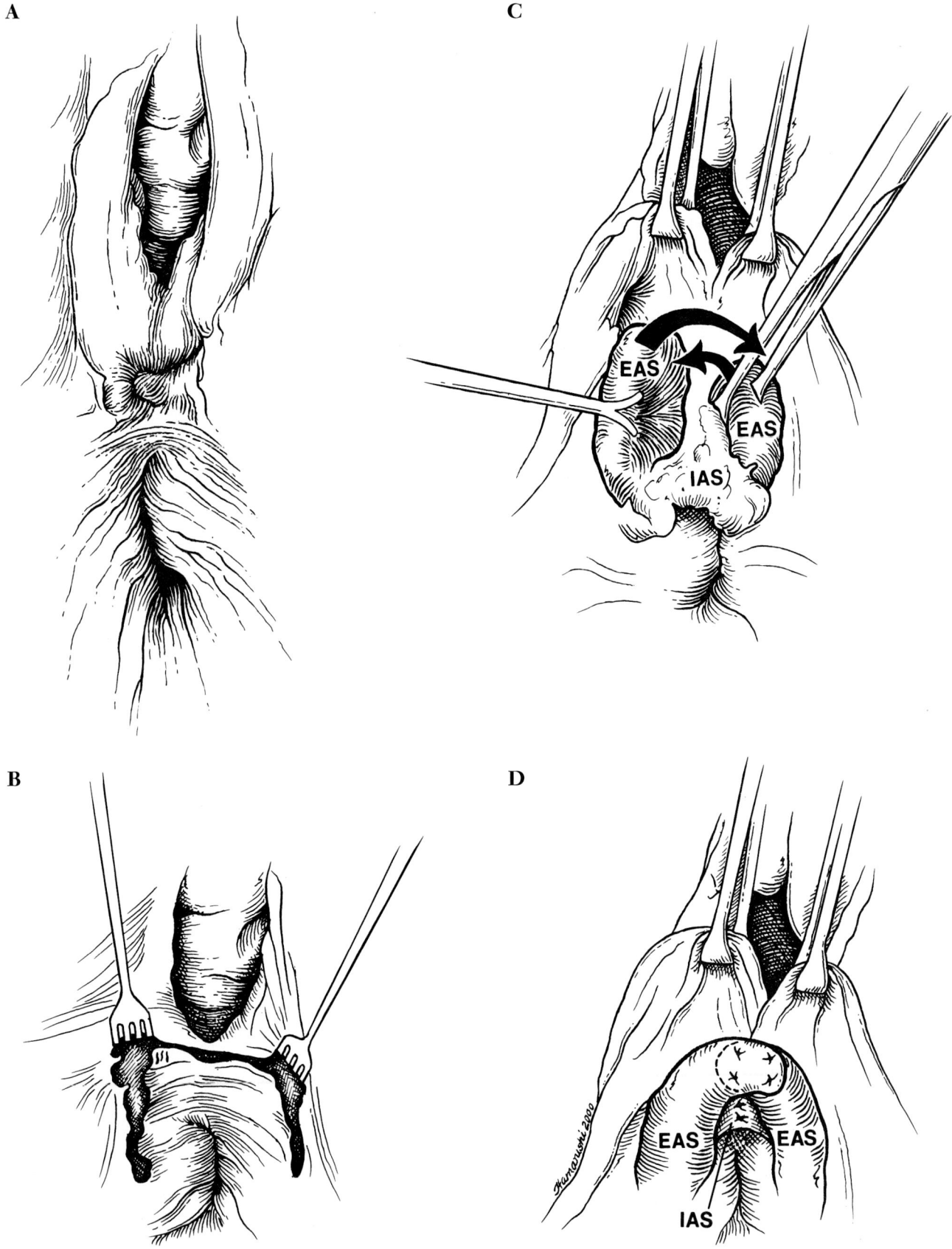

FIGURE 20-25 Sphincter drawing (4). Overlapping sphincteroplasty (A-D).

TABLE 20-9
Etiology of Rectovaginal Fistula

Category	Condition	Mechanism
Traumatic		
Obstetric	Prolonged 2nd stage of labor	Pressure necrosis of rectovaginal septum
	Midline episiotomy	Extension directed into rectum
	Perineal lacerations	
Foreign body	Vaginal pessaries	Pressure necrosis
	Violent coitus	Mechanical perforation
	Sexual abuse	Mechanical perforation
Latrogenic	Hysterectomy	Injury to anterior rectal wall
	Stapled colorectal anastomosis	Staple line includes vagina
	Transanal excision of anterior rectal tumor	Deep margin of resection into vagina
	Enemas	Mechanical perforation
	Anorectal surgery such as incision and drainage of intramural abscesses	Mechanical perforation
Inflammatory	Crohn's disease	Transmural inflammation-perforation
	Pelvic radiation	Early-tumor necrosis
	Pelvic abscess	Late-transmural inflammation
	Perirectal abscess	
Neoplastic	Rectal	Local tumor growth into neighboring structure
	Cervical	
	Uterine	
	Vaginal	
	Primary or recurrent tumors	

From Atlas of clinical gynecology, Stenchever MA and Benson JT, editors, New York, 2000, McGraw-Hill.

inflammatory bowel disease, a colonoscopy is warranted. A rectal examination is important to determine the integrity of the anal sphincters, the quality of the tissues surrounding the fistula, and to palpate for abscesses and other masses. Metholene blue mixed in lubricant can help identify the fistula. If still not identified, a dilute metholene blue enema with a tampon in the vagina may help in isolating the fistula. If the vaginal orifice is found, but not the rectal opening, insertion of an angiocath with a squirting of hydrogen peroxide can show bubbling on the rectal side.

An office anoscopy or proctoscopy may also help to evaluate the surrounding tissues. In general, a mature epitheliazlied fistula that is not infected is not painful on digital examination. If the exam in the office is not successful in locating the fistula or is too painful for the patient, she should be taken to the operating room for exam under anesthesia. If the fistula has still not been identified, filling the vagina with water and insufflating the rectum should produce bubbling in the vagina that can be traced to the opening. A barium enema may also be helpful for identifying high fistulas. A vaginogram using dilute barium solution may also help identify a fistula.

Surgical management of an anovaginal or anoperineal fistula is managed with opening of the fistula tract, curetting the tract, and leaving the tract open to heal secondarily. Excision of the tract and primary closure will result in recurrent fistula formation in most cases.

Many surgical procedures have been described for management of RVF. Regardless of the procedure chosen, basic surgical principles must be followed. The tissue must be healthy, well vascularized, and free of infection and induration. This may require waiting for up to 3 months following the original trauma or surgery for complete healing. If there is significant fecal contamination, prior radiation, or persistent abscess, a diverting colostomy should be considered. After a colostomy, a delay of 8 to 12 weeks is generally required for the inflammation and cellulites around the fistula to heal. At the time of repair, a Martius fat pad graft can be used to increase the vascular supply to the area. Preoperatively, the patient should have a complete mechanical bowel prep starting several days before the surgery to prevent liquid stool from contaminating the field. Some surgeons may place the patient on a liquid diet several days before surgery with no mechanical bowel prep except enemas until clear the night before surgery. The goal is to have no liquid stool in the rectum and to have her first postoperative bowel movement, several days after surgery, be soft, but formed. Antibiotic bowel prophylaxis is warranted.

Other surgical principles include excision of the entire fistulous tract, wide mobilization of the rectal tissue, and broad tissue to tissue closure without tension. The rectal side is the high pressure side and requires the attention to repair. The vaginal side may be closed or left open to drain if indicated and should close spontaneously. A delayed-absorbable suture, such as a 3-0 polysorb, is used on all layers. Permanent suture is not used.

Both transvaginal and transrectal repairs have been described, but gynecologists, generally, prefer the transvaginal approach. Depending on the location and the need to repair the anal sphincters, an uncomplicated fistula can be repaired similar to a fourth-degree laceration as a perineoproctotomy with layer closure. After cutting from the perineal body, through the sphincters and to the fistulous tract, care must be taken to excise the tract and any surrounding scar tissue. A two-layered closure of the rectum and anal canal is then performed as in a fourth-degree closure. Care should be given to closing the EAS.

To preserve an intact sphincter, the RVF can be cored out by placing a pediatric Foley transvaginally and filling the balloon on the rectal side and then using the Foley for traction by pulling upward. After excision, depending on the size, a small fistula can be closed with two-layer purse string sutures or with an interrupted two-layer closure.

Transrectal repairs, preferred by many colorectal surgeons, generally involve the development of rectal mucosal flaps, mobilized and brought down or lateral to cover the excised fistula site. In 23 patients treated at the Cleveland Clinic with rectal advancement flaps, fistulas were successfully cured in 77% of the patients with obstetric or surgical injury and 60% of the patients with Crohn's disease.

Postoperatively, the patient's diet and medications should be managed to keep her bowel movements soft, but formed. In most cases, a clear liquid diet is continued for the first 3 days after surgery followed by a low-residue diet. Broad-spectrum antibiotics should be continued for 2 weeks.

Sitz baths, two or three times a day, followed by the use of a blow dryer or heat lamp, keeps the area clean and dry.

KEY POINTS

- Femoral hernias are more common in females than in males, whereas inguinal hernias are more common in males.

- Congenital fascial defects at the umbilicus generally close within the first 3 years of life.

- In the female, large hernias, hernias that continuously have intraabdominal contents, hernias that cause continuing discomfort, and hernias that have been incarcerated should be operatively repaired.

- In the repair of abdominal wall hernias, fascia should be sutured with nonabsorbable material.

- Urethroceles and cystoceles are more common in women with a gynecoid pelvis than in those with android or anthropoid types.

- Urinary incontinence is usually noted with loss of support of the urethra and bladder neck.

- After cystocele repair, bladder drainage for 1 to 5 days is generally necessary before normal voiding can be anticipated.

- Bladder drainage after cystocele repair may be with a transurethral or suprapubic catheter.

- When an enterocele is present, the sac must be dissected free and ligated at its neck to prevent recurrence.

- Descensus of the uterus and cervix is graded as first degree (prolapse into the upper vagina), second degree (prolapse to or near the introitus), and third degree, or complete (prolapse through the introitus).

- Prolapse of the vaginal stump at some time after hysterectomy has been reported in 0.1% to 18.2% of patients.

- Vaginal prolapse after hysterectomy includes a mixture of cystocele, rectocele, and enterocele in 72% of cases.

- Vaginal vault prolapse can be repaired abdominally or vaginally.

- Vaginal vault prolapse repair using fixation to the sacrospinous ligament will have a success rate approaching 100%, but recurrence rate necessitating reoperation may be as high as 33%.

- Estimates of fecal incontinence range from 2% to 11% of community dwelling women older than 64 years of age.

- Over 30% of women reporting urinary incontinence also report fecal incontinence, known as dual incontinence.

- The IAS, under autonomic control, maintains the high pressure zone or continence zone and, along with the EAS, keeps the anal canal closed.

- The EAS provides the voluntary squeeze pressure that prevents incontinence with increasing rectal or abdominal pressure. The EAS is innervated by the hemorrhoidal branch of the pudendal nerve from the S_2-S_4 nerve roots.

- Incontinence secondary to denervation has been designated as idiopathic and represents 80% of patients with fecal incontinence.

- A common cause of fecal incontinence is damage to the anal sphincter at the time of vaginal delivery with or without neuronal injury. This type of incontinence is often referred to as anal incontinence.

- The incidence of occult external anal sphincter disruption after vaginal delivery determined by endoanal ultrasound ranges from 11% to 35%. The chance of muscular injury is increased with midline episiotomy, instrumented delivery, and vaginal delivery of larger infants.

- Approximately one in ten women will develop some fecal incontinence or fecal urgency after one vaginal delivery.

- At a tertiary colorectal referral clinic, a prospective study showed that further evaluation, including radiologic and physiologic tests, altered the final diagnosis or the cause of fecal incontinence in 19% of cases.

- Sixty to 70% of patients with fecal incontinence secondary to an abnormal pelvic floor will have a 90% reduction in incontinence with biofeedback.

- Overlapping anterior anal sphincteroplasty provides symptomatic control of incontinence in 60% to 80% of patients.

- It is estimated that 0.1% of vaginal births will result in a rectovaginal fistula.

BIBLIOGRAPHY

American Journal of Obstetrics and Gynecology: The standardization of terminology of female pelvic organ prolapse and pelvic floor dysfunction. (Clinical Opinion.) 1996.

Beecham CT: Classification of vaginal relaxation, Am J Obstet Gynecol 136:957, 1980.

Beecham CT and Beecham JB: Correction of prolapsed vagina or enterocele with fascia, Obstet Gynecol 42:542, 1973.

Benson JT, Lucente V, and McCellan E: Vaginal versus abdominal reconstructive surgery for the treatment of pelvic support defects: a prospective randomized study with long-term outcome evaluation, Am J Obstet Gynecol 175:1418, 1996.

Birnbaum EH, Stamm L, Rafferty JF, Fry RD, Kogner IJ, Fleshman JW: Pudendal nerve terminal motor latency influences: surgical outcome and treatment of rectal diseases. Dis Colon Rectum 39:1215, 1996.

Brooks DC: A prospective comparison of laparoscopic and tension-free open herniorrhaphy, Arch Surg 129:361, 1994.

Deans GT, Wilson MS, Royston CM, and Brough WA: Recurrent inguinal hernia after laparoscopic repair: possible cause and prevention, Br J Surg 82:539, 1995.

Denehy TR, Choe JY, Gregori CA, and Breen JL: Modified Le Fort partial colpocleisis with Kelly urethral plication and posterior colpoperineoplasty in the medically compromised elderly: a comparison with vaginal hysterectomy, anterior colporrhaphy, and posterior colpoperineoplasty, Am J Obstet Gynecol 173:1697, 1995.

Glassow F: Inguinal and femoral hernia in women, Int Surg 57:34, 1972.

Halverson K and McVay CB: Inguinal and femoral hernioplasty: a 22 year study of author's methods, Arch Surg 101:127, 1970.

Kauppila O, Punnonen R, and Teisala K: Operative technique for the repair of posthysterectomy vaginal prolapse, Ann Chir Gynaecol 75:242, 1986.

Kavic MS: Laparoscopic hernia repair: three-year experience, Surg Endosc 9:12, 1995.

Keating JP, Stewart PJ, Eyers AA, Warner D, Bokey EL: Are special investigations of value in the management of patients with fecal incontinence? Dis Colon Rectum 40:896, 1997.

Kohli N, Sze EHM, Roat TW, and Karram M: Incidence of recurrent cystocele after anterior colporrhaphy with and without concomitant transvaginal needle suspension, Am J Obstet Gynecol 175:1476, 1996.

Kovac SR and Cruikshank SH: Successful pregnancies and vaginal deliveries after sacrospinous uterosacral fixation in five of nineteen patients, Am J Obstet Gynecol 168:1778, 1993.

Kuhn RJ and Hollyock VE: Observations on the anatomy of the recto-vaginal pouch and septum, Obstet Gynecol 59:445, 1982.

Lind LR, Choe J, and Bhatia N: An in-line suturing device to simplify sacrospinous vaginal vault suspension, Obstet Gynecol 89:129, 1997.

McCall ML: Posterior culdeplasty—surgical correction of enterocele during vaginal hysterectomy: a preliminary report, Obstet Gynecol 10:595, 1957.

Meeks GR, Washburne JF, McGehee RP, and Wiser WL: Repair of vaginal vault prolapse by suspension of the vagina to iliococcygeus (prespinous) fascia, Am J Obstet Gynecol 171:1444, 1994.

Miyazaki FS: Miya hook ligature carrier for sacrospinous ligament suspension, Obstet Gynecol 70:286, 1987.

Morley GW and DeLancey JO: Sacrospinous ligament fixation for eversion of the vagina, Am J Obstet Gynecol 158:872, 1988.

Nichols DH: Transvaginal sacrospinous fixation, Pelvic Surgeon 1:10, 1981.

Panton ON and Panton RJ: Laparoscopic hernia repair, Am J Surg 167:535, 1994.

Paraiso MF, Ballard LA, Walters MD, et al: Pelvic support defects and visceral and sexual function in women treated with sacrospinous ligament suspension and pelvic reconstruction, Obstet Gynecol 175:1423, 1996.

Pasley WW: Sacrospinous suspension: a local practitioner's experience, Am J Obstet Gynecol 173:440, 1995.

Podratz KC, Ferguson LK, Hoverman VR, et al: Abdominal sacral colpopexy for posthysterectomy vaginal vault descensus, J Pelvic Surg 1:18, 1995.

Ramshaw BJ, Tucker JG, Mason EM, et al: A comparison of transabdominal preperitoneal (TAPP) and total extraperitoneal approach (TEPA) laparoscopic herniorrhaphies, Am Surg 61:279, 1995.

Randall CI and Nichols DH: Surgical treatment of vaginal inversion, Obstet Gynecol 38:327, 1971.

Richter K: Massive eversion of the vagina: pathogenesis, diagnosis and therapy of the "true" prolapse of the vaginal stump, Clin Obstet Gynecol 25:897, 1982.

Richter K and Albrich W: Long-term results following fixation of the vagina on the sacrospinal ligament by the vaginal root (vaginae fixatio sacrospinalis vaginalis), Am J Obstet Gynecol 141:811, 1981.

Ridley JH: Evaluation of the colpocleisis operation: a report of 58 cases, Am J Obstet Gynecol 113:1114, 1972.

Schlesinger RE: Vaginal sacrospinous ligament fixation with the Autosuture Endostitch device, Am J Obstet Gynecol 176:1358, 1997.

Schwartz SI, Shires GT, Spencer FC, and Storer EH: Principles of surgery, ed 4, New York, 1984, McGraw-Hill Book Co.

Seigworth GR: Vaginal vault prolapse with eversion, Obstet Gynecol 54:255, 1979.

Sharp TR: Sacrospinous suspension made easy, Obstet Gynecol 82:873, 1993.

Snyder TE and Krantz KE: Abdominal-retroperitoneal sacral colpopexy for the correction of vaginal prolapse, Obstet Gynecol 77:944, 1991.

Strohbehn K, Jakary JA, and Delancey JO: Pelvic organ prolapse in young women, Obstet Gynecol 90:33, 1997.

Sweiger M: Method for determining individual contributions of the voluntary and involuntary anal sphincter to resting tone. Dis Colon Rectum 22:415, 1979.

Symmonds RE: Relaxation of pelvic supports. In Benson RC, editor: Current obstetric and gynecologic diagnosis and treatment, ed 5, Los Altos, Calif, 1984, Lange Medical Publications.

Symmonds RE, Williams TJ, Lee RA, and Webb MJ: Posthysterectomy, enterocele and vaginal vault prolapse, Am J Obstet Gynecol 140:852, 1981.

Sze EHM and Karram MM: Transvaginal repair of vault prolapse: a review, Obstet Gynecol 89:466, 1997.

Sze EHM, Kohli N, Miklos JR, et al: Computed tomography comparison of bony pelvic dimensions between women with and without genital prolapse, Obstet Gynecol 93:229, 1999.

Thill RH and Hopkins WM: The use of Mersilene mesh in adult inguinal and femoral hernia repairs: a comparison with classic techniques, Am Surg 60:553, 1994.

Thomas AG, Brodman ML, Dottino PR, et al: Manchester procedure vs vaginal hysterectomy for uterine prolapse: a comparison, J Reprod Med 40:299, 1995.

Thornton WN Jr. and Peters WA: Repair of vaginal prolapse after hysterectomy, Am J Obstet Gynecol 147:140, 1983.

Tucker JG, Wilson RA, Ramshaw BJ, et al: Laparoscopic herniorrhaphy: technical concerns in prevention of complications and early recurrence, Am Surg 61:36, 1995.

Valaitis SR and Stanton SL: Sacrocolpopexy: a retrospective study of a clinician's experience, Br J Obstet Gynaecol 101:518, 1994.

Veronikis DK and Nichols DH: Ligature carrier specifically designed for transvaginal sacrospinous colpopexy, Obstet Gynecol 89:478, 1997.

Webb MJ, Aronson MP, Ferguson LK, and Lee RA: Posthysterectomy vaginal vault prolapse: primary repair in 693 patients, Obstet Gynecol 92:281, 1998.

Weber AM, Walters MD, and Piedmonte MR: Sexual function and vaginal anatomy in women before and after surgery for pelvic organ prolapse and urinary incontinence, Am J Obstet Gynecol 182:1610, 2000.

Wexner SD, Marchetti F, Jagelman DG: The role of sphincteroplasty for fecal incontinence re-evaluated: a prospective physiologic and functional review. Dis Colon Rectum 34:22, 1991.

Wilson DE, Noseworthy TW, and Grace MG: Caremap management in low-severity surgery: a comparative trial, J Am Coll Surg 181:49, 1995.

Zacharin RF: Pulsion enterocele: review of functional anatomy of the pelvic floor, Obstet Gynecol 55:135, 1980.

Zimmerman LM and Anson BJ: The anatomy of surgery of hernia, Baltimore, 1953, Williams & Wilkins.

Fecal Incontinence

Aronson MP, Lee RA, and Berquist TH: Anatomy of anal sphincters and related structures in continent women studied with magnetic resonance imaging, Obstet Gynecol 76:846, 1990.

Baeten CG, Bailey HR, Bakka A, et al: Safety and efficacy of dynamic graciloplasty for fecal incontinence: report of a prospective, multicenter trial. Dynamic Graciloplasty Therapy Study Group, Dis Colon Rectum 43:743, 2000.

Bartolo DCC, Roe AM, Locke-Edmunds JC, et al: Flap-valve theory of anorectal continence, Br J Surg 73:1012, 1986.

Birnbaum EH, Stamm L, Rafferty JE, et al: Pudendal nerve terminal motor latency influences: surgical outcome in treatment of rectal prolapse, Dis Colon Rectum 39:1215, 1996.

Browning GG and Motson RW: Anal sphincter injury: management and results of Parks sphincter repair, Ann Surg 199:

Burhenne HJ: Intestinal evaluation study: a new roentgenologic technique. Radiol Clin 33:79, 1964.

Burnett SJD, Speakman CTM, Kamm MA, et al: Confirmation of endosonographic detection of external anal sphincter defects by simultaneous electromyographic mapping, Br J Surg 78:448, 1991.

Chen AS, Luchtefeld MA, Senagore AJ, et al: Pudendal nerve latency: does it predict outcome of anal sphincter repair? Dis Colon Rectum 41:1005, 1998.

Ctercteko GC, Fazio VW, Jagelman DG, et al: Anal sphincter repair: a report of 60 cases and a review of the literature, Aust N Z J Surg 58:703, 1988.

Dhaenes G, Emblem R, and Ganes T: Fibre density in idiopathic ano-rectal incontinence, Electromyogr Clin Neurophysiol 35:285, 1995.

Donnelly V, Fynes M, Campbell D, et al: Obstetric events leading to anal sphincter damage, Obstet Gynecol 92:955, 1998.

Engel AF, Kamm MA, Sultan AH, et al: Anterior anal sphincter repair in patients with obstetric trauma, Br J Surg 81:1231, 1994.

Engel AF, van Baal SJ, and Brummelkamp WH: Late results of anterior sphincter plication for traumatic faecal incontinence, Eur J Surg 160:633, 1994.

Fang DT, Nivatvoongs S, Vermeulen FD, et al: Overlapping sphincteroplasty for acquired anal incontinence, Dis Colon Rectum 27:720, 1984.

Felt-Bersma RJ, Cuesta MA, and Koorevaar M: Anal sphincter repair improves anorectal function and endosonographic image: a prospective clinical study, Dis Colon Rectum 39:878, 1996.

Fenner DE, Kriegshauser JS, Lee HH, et al: Anatomic and physiologic measurements of the internal and external anal sphincters in normal females, Obstet Gynecol 91:369, 1998.

Fleshman JW, Dreznik Z, Fry RD, Kodner IJ: Anal sphincter repair for obstetric injury: manometric evaluation of functional results. Dis Colon Rectum 34:1061, 1991.

Fleshman JW, Peters WR, Shemesh EI, et al: Anal sphincter reconstruction: anterior overlapping muscle repair, Dis Colon Rectum 34:739, 1991.

Fynes MM, Donnelly V, Behan M, O'Connell PR, O'Herlihy C: Effect of second vaginal delivery on anorectal physiology and faecal incontinence: a prospective study. Lancet 354:983, 1999.

Gilliland R, Altomare DF, Moreira H Jr, et al: Pudendal neuropathy is predictive of failure following anterior overlapping sphincteroplasty, Dis Colon Rectum 41:1516, 1998.

Gosling JA, Dixson JS, Critchley HD, and Thompson SA: A comparative study of the human external sphincter and periurethral levator ani muscles, Br J Urol 53:35, 1981.

Henry MM, Parks AG, and Swash M: The pelvic floor musculature in the descending perineum syndrome, Br J Surg 69:470, 1982.

Howard D, DeLancey JO, and Burney RE: Fistula-in-ano after episiotomy, Obstet Gynecol 93:800, 1999.

Jackson SL, Weber AM, Hull TL, et al: Fecal incontinence in women with urinary incontinence and pelvic organ prolapse, Obstet Gynecol 89:423, 1997.

Jacobs PPM, Scheuer M, Kuijpers JHC, and Vingerhoets MH: Obstetric fecal incontinence: role of pelvic floor denervation and results of delayed sphincter repair, Dis Colon Rectum 33:494, 1990.

Jensen LL and Lowry AC: Biofeedback: a viable treatment option for anal incontinence, Dis Colon Rectum 34:SupplP6. Abstract, 1991.

Jones IT, Fazio VW, and Jagelman DG: The use of transanal rectal advancement flaps in the management of fistulas involving the anorectum, Dis Colon Rectum 30:919, 1987.

Jorge JM, Wexner SD: Etiology and management of fecal incontinence. Dis Colon Rectum 36:77, 1993.

Keating JP, Stewart PJ, Eyers AA, et al: Are special investigations of value in the management of patients with fecal incontinence? Dis Colon Rectum 40:896, 1997.

Khullar V, Damiano R, Toozs-Hobson P, and Cardozo L: Prevalence of faecal incontinence among women with urinary incontinence, Br J Obstet and Gynaecol 105:1211, 1998.

Kiff ES, Barnes PRH, and Swash M: Evidence of pudendal neuropathy in patients with perineal descent and chronic straining at stool, Gut 25:1279, 1984.

Kiff ES and Swash M: Slowed conduction in the pudendal nerves in idiopathic (neurogenic) faecal incontinence, Br J Surg 71:614, 1984.

Laurberg S, Swash M, and Henry MM: Delayed external sphincter repair for obstetric tear, Br J Surg 75:786, 1988.

Law PJ, Kamm MA, and Bartram CI: A comparison between electromyography and anal endosonography in mapping external anal sphincter defects, Dis Colon Rectum 33:370, 1990.

Leigh RJ, Turnberg LA: Faecal incontinence: the unvoided symptom. Lancet 1:1349, 1982.

Londono-Schimmer EE, Garcia-Duperly R, Nicholls RJ, et al: Overlapping anal sphincter repair for faecal incontinence due to sphincter trauma: five year follow-up functional results, Int J Colorectal Dis 9:110, 1994.

MacArthur C, Bick DE, and Keighley MRB: Faecal incontinence after childbirth, Br J Obstet Gynaecol 104:46, 1997.

Madoff RD, Baeten CGMI, Christiansen J, et al: Standards for anal sphincter replacement, Dis Colon Rectum 43:135, 2000.

Madoff RD, Williams JG, and Caushaj PF: Fecal incontinence, N Engl J Med 326:1002, 1992.

Miller R, Orrom WJ, Cornes H, et al: Anterior sphincter plication and levatroplasty in the treatment of faecal incontinence, Br J Surg 75:1058, 1989.

Neill ME, Parks AG, and Swash M: Physiological studies of the anal sphincter musculature in faecal incontinence and rectal prolapse, Br J Surg 68:531, 1981.

Neill ME and Swash M: Increased motor unit fibre density in the external anal sphincter muscle in anorectal incontinence: a single fibre EMG study, J Neurol Neurosurg Psychiatry 43:343, 1980.

Nelson R, Norton N, Cautley E, and Furner S: Community-based prevalence of anal incontinence, JAMA 274:559, 1995.

Nikiteas N, Korsgen S, Kumar D, and Keighley MR: Audit of sphincter repair: factors associated with poor outcome, Dis Colon Rectum 39:1164, 1996.

Obstetrics and gynecology clinics of North America: Bump RC and Cardiff GW, editors, Urogynecology and pelvic floor dysfunction, Philadelphia, 1998, WB Saunders, p 25.

Oliverira L, Pfeifer J, and Wexner SD: Physiological and clinical outcome of anterior sphincteroplasty, Br J Surg 83:502, 1996.

Parks AG: Anorectal incontinence, Proc R Soc Med 68:681, 1975.

Parks AG, Swash M, and Urich H: Sphincter denervation in anorectal incontinence and rectal prolapse, Gut 18:656, 1977.

Pescatori M, Anastasio G, Bottini C, Mentasti A: New grading and scoring for anal incontinence: evaluation of 335 patients. Dis Colon Rectum 35:482, 1992.

Pickrell KL, Broadbent IR, Masters FW, and Metzger JT: Constitution of a rectal sphincter and restoration of anal incontinence by transplanting the graulis? muscle. A report of four cases in children, Ann Surg 135:853, 1952.

Rasmussen OO, Puggaard L, and Christiansen J: Anal sphincter repair in patients with obstetric trauma: age affects outcome, Dis Colon Rectum 42:193, 1999.

Rieger NA, Schloithe A, Saccone G, and Wattchow D: A prospective study of anal sphincter injury due to childbirth, Scand J Gastroenterol 33:950, 1998.

Rieger NA, Wattchow DA, Sarre RG, et al: Prospective trial of pelvic floor retraining in patients with fecal incontinence, Dis Colon Rectum 40:821, 1997.

Ryhammer AM, Bek KM, and Laurberg S: Multiple vaginal deliveries increase the risk of permanent incontinence of flatus and urine in normal premenopausal women, Dis Colon Rectum 38:1206, 1995.

Sagar PN and Pemberton JH: Anorectal and pelvic floor function. Relevance of continence, incontinence, and constipation, Gastroenterol Clin North Am 25:163, 1996.

Signorello LB, Harlow BL, Chekos AK, and Repke JT: Midline episiotomy and anal incontinence: retrospective cohort study, BMJ 320:86, 2000.

Simmang C, Birnbaum EH, Kodner IJ, et al: Anal sphincter reconstruction in the elderly: does advancing age affect outcome? Dis Colon Rectum 37:1065, 1994.

Sitzler PJ and Thomson JP: Overlap repair of damaged anal sphincter: a single surgeon's series, Dis Colon Rectum 398:1356, 1996.

Smith ARB, Hosker GL, and Warrell DW: The role of partial denervation of the pelvic floor in the aetiology of genitourinary prolapse and stress incontinence of urine: a neurophysiological study, Br J Obstet Gynaecol 96:24, 1989.

Snooks SJ, Barnes PRH, and Swash M: Damage to the innervation of the voluntary anal and periurethral sphincter musculature in incontinence: an electrophysiological study, J Neurol Neurosurg Psychiatry 47:1269, 1984.

Snooks SJ, Setchell M, Swash M, and Henry MM: Injury to innervation of pelvic floor sphincter musculature in childbirth, Lancet 2:546, 1984.

Snooks SJ and Swash M: Abnormalities of the innervation of the urethral striated sphincter in incontinence, Br J Urol 56:401, 1984.

Sultan AH, Kamm MA, Hudson CN, and Bartram CI: Third degree obstetric anal sphincter tears: risk factors and outcome of primary repair, BMJ 308:887, 1994.

Sultan AH, Kamm MA, Hudson CN, et al: Anal-sphincter disruption during vaginal delivery, N Engl J Med 329:1905, 1993.

Swash M: Histopathology of pelvic floor muscles. In Henry MM and Swash M, editors, Coloproctology and the pelvic floor, ed 1, London, 1985, Butterworths, p 129.

Swash M, Snooks SJ, and Henry MM: Unifying concept of pelvic floor disorders and incontinence, J R Soc Med 78:906, 1985.

Sweiger M: Method for determining individual contributions of voluntary and involuntary anal sphincters to resting tone, Dis Colon Rectum 22:415, 1979.

Taverner D and Smiddy FG: An electromyographic study of the normal function of the external anal sphincter and pelvic diaphragm, Dis Colon Rectum 2:153, 1959.

Tetzschner T, Sorensen M, Rasmussen OO, et al: Pudendal nerve damage increases the risk of fecal incontinence in women with anal sphincter rupture after childbirth, Acta Obstet Gynaecol Scand 74:434, 1995.

Toglia MR: Anal incontinence: an under recognized, under treated problem, The Female Patient 21:27, 1996.

Toglia MR and DeLancey JOL: Anal incontinence and the obstetrician-gynecologist, Obstet Gynecol 84:731, 1994.

Varma A, Gunn J, Gardiner A, et al: Obstetric anal sphincter injury: prospective evaluation of incidence, Dis Colon Rectum 42:1537, 1999.

Varma A, Gunn J, Lindow S, and Duthie GS: Do routinely measured delivery variables predict anal sphincter outcome? Dis Colon Rectum 42:1261, 1999.

Venkatesh KS, Ramanujham PS, Larson DM, and Haywood MA: Anorectal complications of vaginal delivery, Dis Colon Rectum 32:1039, 1989.

Wexner JJM: Etiology and management of fecal incontinence, Dis Colon Rectum 36:77, 1993.

Wexner SD, Marchett F, and Jagelman DG: The role of sphincteroplasty for fecal incontinence reevaluated: a prospective physiologic and functional review, Dis Colon Rectum 34:22, 1991.

Wong WD, Jensen LL, Bortolo DC, and Rothenberger DA: Artificial anal sphincter, Dis Colon Rectum 39:1345, 1996.

Womack NRT, Morrison JFB, and Williams NS: Prospective study of the effects of postnatal repair in neurogenic faecal incontinence, Br J Surg 7:52, 1988.

Wunderlich M and Swash M: The overlapping innervation of the two sites of the external anal sphincter by the pudendal nerves, J Neurol Sci 5:109, 1983.

Yoshioka K and Keighley MR: Sphincter repair for fecal incontinence, Dis Colon Rectum 32:39, 1989.

Zetterstrom J, Lopez A, Norman M, et al: Anal sphincter tears at vaginal delivery: risk factors and clinical outcome of primary repair, Obstet Gynecol 94:21, 1999.

Zetterstrom J, Mellgren A, Jensen LL, et al: Effect of delivery on anal sphincter morphology and function, Dis Colon Rectum 42:1253, 1999.

Urogynecology

Physiology of Micturition, Diagnosis of Voiding Dysfunction and Incontinence: Surgical and Nonsurgical Treatment

KEY TERMS AND DEFINITIONS

Cystometry. Method for measuring pressure volume relationships of the bladder.

Detrusor Instability (Dyssynergia). Involuntary contraction of the bladder during distention with urine or other fluids.

Detrusor Pressure. Component of intravesical pressure created by forces in the bladder wall.

Extraurethral Incontinence. The loss of urine through channels other than the urethra.

Flow Rate. Volume of urine expelled via the urethra per unit time expressed in milliliters.

Genuine Stress Incontinence. Condition of immediate involuntary loss of urine when intravesical pressure exceeds the maximum urethral pressure in the absence of detrusor activity.

Incontinence. A condition in which involuntary loss of urine is a social or hygienic problem and one that can be objectively demonstrated.

Interstitial Cystitis. A complex inflammatory condition of the bladder of poorly understood etiology and pathophysiology that is usually associated with altered epithelial permeability, mast cell activation, and an upregulation of secondary afferent nerves.

Intraabdominal Pressure. Pressure surrounding the bladder.

Intravesical Pressure. Pressure within the bladder.

Intrinsic Sphincter Dysfunction. A form of stress urinary incontinence in which the defect is an intraurethral pressure of less than 20 cm of water.

Kegel Exercises. Isometric contractions of the pubococcygeus muscles to improve control of continence.

Osteitis Pubis. An inflammation of the periosteum of the pubic bone, often occurring after suprapubic urethral suspension procedures.

Osteomyelitis Pubis. An infection of the pubic bone, which may occur after pelvic operations.

Overflow Incontinence. Involuntary loss of urine when intravesical pressure exceeds the maximum urethral pressure secondary to an elevation of intravesical pressure associated with bladder distention but in the absence of detrusor activity.

Posterior Urethral Angle (PUV). The angle formed by the posterior aspect of the urethra and the bladder. It is generally less than 120 degrees in continent women.

Reflex Incontinence. The involuntary loss of urine caused by abnormal reflex activity in the spinal cord in the absence of the sensation that is usually associated with the desire to micturate.

Residual Urine. Volume of urine remaining in the bladder immediately after completion of micturition.

Stress (Valsalva) Leak Point Pressure Test. This test measures the intravesical pressure necessary to overcome urethral resistance under stress (cough or strain).

Trigone (Bladder). The area of the floor of the urinary bladder that forms a triangle with the urethral opening at the apex and the ureteral openings at the ends of the base.

Trigonitis. Inflammation of the trigone.

Urethral Closure Pressure Profile. Intraluminal pressure along the length of the urethra with the bladder at rest.

Urethral Syndrome. An inflammatory condition of the urethra in which bacterial cultures are found to be negative. In many cases *Chlamydia* can now be cultured.

Urge Incontinence. The involuntary loss of urine associated with a strong desire to void. This may be divided into motor urge incontinence, which is associated with uninhibited detrusor contractions, and sensory urge incontinence, which is not caused by uninhibited detrusor contractions.

The gynecologist frequently consults on and treats urologic problems in the female patient. Perhaps the most commonly seen of these problems involves infection and inflammation of the lower tract (urethritis, trigonitis, and cystitis). However, many women suffer from some degree of urinary incontinence. In a telephone interview study of 851 women ages 18 and older selected at random in Australia, 267 (31%) stated that they had noted some degree of incontinence during the preceding 12 months, and 142 (12%) suffered two or more regular episodes of leakage per month. Daily incontinence was reported by 5%, and 2.3% were incontinent often or continuously.

This condition increases in incidence with age, and because the number of older women in our population is growing, it is likely that this problem will grow in magnitude with time. At a conference of the National Association of Retired People, Teasdale et al. learned (by questionnaire) that 33% of the total responders experienced some form of urinary incontinence. Women accounted for 75% of the respondents, representing 168 individuals. Of these, 118 complained of dribbling, 13 of spontaneous large losses of urine, and 37 of both dribbling and large losses. Of women over age 60 who are not institutionalized, 15% to 30% report experiencing incontinence, with 25% to 30% of these reporting frequent episodes. The older the woman, the higher the incidence of incontinence.

Continence depends on a number of factors, including the neurologic control of micturition, the anatomic relationships of the urinary tract, and the specific effects of a number of systemic, infectious, and neoplastic conditions. This chapter considers the physiology of micturition and the diagnosis and treatment of pathologic entities that affect the female urologic system, and it offers suggestions on diagnosis and management of urinary incontinence.

PHYSIOLOGY OF MICTURITION

A number of factors are in play to maintain continence. Basically these involve those that maintain a urethral closure mechanism and those that affect detrusor function. In the final analysis it is the balance between urethral closure and detrusor function that determines whether micturition occurs or continence is maintained.

The factors affecting the urethral closure mechanism primarily involve urethral tone and include the basic elasticity of the urethra, the presence of smooth and voluntary (striated) muscle, the vascular component supplying the urethra, and the presence of alpha receptors from the sympathetic nervous system, which when stimulated cause contraction of the urethral sphincter.

Bladder detrusor contractility is stimulated by the activity of the parasympathetic nervous system mediated through the neurotransmitter acetylcholine. This stimulates receptors in the bladder wall, which then activate detrusor contraction. Sympathetic nervous system beta receptors within the bladder cause bladder relaxation when stimulated. Bladder contraction may also be affected by irritation and inflammation of the bladder wall, causing uncoordinated contractions.

The act of voiding is under the control of four basic autonomic and somatic nervous system feedback loops. The first loop (loop I) involves a circuit from the cerebral cortex to the brainstem, which inhibits micturition by modifying sensory stimuli emanating from loop II. Loop II, which originates in the sacral micturition center (S2 through S4) and the detrusor muscle wall itself, represents sensory fibers to the brainstem, where modulation of the stimuli by loop I takes place. If cerebral inhibition is not imposed (loop I), the stimuli are returned to the sacral micturition center as a response to the bladder filling, allowing activation of loop III. Loop III involves sensory flow from the bladder wall to the sacral micturition center with returning motor fibers to the urethral sphincter striated muscle, which allows the voluntary relaxation of the urethral sphincter as the detrusor contracts. Loop IV originates in the frontal lobe of the cerebral cortex and runs to the sacral micturition center and then to the urethral striated muscle, allowing urethral voluntary muscles to relax and thus leading to the initiation of voiding. Figure 21-1 demonstrates these four loops as visualized by Williams and Fitzhugh. Table 21-1 summarizes the important aspects of each loop as reviewed by Ostergard.

Both the parasympathetic and sympathetic nervous systems function with the central nervous system in these feedback loops. Basically, the parasympathetic system is involved in the act of voiding via nuclei in S2 through S4 (micturition center). Contraction of the detrusor muscle puts pressure on the bladder neck and the proximal urethra, contributing to the relaxation of the urethral sphincter. As mentioned, the parasympathetic system mediates its activity through the neurotransmitter acetylcholine,

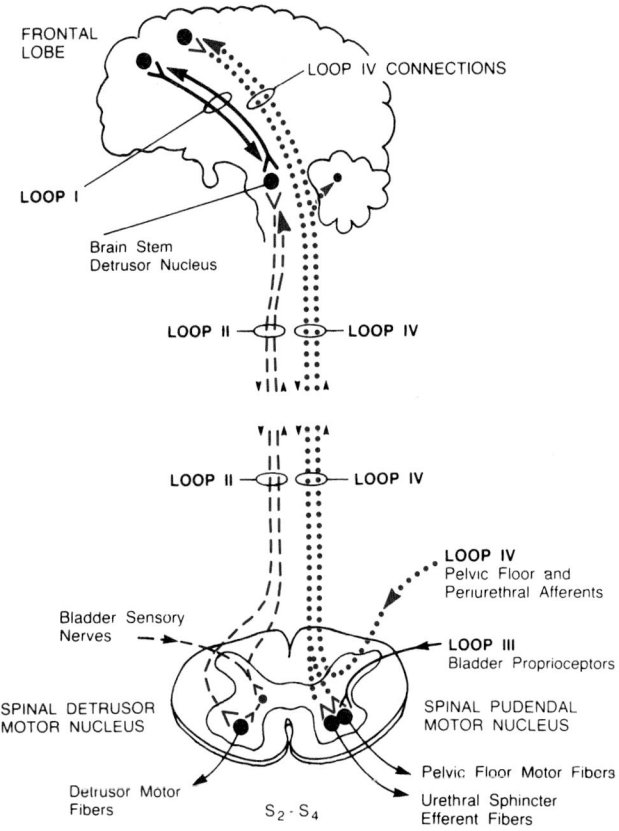

FIGURE 21-1 Central nervous system feedback loops. (From Williams ME and Fitzhugh CP: Ann Intern Med 97:895, 1982.)

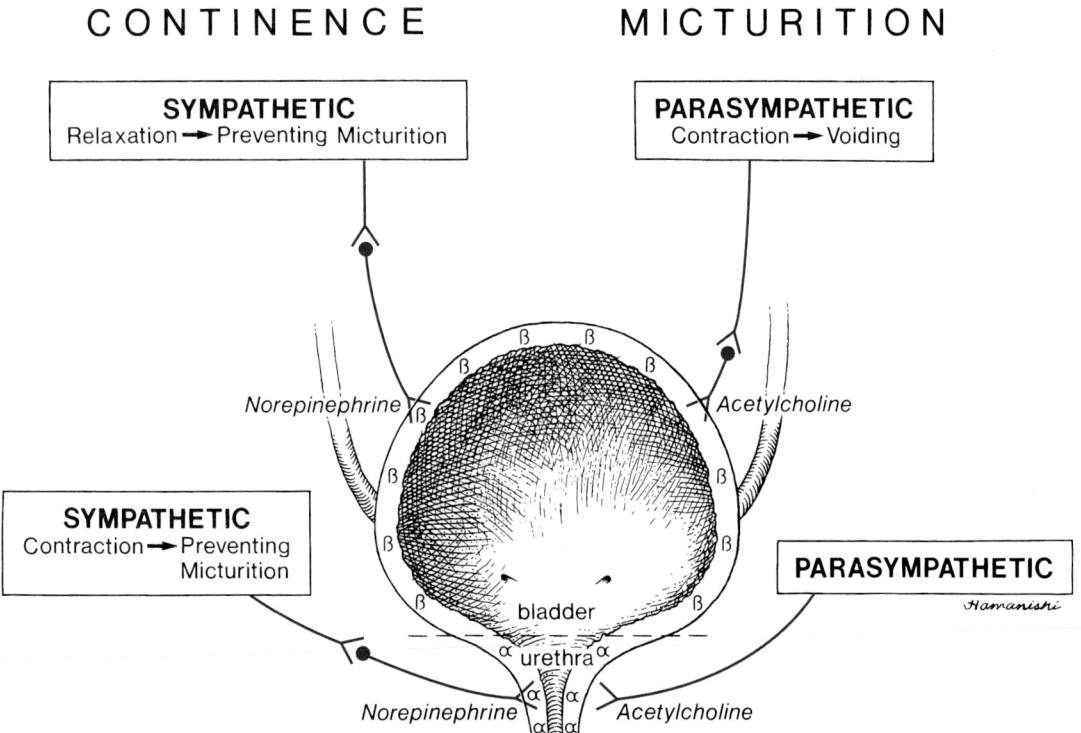

FIGURE 21-2 The innervation of the bladder and urethra. Parasympathetic fibers arising in S2 through S4 have long preganglionic fibers and pelvic ganglia close to the bladder and urethra. These parasympathetic fibers excrete acetylcholine. Sympathetic fibers that have long postganglionic fibers discharge norepinephrine to beta receptors, primarily in the bladder, and alpha receptors, primarily in the urethra. (Redrawn and modified from Raz S: Urol Clin North Am 5:323, 1978.)

TABLE 21-1
Neurologic Control of Micturition: Clinical Considerations on Central Nervous System Reflex Loops

Loop	Origin	Termination	Function	Associated Conditions
I	Frontal lobe	Brainstem	Coordinates volitional control of micturition	Parkinson's disease, brain tumors, trauma, cerebrovascular disease, MS, lower urinary tract disease
II	A. Brainstem B. Bladder wall	Sacral micturition center Brainstem	Detrusor muscle contraction to empty bladder	Spinal cord trauma, MS, spinal cord tumors
III	Sensory afferents of detrusor muscle	Striated muscle of urethral sphincter via pudendal motor nervous and micturition center	Allows relaxation of urethral sphincter in synchrony with detrusor contraction	MS, spinal cord trauma or tumors, diabetic neuropathy, local urinary tract disease
IV	Frontal lobe	Pudendal nucleus	Volitional control of striated external urethral sphincter	Cerebral or spinal trauma or tumor, MS, cerebrovascular disease, lower urinary tract disease

Modified from Ostergard DR: Obstet Gynecol Surv 34:417, 1979.

directly stimulating receptors in the bladder wall. The sympathetic system, on the other hand, basically acts to prevent micturition. Via this system norepinephrine is secreted, stimulating both alpha- and beta-adrenergic receptors. The bladder contains primarily beta receptors, stimulation of which causes relaxation of the detrusor muscle. The urethra contains primarily alpha receptors. Stimulation of these alpha receptors causes contraction of the urethral sphincter. Thus the overall effect is to prevent micturition (Figure 21-2). Because estrogen seems to stimulate alpha receptors and progesterone seems to stimulate beta receptors, these hormones play a role in maintaining continence in women in their reproductive years and in women receiving replacement hormone therapy who are postmenopausal.

Because the neurogenic control of micturition is so complex and depends on the interaction of so many factors, it is understandable that a host of general systemic diseases or diseases involving the nervous system may affect bladder control. These include, but are not limited to, demyelinating diseases (such as multiple sclerosis), diabetes mellitus, vascular diseases, and central nervous system trauma and tumors. In addition, medications that have an effect on the central or autonomic nervous systems may affect bladder control. Compounds with atropine-like effects may interfere with the initiation of micturition, whereas those with cholinergic effects may cause bladder irritability (Table 21-2). An appendix to this chapter (pp. 000-000) contains an exhaustive list developed by Ostergard of agents that affect bladder function.

With the neurologic principles of micturition in mind, it is appropriate to assess other factors that may influence continence. Asmussen and Ulmsten noted that the bladder

and the urethra are essentially a functional unit, with the bladder's subfunction to store urine and the urethra's to allow it to pass. For urine to pass through the urethra, the maximum urethral pressure must be lower than the intravesical pressure. Intravesical pressure depends on (1) the volume of fluid in the bladder, (2) the part of the intraabdominal pressure transmitted to the bladder, and (3) the tension in the bladder wall related to muscular and nervous system activity. The resting pressure in the bladder is between 20 and 30 cm water.

The intraurethral pressure depends on (1) the striated muscle fibers of the urethral wall, (2) smooth muscle fibers of the urethral wall, (3) the vascular content of the urethral submucosal cavernous plexus, (4) the passive elasticity of the urethral wall, and (5) the part of the intraabdominal pressure transmitted to the urethra.

Anatomically the exact border between the bladder and urethra is difficult to determine. The functional length of the urethra, however, is that part in which the urethral pressure exceeds the bladder pressure. Asmussen and Ulmsten have noted that the urethral closure pressure (UCP) is defined as the maximum urethral pressure minus the bladder pressure. For continence to be present the UCP must be greater than the bladder pressure. Urethral pressure varies with age, increasing up to the age of 20 and then gradually decreasing until menopause. However, after menopause the fall of this pressure is more rapid. Asmussen, Ulmsten, and Henriksson have demonstrated that the highest pressure zone in the urethra is about midpoint in the functional urethral length, and Westby et al. have located this zone at about 0.5 cm proximal to the urogenital diaphragm. Most of the functional urethral length is, indeed, above the urogenital diaphragm (Figure 21-3). Asmussen and Ulmsten and Gosling et al. have

TABLE 21-2
Some Common Drugs That Affect Continence and Micturition (See Appendix for Additional Information)

Sympathetic (relaxes bladder; controls urethral sphincter)

Drug	Action
Dopamine	Alpha adrenergic stimulator
Ethylphenylephrine	Alpha adrenergic stimulator
Methamphetamine	Alpha adrenergic stimulator
Norepinephrine	Alpha adrenergic stimulator
Phenylephrine	Alpha adrenergic stimulator
Albuterol	Beta adrenergic stimulator
Ethylnorepinephrine	Beta adrenergic stimulator
Isoproterenol	Beta adrenergic stimulator
Methoxyphenamine	Beta adrenergic stimulator
Terbutaline	Beta adrenergic stimulator

Parasympathetic (stimulates bladder contraction; relaxes urethral sphincter)

Drug	Action
Pilocarpine	Stimulates acetylcholine
Pralidoxime	Stimulates acetylcholine
Pyridostigmine	Stimulates acetylcholine

Sympathetic blockers

Drug	Action
Guanethidine	Adrenergic blocker
Hydralazine	Adrenergic blocker
Methyldopa	Adrenergic blocker
Reserpine	Adrenergic blocker

Parasympathetic blockers

Drug	Action
Anisotropine	Parasympathetic inhibitor
Atropine	Parasympathetic inhibitor
Clidinium	Parasympathetic inhibitor
Homatropine	Parasympathetic inhibitor
Papaverine	Parasympathetic inhibitor
Scopolamine	Parasympathetic inhibitor

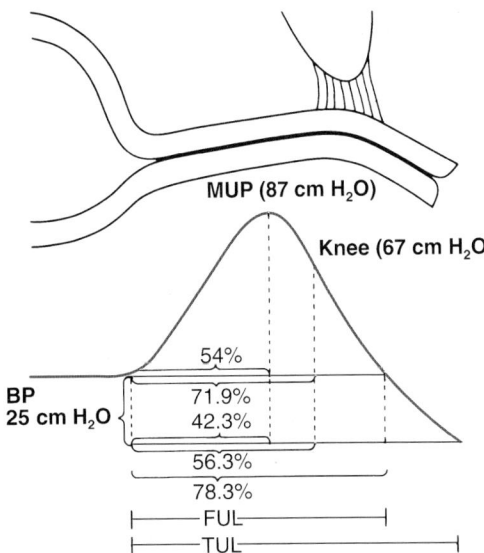

FIGURE 21-3 The location of maximum urethral pressure in relation to the urogenital diaphragm (average value of 25 normal women). KNEE indicates the location of the urogenital diaphragm seen on x-ray film and transformed to the pressure curve. (From Asmussen M and Ulmsten U: On the physiology of continence and pathophysiology of stress incontinence in the female. In Controversies in gynecology and obstetrics, vol 10, Basel, 1983, Karger, S, AG, pp. 32-50.)

pointed out that the submucosal cavernous plexus of vessels, the bulk of the smooth and striated muscle, and the bulk of the autonomic nerve supply are most prominent in the area in which they record the maximum urethral pressure. Because the urethral pressure displays high pressure zone oscillations that are synchronous with the heartbeat, the submucosal cavernous plexus is probably important in helping to maintain continence (Figure 21-4). Indeed, this structure is under the control of estrogen. Enhorning and also Asmussen and Ulmsten have demonstrated that urethral pressure can oscillate as much

as 25 cm of water in young women but seldom more than 5 cm water in postmenopausal women. The cavernous plexus is thicker walled and less elastic in older women. Thus not only are the epithelium of the bladder and the bladder neck dependent on hormone stimulation, but so probably is the vascular system of these areas.

Because the maximum urethral pressure area under normal circumstances lies above the urogenital diaphragm and because intraabdominal pressure likely affects both the bladder and this area of the urethra equally, if normal anatomic relationships are maintained, a sudden intraabdominal pressure increase should not, under normal circumstances, cause incontinence. On the other hand, if the functional urethra is displaced from its usual anatomic relationships, it may be excluded from the effect of increased intraabdominal pressure and therefore be susceptible to it. This problem will be addressed further in the discussion of stress incontinence.

DeLancey made some interesting observations on functioning periurethral anatomy by studying serial histologic sections of intact pelvic viscera and surrounding tissue, as well as by dissecting 22 fresh and embalmed cadavers. Because the length of the urethra varies from woman to woman, topography of urethral and periurethral structures was expressed in terms of the location along the urethra using percentages of the total urethra. DeLancey considered the zero location as that point in which the urethra leaves the bladder lumen and the

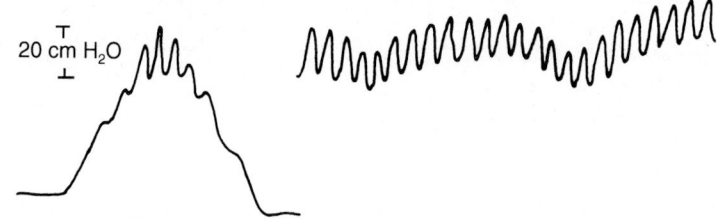

20 cm H₂O

FIGURE 21-4 The maximum urethral pressure shows great variation synchronously with the heartbeat. Variations of 20 cm H₂O as shown in the curve are not uncommon. (From Asmussen M and Ulmsten U: On the physiology of continence and pathophysiology of stress incontinence in the female. In Controversies in gynecology and obstetrics, vol 10, Basel, 1983, Karger, S, AG, pp. 32-50.)

TABLE 21-3
Topography of Urethral and Paraurethral Structures*

Approxiamate Location†	Region of the Urethra	Paraurethral Structures
0–20	Intramural urethra	Urethral lumen traverses the bladder wall
20–60	Midurethra	Striated urethral sphincter muscle Pubourethral ligament Vaginolevator attachment
60–80	Urogenital diaphragm	Compressor urethrae muscle Urethrovaginal sphincter muscle
80–100	Distal urethra	Bulbocavernosus muscle

From DeLancey JO: Obstet Gynecol 68:91, 1986. Reprinted with permission from The American College of Obstetricians and Gynecologists.

*Smooth muscle of the urethra was not considered.

†Expressed as a percentile of total urethral length.

100th percentile as that point in which the urethra terminates on the perineum. From the standpoint of functional anatomy there is excellent agreement among the measurements made from each of his specimens when percentiles were used. Table 21-3 depicts these anatomic relationships. It can be seen that the intramural urethra represents approximately 20% of the length of the urethra. The portion of the urethra encircled by striated urethral sphincter muscle and associated with the pubourethral ligament and vaginal levator attachment concerns the midurethra, that is, that portion which is from the 20th to 60th percentile along the total length. The 60th to 80th percentile of the urethral length passes through the urogenital diaphragm and is under the influence of the urethrovaginal sphincter muscles. Finally, the last 20%, or distal urethra, traverses the bulbocavernosus muscles. These urethral landmarks are depicted in Figure 21-5, which highlights the actual ranges and values found in DeLancey's study. The actual anatomic relationships are depicted in Figure 21-6. DeLancey's observations help to correlate the anatomic relationships to the physiologic observations that others have made.

In a subsequent paper, DeLancey pointed out that additional anatomic factors may influence continence. Using serial histologic sections from 8 female cadavers and the dissections of 34 other cadavers, he noted that the proximal urethra gets added support because the anterior vagina is attached to the muscles of the pelvic diaphragm and to the arcus tendineus fasciae pelvis. Contraction of the pelvic diaphragm thus pulls the vagina against the posterior surface of the urethra, helping to close it. At rest the urethra is supported by both its attachment to the arcus tendineus fasciae pelvis and the tone of the pelvic diaphragm muscles. The distal urethra in the region of the urogenital diaphragm is supported by two striated muscle arches, the compressor urethrae and urethrovaginal sphincter. These muscles help to compress the distal urethra, helping to maintain continence during a cough. Collagen is extremely important in maintaining the strength of the support structures of the urethra and the vagina. Estrogen contributes greatly to the development of collagen and therefore plays a role in this aspect of continence as well.

The U.S. Department of Health and Human Services, Agency for Health Care Policy and Research published a clinical practice guideline on urinary incontinence in adults.

URETHRAL LANDMARKS

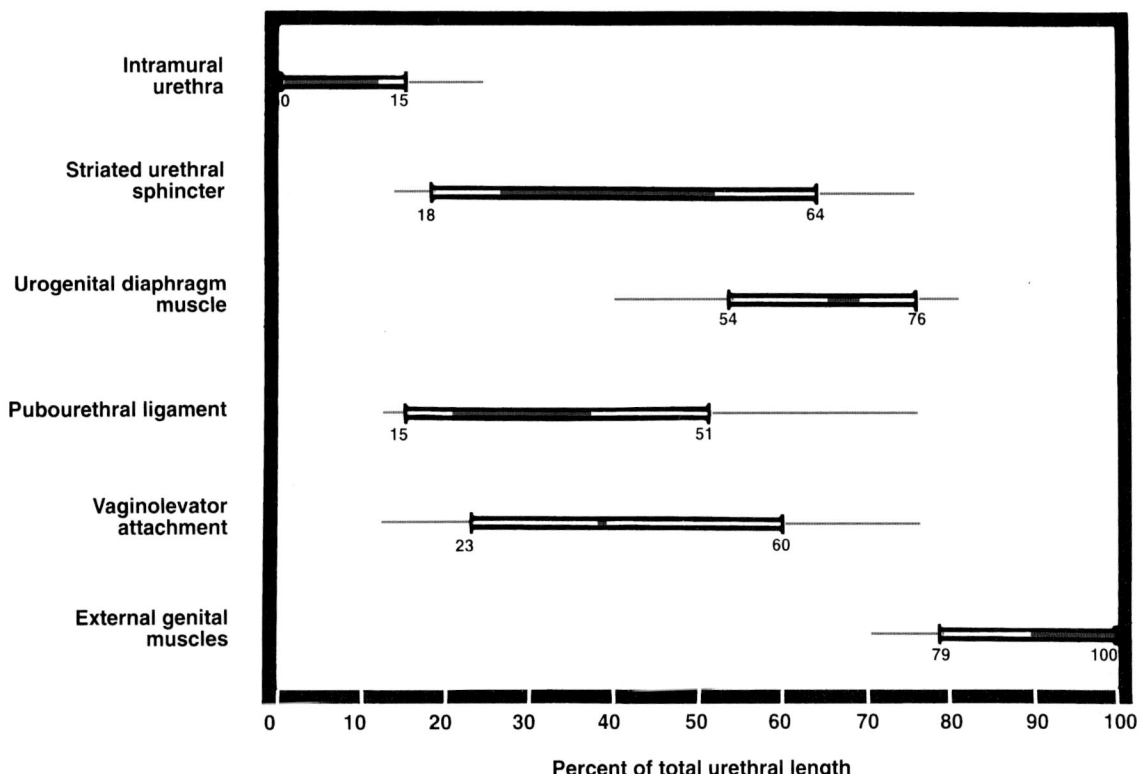

FIGURE 21-5 Average spatial distribution of periurethral structures, as well as the range of values found. Urogenital diaphragm muscles are the compressor urethrae and urethrovaginal sphincter. (From DeLancey JO: Obstet Gynecol 68:91, 1986. Reprinted with permission from The American College of Obstetricians and Gynecologists.)

Risk Factors Associated with Incontinence

Immobility
Medication use
History of smoking
Delirium
High-impact activities (includes heavy lifting or strenuous athletic endeavors)
Pelvic muscle weakness
Pregnancy/childbirth history
Cognitive status
Obesity
History of fecal impaction
History of low fluid intake
Diabetes mellitus
Stroke
Hypoestrogen state
Racial status
History of childhood nocturnal enuresis

The box above lists the currently known risk factors that are associated with incontinence, summarizing the work of several authors. Most of these have been alluded to in this chapter, but a few warrant specific mention. Bump and McClish compared risk factors and determinants of genuine stress incontinence between smokers and nonsmokers using a case-control method. Seventy-one smokers and 118 non-smokers were compared following a complete urogynecologic evaluation. Smokers were found to have stronger urethral sphincters and generated greater increase in bladder pressure with coughing but had similar findings with respect to urethral mobility and pressure transmission ratios when compared with nonsmokers. Genuine stress incontinence developed in smokers despite their stronger urethral sphincter findings, probably due to more violent coughing leading to earlier development of anatomic and pressure transmission defects.

A second area of interest involves racial differences with respect to the presence of urinary incontinence and other pelvic relaxation problems. Bump pointed out that black women with urinary incontinence have a different distribution of symptoms and have different reasons for their incontinence than do white women. The black women had a significantly lower prevalence of pure genuine stress incontinence than did the white women. These conclusions were based on a study of 200 consecutive women, 54 of whom were black, referred for evaluation of urinary stress incontinence or pelvic organ prolapse. The findings may possibly relate to a difference in collagen and connective tissue in individuals of the two races.

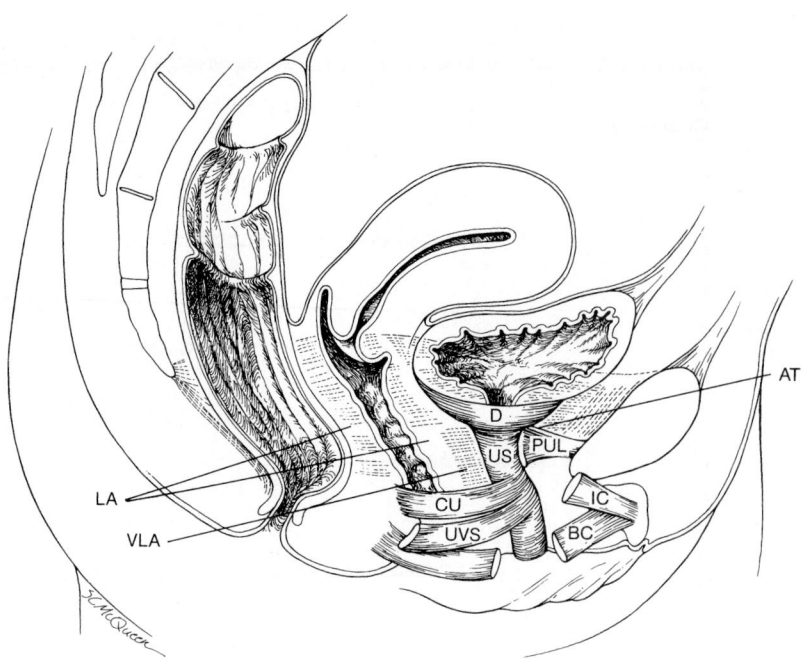

FIGURE 21-6　Interrelationships of approximate location of periurethral structures. Levator ani muscles are shown as light lines running deep to the pelvic viscera. The vaginal levator attachment is shown as a darker area. *VLA,* vaginal levator attachment; *LA,* levator ani muscles; *D,* detrusor muscle; *US,* urethral sphincter; *CU,* compressor urethrae; *UVS,* urethrovaginal sphincter; *AT,* arcus tendineus fasciae pelvis; *PUL,* pubourethral ligament; *IC,* ischiocavernosus muscle; and *BC,* bulbocavernosus muscle. (Redrawn from DeLancey JO: Obstet Gynecol 68:91, 1986. Reproduced with permission from The American College of Obstetricians and Gynecologists.)

DIAGNOSTIC PROCEDURES

Useful testing can be done in the gynecologist's office without the need for sophisticated equipment. These procedures are described next and their benefits noted. Their description is followed by a discussion of more sophisticated diagnostic techniques requiring specialized equipment.

Urine Analysis and Culture

A simple urine analysis and urine culture may give a great deal of information. The presence of white blood cells or red blood cells and bacteria in a catheterized or clean voided sample (in which the perineum around the urethra is appropriately prepared with an antiseptic solution) may suggest urethritis, a diverticulum that is infected, trigonitis, or cystitis. Their presence may also suggest an infection in the upper urinary tract, such as pyelonephritis. Chronic infection in the lower tract may be associated with urgency, frequency, dysuria, and even incontinence. In such instances the urine analysis and urine culture may be diagnostic. Several dipstick methods are available to detect bacteriuria and pyuria. The accuracy of these methods is quite variable, but they do have some use in screening patients who are incontinent or who have symptoms suggestive of infection. In every case a culture should be

obtained both to identify the specific organism involved and to verify the presence of an infection.

Test for Residual Urine

This simple procedure can be extremely helpful in the evaluation of a patient with cystocele or overflow incontinence. The patient is asked to void, and a catheter is inserted within no more than 10 to 15 minutes thereafter. The urine remaining in the bladder is measured and may be sent for analysis and culture. Under normal circumstances the amount of residual urine should be less than 50 ml after the patient has voided at least 100 to 150 ml. Large amounts of residual urine suggest overflow incontinence resulting from inadequate bladder emptying.

Office Cystometrics

Bladder capacity and bladder function may be measured with sophisticated tools, which are discussed later. Nevertheless it is possible to gain a great deal of information about bladder capacity and bladder function with a relatively simple apparatus. If after a catheter is inserted to check for residual urine, the catheter is left in place and attached to a graduated Asepto syringe without bulb, it is possible to pour sterile saline into the syringe and measure the amount of saline that first causes the patient to have the urge to void. This urge should normally occur after 150 to 200 ml of saline have been infused. However, normal women should be able to continue to maintain continence at that level, with a strong, normally uncontrollable urge to void usually occurring when 400 to 500 ml have been instilled. Thus a normal bladder first transmits an urge to void at 150 to 200 ml, and functional capacity is reached at 400 to 500 ml. Most women can maintain continence with larger volumes, but this is usually accomplished with a great deal of conscious effort.

Stress (Bonney) Test

If a bladder has been previously filled to measure capacity, it should then be emptied to about 250 ml of saline, or if the bladder is empty, 250 ml of saline should be instilled. The catheter is then removed, and the patient is asked to cough while in the recumbent position. If urine spurts from the urethral meatus, stress incontinence may be present. The bladder neck should be gently elevated with the finger or an instrument such as a Kelly clamp, and the patient should be asked to cough once again. Care should be taken not to compress the urethra, thereby mechanically occluding it. If urine no longer spurts from the urethra when the bladder neck is supported, this suggests that the bladder neck separation from the pubic symphysis may be responsible for the incontinence, and an appropriate operative repair could be expected to produce continence.

Migliorini and Glenning questioned the value of this test because they noted that a group of women with urethral sphincter weakness demonstrated by urodynamic studies were still incontinent even when the bladder neck was elevated (Bonney test). Bhatia and Bergman had previously reached a similar conclusion, stating that they believed the test restored continence by obstructing the urethra and urethrovesicle junction. However, Miyazaki studying 37 patients with genuine stress incontinence was able to demonstrate that the Bonney test does not work by direct urethral compression, but instead appears to produce continence by restoring the anterior vaginal wall hammock. But it is often noted that patients who have had successful operations to elevate the bladder neck for the treatment of stress incontinence will show obstructive patterns on postoperative urodynamic studies. For the practitioner who is trying to judge clinically whether the replacement of the urethrovesicle junction behind the pubic symphysis will aid continence, the test may still be useful.

Because urine loss with cough should be immediate if stress incontinence is the problem, it may be possible to detect evidence of detrusor instability by observing the time of the spurt of urine in the Bonney test. Classically the detrusor reacts a few seconds after the stimulus; therefore a spurt that occurs after a delay after a cough suggests the presence of a detrusor instability.

After the Bonney test is performed in a recumbent patient, it should be repeated with the patient standing. Frequently the patient will appear to be continent with stress while lying down but may demonstrate incontinence when the influence of gravity on the pelvic organs is brought into play in the standing position.

Thus with the urine analysis, urine culture, tests for residual urine, information about the amount of urine required to cause the first urge to void, information concerning general bladder capacity, and the Bonney test in both the recumbent and the standing positions, the physician will have a great deal of information concerning the etiology of the patient's urinary problem. More sophisticated urodynamic evaluations using specific and often costly equipment should be performed by individuals who are trained and experienced in these tests. A short discussion of these procedures and the equipment involved follows.

Urethroscopy

Urethroscopy is excellent for visualizing the urethra and therefore offers information about inflammatory processes within the urethra, urethral diverticula, other anatomic defects, and estrogenic effects and permits some estimate of urethral tone. The use of a gas medium such as carbon dioxide is appropriate for these studies. Although the equipment used for performing gas urethroscopy makes it possible to measure pressures within the urethra and the bladder, caution must be exercised because a rapid instillation of carbon dioxide into the lower urinary tract may stimulate detrusor contraction, which may in itself lead to reflex opening of the vesical neck, thus giving false information about the bladder neck and the urethral sphincter.

A variety of equipment is available for this procedure. Relatively inexpensive apparatuses can be used for urethroscopy, as well as for cystometry and uroflowmetry.

Cystoscopy and Cystometry

Cystoscopy may be performed using a water system or a carbon dioxide gas system. The water system is probably best used for diagnosis of detrusor hyperactivity because it does not cause the reflex irritability of the detrusor muscle that has been observed with the gas system. In either case the bladder may be visualized and the presence of inflammation or benign or malignant processes noted.

In attempting to understand the basis of anatomic urinary stress incontinence, the practitioner must realize that what must be determined is the relationship between the simultaneous intraurethral and intravesical pressures (Figure 21-7). For greatest accuracy these must be measured with the patient in the standing and reclining positions, at rest and with straining. The ideal means of evaluating a patient for stress incontinence is to use a multichannel recorder that permits pressure determinations at two points within the urethra (proximal and midpoint to distal), one within the bladder, and one intraabdominally as recorded by an intrarectal sensor or by a sensor within the vagina if the vagina is in a relatively normal position (not prolapsed). Should intraabdominal stress be transmitted equally to the bladder and the urethra and should the intravesical pressure be less than the urethral closing pressure, one would expect closing pressure to be overcome and stress incontinence to be demonstrated if an intraabdominal pressure increase is transmitted to the bladder but not to the urethra.

Multiple-channel devices involve more expensive equipment and require continuous maintenance. It is possible to add a video urodynamic system to the multichannel recorders, making it possible to identify reflux into the ureters under pressure situations. The video system also makes it possible to actually observe the act of micturition and the effect of stress. Because the data obtained by multichannel pressure recordings plus the ability to actually visualize the patient micturate offer the most accurate diagnostic information that the clinician can obtain, this technique is considered the standard against which other tests are measured.

Simple or multichannel cystometry makes it possible to diagnose unstable bladder or detrusor instability, detrusor hyperreflexia, detrusor sphincter dyssynergia, detrusor hyperactivity with impaired contractility, hypermobility of the bladder neck, intrinsic sphincter deficiency, and neurogenic sphincter deficiency. Video urodynamics is useful for determining detrusor hyperactivity with

impaired contractility, hypermobility of the bladder neck, and overflow from outlet obstruction.

INFECTIONS OF THE LOWER URINARY TRACT

Infections of the urethra and bladder are almost always associated with some combination of the following: frequency, urgency, dysuria, pyuria, hematuria, acute or chronic pelvic pain, backache, and at times fever. As many as 20% of all women develop urinary tract infections at some time during their life, and by age 70 as many as 10% of women will have chronic urinary tract infections. At times incontinence is associated with acute and chronic infections. Although *Escherichia coli* is the cause of most of the infections, a myriad of organisms including *Enterobacter, Klebsiella, Pseudomonas, Proteus, Streptococcus faecalis, Morganella, Staphylococcus,* and *Chlamydia* are often found. The presence of bacteria in the urine (bacteriuria) does not necessarily prove clinical infection. Bacteriuria is fairly common in women, especially older women. For instance, cumulative data from several studies suggest that 20% of women over 65 years of age will demonstrate bacteriuria, but the percentage increases from about 15% in the 65- to 70-year group to 20% to 50% for women over age 80. Bacteriuria is quite common in women who are on chronic catheterization and in women in nursing homes who are chronically incontinent.

The presence of at least 100,000 organisms per milliliter of urine is generally accepted as evidence for a clinical infection. In cases of urethritis and trigonitis the presence of as few as 100 organisms per milliliter may indicate an infection because of the dilution of bladder urine. White blood cells are always seen in the urine (pyuria) when urinary tract infection occurs, and red blood cells may be present in microscopic or macroscopic numbers. Hematuria is common in acute infections.

Many explanations have been offered as to why the female urinary tract is vulnerable to infection. These include the fact that the female urethra is short, thereby allowing easier access of bacteria to the bladder; the proximity of the vulva, vagina, and rectum to the opening of the urethra; poor hygiene, including the habit in some women of wiping toward the urethra after a bowel movement; the effects of sexual intercourse on the entrance of bacteria into the urethra and the lower urinary tract; and the effect of loss of estrogen on the reproductive tract of elderly women. To this list it is probably appropriate to add personal immunologic variations that may make one woman more susceptible to certain bacteria than other women. This is particularly true for older women, since immunologic competency diminishes with age.

Additional circumstances that may be responsible for infections in women include the dilation of the urinary tract in pregnancy, urinary tract obstruction, ureteral

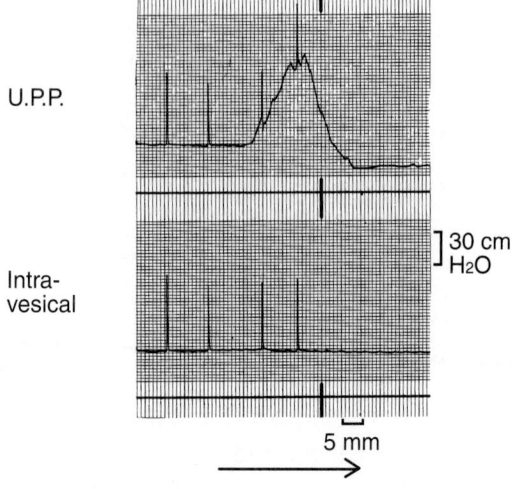

FIGURE 21-7 Simultaneous recordings of urethra and intravesical pressures during coughing. Stress produces a parallel increase of bladder and urethral pressure because the intraabdominal position of the bladder and proximal two thirds of the urethra are displayed. (From Raz S: Urol Clin North Am 5:323, 1978.)

reflux, and situations of urinary tract relaxation. Other causes of urinary tract infections in both men and women are the need for frequent catheterization, instrumentation, the loss of resistance that occurs in general systemic disease, and overdistention of the bladder in neurogenic conditions where stasis becomes a problem.

Urethritis

Patients with urethritis generally have the typical findings of lower urinary tract infection, which include dysuria, frequency, and urgency. They often have a urethra that is tender to palpation. Under certain circumstances it may be possible to express pus from the urethra; this is particularly common in acute infections with the gonococcus or *Chlamydia*. In these situations the infection involves not only the urethra but also the periurethral glands. Frequently, significant pyuria is noted in a clean-catch urine sample, particularly that taken early in the voiding. The urine should be inspected, since *Trichomonas* infestation is frequently noted in such instances.

Pus expressed from the urethra should be submitted for culture and for smear with Gram stain. Intracellular diplococci are suggestive of gonorrhea. *Neisseria gonorrhoeae* or *Chlamydia* is usually cultured in such situations. Urine obtained by the clean-catch method should also be cultured.

If no specific organism is identified on smear, a broad-spectrum coverage such as a sulfa preparation or nitrofurantoin (Macrodantin), 50 or 100 mg three or four times a day, should be prescribed for 10 days. If *Chlamydia* is suspected, tetracycline should be prescribed for at least 10 days. If gonorrhea is diagnosed, the current recommended treatment consists of ceftriaxone 250 mg intramuscularly (single dose) plus doxycycline 100 mg by mouth two times a day for 7 days. An alternative therapy is spectinomycin 2 g intramuscularly (single dose) followed by doxycycline. Penicillin is no longer the drug of choice because of the many penicillin-resistant strains of gonococcus now present.

Urethral Syndrome

The so-called *urethral syndrome* is characterized by the same symptoms of dysuria, frequency, urgency, and pain that are seen with urethritis, but generally the symptoms are of long standing, and no specific organism can be identified. Classically, urethroscopy has revealed a reddened, chronically inflamed urethra with spasm at the bladder neck. This condition is quite common and may affect as many as 20% to 30% of all women at one time or another. The etiology is unknown, but there are many theories, including allergic, immunologic, infectious, neurologic, atrophic, and psychogenic causes. Some feel the problem resides in the paraurethral glands and that infection with such organisms as mycoplasma, uroplasma, or

Chlamydia might be responsible. The incidence of these infections, however, has been about the same as in populations of women without the syndrome. Nevertheless, such organisms should be sought and eradicated with appropriate antibiotic therapy when they are found, since this may alleviate symptoms in such cases.

Recently, Gittes and Nakamura drew attention to the fact that the periurethral glands, analogous to the prostate in the male, might be inflamed clinically just as can the prostate. They suggested treating patients with urethral syndrome in the same fashion that men with prostatitis are treated. Baerheim et al. compared the success of treatment with antibacterial therapy in 51 patients with acute lower urinary tract infection and 58 patients with acute urethral syndrome and found improvement by 3 days in about half of each group.

Because the etiology in most cases is unknown, various therapies have been devised with varying success. These include dilation of the urethra with progressive dilators, antispasmodics, estrogen (in postmenopausal women), and more recently, cryosurgery. Sand et al., in a randomized cross-over trial, compared cryosurgery using a specially designed cryoprobe with dilation and massage of the urethra in 24 patients diagnosed as having the urethral syndrome. Of the patients first treated with cryosurgery, 91% achieved relief of their symptoms, compared with 33% of patients first treated with dilation and massage. When cross-over of the failures occurred, 75% of women treated with cryosurgery were relieved of symptoms, compared with none of the cryotherapy failures who were then treated with dilation and massage.

Patients diagnosed as having the urethral syndrome deserve a careful evaluation before specific therapy is determined.

Cystitis

Cystitis is perhaps the most common of the urinary tract infections. It is diagnosed when a clean-catch urine sample or catheterized specimen has a bacteria concentration of 100,000 or more per milliliter of urine and when the patient suffers the symptoms of dysuria, frequency, urgency, and pain. White blood cells are almost always seen in large numbers in the urine, as are bacteria. Red blood cells are frequently present in microscopic numbers, but gross hematuria may occur as a result of extravasation of blood across dilated and inflamed capillaries. If the bladder is visualized, it is noted to be uniformly reddened and inflamed. Treatment involves obtaining a culture and beginning the patient on a general antibiotic regimen of sulfa or nitrofurantoin, although a variety of other antibiotics could be used as substitutes for general therapy. These include tetracycline, ampicillin, cephalosporin, nalidixic acid (NegGram), or one of the quinolines such as oflaxin or norfloxacin. When results of the culture are reported, the antibiotic may be changed if the organisms noted are not sensitive to the antibiotic in use. Treatment should be continued for 10 days, although shorter periods are appropriate for certain antibiotics, and the patient should remain well hydrated and should be encouraged to continue treatment even though symptoms generally disappear within 48 hours. Infections frequently recur and become chronic because they are not adequately eradicated. This may result from physician error (treating with too low a dose of antibiotic or for too short a period of time) or patient error (not taking the medication as prescribed). The latter occurrence is generally suspected when the same organism is continuously cultured.

Recurrent infections of different organisms should alert the physician to the need for a more complete evaluation of the urinary tract, including intravenous pyelogram (seeking structural abnormalities of the bladder, kidney, and/or ureters). Occasionally, continuous antibiotic therapy at lower doses for more prolonged periods is necessary to ensure that the patient is no longer infected.

Frequent catheterizations or manipulation of the lower urinary tract often causes urinary tract infections. An indwelling catheter for 24 hours leads to bacteriuria in as many as 50% of patients. When left in place for 96 hours, an indwelling catheter causes bacteriuria in nearly 100% of patients. Many physicians suggest prophylactic antibiotics in patients who must continue catheter use, but no good evidence supports this thesis. Certainly a patient with an indwelling catheter should be monitored for the possibility of bacteriuria and urinary tract infections, be kept well hydrated, and have a urine culture when the catheter is removed. Postoperative and debilitated patients are at greatest risk.

Physicians can counsel their patients about preventive measures by instructing them on proper hygiene. This consists of cleansing the vulvar region at least daily, wiping the rectum away from the urethra, and encouraging good hygiene with respect to coitus. In women who develop frequent urinary tract infections secondary to coitus, one technique is to encourage voiding immediately after intercourse. This tends to wash out bacteria that have entered the urethra before they can cause an infection. Elderly sexually active women may benefit from either external or systemic estrogen therapy.

Interstitial Cystitis

Interstitial cystitis is a complex inflammatory condition of the bladder. The etiology and pathophysiology is poorly understood and most likely multifactorial. It is usually associated with an altered epithelial permeability, mast cell activation, and an upregulation of sensory afferent nerves. It is a common disease seen in females more often than males, but the incidence is really not known, although it has been estimated to be as high as 500 per 100,000.

Symptoms of interstitial cystitis are urgency, frequency, and bladder pain without evidence for infection. It is often confused with other bladder conditions, pelvic inflammatory disease, and endometriosis. The patient will usually void frequently and a voiding diary will often demonstrate frequent voiding of less than 150 ml each and with as many as 20 or more voidings per day.

On cystoscopy, the bladder frequently appears normal during filling, but with distention, characteristic petechial hemorrhages resembling glomeruli usually appear. Oozing of blood is often seen. If a biopsy is taken, ulcers with granulation tissue, mucosal hemorrhage, monocytic infiltration, and mast cells in the lamina propia and detrussor muscle are often seen. Parson has proposed that the changes are related to a defective or altered glycoaminoglycan mucus layer which results in altered bladder permeability. However, investigations to date do not show whether this alteration is cause or effect. Some authors feel that these changes are the result of an autoimmune disease. The presence of immunoglobulins and complement in the bladder wall and the increase in interleukin-6 in the urine of patients may support this.

There are many treatments available, but few have been uniformly helpful. Patients are encouraged to see the problem as a chronic one that is not malignant and to try to reduce stress, encourage family support, and avail themselves of the writings and support of the Interstitial Cystitis Foundation. They should be instructed to avoid acidic, alcoholic, and carbonated beverages, spicy foods, coffee, tea, and chocolate, all of which have been associated with increased pain in patients with interstitial cystitis. Bladder retraining to increase the interval between voiding may help and antidepression medications may be useful in appropriate patients.

Standard medical therapy has included DMSO instillation often accompanied by heparin, steroids, or local anesthetics. DMSO is an antiinflammatory agent that acts as a bladder anesthetic, relaxes muscles, causes mast cell inhibition, and may dissolve collagen.

Heparin has been used by bladder instillation for 1 hour, three times a week. Recently, a heparin analogue, pentosan polysulfate sodium (Elmiron), has been given 100 mg three times a day orally with some reported improvement. Often DMSO is given as a single treatment followed by heparin therapy for up to 1 year.

Since interstitial cystitis is a complex disease, it is best treated by experienced physicians with the expertise and patience to deal with the patient and her needs over a prolonged period of time.

Urethral Diverticulum

Etiology

Urethral diverticula occur in perhaps as many as 3% to 4% of all women sometime during their lifetime. Age distribution in published reports ranges from 19 to 76 years, but the majority of diverticula seem to occur between the ages of 30 and 50. Andersen has suggested that the disease occurs more frequently in blacks, with a ratio perhaps as high as 6 to 1.

A variety of etiologies have been suggested, including congenital, acute and chronic inflammatory, and traumatic. The congenital theory stems from the fact that cases have been reported in children and neonates. Evidence for acute and chronic infection stems from the fact that several observers have noted infection and obstruction of periurethral glands, which result in the formation of retention cysts that, when repeatedly infected, may rupture into the lumen of the urethra, giving rise to the diverticulum. Several authors have suggested that the gonococcus is the cause of this, but *E. coli* and other organisms have been found in such processes. Urethral trauma from multiple catheterizations or from childbirth has also been suggested as an etiologic factor. However, many women with diverticula have neither been catheterized nor given birth. The infectious etiology is probably the most common.

Symptoms and Signs

The usual symptoms and signs of a patient with diverticulitis include urgency, frequency, dysuria, and dyspareunia. Frequently a history of recurrent urinary tract infection, dribbling, and incontinence is noted. Occasionally, hematuria occurs. In a series reported from the Mayo Clinic, Lee noted that a palpable, tender, suburethral mass was present in 51 of 85 patients (60%) and that protrusion of the diverticulum from the vaginal introitus occurred in 4 patients. Occasionally, patients have urinary stones within the diverticula.

Diagnosis

Diagnosis is generally suspected by physical examination and confirmed by cystourethroscopy or voiding cystourethrogram. At times it may be necessary to use a double-catheter balloon technique that essentially closes the urethra at each end and forces contrast medium into the diverticulum under pressure during cystogram.

Management

A variety of procedures have been suggested for the management of urethral diverticula. Lapides has suggested a technique for transurethral marsupialization that involves the resection of the roof of the diverticulum, using transurethral electrocautery. Essentially this technique enlarges the orifice of the diverticulum by incising its roof. Spence and Duckett reported a marsupialization technique in which the diverticulum was opened and sutured to the vaginal epithelial surface. Generally this leads to a fistula and requires secondary closure, making this technique useful in only rare circumstances.

A classic operative approach uses urethroscopy to identify the location of the diverticulum. It is important at this point to note the presence of multiple diverticula. In Lee's report from the Mayo Clinic the diverticulum was noted coming from the distal third of the urethra in only 10 of the 85 patients, whereas 38 patients demonstrated an origin from the middle third and 13 from the proximal third, including the bladder neck. Lee noted multiple diverticula in 18 of his 85 patients.

After the diverticulum is identified and evaluated, an incision is made in the anterior vaginal wall and the diverticulum is dissected free of the pubocervical fascia. The diverticulum's attachment to the urethra is noted, it is excised by sharp dissection, and the urethral wall is closed with a row of interrupted 4-0 catgut or polyglycol sutures. The closure line is generally in the longitudinal axis. Occasionally, however, a transverse closure is necessary because of the nature of the attachment. The pubocervical fascia is then reinforced with a row of 3-0 polyglycol reabsorbable interrupted sutures. Hemostasis is scrupulously secured with electrocautery, and the vaginal incision is closed with catgut or polyglycol sutures (Figure 21-8).

Most diverticula emanate from the ventral wall of the urethra. Occasionally, however, the diverticulum is noted to be arising from the lateral wall of the urethra or even from the anterior wall. In such cases the dissection must be carefully carried to the base of the diverticulum and the procedure carried out as stated. In cases of diverticula arising from the dorsal wall of the urethra, it is appropriate to simply excise the diverticulum at its neck and allow the tissue of the urethra to retract. In all cases a No. 16 or 18 Foley catheter is left in place for 6 or 7 days.

Several nuances have been offered to make dissection and subsequent repair easier. One of these is placing a ureteral catheter into the diverticulum and allowing it to coil so that the diverticulum is more easily observable during dissection. Other surgeons have attempted to dilate the neck of the diverticulum before beginning the excision and occasionally have even tried to pack foreign substances such as gauze through the neck to make the dissection easier.

Complications

Major complications of this procedure include urethrovaginal fistula formation, recurrence of the diverticulum, and stricture of the urethra.

In a study from the Mayo Clinic, MacKinnon et al. reported on 140 patients treated operatively, 7 of whom (5%) developed urethrovaginal fistulas. In Lee's report of a later study from the Mayo Clinic, only one patient developed a fistula. In another series, Spraitz and Welch, reporting on 94 patients repaired, found 4 with urethrovaginal fistulas.

Recurrence of diverticula is reported in about 5% to

10% of patients in various series. If the diverticulum recurs within the first few months after operation, it may represent a second diverticulum that was overlooked or an inappropriate repair of the diagnosed diverticulum. If the diverticulum occurs after 1 year, it is probably a new lesion.

Stricture of the urethra has rarely been reported in any of the operative series. It is a theoretic possibility.

Other complications involve stress incontinence, which may be related to the dissection of the bladder neck away from its usual location, and the development of the urethral syndrome, probably caused by continuing inflammation and irritation. These conditions generally respond to appropriate specific therapy.

Urolithiasis

Urinary tract stones may occur in patients of either sex and at any age. They may be related to metabolic abnormalities, such as gout or errors of calcium metabolism, but usually they relate to chronic infection and stasis of urine. Risk factors for calculi in women include pregnancy, during which time the urinary tract becomes dilated and stasis is more common; large cystoceles; and obstruction of outflow secondary to anatomic variations or external pressure from other organs.

A variety of management techniques are available, including observation awaiting spontaneous passage, endoscopic removal, surgical removal, and the destruction of the stone with the lithotriptor. The principal considera-

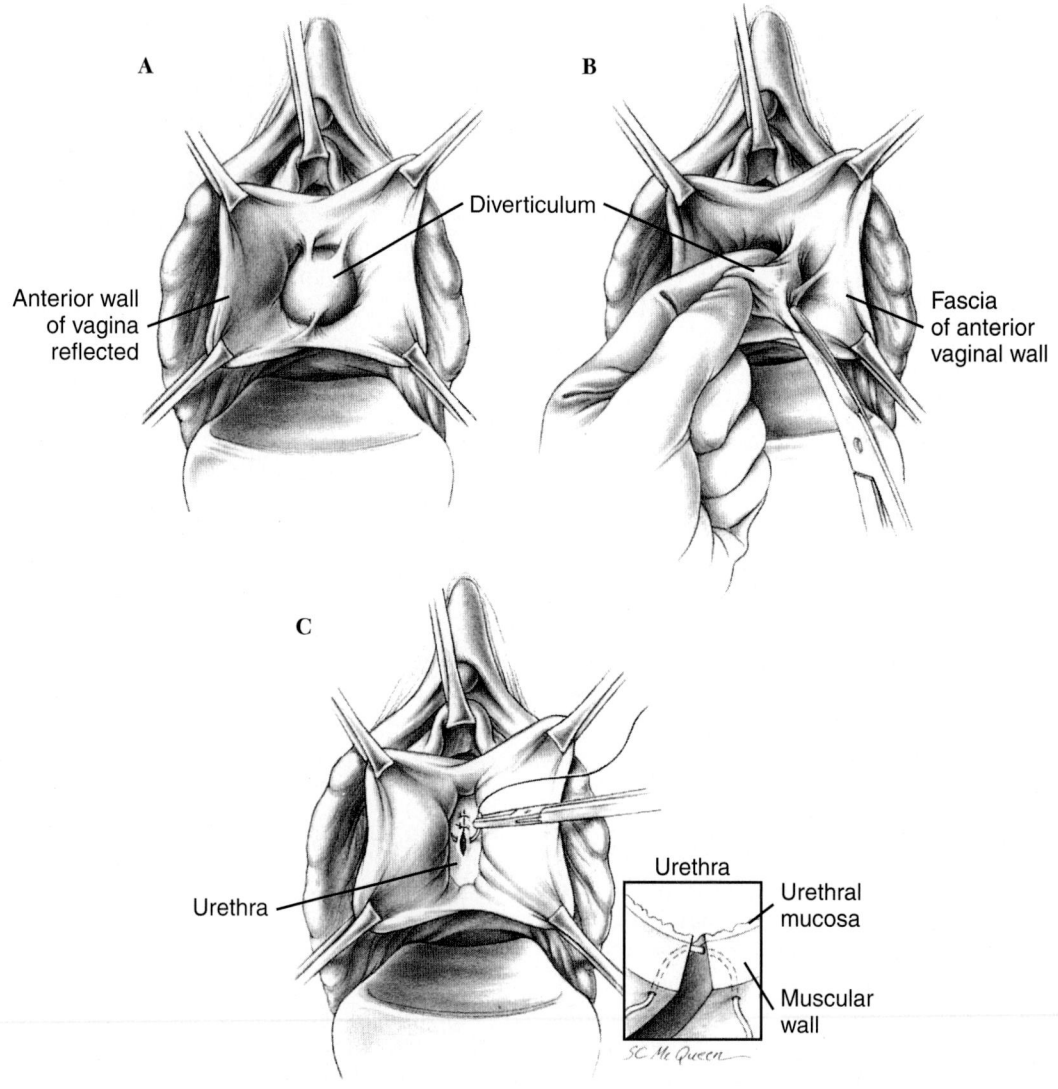

FIGURE 21-8 Resection of urethral diverticulum. **A,** Diverticulum exposed with vaginal lining and endopelvic fascia retracted. **B,** Fingers hold diverticulum on traction, which aids in dissection and identification of ostium. **C,** After complete resection of diverticulum, urethra is closed with fine, uninterrupted, extramucosal sutures. (Redrawn from Lee RA: Obstet Gynecol 61:52, 1983. Reprinted with permission from The American College of Obstetricians and Gynecologists.)

tion, however, should be the correction of the basic problem that caused the stone.

GENUINE STRESS INCONTINENCE

Genuine stress incontinence occurs when increased intraabdominal pressure is not transmitted equally to the bladder and the functional urethra. If intraabdominal pressure plus bladder pressure is sufficient to overcome urethral closing pressure, incontinence will occur. The real problem is the fact that the bladder neck, the base of the bladder, and the proximal urethra are no longer adequately supported. This may result from a separation of the supports that hold the upper vagina and urethra to the pubic symphysis, from a relaxation of pelvic fascia and musculature secondary to childbearing or the aging process, from some sort of trauma, or from an altered connective tissue metabolism causing decreased collagen production. Because the proximal two thirds of the urethra normally is an intraabdominal structure, an increased intraabdominal pressure would normally be exerted against it as well as the bladder. However, with a change in the anatomic relationships of this portion of the urethra, its intraabdominal position may be lost, thereby making it bear the brunt of such pressure rather than allowing it this degree of protection.

Over the years urethral length has been implicated as a related factor in stress incontinence. Lapides et al. measured urethral length using calibrated intraurethral catheters before and after operative correction of stress incontinence and found the urethra was shorter in cases of incontinence. However, during their procedure, downward traction was exerted to give the most meaningful measurement. Because the bladder neck in such women frequently funnels, accuracy of the measurements by Lapides et al. has been considered suspect. Other studies by multiple investigators using bead-chain urethrocystography have failed to show any change in urethral length before or after standard repair procedures. Thus it seems that, except for the most unusual circumstances, anatomic urethral length is not a major factor in stress incontinence.

The importance of a posterior urethrovesical angle in maintaining continence was first discussed by Jeffcoate and Roberts using urethrocystographic techniques in both continent and incontinent women. They concluded that a normal posterior urethrovesical angle (PUV) of less than 120 degrees was an important aspect of the continence mechanism, because such an angle was characteristically greater than 120 degrees in patients suffering from stress incontinence. This point has been verified by several authors since then. It has been noted that the relationship of the bladder neck and urethra to the pubic symphysis is not the major anatomic feature of the etiology of stress incontinence, because many patients with bladder descent but with a normal PUV angle were continent, whereas

some incontinent women had bladders and urethras appropriately positioned to the pubic symphysis but had lost their PUV. Normal continent women demonstrate a bladder base nearly parallel to the horizontal in a standing position and have a sharply defined PUV angle of 90 to 100 degrees. When such bladders are visualized by cystourethrography, it is noted that the angle is maintained even with cough, and funneling does not occur. Most women with stress incontinence usually demonstrate near complete loss of the PUV angle and funneling and posterior descent of the vesical neck.

In the past Green and others have attempted to grade the severity of stress incontinence by the amount of loss of PUV angle. They defined type I loss as showing complete or almost complete loss of PUV angle but with the angle of inclination to the vertical of the urethral axis as being normal (10 to 30 degrees) or at least 45 degrees in the lateral standing–straining configuration, as measured by urethrocystogram. They define a type II defect as representing loss of the PUV angle, with an abnormal angle of inclination to the vertical of the urethral axis generally of 45 to 90 degrees. In 1971 the concept of a saline-moistened Q-tip test was introduced to differentiate these two types of defects. This test involved placing a Q-tip into the urethra and observing the angle the urethra made with the horizontal in the relaxed and voiding positions. Montz and Stanton reevaluated the Q-tip test and discovered that 32% of patients with a positive Q-tip test had either pure detrusor instability or pure sensory urgency after a complete urologic workup. Further, 29% of the patients who had a negative Q-tip test were finally diagnosed as having pure genuine stress incontinence. Although these authors noted that the Q-tip test was more likely to be positive in younger patients with a cystourethrocele who had undergone minimal bladder neck repair, they believed that the Q-tip test was not sensitive enough to differentiate stress incontinence from other forms of incontinence and recommended that more sensitive and specific urodynamic investigations be carried out in incontinent women.

Other investigators have noted similar findings and have concluded that the Q-tip test suggests defects in the anterior vaginal wall supports but not a specific urologic diagnosis. The test also quantifies the mobility of the bladder neck and proximal urethra in both continent and incontinent women with and without pelvic support relaxation but offers no additional information about incontinence to that noted by history or physical examination.

A second test developed to help identify abnormalities of the bladder neck was the bead-chain cystourethrogram. This involved placing a sterile bead chain through the urethra into the bladder and x-raying the patient during the resting stage and during voiding. However, Fantl et al. demonstrated that 83 cystourethrograms interpreted by 3 radiologists using 5 specific radiologic landmarks failed to identify any agreement in interpretation, with a variation in interpretation of from 19.3% to 54.2%. Further, Fantl's group could find no statistically significant difference in the distribution of radiographic characteristics between patients with stress incontinence and detrusor instability.

Bladder neck funneling and position can be evaluated by perineal ultrasound, and this test may have many useful applications in the future. Ultrasound examination of the urethral sphincter may also be helpful in measuring length, thickness, and striated muscle volume. Athanasiou et al. using three-dimensional ultrasound have shown that women with stress urinary incontinence had significantly shorter, thinner, and smaller volumes of striated muscle in their urethras than did continent women of comparable ages and parity.

It is well accepted today that the degree of loss of PUV angle is not as critical as the position of the bladder neck within the abdominal cavity, and Green's classification is no longer used in most centers.

Confusion in diagnosis is commonly caused by the presence of a cystocele. A cystocele is a herniation of the bladder into the vagina and is visualized with the patient in the lithotomy position as a bulge of the anterior vaginal wall. Most patients with cystoceles, however, have well-supported bladder necks and are continent. At times the anatomic defect involves the urethra and the bladder neck as well, forming a cystourethrocele. In such cases, in addition to the presence of the cystocele, the bladder neck is also displaced. Whereas the patient with a cystocele rarely has stress incontinence, the patient with the cystourethrocele frequently has stress incontinence.

Recently, several authors have described the stress leak point pressure test. Instead of measuring the intravesical pressure needed to overcome passive urethral resistance, this test measures the intravesical pressure necessary to overcome urethral resistance under stress (cough or strain). Swift and Ostergard studied 108 consecutive patients prospectively using history, physical examination, cough stress test, and single multichannel urodynamics. Sixty-five patients (60%) were found to have genuine stress incontinence. They noted that urine loss with cough during multichannel studies had a 91% sensitivity and 100% specificity, while positive stress leak point pressure determination had a 78% sensitivity and was 100% specific. They compared this with several other observations relating to stress urinary incontinence and concluded that urine loss with cough during multichannel urodynamics was the best examination for diagnosing genuine stress incontinence in their population. Sultana studied 56 women with genuine stress incontinence urodynamically and found that 40 subjects demonstrated a leak on Valsalva maneuver. In these, maximum urethral closure pressure and leak point pressures were related significantly ($P < 0.001$). This relationship was strongest between leak point pressures up to 120 cm of water and absolute vesical pressure with Valsalva rather than with the change in vesical pressure. The leak point pressure test has a sensitivity for predicting low urethral pressure of 100%. Swift and Ostergard also demonstrated the use of this test in determining stress incontinence secondary to low pressure urethra. Norton and Baker demonstrated that this test could be influenced by postural changes.

Recently, the possibility of trauma, by obstetrical delivery or other traumatic experience, has been implicated in the etiology of genuine stress incontinence. Meyer et al. studied 149 patients during pregnancy and 9 weeks postpartum. They found that 36% of women who were delivered by forceps and 21% who delivered spontaneously suffered from urinary incontinence. Bladder neck mobility was significantly increased after all vaginal births, but bladder neck position at rest was only lowered in the forceps group. Women who underwent cesarean delivery were unaffected. On the other hand, Nygaard studying female American Olympic athletes could not find a difference between the low impact (swimmers) and the high impact (gymnasts and track and field performers) athletes with respect to the development of stress incontinence later in life.

Management

Before considering the operative approaches to the treatment of stress incontinence, it is reasonable to discuss other means of management. The first of these is directed toward the strengthening of the levator ani and pubococcygeal muscles. This can be effected by isometric exercises as described by Kegel. Although a number of modifications of these exercises exist, one useful application is to teach the patient to contract these muscles for the count of 10, 5 to 10 times, and to repeat this series several times a day. Interestingly, Kegel in 1956 suggested that the patient contract her pubococcygeal muscles 5 times on waking, 5 times on rising, and 5 times every half hour throughout the day. The patient can be instructed on how to contract these muscles by being told to attempt to stop the urinary stream while she is voiding. After she learns which muscles to contract, she may perform the exercises at any time without any relationship to voiding. These exercises improve the muscular supports of the bladder neck, and in some cases this may be enough to overcome the anatomic weakness that led to the stress incontinence.

Several studies have been performed to demonstrate the ability of patients to overcome stress incontinence by performing pelvic floor exercises. Henalla et al. used a form of pelvic floor exercise under the direction of physical therapists in two different hospitals. Using a perineal pad weighing test to assess the quantity of urine lost during exercise before and after 3 months of therapy, they found that 67% of patients achieved either complete continence or a significant improvement of symptoms. Although the severity of the symptoms before therapy and the patient's age had no effect on outcome, the treatment was noted to be more effective when the symptoms were present for less than a year. Tchou et al. performed urodynamic evaluations on 14 patients before and after pelvic floor exercise therapy. Of these, nine experienced a reversion of their urinary stress test to negative, and all subjects reported an improvement in symptoms. Henalla et al. in a different study divided 104 patients with stress incontinence into four groups. The first group ($N = 26$) was treated with pelvic floor exercises; the second group ($N = 25$) was treated with a course of 10 interferential (electric current) treatments over a 10-week period (one per week); the third group ($N = 24$) was treated with vaginal conjugated estrogen cream, 2 g per night for 12 weeks (1.25 mg conjugated estrogen/2 g dose); and the fourth group ($N = 25$) was given no treatment and served as a control group. The groups were evaluated before and after therapy (after 3 months) with a perineal pad weighing test, and all 100 were available for questionnaire evaluation 9 months after therapy. A total of 65% (17) of the pelvic floor exercise group, 32% (8) of the interferential group, 12% (3) of the estrogen-treated group, and none of the controls were found either cured or improved.

Many patients enjoy a prolonged relief even after stopping pelvic floor muscle exercise. Bø and Talseth studied 23 women who participated in a 6-month intensive pelvic floor muscle exercise routine and noted that 5 years later 75% demonstrated no leakage during a stress test and 70% were satisfied with their continence. Seventy percent of these patients were still exercising their pelvic muscles at least once a week and demonstrated pelvic floor muscle strength. Nygaard noted similar findings. These authors noted improvement of incontinence not only in patients with stress incontinence but also in those with urge and mixed urinary incontinence.

It is important to be sure that the patient is aware of how to perform the exercises correctly. In a study by Bump et al. in which l47 women were given either simple verbal or written instructions, 23 (49%) had an ideal Kegel effort signified by an increase in force of the urethral closure, while 12 subjects (25%) were performing the technique poorly and in such a way that incontinence might be promoted. These authors recommended a demonstration approach rather than a written or verbal approach.

A variation in pelvic muscle training is the use of vaginal cones. This involves a set of cones of increasing weight that require pelvic muscle contraction to hold them within the vagina. Peattie et al. demonstrated an improvement in 70% of 30 premenopausal women with stress incontinence after only 1 month of exercise. A correlation was noted between decreased urine loss and the ability to retain cones of increased weight.

Pelvic floor electrical stimulation has also been used and shown to be of value in improving pelvic floor muscle strength and decreasing symptoms of stress incontinence. Sand et al. conducted a multicenter prospective, randomized, double-blind placebo control, 15-week trial comparing the use of a pelvic floor stimulation with a sham device. Thirty-five women used the active unit, and 17 used the sham device. All were followed by urodynamic testing. Significant improvement from the baseline was found in the study patients but not in the controls, with respect to numbers of leakage episodes per day and per week, pad studies, and vaginal muscle strength.

In postmenopausal women, estrogen therapy may increase the vasculature and the tone of the bladder neck, thereby increasing urethral closing pressure and again overcoming the effects that have led to mild degrees of stress incontinence. Estrogen also has a positive effect on pelvic supports in many women, by improving collagen production, and the combination of estrogen and Kegel exercises may occasionally be all that some women require to overcome their stress incontinence (see box below).

Other drugs and combinations of drugs have been studied to determine whether nonoperative therapy could aid stress incontinent women. In a study of 30 stress incontinent women using clinical and urodynamic assessment, Kiesswetter et al. compared continence profiles after treatment with an alpha-adrenergic stimulant, midodrine; a cholinesterase inhibitor, distigmine bromide; a tricyclic antidepressant, imipramine; or an estriol, triodurin. In each case the patients were treated for 4 weeks and reevaluated. Finally, a suspensory sling operation was performed. After a successful sling operation the profile for continence as outlined by the authors increased 45% compared with an increase of 9% for midodrine, 8.9% for imipramine, and 7.9% for the combination of estriol and distigmine bromide. The urethral pressures showed an increase of mean value of 8.1% after operation, 8.3% after midodrine, 7.9% after imipramine, 3.5% after estriol, and 3.5% after distigmine bromide. The authors believed that estriol plus midodrine and estriol plus imipramine were favored subjectively by the patients over single-drug therapy, but little difference was noted in urodynamic assessment to show the advantage of one drug or combination over another. Although imipramine is a tricyclic antidepressant, it has alpha-adrenergic enhancement characteristics. Other alpha-adrenergic drugs such as phenylpropanolamine may be useful in treating genuine stress incontinence because of their action on the alpha receptors in the bladder neck and urethra causing muscle contraction. Table 21-4 is a summary by Corlett of classes of other agents that may affect urinary function or therapy.

Methods of Pelvic Muscle Strengthening

Kegel exercises
   Isometric with vaginal cones (weights)
Electrical stimulation of pelvic floor

TABLE 21-4
Drugs with Possible Effects on the Lower Urinary Tract

Class	Possible Side Effects	Drug and Usual Indication	Action
Antihypertensives	Incontinence	Reserpine—hypertension Methyldopa—hypertension	Pharmacologic sympathectomy by depleting catecholamines
Dopaminergic agonists	Bladder neck obstruction	Bromocriptine—galactorrhea Levodopa—Parkinson's disease	Increased urethral resistance and decreased detrusor contractions
Cholinergic agonists	Decreased bladder capacity and increased intravesical pressure	Digitalis—cardiotropic	Increased bladder wall tension
Neuroleptics	Incontinence	Major tranquilizers: prochlorperazine, promethazine, trifluoperazine, chlorpromazine, haloperido	Dopamine receptor blockade, with internal sphincter relaxation
β-Adrenergic agents	Urinary retention	Isoxsuprine—vasodilator Terbutaline—bronchodilator Ritodrine—tocolytic agent	Inhibited bladder muscle contractility
Xanthines	Incontinence	Caffeine	Decreased urethral closure pressure

From Corlett RC: Female Patient 10:20, 1985.

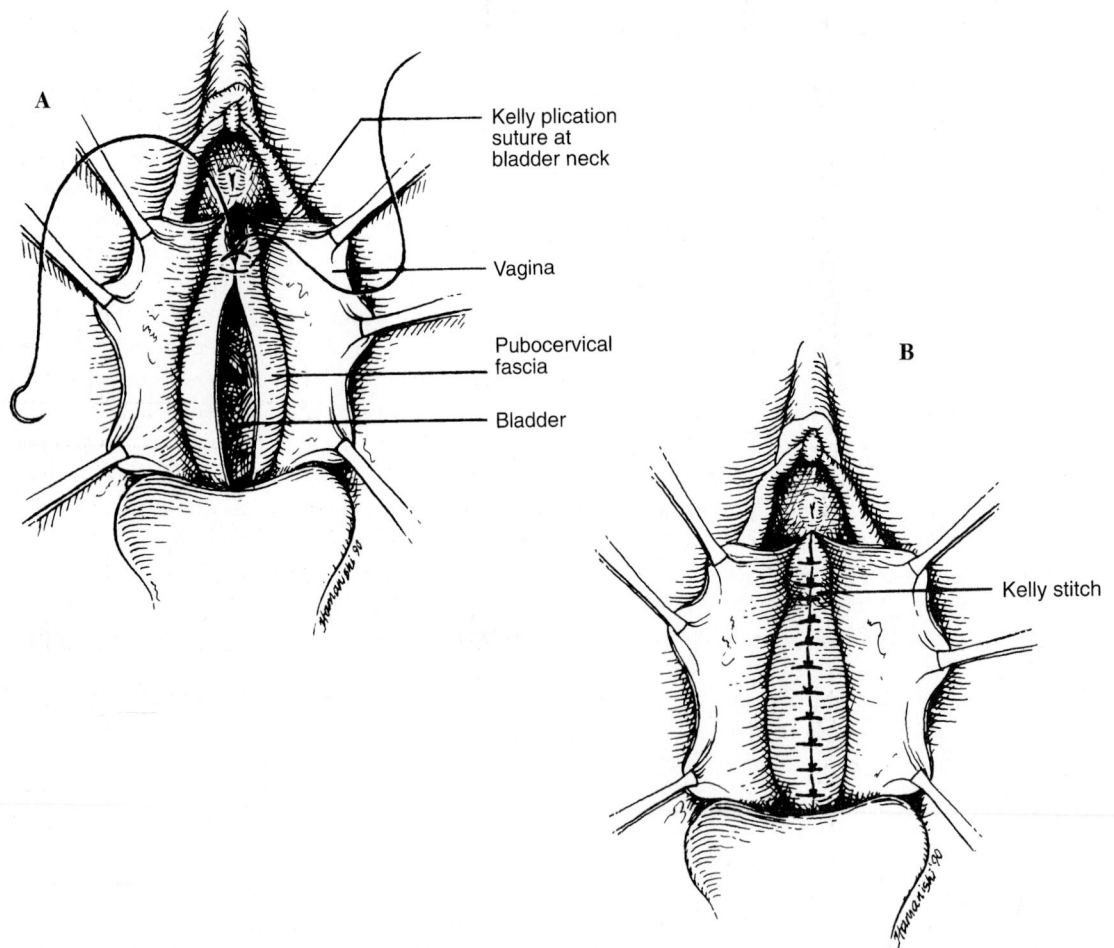

FIGURE 21-9 Cystourethrocele repair. **A,** Appearance of cystourethrocele after plication of bladder neck and repair of cystocele; cut edge of vagina is held apart above repair. **B,** Repair of vagina over cystocele is noted. (Redrawn from Symmonds RE: Relaxation of pelvic supports. In Benson RC, ed: Current obstetric and gynecologic diagnosis and treatment, ed 5, Los Altos, Calif, 1984, Lange Medical Publications.)

Before the 1950s the operative approach to treat stress incontinence primarily involved vaginal procedures, which included plication of the bladder neck (Kelly procedure) with anterior colporrhaphy to reduce a cystocele. However, after Green attempted to grade the degree of PUV angle loss in such patients, it was demonstrated by Bailey and others that the success rate using the vaginal approach varied according to the etiology. Patients showing an almost complete loss of PUV angle had a 90% success rate when followed for 5 to 10 years after a bladder neck plication and anterior colporrhaphy, but only 50% of patients with lesser PUV angle loss remained continent over that period. However, after the introduction of suprapubic urethrovesical suspension operations, the 5-year cure rate for these latter patients surpassed 90% in most series. Bergman and Giovanni and Harris et al. have published data demonstrating that the retropubic urethropexy operations have a higher cure rate than do anterior colporrhaphies of various types when the patients are followed long term. However, the latter authors point out correctly that genuine stress incontinence is a complex problem and that anterior colporrhaphy is often used in patients with pelvic floor defects. In this respect, comparing the results of operations may be inappropriate because the etiology of the problem may be different in the various groups.

It thus seemed important to determine the type of anatomic defect the patient had and to design appropriate operative management. For the patient with a definite relaxation of the anterior vaginal wall and a bladder neck that is displaced into the lower pelvis, an anterior colporrhaphy with bladder neck plication is appropriate. This is frequently performed in conjunction with a vaginal hysterectomy if there is evidence for uterine prolapse, and a posterior colporrhaphy, because such patients frequently have relaxation of the support structures of both anterior and posterior vaginal walls. The decision whether to perform a vaginal hysterectomy and posterior wall repair depends on the circumstances of the patient and does not modify the success rate of the anterior colporrhaphy and bladder neck plication in treating stress incontinence.

The anterior colporrhaphy is carried out by incising the vaginal mucosa in the midline and separating the pubocervical fascia from the vaginal mucosa by blunt and sharp dissection. The dissection is carried to the area of the bladder neck, and the first plication suture is placed on either side of the bladder neck using a 0 or 2-0 polyglycol suture. The slowly absorbable suture is ideal for this type of repair. Bladder plication is then continued from the area of the bladder neck to reduce an existing cystocele (Figure 21-9). In a patient with a displaced bladder neck and a cystourethrocele, it is often useful to place sutures in paravaginal tissue lateral to the bladder neck and fix this area to the pubic symphysis during the vaginal procedure. The vaginal tissue parallel to the bladder neck is identified and sutured with a polyglycol suture that is placed into the pubic symphysis. One suture on each side frequently suffices; the procedure requires a certain amount of dexterity, but the operator can quickly achieve this with practice.

Modifications of this procedure have been described. Special needles have been developed by Pereyra that can be used to guide sutures from the paravaginal tissue through the space of Retzius. Nonabsorbable material is used, and the suture is tied over the rectus fascia just above the bladder neck. This is carried out through a small suprapubic incision. It is appropriate to follow the steps of this procedure under direct urethrocystoscopy to avoid injuring the bladder neck during the needle placement. Stamey's modification of the Pereyra procedure uses a small tube of Dacron material to buttress the suture, thereby keeping it from pulling through. Stamey reports about 3% of the patients in his series required a removal of the suprapubic suture because of pain or infection.

In assessing the long-term success rate of the use of the modified Pereyra procedure in patients with recurrent stress urinary incontinence, Holschneider et al. studied 54 patients. These women were divided into two groups. Group 1 comprised those individuals with no risk factors, which include evidence for detrusor instability, low pressure urethra, fibrotic urethra, a negative Q-tip test, and neurogenic incontinence. Group 2 comprised individuals who had such risk factors. Of the 38 patients in group 1, 81.6% demonstrated continence after a mean follow-up period of 36.3 months. On the other hand, the 16 patients in group 2 demonstrated only a 43.8% cure rate, and the mean time to the recurrence of incontinence in those who failed in this group was 6.8 months. These authors noted an intraoperative complication rate of 7.4% for both groups, with the complications involving suture in the bladder and hemorrhage, and a postoperative complication rate of 25.9%, in which infection most often was the complication. Also, 33.3% of these patients suffered late postoperative complications, which included detrusor instability and obstructive voiding dysfunction.

Appropriate therapy for patients with bladder neck displacement, without significant anterior vaginal wall relaxation but with incontinence, in most instances is by a suprapubic approach. The Marshall-Marchetti-Krantz suprapubic urethrovesical suspension operation was first reported in 1949 and has been the mainstay of many surgeons attempting to alleviate stress incontinence in such patients. The procedure may be done by itself or in conjunction with other abdominal procedures, such as an abdominal hysterectomy. The space of Retzius is entered, the bladder neck is identified generally with a 30-ml bulb Foley catheter in the bladder, and the paravaginal tissue adjacent to the bladder neck is identified and sutured to the pubic symphysis using two or three interrupted sutures on each side of the bladder neck. Again, 0 or 2-0 polyglycol suture is ideal for this procedure, but some operators prefer nonabsorbable suture. The operator must be careful not to place undue stress on the bladder neck. Stress can generally be assessed by placing one hand in the vagina and palpating the tension on the bladder neck at the time the sutures are tied (Figure 21-10). The patient is followed for 2 to 5 days with continuous catheter drainage. In most cases, after removal of the catheter, the patient will void. Occasionally, voiding is delayed and the patient may need to be discharged with an indwelling catheter in the bladder to be checked 1 week hence. It is usual to check a patient for residual urine after she voids; residuals of less than 100 to 150 ml, after the patient voids at least 200 ml, are considered acceptable. Larger residuals should signal continuing catheterization for 48 to 72 hours or the use of intermittent self-catheterization.

A rare (1% to 2%) but painful complication of the Marshall-Marchetti-Krantz procedure is osteitis pubis. This condition is an inflammatory reaction in the periosteum of the pubic bone more often associated with permanent suture material. This complication after suprapubic cystotomy was first reported in 1923 by Legueu and Rochet. The next year Beer described six patients with pubic symphysis periostitis after suprapubic procedures. Pain is the major symptom, but patients usually demonstrate a "waddling gait."

Kammerer-Doak et al. reviewed the Mayo Clinic experience with 2030 Marshall-Marchetti-Krantz procedures performed between 1980 and 1994. There were 15 cases of osteitis pubis (0.74%) occurring an average of 69 days postoperative (range 10-459 days). Conserva-

tive therapy relieved symptoms in 47% and seven of the remaining patients needed surgical intervention including suture removal (57%) and symphyseal debridement (86%). In five cases bone cultures were positive.

It is important to differentiate this condition from true osteomyelitis. The latter condition, seen occasionally after radical pelvic operations and other pelvic procedures, involves infection of the bone and is often associated with positive blood cultures. Hoyme et al. reviewed this subject in relation to radical gynecologic operations. Treatment of osteomyelitis often involves prolonged antibiotic therapy and surgical debridement. Treatment of osteitis pubis includes antibiotics and analgesics and may require the removal of permanent sutures.

In 1961 Burch advocated a modification of the suprapubic bladder neck suspension by suspending the vaginal wall to Cooper's ligament (Figure 21-11). The original description uses 2-0 chromic catgut suture, but polyglycol or nonabsorbable sutures are probably more appropriate now. Postoperative care similar to that described for the Marshall-Marchetti-Krantz operation is appropriate. At times patients have difficulty voiding for prolonged periods, and the occasional patient may report that she needs to rise off the commode to a semistanding position to void.

Both the Marshall-Marchetti-Krantz and Burch procedures have their advocates. When properly performed, each procedure produces a long-term cure in more than 80% of patients with stress incontinence. Feyereisl et al.

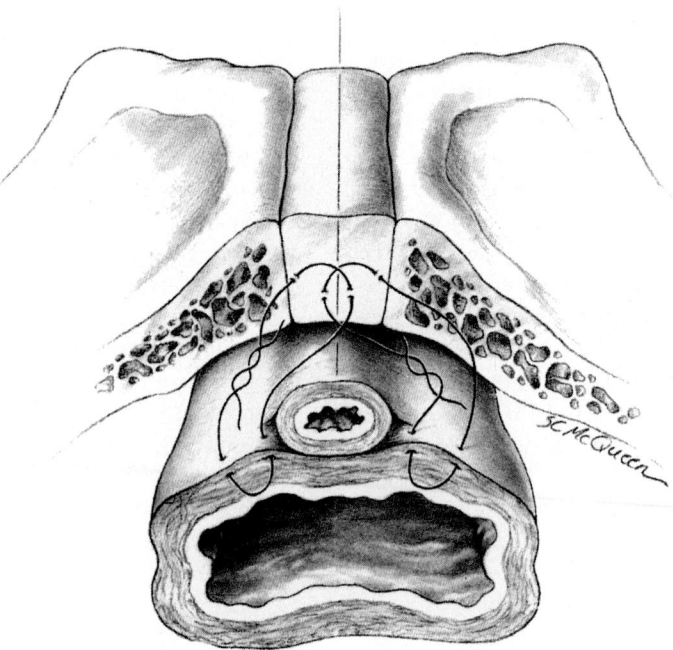

FIGURE 21-10 Demonstration of the relative position of a pair of sutures adjacent to the urethra securely placed into the pubic symphysis. (Redrawn from Buchsbaum HJ and Schmidt JD, eds: Gynecologic and obstetric urology. Reprinted with permission from WB Saunders Co, Philadelphia, 1982.)

reported a long-term success rate of 81.6% in 87 women carefully evaluated preoperatively for stress urinary incontinence. Their follow-up was between 5 and 10 years. Colombo et al. performed a prospective randomized clinical trial using the Burch and Marshall-Marchetti-Krantz procedures. The follow-up was 2 to 7 years. These authors reported subjective and objective cure rates of 92% and 80% respectively for the Burch procedure and 85% and 65% for the Marshall-Marchetti-Krantz procedure. These differences were not statistically significant. In a recent review of English language articles concerning the Burch procedures, Dainer et al. noted that the success rate reported varied from 85.2% at 1 year, 89.8% at 5.10 years to 69% at 10 to 20 years. Frequently, failures can be resolved by performing the same procedure again, indicating that the problem was technical performance of the procedure rather than a failure of the type of procedure.

Herbertsson and Iosif studied 72 women who had undergone retropubic colpourethrocystopexy between 1979 and 1982 for genuine stress incontinence. Follow-up urodynamic studies were performed in 1989 and 1990. The surgical cure rate was considered to be 90.3%, but five of the seven patients who were considered failures felt that their symptoms had improved. Thirty-eight of the patients were found on urodynamic studies to have an incompetent bladder neck. But 31 of these 38 patients were still continent. The authors concluded that this type of surgical approach to genuine stress urinary incontinence was most appropriate.

The Burch procedure can also be performed laparoscopically. Saidi et al. have reported comparable 12-month cure rates in 70 patients undergoing laparoscopic procedures (91.4%) and 87 patients undergoing open procedures (92%). The laparoscopic procedures had a somewhat shorter operative time and a much shorter hospital stay. Ross followed 48 consecutive patients who underwent laparoscopic Burch procedures and found a cure rate of 93% and 89% at 1 and 2 years using multichannel urodynamic studies.

Shull and Baden reported on 149 consecutive patients who were assessed anatomically and found to have a paravaginal defect causing stress urinary incontinence. In such cases they performed an abdominal repair in which the anterior vaginal wall was sutured with permanent suture to the white line bilateral. In follow-up for as long as 48 months, 97% of the patients remained continent. However, 6% suffered vaginal cuff prolapse, 5% developed an enterocele in addition to cuff prolapse, and 5% redeveloped the cystocele after the operation. When, on anatomic examination, the paravaginal fascial defect is noted, this operation has good application as an alternative to other described procedures. It may also be utilized in conjunction with other procedures when multiple anatomic defects are identified. It can be performed abdominally or vaginally.

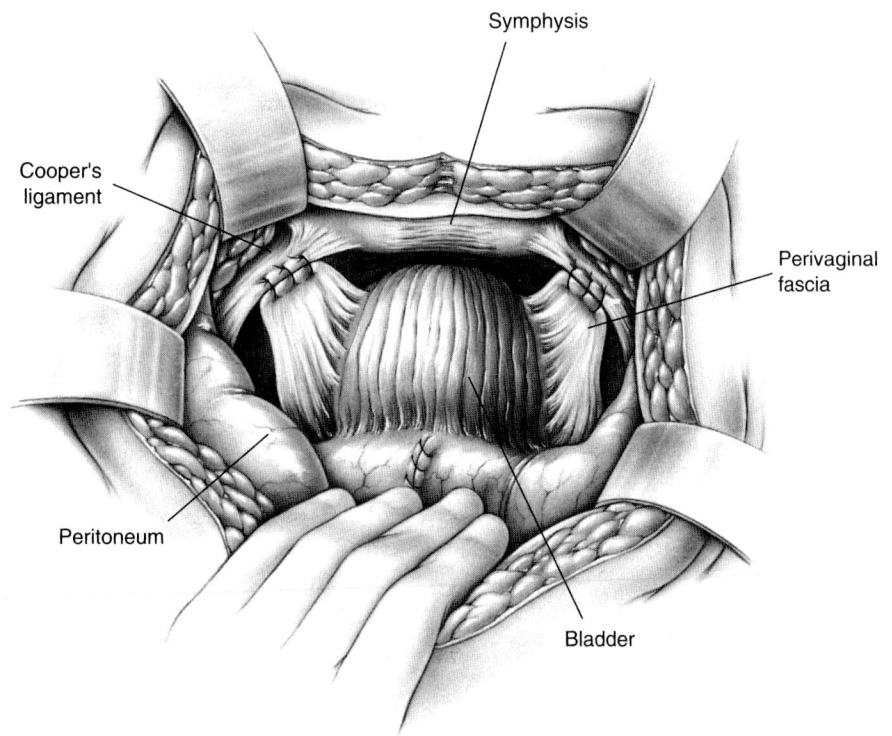

FIGURE 21-11 Burch procedure. The lateral edges of the vagina have been sutured to Cooper's ligament. (Redrawn from Burch JC: Am J Obstet Gynecol 81:281, 1961.)

Urethral Sphincter Dysfunction

Sand et al. offered some insight into why at least some retropubic urethropexy procedures fail. In a study of 86 patients who were evaluated preoperatively and postoperatively with urodynamic studies, they noted that in women under 50 years of age there was a significant risk of failure if the preoperative urethral closure pressure was less than 20 cm H₂O. Although low urethral closure pressure was found to be an independent risk factor in women under age 50, it was not found to be so in women over age 50.

In 1981 McGuire noted the loss of intrinsic urethral tone in a number of women, particularly those with a history of pelvic trauma, radiation, underlying neurologic conditions, or scarring of the urethral sphincter. At first this was called Type III incontinence but is currently referred to as *intrinsic sphincter dysfunction.*

Recently, Horbach and Ostergard retrospectively evaluated 263 consecutive patients undergoing a complete urodynamic evaluation because of urinary leakage. Intrinsic sphincter dysfunction was defined as maximum urethral closure of 20 cm of water or less in the sitting position at maximum cystometric capacity. One hundred and thirty-two women (50.2%) were found to have intrinsic sphincter dysfunction. Women in this group tended to be older and were more likely to have undergone a hysterectomy and at least one antiincontinence procedure compared with those women with continence problems who had normal urethral pressure. By multivariant analysis, they noted that age greater than 50 was the only independent variable that could predict the presence of intrinsic sphincter dysfunction in women with stress urinary incontinence.

At present, treatment for urinary stress incontinence caused by intrinsic urethral dysfunction consists of one of the following: periurethral bulk substance injections, urethral sling procedure, or the use of an artificial sphincter device. A number of substances have been used for periurethral bulk injection. These have included the individual's blood or fat, Teflon, and more recently, beef collagen. Injection of blood or fat has given only transient relief, and the use of Teflon has resulted in several complications, primarily caused by the wandering of the Teflon to distant sites. Currently, GAX-collagen has been used as a urethral bulking agent. This is a cross-linked glutaraldehyde bovine dermal collagen first used by Appell and McGuire et al., who reported a high success rate. This agent has a relatively high incidence of hypersensitivity reaction, and therefore the patient should be skin tested before its use. Without hypersensitivity it appears to be a relatively safe, effective, and minimally invasive means of supporting the upper urethral sphincter, and several centers are now using it for this purpose. Long-term follow-up will be required to determine whether this therapy will have lasting benefits. To date,

it seems to have a positive effect for at least 2 years, and it is possible to reinject patients.

A variety of sling procedures, including the use of fascia lata, anterior rectus fascial tissue, and inert materials such as Mersilene, can be used. These procedures mobilize the bladder neck, often by a vaginal or vaginal and abdominal approach, and allow the interposition of a strip of material under the urethra surrounding the bladder neck, which is attached to the anterior rectus sheath. This creates a pulley effect and with intraabdominal stress, contraction of the abdominal wall muscles allows the "pulling up" effect on the bladder neck. This procedure is generally effective in creating continence.

The surgeon must exercise care in determining the tension to be applied on the bladder neck when the sling is fixed. Making it too tight may interfere with voiding and may actually damage the bladder neck; making it too loose will abrogate its effectiveness. Generally with a No. 16 or 18 Foley catheter in the urethra it should be possible for the surgeon to judge the tension so that the sling fits comfortably against the urethra without compressing it. Concomitant cystoscopy may also be used.

Beck et al. reported their results in treating 170 patients over 22 years with a fascia lata sling procedure. These patients had undergone one or more unsuccessful attempts to correct their stress urinary incontinence. In all patients an intraurethral pressure of 80 to 90 cm of water was created at the site of the sling. Their success rate in curing the stress urinary incontinence was 98.2%, with 100% success noted in their last 148 cases. The most troublesome postoperative problem was delayed voiding, which averaged 59.6 days. Others, including the chapter author, have had similar experiences with this procedure.

Although an anterior rectus sheath fascial sling procedure is probably as effective as a Marshall-Marchetti-Krantz or Burch procedure, it involves a greater degree of dissection, as well as entry into the vagina with the potential risk of ascending infection. Thus sling procedures are generally reserved for patients with intrinsic urethral deficiency and not used as primary therapy for genuine stress urinary incontinence. Fascia lata slings are being placed in many centers and can be performed vaginally in a relatively short operative time. Autologus fascia lata is more effective than irradiated and freeze-dried donor fascia lata, with the use of the latter type leading to a high degree of graft degeneration and, thus, procedure failure.

The use of the artificial urinary sphincter is a relatively new procedure that may be a viable option for some women and will generally produce continence. Artificial urinary sphincters are generally placed by an abdominal and vaginal surgical approach. Expulsion of these devices is a potential side effect. The artificial sphincter consists of a cuff surrounding the urethra. The device is controlled by a pressure balloon placed in the

TABLE 21-5
Treatment Outcomes for Intrinsic Deficiency
(Combined Multiple Studies)

Outcome	Collagen	Sling	Artificial Sphincter
Cured	69%	84%	92%
Improved	25%	6%	4%
Cured or improved	94%	95%	96%
Complications	—	31%	32%

space of Retzius. The patient controls the device by releasing pressure when she wishes to void and reestablishing pressure when she wishes to be continent. Diokno et al. reported a 91% success rate in 32 patients in whom they implanted the device. Other authors have reported similar results.

Table 21-5 summarizes the overall long-term care and improvement rate in multiple studies published before 1995 as summarized by the U.S. Department of Health and Human Services, Agency for Health Care Policy and Research.

Urodynamic Studies After Retropubic Urethropexy for Stress Incontinence

In a study of 29 women with stress incontinence investigated urodynamically before and after Marshall-Marchetti-Krantz operation by Beisland et al., no major changes in the urethral pressure profile could be demonstrated. The authors did note a good correlation between clinical results and the changes in transmission of increased abdominal pressure to the urethra. The operative procedure did not seem to increase the urethral pressure. Those patients with low maximal urethral pressure preoperatively continued to have insufficient urethral sphincter function after the operation. Indeed the operation in some cases may have caused injury to the sphincter because of excessive dissection around the urethra.

In a study of 25 women after Burch colposuspension in which 88% had objective evidence of cure, an increase in voiding difficulty and urodynamic evidence of outflow obstruction was seen 6 months after the procedure. Beisland et al. also noted that the Burch procedure, like the Marshall-Marchetti-Krantz operation, does not induce any significant change in resting urethral profile; they believed the changes noted were probably a mechanical obstruction of the bladder neck.

Recently, van Geelen et al. investigated the urodynamic effects of both anterior vaginal wall and Burch procedures. There were no changes in resting urethral pressure profiles in either group of patients after sur-

gery. Pressure transmission rates in the proximal urethra were increased in women treated successfully with the Burch procedure in supine, sitting, and standing positions, but in women unsuccessfully relieved of their incontinence, no significant increase in pressure transmission could be noted. In those women treated successfully with an anterior repair, a significant increase in pressure was observed in the midurethra in the sitting position and in the proximal urethra in the standing position. The authors concluded that the Burch procedure was more effective than an anterior repair in correcting genuine stress incontinence.

Some authors have suggested that the chance of curing genuine stress incontinence with a surgical procedure was increased by performing a hysterectomy as well. Van Geelen et al. did not note this in their study, and in a recent report by Langer et al. no differences were found in the cure rate of 45 patients, of whom 22 underwent a Burch procedure without hysterectomy and 23 underwent a Burch procedure with hysterectomy.

It is difficult to compare the results obtained in curing stress incontinence with different procedures. Differences in techniques and skills of operators and variations in patient selection methods make different procedures difficult to compare. In a large study of 680 surgically treated patients reported by Park and Miller, the Marshall-Marchetti-Krantz procedure and Kelly plication were noted to be equally successful in correcting stress incontinence after 3 years (69% and 66%, respectively). Patients who underwent the Pereyra procedure as their primary repair had a 41% success rate after 3 years. Still, the reader must remember that differences in the groups and in the skills of the surgeons involved may have played a role in the outcomes.

DETRUSOR INSTABILITY

Walter and Olesen studied 303 patients complaining of urinary incontinence and discovered that 43% had stress incontinence, 21% urge incontinence, and 36% both urge and stress incontinence. Most patients with urge incontinence suffer from detrusor instability. This condition is generally chronic and is associated with an urgency-frequency problem often accompanied by painless urine loss. Generally a large volume of urine is lost; leakage may occur in any position and often with a change in position. Stress secondary to running, walking, coughing, sneezing, or laughing may trigger this type of incontinence, but it is generally delayed until several seconds after the stress has occurred. Stress incontinence frequently disappears during the night, but urge incontinence continues, often with nocturia. Patients are often unable to stop their stream during the act of voiding, whereas women with stress incontinence can accomplish this.

Detrusor instability is the result of sudden, spontaneous detrusor muscle activity and has previously been termed *detrusor dyssynergia* or *detrusor irritability*. Some 50% to 80% of patients have an underlying functional or psychosomatic component. Patients, however, may suffer from generalized diseases affecting the bladder or its innervation. When an involuntary loss of urine is associated with a sudden and strong desire to void (urgency), this function is called *urge incontinence*. This is due to overactivity of the detrusor muscle and is more appropriately termed *detrusor instability*. If a neurologic disorder, such as stroke, Parkinson's disease, or other CNS pathology is present, the term *detrusor hyperreflexia* is frequently used. In the elderly, often detrusor muscle strength is decreased and the urgency is accompanied by urinary retention. Dribbling often results.

The loss of urine is probably triggered by sudden, uninhibited stimulation of receptors in the bladder wall. These may be hyperreactive for emotional reasons or may be a result of acute or chronic irritation. The problem may also be caused by the breakdown of normal neurologic and inhibitory reflexes. Frequently such patients demonstrate symptoms of chronic anxiety.

A study of 86 women with genuine stress incontinence was reported by Sands et al. Of these, 20 (23.3%) also had unstable detrusor function preoperatively. Of these 20, 11 (55%) had stable detrusor function after retropubic urethropexy, whereas 5 of the 66 (7.6%) patients who had stable detrusor function preoperatively developed unstable detrusors postoperatively. Overall, women with both stress incontinence and unstable detrusors experienced a cure rate of only 30% with surgery. No relationship could be found in preoperative symptoms, age, history of previous procedures, and cystometric parameters between those who were cured and those who were not. In addition, none of these criteria could predict which patient who was detrusor stable before surgery would develop instability after surgery. Risks of developing detrusor instability after surgery must be recognized and may require further medical therapy.

Diagnosis

Electronic urethrocystometry and fluid cystometrographic techniques allow the detection of spontaneous involuntary pressure changes within the bladder, which are noted as the bladder fills. These techniques are also useful in detecting patients with true stress incontinence who have an urgency (detrusor dyssynergic) component to their incontinence. It is important that in such cases both problems be treated, or it is not likely that incontinence will be cured.

Management

Operative procedures are useless in treating urgency incontinence. In fact, they can be expected to have no influence on the problem at all. In those patients who have stress incontinence and detrusor dyssynergia, an operation may have a place in the specific therapy. However, if the major part of the problem seems to be detrusor instability, this should be treated first, as an operative procedure frequently may not be necessary. Likewise, patients who have undergone an operation for stress urinary incontinence and continue to be incontinent should be evaluated for detrusor dyssynergia. Bates et al. demonstrated that a high percentage of such failures will be found on urethrocystometric studies to have detrusor dyssynergia.

Because the majority of patients with detrusor instability have psychosomatic problems, retraining or bladder drills may be of use. This should take the form of bladder retraining, which involves a programmed progressive lengthening of the period between voiding with or without the addition of biofeedback techniques. In a study Millard and Oldenburg demonstrated improvement in 74% of women with detrusor instability using such techniques. Cystometric studies performed on these patients revealed a reversion to stable bladder function. But compliance with bladder retraining by patients is often a problem. Visco studied 123 women who were offered bladder retraining and found that 55% either never started treatment or were noncompliant. They noted that women who were given concurrent pharmacological therapy had an 87% compliance rate, compared to a 53% rate in those who started training and did not complete it and who were not given medication.

Postmenopausal women may benefit from estrogen therapy; estrogen not only improves the vasculature of the bladder neck and the mucosa of the urethra and trigone but also has an alpha-adrenergic stimulating capacity that may help overall urinary control.

Anticholinergic drugs or beta-adrenergic drugs may be useful. The following may be tried: propantheline (Pro-Banthine) at doses of 15 to 30 mg 4 times a day, oxybutynin chloride (Ditropan) 5 mg every 8 to 12 hours, flavoxate (Urispas) 200 mg every 6 hours, tolterodine tartrate (Detrol) 2 mg 2 times a day, imipramine (Tofranil) 50 mg every 8 hours, or ephedrine sulfate 25 mg every 6 hours. At times these medications in conjunction with bladder retraining have greater efficacy than either alone.

Terodiline is a calcium antagonist that has been used extensively worldwide to treat detrusor instability. It is not currently available in the United States, but in a multicenter, randomized, placebo-controlled trial recently completed, Norton et al. reported that this agent decreased the mean number of incontinent episodes per week in 70% of women treated compared with a 9% reduction in the placebo group. All women were diagnosed before treatment as having urinary frequency and urge incontinence. The medication was found to be well tolerated in these individuals. Thus new approaches to medical therapy may be available in the near future.

TRUE INCONTINENCE

True incontinence is a loss of urine without abnormal bladder function. This is generally caused by fistulas or by other damage to the urinary tract. Such damage may occur congenitally or secondary to trauma.

OVERFLOW INCONTINENCE

Overflow incontinence occurs when a bladder is overdistended because of its inability to empty. The problem may be caused by a neurologic disorder that interferes with normal bladder reflexes or by partial obstruction of the urethra. Typically the patient complains of voiding small amounts and still having the feeling that there is urine in the bladder. In addition, the patient frequently loses small amounts of urine without any control. This condition is commonly seen in patients with multiple sclerosis, diabetic neuropathy, and trauma or tumors of the central nervous system. A complete general medical and urologic workup is necessary to clarify the patient's condition. Therapy directed at the primary cause may be beneficial. Often the patient must be trained in techniques of intermittent self-catheterization.

KEY POINTS

- As many as 30% of all women may suffer from some degree of urinary incontinence during their lifetime.

- Continence is determined by the balance between those forces that maintain urethral closure and those that affect detrusor function.

- Parasympathetic nervous system activity via the neurotransmitter acetylcholine stimulates receptors in the bladder wall to activate detrusor contraction.

- Anticholinergic agents decrease detrusor activity.

- Sympathetic nervous system receptors in the bladder are mostly beta receptors and when stimulated cause relaxation.

- Sympathetic nervous system receptors in the urethra are basically alpha receptors. Stimulation causes contraction.

- The highest pressure zone in the urethra is about midpoint in the functional urethra, which is roughly 0.5 cm proximal to the urogenital diaphragm.

- Resting pressure within the bladder is between 20 and 30 cm of water.

- A normal bladder transmits a voiding urge at 150 to 200 ml volume, and functional capacity is generally 400 to 500 ml.

- About 20% of all women will develop urinary infections at some time in their life, and by age 70 as many as 10% of women will have chronic urinary tract infections.

- Bacterial counts of 100,000 or greater per milliliter of urine usually indicate a urinary tract infection. *Escherichia coli* is the most common organism seen.

- Bacterial counts of 100 per milliliter may be seen in patients with urethritis.

- Interstitial cystitis is an inflammatory condition of the bladder that is not related to infection and is associated with altered epithelial permeability, mast cell activation, and an upregulation of sensory afferent nerves.

- Some 3% to 4% of all women will suffer from urethral diverticula, with the majority of cases occurring between the ages of 30 and 50. Most urethral diverticula originate in the middle third of the urethra, but diverticula may occur from any area of the urethra and may be multiple.

- Urethral syndrome can occur in as many as 20% to 30% of women and should not be diagnosed until all infectious organisms have been discounted.

- Some 75% to 80% of women with urinary incontinence suffer from stress incontinence.

- The long-term cure rate for Marshall-Marchetti-Krantz and Burch procedures is usually greater than 80% in properly selected patients.

- Osteitis pubis occurs in 1% to 2% of suprapubic suspension operations.

- Intrinsic urethral sphincter deficiency is seen in women past age 50 and in individuals with a history of urethral and bladder neck surgery or radiation. Intraurethral pressure is generally less than 20 cm of water.

- Intrinsic urethral sphincter dysfunction is best treated by periurethral collagen injection, a sling procedure, or instillation of an artificial urethral sphincter.

- Long-term (over 3 years) follow-up of patients who underwent Kelly plication of the bladder neck and those who underwent retropubic urethropexy showed the two procedures had about the same success rate.

- About 20% of women with urinary incontinence suffer from detrusor instability.

- Some 50% to 80% of patients with detrusor dyssynergia have an underlying functional or psychosomatic component.

- Operative procedures are of no value in treating detrusor dyssynergia unless there is a stress incontinence component as well.

- An indwelling catheter for more than 24 hours leads to urinary tract infection in about 50% of cases and in nearly 100% after 96 hours.

BIBLIOGRAPHY

American Uro-Gynecologic Society: Periurethral bulking agents, Quarterly Report: XII, 1994.

Andersen MTF: The incidence of diverticula in the female urethra, J Urol 98:96, 1967.

Appell RA: New developments: injectables for urethral incompetence in women, Int Urogynecol J 1:117, 1990.

Appell RA, Macaluso JN Jr, Deutsch JS, et al: Endourologic control of incontinence with GAX collagen: the LSU experience, J Endourol 6:275, 1992.

Arnold EP, Webster JR, Loose H, et al: Urodynamics of female incontinence: factors influencing the results of surgery, Am J Obstet Gynecol 117:805, 1973.

Asmussen M and Ulmsten U: A new technique for measurement of the urethra pressure profile, Acta Obstet Gynecol Scand 55:167, 1976.

Asmussen M and Ulmsten U: Simultaneous urethrocystommetry with a new technique, Scand J Urol Nephrol 10:7, 1976.

Asmussen M and Ulmsten U: On the physiology of continence and pathophysiology of stress incontinence in the female. In Controversies in gynecology and obstetrics, vol 10, Basel, 1983, Karger, S, AG.

Athanasiou S, Khullar V, Boos K, Salvatore S, and Cardoza L: Imaging the urethral sphincter with three dimensional ultrasound. Obstet Gynecol 94:295, 1999.

Baerheim A, Digranes A, and Hunskaar S: Equal symptomatic outcome after antibacterial treatment of acute lower urinary tract infection and the acute urethral syndrome in adult women. Scand J Prim Health Care 17:170, 1999.

Bailey KV: A clinical investigation into uterine prolapse with stress incontinence. Treatment by modified Manchester colporrhaphy, J Obstet Gynaecol Br Comm Part I, 61:291, 1954; Part II, 63:663, 1956; Part III, 70:947, 1963.

Barnett RM: The modern Kelly plication, Obstet Gynecol 34:667, 1969.

Bates CP, Bradley W, Glen E, et al: First report of the standardization of terminology of lower urinary tract function, J Urol 48:39, 1976.

Bates P, Bradley WE, Glen E, et al: The standardization of terminology of lower urinary tract function, J Urol 121:551, 1979.

Bates CP, Loose H, and Stanton SLR: The objective study of incontinence after repair operations, Surg Gynecol Obstet 136:17, 1973.

Beck RP and Maughan GB: Simultaneous intraurethral and intravesical pressure studies in normal women and those with stress incontinence, Am J Obstet Gynecol 89:746, 1964.

Beck RP, McCormick S, and Nordstrom L: The fascia lata sling procedure for treating recurrent genuine stress incontinence of urine, Obstet Gynecol 72:699, 1988.

Beer E: Periostitis of the symphysis and descending rami of the pubes following suprapubic operations, Int J Med 37:224, 1924.

Beisland HO, Fossberg E, and Sander S: Urodynamic studies before and after retropubic urethropexy for stress incontinence in females, Surg Gynecol Obstet 155:333, 1982.

Bergman A and Giovanni E: Three surgical procedures for genuine stress incontinence: five year follow-up of a prospective randomized study, Am J Obstet Gynecol 173:66, 1995.

Bhatia NN and Bergman A: Urodynamic appraisal of the Bonney test in women with stress urinary incontinence, Obstet Gynecol 62:696, 1983.

Bhatia NN and Ostergard DR: Urodynamics in women with stress urinary incontinence, Obstet Gynecol 60:552, 1982.

Blaivas JG and Jocobs BZ: Pubovaginal fascial sling for the treatment of complicated stress urinary incontinence, J Urol 145:1214, 1991.

Bø K and Talseth T: Long-term effect of pelvic floor muscle exercise 5 years after cessation of organized training, Obstet Gynecol 87:261, 1996.

Burgio KL, Matthews KA, Engel BT, et al: Prevalence, incidence and correlates of urinary incontinence in healthy middle aged women, J Urol 146:1255, 1991.

Buchsbaum HJ and Schmidt JD, eds: Gynecologic and obstetric urology. Philadelphia, 1982, WB Saunders Co.

Bump RC: Racial comparisons and contrasts in urinary incontinence and pelvic organ prolapse, Obstet Gynecol 81:421, 1993.

Bump RC, Hurt WG, Fantl JA, and Wyman JF: Assessment of Kegel pelvic floor muscle exercise performance after brief verbal instruction, Am J Obstet Gynecol 165:322, 1991.

Bump RC and McClish DM: Cigarette smoking and pure genuine stress incontinence of urine: a comparison of risk factors and determinants between smokers and nonsmokers, Am J Obstet Gynecol 170:579, 1994.

Burch JC: Cooper's ligament urethrovesical suspension for stress incontinence, Am J Obstet Gynecol 100:764, 1968.

Caputo RM and Benson JT: The Q-tip test and urethrovesical junction mobility, Obstet Gynecol 82:892, 1993.

Cherney C and Boscia JA: Asymptomatic bacteriuria in the elderly, Geriat Med 7:46, 1988.

Colombo M, Scalambrino S, Maggioni A, and Milani R: Burch colposuspension versus modified Marshall-Marchetti-Krantz urethropexy for primary genuine stress urinary incontinence: a prospective, randomized clinical trial, Am J Obstet Gynecol 171:1573, 1994.

Corlett RC: Gynecologic urology. I. Urinary incontinence, Female Patient 10:20, 1985.

DeLancey JO: Correlative study of periurethral anatomy, Obstet Gynecol 68:91, 1986.

DeLancey JO: Structural aspects of the extrinsic continence mechanism, Obstet Gynecol 72:296, 1988.

Diokno AC, Brock BM, Brown HB, and Herzog AR: Prevalence of urinary incontinence and other neurologic symptoms in the non-institutionalized elderly, J Urol 136:1022, 1986.

Diokno AC and Taub ME: Experience with the artifical urinary sphincter at Michigan, J Urol 116:496, 1988.

Dwyer PL and Teele JS: Prazosin: a neglected cause of genuine stress incontinence, Obstet Gynecol 79:117, 1992.

Enhorning G: Simultaneous recording of intravesical and intraurethral pressure, Acta Chir Scand Suppl 276:1, 1971.

Falconer C, Ekman G, Malmström A, and Ulmsten U: Decreased collagen synthesis in stress-incontinent women, Obstet Gynecol 84:583, 1994.

Fantl JA, Beachley MC, Bosch HA, et al: Bead-chain cystourethrogram: an evaluation, Obstet Gynecol 58:237, 1981.

Fernie GR, Jewett MAS, Halsall P, et al: Urodynamic characterization of incontinence in the elderly by bladder volume, J Urol 129:772, 1983.

Feyereisl J, Dreher E, Haenggi W, et al: Long-term results after Burch colposuspension, Am J Obstet Gynecol 171:647, 1994.

Fitzgerald MP, Mollenhauer J, Bitterman P, and Brubaker L:

Functional failure of fascia lata allographs. Am J Obstet Gynecol 181:1339, 1999.

Fossberg E, Veisland HO, and Lundgren RA: Stress incontinence in females: treatment with phenylpropanolamine: a urodynamic and pharmacological evaluation, Urol Int 38:293, 1983.

Frewen WK: Urgency incontinence, J Obstet Gynaecol Br Comm 79:77, 1972.

Gillespie WA, Henderson EP, Linton KB, and Smith PJB: Microbiology of the urethral (frequency and dysuria) syndrome: a controlled study with a 5-year review, Br J Urology 64:270, 1989.

Gittes RF and Nakamura RM: Female urethral syndrome. A female prostatitis? Invest J Med 164:435, 1996.

Gosling JA, Dixon JS, Critchley HO, and Thompson SA: Comparative studies of the human external sphincter and periurethral levator ani muscles, Br J Urol 53:35, 1981.

Green TH Jr: Development of a plan for diagnosis and treatment of urinary stress incontinence, Am J Obstet Gynecol 83:632, 1962.

Green TH Jr: The problem of urinary stress incontinence in the female: an appraisal of its current status, Obstet Gynecol Surv 23:603, 1968.

Green TH Jr: Urinary stress incontinence differential diagnosis pathophysiology and management, Am J Obstet Gynecol 122:368, 1975.

Hajj SN: Female urinary incontinence: a dynamic evaluation, J Reprod Med 23:33, 1979.

Harris RL, Yancey CA, Wiser WL, et al: Comparison of anterior colporrhaphy and retropubic urethropexy for patients with genuine stress urinary incontinence, Am J Obstet Gynecol 173:1671, 1995.

Henalla SM, Hutchins CJ, Robinson P, and MacVicar J: Nonoperative methods in the treatment of female genuine stress incontinence of urine, Br J Obstet Gynaecol 9:222, 1989.

Henalla SM, Kirwan P, Castleden CM, et al: The effect of pelvic floor exercises in the treatment of genuine urinary stress incontinence in women at two hospitals, Br J Obstet Gynaecol 95:602, 1988.

Henriksson L and Ulmsten U: Urodynamic evaluation of the effects of abdominal urethrocystopexy and vaginal sling urethroplasty in women with stress incontinence, Am J Obstet Gynecol 131:77, 1978.

Herbertsson G and Iosif CS: Surgical results and urodynamic studies 10 years after retropubic colpourethrocystopexy, Acta Obstet Gynecol Scand 72:298, 1993.

Hilton P and Stanton SL: A clinical and urodynamic assessment of the Burch colposuspension for genuine stress incontinence, Br J Obstet Gynaecol 90:934, 1983.

Hilton P and Stanton SL: Urethral pressure measurements by microtransducer: the results of symptom-free women and in those with genuine stress incontinence, Br J Obstet Gynaecol 90:919, 1983.

Hilton P and Stanton SL: Use of intravaginal oestrogen cream in genuine stress incontinence, Br J Obstet Gynaecol 90:940, 1983.

Hodgkinson CP: Relationships of the female urethra and bladder in urinary stress incontinence, Am J Obstet Gynecol 65:506, 1953.

Hodgkinson CP, Ayers MA, and Drukker BH: Dyssynergic detrusor dysfunction in the apparently normal female, Am J Obstet Gynecol 87:717, 1963.

Hodgkinson CP and Cobert N: Direct urethrocystommetry, Am J Obstet Gynecol 79:648, 1960.

Hodgkinson CP, Drukker BH, and Hershey GJG: Stress urinary incontinence in the female. VIII. Etiology significance of the short urethra, Am J Obstet Gynecol 86:16, 1963.

Holschneider CH, Solh S, Lebherz TB, and Montz FJ: The modified Pereyra procedure in recurrent stress urinary incontinence: a 15-year review, Obstet Gynecol 83:573, 1994.

Holst K and Wilson PD: The prevalence of female urinary incontinence and reasons for not seeking treatment, N Z Med J 101:758, 1988.

Horbach NS and Ostergard DR: Predicting intrinsic urethral sphincter dysfunction in women with stress urinary incontinence, Obstet Gynecol 84:188, 1994.

Hoyme UB, Tamimi HK, Eschenbach DA, et al: Osteomyelitis pubis after radical gynecologic operations, Obstet Gynecol 63:47S, 1984.

Jeffcoate TNA and Roberts H: Observations of stress incontinence of urine, Am J Obstet Gynecol 64:721, 1952.

Kammerer-Duak DN, Cornella JL, Margrina JF, Stanhope CR, and Smilack J: Osteitis pubis after Marshall-Marchetti-Krantz urethropexy: a pubic osteomyelitis. Am J Obstet Gynecol 179:586, 1998.

Karram MM and Bhatia NN: The Q-tip test: standardization of the technique and its interpretation in women with urinary incontinence, Obstet Gynecol 71:807, 1988.

Karram MM, Rosenzweig BA, and Bhatia NN: Artificial urinary sphincter for recurrent/severe stress incontinence in women: urogynecologic perspective, J Reprod Med 38:791, 1993.

Kegel AH: Stress incontinence of urine in women: physiologic treatment, J Int Coll Surg 25:487, 1956.

Kiesswetter H, Hennrich F, and Englisch M: Clinical and urodynamic assessment of pharmacologic therapy of stress incontinence, Urol Int 38:58, 1983.

Korn AP: Does use of permanent suture material affect outcome of the modified Pereyra procedure? Obstet Gynecol 83:104, 1994.

Koziol JA: Epidemiology of interstitial cystitis. Urol Clin North Am 21:7, 1994.

Kujansuu E: The effect of pelvic floor exercises on urethral function in female stress incontinence and urodynamic study, Ann Chir Gynaecol 72:28, 1983.

Langer R, Ron-El R, Neuman M, et al: The value of simultaneous hysterectomy during Burch colposuspension for urinary stress incontinence, Obstet Gynecol 72:866, 1988.

Lapides J: Transurethral treatment of urethral diverticula in women, Trans Am Assoc Genitourin Surg 70:135, 1978.

Lapides J, Ajemian EP, Stewart BH, et al: Physiopathology of stress incontinence, Surg Gynecol Obstet 111:224, 1960.

Lee RA: Diverticulum of the female urethra: postoperative complications and results, Obstet Gynecol 61:52, 1983.

Lentz SS: Osteitis pubis: a review, Obstet Gynecol Surv 50:310, 1995.

Low JA: Clinical characteristics of patients with demonstrable urinary incontinence, Am J Obstet Gynecol 88:322, 1964.

MacKinnon M, Pratt JH, and Pool TL: Diverticulum of the female urethra, Surg Clin North Am 39:953, 1959.

Marchetti AA, Marshall VF, and Shultis LD: Simple vesicourethral suspension for stress incontinence of urine, Am J Obstet Gynecol 74:57, 1957.

Matilla J: Vascular immunopathology in interstitial cystitis. Clin Immunol Immunopathol 23:648, 1982.

McGuire EJ: Urodynamic findings in patients after failure of stress incontinence operations, Prog Clin Biol Res 78:351, 1981.

McGuire EJ and Appell RA: Collagen injection for the dysfunctional urethra, Contemp Urol 3:11, 1991.

McGuire EJ, Wang SC, Appell RA, et al: Treatment of urethral continence by collagen injection, J Urol 143:224A, 1990.

Meyer S, Schreyer A, DeGrandi P, and Hohlfeld P: The effects of birth on urinary continence mechanisms and other pelvic floor characteristics. Obstet Gynecol 92:613, 1998.

Migliorini GR and Glenning PP: Bonney's test—fact or fiction? Br J Obstet Gynaecol 94:157, 1987.

Millard RJ and Oldenburg BF: The symptomatic urodynamic and psychodynamic results of bladder reeducation programs, J Urol 130:715, 1983.

Miyazaki FS: The Bonney test: a reassessment. Am J Obstet Gynecol 177:1322, 1997.

Mohr JA, Rogers J Jr, Brown TN, et al: Stress urinary incontinence: the simple and practical approach to diagnosis and treatment, J Am Geriatr Soc 31:476, 1983.

Montz FJ and Stanton SL: Q-tip test in female urinary incontinence, Obstet Gynecol 67:258, 1986.

Muellner SR and Fleischner FG: Normal and abnormal micturition study of the bladder behavior by means of fluoroscopy, J Urol 61:233, 1949.

Nichols DH: A Mersilene mesh gauze hammock for severe urinary stress incontinence, Obstet Gynecol 41:88, 1973.

Norton PA and Baker JE: Postural changes can reduce leakage in women with stress urinary incontinence, Obstet Gynecol 84:770, 1994.

Norton P, Karram M, Wall L, et al: Randomized double-blind trial of Terodiline in the treatment of urge incontinence in women, Obstet Gynecol 84:386, 1994.

Nygaard IE: Does prolonged high-impact activity contribute to later urinary incontinence? A retrospective cohort study of female Olympians. Obstet Gynecol 90:718, 1997.

Nygaard IE, Kreder KJ, Lepic MM, et al: Efficacy of pelvic floor muscle exercises in women with stress, urge, and mixed urinary incontinence, Am J Obstet Gynecol 174:120, 1996.

Ostergard DR: The effect of drugs on the lower urinary tract, Obstet Gynecol Surv 34:424, 1979.

Ostergard DR: The neurologic control of micturition and integral voiding reflexes, Obstet Gynecol Surv 34:417, 1979.

Owens RG, Kohlt N, Wynne J, Roat T, and Karram MM: Long term results of a fascia lata suburethral patch sling for severe stress urinary incontinence. J Pelvic Surg 5:196, 1999.

Park GS and Miller EJ Jr: Surgical treatment of stress urinary incontinence: a comparison of the Kelly plication, Marshall-Marchetti-Krantz, and Pereyra procedures, Obstet Gynecol 71:575, 1988.

Parsons CL: The therapeutic role of sulfated polysaccharides in the urinary bladder. Urol Clin North Am 21:93, 1994.

Parsons CL, Benson G, Childs SJ, et al: A quantitatively controlled method to prospectively study interstitial cystitis and demonstrate the efficacy of pentosanpolysulfate. J Urol 150:845, 1993.

Parsons LL: Interstitial cystitis. In Kurol ED and McGuire EJ, eds: Female urology, Philadelphia, 1994, Lippincott.

Peattie AB, Plevnik S, and Stanton SL: Vaginal cones: a conservative method of treating genuine stress incontinence, Br J Obstet Gynaecol 95:1049, 1988.

Pereyra AJ: A simplified surgical procedure for the correction of stress incontinence in women, West J Surg 67:223, 1959.

Pereyra AJ and Lebherz TB: Combined urethrovesical suspension and vaginal urethroplasty for correction of stress incontinence, Obstet Gynecol 30:537, 1967.

Perez-Marrero R, Emerson LE, Feltis JT: A controlled study of dimethyl sulfoxide in interstitial cystitis. J Urol 140:36, 1988.

Rosamilia A and Dwyer PL: Interstitial cystitis and the gynecologist. Obstet Gynecol Survey 53:309, 1998.

Ross JW: Multichannel urodynamic evaluation of laparoscopic Burch Colposuspension for genuine stress incontinence. Obstet Gynecol 91:55, 1998.

Rudd T: Urethral pressure profile in continent women from childhood to old age, Acta Obstet Gynecol Scand 59:331, 1979.

Saidi MH, Gallagher MS, Skop IP, Saidi JA, Sadler RK, and Diaz KE: Extraperitoneal laparoscopic colposuspension: short-term cure rate, complications, and duration of hospital stay in comparison with Burch Colposuspension. Obstet Gynecol 92:619, 1998.

Sand PK, Bowen LW, Ostergard DR, et al: The effect of retropubic urethropexy on detrusor stability, Obstet Gynecol 71:818, 1988.

Sand PK, Bowen LW, Ostergard DR, et al: Cryosurgery versus dilation and massage for the treatment of recurrent urethral syndrome, J Repro Med 34:499, 1989.

Sand PK, Bowen LW, Panganiban R, and Ostergard DR: The low pressure urethra as a factor in failed retropubic urethropexy, Obstet Gynecol 69:399, 1987.

Sand PK, Richardson DA, Staskin DR, et al: Pelvic floor electrical stimulation in the treatment of genuine stress incontinence: a multicenter, placebo-controlled trial, Am J Obstet Gynecol 173:72, 1995.

Sant GR and LaRock DR: Standard intravesicle therapies for interstitial cystitis. Urol Clin North Am 21:73, 1994.

Schaer GN, Koechli OR, Schuessler B, and Haller U: Improvement of perineal sonographic bladder neck imaging with ultrasound contrast medium, Obstet Gynecol 86:950, 1995.

Schaer GN, Koechli OR, Schuessler B, and Haller U: Perineal ultrasound for evaluating the bladder neck in urinary stress incontinence, Obstet Gynecol 85:220, 1995.

Shull BL and Baden WF: A six-year experience with paravaginal defect repair for stress urinary incontinence, Am J Obstet Gynecol 160:1432, 1989.

Sjoberg B and Nyman CR: Hydrodynamics of micturition in stress incontinent women: comparisons of pressure and flow at different micturition volumes in stress incontinent and continent women, Scand J Urol Nephrol 16:1, 1982.

Spence HM and Duckett JW Jr: Diverticulum of the female urethra: clinical aspects and presentation of a simple operative technique for cure, J Urol 104:432, 1970.

Spraitz AF Jr and Welch JS: Diverticulum of the female urethra, Am J Obstet Gynecol 91:1013, 1965.

Stamey TA: Endoscopic suspension of the vesical neck for urinary incontinence in females: report of 203 consecutive cases, Ann Surg 192:465, 1980.

Sultana CJ: Urethral closure pressure and leak-point pressure in incontinent women, Obstet Gynecol 86:839, 1995.

Swift SE and Ostergard DR: A comparison of stress leak-point pressure and maximal urethral closure pressure in patients with genuine stress incontinence, Obstet Gynecol 85:704, 1995.

Swift SE and Ostergard DR: Evaluation of current urodynamic testing methods in the diagnosis of genuine stress incontinence, Obstet Gynecol 86:85, 1995.

Tchou DCH, Adams C, Varner RE, and Denton B: Pelvic-floor musculature exercises in treatment of anatomical urinary stress incontinence, Phys Ther 68:652, 1988.

Teasdale TA, Taffet GE, Luchi RJ, and Adam E: Urinary incontinence in a community-residing elderly population, J Am Geriatr Soc 36:600, 1988.

Te Linde RW: Urethral sling operation, Clin Obstet Gynecol 6:206, 1963.

US Department of Health and Human Services, Public Health Service Agency for Health Care Policy and Research: Urinary incontinence in adults, April, 1995.

Van Geelen JM, Theeuwes AGM, Eskes TKAB, and Martin CB Jr: The clinical and urodynamic effects of anterior vaginal repair and Burch colposuspension, Am J Obstet Gynecol 159:137, 1988.

Vesey SG, Rivett A, and O'Boyle PJ: Teflon injection in female stress incontinence: effect on urethral pressure profile and flow rate, Br J Urol 62:39, 1988.

Visco AG, Weidner AC, Cundiff GW, and Bump RC: Observed patient compliance with a structured outpatient bladder retraining program. Am J Obstet Gynecol 181:1392, 1999.

Walter S and Olesen KP: Urinary incontinence in genital prolapse in the female: clinical urodynamic and radiologic examinations, Br J Obstet Gynaecol 89:393, 1982.

Walters MD and Diaz K: Q-tip test: a study of continent and incontinent women, Obstet Gynecol 70:208, 1987.

Walters MD and Shields LE: The diagnostic value of history, physical examination, and the Q-tip cotton swab test in women with urinary incontinence, Am J Obstet Gynecol 159:145, 1988.

Weinberger MW and Ostergard DR: Long-term clinical and urodynamic evaluation of the polytetrafluoroethylene suburethral sling for treatment of genuine stress incontinence, Obstet Gynecol 86:92, 1995.

Westby M, Asmussen M, and Ulmsten U: Localization of maximum intraurethral pressure related to urogenital diaphragm in the female subject as studied by simultaneous urethrocystommetry and voiding urethrocystography, Am J Obstet Gynecol 144:408, 1982.

Williams ME and Fitzhugh CP: Urinary incontinence in the elderly, Ann Intern Med 97:895, 1982.

Young SB, Rosenblatt PL, Pingeton DM, et al: The Mersilene mesh suburethral sling: a clinical and urodynamic evaluation, Am J Obstet Gynecol 173:1719, 1995.

APPENDIX

Drugs That Affect Bladder Functions

Generic Name	Trade Name	Generic Name	Trade Name
Drugs affecting sympathetic nervous system		*General adrenergic stimulators—cont'd*	
Alpha-adrenergic blockers		Tramazoline	—
		Tuaminoheptane	Taumine
Azapetine	Ilidar	Tymazoline*	Pernazene
Dihydroergotoxine	Hydergine	Xylometazoline	Otrivin
Ergot alkaloids	—		
Phenothiazines	(Various; see p. 000: Drugs Affecting Autonomic Nervous System—Causing Retention)	*Alpha-adrenergic stimulators*	
		Amidephrine	—
Phentolamine	Regitine	Cyclopentamine	Clopane
Piperoxan	Benodaine	Dopamine	Intropin
Tolazoline	Priscoline	Etafedrine	—
		Ethylphenylephrine	Effortil
Beta-adrenergic blockers		Hydroxyamphetamine	Paredrine
		Metaraminol	Aramine
Alprenolol	—	Methamphetamine	Desoxyn; Efroxine, Methedrine, Norodin, Synodroy
Butidrine	—		
Butoxamine	—	Methoxamine	Vasoxyl
Dichloroisoproterenol	Alderlin, Nethalide, Pronethalol	Methylhexaneamine	Forthane
Isopropylmethoxamine	—	Nordefrin	Cobefrin
Ko692	—	Norepinephrine	Levarterenol
LB-46	Prinololol	Novadral	—
M 1999	Sotalol	Phenylephrine	Neo-Synephrine, Isophrin, Synasal, Alconefrin Biomydrin, Isohalent Improved
Oxprenolol	—		
Practolol	Eraldin		
		Phenylpropylmethylamine	Vonedrine
General adrenergic stimulators		Propylhexedrine	Benzedrex
		Tyramine	—
Adrenalone	Kephrine		
Aminorex*	—	*Beta-adrenergic stimulators*	
—	Aranthol		
Benzphetamine	Didrex	Albuterol	Proventil, Ventolin
Chlorphentermine	Pre-Sate	Bamethan*	—
Clortemine	Voranil	Chlorprenaline	—
Cyclopantamine	Clopane	Dioxethedrine	—
Deoxyepinephrine	Epinine	Etafedrine	—
Dextroamphetamine	Dexedrine	Ethylnorepinephrine	Butanefrine, Bronkephrine
Diethylpropion	Tenuate, Tepanil	Hydroxyephedrine	—
Epinephrine	—	Isoethamine	—
Ethylnorepinephrine	Bronkephrine	Isoproterenol	Aludrine, Isuprel, Norisodrine
Fenfluramine	Pondimin	Methoxyphenamine	Orthoxine
Hydroxyamphetamine	Paredrine	Nylidrin	Arlidin
H1032*	—	Protokylol	Caytine
Isometheptene	Octin	Salbutanal	—
Levamphetamine	Ad-Nil, Amodril, Cydril, Maigret	Soterenol	—
Mazindol	Sanorex	Terbutaline	Bricamyl
Mephentermine	Wyamine		
Methamphetamine	Dexoxyn	*Adrenergic neuron blockers*	
Methylaminoheptane	Oenethyl		
Methylhexamine	Forthane	Alseroxylon	Rautensin, Rauwiloid
Naphazoline	Privine	Bethanidine	Esbatal
Oxymetazoline	Afrin	Bretylium	Darenthin
Phedrazine*	—	Debrisoquin	Declinax
Phendimetrazine	Dietrol, Plegine	Deserpidine	Harmonyl
Phenmetrazine	Preludin	Guanadrel	—
Phentermine	Ionamin, Wilpo	Guanethidine	Ismelin
Pholedrine	Paredrinal	Guanoclor	Vatensol
Propylhexedrine	Benzedrex	Guanoxan	Envacar
Pseudoephedrine	Sudafed, Ro-Fedrin	Hydralazine	Apresoline
Racephedrine	—	Methyldopa	Aldomet
Synephrine*	—	Methyldopate	Aldomet Ester
Tenaphtoxaline*	—	Nialamide	—
Tetrahydrozoline	Tyzine	Pargyline	Eutonyl

Continued

Drugs That Affect Bladder Functions

Generic Name	Trade Name	Generic Name	Trade Name
Adrenergic neuron blockers—cont'd		*Inhibitors—cont'd*	
Prazosin	Minipress	Tincture of belladonna	—
Rauwolfia	Hyperloid, Raudixin, Rauja, Raulfin, Rautina, Rauval, Venibar	Tricyclamol	Elorine
		Tridihexethyl	Pathilon
Rescinnamine	Cinatabs, Moderil	Tropicamide	Mydriacyl
Reserpine	Lemiserp, Rau-Sed, Resercen, Reserpoid, Rolserp, Sandril, Serpasil, Sertina, Vio-Serpine	Valethamate	Murel
		Drugs affecting sympathetic and parasympathetic nervous system—ganglionic blockers	
Syrosingopine	Singoserp		
Tranylcypromine	—	Azamethonium	Pendiomid
Veratrum alkaloids	Unitensin, Veralba, Veriloid, Vertairs	Chlorisondamine	Ecolid
		Hexamethonium	—
Drugs affecting parasympathetic nervous system		Mecamylamine	Inversine
Stimulators		Methaphan	Arfonad
		Pentolium	Ansolysen
Ambenonium	Mytelase	Sparteine	Spartocin, Tocosamine
Carbachol	Carcholin, Isopto Carbachol	Trimethidinium	Ostensin
Echothioplate	Phospholine		
Demecarium	Humorsol	*Drugs affecting autonomic nervous system*	
Edrophonium	Tensilon	*Causing retention*	
Isoflurophate	Floropryl		
Methacholine	Mecholyl	Acetophenazine	Tindal
Pilocarpine	Pilocar	Amitriptyline	Elavil
Pralidoxime	Protopam	Amphotericin B	Fungizone
Pyridostigmine	Mestinon	Benztropine	Cogentin
		Biperiden	Akineton
Inhibitors		Bromodiphenhydramine	Ambodryl
		Brompheniramine	Dimetane
Adiphenine	Trasentine	Butaperazine	Repoise
Alverine	Prafenil, Spacolin	Carbinoxzmine	Clistin
Anisotropine	Valpin	Carphenazine	Proketazine
Atropine	—	Chlorpheniramine	Chlor-Trimeton, Histaspan, Teldrin
Belladonna extract	—	Chlorphenoxamine	Systral, Phenoxene
Carbofluorene	Pavatrine	Chlorpromazine	Thorazine
Clidinium	Librax, Quarzan	Chlorprothixene	Taractan
Cyclopentolate	Cyclogyl	Cycrimine	Pagitane
Diphemanil	Prantal	Deanol	Deaner
Ethaverine	Ethaquin, Laverin, Neopavrin	Desipramine	Norpramin, Pertofrane
Eucatropine	Euphthalmine	Dexbrompheniramine	Disomer
Glycopyrrolate	Robinul	Dexchlorpheniramine	Polaramine
Hexocyclium	Tral	Dimethindene	Forhistal, Triten
Homatropine hydrobromide	—	Diphenhydramine	Benadryl
Homatropine methylbromide	Homapin, Malcotran, Mesopin, Novatrin	Diphenylpyraline	Diafen, Hispril
		Doxepin	Adapin, Sinequan
Hyoscyamine sulfate	Levsin	Doxylamine	Decapryn
Isometheptene	Isometene, Octin	Droperidol	Inapsine
Mepenzolate	Cantil	Ethopropazine	Parsidol
Methixene	Trest	Fluphenazine	Prolixin, Permitil
Methscopolamine bromide	Pamine	Haloperidol	Haldol
Methylatropine nitrate (atropine methylnitrate)	Metropine	Imipramine	Tofranil, Presamine
		Isocarboxazid	Marplan
Oxyphenonium	Antrenyl	Mepazine	—
Papaverine	Cerespan, Pap-Kaps, Pavabid, Pavacap, Pavacen, Pavarine, Pavatest, Paveril, Vasal, Vaso-span	Mesoridazine	Serentil
		Metaxalone	Skelaxin
		Methapyrilene	Histadyl
		Methdilazine	Tacaryl
Pentapiperium	Quilene	Methylphenidate	Ritalin
Penthienate	Monodral	Methysergide	Sansert
Pipenzolate	Piptal	Molindone	Moban
Piperidolate	Dactil	Nortriptyline	Aventyl
Poldine	Nacton	Orphenadrine	Norflex
Scopolamine	—	Perphenazine	Trilafon
Thihexinol	Sorboquel	Phenelzine	Nardil
Thiphenamil	Trocinate		

Drugs That Affect Bladder Functions

Generic Name	Trade Name	Generic Name	Trade Name
Causing retention—cont'd		*Causing retention—cont'd*	
Phenindamine	Thephorin	Tripelennamine	Pyribenzamine
Piperacetazine	Quide	Triprolidine	Actidil
Pipradrol	Meratran	*Causing miscellaneous urologic symptoms*	
Prochlorperazine	Compazine	*Frequency*	
Procyclidine	Kemadrin		
Promazine	Sparine	Dantrolene	Dantrium Triavil (mixture)
Promethazine	Phenergan	Iron Sorbitex	Jectofer Etrafon (mixture)
Protriptyline	Vivactil		
Pyrilamine	—	*Incontinence*	
Rotoxamine	Turiston	Estrogens	—
Thiopropazate	Dartal	Hydroxystilbamidine	—
Thioridazine	Mellaril		
Thiothixene	Navane	*Urgency*	
Tranylcypromine	Parnate	Disodium Edetate	Endrate
Trifluoperazine	Stelazine		
Triflupromazine	Vesprin	*Frequency, retention, and incontinence*	
Trihexyphenidyl	Artane, Pipanol, Tremin	Levodopa	Bendopa, Dopar, Larodopa, Levodopa
Trimeprazine	Temaril	Levopropoxyphene	Novrad

Combined Preparation Drugs

Drugs affecting sympathetic nervous system

Actifed-C Expectorant	Duovent		
Acutuss	Dylephrine		
Acutuss Expectorant	Ephed-Organidin		
with Codeine	Ephedrine and Chlorcyclizine		
Aerolone Compound	Ephedrine and Nembutal		
Amesec	Ephedrine and Seconal Sodium		
Amodrine	Ephoxamine		
Asbron	Glynazan/EP		
Ayrcap	Hyadrine		
AyrLiquid	Hydryllin with Racephedrine		
Bihisdin	Hydrochloride		
Brondilate	Iso-Tabs		
Bronkometer	Isuprel Compound		
Bronkosol	Lufyllin-EP		
Bronkotabs	Marax		
Calcidrine Syrup	Neo-Vadrin		
Cerose Expectorant	Norisodrine with Calcium Iodide		
Chlor-Trimeton Expectorant	Novalene		
with Codeine	NTZ		
Citra	Numa		
Colrex Compound	Orthoxine and Aminopylline		
Copavin	Pyracort		
Copavin Compound	Quadrinal		
Coricidin Nasal Mist	Tedral		
Co-Xan	Tedral-25		
Dainite	Tedral Anti-H		
Dainite-KI	Thalfed		
Deltasmyl	Triaminicin		
Duo-Medihaler			

Drugs inhibiting sympathetic nervous system

Aldoclor	Naquival
Aldoril	Nyomin
Butiserpazide	Oreticyl
Diupres	Protalba-R
Diutensen	Rautrax
Enduronyl	Rawiloid + Veriloid
Esimil	Regroton
Eutron	Renese-R
Exna-R	Salutensin
Hydromox-R	Sandril with Pyronil
Hydropres	Serpasil-Esidrix
Maxitate with Rauwolfia	Singoserp-Esidrix
Metatensin	

Drugs inhibiting parasympathetic nervous system

Belbarb	Kolantyl
Belladenal	Levsin with Phenobarbital
Bellergal	Milpath
Butibel	Nolamine
Cantil with Phenobarbital	Pamine
Chardonna	Pathibamate
Combid	Pathilon with Phenobarbital
Daricon-PB	Phenobarbital and Belladonna
Donnatal	Probanthine with Dartal
Donphen	Probanthine with Phenobarbital
Enarax	Robinul-PH
Histalet	Sidonna
Hybephen	Trasetine-phenobarbital
Kinesed	Valpin-PB

From Ostergard DR: Obstet Gynecol Surv 34:424, 1979.

Infections of the Lower Genital Tract

Vulva, Vagina, Cervix, Toxic Shock Syndrome, HIV Infections

KEY TERMS AND DEFINITIONS

Bubo. An enlarged and inflamed lymph node, particularly in the axilla or groin, caused by infections such as plague, syphilis, gonorrhea, lymphogranuloma venereum, and/or tuberculosis.

Calymmatobacterium Granulomatis. The gram-negative, nonmotile rod that causes granuloma inguinale.

Clue Cells. Epithelial cells with clusters of bacteria adherent to their external surfaces, obscuring their normal, fine border. They have a granular or stippled appearance and are associated with bacterial vaginosis.

Condyloma Acuminatum. A sexually transmitted viral disease of the vulva, vagina, cervix, and rectum caused by the human papillomavirus.

Condyloma Latum. The large, raised, flattened, grayish white lesions of secondary syphilis, most often found on the vulva.

Dark-Field Microscopy. A technique used to identify the spirochetes of syphilis, *Treponema pallidum.*

Donovan Bodies. The pathognomonic clusters of dark-staining bacteria (bipolar in appearance) found in the cytoplasm of large mononuclear cells in patients with granuloma inguinale.

Forme Fruste. A mild form of a disease.

Groove Sign. A depression between groups of inflamed nodes producing a double genitocrural fold in patients with lymphogranuloma venereum.

Gumma. An infectious granuloma characteristic of late or tertiary syphilis.

HIV. The human immunodeficiency virus, responsible for acquired immune deficiency syndrome (AIDS). It is an RNA virus of the retrovirus family.

Koilocytosis. The histologic appearance of cells with perinuclear halos consistent with HPV infection.

Mucopurulent Cervicitis. This inflammatory condition is diagnosed by gross visualization of yellow mucopurulent material or the presence of 10 or more polymorphonucleocytes per high-powered field on Gram stain of the endocervix.

Nit. The egg of the crab louse.

Podophyllin. A topical resin mixed with benzoin and alcohol used to treat the lesions of condyloma acuminatum.

Prozone Phenomenon. A false-negative VDRL or RPR caused by an excess of anticardiolipin antibody in the serum.

Sexually Transmitted Disease (STD). A term used to describe an infection acquired primarily through sexual contact; venereal disease.

Toxin 1. The toxin involved in producing the signs and symptoms of toxic shock syndrome. It is a small protein with a molecular weight of 22,000. Its primary effects are the production of increased vascular permeability and profuse leaking of fluid from the intravascular space to the extravascular space.

Western Blot Test. A technique to identify antibodies to a protein of a specific molecular weight. This test is more specific than the ELISA test for AIDS.

Whiff Test. A test used clinically. The smell of vaginal discharge after the addition of 10% potassium hydroxide. A positive sample associated with either bacterial vaginosis or *Trichomonas* infections will give off a fishy or aminelike smell.

Word Catheter. A short catheter with an inflatable Foley balloon used to help develop a fistulous tract from a Bartholin's duct to the vestibule.

The Centers for Disease Control (CDC) regularly revises its treatment protocols for sexually transmitted diseases. The recommendations and medications in this edition are based on the 1998 CDC guidelines. Readers are urged to consult any updates in CDC guidelines, since bacterial sensitivities and epidemiologic concerns may lead to changes in treatment protocols. The latest information may be found on the CDC Internet site: http://www.cdc.gov/.

The discussion of infectious diseases of the female genital tract is divided into two chapters. Infections involving the vulva, vagina, and cervix are discussed in this chapter, and infections involving the uterus, oviducts, and ovaries are discussed in Chapter 23. This separation has been made only to be similar to other chapters of the book and for clarity of presentation. The female genital tract has anatomic and physiologic continuity. Thus infectious agents that colonize and involve one organ often infect adjacent organs. To understand the pathophysiology and natural history of infectious diseases of the genital tract, one must keep this continuity in mind.

The symptoms caused by infections of the lower genital tract produce the most common conditions seen by gynecologists. Therefore the focus of this chapter is on clinical presentation and differential diagnosis of vulvitis, vaginitis, and cervicitis.

Toxic shock syndrome, acquired immune deficiency syndrome (AIDS), and syphilis are discussed in this chapter also. Although the most devastating pathologic processes from these diseases occur in sites other than the genital tract, often they obtain entry into the body through the vulvar, rectal, vaginal, or cervical epithelium.

Many of the infections discussed in this chapter may be acquired through sexual contact and are termed sexually transmitted diseases (STDs). The prevalence of STD infections in the United States currently is estimated to be 12 million individuals with approximately 3 million of these infections occurring in teenagers. STDs often coexist—for example, vulvar herpes and condyloma acuminatum or infections of *Chlamydia trachomatis* and *Neisseria gonorrhoeae*. When one disease is suspected, appropriate diagnostic methods must be used to detect other infections. This principle cannot be overemphasized.

INFECTIONS OF THE VULVA

The skin of the vulva is composed of a stratified squamous epithelium containing hair follicles and sebaceous, sweat, and apocrine glands. The subcutaneous tissue of the vulva also contains specialized structures such as the Bartholin glands. Similar to skin elsewhere on the body, the vulvar area is subject to both primary and secondary infections. The three most prevalent primary viral infections of the vulva are herpes genitalis, condyloma acuminatum, and molluscum contagiosum. However, symptoms from secondary infections of the vulva caused by organisms that produce vulvovaginitis are among the most common of all gynecologic conditions. To understand the differential diagnosis of vulvar infections, one must consider that vulvar skin is also sensitive to hormonal, metabolic, and allergic influences.

Vulvar itching or burning of acute onset and short duration suggests infection or a contact dermatitis. Approximately 10% of outpatient visits to gynecologists are for vulvar pruritus. The signs of erythema, edema, and superficial skin ulcers of the vulva also suggest infection. Skin fissures and excoriation may be signs of primary infection, may be caused by the patient's scratching as a result of irritation from a vaginal discharge, or may be the manifestation of a primary dermatologic disease.

Acute Bacterial Cystitis

Dysuria, urgency, and urinary frequency are the classic symptoms of infections of the lower urinary tract. It is estimated that 10% to 20% of adult women experience symptoms of dysuria and urinary frequency each year. An individual woman's lifetime risk of developing at least one urinary tract infection is approximately 50%. The highest incidence of acute bacterial cystitis is found in women during their early 20s. Urinary tract infections are the most common bacterial infection experienced by mature women. Reproductive-aged women are prone to ascending infections because of the shortness of the female urethra and the fact that the distal one third of the urethra is often colonized by bacteria from the vulvar vestibule. In postmenopausal women the lack of estrogenic effect on urovaginal epithelium and sometimes the presence of residual urine after voiding predisposes them to infection. Independent risk factors for the development of acute bacterial cystitis include sexual intercourse, use of a vaginal diaphragm and/or spermicide, previous urinary tract infection, recent exposure to antibiotics, and concurrent diagnosis of bacterial vaginosis. Basic science studies have demonstrated that vaginal and uroepithelial cells have an increased susceptibility to adherence by *E. coli* in some women.

Acute bacterial cystitis is characterized by multiple symptoms, including dysuria, urgency, and frequent voiding. It is usually abrupt in onset. Suprapubic tenderness is a specific sign for acute bacterial cystitis; however, it is not present in the majority of patients. The differential diagnosis of an adult woman with dysuria includes acute cystitis, acute urethritis, or vulvovaginitis. Table 22-1 lists characteristic features that help to differentiate the three most common causes of dysuria in adult women.

The patient's perception of the anatomic site of the dysuria may be helpful. Vulvovaginitis tends to produce "external" dysuria in contrast to a deeper "internal" dysuria associated with cystitis. In general, women with urethritis have more chronic symptoms, with a gradual onset and less urgency, than do women with acute bacterial cystitis. The most common pathogens causing acute urethritis are *C. trachomatis* and *N. gonorrhoeae*. Postmenopausal women often

TABLE 22-1

Major Infectious Causes of Acute Dysuria in Women

Condition	Pathogen	Pyuria	Hematuria	Urine Culture* cfu/mL	Symptoms, Signs, and Factors
Cystitis	E. coli, S. saprophyticus, proteus sp., Klebsiella sp.	Usually	Sometimes	10^2 to $\geq 10^5$	Abrupt onset, severe symptoms, multiple symptoms (dysuria, increased frequency and urgency), suprapubic or low back pain; suprapubic tenderness on examination
Urethritis	C. trachomatis, N. gonorrhoeae, herpes simplex virus	Usually	Rarely	$<10^2$	Gradual onset, mild symptoms, vaginal discharge or bleeding (due to concomitant cervicitis), lower abdominal pain, new sexual partner; cervicitis or vulvovaginal herpetic lesions on examination
Vaginitis	Candida species, Trichomonas vaginalis	Rarely	Rarely	$<10^2$	Vaginal discharge or odor, pruritus, dyspareunia, external dysuria, no increased frequency or urgency; vulvovaginitis on examination

From Stamm WE and Hooton TM: N Engl J Med 329:1328, 1993.

*Values indicate colony-forming units (cfu) per milliliter of urine.

experience similar symptoms related to estrogen deficiency without significant bacterial colonization of the bladder.

The most common cause of acute bacterial cystitis is ascending infection from the introitus and distal urethra. The pathogens most frequently involved in uncomplicated lower urinary tract infections are *Escherichia coli* (approximately 80%) and *Staphylococcus saprophyticus* (approximately 5% to 15%). There is increasing resistance of urinary tract pathogens with 25% to 50% of bacterial isolates being resistant to sulfanilamides, amoxicillin, tetracycline, and first-generation cephalosporins. The prevalence of resistance to trimethoprim and trimethoprim/sulfamethoxazole

has increased to approximately 20% in some geographic areas (Figure 22-1).

There are varying diagnostic steps in the laboratory work-up of the woman who has the classic symptoms of acute cystitis. The first step is to demonstrate pyuria by microscopic examination of the urine. Pyuria is demonstrated in the vast majority of episodes of acute bacterial cystitis and gross hematuria identified in approximately 20%. Alternatively, the leukocyte esterase dip stick has a reported sensitivity of approximately 85% in the detection of white blood cells in the urine. In women with classic symptoms and confirmation of pyuria, it is not necessary

Percentages of urinary isolates from women with acute uncomplicated cystitis resistant to selected antimicrobial agents*

	1992 E coli (n=567)	1992 All (n=653)	1993 E coli (n=931)	1993 All (n=1081)	1994 E coli (n=967)	1994 All (n=1127)	1995 E coli (n=691)	1995 All (n=807)	1996 Ecoli (n=580)	1996 All (n=674)
Ampicillin†	26	29	29	32	31	33	32	34	34	38
Cephalothin†	20	20	25	24	38	37	32	32	28	28
Ciprofloxacin hydrochloride	0.2	0.3	0	0.2	0.1	1	0	0.3	0.2	0.3
Gentamicin	2	2	1	1	1	1	0.4	0.4	1	1
Nitrofurantoin	1	7	1	6	2	9	1	7	0.2	6
Sulfamethoxazole	22	21	25	24	26	24	25	22	27	26
Trimethoprim-sulfamethoxazole†	9	8	10	9	9	9	12	12	18	16
Trimethoprim†	9	9	10	9	10	9	12	12	18	16

*Percentages reflect the number of isolates tested with each antimicrobial agent; this may be less than the total number for each column. E coli indicates *Escherichia coli*.

†There was a significant increasing linear trend in resistance from 1992 to 1996 for *E coli* and all isolates: ampicillin ($P<.002$), cephalothin ($P<.001$), trimethoprim ($P<.001$), and trimethoprim-sulfanmethoxazole ($P<.001$), using the test χ^2 for linear trend.

FIGURE 22-1 Percentages of urinary isolates from women with acute uncomplicated cystitis resistant to selected antimicrobial agents. (From Gupta K, Scholes D, and Stamm WE: JAMA 281:736, 1999.)

to perform a urine culture. However, if the patient has been treated for similar symptoms in the past, a clean-voided urine culture should be obtained. Indications for urine cultures include patients with a complicated history, urinary tract infections within the past month, urinary symptomatology that has been present more than 7 days, cystitis in a woman over age 65, pregnancy, or intercurrent diseases such as diabetes mellitus or immunosuppression.

To obtain accurate estimates of the number of bacteria per milliliter, it is important to culture the urine within 2 hours or to refrigerate the specimen until it is sent to the laboratory. The gold standard of more than 10^5 uropathogens per milliliter had been the criterion used to make the diagnosis of significant bacteriuria in asymptomatic women. However, bacterial concentrations of as few as 10^2 per milliliter are accepted as bacteriologic confirmation of cystitis in symptomatic women.

For the first episode of acute, uncomplicated cystitis the current treatment of choice is 3 days of oral therapy with trimethoprim/sulfamethoxazole, trimethoprim alone, or one of the quinolones such as ciprofloxacin or norfloxacin (Table 22-2). Compared with the traditional 7 to 14 days of therapy, the advantages of 3-day therapy are simplicity, better patient compliance, lower cost, and reduction of side effects such as diarrhea and vaginitis. With appropriate antibiotic therapy it takes approximately 24 hours for the symptoms of acute bacterial cystitis to resolve. In a community where resistance to trimethoprim is greater than 25%, treatment with a quinolone such as 250 mg bid of ciprofloxacin is appropriate. Obviously standard empiric regimens for acute bacterial cystitis should be reassessed periodically because of changing patterns of resistance to antibiotics. Women with chronic infections, systemic manifestations of infection, renal disease, anatomic abnormalities of the urinary tract, pregnancy, or diabetes mellitus should be given more prolonged oral therapy for a minimum of 7 to 14 days. Failure to respond necessitates quantitative culture of the urine for bacteria and also culture of the endocervix and urethra for *Chlamydia* and gonorrhea organisms. In the past, single-dose therapy was a popular regimen because of the convenience and simplicity. However, the rates of recurrence and failure with single-dose therapy were found to be unacceptable.

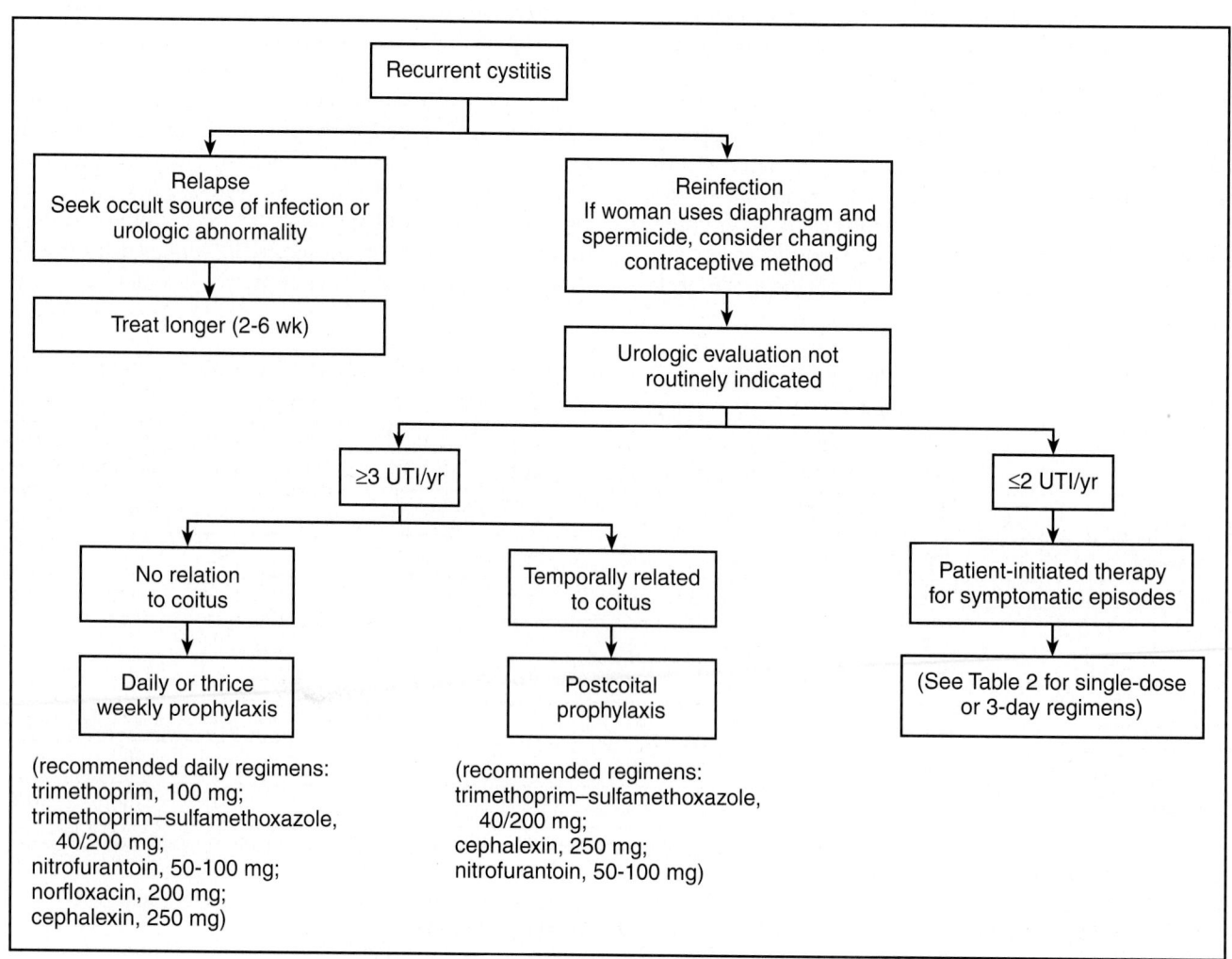

FIGURE 22-2 Strategies for managing recurrent cystitis in women. (From Stamm WE and Hooton TM: N Engl J Med 329:1328, 1993).

Persistent or recurrent cystitis following the initial infection presents in approximately 20% of women (Figure 22-2). It is important to differentiate whether the infection is a relapse or a reinfection. More than 90% of recurrences in young women are exogenous reinfection with new isolates arising from local flora. Behavioral modification has become popular for preventing recurrent acute cystitis. Possible modifications in lifestyle include discontinuing use of a diaphragm for contraception, increasing oral fluid intake, voiding frequently, voiding immediately after intercourse, double voiding, and drinking cranberry juice. Approximately 75% of episodes of acute bacterial infection in women with recurrent cystitis occur within 24 hours of coitus. These women are excellent candidates to be treated with prophylactic antibiotics. The type of prophylaxis depends on the individual patient's history whether broad-spectrum antibiotics are prescribed continuously, postcoitally, or when the patient believes she is developing an infection. The broad-spectrum antibiotics that are most commonly chosen for low-dose antibiotic prophylaxis are trimethoprim, trimethoprim/sulfamethoxazole, nitrofurantoin, or a cephalosporin. Prophylaxis may be given for months without significant emergence of antibiotic-resistant bacteria.

Complicated lower urinary tract infections are those caused by antibiotic-resistant bacteria and those infections that occur in women with anatomic or functional abnormalities of the urinary tract. There are many different organisms that may be cultured in complicated cystitis, including *Escherichia coli, Enterococcus faecalis, Proteus mirabilis, Staphylococcus epidermidis, Staphylococcus aureus, Klebsiella, Pseudomonas, Enterobacter,* and *Serratia*. The quinolones currently are the drugs of choice for empiric therapy of complicated cystitis, primarily because of their broad antibacterial spectrum.

Infections of Bartholin's Glands

Bartholin's glands normally are two rounded, pea-sized glands deep in the perineum. They are located at the entrance of the vagina at 5 and 7 o'clock. A normal Bartholin's gland cannot be palpated. The Bartholin's ducts are approximately 2 cm in length and they open in a groove between the hymen and labia minora in the posterior lateral wall of the vagina. Approximately 2% of adult women develop enlargements of one or both glands, of which there are three common causes. The most common cause is cystic dilation of Bartholin's duct (Figure 22-3). Subsequently, symptomatic enlargement of Bartholin's glands may be related to adenitis or abscess formation. Mechanical obstruction of the duct usually precedes overt infection. The most serious sequela of infection is a polymicrobial, necrotizing subcutaneous infection, especially in diabetic women. In women over the age of 40, enlargement may be caused by the rare adenocarcinoma of Bartholin's glands. More than 85% of women who develop enlargement of the Bartholin's glands do so during their reproductive years. The mean age of discovery of a Bartholin's gland carcinoma is 50.

The etiology of a Bartholin's duct cyst is obstruction of

TABLE 22-2
Recommended Three-Day Regimens for Acute Uncomplicated Cystitis in Young Women

Drug	Dosage
Trimethoprim/sulfamethoxazole	160/180 mg q12h
Trimethoprim	100 mg q12h
Quinolones	
Ciprofloxacin	250 mg q12h
Enoxacin	400 mg q12h
Lomefloxacin 4	400 mg q24h
Norfloxacin	400 mg q12h
Ofloxacin	200 mg q12h

From Sweet RL and Gibbs RS: Infectious diseases of the female genital tract, ed 3, Baltimore, 1995, Williams & Wilkins.

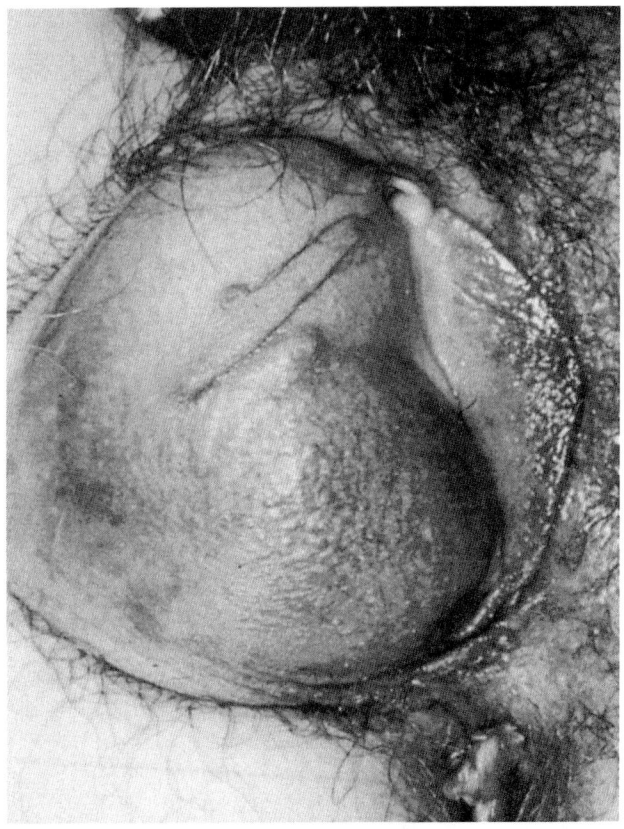

FIGURE 22-3 Bartholin's abscess. Mass is tender and fluctuant and is situated on lower lateral aspect of labium minus at 5 o'clock. (From Kaufman RH: Cystic tumors. In Kaufman RH and Faro S, editors: Benign diseases of the vulva and vagina, ed 4, St. Louis, 1994, Mosby–Year Book, Inc.)

the duct secondary to nonspecific inflammation or trauma. Histologically, the Bartholin's ducts are lined by transitional epithelium. These ducts are easily obstructed, usually near the distal orifice. Following obstruction, there is continued secretion of glandular fluid, which results in the cystic dilation. Years ago bilateral enlargement of Bartholin's glands was believed to be a pathognomonic sign of gonococcal infection. This is no longer true. Unilateral or bilateral Bartholin's gland infection in the majority of cases is not caused by a sexually transmitted disease. Lee et al. obtained bacterial cultures of fluid from Bartholin's duct cysts and abscesses. More than 80% of cultures from cysts were sterile, as were one in three cultures from Bartholin's abscesses. Brook reported positive cultures from 26 of 28 patients. He reported a total of 67 bacterial isolates, 43 of which were anaerobic and 24 of which were aerobic and facultative anaerobic organisms. In summary, positive cultures from Bartholin's gland abscesses are often polymicrobial and contain a wide range of bacteria similar to the normal flora of the vagina.

The differential diagnosis of Bartholin's gland cysts includes mesonephric cysts of the vagina and epithelial inclusion cysts. Mesonephric cysts are generally more anterior and cephalad in the vagina, whereas epithelial inclusion cysts are more superficial. Rarely, a lipoma, fibroma, hernia, or hydrocele may be confused with a Bartholin's duct cyst. Bartholin's duct cysts are found in the labia majora, whereas Bartholin's glands are at the base of the labia minora.

Most women with Bartholin's duct cysts are asymptomatic. The cysts may vary from 1 to 8 cm in diameter, and they are usually unilateral, tense, and nonpainful. The majority of cysts are unilocular. However, occasionally in chronic or recurrent cysts there are multiple compartments.

An abscess of a Bartholin's gland tends to develop rapidly over 2 to 4 days. Symptoms include acute vulvar pain, dyspareunia, and pain during walking. Local symptoms of acute pain and tenderness are secondary to rapid enlargement, hemorrhage, or secondary infection. The signs are those of a classic abscess: erythema, acute tenderness, edema, and occasionally cellulitis of the surrounding subcutaneous tissue. Without therapy, most abscesses tend to rupture spontaneously by the third or fourth day.

The treatment of infections or enlargement of Bartholin's glands depends on their symptomatology. Asymptomatic cysts in women under the age of 40 do not need treatment. The therapy for acute adenitis without abscess formation is broad-spectrum antibiotics and frequent hot sitz baths.

The treatment of choice for a symptomatic cyst or abscess is the development of a fistulous tract from the dilated duct to the vestibule. Simple incision and drainage of a Bartholin's gland abscess are complicated by a tendency for the abscess to recur. The classic surgical treatment is to develop a fistulous tract to "marsupialize" the duct. After an elliptical wedge of tissue has been removed, the remaining edges of the duct or abscess are everted and sutured to the surrounding skin with interrupted sutures. This forms an epithelialized pouch that provides drainage for the gland. The recurrence rate following marsupialization is approximately 5% to 10%. An alternative surgical approach is to insert a Word catheter (a short catheter with an inflatable Foley balloon) through a stab incision into the abscess and leave it in place for 4 to 6 weeks (Figure 22-4). During this period a tract of epithelium will form. One may use a carbon dioxide laser to produce a neostoma in a Bartholin's duct cyst. All of the previously mentioned operations may be performed with local anesthesia. Antibi-

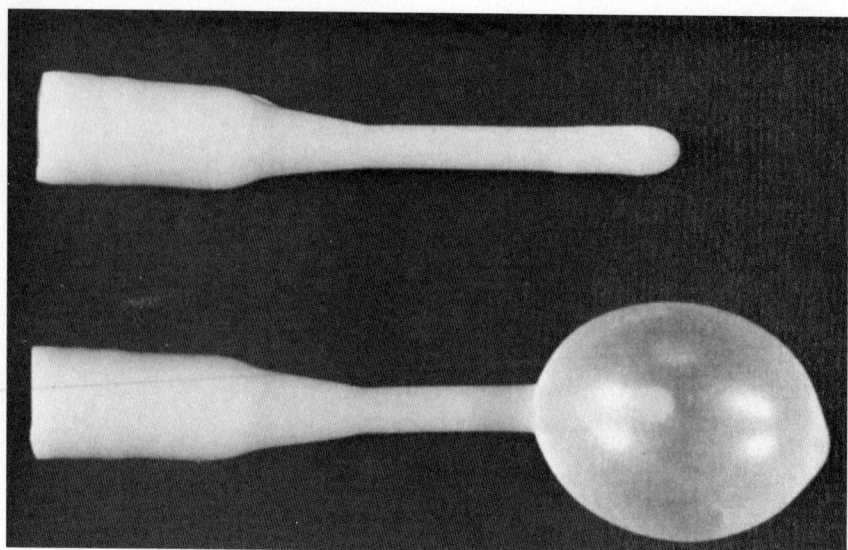

FIGURE 22-4 Word catheters before and after inflation. They are used to develop a fistula from Bartholin's cyst or abscess to vestibule. (From Friedrich EG: Vulvar disease, ed 2, Philadelphia, 1983, WB Saunders Co.)

otics are not necessary unless there is an associated cellulitis surrounding the Bartholin's gland abscess.

Excision of a Bartholin's duct and gland is indicated for persistent deep infection, multiple recurrences of abscesses, or enlargement of the gland in women over the age of 40. Excision or biopsy for gland enlargement in women over 40 is performed to diagnose adenocarcinoma of Bartholin's gland. Removal of a Bartholin's gland for recurrent infection should be performed when the infection is quiescent. Because of the richness of the vascular supply to the region, including the vestibular bulbs directly below Bartholin's gland, excision is a more formidable task than one would expect. It is best to have either regional block or general anesthesia for excision. Removal of a Bartholin's gland is often accompanied by morbidity, including intraoperative hemorrhage, hematoma formation, fenestration of the labia, postoperative scarring, and associated dyspareunia. Bartholin's gland secretions are not important for providing lubrication during sexual intercourse. Mucinous secretions from Bartholin's glands do provide moisture for the epithelium of the vestibule but are not important for vaginal lubrication.

Pediculosis Pubis and Scabies

The skin of the vulva is a frequent site of infestation by animal parasites, the two most common being the crab louse and the itch mite. Lice are insects and scabies mites are arachnids; both are arthropods. Ideally, early diagnosis and treatment are of the utmost importance to control parasitic infection. However, because many women experience embarrassment, guilt, and anxiety over the potential diagnosis of this infection, delay in diagnosis often interferes with ideal treatment.

Pediculosis pubis is an infestation by the crab louse, *Phthirus pubis*. The crab louse is also called the pubic louse and is a different species than the body or head louse. The louse is transmitted usually by close contact, although it may be acquired from towels or bedding. Lice in the pubic hair are the most contagious of all sexually transmitted diseases. It is estimated that over 90% of sexual partners are infected following a single exposure. *P. pubis* is generally confined to the hairy areas of the vulva. It may occasionally be found in other areas such as the eyelids. The major nourishment of the louse is human blood. Body lice predominately infect schoolchildren and, secondarily, their mothers, by direct contact. Schools and playgrounds are the major reservoir. In contrast pubic lice are typically transmitted by direct sexual contact. However, nonsexual transmission of pubic lice has been documented.

There are three stages in the louse's life cycle: egg (nit), nymph, and adult. The entire life cycle is spent on the host. Eggs are deposited at the base of hair follicles. The adult parasite is approximately 1 mm long and dark gray when its alimentary tract is not filled with blood (Figure 22-5).

Of clinical importance for diagnosis is the fact that the louse moves slowly.

Scabies is a parasitic infection of the itch mite, *Sarcoptes scabiei*. There is a centuries-old belief that an outbreak of scabies portends the beginning of a war. The medical corollary is that epidemic outbreaks of scabies tend to occur approximately every 20 to 30 years. Similar to the crab louse, it is transmitted by close contact. Unlike louse infestation, scabies is an infection that is widespread over the body without a predilection for hairy areas. The adult female itch mite digs a burrow just beneath the skin. She lays eggs in this home during her life span of approximately 1 month. The adult itch mite is usually less than 0.5 mm long, approximately the size of a grain of sand. Unlike the crab louse, an itch mite travels rapidly over skin and may move up to 2.5 cm in 1 minute. Mites are able to survive for only a few hours away from the warmth of skin.

The predominant clinical symptom of louse infestation is constant itching in the pubic area, which is secondary to allergic sensitization. It is estimated that it takes a minimum of 5 days following initial infection to develop allergic sensitization. Usually, initial sensitization takes several weeks to develop. The incubation period for pediculosis is approximately 30 days. Pruritus may occur within 24 hours after a reinfection. Examination of the vulvar area without magnification demonstrates eggs and adult lice and "pepper grain" feces adjacent to the hair shafts (Figure 22-6). The tiny rough spots visualized with the naked eye are the alimentary tracts of lice filled with human blood. The vulvar skin may become secondarily irritated or infected by constant scratching. For definitive diagnosis one can make a microscopic slide by scratching the skin papule with a needle and placing the crust under a drop of mineral oil. The louse's body looks like that of a miniature crab with six legs that have claws on them.

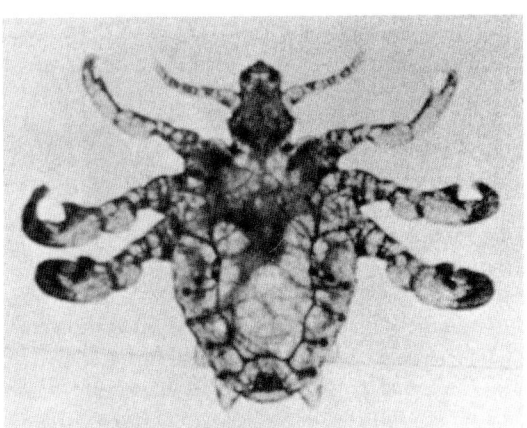

FIGURE 22-5 Pubic louse, *Phthirus pubis*, after blood meal. (From Billstein S: Human lice. In Holmes KK, Mårdh PA, Sparling PF, et al, editors: Sexually transmitted diseases, New York, 1984, McGraw-Hill Book Co.)

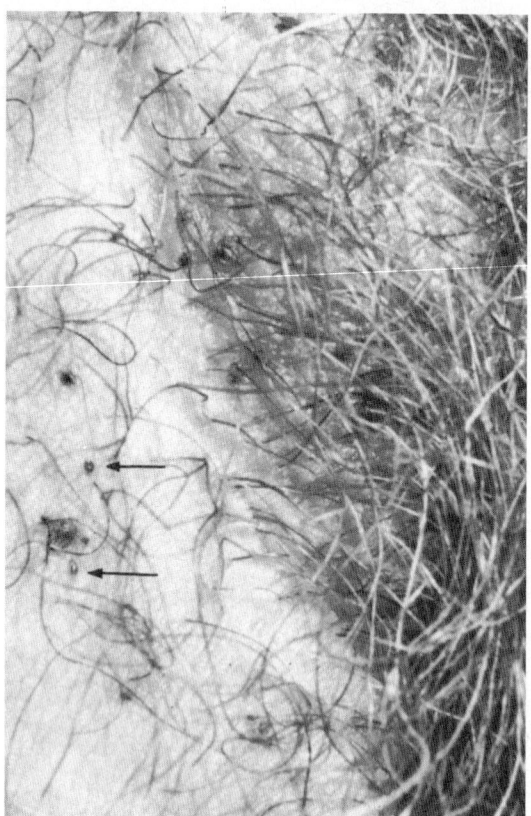

FIGURE 22-6 Crab lice and nits of pediculosis pubis *(arrows.)* (From Kaufman RH: Miscellaneous vulvar disorders. In Kaufman RH and Faro S, editors: Benign diseases of the vulva and vagina, ed 4, St. Louis, 1994, Mosby–Year Book, Inc.)

The predominant clinical symptom of scabies is severe but intermittent itching. Generally, more intense pruritus occurs at night when the skin is warmer and the mites are more active. Initial symptoms usually present approximately 3 weeks after primary infestation. Scabies may present as papules, vesicles, or burrows. However, the pathognomonic sign of scabies infection is the burrow in the skin. The burrow usually has the appearance of a twisted line on the skin surface, with a small vesicle at one end. Any area of the skin may be infected, with the hands, wrists, breasts, vulva, and buttocks being most commonly involved. A handheld magnifying lens is helpful for examining suspicious areas. Microscopic slides may be made by use of mineral oil and a scratch technique (Figure 22-7). Mites lack lateral claw legs but have two anterior triangular hairy buds. Scabies infections are common in approximately 2% to 4% of women with HIV. Scabies has been termed the *great dermatologic imitator,* and the differential diagnosis includes virtually all dermatologic diseases that cause pruritus.

The treatment of pediculosis pubis or scabies involves an agent that kills both the adult parasite and the eggs. The therapy currently recommended by the CDC for pediculosis pubis involves the use of permethrin (Nix Creme), lindane (Kwell), or pyrethrins with piperonyl butoxide. Per-

methrin is available as a 1% cream rinse. It should be applied to affected areas and washed off after 10 minutes. Lindane 1% is recommended as a shampoo. It should be applied for 4 minutes to the affected area and subsequently thoroughly washed off. An alternative is pyrethrin with piperonyl butoxide applied to the affected area and washed off in 10 minutes. None of the regimens should be applied to the eyelids. Permethrin is more expensive than lindane, and it has less potential for toxicity in the event of inappropriate use. Seizures have been reported when lindane was applied immediately after a bath or in women with extensive dermatitis. Lindane is not recommended for pregnant or lactating women, or for children under age 2. Women should be reevaluated after 7 days if symptoms persist. Retreatment may be necessary if lice are found or if eggs are observed at the hair-skin junction.

The CDC recommendation for scabies is permethrin cream 5% applied to all areas of the body from the neck down and washed off after 8 to 14 hours. Alternate regimens include lindane 1% 1 oz. of lotion or 30 g of cream applied thinly to all areas of the body from the neck down and thoroughly washed off after 8 hours. The second alternative is sulfur 6% precipitated in ointment applied thinly to all areas nightly for 3 nights. Previous applications should be washed off before new applications are applied, and the patient should thoroughly wash off 24 hours after the last application. Resistance to lindane has been reported in some parts of the United States. Patients with scabies have intense pruritus that may persist for many days following effective therapy. An antihistamine will help to alleviate this symptom. Similar to pediculosis pubis, women should be examined 1 week following initial therapy and retreated with an alternative regimen if live mites are observed.

To avoid reinfection by either pediculosis pubis or scabies, treatment should be prescribed for sexual contacts within the previous 6 weeks and other close household contacts. Those individuals with close physical contact should be treated at the same time as the infected woman whether or not they have symptoms. Obviously, clothing and bedding should be decontaminated. Most importantly, women and physicians alike should not confuse the 1% cream rinse of permethrin dosage recommended for pubic lice with the permethrin cream 5% being recommended for scabies.

Ivermectin (single low dose of 200 ug/kg or 0.8% topical solution) is a new therapeutic treatment for scabies. Randomized clinical trials comparing ivermectin and currently recommended therapies are just beginning to be published.

Molluscum Contagiosum

Molluscum contagiosum in adults is an asymptomatic viral disease primarily of the vulvar skin. In contrast, molluscum contagiosum in children may present over the entire body. Molluscum contagiosum is a common generalized skin disease in adults with immunodeficiency, especially

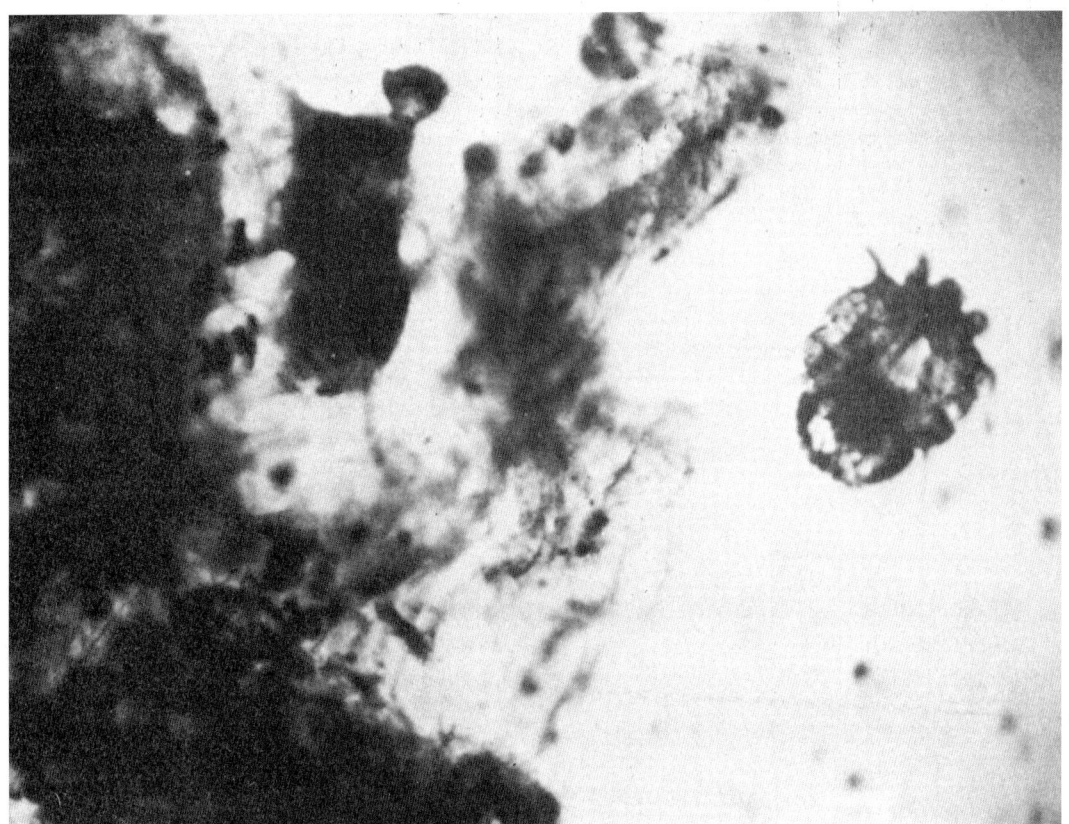

FIGURE 22-7 Skin scrapings of unexcoriated papules fortuitously disclose adults, larvae, eggs, and fecal pellets, any of which would be diagnostic of scabies. (From Orkin M and Howard IM: Scabies. In Holmes KK, Mårdh PA, Sparling PF, et al, editors: Sexually transmitted diseases, New York, 1984, McGraw-Hill Book Co.)

HIV infection. This benign skin disease is caused by the poxvirus and is spread by close contact. Poxvirus does not grow on mucous membranes. The pox virus cannot be grown in culture other than human skin as its host. In the vulvar region, the lesions of molluscum contagiosum and condyloma acuminata often coexist, which makes identification of the gross lesions a challenge. The characteristic skin lesion of molluscum contagiosum is an umbilicated papule. Unlike most sexually transmitted diseases, poxvirus is only mildly contagious. The disease is also acquired via nonsexual contact. The prevalence of the disease has increased rapidly over the past 20 years. The incubation period is 2 to 7 weeks. Many of the skin lesions result from autoinoculation. When the umbilicated papules are secondarily infected they resemble furuncles.

The small nodules or domed papules of molluscum contagiosum are usually 1 to 5 mm in diameter (Figure 22-8). A descriptive name for the small nodule is the "water wart." Close inspection reveals that many of the more mature nodules have an umbilicated center. Characteristically, an infected woman will have 1 to 20 solitary lesions randomly distributed over the vulvar skin. A crop of new nodules will persist from several months to years. If the diagnosis cannot be made by simple inspection, the white, waxy material from inside the nodule should be

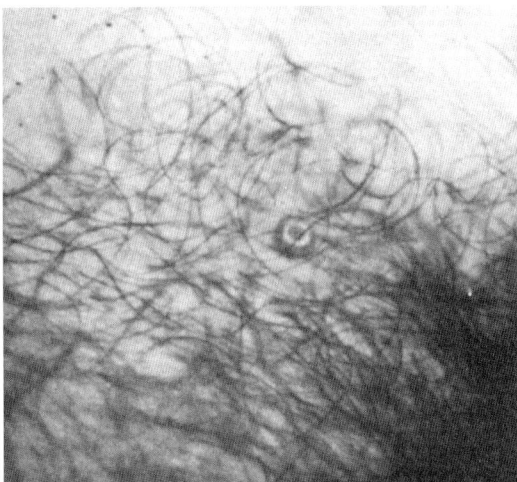

FIGURE 22-8 Papule of molluscum contagiosum with umbilicated center. (From Brown ST: Molluscum contagiosum. In Holmes KK, Mårdh PA, Sparling PF, et al, editors: Sexually transmitted diseases, New York, 1984, McGraw-Hill Book Co.)

expressed on a microscopic slide. The finding of intracytoplasmic molluscum bodies with Wright's or Giemsa stain confirms the diagnosis (Figure 22-9). The major complication of molluscum contagiosum is bacterial superinfection.

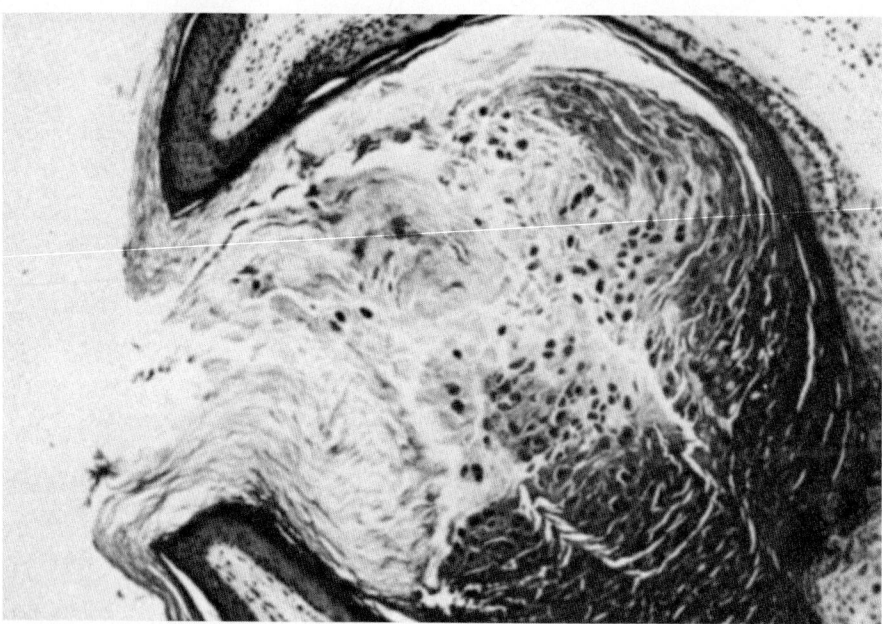

FIGURE 22-9 Papule of molluscum contagiosum with plug of acanthotic and hyperkeratolytic epidermis containing numerous intracytoplasmic inclusions opening to the surface through an apical hole. (H&E stain; ×75.) (From Brown ST: Molluscum contagiosum. In Holmes KK, Mårdh PA, Sparling PF, et al, editors: Sexually transmitted diseases, New York, 1984, McGraw-Hill Book Co.)

Molluscum contagiosum is usually a self-limiting infection; however, treatment of individual papules will decrease transmission and autoinoculation of the virus. Treatment of individual papules is initiated with injection of a local anesthetic with a small subdermal wheal of 1% lidocaine (Xylocaine). The caseous material is then evacuated and the nodule excised with a sharp dermal curet. The base of the papule is subsequently chemically treated with either ferric subsulfate (Monsel's solution) or 85% trichloroacetic acid. An alternative chemical method abrades smaller lesions using tincture of iodine on the end of a pointed orange stick. As an alternative the base of the papule may be treated with cryosurgery or electrocautery. In the future molluscum contagiosum may be treated by local cytokine stimulators and topical antiviral agents.

Condyloma Acuminatum

Condyloma acuminatum is a sexually transmitted viral disease of the vulva, vagina, rectum, and cervix caused by the human papillomavirus (HPV). It is frequently discovered in women concurrently with other sexually transmitted diseases. Synonyms for vulvar condylomata acuminata include genital, venereal, or anogenital warts. In the past few years this disease has reached epidemic levels. HPV is the most common viral sexually transmitted disease (Figure 22-10). It presents as a clinically recognizable macroscopic lesion in 30% of infected women and as an asymptomatic, unrecognized subclinical infection in the remaining 70%. Recent advances in DNA hybridization have demonstrated that the majority of HPV infections are subclinical. Thus the prevalence of the disease depends

on the sophistication of the technique used to diagnose subclinical infection, such as cytology, colposcopy, or molecular probes of biopsy material. It is estimated that in the past 20 to 25 years the number of infected individuals has increased approximately 700%. The prevalence of HPV varies widely depending on the population studied. However, it is as high as 50% in sexually active teenagers with multiple partners. The increasing incidence and the awareness of the relationship between HPV infection and early lower genital tract intraepithelial neoplasia and invasive squamous cell carcinoma have been the stimuli for expanding research efforts into this complex group of viruses.

More than 70 subtypes of HPV, which differ from one another in their individual genomes, have been identified. At least 25 different subtypes of HPV have been involved in genital infection. Of the most common HPV subtypes, numbers 16 and 18 are high risk to be associated with aneuploid, premalignant, or malignant lesions of the female genital tract. Types 6 and 11 are more commonly associated with benign, euploid lesions (Table 22-3). Women may be infected simultaneously with more than one HPV type. Sexual intercourse is the usual method of transmitting genital HPV infection. Autoinoculation definitely occurs because HPV DNA has been demonstrated on the fingers of women with genital warts suggesting the possibility of this secondary means of inoculation. The virus can be shed from both macroscopic and microscopic lesions. It is highly contagious, with 25% to 65% of sexual partners developing the infection. Oriel discovered that 60% of adults develop the disease following intercourse with a partner who was actively shedding the virus.

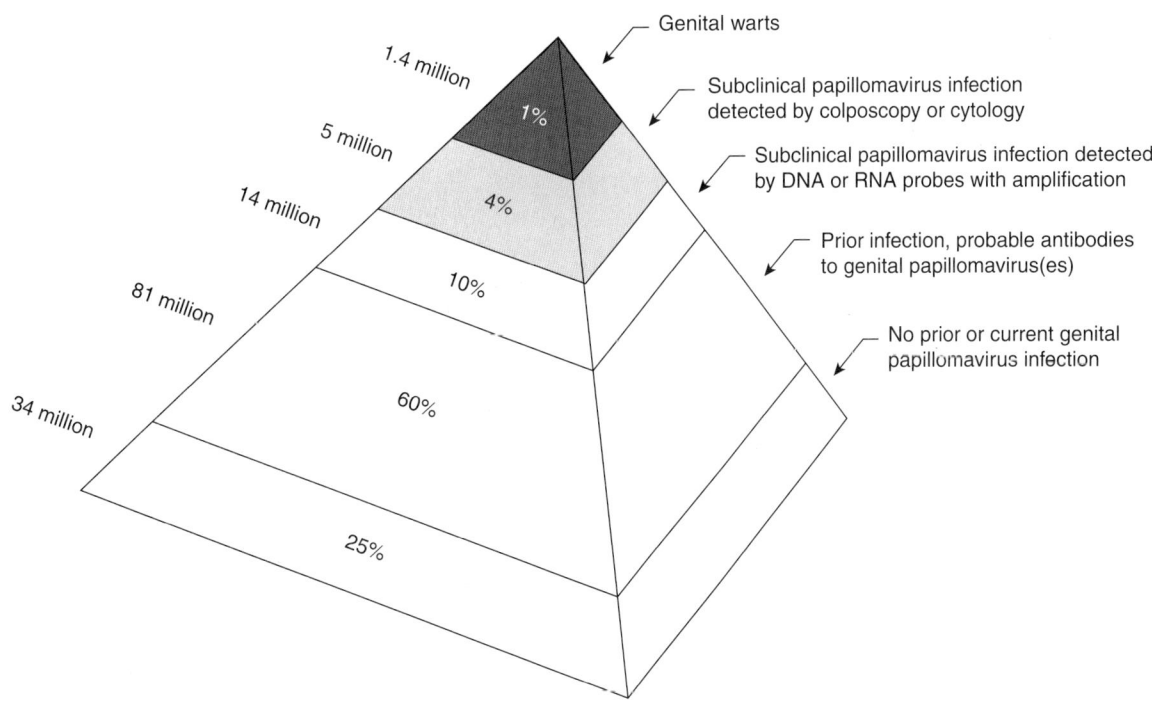

1.4 million — Genital warts

5 million — Subclinical papillomavirus infection detected by colposcopy or cytology

14 million — Subclinical papillomavirus infection detected by DNA or RNA probes with amplification

81 million — Prior infection, probable antibodies to genital papillomavirus(es)

34 million — No prior or current genital papillomavirus infection

1%
4%
10%
60%
25%

FIGURE 22-10 Estimated prevalence of genital HPV infection among sexually active men and women 15 to 49 years of age in the United States. (From Koutsky LA and Kiviat NB: Genital human papillomavirus. In Holmes KK, Sparling F, Mårdh PA, et al, editors: Sexually transmitted diseases, New York, 1999, McGraw Hill.)

TABLE 22-3
HPV Types of Relative Cancer Risk

HPV Type	Cancer Risk*
6/11, 42–44	Low to none
31, 33, 35, 39, 51, 52, 53, 55, 58, 59, 63, 66, 68	Intermediate
16/18, 45, 56	High

From Ferenczy A: Am J Obstet Gynecol 172:1331, 1995.
*Cervical cancer.

Unlike most sexually transmitted diseases, studies have demonstrated no benefit in the use of condoms to prevent transmission of HPV. The average incubation period is 3 months, with a wide range of 1 to 8 months. As with other sexually transmitted diseases, peak incidence occurs between the ages of 15 and 25 years.

Dermatologically, there are four morphologic types of genital warts: cauliflower-shaped condyloma acuminata, smooth papular (1 to 4 mm papules), keratotic (resembling a seborrheic keratosis), and flat. In the majority of women, the diagnosis of overt condyloma acuminatum can be made by direct inspection. Condyloma acuminata–type warts tend to occur primarily on moist surfaces. Indications to perform a biopsy include the rare situations when lesions do not respond to standard therapy; the condition accelerates during therapy; the woman is immunocompromised; or when growths are pigmented, indurated, fixed, or ulcerated. Type-specific HPV nucleic acid tests are not indicated, nor are they of benefit in the diagnosis or management of visible genital warts. Pedunculated warts are friable and tend to bleed following minor trauma. Initial infections usually begin in the vestibule and adjacent areas of the labia. However, adjacent, moist epithelium may be involved with condyloma, including the vagina, cervix, urethra, bladder, and rectum (Table 22-4). Initial lesions are pedunculated, soft papules approximately 2 to 3 mm in diameter and 10 to 20 mm long. They may occur as a single papule or in clusters. The infection progresses by means of autoinoculation. As adjacent lesions coalesce, many different presentations may evolve (Figure 22-11). Lesions vary from pinhead-sized papules to large cauliflower-like masses that may grow to several centimeters in diameter. Uncomplicated condylomata acuminata are usually asymptomatic. Depending on size and location, some warts are symptomatic producing pain, itching, tendency to bleed when friable, and an odor when secondarily infected. Condylomata in the cervix tend to be flat and sometimes bleed on contact. The presence of condylomata of the cervix, especially subclinical disease, is generally discovered by colposcopic examination. Perianal warts occur in approximately 20% of women with condyloma acuminatum. Subclinical HPV infection of the cervix, vagina, or vulva may be discovered by applying 3% to 5% acetic acid to the epithelium. Often, HPV-infected cells appear shiny white in color, with the area of infection having irregular borders and sometimes satellite lesions. However, application of acetic acid is not a specific test for HPV infection. Thus, in a low-risk population, many false positives will be encountered if one uses this test for screening. Vaginal condylomata are identified in approximately one of three women with vulvar disease. Subclinical infection is often discovered by routine cytology, with koilocytosis (cells with perinuclear halos) being the classic

finding. If the pap smear demonstrates nuclear atypia, delayed maturation, hyperkeratosis, parakeratosis, and koilocytosis, there is a strong indication that HPV infection is present. In sophisticated DNA studies, 10% of women with normal smears have HPV identified, while greater than 90% of abnormal cytologic smears are positive for HPV DNA. Common benign skin lesions to consider in the differential diagnosis of condyloma acuminata are micropapillomatosis labialis, seborrheic keratosis, nevi, and other STDs such as condyloma lata and molluscum contagiosum and neoplasms such as giant condyloma or bowenoid papulosis, or squamous cell carcinoma. Research efforts are progressing toward the development of a safe vaccine.

Several conditions are known to predispose women to infection with HPV. They include immunosuppression, diabetes, pregnancy, and local trauma. Often, preexisting vulvovaginitis has provided the moist, excoriated skin on which the HPV colonizes. The vulvovaginitis should be treated as part of the therapeutic plan for condyloma acuminatum.

The management of the individual woman depends on the location, size, and extent of the condyloma and whether the woman is pregnant. Most clinicians attempt to treat the patient until the macroscopic lesions disappear. The most important priority is to remove symptomatic

---

TABLE 22-4
Anatomic Distribution of Anogenital HPV Infections* in Female Patients

Site	Percentage†
Cervix	70
Vulva	25
Vagina	10
Anus	20

From Ferenczy A: Am J Obstet Gynecol 172:1331, 1995.

*Including subclinical lesions.

†Total exceeds 100% because of the multicentric distribution of HPV infection.

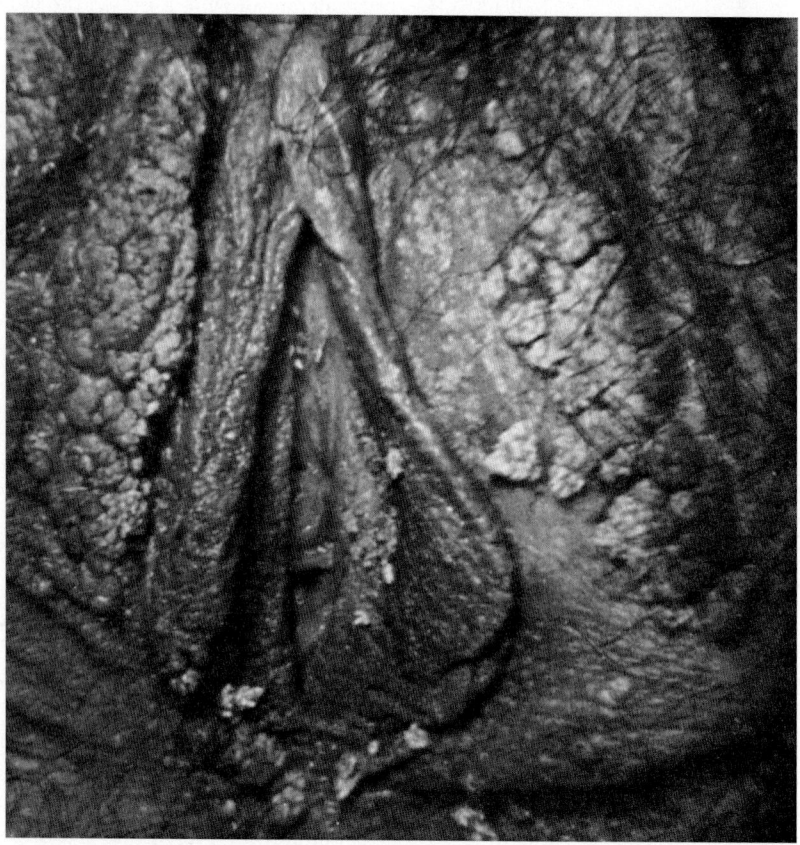

FIGURE 22-11   Condyloma acuminatum. Often small, younger lesions are present with larger, older lesions. (From Friedrich EG: Vulvar disease, ed 2, Philadelphia, 1983, WB Saunders Co.)

growths. No present therapy of HPV eliminates subclinical infection from the surrounding epithelium. Untreated condyloma usually resolve. However, some remain unchanged and some increase in size. There is no evidence that treatment changes infectivity or the natural history of the disease. Serial HPV DNA testing has delineated the natural history of HPV. Almost all low-risk HPV infections and two thirds of high-risk HPV infections are eradicated over a 24-month period. There is a wide range of therapeutic choices, including chemical, cautery, and immunologic therapy. The Centers for Disease Control recommended treatments for external genital warts are subdivided into patient-applied therapies and provider-administrated therapies (box this page). None of the various treatment regimens is more effective than other acceptable treatments. However, warts located on moist surfaces and in intertriginous areas respond faster to topical treatment than do warts on drier surfaces. Approximately two thirds of women notice moderate burning and pain in the areas that are being treated. Data from randomized clinical trials is presented in Table 22-5. Complications rarely occur unless the treatment is overzealous, which results in ulcerated or infected areas of vulvar skin.

Another chemical alternative is topical 5-fluorouracil/epinephrine/bovine collagen gel. The preparation is injected directly into the base of the wart. This therapy requires frequent visits and the lack of superior efficacy makes it difficult to justify its routine use.

Lesions larger than 2 to 3 cm are best treated by cryotherapy, electrocautery, or laser therapy. It is sometimes best to surgically shave the condyloma and then apply thermal injury to the virus in the base of the lesion. The woman should be advised that changes in skin pigmentation are common following ablative therapy.

To date, effective treatment of condyloma acuminatum with systemic immunotherapy by itself has been disappointing. Interferon, because of its antiviral and antiproliferative properties, was postulated to be an ideal drug to treat HPV infection. Regretfully, interferons, when given parenterally, may result in severe systemic symptoms similar to a viral illness in some women. Interferon treatment of HPV has been accomplished by topical creams and direct injection into the condylomata. Local application exerts antiviral activity by stimulating a focal immune response.

Recurrences usually present within 3 months of success-

External Genital Warts

Recommended Treatments

Patient-Applied:
Podofilox 0.5% solution or gel. Patients may apply podofilox solution with a cotton swab, or podofilox gel with a finger, to visible genital warts twice a day for 3 days, followed by 4 days of no therapy. This cycle may be repeated as necessary for a total of four cycles. The total wart area treated should not exceed 10 cm^2, and a total volume of podofilox should not exceed 0.5 ml per day. If possible, the health care provider should apply the initial treatment to demonstrate the proper application technique and identify which warts should be treated. *The safety of podofilox during pregnancy has not been established.*

OR

Imiquimod 5% cream. Patients should apply imiquimod cream with a finger at bedtime, 3 times a week for as long as 16 weeks. The treatment area should be washed with mild soap and water 6 to 10 hours after the application. Many patients may be clear of warts by 8 to 10 weeks or sooner. *The safety of imiquimod during pregnancy has not been established.*

Provider-Administered:
Cryotherapy with liquid nitrogen or cryoprobe. Repeat applications every 1 to 2 weeks.

OR

Podophyllin resin 10% to 25% in compound tincture of benzoin. A small amount should be applied to each wart and allowed to air dry. To avoid the possibility of complications associated with systemic absorption and toxicity, some experts recommend that application be limited to ≤ 0.5 ml of podophyllin or ≤ 10 cm^2 of warts per session. Some experts suggest that the preparation should be thoroughly washed off 1 to 4 hours after application to reduce local irritation. Repeat weekly if necessary. *The safety of podophyllin during pregnancy has not been established.*

OR

TCA or BCA 80% to 90%. Apply a small amount only to warts and allow to dry, at which time a white "frosting" develops; powder with talc or sodium bicarbonate (i.e., baking soda) to remove unreacted acid if an excess amount is applied. Repeat weekly if necessary.

OR

Surgical removal either by tangential scissor excision, tangential shave excision, curettage, or electrosurgery.

Alternative Treatments

Intralesional interferon,

OR

Laser surgery.

From CDC: MMWR 47:89, 1998.

TABLE 22-5
Clearance and Recurrence Rates with Different Treatment Modalities for External Genital Warts

Treatment	Clearance Rates (%)		Recurrent Rates
	End of Treatment	3 Months or More	
Cryotherapy	63–88	63–92	0–39
Electrocautery/electrotherapy	93–94	78–91	24
Interferon			
Intralesional	19–62	36–62	0–33
Systemic	7–51	18–21	0–23
Topical	6–90	33	6
Laser therapy	27–89	39–86	<7–45
LEEP	≤90	—	—
Podophyllin*	32–79	22–73	11–65
Podophyllotoxin (Podofilox)	42–88	34–77	10–91
Surgical/scissor excision	89–93	36	0–29
Trichloroacetic acid	50–81	70	36
5-fluorouracil	10–71	37	10–13

*Studies using more than one treatment strength have been grouped together.

LEEP = loop electrocautery excision procedure.

From Beutner KR, Wiley DJ: Recurrent external genital warts: A literature review. Papillomavirus Report 8:69-74, 1997; with permission.

From Maw RD: Dermatologic Clinics 16:829, 1998.

TABLE 22-6
Clinical Features of Genital Ulcers

	Syphilis	Herpes	Chancroid	Lymphogranuloma Venereum	Donovanosis
Incubation period	2–4 weeks (1–12 weeks)	2–7 days	1–14 days	3 days–6 weeks	1–4 weeks (up to 6 months)
Primary lesion	Papule	Vesicle	Papule or pustule	Papule, pustule, or vesicle	Papule
Number of lesions	Usually one	Multiple, may coalesce	Usually multiple, may coalesce	Usually one	Variable
Diameter (mm)	5–15	1–2	2–20	2–10	Variable
Edges	Sharply demarcated, elevated, round or oval	Erythematous	Undermined, ragged, irregular	Elevated, round or oval	Elevated, irregular
Depth	Superficial or deep	Superficial	Excavated	Superficial or deep	Elevated
Base	Smooth, nonpurulent	Serous, erythematous	Purulent	Variable	Red and rough ("beefy")
Induration	Firm	None	Soft	Occasionally firm	Firm
Pain	Unusual	Common	Usually very tender	Variable	Uncommon
Lymphadenopathy	Firm, nontender, bilateral	Firm, tender, often bilateral	Tender, may suppurate, usually unilateral	Tender, may suppurate, loculated, usually unilateral	Pseudoadenopathy

From Holmes KK, Mårdh PA, Sparling PF, et al, editors: Sexually transmitted diseases, ed 2, New York, 1990, McGraw-Hill Book Co.

TABLE 22-7
Laboratory Tests for the Diagnosis of Genital Ulcer Adenopathy Syndrome

	Syphilis	Herpes	Chancroid	Lymphogranuloma Venereum	Donovanosis
Microscopy	Dark-field examination	Antigen detection	Gram stain has low sensitivity and specificity	Not available	Giemsa- or Wright-stained tissue smears and sections
Culture	Not available	Cell culture	Sensitive, selective media available	Cell culture	Not available
Serology	RPR/VDRL, FTA-ABS, MHA-TP	Rarely useful (primary herpes)	Experimental	Complement fixation, immunofluorescent antibody tests	Not available

From Holmes KK, Mårdh PA, Sparling PF, et al, editors: Sexually transmitted diseases, ed 2, New York, 1990, McGraw-Hill Book Co.

ful treatment of the initial treatment. In the near future, hopefully a prophylactic HPV vaccine will be successful in providing protection prior to initial sexual activity. An adequate vaccine will depend directly on the identification of a common antigenic epitope against the most common HPV subtypes.

Genital Ulcers

Herpes, granuloma inguinale (donovanosis), lymphogranuloma venereum, chancroid, and syphilis all may present as ulcerations in the genital area. However, their etiologies, disease courses, and treatments are different. Table 22-6 lists some of their major characteristics. Table 22-7 contrasts the major laboratory tests used in the differential diagnosis of genital ulcers. Physicians must always consider the possibility of more than one sexually transmitted disease concurrently infecting an individual.

Genital Herpes

Genital herpes is a recurrent, incurable, sexually transmitted disease that has reached epidemic proportions. Regretfully, there is no cure for this viral disease. Judging by either incidence or prevalence, it is among the most frequently encountered sexually transmitted diseases, with somewhere between 500,000 and 2 million new cases of herpes estimated to occur per year. The prevalence of genital herpes infection is estimated to be between 45 and 60 million individuals in the United States. Tragically, approximately 80% of the individuals are unaware they are infected. Herpes is highly contagious, with 75% of sexual partners of infected individuals contracting the disease. Genital herpes is most frequently transmitted by individuals who are asymptomatic and unaware that they have the infection at the time of transmission. A seroepidemiologic survey of the prevalence of

herpes simplex virus type II infection found a prevalence of 18% in women ages 35 to 50. It has been hypothesized that the ulceration associated with herpes genital infection may facilitate infection with the human immunodeficiency virus.

Corey and Handsfield stress the often misunderstood aspect of genital herpes is that transmission can occur in long-standing monogamous relationships. Similarly, seropositivity for HSV-2 is associated with viral shedding from the reproductive tract even in women with no reported history of genital herpes. Recent evidence suggests that viral shedding from asymptomatic individuals may occur as frequently as 1 in 5 days. Thus some infectious disease specialists consider herpes a persistent rather than a intermittent disease. It is important that the woman understand the natural history of disease with emphasis on probability of recurrent attacks, the effect of antiviral agents, and the risks of neonatal infection.

Recurrent genital herpes is not a debilitating physical disease, yet it may present an overwhelming psychologic burden (Figure 22-12). To the individual patient there is an immense sense of social isolation and a reluctance to initiate a sexual relationship. This can result in a decrease in self-esteem, depression, and, most important, a feeling of loss of control due to the inability to predict the time of the next recurrence. Luby and Klinge and Bierman have excellent reviews of the psychologic fears and anxieties created by herpes and the perception of its being "an incurable disease."

There are two distinct types of herpes simplex virus—type I (HSV-I) and type II (HSV-II). As a broad generalization, HSV-I tends to infect epithelium above the waist, and HSV-II tends to cause ulceration below the waist. However, depending on the series, HSV-I may cause lower genital tract infections between 13% and 40% of the time. From a molecular biologic standpoint the classification of HSV-I and HSV-II is an oversimplification.

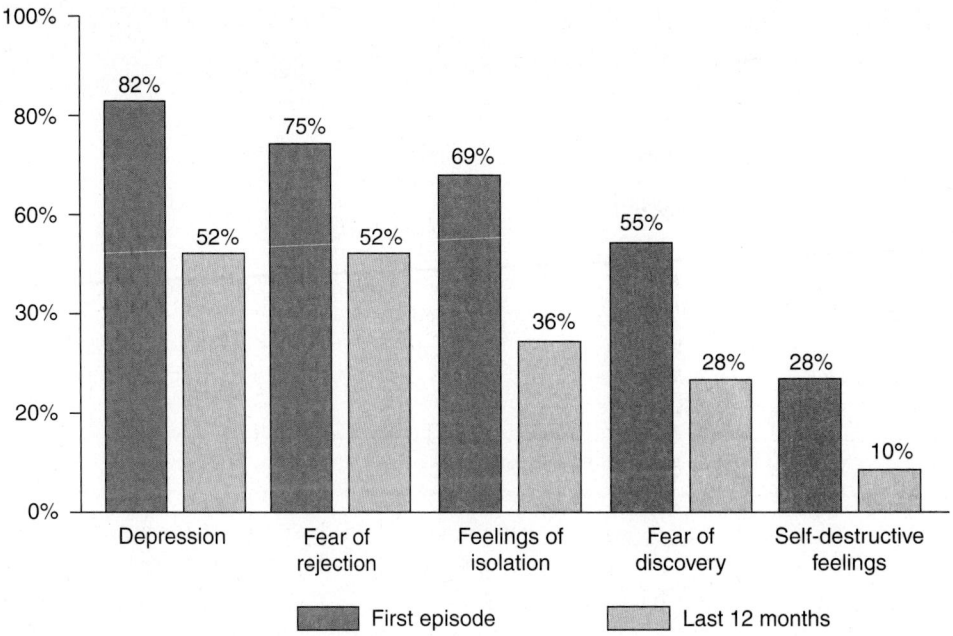

FIGURE 22-12 Frequently reported psychologic sequelae by patients with genital herpes. (From AMA: Genital herpes: a clinician's guide to diagnosis and treatment, part I, AMA Continuing Education Program, Evans, RM and Brakl MJ, editors, 1997.)

Multiple strains of each virus have been discovered. Interestingly, approximately two thirds of newly acquired HSV-1 infections are symptomatic. In contrast only 40% of newly acquired HSV-2 infections are symptomatic. From a clinical standpoint the only important difference is that the frequency of recurrence is 4 times greater following a primary infection with HSV-II in comparison to HSV-I.

The primary infection by herpes is both a local and a systemic disease (Figure 22-13). The majority of initial genital infections occur in women between the ages of 15 and 35. The incubation period is between 3 and 7 days, with an average of 6 days. Often the patient experiences paresthesias of the vulvar skin before papules and subsequent vesicle formation. Usually there are multiple vesicles that become shallow, superficial ulcers over a large area of the vulva. There is often simultaneous involvement of the vagina and cervix (Figure 22-14). Patients experience multiple crops of ulcers for 2 to 6 weeks. Often the ulcers coalesce; however, the ulcers heal spontaneously without scarring. Viral shedding may occur for 2 to 3 weeks after vulvar lesions appear. During primary infections, positive cultures for herpesvirus may be obtained from the cervix in 75% of women and from the urine in 50% of women The majority of symptomatic women have severe vulvar pain, tenderness, and inguinal adenopathy. Nevertheless, subclinical primary herpes infection is common. Regional lymphadenopathy usually develops during primary genital infections.

Systemic symptoms, including general malaise and fever, are experienced by 70% of women during the primary infection. Rarely there is central nervous system infection, with the reported mortality from herpes encephalitis being approximately 50%. Primary infections of the urethra and bladder may result in acute urinary retention, necessitating catheterization. The symptoms of vulvar pain, pruritus, and discharge peak between days 7 and 11 of the primary infection. The average woman experiences severe symptoms for approximately 14 days. Approximately 10% of women with primary infection have symptoms severe enough to require hospitalization. Indications for hospitalization include severe headache, central nervous system involvement, extreme pain, difficulty in walking, and severe pain on urination or acute urinary retention. Occasionally a primary pelvic infection is subclinical.

Recurrent genital herpes is a local disease, and the symptoms are much less severe than the primary outbreak. Many women develop asymptomatic recurrences. In 50% of women the first recurrence occurs within 6 months of the initial infection. Corey et al. estimates that if a woman's initial genital infection was HSV-II she has an approximately 80% chance of having a recurrence within 12 months. Women whose primary HSV-II infection was severe have recurrences approximately twice as often, with a shorter time to recurrence intervals compared with women with milder initial episodes of the disease. On the average a woman will have four recurrences during the first year. In contrast, if the initial pelvic

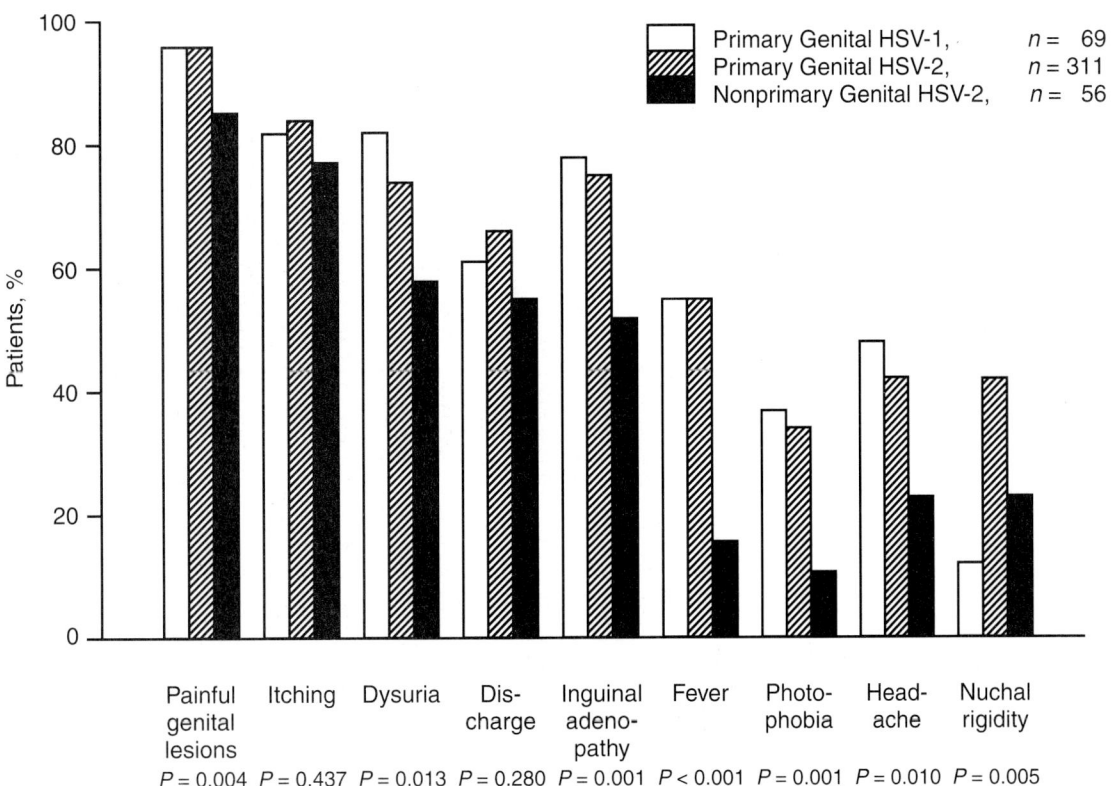

FIGURE 22-13 Frequency of clinical signs and symptoms of first-episode genital herpes by viral type and evidence of previous herpes simplex virus type 1 (HSV-1) exposure. *P* values are based on chi square differences among the three groups. (From Benedetti J, Corey L, and Ashley R: Ann Intern Med 121:847, 1994.)

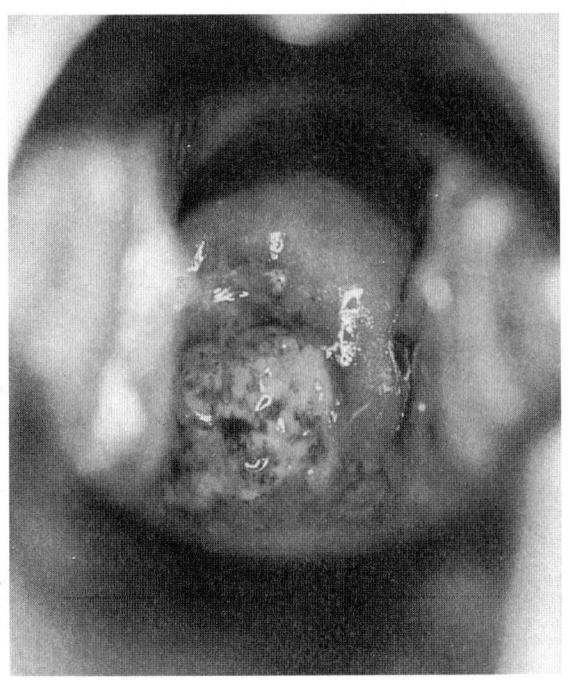

FIGURE 22-14 Primary herpes involving cervix. Necrotic exophytic mass is seen on posterior lip. This was clinically thought to be invasive carcinoma. Herpes simplex virus culture was positive. Lesion spontaneously disappeared. (From Kaufman RH and Faro S: Clin Obstet Gynecol 28:154, 1985.)

infection was HSV-I, there is a 55% chance of a recurrence within 1 year, with the average rate of recurrence slightly less than one episode. There is a general clinical opinion that recurrences are frequently related to the onset of a menstrual period or emotional stress. To generalize, most clinical manifestations of recurrent infection are half as severe as those of primary infections. That is, vulvar involvement is usually unilateral, recurrent attacks last an average of 7 days, and viral shedding occurs for approximately 5 days. The ability to successfully culture herpesvirus from the cervix during that period varies from 20% to 60%, depending on the study cited. Recurrent herpetic ulcers are small—1 to 5 mm in diameter (Figure 22-15). A common feature of recurrence is a prodromal phase of sacroneuralgia, vulvar burning, tenderness, and pruritus for a few hours to 5 days before vesicle formation. The probability and frequency of recurrence of herpes is related to the HSV serotype. Extragenital sites of recurrent infection are common.

The herpesvirus resides in a latent phase in the dorsal root ganglia of S-2, S-3, and S-4. Corey et al. reviewed two hypotheses regarding the etiology of recurrent attacks. The "ganglion trigger theory" proposes a constant viral replication in the privileged immune site of the dorsal root ganglia.

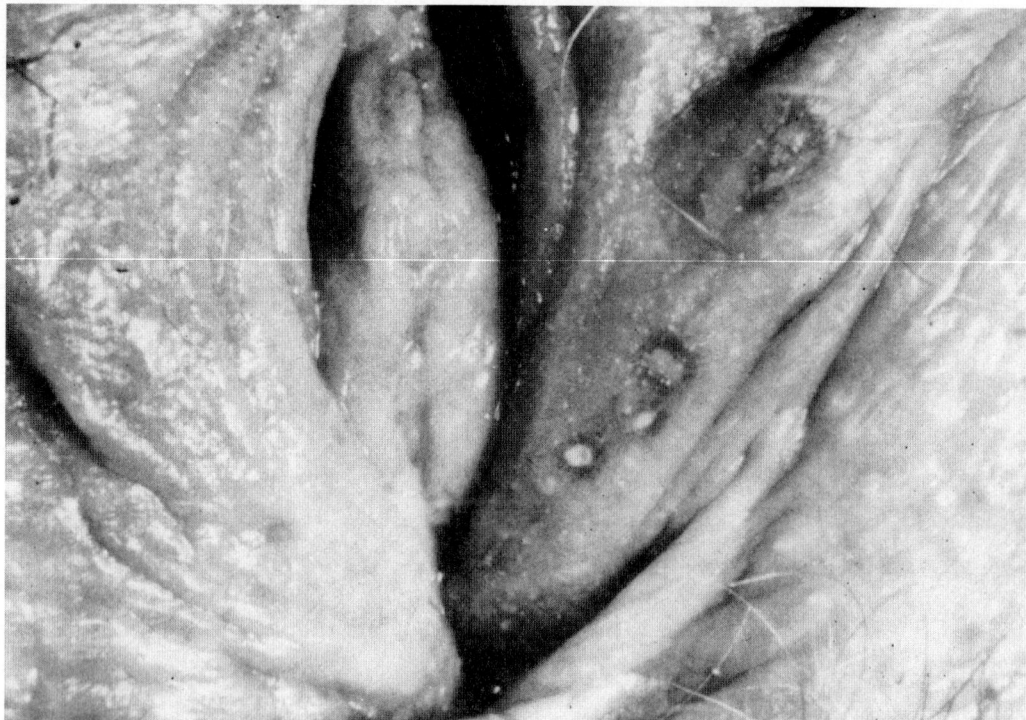

FIGURE 22-15 Recurrent herpes genitalis. Superficial ulcers are noted following rupture of vesicles. (From Kaufman RH and Faro S: Clin Obstet Gynecol 28:156, 1985.)

Unknown stimuli, possibly hormonal, trigger the release of virus, which travels in a retrograde fashion via the peripheral nerves to the female genital organs. The alternate "skin trigger theory" proposes a regular production and retrograde flow of virus from the nerve ganglion down the sensory axon. Normally, local immunity inactivates the virus and recurrence results from a local immunologic defect.

The clinical diagnosis of genital herpes usually can be made by simple clinical inspection. Women come to the physician when they develop symptoms from vulvar ulcers. Herpetic ulcers are painful when touched with a cotton-tipped applicator, whereas the ulcers of syphilis are painless. Of the laboratory tests, viral cultures of the lesions are the most accurate in confirming the diagnosis. The estimated failure rate (false negative) for a culture of the herpesvirus from a recognized lesion is between 10% and 20%. Most herpesvirus cultures will become positive within 2 to 4 days of inoculation. Rapid direct fluorescent antibody tests or cytologic studies are less reliable than viral cultures because approximately one in four are false negatives. The sensitivity and specificity of the ELISA test is competitive with any other detection technique in populations with a high prevalence of herpetic infection. The most accurate and newest technique to identify herpesvirus is the polymerase chain reaction test. Serologic tests are only helpful in determining whether a patient has been infected in the past with herpesvirus. Western blot assay for antibodies to herpes is the most specific method to diagnosis recurrent herpes, as well as recent unrecognized or subclinical infection. Obviously, appropriate screening tests for other sexually transmitted diseases should be obtained, as they may coexist with herpes.

If the patient does not require hospitalization, first episodes of genital herpes infections may be treated with oral medication. Three antiviral drugs have been proven to provide clinical benefit for women with genital herpes: acyclovir, valacyclovir, and famciclovir. The CDC recommends four different antiviral regimens for the first clinical episode of genital herpes. They are acyclovir 400 mg orally three times a day for 7 to 10 days, or acyclovir 200 mg orally five times a day for 7 to 10 days, famciclovir 250 mg three times a day for 7-10 days, or valacyclovir 1 g orally twice a day for 7-10 days. Oral therapy should be extended beyond 10 days if there is not a complete healing. Women whose first episode involves proctitis or oral infection usually are given higher doses of acyclovir such as 400 mg orally five times a day. Acyclovir significantly reduced the median duration of viral shedding, time to crusting and healing of lesions, and the duration of both constitutional symptoms and local pain as compared with times for control subjects. The clinical course of the disease was shortened approximately 1 week. Treating the woman with oral acyclovir for 7 to 10 days during the primary herpetic infection does not influence viral latency—that is, either the frequency of or time to first recurrence.

Many experts are using higher doses of acyclovir to treat herpetic infections in women with immunodeficiencies, especially HIV.

Topical acyclovir in a 5% ointment is sometimes prescribed for primary episodes. However, because of the possibility of spreading the infection with topical medication, the oral drug is preferred. Topical acyclovir therapy is definitely less effective than therapy with the oral preparation and its use should be discouraged.

The treatment of choice for either severe primary genital herpes requiring hospitalization or herpes genitalis in an immunosuppressed woman is intravenous acyclovir (5 to 10 mg/kg every 8 hours for approximately 5 to 7 days). The drug is given as an infusion over approximately 1 hour. Acyclovir (Zovirax) is an antiviral agent that is a purine nucleoside analogue. The drug is concentrated in cells infected with virus and produces its desired action by the inhibition of viral DNA synthesis. The pharmacology of intravenous acyclovir is similar to that of aminoglycosides, although they do not share similar structures. Care must be taken that the patient has normal renal function. Side effects of intravenous acyclovir include local phlebitis and a transient increase in serum creatinine levels in 15% of cases. The dosage of antiviral drugs for ambulatory HIV-infected women is most controversial. However, it definitely has been demonstrated that immunocompromised women benefit from an increased dosage of antiviral drugs. Resistance of the herpes simplex viral strain to acyclovir should be suspected if lesions persist in women with HIV receiving acyclovir. Alternative antiviral therapy should be given by an expert in the field because strains resistant to acyclovir usually also are resistant to valacyclovir and famciclovir.

The major concerns of women with recurrent genital herpes are the rate of recurrence and possible transmission of the disease to their sexual partners. Women should be instructed to abstain from sexual intercourse from the time of prodromal symptoms or the time that lesions appear until the time that all lesions have completely reepithelialized. Active viral shedding may occur from the time of the prodromal period and does occur in women with ulcers even though the ulcers have crusted over. Episodic oral acyclovir therapy has been shown to be beneficial in reducing the duration of ulcerative lesions and in reducing the time that the virus can be isolated from these lesions. The recommended dose of acyclovir is 400 mg orally three times per day for 5 days (see boxes at right). It is interesting that patient-initiated therapy has been found to be superior to therapy ordered by a physician because patients initiate therapy earlier in the course of their recurrence. The antiviral medication should be started as early as possible during the prodrome and definitely within 24 hours of the appearance of lesions.

Patients with frequent episodes of recurrent genital herpes may be successfully treated with daily prophylactic suppressive oral acyclovir. The primary goals of continu-

---

Recommended Regimens for Episodic Recurrent HSV Infection

Acyclovir 400 mg orally three times a day for 5 days,
OR
Acyclovir 200 mg orally five times a day for 5 days,
OR
Acyclovir 800 mg orally twice a day for 5 days,
OR
Famciclovir 125 mg orally twice a day for 5 days,
OR
Valacyclovir 500 mg orally twice a day for 5 days.

From CDC 1998 Guidelines for Treatment of Sexually Transmitted Diseases, MMWR 47:23, 1997

Recommended Regimens for Daily HSV Suppressive Therapy

Acyclovir 400 mg orally twice a day,
OR
Famciclovir 250 mg orally twice a day,
OR
Valacyclovir 250 mg orally twice a day,
OR
Valacyclovir 500 mg orally once a day,
OR
Valacyclovir 1000 mg orally once a day.

From CDC 1998 Guidelines for Treatment of Sexually Transmitted Diseases, MMWR 47:23, 1997.

---

ous suppressive therapy are to limit the severity and number of recurrences as well as to give the woman a sense of control over her disease. Douglas et al. studied 91 women given 200-mg acyclovir tablets (two to five tablets daily) for 4 months and 47 placebo recipients. The median time to first clinical recurrence was 120 days in the acyclovir group versus 18 days in women receiving the placebo. Alternative studies have used a dosage of 400 mg twice a day with improved patient compliance (see boxes this page). This regimen resulted in a 53% reduction in the number of clinical recurrences and a 71% reduction in viral-positive (by culture) recurrences. After acyclovir had been discontinued, the recurrence rate returned to the same frequency as the pretreatment rate. Mertz et al. have published studies of a chronic daily oral acyclovir regimen for as long as 24 months. The average number of recurrences was 1.8 per year in those subjects taking acyclovir, while the placebo group averaged 11.4 recurrences per year. It is important to emphasize that daily suppressive therapy with acyclovir may reduce, but does not eliminate asymptomatic viral shedding. Studies suggest that all three viral agents are equal in efficacy. However, famciclovir and valacyclovir potentially will have greater patient compliance for prolonged therapy. At the present time, there is not enough data to recommend giving famciclovir or valacyclovir for a period of more than 12 months.

Acyclovir is a drug with relatively minimal toxicity, and recent reports have documented daily use for as long as 6 years helping to establish the long-term safety of the drug. However, the CDC recommends that acyclovir should be discontinued after 12 months of suppressive therapy to determine the subsequent rate of recurrence for each individual woman. Even if herpes is not treated over time, clinical recurrences tend to dramatically decrease in number.

A vaccine would be the logical approach for optimum prevention of herpes. There have been extensive attempts to develop a safe vaccine. During the past 20 years, six different types of genital herpes vaccines have been developed. Presently, several of these are undergoing preliminary clinical trials. Expectations are that the vaccines may protect an individual from developing symptomatic genital herpes and may reduce or prevent latent infection, thus hopefully diminishing the risk of transmission.

Granuloma Inguinale (Donovanosis)

Granuloma inguinale, also known as donovanosis, is a chronic, ulcerative, bacterial infection of the skin and subcutaneous tissue of the vulva. Rarely the vagina and cervix are involved in advanced, untreated cases. Granuloma inguinale is common in tropical climates such as New Guinea and the Caribbean islands, but fewer than 20 cases are reported each year in the United States.

This chronic disease is caused by an intracellular gramnegative, nonmotile, encapsulated rod—*Calymmatobacterium granulomatis*. This bacterium shares common antigens with *Klebsiella* and *Escherichia coli*. It cannot be cultured on standard media, and serologic tests are nonspecific. This disease can be spread both as a sexually transmitted disease and through close, nonsexual contact. However, it is not highly contagious, and chronic exposure is usually necessary to contract the disease. The incubation period is extremely variable—from 1 to 12 weeks. The mildly contagious disease is found in 1% to 52% of sexual partners of women with the disease. However, it is also found in young children and elderly women, who are not sexually active. Thus some experts hypothesize that the disease may be secondary to autoinoculation following trauma to the infected area.

The initial growth of granuloma inguinale is an asymptomatic nodule. The skin over the nodule ulcerates, and the characteristic lesion is a beefy-red ulcer with fresh granulation tissue. The area around the lesions is highly vascular, thus the ulcers bleed easily when touched. Usually there are multiple nodules and, subsequently, multiple ulcers of the vulva. Adjacent areas of ulceration grow and coalesce and, if not treated, will eventually destroy the normal vulvar architecture. The ulcers are painless unless secondarily infected. Adenopathy is not a prominent feature unless there is a superimposed infection. Vulvar edema, especially of the labia, is a common feature of the disease. If untreated, the chronic form of the disease is characterized by scarring and lymphatic obstruction, which produces marked enlargement of the vulva.

In endemic areas the disease is usually diagnosed by its clinical manifestations. The diagnosis is established by identifying Donovan bodies in smears and specimens taken from the ulcers (Figure 22-16). Both the deep aspects of the ulcer crater and the fresh edge of an expanding lesion should be sampled. The pathognomonic Donovan bodies are clusters of dark-staining bacteria with a bipolar (safety pin) appearance found in the cytoplasm of large mononuclear cells (Figure 22-17). Special silver

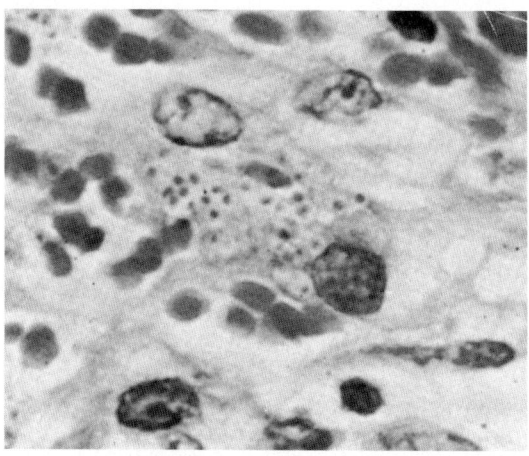

FIGURE 22-16 Donovanosis. Biopsy specimen shows intracytoplasmic Donovan bodies. (H&E stain.) (From Hart G: Donovanosis. In Holmes KK, Mårdh PA, Sparling PF, et al, editors: Sexually transmitted diseases, New York, 1984, McGraw-Hill Book Co.)

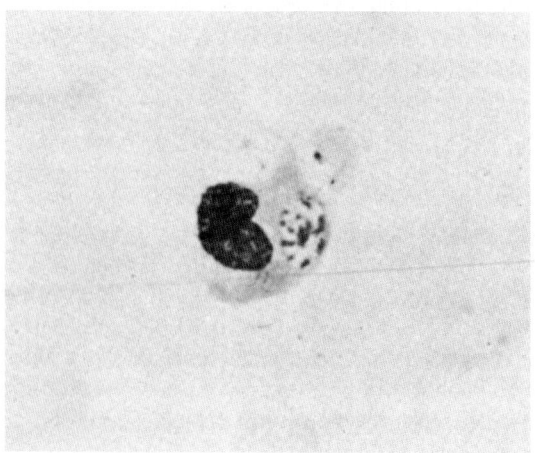

FIGURE 22-17 Donovanosis. Crust preparation from biopsy specimen shows single cell with many intracytoplasmic Donovan bodies. (Giemsa stain.) (From Hart G: Donovanosis. In Holmes KK, Mårdh PA, Sparling PF, et al, editors: Sexually transmitted diseases, New York, 1984, McGraw-Hill Book Co.)

stains highlight the Donovan bodies. However, even a brief period of previous antibiotic therapy may result in an absence of Donovan bodies in women who have granuloma inguinale. The differential diagnosis includes lymphogranuloma venereum, vulvar carcinoma, syphilis, chancroid, genital herpes, amebiasis, and other granulomatous diseases.

Granuloma inguinale may be managed by a wide range of oral broad-spectrum antibiotics. The CDC recommends trimethoprim/sulfamethoxazole one double strength tablet orally twice a day for a minimum of 3 weeks or doxycycline 100 mg orally twice a day for a minimum of 3 weeks. Alternative antibiotic regimens are ciprofloxacin 750 mg orally twice a day for a minimum of 3 weeks or erythromycin base 500 mg orally four times a day for a minimum of 3 weeks. Tetracycline is no longer recommended because many strains of the bacteria have developed resistance. The initial response to antibiotic therapy should be apparent within the first 7 days. However, optimal clinical response usually takes 3 to 5 weeks to ensure that the lesions have healed completely. It is best to continue antibiotics until a complete clinical response is noted with healing of the ulcerative lesions. Alternative antibiotic therapy such as an aminoglycoside has been used in refractory cases. Rarely, medical therapy fails and surgical excision is required. Coinfection with another sexually transmitted pathogen is a distinct possibility. Sex partners of women who have granuloma inguinale should be examined if they have had sexual contact during the 60 days preceding the onset of symptoms.

Lymphogranuloma Venereum

Lymphogranuloma venereum (LGV) is a chronic infection of lymphatic tissue produced by *Chlamydia trachomatis.* It is found most commonly in the tropics. Cases occur infrequently in the United States, with fewer than 150 new cases being reported each year. The majority of cases are reported to occur in men. In most series the ratio of males to females with the disease is approximately 5:1. The vulva is the most frequent site of infection in women, but the urethra, rectum, and cervix may also be involved. Subclinical infection is common. Studies have demonstrated positive complement fixation tests in more than 50% of prostitutes without demonstrable disease. This sexually transmitted disease is produced by serotypes L_1, L_2, and L_3 of *C. trachomatis.* These serotypes are similar to the serotypes that produce trachoma. The incubation period is between 3 and 30 days.

There are three distinct phases of vulvar and perirectal LGV. The primary infection is a shallow, painless ulcer of the vestibule or labia. Occasionally this ulcer is near the urethra or rectum. The ulcer heals rapidly without therapy. The patient usually consults a physician during the secondary phase of the disease, which begins 1 to 4 weeks after the primary infection. The secondary phase is marked by painful adenopathy in the inguinal and perirectal areas. Two thirds of women have unilateral adenopathy, and half have systemic symptoms, including general malaise and fever. When the disease is not treated, the infected nodes become increasingly tender, enlarged, matted together, and adherent to overlying skin, forming bubos (tender lymph nodes). A classic clinical sign of LGV is the double genitocrural fold or "groove sign" (Figure 22-18), a depression between groups of inflamed nodes. The groove sign develops in approximately 20% of women with LGV. Within 7 to 15 days the bubo will rupture spontaneously and form multiple draining sinuses and fistulas. These are classic signs of the tertiary phase of the infection. Extensive tissue destruction of the external genitalia and anorectal region may occur during the tertiary phase. This tissue destruction and secondary extensive scarring and fibrosis may result in elephantiasis, multiple fistulas, and stricture formation of the anal canal and rectum.

Diagnosis is established by culture of pus or aspirate from a tender lymph node. With the recent development of monoclonal antibodies for *Chlamydia,* the diagnosis may be confirmed with this technique using fluid aspirated from an infected node. The complement fixation antibody titer is the most frequently used serum method for diagnosis. Antibody titers greater than 1:64 are indicative of active infection. The antibody test will cross-react with other *Chlamydia* infections. However, mucosal *Chlamydia* infections usually are associated with low

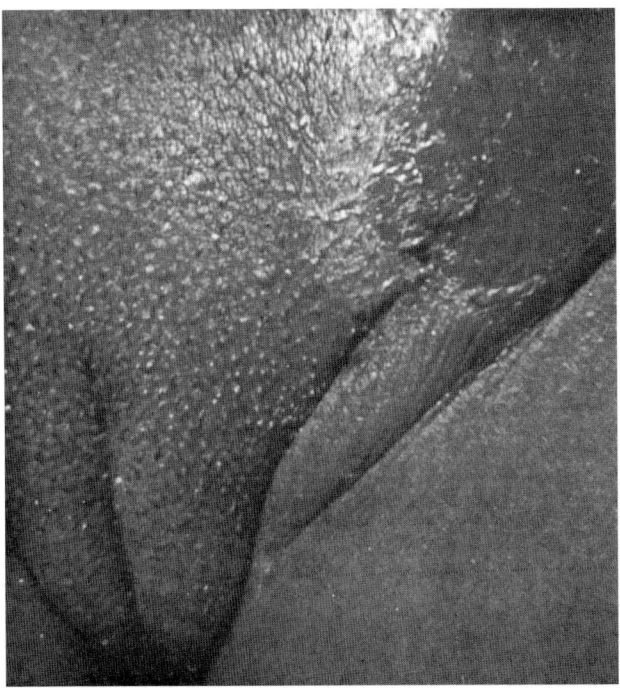

FIGURE 22-18 Lymphogranuloma venereum bubo with "groove" sign. (From Friedrich EG: Vulvar disease, ed 2, Philadelphia, 1983, WB Saunders Co.)

titers. The Frei skin test has been abandoned because of its low sensitivity. The differential diagnosis of LGV includes syphilis, chancroid, granuloma inguinale, bacterial lymphadenitis, vulvar carcinoma, genital herpes, and Hodgkin's disease.

The CDC recommends doxycycline 100 mg bid for at least 21 days as the preferred treatment. The alternative choice for therapy is erythromycin base 500 mg four times daily orally for 21 days. Antibiotic therapy cures the bacterial infection and prevents further tissue destruction. However, fluctuant nodes should be aspirated to prevent sinus formation. Rarely incision and drainage of infected nodes are necessary to alleviate inguinal pain. The late sequelae of the destructive tertiary phase of LGV often require extensive surgical reconstruction. It is important to administer antibiotics during the perioperative period.

Chancroid

Chancroid is a sexually transmitted, acute, ulcerative disease of the vulva. The soft chancre of chancroid is always painful and tender. In comparison, the hard chancre of syphilis is usually asymptomatic. The clinical importance of chancroid is enhanced by recent reports that the genital ulcers of chancroid facilitate the transmission of HIV infection. Chancroid is a common disease in developing countries, but until the early 1980s it was rarely discovered in the United States. Recently there has been a substantial decline in reported cases in the United States, with only 243 reported in 1997. Epidemiologic studies suggest that men and women prostitutes constitute a core transmitter group for genital ulcer disease. The disease is more common in males than females, with the male-to-female ratio varying from 5:1 to 10:1 in most series.

Chancroid is caused by *Haemophilus ducreyi,* a highly contagious, small, gram-negative rod. *H. ducreyi* is a nonmotile, facultative anaerobe. This bacterium on Gram stain exhibits a classic appearance of streptobacillary chains, or what has been described as an extracellular "school of fish." The incubation period is short—usually 3 to 6 days. Tissue trauma and excoriation of the skin must precede initial infection because *H. ducreyi* is unable to penetrate and invade normal skin.

Women with chancroid who consult a physician have solitary or multiple ulcers, most commonly of the vulvar vestibule and rarely of the vagina or cervix. The initial lesion is a small papule. Within 48 to 72 hours the papule evolves into a pustule and subsequently ulcerates. Multiple papules and ulcers may be in different phases of maturation secondary to autoinoculation. The extremely painful ulcers are shallow with a characteristic ragged edge. The ulcers have a dirty, gray, necrotic, foul-smelling exudate, and there is an absence of induration at the base (the soft chancre). Approximately 50% of women develop acutely tender inguinal adenopathy, a bubo, usually within the first 2 weeks of an untreated infection. In most cases the inguinal adenopathy is unilateral, on the same side of the vulva as the preponderance of infection. Nodes that are fluctuant should be treated by needle aspiration to prevent rupture of the abscess or, if greater than 5 cm in diameter, treated by incision and drainage.

The diagnosis is made by Gram stain and culture of purulent material or by aspiration of tender lymph nodes. *H. ducreyi* may be difficult to grow in culture, depending on the experience of the bacteriology laboratory. Sometimes the clinical diagnosis is made in a woman with painful vulvar ulcers after the differential diagnosis of syphilis and herpes simplex infections have been excluded. Tissue biopsy helps to differentiate chancroid from the other common sexually transmitted diseases that produce vulvar ulcers, including genital herpes, syphilis, lymphogranuloma venereum, and donovanosis. A sensitive and specific polymerase chain reaction (PCR) test for *H. ducreyi* recently has been developed.

Because of antibiotic resistance to tetracyclines and sulfonamides, the CDC recommends azithromycin 1 g orally in a single dose or ceftriaxone 250 mg intramuscularly in a single dose, or ciprofloxacin 500 mg orally twice a day for 3 days or erythromycin base 500 mg orally four times a day for 7 days. All four regimens are effective for treatment of chancroid in HIV-infected women. Large ulcers may require 2 to 3 weeks to heal with clinical resolution of lymphadenopathy slower than that of ulcers. Sexual partners should be treated in a similar fashion. *H. ducreyi* is very sensitive to quinolones, but they are contraindicated in pregnancy.

Successful antibiotic therapy results in both symptomatic and objective improvement within 5 to 7 days of initiating therapy. Following therapy, symptomatic improvement in ulcers occurs within 3 days. Objective improvement occurs within 7 days. Bubos respond at a slower rate than do skin ulcers. Approximately 10% of women whose ulcers initially heal have a recurrence at the same site. Women with HIV infection have an increased rate of failure to the standard treatments for chancroid and therefore often require more prolonged therapy. Approximately 20% of patients with chancroid in large urban areas in the United States are concurrently infected with herpes simplex virus, *Treponema palladium,* and/or HIV. Often, *H. ducreyi* is resistant to multiple antibiotics. Therefore, susceptibility testing of bacterial isolates should be performed on patients who do not respond to therapy.

Syphilis

Syphilis is a chronic, complex systemic disease produced by the spirochete *Treponema pallidum.* The infection initially involves mucous membranes. Syphilis remains one of the important sexually transmitted diseases in the United States. The incidence of primary and secondary syphilis in the United States peaked in 1990. The CDC estimates there were 3.2 cases reported per 100,000 people in the United States in 1998. This is the lowest rate since surveillance began in 1941. However, syphilis remains a devastating disease. Early syphilis is a cofactor in the transmission and acquisition of HIV. Epidemiologists speculate that only one out of four new cases of syphilis is reported. Even with mandatory screening, congenital syphilis continues to be a public health problem. The mothers experiencing the tragedy of stillbirth or neonatal death from syphilis usually have not received prenatal care. Syphilis should be included in the differential diagnosis of all genital ulcers and cutaneous rashes of unknown etiology.

Sir William Osler emphasized that syphilis was the great imitator of clinical medicine. He taught that if a physician had mastered all the systemic manifestations of syphilis, he would understand clinical medicine.

T. pallidum is an anaerobic, elongated, tightly wound spirochete. Because of its extreme thinness, it is difficult to detect by light microscopy. Therefore, the presence of spirochetes is diagnosed by use of specially adapted techniques—dark-field microscopy or direct fluorescent antibody tests (Figure 22-19). These organisms have the ability to penetrate either skin or mucous membranes.

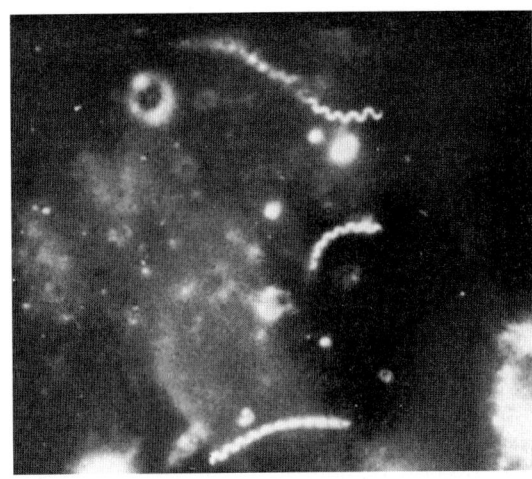

FIGURE 22-19 Dark-field microscopic appearance of *T. pallidum.* (From Larsen SA, McGrew BE, Hunter EF, et al: Syphilis serology and dark field microscopy. In Holmes KK, Mårdh PA, Sparling PF, et al, editors: Sexually transmitted diseases, New York, 1984, McGraw-Hill Book Co.)

TABLE 22-8
Potential Causes of False Positive Serologic Tests for Syphilis

	Infectious Causes	Noninfectious Causes
Reaginic or nontreponemal tests (RPR, VDRL)		
Bacterial	Pneumococcal pneumonia	Pregnancy
	Scarlet fever	Chronic liver disease
	Leprosy	Advanced cancer
	Lymphogranuloma venereum	Intravenous drug use
	Relapsing fever	Multiple myeloma
	Bacterial endocarditis	Advancing age
	Malaria	Connective-tissue disease
	Rickettsial disease	Multiple blood transfusions
	Psittacosis	
	Leptospirosis	
	Chancroid	
	Tuberculosis	
	Mycoplasmal pneumonia	
	Trypanosomiasis	
Viral	Vaccinia (vaccination)	
	Chickenpox	
	HIV	
	Measles	
	Infectious mononucleosis	
	Mumps	
	Viral hepatitis	
Treponemal tests (FTA-ABS, MHA-TP)	Lyme disease	Systemic lupus erythematosus
	Leprosy	
	Malaria	
	Infectious mononucleosis	
	Relapsing fever	
	Leptospirosis	

From Hook EW III and Marra CM: N Engl J Med 326:1060, 1992.

The incubation period is between 10 and 90 days, with the average being 3 weeks. They replicate every 30 to 36 hours, which accounts for the comparatively long incubation period.

Syphilis is a moderately contagious disease. Approximately 3% to 10% of patients contract the disease from a single sexual encounter with an infected partner. Similar studies have documented that 30% of individuals become infected during a 1-month exposure to a sexual partner with primary or secondary syphilis. Patients are contagious during primary, secondary, and probably the first year of latent syphilis.

Serologic tests have been the foundation of screening programs to detect early syphilis, and there are two types of serologic tests—the nonspecific, nontreponemal and the specific, antitreponemal antibody tests. The nonspecific tests such as the VDRL (Venereal Disease Research Laboratories) slide test and the RPR (rapid plasma reagin) card test are inexpensive and easy to perform. They are used as screening tests for the disease and also as an index of response to treatment. These tests evaluate the patient's serum for the presence of reagin antibodies as they react with an antigen from beef heart. Quantitative nontreponemal antibody titers usually correlate with the activity of the disease. Approximately 1% of patients have technical or biologic false positive results with the nonspecific tests. Many conditions produce biologic false positive results, including a recent febrile illness, pregnancy, immunization, chronic active hepatitis, malaria, sarcoidosis, intravenous drug use, HIV infection, advancing age, acute herpes simplex, and autoimmune diseases such as lupus erythematosus or rheumatoid arthritis. Biologic false positive serum tests usually are associated with extremely low titers (<1:8). A false negative result is a possibility, occurring in approximately 1% to 2% of tests. This negative reaction occurs in women in whom there is an excess of anticardiolipin antibody in the serum—termed the *prozone phenomenon.*

If a nonspecific test result is positive, the significance of this result must be confirmed by a specific antitreponemal test. Specific tests are more sensitive; however, occasionally they may produce false-positive results. Most false-positive results occur among women with lupus erythematosus (Table 22-8). The standard for specific tests had been the TPI (*Treponema* immobilization test). It has largely been replaced by the FTA-ABS (fluorescent-labeled *Treponema* antibody absorption) and the MHA-TP (microhemagglutination assay for antibodies to *T. pallidum*). The MHA-TP does not have as high a rate of false-positive results as the FTA-ABS. A woman with a positive reactive treponemal test usually will have this positive reaction for her lifetime regardless of treatment or the activity of the disease.

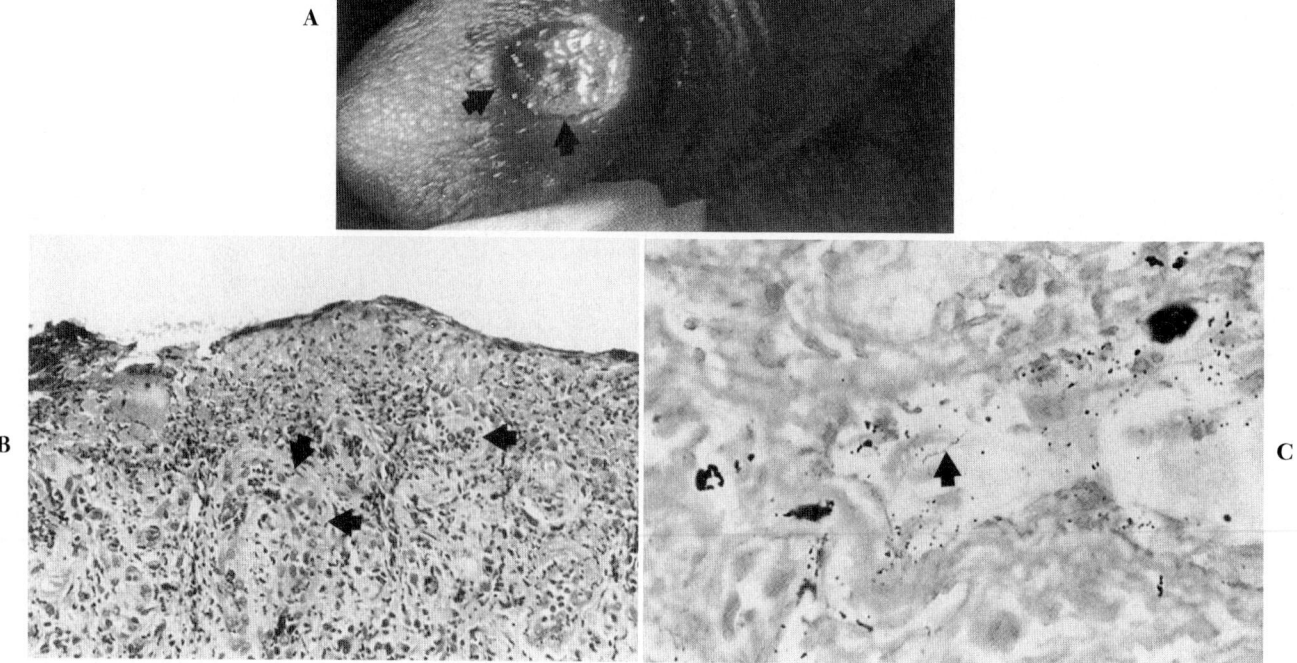

FIGURE 22-20 Primary syphilis. **A** shows a primary chancre of syphilis, which began as a papule, eroded and developed into a painless ulcer (*arrows*) with raised, firm, indurated borders and a clean smooth base. Histologically, it is characterized by superficial ulceration, plasma-cell infiltrates, endarteritis, and endothelial proliferation (**B**, *arrows*). In **C** silver staining reveals a spirochete 6 to 15 m in length with regularly spaced spiral coils (*arrow*). From Wong TY and Mihm MC, Jr: N Engl J Med 331:1492, 1994.)

Clinically, syphilis is divided into primary, secondary, and tertiary stages. The classic finding of primary syphilis is a hard chancre (Figure 22-20). The chancre is a painless ulcer, with an indurated base that develops at the site of entry of the spirochete. The spirochetes of *T. pallidum* usually enter the body only through ulcerations or minute traumatic defects in the mucous membranes or skin. Most often the chancre is solitary, painless, and found on the vulva, vagina, or cervix. The characteristic chancre is a red, round ulcer with firm, well-formed, raised edges, with a nonpurulent clean base and yellow-gray exudate. During the first week of clinical disease, the woman develops regional adenopathy that is nontender and firm. An increase in extragenital primary lesions has been reported, including lesions of the mouth, anal canal, and nipple of the breast. Approximately 5% of chancres occur in extragenital locations. A primary chancre develops approximately 3 weeks after sexual contact with an infected partner. The incubation period for primary syphilis may vary widely, from 10 to 100 days. The ulcer heals spontaneously within 2 to 6 weeks without antibiotic treatment. Confirmation that the ulcer is primary or secondary syphilis depends on identification of *T. pallidum* by dark-field microscopy from wet smears of the ulcer. Special preparations must be made to obtain suitable smears. It is important to clean and abrade the ulcer with gauze before obtaining the serum for the slides. Primary chancres of the cervix or the vagina will often fail to produce symptoms and thus will go undiscovered. Therefore, syphilis is not frequently diagnosed in the primary stage in women.

Serologic tests for syphilis generally become positive 4 to 6 weeks after exposure—thus 1 to 2 weeks after development of the chancre. At the time of dark-field identification of *T. pallidum* from a primary chancre, approximately 70% of women will have a positive serologic test. If the serologic test result remains negative for 3 months, it is unlikely that the ulcer was syphilis.

Secondary syphilis is the result of hematogenous dissemination of the spirochetes and is a systemic disease. If primary syphilis is untreated, approximately 50% of infections progress to secondary syphilis and the other 50% become latent infections. The stages are not exclusive with approximately 25% of women still having a primary chancre when the secondary lesions appear. Secondary syphilis develops between 6 weeks and 6 months (with an average of 9 weeks) after the primary chancre. During an attack of secondary syphilis, which if untreated will last 2 to 6 weeks, there is a multitude of systemic symptoms depending on the major organs involved. The classic rash of secondary syphilis is red macules and papules over the palms of the hands and the soles of the feet (Figure 22-21). Vulvar lesions include mucous patches and condyloma latum associated with painless lymphadenopathy. The vulvar lesions of condyloma latum are large, raised, flattened, grayish-white areas (Figure 22-22). On wet surfaces of the vulva, soft papules that often coalesce form ulcers. These ulcers are larger than herpetic ulcers and are not tender unless secondarily infected. A woman with syphilis is most infectious during the first 1 to 2 years of her disease with decreasing infectivity thereafter.

The latent stage of syphilis follows the secondary stage and varies in duration from 2 to 20 years. During the latency period, a woman has a positive serology without symptoms or signs of her disease. The majority of women who are diagnosed as having syphilis are discovered by positive blood tests during the latent stage of the disease.

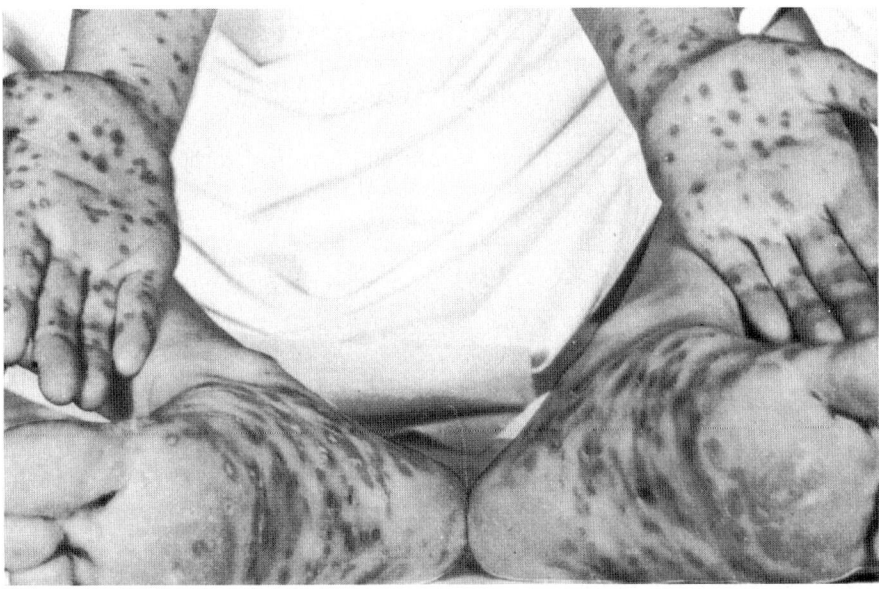

FIGURE 22-21   Rash of secondary syphilis. Red maculopapular lesions involve palms and soles. (From Kissane JM: Bacterial diseases. In Kissane JM, editor: Anderson's pathology, St Louis, 1985, Mosby–Year Book, Inc.)

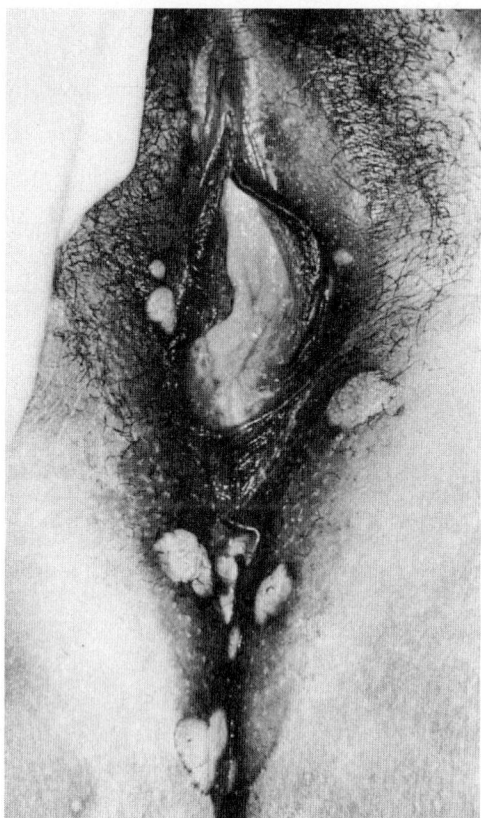

FIGURE 22-22 Multiple lesions of condylomata lata on vulva and perineum. Dark-field microscopic findings were positive. (From Faro S: Sexually transmitted diseases. In Kaufman RH and Faro S, editors: Benign diseases of the vulva and vagina, ed 4, St. Louis, 1994, Mosby–Year Book, Inc.)

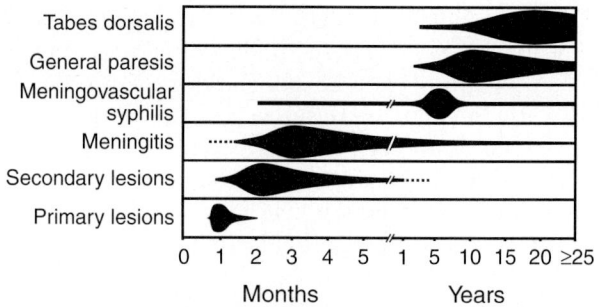

FIGURE 22-23 Approximate time course of the clinical manifestations of early syphilis and neurosyphilis. Shaded areas corresponding to each syndrome represent the approximate proportion of patients with the syndrome specified and do not indicate the proportion of all patients with syphilis who have that syndrome. (From Hook EW III and Marra CM: N Engl J Med 326:1060, 1992.)

All women who have been sexually active with latent syphilis should have a pelvic exam to potentially discover lesions involving the vagina or cervix. Women with latent syphilis should have quantitative nontreponemal serologic tests 6, 12, and 24 months following therapy. During the first 3 to 4 years of the latent phase an individual may experience relapses of secondary syphilis. Women with syphilis in the primary or secondary stages and during the first year of latent syphilis are believed to be infectious.

The tertiary phase of syphilis is devastating in its potentially destructive effects on the central nervous, cardiovascular, and musculoskeletal systems. Tertiary syphilis develops in approximately 33% of patients who are not appropriately treated during the primary, secondary, or latent phases of the disease (Figure 22-23). The manifestations of late syphilis include optic atrophy, tabes dorsalis, generalized paresis, aortic aneurysm, and gummas of the skin and bones. A gumma is similar to a cold abscess with a necrotic center and the obliteration of small vessels by endarteritis.

Parenteral penicillin G is the drug of choice for syphilis. *T. pallidum* is exquisitely sensitive to penicillin. However, because of the slow replication time of the spirochete, blood levels must be maintained for 7 to 14 days. The CDC recommends 2.4 million units of benzathine penicillin G intramuscularly in one dose for early syphilis (primary and secondary syphilis and the first year of latent syphilis). Patients who are allergic to penicillin should receive oral tetracycline 500 mg every 6 hours for 14 days or doxycycline 100 mg orally twice a day for 2 weeks. Standard treatment protocols for syphilis are detailed in the box on the opposite page. Approximately 60% of women develop an acute febrile reaction associated with flulike symptoms such as headache and myalgia within the first 24 hours after parenteral penicillin therapy for early syphilis. This response is termed the "Jarisch-Herxheimer" reaction.

All women with early syphilis should be reexamined clinically and serologically at 6 months and 12 months following therapy. With successful therapy in early syphilis, the titer should decline fourfold in 6 months and become negative within 12 months. Women who have a sustained fourfold increase in nontreponemal test titers have failed treatment or become reinfected. They should be retreated and evaluated for concurrent HIV infection. When women are retreated the recommendation is three weekly injections of benzathine penicillin G 2.4 million units IM. For long-term follow-up the same serologic tests should be ordered. Optimally, the test should be obtained from the same laboratory. The VDRL and RPR are equally valid, but RPR titers tend to be slightly higher than VDRL titers. With successful treatment the VDRL titer will become nonreactive or at most be reactive with a lower titer within 1 year. There is a 1% to 2% chance that the patient will not exhibit a fourfold titer decline, and these cases are considered therapeutic failures. They should be treated once again. Patients with syphilis lasting longer than 1 year should have quantitative VDRL titers for 2 years following therapy because their titers will decline more slowly. A specific test for syphilis, such as the FTA-ABS, remains reactive indefinitely. In summary, all women with a first attack of primary syphilis should have a negative nonspecific serology within 1 year and women treated for secondary syphilis should have a negative serology within 2 years. If they are not, treatment failure, reinfection, and concurrent HIV infection should be investigated.

Centers for Disease Control Recommended Treatment of Syphilis (1998)

Early Syphilis (Primary, Secondary, and Early Latent Syphilis of Less Than 1 Year's Duration)

Recommended Regimen:
Benzathine penicillin G, 2.4 million units intramuscularly, one dose

Alternative Regimen (Penicillin-Allergic Nonpregnant Patients):
Doxycycline 100 mg orally 2 times a day for 2 weeks
   OR
Tetracycline 500 mg orally 4 times a day for 2 weeks

Late Latent Syphilis of More Than 1 Year's Duration, Gummas, and Cardiovascular Syphilis

Recommended Regimen:
Benzathine penicillin G, 7.2 million units total, administered as 3 doses of 2.4 million units intramuscularly at 1-week intervals

Alternative Regimen (Penicillin-Allergic Nonpregnant Patients):
   Doxycycline 100 mg orally 2 times a day for 2 weeks if <1 year; otherwise, for 4 weeks
   OR
   Tetracycline 500 mg orally 4 times a day for 2 weeks if <1 year; otherwise, for 4 weeks

Neurosyphilis

Recommended Regimen:
   Aqueous crystalline penicillin G, 18 to 24 million units daily, administered as 3 to 4 million units intravenously every 4 hours, for 10 to 14 days

Alternative Regimen:
   Procaine penicillin 2.4 million units intramuscularly daily, for 10 to 14 days
   PLUS
   Probenecid 500 mg orally 4 times a day for 10 to 14 days

Syphilis in Pregnancy

Recommended Regimen:
   Penicillin regimen appropriate for stage of syphilis. Some experts recommend additional therapy (e.g., a second dose of benzathine penicillin 2.4 million units intramuscularly) 1 week after the initial dose, for those who have primary, secondary, or early latent syphilis.

Alternative Regimen (Penicillin Allergy):
   Pregnant women with a history of penicillin allergy should be skin tested and desensitized

Syphilis Among HIV-Infected Patients

Primary and Secondary Syphilis
   Recommended benzathine penicillin G 2.4 million units intramuscularly. Some experts recommend additional treatments, such as 3 weekly doses of benzathine penicillin G, as in late syphilis. Penicillin-allergic patients should be desensitized and treated with penicillin

Latent Syphilis (Normal CSF Examination)
   Benzathine penicillin G 7.2 million units as 3 weekly doses of 2.4 million units each

From CDC 1998 Guidelines for Treatment of Sexually Transmitted Diseases, MMWR 47:28, 1997.

Syphilis often involves the central nervous system. The diagnosis is complicated, and there is no established diagnostic test that is a gold standard for neurosyphilis. All women with suspected neurosyphilis should be tested for HIV infection. The diagnosis of neurosyphilis is made on a combination of clinical findings, reactive serologic tests, and abnormalities of cerebrospinal fluid, serology, cell count, or protein. Infection of the central nervous system by spirochetes may occur during any stage of syphilis. Women should undergo a cerebral spinal fluid examination if they develop neurologic or ophthalmologic signs or symptoms, evidence of active tertiary syphilis, treatment failures, and HIV infection with late latent syphilis or syphilis of an unknown duration. For the treatment for neurosyphilis, the CDC recommends aqueous crystalline penicillin G 18 to 24 million units a day, administered as 3 to 4 million units IV every 4 hours for 10 to 14 days. An alternative regimen is procaine penicillin 2.4 million units IM a day, plus probenecid 500 mg orally four times a day, for 10 to 14 days. The duration of both of these regimens for neurosyphilis are shorter than that of the regimen used for late syphilis in the absence of neurosyphilis. Therefore, some experts administer benzathine penicillin, 2.4 million units IM, after completion of either regimen to provide comparable total duration of therapy.

Concurrent HIV infection should be considered in patients with syphilis. It is important for all women with syphilis to be tested for HIV infection. Simultaneous syphilis and HIV infection alters the natural history of syphilis, with earlier involvement of the central nervous system. Women with HIV infection may have a slightly increased rate of treatment failure with currently recommended regimens. Similarly, they may exhibit unusual serologic responses. Most often serologic titers are higher than expected. However, false-negative serologic tests or delayed appearance of seroreactivity has been reported. Nevertheless, the CDC's recommendation for treating early syphilis is the same for women whether or not they are concurrently infected with HIV. Following penicillin treatment for syphilis, women with HIV should be followed with quantitative titers at more frequent intervals, for example 3, 6, 9, 12, and 24 months following therapy.

Sexual partners of women with syphilis in any stage should be evaluated both clinically and serologically. The time intervals used to identify an at-risk sex partner are 3 months plus duration of symptoms for primary syphilis, 3 months plus duration of symptoms for secondary syphilis, and 1 year for early latent syphilis. Individuals who are exposed within the 90 days preceding the diagnosis of primary, secondary, or early latent syphilis in their sexual partners should be treated presumptively because they may be infected even if seronegative.

Two years ago, the complete sequencing of the genome of the *T. pallidum* was reported. Hopefully, further basic science research will result in the development of new diagnostic tests and novel therapies to prevent and/or treat the disease.

Vulvar Irritation Caused by Vaginitis

Anatomic distribution of symptoms occasionally creates a semantic misinterpretation of the clinical reality. This is true for vulvar disease. The first symptom of vaginal infection is often vulvar pruritus, and the first sign of vaginal infection may be secondary erythema and edema of the vulvar skin. Sometimes, self-medication for a vaginal infection may produce irritation of the vulva. Women whose chief complaint is vaginal itching or burning may have symptoms because of irritation of the vestibule and adjacent vulvar epithelium. The sensory nerve endings are more numerous in the vulvar skin than in the vagina. The presence of excessive vaginal fluid is not appreciated until the fluid flows from the vagina onto the vulva.

A semantic compromise is to term most vaginal infections as vulvovaginitis. This is especially true with candidiasis. There is a separate clinical entity of primary cutaneous candidiasis, but it is rare and is most often found in women with diabetes mellitus. The skin involvement of primary candidiasis is most prominent on the labia and the genitocrural folds. In this condition, the vulva appears beefy red, the labia are edematous, and the skin of the vulva has fissures and often small vesicles and pustules.

The differential diagnosis for women with symptoms of vulvovaginitis is complex. Discharge, burning, and pruritus are the common symptoms, and signs of vulvar irritation include erythema and excoriation of the vulvar skin. Dis-

charge may be caused by either a cervical or vaginal infection. Vulvar irritation may be produced by primary or secondary infections, a primary skin irritant, or contact dermatitis. Physiologic fluids such as urine and normal cervical secretions and vaginal fluid may cause maceration of the vulvar skin when the epithelium remains constantly moist, such as in the situation produced by tight-fitting synthetic fabric undergarments, especially panty hose.

The clinical symptoms of vulvovaginitis are usually not helpful in establishing the etiology. A careful history for contact allergens must be obtained. Sometimes vaginal spermicides, soaps, perfumes, and feminine hygiene sprays will cause skin irritation. The cervical and vaginal secretions should be examined under the microscope for infection. The diagnosis of primary vulvar skin infections should be entertained.

First and foremost in alleviating the symptoms of vulvovaginitis is emphasis on keeping the vulvar skin dry. The patient should be encouraged to wear loose-fitting cotton undergarments. Treatment of vaginal infection is important and will be discussed in the next section.

VAGINITIS

Vaginal discharge is the most common symptom in gynecology. Other symptoms associated with vaginal infection include superficial dyspareunia, dysuria, odor, and vulvar burning and pruritus. There are three common infections of the vagina—one produced by a fungus (candidiasis), another by a protozoon *(Trichomonas),* and the third a synergistic bacterial infection (bacterial vaginosis). Relative prevalence differs depending on the population studied. However, in a group of middle-class women in the reproductive range, bacterial vaginosis represents approximately 50% of cases, whereas candidiasis and *Trichomonas* infection each constitute approximately 25% of cases. Vaginal discharge resulting from viral infections such as herpes was discussed earlier in the chapter. Vaginitis in prepubertal and postmenopausal women is discussed in chapters dedicated to gynecologic problems in those age groups (Chapters 12 and 42). Atrophic vaginitis, secondary to low levels of circulating estrogens, predisposes women to secondary infection due to the thin atrophic lining of the vaginal canal.

The vaginal environment has been described as both a dynamic and a delicate ecosystem. The normal vaginal pH is approximately 4.0 in premenopausal women. The maintenance of an optimum pH balance involves a complex interplay of hormonal, microbiologic, and other unknown factors. In reproductive-age women, estrogen stimulates the glycogen content of vaginal epithelial cells. The glycogen is metabolized to lactic acid and other short-chain organic acids, principally by the lactobacilli but also by other vaginal bacteria and enzymes. This interplay maintains the acidic environment of the vagina at a pH of approximately 4.0, which in turn limits the growth of potentially pathogenic bacteria and protozoa.

One of the most helpful diagnostic aids in the differential diagnosis of vaginitis is to measure vaginal acidity with pH indicator paper. A vaginal pH of greater than 5.0 indicates bacterial vaginosis or *Trichomonas* infection or possibly an atrophic vaginal discharge. A vaginal pH of less than 4.5 represents either a physiologic discharge or a fungal infection. Cervical mucus, vaginal fluids produced during sexual excitement, and semen are all of a neutral or basic pH and may temporarily change the normal acidity. Semen has been found to buffer vaginal acidity for 6 to 8 hours following intercourse. Douching has little effect on vaginal pH. Vaginal pH is slightly higher in postmenopausal women than in premenopausal women. Maintenance of a normal vaginal ecosystem depends on an appropriate concentration of *Lactobacillus acidophilus*.

Normal physiologic vaginal discharge consists of cervical and vaginal epithelium, normal bacterial flora, water, electrolytes, and other chemicals. The quantitative concentration of bacterial organisms is 10^8 to 10^9 colonies per milliliter of vaginal fluid. Larsen and Galask, as well as Bartlett and Polk, have published extensive reviews of both qualitative and quantitative studies of normal bacterial flora of the vagina. Bartlett and Polk serially sampled women throughout the same cycle. They discovered that the concentration of anaerobic and aerobic bacteria varied considerably during the menstrual cycle. Qualitatively the number of bacterial species varied from 17 to 29. Anaerobic bacteria were quantitatively the most prevalent—5 times more common than aerobic bacteria.

Lactobacillus, an aerobic gram-positive rod, is found in 62% to 88% of asymptomatic women. Other common aerobic bacteria found in the vagina are diphtheroids, streptococci, *Staphylococcus epidermidis*, and *Gardnerella vaginalis*. The most common gram-negative bacillus is *E. coli*. Anaerobic bacteria have been detected in approximately 80% of women, the most prevalent being *Peptococcus*, *Peptostreptococcus*, and *Bacteroides* species (Table 22-9). *Candida* species and mycoplasmas are also common inhabitants of asymptomatic women.

The clinical diagnosis of the etiology of vaginitis depends on examination of the vaginal secretions under the microscope and measurement of vaginal pH. Nevertheless it is helpful to generalize about the classic characteristics of normal secretions and the three common vaginal infections (Table 22-10).

TABLE 22-9
Bacterial Vaginal Flora among Asymptomatic Women without Vaginitis

Organism	Range of Recovery (%)
Facultative organisms	
Gram-positive rods	
Lactobacilli	50–75
Diphtheroids	40
Gram-positive cocci	
Staphylococcus epidermidis	40–55
Staphylococcus aureus	0–5
Beta-hemolytic streptococci	20
Group D streptococci	35–55
Gram-negative organisms	
Escherichia coli	10–30
Klebsiella sp.	10
Other organisms	2–10
Anaerobic organisms	
Peptococcus sp.	5–65
Peptostreptococcus spp.	25–35
Bacteroides spp.	20–40
Bacteroides fragilis	5–15
Fusobacterium sp.	5–25
Clostridium sp.	5–20
Eubacterium sp.	5–35
Veillonella sp.	10–30

From Eschenbach DA: Clin Obstet Gynecol 26:187, 1983.

TABLE 22-10
Appearance of Vaginal Discharge

	Normal	Bacterial Vaginosis	Trichomoniasis	Candidiasis
Discharge present at introitus	No	Yes	Yes	No
Color	White	Gray	Yellow-gray	White
Viscosity	High	Low	Low	High
Consistency	Floccular	Homogenous	Homogenous	Floccular
Presence in vagina	Dependent portion	Adherent to vaginal walls	Adherent to vaginal walls	Adherent to vaginal walls

From Eschenbach DA: Clin Obstet Gynecol 26:186, 1983.

Normal vaginal secretions are white, floccular or curdy, and odorless. In a woman with a normal or physiologic discharge it is important to note that the vaginal discharge is present only in the dependent portions of the vagina. Pathologic discharges usually involve the anterior and lateral walls of the vagina. If the vaginal discharge is white and curdy, fungal infections are more likely. Gray-white discharges that are thin and usually profuse suggest a differential diagnosis of *Trichomonas* or bacterial vaginosis. Vaginal discharges that have a foul odor are usually caused by either *Trichomonas* or bacterial vaginosis. The offensive odor secondary to necrotic gynecologic tumors of the lower genital tract may be minimized by treating the woman topically for bacterial vaginosis.

During the next few years research will emphasize local changes in substances that afford nonspecific protection from vaginal infection, such as lysozymes, lactoferrin, zinc, fibronectin, and complement. A recent report by Giraldo et al. has demonstrated that the expression of heat shock proteins in the vagina is an early indication of an altered vaginal environment and a marker of susceptibility to the development of symptomatic vaginitis.

Bacterial Vaginosis

Bacterial vaginosis refers to a condition in which high concentrations of anaerobic bacteria predominate in the vaginal flora by replacing the normal lactobacillus. Bacterial vaginosis is the most prevalent cause of vaginitis with a prevalence of approximately 12%. Though it may be a sexually transmitted disease, it is not invariably so. Multiple sexual partners are a risk factor for the development of bacterial vaginosis and some bacteria associated with the syndrome have been cultured from male partners. Conversely, bacterial vaginosis, is common in women who are not sexually active, and most studies have not demonstrated an improvement in cure rate following treatment of the male partner. Histologically there is an absence of inflammation in biopsies of the vagina, thus the term *vaginosis* rather than vaginitis. Bacterial vaginosis has been associated with upper tract infections, including endometritis, pelvic inflammatory disease, postoperative vaginal cuff cellulitis, and multiple complications of infection during pregnancy, such as preterm rupture of the membranes and endomyometritis.

Concepts of the etiology of this disease have changed over the past few years. An associated semantic debate concerning the best descriptive name for the type of vaginitis caused by one or more bacteria has accompanied the changing concepts. Thirty years ago the offending organism was called *Haemophilus* or *Corynebacterium vaginale.* Subsequently a specific species was named after Herman Gardner and called *Gardnerella vaginalis.* The latter is classified as a gram-negative, small bacillus. In practice the organism is a coccobacillus that is gram variable (sometimes gram positive, sometimes gram negative),

depending on the age of the cultures. As more sophisticated culture techniques have been developed, it is apparent that *G. vaginalis* may be recovered from the vaginas of 30% to 40% of asymptomatic women. Similarly, *G. vaginalis* may be cultured from 40% of women who have been successfully treated for bacterial vaginosis.

Holmes and Eschenbach and their colleagues from Seattle proposed that nonspecific vaginitis was a symbiotic and synergistic condition due to many anaerobic bacteria and *Gardnerella*, all contributing to produce the clinical symptoms. They discovered that the prevalence and concentration of *Gardnerella* organisms were increased from 10^4 bacteria per milliliter in asymptomatic women to 10^7 bacteria per milliliter in symptomatic women. Concentrations of anaerobic bacteria increased tenfold in symptomatic women. The name of the infection was changed from nonspecific vaginitis to bacterial vaginosis. Associated with the increase in anaerobic bacteria was a decrease in the concentration of lactobacilli and also the absence or dramatic decrease in the presence of lactobacilli species that produce hydrogen peroxide. To further complicate the picture, several groups have described the association of vaginal *vibrios* in approximately 50% of symptomatic women. These small, curved anaerobic rods are from the *Mobiluncus* group, and most likely they are part of the bacterial synergism that produces the clinical symptoms. In summary, bacterial vaginosis is a condition that results when high concentrations of anaerobic bacteria replace the normal H_2O_2-producing lactobacillus species in the vagina.

Women with bacterial vaginosis have the most uniform spectrum of symptoms of all the types of infectious vaginitis (Table 22-11). The most frequent symptom is an unpleasant vaginal odor, which patients describe as "musty" or "fishy." The odor is often sensed following intercourse, when the alkaline semen results in a release of aromatic amines.

The vaginal discharge associated with bacterial vaginosis is thin and gray-white. The consistency of the discharge is similar to a thin paste made from flour. Speculum examination reveals that the discharge is mildly adherent to the vaginal walls, in contrast to a physiologic discharge, which is discovered in the most dependent areas of the vagina. The vaginal discharge is frothy in approximately 10% of women, and it is rare to have associated pruritus or vulvar irritation.

The diagnosis of bacterial vaginosis is confirmed by a saline wet smear. The classic findings on wet smear are clumps of bacteria and "clue cells," which are vaginal epithelial cells with clusters of bacteria adherent to their external surfaces (Figure 22-24). The bacteria give the clue cells a granular or stippled appearance by obscuring their cellular borders. The percentage of clue cells may vary widely, ranging from 2% to 50% of infected women. The wet smear also demonstrates a comparative lack of inflammatory cells and lactobacilli. Leukocytes are not nearly as frequent as epithelial cells underneath the microscope. If

TABLE 22-11
Major Categories of Vaginitis

	C. albicans	*C. glabrata*	*Gardnerella*	*Trichomonas*
Symptom	Itch	Burn	Odor	Discharge
Mucosal erythema*	+++	+	None	Variable
pH	4–5	4–5	5–6	6–7
Wet smear	Budding filaments	Spores only	Clue cells	Many white blood cell protozoa

From Friedrich EG: Am J Obstet Gynecol 152:248, 1985.

*Degree of severity; +, mild; +++, severe.

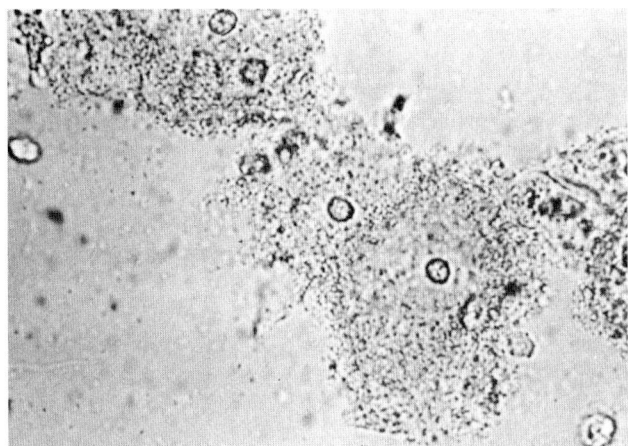

FIGURE 22-24   Vaginal epithelial cells from woman with bacterial vaginosis. These are typical clue cells, being heavily covered by coccobacilli, with loss of distinct cell margins. (×400.) (From Holmes KK: Lower genital tract infections in women: cystitis/urethritis, vulvovaginitis, and cervicitis. In Holmes KK, Mårdh PA, Sparling PF, et al, editors: Sexually transmitted diseases, New York, 1984, McGraw-Hill Book Co.)

inflammatory cells are visualized on wet smear, there is usually associated cervical infection with *N. gonorrhea, C. trachomatis* or *Trichomonas vaginalis*, infection. In experimental studies where vaginal biopsies have been performed in women with bacterial vaginosis, there is no histologic evidence of vaginal inflammation.

In summary, the Seattle group has established four criteria for the diagnosis of bacterial vaginosis: (1) a homogeneous vaginal discharge is present; (2) the vaginal discharge has a pH equal to or greater than 4.5; (3) the vaginal discharge has an aminelike odor when mixed with potassium hydroxide; and (4) a wet smear of the vaginal discharge demonstrates clue cells greater in number than 20% of the number of the vaginal epithelial cells. For the clinician three of the four criteria is sufficient for a presumptive diagnosis. Ironically, 50% of women who have three of the four clinical criteria for bacterial vaginosis are asymptomatic. If readily available, a Gram stain of vaginal secretion is an excellent diagnostic method. There are subtle differences in the prevalence of bacterial vaginosis depending whether clinical criteria or Gram stain is used as the gold standard for diagnosis. Recently, a rapid colorimetric test that detects proline iminopeptidase has been developed for office use. Enzyme levels in vaginal fluid are elevated in women with bacterial vaginosis.

The vaginal pH associated with bacterial vaginosis is 5.0 to 6.0. When 10% potassium hydroxide is placed on the vaginal speculum or a glass slide containing vaginal secretions, an aromatic amine will be vaporized. A positive "whiff test" may be obtained with either bacterial vaginosis or *Trichomonas* infection. It is usually more prominent with bacterial infections because of the amount of anaerobic metabolism. The common aromatic amines are cadaverine and putrescine, both of which result from anaerobic metabolism. The *Gardnerella* organism may be recovered from approximately 90% of male partners. Women with multiple sexual partners are in a high-risk group for the disease. It has been postulated that the associated increased prevalence and concentration of anaerobic bacteria in the vagina may also predispose certain women to upper tract pelvic infection.

The treatment for bacterial vaginosis is metronidazole (Protostat, Flagyl), 500 mg twice daily for 7 days. Metronidazole has excellent activity against anaerobic bacteria, and its hydroxy metabolite is active against *G. vaginalis*. Pfeifer et al. found clinical cures in 80 of 81 women treated with metronidazole but mediocre response to ampicillin, tetracycline, or sulfa cream. More important, facultative *Lactobacillus* organisms return after treatment with metronidazole but not with ampicillin. Most investigators report a cure rate of approximately two out of three women with a 1-week course of ampicillin 500 mg every 6 hours. Blackwell et al. have contrasted treatment of 7 days of metronidazole with a regimen of 2 g of metronidazole divided over 12 hours. They described a 95% cure rate with 7 days versus a 75% cure rate with single-day therapy. Purdon et al. found similar results, with 67% of women treated with single-day therapy and 86% of patients cured receiving the 7-day course. However, a metaanalysis by Lugo-Miro et al. determined that single-dose therapy resulted in a 72% cure versus a 78% cure with a 7-day regimen. Women who are allergic to metronidazole, or resistant cases, should be treated with oral clindamycin 300 mg every 12 hours for 7 days. Alternate treatment regimens to metronidazole or clindamycin include amoxicillin 500 mg plus clavulanic acid (Augmentin) every 8 hours for 7 days or cephradine 500 mg every 6 hours for 7 days. The FDA has approved oral metronidazole 750 mg once daily for 7 days for treatment of bacterial vaginosis.

As alternative treatments to oral antibiotics, the CDC recommends topical vaginal therapy with either clindamycin cream or metronidazole gel. Topical therapy is popular with both clinicians and patients. As bacterial vaginosis is a superficial mucosal infection, topical therapy should be as efficacious as systemic therapy and produce fewer side effects. Clindamycin 2% cream is prescribed as 1 vaginal applicator at bedtime for 7 days. The recommended new regimen of topical metronidazole gel 0.75% is 1 applicator (5 g) once a day for 5 days rather than the traditional twice-a-day therapy. Compliance is better with the once-a-day regimens.

Bump et al. have added to the therapeutic dilemma by a study of prevalence and persistence of *G. vaginalis* in asymptomatic women over a 6-month period. They believe that the *Gardnerella* bacterium is indigenous flora and is often transient. They advise not treating a patient unless she exhibits symptoms.

Concurrent treatment of the male partner is controversial. The literature is divided on this subject. We favor treating the male partner if there is recurrent vaginitis or any suspicion of associated upper genital tract infection.

Trichomonas Vaginal Infection

Trichomonas vaginalis is a unicellular protozoon that inhabits the vagina and lower urinary tract, especially Skene's ducts in the female. It is estimated that there are between 2.5 and 3 million cases of vaginitis secondary to *Trichomonas* infection in the United States each year. The prevalence of the disease remains high despite the availability of effective treatments since the early 1960s. *Trichomonas* vaginal infection is the most prevalent nonviral, nonchlamydial sexually transmitted disease of women. *Trichomonas* is the etiologic factor for approximately one in four episodes of infectious vaginitis.

Many women who harbor *Trichomonas* in their vaginal secretions are free of symptoms. McLellan et al. discovered that only one out of two women with positive vaginal cultures had symptoms of a vaginal discharge. In the same study only one out of six women complained of vulvar pruritus. Positive wet smears or cultures for *Trichomonas* are reported in 3% to 10% of asymptomatic gynecology patients, with a much higher percentage being found in women attending a sexually transmitted disease clinic. Trichomoniasis is definitely a sexually transmitted disease, with the protozoa being isolated from 30% to 40% of male partners of women with a positive culture and approxi-

mately 85% of female partners of a male with a positive culture. *T. vaginalis* is a highly contagious sexually transmitted disease. Following a single sexual contact, at least two thirds of both male and female sexual partners become infected. The incubation period for *Trichomonas* infection is 4 to 28 days. *Trichomonas* is a hardy organism and will survive for up to 24 hours on a wet towel and up to 6 hours on a moist surface. However, experimental studies have established that successful vaginal infection depends on the deposition of an inoculum of several thousand organisms. Thus it is unlikely that infection may be related to exposure from infected towels or swimming pools.

Trichomonas vaginitis is caused by the anaerobic, flagellated protozoon, *T. vaginalis* (Figure 22-25). There are other species of *Trichomonas* that reside in the oral pharynx and rectum. These species are site specific and do not produce disease in the vagina. *T. vaginalis* resides in the paraurethral glands of both the male and female. When a woman is treated with topical medication, reinfection occurs not only from an infected partner but also from the patient's own urethra and Skene's ducts.

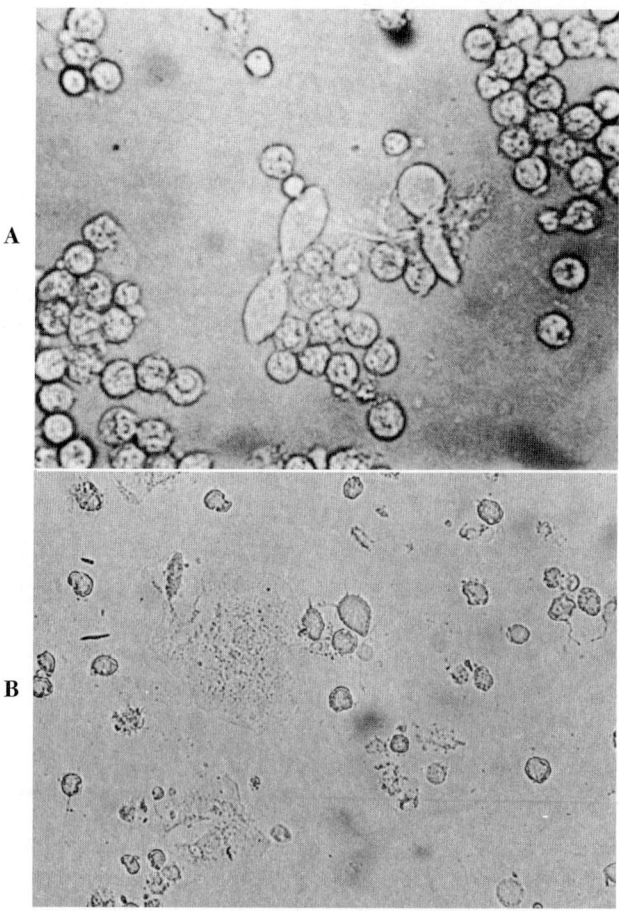

FIGURE 22-25 A and **B,** Trichomonads in wet mount prepared with physiologic saline. (**A** from Faro S: Trichomoniasis. In Kaufman RH and Faro S, editors: Benign diseases of the vulva and vagina, ed 4, St. Louis, 1994, Mosby–Year Book, Inc. **B** from Friedrich EG: Vulvar disease, ed 2, Philadelphia, 1983, WB Saunders Co.)

T. vaginalis is a unicellular protozoon that is normally fusiform in shape. This organism exists only in the trophozoite form or vegetative cell. It is slightly larger than a white blood cell. Three to five flagella extend from one end of the organism. The flagella provide the active movement of the protozoon, with the direction of motion usually toward the end with the flagella. The *Trichomonas* organism assumes a spherical shape in an acidic environment (Figure 22-26). Motion is then restricted to waves of the undulating membrane of the protozoon.

Vaginitis from *Trichomonas* is a disease primarily of women in the reproductive years. The normal highly acidic vaginal environment is resistant to *Trichomonas* infection. When lactobacilli predominate in the vaginal fluid, a woman will not develop symptoms. However, menstrual blood, semen, or other vaginal pathogens that transform the vaginal pH to a more basic level favor the growth of *Trichomonas* organisms.

Trichomonas produces a wide variety of patterns of vaginal infection. Women may or may not have symptoms and signs of acute or chronic infection. The primary symptom of *Trichomonas* vaginal infection is profuse vaginal discharge. The volume of discharge associated with symptomatic *Trichomonas* infection is the most abundant of common vaginal infections. Patients often complain that the copious discharge makes them feel "wet." The discharge may be white, gray, yellow, or green. The classic discharge of *Trichomonas* infection has been termed "frothy" (with bubbles) and often has an unpleasant odor.

However, a frothy discharge is only noted in 10% to 25% of women with proven *Trichomonas* infection. This discharge is not diagnostic, because it may be seen also with bacterial vaginosis.

Associated with the acute vaginal discharge are erythema and edema of the vulva and vagina. Approximately 50% of symptomatic women detect abnormal vaginal odor and experience vulvar pruritus. The classic sign of a strawberry appearance of the upper vagina and cervix is rare and is noted in less than 10% of women. Approximately 25% of women experience vulvar pruritus. Vulvar skin involvement is limited to the vestibule and labia minora, which helps to distinguish it from the more extensive vulvar involvement of *Candida* vulvovaginitis. Often women with chronic infection have a malodorous discharge as their only complaint. Dysuria is a symptom in approximately one out of five women with symptomatic *Trichomonas* infection.

The diagnosis of *Trichomonas* vaginal infection is confirmed by examination of vaginal fluid mixed with physiologic saline under the microscope (see Figure 22-25). To optimally visualize *Trichomonas* organisms, it is best to use high power and dampen the condenser to produce the greatest contrast. Trichomonads are best discovered in an area of the wet smear with relatively few white blood cells. If the wet smear is fresh and warm, the organisms will exhibit forward motion. If the slide is cold, if the organisms are surrounded by white blood cells, or if the saline is too hypertonic, the *Trichomonas* organisms will

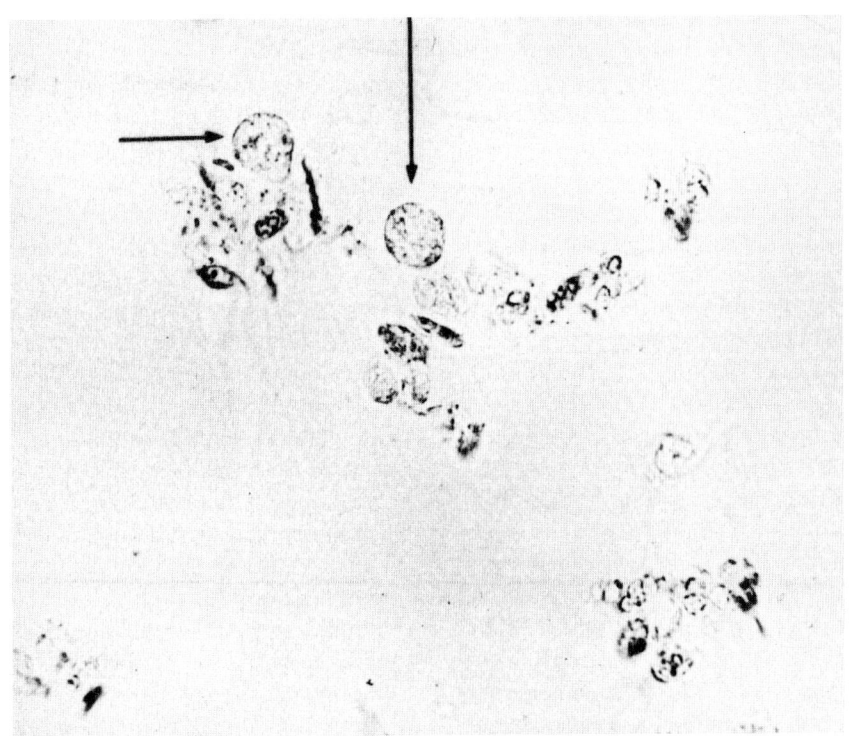

FIGURE 22-26   "Balled-up" trichomonads *(arrows)* in urinary sediment. (From Faro S: Trichomoniasis. In Kaufman RH and Faro S, editors: Benign diseases of the vulva and vagina, ed 4, St. Louis, 1994, Mosby–Year Book, Inc.)

assume an ovoid configuration and exhibit minimal motion. The wet smear usually contains a large number of inflammatory cells and many vaginal epithelial cells. The only other vaginitis with an abundance of white blood cells is atrophic vaginitis. The epithelial cells are normal in appearance and have distinct edges. It is postulated that *Trichomonas* excretes a cytotoxic substance that lyses intracellular bridges. This may explain the large number of normal epithelial cells on wet smear seen with severe infection.

The accuracy of diagnosis by wet smear varies widely throughout the literature. If the patient is symptomatic, the sensitivity of a saline wet preparation is 80% to 90%. Therefore a culture for *Trichomonas* is rarely indicated. Attempts to diagnose *T. vaginalis* infection by Papanicolaou smear results in an error rate of at least 50%. There is a large number of both false-positive and false-negative reports. A complementary laboratory test to the wet smear is the measurement of pH of the vaginal fluid with colorimetric paper. The vaginal pH associated with *T. vaginalis* is between 5.0 and 7.0. Microscopic examination of a spun urine specimen improves the detection rate of *T. vaginalis* over microscopic examination of only a vaginal wet smear. Krieger et al. has reported a comparison study of direct wet-mount Pap smear slides, fluorescein-conjugated monoclonal antibodies, and two culture media. In this study he used the culture results as the gold standard and found that the wet mount discovered 60%, Pap smears 56%, and the monoclonal antibodies 86% of infections. Importantly, the Pap smear also identified seven women who were false positives and 18 who were suspicious for *Trichomonas* in which the cultures were negative. The fluorescein-conjugated monoclonal antibody test and another rapid test using DNA probes are both new tests for the office diagnosis of *Trichomonas* infection. A polymerase chain reaction assay to detect *Trichomonas vaginalis* has been developed. Preliminary studies have found that this new assay, even when used with a self-administered tampon sampling method, compares favorably with culture results using Diamond's media.

Metronidazole (Flagyl, Protostat) is the treatment of choice for *T. vaginalis* infection. Metronidazole is marketed in the United States as 250, 375, 500, and 750 mg tablets and an intravenous preparation for severe anaerobic infections. The drug is completely absorbed orally and has a half-life of 8 hours. Phenobarbital decreases the serum concentration approximately 50% by activating liver enzymes. There are two standard treatment regimens, which yield similar results of an approximately 90% cure rate. Single-day therapy is 1 g of metronidazole in the morning and another 1 g at night. Often a single oral dose of 2 g is prescribed. However, the incidence of nausea is higher than the twice-a-day regimen. Alternative therapy is 500 mg every 12 hours for 7 days. Single-day therapy is preferable, because it is less expensive and has fewer side effects and greater patient compliance.

The major side effects of metronidazole therapy include nausea, vomiting, a metallic taste, and secondary *Candida* infections. Nausea is the most frequent complication and is experienced by 5% of women. Patients should be warned that metronidazole inhibits ethanol metabolism. Therefore, they may experience a disulfiram-like reaction if the two drugs are used concurrently. Several reports have noted an association between chronic high-dose metronidazole treatment and pulmonary cancers in mice. However, studies of humans have not confirmed any relationship between metronidazole therapy and oncogenesis.

The asymptomatic female who has *Trichomonas* identified in the lower genital urinary tract definitely should be treated. Extended follow-up studies have shown that one out of three asymptomatic females will become symptomatic within 3 months. Furthermore, there is speculation that *Trichomonas* may be a vector for viral or bacterial pelvic infections. Obviously, all sexually transmitted diseases have common epidemiologic backgrounds, and finding one dictates appropriate studies to rule out colonization or infection with another sexually transmitted disease. Frequently, vaginal infections are a mixed infection, with *Trichomonas* and bacterial vaginosis occurring simultaneously in the same individual. Metronidazole gel has been approved for the treatment of bacterial vaginosis, but it is inferior to oral therapy for the treatment of *Trichomonas*.

One of the continuing debates regarding therapy is treatment of the asymptomatic male partner. Gardner and Dukes documented a 2.5-fold greater reinfection rate when the sexual partner was not treated. Some physicians elect to treat the male partner only when the vaginitis is recurrent. We believe that *Trichomonas* infection should be treated in a similar fashion to any sexually transmitted disease. Thus it is our practice to treat male sexual partners with 2 g of metronidazole (single-day therapy). Trichomoniasis in males is usually asymptomatic. Some men report the symptoms and signs of urethritis.

Women who have recurrence have in most cases either been reinfected or complied poorly with therapy. Recently a few resistant strains of *Trichomonas* have been documented. These resistant cases usually respond to metronidazole 500 mg twice a day for 7 days. If this regimen is not successful, the woman should be treated with a single 2 g dose of metronidazole once a day for 5 days. A clue to a woman with resistant strains of *Trichomonas* is that when a wet smear is obtained 3 to 5 days after therapy, the *Trichomonas* organisms are larger and plumper than normal.

There are two alternatives if a woman is allergic to metronidazole. It is possible to desensitize the woman to metronidazole or, alternatively, use topical clotrimazole, an imidazole derivative. Clotrimazole is a less than ideal drug for *Trichomonas* for its efficacy cures only two out of three women. Friedrich has advocated douching with hypertonic (20%) saline solution to reduce the vaginal inoculum.

Candida Vaginitis

Candida vaginitis (Figure 22-27) is produced by a ubiquitous, airborne, gram-positive fungus. Greater than 75% of cases are caused by *Candida albicans*, with 5% to 20% of vaginal fungal infections produced by *C. glabrata* or *C. tropicalis*. The percentage of infections related to the latter two species has increased in recent years. *Candida* species are part of the normal flora of approximately 25% of women, being a commensal saprophytic organism on the mucosal surface of the vagina. Its prevalence in the rectum is three to four times greater and in the mouth two times greater than in the vagina. When the ecosystem of the vagina is disturbed, *C. albicans* becomes an opportunistic pathogen. Lactobacilli inhibit the growth of fungi in the vagina. However, when the relative concentration of lactobacilli declines, rapid overgrowth of *Candida* species occurs. Following the traditional 10 to 14 days of oral broad-spectrum antibiotics, the percentage of women who have vaginal colonization with *Candida* increases threefold.

Vulvovaginal candidiasis has a variety of names, such as "moniliasis." This term is semantically incorrect, because the name is reserved for plant pathogens. Candidiasis is also often referred to as a yeast infection because of its similarity to true yeast cells.

Candida vaginitis has several features unlike those of protozoal or bacterial vaginitis. *Candida* is rarely found in a mixed infection with *Trichomonas* or bacterial vaginosis. *Candida* vulvovaginitis is not usually associated with other sexually transmitted diseases and is not seen more frequently in STD clinics. However, vaginal candidiasis often becomes symptomatic following successful treatment of *Trichomonas* or bacterial vaginosis. Unlike other vaginal infections, there is no direct relationship between the number of organisms and the patient's signs and symptoms. Some women with a small amount of yeast may have extensive symptoms. It has been postulated that such patients may be hypersensitive to the fungus. Also, candidiasis is not considered a sexually transmitted disease. However, 10% of male partners have concomitant symptomatic penile infection. Treatment of the male partners does not reduce the recurrence rate.

Vaginitis caused by fungal infection is primarily a disease of the childbearing years. It is estimated that three out of four women will have at least one episode of vulvovaginal candidiasis during their lifetime. The greatest enigma of this condition is the recurrence rate after an apparent cure, varying from 20% to 80%. Approximately 3% to 5% of these women experience recurrent vulvovaginal candidiasis.

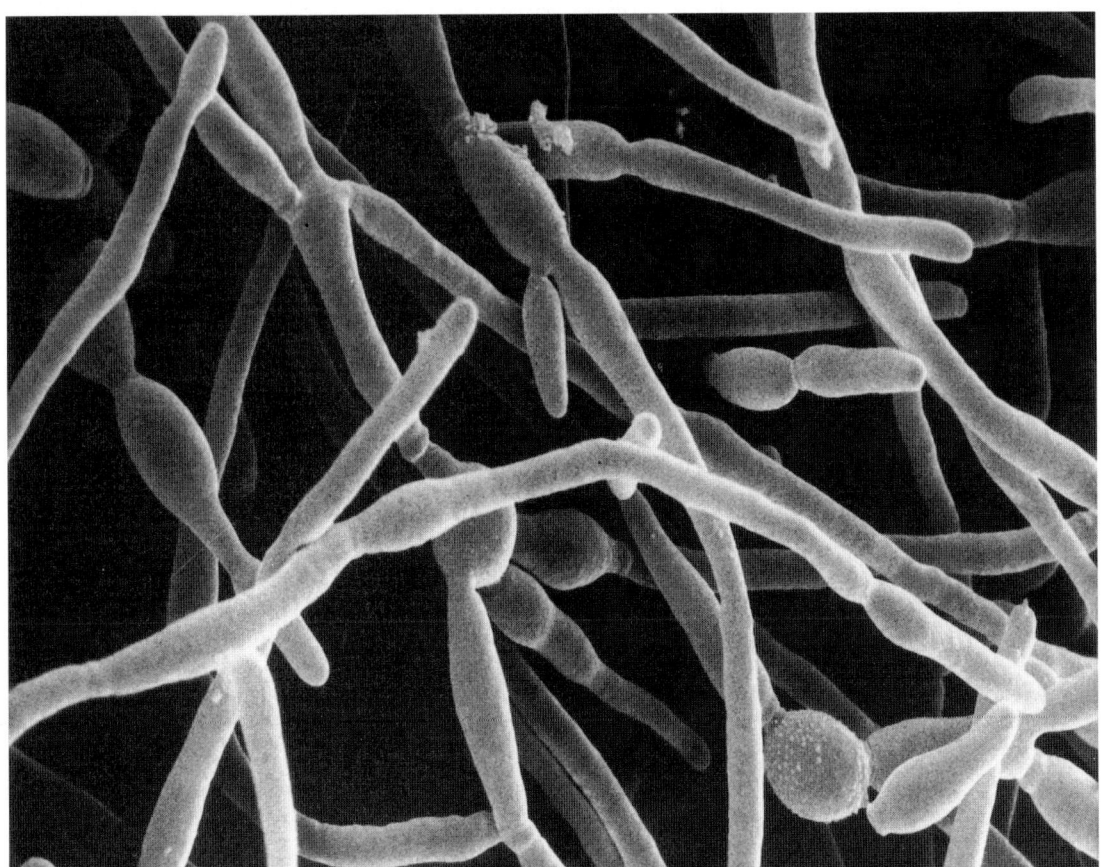

FIGURE 22-27   A scanning electron micrograph shows a pure culture of *Candida albicans* (×6030). (From Phillips DM: N Engl J Med 328:1322, 1993.)

C. albicans is responsible for 80% to 95% of vaginal fungal infections. The organisms develop both filamentous (hyphae and pseudohyphae) and ovoid forms, termed *conidia, buds, or spores*. In contrast, *C. glabrata* does not produce filamentous forms. Merkus et al. and Montes and Wilborn have reported studies of the pathophysiology of *Candida* infections as viewed with the electron microscope. The filamentous forms of *C. albicans* have the ability to penetrate the mucosal surface and become intertwined with the host cells (Figure 22-28). This results in secondary hyperemia and limited lysis of tissue near the site of infection.

C. albicans, although normally not pathogenic, may overgrow in the vagina because of a number of well-established host factors that enhance growth of the fungus. Hormonal factors, depressed cell-mediated immunity, and antibiotic use are the three most important. The hormonal changes associated with both pregnancy and menstruation favor growth of the fungus. The prevalence of *Candida* vaginitis increases throughout pregnancy, probably as a result of the high estrogen levels. The literature was initially mixed with respect to the relationship between oral contraceptives and candidiasis. Oriel et al. discovered more positive cultures, but fewer symptoms, in women taking oral contraceptives. Presently, with low-dose estrogen oral contraceptives, there is no increase in the incidence of fungal vaginitis. Women tend to report recurrent episodes of vaginitis immediately preceding and immediately following their menstrual periods. Broad-spectrum antibiotics, especially those that destroy lactobacilli (penicillin, tetracycline, cephalosporins), are notorious for precipitating acute episodes of *C. albicans* vaginitis. Women with diabetes mellitus, or even a low renal threshold for sugar, have a higher incidence of vaginal and vulvar candidiasis. Obesity and debilitating disease are other predisposing factors.

Probably the most important host factor is depressed cell-mediated immunity. Women who take exogenous corticosteroids and women with AIDS often experience recurrent *Candida* vulvovaginitis. For years authors have written of an X-factor that predisposed certain women to recurrent vaginitis. This X-factor is most likely a subtle defect in cell-mediated immunity.

Since fungal vaginitis usually presents as a vulvovaginitis, the predominant symptom is pruritus. Depending on the degree of vulvar skin involvement, pruritus may be accompanied by vulvar burning, external dysuria, and dyspareunia. The vaginal discharge is white or whitish-gray, highly viscous, and described as granular or floccular. It does not have an odor. The amount of discharge is highly variable. The vulvar signs include erythema, edema, and excoriation. With extensive skin involvement, pustules may extend beyond the line of erythema. During speculum examination a cottage cheese–type discharge is often visualized with adherent clumps and plaques (thrush patches) attached to the walls of the vagina. These clumps or raised plaques are usually white or yellow. The pH of the vagina associated with this infection is below 4.5.

The diagnosis is established by obtaining a wet smear of vaginal secretion and mixing this with 10% to 20% potassium hydroxide (Figure 22-29). The alkali rapidly lyse both red blood cells and inflammatory cells. It is important always to use a coverslip, because potassium hydroxide will destroy the glass lens of the microscope. Active disease is associated with filamentous forms, mycelia and/or pseudohyphae, rather than spores. However, it may be necessary to search the slide and scan many different microscopic fields to identify hyphae or pseudohyphae. The average concentration of organisms is 10^3 to 10^4 per milliliter, but as stated previously, there is no direct relationship between the concentration of the organism and the severity of the signs and symptoms. The microscopic diagnosis of fungal infection has a sensitivity of approximately 65%. A negative smear does not exclude *Candida* vulvovaginitis. The diagnosis can be established by culture with either Nickerson or Sabouraud medium. These cultures will become positive in 24 to 72 hours and are a simple office procedure, because they can be grown at room temperature. A concentration of 10^3 organisms per milliliter is required to obtain a positive laboratory culture. Thus a culture following treatment may be negative while the woman continues to have residual organisms in the vagina. A 2-minute test, which is a slide latex agglutination method, has been developed. The sensitivity of this test is approximately 70% to 75%. The differential diagnosis includes other common causes of vaginitis such as bacterial vaginosis, Trichomonas, and atrophic vaginitis. Also, one should consider noninfectious conditions such as allergic reactions, contact dermatitis, chemical irritants, and rare diseases such as lichens planus.

The treatment of choice for *Candida* vaginitis is the topical application of one of the synthetic imidazoles—miconazole (Monistat), clotrimazole (Lotrimin, Mycelex), butoconazole (Femstat), tioconazole (Vagistat), or one of the triazoles, such as the topical terconazole (Terazol) or the oral medication fluconazole (Diflucan). The topical preparations are marketed in an array of carrier vehicles, primarily as suppositories or creams. They exert their action by changing the permeability of the surface membrane of the fungus. Several comparative studies have documented equal effectiveness between the traditional 7-day therapy and the 3-day therapy. The 3-day or 1-day therapy is less expensive and provides improved patient compliance. Symptom cure rates are greater than 90%; however, approximately 20% of women will have positive cultures when followed for 4 to 6 weeks after therapy. Marketing studies demonstrate that most practitioners prefer the traditional 7 days of therapy and are reluctant to change their prescribing habits to a shorter course of therapy. Many of the intravaginal antifungal agents are oil based, which may result in weakness in latex condoms and diaphragms. Several of the intravaginal azole preparations are now available without prescription.

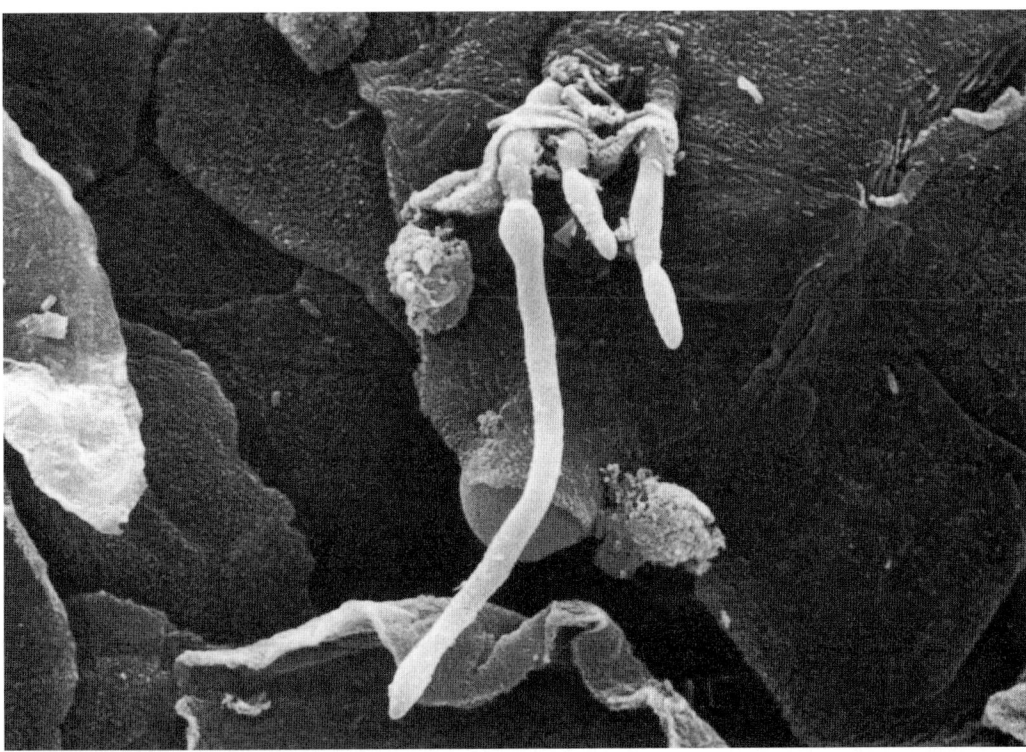

FIGURE 22-28 Scanning electron microscopy of intraluminal debris of specimen of vaginal wall taken from patient with vaginal candidiasis (×3,500). Hyphae of *C. albicans* penetrate epithelial layers of vaginal surface. (From Merkus JMWM, Bisschop MPJM, and Stolte LAM: Obstet Gynecol Surv 40:499, 1985. Copyright 1985 by Williams & Wilkins.)

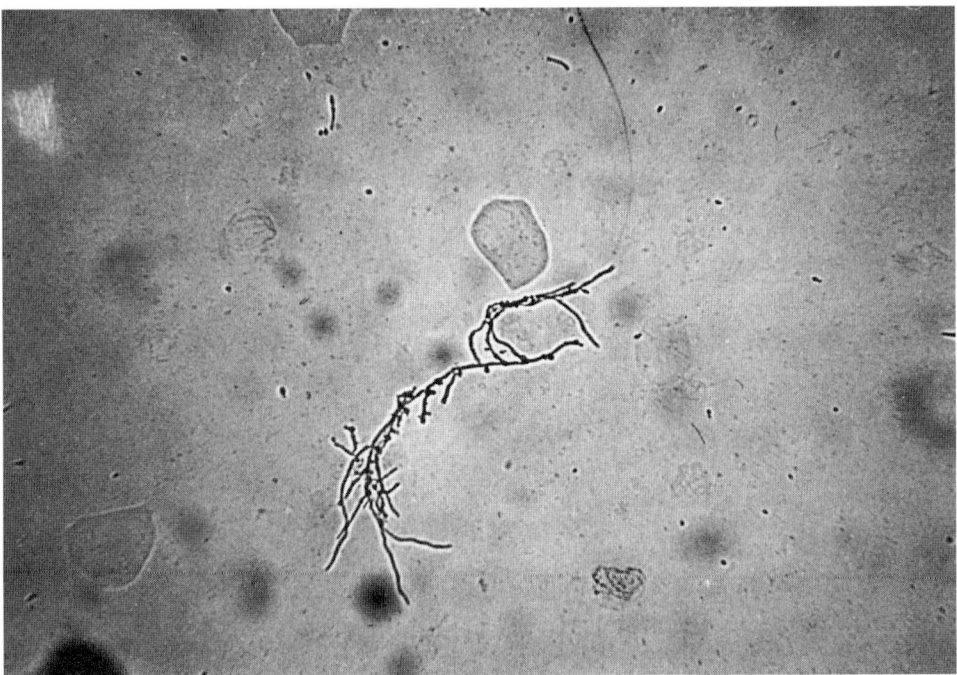

FIGURE 22-29 Microscopic appearance of vaginal smear in a case of vaginal candidiasis. Potassium hydroxide preparation; yeast cells and pseudomycelia (×320). (From Merkus JMWM, Bisschop MPJM, and Stolte LAM: Obstet Gynecol Surv 40:495, 1985. Copyright 1985 by Williams & Wilkins.)

Obviously, women whose symptoms persist after using an over-the-counter preparation or have a recurrence of symptoms within a few weeks should seek medical care. The majority of women prefer oral therapy rather than topical preparations. Fluconazole (Diflucan) has a prolonged plasma half-life. Thus it is prescribed as a single oral tablet of 150 mg, which produces therapeutic concentrations in vaginal secretions for a minimum of 72 hours. Comparative studies have found equal effectiveness between single-dose oral therapy with fluconazole and topical therapy. Fluconazole has the possibility of drug interactions with multiple other drugs. Most importantly it may produce significant hypoglycemia in women taking oral medications for diabetes.

Before the introduction of synthetic imidazoles, polyenes, primarily nystatin (Mycostatin), were the standard therapy. Nystatin was prescribed for 10 to 14 days and resulted in clinical cure rates of approximately 80%. Povidone-iodine douche has been used for years, but when used alone it is only 60% effective.

A new term recently has been developed: "complicated" vulvovaginal candidiasis. Included in this classification is severe local or recurrent disease in a woman who is immunocompromised or whose infection is caused by a less susceptible fungal pathogen such as *C. glabrata*. Women with complicated vulvovaginal candidiasis require a longer duration of therapy, at least 10 to 14 days with a topical or oral azole.

One of the most perplexing problems in clinical gynecology is recurrent vaginal infection caused by *C. albicans*. Often it is difficult to distinguish a relapse from a reinfection. Recurrent vulvovaginal candidiasis is defined as four or more episodes of symptomatic lower tract infection within 12 months. It is important first to confirm that the woman's symptoms are not the result of drug sensitivity. Some investigators hypothesize that an allergic response of the vagina may be a predisposing factor to recurrent infections. A screening test for diabetes should be performed. The vaginal discharge should be cultured and the identity of the fungus species determined. Women with recurrent vulvovaginal candidiasis are three times more likely to be asymptomatic carriers of *Candida* in their vagina than women who do not have a history of frequent episodes of vaginitis. Horowitz et al. have demonstrated a twofold rate of recurrence with *C. tropicalis*, because this organism is not as susceptible to the imidazoles as *C. albicans*. Similarly, *C. glabrata* infections are often resistant to imidazoles. The latter fungus produces a clinical syndrome of vulvar burning with little to no vaginal discharge. Both *C. tropicalis* and *C. glabrata* may be treated with topical gentian violet.

Sobel and Eschenbach have each reported clinical trials for recurrent or persistent vulvovaginal candidiasis using ketoconazole (400 mg daily), an oral preparation. Both studies reported greater than 50% recurrence rates after the drug was discontinued. Liver toxicity is a worrisome side effect of ketoconazole; thus it is unlikely that it will be prescribed for long periods for vaginal infection. It is estimated that ketoconazole produces hepatic toxicity in approximately one out of every 12,500 exposed patients. Treatment of the male partner and elimination of *Candida* species from the gastrointestinal tract have not been beneficial in alleviating the problem.

Potential therapy for recurrent disease includes gentian violet, boric acid, povidone-iodine douching, and dietary changes. Painting the vagina with 1% gentian violet is messy, and patients must be warned to wear a minipad so that their clothes will not be stained. The vagina should be treated with gentian violet 4 times at intervals of approximately 7 days. Treating the patient at more frequent intervals may result in the development of a chemical "burn." Van Slyke et al. recommended that 600 mg boric acid in gelatin capsules be placed high in the vagina twice a day. Boric acid is toxic when taken orally. However, studies have demonstrated minimal absorption following placement in the vagina. Douching with povidone-iodine is sometimes helpful as adjunctive therapy to other methods. There are anecdotal reports of successful therapy with instructions to restrict sugar in the diet. For years there have been anecdotal reports of successful therapy using intravaginal or oral yogurt preparations. An article by Hilton et al. in the *Annals of Internal Medicine* documented an approximately threefold decrease in both *Candida* colonization and reinfection in women who ingested 8 ounces of yogurt containing *Lactobacillus acidophilus*. One caveat: Hughes and Hillier have discovered that only 4 out of 16 commercially available over-the-counter yogurt products contained the appropriate *Lactobacillus acidophilus* that produced hydrogen peroxide.

Optimal treatment of recurrent vaginal infections related to *C. albicans* often involves therapy similar to treating recurrent urinary tract infections. The patient must be provided with enough medication so that she is able to self-treat at the first suggestion of recurrent symptoms or signs. Prophylactic treatment is often beneficial either immediately before or following menses or at the first sign of recurrence.

TOXIC SHOCK SYNDROME

Toxic shock syndrome (TSS) is an acute, febrile illness produced by a bacterial exotoxin, with a fulminating downhill course involving dysfunction of multiple organ systems. The cardinal features of the disease are the abrupt onset and the rapidity with which the clinical signs and symptoms may present and progress. It is not unusual for the syndrome to develop from a site of bacterial colonization rather than from an infection. A woman with TSS may develop rapid onset of hypotension associated with multiorgan system failure. TSS was first described in 1978 by Todd as a sometimes fatal sequela of *Staphylococ-*

cus aureus infection in children. In the early 1980s more than 95% of the reported cases of TSS were diagnosed in previously healthy, young (<30 years), menstruating females. *S. aureus* has been isolated from the vagina in more than 90% of these cases.

Presently, approximately 50% of cases of TSS are related to menses. In cases of menses-related TSS there is a history of the presence of a foreign body in the vagina, usually a tampon or diaphragm. Nonmenstrual TSS may be a sequela of focal staphylococcal infection of the skin and subcutaneous tissue, often following a surgical procedure. In the past few years it has been recognized that occasionally severe postoperative infections by *Streptococcus pyrogenes* produce a similar "streptococcal toxic shock-like syndrome." TSS related to a surgical wound occurs early in the postoperative course, usually within the first 48 hours.

There are three requirements for the development of classical TSS: (1) the woman must be colonized or infected with *S. aureus,* (2) the bacteria must produce TSS toxin 1 (TSST-1) and/or related toxins, and (3) the toxins must have a route of entry into the systemic circulation. The majority of strains of *S. aureus* are unable to produce TSS toxin 1. Interestingly, approximately 85% of adult females have antibodies against TSST-1

The mortality of reported cases is high—2% to 8%. If an individual woman continues to use tampons when the vagina is colonized with *S. aureus,* there is a significant chance of a recurrence. It has been reported that one woman experienced five episodes of the disease. There appears to be no pattern to these recurrent episodes. Interestingly, women with menstrual-related TSS do not respond immunologically to TSST-1 as do women with nonmenstrual-related TSS. It is very rare for a woman with nonmenstrual TSS to have a recurrence.

The signs and symptoms of TSS are produced by the exotoxin named toxin 1. Toxin 1 is a simple protein with a molecular weight of 22,000. It is accepted as the underlying cause of the disease. The current hypothesis is that toxins act as "superantigens" and facilitate the release of tumor necrosis factor, interleukins, and other cytokines, and also induce a suppression of some immune responses. Pathophysiologically, superantigens are able to bypass some of the steps of the typical immune response sequence. The primary effects of toxin 1 are to produce increased vascular permeability and thus profuse leaking of fluid (capillary leak) from the intravascular compartment into the interstitial space and associated profound loss of vasomotor tone resulting in decreased peripheral resistance.

Studies of the bacteriology of the vagina of normal menstruating females have documented that 5% to 17% of women are colonized with *S. aureus.* Approximately 5% test positive when the culture is obtained at midcycle, and the percentage increases to 10% to 17% during the menses. Rarely are blood cultures positive for *S. aureus* in a woman with TSS. Thus the exotoxin is believed to be absorbed directly from the vagina. It is possible that microulcerations produced by use of tampons facilitate the toxin's entry into the systemic circulation. The risk of nonmenstrual TSS is definitely increased in women who use barrier contraceptives such as the diaphragm, cervical cap, or a sponge containing nonoxynol 9.

Because of the severity of the disease, gynecologists should have a high index of suspicion for TSS in a woman who has an unexplained fever and a rash during or immediately following her menstrual period. The syndrome has a wide range of symptoms. The varying degree of severity of both symptoms and signs depends on the magnitude of involvement of individual organs. Most women experience a prodromal flulike illness for the first 24 hours. Between days 2 and 4 of the menstrual period, the patient experiences an abrupt onset of a high temperature associated with headache, myalgia, sore throat, vomiting, diarrhea, a generalized skin rash, and often hypotension. It is important to consider that not all women with TSS experience the full-blown manifestations of the disease. The rigid criteria developed by the CDC are used for epidemiologic studies. Clinically, many women present with a "forme fruste" of TSS, with low-grade fever and dizziness rather than hypotension.

Case Definition of Toxic Shock Syndrome

1. Fever (temperature 38.9° C, 102° F)
2. Rash characterized by diffuse macular erythroderma
3. Desquamation occurring 1-2 weeks after onset of illness (in survivors)
4. Hypotension (systolic blood pressure ≤90 mm Hg in adults) or orthostatic syncope
5. Involvement of three or more of the following organ systems:
   a. Gastrointestinal (vomiting or diarrhea at onset of illness)
   b. Muscular (myalgia or creatine phosphokinase level twice normal)
   c. Mucous membrane (vaginal, oropharyngeal, or conjunctival hyperemia)
   d. Renal (BUN or creatinine level ≥ twice normal or ≥5 WBC per HPF in absence of urinary tract infection)
   e. Hepatic (total bilirubin, SGOT, or SGPT twice normal level)
   f. Hematologic (platelets ≤ 100,000/mm³)
   g. Central nervous system (disorientation or alterations in consciousness without focal neurologic signs when fever and hypotension absent)
   h. Cardiopulmonary (adult respiratory distress syndrome, pulmonary edema, new onset of second- or third-degree heart block, myocarditis)
6. Negative throat and cerebrospinal fluid cultures (a positive blood culture for *S. aureus* does not exclude a case)
7. Negative serologic tests for Rocky Mountain spotted fever, leptospirosis, rubeola

From Toxic shock syndrome—United States, 1970–1982, MMWR 31:201, 1982.

The most characteristic manifestations of TSS are the skin changes. During the first 48 hours the skin rash appears similar to an intense sunburn. During the next few days the erythema will become more macular and look like a drug-related rash. From days 12 to 15 of the illness, there is a fine, flaky, desquamation of skin over the face and trunk with sloughing of the entire skin thickness of the palms and soles. The vaginal mucosa is hyperemic during the initial phase of the syndrome. During pelvic examination, patients complain of tenderness of the external genitalia and vagina. Myalgia, vomiting, and diarrhea are experienced by more than 90% of women with TSS (see the box on p. 679). Many abnormal laboratory findings are associated with the disease, and again they reflect the severity of involvement of individual organ systems (see the box below). The differential diagnosis of toxic shock syndrome includes Rocky Mountain spotted fever, streptococcal scarlet fever, and leptospirosis.

The management of a classic case of severe TSS demands an intensive care unit and the skills of an expert in critical care medicine. The first priority is to eliminate the hypotension produced by the exotoxin. Copious amounts of intravenous fluids are given while pressure and volume dynamics are monitored with a pulmonary artery catheter. Mechanical ventilation is required for women who develop adult respiratory distress syndrome.

Laboratory Abnormalities in Early Toxic Shock Syndrome*

Present in >85% of Patients
Coagulase-positive staphylococci in cervix or vagina
Immature and mature polymorphonuclear cells >90% of WBCs
Total lymphocyte count <650/mm³
Total serum protein level <5.6 mg/dl
Serum albumin level <3.1 g/dl
Serum calcium level <7.8 mg/dl
Serum creatinine clearance >1.0 mg/dl
Serum bilirubin value >1.5 mg/dl
Serum cholesterol level ≤120 mg/dl
Prothrombin time >12 seconds

Present in >70% of Patients
Platelet count <150,000/mm³
Pyuria >5 WBCs per high-power field
Proteinuria ≥2
(BUN) >20 mg/dl
Aspartate aminotransferase (formerly SGOT) > 41 U/L

From Chesney PJ, Davis JP, Purdy WK, et al: Clinical manifestations of toxic shock syndrome, JAMA 246:746, 1981. Copyright 1981, American Medical Association.

*Results were available for at least 18 patients per category with the following exceptions: cervicovaginal cultures (12 patients), cholesterol level (15 patients), and prothrombin time (14 patients).

When the patient is initially admitted to the hospital, it is important to obtain cervical, vaginal, and blood cultures for *S. aureus*. Although there is no controlled series documenting its efficacy, it is prudent to wash out the vagina with saline or dilute iodine solution to diminish the amount of exotoxin that may be absorbed into the systemic circulation.

Women with TSS should be treated with a beta-lactamase-resistant antistaphylococcal antibiotic for 10 to 14 days. Possible antibiotic choices include beta-lactamase-resistant penicillins (oxacillin, methicillin, or nafcillin), clindamycin and gentamicin, vancomycin, and aminoglycosides. If the diagnosis is questionable, it is best to include the use of an aminoglycoside to obtain coverage for possible gram-negative sepsis. Antibiotic therapy probably has little effect on the course of an individual episode of TSS. However, Helgerson et al. have found that antibiotics definitely decrease the risk of recurrence of TSS. In their series only one recurrent case of TSS was documented among 53 different women. The reported risk of recurrence without antibiotic therapy is approximately 33%. If the underlying etiology of toxic shock syndrome is a skin infection, the infected site should be drained and debrided.

For severe cases of TSS, Todd et al. have recommended early administration of pharmacologic doses of parenteral corticosteroids. However, most centers no longer give corticosteroids. Infusions of vasopressors are titrated to obtain optimal perfusion pressures. Others have advocated naloxone (Narcan) for treatment of severe hypotension. Recent reports suggest that intravenous immunoglobulins may be beneficial.

In summary, the treatment of TSS depends on the severity of involvement of individual organ systems. Not all patients develop a temperature of greater than 38.9° C and hypotension. Thus clinicians should be aware of the "forme fruste" manifestations of the syndrome. The foundation of treatment of the disease is prompt and aggressive management because of the rapidity with which the disease may progress.

It is possible to decrease the incidence of TSS by a change in use of catamenial products. Women should be encouraged to change tampons every 4 to 6 hours. The intermittent use of external pads is also good preventive medicine. Women will usually accept the recommendation to wear external pads during sleep. The incidence of TSS has decreased dramatically with the removal of superabsorbing tampons from the market. A study by Tierno and Hanna reported that all-cotton tampons are the safest choice to avoid menstrual toxic shock syndrome.

Lastly, there are cases of streptococcal toxic shock-like syndrome that are secondary to life-threatening infections with group A streptococcus (*Streptococcus pyogenes*). Several different exotoxins have been identified and M-type 1 and 3 are the two most common serotypes. In gynecology the majority of these cases involve massive subcutaneous postoperative infections. One of the most distinguishing characteristics of a necrotizing skin infection is the intense localized pain in the involved area. Elderly women and women who are diabetic or immunocompromised are at much greater risk to develop invasive streptococcal infection and streptococcal toxic shock–like syndrome. The mortality rate is approximately 30% when TSS is secondary to group A streptococcal infections.

ACQUIRED IMMUNE DEFICIENCY SYNDROME

Acquired immune deficiency syndrome (AIDS) is the advanced disease state manifestation of a viral infection by the human immunodeficiency virus (HIV). This virus has a predilection for cells of the immune system, specifically "helper" lymphocytes (lymphocytes with CD_4 marker) and monocytes. Infection of these cells leads to a breakdown of the body's immune system, particularly cell-mediated immunity. Clinically, the AIDS patient is affected by a series of opportunistic infections and neoplasms that are eventually lethal. The virus may also infect cells of other organ systems, such as the central nervous system, producing AIDS dementia complex; and cells of the gastrointestinal tract, producing malabsorption, weight loss, and diarrhea.

The disease was first recognized in 1981 in a small cluster of patients with an unexplained defect of cellular immunity and *Pneumocystis carinii* pneumonia. The etiologic agent, human immunodeficiency virus, was identified in 1983. By the end of 1991, 10 years after the disease's first description, the CDC had estimated that approximately 1.5 million people in the United States were infected by HIV. Current estimates are that approximately one in every 300 individuals in the United States is infected. Initially, the disease predominately affected homosexual men. It is now a disease of heterosexual contact as well. AIDS is ubiquitous and has been reported from every state in the United States and from every continent. The region of the United States with the highest rate of infection is the Northeast. AIDS is one of the five leading causes of death in reproductive age women. It is also found in postmenopausal women. Studies have found that the prevalence of HIV in the United States ranges from as little as 0.02% in blood donors and university students to as much as 6.3% of individuals in urban sexually transmitted disease clinics.

In the United States high-risk populations for AIDS include homosexual men, intravenous drug users and their sexual partners, and hemophiliacs. Transmission of the virus occurs by both horizontal and vertical routes. There are three primary methods of contracting the virus: intimate sexual contact, use of contaminated needles or blood products, and perinatal transmission from mother to child. When there is transmission of the virus through contamination of bodily fluids, it is more commonly virus within the cellular portion of the inoculum rather than free virus that leads to infection. The further advanced a person's disease state, the more viral particles present and the more infectious the inoculum becomes. However, individuals in the acute phase of the disease also are highly contagious because of the viremia that occurs at that time.

HIV is a lentivirus in the family of retroviruses. These RNA viruses contain reverse transcriptase, which translates viral RNA into DNA. Subsequently, this DNA is incorporated into the DNA of the host cell. Pseudonyms for HIV include human T cell leukemia virus (HTLV-3), lymphadenopathy virus (LAV), and AIDS-related virus (ARV). HIV primarily infects and affects T_4, or helper, lymphocytes with a CD_4 marker on the cell surface. This protein marker is the primary receptor for the virus. Current theory is that infectious strains of the virus attach to dendritic-Langerhan's cells in the cervicoepithelium. Susceptible cells have a CCR_5 receptor (a chemokine) that will bind the infectious strain of the virus and the CD_4 lymphocyte. Subsequently, the CD_4 lymphocyte carries the virus into the lymph nodes. Over the next several days, the virus is disseminated throughout the body (Figure 22-30). Genital ulcers and mucosal tears facilitate passage of the virus across the vaginal epithelium, and increase the potential of infection.

In the body the virus can also attach and infect cells that may lack the CD_4 marker, including monocytes, fibroblasts, neurons, and renal, hepatic, intestinal, and other cells. Once the virus is incorporated into the cell, the RNA of the viral core is translated into DNA and incorporated into the host's genome. In some cells, the virus then may lie dormant—the CD_4 memory cells. In other cells, the virus may induce the production of new viral proteins and new virus. For most human cells the production of new virus is a cytotoxic process.

There are two subtypes of HIV: HIV-1 and HIV-2. HIV-2 is found primarily in humans in West Africa. Both HIV viruses have a similar lipid outer coat and similar RNA that codes for three genes. The viruses differ slightly in the products of these genes. In addition, there are multiple strains of HIV-1 virus. The strains differ in the various regulatory proteins that they code. Since vaccines are usually directed against specific proteins, the multiple strains of HIV make the development and production of a vaccine very difficult. HIV mutates and develops into new strains within an individual after he or she is infected. As HIV mutates, it may become more infectious or more pathologic to specific tissues, such as the CNS. The mutation to more pathogenic strains of HIV is one mechanism by which a patient may progress into the advanced disease state of AIDS.

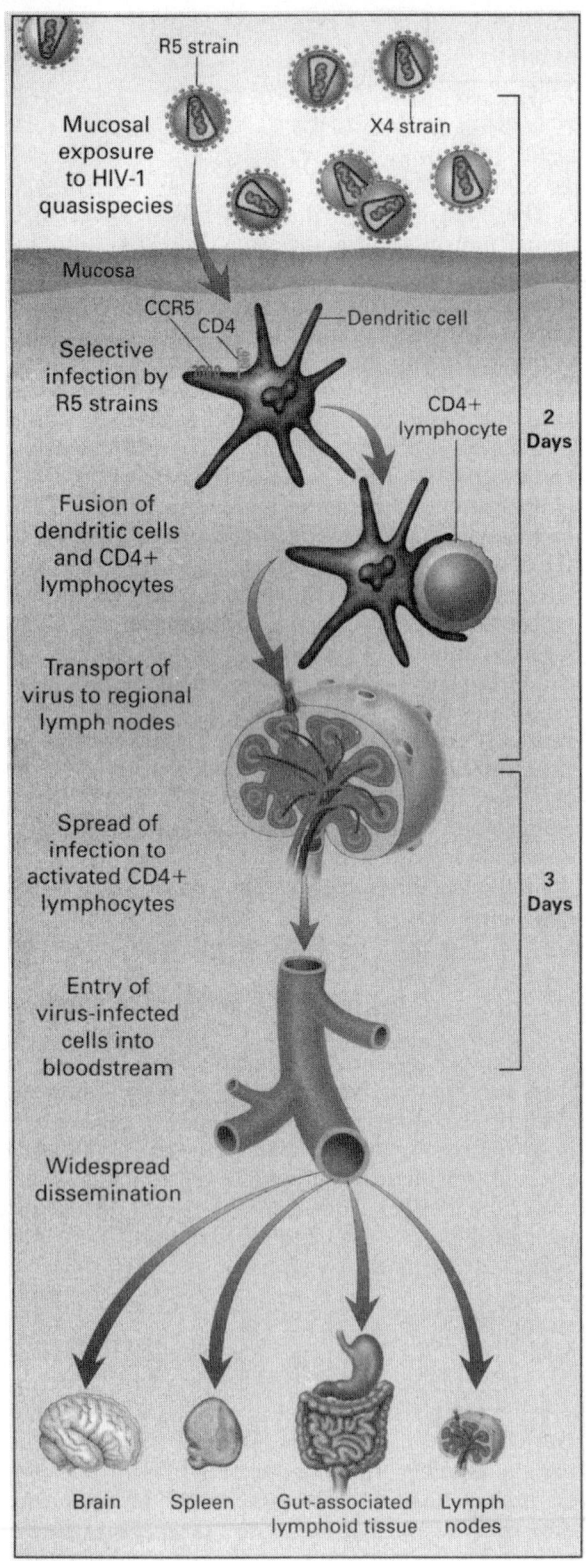

R5 strain

X4 strain

Mucosal exposure to HIV-1 quasispecies

Mucosa

CCR5
CD4 — Dendritic cell

Selective infection by R5 strains

CD4+ lymphocyte

2 Days

Fusion of dendritic cells and CD4+ lymphocytes

Transport of virus to regional lymph nodes

Spread of infection to activated CD4+ lymphocytes

3 Days

Entry of virus-infected cells into bloodstream

Widespread dissemination

Brain   Spleen   Gut-associated lymphoid tissue   Lymph nodes

FIGURE 22-30 Early events in transmucosal HIV-1 infection. The arrows indicate the path of the virus. The viral-envelope protein binds to the CD$_4$ molecule on dendritic cells. Entry into the cells requires the presence of CCR$_5$, a surface chemokine receptor. Dendritic cells, which express the viral coreceptors CD$_4$ and CCR$_5$, are selectively infected by R$_5$ (macrophage-tropic) strains. Within 2 days after mucosal exposure, virus can be detected in lymph nodes. Within another 3 days, it can be cultured from plasma. (From Kahn JO and Walker BD: N Engl J Med 339: 33, 1998.)

Among the proteins made by HIV virus is a core protein, P$_{24}$, which is measured clinically as a serum marker. Other proteins made by the virus are responsible for down-regulation of the virus and inhibition of viral replication. Escape from viral regulatory proteins by mutating strains of HIV is another factor responsible for the progression of the disease.

The CDC has classified HIV infection according to a patient's symptomatology combined with the CD$_4$ lymphocyte count (Table 22-12). Three groups of patients have been described. *Category A* comprises individuals who are in the initial viremic period and have CD$_4$ counts greater than 200 cells per microliter. The initial viremia may last for up to 6 weeks, during which time high levels of free virus may be found in the blood, as well as in the CNS (Figure 22-31). During this time, the acute phase, antibodies to HIV are at a low level. The infected individual may be asymptomatic or may suffer an acute, mononucleosis-like illness. Up to 80% of infected patients experience fever, fatigue, and a maculopapular rash (Table 22-13). The viral exanthem is transient and occurs primarily over the trunk. The viral antigen p24 and viral RNA will be positive during this time; however the antibody will be negative. Thus the standard test for AIDS will be negative. After 4 to 10 weeks, HIV antibody levels begin to rise and viral antigen levels decline. Individuals at this time enter into an intermediate latency period. The period of latency may last for 10 years or more with rare, intermittent viremic spikes. This is a period of clinical latency. During this time, the immune system is actively challenging and attempting to eradicate the virus. Concurrently, the virus is mutating. There is a gradual and variable decline in CD$_4$ lymphocytes. Current therapeutic interventions have changed dramatically the natural history of the disease. Debate exists as to when during clinical latency anti-HIV treatment should be initiated. Ninety-nine percent of HIV-infected individuals are in the latency period. During this asymptomatic period, 2% to 10% of individuals per year will undergo progression of disease. Individuals in category B are symptomatic but not from the initial viremia and not with full-blown AIDS. These individuals have CD$_4$ counts greater than 200 cells per microliter. The diseases of category B include problems such as cervical dysplasia (but not invasive carcinoma), chronic diarrhea, pelvic inflammatory disease, or idiopathic thrombocytopenia purpura. Category C disease is clinical AIDS or a CD$_4$ count less than 200 cells per microliter. Clinical AIDS may be manifested by opportunistic infection, malignancy, or central nervous system symptoms (see the box on p. 684). The progression from category B to category C disease is characterized by a gradual rise in viral proteins and free virus in blood and secretions, as well as a decline in the CD$_4$ lymphocyte count. A normal count is greater than 800 cells per microliter. A CD$_4$ count of less than 200

TABLE 22-12

1993 Revised Classification System for HIV Infection and Expanded AIDS Surveillance Case Definition for Adolescents and Adults*

CD$_4$+ T-cell categories	Clinical Categories		
	(A) Asymptomatic, Acute (primary) HIV or PGL†	**(B)** Symptomatic, Not (A) or (C) Conditions‡	**(C)** AIDS-Indicator Conditions
(1) ≥500/µL	A1	B1	C1
(2) 200–499/µL	A2	B2	C2
(3) <200/µL AIDS-indicator T-cell count	A3	B3	C3

From MMWR 41:1, 1992.

*Persons with AIDS-indicator conditions (Category C) as well as those with CD$_4$+ T-lymphocyte counts <200/µL (Categories A3 or B3) will be reportable as AIDS cases in the United States and territories, effective Jan. 1, 1993.

†PGL, persistent generalized lymphadenopathy. Clinical Category A includes acute (primary) HIV infection (29,30).

‡See text for discussion.

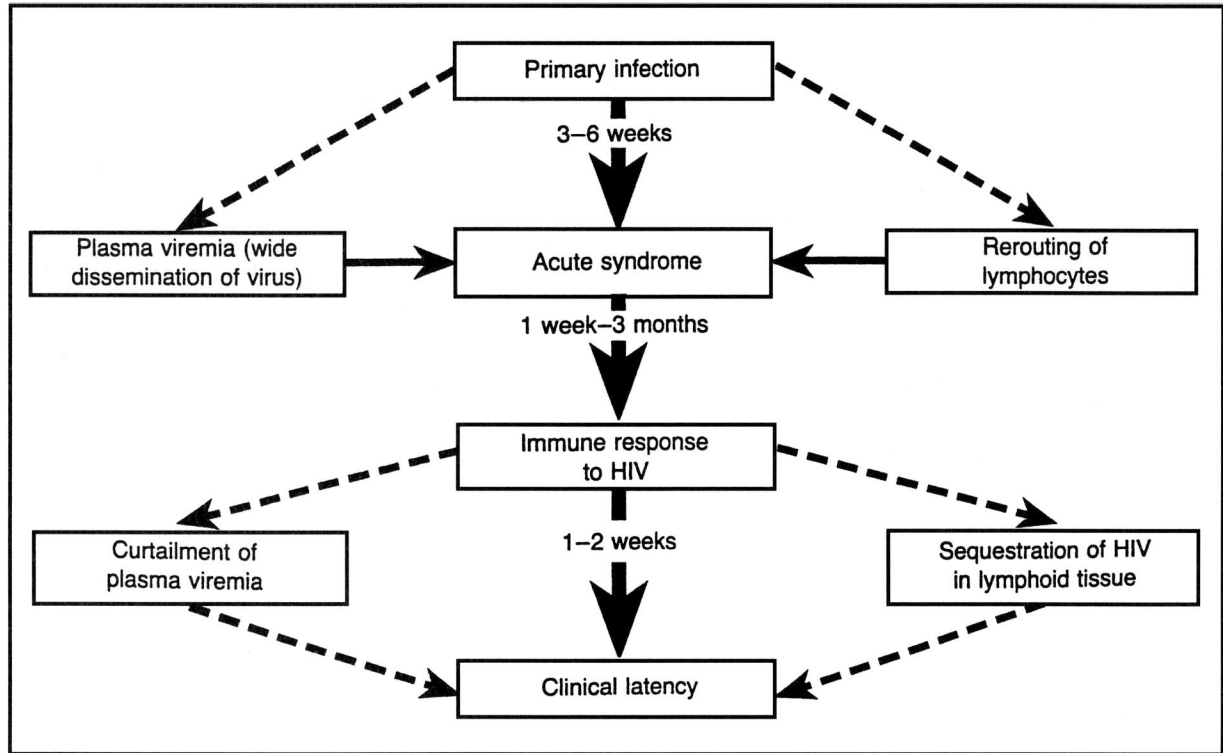

FIGURE 22-31 The progression of HIV infection from primary infection through the acute HIV syndrome to the stage of clinical latency. (From Pantaleo G, Graziosi C, Fauci AS: N Engl J Med 328:327, 1993.)

cells per microliter is usually associated with opportunistic infections (Figure 22-32).

There are two very rare patterns of HIV infection. One is an initial high level of antibody with a low-level viremia. There is subsequent loss of detectable viral anti-gen in the blood and later loss of circulating antibody. In these rare cases there are still low levels of viral DNA within lymphocytes. The small levels are only detected by the extremely sensitive and specific polymerase chain reaction (PCR) technique. The second rare pattern of

TABLE 22-13
Frequency of Symptoms and Findings Associated with Acute HIV-1 Infection

Symptom or Finding	Percentage of Patients
Fever	>80–90
Fatigue	>70–90
Rash	>40–80
Headache	32–70
Lymphadenopathy	40–70
Pharyngitis	50–70
Myalgia or arthralgia	50–70
Nausea, vomiting, or diarrhea	30–60
Night sweats	50
Aseptic meningitis	24
Oral ulcers	10–20
Genital ulcers	5–15
Thrombocytopenia	45
Leukopenia	40
Elevated hepatic-enzyme levels	21

From Kahn JO and Walker BD: N Engl J Med 339:33, 1998.

HIV infection is a low-level viral antigenemia with a prolonged (1 to 4 years) period of minimal HIV antibody production. The subject is thus infectious but may test negative for HIV antibody.

The duration of the latency period is affected not only by the regulatory genes and the degree of the viral mutation but also by host immunity. Host immunity is primarily via production of antibody against the HIV virus and via CD_8 cell, or killer lymphocyte, activity against infected CD_4 cells. When the host mechanisms are overwhelmed, the last stage of the disease, clinical AIDS, begins.

The symptoms of clinical AIDS are caused by a decline in the number and quality of the CD_4 lymphocytes. The CD_4 lymphocyte modulates almost all immune functions in the human immune system. Monocytes are also infected by HIV. These cells circulate throughout the body and then migrate after 1 to 4 days into peripheral tissues, including the CNS, carrying the virus with them.

As patients enter into an active disease state and the CD_4 count drops, general systemic symptoms often develop. The patient may experience leukoplakia, thrush, weight loss, diarrhea, fever, fatigue, and thrombocytopenia. Patients with CD_4 counts between 500 and 800 cells per microliter are more susceptible to community-acquired pneumonia, gastroenteritis, and general viral infections. As the CD_4 count drops below 500, patients may develop malignancies such as Kaposi's sarcoma and lymphoma.

Conditions Included in the 1993 AIDS Surveillance Case Definition

Candidiasis of bronchi, trachea, or lungs
Candidiasis, esophageal
Cervical cancer, invasive*
Coccidioidomycosis, disseminated or extrapulmonary
Cryptococcosis, extrapulmonary
Cryptosporidiosis, chronic intestinal (>1 month's duration)
Cytomegalovirus disease (other than liver, spleen, or nodes)
Cytomegalovirus retinitis (with loss of vision)
Encephalopathy, HIV-related
Herpes simplex: chronic ulcer(s) (>1 month's duration); or bronchitis pneumonitis, or esophagitis
Histoplasmosis, disseminated or extrapulmonary
Isosporiosis, chronic intestinal (>1 month's duration)
Kaposi's sarcoma
Lymphoma, Burkitt's (or equivalent term)
Lymphoma, immunoblastic (or equivalent term)
Lymphoma, primary, of brain
Mycobacterium avium complex or *M. kansasii*, disseminated or extrapulmonary
Mycobacterium tuberculosis, any site (pulmonary* or extrapulmonary)
Mycobacterium, other species or unidentified species, disseminated extrapulmonary
Pneumocystis carinii pneumonia
Pneumonia, recurrent*
Progressive multifocal leukoencephalopathy
Salmonella septicemia, recurrent
Toxoplasmosis of brain
Wasting syndrome due to HIV

From MMWR 41:1, 1992.

*Added in the 1993 expansion of the AIDS surveillance case definition.

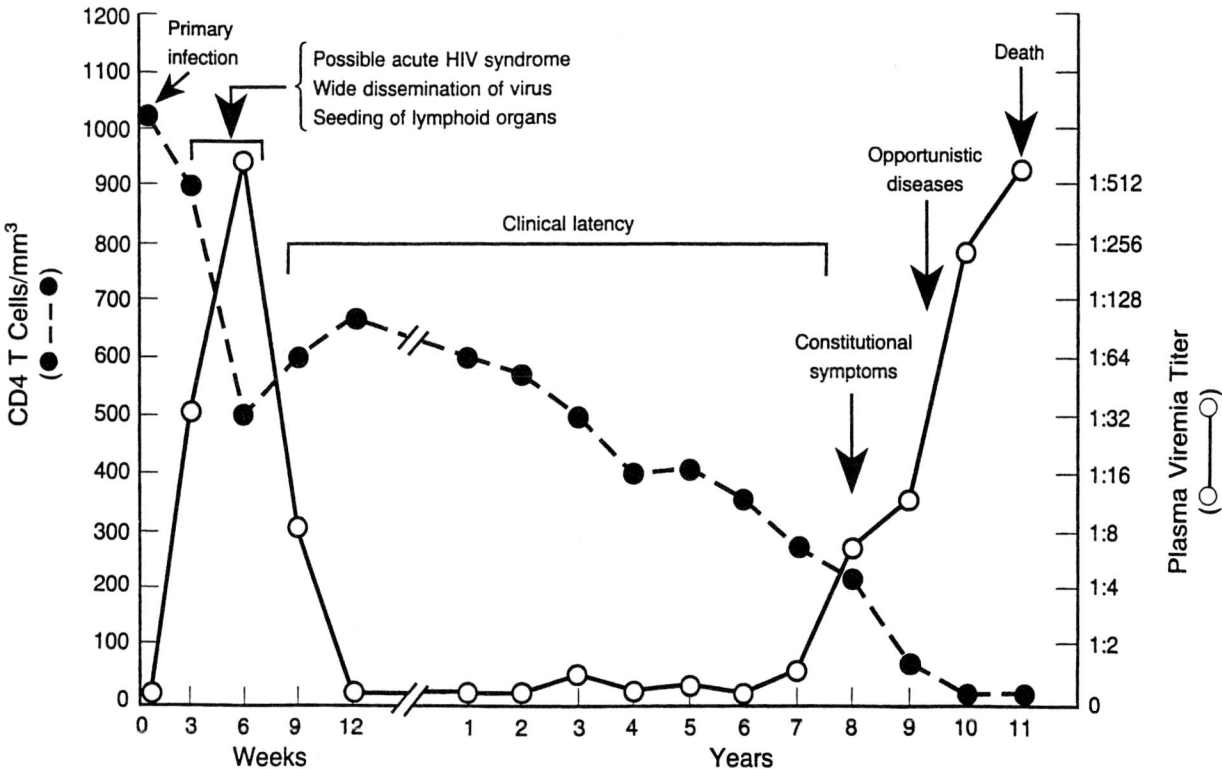

FIGURE 22-32 Typical course of HIV infection. (From Pantaleo G, Graziosi C, and Fauci AS: N Engl J Med 328:327, 1993.)

Before the AIDS epidemic, Kaposi's sarcoma was an extremely rare neoplasm of connective tissue and blood cells. It is usually a slow-growing cancer involving purple or reddish nodules or plaques on the skin and epithelium of the gastrointestinal tract. Kaposi's sarcoma associated with AIDS may involve lymph nodes and occasionally has a rapid downhill course. However, most individuals with Kaposi's sarcoma usually die of opportunistic infections. Kaposi's sarcoma is found much more commonly in men than in women. Twenty-three percent of male homosexual patients with AIDS develop Kaposi's sarcoma, compared with 3% of male heterosexual AIDS victims and 1% of women with the disease. As the CD_4 count drops below 200 cells per milliliter, opportunistic infections are found with increasing frequency. *P. carinii* pneumonia has been a common infection in AIDS patients. Trimethoprim/sulfamethoxazole and pentamidine have been found to be effective prophylactic agents in decreasing the incidence of this pneumonia. The clinical course in patients who develop *P. carinii* pneumonia varies from intermittent, slowly progressive disease to a fulminating infection with respiratory collapse and death in a few days.

Other common opportunistic infections in AIDS patients are listed in the box on this page, including disseminated viral, fungal, parasitic infections, as well as disseminated bacterial infections. Symptomatic infections with the following organisms are less common—*Listeria monocytogenes, Nocardia asteroides;* viruses—Epstein-Barr virus, adenovirus.

Common Opportunistic Infections in AIDS Patients

Bacteria
Mycobacterium tuberculosis
Mycobacterium avium-intracellulare
Mycobacterium fortuitum
Salmonella sp.
Legionella pneumophila

Fungi
Cryptococcus carinii
Candida sp.
Aspergillus sp.
Histoplasma capsulatum
Coccidioides immitis

Parasites
Pneumocystis carinii
Toxoplasma gondii
Cryptosporidium sp.
Isospora belli
Strongyloides stercoralis

Viruses
Cytomegalovirus
Herpes simplex virus
Varicella-zoster virus
JC virus (progressive multifocal leukoencephalopathy)

From Curran JW, Gold J, and Jaffe HW: The acquired immunodeficiency syndrome (AIDS). In Holmes KK, Mårdh PA, Sparling PF, et al, editors: Sexually transmitted diseases, ed 2, New York, 1990, McGraw-Hill Book Co.

Patients with AIDS often develop symptoms involving the CNS. One third of patients with HIV infection will initially present with CNS symptoms, and 80% to 90% of all AIDS patients eventually develop some aspect of the AIDS dementia complex (ADC) during their disease course. This syndrome is characterized by acute and subacute meningoencephalitis, peripheral neuropathy, cortical atrophy, dementia, memory loss, and a variety of psychiatric dysfunctions. Patients who present with CNS symptoms must be evaluated for infection, since many of the opportunistic infections of AIDS involve the CNS.

The screening test for AIDS is an enzyme-linked immunosorbent assay (ELISA) that tests for antibodies against the HIV virus. There are biologic false-positive and false-negative results related to nonspecific test factors and infections by viruses with similar antigens. The sensitivity of the ELISA test is approximately 95%, and the specificity is 99.7%. Thus, in a population group with a low disease prevalence for AIDS, of 100 positive ELISA tests, 99% may be false positive, with 1 true positive result. False-positive results are more common in multiparous women and women taking oral contraceptives. A more specific assay, the Western blot technique, is used to investigate individuals with persistently positive ELISA tests. The Western blot technique identifies antibodies to proteins of a specific molecular weight; it is, therefore, more specific than the ELISA test. The most specific test is the polymerase chain reaction (PCR), which tests specifically for HIV RNA molecules/ml.

Management of HIV has evolved around two themes: prevention and chemotherapy. From the clinician's perspective the major aspect of prevention involves education and contraceptive counseling. Education efforts should emphasize modes of transmission of the virus. "Safe sex," a term used frequently in the lay press, is a misnomer. "Safer sex" to avoid HIV infection includes the use of condoms and spermicides. Condom use will prevent HIV infection in the great majority of cases. It is not 100% effective, however. Latex condoms rather than "natural membrane" condoms should be used. Condoms made from animal intestines will not prevent viral transmission. The additional use of nonoxynol 9 will afford more protection against the HIV virus, as well as being more effective than condoms alone as a contraceptive agent. Nonoxynol 9 can be found in spermicides, foam, some condoms, and spermicidal gels. This agent destroys HIV. Education should also include information about risk factors that increase the likelihood of acquiring the infection, including sex when the individual has ulcers or abrasions or is sexually promiscuous. Many authors have emphasized that all patients should receive counseling about safe sex practices.

The treatment of AIDS currently focuses on chemotherapeutic agents that attack the virus' life cycle (Figure 22-33). A detailed description of chemotherapy protocols for HIV is beyond the scope of this text. However, general principles may be valuable to the reader.

The CDC has stated that the treatment of HIV involves "a complex array of behavioral, psychosocial, and medical facilities." Anti-HIV chemotherapy necessitates multiple drugs that have drug interactions and complicated side effects. Thus physicians trained and experienced in HIV management should be prescribing therapies.

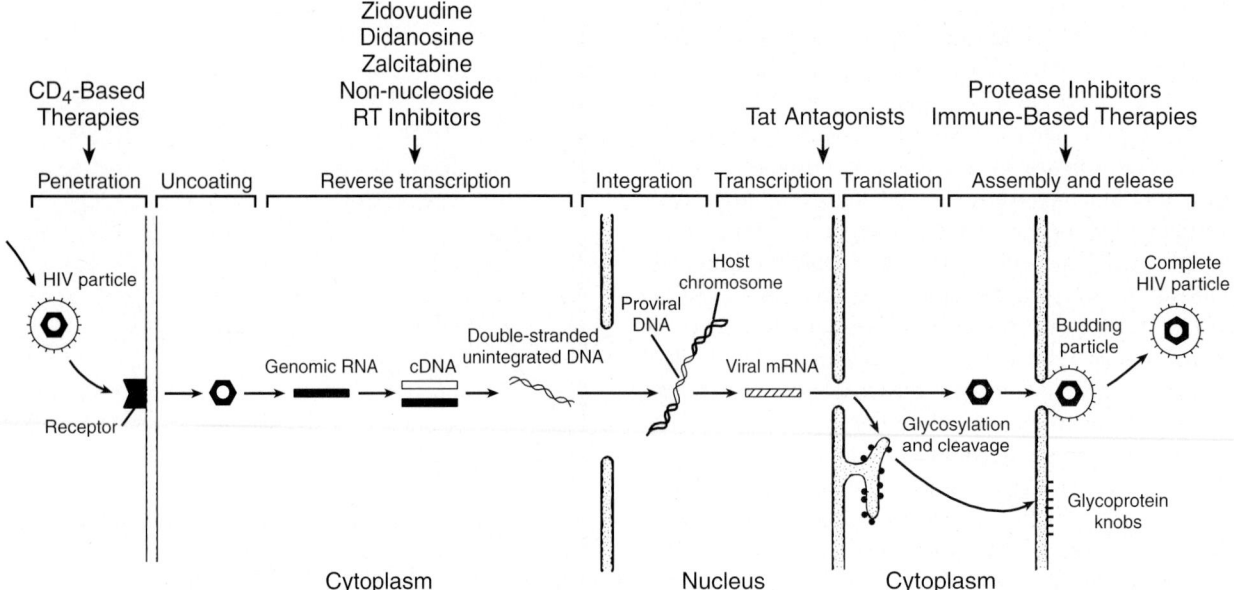

FIGURE 22-33 Diagram of the replicative cycle of HIV-1, showing the sites of action of antiviral agents. Various antiviral agents are shown at the top. RT denotes reverse transcriptase; cDNA, complementary DNA; and mRNA, messenger RNA. (From Hirsch MS and D'Aquila RT: N Engl J Med 328:1686, 1993.)

The classes of anti-HIV drugs include the nucleoside reverse transcriptase inhibitors (NPTI) of which zidovudine is the most well known; the nonnucleoside reverse transcriptase inhibitors (NNPTI); and protease inhibitors. The combinations of these drugs have been remarkably effective in increasing CD_4 counts and reducing viral loads. The plasma viral RNA measurements often are reduced to nondetectable levels. Monotherapy is not used in treating HIV because single drug regimens hasten the development of drug resistance. Combination therapy has been given the acronym HAART (highly active antiretroviral therapy).

Patients who begin chemotherapy for AIDS must be prepared to remain on the drugs for the rest of their lives; thus counseling is invaluable. Second-line treatments after viral mutations "break through" existing drugs include immunosuppressants such as hydroxyurea and cyclosporin. Also multidrug-resistant therapies may be used for second-line treatment and may include a combination of up to 9 first-line drugs. Combination therapy using simultaneous multiple-drug regimens is the most effective method of controlling the disease. Vaccine development for HIV is a difficult goal. The multiple strains of HIV-1 virus have been important impediments to the development of the vaccine.

For the gynecologist there are special concerns for the patient who has HIV infection because the virus and its immunosuppressive effects lead to an increase in gynecologic infections. Any ulcerative process increases susceptibility to HIV infection. Nonulcerative sexually transmitted diseases also may increase the likelihood of HIV transmission. Because of the susceptibility to generalized systemic infections, patients with HIV frequently present with vaginal symptoms. Genital herpes is a common problem for patients with HIV infection. Acyclovir can be used safely with this disease and does not interfere with zidovudine. Acyclovir dosages may need to be increased when treating acute herpetic infection in HIV patients, from 200 mg to 400 mg 5 times a day. Dosages greater than 200 mg 3 times a day are often necessary for suppressive therapy. Vaginal candidal infections are a frequent problem in patients with HIV infection, and recurrent candidiasis may be the presenting symptom of AIDS. Chronic antifungal suppression is often necessary. The development of mucocutaneous candidiasis is a marker for disease progression.

Primary syphilis increases the susceptibility to HIV infection. In addition, the effect of HIV on syphilis, because of the generalized immunosuppression, may be a more rapid progression of disease and a relative refractory response to standard antibiotic treatment. Syphilis appears more commonly as secondary syphilis in the HIV-infected patient. For early syphilis the treatment is the same as for individuals without HIV. However, serum markers should be retested at monthly intervals until a twofold dilution is seen. If there is not a twofold dilution, or if there is an increase in antisyphilis titer, then the patient should be considered refractory to treatment and the patient's CSF should be examined. Any patient with syphilis of unknown duration or latent syphilis should have a CSF examination. The CDC has recommended that neurosyphilis be considered in the differential diagnosis of neurologic disease in HIV-positive patients.

Several studies have noted an increase in human papillomavirus (HPV) infection among HIV-positive patients. Widespread HPV infections throughout the lower genital tract have been noted by several authors. An increased incidence of abnormal Pap smears with HPV-related atypia has also been noted among HIV-infected women. Several investigators have documented an increase in cervical intraepithelial neoplasia (CIN) among HIV patients. In one study Sun et al. noted that in seropositive HIV women the incidence of HPV infection was 60% compared with 36% of seronegative controls. Women with HPV and HIV were more likely to have CIN and VIN than women with HPV who do not have HIV. One study found a 7.3 times increased risk of condyloma and a 3 times increased risk of VIN in HIV positive women. In 1993 the CDC included invasive cervical cancer as one of the malignancies that places a patient in category C—full-blown AIDS. Patients with HIV infection and concomitant HPV infection should be screened carefully for CIN and VIN. Some authors suggest more frequent Pap smears in women who are HIV positive. Because of a more frequent occurrence and more rapid progression of dysplasia in women who are HIV positive, false-negative Pap smears are a concern. Some authors recommend regular colposcopy in addition to cytology for women with a history of CIN who are HIV positive. Cryotherapy is discouraged as a management of CIN in these patients. Women with normal CD_4 counts and two negative Pap smears can be followed with yearly cytology. All other women should be seen at least every 6 months.

Clinicians are legitimately concerned when treating patients with HIV infection about becoming infected themselves. Medical ethics dictate that patients be treated without prejudice for their disease. The American College of Obstetricians and Gynecologists has restated that it is unethical to refuse to "accept or continue to care" for persons solely on the basis of their HIV status. However, it is also in a physician's interest to take adequate precautions from becoming infected. Since over 90% of HIV-infected individuals are asymptomatic, and many patients do not know that they are HIV positive, we advise precautions be taken at all times. The CDC has recommended "universal blood and body fluid precautions" to minimize the risk of HIV infections. These are summarized in the box on page 688. Infection may occur after exposure to contaminated substances, body fluids, or secretions through any break in the skin. Abrasions or cuts on the hands, arms, or face, as well as ulcers on the mucous membrane, are susceptible sites for infection. Thus gowns and face and eye protection are advisable in all cases.

Universal Blood and Body Fluid Precautions

1. All blood and body fluids from all patients should be considered potentially infectious for HIV.
2. Barrier precautions such as masks and gowns should be used whenever contact with body fluids is anticipated.
3. Gloves should be worn when touching mucous membranes or nonintact skin, handling blood or body fluids, or touching surfaces contaminated with fluids.
4. Gloves and/or gowns should be changed after each contact.
5. Eyes, mouth, and nose should be protected by face shields, masks, and/or goggles during any procedure that may involve splashing of body fluids.
6. All blood and body fluids should be washed from hands and other skin surfaces immediately and completely even after gloves have been worn.
7. Never recap, bend, or break needles by hand or attempt to remove needles from disposable syringes.
8. Puncture-resistant disposable containers should be available and nearby at all times and, if possible, at every work site.
9. Resuscitation bags or mouthpieces should be available for emergency resuscitation in all appropriate places.

During operative procedures, studies have suggested that approximately 10% of gloves will be punctured. Double gloving decreases that rate by 60% to 80%. Thus double gloving will allow an individual only a 2% to 4% risk of hand contamination during any surgical case. The greatest risk of glove perforation occurs in surgeries longer than 3 hours with greater than 300 mL blood loss. If a needle puncture occurs through the skin, HIV infection may also occur. It is estimated that seroconversion will occur in 0.03% to 0.9% of hollow needle punctures. Thus HIV infection is extremely rare from a needle puncture. It is estimated that by the end of 1991, there were fewer than 50 health care workers who have developed HIV infection from exposures related to medical care. This is to be contrasted with a study from San Francisco General Hospital that indicated that cutaneous and parenteral exposures during surgeries occurred in 6.4% of cases despite precautions. The low number of reported HIV conversions compared with the high number of exposures is indicative of the difficulty of becoming infected from slight exposure.

Clinicians are often asked about the risk of developing AIDS from transfusion. In 1985 routine screening of all blood products for HIV was instituted in the United States. The current risk of developing HIV infection from blood transfusion is estimated to be 1:1,000,000 units transfused.

CERVICITIS

With the current and ongoing epidemic of sexually transmitted diseases, cervical infections have drawn increasing interest from both clinicians and epidemiologists. The cervix is a potential reservoir for *Neisseria gonorrhoeae, Chlamydia trachomatis,* herpes simplex virus, human papillomavirus, and *Mycoplasma* species. Often the patient is asymptomatic, even though the cervix is colonized with either gonorrheal or chlamydial organisms. The cervix acts as a barrier between the abundant bacterial flora of the vagina and the bacteriologically sterile endometrial cavity

and oviducts. Viral infections of the cervix such as herpes simplex and human papillomavirus are frequently associated with the development of cervical intraepithelial neoplasia. Bacterial infection of the endocervix becomes a major reservoir for sexual and perinatal transmission of pathogenic microorganisms. Primary cervical infection may result in secondary ascending infections including pelvic inflammatory disease and perinatal infections of the membranes, amniotic fluid, and parametria. Ectocervicitis is most frequently secondary to acute infection by herpes simplex virus, *T. vaginalis,* and *C. albicans.*

The semantics of cervical infections have recently been dramatically revised. Colposcopy has demonstrated that the redness that was believed to be inflammation is often the capillary bed below an area of ectopic columnar epithelia (ectopy). Cervicitis used to be diagnosed erroneously when the clinician was viewing an area of metaplasia or erosion. Therefore descriptive clinical terms such as *acute cervicitis, chronic cervicitis,* and *follicular* and *hypertrophic cervicitis* have been abandoned. In a similar fashion the histologic diagnosis of chronic cervicitis is so prevalent that it should be considered the norm for parous women of reproductive age. Current terminology emphasizes the site of cervical infection. Endocervicitis is usually secondary to bacterial infection with either *C. trachomatis* or *N. gonorrhoeae.* The most common site of *Chlamydia* infection in the female reproductive tract is the columnar cells of the endocervix. Ectocervical infections are generally either a virus or *Trichomonas vaginalis.* The histopathology of endocervicitis is characterized by a severe inflammatory reaction in the mucosa and submucosa. The tissues are infiltrated with a large number of polymorphonuclear cells and monocytes, and occasionally there is associated epithelial necrosis. Physiologically, there is a resident population of a small number of leukocytes in the normal cervix. Thus the emphasis is on a severe inflammatory reaction by a large number of polymorphonuclear cells.

The pathophysiologic relationship between cervical mucus and both lower and upper genital tract infections is beginning to be elucidated. Mucus is much more than a simple physical barrier; it exerts a definite bacteriostatic effect. Mucus may also act as a competitive inhibitor with bacteria for receptors on the endocervical epithelial cells. Cervical mucus also contains antibodies and inflammatory cells that are active against various sexually transmitted organisms. The present debate concerning the effect of oral contraceptives on the prevalence of serious upper tract pelvic infection may yield insight into the pathophysiology of cervical infection. Women taking oral contraceptives have a twofold to threefold increase in incidence of positive endocervical cultures for *C. trachomatis*. There are several hypotheses to explain this association. The cervical ectopy produced by oral contraceptives may preferentially facilitate adherence of *Chlamydia* organisms (Figure 22-34). Cultures of *Chlamydia* may be more productive from smears of columnar cells. The higher prevalence may simply reflect a higher isolation rate. It may relate to differences in sexual activity.

The cervix may become infected by a wide variety of viral, protozoal, and fungal organisms. Most of the sexually transmitted diseases may produce ulcerative lesions of the cervix. However, the principal infections of the cervix are caused by *N. gonorrhoeae, C. trachomatis,* herpes simplex, and human papillomavirus. This section will focus on mucopurulent cervicitis and techniques to diagnose common cervical infections.

Mucopurulent Cervicitis

During the past 10 years, the diagnosis of cervicitis has changed from a vague to a distinct clinical condition. Brunham et al. have described objective criteria to diagnose endocervical infections. They suggested the term *mucopurulent cervicitis* for the clinical diagnosis of active cervical infection. Two simple, definitive, objective criteria have been developed to establish this diagnosis—gross visualization of yellow mucopurulent material on a white cotton swab and the presence of 10 or more polymorphonuclear leukocytes per microscopic field (magnification × 1000) on Gram-stained smears obtained from the endocervix. An alternative clinical criteria that may be adopted is erythema and edema in an area of cervical ectopy, and/or associated with bleeding secondary to endocervical ulceration, or friability when the endocervical smear is obtained. In their original study, the Seattle group discovered that 40% of patients with sexually transmitted diseases had mucopurulent cervicitis (24% diagnosed by grossly visualized purulent material and 16% without mucopus but positive Gram stains of cervical mucus). However, the sensitivity, specificity, and positive predictive value of objective criteria have varied markedly in follow-up studies.

The prevalence of mucopurulent cervicitis depends on

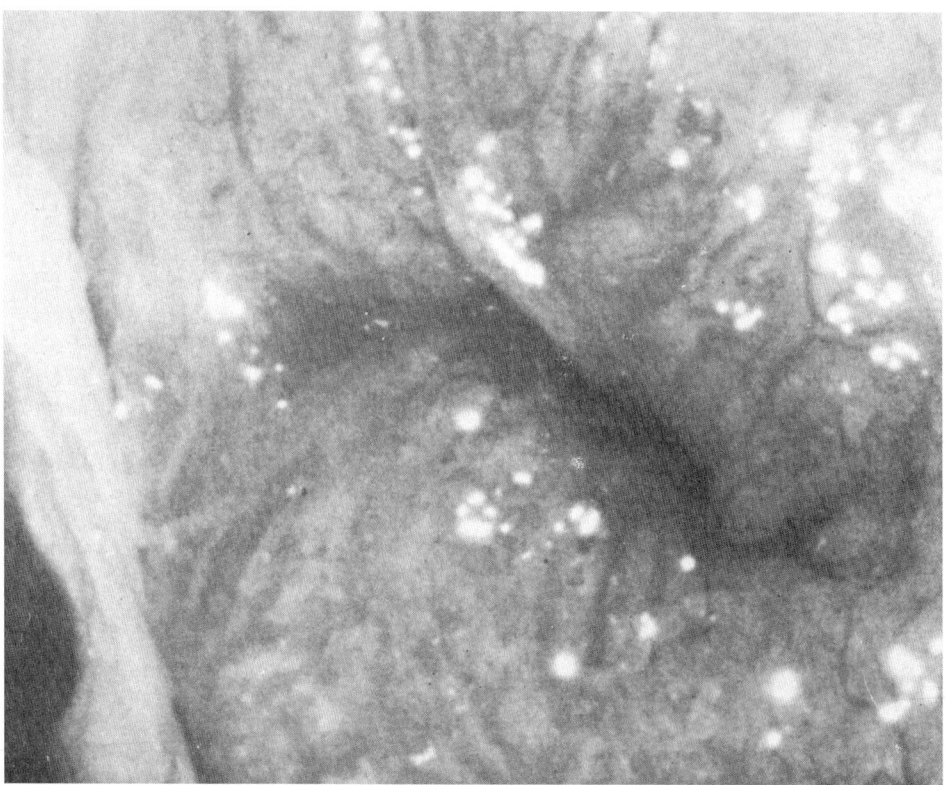

FIGURE 22-34 Colpophotograph of cervix infected with *Chlamydia trachomatis*, showing proliferation and dilation of subepithelial capillaries in zone of ectopy. (From Holmes KK: Lower genital tract infections in women: cystitis/urethritis, vulvovaginitis, and cervicitis. In Holmes KK, Mårdh PA, Sparling PF, et al, editors: Sexually transmitted diseases, New York, 1984, McGraw-Hill Book Co.)

the population being studied. Approximately 30% to 40% of women attending clinics for sexually transmitted diseases and 8% to 10% of women in university student health clinics have the condition. Greater than 60% of women with this disease are asymptomatic. Symptoms that suggest cervical infection include vaginal discharge, deep dyspareunia, and postcoital bleeding. The physical signs of a cervical infection are a cervix that is hypertrophic and edematous.

C. trachomatis is the cause of cervical infection in most women with mucopurulent cervicitis (Figure 22-35). In the initial study in Seattle, *Chlamydia* organisms were isolated from specimens of 20 of 40 women with mucopurulent cervicitis but only 2 of 60 without mucopurulent cervicitis. Mucopurulent cervicitis is present in approximately 40% to 60% of women in whom no cervical pathogen can be identified. Thus this condition often persists following adequate broad-spectrum antibiotic therapy. The presence of active herpes infection is correlated with ulceration of the exocervix but not with mucopus. *N. gonorrhoeae* was frequently isolated in this study, but its presence was not statistically significantly associated with either mucopus or 10 or more inflammatory cells per high-powered field. The mean number of inflammatory cells with positive gonorrheal cultures was 1.9 per high-powered field. Regardless of the results of the Seattle

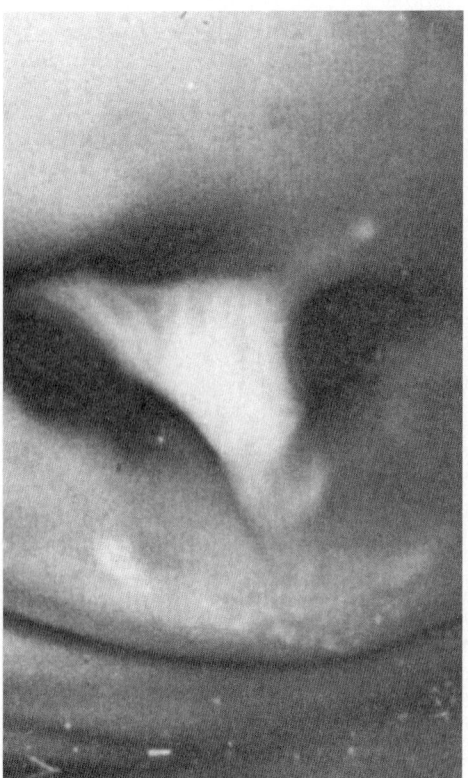

FIGURE 22-35 Mucopurulent cervicitis caused by *C. trachomatis*. (From Holmes KK, Mårdh PA, Sparling PF, et al, editors: Sexually transmitted diseases, ed 2, New York, 1990, McGraw-Hill Book Co.)

study, most authorities believe that gonorrhea is an important cause of mucopurulent cervicitis. However, the majority of women who have lower reproductive tract infections by *C. trachomatis* or *N. gonorrhoeae* do not have mucopurulent cervicitis. The corollary is that the majority of women who have mucopurulent cervicitis are not infected by *C. trachomatis* or *N. gonorrhoeae*.

Special care must be taken in obtaining the cervical smears to establish a diagnosis of mucopurulent cervicitis. Initially a large cotton swab is used to absorb the vaginal secretions from the upper vagina and wipe away the mucus from the exocervix. Next a small white cotton swab is inserted into the endocervical canal. It is inspected grossly for the presence of yellow purulent material, gross pus from the endocervix being similar to the purulent urethral discharge in a male. Subsequently, the swab is rolled on a glass slide, and the slide is dried and Gram stained. The slide is scanned to identify strands of cervical mucus containing areas of inflammatory cells. If 10 or more polymorphonuclear leukocytes are seen at a magnification of 1000, a positive diagnosis has been made. A culture for gonorrheal organisms should also be obtained, as the two organisms will be found simultaneously in approximately one third of cervical infections. Menstruation or the presence of vaginal squamous cells destroys the validity of the slide. Endocervical leukocytes are a normal physiologic response to the deposition of sperm in the cervical canal. Therefore, if sperm are present, leukocyte presence indicates only a physiologic response of the cervix and not a pathologic reaction.

The treatment of choice for mucopurulent cervicitis if *N. gonorrhoeae* is not found on Gram stain or endocervical culture is oral doxycycline 100 mg twice a day for 7 days or azithromycin 1 g orally in a single dose (see box on opposite page). Clinical studies have demonstrated that azithromycin and doxycycline are equally effective. However, azithromycin is the drug of choice in women who are likely to have minimal follow-up and poor compliance because it provides a single dose of therapy that may be directly observed. Alternative regimens include ofloxacin 300 mg orally 2 times a day for 7 days, or erythromycin base 500 mg orally 4 times a day for 7 days, or erythromycin ethylsuccinate 800 mg orally 4 times a day for 7 days. The male partner should receive identical therapy. Obviously, if the Gram stain or culture is positive for gonorrhea, tetracycline treatment alone is not sufficient because of the possibility of tetracycline-resistant *N. gonorrhoeae*. Thus the patient should be treated with ceftriaxone, 125 mg intramuscularly, or cefixime 400 mg orally in a single dose, or ciprofloxacin 500 mg orally in a single dose, or ofloxacin 400 mg orally. Routine dual therapy for gonococcal and chlamydial infections is indicated if the women come from a population in which chlamydial infections are found simultaneously with 20% to 40% of gonococcal infections. The cost of therapy for chlamydia is much less than the cost of testing. The CDC recommends doxycycline 100 mg orally twice a day for 7

Recommended Regimens for Treatment of Chlamydial Infection

Recommended Regimens
Azithromycin 1 g orally in a single dose,
OR
Doxycycline 100 mg orally twice a day for 7 days.

Alternative Regimens
Erythromycin base 500 mg orally four times a day for 7 days,
OR
Erythromycin ethylsuccinate 800 mg orally four times a day for 7 days,
OR
Ofloxacin 300 mg orally twice a day for 7 days.

From CDC 1998 Guidelines for Treatment of Sexually Transmitted Diseases, MMWR 47:54, 1997.

---

days or azithromycin 1 g orally in a single dose for possible coinfection with *C. trachomatis*. Women treated for chlamydia should be instructed to abstain from sexual intercourse for 7 days after single-dose therapy or until completion of the 7-day regimen.

The genital mycoplasmas, *Mycoplasma hominis* and *Ureaplasma urealyticum*, are frequently isolated from both the vagina and endocervix. Colonization rates as high as 75% have been reported. The exact role of genital mycoplasmas in producing either bacterial vaginosis or active cervical infection is unclear. Paavonen and Wolner-Hanssen reported that genital mycoplasmas do not produce mucopurulent cervicitis.

The key teaching point is that many women harboring sexually transmitted pathogens in the cervix are asymptomatic.

Detection of Pathogenic Cervical Bacteria

Neisseria Gonorrhoeae

The diagnosis of cervical infection from *N. gonorrhoeae* is made by culture of the endocervical mucus. The majority of women who are colonized with gonorrhea are asymptomatic. Therefore, it is important to routinely screen women at high risk for gonorrheal infection with cultures of mucus from the endocervical canal. Screening of high-risk individuals is the primary way to control the disease. Gram staining of the endocervical mucus has a sensitivity of only 50% to 60% and a specificity of approximately 95% in asymptomatic women. Thus culture of endocervical mucus directly on modified Thayer-Martin containing antibiotics or similar selective media is the diagnostic standard. A dry cotton swab should be rotated deep in the endocervical canal for 15 to 20 seconds. A single endocervical culture will detect approximately 85% of cervical infections. A culture from a second consecutive endocervi-

cal cotton swab will increase detection approximately 7% to 10%. If a separate rectal swab specimen is cultured, the accuracy of diagnosing gonorrhea increases to 93%. Additional cultures of the pharynx, urethra, and ducts of accessory sex glands may be obtained depending on the patient's symptoms and sexual habits. Culture of the urethra gives the highest yield in women who previously have had an abdominal or vaginal hysterectomy. Although transport media are available, it is important for the culture to reach the laboratory within 24 hours or there will be a loss of sensitivity. Growth of *N. gonorrhoeae* in culture is best at 37° C and in an environment between 2% and 10% carbon dioxide.

Recently, reliable nonculture assays for gonorrhea have been developed. These tests are valuable for clinics that are located a considerable distance from their bacteriologic laboratory and thus the culture cannot be performed within 24 hours. One of these tests is a nonamplified DNA-probe test, which has a sensitivity ranging from 89% to 97% and a specificity of 99%. Another test, the ligase chain reaction assay, has been extensively tested and is excellent for screening urine specimens for *N. gonorrhoeae*. The ligase chain reaction assay is equally sensitive to culture methods when using endocervical swabs. Screening of urine is especially practical in young teenagers who are not cooperative or who are frightened by pelvic exams.

It is important to test positive cultures for sensitivity to penicillin and other antibiotics. The treatment for gonococcal urethritis and cervicitis recommended by the CDC changes periodically. These changes are based on the increasing trends of the development of antibiotic-resistant *N. gonorrhoeae*, including penicillinase-producing *N. gonorrhoeae*, tetracycline-resistant *N. gonorrhoeae*, fluoroquinolones-resistant *N. gonorrhoeae*, and strains with chromosomally mediated resistance to multiple antibiotics, including penicillin and spectinomycin. In 1995 penicillinase-producing strains of *N. gonorrhoeae* caused approximately 13% of gonorrheal infections in the United States. The genetic-resistant strains have a prevalence of 15% to 20% in major urban areas in the Northeast. Two other considerations are given high priority when choosing an antibiotic: single-dose efficacy and simultaneously treating coexisting chlamydial infection. *C. trachomatis* has been found to simultaneously colonize women with gonorrhea in almost 50% of cases. The present recommended parenteral regimen is ceftriaxone, 125 mg intramuscularly one time. Alternatively, cefixime, ciprofloxacin, or ofloxacin may be given in a single oral dose. These regimens have documented cure rates of greater than 95% in uncomplicated anogenital gonorrhea. Ceftriaxone or ofloxacin cure greater than 90% of pharyngeal gonorrhea. For patients who are allergic or intolerant to cephalosporins and quinolones, the number-one alternative is spectinomycin, 2 g intramuscularly in a single dose (see the box on page 692). In addition to the antibiotics for gonorrhea, the CDC recommends treating with oral doxycycline, 100 mg twice daily for 7 days, or azithromycin 1 g orally in a single dose, because almost 50% of patients with gonorrhea have coexisting chlamydial infection (see box this page).

If the woman is asymptomatic, follow-up cultures are no longer recommended by the CDC as a test of cure for lower tract infections (uncomplicated gonorrhea). Women with positive cultures for gonorrhea should have a serologic test for syphilis in 4 to 6 weeks, even though patients with incubating syphilis are usually cured by antibiotic combinations of ceftriaxone and tetracycline. Similarly, patients should be offered informed consent and testing for HIV infection.

Chlamydia Trachomatis

For years the gold standard of techniques used to identify *C. trachomatis* infection was isolation of this intracellular organism in tissue culture. Recently introduced to clinical practice are a polymerase chain reaction (PCR) assay and a deoxyribonucleic acid (DNA) probe assay. Both tests are essentially equivalent to standard tissue culture in terms of sensitivity and specificity, and positive and negative predictive value. They are rapidly replacing culture techniques even in populations in which the prevalence of the disease is low and the women are asymptomatic. Because *C. trachomatis* is an obligatory intracellular organism, it is mandatory to obtain epithelial cells to maximize the percentage of positive cultures. A dacron, rayon, or calcium alginate swab is placed in the endocervical canal. It is rotated for 15 to 20 seconds to gently abrade the columnar epithelium. The cytobrush, which was developed primarily to enhance sampling of endocervical cells for cytology, has been discovered to be the optimal instrument for appropriate sampling of *Chlamydia* as well. The swab is placed in an antibiotic-containing transport medium and stored at 4° C. A specimen that is predominately a mucopurulent discharge or from a cotton-tipped swab with a wooden stick are not adequate to produce a positive culture. It is important to inoculate the definitive culture within 24 hours. Freezing and thawing of the transport medium decrease the eventual yield of positive cultures. Cultures are incubated on McCoy cell monolayers. Subsequently, in approximately 48 to 72 hours, the monolayers are stained and examined microscopically for inclusions. The exact sensitivity of culture techniques is not known. Most experts estimate the sensitivity to be approximately 75%, depending primarily on the adequacy of sampling infected epithelial cells. Laboratories that routinely add a blind second passage following negative cultures may identify approximately 15% of additional infections.

Rapid, simple, and sensitive methods to detect chlamydial antigens have been introduced. These tests are less expensive than culture and are most appropriate for screening when the prevalence of infection exceeds 10%. One test uses fluorescein-conjugated monoclonal antibodies to detect elementary bodies of *C. trachomatis*. This slide test may be performed on endocervical smears and takes less than 30 minutes to complete. Tam et al. and Stamm et al. have published large series comparing this monoclonal antibody test with traditional tissue culture methods. For women the rapid slide test (MicroTrak, Syva) has a sensitivity of 86% to 93% and a specificity of 93% to 99%. False-positive and false-negative results were discovered in slide specimens containing a limited number of

---

Centers for Disease Control Recommended Treatment of Uncomplicated Gonococcal Infections of the Cervix, Urethra, and Rectum in Adults (1997)

Recommended Regimens:
  Cefixime 400 mg orally in a single dose
    OR
  Ceftriaxone 125 mg intramuscularly in a single dose
    OR
  Ciprofloxacin 500 mg orally in a single dose,
    OR
  Ofloxacin 400 mg orally in a single dose
    PLUS
  Azithromycin 1 gram orally in a single dose,
    OR
  Doxycycline 100 mg orally 2 times a day for 7 days

Alternative Regimens:
  1. Spectinomycin 2 g intramuscularly in a single dose
  2. Injectable cephalosporins such as ceftizoxime 500 mg intramuscularly, cefotaxime 500 mg intramuscularly, cefotetan 1 g intramuscularly, cefoxitin 2 g intramuscularly with probenecid 1 g orally, all as a single dose
  3. Other quinolones such as enoxacin 400 mg orally, lomefloxacin 400 mg orally, or norfloxacin 800 mg orally, all as a single dose

From CDC: MMWR 47:60, 1997

organisms. This slide test is approximately one third as expensive as cell culture techniques. There is only one major drawback to the direct test. There is a subjective assessment in reading the immunofluorescence, which necessitates several hours of training by laboratory personnel. The second method uses the ELISA assay (Chlamydiazyme, Abbot Laboratories), takes about 3 to 4 hours, requires a spectrophotometer, and has a sensitivity and specificity similar to the fluorescent monoclonal antibody test. A limitation of the ELISA method is the false positives that result from nonspecific binding or cross reactivity to other antigens. Gen-probe PACE-2 is a diagnostic test that uses DNA hybridization to detect chlamydia. Its sensitivity and specificity for endocervical and urethral specimens is similar to the other two rapid tests. Regretfully, the sensitivity of these methods for screening urine specimens has been approximately 50% as compared to culture.

Newer techniques have been introduced into clinical practice to rapidly detect *C. trachomatis* directly from swabs from the cervix or vaginal introitus. They are DNA amplification techniques using polymerase chain reaction or ligase chain reaction. Clinical studies have found them to be essentially equivalent to standard tissue culture. Both tests are simple, convenient, and reliable even in low-risk populations. For screening, a urine sample can be used for testing, which avoids the painful urethral swab method. In summary, the selection of the most appropriate diagnostic test for detecting lower genital tract infection with *Chlamydia* primarily depends on the prevalence of *C. trachomatis* in the population to be tested and whether the sample is a smear or from a urine specimen. PCR, DNA probe assays, and cell culture are most appropriate for screening low-risk populations. If the prevalence of infection is greater than 10%, then either the fluorescent monoclonal antigen test or the ELISA test are appropriate screening tools.

Attempts have been made to diagnose chlamydial cervical infection from routine Pap smears. However, at best this is a nonsensitive, nonspecific method to judge acute cervical inflammation and will be positive in only approximately one out of four infected females.

KEY POINTS

- The prevalence of STD infections in the United States currently is estimated to be 12 million individuals with approximately 3 million of these infections occurring in teenagers.

- The three most prevalent primary viral infections of the skin of the vulva are genital herpes, condyloma acuminatum, and molluscum contagiosum.

- Acute bacterial cystitis is characterized by abrupt onset and multiple symptoms, including dysuria, urgency, and frequent voiding. Suprapubic tenderness is a specific sign for acute bacterial cystitis; however, it is not present in the majority of patients.

- The differential diagnosis of adult women with dysuria includes acute cystitis, acute urethritis, or vulvovaginitis.

- The most frequent pathogens involved in uncomplicated lower urinary tract infection are *Escherichia coli* (approximately 80%) and *Staphylococcus saprophyticus* (approximately 5% to 15%).

- For the first episode of acute, uncomplicated cystitis the current treatment of choice is 3 days of oral therapy with trimethoprim/sulfamethoxazole, trimethoprim alone, or one of the quinolones such as ciprofloxacin or norfloxacin.

- More than 90% of recurrences in young women are exogenous reinfection with new isolates arising from local flora.

- A normal Bartholin's gland cannot be palpated. Approximately 2% of adult women develop enlargement of both Bartholin's glands.

- The treatment of choice for a symptomatic Bartholin's cyst or abscess is the development of a fistulous tract from the dilated Bartholin's duct to the vestibule.

- Excision of Bartholin's duct and gland is indicated for persistent deep infection, multiple recurrences of abscesses, or enlargement of the gland in a woman over the age of 40. Removal of a Bartholin's gland for recurrent infection should be performed when the infection is quiescent.

- Pediculosis pubis, an infestation by the crab louse *Phthirus pubis,* is characterized by constant itching, predominantly vulvar involvement, and the finding of eggs and lice by visual inspection. It may be treated by topical application of 1% permethrin cream rinse (Nix) or 1% lindane shampoo (Kwell).

- Scabies, an infection by the itch mite *Sarcoptes scabiei,* is characterized by intermittent pruritus, most commonly in the hands, wrists, breasts, vulva, and buttocks. It is diagnosed by a scraping of the papules, vesicles, or burrows in which the mites live and inspection under the microscope. It may be treated by topical application of 5% permethrin cream (Nix) or 1% lindane lotion or 30 g of cream.

- Permethrin is more expensive than lindane, and permethrin has less potential for toxicity in the event of inappropriate use. Seizures have been reported when lindane was applied immediately after a bath or in women with extensive dermatitis. Lindane is not recommended during pregnancy or for lactating women or children under the age of 2.

- Molluscum contagiosum in adults is an asymptomatic viral disease primarily of the vulvar skin. It is a common generalized skin disease in adults with immunodeficiency, especially HIV infection.

- Condyloma acuminatum presents as a clinically recognizable macroscopic lesion in 30% of infected women and as a subclinical infection in 70% of women.

- Condyloma acuminatum is a sexually transmitted disease spread by skin-to-skin contact. It is caused by the human papillomavirus (HPV). Autoinoculation also occurs. It is a highly contagious disease.

- Dermatologically, there are four morphologic types of genital warts: the cauliflower-shaped condyloma acuminata, smooth papular (1 to 4 mm papules), keratotic (resembling a seborrheic keratosis), and flat. Condyloma acuminata–type warts tend to occur primarily on moist surfaces.

- Vaginal condyloma are identified in approximately one of three women with vulvar disease.

- No present therapy of HPV eliminates subclinical infection from the surrounding epithelium.

- Genital herpes is a recurrent, incurable, sexually transmitted disease that has reached epidemic proportions. Tragically, approximately 80% of the individuals are unaware they are infected.

- Genital herpes is most frequently transmitted by individuals who are asymptomatic and unaware that they have the infection at the time of transmission.

- From a clinical standpoint the important difference between HSV-1 and HSV-2 is that the frequency of recurrence is 4 times greater following a primary infection with HSV-2 compared with HSV-1.

- The primary infection by herpes is both a local and a systemic disease. The majority of symptomatic women have severe vulvar pain, tenderness, and inguinal adenopathy. However, subclinical primary herpes infection is common.

- Oral acyclovir has been shown to be beneficial in reducing the duration of herpetic ulcerative lesions and in reducing the time that the virus can be isolated from these lesions.

- Patients with frequent episodes of recurrent genital herpes may be successfully treated with prophylactic oral acyclovir. The primary goals of continuous suppressive therapy are to limit the severity and number of occurrences as well as to give the woman a sense of control over her disease.

- Granuloma inguinale, also known as donovanosis, is a chronic, ulcerative, bacterial infection of the skin and subcutaneous tissue of the vulva.

- Granuloma inguinale may be managed by a wide range of oral broad-spectrum antibiotics.

- Lymphogranuloma venereum (LGV) is a sexually transmitted disease produced by serotypes L_1, L_2, and L_3 of *C. trachomatis*.

- The treatment for lymphogranuloma venereum is oral doxycycline, 100 mg twice a day for 3 weeks. An alternative regimen is erythromycin base 500 mg every 6 hours for 3 to 6 weeks.

- Chancroid is a sexually transmitted, acute, ulcerative disease of the vulva. The soft chancre of chancroid is always painful and tender. In comparison, the hard chancre of syphilis is usually asymptomatic.

- Syphilis is a chronic complex systemic disease produced by the spirochete *Treponema pallidum*.

- Early syphilis is a cofactor in the transmission and acquisition of HIV.

- Dark-field microscopy rather than normal light microscopy is used for detection of syphilis because of the extreme thinness of the spirochete *Treponema pallidum*.

- Quantitative nontreponemal antibody titers usually correlate with the activity of syphilis.

- Nonspecific tests for syphilis, the VDRL and RPR, have a 1% false positive rate. Many conditions produce biologic false-positive results, including a recent febrile illness, pregnancy, immunization, chronic active hepatitis, malaria, sarcoidosis, intravenous drug use, and autoimmune diseases such as lupus erythematosus or rheumatoid arthritis. Therefore, specific tests such as the TPI, FTA-ABS, and MHA-TP must be employed when a positive nonspecific test result is encountered.

- A woman with a positive reactive treponemal test usually will have this positive reaction for her lifetime regardless of treatment or the activity of the disease.

- The characteristic chancre of primary syphilis is a red, round ulcer with firm, well-formed, raised edges, with a nonpurulent clean base and yellow-gray exudate. During the first week of clinical disease, the woman develops regional adenopathy that is nontender and firm.

- A woman with syphilis is most infectious during the first 1 to 2 years of her disease with decreasing infectivity thereafter.

- Tertiary syphilis develops in approximately 33% of patients who are not appropriately treated during the primary, secondary, or latent phases of the disease.

- Concurrent HIV infection should be considered in patients with syphilis. It is optimal for all women with syphilis to be tested for HIV infection.

- Sexual partners of women with syphilis in any stage should be evaluated both clinically and serologically.

- In middle-class women in the reproductive age range, bacterial vaginosis represents approximately 50% of vaginitis, while candidiasis and *Trichomonas* infection represent approximately 25% each.

- The normal vaginal environment is a dynamic and delicate ecosystem, with a pH of approximately 4.0 in premenopausal women.

- A vaginal pH of greater than 5.0 indicates atrophic vaginitis, bacterial vaginosis, or *Trichomonas* infection, whereas a vaginal pH of less than 4.5 in a symptomatic woman is either a physiologic discharge or fungal infection.

- Bacterial vaginosis results when high concentrations of anaerobic bacteria replace the normal H_2O_2-producing lactobacillus species in the vagina. Histologically, there is an absence of inflammation in biopsies of the vagina.

- The classic criteria for the diagnosis of bacterial vaginosis are (1) a homogeneous vaginal discharge is present; (2) the vaginal discharge has a pH equal to or greater than 4.5; (3) the vaginal discharge has an aminelike odor when mixed with potassium hydroxide; and (4) a wet smear of the vaginal discharge demonstrates clue cells greater in number than 20% of the number of the vaginal epithelial cells.

- Ironically, 50% of women who have three of the four clinical criteria for bacterial vaginosis are asymptomatic.

- The recommended regimen of treatment for bacterial vaginosis is oral metronidazole (Flagyl), 500 mg twice daily for 7 days. An alternative regimen is metronidazole 2 g orally in a single dose.

- *Trichomonas* vaginal infection is the most prevalent nonviral, nonchlamydial sexually transmitted disease of women. *Trichomonas* is the etiologic factor for approximately one in four episodes of infectious vaginitis.

- *T. vaginalis* is a highly contagious sexually transmitted disease. Following a single sexual contact, at least two thirds of both male and female sexual partners become infected.

- Dysuria is a symptom in approximately one of five women with symptomatic *Trichomonas* infection.

- The asymptomatic female who has *Trichomonas* identified in the lower female genital urinary tract definitely should be treated. Extended follow-up studies have shown that one in three asymptomatic females will become symptomatic within 3 months.

- *Candida* vaginitis is produced by a ubiquitous, airborne, gram-positive fungus. The vast majority of cases are caused by *Candida albicans,* with 5% to 20% of vaginal fungal infections produced by *C. glabrata* or *C. tropicalis.*

- *Candida* species are part of the normal flora of approximately 25% of women, being a commensal saprophytic organism on the mucosal surface of the vagina. When the ecosystem of the vagina is disturbed, *Candida* becomes an opportunistic pathogen.

- Recurrent vulvovaginal candidiasis is defined as four or more episodes of symptomatic lower tract infection within 12 months.

- Toxic shock syndrome (TSS) is an acute, febrile illness, produced by a bacterial exotoxin with a fulminating downhill course involving dysfunction of multiple organ systems.

- Approximately 50% of cases of TSS are related to menses, and 50% are not. Severe postoperative infections by *Streptococcus pyogenes* may produce a similar toxic shock syndrome.

- Because of the severity of the disease, gynecologists should have a high index of suspicion for TSS in a woman who has an unexplained fever and a rash during or immediately following her menstrual period.

- The initial rash of TSS over the first 48 hours is similar in appearance to an intense sunburn. Over the next several days it evolves into a macular rash with fine, flaky desquamation over the face and trunk and sloughing of the entire skin thickness over the palms and soles.

- The differential diagnosis of toxic shock syndrome includes Rocky Mountain spotted fever, streptococcal scarlet fever, and leptospirosis.

- Current estimates are that approximately one in every 300 individuals in the United States is infected with HIV.

- There are three primary methods of contracting HIV: intimate sexual contact; use of contaminated needles or blood products, especially in hemophiliacs; and perinatal transmission from mother to child.

- The immune defects of AIDS are caused by infection of CD_4 lymphocytes (helper T cells) by the HIV virus.

- Both ulcerative and nonulcerative sexually transmitted diseases increase the likelihood of HIV transmission.

- Bacterial infection of the endocervix becomes a major reservoir for sexual and perinatal transmission of pathogenic microorganisms.

- Sperm-induced leukocyte presence in the endocervical mucus is a physiologic response.

- The most common site of *Chlamydia* infection in the female reproductive tract is the columnar cells of the endocervix.

- Symptoms that suggest cervical infection include vaginal discharge, deep dyspareunia, and postcoital bleeding. *Chlamydia trachomatis* is the major etiologic agent in women with mucopurulent cervicitis.

- The majority of women who have lower reproductive tract infections by *C. trachomatis* or *N. gonorrhoeae* do not have mucopurulent cervicitis. The corollary is the majority of women who have mucopurulent cervicitis are not infected by *C. trachomatis* or *N. gonorrhoeae*.

- Routine dual therapy for gonococcal and chlamydial infections is indicated if the woman comes from a population in which chlamydial infections are found simultaneously with 20% to 40% of gonococcal infections.

- Many women harboring sexually transmitted pathogens in the cervix are asymptomatic.

- Culture is the standard technique for diagnosis of *Neisseria gonorrhoeae* because Gram stain smears are positive for only 50% of women with positive cultures. Culture of a second consecutive endocervical cotton swab will increase detection of *Neisseria gonorrhoeae* by approximately 7% to 10%.

- If the woman is asymptomatic, follow-up cultures are no longer recommended by the CDC as a test of cure for lower tract infections (uncomplicated gonorrhea).

- For detection of *N. gonorrhoeae*, culture of the urethra gives the highest yield in women who previously have had an abdominal or vaginal hysterectomy.

- Newer techniques have been introduced into clinical practice to rapidly detect *C. trachomatis* directly from swabs from the cervix or vaginal introitus. They are DNA amplification techniques using polymerase chain reaction or ligase chain reaction. Clinical studies have found them to be essentially equivalent to standard tissue culture.

BIBLIOGRAPHY

Abulafia O and Sherer DM: Bartholin gland abscess: sonographic findings, J Clin Ultrasound 25:47, 1997.

American Medical Association: Genital herpes: a clinician's guide to diagnosis and treatment, part I, Evans RM and Brakl MJ, eds, AMA Continuing Medical Education Program, 1997.

American Medical Association: Genital herpes: a clinician's guide to diagnosis and treatment, part II, Evans RM and Brakl MJ, eds, AMA Continuing Medical Education Program, 1997.

American Medical Association: External genital warts: diagnosis and treatment, Evans RM and Wiley D, eds, AMA Continuing Medical Education Program, 1997.

Andersen PG, Christensen S, Detlefsen GU, and Kern-Hansen P: Treatment of Bartholin's abscess: marsupialization versus incision, curettage and suture under antibiotic cover. A randomized study with 6 months' follow-up, Acta Obstet Gynecol Scand 71:59, 1992.

Antonelli N, Diehl SJ, and Wright JW: A randomized trial of intravaginal nonoxynol 9 versus oral metronidazole in the treatment of vaginal trichomoniasis, Am J Obstet Gynecol 182:1008, 2000.

Armstrong DKB, Maw RD, Dinsmore WW, et al: A randomized, double-blind, parallel group study to compare subcutaneous interferon alpha-2a plus podophyllin with placebo plus podophyllin in the treatment of primary condylomata acuminata, Genitourin Med 70:389, 1994.

Arav-Boger R, Leibovici L, and Danon YL: Urinary tract infections with low and high colony counts in young women: spontaneous remission and single-dose vs multiple-day treatment, Arch Intern Med 154:300, 1994.

Augenbraun M, Feldman J, Chirgwin K, et al: Increased genital shedding of herpes simplex virus Type 2 in HIV-seropositive women, Ann Intern Med 123:845, 1995.

Avorn J, Monane M, Gurqitz JH, et al: Reduction of bacteriuria and pyuria after ingestion of cranberry juice, JAMA 271:751, 1994.

Barbosa C, Macasaet M, Brockmann S, et al: Pelvic inflammatory disease and human immunodeficiency virus infection, Obstet Gynecol 89:65, 1997.

Barbosa-Cesnik CT, Gerbase A, and Heymann D: STD vaccines—an overview, Genitourin Med 73:336, 1997.

Barrasso R, De Brux J, Croissant O, and Orth G: High prevalence of papillomavirus-associated penile intraepithelial neoplasia in sexual partners of women with cervical intraepithelial neoplasia, N Engl J Med 317:916, 1987.

Bartlett JG and Polk R: Bacterial flora of the vagina: quantitative study, Rev Infect Dis 6:S67, 1984.

Benedetti J, Corey L, and Ashley R: Recurrence rates in genital herpes after symptomatic first-episode infection, Ann Intern Med 121:847, 1994.

Beneditti JK, Zeh J, and Corey L: Clinical reactivation of genital herpes simplex virus infection decreases in frequency over time, Ann Intern Med 131:14, 1999.

Berkley SF, Hightower AW, Broome CV, and Reingold AL: The relationship of tampon characteristics to menstrual toxic shock syndrome, JAMA 258:917, 1987.

Bierman SM: Recurrent genital herpes simplex infection: a trivial disorder, Arch Dermatol 121:513, 1985.

Blackwell AL, Phillips I, Fox AR, et al: Anaerobic vaginosis (non-specific vaginitis): clinical, microbiological, and therapeutic findings, Lancet 2:1379, 1983.

Blake DR, Duggan A, and Joffe A: Use of spun urine to enhance detection of *Trichomonas vaginalis* in adolescent women, Arch Pediatr Adolesc Med 153:1222, 1999.

Boeke AJP, Dekker JH, and Peerbooms PGH: A comparison of yield from cervix versus vagina for culturing *Candida albicans* and *Trichomonas vaginalis*, Genitourin Med 69:41, 1993.

Bonnez W, Elswick RK Jr, Bailey-Farchione A, et al: Efficacy and safety of 0.5% podofilox solution in the treatment and suppression of anogenital warts, Am J Med 96:420, 1994.

Bornstein J, Pascal B, and Abramovici H: The common problem of vulvar pruritus, Obstet Gynecol Surv 48:111, 1993.

Bozbora A, Erbil Y, Berber E, et al: Surgical treatment of granuloma inguinale, Br J Dermatol 138:1079, 1998.

Britigan BE, Cohen MS, and Sparling PF: Gonococcal infection: a model of molecular pathogenesis, N Engl J Med 312:1683, 1985.

Brook I: Aerobic and anaerobic microbiology of Bartholin's abscess, Surg Gynecol Obstet 169:32, 1989.

Brown ST, Nalley JF, and Kraus SJ: Molluscum contagiosum, Sex Transm Dis 8:227, 1981.

Brown TJ, Yen-Moore A, and Tyring SK: An overview of sexually transmitted diseases, part I, J Am Acad Dermatol 41:511, 1999.

Brown TJ, Yen-Moore A, and Tyring SK: An overview of sexually transmitted diseases, part II, J Am Acad Dermatol 41:661, 1999.

Brunham RC, Paavonen J, Stevens CE, et al: Mucopurulent cervicitis—the ignored counterpart in women of urethritis in men, N Engl J Med 311:1, 1984.

Bump RC, Zuspan FP, Buesching WJ, et al: The prevalence, six-month persistence and predictive values of laboratory indica-

tors of bacterial vaginosis (nonspecific vaginitis) in asymptomatic women, Am J Obstet Gynecol 150:917, 1984.

Buntin DM, Rosen T, Lesher JL, et al: Sexually transmitted diseases: bacterial infections, J Am Acad Dermatol 25:287, 1991.

Catanzarite VA, Piacquadio KM, Stanco LM, et al: Preventing transmission of AIDS and hepatitis in obstetric-care providers, Contemp OB/GYN 44:39, 1999.

Cates W Jr and Wasserheit JN: Genital chlamydial infections: epidemiology and reproductive sequelae, Am J Obstet Gynecol 164:1771, 1991.

Cavannah DK and Ballas ZK: Pseudoephedrine reaction presenting as recurrent toxic shock syndrome, Ann Intern Med 119:302, 1993.

Centers for Disease Control: 1998 Guidelines for treatment of sexually transmitted diseases, MMWR 47:1, 1997.

Centers for Disease Control: 1993 revised classification system for HIV infection and expanded surveillance case definition for AIDS among adolescents and adults, MMWR 41:1, 1992.

Centers for Disease Control: Sexually transmitted diseases treatment guidelines, MMWR 42:56, 1993.

Centers for Disease Control: Update: acquired immunodeficiency syndrome—United States, 1994, MMWR, 44:64, 1995.

Centers for Disease Control: Update: AIDS among women—United States, 1994, Arch Dermatol 131:395, 1995.

Centers for Disease Control: First 500,000 AIDS cases—United States, 1995, MMWR 44:849, 1995.

Chiasson MA, Ellerbrock TV, Bush TJ, et al: Increased prevalence of vulvovaginal condyloma and vulvar intraepithelial neoplasia in women infected with the human immunodeficiency virus, Obstet Gynecol 89:690, 1997.

Chesney PJ: Clinical aspects and spectrum of illness of toxic shock syndrome: overview, Rev Infect Dis 11:S1, 1989.

Chesney PJ, Davis JP, Purdy WK, et al: Clinical manifestations of toxic shock syndrome, JAMA 246:741, 1981.

Chin KM, Sidhu JS, Janssen RS, and Weber JT: Invasive cervical cancer in human immunodeficiency virus–infected and uninfected hospital patients, Obstet Gynecol 92:83, 1998.

Cho JY, Ahn MO, and Cha KS: Window operation: an alternative treatment method for Bartholin gland cysts and abscesses, Obstet Gynecol 76:886, 1990.

Chosidow O: Scabies and pediculosis, Lancet 355:819, 2000.

Chouela EN, Abeldaño AM, Pellerano G, et al: Equivalent therapeutic efficacy and safety of Ivermectin and Lindane in the treatment of human scabies, Arch Dermatol 135:651, 1999.

Collier AC and Schwartz MA: Strategies for second-line antiretroviral therapy in adults with HIV infection, Advan Exper Med Biol 458:239, 1999.

Coodley GO, Coodley MK, and Thompson AF: Clinical aspects of HIV infection in women, J Gen Intern Med 10:99, 1995.

Condylomata International Collaborative Study Group: Recurrent condylomata acuminata treated with recombinant interferon alfa-2a: a multicenter double-blind placebo-controlled clinical trial, JAMA 265:2684, 1991.

Corey L, Adams HG, Brown ZA, et al: Genital herpes simplex virus infections: clinical manifestations, course, and complications, Ann Intern Med 98:958, 1983.

Corey L and Handsfield HH: Genital herpes and public health: addressing a global problem, JAMA 283:791, 2000.

Cox NH: Permethrin treatment in scabies infestation: importance of the correct formulation, BMJ 320:37, 2000.

Croen KD, Ostrove JM, Dragovic L, and Straus SE: Characterization of herpes simplex virus type 2 latency-associated transcription in human sacral ganglia and in cell culture, J Infect Dis 163:23, 1991.

Davis JP, Vergeront JM, Amsterdam LE, et al: Long-term effects of toxic shock syndrome in women: sequelae, subsequent pregnancy, menstrual history, and long-term trends in catamenial product use, Rev Infect Dis 11:S50, 1989.

del Giudice P: Ivermectin: a new therapeutic weapon in dermatology? Arch Dermatol 135:705, 1999.

Desrosiers RC: Strategies used by human immunodeficiency virus that allow persistent viral replication, Nature Med 7:723, 1999.

Donders GGG, Bosmans E, Dekeesmaecker A, et al: Pathogenesis of abnormal vaginal bacterial flora, Am J Obstet Gynecol 182:872, 2000.

Douglas JM, Critchlow C, Benedetti J, et al: A double-blind study of oral acyclovir for suppression of recurrences of genital herpes simplex virus infection, N Engl J Med 310:1551, 1984.

Droegemueller W, Adamson DG, Brown D, et al: Three-day treatment with butoconazole nitrate for vulvovaginal candidiasis, Obstet Gynecol 64:530, 1984.

Eckert LO, Watts DH, Koutsky LA, et al: A matched prospective study of human immunodeficiency virus serostatus, human papillomavirus DNA, and cervical lesions detected by cytology and colposcopy, Infect Dis Obstet Gynecol 7:158, 1999.

Ellerbrock TV, Bush TJ, Chamberland ME, and Oxtoby MJ: Epidemiology of women with AIDS in United States, 1981 through 1990: a comparison with heterosexual men with AIDS, JAMA 265: 2971, 1991.

Erbelding EM, Vlahov D, Nelson KE, et al: Syphilis serology in human immunodeficiency virus infection: evidence for false-negative fluorescent treponemal testing, J Infect Dis 176:1397, 1997.

Eschenbach DA: History and review of bacterial vaginosis, Am J Obstet Gynecol 169:441, 1993.

Eschenbach DA, Hillier S, Critchlow C, et al: Diagnosis and clinical manifestations of bacterial vaginosis, Am J Obstet Gynecol 158:819, 1988.

Eschenbach DA, Hummel D, and Gravett MG: Recurrent and persistent vulvovaginal candidiasis: treatment with ketoconazole, Obstet Gynecol 66:248, 1985.

Faber BM: The diagnosis and treatment of scabies and pubic lice, Prim Care Update Ob/Gyns 3:20, 1996.

Farley DE, Katz VL, and Dotters DJ: Toxic shock syndrome associated with vulvar necrotizing fasciitis, Obstet Gynecol 82:660, 1993.

Faro S: Systemic vs. topical therapy for the treatment of vulvovaginal candidiasis, Infect Dis Obstet Gynecol 1:202, 1994.

Faro S: A review of Famciclovir in the management of genital herpes, Infect Dis Obstet Gynecol 6:38, 1998.

Feldman JG, Chirgwin K, Dehovitz JA, and Minkoff H: The association of smoking and risk of condyloma acuminatum in women, Obstet Gynecol 89:346, 1997.

Ferenczy A: Epidemiology and clinical pathophysiology of condylomata acuminata, Am J Obstet Gynecol 172:1331, 1995.

Fife KH, Crumpacker SC, Mertz GJ, et al: Recurrence and resistance patterns of herpes simplex virus following cessation of ≥6 years of chronic suppression with acyclovir, J Infect Dis 169:1338, 1994.

Fineberg HV: Education to prevent AIDS: prospects and obstacles, Science 239:592, 1988.

Fischbach F, Petersen EE, Weissenbacher ER, et al: Efficacy of clindamycin vaginal cream versus oral metronidazole in the treatment of bacterial vaginosis, Obstet Gynecol 82:405, 1993.

Fong IW, Bannatyne RM, and Wong P: Lack of in vitro resistance of Candida albicans to ketoconazole, itraconazole and clotrimazole in women treated for recurrent vaginal candidiasis, Genitourin Med 69:44, 1993.

Freedberg KA and Samet HJ: Think HIV: why physicians should lower their threshold for HIV testing, Arch Intern Med 159:1994, 1999.

Friedman-Klein A: Management of condylomata acuminata with Alferon N injection, interferon alfa-n3 (human leukocyte derived), Am J Obstet Gynecol 172:1359, 1995.

Friedrich EG: Vulvar disease, ed 2, Philadelphia, 1983, WB Saunders Co.

Fu YL, Hu YX, Ling HL, et al: Human papillomaviruses and papillomatosis lesions of the female lower genital tract, Infect Dis Obstet Gynecol 1:235, 1994.

Furtado MR, Callaway DS, Phair JP, et al: Persistence of HIV-1 transcription in peripheral-blood mononuclear cells in patients receiving potent antiretroviral therapy, N Engl J Med 340:1614, 1999.

Galgiani JN: Fluconazole, a new antifungal agent, Ann Intern Med 113:177, 1990.

Gall SA: Human papillomavirus infection and therapy with interferon, Am J Obstet Gynecol 172:1354, 1995.

Gallant JE: Strategies for long-term success in the treatment of HIV infection, JAMA 283:1329, 2000.

García-Closas M, Herrero R, Bratti C, et al: Epidemiologic determinants of vaginal pH, Am J Obstet Gynecol 180:1060, 1999.

Gardner HL and Dukes CD: Clinical and laboratory effects of metronidazole, Am J Obstet Gynecol 89:990, 1964.

Gaydos CA, Howell MR, Pare B, et al: Chlamydia Trachomatis infections in female military recruits, N Engl J Med 339:739, 1998.

Giraldo P, Neuer A, Riberio-Filho A, et al: Detection of human 70-kD and 60-kD heat shock proteins in the vagina: relation to microbial flora, vaginal pH, and method of contraception, Infect Dis Obstet Gynecol 7:23, 1999.

Giraldo P, von Nowaskonski A, Gomes FAM, et al: Vaginal colonization by Candida in asymptomatic women with and without a history of recurrent vulvovaginal candidiasis, Obstet Gynecol 95:413, 2000.

Goldberg LH, Kaufman R, Kurtz TO, et al: Long-term suppression of recurrent genital herpes with acyclovir: a 5-year benchmark, Arch Dermatol 129:582, 1993.

Goldie SJ, Weinstein MC, Kuntz KM, and Freedberg KA: The costs, clinical benefits, and cost-effectiveness of screening for cervical cancer in HIV-infected women, Ann Intern Med 130:97, 1999.

Goldman P: Metronidazole, N Engl J Med 303:1212, 1980.

Goldmeier D and Hay P: A review and update on adult syphilis, with particular reference to its treatment, Int J STD AIDS 4:70, 1993.

Goldschmidt RH and Dong BJ: Treatment of AIDS and HIV-related conditions—1999, JABFP 12:71, 1999.

Gordon SM, Eaton ME, George R, et al: The response of symptomatic neurosyphilis to high-dose intravenous penicillin G in patients with human immunodeficiency virus infection, N Engl J Med 331:1469, 1994.

Gottlieb SL and Myskowski PL: Molluscum contagiosum, Int J Dermatol 33:453, 1994.

Graham BS and Wright PF: Drug therapy: candidate AIDS vaccines, N Engl J Med 333:1331, 1995.

Greene WC: The molecular biology of human immunodeficiency virus type I infection, N Engl J Med 324:308, 1991.

Gupta K, Scholes D, and Stamm WE: Increasing prevalence of antimicrobial resistance among uropathogens causing acute uncomplicated cystitis in women, JAMA 281:736, 1999.

Gwinn M, Pappaioanou M, George JR, et al: Prevalence of HIV infection in childbearing women in the United States: surveillance using newborn blood samples, JAMA 265:1704, 1991.

Harmanli OH, Cheng GY, Nyirjesy P, et al: Urinary tract infections in women with bacterial vaginosis, Obstet Gynecol 95:710, 2000.

Hart G: Donovanosis, Clin Infect Dis 25:24, 1997.

Hatch KD: Clinical appearance and treatment strategies for human papillomavirus: a gynecologic perspective, Am J Obstet Gynecol 172:1340, 1995.

Havlir DV, Marschner IC, Hirsch MS, et al: Maintenance antiretroviral therapies in HIV-infected subjects with undetectable plasma HIV RNA after triple-drug therapy, N Engl J Med 339:1261, 1998.

Heaton CL: Clinical manifestations and modern management of condylomata acuminata: a dermatologic perspective, Am J Obstet Gynecol 172:1344, 1995.

Helgerson SD, Mallery BL, and Foster LR: Toxic shock syndrome in Oregon, JAMA 252:3402, 1984.

Herrington CS: Human papillomaviruses (HPV) in gynaecological cytology: from molecular biology to clinical testing, Cytopathology 6:176, 1995.

Hill GB and Livengood CH III: Bacterial vaginosis-associated microflora and effects of topical intravaginal clindamycin, Am J Obstet Gynecol 171:1198, 1994.

Hillier SL: Diagnostic microbiology of bacterial vaginosis, Am J Obstet Gynecol 169:455, 1993.

Hillier SL, Krohn MA, Klebanoff SJ, and Eschenbach DA: The relationship of hydrogen peroxide–producing lactobacilli to bacterial vaginosis and genital microflora in pregnant women, Obstet Gynecol 79:369, 1992.

Hillier S, Krohn MA, Watts DH, et al: Microbiologic efficacy of intravaginal clindamycin cream for the treatment of bacterial vaginosis, Obstet Gynecol 76:407, 1990.

Hillier SL, Lipinski C, Briselden AM, and Eschenbach DA: Efficacy of intravaginal 0.75% metronidazole gel for the treatment of bacterial vaginosis, Obstet Gynecol 81:963, 1993.

Hilton E, Isenberg HD, Alperstein P, et al: Ingestion of yogurt containing *Lactobacillus acidophilus* as prophylaxis for candidal vaginitis, Ann Intern Med 116:353, 1992.

Hines JF, Ghrim S, Schlegel R, and Jenson AB: Prospects for a vaccine against human papillomavirus, Obstet Gynecol 86:860, 1995.

Hoge CW, Schwartz B, Talkington DF, et al: The changing epidemiology of invasive group A streptococcal infections and the emergence of streptococcal toxic shock-like syndrome: a retrospective population-based study, JAMA 269:384, 1993.

Holmes KK, Mårdh PA, Sparling PF, et al, editors: Sexually transmitted diseases, ed 3, New York, 1999, McGraw-Hill Book Co.

Hook EW III and Marra CM: Acquired syphilis in adults, N Engl J Med 326:1060, 1992.

Hook EW III, Spitters C, Reichart CA, et al: Use of cell culture and a rapid diagnostic assay for *Chlamydia trachomatis* screening, JAMA 272:867, 1994.

Horowitz BJ, Edelstein SW, and Lippman L: *Candida tropicalis* vulvovaginitis, Obstet Gynecol 66:229, 1985.

Howard RJ: Human immunodeficiency virus testing and the risk to the surgeon of acquiring HIV, Surgery 171:22, 1990.

Hughes VL and Hillier SL: Microbiologic characteristics of Lactobacillus products used for colonization of the vagina, Obstet Gynecol 75:244, 1990.

Hutchison CM, Hook EW III, Shepherd M, et al: Altered clinical presentation of early syphilis in patients with human immunodeficiency virus infection, Ann Intern Med 121:94, 1994.

Ioannidis JPA, Cappelleri JC, Lau J, et al: Early or deferred zidovudine therapy in HIV-infected patients without an AIDS-defining illness, Ann Intern Med 122:856, 1995.

Jeremias J, Draper D, Ziegert M, et al: Detection of *Trichomonas vaginalis* using the polymerase chain reaction in pregnant and non-pregnant women, Infect Dis Obstet Gynecol 2:16, 1994.

Joesoef MR and Schmid GP: Bacterial vaginosis: review of treatment options and potential clinical indications for therapy, Clin Infect Dis 20(S1):S72, 1995.

Joesoef MR, Schmid GP, and Hillier SL: Bacterial vaginosis: review of treatment options and potential clinical indications for therapy, Clin Infect Dis 28(S1):S57, 1999.

Johnson JR and Stamm WE: Urinary tract infections in women: diagnosis and treatment, Ann Intern Med 111:906, 1989.

Johnstone FD, McGoogan E, Smart GE, et al: A population-based, controlled study of the relation between HIV infection and cervical neoplasia, Br J Obstet Gynaecol 101:986, 1994.

Joseph AK and Rosen T: Laboratory techniques used in the diagnosis of chancroid, granuloma inguinale, and lymphogranuloma venereum, Dermatol Clin 12:1, 1994.

Kahn JO and Walker BD: Acute human immunodeficiency virus type 1 infection, N Engl J Med 339:33, 1998.

Kain KC, Schulzer M, and Chow AW: Clinical spectrum of nonmenstrual toxic shock syndrome (TSS): comparison with menstrual TSS by multivariate discriminate analyses, Clin Infect Dis 16:100, 1993.

Kaplowitz LG, Baker D, Gelb L, et al: Prolonged continuous acyclovir treatment of normal adults with frequently recurring genital herpes simplex virus infection, JAMA 265:747, 1991.

Kaufman RH and Faro S: Benign diseases of the vulva and vagina, ed 4, St. Louis, 1994, Mosby–Year Book, Inc.

Koelle DM, Benedetti J, Langenberg A, and Corey L: Asymptomatic reactivation of herpes simplex virus in women after the first episode of genital herpes, Ann Intern Med 116:433, 1992.

Koutsky LA, Stevens CE, Holmes KK, et al: Underdiagnosis of genital herpes by current clinical and viral-isolation procedures, N Engl J Med 326:1533, 1992.

Kovacs JA and Masur H: Prophylaxis against opportunistic infections in patients with human immunodeficiency virus infection, N Engl J Med 342:1416, 2000.

Krebs HB and Helmkamp F: Chronic ulcerations following topical therapy with 5-fluorouracil for vaginal human papillomavirus-associated lesions, Obstet Gynecol 78:205, 1991.

Krebs HB and Helmkamp F: Treatment failure of genital condylomata acuminata in women: role of the male sexual partner, Am J Obstet Gynecol 165:337, 1991.

Krieger JN, Jenny C, Verdon M, et al: Clinical manifestations of trichomoniasis in men, Ann Intern Med 118:844, 1993.

Krieger JN, Tam MR, Stevens CE, et al: Diagnosis of trichomoniasis: comparison of conventional wet-mount examination with cytologic studies, cultures, and monoclonal antibody staining of direct specimens, JAMA 259:1223, 1988.

Kunin CM: Urinary tract infections in females, Clin Infect Dis 18:1, 1994.

Kunin CM, White LV, and Hua TH: A reassessment of the importance of "low-count" bacteriuria in young women with acute urinary symptoms, Ann Intern Med 119:454, 1993.

Langenberg A, Burke RL, Adair SF, et al: A recombinant glycoprotein vaccine for herpes simplex type 2: safety and efficacy, Ann Intern Med 122:889, 1995.

Langenberg AGM, Corey L, Ashley RL, et al: A prospective study of new infections with herpes simplex virus type 1 and type 2, N Engl J Med 341:1432, 1999.

Larsen B and Galask RP: Vaginal microbial flora: composition and influences of host physiology, Ann Intern Med 96:926, 1982.

Larsen B and White S: Antifungal effect of hydrogen peroxide on catalase-producing strains of *Candida spp.*, Infect Dis Obstet Gynecol 3:73, 1995.

Larsson PG: Bacterial vaginosis: diagnosis, treatment and significance in gynecological practice, Acta Obstet Gynecol Scand 71:560, 1992.

Lazarus HM, Belanger R, Candoni A, et al: Intravenous penciclovir for treatment of herpes simplex infections in immunocompromised patients: results of a multicenter, acyclovir-controlled trial, Antimicrob Agents Chemother 43:1192, 1999.

Lee YH, Rankin JS, Alpert S, et al: Microbiological investigation of Bartholin's gland abscesses and cysts, Am J Obstet Gynecol 129:150, 1977.

Livengood CH III, McGregor JA, Soper DE, et al: Bacterial vaginosis: efficacy and safety of intravaginal metronidazole treatment, Am J Obstet Gynecol 170:759, 1994.

Livengood CH III, Soper DE, Sheehan KL, et al: Comparison of once-daily and twice-daily dosing of 0.75% metronidazole gel in the treatment of bacterial vaginosis, Sex Transmit Dis 26:137, 1999.

Lossick JG and Kent HL: Trichomoniasis: trends in diagnosis and treatment, 165:1217, 1991.

Louv WC, Austin H, Perlman J, and Alexander WJ: Oral contraceptive use and the risk of chlamydial and gonococcal infections, Am J Obstet Gynecol 160:396, 1989.

Lowy FD: *Staphylococcus aureus* infections, N Engl J Med 339:520, 1998.

Luby ED and Klinge V: Genital herpes: a pervasive psychosocial disorder, Arch Dermatol 121:494, 1985.

Lugo-Miro VI, Green M, and Mazur L: Comparison of different metronidazole therapeutic regimens for bacterial vaginosis: a meta-analysis, JAMA 268:92, 1992.

Lytle CD, Carney PG, Vohra S, et al: Virus leakage through natural membrane condoms, Sex Transm Dis 17:58, 1990.

MacDermott RIJ: Bacterial vaginosis, Br J Obstet Gynaecol 102:92, 1995.

Madico G, Quinn TC, Rompalo A, et al: Diagnosis of *Trichomonas vaginalis* infection by PCR using vaginal swab samples, J Clin Microbiol 36:3205, 1998.

Mårdh PA: The vaginal ecosystem, Am J Obstet Gynecol 165:1163, 1991.

Manders SM: Toxin-mediated streptococcal and staphylococcal disease, J Am Acad Dermatol 39:383, 1998.

Markowitz M, Saag M, Powderly WG, et al: A preliminary study of ritonavir, an inhibitor of HIV-1 protease, to treat HIV-1 infection, N Engl J Med 333:1534, 1995.

Marlière V, Roul S, Labrèze C, and Taïeb A: Crusted (Norwegian) scabies induced by use of topical corticosteroids and treated successfully with ivermectin, J Pediatr 135:122, 1999.

Martin DH and DiCarlo RP: Recent changes in the epidemiology of genital ulcer disease in the United States: the crack cocaine connection, Sex Transm Dis 21(S2):S76, 1994.

Martin DH, Mroczkowski TF, Dalu ZA, et al: A controlled trial of a single dose of azithromycin for the treatment of chlamydial urethritis and cervicitis, N Engl J Med 327:921, 1992.

Maskell R: Broadening the concept of urinary tract infection, Br J Urol 76:2, 1995.

Matta H, Thompson AM, and Rainey JB: Does wearing two pairs of gloves protect operating theatre staff from skin contamination? Br Med J 297:597, 1988.

Maunder JW: Lice and scabies: myths and reality, Sex Transmit Dis 16:843, 1998.

Maw RD: Treatment of anogenital warts, Dermatol Clin 16:829, 1998.

McCarty JM: Azithromycin (Zithromax), Infect Dis Obstet Gynecol 4:215, 1996.

McLachlin CM: Pathology of human papillomavirus in the female genital tract, Curr Opin Obstet Gynecol 7:24, 1995.

McLellan R, Spence MR, Brockman M, et al: The clinical diagnosis of trichomoniasis, Obstet Gynecol 60:30, 1982.

Meikle SF, Zhang X, Marine WM, et al: *Chlamydia trachomatis* antibody titers and hysterosalpingography in predicting tubal disease in infertility patients, Fertil Steril 62:305, 1994.

Merkus JMWM, Bisschop MPJM, and Stolte LAM: The proper nature of vaginal candidosis and the problem of recurrence, Obstet Gynecol Surv 40:493, 1985.

Mertz GJ, Benedetti J, Ashely R, et al: Risk factors for the sexual transmission of genital herpes, Ann Intern Med 116:197, 1992.

Mertz GJ, Eron L, Kaufman R, et al: Prolonged continuous versus intermittent oral acyclovir treatment in normal adults with frequently recurring genital herpes simplex virus infection, Am J Med 85(suppl 2A):14, 1988.

Mertz GJ, Jones CC, Mills J, et al: Long-term acyclovir suppression of frequently recurring genital herpes simplex virus infection: a multicenter double-blind trial, JAMA 260:201, 1988.

Milsom I, Arvidsson L, Ekelund P, et al: Factors influencing vaginal cytology, pH and bacterial flora in elderly women, Acta Obstet Gynecol Scand 72:286, 1993.

Montes LF and Wilborn WH: Fungus-host relationship in candidiasis, Arch Dermatol 121:119, 1985.

Moore P: Diagnosing and treating scabies, Practitioner 238:632, 1994.

Moscicki AB, Shiboski S, Broering J, et al: The natural history of human papillomavirus infection as measured by repeated DNA testing in adolescent and young women, J Pediatr 132:277, 1998.

Mroczkowski TF and Martin DH: Genital ulcer disease, Dermatol Clin 12:753, 1994.

Nahas GT, Goldstein BA, Zhu WY, et al: Comparison of Tzanck smear, viral culture, and DNA diagnostic methods in detection of herpes simplex and varicella-zoster infection, JAMA 268:2541, 1992.

Nandwani R and Evans DTP: Are you sure it's syphilis? A review of false positive serology, Int J STD AIDS, 6:241, 1995.

Neri A, Rabinerson D, and Kaplan B: Bacterial vaginosis: drugs versus alternative treatment, Obstet Gyncol Surv 49:809, 1994.

Neu HC: Urinary tract infections, Am J Med 92(S4A):63S, 1992.

Nilsen AE, Aasen T, Halsos AM, et al: Efficacy of oral acyclovir in the treatment of initial and recurrent genital herpes, Lancet 2:571, 1982.

Nuovo GJ and Pedemonte BM: Human papillomavirus types and recurrent cervical warts, JAMA 263:1223, 1990.

Nyirjesy P, Seeney SM, Grody MHT, et al: Chronic fungal vaginitis: the value of cultures, Am J Obstet Gynecol 173:820, 1995.

Oriel JD: Natural history of genital warts, Br J Vener Dis 47:1, 1971.

Oriel JD: The increase in molluscum contagiosum, Br Med J 294:74, 1987.

Oriel JD, Partridge BM, Denny MJ, et al: Genital yeast infections, Br Med J 4:761, 1972.

Ortiz-Zepeda C, Hernandez-Perez E, and Marroquin-Burgos R: Gross and microscopic features in chancroid: a study in 200 new culture-proven cases in San Salvador, Sex Trans Dis 21:112, 1994.

Paavonen J and Wolner-Hanssen P: *Chlamydia trachomatis:* a major threat to reproduction, Hum Reprod 4:111, 1989.

Pantaleo G, Graziosi C, and Fauci AS: The immunopathogenesis of human immunodeficiency virus infection, N Engl J Med 328:327, 1993.

Patterson BA, Garland SM, Bowden FJ, et al: The diagnosis of *Trichomonas vaginalis:* new advances, Int J STD AIDS 10:68, 1999.

Pearlman MD, Yashar C, Ernst S, and Solomon W: An incremental dosing protocol for women with severe vaginal trichomoniasis and adverse reactions to metronidazole, Am J Obstet Gynecol 174:934, 1996.

Peipert JF, Montagno AB, Cooper AS, and Sung CJ: Bacterial vaginosis as a risk factor for upper genital tract infection, Am J Obstet Gynecol 177:1184, 1997.

Peterman TA and Curran JW: Sexual transmission of human immunodeficiency virus, JAMA 256:2222, 1986.

Peters WA III: Bartholinitis after vulvovaginal surgery, Am J Obstet Gynecol 178:1143, 1998.

Pfeifer TA, Forsyth PS, Durfee MA, et al: Nonspecific vaginitis: role of *Haemophilus vaginalis* and treatment with metronidazole, N Engl J Med 298:1429, 1978.

Phillips DM: *Candida albicans,* N Engl J Med 328:1322, 1993.

Phillips RS, Hanff PA, Holmes MD, et al: *Chlamydia trachomatis* cervical infection in women seeking routine gynecologic care: criteria for selective testing, Am J Med 86:515, 1989.

Piper JM, Mitchel EF, and Ray WA: Prenatal use of metronidazole and birth defects: no association, Obstet Gynecol 82:348, 1993.

Potter J: Should sexual partners of women with bacterial vaginosis receive treatment? Br J Gen Pract 49:913, 1999.

Priestley CJF, Jones BM, Dhar J, and Goodwin L: What is normal vaginal flora? Genitourin Med 73:23: 1997.

Purdon A, Hanna JH, Morse PL, et al: An evaluation of single-dose metronidazole treatment of *Gardnerella vaginalis,* Obstet Gynecol 64:271, 1984.

Quinn TC, Wawer MJ, Sewankambo N, et al: Viral load and heterosexual transmission of human immunodeficiency virus type 1, N Engl J Med 342:921, 2000.

Ravot E, Lisziewicz J, and Fori F: New uses for old drugs in HIV infection, Drugs 58:953, 1999.

Raz R and Stamm WE: A controlled trial of intravaginal estriol in postmenopausal women with recurrent urinary tract infections, N Engl J Med 329:753, 1993.

Redondo-Lopez V, Lynch M, Schmitt C, et al: *Torulopsis glabrata* vaginitis: clinical aspects and susceptibility to antifungal agents, Obstet Gynecol 76:651, 1990.

Reed BD: Risk factors for *Candida* vulvovaginitis, Obstet Gynecol Surv 47:551, 1992.

Reef SE, Levine WC, McNeil MM, et al: Treatment options for vulvovaginal candidiasis, 1993, Clin Infect Dis 20(S1):S80, 1995.

Richart RM and Nuovo GJ: Human papillomavirus DNA in situ hybridization may be used for the quality control of genital tract biopsies, Obstet Gynecol 75:223, 1990.

Richens J: The diagnosis and treatment of donovanosis (granuloma inguinale), Genitourin Med 67:441, 1991.

Ridgway GL and Taylor-Robinson D: Current problems in microbiology. I. Chlamydial infections: which laboratory test? J Clin Pathol 44:1, 1991.

Rigg D, Miller MM, and Metzger WJ: Recurrent allergic vulvovaginitis: treatment with *Candida albicans* allergen immunotherapy, Am J Obstet Gynecol 162:332, 1990.

Rolfs RT: Treatment of syphilis, 1993, Clin Infect Dis 20(S1):S23, 1995.

Rolfs RT, Joesoef MR, Hendershot EF, et al: A randomized trial of enhanced therapy for early syphilis in patients with and without human immunodeficiency virus infection, N Engl J Med 337:307, 1997.

Rooney JF, Straus SE, Mannix ML, et al: Oral acyclovir to suppress frequently recurrent herpes labialis: a double-blind, placebo-controlled trial, Ann Intern Med 118:268, 1993.

Rosen DJD, Margolin ML, Menashe Y, and Greenspoon JS: Toxic shock syndrome after loop electrosurgical excision procedure, Am J Obstet Gynecol 169:202,1993.

Rosen T and Brown TJ: Genital ulcers: evaluation and treatment, Sex Transm Dis 16:673, 1998.

Ross RA, Lee MT, and Onderdonk AB: Effect of *Candida albicans* infection and clotrimazole treatment on vaginal microflora in vitro, Obstet Gynecol 86:925, 1995.

Rowland-Jones S: The role of chemokine receptors in HIV infection, Sex Transm Infect 75:148, 1999.

Sacks SL: Famciclovir (FAMVIR), Infect Dis Obstet Gynecol 5:3, 1997.

Sanguineti A, Carmichael K, and Campbell K: Fluconazole-resistant *Candida albicans* after long-term suppressive therapy, Arch Intern Med 153:1122, 1993.

Sasadeusz JJ and Sacks SL: Herpes latency, meningitis, radiculomyelopathy and disseminated infection, Genitourin Med 70:369, 1994.

Schacker T, Hu H, Koelle DM, et al: Famciclovir for the suppression of symptomatic and asymptomatic herpes simplex virus reactivation in HIV-infected persons: a double-blind, placebo-controlled trial, Ann Intern Med 128:21, 1998.

Schmid GP, Sanders LL, Blount JH, et al: Chancroid in the United States: reestablishment of an old disease, JAMA 258:3265, 1987.

Schneider A, Sterzik K, Buck G, and DeVilliers EM: Colposcopy is superior to cytology for the detection of early genital human papillomavirus infection, Obstet Gynecol 71:236, 1988.

Schulte JM and Schmid GP: Recommendations for treatment of chancroid, 1993, Clin Infect Dis 20(S1):S39, 1995.

Schwarcz SK, Zenilman JM, Schnell D, et al: National surveillance of antimicrobial resistance in Neisseria gonorrhoeae, JAMA 264:1413, 1990.

Schwartz B, Gaventa S, Broome CV, et al: Nonmenstrual toxic shock syndrome associated with barrier contraceptives: report of a case-controlled study, Rev Infect Dis 11:S43, 1989.

Schwebke JR: Diagnostic methods for bacterial vaginosis, Int J Gynecol Obstet 67:S21, 1999.

Schwebke JR, Schulien MB, and Zajackowski M: Pilot study to evaluate the appropriate management of patients with coexistent bacterial vaginosis and cervicitis, Infect Dis Obstet Gynecol 3:119, 1995.

Severson JL and Tyring SK: Relation between herpes simplex viruses and human immunodeficiency virus infections, Arch Dermatol 135:1393, 1999.

Shah PN, Kell PD, and Barton SE: Gynaecological disorders and human immunodeficiency virus infection, Int J STD AIDS 5:383, 1994.

Shimizu Y: Streptococcal toxic shock-like syndrome, Intern Med 39:195, 2000.

Sjöberg I and Hakansson S: Endotoxin in vaginal fluid of women with bacterial vaginosis, Obstet Gynecol 77:265, 1991.

Smith JR, Kitchen VS, Botcherby M, et al: Is HIV infection associated with an increase in the prevalence of cervical neoplasia? Br J Obstet Gynaecol 100:149, 1993.

Smith KL, Yeager J, and Skelton H: Molluscum contagiosum: its clinical, histopathologic, and immunohistochemical spectrum, Int J Dermatol 38:664, 1999.

Sobel JD: Management of recurrent vulvovaginal candidiasis with intermittent ketoconazole prophylaxis, Obstet Gynecol 65:435, 1985.

Sobel JD: Vaginitis, N Engl J Med 337:1896, 1997.

Sobel JD, Brooker D, Stein GE, et al: Single dose fluconazole compared with conventional clotrimazole topical therapy of Candida vaginitis, Am J Obstet Gynecol 172:1263, 1995.

Sobel JD and Chaim W: Treatment of Torulopsis glabrata vaginitis: retrospective review of boric acid therapy, Clin Infect Dis 24:649, 1997.

Sobel JD, Faro S, Force RW, et al: Vulvovaginal candidiasis: epidemiologic, diagnostic, and therapeutic considerations, Am J Obstet Gynecol 178:203, 1998.

Sobel JD, Schmitt C, and Meriwether C: Clotrimazole treatment of recurrent and chronic candida vulvovaginitis, Obstet Gynecol 73:330, 1989.

Soll DR, Morrow B, Srikantha T, et al: Developmental and molecular biology of switching in Candida albicans, Oral Surg Oral Med Oral Pathol 78:194, 1994.

Sonnex C: The amine test: a simple, rapid, inexpensive method for diagnosing bacterial vaginosis, Br J Obstet Gynaecol 102:160, 1995.

Sonnex C, Strauss S, and Gray JJ: Detection of human papillomavirus DNA on the fingers of patients with genital warts, Sex Transm Infect 75:317, 1999.

Soper DE: Bacterial vaginosis and trichomoniasis: epidemiology and management of recurrent disease, Infect Dis Obstet Gynecol 2:242, 1995.

Soper DE: Gynecologic sequelae of bacterial vaginosis, Int J Gynecol Obstet 67:S25, 1999.

Spinillo A, Capuzzo E, Egbe TO, et al: Torulopsis glabrata vaginitis, Obstet Gynecol 85:993, 1995.

Spitzer M: Lower genital tract intraepithelial neoplasia in HIV-infected women: guidelines for evaluation and management, Obstet Gynecol Surv 54:131, 1999.

Spruance SL, Stewart JCB, Rowe NH, et al: Treatment of recurrent herpes simplex labialis with oral acyclovir, J Infect Dis 161:185, 1990.

Staary A, Schuh E, Kerschbaumer M, et al: Performance of transcription-mediated amplification and ligase chain reaction assays for detection of chlamydial infection in urogenital samples obtained by invasive and noninvasive methods, J Clin Microbiol 36:2666, 1998.

Stamm WE and Hooton TM: Management of urinary tract infections in adults, N Engl J Med 329:1328, 1993.

Stanberry LR: Control of STDs—the role of prophylactic vaccines against herpes simplex virus, Sex Transm Dis 74:391, 1998.

Stapleton A, Latham RH, Johnson C, and Stamm WE: Postcoital antimicrobial prophylaxis for recurrent urinary tract infection: a randomized, double-blind, placebo-controlled trial, JAMA 264:703, 1990.

Stapleton A and Stamm WE: Prevention of urinary tract infection, Infect Dis Clin North Am 11:719, 1997.

Stern JE, Givan AL, Gonzalez JL, et al: Leukocytes in the cervix: a quantitative evaluation of cervicitis, Obstet Gynecol 91:987, 1998.

St Louis ME and Wasserheit JN: Elimination of syphilis in the United States, Science 281:353, 1998.

Stone KM and Whittington WL: Treatment of genital herpes, Rev Infect Dis 12:S610, 1990.

Straus SE, Croen KD, Sawyer MH, et al: Acyclovir suppression of frequently recurring genital herpes: efficacy and diminishing need during successive years of treatment, JAMA 260:2227, 1988.

Strausbaugh LJ: Toxic shock syndrome: are you recognizing its changing presentations? Postgrad Med 94:107, 1993.

Sumners D, Kelsey M, and Chait I: Psychological aspects of lower urinary tract infections in women, BMJ 304:17, 1992.

Sun XW, Ellerbrock TV, Lungu O, et al: Human papillomavirus infection in human immunodeficiency virus-seropositive women, Obstet Gynecol 85:680, 1995.

Sun XW, Ferenczy A, Johnson D, et al: Evaluation of the hybrid capture human papillomavirus deoxyribonucleic acid detection test, Am J Obstet Gynecol 173:1432, 1995.

Sweet RL: New approaches for the treatment of bacterial vaginosis, Am J Obstet Gynecol 169:479, 1993.

Sweet RL: The enigmatic cervix, Dermatol Clin 16:739, 1998.

Sweet RL and Gibbs RS: Infectious diseases of the female genital tract, ed 3, Baltimore, 1995, Williams & Wilkins.

Sykes NL Jr: Condyloma acuminatum, Int J Dermatol 34:297, 1995.

Tam MR, Stamm WE, Handsfield H, et al: Culture-independent diagnosis of Chlamydia trachomatis using monoclonal antibodies, N Engl J Med 310:1146, 1984.

Tam MT, Yngbluth M, and Myles T: Gram stain method shows better sensitivity than clinical criteria for detection of bacterial vaginosis in surveillance of pregnant, low-income women in a clinical setting, Infect Dis Obstet Gynecol 6:204, 1998.

Testa GM: The urethral syndrome: why what we do works, or doesn't, Med J Aust 157:549, 1992.

Tice AD: Short-course therapy of acute cystitis: a brief review of therapeutic strategies, J Antimicrob Chemother 43(SA):85, 1999.

Tidwell BH, Lushbaugh WB, Laughlin MD, et al: A double-blind placebo-controlled trial of single-dose intravaginal versus single-dose oral metronidazole in the treatment of trichomonal vaginitis, J Infect Dis 170:242, 1994.

Tierno PM and Hanna BA: Propensity of tampons and barrier contraceptives to amplify *Staphylococcus aureus* toxic shock syndrome toxin-1, Infect Dis Obstet Gynecol 2:140, 1994.

Todd JK, Ressman M, Caston SA, et al: Corticosteroid therapy for patients with toxic shock syndrome, JAMA 252:3399, 1984.

Turrentine M and Gonik B: Herpes simplex virus, Curr Opin Obstet Gynecol 6:377, 1994.

Tyring SK: Interferons: biochemistry and mechanisms of action, Am J Obstet Gynecol 172:1350, 1995.

Usha V and Nair TVG: A comparative study of oral ivermectin and topical permethrin cream in the treatment of scabies, J Am Acad Dermatol 42:236, 2000.

Uvin SC and Caliendo AM: Cervicovaginal human immunodeficiency virus secretion and plasma viral load in human immunodeficiency virus-seropositive women, Obstet Gynecol 90:739, 1997.

van Heusden AM, Merkus HMWM, Euser R, and Verhoeff A: A randomized, comparative study of a single oral dose of fluconazole versus a single topical dose of clotrimazole in the treatment of vaginal candidosis among general practitioners and gynaecologists, Eur J Obstet Gynecol Reprod Biol 55:123, 1994.

Van Slyke KK, Michel VP, and Rein MF: Treatment of vulvovaginal candidiasis with boric acid powder, Am J Obstet Gynecol 141:145, 1981.

Vejtorp M, Bollerup AC, Vejtorp L, et al: Bacterial vaginosis: a double-blind randomized trial of the effect of treatment of the sexual partner, Br J Obstet Gynaecol 95:920, 1988.

Von Gruenigen VE, Coleman RL, Li AJ, et al: Bacteriology and treatment of malodorous lower reproductive tract in gynecologic cancer patients, Obstet Gynecol 96:23, 2000.

Von Krogh G and Hellberg D: Self-treatment using a 0.5% podophyllotoxin cream of external genital condylomata acuminata in women: a placebo-controlled, double-blind study, Sex Transm Dis 19:170, 1992.

Wain AM: Metronidazole vaginal gel 0.75% (MetroGel-Vaginal): a brief review, Infect Dis Obstet Gynecol 6:3, 1998.

Wald A, Zeh J, Selke S, et al: Reactivation of genital herpes simplex virus type 2 infection in asymptomatic seropositive persons, N Engl J Med 342:844, 2000.

Wallin KL, Wiklund F, Ågnström T, et al: Type-specific persistence of human papillomavirus DNA before the development of invasive cervical cancer, N Engl J Med 341:1633, 1999.

Wang J: Trichomoniasis, Prim Care Update 7:148, 2000.

Warren JW, Abrutyn E, Hebel JR, et al: Guidelines for antimicrobial treatment of uncomplicated acute bacterial cystitis and acute pyelonephritis in women, Clin Infect Dis 29:745, 1999.

Washington AE, Gove S, Schachter J, et al: Oral contraceptives, *Chlamydia trachomatis* infection, and pelvic inflammatory disease, JAMA 253:2246, 1985.

Waugh MA: Molluscum contagiosum, Dermatol Clin 16:839, 1998.

Weber JT and Johnson RE: New treatments for *Chlamydia trachomatis* genital infection, Clin Infect Dis 20(S1):S66, 1995.

Williams LA, Klausner JD, Whittington WLH, et al: Elimination and reintroduction of primary and secondary syphilis, Am J Public Health 89:1093, 1999.

Winberg J, Herthelius-Elman M, Möllby R, and Nord CE: Pathogenesis of urinary tract infection: experimental studies of vaginal resistance to colonization, Pediatr Nephrol 7:509, 1993.

Wisenfeld HC, Heine RP, Rideout A, et al: The vaginal introitus: a novel site for *Chlamydia trachomatis* testing in women, Am J Obstet Gynecol 174:1542, 1996.

Witkin SS, Inglis SR, and Polaneczky M: Detection of *Chlamydia trachomatis* and *Trichomonas vaginalis* by polymerase chain reaction in introital specimens from pregnant women, Am J Obstet Gynecol 175:165, 1996.

Wong TY and Mihm MC Jr: Primary syphilis, N Engl J Med 331:1492, 1994.

Word B: Office treatment of cyst and abscess of Bartholin's gland duct, South Med J 61:514, 1968.

Working Group on Severe Streptococcal Infections: Defining the group A streptococcal toxic shock syndrome: rationale and consensus definition, JAMA 269:390, 1993.

Workowski KA, Lampe MF, Wong KG, et al: Long-term eradication of *Chlamydia trachomatis* genital infection after antimicrobial therapy: evidence against persistent infection, JAMA 270:2071, 1993.

Wright TC Jr, Ellerbrock TV, Chiasson MA, et al: Cervical intraepithelial neoplasia in women infected with human immunodeficiency virus: prevalence, risk factors, and validity of Papanicolaou smears, Obstet Gynecol 84:591, 1994.

Young DC, Craft S, Day MC, et al: Comparison of Abbott LCx *Chlamydia trachomatis* assay with Gen-Probe PACE2 and culture, Infect Dis Obstet Gynecol 8:112, 2000.

Young H: Syphilis: new diagnostic directions, Int J STD AIDS, 3:391, 1992.

Zhang L, Ramratnam B, Tenner-Racz K, et al: Quantifying residual HIV-1 replication in patients receiving combination antiretroviral therapy, N Engl J Med 340:1605, 1999.

Infections of the Upper Genital Tract
Endometritis, Acute and Chronic Salpingitis

KEY TERMS AND DEFINITIONS

Atypical or Silent Pelvic Inflammatory Disease. Relatively asymptomatic inflammation of the upper genital tract.

Canaliculus. A small, canal-like opening forming a channel for ascension of bacteria from the lower to the upper genital tract.

Commensal Bacteria. An organism that may exist in the genital tract without actually causing disease.

Fitz-Hugh–Curtis Syndrome. A syndrome of perihepatic inflammation that develops in 5% to 10% of women with acute pelvic inflammatory disease, originating from transperitoneal or vascular dissemination of either *Neisseria gonorrhoeae* or *Chlamydia trachomatis*.

Hydrosalpinx. A collection of watery, sterile fluid in the fallopian tube, secondary to tubal obstruction an end stage of a pyosalpinx.

Multidrug Resistant Tuberculosis. Infection from *Mycobacterium tuberculosis* that is resistant to two or more antituberculin drugs, including isoniazid.

Nonoxynol-9. A chemical detergent used in spermicidal preparations that is also bactericidal and viricidal.

Penicillinase-Producing Gonorrhea. Strains of *N. gonorrhoeae* that become resistant to penicillin by acquiring a resistance factor plasmid that enables the gonococcus to produce an enzyme that destroys penicillin.

Pelvic Inflammatory Disease. A nonspecific term that most commonly refers to inflammation caused by infection in the upper genital tract; often used synonymously with the term *acute salpingitis*.

Tuboovarian Complex. A collection of pus within an anatomic space created by adherence of adjacent organs, involving the oviducts, ovaries, and sometimes the intestines.

This chapter considers upper genital tract infections. The primary focus is on acute pelvic inflammatory disease, which is one of the major manifestations of sexually transmitted diseases. This discussion considers the epidemiology, diagnosis, and treatment of acute pelvic inflammatory disease. There are three major sequelae of PID—ectopic pregnancies, chronic pain, and infertility: this chapter will also consider uncommon causes of upper genital tract infection, such as tuberculosis and actinomycosis. For more detail of the infections with *Neisseria*

gonorrhoeae and *Chlamydia trachomatis*, the reader is referred to Chapter 22.

The Centers for Disease Control (CDC) regularly revises its treatment protocols for sexually transmitted diseases. The recommendations and medications in this edition are based on the 1998 CDC guidelines. Readers are urged to consult any updates in CDC guidelines, since bacterial resistance to antibiotics and epidemiologic concerns may lead to changes in treatment protocols. This information may be accessed online at www.cdc.gov/publications.htm.

ENDOMETRITIS

Nonpuerperal endometritis is an obscure, chronic infection of the lining of the uterus. The obstetric counterpart of an acute endometritis that develops following a delivery or an abortion is a considerably more common problem. Since acute pelvic inflammatory disease is an ascending infection along the mucosa of the reproductive tract, endometritis must be an intermediate state of ascending infection from the endocervical canal. The temporal development of endometritis has not been studied extensively in women with either mucopurulent cervicitis or acute pelvic inflammatory disease. Many of the pertinent clinical questions remain unanswered, such as the time it takes for an ascending infection to colonize various areas of the upper genital tract.

Endometritis is often undiagnosed unless there is a high degree of suspicion by both the clinician and the pathologist. Paavonen et al. found that 72% of women with laparoscopically proven acute pelvic inflammatory disease had associated histologic evidence of endometritis. Similar studies have found that 40% of women with mucopurulent cervicitis and 58% of women with positive endocervical cultures for either *C. trachomatis* or *N. gonorrhoeae* have concomitant endometritis.

The pathophysiology of endometritis is straightforward. A cervical infection leads to canalicular spread of organisms from the endocervix to the endometrium and subsequently to the endosalpinx. Microorganisms that have been commonly associated with chronic bacterial endometritis include *C. trachomatis, N. gonorrhoeae,* and *Streptococcus agalactiae.* Paavonen et al. found a correlation between serum antibody levels of *Mycoplasma hominis* and *C. trachomatis* and the prevalence of endometritis. Recent studies have emphasized that organisms that produce bacterial vaginosis may also produce plasma cell endometritis even in women without symptoms of upper tract disease. Preliminary observations suggest an increased frequency and severity of plasma cell endometritis in HIV-infected women.

Many women with chronic endometritis are asymptomatic. Interestingly, women with unrecognized endometritis are more than four times more likely to be using oral contraceptives than women with recognized endometritis. Møller et al., in a study of women undergoing hysterectomy, found microorganisms in the uteri of 24 of 99 women. Conversely, when endometritis coexists with acute pelvic inflammatory disease, it is difficult to differentiate whether inflammation of the oviducts or of the endometrium is producing the pelvic symptoms. The classic symptom of chronic endometritis is intermenstrual vaginal bleeding. Some women experience menorrhagia. Other women complain of a dull, constant lower abdominal pain. Chronic endometritis is a rare cause of infertility.

The diagnosis of chronic endometritis is established by endometrial biopsy and culture. It is possible to have a positive endometrial culture and at the same time a negative endocervical culture. The classic histologic finding of chronic endometritis is an inflammatory reaction of monocytes and plasma cells in the endometrial stroma. In severe cases, diffuse inflammatory infiltrates of lymphocytes and plasma cells are seen throughout the endometrial stroma. This may be associated with lymphoid follicles and stromal necrosis. No histopathologic correlation has been found between the presence of small numbers of polymorphonuclear leukocytes and chronic endometritis. During menses, it is normal to see polymorphonuclear leukocytes in the endometrium.

The ideal treatment of chronic endometritis is oral ofloxacin, 400 mg twice daily for 14 days plus metronidazole, 500 mg twice daily for 14 days. With the presence of concurrent bacterial vaginosis, treatment with agents that have anaerobic coverage is definitely indicated. Many women will have clinically persistent endometritis following treatment of acute pelvic inflammatory disease if they are not given or do not complete an antichlamydial antibiotic regimen.

PELVIC INFLAMMATORY DISEASE

Pelvic inflammatory disease is a gynecologic condition that lacks a precise definition. The term is used most commonly to refer to inflammation caused by an infection in the upper genital tract not associated with pregnancy or intraperitoneal pelvic operations. Thus it may include infection of *any or all* of the following anatomic locations: the endometrium (endometritis), the oviducts (salpingitis), the ovary (oophoritis), the uterine wall (myometritis), the uterine serosa and broad ligaments (parametritis), and the pelvic peritoneum. Many authors prefer the term *salpingitis* because infection of the oviducts is the most characteristic and common component of pelvic inflammatory disease. Importantly, most long-term sequelae of pelvic inflammatory disease result from destruction of the tubal architecture by the infection. In most clinical situations the terms acute *salpingitis* and *pelvic inflammatory disease* are used synonymously to describe an acute infection. *Chronic pelvic inflammatory disease* is a term that has largely been abandoned because the long-term sequelae of acute infection, such as adhesions and hydrosalpinx, are bacteriologically sterile. Pelvic infections are not active for several weeks or months with the exception of chronic colonization by *C. trachomatis* or infection with rare organisms, such as tuberculosis or actinomycosis.

The present epidemic of sexually transmitted diseases and corresponding pelvic inflammatory disease is a major public health concern. However, the incidence of the disease has started to decline over the past few years. In the United States the most recent estimates of the direct costs of pelvic inflammatory disease and its sequelae are $1.88 billion per year in 1998 dollars. This report by Rein et al. was published in March 2000. A report in 1991 projected by the year 2000, the direct and indirect costs from PID would be $10 billion annually. Two factors affect the decrease in financial burden: the fewer cases of acute pelvic inflammatory disease and the recent change from inpatient to less expensive outpatient management of the diseases. Presently, it is estimated that there are approximately 1 million cases of acute pelvic inflammatory disease a year in this country. Acute pelvic inflammatory disease is the most common gynecologic condition that results in hospitalization of women of reproductive age in the United States. To reduce the medical impact of acute pelvic inflammatory disease, emphasis must be placed on aggressive therapy for lower genital tract infection and early diagnosis and treatment of upper genital tract infection. Public health emphasis also must be placed on primary prevention involving attempts to prevent exposure and acquisition of sexually transmitted disease. This includes teaching adolescents safe sex practices and promoting use of condoms and chemical barrier methods. Secondary prevention of pelvic inflammatory disease involves universal screening of women at high risk for chlamydia and gonorrhea; screening for active cervicitis; increasing use of sensitive tests to diagnose lower genital infection; treatment of sexual partners; and education to prevent recurrent infection.

Acute pelvic inflammatory disease results from ascending infection from the bacterial flora of the vagina and cervix in more than 99% of cases. This ascending infection occurs along the mucosal surface, where the bacteria colonize and infect the endometrium and fallopian tubes. Acute pelvic inflammatory disease is rare in the woman without menstrual periods, such as the pregnant, premenarchal, or postmenopausal woman. The process sometimes extends to the surface of the ovaries and nearby peritoneum and rarely into the adjacent soft tissues, such as the broad ligament and pelvic blood vessels. In less than 1% of cases, acute pelvic inflammatory disease results from transperitoneal spread of infectious material from a perforated appendix or intraabdominal abscess. Hematogenous and lymphatic spread to the tubes or ovaries is another remote possibility. Acute pelvic inflammatory disease is usually a polymicrobial infection that is a mixture of aerobic and anaerobic bacteria clinically appearing as a complex infection. Therapeutic strategies and regimens are broad spectrum, seeking to suppress aerobic and anaerobic organisms. More than 20 species of microorganisms have been cultured from direct aspiration of purulent material from infected tubes. Acute PID is unlike an infection in many other areas of the body, which usually is caused predominantly by one species of microorganism.

Annually, acute pelvic inflammatory disease occurs in 1% to 2% of all young, sexually active women. It is the most common serious infection of women aged 16 to 25. Approximately 85% of infections are spontaneous in sexually active females. The other 15% of infections develop following procedures that break the cervical mucus barrier, allowing the vaginal flora the opportunity to colonize the upper genital tract. These procedures include endometrial biopsy, curettage, intrauterine device insertion, hysterosalpingography, and hysteroscopy. For emphasis, pelvic inflammatory disease is extremely rare in women who are either amenorrheic or not sexually active. When pelvic inflammatory disease is found in the postmenopausal woman associated conditions such as genital malignancies, diabetes, and/or concurrent intestinal diseases, such as diverticulitis, appendicitis, or carcinoma are usually discovered.

One in four women with acute pelvic inflammatory disease experiences medical sequelae. Conversely, many women with sequelae of the disease, such as infertility related to tubal obstruction, do not have a history of having had the symptoms or signs of an acute infection. Following acute pelvic inflammatory disease, the rate of ectopic pregnancy increases sixfold to tenfold, and the chance of developing chronic pelvic pain increases fourfold. In the United States each year 26,100 ectopic pregnancies and 90,000 new cases of chronic abdominal pain are directly related to pelvic inflammatory disease (Table 23-1). The incidence of infertility following acute pelvic inflammatory disease varies

---

TABLE 23-1

Incidence of Acute PID and Associated Sequelae for Women Aged 15 to 44 Years

| | Pelvic Inflammatory Disease | | | | |
Age (years)	Number of Hospitalized Cases	Number of Outpatient Cases	Number of Surgical Procedures	Number of Ectopic Pregnancies	Number of Infertile Women
15–19	42,000	158,000	—	4100	—
20–24	72,100	271,300	—	7050	—
25–29	62,700	236,000	—	6150	—
30–34	43,200	162,600	—	4200	—
35–39	26,700	100,400	—	2600	—
40–44	20,500	77,100	—	2000	—
TOTAL	267,200	1,005,400	118,900	26,100	200,000

From Washington AE, Arno PS, and Brooks MA: JAMA 255:1736, 1986. Copyright 1986, American Medical Association.

widely (6% to 60%) depending on the severity of the infection, the number of episodes of infection, and the age of the patient. Weström reported that hospitalized patients have an incidence of infertility due to tubal obstruction of 11.4% after one episode of pelvic inflammatory disease, 23.1% after two episodes, and 54.3% after three or more episodes. Women with one episode of acute pelvic inflammatory disease are also more susceptible to developing a subsequent infection. It is difficult to distinguish whether this tendency is related primarily to mucosal damage or to reinfection by a potentially infected mate. Grimes has estimated that 0.29 deaths per 100,000 women aged 15 to 44 are directly related to pelvic inflammatory disease.

The clinical symptoms and signs of acute pelvic inflammatory disease vary considerably and are usually nonspecific. Importantly, some patients may have very little symptomatology, a condition called *silent* or *asymptomatic PID*.

Ideally, laparoscopy with direct visualization of the internal female organs would not only improve the diagnostic accuracy but also afford the opportunity for direct cultures of purulent material, which might help to establish optimum therapy. Although laparoscopy is being used more extensively in the early diagnosis of acute pelvic inflammatory disease, in practice most women do not undergo this procedure because of the expense. Needle laparoscopy offers a less expensive alternative. However, this procedure has not gained wide acceptance in the outpatient setting.

In summary, the CDC has emphasized that physicians should aggressively treat women if there is any suspicion of the disease, since the sequelae are so devastating and the clinical diagnosis made from symptoms, signs, and laboratory data is often incorrect.

Etiology

Acute pelvic inflammatory disease is usually a polymicrobial infection caused by organisms ascending from the vagina and cervix along the mucosa of the endometrium to infect the mucosa of the oviduct. Two classic sexually transmitted organisms, *N. gonorrhoeae* and *C. trachomatis,* cause acute pelvic inflammatory disease in the majority of cases. These two organisms coexist in the same individual 25% to 50% of the time. Endogenous aerobic and anaerobic bacteria that originated from the normal vaginal flora are cultured from tubal fluid in approximately 50% of cases. The tubal culture also is positive for *N. gonorrhoeae, C. trachomatis,* or both in approximately one half of the tubal infections in which normal vaginal flora are present. Direct cultures have proved that tubal infections are usually polymicrobial throughout the active infectious process. Sweet discovered an average of seven different species in his series of intraabdominal cultures performed via the laparoscope. However, the type and number of species vary depending on the stage of the disease when the culture is obtained. For example, gonorrheal organisms are fre-

quently cultured during the first 24 to 48 hours of the disease but are often absent later. Similarly, later in the disease process, anaerobic bacteria tend to predominate.

It used to be common practice to divide pelvic inflammatory disease into gonococcal and nongonococcal disease depending on the recovery of *N. gonorrhoeae* from the endocervix. Laparoscopic studies have demonstrated a correlation of no better than 50% between endocervical and tubal cultures. Thus endocervical cultures are a crude index at best of the specific cause of upper genital tract infection.

Multiple studies have demonstrated a wide range of positive cultures from women with acute pelvic inflammatory disease. The organisms differ depending on the geographic location of the study, the prevalence of lower genital tract disease, the population studied, the duration of symptoms, the severity of the disease, and the number of previous episodes of acute pelvic inflammatory disease.

Because of the virulence of *N. gonorrhoeae* in both in vitro and in vivo studies, its major role in pelvic inflammatory disease is well established. Approximately 20% of women with cervical infection by *N. gonorrhoeae* subsequently develop acute pelvic inflammatory disease. Approximately 50% of women with endocervical cultures positive for *N. gonorrhoeae* at the time of acute pelvic inflammatory disease will have the same organism cultured from the fallopian tubes. If *N. gonorrhoeae* is the only organism cultured from the tubes, a patient will usually respond rapidly to treatment.

The virulence of the strain or colony type of *N. gonorrhoeae* helps to predict the incidence of upper genital tract infection. Transparent colonies of *N. gonorrhoeae* on culture medium attach more readily to epithelial cells and thus produce tubal infection more frequently than opaque-appearing colonies. Immunologic studies have demonstrated that an antibody against the outer membrane protein of the gonococcus develops in approximately 70% of women following severe pelvic infection. The lack of significant antibody titers may help explain why teenagers are more likely to develop upper genital tract disease than women in their late 20s.

There is an extremely wide variation in the recovery rates of *N. gonorrhoeae* depending on the geographic location of the study (Table 23-2). The highest recovery rates occur in young, urban women in the United States.

The gonococcus produces an intense inflammatory reaction in the tubes, which causes narrowing or occlusion of the tubal lumen because of the presence of necrotic debris and purulent material. This cellular destruction is much more extensive than the reaction associated with a chlamydial infection.

C. trachomatis is an intracellular, sexually transmitted bacterial pathogen. A report from Edinburgh found a ratio of chlamydial to gonococcal PID diagnosed by laparoscopy of 4:1. However, there is a widespread difference in isolation rates depending on the series and the geographic location (Table 23-3). One of the primary reasons that chlamydial

TABLE 23-2

Comparison of *C. trachomatis* and *N. gonorrhoeae* Cervical Isolation and *N. gonorrhoeae* Tubal Isolation among Women with Acute PID

| First Author of Study | No. of Patients | Cervical Infection | | Tubal/Peritoneal Infection* |
		C. trachomatis	*N. gonorrhoeae*	*N. gonorrhoeae*
Henry-Suchet	17	6/16 (38%)	0/4	1/4 (25%)
Møller	166	37 (22%)	9 (5%)	
Mårdh	60	23 (38%)	4 (5%)	
Gjønnaess	65	26/56 (46%)	5 (8%)	0/65
Mårdh	63	19/53 (36%)	11 (17%)	1/14 (7%)
Adler	78	4 (5%)	14 (18%)	
Ripa	206	52/156 (33%)	39 (19%)	
Osser	209	52/111 (47%)	41 (20%)	
Paavonen	106	27 (25%)	27 (25%)	
Paavonen	101	32 (32%)	25 (25%)	
Paavonen	228	69 (30%)	60 (26%)	
Eilard	22	6 (27%)	7 (32%)	1/22 (5%)
Bowie	43	22 (51%)	15 (35%)	
Eschenbach	204	20/100 (20%)	90 (44%)	7/54 (13%)
Sweet	39	2 (5%)	18 (46%)	8/35 (23%)
Cunningham	104		56 (54%)	30/104 (29%)
Thompson	30	3 (10%)	24 (80%)	10/30 (33%)
TOTAL	1741	400/1365 (29%)	445/1728 (26%)	58/328 (18%)

From Eschenbach DA: Acute pelvic inflammatory disease, vol 1. In Gynecology and obstetrics, Philadelphia, 1985, Harper & Row, Publishers, p. 8.

*Isolation of *N. gonorrhoeae* from the peritoneum of the total number of women studied.

TABLE 23-3

Chlamydia trachomatis in Acute Pelvic Inflammatory Disease

| Study (ref) | No. of Patients | Isolation Rate of *C. trachomatis* | | |
		Endocervix (%)	Upper Genital and Peritoneal Cavity (%)	Fourfold Rise in Serum Antibodies (%)
Eilard et al. (129)	22	6 (27)	2 (9)[a]	5 (23)
Mårdh et al. (130)	53	19 (37)	6/20 (30)[a]	
Treharne et al. (131)	143			88 (62)[b]
Paavonen et al. (132)	106	27 (26)		19/72 (26)
Paavonen (133)	228	68 (30)		32/167 (19)
Mårdh et al. (134)	60	23 (38)		24/60 (40)
Ripa et al. (135)	206	52/156 (33)		118 (57)[c]
Gjønnaess et al. (136)	56	26 (46)	5/42 (12)[a]	26/52 (46)
Møller et al. (137)	166	37 (22)		34 (21)
Osser and Persson (138)	111	52 (47)		37/72 (51)
Eschenbach et al. (87)	100	20 (20)	1/54 (2)[d]	15/74 (20)
Sweet et al. (105)	37	2 (5)	0[a]	5/22 (23)
Thompson et al. (98)	30	3 (10)	3 (10)[e]	
Sweet et al. (35)	71	10 (14)	17 (24)[f]	
Wasserheit et al. (36)	22	10 (45)	8 (36)[f]	
Kiviat et al. (139)	55	12 (22)	12 (22)[f]	
Brunham et al. (90)	50	7 (14)	4 (8)[e]	20 (40)
Landers et al. (108)	148	41 (28)	32 (22)[f]	
Soper et al. (86)	84	13 (15)	1 (1)[e]	
			6 (7)[f]	
Kiviat et al. (140)	69		16 (23)	

From Sweet RL and Gibbs RS: Infectious diseases of the female genital tract, ed 3, Baltimore, 1995, Williams & Wilkins.

[a]Fallopian tube.

[b]Chlamydial IgG ≥ 1:64; 23% had IgM = 1:8.

[c]Chlamydial IgG ≥ 1:64; fourfold rise in 28/80 (35%).

[d]Culdocentesis.

[e]Exudate from fallopian tube.

[f]Fallopian tube and/or endometrial cavity.

organisms were not recovered in early studies in the United States was the reluctance to perform a biopsy of the fallopian tubes to obtain culture material. Recently, *Chlamydia* has become more prevalent than gonorrhea. From 20% to 40% of sexually active women have antibodies against *C. trachomatis*. From 10% to 30% of women with acute pelvic inflammatory disease who do not have cultures positive for *Chlamydia* have evidence of acute chlamydial infection by serial antibody titer testing. Overall, *Chlamydia* is involved in at least 40% of women who are hospitalized with PID. Approximately 30% of women with documented acute cervicitis secondary to chlamydia subsequently develop acute pelvic inflammatory disease. Studies have shown upper tract chlamydial infection increases the risk of an ectopic pregnancy from 3 to 6 times compared with women without chlamydial infection.

C. trachomatis infection of either the lower or upper genital tract is seen most frequently in young women who are sexually active. Clinically, *Chlamydia* produces a mild form of salpingitis with an insidious onset. Whereas gonorrhea remains in the fallopian tubes for at most a few days in untreated patients, *Chlamydia* may remain in the fallopian tubes for months after initial colonization of the upper genital tract.

Sophisticated polymerase chain reaction, in situ hybridization, and electron microscopy studies demonstrate persistence of the *C. trachomatis* in the fallopian tubes for years. Whether this represents persistent or recurrent infection of the upper genital tract is unknown. In experimental studies the salpingitis produced by *Chlamydia* is confined to the tubal mucosa. Most likely *Chlamydia* produces a disruption of the tubal mucosa by an immunopathologic mechanism rather than by a direct cytotoxicity, as is the case with *N. gonorrhoeae*. A host cell-mediated immune response to a chlamydial heat shock protein produces the disruption of the tubal mucosa. Recent basic research has demonstrated a genetic modulation of the immune response to *C. trachomatis* infection with an increased risk in women with HLA-1. Preliminary evidence suggests that the specific chlamydial strain also may be an important variable.

The past decade has produced a clinical awareness of a syndrome called *atypical* or *silent PID*. This is an asymptomatic, or relatively asymptomatic, inflammation of the upper genital tract often associated with chlamydial infection. The sequelae of repeated asymptomatic chlamydial infections is tubal infertility and ectopic pregnancy. Some investigators believe that atypical PID may be the more common form of upper tract infection, and symptomatic PID may be but the "tip of the iceberg." As many as 40% of women with cervicitis without upper tract symptoms will also have endometritis noted on endometrial biopsy. Studies of women with tubal infertility have noted that many women, though not diagnosed as having had overt PID, have had symptoms of acute pelvic pain.

The role of genital mycoplasmas in the etiology of acute pelvic inflammatory disease is unclear. Cervical cultures positive for both *Mycoplasma hominis* and *Ureaplasma urealyticum* may be obtained from the majority of young, sexually active women. The rate of isolation of genital mycoplasmas from the cervix is approximately 75% and similar in populations of women who are sexually active both with and without pelvic inflammatory disease.

Direct tubal cultures demonstrated *M. hominis* in 4% to 17% and *U. urealyticum* in 2% to 20% of women with acute pelvic inflammatory disease. However, serologic studies in women with acute pelvic inflammatory disease have demonstrated that only one woman in four develops a significant rise in antibody titers to these organisms. Experimental inoculation of the cervix of the Grivet monkey demonstrated that the route of spread of mycoplasmas is via the parametria rather than the mucosa. Thus the primary upper genital tract infection is in the parametria and the tissue surrounding the tubes, not in the tubal lumen. This fact may help to explain the low success rate of direct tubal cultures. Histologically, *Mycoplasma* does not appear to produce damage to the tubal mucosa. These organisms are not highly pathogenic. A recent study by Chatwani et al. demonstrated that the presence of genital mycoplasmas does not change the clinical presentation and clinical course of acute pelvic inflammatory disease. The investigators found that both *M. hominis* and *U. urealyticum* may colonize or persist in the endometrial cavity after complete recovery from acute pelvic inflammatory disease. In summary, in vitro and in vivo studies suggest that *Mycoplasma* may be a commensal bacterium rather than a pathogen in the oviducts.

The endogenous aerobic and anaerobic flora of the vagina frequently ascend to colonize and infect the upper reproductive tract. Direct cultures of purulent material from the tubal lumen or posterior cul-de-sac have demonstrated a wide range of organisms (Table 23-4). The most common aerobic organisms are nonhemolytic *Streptococcus*, *Escherichia coli*, group B *Streptococcus*, and coagulase-negative *Staphylococcus*. Anaerobic organisms tend to predominate over aerobes, and the most common anaerobic organisms are *Bacteroides* species, *Peptostreptococcus*, and *Peptococcus*. Anaerobic organisms are almost ubiquitous in pelvic abscesses associated with acute pelvic inflammatory disease. Tuboovarian complexes and abscesses are more common in women with concurrent bacterial vaginosis or HIV infection. Presently there is a controversy as to which species of *Bacteroides* is the predominant agent in acute disease. Some investigators have discovered primarily *Bacteroides fragilis*, whereas others believe *Bacteroides bivius* is the most important anaerobe. The finding of concurrent bacterial vaginosis and pelvic inflammatory disease, as well as the association of bacterial vaginosis with endometritis, serve to emphasize the contributory role of these organisms in the pathogenesis of PID. In some women, no organism will be cultured from the fallopian tubes.

TABLE 23-4
Nongonococcal, Nonchlamydial Bacteria Recovered from the Upper Genital Tract of Patients
with Acute Salpingitis at San Francisco General Hospital (*N* = 188)

Bacteroides spp.	88	*G. vaginalis*	121
B. bivius	72	*E. coli*	25
B. disiens	25	Nonhemolytic streptococci	49
Other *Bacteroides*	99	Group B streptococci	29
Peptostreptococcus asaccharolyticus	93	α-Hemolytic streptococci	45
Peptostreptococcus anaerobius	71	Coagulase-negative staphylococci	72

From Sweet RL and Gibbs RS: Infectious diseases of the female genital tract, ed 3, Baltimore, 1995, Williams & Wilkins.

Risk Factors

Risk factors are important considerations in both the clinical management and prevention of upper genital tract infections. The woman who is classically at highest risk is the menstruating teenager who has multiple sexual partners, does not use contraception, and lives in an area with a high prevalence of sexually transmitted disease. There is a strong correlation between the incidence of sexually transmitted disease and acute pelvic inflammatory disease in any given population. The age distribution of uncomplicated sexually transmitted disease is usually the same as that for acute pelvic inflammatory disease.

In epidemiologic studies, age at first intercourse, marital status, and number of sexual partners are all gross indicators of the frequency of exposure to sexually transmitted diseases. Having multiple sexual partners increases the chance of acquiring acute pelvic inflammatory disease approximately fivefold. The frequency of intercourse with a monogamous partner is not a risk factor.

The incidence of acute pelvic inflammatory disease decreases with advancing age. Acute pelvic inflammatory disease is a condition of young females, with 75% of cases occurring in women less than 25 years of age. The risk that a sexually active adolescent female will develop acute pelvic inflammatory disease is 1 in 8. This risk factor decreases to 1 in 80 for women over the age of 25. Obviously the sexual habits of teenagers, including contact with multiple partners and lack of contraception, predispose them to sexually transmitted diseases and, correspondingly, acute pelvic inflammatory disease. Younger age also increases the incidence of acute pelvic inflammatory disease. For unknown reasons young women with colonization of the cervix by *Chlamydia* have a higher incidence of upper genital tract infection than older women do. A hypothesis to explain the increased infection rate in teenagers includes the comparative lack of antibody protection and the wider area of cervical columnar epithelium, which allows colonization by *C. trachomatis* and *N. gonorrhoeae*.

Stone et al. have tabulated (Table 23-5) both proven and hypothetical methods of preventing sexually trans-

mitted disease and acute pelvic inflammatory disease. Both clinical and laboratory studies have documented that the use of contraceptives changes the relative risk of developing acute pelvic inflammatory disease. Weström has developed an arbitrary risk rating scale in which the risk of developing acute pelvic inflammatory disease in sexually active women not using contraception is assigned a score of 1. The corresponding risk among women using oral contraceptives is 0.3; among women using a barrier method of contraception it is 0.4.

Barrier methods—condoms, diaphragms, and spermicidal preparations—are effective both as mechanical obstructive devices and as chemical barriers. Nonoxynol 9, the material ubiquitous in spermicidal preparations, is both bactericidal and viricidal. Laboratory tests have demonstrated that Nonoxynol 9 kills *N. gonorrhoeae*, genital *Mycoplasma* species, *Trichomonas vaginalis*, *Treponema pallidum*, herpes simplex virus, and human immunodeficiency virus (HIV). The porosity of latex in condoms is more than 1000 times smaller than viral particles. Thus routine condom use prevents deposition and transmission of infected organisms from the semen to the endocervix. In contrast, frequent vaginal douching increases the relative risk of PID threefold to fourfold over women who douche less frequently than once a month.

Oral contraceptive use has two different effects: a lower incidence of acute pelvic inflammatory disease and a milder form of upper genital tract infection when it does occur. The decrease in incidence of upper genital tract infection is believed to be secondary to thicker cervical mucus produced by the progestin component of oral contraceptives, which inhibits sperm and bacterial penetration. The decrease in duration of menstrual flow accompanying oral contraceptive use theoretically creates a shorter interval for bacterial colonization of the upper tract. Wølner-Hanssen et al. correlated laparoscopic findings of women with acute pelvic inflammatory disease and contraceptive use in a case-controlled study. Not only was there less pelvic inflammatory disease in the oral contraceptive group, but also the spread of inflammation to the fallopian tubes seemed to be inhibited in oral contraceptive users (Table 23-6). Washington et al. have urged cau-

TABLE 23-5
Methods of Preventing STDs, Mechanisms of Action, and Efficacy

Method	Mechanism	Efficacy in Prevention of STDs
Behavioral		
Monogamy	Decreases likelihood of exposure to infected persons	Not well studied; theoretic efficacy
Reducing number of partners	Decreases likelihood of contact with infectious agents	
Avoiding certain sexual practices		
Inspecting and questioning partners		
Barriers		
Condom	Protects partner from direct contact with semen, urethral discharge, or penile lesion Protects wearer from direct contact with partner's mucosal secretions	Effective in vitro barrier to chlamydiae, CMV, HSV, and HIV Appears to decrease risk of acquiring urethral/cervical GC, PID, cervical cancer, and male urethral *Ureaplasma* colonization Effect on risk of acquiring NGU not established
Spermicide	Chemically inactivates infectious agents	Nonvaginal use has not been studied Inactivates gonococci, syphilis spirochetes, trichomonads, HSV, ureaplasmas, and HIV in vitro Appears to decrease risk of acquiring cervical GC, PID, and cervical cancer; chlamydiae studies in progress
Diaphragm/spermicide	Mechanical barrier covers cervix Used with spermicides	Diaphragm alone has not been studied Appears to decrease risk of acquiring cervical GC and PID
Vaccines	Induce antibody response that renders host immune to disease	Commercially available hepatitis B vaccine is safe and effective Results of clinical trials of gonococcal and herpes simplex vaccines not encouraging Gonococcal, HIV, and HSV vaccines research in progress
Oral antibiotics		
Penicillin	Kill infectious agent on or shortly after exposure before infection is established	No studies among women or civilian men
Sulfathioazole		Appears to decrease risk of acquiring GC and hard and soft chancres, but use not recommended
Tetracycline analogues		
Local		
Postcoital urination	Flushes infectious agents out of urethra and washes infectious agents of genital skin and mucous membrane	Poorly studied
Postcoital washing		
Postcoital antiseptic douching	Inactivates and washes infectious agents out of vagina	Poorly studied

From Stone KM, Grimes DA, and Magder LS: JAMA 255:1763, 1986. Copyright 1986, American Medical Association. *CMV,* Cytomegalovirus; *HSV,* herpes simplex virus; *HIV,* human immunodeficiency virus; *GC,* gonorrhea; *PID,* pelvic inflammatory disease; *NGU,* nongonococcal urethritis.

TABLE 23-6

Comparison of Laparoscopic Findings with Type of Contraceptive Use in 738 Women with Signs and Symptoms Suggestive of Acute Salpingitis

Laparoscopic Findings	Contraceptive Method*		
	Oral Contraceptive (%)	Intrauterine Device (%)	Reference† (%)
Salpingitis	171 (59.8)	183 (80.6)	190 (84.4)
Nonsalpingitis	115 (40.2)	44 (19.4)	35 (15.6)

From Wølner-Hanssen P, Svensson L, Mårdh PA, et al: Obstet Gynecol 66:234, 1985. Reprinted with permission from the American College of Obstetricians and Gynecologists.

*Relative risk of oral contraceptive use versus reference = 0.27 χ^2_1 = 36.9, $P < 0.0001$; relative risk of IUD use versus reference = 0.77 (95% confidence interval 0.47 to 1.26, χ^2_1 = 1.1, $P = 0.28$); and relative risk of oral contraceptive versus IUD use = 0.36 (95% confidence interval 0.24 to 0.54, χ^2_1 = 25.7, $P < 0.0001$).

†Reference = barrier methods or no contraception.

tion in the conclusion that oral contraceptives protect against all forms of acute pelvic inflammatory disease. A twofold to threefold increase in the prevalence of endocervical infection by *C. trachomatis* has been demonstrated in multiple epidemiologic studies of women using oral contraceptives. Whether the colonization of the endocervix results in more upper genital tract disease is presently being studied.

Twenty to thirty years ago, multiple case-controlled studies reported an increased risk of acute pelvic inflammatory disease in women who were using an IUD. There has been just criticism of these early epidemiologic studies for their selection of control groups and the bias of including women with Dalkon Shields in their statistics. The increase in risk for PID occurs only at the time of insertion of the IUD and in the first three weeks after placement. An analysis from the World Health Organization found the rate of PID to be 9.7 per 1000 woman-years for the first 20 days after insertion compared with 1.4 per 1000 woman-years for the next 8 years of follow-up.

Acute salpingitis occurring in a woman with a previous tubal ligation is extremely rare, and when it does occur, the symptoms of the infection are less severe. Phillips and D'Ablaing reported the incidence of acute pelvic inflammatory disease developing in the proximal stump of previously ligated fallopian tubes as 1 in 450 women hospitalized for acute salpingitis (Figure 23-1).

Epidemiologic studies have documented that previous acute pelvic inflammatory disease is a definite risk factor for future attacks of the disease. Approximately 25% of women with acute pelvic inflammatory disease subsequently develop another acute tubal infection. Ten years

ago this reinfection was believed to be "chronic infection" or exacerbations of a "latent" tubal process. Direct cultures have proven that the disease is another primary infection. The microscopic tubal damage produced by the initial upper genital tract infection may facilitate repeat infection. This increased risk may be related to the sexual habits of the woman involved or to an untreated male partner. Studies have documented that greater than 80% of male contacts are not treated. Approximately 50% of men with sexually transmitted diseases are free of symptoms, and thus they do not seek treatment.

Transcervical penetration of the cervical mucus barrier with instrumentation of the uterus is a risk factor, for it may initiate "iatrogenic" acute pelvic inflammatory disease. Approximately 1 million first-trimester abortions are performed each year in the United States. The incidence of upper genital tract infection associated with this procedure is approximately 1 in 200 cases. Recent practice has emphasized the use of prophylactic antibiotics in high-risk cases to attempt to decrease the incidence of associated acute pelvic inflammatory disease. Women with concurrent bacterial vaginosis have a higher risk for postabortal infection and thus should be treated with oral antibiotics with anaerobic coverage.

A growing area of research involves identification of changes in the virulence of organisms and the host's response to the organisms. The change in virulence of an organism is another risk factor for pelvic inflammatory disease and may explain why some lower tract infections progress to upper tract disease while others do not. The gonococcus possesses different factors that may become activated in certain environments to increase the virulence of the organism. Similarly, other organisms that are usu-

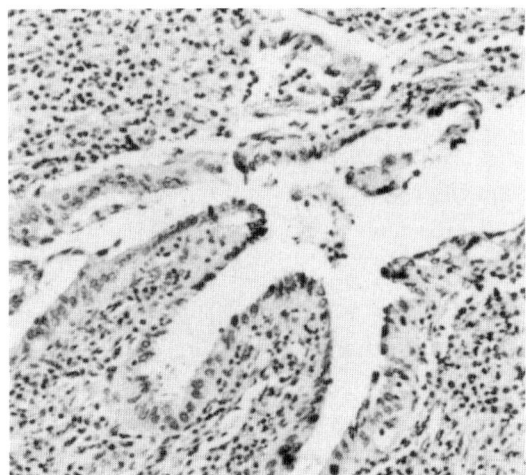

FIGURE 23-1 Tubal mucous membrane of proximal stump with lamina propria extensively infiltrated by numerous acute and chronic inflammatory cells in woman with a previous tubal ligation. (From Phillips AJ and D'Ablaing G: Obstet Gynecol 67:56S, 1986. Reprinted with permission from the American College of Obstetricians and Gynecologists.)

ally of low virulence may possess factors that affect their virulence and pathogenicity. Both bacterial virulence factors, such as hemolysin enzymes and proteases, and bacterial defense mechanisms that inhibit host responses may become activated under varying microenvironments.

In summary, the primary emphasis in disease prevention is the treatment of sexual partners of women with acute pelvic inflammatory disease. The male partner is frequently asymptomatic and should be treated empirically with antibiotics against both *Chlamydia* and gonorrhea.

Symptoms and Signs

Patients with acute pelvic inflammatory disease present with a wide range of nonspecific clinical symptoms and signs. Thus the diagnosis of acute pelvic inflammatory disease even by experienced clinicians is imprecise. Many women have mild, nonspecific pelvic symptoms that are overlooked by both the woman and her physician. The severity of the clinical presentation of acute PID varies from being asymptomatic to a woman with diffuse peritonitis and a life-threatening illness. Since the diagnosis is usually based on clinical criteria, there is both a high false positive rate and a high false negative rate. The differential diagnosis of acute pelvic inflammatory disease includes lower genital tract pelvic infection, ectopic pregnancy, torsion or rupture of an adnexal mass, acute appendicitis, gastroenteritis, and endometriosis.

Laparoscopic studies of women with a clinical diagnosis of acute pelvic inflammatory disease have established the inadequacy of diagnosis by the usual criteria of history and physical and laboratory examination. In these studies approximately 20% to 25% of women had no identifiable intraabdominal or pelvic disease. Another 10% to 15% of patients were found to have other pathologic conditions, such as ectopic pregnancy, acute appendicitis, or torsion of the adnexa. In one of these studies Jacobson reported a series of 814 women in whom laparoscopy was performed because of clinically suspected acute pelvic inflammatory disease. The clinical diagnosis was confirmed at laparoscopy in 532 women (65%). This study also documented the laparoscopic findings in 98 women with a false positive clinical diagnosis of acute pelvic inflammatory disease and 91 cases of false negative clinical diagnosis of acute pelvic inflammatory disease (Tables 23-7 and 23-8). Another interesting finding of laparoscopic studies is the lack of correlation between the number and intensity of symptoms, signs and degree of abnormality of laboratory values, and the severity of tubal inflammation. Women with *C. trachomatis* infections may exhibit minor symptoms but have a severe inflammatory process visualized by laparoscopic examination. Criteria for establishing the severity of acute pelvic inflammatory disease by laparoscopic examination are listed in Table 23-9.

TABLE 23-7
Laparoscopic Findings in Patients with False Positive Clinical Diagnosis of Acute PID but with Pelvic Disorders Other Than PID

Laparoscopic Finding	No.
Acute appendicitis	24
Endometriosis	16
Corpus luteum bleeding	12
Ectopic pregnancy	11
Pelvic adhesions only	7
Benign ovarian tumor	7
Chronic salpingitis	6
Miscellaneous	15
TOTAL	98

From Jacobson LJ: Am J Obstet Gynecol 138:1006, 1980

TABLE 23-8
Preoperative Diagnoses in Patients with False Negative Clinical Diagnosis of Acute PID Prior to Laparoscopy/Laparotomy

Clinical Diagnosis	Visual Diagnosis: Acute PID (No.)
Ovarian tumor	20
Acute appendicitis	18
Ectopic pregnancy	16
Chronic salpingitis	10
Acute peritonitis	6
Endometriosis	5
Uterine myoma	5
Uncharacteristic pelvic pain	5
Miscellaneous	6
TOTAL	91

From Jacobson LJ: Am J Obstet Gynecol 138:1006, 1980

TABLE 23-9
Severity of Disease by Laparoscopic Examination

Severity	Findings
Mild	Erythema, edema, no spontaneous purulent exudate*; tubes freely movable
Moderate	Gross purulent material evident; erythema and edema more marked; tubes may not be freely movable, and fimbria stoma may not be patent
Severe	Pyosalpinx or inflammatory complex
	Abscess†

From Hager WD, Eschenbach DA, Spence MR, et al: Obstet Gynecol 61:114, 1983. Reprinted with permission from the American College of Obstetricians and Gynecologists.

*The tubes may require manipulation to produce purulent exudate.

†The size of any pelvic abscess should be measured.

Historically, the diagnosis of acute pelvic inflammatory disease was not established unless the patient had the triad of fever, elevated erythrocyte sedimentation rate, and adnexal tenderness or a mass. Only 17% of laparoscopically identified cases have this classic triad. Jacobson described the reverse logic that has been applied to the syndrome of acute pelvic inflammatory disease. He points out that the disorder had been made to fit the criteria established for it and not vice versa, as is usually the clinical practice. Thus reliance on stringent clinical criteria for establishing the diagnosis of the disease would result in the majority of cases being overlooked and not treated. Obviously, more frequent and liberal use of diagnostic laparoscopy is an important advance in the management of the disease. Laparoscopy allows precise diagnosis and also the opportunity to collect culture material from the site of the infection. However, in practice the majority of women with acute pelvic inflammatory disease do not undergo laparoscopy because of the expense of this invasive technique.

Hager et al. have established clinical criteria for acute pelvic inflammatory disease (Table 23-10). These uniform criteria were adopted by the Obstetrical and Gynecologic Infectious Disease Society. Hadgu et al. published a multivariate logistic regression analysis of symptoms, signs, and laboratory findings of women laparoscopically diagnosed as having their first episode of acute pelvic inflammatory disease. This mathematic model correctly predicted 87% of cases and had an overall correct classification rate of 76%. The frequencies of various symptoms, signs, and laboratory data from this series of 414 women are depicted in Tables 23-11 and 23-12. In 1993 the CDC established the latest list of clinical criteria, which is the current standard to initiate empiric treatment of acute PID (see the box on p. 720).

TABLE 23-10
Acute Salpingitis: Clinical Criteria for Diagnosis

Criteria

Abdominal direct tenderness, with or without rebound tenderness
Tenderness with motion of cervix and uterus
Adnexal tenderness

} All 3 necessary for diagnosis

plus

Gram stain of endocervix—positive for gram-negative, intracellular diplococci
Temperature (>38° C)
Leukocytosis (>10,000)

Purulent material (white blood cells present) from peritoneal cavity by culdocentesis or laparoscopy
Pelvic abscess or inflammatory complex on bimanual examination or on sonography

} 1 or more necessary for diagnosis

From Hager WD, Eschenbach DA, Spence MR, et al: Obstet Gynecol 61:114, 1983. Reprinted with permission from the American College of Obstetricians and Gynecologists

Pain in the lower abdomen and pelvis is by far the most frequent symptom of acute pelvic inflammatory disease. In all large series, more than 90% of women present with diffuse bilateral lower abdominal pain. This pain is usually described as constant and dull. On occasion the pain may become cramping, and it is accentuated by motion or sexual

TABLE 23-11
Frequency of Various Symptoms as Reported by Patients in Acute PID and Visually Normal Groups (first-time PID patients)

| | Laparoscopic Diagnosis | | | | |
| | Acute PID (No. = 414) | | Normal (No. = 138) | | |
Symptom	Number	Percent	Number	Percent	P Value
Lower abdominal pain	411	99.3	135	97.8	NS
Vaginal discharge	287	69.3	85	61.6	NS
Temperature ≥38° C	142	34.4	34	24.6	0.05
Irregular bleeding	165	40.0	54	39.1	NS
Urinary symptoms	82	19.8	29	21.0	NS
Vomiting	43	10.4	13	9.4	NS
Protitis symptoms	30	7.3	4	2.9	NS
Other	33	8.0	8	5.8	NS

From Hadgu A, Weström L, Brooks CA, et al: Am J Obstet Gynecol 155:956, 1986.

TABLE 23-12

Frequency of Various Objective Findings at Admission in Acute PID and Visually Normal Groups

Clinical Findings at Admission	Laparoscopic Diagnosis				P Value
	Acute PID (No. = 414)		Normal (No. = 138)		
	Number	Percent	Number	Percent	
Bimanual examination					
Marked tenderness	193	95.4	128	92.8	NS
Palpable mass or swelling	198	47.8	36	26.1	0.001
Erythrocyte sedimentation rate > 15 mm/hr	336	81.2	78	56.5	0.001
Abnormal vaginal discharge	337	81.4	80	58.0	0.001
Fever (38° C)	146	35.3	21	15.2	0.001

From Hadgu A, Weström L, Brooks CA, et al: Am J Obstet Gynecol 155:956, 1986.

activity. Generally the pain is of short duration, usually less than 7 days. If the pain has been present for longer than 3 weeks, it is unlikely that the patient has acute pelvic inflammatory disease. Approximately 75% of patients with acute pelvic inflammatory disease have an associated endocervical infection or a coexistent purulent vaginal discharge. Abnormal uterine bleeding, especially spotting or menorrhagia, is noted in about 40% of patients. The presence of abnormal uterine bleeding often leads to a suspected diagnosis of ectopic pregnancy. Nausea and vomiting are relatively late symptoms in the course of the disease.

When one compares the frequency of individual symptoms and signs between women with laparoscopically proven acute pelvic inflammatory disease and those without the disease, there is no significant difference with the exception of fever (Figure 23-2). Acute pelvic inflammatory disease often occurs with minimum symptoms. Most studies have found that approximately 50% of women who are infertile as a result of tubal obstruction do not remember ever having symptoms of acute pelvic infection.

The symptoms of acute pelvic infection secondary to *N. gonorrhoeae* are of rapid onset, and the pelvic pain usually begins a few days after the onset of a menstrual period. Acute pelvic infection caused by *C. trachomatis* alone often may have an indolent course with slow onset, less pain, and less fever.

Five to ten percent of women with acute pelvic inflammatory disease develop symptoms of perihepatic inflammation—the Fitz-Hugh–Curtis syndrome. The condition is often mistakenly diagnosed as either pneumonia or acute cholecystitis. Persistent symptoms and signs include right upper quadrant pain, pleuritic pain, and tenderness in the right upper quadrant when the liver is palpated. The pain may radiate to the shoulder or into the back. Liver transaminases may be elevated. Fitz-Hugh–Curtis syndrome develops from transperitoneal or vascular dissemination of either the gonococcus or *Chlamydia* organism to

produce the perihepatic inflammation. Currently, *Chlamydia* produces the majority of cases. Other organisms, including anaerobic streptococci and coxsackievirus, have also been associated with this syndrome. Laparoscopy may be useful in the diagnosis of this syndrome. The liver capsule will appear inflamed, with classic "violin" string adhesions to the parietal peritoneum beneath the diaphragm. Women with perihepatitis have a higher prevalence of moderate to severe pelvic adhesions and a higher prevalence and higher titers of antibodies to the chlamydial heat-shock protein-60. Treatment is the same as the treatment for acute salpingitis.

Women with laparoscopically confirmed acute pelvic inflammatory disease are often afebrile. Only one out of three women with acute pelvic inflammatory disease presents with a temperature greater than 38° C. In a study of women with biopsy-proven acute chlamydial salpingitis, only 20% had a fever. Lower abdominal and pelvic tenderness during examination is the hallmark of acute pelvic inflammatory disease. Most women with acute pelvic inflammatory disease have tenderness to direct palpation in the lower abdomen and sometimes may have rebound tenderness. Bilateral tenderness of the parametria and adnexa is usually discovered during pelvic examination. This tenderness is especially noted with movement of the uterus or cervix during the pelvic examination. An ill-defined adnexal fullness is frequently noted. This may represent edema, inflammatory adhesions to either the small or large intestine, or an adnexal complex or abscess. The incidence of true adnexal abscess is approximately 10% in women with acute pelvic inflammatory disease.

Diagnosis

Direct visualization via the laparoscope is the most accurate method of diagnosis of acute pelvic inflammatory disease. Laparoscopy is also indispensable in the clinical

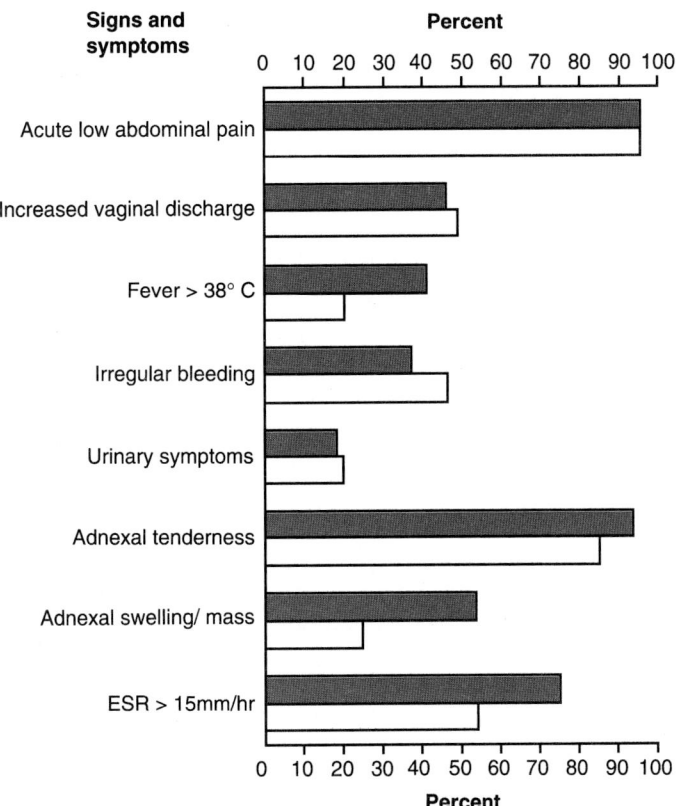

FIGURE 23-2 Comparison of frequency of symptoms, signs, and laboratory findings between patients with acute pelvic inflammatory disease (PID) *(blue bars)* and suspected PID without pelvic pathology *(open bars)* by laparoscopic examination. (From Jacobson LJ: Am J Obstet Gynecol 138:1008, 1980.)

research of the disease. Obviously, there are several presentations of acute PID in which laparoscopy or laparotomy is strongly indicated, such as impending septic shock, acute surgical abdomen, and in a complicated differential diagnosis in a postmenopausal woman. Women who undergo laparoscopy to confirm the diagnosis of acute PID have the additional advantage of concurrent operative procedures such as lysis of adhesions, potential drainage of an abscess, and irrigation of the pelvic cavity. To date, operative laparoscopy during acute infection has not been proven to reduce the prevalence of long-term sequelae. Nevertheless the diagnosis of the majority of episodes of acute pelvic inflammatory disease is made on the basis of clinical history and physical examination. As emphasized previously, the disease should be diagnosed with a minimum of suspicion, with the knowledge that overtreatment is preferable to missed diagnosis. Acute pelvic inflammatory disease should be included in the differential diagnosis of any sexually active young woman with pelvic pain. Laboratory tests may be obtained, but their results lack sufficient sensitivity and specificity to make them an important factor in establishing the diagnosis. For example, the criteria of the infectious disease society (see Table 23-10) assign a minor role to positive laboratory data. Since clinical

symptoms and signs are nonspecific for the disease, when the diagnosis is based on clinical criteria, there is a high percentage of both false positive and false negative rates. Because of the long-term sequelae of the disease, most clinicians maintain a low threshold in entertaining a diagnosis of acute pelvic inflammatory disease, readily accepting that they are treating many women who actually do not have pelvic infection, in order not to omit treating women with early or mild disease. For the CDC guidelines for diagnosis of acute PID, see the box on page 720.

Leukocytosis is not a reliable indicator of acute pelvic inflammatory disease, nor does it correlate with the need for hospitalization or the severity of tubal inflammation. Less than 50% of women with acute pelvic inflammatory disease have a white blood cell count of greater than 10,000 cells per milliliter. For years, erythrocyte sedimentation rate was a standard laboratory test for women with acute pelvic inflammatory disease. This laboratory test is nonspecific. The sedimentation rate is elevated, greater than 15 mm per hour, in approximately 75% of women with laparoscopically confirmed acute pelvic infection. However, 53% of women with pelvic pain and visually normal pelvic organs have an elevated erythrocyte sedimentation rate. Similarly, the sedimentation rate is a

CDC Guidelines for Diagnosis of Acute PID Clinical Criteria for Initiating Therapy

Minimum Criteria

Empiric treatment of PID should be initiated in sexually active young women and others at risk for STDs if all the following minimum criteria are present and no other cause(s) for the illness can be identified:

Lower abdominal tenderness
Adnexal tenderness
Cervical motion tenderness

Additional Criteria

More elaborate diagnostic evaluation often is needed, because incorrect diagnosis and management might cause unnecessary morbidity. These additional criteria may be used to enhance the specificity of the minimum criteria

Routine Criteria for Diagnosing PID:
Oral temperature >38.3° C
Abnormal cervical or vaginal discharge
Elevated erythrocyte sedimentation rate
Elevated C-reactive protein
Laboratory documentation of cervical infection with *N. gonorrhoeae* or *C. trachomatis.*

Definitive Criteria for Diagnosing PID:
Histopathologic evidence of endometritis on endometrial biopsy
Transvaginal sonography or other imaging techniques showing thickened fluid-filled tubes with or without free pelvic fluid or tuboovarian complex
Laparoscopic abnormalities consistent with PID

Although initial treatment decisions can be made before bacteriologic diagnosis of *C. trachomatis* or *N. gonorrhoeae* infection, such a diagnosis emphasizes the need to treat sex partners.

From Centers for Disease Control and Prevention: 1998 Guidelines for treatment of sexually transmitted diseases, MMWR 47:80, 1997.

Recently, *C. trachomatis* has surpassed *N. gonorrhea* as the most prevalent sexually transmitted bacteria-producing upper tract infection in the developed world. A positive Gram-stained smear of the endocervical mucus is nonspecific, and a negative smear does not rule out upper tract infection. A saline prep and pH of vaginal secretions for bacterial vaginosis should also be obtained. Peipert has reported that the presence of an increased number of vaginal white blood cells is the most sensitive laboratory indicator of acute pelvic inflammatory disease. However, he concluded that no one diagnostic laboratory test is pathognomonic for upper genital tract infection. Most importantly, combinations of positive tests improved diagnostic specificity and positive predictive value. However, this results in a diminution of sensitivity and negative predictive value (Table 23-13).

Some clinicians perform an endometrial biopsy looking for evidence of endometritis. Pragmatically, because of the time delay between biopsy and the final histopathologic report, this test is primarily used in research protocols rather than in clinical practice. It is important to realize that although the majority of women with acute salpingitis have coexisting endometritis, the converse that the majority of women with endometritis have salpingitis has not been established. In one investigation of women with biopsy-proven endometritis, the accuracy of coexistent acute pelvic inflammatory disease confirmed by laparoscopy had a sensitivity of 89% and a specificity of 87%.

The percentage of American women with acute PID who also are infected with HIV has been estimated to be 6% to 22%. Most studies demonstrate that women with acute PID and HIV infection have a higher incidence of adnexal masses. However, the acute pelvic infection responds to antibiotic therapy in a similar fashion as in women who are not infected with HIV. Because acute pelvic inflammatory disease is usually secondary to a sexually transmitted disease, it is ideal to examine, culture, and smear urethral secretions from the male partner. Often this step is not performed for a variety of nonmedical reasons. The Centers for Disease Control continues to emphasize the importance of treating partners of women with sexually transmitted disease.

Ultrasonography is of limited value for patients with mild or moderate pelvic inflammatory disease due to its low sensitivity. However, vaginal ultrasonography is helpful in documenting an adnexal mass and differentiating between a tuboovarian abscess and a tuboovarian complex (Figure 23-3). Ultrasonography is also a noninvasive diagnostic aid for patients who are so tender during pelvic examination that the physician cannot determine the presence or absence of a pelvic mass. Though ultrasonography is neither specific nor sensitive in distinguishing the etiology of a pelvic mass, findings of dilated and fluid-filled tubes, free peritoneal fluid, and adnexal masses may be confirmatory of symptoms and

crude indicator of severity of disease and is no longer used to guide therapy. Some investigators obtain C-reactive protein levels. We have not found that these levels change clinical management.

Women with acute pelvic inflammatory disease should have a sensitive test for human chorionic gonadotrophin to help in the differential diagnosis of ectopic pregnancy. About 3 to 4 of every 100 women who are admitted to a hospital with a diagnosis of acute pelvic infection have an ectopic pregnancy.

Because most cases of upper genital tract infection are preceded by lower genital tract infection, it is important to examine the endocervical mucus for inflammatory cells, culture for both *N. gonorrhoeae* and *C. trachomatis,* and have the laboratory perform a Gram stain. *C. trachomatis* is the most prevalent causative pathogen.

TABLE 23-13
Diagnostic Test Characteristics of Laboratory Tests for the Diagnosis of Acute Upper Genital Tract Infection

Test	Sensitivity (%)	Specificity (%)	Prevalence 30%		Prevalence 60%	
			NPV (%)	PPV (%)	NPV (%)	PPV (%)
Entire cohort (N = 120)						
ESR	70	52	80	38	54	69
CRP	71	66	84	47	60	76
WBC	57	88	83	67	58	88
Vaginal WBC	78	39	80	35	54	66
Classical PID (N = 70)						
ESR	72	53	82	40	56	70
CRP	76	59	85	44	62	74
WBC	66	80	85	59	61	83
Vaginal WBC	87	38	87	38	66	68
Nonclassical PID (N = 50)						
ESR	64	51	77	36	49	66
CRP	58	73	80	48	54	76
WBC	38	97	78	84	51	95
Vaginal WBC	62	41	72	31	42	61

From Peipert et al: Obstet Gynecol 87:733, 1996. Reprinted with permission from the American College of Obstetricians and Gynecologists.

NPV = negative predictive value; PPV = positive predictive value; ESR = erythrocyte sedimentation rate; CRP = C-reactive protein; WBC = white blood cell count.

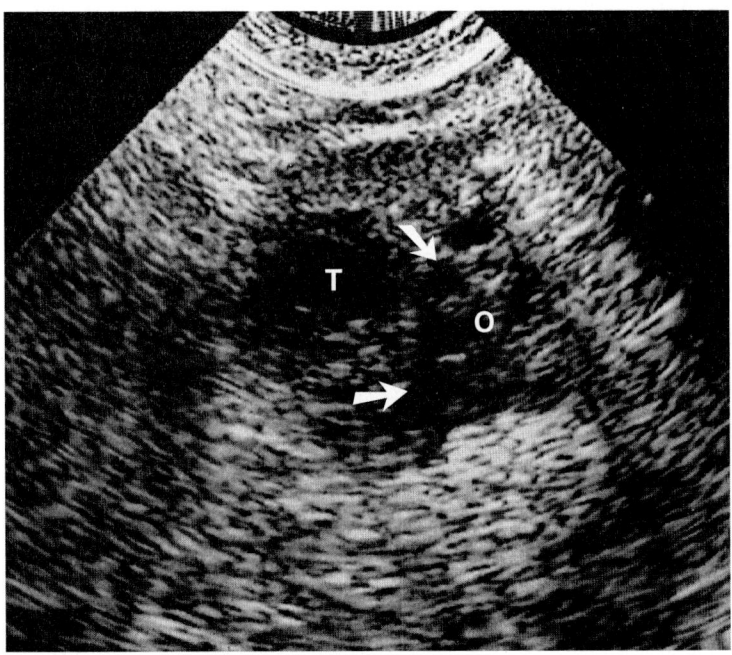

FIGURE 23-3 Cross-section of an adnexal mass suggestive of tuboovarian complex. The slightly dilated and fluid-filled tube *(T)* is seen very close to the ovary *(O)*. The ovarian part of the complex can be recognized by the presence of follicles *(arrows)*. Endometrial biopsy showed plasma cell endometritis. (From Cacciatore B, Leminen A, Ingman-Friberg S, et al: Obstet Gynecol 80:912, 1992.)

physical signs (Figures 23-4, 23-5, and 23-6). Thus vaginal ultrasound does have a high positive predictive value when used in a high-risk population.

Laparoscopy, as already noted, is the gold standard in the diagnosis of acute pelvic inflammatory disease. Direct visualization of the pelvic organs is the most accurate method of diagnosis. The appearance of the pelvic organs may vary from red, indurated, edematous oviducts, to pockets of purulent material, to a large pyosalpinx or tuboovarian abscess. In recent years there has been increasing

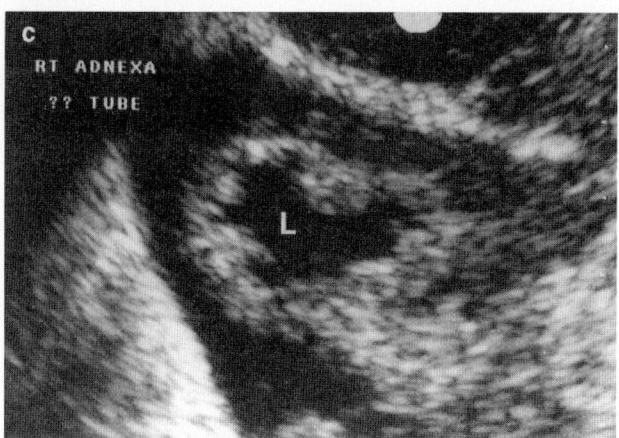

FIGURE 23-4 Transvaginal sonographic image of acute salpingitis. The central sonolucent fluid in the lumen (L) and the thickened endosalpingeal folds render this the "cogwheel" appearance. (From Timor-Tritsch IE, Lerner JP, Monteagudo A, et al: Ultrasound Obstet Gynecol 12:56, 1998.)

use of the laparoscope in women with acute pelvic pain. Laparoscopy is definitely indicated for patients who are not responding to therapy, both to confirm the diagnosis and to obtain cultures of purulent material.

Management

The two most important goals of the medical therapy of acute pelvic inflammatory disease are the resolution of symptoms and the preservation of tubal function. Antibiotic therapy should be started as soon as cervical cultures have been obtained and the diagnosis is suspect. Early diag-

nosis and early treatment will help reduce the number of women who suffer from the long-term sequelae of the disease. Women who are not treated in the first 72 hours following the onset of symptoms are three times as likely to develop tubal infertility or ectopic pregnancy as compared to those who are treated early in the disease process. The CDC recommends empiric treatment of PID in sexually active young women and others at risk for sexually transmitted diseases if all of the following minimum criteria are present and no other cause(s) for the illness can be identified: lower abdominal tenderness, adnexal tenderness, and cervical motion tenderness. Both animal and human studies have suggested that early antibiotic treatment improves long-term fertility. In the management of acute pelvic inflammatory disease, one should not forget the treatment of the male partner and education for the prevention of the disease, including the use of proper contraceptives, which help to reduce the rate of upper genital tract infection.

The choice of antibiotic therapy for most infectious diseases is usually based on culture and sensitivity of bacteria obtained directly from the site of the infection. Pragmatically, direct culture from the fallopian tube is rarely obtained before instituting empiric antibiotic treatment. Because most cases of pelvic inflammatory disease are polymicrobial, broad-spectrum antibiotic coverage is indicated. Empirical antibiotic protocols should cover a wide range of bacteria, including *N. gonorrhoeae, C. trachomatis,* anaerobic rods and cocci, gram-negative aerobic rods and gram-positive aerobes (Table 23-14). Selection of one antibiotic protocol over another may be influenced by the clinical history. For example, acute pelvic inflammatory disease following an operative procedure is usually caused by endogenous flora of the vagina, whereas acute pelvic

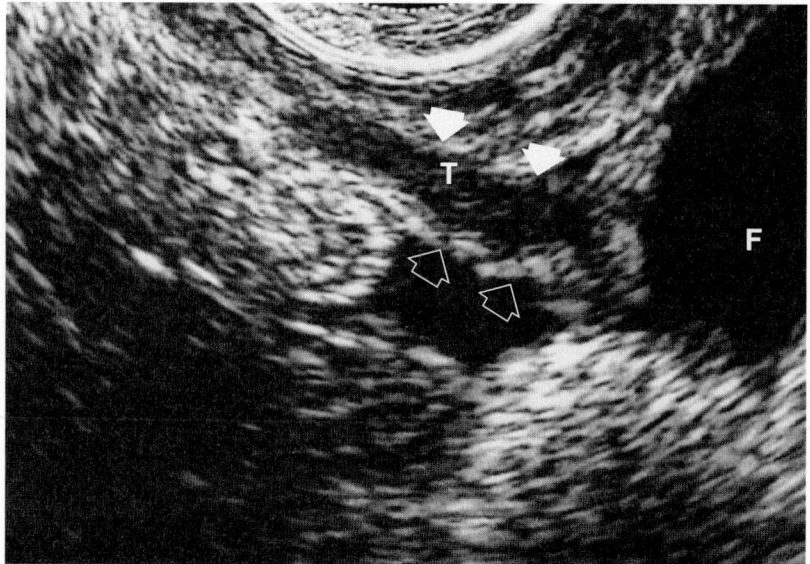

FIGURE 23-5 Longitudinal section of a slightly dilated and fluid-filled tube *(T)*. Its walls are slightly thickened *(arrows)*. Endometrial biopsy showed plasma cell endometritis. F = free fluid. (From Cacciatore B, Leminen A, Ingman-Friberg S, et al: Obstet Gynecol 80:912, 1992.)

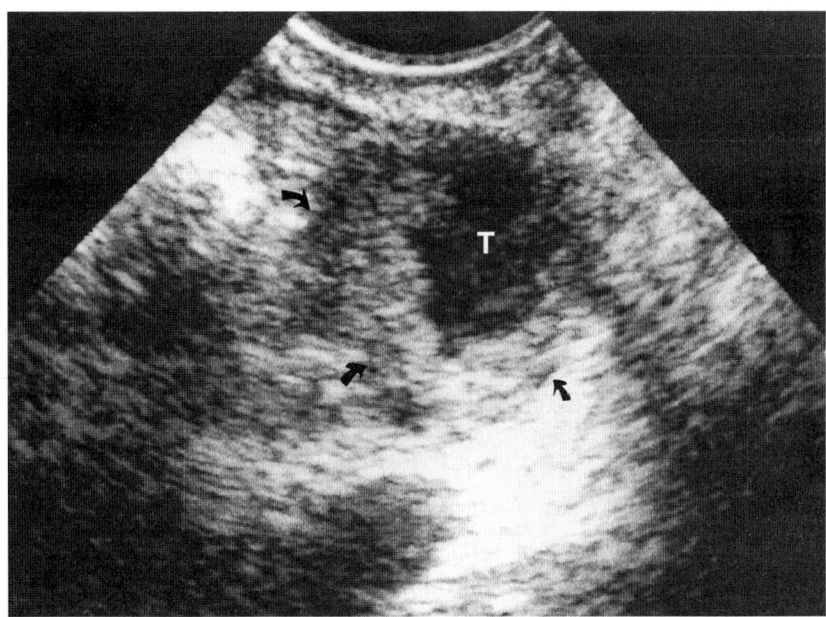

FIGURE 23-6   Cross-section of a dilated and fluid-filled fallopian tube *(T)*. The wall is thickened and irregular in shape *(arrows)*. Endometrial biopsy showed plasma endometritis. (From Cacciatore B, Leminen A, Ingman-Friberg S, et al: Obstet Gynecol 80:912, 1992.)

TABLE 23-14
Microorganisms Isolated from the Fallopian Tubes of Patients with Acute Pelvic Inflammatory Disease

Type of Agent	Organism
Sexually transmitted disease	*Chlamydia trachomatis*
	Neisseria gonorrhoeae
	Mycoplasma hominis
Endogenous agent aerobic or facultative	*Streptococcus* species
	Staphylococcus species
	Haemophilus species
	Escherichia coli
Anaerobic	*Bacteroides* species
	Peptococcus species
	Peptostreptococcus species
	Clostridium species
	Actinomyces species

From Weström L: Sex Transm Dis 11:439, 1984.

inflammatory disease in a 19-year-old college student is almost invariably secondary to *C. trachomatis.*

A failure of outpatient oral therapy may be related to noncompliance, reinfection, or inadequate antibiotic coverage for penicillinase-producing or chromosomally mediated resistant *N. gonorrhoeae* or facultative or anaerobic organisms involved in upper genital tract infection that are resistant to the drug prescribed. Thus culture with sensitivity testing is imperative. Inpatient failure rates for resolution of acute symptoms with intravenous antibiotics are approximately 5% to 10%.

A variety of oral and parenteral antibiotic regimens have been effective in achieving short-term clinical and microbiologic cures in randomized clinical trials. However, there is a paucity of data comparing the effect of various protocols on the incidence of long-term complications and elimination of bacterial infection in both the endometrium and fallopian tubes. The CDC has published recommendations of outpatient treatment of PID. Regimen A is ofloxacin 400 mg orally twice a day for 14 days plus metronidazole 500 mg orally twice a day for the same 14 days. Oral ofloxacin is effective as a single agent against both *N. gonorrhoeae* and *C. trachomatis.* Metronidazole is added to this regimen because of the lack of anaerobic coverage with ofloxacin. Regimen B is ceftriaxone 250 mg IM once or cefoxitin 2 g IM plus probenecid 1 g orally in a single dose concurrently once, or another parenteral third-generation cephalosporin such as ceftizoxime or cefotaxime. Regimen B also includes doxycycline 100 mg orally twice a day for 14 days with the cephalosporin. The optimal cephalosporin choice for regimen B is not known. Ceftizoxime has unparalleled coverage against *N. gonorrhoeae;* cefotaxime has better anaerobic coverage. Regimen B is less expensive than regimen A. The clinician should individualize the choice of regimens depending on his or her estimate of the need for anaerobic coverage. Obviously, if the woman has bacterial vaginosis, prolonged coverage with metronidazole is preferable. To date there is not data regarding the use of oral cephalosporins for the treatment of pelvic inflammatory disease. The CDC makes a special notation of the fact there is little data concerning long-term outcomes with outpatient therapy.

Alternative oral regimens that may be recommended by the CDC in the future include amoxicillin/clavulanic acid plus doxycycline for 14 days. Ongoing trials are evaluating the gastrointestinal side effects associated with this regimen. Other investigators are studying the use of azithromycin for the treatment of acute pelvic inflammatory disease (see the box below).

It is important to reexamine women within 48 to 72 hours of initiating outpatient therapy to evaluate the response of the disease to oral antibiotics. The patient should be hospitalized when the therapeutic response is not optimal. If the disease is responding well, approximately 4 to 6 weeks after therapy the endocervix should be cultured to test for microbiologic cure.

Ideally, every young woman with acute pelvic inflammatory disease would be hospitalized for the first few days of antibiotic treatment. In the United States, for economic reasons, 75% to 80% of women with acute pelvic inflammatory disease are not hospitalized. Nevertheless, it is important to develop a list of criteria or indications for hospitalization (see the box at right, above). If possible, adolescent young women should be hospitalized with their first episode of acute pelvic inflammatory disease. This would ensure maximum levels of antibiotics in the hope of preventing microscopic tubal damage. An almost absolute indication for hospitalization is an adnexal mass. Outpatient therapy does not provide high enough levels of appropriate antibiotics to successfully penetrate an abscess cavity. The association of a viable pregnancy and pelvic inflammatory disease, without a foreign body being inserted into the uterus, is a rare event. However, the second-trimester uterus is a fertile ground for severe pelvic infection, since infection does not become localized. A patient may develop widespread signs and symptoms of sepsis before the subtle inflammatory changes in the pelvis are recognized.

Indications for Hospitalizing Patients with Acute Pelvic Inflammatory Disease

Presence of tuboovarian complex or abscess
Pregnancy
All adolescents (compliance with therapy unpredictable)
Immunodeficient (has HIV infection with low CD4 counts, taking immunosuppressive therapy, or has another disease)
Uncertain diagnosis and surgical emergencies
Gastrointestinal symptoms (nausea and vomiting)
History of operative or diagnostic procedures
Inadequate response to outpatient therapy
Peritonitis in upper quadrants
Presence of an intrauterine device

Modified from Centers for Disease Control and Prevention: 1998 Guidelines for treatment of sexually transmitted diseases, MMWR 47:81, 1997.

Women for whom the definitive diagnosis of acute pelvic inflammatory disease is questionable are best admitted to the hospital. Any large series of 100 consecutive suspected cases of pelvic inflammatory disease will include 3 or 4 patients with ectopic pregnancy and 3 or 4 patients with acute appendicitis. Both the wide clinical spectrum of pelvic inflammatory disease and the difficulty of establishing a correct diagnosis without direct visualization of the pelvic organs are uncertainties that are best clarified in the hospital. The foundation of outpatient therapy of acute pelvic inflammatory disease is broad-spectrum oral antibiotics. If the patient presents with gastrointestinal symptoms, such as nausea and vomiting, there is a good chance that she will not be able to tolerate oral medications. Acute peritonitis in the right upper quadrant, especially liver tenderness without hepatomegaly, is another indication for hospital admission.

Acute pelvic inflammatory disease associated with the presence of an IUD is usually more advanced at the time of diagnosis than infection without a foreign body. Both patient and physician delays in diagnosis are not unusual. Often women misinterpret the early signs and symptoms of an infection as being related to the IUD. Pelvic infections with an IUD in place and pelvic infections following operative or diagnostic procedures often are due to anaerobic bacteria. Thus it is best to hospitalize these patients and use intravenous antibiotics. The IUD should be removed and cultured as soon as appropriate levels of intravenous antibiotics have been obtained. Concurrent immunodeficiency, especially HIV infection with a low CD4 count is another important criterion for hospitalization. If a therapeutic response or compliance with oral medications has not been optimal or is questionable, or if follow-up in 72 hours is not possible, then the patient should be admitted for intravenous antibiotic therapy.

In 1998 the CDC published its most recent guidelines for inpatient treatment of acute pelvic inflammatory dis-

---

Centers for Disease Control Ambulatory Management of Acute PID

Oral Regimen A
Ofloxacin 400 mg orally twice a day for 14 days,
PLUS
Metronidazole 500 mg orally twice a day for 14 days.

Oral Regimen B
Ceftriaxone 250 mg IM once,
OR
Cefoxitin 2 g IM plus **Probenecid** 1 g orally in a single dose concurrently once,
OR
Other parenteral third-generation **cephalosporin** (e.g., **ceftizoxime** or **cefotaxime**)
PLUS
Doxycycline 100 mg orally twice a day for 14 days. (Include this regimen with one of the above regimens.)

From Centers for Disease Control and Prevention: 1998 Guidelines for treatment of sexually transmitted diseases, MMWR 47:83, 1997.

ease. Its recommendations have been widely accepted, with only minor modifications. Its protocols stress the polymicrobial etiology of acute pelvic infection, the increasing importance of *C. trachomatis,* and the emergence of penicillin-resistant *N. gonorrhoea.* Thus each protocol includes at least two antibiotics (see the box below). With intravenous protocols the CDC recommends that intravenous antibiotics be continued at least 24 hours after substantial improvement in the patient. When the patient has a mass, we add ampicillin to clindamycin and gentamicin. However, for patients without a mass, we switch to oral antibiotics when the symptoms have diminished and the patient has been afebrile for 24 hours. In both regimens doxycycline is continued for a total of 14 days.

Regimen A (see the box on this page) is a combination of doxycycline and intravenous cefoxitin. It is excellent for community-acquired infection because it treats both gonorrhea and chlamydial infection. Doxycycline and cefoxitin provide excellent coverage for *N. gonorrhoeae, C. trachomatis,* and also penicillinase-producing *N. gonorrhoeae.* Cefoxitin is an excellent antibiotic against *Peptococcus, Peptostreptococcus,* and *E. coli.* The disadvantage of this combination is that the two drugs are less than ideal for a pelvic abscess or for anaerobic infections. To date cefotetan has been found equally as effective as cefoxitin.

Centers for Disease Control Inpatient Management of Acute PID

Parenteral Regimen A
Cefotetan 2 g intravenously every 12 hours, or cefoxitin 2 g intravenously every 6 hours plus doxycycline 100 mg intravenously or orally every 12 hours. Parenteral therapy may be discontinued 24 hours after a patient improves clinically, and oral therapy with doxycycline (100 mg twice a day) should continue for a total of 14 days. When tuboovarian abscess is present, many health care providers use clindamycin or metronidazole with doxycycline for continued therapy rather than doxycycline alone, because it provides more effective anaerobic coverage.

Parenteral Regimen B
Clindamycin 900 mg intravenously every 8 hours plus gentamicin loading dose intravenously or intramuscularly (2 mg/kg) followed by maintenance dose (1.5 mg/kg) every 8 hours. Single daily dosing may be substituted.

Alternative Parenteral Regimens
Ofloxacin 400 mg intravenously every 12 hours plus metronidazole 500 mg intravenously every 8 hours or ampicillin/sulbactam 3 g intravenously every 6 hours, plus doxycycline 100 mg intravenously or orally every 12 hours. Or ciprofloxacin 200 mg intravenously every 12 hours, plus doxycycline 100 mg intravenously or orally every 12 hours, plus metronidazole 500 mg intravenously every 8 hours.

From Centers for Disease Control and Prevention: 1998 Guidelines for treatment of sexually transmitted diseases, MMWR 47:82, 1997.

There is no clinically significant difference in bioavailability of doxycycline whether it is given by the oral or intravenous route. Thus doxycycline should be administered orally whenever possible because of the marked superficial phlebitis produced by intravenous infusion.

Doxycycline should be included in the regimen of follow-up oral therapy. Sweet observed 17 women with pelvic inflammatory disease who initially had endometrial cultures positive for *Chlamydia.* Clinically, 16 of 17 women responded to treatment with cephalosporins alone. However, posttreatment endometrial cultures remained positive for *Chlamydia* in 12 of 13 women. Therefore without tetracycline or erythromycin a patient may appear free of symptoms but may still be harboring *Chlamydia.* Antibiotics active against *C. trachomatis* must be present in effective dosages for at least 7 days for both clinical and microbiologic cures. *C. trachomatis* has a 48- to 72-hour life cycle inside of the mucosal cell. Thus prolonged therapeutic levels of the antichlamydial antibiotic are imperative.

Regimen B is a combination of clindamycin and an aminoglycoside (gentamicin). Regimen B has the advantage of providing excellent coverage for anaerobic infections and facultative gram-negative rods. Therefore it is preferred for patients with an abscess, IUD-related infections, and pelvic infections after a diagnostic or operative procedure. We prefer triple coverage with the addition of ampicillin. Studies have demonstrated that high intravenous levels of clindamycin, such as 900 mg every 8 hours, provide activity against 90% of bacterial strains of *Chlamydia.* Most infectious disease experts recommend the use of a single daily dose of gentamicin rather than a dose given every 8 hours. The initial once daily aminoglycoside dose is based on nomograms that take into consideration adjusted body weight and creatinine clearance. To monitor the level of the aminoglycoside, a single random serum level may be obtained between 6 and 14 hours after the first dose. This level is compared to the Hartford Hospital nomogram as described by Nicolau et al. Serum creatinines are obtained every 48 to 72 hours and serum aminoglycoside levels are reevaluated every 5 to 7 days or at more frequent intervals if the serum creatinine level changes appreciably. The advantages of a once daily aminoglycoside program are decreased toxicity, increased efficacy, and a decreased cost. The incidence of aminoglycoside toxicity is 2% to 3%, and approximately 25% of women require an adjustment in their intravenous dosage. Aztreonam, a monobactam, has an antibiotic spectrum similar to that of the aminoglycosides but without renal toxicity. However, it is much more expensive. It may be given in a dose of 2 g intravenously every 8 hours. Also, a third-generation cephalosporin may be used instead of an aminoglycoside in a patient with renal disease. Parenteral antibiotic therapy may be discontinued when the woman has been afebrile for 24 hours. We prefer clindamycin 450 mg orally four times a day for follow-up oral therapy instead of doxycycline because of the more efficacious anaerobic coverage. Alternative inpatient regimens include ampicillin/sulbactam plus doxycycline for they would have excellent anaerobic coverage and thus would be a good choice for women with a tuboovarian complex. Similarly the combination of ofloxacin plus either clindamycin or metronidazole or ciprofloxacin plus both doxycycline and metronidazole would provide excellent broad-spectrum coverage. Ciprofloxacin has poor coverage against *C. trachomatis* and a limited anaerobic spectrum. Thus both doxycycline and metronidazole should be given with ciprofloxacin.

In summary, neither regimen is uniformly effective for all patients. To date there are insufficient clinical data to suggest superiority of one regimen over another, either with respect to initial response or subsequent fertility. Hemsell et al., in a prospective open-label study, evaluated cefoxitin and doxycycline, cefotetan and doxycycline, and clindamycin and gentamicin for clinical response and duration of therapy. Outcomes were similar in the three groups. Walker et al. evaluated multiple-drug studies in a meta-analysis of PID treatments. Cure rates ranged from 75% to 95%. As would be expected, broad-spectrum coverage had the highest cure rates, and trials using metronidazole or doxycycline alone had cure rates of less than 80%.

Operative treatment of acute pelvic inflammatory disease has decreased markedly in the past 15 years. Operations are restricted to life-threatening infections, ruptured tuboovarian abscesses, laparoscopic drainage of a pelvic abscess, persistent masses in some older women for whom future childbearing is not a consideration, and removal of a persistent symptomatic mass. Because of the techniques of in vitro fertilization, every effort is made to perform conservative surgery and preserve ovarian and uterine function in women who have not completed their families. Unilateral removal of a tuboovarian complex or an abscess is a frequent conservative operation for acute pelvic inflammatory disease. Similarly, drainage of a cul-de-sac abscess via percutaneous drainage or a culpotomy incision results in preservation of the reproductive organs.

Percutaneous aspiration or drainage of pelvic abscesses may be accomplished under ultrasonic or computer tomography guidance. Percutaneous aspiration may be transvaginal or transabdominal. This technique has shown excellent results. In one small randomized trial early transvaginal drainage and intensive antibiotic therapy were compared to intensive antibiotic therapy alone. A favorable short-term outcome occurred in 90% of those who underwent ultrasound-guided transvaginal drainage in contrast to 65% of the control group. However, fertility and ectopic pregnancy rates after percutaneous drainage are unknown at this time. Long-term recurrence and sequelae need to be evaluated before this technique is accepted as a therapeutic standard. Obviously, a strong contraindication to percutaneous aspiration is any suspicion of an infected carcinoma in the differential diagnosis. Laparoscopic aspiration of tuboovarian complexes is another alternative. This procedure has shown good results but does not have greater benefit than percutaneous ultrasound-guided aspiration of abscess cavities. Laparoscopic aspiration obviously carries more operative risks than ultrasound-guided aspiration.

Rigorously defined, an abscess is a collection of pus within a newly created space. In contrast, a tuboovarian complex is a collection of pus within an anatomic space created by adherence of adjacent organs. Clinically, these two conditions are treated in similar fashions. Landers and Sweet published a large series of 232 women with tuboovarian abscesses or complexes initially treated conservatively with antibiotics (Tables 23-15 and 23-16).

Unilateral tuboovarian abscesses were discovered in 164 (71%) of the women. Seven women (3%) suffered acute rupture of their tuboovarian abscesses. There was no statistical difference between the incidence of unilateral tuboovarian abscess in women with IUDs and those without IUDs. Landers and Sweet described a 20% rate of early treatment failure after 48 to 72 hours of antibiotic therapy as a result of persistent pain or enlargement of the tuboovarian abscess or complex. In addition, 31%

TABLE 23-15

Epidemiologic Correlates of Tuboovarian Abscesses (TOAs) Diagnosed Clinically and Those of TOAs Confirmed Surgically

Patient Category (No. of Patients)	No. of Patients (%) with Indicated Epidemiologic Correlate			
	Nulliparous	Prior History of Gonorrhea	Prior History of Salpingitis	IUD Usage
TOA clinically diagnosed only (160)	90 (56)	48 (30)	52 (32.5)	53 (33)
TOA surgically confirmed (72)	30 (42)	23 (32)	24 (33)	23 (32)
TOA not excised (20)	9 (45)	6 (30)	6 (30)	4 (20)
TOA excised (52)	21 (40)	17 (33)	18 (35)	19 (36)
TOTAL (232)	120 (52)	71 (31)	76 (33)	76 (33)

From Landers DV and Sweet RL: Rev Infect Dis 5:878, 1983.

TABLE 23-16
Presenting Symptoms and Findings among
232 Patients with Tuboovarian Abscess

Symptom/Finding	No. of Patients in Indicated Group (%) with Presenting Symptom or Finding	
	Medically Treated (No. = 175)	Surgically Treated (No. = 57)
Acute pain	158 (90)	48 (84)
Chronic pain	29 (17)	14 (25)
Fever/chills	86 (49)	31 (53)
Vaginal discharge	53 (30)	11 (19)
Abnormal uterine bleeding	37 (21)	11 (19)
Nausea	44 (25)	17 (30)
Vomiting	23 (13)	13 (23)
Temperature > 100° F	102 (58)	37 (65)
White blood cell count >10,000/mm³	114 (72)	44 (77)

From Landers DV and Sweet RL: Rev Infect Dis 5:879, 1983.

required an operation several weeks to months following their acute infections. The most interesting findings brought to light from this study was that even though women had prior tuboovarian abscesses, 14% subsequently experienced an intrauterine pregnancy.

Abscesses caused by acute pelvic inflammatory disease contain a mixture of anaerobes and facultative or aerobic organisms (Figure 23-7). The environment of an abscess cavity results in a low level of oxygen tension. Therefore anaerobic organisms predominate and have been cultured from 60% to 100% of reported cases. Basic investigations have discovered that clindamycin penetrates the human neutrophil, and it is possible that this property facilitates the level of clindamycin within the abscess. Clindamycin is also stable in the abscess environment, which is not true of many other antibiotics. Thus a combination of clindamycin and an aminoglycoside is considered the standard for treatment of a tuboovarian abscess. This combination does not treat the enterococcus, and ampicillin should be added if there is suspicion that this organism is involved. Metronidazole alone is an effective alternative to clindamycin for anaerobic infections but does not provide gram-negative coverage. If abscesses do not respond to parenteral broad-spectrum antibiotics, drainage is imperative.

Postmenopausal women with suspected pelvic inflammatory disease should have appropriate imaging studies to rule out other concurrent diseases, especially malignancies. The bacterial etiology in postmenopausal women is not usually a sexually transmitted microorganism, but rather bacteria from the intestinal tract or normal vaginal flora. The disease process involves tuboovarian complexes and abscesses. Medical treatment should emphasize broad-spectrum antibiotic regimens with adequate anaerobic coverage. Operative intervention in a postmenopausal woman should be considered early in the disease, especially if the condition does not rapidly improve with medical therapy.

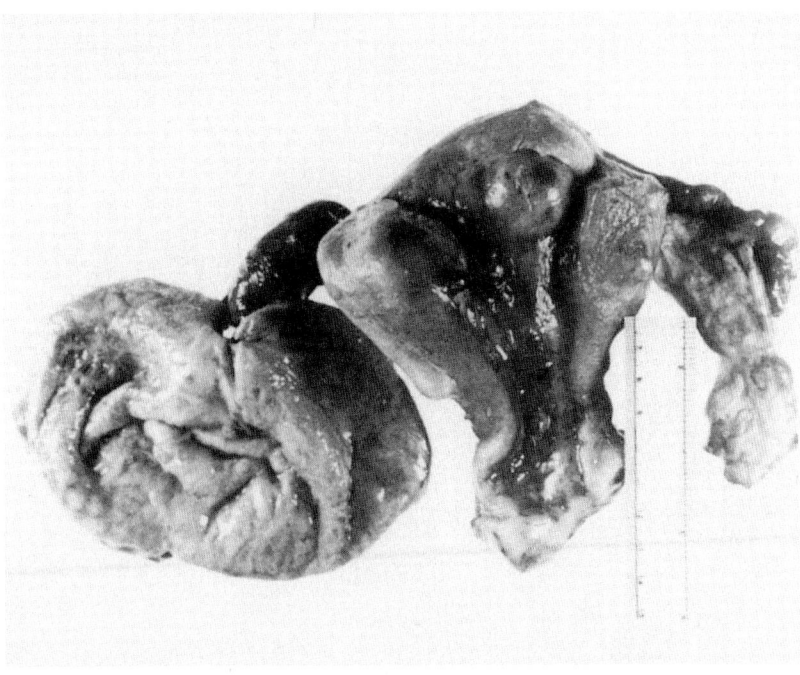

FIGURE 23-7 Pyosalpinx. Right tube is markedly enlarged and contains 50 ml of creamy pus. Tubal wall is thickened. (From Janovski NA, ed: Color atlas of gross gynecologic and obstetric pathology, New York, 1969, McGraw-Hill, Inc., p. 131.)

Sequelae

Before antibiotic therapy, the mortality associated with acute pelvic inflammatory disease was 1%. Grimes has estimated that there is presently one death every other day in the United States directly related to pelvic inflammatory disease. Most of these deaths result from rupture of tuboovarian abscesses. The mortality today is 5% to 10% for ruptured tuboovarian abscesses even with modern medical and operative therapy.

Recurrent acute pelvic inflammatory disease is experienced by approximately 25% of women. Younger women become reinfected twice as often as older women. A great challenge to health care providers is to educate women with pelvic inflammatory disease to reduce their chances of a second episode of infection. It is essential and imperative that preventive medicine include treatment and education of the male partner. Selection of contraceptives that will reduce the chance of upper genital tract infections and liberal prescriptions for treatment of lower genital tract disease for these women are also important. Because sequelae to PID, both overt and silent, are related to the number of infections, prevention cannot be overemphasized. Because the majority of PID in the United States is related to sexually transmitted diseases, increased attention to partner treatment and education is appropriate.

The number of ectopic pregnancies has increased threefold to fivefold over the past 25 years. This increased rate is directly parallel and proportional to the epidemic of sexually transmitted diseases and acute pelvic inflammatory diseases. Histologic studies estimate that approximately 50% of ectopic pregnancies occur in oviducts damaged by previous salpingitis (Figure 23-8). The microscopic tubal damage either retards transport of or entraps a fertilized ovum, thereby producing implantation in the tube rather than the endometrial cavity. Weström, in a long-term follow-up of women with acute salpingitis in Sweden, confirmed by laparoscopy, documented an ectopic pregnancy rate of 9.1% among 1732 women. In a control group the ectopic pregnancy rate was 1.4% (Table 23-17).

Studies have found an increased prevalence of developing chronic pain after an acute episode of PID. One study found the chance that a woman will develop chronic pelvic pain following acute salpingitis to be 4 times greater than the risk for control subjects. Approximately 20% of women with acute pelvic infections subsequently developed chronic pelvic pain, versus approximately 5% among controls without pelvic infection. Other studies have found similar results (Table 23-18). Among women with chronic pelvic pain, approximately two out of three are involuntarily infertile, and a similar percentage have deep dyspareunia. In a study from Oxford of 1355 women with PID and 10,507 controls, chronic abdominal pain developed 10 times more commonly in subjects who had PID (Table 23-19). Chronic pelvic pain may be caused by a hydrosalpinx, a collection of sterile, watery fluid in the fallopian tube. A hydrosalpinx is the end-stage development of a pyosalpinx.

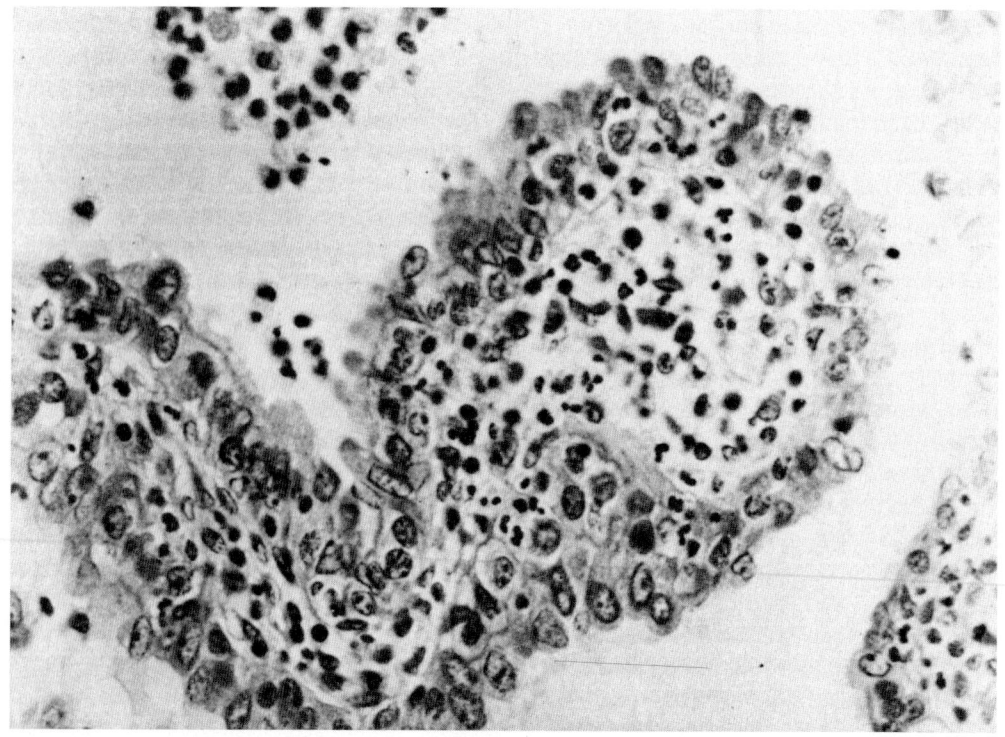

FIGURE 23-8 Microscopic appearance of salpingitis. (From Gompel C and Silverberg SG, eds: Pathology in gynecology and obstetrics, ed 2, Philadelphia, 1977, JB Lippincott Co., p. 253.)

TABLE 23-17
Summary of the Reproductive Events
After Index Laparoscopy in the Total Sample
of 1732 Patients and 601 Control Subjects

Category	Patients No. (%)	Control Subjects No. (%)
Total No. followed	1732	601
Avoiding pregnancy	370 (21.4)	144 (24.0)
Not pregnant for unknown reasons*	53 (3.1)	6 (1.0)
Attempting pregnancy	1309	451
Pregnant	1100 (80.8)	439 (96.1)
First pregnancy ectopic	100 (9.1)	6 (1.4)
Not pregnant	209 (16.0)	12 (2.7)
Completely examined	162	3
with proved TFI	141	0
with nTFI (other cause of infertility)	21	3
Incompletely examined	47	9

From Weström L et al: Sex Transm Dis 19:185, 1992.

TFI, tubal factor infertility; nTFI, nontubular factor infertility.

*Reporting no use of contraceptive and not consulting for infertility.

Chronic pain often develops in a woman even though she may have had a normal pelvic examination when examined 4 to 8 weeks following her acute infection. The pain may be related to adhesions surrounding the ovary (Table 23-20). The hypothesis has been advanced that the chronic dull pain is secondary to menstrual cycle–related changes in the volume of the ovary, which produce tension in the surrounding adhesions. All women with chronic pelvic pain believed to be caused by acute pelvic inflammatory disease should undergo laparoscopy to establish the diagnosis and rule out other diseases, such as endometriosis. Often, conservative surgery for this sequela via either laparoscopy or celiotomy is successful.

Acute pelvic infection is one of the major causes of female infertility. Epidemiologic studies estimate that between 4% and 13% of women either are infertile or have an operative procedure secondary to acute pelvic inflammatory disease.

The sequelae of infections vary from a damaged yet patent oviduct, to peritubular and periovarian adhesions that may hinder ovum pickup, to complete tubal obstruction. Tubal obstructions that are secondary to infection are commonly found at the fimbrial end or the cornual region of the oviduct. An alarming factor that has been documented with chlamydial infection is the tubal damage from subacute pelvic inflammatory disease. Patton et al. found essentially equally severe tubal damage, adhesion, degeneration of endosalpingeal structures, and cilia dysfunction in women with acute chlamydial PID and women with silent chlamydial infection.

Weström followed a large cohort of women with pelvic inflammatory disease in southern Sweden from 1960 through 1984. He discovered that the infertility rate was significantly lower in the younger women than in older women, following a single episode of infection (Table 23-21). The milder the episode of acute pelvic inflammatory disease the less likely a woman was to suffer tubal obstruction and infertility. The infertility rate also increased directly with the number of episodes of acute pelvic infection. These data are not surprising, because the prevalence of long-term sequelae is directly proportional to the number and severity of the episodes of acute pelvic inflammatory disease. Lepine et al.

TABLE 23-18
Frequency and Predictors of Long-Term Sequelae of Acute Pelvic Inflammatory Disease

Sequela	Frequency (No. and %)	Risk Factor	Univariate Analysis		Multivariate Analysis p Value
			P	Relative Risk and 95% Confidence Interval	
Involuntary infertility	17/42 (40%)	History of pelvic inflammatory disease	0.05	1.8 (1.0–3.3)	0.05
		Age at time of first sex	0.04	0.39	
		≥2 days of pain before therapy	0.02	2.0 (1.1–3.6)	0.07
Chronic pelvic pain	12/51 (24%)	History of pelvic inflammatory disease	0.03	1.5 (1.0–2.2)	
Pelvic inflammatory disease after index episode	22/51 (43%)	History of pelvic inflammatory disease	0.06	1.7 (0.9–3.1)	0.02
		Mean No. of days of pain before therapy	0.04	—	0.04
		Age at time of first sex	0.0008	—	0.01
Ectopic pregnancy	2/51 (2.4%)	*			

From Safrin S et al: Am J Obstet Gynecol 166:1300, 1992.

*Risk analysis not performed because of small numbers involved.

TABLE 23-19
Standardised (Indirect Standardisation) First Event Rates Per 1000 Woman-Years for Specified Outcomes After Admission with Either Acute Pelvic Inflammatory Disease (PID) or a Control Event in Cohorts of Women in the Oxford Record Linkage Study Followed from 1970 to 1985. Number of Women Shown in Parentheses

Outcome Condition	Women with PID N = 1200	Women with Control Conditions N = 10,507	Relative Risk
Nonspecific abdominal pain	16.7 (155)	1.7 (158)	9.8
Gynaecologic pain	3.6 (38)	0.8 (70)	4.5
Endometriosis	2.2 (18)	0.4 (34)	5.5
Hysterectomy	18.2 (152)	2.3 (204)	7.9
Ectopic pregnancy	1.9 (19)	0.2 (14)	9.5

From Buchan H et al: Br J Obstet Gynaecol 100:558, 1993.

TABLE 23-20
Associations Between a History of Acute Pelvic Inflammatory Disease and Adnexal Adhesions, Distal Tubal Occlusion, and/or Perihepatic Adhesions

Laparoscopic Findings	Pelvic Inflammatory Disease Yes (N = 22)	No (N = 90)	OR	95% CI	P
Distal tubal occlusion	4 (18.2%)	7 (7.8%)	2.6	0.7–10.0	0.14
Tubal adhesions	8 (36.4%)	21 (23.3%)	1.9	0.7–5.1	0.16
Ovarian adhesions	9 (40.9%)	21 (23.3%)	2.3	0.9–6.5	0.08
Perihepatic adhesions	3/21 (14.3%)	2/84 (2.4%)	6.8	1.1–43.9	0.05
Any adhesions	11 (50.0%)	25 (27.8%)	2.6	1.0–6.8	0.04

From Wølner-Hanssen P: Obstet Gynecol 86:321, 1995.

OR, odds ratio; CI, confidence interval.

TABLE 23-21
Percent and Number of Patients Attempting to Conceive Who Had Tubal Factor Infertility by Age, Number of Acute Pelvic Inflammatory Disease Episodes, and Severity of Pelvic Inflammatory Disease*

No. of Episodes of PID	Age (Years) <25 %	<25 (n/N)	≥25 %	≥25 (n/N)	Total %	Total (n/N)
One	7.7	(59/771)	9.1	(20/220)	8.0	(79/991)
Mild	0.8	(2/241)	0.0	(0/71)	0.6	(2/312)
Moderate	6.4	(23/361)	5.6	(5/89)	6.2	(28/452)
Severe	20.1	(34/169)	25.0	(15/60)	21.4	(49/229)
Two	18.4	(29/158)	25.9	(7/27)	19.5	(36/185)
Three or more	37.7	(23/61)	75.0	(3/4)	40.0	(26/65)
TOTAL	11.2	(111/990)	12.0	(30/251)	11.4	(141/1241)

From Weström L et al: Sex Transmit Dis 19:185, 1992.

PID, pelvic inflammatory disease; n, total number of cases followed; N, total number of evaluable cases.

*Excluding those with nontubal factor infertility and with incomplete infertility examinations.

recently reported additional data from the world's largest and longest prospective cohort study of women with acute pelvic inflammatory disease. The authors, from Lund, Sweden, found that increasing severity of the initial episode of acute pelvic infection correlates with a longer low-term probability of live birth. The cumulative proportion of women achieving a live birth after 12 years was 90% for women whose initial infection was mild, 82% for women with moderate disease, and 57% for women with severe pelvic inflammatory disease. Subsequent episodes of pelvic infection had a greater impact on women whose initial episode was judged as severe compared to those with milder disease.

ACTINOMYCES INFECTION

Actinomyces is a rare cause of upper genital tract infection. *Actinomyces israelii* is the most common species found and is a gram-positive anaerobic bacteria, which is difficult to culture. To successfully culture this organism, an anaerobic environment must be maintained for 2 to 3 weeks.

A. israelii is discovered either by histologic examination or culture from women with tuboovarian abscesses. There are many large series of tuboovarian abscesses without a single case of *A. israelii* described. Most cases described have been in women chronically wearing an IUD for an average of 8 years. Usually *A. israelii* is part of a polymicrobial infection, and whether its role is primary or secondary in the infectious process is unknown.

There is a controversy as to the significance of discovering actinomycetes on a Papanicolaou smear of women wearing an IUD. Burkman et al. reported that women with a positive smear had a 3.5-fold risk of hospitalization for acute pelvic inflammatory disease. These investigators found that when women developed acute infections, there was a higher tendency to develop tuboovarian abscesses. Other investigations have disagreed with this hypothesis. The contrasting, relatively high detection rate of actinomyces observed on Papanicolaou smears from IUD users, and extreme rarity of subsequent development of pelvic actinomycosis, leads most experts to conclude that progression to upper tract infection is highly unlikely to be related. Most clinicians who find a woman with an IUD and actinomycetes on Pap smear will remove the IUD. Some clinicians will also treat with antibiotics. Chatwani and Amin-Hanjani, reporting a retrospective analysis of 173 asymptomatic women with IUDs and *Actinomyces,* found on Pap smear that *Actinomyces* resolved at the same rate when the IUD was removed, whether or not antibiotics were used.

Actinomycetes may produce a chronic endometritis with an associated foul-smelling discharge. The clinical infection may be manifest by widespread adhesions, induration, and fibrosis. The diagnosis of *Actinomyces*

infection is usually not made until a tuboovarian abscess is examined by the pathologist. Then the classic "sulfur granules" are observed histologically along with gram-positive filaments.

Although much has been written about chronic draining sinuses with *Actinomyces* infection, this complication is unusual in gynecology. However, when this organism is present in a tuboovarian abscess, the patient should receive oral penicillin for 12 weeks following an operative procedure.

TUBERCULOSIS

Tuberculosis of the upper genital tract, primarily chronic salpingitis and chronic endometritis, is a rare disease in the United States. To date most gynecologists will not have encountered a single case. However, pulmonary tuberculosis is steadily increasing in the United States, and it is likely that the incidence of pelvic tuberculosis also will rise. Tuberculosis is a frequent cause of chronic pelvic inflammatory disease and infertility in other parts of the world. Thus it should be suspected in immigrants, especially those from Asia, the Middle East, and Latin America. Though the disease is usually found in premenopausal women, it will occur in postmenopausal women 10% of the time.

Pelvic tuberculosis may be produced by either *Mycobacterium tuberculosis* or *Mycobacterium bovis.* The primary site of infection for tuberculosis is usually the lung. Early in the course of pulmonary infection the bacteria spread hematogenously, and the infection becomes located in the oviduct. Subsequently the bacilli usually spread to the endometrium and less commonly to the ovaries. However, the oviducts are the primary and predominant site of pelvic tuberculosis. In developing countries without pasteurization of milk, bovine tuberculosis produces primary infections in the human gastrointestinal tract. Subsequent lymphatic or hematogenous dissemination results in pelvic tuberculosis. Autopsy studies published 25 years ago demonstrated that between 4% to 12% of women who died of pulmonary tuberculosis concurrently had evidence of upper genital tract infection. In a recent large study from India, 117 women had tubal blockage secondary to tuberculosis. When these women underwent laparoscopy, the findings were 50% simple tubal blockage, 15% tuboovarian masses, and 24% a frozen pelvis.

In general, extrapulmonary tuberculosis may present as either an insidious or as a rapidly progressing disease. The clinical symptoms and signs of pelvic tuberculosis are similar to the chronic sequelae of nontuberculous acute pelvic inflammatory disease. The predominant presentations of this chronic infection are infertility and abnormal uterine bleeding. Mild to moderate chronic abdominal and pelvic pain occur in 35% of women with the disease. Advanced cases are often accompanied by ascites. Some

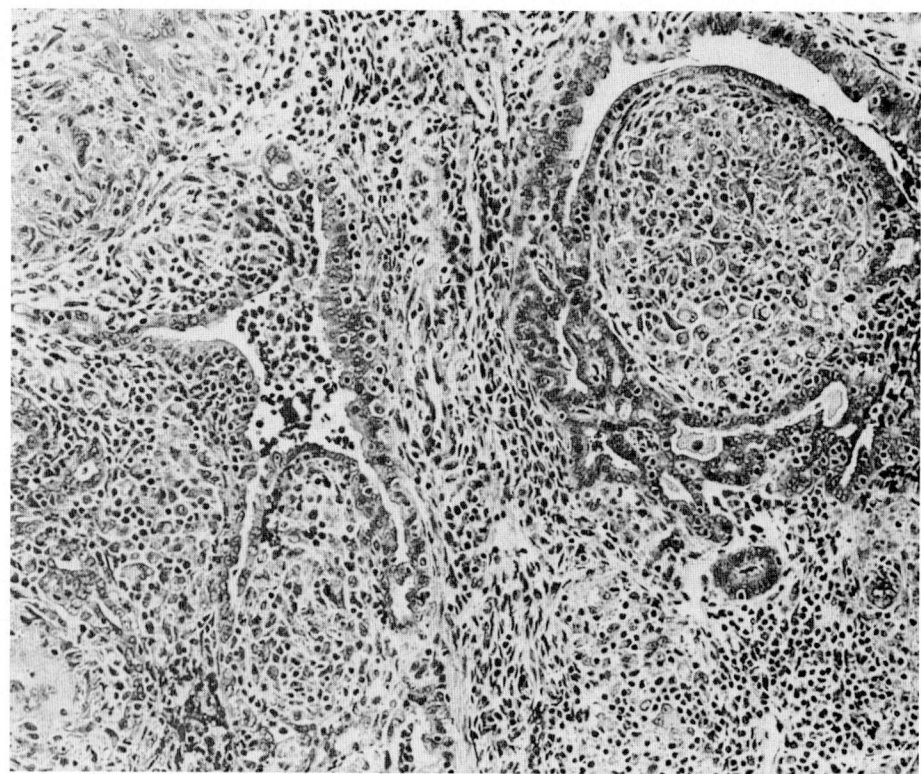

FIGURE 23-9 Tuberculous salpingitis: Langhans' giant cell granuloma. (From Gompel C and Silverberg SG, eds: Pathology in gynecology and obstetrics, ed 2, Philadelphia, 1977, JB Lippincott Co., p. 258.)

women may be asymptomatic. The findings at pelvic examination are normal in approximately 50% of cases. The remaining patients have mild adnexal tenderness and bilateral adnexal masses, with an inability to manipulate the adnexa because of scarring and fixation.

Tuberculous salpingitis may be suspected when a patient is not responding to conventional antibiotic therapy for acute bacterial pelvic inflammatory disease. Results of a tuberculin skin test will be positive. However, approximately one in three women does not have evidence of pulmonary tuberculosis on chest x-ray films. The diagnosis may be established by performing an endometrial biopsy late in the secretory phase of the cycle. A portion of the endometrial biopsy should be sent for culture and animal inoculation, while the remaining portion should be examined histologically. The findings of classic giant cells, granulomas, and caseous necrosis confirm the diagnosis (Figure 23-9). Approximately two out of three women with tuberculous salpingitis will have concomitant tuberculous endometritis. Pelvic tuberculosis may not be diagnosed until laparotomy or celiotomy, when the characteristic changes may be visualized. The distal ends of the oviduct remain everted, producing a "tobacco pouch" appearance. When the diagnosis has been established, the patient should have a chest x-ray examination, intravenous pyelogram, serial gastric washings, and urine cultures for tuberculosis.

Approximately 10% of women with pelvic tuberculosis have concomitant urinary tract tuberculosis.

The treatment of pelvic tuberculosis is medical. Not uncommonly patients will be admitted to the hospital for initiation of therapy, for observation, and to ensure appropriate compliance. Initial therapy in a patient with newly diagnosed tuberculosis usually will include five drugs because of the emergence of multidrug-resistant organisms. Multidrug resistant (MDR) tuberculosis is defined as infection from a strain of *M. tuberculous* that is resistant to two or more agents, including isoniazid. The mortality in HIV-negative patients who develop MDR infection may be as high as 80%. Often, health care workers become infected during outbreaks of MDR tuberculosis. The CDC has recommended starting a patient on multidrug regimens until the patient's culture results yield specific sensitivity. At that time medications may be decreased to two or three agents. Patients who have infection from MDR strains are usually kept on five drug regimens. Operative therapy for pelvic tuberculosis is reserved for women with persistent pelvic masses, some women with resistant organisms, women over age 40, and women whose endometrial cultures remain positive. Although the major sequelae of pelvic tuberculosis is infertility, occasionally a woman will become pregnant following medical therapy.

KEY POINTS

- The Centers for Disease Control (CDC) regularly revises its treatment protocols for sexually transmitted diseases. This information may be accessed online at www.cdc.gov/publications.htm.

- Studies have emphasized that organisms that produce bacterial vaginosis may also produce histologic endometritis even in women without symptoms of upper tract disease.

- The diagnosis of chronic endometritis is established by the finding of plasma cells on endometrial biopsy.

- During menses, it is normal to see scattered polymorphonuclear leukocytes in an endometrial biopsy.

- Pelvic inflammatory disease may include infection of *any or all* of the following anatomic locations: the endometrium (endometritis), the oviducts (salpingitis), the ovary (oophoritis), the uterine wall (myometritis), the uterine serosa and broad ligaments (parametritis), and the pelvic peritoneum.

- Approximately one in four women with acute pelvic inflammatory disease experiences further medical sequelae including recurrent acute pelvic inflammatory disease, ectopic pregnancy, and chronic pelvic pain.

- The CDC has emphasized that physicians should aggressively treat women if there is any suspicion of the disease, since sequelae are so devastating and the clinical diagnosis made from symptoms, signs, and laboratory data is often incorrect.

- Acute pelvic inflammatory disease is usually caused by a polymicrobial infection of organisms ascending from the vagina and cervix, traveling along the mucosa of the endometrium to infect the mucosa of the oviduct. The primary bacterial organisms cultured from tubal fluid and mucosa include *Neisseria gonorrhoeae, Chlamydia trachomatis,* and endogenous aerobic and anaerobic bacteria.

- Approximately 20% of women with cervical infection by gonorrhea subsequently develop pelvic inflammatory disease. The virulence of the strain of *N. gonorrhoeae* helps to predict the incidence of upper genital tract infection.

- *C. trachomatis* is the most prevalent organism causing pelvic inflammatory disease. The salpingitis it produces is usually insidious in onset.

- Approximately 30% of women with documented acute cervicitis secondary to chlamydia subsequently develop acute pelvic inflammatory disease.

- Studies of women with tubal infertility have noted that many women, though not diagnosed as having had overt PID, have had symptoms of pelvic pain. Some investigators believe that atypical or silent PID may be the more common form of upper tract infection, and symptomatic PID may be but the "tip of the iceberg."

- Anaerobic organisms are almost ubiquitous in pelvic abscesses associated with acute pelvic inflammatory disease. Tuboovarian complexes and abscesses are more common in women with concurrent bacterial vaginosis or HIV infection.

- There is a strong correlation between the incidence of sexually transmitted disease within a population and the incidence of acute pelvic inflammatory disease.

- In epidemiologic studies, age at first intercourse, marital status, and number of sexual partners are all gross indicators of the frequency of exposure to sexually transmitted diseases. Having multiple sexual partners increases the chance of acquiring acute pelvic inflammatory disease approximately fivefold.

- Acute pelvic inflammatory disease is a condition of young menstruating women, with 75% of cases occurring in women younger than 25 years of age. The risk for a sexually active adolescent female is 1 in 8. This decreases to 1 in 80 for women over the age of 25.

- When pelvic inflammatory disease is found in the postmenopausal woman, genital malignancies, diabetes, and/or concurrent intestinal disease is usually found.

- Oral contraceptive use provides some protection against the development of pelvic inflammatory disease. One mechanism may be the thickening of cervical mucus caused by the progestin component of the oral contraceptives. The other may be the decrease in the duration of menstrual flow, which creates a shorter interval for bacterial colonization of the upper genital tract.

- The increase in risk for PID occurs only at the time of insertion of the IUD and in the first three weeks after placement.

- Acute salpingitis occurring in a woman with a previous tubal ligation is rare and when it does occur presents with less severe symptoms.

- Approximately 20% to 25% of women have no identifiable intraabdominal or pelvic disease by laparoscopy when diagnosed as having acute pelvic inflammatory disease on the basis of history, physical, and laboratory examination.

- Pain in the lower abdomen and pelvis is the most frequent symptom of acute pelvic inflammatory disease, and in all large series more than 90% of women with the diagnosis have some type of abdominal pain.

- Seventy-five percent of patients with acute pelvic inflammatory disease have an associated endocervical infection or a coexistent purulent vaginal discharge.

- Nausea and vomiting are comparatively late symptoms in the course of acute pelvic inflammatory disease.

- From 5% to 10% of women with acute pelvic inflammatory disease develop perihepatic inflammation, Fitz-Hugh–Curtis syndrome.

- Approximately one third of women with acute pelvic inflammatory disease present with a temperature greater than 38°C.

- The incidence of adnexal abscess is approximately 10% in women with acute pelvic inflammatory disease.

- Acute PID should be diagnosed with a minimum of suspicion with the knowledge that overtreatment is preferable to missed diagnosis.

- Acute pelvic inflammatory disease should be included in the differential diagnosis of any sexually active young woman with pelvic pain.

- Because acute pelvic inflammatory disease has a wide range of nonspecific clinical symptoms, there is both a high false positive rate and a high false negative rate when the diagnosis is based on clinical findings and laboratory results.

- Less than 50% of women with acute pelvic inflammatory disease have a white blood cell count of greater than 10,000 cells per milliliter.

- Most studies demonstrate that women with acute PID and HIV infection have a higher incidence of adnexal masses. However, the acute pelvic infection responds to antibiotic therapy in a similar fashion as in women who are not infected with HIV.

- Though ultrasonography is neither specific nor sensitive in distinguishing the etiology of a pelvic mass, findings of dilated and fluid-filled tubes, free peritoneal fluid, and adnexal masses may be confirmatory of symptoms and physical signs. Vaginal ultrasound does have a high positive predictive value when used in a high-risk population.

- Laparoscopy is the optimum method to accurately establish the diagnosis of acute pelvic inflammatory disease.

- Women who are being treated as outpatients for acute pelvic inflammatory disease should be reexamined within 48 to 72 hours of initiation of therapy to evaluate the response of the disease to oral antibiotics.

- Indications for hospitalization for treatment of PID include presence of tuboovarian complex or abscess, pregnancy, adolescents, concurrent HIV infection, uncertain diagnosis, gastrointestinal symptoms, peritonitis in upper quadrants, history of operative or diagnostic procedures, and inadequate response to outpatient therapy.

- There is no clinically significant difference in bioavailability of doxycycline whether it is given by the oral or intravenous route. Thus doxycycline should be administered orally whenever possible because of the marked superficial phlebitis produced by intravenous infusion.

- Antibiotics against *C. trachomatis* must be present in effective dosages for at least 7 days for both clinical and microbiologic cures. *C. trachomatis* has a 48- to 72-hour life cycle inside of the mucosal cell. Thus prolonged therapeutic levels of the antichlamydial antibiotic are imperative.

- The advantages of a once daily aminoglycoside program are decreased toxicity, increased efficacy, and a decreased cost.

- Surgical treatment for acute pelvic inflammatory disease is restricted to life-threatening infections, ruptured tuboovarian abscesses, laparoscopic drainage of a pelvic abscess, persistent masses in some older women for whom future childbearing is not a consideration, and removal of a persistent symptomatic mass. Unilateral removal of a tuboovarian complex or abscess is a frequent conservative operation for acute pelvic inflammatory disease for women desiring future childbearing.

- Recurrent acute pelvic inflammatory disease is experienced by approximately 25% of women. The chance that a woman will develop chronic pelvic pain following acute pelvic inflammatory disease is 4 times greater than is the risk for control subjects.

- Because sequelae of acute pelvic inflammatory disease are related to the number of infections, prevention cannot be overemphasized.

- *Actinomyces* is a rare cause of upper genital tract infection. *Actinomyces israelii* is the most common species found and is a gram-positive anaerobe, which is difficult to culture.

- Pelvic tuberculosis may be produced by either *Mycobacterium tuberculosis* or *Mycobacterium bovis*. The primary sites of infection are the lung and the gastrointestinal tract.

- The predominant presentations of tuberculous salpingitis are infertility and abnormal uterine bleeding.

- Because of the emergence of multidrug-resistant strains, the CDC has recommended starting a patient on multidrug regimens until the patient's culture results yield specific sensitivity.

BIBLIOGRAPHY

Abbul SB, Muskin EP, and Shofer FS: Pelvic inflammatory disease in patients with bilateral tubal ligation, Am J Emerg Med 15:271, 1997.

Aboulghar MA, Mansour RT, and Serour GI: Ultrasonographically guided transvaginal aspiration of tuboovarian abscesses and pyosalpinges: an optional treatment for acute pelvic inflammatory disease, Am J Obstet Gynecol 172:1501, 1995.

Abu-Rustum RS: Imipenem and cilastatin sodium, Prim Care Update Ob/Gyns 4:21, 1997.

Ahmad MM: IUDs and actinomyces, IPPF Med Bul 21:3, 1987.

Amin-Hanjani S and Chatwani A: Endometrial cultures in acute pelvic inflammatory disease, Infect Dis Obstet Gynecol 3:56, 1995.

Anthony SJ and Lopez P: Genital amebiasis: historical perspective on an unusual disease presentation, Urology 54:952, 1999.

Askienazy-Elbhar M and Henry-Suchet J: Persistent "silent" *Chlamydia trachomatis* female genital tract infections, Infec Dis Obstet Gynecol 7:31, 1999.

Baker DA: Re-emergence of tuberculosis, Curr Opin Obstet Gynecol 6:373, 1994.

Boardman LA, Peipert JF, Brody JM, et al: Endovaginal sonography for the diagnosis of upper genital tract infection, Obstet Gynecol 90:54, 1997.

Bowie WR: Antibiotics and sexually transmitted diseases, Infect Dis Clin North Am 8:841, 1994.

Buchan H, Vessey M, Goldacre M, and Fairweather J: Morbidity following pelvic inflammatory disease, Br J Obstet Gynaecol 100:558, 1993.

Burkman R, Schlesselman S, McCaffrey L, et al. The relationship of genital tract actinomycetes and the development of pelvic inflammatory disease, Am J Obstet Gynecol 143:585, 1982.

Bukusi EA, Cohen CR, Stevens CE, et al: Effects of human immunodeficiency virus 1 infection on microbial origins of pelvic inflammatory disease on efficacy of ambulatory oral therapy, Am J Obstet Gynecol 181:1374, 1999.

Cacciatore B, Leminen A, Ingman-Friberg S, et al: Transvaginal sonographic findings in ambulatory patients with suspected pelvic inflammatory disease, Obstet Gynecol 80:912, 1992.

Cates W, Joesoef MR, and Goldman MB: Atypical pelvic inflammatory disease: can we identify clinical predictors? Am J Obstet Gynecol 169:341, 1993.

Centers for Disease Control: 1998 Guidelines for treatment of sexually transmitted diseases, MMWR 44:1,1997.

Chan Y, Parchment W, Skurnick JH, et al: Epidemiology and clinical outcome of patients hospitalized with pelvic inflammatory disease complicated by tubo-ovarian abscess, Infect Dis Obstet Gynecol 3:135, 1995.

Chatwani A and Amin-Hanjani S: Management of intrauterine device-associated actinomycosis, Infect Dis Obstet Gynecol 1:130, 1993.

Chatwani A, Harmanli OH, Nyirjesy P, and Reece EA: Significance of genital mycoplasmas in pelvic inflammatory disease: innocent bystander, Infec Dis Obstet Gynecol, 4:263, 1996.

Chow JM, Yonekuram L, Richwald GA, et al: The association between *Chlamydia trachomatis* and ectopic pregnancy, JAMA 263:3164, 1990.

Cohen CR and Brunham RC: Pathogenesis of chlamydia induced pelvic inflammatory disease, Sex Transm Infect 75:21, 1999.

Cohen CR, Sinei S, Reilly M, et al: Effects of human immunodeficiency virus type 1 infection upon acute salpingitis: a laparoscopic study, J Infec Dis 178:1352, 1998.

Corsi PJ, Johnson SC, Gonik B, et al: Transvaginal ultrasound-guided aspiration of pelvic abscesses, Infec Dis Obstet Gynecol 7:216, 1999.

Dan BB: Sex, lives, and Chlamydia rates, JAMA 263:3191, 1990.

Davis JD: Aztreonam, Prim Care Update Ob/Gyns 4:61, 1997.

Devine PA: Extrapelvic manifestations of gonorrhea, Prim Care Update Ob/Gyns 5:233, 1998.

Dieterie S, Rummel C, Bader LW, et al: Presence of the major outer-membrane protein of Chlamydia trachomatis in patients with chronic salpingitis and salpingitis isthmica nodosa with tubal occlusion, Fertil Steril 70:/74, 1998.

Dodson MG and Faro S: The polymicrobial etiology of acute pelvic inflammatory disease and treatment regimens, Rev Infect Dis 7:S696, 1985.

Eschenbach DA, Wölner-Hanssen P, Hawes SE, et al: Acute pelvic inflammatory disease: associations of clinical and laboratory findings with laparoscopic findings, Obstet Gynecol 89:184, 1997.

Farley TMM, Rosenberg MJ, Rowe PJ, et al: Intrauterine devices and pelvic inflammatory disease: an international perspective, Lancet 339:785, 1992.

Faro S, Martens M, Maccato M, et al: Vaginal flora and pelvic inflammatory disease, Am J Obstet Gynecol 169:470, 1993.

Fiorino AS: Intrauterine contraceptive device-associated actinomycotic abcess and actinomyces detection on cervical smear, Obstet Gynecol 87:142, 1996.

Fleenor-Ford A, Hayden MK, and Weinstein RA: Vancomycin-resistant enterococci: implications for surgeons, Surg 125:121, 1999.

Garland SM and Kelly VN: Role of genital mycoplasmas in bacteremia: should we be routinely culturing for these organisms? Infec Dis Obstet Gynecol 4:329, 1996.

Gérard HC, Branigan PJ, Balsara GR, et al: Viability of Chlamydia trachomatis in fallopian tubes of patients with ectopic pregnancy, Fertil Steril 70:945, 1998.

Gilbert DN, Lee BL, Dworkin RJ, et al: A randomized comparison of the safety and efficacy of once-daily gentamicin or thrice-daily gentamicin in combination with ticarillin-clavulanate, Am J Med 105:182, 1998.

Grimes DA: Deaths due to sexually transmitted diseases, JAMA 255:1727, 1986.

Hadgu A, Weström L, Brooks CA, et al: Predicting acute pelvic inflammatory disease: a multivariate analysis, Am J Obstet Gynecol 155:954, 1986.

Haeusler G, Tempfer C, Lehner R, et al: Fallopian tissue sampling with a cytobrush during hysteroscopy: a new approach for detecting tubal infection, Fertil Steril 67:580, 1997.

Hager WD, Eschenbach DA, Spence MR, et al: Criteria for diagnosis and grading of salpingitis, Obstet Gynecol 61:113, 1983.

Hemsell DL, Little BB, Faro S, et al: Comparison of three regimens recommended by the Centers for Disease Control and Prevention for the treatment of women hospitalized with acute pelvic inflammatory disease, Clin Infect Dis 19:720, 1994.

Hillier SL, Kiviat NB, Hawes SE, et al: Role of bacterial vaginosis-associated microorganisms in endometritis, Am J Obstet Gynecol 175:435, 1996.

Hillis SD, Owens LM, Marchbanks PA, et al: Recurrent chlamy-dial infections increase risks of hospitalization for ectopic pregnancy and pelvic inflammatory disease, Am J Obstet Gynecol 176:103, 1997.

Holmes KK, Mrdh PA, Sparling PF, and Wiesner PJ, eds: Sexually transmitted diseases, ed 2, New York, 1990, McGraw Hill, Inc.

Irwin KL, Moorman AC, O'Sullivan MJ, et al: Influence of human immunodeficiency virus infection on pelvic inflammatory disease, Obstet Gynecol 95:525, 2000.

Jackson SL and Soper DE: Pelvic inflammatory disease in the postmenopausal woman, Infec Dis Obstet Gynecol 7:248, 1999.

Jacobson LJ: Differential diagnosis of acute pelvic inflammatory disease, Am J Obstet Gynecol 138:1006, 1980.

Jacobs RF: MultipleBdrug-resistant tuberculosis, Clin Infect Dis 19:1, 1994.

Jamieson DJ, Duerr A, Macasaet MA, et al: Risk factors for a complicated clinical course among women hospitalized with pelvic inflammatory disease, Infec Dis Obstet Gynecol 8:88, 2000.

Jana N, Vasishta K, Saha SC, and Ghosh K: Obstetrical outcomes among women with extrapulmonary tuberculosis, N Engl J Med 341:645, 1999.

Janovski NA, ed: Color atlas of gross gynecologic and obstetric pathology, New York, 1969, McGraw-Hill, Inc.

Jossens MOR, Schachter J, and Sweet RL: Risk factors associated with pelvic inflammatory disease of differing microbial etiologies, Obstet Gynecol 83:989, 1994.

Kamwendo F, Forslin L, Bodin L, and Danielson D: Programmes to reduce pelvic inflammatory disease—the Swedish experience, Lancet 351:25, 1998.

Kerr-Layton JA, Stamm CA, Peterson LS, and McGregor JA: Chronic plasma cell endometritis in hysterectomy specimens of HIV-infected women: a retrospective analysis, Infec Dis Obstet Gynecol 6:186, 1998.

Korn AP, Bolan G, Padian N, et al: Plasma cell endometritis in women with symptomatic bacterial vaginosis, Obstet Gynecol 85:387, 1995.

Korn AP, Hessol NA, Padian NS, et al: Risk factors for plasma cell endometritis among women with cervical Neisseria gonorrhoeae, cervical Chlamydia trachomatis, or bacterial vaginosis, Am J Obstet Gynecol 178:987, 1998.

Landers DV and Sweet RL: Tubo-ovarian abscess: contemporary approach to management, Rev Infect Dis 5:876, 1983.

Landers DV, Wölner-Hanssen P, Paavonen J, et al: Combination antimicrobial therapy in the treatment of acute pelvic inflammatory disease, Am J Obstet Gynecol 164:849, 1991.

Larsen B: Virulence attributes of low-virulence organisms, Infect Dis Obstet Gynecol 2:95, 1994.

Larsson PG, Platz-Christensen JJ, Thejls H, et al: Incidence of pelvic inflammatory disease after first-trimester legal abortion in women with bacterial vaginosis after treatment with metronidazole: a double-blind randomized study, Am J Obstet Gynecol 166:100, 1992.

Lepine LA, Hillis SD, Marchbanks PA, et al: Severity of pelvic inflammatory disease as a predictor of the probability of live birth, Am J Obstet Gynecol 178:977, 1998.

Lippes J: Pelvic actinomycosis: a review and preliminary look at prevalence, Am J Obstet Gynecol 180:265, 1999.

Livengood CH III, Hill GB, and Addison WA: Pelvic inflammatory disease: findings during inpatient treatment of clinically severe, laparoscopy-documented disease, Am J Obstet Gynecol 166:519, 1992.

Mann SN, Smith JR, and Barton SE: Pelvic inflammatory disease, Internat J STD AIDS 7:315, 1996.

McCormack WM: Pelvic inflammatory disease, N Engl J Med 330:115, 1994.

McGregor JA, Crombleholme WR, Newton E, et al: Randomized comparison of ampicillin-sulbactam to cefoxitin and doxycycline or clindamycin and gentamicin in the treatment of pelvic inflammatory disease or endometriosis, Obstet Gynecol 83:998, 1994.

McNeeley SG, Hendrix SL, Mazzoni MM, et al: Medically sound, cost-effective treatment for pelvic inflammatory disease and tuboovarian abscess, Am J Obstet Gynecol 178:1272, 1998.

Møller BR, Kristiansen FV, Thorsen P, et al: Sterility of the uterine cavity, Acta Obstet Gynecol Scand 74:216, 1995.

Money DM, Hawes SE, Eschenbach DA, et al: Antibodies to the chlamydial 60 kd heat-shock protein are associated with laparoscopically confirmed perihepatitis, Am J Obstet Gynecol 176:870, 1997.

Monif GRG: Abscesses occurring after acute salpingitis, Contemp OB/GYN 37:55, 1992.

Monif GRG: The great douching debate: to douche or not to douche, Obstet Gynecol 94:630, 1999.

Munday PE: Clinical aspects of pelvic inflammatory disease, Hum Reprod 12 (suppl):121, 1997.

Ness RB, Keder LM, Soper DE, et al: Oral contraception and recognition of endometritis, Am J Obstet Gynecol 176:580, 1997.

Nicolau D, et al: Experience with a once-daily aminoglycoside program administered to 2,184 adult patients, Antimicrob Agent Chemother 39:650, 1995.

Paavonen J: Pelvic inflammatory disease: from diagnosis to prevention, Sex Transmit Dis 16:747, 1998.

Paavonen J, Kiviat N, Brunham RC, et al: Prevalence and manifestations of endometritis among women with cervicitis, Am J Obstet Gynecol 152:280, 1985.

Padian NS and Washington AE: Pelvic inflammatory disease: a brief overview, Ann Epidemiol 4:128, 1994.

Panoskaltsis TA, Moore DA, Haidopoulos DA, and McIndoe AG: Tuberculous peritonitis: part of the differential diagnosis in ovarian cancer, Am J Obstet Gynecol 182:740, 2000.

Parikh FR, Nadkarni SG, Kamat SA, et al: Genital tuberculosis—a major pelvic factor causing infertility in Indian women, Fertil Steril 67:497, 1997.

Patton DL, Moore DE, Spadoni LR, et al: A comparison of the fallopian tube's response to overt and silent salpingitis, Obstet Gynecol 73:622, 1989.

Paukku M, Puolakkainen M, Paavonen T, and Paavenen J: Plasma cell endometritis is associated with *Chlamydia trachomatis* infection, Am J Clin Pathol 112:211, 1999.

Pavletic AJ, Wölner-Hanssen P, Paavonen J, et al: Infertility following pelvic inflammatory disease, Infec Dis Obstet Gynecol 7:145, 1999.

Peipert JF, Boardman LA, and Sung CJ: Performance of clinical and laparoscopic criteria for the diagnosis of upper genital tract infection, Infec Dis Obstet Gynecol 5:291, 1997.

Peipert JF, Montagno AB, Cooper AS, and Sung CJ: Bacterial vaginosis as a risk factor for upper genital tract infection, Am J Obstet Gynecol 177:1184, 1997.

Peipert JF, Ness RB, Soper DE, and Bass D: Association of lower genital tract inflammation with objective evidence of endometritis, Infec Dis Obstet Gynecol 8:83, 2000.

Peipert JF and Soper DE: Diagnostic evaluation of pelvic inflammatory disease, Infect Dis Obstet Gynecol 2:38, 1994.

Peipert JF, Sweet RL, Walker CK, et al: Evaluation of ofloxacin in the treatment of laparoscopically documented acute pelvic inflammatory disease (salpingitis), Infec Dis Obstet Gynecol 7:138, 1999.

Perdigon PL: Imaging techniques for diagnosis of serious intraabdominal and pelvic infections, Prim Care Update Ob/Gyns 6:115, 1999.

Perez-Medina T, Huertas MA, and Bajo JM: Early ultrasound-guided transvaginal drainage of tubo-ovarian abscesses: a randomized study, Ultrasound Obstet Gynecol 7:435, 1996.

Peterson HB, Galaqid EI, and Zenilman JM: Pelvic inflammatory disease: review of treatment options, Rev Infect Dis 12(S6):S656, 1990.

Phillips AJ and D'Ablaing G: Acute salpingitis subsequent to tubal ligation, Obstet Gynecol 67:55S, 1986.

Reed SD, Landers DV, and Sweet RL: Antibiotic treatment of tuboovarian abscess: comparison of broad-spectrum β-lactam agents versus clindamycin-containing regimens, Am J Obstet Gynecol 164:1556, 1991.

Rein DB, Kassler WJ, Irwin KL, and Rabiee L: Direct medical cost of pelvic inflammatory disease and its sequelae: decreasing, but still substantial, Obstet Gynecol 95:397, 2000.

Richter HE, Holley RL, Andrews WW, et al: The association of interleukin 6 with clinical and laboratory parameters of acute pelvic inflammatory disease, Am J Obstet Gynecol 181:940, 1999.

Rodvold KA, Danziger LH, and Quinn JP: Single daily doses of aminoglycosides, Lancet 350:1412, 1997.

Safrin S, Schachter J, Dahrouge D, and Sweet RL: Long-term sequelae of acute inflammatory disease: a retrospective cohort study, Am J Obstet Gynecol 166:1300, 1992.

Schaefer G: Female genital tuberculosis, Clin Obstet Gynecol 19:223, 1976.

Scholes D, Daling JR, Stergachis A, et al: Vaginal douching as a risk factor for acute pelvic inflammatory disease, Obstet Gynecol 81:601, 1993.

Sellers J, Mahony J, Goldsmith C, et al: The accuracy of clinical findings and laparoscopy in pelvic inflammatory disease, Am J Obstet Gyneol 164:113, 1991.

Shulman A, Maymon R, Schapiro A, and Bahary C: Percutaneous catheter drainage of tubo-ovarian abscesses, Obstet Gynecol 80:555, 1992.

Soper DE: Pelvic inflammatory disease, Infect Dis Clin North Am 8:821, 1994.

Soper DE: The semantics of pelvic inflammatory disease, Sex Transmit Dis 22:342, 1995.

Soper DE: Pelvic inflammatory disease (PID), Infec Dis Obstet Gynecol 4:62, 1996.

Soper DE, Brockwell NJ, and Dalton HP: False-positive cultures of the cul-de-sac associated with culdocentesis in patients undergoing elective laparoscopy, Obstet Gynecol 77:134, 1991.

Soper DE, Brockwell NJ, Dalton HP, and Johnson D: Observations concerning the microbial etiology of acute salpingitis, Am J Obstet Gynecol 170:1008, 1994.

Stacey CM, Munday PE, Taylor-Robinson D, et al: A longitudinal study of pelvic inflammatory disease, Br J Obstet Gynaecol 99:994, 1992.

Stamm WE: *Chlamydia trachomatis* infections: progress and problems, J Infec Dis 179 (suppl):S380, 1999.

Stevens HA: Clindamycin, Prim Care Update Ob/Gyns 4:251, 1997.

Stone KM, Grimes DA, and Magder LS: Primary prevention of sexually transmitted diseases, JAMA 255:1763, 1986.

Sweet RL, Blankfort-Doyle M, Robbie MO, et al: The occurrence of chlamydial and gonococcal salpingitis during the menstrual cycle, JAMA 255:2062, 1986.

Sweet RL and Gibbs RS: Infectious diseases of the female genital tract, ed 3, Baltimore, 1995, Williams & Wilkins.

Teisala K, Heinonen PK, and Punnonen R: Laparoscopic diagnosis and treatment of acute pyosalpinx, J Reprod Med 35:19, 1990.

Teisala K, Heinonen PK, and Punnonen R: Transvaginal ultrasound in the diagnosis and treatment of tubo-ovarian abscess, Br J Obstet Gynaecol 97:178, 1990.

Telenti A and Iseman M: Drug-resistant tuberculosis: what do we do now? Drugs 59:171, 2000.

Toglia MR and Schaffer JI: Tubo-ovarian abscess formation in users of intrauterine devices remote from insertion: a report of three cases, Infec Dis Obstet Gynecol 4:85, 1996.

Toth A, O'Leary WM, and Ledger W: Evidence for microbial transfer by spermatozoa, Obstet Gynecol 59:556, 1982.

Toub DB, Goff BA, and Muntz HG: Tuberculous endometritis presenting as postmenopausal bleeding: a case report, J Reprod Med 36:616, 1991.

Walker CK, Kahn JG, Washington AE, et al: Pelvic inflammatory disease: metaanalysis of antimicrobial regimen efficacy, J Infect Dis 168:969, 1993.

Walker CK, Workowski KA, Washington AE, et al: Anaerobes in pelvic inflammatory disease: implications for the Centers for Disease Control and Prevention's Guidelines for Sexually Transmitted Diseases, Clin Infec Dis 28 (suppl):S29, 1999.

Walsh T, Grimes D, Frezieres R, et al: Randomized controlled trial of prophylactic antibiotics before insertion of intrauterine devices, Lancet 351:1005, 1998.

Walters MD, Eddy CA, Gibbs RS et al: Antibodies to *Chlamydia trachomatis* and risk for tubal pregnancy, Am J Obstet Gynecol 159:942, 1988.

Walters MD and Gibbs RS: A randomized comparison of gentamicin-clindamycin and cefoxitin-doxycycline in the treatment of acute pelvic inflammatory disease, Obstet Gynecol 75:867, 1990.

Washington AE, Gove S, Schachter J, et al: Oral contraceptives, *Chlamydia trachomatis* infection, and pelvic inflammatory disease, JAMA 253:2246, 1985.

Weström L: Incidence, prevalence, and trends of acute pelvic inflammatory disease and its consequences in industrialized countries, Am J Obstet Gynecol 138:880, 1980.

Weström L: Introductory address: treatment of pelvic inflammatory disease in view of etiology and risk factors, Sex Transm Dis 11:437, 1984.

Weström L: Pelvic inflammatory disease and other sexually transmitted diseases, Curr Opin Obstet Gynecol 1:5, 1989.

Weström L, Joesoef R, Reynolds G, et al: Pelvic inflammatory disease and fertility: a cohort study of 1,844 women with laparoscopically verified disease and 657 control women with normal laparoscopic results, Sex Transmit Dis 19:185, 1992.

Wølner-Hanssen P: Silent pelvic inflammatory disease: is it overstated? Obstet Gynecol 86:321, 1995.

Wølner-Hanssen P, Eschenbach DA, Paavonen J, et al: Association between vaginal douching and acute pelvic inflammatory disease, JAMA 263:1936, 1990.

Wølner-Hanssen P, Svensson L, Mrdh PA, et al: Laparoscopic findings and contraceptive use in women with signs and symptoms suggestive of acute salpingitis, Obstet Gynecol 66:233, 1985.

Preoperative Counseling and Management

Patient Evaluation, Informed Consent, Infection Prophylaxis, Avoidance of Complications

KEY TERMS AND DEFINITIONS

Antisialagogue. An agent that decreases the production and amount of saliva.

Effective Period of Prophylactic Antibiotics. The first 3 hours of decreased tissue resistance following a surgical insult. Prophylactic antibiotics must be at the site of damaged tissue during this interval.

Informed Consent. An agreement by the patient that she understands the following: the nature and extent of the disease process, the nature and extent of the contemplated operation, the anticipated benefits and results of the surgery including a conservative estimate of successful outcome, the risks and potential complications of the operative procedure, and alternative methods of therapy.

Minidose Heparin. A low dose of heparin given subcutaneously both preoperatively and postoperatively as a prophylactic agent to decrease the incidence of venous thrombosis. The dosage and frequency of heparin injections depend on whether fractionated or unfractionated heparin is given and the ponderal index of the woman.

Nosocomial Infection. An infection acquired in a hospital.

Prophylactic Antibiotics. The administration of antibiotics to patients without evidence of infection to prevent postoperative morbidity related to infection.

Preoperative evaluation is a challenge to the gynecologist, for it involves both the art and the science of clinical medicine. Excellent preparation for the operation facilitates a successful end result. Optimum preparation involves two personality traits: compulsive attention to detailed planning and a deep empathy for the patient. For the gynecologist, preoperative planning can be divided into three basic aspects: obtaining preoperative information, reducing the patient's anxieties and fears, and obtaining informed consent. Francis D. Moore states that the first aphorism of preoperative preparation is to avoid "surprises." This dictum should be applied to protect both the patient and the physician.

The gynecologist, as leader of the surgical team, has an obligation to prepare the patient, her family, and the hospital personnel, including nurses, anesthesiologists, and the operating room team, concerning the anticipated details surrounding the surgical procedure. The majority of gynecologic operations are elective and thus allow sufficient time to prepare. However, even in emergency situations, preoperative preparation should be as detailed as possible because shortcuts during an emergency can result in further compromise to the patient.

For the patient, there are no small, insignificant, or minor operations. Almost any operation is a major event in her life. Associated with an elective operation are the anxiety and apprehension of the anticipated surgical procedure coupled with the ambivalence of deciding whether to have the operation. To help her decide, it is important for the physician to outline the natural history of the gynecologic disease so that the patient is able to understand the benefits of surgery. Most women have questions concerning the return of normal body functions and the cosmetic changes produced by the operation; these questions must be answered. Questions concerning the woman's perception of the operation's impact on her sexuality must be discussed. Recent prospective studies have documented that sexual function is most likely to remain the same or improve following gynecologic surgery for benign disease. As always, the physician is an educator. His or her goal should be to outline for the patient the reason and approximate time frame for each preoperative step and procedure. If the patient is ambivalent concerning the need for a surgical procedure, this often may be resolved by suggesting that she seek another professional opinion. Many third-party payer programs insist that patients obtain a second opinion before elective gynecologic operations.

There are not many events that assault human dignity as much as the events surrounding an elective operation. The woman is stripped of her clothing, bombarded with questions, and sometimes shaved of her pubic hair. It is important for the physician to protect the patient's privacy and human dignity during the preoperative period. The gynecologist must appreciate that the preoperative period is one of great psychologic stress for the patient. The time of the anticipated surgical procedure is a catalyst for emotional responses ranging from vulnerability and helplessness to the grief produced by anticipated loss of a reproductive organ. The physician-patient relationship is far more than the legally described contractual one. An important aspect of the relationship is the physician's encouragement of the patient to be a partner in the mutual goal of a return to normal function. The understanding and trust built between the patient and physician during the preoperative period will help the patient to build confidence and cope with the stress of the postoperative period.

One of the most important aspects of the preoperative preparation is a discussion with the physician before the procedure. Ideally the physician, the patient, and her family have a private meeting. During this time, it is important for the physician to answer all the patient's questions, as well as those of her family. It is acceptable to answer a question with the statement, "I don't know." Patients admire the honesty this response expresses. The gynecologist must remember that just as he or she studies the patient for both verbal and nonverbal information, so does the patient watch the gynecologist. Gentleness and patience are essential for the gynecologist to display at this time. Sincere interest may be reinforced by eye-to-eye contact and a gentle touch of the hands.

A thorough and detailed history and physical examination, considering the entire patient, not just the pelvis, detect approximately 90% of the facts pertinent to the surgical procedure. Multiple studies have demonstrated that the most significant risk factors for postoperative morbidity are preoperative conditions. Preoperative laboratory screening tests discover fewer than 10% of significant surgical risk factors. It is an established surgical axiom that operative morbidity and mortality are directly proportional to preexisting conditions. Known or unsuspected medical illnesses may affect the operation, anesthesia, and postoperative course and in rare instances may preclude the procedure altogether. Also, it is important to evaluate the influence of gynecologic disease on other organ systems. For example, is a pelvic mass producing obstruction of the ureters?

This chapter outlines the preoperative preparations for gynecologic operations for benign disease. Emphasis is placed on obtaining a standard complete history, performing an adequate physical examination, and educating the patient and family (including obtaining informed consent). Special considerations for women with concurrent common medical disease are also included. Two recurrent themes are stressed in the chapter: avoiding surprises during each step in the preoperative period and alleviating the patient's fears and anxiety. This chapter is not intended to be an exhaustive discussion of all medical and surgical conditions that may have some impact on preoperative planning. Rather, the focus is on common preoperative problems encountered in benign gynecologic surgery. Cost containment strategies have placed increasing emphasis on same-day admission for almost all major gynecologic operations regardless of the woman's age. This practice has abruptly changed the timing of many preoperative events. Laboratory tests, electrocardiograms, and x-ray examinations are performed on an outpatient basis the week before surgery. Even preparation of the large intestine must be performed at home.

Not many events in a person's life are as depersonalizing or anxiety-producing as the 24 hours prior to the beginning of the surgical operation. Two considerations are helpful to women who must run this hospital gauntlet. It is important to give the patient a specific list of instructions for the 24 hours prior to surgery. Second, the patient needs a drug that will help relieve anxiety, such as diazepam 10 mg, to be taken the night before surgery. Often the latter is ordered by the anesthesiologist. The financial realities of current medical practice place a significant burden of preparation for the operation on the woman herself. Obviously, she needs to be educated concerning the specifics of this challenge and the education reinforced by a specific list of do's and don'ts. The two primary goals of preoperative preparation are to reduce the morbidity of the operative procedure and to shorten the length of time necessary for each phase of the recovery process.

PREOPERATIVE HISTORY

A detailed complete history not only obtains information but also helps to relieve the patient's fears and anxieties. When the history is obtained in an unhurried manner, the process is reassuring to the patient. The patient should perceive the gynecologist as a gentle and reassuring clinician rather than as a detective trying to rapidly solve a crime.

The extent and depth of the general history are modified to a minor degree by the age and general health of the woman and the operation contemplated. However, even minor operations may have major complications. Therefore it is best to be overprepared. The possibility of degenerative multiple organ disease necessitates a meticulous review before any surgical procedure in geriatric patients. Even for an emergency operation a detailed history is important.

For elective operations the preoperative history usually is taken on two separate occasions. Studies have documented that patients often omit important medical information particularly when under stress. Repetitive history taking does provide additional information and helps to decrease the risk of omission of significant historical information. The interview occurs initially in the physician's office several weeks before the operation and is repeated 1 to 7 days before the procedure is done. The initial interval is valuable, for it gives the patient an opportunity to reconsider her decision. Similarly, the physician uses the time to collect necessary information, such as records of previous surgical procedures. In reviewing the history the second time, often the patient recalls important information that she omitted during the initial history. For example, she may have recently talked to a sister who has a history of excessive bleeding during an operation.

There are two purposes in obtaining a detailed and comprehensive history from the patient. The first is to put the patient at ease; the second is to cover a formalized and extremely thorough set of questions. The two processes demand time and gentle consideration of the patient's anxiety. It is best to let the woman offer her perspective first. Subsequently the physician may direct the questions to a standard format. Obviously the format must be covered in a systematic manner so that essential areas are not omitted. Many gynecologists have the woman complete a standardized historical questionnaire prior to the outpatient appointment.

Although this chapter does not review all the components of a complete history (see Chapter 6), it is advantageous to group questions under the specific organ systems: pulmonary, cardiovascular, renal, hepatic, metabolic, endocrine, neurologic, hematologic, and immunologic. Several specific questions should be included to fill any holes and to cross-check on the review of symptoms. These questions cover problems with surgery, anesthesia, or bleeding in the patient or her family.

The next general category is drug allergy and current medications. Questions must be constructed so as to include both prescribed and over-the-counter medications. Approximately 0.5% of the general population and 1.5% of women over the age of 55 are receiving continuous glucocorticoids. Thus a specific question about glucocorticoid therapy for chronic medical problems is essential. It is important to inquire regarding over-the-counter vitamins, nutritional, and herbal supplements because of the increasing incidence of interactions with drugs.

Many women do not consider aspirin or oral contraceptives as medication; therefore specific questions regarding these substances are needed. General questions regarding smoking, alcohol, exercise tolerance, and recent upper respiratory infections are often grouped together. Specific questions should be directed toward sensitivity to iodine or latex. Latex allergy is directly responsible for 12% of the perioperative anaphylactic reactions in adult patients and for 70% in children.

The woman's contraceptive history, including any recent change, must be known. Over the years there has been no greater embarrassment in the operating room than the realization that a recent contraceptive practice has been abandoned and the patient is pregnant. Included with the contraceptive history are key questions concerning possible exposure to the human immunodeficiency virus (HIV). Also, the physician should estimate the probability of blood transfusion and together with the patient decide whether autologous blood should be donated for possible transfusion. Many women and their families are deeply concerned about the potential risk of acquiring human immunodeficiency virus via allogeneic blood. Presently the risk of an HIV-contaminated unit of donated blood passing through screening tests and infecting the woman is approximately one in 1,000,000 units of blood. Etchason et al., using a decision analysis model to assess the cost effectiveness of autologous blood donation, found considerable additional cost ($68 to $4783) per unit of blood. Managed care programs will struggle with this ethical dilemma. Lastly, there is no evidence that blood from directed donors, selected by the patient, is safer than blood from volunteer donors. With the length of life increasing, more elderly women are candidates for gynecologic surgery. Age is an important risk factor.

PHYSICAL EXAMINATION

The preoperative physical examination should answer three basic questions: Has the primary gynecologic disease process changed since the initial diagnosis? What is the impact of the primary gynecologic disease on other organ systems? What deficiencies in other organ systems may affect the proposed surgery and hospitalization? A pelvic examination performed the day before surgery may demonstrate that a myoma has undergone acute degeneration or an ovarian cyst may have ruptured and "disappeared." Pelvic masses adherent to the large intestine suggest the necessity of mechanical cleansing of the bowel before surgery. A patient with cardiac murmurs secondary to valvular heart disease needs antibiotic prophylaxis against subacute bacterial endocarditis. Often the morbidly obese woman has impairments in the function of the circulatory and respiratory systems.

The most important feature of the preoperative physical is that it should be performed in a thorough and compulsive manner. The gynecologist should use the same sequence every time to help focus attention on the evaluation of each organ system.

The physical examination is best performed in the physician's office. To diminish the patient's anxiety, the physical examination should not be performed in silence. Conversation with the patient may involve further history taking or questions and answers about the proposed operation. Gentle palpation is important. A gentle touch helps to build the trust and confidence that are the foundation of the physician-patient relationship.

Two important axioms should be stressed. First, in emergency situations it is imperative to perform a complete physical examination. This examination should include an evaluation of the blood pressure and pulse in both the recumbent and sitting positions; orthostatic hypotension and tachycardia are crude indexes of a decrease in circulating intravascular volume. Second, it is important to perform a pelvic and rectal examination the day before the operation and again in the operating room immediately before the surgical incision. Pelvic masses sometimes change in size when the bladder and gastrointestinal tracts are empty. These measures help avoid surprises.

LABORATORY PROCEDURES

The general purpose of preoperative laboratory procedures is to identify conditions that will alter or aid in perioperative management. Specifically, screening tests are used to find unsuspected, asymptomatic diseases that may affect, alter, or postpone the anticipated surgical procedure. Preoperative laboratory tests also help to establish the extent of known disease that may influence the scheduling of elective surgery. Gynecologists should individualize their preoperative approach to patients and select specific tests for each patient. The downside of multiple routine preoperative testing is that it increases the likelihood of false-positive results, especially if the disease has a low prevalence in the population being tested. A false-positive test has many negative features, including anxiety for the patient, additional testing, financial cost, and often delays scheduling the operation. Sometimes special imaging procedures are used to determine the effects of pelvic disease on other organ systems.

Presently there is an extensive debate over which preoperative laboratory procedures should be standard. Attention has been drawn to the cost-benefit ratio of preoperative screening. Although the cost of each individual test is usually low, the aggregate costs are substantial. Often the cost argument is overcome by the individual gynecologist's concern to practice defensive medicine in the present medicolegal climate. Many preoperative laboratory tests are ordered simply by convention, for years being standard orders in an individual's or hospital's practice.

Kaplan et al. have retrospectively studied the usefulness of preoperative laboratory procedures. They estimate that 60% of the routinely ordered tests, such as differential cell count, platelet count, and 12-factor automated multiple analyses, would not have been performed if tests had been ordered only for an indication discovered by history or physical examination. Most important, only 0.22% of these tests demonstrated an abnormality that might influence perioperative management (Figure 24-1). The final conclusion in their assessment of 2000 patients undergoing elective operations was that in the absence of specific indications, routine preoperative laboratory tests do not significantly contribute to patient care and could be eliminated. The Mayo Clinic does not perform any routine preoperative clinic screening test on patients younger than 40 years who have been assessed as healthy by history and physical exam.

Two of the most important considerations in the choice of preoperative tests are the age of the patient and the extent of the surgical procedure. Preoperative laboratory procedures should be determined in each patient based on the findings of both a complete history and a physical examination. Women who benefit from preoperative testing have significant risk factors or positive findings discovered during the complete history and physical exam. Most important, abnormal results from any laboratory test should result in some change in perioperative management. Regretfully, unexpected abnormalities in many standard preoperative laboratory tests are frequently overlooked or ignored. Studies have found that between 30% and 60% of unexpected abnormalities detected by preoperative laboratory tests are not actually noted or investigated prior to surgery.

Preoperative complete blood count and urinalysis are required by nearly all hospitals. By far the most important of these for gynecologists is the test for anemia. A woman should not be admitted for elective gynecologic surgery with a low hematocrit level that will necessitate transfusion during the perioperative period, unless a delay in surgery is contraindicated or medical therapy to improve the hematocrit level has been unsuccessful. The results of the urinalysis, white blood cell count, and differential count rarely alter management. Before major gynecologic surgery, with an anticipated potential blood loss of greater than 750 ml, a blood sample should be sent to the blood bank for typing and screening for unusual antibodies. This should replace the expensive routine typing and cross-match. However, it is important that the blood bank have the capability of providing cross-matched blood within a reasonable period of time if serious intraoperative bleeding does occur. Routine preoperative type and screen for uncomplicated abdominal or vaginal hysterectomy is not cost effective. Also, routine clotting studies are not cost effective and rarely provide useful clinical information unless indicated by history and physical examination (Table 24-1).

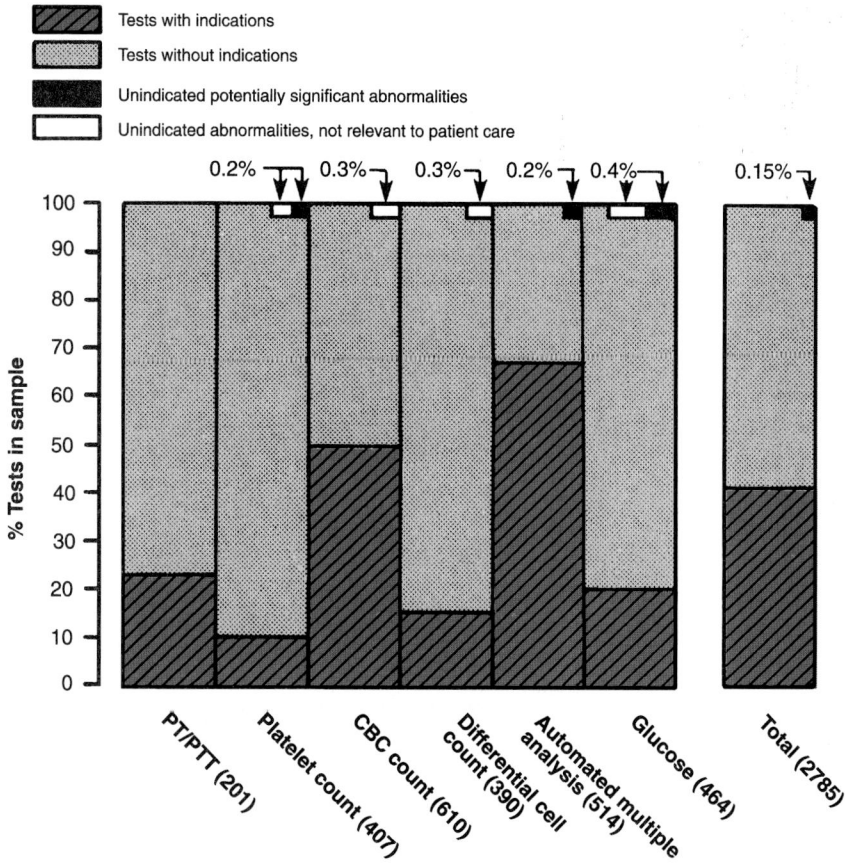

FIGURE 24-1 Proportions of indicated and unindicated preoperative tests, drawn to scale. Numbers in parentheses represent sample sizes used. *PT/PTT*, Prothrombin time/partial thromboplastin time; *CBC*, complete blood cell. Automated multiple analysis is six factor. (From Kaplan EB, Scheiner LB, Boeckmann AJ, et al: JAMA 253:3578, 1985.)

TABLE 24-1

Comparison of the Clinical Characteristics of Platelet and Clotting Factor Disorder

	Platelet Disorder	Clotting Factor Disorder
Site of bleeding	Skin Mucous membrane (nasal, oral, vaginal, gastro-intestinal, etc.)	Deep/soft tissue (e.g., muscles, joints)
Bleeding after cuts and scratches	Yes	No
Petechiae	Yes	No
Ecchymoses	Small, superficial	Large, deep (often palpable)
Hemarthroses	Rare	Common
Bleeding after surgery	Immediate, usually mild	Delayed (several hours or 1–2 days), then severe

From Clarke-Pearson DL: Obstet Gynecol Forum 6:2, 1992.

It is beneficial to order limited blood screening tests in women over age 40 or in women who have positive family histories or questionable past histories of hepatic or renal disease. A preoperative creatinine or BUN is especially important if the patient is going to be treated with antibiotics excreted by the kidneys. A test for human chorionic gonadotrophin may be appropriate, depending on contraceptive and sexual history. A pregnancy test should almost always be obtained if the patient is a teenager. Menstrual history is at best an imperfect indication of an early pregnancy. Serum electrolytes are ordered in women taking diuretics or for those with a history of renal disease or heart disease. Also, serum electrolytes should be evaluated for patients with vomiting, diarrhea, ileus, bowel obstruction, or any condition that affects water or electrolyte balance.

The tradition of ordering chest x-ray films on all patients has been seriously questioned. Roizen performed a detailed cost analysis of routine chest x-ray films and determined the practice was not cost effective unless the patient was over age 75 or had known pulmonary or cardiac disease. Rucker et al., in a similar study, concluded that a history and physical examination are sufficient to screen patients and chest x-ray films need be ordered only for patients with positive findings. In the latter study of 368 patients without risk factors, only one had a positive chest x-ray finding, and that finding did not alter the surgical procedure. A meta-analysis of studies of routine preoperative chest radiographs demonstrated that false-positive results leading to invasive procedures and associated morbidity were more frequent than the discovery of new findings leading to a change in management.

A baseline preoperative electrocardiogram has been found to be cost effective in asymptomatic patients only after age 60 in women without a history of cardiac disease or significant risk factors. It sometimes detects a recent asymptomatic myocardial infarction or serious cardiac arrhythmias.

The results of screening tests should be reviewed during the office visit just before hospitalization. These include a recent Pap smear on all patients and mammography, depending on the patient's age and risk factors. Testing the stool for occult blood in women over age 50 detects bleeding from a colon cancer in approximately 2 of 1000 asymptomatic women.

At the conclusion of a complete history, physical examination, and screening laboratory procedures, the gynecologist should determine whether consultation with other specialists is necessary. This decision should be based on the seriousness of the concurrent disease and the complexity of the proposed operation.

PATIENT-FAMILY EDUCATION AND INFORMED CONSENT

One of the primary responsibilities of the gynecologic surgeon is to educate the patient and her family about the anticipated surgical procedure and hospitalization. Giving this information is both an ethical and legal responsibility. Informed consent is an important principle to ensure that the woman's right to self-determination is respected. The ethical concept of the process of informed consent includes two important components: free consent and comprehension. More important, in most circumstances the patient and her family want to know about the operation. Similar to the history and physical examination, educational discussions should take place on at least two occasions. Throughout the educational process, questions from the patient or family should be welcomed. The patient and family should be informed about the potential use of intravenous fluids, urinary catheters, and monitoring equipment. Often physicians take these devices for granted, not realizing such equipment may cause anxiety and fears in laypersons not familiar with modern postoperative care.

Educating the patient is a great step in relieving anxiety. If the patient is aware of the sequence of events, the stress of this time becomes more tolerable. It is difficult to overeducate the patient on details of the preoperative area, the operating room, and recovery room routines. Psychologic preparation of the family is equally important, and arrangements should be made for a specific location for a meeting with family members immediately following the operation. An informed family is one of the surgeon's greatest assistants. An uninformed family will often harass the entire health care delivery team.

Few concepts bring more ambivalence and concern to the physician than the doctrine of informed consent. In the present medicolegal climate, the absence of informed consent is cited as a major problem in many lawsuits. Some critics have pointed out that true informed consent would involve sending the patient to medical school and then through several hours of intensive discussion.

It is important to differentiate the concepts of consent and informed consent. Consent involves a simple yes-or-no decision, while informed consent is an educational process. If a gynecologist were to operate without consent, he or she would be vulnerable to charges of assault and battery. The right of an adult woman to have final authority to consent to an operation has over 200 years of legal precedent. The preoperative consent form that is standard in most hospitals simply documents that consent, hopefully informed consent, has been obtained.

To obtain informed consent, the surgeon must explain to the patient in understandable terms the following: the nature and extent of the disease process; the nature and extent of the contemplated operation; the anticipated benefits and results of the surgery, including a conservative estimate of successful outcome; the risks and potential complications of the operative procedure; alternative methods of therapy; and any potential changes in sexual function. The gynecologist should also discuss with the patient what the operation will not accomplish. Many patients expect surgery to magically cure a large constellation of symptoms. Questions from the patient should be encouraged and welcomed. After being educated and considering the information, the patient acquires an understanding of the risks and benefits of the proposed procedures and may make a "fully informed" decision and give informed consent for the operation to be performed.

The possibility of unanticipated pathologic conditions should be discussed with the patient and permission obtained on the written consent form for the most extensive operative procedure that may be necessary. Patients readily accept the necessity of freedom of judgment by the gynecologist during the operation as to the extent of the operative procedure, depending on what is discovered during surgery. For example, permission to remove both fallopian tubes and ovaries along with the uterus should be obtained in the event that extensive adnexal disease is an unanticipated finding.

One of the greatest dilemmas in the doctrine of informed consent is the extent and depth of discussions concerning potential complications of an operation. Attorneys who specialize in defending gynecologists in medical malpractice litigation strongly advise discussing all major complications, including death from surgery and rare, serious complications, such as urinary tract fistulas following hysterectomy. Studies have documented that approximately 70% of patients do not read the consent form before signing it. Ideally, to protect the gynecologist, the final discussion of the informed consent process should be witnessed by a family member and another member of the health delivery team. Highlights of this discussion should be documented by a paragraph written by the gynecologist in the progress notes of the chart.

Regretfully the patient may be overwhelmed by multiple caregivers' perceived "obligation" to give information. The excessive and conflicting information provided by physicians, nurses, and other caring individuals in the typical tertiary-care hospital may confuse and increase the fears of the woman and her family. Adding to this problem is the abundance of conflicting nonpeer-reviewed information available via the lay press and the Internet. In summary, a caring gynecologist must not only educate the patient, but be prepared to discuss other information that the woman has received.

PREOPERATIVE PREPARATION

Rarely a woman is admitted to the hospital prior to the operation. The preoperative orders should communicate the gynecologist's preoperative preparation for his or her patient. To avoid omissions, it is important to develop a systematic method of writing preoperative orders. The orders should be individualized depending on the previous history and physical examination obtained as an outpatient, the patient's age, and the extent of the proposed surgical procedure. Unusual or infrequent orders should be written in specific detail to avoid confusion by nursing and other hospital personnel. Because of the increasing emphasis on same-day admission to the hospital, most procedures and orders are accomplished on an outpatient basis. Therefore it is important to give the patient a specific list of instructions for the 24 hours before surgery.

The first two or three lines of the order sheet should include the proposed operation, and a list of the patient's diseases. Further orders are subdivided into four broad categories: general measures, medication, laboratory tests, and preventive therapies.

General measures include orders for activity, diet, and vital signs. The patient should have nothing more than clear liquids during the 2 to 4 hours prior to elective surgery. If the patient's operation is not scheduled until the middle of the afternoon, it is acceptable for the patient to have an early liquid breakfast. Interestingly the extent of preoperative anxiety does not influence gastric fluid volume or acidity.

The second category of orders is for medications. When prophylactic antibiotics are ordered, the time of injection should ensure that significant blood and tissue levels will be present at the time of bacterial contamination during the surgical procedure. An additional subgroup is special medications for specific medical illness. It is presumed that the anesthesiologist will write orders for preoperative medication to alleviate anxiety and reduce tracheobronchial secretions.

The third major group of orders involves preoperative laboratory tests. This group includes standard laboratory tests and specifically indicated laboratory tests.

The fourth and last group of orders involves preventive therapies. Thrombophlebitis remains a major complication of gynecologic surgery. Patients should wear graded compression elastic stockings to help overcome venous stasis. Prophylactic subcutaneous heparin and/or intermittent pneumatic leg compression devices are indicated in women at moderate and high risk for thromboembolic disease. Because the lower intestinal tract should be empty before an operation, it is appropriate to order an enema to cleanse the lower intestine. Patients who have been NPO for a prolonged period or who have lost fluid from cleansing of the gastrointestinal tract should be given intravenous fluids before induction of anesthesia to ensure proper hydration. One of the time-honored traditions in gynecologic surgery has been douching the evening before the operation. The medical value of this habit is unproved. If removal of hair is necessary for the operation, it should be clipped immediately before the operation.

CONSULTATION WITH THE ANESTHESIOLOGIST

The preoperative interaction between the patient and the anesthesiologist in a preoperative screening clinic is most important. For the patient, both the reassurance of meeting the anesthesiologist and their exchange of information greatly alleviate anxiety. For the anesthesiologist, it is an opportunity to obtain necessary medical information, evaluate the patient, determine the risk of the perioperative period, and write preoperative medication orders. This meeting had traditionally occurred the afternoon or evening before surgery. However, with emphasis on cost containment and greater use of outpatient facilities, and with admission to the hospital the morning of the operation, this meeting frequently occurs in an outpatient clinic several days before surgery. Recently, anesthesiologists have assumed more responsibility for postoperative pain management, primarily using epidural narcotics. This subject should be discussed with the patient. Roizen has emphasized that recovery is more rapid when a patient's concerns are addressed and when she knows what to expect regarding postoperative therapy for pain.

Anesthesiologists classify surgical procedures according to the patient's risk of mortality. Dripps, in 1961, first published guidelines to determine the risk of death related to major operative procedures. This Physical Status Scale (Table 24-2) has been adopted by the American Society of Anesthesiologists. An emergency operation doubles the mortality risks for classes 1, 2, and 3; produces a slightly increased risk in class 4; and does not change the risk in class 5. Hirsch is of the opinion that 5% to 10% of the total perioperative mortality rate is directly related to anesthetic problems. The majority of deaths due to anesthesia are ascribable to human error. The most common serious morbidity associated with elective surgery are cardiovascular complications. A recent report found that evaluations by anesthesiologists in a preoperative clinic provide information leading to changes in management for more than 15% of healthy patients. In this report, the most common medical conditions of concern were gastric reflux, insulin-dependent diabetes mellitus, asthma, and anticipated difficulties in intubation.

A problem frequently encountered by both gynecologists and anesthesiologists is whether to continue or interrupt medications that the patient is taking. If the drug is prescribed for a medical illness, it is best to continue the drug through the perioperative period. The physician must determine whether the drug will adversely affect the course of either the anesthesia or the surgery and whether it will interact with other drugs to be given during the procedure. It is acceptable to have the patient take oral medications the morning of surgery. The 30 to 60 ml of water needed to swallow the oral medication is negligible compared with gastric fluid volumes. Roizen has listed several drugs as special exceptions to routine administration before the operation, for they interfere or interact with either anesthesia or surgery. This list includes monoamine oxidase inhibitors, nicotinic acid, insulin, metformin, corticosteroids, and anticoagulants.

TABLE 24-2
Dripps—American Society
of Anesthesiologists Classification

Class	Description
1	A normal healthy patient
2	A patient with mild to moderate systemic disease
3	A patient with severe systemic disease with limited activity but not incapacitated
4	A patient with incapacitating, constantly life-threatening systemic disease
5	A moribund patient not expected to survive 24 hours with or without operation

Modified from Anesthesiology 24:111, 1963. From Jewell ER and Persson AV: Surg Clin North Am 65:3, 1985.

The primary goals of preoperative medication are to relieve anxiety and produce sedation. Many patients desire amnesia. This may not be a reasonable goal for early discharge following the operation. Sedation is easy to accomplish; however, relief of anxiety does not invariably accompany sedation. Narcotics and sedatives should be used with caution in patients with chronic respiratory or liver disease. Recently, a task force of the American Society for Anesthesiologists recommended against the routine prophylactic use of anticholinergics, antihistamines, and H2 receptor antagonists to reduce the incidence of pulmonary aspiration.

PROPHYLACTIC ANTIBIOTICS

The use of prophylactic antibiotics in gynecologic surgical procedures has become standard practice when a clinically significant risk of postoperative infection exists. Wound infections and pelvic cellulitis, although infrequent, are important causes of postoperative morbidity. Gynecologic operations produce both hypoxic tissue and collections of bloody and serous fluids, both of which are excellent culture media. Rigidly defined, prophylactic antibiotic use involves the administration of antibiotics to women without evidence of pelvic infection to prevent postoperative morbidity related to infection. The major use of prophylactic antibiotics is in operations such as vaginal hysterectomy, following which there is potential for a high incidence of postoperative pelvic cellulitis. The goal of antibiotic therapy is to prevent infection by the endogenous flora of the lower female reproductive tract. Prophylactic antibiotics are given occasionally when the incidence of postoperative infection is low but the results of the surgical procedure would be severely compromised if an infection did occur, such as with reconstructive operations on the fallopian tubes. Approximately 40% of all antibiotics used in hospitals are ordered as prophylaxis.

The use of prophylactic antibiotics in gynecologic surgery has been the subject of much debate. As in any discussion of preventive medicine, one has to evaluate the benefits, risks, and costs. In general, the use of prophylactic antibiotics results in fewer operative site infections (abdominal wound and pelvic cellulitis), reduced febrile morbidity, and shorter hospital stays. The major risk of allergic or toxic reactions is small, especially with a short course of prophylactic antibiotics. The increased cost of the antibiotics is justified by a lower total cost from a shorter hospitalization. Certainly the economic costs of prolonged hospitalization for even a minor postoperative infection are substantial.

The foundation of our understanding of prophylactic antibiotics is the classic research of John Burke published in 1961. He stressed the fact that maximum antibacterial activity in subcutaneous wounds results from a combination of host resistance and antibiotics. His experimental studies proved that the antibiotic must be present in damaged tissue at the time of contamination with bacteria or shortly thereafter. Burke termed the first 3 hours of decreased tissue resistance following a surgical insult as the *effective period.* He found that there was no protective effect in preventing the development of subcutaneous wound infections if the antibiotics were given later than 3 hours following bacterial contamination.

Subsequent studies have documented two other important facts concerning prophylactic antibiotics in gynecology. First, the goal of prophylactic antibiotics is to reduce the total number of bacteria present in the operative site. It is not necessary to kill all of the bacteria. Second, for prophylaxis to be successful, adequate tissue levels of antibiotics need to be maintained only for the duration of the operation. The normal endogenous vaginal flora has 1 $\times$ 10^8 bacteria per milliliter of vaginal secretions, consisting of a wide spectrum of both aerobic and anaerobic organisms. Thus, theoretically, the choice of a single antibiotic for prophylaxis in gynecology is a most difficult one. Ideally the drug chosen as a prophylactic antibiotic should be nontoxic, inexpensive, and effective against most organisms encountered in the endogenous flora. Multiple reports have documented a linear relationship between the incidence of bacterial vaginosis and the incidence of postoperative pelvic infection. Therefore, a woman should not have an elective hysterectomy if bacterial vaginosis is discovered during the 2 weeks prior to surgery. It is important for the gynecologist to identify women with bacterial vaginosis. Following treatment, the vaginal ecosystem should return to normal prior to the operation.

There is abundant literature supporting the use of prophylactic antibiotics in gynecology. More than 50 studies summarize the data from women who received prophylactic antibiotics for vaginal hysterectomy. The results of these studies show that the incidence of febrile morbidity was reduced from 40% to 15% and the incidence of pelvic infection from 25% to 5%. The results of more than 30 studies of women having abdominal hysterectomies are not as decisive. Some studies demonstrated no significant improvement, whereas positive studies demonstrated less dramatic declines in febrile morbidity, pelvic infection, and wound infection. The average reduction in febrile morbidity was 12%, and the average reduction in operation site infection, 5%. In many studies it is difficult to determine whether the investigators equated postoperative fever with postoperative infection.

No center or expert has demonstrated the specific antibiotic of choice for prophylaxis in gynecology. It is most difficult to compare one prophylactic antibiotic with another. Not only are there differences in methodology between studies but also differences in terminology between definitions of febrile morbidity and documented

pelvic infections. However, there are not significant differences in outcome no matter which single broad-spectrum antibiotic is used. Presently, first- or second-generation cephalosporins are the most popular choice for prophylactic antibiotics in gynecology (e.g., a single dose of first-generation cefazolin [Kefzol], 1 to 2 g intramuscularly or intravenously 30 minutes before the operation, or second-generation cefoxitin [Mefoxin], 1 to 2 g intramuscularly or intravenously immediately before the operation). A meta-analysis by Tanos and Rojansky suggests a significant reduction in the incidence of infection, but not postoperative fever, with the use of prophylactic cephalosporins by the intravenous rather than the intramuscular route (odds ratio [OR], 0.66, CI, 0.5 to 0.9). Often nursing personnel give prophylactic antibiotics prematurely by optimistically anticipating when the patient will go to the operating room. This practice may result in lower than desirable antibiotic levels during the time of bacterial contamination. Some hospitals have developed standard protocols to ensure that prophylactic antibiotics are given at the appropriate time.

With the wide spectrum of bacteria involved in the constantly changing ecologic system of the vagina, a single antibiotic does not have the spectrum to be bactericidal or bacteriostatic against all the bacteria present. The important feature sought in a prophylactic antibiotic is an ability to reduce the total number of bacteria present in the bacterial inoculum; it does not have to affect all organisms. A reduction in overall number allows the woman's natural defense mechanisms to eradicate the remaining bacteria.

Recent emphasis has focused on an extremely short duration of therapy for prophylactic antibiotics. Comparative studies have documented that single-dose therapy is as effective as 24 hours of antibiotics. No advantage exists to continuing prophylactic antibiotics beyond the immediate operative period. This short duration of administration also reduces cost and complications. The incidence of serious complications, such as drug allergy and resistant bacteria, is directly related to the length of administration of the antibiotic. With prophylactic antibiotics the major concern is the potential threat of increasing bacterial resistance. This results in two problems: more nosocomial infections with resistant organisms and alterations of the normal vaginal flora. If infection does develop following prolonged use of prophylactic antibiotics, one must obtain cultures and select antibiotic coverage different from the antibiotic used for prophylaxis. Other potential complications from prophylactic antibiotics are antibiotic-associated diarrhea and/or colitis or the more serious pseudomembranous enterocolitis often secondary to *Clostridium difficile* infection. This complication usually follows chronic use of antibiotics, but rarely it may occur after a short exposure to antibiotics. Antibiotic therapy any time in the previous 6 weeks may be responsible for precipitating the onset of this disease.

Many factors affect the risk of postoperative infection. The most important include the length of the operation, whether the woman is premenopausal or postmenopausal, obesity, low socioeconomic status, malnutrition, immunosuppression, the use of prophylactic antibiotics, and the operative approach. Most studies have not documented that prophylactic antibiotics decrease the incidence of serious pelvic infections such as pelvic abscess. However, since this is a rare complication, the studies performed to date are not large enough to eliminate a beta error. Some studies have questioned the benefits of prophylactic antibiotics in operative procedures that last more than 3½ hours.

A randomized clinical trial reported by Greif et al. studied supplemental perioperative oxygen in 500 patients undergoing operations involving the large bowel. The authors discovered the administration of supplemental oxygen during the operation and in the first 2 hours of the perioperative period resulted in a 50% reduction in the incidence of wound infection. If this initial report is confirmed by subsequent studies, supplemental oxygen use quickly will become the standard because the cost and risk are not major factors.

In summary, prophylactic antibiotics are routinely ordered for vaginal or abdominal hysterectomies and gynecologic operations that carry a substantial risk of postoperative infection. The most popular choice is a first- or second-generation cephalosporin, such as cefazolin or cefoxitin. Preferentially the prophylactic antibiotics should be administered intravenously (Figure 24-2). Whatever broad-spectrum antibiotic is selected, the gynecologist must know the pharmacokinetics of the drug. The half-life of the antibiotic is important in selecting the proper timing and route of preoperative administration and the possible necessity of an intraoperative dose for longer operations. The amount of antibiotic bound to plasma proteins is important, for it determines the concentration of free antibiotic in the tissues (Table 24-3). The antibiotic selected should be active against the majority of endogenous flora of the vagina. The drug should be present at the time of surgical insult, and it should be used only during the time of the operative procedure. Obviously, prophylactic antibiotics are helpful, but they should not be exchanged or substituted for meticulous surgical technique. Most importantly antibiotic prophylaxis should not be used indiscriminately because of the increasing problem with selection of resistant bacteria.

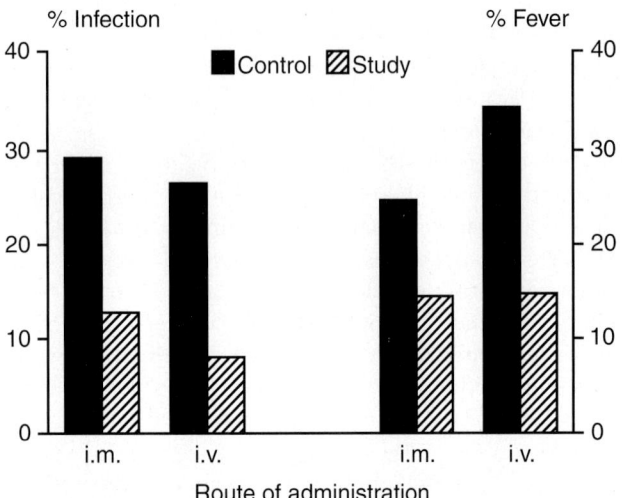

FIGURE 24-2   Prevalence of infection and febrile morbidity in the study and control group by route of administration. i.m., intramuscularly; i.v., intravenously. (From Tanos V and Rojansky N: J Am Coll Surg 179:593, 1994.)

TABLE 24-3
Pharmacologic Properties of Cephalosporins

	Peak Serum Concentration (µg/mL)		Half-Life (minutes)	Protein Binding (%)
	Intravenous*	Intramuscular†		
Parenteral (1g dose)				
Cephalothin	15	20	40	70
Cephapirin	15	20	40	45
Cephradine	15	15	20	10
Cefazolin	80	60	100	80
Cefamandole	55	25	40	80
Cefoxitin	30	20	40	70
Cefotaxime	50	20	60	40
Moxalactam	90	25	120	50

From Thompson RL and Wright AJ: Mayo Clin Proc 58:82, 1983.

*At 30 minutes after rapid infusion.

†At 30 minutes after intramuscular injection.

THROMBOEMBOLIC DISEASE

Thrombophlebitis of either the pelvic or the leg veins is a frequent complication of gynecologic surgery (Table 24-4). Using sophisticated I^{125} fibrinogen scanning techniques, approximately 15% of women having surgery for a benign disease and approximately 22% of women having surgery for malignant disease develop thrombophlebitis. Most alarming, Moser et al. discovered that almost 40% of patients with deep venous thrombophlebitis and no symptoms of pulmonary embolus had documented evidence of a pulmonary embolus by ventilation perfusion studies of the lung. Classically the three major pathophysiologic changes that facilitate the development of thrombophlebitis and pulmonary embolus are venous injury, circulatory stasis, and hypercoagulable conditions. John Bonnar from Dublin, Ireland, is the world's leading authority in the field of venous thromboembolism in obstetrics and gynecology. Bonnar defines thrombosis as "the process by which liquid blood flowing through the venous system turns into a solid mass of fibrin, platelets and cells within the vein." He underlines the two potential serious outcomes associated with thrombosis: pulmonary embolus early in the course of the disease and the chronic complication of post-thrombotic venous insufficiency, which may greatly impair the quality of a woman's life. Many aspects of pelvic surgery predispose the woman to develop thrombophlebitis, including venous stasis, surgical injury to the walls of large veins, and often associated anaerobic infection.

Because of the significant morbidity and mortality associated with a postoperative pulmonary embolus, every effort should be made to reduce the incidence of thrombophlebitis. Approximately 40% of deaths following gynecologic surgery are directly or indirectly related to pulmonary emboli. Although the initial venous injury most often occurs at the time of the operation, approximately 15% of symptomatic emboli do not occur until the first week following discharge from the hospital.

During the preoperative period the patient should be evaluated for factors that place her at increased risk for thromboembolic disease. Such factors include a history of previous thrombophlebitis or embolus, family or personal history of hypercoagulability (thrombophilic state), malignant disease, previous radiation therapy, congestive heart failure, morbid obesity, venous disease, edema of the legs, active pelvic infection, age, current use of oral contraceptives or hormone replacement therapy up to the time of the operation, and length of preoperative hospitalization (Table 24-5). Lengthy surgical procedures, especially associated with profuse bleeding, are also significant risk factors.

Various means are used to prevent thromboembolic disease. Ideally, the first prophylactic measure to reduce the incidence of embolic disease is to discontinue oral contraceptives or hormone replacement therapy 4 weeks before *major* elective operations. The increase in absolute risk is very small. Thus, pragmatically the risk avoided by stopping oral contraceptives must be weighted against the possible risk of an unwanted pregnancy. Other simple prophylactic measures include elastic stockings, early ambulation, and leg exercises in bed. Support hose should be thigh high so as to avoid venous stasis at the knee. The appearance of the support hose also serves a teaching function to remind women and nursing personnel of the importance of ambulation and exercise to prevent venous stasis.

Randomized clinical trials have demonstrated that either pharmacologic agents, such as low-dose heparin, and/or mechanical methods, such as intermittent pneumatic compression of the legs, are effective in preventing thrombophlebitis. The key decision for the prophylaxis of thromboembolic diseases is whether to order prophylactic mini-heparin, or pneumatic inflated sleeve devices, or a

TABLE 24-4
Incidence of Venous Thrombosis After Gynecologic Operations with I-Fibrinogen Scanning

Reference	No. of Patients	Type of Operation	Incidence of Leg Vein Thrombosis
Adolf et al.	75	Major	29
Ballard et al.	55	Major benign disease	29
Clayton et al.	231	Major	16
Endl and Auinger	43	Major	37
Walsh et al.	100	Vaginal hysterectomy	7
	117	Abdominal hysterectomy	13
	23	Wertheim's operation	25
	22	Other malignant disease	45

From Bonnar J: Clin Obstet Gynecol 28:433, 1985.

TABLE 24-5
Assessment of Risk of Venous Thromboembolism in Gynecologic Patients

Thromboembolic Complications	Low Risk (Under 40 years; operative procedures less than 30 minutes; no immobilization)	Moderate Risk (Over 40 years; estrogen therapy; operative procedures more than 30 minutes; varicose veins; obesity; postoperative infection)	High Risk (Previous thromboembolism; abdominal or pelvic operation for malignant disease; immobilization)
Calf vein thrombosis	<3%	10%–30%	30%–60%
Proximal vein thrombosis	<1%	2%–8%	6%–12%
Pulmonary embolism	<0.01%	0.1%–0.7%	1%–2%

From Bonnar J: Clin Obstet Gynecol 28:435, 1985.

combination of both. It is our practice to evaluate the severity of risk and then select the most appropriate method, taking into consideration the side effects and cost. Women are categorized into low-, moderate-, or high-risk groups depending on their risk assessment profile (Table 24-6). Current recommendations to prevent or diminish the thrombophlebitis risk for each group are listed in the box. Obviously, women at high risk should have both pharmacologic and mechanical prophylaxis. Some women are transiently anticoagulated by the mini-heparin dose of 5000 units of unfractionated heparin every 8 to 12 hours and thus may experience excessive bleeding during or following the operative procedure. This complication is experienced by approximately 2% of women. Obese or extremely thin patients should have their dosage of subcutaneous heparin adjusted according to activated partial thromboplastin time.

Thromboprophylaxis in the Gynecologic Patient

1. In the low-risk group, provide early mobilization and attention to hydration.
2. In the moderate-risk group, administer 5000 U/12 h standard heparin subcutaneously, 20 mg/d low-molecular-weight subcutaneously, 20 mg/d low-molecular-weight heparin enoxaparin subcutaneously, 2500 U/d dalteparin, or intermittent pneumatic calf compression.
3. In the high-risk group, administer 5000 U/8 h standard heparin subcutaneously, 40 mg/d low-molecular-weight heparin enoxaparin subcutaneously, or 5000 U/d dalteparin, in conjunction with a mechanical method such as graduated elastic compression stockings or intermittent pneumatic calf compression for ≥5 days.

From Bonnar J: Can more be done in obstetric and gynecologic practice to reduce morbidity and mortality associated with venous thromboembolism? Am J Obstet Gynecol 180:784, 1999.

Collins et al. performed a meta-analysis, reviewing more than 70 randomized trials of perioperative subcutaneous heparin in more than 16,000 general surgery, orthopedic, and urologic patients. This study demonstrated that subcutaneous heparin prevents approximately two thirds of deep venous thrombosis and 50% of all deaths from pulmonary emboli. The most striking data in this study related the reduction in death directly to pulmonary emboli, with 19 deaths in the patients given perioperative heparin and 55 deaths in the control group.

Low-molecular heparins are superior to standard unfractionated heparin, for they have a longer half-life, almost 100% bioavailability, dose-independent clearance, and thus a more consistent anticoagulation effect from dose to dose. Therefore most studies report significantly fewer hemorrhagic complications with low-molecular-weight heparins compared with unfractionated heparin. Importantly, the incidence of heparin-induced thrombocytopenia is significantly lower in patients given prophylaxis with low-molecular-weight heparin than those receiving unfractionated heparin. However, in some managed care protocols, low-molecular-weight heparin is reserved for the high-risk or difficult-to-manage woman because it is approximately 10 to 20 times as expensive as unfractionated heparin.

The primary alternative to anticoagulation is intermittent pneumatic calf compression modalities, which include graduated elastic compression stockings and air pumps. Together these devices not only prevent stasis and the endothelial injury that may occur with extreme venous distention but also stimulate the fibrinolytic system. In one meta-analysis of 11 randomized clinical trials, there was an almost 70% reduction in incidence of deep venous thrombosis in patients using intermittent pneumatic calf compression. Compression stockings are relatively inexpensive, and their only down side is poorly fitting stockings that produce a tourniquet effect at the knee. Intermittent pneumatic compression devices are equal in cost and

---

TABLE 24-6
Risk Assessment Profile for Thromboembolism
in Gynecologic Surgery

Low risk, early mobilization and hydration

- Minor surgery (<30 min) with no other risk factors
- Major surgery (<30 min) but with age <40 y and no other risk factors

Moderate risk, consider ≥1 of a variety of prophylactic measures

- Minor surgery (<30 min) in patients with a personal or family history of deep vein thrombosis, pulmonary embolism, or thrombophilia
- Major surgery (>30 min)
- Laparoscopic extended surgery
- Obesity (>80 kg)
- Gross varicose veins
- Current infection
- Immobility before operation (>4 d)
- Major current illness (e.g., heart or lung disease, cancer, inflammatory bowel disease, nephrotic syndrome, malignancies other than gynecologic)
- Heart failure or recent myocardial infarction

High risk, heparin prophylaxis with or without leg stockings

- Presence of ≥3 moderate risk factors from moderate risk list
- Major pelvic or abdominal surgery for gynecologic cancer
- Major surgery (>30 min) in patients with personal or family history of previous deep vein thrombosis, pulmonary embolism, or thrombophilia; paralysis or immobilization of lower limbs

---

From Bonnar J: Can more be done in obstetric and gynecologic practice to reduce morbidity and mortality associated with venous thromboembolism? Am J Obstet Gynecol 180:784, 1999.

---

effectiveness to subcutaneous heparin. They should be used intraoperatively and for the entire hospitalization. Complications or side effects are extremely rare, but injuries to the common peroneal nerve and compartment syndrome have been reported. Both nursing personnel and patients must be educated as to the benefits of the devices or their compliance with this mechanical method is poor. Authors of randomized clinical trials in gynecology comparing low-dose heparin and intermittent pneumatic compression devices favor the choice of the mechanical method. This decision is primarily based on the difference in bleeding complications between the two regimens.

GASTROINTESTINAL TRACT

Gastrointestinal symptoms are rare in women being evaluated for elective operations for benign gynecologic conditions. However, if the patient has such symptoms, the gynecologist should consider preoperative endoscopy and/or radiologic studies of the gastrointestinal tract. The impact of nausea, vomiting, or diarrhea on serum electrolytes and also on the nutritional status of the patient needs to be evaluated.

In this era of cost containment, a barium enema or flexible colonoscopy need not be routinely performed on all patients with adnexal masses. These tests do help to establish the differential diagnosis among diverticulitis, carcinoma of the colon, and endometriosis. Therefore a barium enema or endoscopy are indicated for benign disease if there is a left-sided adnexal mass in a woman over age 40, a positive stool guaiac test, or bowel symptoms. Again, the evaluation of each patient must be individualized in an attempt to determine if a primary gynecologic process is pressing on the bowel or directly invading the large intestine.

Proper mechanical cleansing of the gastrointestinal tract is important before every elective gynecologic operation. The patient should not have eaten solid food for 6 hours before surgery. Clear liquids are emptied from the stomach within minutes; however, fatty foods greatly delay gastric emptying. Obviously, incomplete preparation of the upper gastrointestinal tract increases the risk of aspiration, which is a serious complication of anesthesia and operations. Recent studies have documented the safety of allowing both inpatients and outpatients to ingest clear liquids up until 2 hours before elective surgery.

A preoperative enema to mechanically empty the large bowel is one of the simplest of preoperative preparations. When properly performed, preoperative enemas hasten the return of normal bowel function postoperatively and help to reduce the incidence of fecal impaction during the immediate postoperative period. Enemas should be given early on the evening before the operation so that most gas and all fluid and stool are properly expelled from the distal colon. If an enema is given the morning of the operation and the colon subsequently is not totally evacuated, the patient is likely to expel the contents during the operation. As stated, the physician and patient must be adaptive, since preoperative preparation often occurs in the outpatient setting.

If there is a suspicion that the operation will necessitate entry into the lumen of the large intestine, both mechanical cleansing and antibiotics to reduce the bacterial count of the colon should be ordered. Colon and rectal surgeons have debated for years about the best methods to accomplish this. Traditionally, mechanical preparation has been accomplished by 3 days of liquid diet, cathartics, and enemas. Almost all gynecologists have modified their mechanical preparation to a single day of an oral gut lavage solution (GoLYTELY or Colyte) (Table 24-7). The solution is isotonic and contains polyethylene glycol in a balanced salt solution. GoLYTELY is ingested at a rate of 1.5 L per hour until diarrheal effluent is clear, usually within 3 to 6 hours. Patients' compliance with GoLYTELY is facilitated if it is chilled. The average woman must ingest 4 L of lavage solution within 4 hours to produce optimal results. Many patients do not accomplish this task in an outpatient setting. Oliveria et al. recently reported a large randomized trial comparing sodium phosphate and polyethylene glycol-based oral lavage solutions. The efficacy of the two preparations was similar. However, there was superior subjective patient tolerance to the 90 ml dose of sodium phosphate. Care must be taken in selecting women who receive oral sodium phosphate because it produces hypokalemia and is contraindicated in women with ascites and renal or heart failure. In summary, the advantages of oral gut lavage are that it is rapid and safe, with negligible water and sodium absorption or intestinal secretion.

There is a great debate as to the most advantageous method of giving prophylactic antibiotics to prepare the large bowel. The majority of colon and rectal surgeons use a combination of both oral and systemic antibiotics. The alternative choices concerning antibiotic coverage have focused on whether to reduce the high bacterial count inside the bowel lumen (neomycin 1 g and erythromycin base 1 g, each given three times the day before the operation) or to use parenteral prophylactic antibiotics so as to obtain high tissue levels before possible contamination by colon bacteria. Because of concern regarding anaerobic infection, some gynecologists substitute metronidazole (500 mg) for each erythromycin dose. We believe both oral and systemic antibiotic prophylaxis are important and both should be utilized (Table 24-8).

TABLE 24-7
GOLYTELY Formulation

Components	Concentration
Polyethylene glycol 4000 (PEG)	59.1 g/L
Sodium sulfate (Na$_2$SO$_4$)	40 mmol/L
Potassium chloride (KCl)	10 mmol/L
Sodium chloride (NaCl)	25 mmol/L
Sodium bicarbonate (NaHCO$_3$)	20 mmol/L
Distilled water*	
Parabens†	
Final osmolarity	280–300 mosm/L

From Beck DE, Harford FJ, and DiPalma JA: Dis Colon Rectum 28:492, 1985.

*Distilled to a final volume of 1000 ml.

†Methylparabens 0.2 g; prophylparabens 0.1 g.

TABLE 24-8
Mechanical and Antibiotic Preparation of Intestine

Day Before the Operation	Day of the Operation
GOLYTELY orally 1.5 L/hour until effluent is clear	Cefoxitin 2 g IV or IM 30 minutes before the operation
Neomycin 1 g and erythromycin base 1 g orally at 2, 4, and 10 PM	

URINARY TRACT

The lower urinary tract is in close anatomic proximity to the pelvic organs. Both benign and malignant gynecologic diseases frequently produce anatomic distortion of the urethra, urinary bladder, or ureters. Similarly gynecologic neoplasias may produce partial or complete obstruction of one or both ureters resulting in hydroureter, or hydronephrosis. Preoperative evaluation may include blood chemistry studies such as a BUN or creatinine, imaging studies such as an IVP or enhanced CT scan, and function studies such as a glomerular filtration rate. In a recent editorial entitled, "Epitaph for the Urogram," Amis predicts in the near future IVP will be replaced by CT urography as the mainstay in imaging of the urinary tract. Two decades ago many gynecologists ordered a routine preoperative intravenous pyelogram (IVP) before all major gynecologic operations in an attempt to identify anatomic or functional abnormalities of the lower urinary tract. Recently, indications for a preoperative IVP have become more restricted in women without pelvic malignancy, endometriosis, or large pelvic masses that extend laterally, such as leiomyomata in the broad ligaments.

An IVP helps to diagnose congenital abnormalities of the urinary tract. Congenital urinary anomalies are rare but are more common in women with congenital anomalies of the reproductive tract. The presence of a pelvic kidney is important information in the differential diagnosis of a large, fixed adnexal mass. The presence of a double ureter is another anomaly discovered by preoperative radiologic studies. Preoperative knowledge of a double ureter is advantageous in anatomic identification of structures in the retroperitoneal spaces.

A preoperative IVP or enhanced CT scan helps to confirm the patency of the lower urinary tract. It is important to establish whether the enlargement, inflammation, or displacement of the gynecologic organs has produced distortion, obstruction, and possibly associated chronic infection of the urinary tract. For example, when a uterus is enlarged to the pelvic brim with myomas, hydronephrosis is noted in approximately one third of patients. Common indications for the preoperative IVP or enhanced CT scan with benign gynecologic disease include cervical myomas, lateral projection of uterine myomas, adnexal masses that are fixed and adherent, endometriosis, and large pelvic masses that produce urinary symptoms. Using these conservative indications, approximately 25% of preoperative IVPs will demonstrate an abnormal finding. However, a preoperative IVP will not give the gynecologist information that will necessarily reduce the incidence of operative injury to the ureters. During the operation the ureters must be identified along their entire course. The exact incidence of ureteral injury associated with benign surgery is unknown, for many injuries do not produce symptoms. However, Symmonds and others have estimated that ureteral injury occurs in 0.5% to 2.5% of all gynecologic operations.

One serious problem with IVPs is an allergic reaction triggered by immunoglobulin E antibodies to the radiologic contrast medium. An imaging study of the kidneys using conventional ionic contrast media has an adverse reaction rate of approximately 8%, and life-threatening reactions occur following 1 in every 1,000 injection. Lasser et al. have reported that in pretreating patients with oral corticosteroids, giving methylprednisolone, 32 mg, 12 hours and 2 hours before the injection of intravenous contrast material significantly reduces the incidence of allergic reaction. This treatment is an alternative to using monomeric, nonionic, iodinated compounds as the contrast media, with a lower incidence of allergic reactions. These compounds are expensive and have an osmolarity approximately 50% less than standard medications. Studies demonstrate a decrease in severe allergic reactions of fivefold to thirtyfold with nonionic compared with ionic contrast media.

Another serious concern in ordering an IVP is the possibility of clinically significant nephrotoxicity being caused by the contrast material. Nephropathy induced by radiocontrast dye is the third most common cause of hospital-acquired acute renal failure. Women with diabetes, existing renal impairment, moderate to severe congestive heart failure, those with reduced effective arterial volume, and women receiving drugs that impair renal function are at high risk for contrast nephrotoxicity. For example, 15% of women with diabetic nephropathy will develop renal failure requiring dialysis despite adequate hydration and the use of low osmolar agents. The pathogenesis of contrast nephrotoxicity is believed to be both direct tubular insult and ischemic injury. Low osmotic, nonionic contrast media are less nephrotoxic than are high osmotic, ionic media in high-risk patients. A recent study of 83 patients with chronic renal insufficiency demonstrated a combination of prophylactic oral administration of the antioxidant acetylcysteine along with hydration was an effective means of preventing further renal damage produced by a nonionic, low osmolality contrast agent.

Insufficient renal function is a major risk factor in elective operations because of the patient's decreased ability to excrete drugs. Women with insufficient renal function do poorly if they develop perioperative infections. Patients with azotemia have a threefold greater risk of adverse drug reactions than women with normal renal function. However, renal insufficiency is very infrequent in an asymptomatic woman under age 40, especially compared with the incidence of unsuspected respiratory disease. The frequency of abnormal serum BUN or creatinine levels is directly dependent on the patient's age. Baseline and interval tests of renal function in women who are going to be treated with aminoglycosides are necessary and valuable studies.

Women with chronic renal insufficiency, diabetes, jaundice, and congestive heart failure, as well as the elderly, are at high risk to develop acute renal failure during the perioperative period. Prior to surgery, these patients should be evaluated to ensure that they have normal blood volume and osmolar status. These women should be carefully monitored to avoid hypotension and nephrotoxins.

RESPIRATORY SYSTEM

Pulmonary complications are the most frequent postoperative morbidity experienced by women following gynecologic operative procedures. The goals of the preoperative assessment of the respiratory system are to identify women at risk for developing postoperative pulmonary complications and to prescribe appropriate preoperative therapy to reduce these risks. Common pulmonary complications include bronchospasm, atelectasis, pneumonia, and exacerbation of underlying chronic lung disease. A rare, but most serious problem, is respiratory failure with prolonged mechanical ventilation usually seen in women with severely diminished pulmonary reserve. Obviously, predicting and preventing postoperative cardiac problems will dramatically reduce postoperative pulmonary morbidity. Only rarely a patient cannot be anesthetized and well oxygenated intraoperatively. The primary goal should be to avoid postoperative pulmonary complications. Similar to the evaluation of other organ systems, the history and physical examination are the most important parts of the pulmonary evaluation. Pulmonary function tests of lung volumes and flow rates are indicated only to evaluate women with history or physical findings suggestive of restrictive or obstructive pulmonary disease.

Preoperative assessment must determine if the patient has the pulmonary reserve to overcome the normal postoperative decrease in pulmonary function. Women who have compromised preoperative pulmonary function are especially susceptible to develop clinically significant postoperative atelectasis, which occurs following approximately 10% of gynecologic operations. Predisposing factors that increase the incidence of atelectasis include morbid obesity, smoking, pulmonary disease, and advanced age. Increased pain, the supine position, abdominal distention, impaired function of the diaphragm, and sedation also contribute to decreased lung volumes and reduced dynamic measurements of pulmonary function for the postoperative patient. The sequence of events that predispose a woman to postoperative pulmonary complications are depicted in Figure 24-3.

Important questions in the history relate to smoking, recent upper respiratory infection, cough, amount of sputum production, degree of dyspnea, wheezing, and most important, exercise tolerance. In women with known respiratory disease, a complete medication history should be obtained, including antibiotics, bronchodilators, mucolytic agents, and corticosteroids. Some women exhibit suppression of their hypothalamic pituitary axis function if they have received low daily doses of either oral or inhaled corticosteroids. Thus, if low daily doses of either oral or inhalation corticosteroids have been taken during the past 6 to 9 months, the patient should receive parenteral hydro-

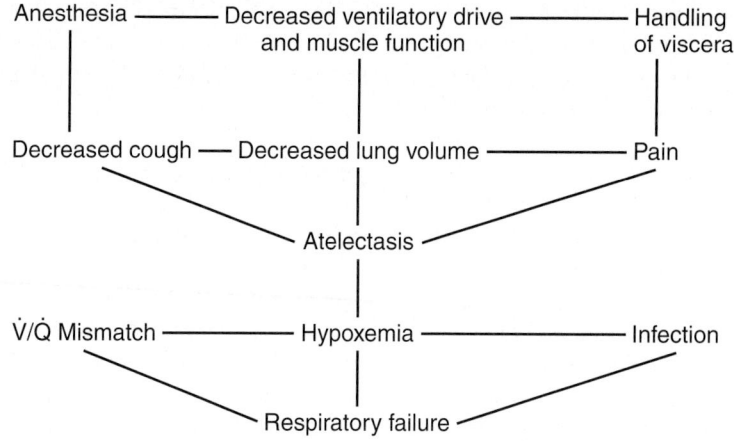

FIGURE 24-3 The administration of anesthesia and handling of viscera precipitate a series of changes that may lead to postoperative pulmonary complications. (From Celli BR: Med Clin North Am 2:309, 1993.)

cortisone to cover potential adrenal insufficiency during the perioperative period. The history should also include questions about exposure to industrial air pollution.

If the woman is currently a smoker, the risk of postoperative pulmonary complications increases approximately fourfold. The basic defense mechanisms of the lungs, such as the ciliary action of the epithelial cells that line the respiratory tract, are significantly impaired by smoking. Even young women with "normal lungs" who smoke half a pack of cigarettes a day are at an increased risk. Ideally, women should stop smoking 8 weeks preoperatively. However, abstinence from cigarettes for 2 to 4 weeks preoperatively is a more practical goal. Providing transdermal nicotine replacement is helpful in alleviating the symptoms of acute nicotine withdrawal. Smoking is most detrimental in women with chronic bronchitis or chronic obstructive pulmonary disease.

Traditionally, anesthesiologists have insisted on at least a 10-day interval between an upper respiratory infection and the date of an elective operation. If the patient has productive sputum, the amount of sputum is estimated, purulent sputum cultured, and appropriate antibiotics given. However, a dramatic change in this practice has affected women without underlying pulmonary disease. Fennelly and Hall state that there is little evidence that anesthesia in adult patients with an upper respiratory tract infection results in respiratory complications.

During the physical examination, special attention should be given to findings of tachypnea, wheezing, rhonchi, rales, decreased breath sounds, and prolonged expiration. Direct observation of exercise tolerance, such as climbing a flight of stairs, is helpful in evaluating the extent of pulmonary reserve. This is a crude index of pulmonary function. Patients with any positive findings on history or physical examination should have a chest x-ray examination and in selected cases arterial blood gases and pulmonary function tests. Preoperative pulmonary function tests should be performed on patients with productive sputum (more than 2 ounces per day), age greater than 65 years, 20 pack-years or

greater smoking history, morbid obesity, asthma, and chronic obstructive pulmonary disease. Women with chronic lung disease often have shunting of blood in the lungs and arterial hypoxemia. Thus preoperative arterial blood gases should be measured. When arterial blood gases are evaluated, the oxygen tension should exceed 65 mm Hg, and the carbon dioxide tension should be less than 45 mm Hg. An elevated arterial CO_2 is an important warning sign because the respiratory drive has become refractory to hypercarbia.

Pulmonary function tests help both to assess the pulmonary reserve and to identify the extent to which the dysfunction is reversible. These tests help to identify women at increased risk for pulmonary problems during the postoperative period. Pulmonary function tests that measure lung volumes and flow rates help to distinguish restrictive defects or a decrease in the amount of lung tis- sue from obstructive defects in which there is a reduction and prolongation of airflow during expiration. The two most common pulmonary function tests used for screening are forced vital capacity and forced expiratory volume in 1 second. A woman with a forced vital capacity volume of less than 50% of the predicted normal for her age and body size should have more extensive testing for significant lung disease. Similarly, the forced expiratory volume in 1 second should be greater than 75% of the predicted normal volume.

Twenty-five million Americans have asthma. Thus this condition is frequently encountered during the preoperative evaluation. Asthma increases the incidence of perioperative respiratory problems approximately fourfold. Asthmatic women are susceptible to perioperative respiratory complications secondary to bronchial hyperresponsiveness, airflow obstruction, and hypersecretion of mucus. Ideally, an asthmatic patient should have elective surgery when she is free of wheezing and has optimal pulmonary status, as measured by pulmonary function tests (peak flow >80% of the predicted or her personal best value).

Preoperative preparation of patients with asthma or other chronic obstructive pulmonary disease includes cessation of smoking; instruction in incentive spirometry, the combination of inhaled ipratropium and an inhaled beta-adrenergic-receptor-agonist, chest physiotherapy, and postural drainage; adequate hydration; sometimes high-dose oral corticosteroids; and antibiotics for purulent sputum for several days before the anticipated surgery. Most authorities advise combining multiple therapeutic regimens to try to reduce the risk of postoperative pulmonary complications. Data does not exist on the advantage of one therapy versus another. Ideally, these women should discontinue smoking at least 8 weeks before surgery. Realistically, only one of four patients will adhere to this recommendation. Improvements in pulmonary function by intensive treatment several days before an operation should be documented by serial pulmonary function tests.

In summary, the major factors in postoperative respiratory morbidity are underlying pulmonary disease and the associated decrease in functional respiratory capacity normally produced by the events surrounding an operation. Prophylactic lung expansion programs are the foundation of effective plans to decrease the risk of postoperative atelectasis in high-risk individuals. Meta-analysis of studies of either incentive spirometer or deep breathing exercises find a decrease in relative risk of pulmonary complications by approximately 50%. Effective pain control by epidural analgesia also reduces the risk of pulmonary complications (Table 24-9).

TABLE 24-9
Risk Reduction Stategies

Preoperative

Encourage cessation of cigarette smoking for at least 8 wk
Treat airflow obstruction in patients with chronic obstructive pulmonary disease or asthma
Administer antibiotics and delay surgery if respiratory infection is present
Begin patient education regarding lung-expansion maneuvers

Intraoperative

Limit duration of surgery to less than 3 hr
Use spinal or epidural anesthesia*
Avoid use of pancuronium
Use laparoscopic procedures when possible
Substitute less ambitious procedure for upper abdominal or thoracic surgery when possible

Postoperative

Use deep-breathing exercises or incentive spirometry
Use continuous positive airway pressure
Use epidural analgesia*
Use intercostal nerve blocks*

From Smetana GW: Preoperative pulmonary evaluation, N Engl J Med 340(12), 1999.

*This strategy is recommended, although variable efficacy has been reported in the literature.

DIABETES MELLITUS

Diabetes mellitus is encountered more frequently in women undergoing gynecologic surgery than any other disease of the endocrine system. The prevalence of diabetes in adult women is approximately 5% in women under the age of 65 and incidence increases rapidly in the older population. Elective operations should be scheduled for the diabetic patient only if she is in nutritional balance and under good diabetic control. Associated electrolyte problems must be recognized and corrected before the operation. The stress of an operation and of anesthesia often produces changes in glucose tolerance and insulin resistance. There is a threefold increase in morbidity and a doubling of mortality if an operation is performed in diabetic patients in poor control.

During the perioperative period the additional release of catecholamines, cortisol, growth hormone, and glucagon may produce hyperglycemia. The combined effects of these three hormones tend to elevate the blood sugar levels by 20 to 40 mg/dL. The principal postoperative complications in diabetic patients are increased operative site infections and wound disruptions. The increase in infection rate is believed to be secondary to a decrease in both cellular and humoral responses to bacteria. Women with diabetes have approximately a fivefold increase in incidence of wound infection compared to age-matched controls. The increased incidence of wound disruptions is due to a decreased tensile strength during healing.

Preoperative evaluation requires meticulous attention to the details of the patient's disease during the history and physical examination. Important questions center on the severity of the diabetes, types of medications, and recent diabetic control, including blood glucose levels. Specific inquiries should be made about the complications of chronic diabetes, especially those affecting the cardiovascular and renal systems. During the physical examination, attention should be directed toward the diagnosis of peripheral neuropathy. Diabetic neuropathy may be the explanation of persistent pain during the perioperative period. Autonomic neuropathy may cause postoperative gastrointestinal or genitourinary dysfunction. Autonomic dysfunction also predisposes the diabetic patient to postural hypotension, cardiac arrhythmias, and cardiac arrest. Preoperative blood studies should include some measurement of recent diabetic control, such as a glycated hemoglobin A1C, and also electrolyte and renal profiles. An electrocardiogram (ECG) and chest x-ray film should be obtained regardless of the woman's age. Special emphasis should be directed to screening for asymptomatic infection, especially in the urinary tract. The major perioperative morbidity in diabetic patients usually results from chronic vascular and end-organ damage, not acute changes in glucose control. Thus the cardiovascular, renal, and central nervous systems should be the focus of concern. In a recent shift in clinical opinion, rigid perioperative control of blood glucose levels is not as beneficial as previously believed.

The risks of hypoglycemia must be balanced against the benefit of rigid control to prevent hyperglycemia. In general, the perioperative glucose level should be maintained between 120 and 200 mg/dL. It is preferable to be in the higher side of this range to avoid hypoglycemia.

The medical sequelae of diabetes mellitus, such as renal and cardiac insufficiency, peripheral neuropathy, and peripheral vascular disease, are related to both the severity and the chronicity of the disease. The patient's history will help to differentiate mild insulin-dependent diabetes from severe insulin-dependent diabetes. When diabetes is treated with oral agents, consideration should be directed to preoperative dosage. Long-acting sulfonylureas have long half-lives and should be discontinued 3 days before surgery. Short-acting sulfonylureas should be discontinued 24 hours before operation. During major elective surgery, mildly diabetic patients are usually treated with small doses of regular insulin.

There are three current rationales of perioperative management of insulin-dependent diabetes. The general goals of all regimens are to avoid ketosis, hypoglycemia, and hyperosmolar conditions. Epidural anesthesia has minimal effects on glucose metabolism, differing from general anesthesia. Therefore, there is a greater risk for hypoglycemia with epidural anesthesia. Women with type I diabetes are much more prone to develop ketoacidosis and hypoglycemia than are women with type II diabetes. The first regimen uses no insulin and no glucose. This method is appropriate only for diabetic women under excellent control whose proposed surgery will have a short operative time, with limited disruption of gastrointestinal function. The second regimen is the administration of one third to one half of a woman's usual insulin dosage given subcutaneously the morning of surgery. An intravenous infusion of 5% dextrose at 125 ml per hour is begun 1 hour before surgery. The availability of rapid bedside measurements of blood sugar allows the adjustment of blood sugar levels by supplemental intravenous regular insulin. Importantly, regular insulin should not be given routinely by intravenous bolus injection. The half-life is only 10 minutes by this method. The third regimen is one of rigid glucose control. The goal of the rigid protocol is to maintain the blood glucose level between 120 to 200 mg/dL throughout the perioperative period. Patients are placed on a continuous intravenous infusion of regular insulin in D5 ½ NS. Lactate is a gluconeogenic precursor. Thus one should be cautious in giving large volumes of lactated Ringer's solution as it may produce hyperglycemia. Levels of blood glucose are obtained at frequent intervals and insulin adjusted until a steady state is obtained. Thereafter the blood glucose level is measured at least every 4 hours. Recently, the use of insulin lispro (Humalog) has facilitated the perioperative management of diabetes. The advantages of this medication are its extremely short onset, peak levels and duration of action, and more predictable subcutaneous absorption. Thus an understanding of the pharmacokinetics of the new analog of human insulin, insulin lispro, as it compares to older preparations, is important (Table 24-10). One last caveat: for obvious reasons elective operations on women with diabetes mellitus should be scheduled early in the morning.

CARDIOVASCULAR DISEASE

The vast majority of women with heart disease who have compensated cardiac function tolerate surgery well. The presence of congestive failure is the single most predictive

---

TABLE 24-10
Pharmacokinetics of Human Insulin

Type	Onset of Action (hrs)	Peak Effect (hrs)	Duration of Action (hrs)
Rapid-Acting			
Insulin Lispro	0.2–0.5	0.5–2	3–4
Insulin injection (regular)	0.5–1	2–3	4–6
Intermediate-Acting			
Isophane insulin suspension (NPH)	1–2	6–8	12–24
Isophane insulin suspension and regular insulin injection (70/30)	0.5–1	2–3 and 6–8	4–6 and 12–24
Isophane insulin suspension and regular insuline injection (50/50)	0.5–1	2–3 and 6–8	4–6 and 12–24
Insulin zinc suspension (Lente)	1–2.5	6–12	18–24
Long-Acting			
Extended insulin zinc suspension (Ultralente)	4–8	10–30	36

From Klocke S: Clin Pharm Rev, [newsletter], Spring 1997.

factor of cardiovascular complications during the perioperative period. If a patient with cardiac disease is not in failure and does not have severe coronary artery disease, she will do as well as a woman without heart disease.

Elective surgery should be scheduled only when a patient is not in cardiac failure and her blood pressure is under proper control. The cardiovascular risks associated with surgery are increased two- to fivefold during an emergency operation. Physiologically, surgery and anesthesia decrease cardiac output by reducing cardiac function and decreasing effective intravascular volume. The stress of surgery results in increased production of catecholamines, cortisol, and antidiuretic hormone. Anesthetic agents depress myocardial function and have varying effects on the autonomic nervous system and peripheral vascular tone. Surgery and anesthesia are an additional burden to a cardiovascular system without adequate reserve. Postoperative cardiac problems are the primary cause of death in approximately 50% of the women who die within 6 weeks following a hysterectomy.

The severity of cardiac disease may be assessed by questions regarding exercise tolerance, dyspnea, chest pain, and orthopnea. Simple questions such as the ability to walk up more than one flight of stairs help to determine the woman's cardiovascular capacity. On physical examination an abnormal heart rate or rhythm, cardiac size, murmurs, and signs of cardiac failure should be noted. A large, appropriately sized blood pressure cuff should be utilized for obese women. Routine ECGs obtained on postmenopausal women may diagnose asymptomatic myocardial infarctions or serious arrhythmias, which will necessitate postponing elective surgery. Conversely, 2 weeks following a documented myocardial infarction, a normal EKG is found in approximately 1 out of 4 women. Preoperative correction of an electrolyte abnormality such as hypokalemia decreases the incidence of cardiac arrhythmias.

The potential dangers of an operation in a woman with multiple premature ventricular contractions (PVCs) are most significant if the PVCs are associated with a decrease in left ventricular function. When women with severe heart disease have major surgery, optimum control of fluid balance and filling pressures are determined by monitoring hemodynamic changes with arterial lines and Swan-Ganz catheters. For example, a preoperative history of pulmonary edema is associated with an approximately 40% chance of developing postoperative congestive heart failure.

Goldman et al. published a classic study predicting perioperative cardiac risk. Their study involved 1001 patients over age 40. By multivariate analysis, they identified factors related to life-threatening cardiac complications. Recently, a committee of the American College of Physicians published an updated cardiac risk index (Table 24-11). Patients can be rated via a numeric score (Table 24-12) as to the risk of cardiac death or significant cardiac morbidity. Statistics in this table should be interpreted in light of the

---

TABLE 24-11
American College of Physicians
Modified Cardiac Risk Index*

Variable	Points, *n*
Coronary artery disease	
Myocardial infarction <6 months earlier	10
Myocardial infarction >6 months earlier	5
Canadian Cardiovascular Society angina classification†	
Class III	10
Class IV	20
Alveolar pulmonary edema	
Within 1 week	10
Ever	5
Suspected critical aortic stenosis	20
Arrhythmias	
Rhythm other than sinus or sinus plus atrial premature beats on electrocardiogram	5
>5 premature ventricular contractions on electrocardiogram	5
Poor general medical status, defined as any of the following: PO_2 < 60 mm Hg, PCO_2 > 50 mm Hg, K^+ level < 3 mmol/L, blood urea nitrogen level > 50 mmol/L, creatinine level > 260 µmol/L, bedridden	5
Age >70 years	5
Emergency surgery	10

From American College of Physicians: Guidelines for assessing and managing the perioperative risk from coronary artery disease associated with major noncardiac surgery, Ann Intern Med 127(4), 1997.

*Class I = 0 to 15 points; class II = 20–30 points; class III = more than 30 points.

†Canadian Cardiovascular Society classification of angina (2): 0 = asymptomatic; I = angina with strenuous exercise; II = angina with moderate exertion; III = angina with walking 1–2 level blocks or climbing 1 flight of stairs or less at a normal pace; IV = inability to perform any physical activity without development of angina.

---

improvements in intensive care that have occurred over the past 25 years.

HYPERTENSIVE DISEASE. Women with controlled essential hypertension in the absence of cardiac or renal complications are not at an increased risk for major problems with elective surgery. However, women with poorly controlled hypertension and a diastolic pressure greater than 110 mm Hg should have more intense medical management of their hypertension before elective surgery. No increased risk of cardiovascular complications from surgery occurs in women with uncomplicated mild to moderate hypertension when the diastolic blood pressure is less than 110 mm Hg. If mild or moderate hypertension is complicated by angina, congestive heart failure, abnormal ECG, left ventricular hypertrophy, or renal insufficiency, the surgery should be postponed until the woman is completely evaluated by a cardiologist. During the induction of anesthesia, there is a potential abrupt

TABLE 24-12
Cardiac Risk Classes for Patients Going to Surgery

Risk Class	Point Score	No or Minor Complications (%)	Life-Threatening Complications* (%)	Cardiac Death (%)
I	0–5	99	0.7	0.2
II	6–12	93	5	2
III	13–25	86	11	2
IV	>26	22	22	56

Modified from Goldman L, Caldera DL, Southwick FS, et al: Medicine 57:357, 1978. From Salem DN, Homans D, McNally JW, et al: Cardiology. In Molitch ME, editor: Management of medical problems in surgical patients, Philadelphia, 1982, FA Davis Co, p 76.

*Myocardial infarction, ventricular tachycardia, pulmonary edema.

rise of blood pressure of 20 to 50 mm Hg. This transient hypertension is experienced during intubation in 6% of normotensive patients and 17% of women with hypertension. Rapid hemodynamic fluctuations are directly related to morbidity in hypertensive women. Major differences between preoperative and intraoperative blood pressures correlate directly with episodes of myocardial ischemia. Perioperative hypotension or hypertension will occur in 20% to 30% of hypertensive women in whom the blood pressure is controlled prior to surgery.

Antihypertensive medication should be continued throughout the perioperative period. The only exception is monoamine oxidase inhibitors, primarily used to treat depression, which should be discontinued for at least 2 weeks before surgery. Discontinuing some antihypertensive agents is potentially harmful. For example, if beta-blockers are withdrawn, patients may develop a hypersensitivity to adrenergic stimulation and an exacerbation of ischemic heart disease. Myocardial infarct, ventricular tachycardia, and abrupt cardiac arrest have all been documented in women in whom beta-blockers have been abruptly discontinued prior to surgery. Similarly, patients taking clonidine develop abrupt hypertensive rebound if the drug is withdrawn. Diuretic therapy need not be discontinued before surgery. Potential hazards of diuretics include a relative hypovolemia and hypokalemia. Although diuretics often produce hypokalemia, and associated arrhythmias are a concern in women with organic heart disease, they are rarely seen in women without significant heart disease.

CORONARY ARTERY DISEASE. Medically significant coronary artery disease is a problem of older women. It is unusual for a premenopausal woman to have ischemic heart disease unless she has diabetes, hyperlipidemia, severe hypertension, or a strong family history of coronary disease. Nevertheless, women over age 50 often have elective gynecologic surgery. Thus considerations of angina and previous myocardial infarctions are essential in planning elective surgery. Taking a detailed cardiovascular history is the most sensitive way to screen for coronary artery disease. Referral to a cardiologist facilitates proper stratification of the cardiac risks for surgery and optimal treatment plans. Women can be stratified on clinical grounds into low-, medium-, and high-risk categories. A recent randomized controlled trial has demonstrated a benefit in survival associated with perioperative use of beta-blockers in patients at high risk secondary to coronary artery disease. Perioperative administration of bisoprolol 1 to 2 weeks prior to surgery reduced the perioperative incidence of both death from cardiac causes and nonfatal myocardial infarct in high-risk patients undergoing vascular surgery.

Unstable angina of less than 3 months duration is a strong contraindication to an elective operation. Conversely, women with stable angina without a previous history of myocardial infarction do not have an increased risk of infarction during operations. Regardless of the duration of angina, the patient should be evaluated by a cardiologist prior to elective surgery. When a woman has had a myocardial infarction, it is important to delay an elective operation for approximately 6 months. The excessive mortality associated with a noncardiac operative procedure within 3 months of an acute myocardial infarct is 27% to 37%. Following a 6-month interval the chance of a reinfarction is 4% to 6% with elective operations. Randomized controlled studies of preoperative percutaneous transluminal coronary stent placement or coronary angioplasty have not been published. To date, revascularization operations on the heart have not been demonstrated to reduce short-term mortality in patients subsequently undergoing noncardiac surgery within 6 months of an acute myocardial infarction. No advantage exists in delaying surgery longer than 6 months, because the woman's risk remains constant for the rest of her life.

The induction of anesthesia is an especially vulnerable time for myocardial ischemia. Myocardial ischemia occurs when the heart has to increase its rate and respond to an increase in systemic blood pressure. Approximately 60% of postoperative myocardial infarctions are not accompa-

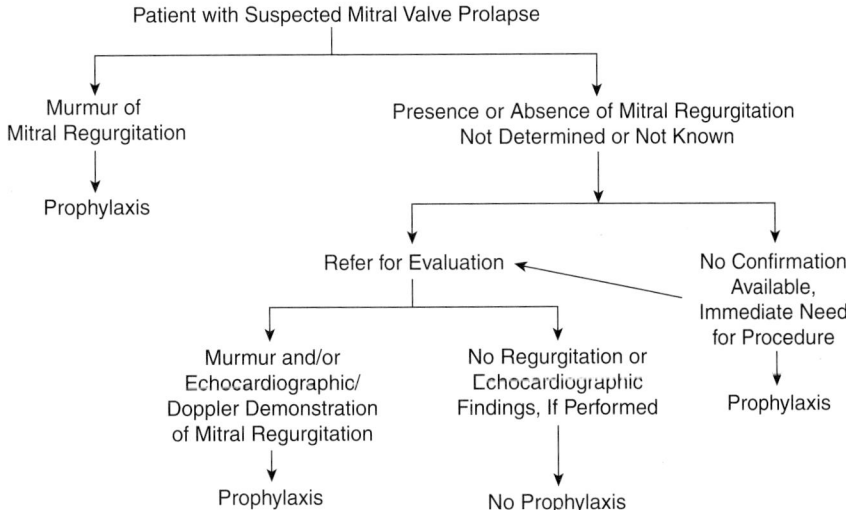

Patient with Suspected Mitral Valve Prolapse

Murmur of Mitral Regurgitation → Prophylaxis

Presence or Absence of Mitral Regurgitation Not Determined or Not Known

Refer for Evaluation

No Confirmation Available, Immediate Need for Procedure → Prophylaxis

Murmur and/or Echocardiographic/ Doppler Demonstration of Mitral Regurgitation → Prophylaxis

No Regurgitation or Echocardiographic Findings, If Performed → No Prophylaxis

FIGURE 24-4 Clinical approach to determination of the need for prophylaxis in patients with suspected mitral valve prolapse. (From Dajani AS, Taubert KA, Wilson W, et al: JAMA 277:1796, 1997.)

nied by chest pain. The woman develops congestive heart failure, arrhythmia, and, in the elderly woman, confusion. The majority of postoperative myocardial infarcts occur during the first 48 hours following surgery. However, it is not unusual for the heart attack to present on the third or fourth postoperative day. Thus women with coronary artery disease should be closely monitored both hemodynamically and electrocardiographically for at least 3 to 4 days postoperatively.

VALVULAR HEART DISEASE. Women with valvular heart disease who are at significant risk during surgery are those with aortic and mitral stenosis. Physiologically, these lesions are similar in that the fixed cardiac output may lead to decompensation secondary to the need for changes in cardiac output during surgical procedures.

The major perioperative consideration in women with valvular heart disease is the use of prophylactic antibiotics to reduce the incidence of subacute bacterial endocarditis developing from a bacteremia associated with the surgical procedure. Even without antibiotic coverage, this is a rare complication. However, because of the substantial morbidity and mortality associated with bacterial endocarditis, antibiotic prophylaxis is the standard of care.

The American Heart Association has updated its recommendations for the prevention of bacterial endocarditis in a paper published in the AMA journal in 1997. Mitral valve prolapse is presently the leading indication for endocarditis prophylaxis. Mitral valve prolapse is a common finding, being diagnosed in 6% to 8% of women having gynecologic surgery. A recent report by Fried documents the prevalence of mitral valve prolapse is considerably lower than previously reported. The prevalence of mitral valve prolapse is highest in young, thin females. The incidence of bacterial endocarditis is threefold to eightfold higher in women with mitral valve prolapse than in the general population. An ad

hoc group of the American Heart Association has developed an algorithm to define when prophylaxis is recommended for patients with mitral valve prolapse (Figure 24-4). Women who are in the high-risk category include those with prosthetic cardiac valves, previous endocarditis, complex cyanotic congenital heart disease, and surgically constructed systemic pulmonary shunts or conduits. Women who are in the moderate-risk category include most other congenital cardiac malformations, acquired valvular dysfunction such as associated with rheumatic heart disease, hypertrophic cardiomyopathy, and mitral valve prolapse with valvular regurgitation and/or thickened leaflets. Women in both the high-risk and moderate-risk categories definitely should receive antibiotics prophylactically to prevent endocarditis. Women in the negligible-risk category for which endocarditis prophylaxis is not recommended include those with an isolated secundum atrial septal defect, previous coronary artery bypass graft surgery, cardiac pacemakers, and previous surgical repair of atrial septal, ventricular septal, or patent ductus arteriosis. An appropriate antibiotic coverage for gynecologic surgery is ampicillin (2 g intramuscularly or intravenously) and gentamicin (1.5 mg/kg of body weight intramuscularly not to exceed 120 mg IM/IV) within 30 minutes of starting the procedure. Depending on the time of expected bacteremia, often the same dosage of both drugs is repeated 6 hours later or amoxicillin 1.0 g orally 6 hours following the parenteral antibiotics. If the woman is allergic to ampicillin, vancomycin (1 g given slowly intravenously) may be substituted.

Special consideration should be given to women with valvular heart disease who are receiving chronic oral anticoagulation. It is preferable to discontinue the oral medication 48 to 72 hours before surgery. There has been a recent change in clinical opinion concerning the need for intravenous heparin in these patients. Kearn and Hirsh postulate that the absolute risk of thromboembolism associated with a few days of perioperative subtherapeutic anticoagulation is generally very low. In contrast, the risk of bleeding associated with perioperative intravenous heparin is often relatively high. Therefore, they believe that the risk/benefit ratio does not favor the use of perioperative heparin. Oral anticoagulants are usually resumed approximately 72 hours postoperatively.

THE MORNING OF THE OPERATION

Preoperative Note

A brief preoperative note helps to serve as a final summary of preoperative preparation. This abbreviated checklist should summarize important findings in the preoperative history, physical examination, and laboratory screening tests. This note is designed to assure that no step has been forgotten and to summarize in a few words pertinent details for other individuals who subsequently attend the patient. The surgeon should make a brief notation that all the patient's questions have been answered and that both patient and physician are in agreement over the proposed operative procedure.

Shaving

Most centers have abandoned the ancient ritual of shaving the abdomen and vulvar areas the day before surgery. Shaving is not necessary unless dense hair presents a mechanical problem in preoperative washing of the skin. Multiple studies have documented a twofold to threefold increase in infection rate directly related to perioperative shaving. Cruse and Foord studied approximately 63,000 operations over a 10-year period and found a 0.9% incidence of infection when patients were not shaved as opposed to 2.5% when they were shaved. Razors produce macroscopic and microscopic nicks and cuts that allow a protective environment for colonization by skin bacteria.

Depilatory agents often produce intense burning if used on the perineum. In general, gynecologists should abandon the humiliating and crude procedure of preoperative shaving. If the hair is mechanically in the way, it should be clipped just before the operation.

Reassurance

Many women are extremely anxious the morning of their operation, and admission to the hospital the morning of surgery usually intensifies their anxiety. In many hospitals this process offers little emotional support to the individual woman but rather gives her the opinion that she is being "herded" in an impersonal fashion. The physical presence of "her" gynecologist when she enters the operating room provides great reassurance. The kindness of touching the woman's hand or standing by her side as the induction of anesthesia begins is greatly appreciated.

Pelvic Examination

After the patient is asleep or the conduction anesthesia has taken effect, the gynecologic surgeon has two important responsibilities: performing the preoperative pelvic examination and supervising the positioning of the patient. A pelvic examination following catheterization and just before surgical incision should be standard practice, regardless of the type or extent of the proposed gynecologic operation. The relaxation of the abdominal wall produced by anesthesia and the advantage of an empty bladder and lower intestinal tract affords the surgeon the optimum environment for performing a pelvic examination. The findings may change the choice of incision or operative approach. Before draping the patient, the gynecologist should make sure that the patient is properly positioned on the operating room table. This is especially true to obtain good exposure in the lithotomy position. Pressure points should be avoided to protect against neuromuscular and skin injury, especially over bony prominences.

KEY POINTS

- For the patient, there are no small, insignificant, or minor operations. Almost any operation is a major event in her life.

- The goals of preoperative planning are to obtain appropriate information, reduce the patient's anxieties and fears, and obtain informed consent.

- The first aphorism of preoperative preparation is to avoid "surprises." This dictum should be applied to protect both the patient and the physician.

- Eye-to-eye contact and gentle touching of the hands are appropriate and effective ways to express the physician's sincere interest in caring for the patient.

- A detailed history and physical examination will detect approximately 90% of the information pertinent to the surgical procedure.

- Surgical morbidity and mortality are directly proportional to the extent of a patient's preexisting medical disease.

- Studies have documented that patients often omit important medical information particularly when under stress. Repetitive history taking does provide additional information and helps to decrease the risk of omission of significant historical information.

- It is important to inquire regarding over-the-counter vitamin, nutritional, and herbal supplements because of the increasing incidence of interactions with drugs.

- Specific questions should be directed toward sensitivity to iodine or latex. Latex allergy is directly responsible for 12% of the perioperative anaphylactic reactions in adult patients and for 70% in children.

- The preoperative physical examination should answer three basic questions: Has the primary gynecologic disease process changed since the initial diagnosis? What is the impact of the primary gynecologic disease on other organ systems? What deficiencies in other organ systems may affect the proposed surgery and hospitalization?

- In emergency situations it is imperative to perform a complete physical examination. This examination should include an evaluation of the blood pressure and pulse in both the recumbent and sitting positions; orthostatic hypotension and tachycardia are crude indexes of a decrease in circulating intravascular volume.

- The choice of which preoperative tests to perform should be based on the age of the patient and the extent of the surgical procedure, as well as on details from the history and physical examination.

- Studies have found that between 30% and 60% of unexpected abnormalities detected by preoperative laboratory tests are not actually noted or investigated prior to surgery.

- Routine preoperative type and screen for uncomplicated abdominal or vaginal hysterectomy is not cost effective.

- A pregnancy test should almost always be obtained if the patient is a teenager.

- Serum electrolyte levels should be evaluated for patients with vomiting, diarrhea, ileus, bowel obstruction, or any condition that affects water or electrolyte balance.

- Routine chest x-ray films are not cost effective unless the patient is over age 75 or has findings in the history or physical examination suggestive of cardiac or respiratory disease.

- A baseline preoperative electrocardiogram is appropriate and cost effective in women over age 60.

- An operation without consent makes the gynecologist vulnerable to charges of assault and battery, except in an emergency.

- Highlights of the discussion regarding informed consent should be documented by a paragraph written by the gynecologist in the progress notes of the chart.

- Oral medications that a woman may be taking for a specific condition or illness may be taken the morning before surgery with 30 to 60 ml of water.

- Antibiotic prophylaxis is effective by reducing the number of bacteria present, not by killing all bacteria. To be effective, the antibiotic must be present at the time of tissue injury or shortly thereafter.

- Prophylactic antibiotics are routinely ordered for vaginal or abdominal hysterectomies and gynecologic operations that carry a substantial risk of postoperative infection. The most popular choice is a first- or second-generation cephalosporin, such as cefazolin or cefoxitin. Preferentially the prophylactic antibiotics should be administered intravenously.

- Using sophisticated I^{125} fibrinogen scanning techniques, approximately 15% of women having surgery for a benign disease and approximately 22% of women having surgery for malignant disease develop thrombophlebitis.

- Approximately 40% of deaths following gynecologic surgery are directly or indirectly related to pulmonary emboli.

- The factors that make a woman at high risk for thromboembolic disease include a previous history of thromboembolic disease, a family or personal history of hypercoagulability (thrombophilic state), malignant disease, previous radiation therapy, congestive heart failure, morbid obesity, venous disease, edema of the legs, active pelvic infection, age, current use of oral contraceptives or hormone replacement therapy up to the time of the operation, and length of preoperative hospitalization.

- Oral contraceptives or hormone replacement therapy should be discontinued 4 weeks before major elective surgery.

- Patients at high risk for thromboembolic disease should be considered as candidates for both mechanical prophylaxis and prophylactic heparin.

- Barium enema or colonoscopy need not be performed routinely on all patients with adnexal masses. These tests are indicated in women over age 40 with left-sided masses, women with positive stool guaiac tests, or women with bowel symptoms.

- If there is a possibility that the pelvic pathology may necessitate entry in the lumen of the large intestine, both mechanical cleansing of the bowel and antibiotics to reduce the bacterial count should be ordered before surgery.

- The average woman must ingest 4 L of lavage solution within 4 hours to produce optimal mechanical preparation of the intestines. Many patients do not accomplish this task in an outpatient setting.

- An imaging study of the kidneys using conventional ionic contrast media has an adverse reaction rate of approximately 8%, and life-threatening reactions occur following 1 in every 1,000 injections.

- Nephropathy induced by radiocontrast dye is the third most common cause of hospital-acquired acute renal failure.

- Pulmonary complications are the most frequent postoperative morbidity experienced by women following gynecologic operative procedures.

- Factors that increase the incidence of atelectasis include morbid obesity, smoking, pulmonary disease, and advanced age.

- Some women exhibit suppression of their hypothalamic pituitary axis function if they have received low daily doses of either oral or inhaled corticosteroids.

- If a woman is currently a smoker, her risk of postoperative pulmonary complications increases approximately fourfold.

- If preoperative arterial blood gases are measured, the oxygen tension should exceed 65 mm Hg, and the carbon dioxide tension should be less than 45 mm Hg.

- Asthma increases the incidence of perioperative respiratory problems approximately fourfold.

- There is a threefold increase in morbidity and a doubling of mortality if surgery is performed on diabetic patients who are in poor glucose control.

- Women with diabetes have approximately a fivefold increase in incidence of wound infection compared to age-matched controls.

- Autonomic neuropathy may cause postoperative gastrointestinal or genitourinary dysfunction. Autonomic dysfunction also predisposes the diabetic patient to postural hypotension, cardiac arrhythmias, and cardiac arrest.

- The perioperative blood glucose levels in diabetic women should be maintained between 120 and 200 mg/dL. It is preferable to be in the higher side of this range to avoid hypoglycemia.

- The use of insulin lispro (Humalog) has facilitated the perioperative management of diabetes. The advantages of this medication are its extremely short onset, peak levels and duration of action, and more predictable subcutaneous absorption.

- Elective operations on diabetic women should be scheduled early in the morning.

- The presence of congestive failure is the single most predictive factor of cardiovascular complications during the perioperative period.

- The cardiovascular risks associated with surgery are increased two- to fivefold during an emergency operation.

- No increased risk of cardiovascular complications from surgery occurs in women with uncomplicated mild to moderate hypertension when the diastolic blood pressure is less than 110 mm Hg.

- The excessive mortality associated with noncardiac surgery within 3 months of an acute myocardial infarction is 27% to 37%.

- The recommended protocol for bacterial endocarditis prophylaxis is ampicillin (2 g intramuscularly or intravenously) and gentamicin (1.5 mg/kg of body weight intramuscularly not to exceed 120 mg IM/IV) within 30 minutes of starting the procedure.

BIBLIOGRAPHY

Aitkenhead AR: Awareness during anaesthesia: what should the patient be told? Anaesthesia 45:351, 1990.

Agnelli G: Anticoagulation in the prevention of pulmonary embolism, Chest 107:S39, 1995.

Almany SL, Mileto L, and Kahn JK: Preoperative cardiac evaluation: assessing risk before noncardiac surgery, Postgrad Med 98:171, 1995.

American College of Obstetricians and Gynecologists: Ethical dimensions of informed consent, ACOG Committee Opinion 108, 1992.

American Society of Anesthesiologists Practice Guidelines: Practice guidelines for preoperative fasting and the use of pharmacologic agents to reduce the risk of pulmonary aspiration: application to health patients undergoing elective procedures, Anesthesiology 90:896, 1999.

Amis ES Jr: Epitaph for the urogram, Radiology 213:639, 1999.

Aspinall ST and Dealler SF: New rapid identification test for *Clostridium difficile*, J Clin Pathol 45:956, 1992.

Barrett BJ: Contrast nephrotoxicity, J Am Soc Nephrol 5:125, 1994.

Bartlett JG: Antibiotic-associated diarrhea, Clin Infect Dis 15:573, 1992.

Beck DE, Harford FJ, and DiPalma JA: Comparison of cleansing methods in preparation for colonic surgery, Dis Colon Rectum 28:491, 1985.

Beck DE and DiPalma JA: A new oral lavage solution vs cathartics and enema method for preoperative colonic cleansing, Arch Surg 126:552, 1991.

Bergqvist D, Burmark US, Flordal PA, et al: Low molecular weight heparin started before surgery as prophylaxis against deep vein thrombosis: 2500 versus 5000 XaI units in 2070 patients, Br J Surg 82:496, 1995.

Bone RC: Ventilation/perfusion scan in pulmonary embolism: "the emperor is incompletely attired," JAMA 263:2794, 1990.

Brasch RC: The case strengthens for allergy to contrast media, Radiology 209:35, 1998.

Burke JF: The effective period of preventive antibiotic action in experimental incisions and dermal lesions, Surgery 50:161, 1961.

Burnand KG, Gaffney PJ, McGuiness CL, et al: The role of monocyte in the generation and dissolution of arterial and venous thrombi, Cardiovas Surg 6:119, 1998.

Burns ER and Lawrence C: Bleeding time: a guide to its diagnostic and clinical utility, Arch Pathol Lab Med 113:1219, 1989.

Caprini JA, Scurr JH, and Hasty JH: Role of compression modalities in a prophylactic program for deep vein thrombosis, Sem Thromb Hemost 14(S1):77, 1988.

Carter CJ: The pathophysiology of venous thrombosis, Prog Cardiovasc Dis 36:439, 1994.

Celli BR: What is the value of preoperative pulmonary function testing? Med Clin North Am 2:309, 1993.

Chalker RB and Celli BR: Special considerations in the elderly patient, Clin Chest Med 14:437, 1993.

Choban PS and Flancbaum L: The impact of obesity on surgical outcomes: a review, J Am Coll Surg 185:593, 1997.

Christian SS and Christian JS: The cephalosporin antibiotics, Prim Care Update Ob/Gyns 4:168, 1997.

Clagett GP: Prevention of postoperative venous thromboembolism: an update, Am J Surg 168:515, 1994.

Clarke-Pearson DL: Preoperative and antenatal evaluation of patients at risk for intraoperative or obstetric hemorrhage, Obstet Gynecol Forum 6:2, 1992.

Clarke-Pearson DL: Prevention of venous thrombosis following gynecologic surgery, J Gynecol Tech 1:11, 1995.

Classen DC, Evans RS, Pestotnik SL, et al: The timing of prophylactic administration of antibiotics and the risk of surgical-wound infection, N Engl J Med 326:281, 1992.

Collins R, Scrimgeour A, Yusuf S, et al: Reduction in fatal pulmonary embolism and venous thrombosis by perioperative administration of subcutaneous heparin, N Engl J Med 318:1162, 1988.

Crapo RO: Pulmonary-function testing, N Engl J Med 331:25, 1994.

Cruse PJ and Foord R: A 10-year prospective study of 62,939 wounds, Surg Clin North Am 60:27, 1980.

Daly E, Vessey MP, Hawkins MM, et al: Risk of venous thromboembolism in users of hormone replacement therapy, Lancet 348:977, 1996.

Davis JM, Demling RH, Lewis FR, et al: The Surgical Infection Society's policy on human immunodeficiency virus and hepatitis B and C infection, Arch Surg 127:218, 1992.

Devereux RB, Frary CJ, Kramer-Fox R, et al: Cost-effectiveness of infective endocarditis prophylaxis for mitral valve prolapse with or without a mitral regurgitant murmur, Am J Cardiol 74:1024, 1994.

Devor M, Barrett-Connor E, Renvall M, et al: Estrogen replacement therapy and the risk of venous thrombosis, Am J Med 92:275, 1992.

Doyle RL: Assessing and modifying the risk of postoperative pulmonary complications, Chest 115:77S, 1999.

Eason EL, Sampalis JS, Hemmings R, and Joseph L: Povidone-iodine gel vaginal antisepsis for abdominal hysterectomy, Am J Obstet Gynecol 176:1011, 1997.

Etchason J, Petz L, Keeler E, et al: The cost effectiveness of preoperative autologous blood donations, N Engl J Med 332:719, 1995.

Fareed J, Hoppensteadt DA, and Walenga JM: Current perspectives on low molecular weight heparins, Semin Thromb Hemost 19(S1):1, 1993.

Fekety R and Shah AB: Diagnosis and treatment of *Clostridium difficile* colitis, JAMA 269:71, 1993.

Fennelly ME and Hall GM: Anaesthesia and upper respiratory tract infections—a non-existent hazard? Br J Anaesth 64:535, 1990.

Ferguson GT and Cherniack RM: Management of chronic obstructive pulmonary disease, N Engl J Med 328:1017, 1993.

Ferguson KJ, Strauss RG, Toy PTCY, et al: Physician recommendation as the key factor in patients' decisions to participate in preoperative autologous blood donation programs, Am J Surg 168:2, 1994.

Ferguson MK: Preoperative assessment of pulmonary risk, Chest 115:58S, 1999.

Fisher QA, Feldman MA, and Wilson MD: Pediatric responsibilities for preoperative evaluation, J Pediatr 125:675, 1994.

Francis JL: Laboratory investigation of hypercoagulability, Semin Thromb Hemost 24:111, 1998.

Freed LA, Levy D, Levine RA, et al: Prevalence and clinical outcome of mitral-valve prolapse, N Engl J Med 341:1, 1999.

Friedel HA and Balfour JA: Tinzaparin: a review of its pharmacology and clinical potential in the prevention and treatment of thromboembolic disease, Drugs 48:638, 1994.

Gal TJ: Pulmonary function testing. In Miller RD, editor: Anesthesia, vol 1, ed 5, Philadelphia, Churchill Livingstone, Inc., 2000.

Gerding DN: Disease associated with *Clostridium difficile* infection, Ann Intern Med 110:255, 1989.

Gilmour IJ: Perioperative respiratory care, Urol Clin North Am 10:65, 1983.

Goldfarb S, Spinler S, Berns JS, and Rudnick MR: Low-osmolality contrast media and the risk of contrast-associated nephrotoxicity, Invest Radiol 28(S5):S7, 1993.

Goldhaber SZ, Morpurgo M, WHO/ISFC Task Force on Pulmonary Embolism: Diagnosis, treatment, and prevention of pulmonary embolism: report of the WHO/International Society and Federation of Cardiology Task Force, JAMA 268:1727, 1992.

Goldman L, Caldera DL, Nussbaum SR, et al: Multifactorial index of cardiac risk in noncardiac surgical procedures, N Engl J Med 297:845, 1977.

Goodnough LT: The implications of cost-effectiveness for autologous blood procurement, Arch Pathol Lab Med 118:333, 1994.

Greif R, Akca O, Horn EP, et al: Supplemental perioperative oxygen to reduce the incidence of surgical-wound infection, N Engl J Med 342:161, 2000.

Haavik PE, Søreide E, Hofstad B, and Steen PA: Does preoperative anxiety influence gastric fluid volume and acidity? Anesth Analg 75:91, 1992.

Hall GM: Insulin administration in diabetic patients—return of the bolus? Br J Anaesth 72:1, 1994.

Handlin DS and Baker T: The effects of smoking on postoperative recovery, Am J Med 93(S1A):32S, 1992.

Hayden SP, Mayer ME, and Stoller JK: Postoperative pulmonary complications: risk assessment, prevention, and treatment, Cleve Clin J Med 62:401, 1995.

Hayhurst MD: Preoperative pulmonary function testing, Respir Med 87:161, 1993.

Helström L, Sörbom D, and Bäckström T: Influence of partner relationship on sexuality after subtotal hysterectomy, Acta Obstet Gynecol Scand 74:142, 1995.

Hirsch IB and Paauw DS: Diabetes management in special situations, Endocrinol Metab Clin North Am 26:631, 1997.

Hirsh RA: An approach to assessing perioperative risk. In Goldman DR, Brown FH, Levy WK, et al, editors: Medical care of the surgical patient, Philadelphia, 1982, JB Lippincott Co.

Holleman DR and Simel DL: Does the clinical examination predict airflow limitation? JAMA 273:313, 1995.

Hollenberg SM: Preoperative cardiac risk assessment, Chest 115:51S, 1999.

Houry S, Georgeac C, Hay JM, et al: A prospective multicenter evaluation of preoperative hemostatic screening tests, Am J Surg 170:19, 1995.

Hovanessian HC: New-generation anticoagulants: the low molecular weight heparins, Ann Emerg Med 34:768, 1999.

Hubbell FA, Greenfield S, Tyler JL, et al: The impact of routine admission chest x-ray films on patient care, N Engl J Med 312:209, 1985.

Jacquet-Davis P: Mitral valve prolapse, Prim Care Update Ob/Gyns 2:1, 1995.

Jick H, Derby LE, Myers MW, et al: Risk of hospital admission for idiopathic venous thromboembolism among users of postmenopausal Oestrogens, Lancet 348981, 1996.

Jones T and Isaacson: Preoperative screening: what tests are necessary? Cleve Clin J Med 62:374, 1995.

Jørgensen LN, Wille-Jørgensen P, and Hauch O: Prophylaxis of postoperative thromboembolism with low molecular weight heparins, Br J Surg 80:689, 1993.

Kallar SK and Everett LL: Potential risks and preventive measures for pulmonary aspiration: new concepts in preoperative fasting guidelines, Anesth Analg 77:171, 1993.

Kaplan EB, Sheiner LB, Boeckmann AJ, et al: The usefulness of preoperative laboratory screening, JAMA 253:3576, 1985.

Kearon C and Hirsh J: Management of anticoagulation before and after elective surgery, N Engl J Med 330:1506, 1997.

Kellerman PS: Perioperative care of the renal patient, Arch Intern Med 154:1674, 1994.

Kelley MA, Carson JL, Palevsky HI, and Schwartz JS: Diagnosing pulmonary embolism: new facts and strategies, Ann Intern Med 114:300, 1991.

Krämer BK, Kammerl M, Schweda F, and Schreiber M: A primer in radiocontrast-induced nephropathy, Nephrol Dial Transplant 14:2830, 1999.

Kreisel D, Savel TG, Silver AL, and Cunningham JD: Surgical antibiotic prophylaxis and *Clostridium difficile* toxin positivity, Arch Surg 130:989, 1995.

Lasser EC, Berry CC, Talner LB, et al: Pretreatment with corticosteroids to alleviate reactions to intravenous contrast material, N Engl J Med 317:845, 1987.

Lavelle-Jones C, Byrne DJ, Rice P, and Cuschieri A: Factors affecting quality of informed consent, BMJ 306:885, 1993.

Lin L, Song J, Kimber N, et al: The role of bacterial vaginosis in infection after major gynecologic surgery, Infec Dis Obstet Gynecol 7:169, 1999.

Ljungqvist O, Thorell A, Gutniak M, et al: Glucose infusion instead of preoperative fasting reduces postoperative insulin resistance, J Am Coll Surg 178:329, 1994.

Macpherson DS: Preoperative laboratory testing: should any tests be "routine" before surgery? Med Clin North Am 77:289, 1993.

Madden S and Porter TF: Deep venous thrombosis: prophylaxis in gynecology, Clin Obstet Gynecol 42:895, 1999.

Mannino DM, Etzel RA, and Flanders WD: Do the medical history and physical examination predict low lung function? Arch Intern Med 153:1892, 1993.

Marks AR, Choong CY, Chir MBB, et al: Identification of high-risk and low-risk subgroups of patients with mitral-valve prolapse, N Engl J Med 320:1031, 1989.

McCray E, Martone WJ, Wise RP, and Culver DH: Risk factors for wound infections after genitourinary reconstructive surgery, Am J Epidemiol 123:1026, 1986.

McIntyre FJ and McCloy R: Shaving patients before operation: a dangerous myth? Ann R Coll Surg Engl 76:3, 1994.

Mittendorf R, Aronson MP, Berry RE, et al: Avoiding serious infections associated with abdominal hysterectomy: a meta-analysis of antibiotic prophylaxis, Am J Obstet Gynecol 169:1119, 1993.

Morcos SK and El Nahas AM: Advances in the understanding of the nephrotoxicity of radiocontrast media, Nephron 78:249, 1998.

Morcos SK, Oldroyd S, and Haylor J: Contrast media-induced nephrotoxicity: a new insight, Clin Radiol 52:573, 1997.

Morris TW: X-ray contrast media: where are we now, and where are we going? Radiology 188:11, 1993.

Moser KM, Fedullo PF, LitteJohn JK, and Crawford R: Frequent asymptomatic pulmonary embolism in patients with deep venous thrombosis, JAMA 271:223, 1994.

Murdoch CJ, Murdoch DR, McIntyre P, et al: The pre-operative ECG in day surgery: a habit? Anaesthesia 54:907, 1999.

Myers ER, Clarke-Pearson DL, Olt GJ, et al: Preoperative coagulation testing on a gynecologic oncology service, Obstet Gynecol 83:438, 1994.

Narr BJ, Warner ME, Schroeder DS, and Warner MA: Outcomes of patients with no laboratory assessment before anesthesia and a surgical procedure, Mayo Clin Proc 72:505, 1997.

National Blood Resource Education Program Expert Panel: The use of autologous blood, JAMA 263:414, 1990.

O'Dwyer G, Mylotte M, Sweeney M, and Egan EL: Experience of autologous blood transfusion in an obstetrics and gynaecology department, Br J Obstet Gynaecol 100:571, 1993.

Oliveira L, Wexner SD, Daniel N, et al: Mechanical bowel preparation for elective colorectal surgery: a prospective, randomized, surgeon-blinded trial comparing sodium phosphate and polyethylene glycol-based oral lavage solutions, Dis Colon Rectum 40:585, 1997.

Palda VA and Detsky AS: Perioperative assessment and management of risk from coronary artery disease, Ann Intern Med 127:313, 1997.

Paluzzi RG: Antimicrobial prophylaxis for surgery, Med Clin North Am 77:427, 1993.

Parfrey PS, Griffiths SM, Barrett BJ, et al: Contrast material–induced renal failure in patients with diabetes mellitus, renal insufficiency, or both: a prospective controlled study, N Engl J Med 320:143, 1989.

Phillips S, Hutchinson S, and Davidson T: Preoperative drinking does not affect gastric contents, Br J Anaesth 70:6, 1993.

Platell C and Hall J: What is the role of mechanical bowel preparation in patients undergoing colorectal surgery? Dis Colon Rectum 41:875, 1998.

Polak JF, Cutter SS, and O'Leary DH: Deep veins of the calf: assessment with Doppler flow imaging, Radiology 171:481, 1989.

Poldermans D, Boersma E, Bax JJ, et al: The effect of bisoprolol on perioperative mortality and myocardial infarction in high-risk patients undergoing vascular surgery, N Engl J Med 341:1789, 1999.

Poller A, McKernan A, Thomson JM, et al: Fixed minidose warfarin: a new approach to prophylaxis against venous thrombosis after major surgery, Br Med J 295:1309, 1987.

Porri F, Lemiere C, Birnbaum J, et al: Prevalence of latex sensitization in subjects attending health screening: implications for a perioperative screening, Clin Experiment Allergy 27:413, 1996.

Porter GA: Effects of contrast agents on renal function, Invest Radiol 28:S1, 1993.

Prather CM and Ortiz-Camacho CP: Evaluation and treatment of constipation and fecal impaction in adults, Mayo Clin Proc 73:881, 1998.

Ransom SB, McNeeley SG, and Malone JM Jr: A cost-effectiveness evaluation of preoperative type-and-screen testing for vaginal hysterectomy, Am J Obstet Gynecol 175:1201, 1996.

Roizen MF: Anesthetic implications of concurrent diseases. In Miller RD, editor: Anesthesia, vol 1, ed 5, Philadelphia, Churchill Livingstone, Inc., 2000.

Roizen MF: Preoperative evaluation of patients with diseases that require special preoperative evaluation and intraoperative management. In Miller RD, editor: Anesthesia, vol 1, ed 2, New York, 1986, Churchill Livingstone, Inc.

Roizen MF: Routine preoperative evaluation. In Miller RD, editor: Anesthesia, vol 1, ed 2, New York, 1986, Churchill Livingstone, Inc.

Roizen MF: More preoperative assessment by physicians and less by laboratory tests, N Engl J Med 342:204, 2000.

Roizen MF, Foss JF, and Fischer SP: Preoperative evaluation. In Miller RD, editor: Anesthesia, vol 1, ed 5, Philadelphia, Churchill Livingstone, Inc., 2000.

Rosenberg RD and Aird WC: Vascular-bed-specific hemostasis and hypercoagulable states, N Engl J Med 340:1555, 1999.

Rust OA and Magann EF: Prophylaxis for subacute bacterial endocarditis in obstetrics and gynecology, Prim Care Update Ob/Gyns 1:183, 1994.

Saint S, Bent S, Vittinghoff E, and Grady D: Antibiotics in chronic obstructive pulmonary disease exacerbations: a meta-analysis, JAMA 273:957, 1995.

Salem M, Tainsh RE Jr, Bromberg J, et al: Perioperative glucocorticoid coverage: a reassessment 42 years after emergence of a problem, Ann Surg 219:416, 1994.

Saltzman AK, Carter JR, Fowler JM, et al: The utility of preoperative screening colonoscopy in gynecologic oncology, Gynecol Oncol 56:181, 1995.

Schackelford DP, Hoffman MK, Kramer PR Jr, et al: Evaluation of preoperative cardiac risk index values in patients undergoing vaginal surgery, Am J Obstet Gynecol 173:80, 1995.

Schein OD, Katz J, Bass EB, et al: The value of routine preoperative medical testing before cataract surgery, N Engl J Med 342:168, 2000.

Silver D: An overview of venous thromboembolism prophylaxis, Am J Surg 161:537, 1991.

Sloand EM, Pitt E, and Klein HB: Safety of the blood supply, JAMA 274:1368, 1995.

Sparrow RA, Hardy JG, and Fentem PH: Effect of "antiembolism" compression hosiery on leg blood volume, Br J Surg 82:53, 1995.

Stagnaro-Green A: Perioperative glucose control: does it really matter? Mt Sinai J Med 58:299, 1991.

Stenchever MA: Too much informed consent? Obstet Gynecol 77:631, 1991.

Strunin L: How long should patients fast before surgery? Time for new guidelines, Br J Anaesth 70:1, 1993.

Sundram CJ: Informed consent for major medical treatment of mentally disabled people, N Engl J Med 318:1368, 1988.

Symmonds RE: Ureteral injuries associated with gynecologic surgery: prevention and management, Clin Obstet Gynecol 19:632, 1976.

Tanos V and Rojansky N: Prophylactic antibiotics in abdominal hysterectomy, J Am Coll Surg 179:593, 1994.

Tepel M, Van Der Giet M, Schwarzfeld C, et al: Prevention of radiographic-contrast-agent-induced reductions in renal function by acetylcysteine, N Engl J Med 343:180, 2000.

Tønnesen H: The alcohol patient and surgery, Alcohol Alcoholism 34:148, 1999.

Toogood JH: Side effects of inhaled corticosteroids, J Allergy Clin Immunol 102:705, 1998.

Waggoner SE, Barter J, Delgado G, and Barnes W: Case-control analysis of *Clostridium difficile*–associated diarrhea on a gynecologic oncology service, Infect Dis Obstet Gynecol 2:154, 1994.

Weitz JI: Low-molecular-weight heparins, N Engl J Med, 337:688, 1997.

Wilcox MH and Spencer RC: *Clostridium difficile* infection: responses, relapses and reinfections, J Hosp Infect 22:85, 1992.

Williams-Russo P, Charlson ME, MacKenzie CR, et al: Predicting postoperative pulmonary complications: is it a real problem? Arch Intern Med 152:1209, 1992.

Wilson AT and Reilly CS: Anaesthesia and the obese patient, Int J Obesity 17:427, 1993.

Younis LT, Miller DD, and Chaitman BR: Preoperative strategies to assess cardiac risk before noncardiac surgery, Clin Cardiol 18:447, 1995.

Zibrak JD and O'Donnell CR: Indications for preoperative pulmonary function testing, Clin Chest Med 14:227, 1993.

Postoperative Counseling and Management

Fever, Respiratory, Cardiovascular, Thromboembolic, Urinary Tract, Gastrointestinal, Wound, Operative Site, Neurologic Injury, Psychologic Sequelae

KEY TERMS AND DEFINITIONS

Adynamic (Paralytic) Ileus. A temporary loss of intestinal peristalsis that may lead to a functional intestinal obstruction.

Antipyretic. A drug or device to lower body temperature.

Atelectasis. Imperfect expansion of the lung.

Biofilm. The adherent layer of bacteria and bacterial by-products that forms around indwelling urinary catheters.

Cuff Cellulitis. One of many terms used for the cellulitis caused by an infection from endogenous bacteria in the serosanguineous fluid that collects in the retroperitoneal space at the vaginal apex.

Duplex Ultrasound. A high-resolution ultrasound technique using real time and Doppler, used as a method to diagnose deep venous thrombosis.

Homans' Sign. Discomfort behind the knee on forced dorsiflexion of the foot; a sign of deep vein thrombophlebitis in the calf.

Impedance Plethysmography. A noninvasive screening method using changes in blood volume, as measured by changes in electrical resistance, for the detection of deep vein thrombosis.

Latzko's Operation. A technique for repair of a fistula at the vaginal apex that includes partial colpocleisis with denudation of the vaginal mucosa surrounding the fistula and subsequent multilayer closure without entering the bladder.

Lymphocyst. A local collection of lymphatic fluid.

Necrotizing Fasciitis. A virulent, rapidly progressing soft tissue infection that is sometimes fatal.

Phlebography (Venography). Radiography of the venous system, a method of detecting deep vein thrombosis.

Shock. A condition in which circulatory insufficiency prevents adequate vascular perfusion of vital organs.

Ventilation/Perfusion Scan (V/Q Scan). A noninvasive imaging technique that is a step in establishing or excluding the diagnosis of pulmonary embolus.

Ventilation Scintigraphy. A technique of injection of small radionuclides of technetium or xenon gas used to detect pulmonary emboli.

Wound Dehiscence. Disruption of any layers of the surgical incision caused by a failure of normal healing. The peritoneum remains intact.

Wound Evisceration. Complete breakdown of the healing process through all levels of the incision, with omentum or bowel presenting through the incision.

Postoperative complications may occur even after minor operations. Often, the woman and her family judge the competence of the gynecologist by the compassion displayed during the immediate postoperative period. The goal of postoperative care is to restore the woman to normal physiologic and psychologic health. Some problems are inherently nonpreventable, and therefore early recognition and treatment are necessary. If minor complications are overlooked, they may evolve into major problems for both the patient and her physician. Many complications increase the duration of the postoperative stay in the hospital. Interestingly, in a study of women readmitted with postoperative complications, approximately 40% had been discharged earlier than the mean length of stay for the corresponding operative procedure.

During the first 24 hours following most major operations, the cardiovascular, renal, and respiratory systems should be monitored closely. If the woman is in good health and has had a gynecologic operation for a benign disease, she may be moved to an inpatient room or discharged after being monitored for 1 to 3 hours in the recovery room. The expert monitoring and skilled assistance of an intensive care unit are preferable for women with coexisting illness or extensive operations for malignancy.

An outline of general guidelines for postoperative orders for a woman following an abdominal hysterectomy is included in the box below. Considerations of cost containment in the postoperative regimen is rapidly influencing clinical care. Flexibility and individual considerations should take precedence over standard orders, but guidelines can help the physician develop his or her own preferences. Individualization is especially important in the postoperative care of geriatric women. Special nursing attention and minimal doses of narcotics help to prevent confusion and disorientation. Ongoing verbal communication with the nursing staff helps eliminate misunderstandings that might result in less than ideal postoperative care.

Two major considerations in the postoperative course are pyrexia and blood loss. The causes of fever encompass the majority of postoperative complications. All gynecologic organs are endowed with a rich blood supply. Thus hemorrhage, hematoma, and seroma formation are frequent postoperative complications.

POSTOPERATIVE FEVER

The exact definition of postoperative febrile morbidity varies greatly among authors. Diurnal fluctuations are characteristic of the daily body temperature patterns of humans. A normal temperature is usually 37.2° C in the morning and 37.7° C overall. Most definitions use a temperature greater than 38° C as the febrile indicator of morbidity. It is not unusual for gynecologic patients to have a mild temperature elevation during the first 72 hours of the postoperative period, especially during the late afternoon or evening. Approximately 75% of patients develop a temperature greater than 37° C, which is usually not associated with an infectious process. Approximately 25% of women after abdominal hysterectomy and 35% following vaginal hysterectomy exhibit febrile morbidity.

The physician's primary goal in examining the postoperatively febrile patient is to determine whether the fever is caused by an infection. Approximately 20% of postoperative fevers are directly related to infection, and 80% are related to noninfectious causes. Some conditions necessitate active intervention, whereas others are self-limiting. Thus it is imperative not to empirically treat a postoperatively febrile patient with broad-spectrum antibiotics; in addition, it is usually unnecessary to give antipyretics to lower the temperature of an adult. As Duff has emphasized, fever is a phylogenic host response to infection in fish, lizards, and in higher mammals, including humans. Fever may be a beneficial response to the host.

Fever is a common postoperative finding, especially a mild temperature elevation during the first 48 to 72 hours following an operation. The pathophysiology of postoperative fever is primarily related to the release of cytokines. The cause of a postoperative fever may be simple and common, such as atelectasis or dehydration, or unusual, such as malignant hyperthermia or septicemia. The temporal relationship of the *onset* of a patient's febrile response to common postoperative complications is depicted in Table 25-1.

Fever is the most common diagnostic problem in the postoperative patient. Common causes of a fever include atelectasis, pneumonia, urinary tract infection, nonseptic phlebitis, wound infection, and operative site infection. Two intraoperative factors that dramatically increase the risk of postoperative fever are an operative time longer than 2 hours and the necessity for intraoperative transfusion.

Sample Postoperative Orders for Abdominal Hysterectomy

1. Admit to recovery area; to postoperative room when awake and vital signs are stable
2. Diagnosis: abdominal hysterectomy for myomas
3. Condition: stable
4. Vital signs: q15min *4, q30min *2, q1h *4, q4h
5. List of allergies
6. I & O (intake and output)
7. Provide incentive spirometer at bedside. Encourage use q2h
8. Ambulate as soon as tolerated
9. IV solutions: 5% dextrose and lactated Ringer's solution 125 ml/h
10. Full liquid diet
11. Medications: PCA (patient-controlled analgesic) pump for narcotics (see Table 25-21 for specific dosage)
12. Foley catheter to gravity drainage
13. Pneumatic compression device and stockings to legs
14. Hematocrit on postoperative days 1 and 3

TABLE 25-1
Time of Usual Onset of Fever for Various Postoperative Complications

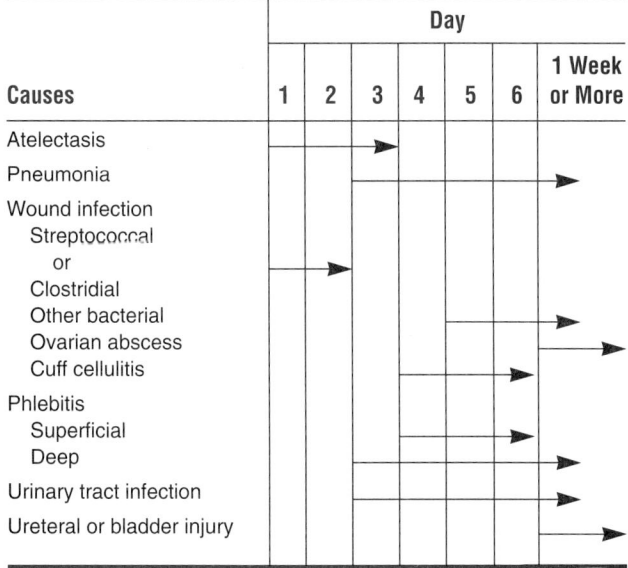

Causes	Day						1 Week or More
	1	2	3	4	5	6	
Atelectasis			→				
Pneumonia							→
Wound infection							
Streptococcal or Clostridial		→					
Other bacterial					→		→
Ovarian abscess						→	→
Cuff cellulitis						→	→
Phlebitis							
Superficial							→
Deep							→
Urinary tract infection							→
Ureteral or bladder injury							→

Workup for Fever

The initial workup for a postoperatively febrile woman should emphasize the most common problems. Medical students memorize the five Ws in the differential diagnosis: wind (atelectasis), water (urinary tract infection), wound (infection or hematoma), walk (superficial or deep vein phlebitis), and wonder drugs (drug-induced fever).

The proper workup of a postoperative fever, similar to that of any problem in gynecology, involves the three classic steps of history, physical examination, and laboratory evaluations, with major emphasis placed on the physical examination. A chart review and history from the patient may highlight preoperative problems that might cause fever: intraoperative complications, such as aspiration of gastric or oral contents; placement of foreign bodies, such as drains; recent infusion of blood products or drugs; and known allergies. The physical examination emphasizes examination of the lungs for atelectasis and pneumonia; the wound and operative site for infection or hematoma formation; the costovertebral angles for tenderness, which might suggest pyelonephritis; and superficial veins in the arms for superficial phlebitis and deep veins in the legs for deep vein phlebitis.

The findings of the history and especially the physical examination and considerations of cost containment all influence the extent of laboratory tests ordered. Ordering a specific list of laboratory tests is unrewarding. The three most commonly ordered laboratory tests are complete blood count, chest roentgenogram, and urinalysis. Other common tests include culture and Gram stains of body fluids, including sputum, urine, and blood. One study of over 300 women who were febrile following hysterectomy did not identify a single positive blood culture. Women with persistent and undiagnosed fevers may need tests of liver function or special imaging studies, such as an intravenous pyelogram, computed tomography (CT), or magnetic resonance imaging (MRI), to detect problems such as compromised ureters, abscesses, or foreign bodies.

Each major complication will be discussed in detail later in the chapter. However, several specific generalizations concerning the type and characteristics of fever patterns should be emphasized. Fever is a common postoperative finding, occurring in approximately 75% of women. Rarely is the cause of the fever a serious infection. Microatelectasis is thought to be the cause of approximately 90% of fevers occurring in the first 48 hours after operation. Patients who develop fever as a result of foreign bodies, such as plastic intravenous lines or Foley catheters, are afebrile for several days, then experience an abrupt temperature spike. In contrast, wound or pelvic infections, which are usually clinically diagnosed from the fourth to seventh postoperative days, usually are associated with a low-grade fever that begins early in the postoperative period. An empiric trial of intravenous heparin for 72 hours is often a diagnostic and therapeutic trial for pelvic thrombophlebitis in refractory cases of postoperative fever of unknown origin.

A patient with a drug-induced fever feels better and does not look as ill as her temperature course indicates. The tachycardia associated with the elevated temperature is usually much less than usually anticipated with a similar temperature secondary to inflammation or infection. The presence of eosinophilia suggests a drug-induced fever. However, it is often a diagnosis of exclusion. Presumptive evidence of a drug-induced fever is established when the fever disappears after discontinuation of the drug. Scientifically, the diagnosis can only be confirmed by challenging the patient with the medication again after the fever has subsided. Clinically, this latter technique is not pragmatic.

Superficial thrombophlebitis often produces an enigmatic fever. Thus it is important to empirically change any intravenous lines that have been in place for longer than 48 hours. The etiology of febrile transfusion reactions is a concern. However, usually the reactions are caused by leukocyte or platelet antibodies. As long as a major blood type incompatibility is not found, treatment may be conservative.

The basic fever workup should be repeated at intervals until the diagnosis is established. The patient should be reexamined and selective laboratory tests reordered. Rare causes of postoperative fever include malignant neoplasms, pulmonary embolus, thyroid storm, and malignant hyperthermia.

It is important to consider that fever is a potential beneficial physiologic response to the patient. Therefore, unless the adult is markedly symptomatic secondary to the elevated temperature, it is not necessary to order an antipyretic medication. Cellular damage only occurs when the core temperature exceeds 41° C. Active cutaneous cooling does not reduce core temperature and may have undesirable effects such as increasing the metabolic rate and activating the autonomic nervous system.

MANAGEMENT OF A FALLING HEMATOCRIT

Bleeding is one of the most feared postoperative complications because it not only prolongs the hospital stay but also in rare cases may lead to the patient's death. Significant arterial bleeding in the first 24 hours often necessitates reoperation. This complication is discussed along with the management of shock and pelvic hematomas later in the chapter.

Vital signs should be ordered at frequent intervals during the first 24 hours to detect hypovolemia secondary to postoperative bleeding. However, following an operation, sizable amounts of unrecognized intraperitoneal or retroperitoneal bleeding sometimes are present without the woman having subjective symptoms or appreciable changes in her vital signs or urine output. However, a consistent orthostatic decrease in blood pressure of greater than 10 mm Hg may indicate a possible decrease of 20% of the blood volume. Thus a hematocrit may be helpful at two intervals during the postoperative course. We prefer a hematocrit at 24 and 72 hours following the operative procedure. A hematocrit drawn 24 hours following an operation may not give a true reflection of postoperative blood loss. The normal physiologic response to the stress of the operation and tissue destruction is a release of increased levels of aldosterone and antidiuretic hormone. The higher levels of aldosterone produce an increase in both sodium and water retention, while increased levels of antidiuretic hormone promote free water retention. Depending on the type and amount of intraoperative and postoperative intravenous fluids, the hematocrit on the first postoperative day may be misleading and reflect fluid changes rather than postoperative hemorrhage. The hematocrit from the third postoperative day is a more valid measurement of postoperative change. Hematocrits should be obtained in a standard fashion so as to eliminate sampling errors. For example, hematocrit samples drawn from central lines or during blood gas determinations often give false values because of the heparin or saline flush solutions.

After the effects of the operative blood loss are subtracted from the preoperative hematocrit, each further reduction in hematocrit of 3 to 5 points reflects a postoperative hemorrhage of approximately 500 ml. The safe level of postoperative anemia is a controversial issue. Certainly it is not identical to the level needed before an operation. Most young, healthy women without complicating medical illness will tolerate hematocrits of 20% to 22% without transfusion. These patients should be observed for orthostatic changes in their vital signs. Women over the age of 60 should be transfused if their hematocrit falls below 28%. Obviously the site of the hematoma should be discovered by abdominal and bimanual examination (see discussions on the diagnosis and management of wound and pelvic hematomas).

In summary, the morbidity and mortality of a surgical procedure is directly related to the amount of intraoperative and postoperative blood loss and not the corresponding level of preoperative anemia.

RESPIRATORY COMPLICATIONS

Alterations of pulmonary function are an expected physiologic change in women having general anesthesia and operations that open the peritoneal cavity. Of importance, respiratory complications directly cause 25% of deaths in women who die during the first 7 postoperative days. Most respiratory problems are secondary to inadequate ventilation by women as they try to minimize acute pain from the operative incision.

Atelectasis

The term *atelectasis* is derived from two Greek words that mean "imperfect expansion." The severity of atelectasis ranges from lack of expansion of a small group of terminal bronchioles and alveoli to complete collapse of a lung. In most patients, atelectasis is the failure to maintain patency of the small pulmonary airways and alveoli. Microatelectasis is a common occurrence, developing during almost all pelvic operations, and it is persistent 24 hours postoperatively in approximately 50% of women. Atelectasis is the most common cause of postoperative fever. Studies have demonstrated that there is no association between fever and the amount of atelectasis diagnosed radiologically. The incidence of atelectasis depends on the number of predisposing risk factors and the vigor with which the clinical diagnosis is established.

Ninety percent of all postoperative respiratory complications are related to atelectasis. The immediate postoperative period is characterized by a decrease in functional residual capacity and lung compliance (Figure 25-1). Thus the work of breathing is increased. Microatelectasis is most common where small airways (less than 1 mm in diameter) become blocked by secretions. When small airways remain closed by a combination of mucus plugs and bronchospasm, the gas distal to the obstruction is absorbed. This process results in atelectasis. These changes occur during the first 72 hours following an operation. When atelectasis becomes progressive and involves a large area of lung tissue, there is an associated decrease in oxygen saturation and a decrease in arterial oxygen pressure (PO_2). This is associated with a normal to low arterial carbon dioxide pressure (PCO_2).

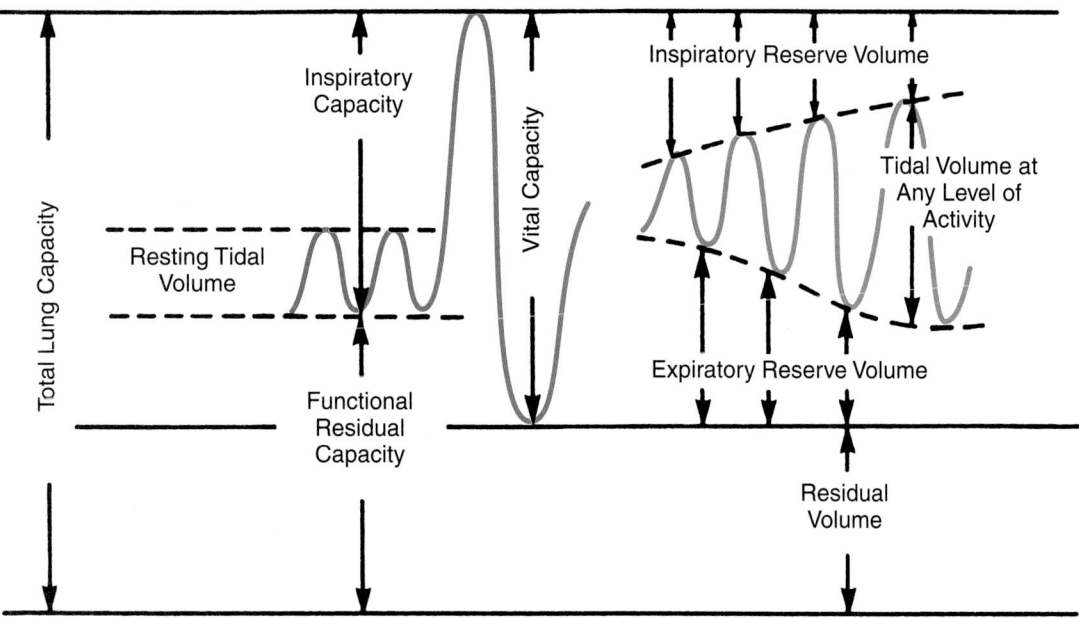

FIGURE 25-1 Graphic illustration of lung volumes and capacities. (From Wellman JJ: Respiratory care in the surgical patient. In Lubin MF, Walker HD, and Smith RB, editors: Medical management of the surgical patient, Stoneham, Mass, 1982, Butterworth Publishers, p 285. Used with permission.)

Wellman has listed both nonpulmonary and pulmonary factors that favor premature airway closure and development of atelectasis (see the box at right). The supine position decreases the functional residual capacity approximately 20% compared with the erect position. Obesity, smoking, age greater than 60 years, prolonged operative time, presence of a nasogastric tube, and coexisting medical conditions, such as cardiac or lung disease and pulmonary infection, all predispose women to atelectasis. In one study, 40% of obese women demonstrated radiologic evidence of atelectasis in their postoperative chest roentgenograms.

In normal breathing there are periodic, involuntary, deep inspirations that help to expand all areas of the lung. Pain, the supine position, and abdominal distention contribute to a pattern of monotonous shallow breathing without spontaneous deep sighs in the postoperative period. Because of the pain of an abdominal incision, chest wall breathing dominates over abdominal breathing. The resultant decrease in the movement of the diaphragm contributes to the development of atelectasis. A further decrease in functional residual capacity, a decrease in surfactant, and a depression of mucociliary transport all contribute to ventilation/perfusion mismatches and reduced ventilation/perfusion ratios. The end results are gas trapping, atelectasis, and vascular shunting. In the majority of individuals, microatelectasis is patchy and localized to small areas. However, the severity of atelectasis varies and may involve a complete lung.

Distribution of pulmonary blood flow is influenced by gravity. A greater proportion of pulmonary blood flows to dependent areas of the lungs in the supine patient. This increased blood flow, combined with the atelectasis in

> **Nonpulmonary and Pulmonary Factors That Favor Premature Airway Closure and Atelectasis**
>
> **Nonpulmonary Factors**
> Supine position
> Obesity
> Increased abdominal girth (ileus, pneumoperitoneum)
> Breathing at low lung volumes
>   Bindings around the chest and abdomen
>   Incisional pain
>   Sedative narcotic drugs
>   Prolonged effect of paralyzing drugs
>   Immobility
>   Excessively high concentrations of oxygen for prolonged periods
>
> **Pulmonary Factors**
> Interstitial edema
> Loss of surfactant with air space instability
> Airway obstruction
>   Inflammation with swelling of bronchial and interbronchial tissue
>   Constriction of bronchial smooth muscle
>   Retained secretions
>
> From Wellman JJ: Respirator care in the surgical patient. In Lubin MF, Walker HK, and Smith RB, editors: Medical management of the surgical patient, Stoneham, Mass, 1982, Butterworth Publishers, p 288. Used with permission.

dependent areas, results in an increased impairment of oxygenation, as well as a decrease in the elimination of carbon dioxide.

The endotracheal tube may contribute to the development of atelectasis. Even correctly placed endotracheal tubes are associated with destruction of cilia in the respiratory tract epithelium. Women with nasogastric tubes have a higher incidence of atelectasis, more commonly related to a decrease in deep breathing than to aspiration of stomach contents.

Atelectasis may present as the classic triad of fever, tachypnea, and tachycardia developing within the first 72 hours following an operation. On physical examination, tubular breathing, decreased breath sounds, and moist inspiratory rales may be heard. These findings are most prominent over the bases of the lung. If the condition progresses, an increase in productive cough and leukocytosis result. Chest x-ray films may demonstrate a patchy infiltrate with elevations of the diaphragm. There may be a corresponding shift of the trachea and mediastinum when atelectasis involves a large segment of the lung.

Atelectasis usually resolves spontaneously by the third to fifth postoperative day. Nevertheless, major efforts are made to prevent atelectasis, especially in high-risk individuals. The foundations of prevention of atelectasis are the encouragement of uneven ventilation and the production of episodes of prolonged inspiration to increase functional residual capacity. Thus the patient is encouraged to walk, take deep breaths, cough, turn from side to side, and remain semierect rather than supine. Early mobilization and ambulation have been documented to be as effective as chest physical therapy in the prevention of pulmonary complications. Keeping pain relief to a level where the woman will be able to cooperate and not have monotonous shallow breathing is also helpful. The most important aid to prevent and treat atelectasis is a simple bedside incentive spirometry device. Many women need encouragement by the hospital staff to use these devices effectively.

In summary, basilar atelectasis is the most common postoperative pulmonary problem experienced by gynecologic patients. If atelectasis does not clear, the woman should be treated with chest physical therapy, intermittent positive pressure breathing, aerosol therapy, or intermittent continuous positive airway pressure by mask. Rarely, bronchoscopy may be indicated to remove large mucus plugs.

Pneumonia

Postoperative pneumonia is commonly associated with atelectasis, because bacterial infections often begin in collapsed areas of the lungs. The infections lead to increased water in the lungs, increased elastic resistance, and decreased lung compliance. In animals the inhalation of infected material does not produce pneumonia without associated atelectasis. In experimental animals the injection of an intravenous bolus of bacteria was found to cause pneumonia in selectively localized areas of the lung that were obstructed. Predisposing factors to the development of pneumonia include chronic pulmonary disease, heavy cigarette smoking, alcohol abuse, obesity, advanced age, nasogastric tubes, long operative procedures, gram-negative bacterial infections, postoperative peritonitis, and debilitating illnesses.

The symptoms and signs of pneumonia are fever, cough, dyspnea, tachypnea, and purulent sputum. The classic physical finding of pneumonia is coarse rales over the infected area. The patient usually has a higher temperature and more systemic toxicity than does a woman with atelectasis. Chest roentgenograms often demonstrate diffuse, patchy infiltrates of the lung. Radiographic diagnoses are approximately 60% accurate for either bacterial or viral pneumonia in women with laboratory-proven pneumonia. Gram stain of the sputum helps to differentiate between bacterial colonization and infection. In cases of pneumonia the smear contains a large number of inflammatory cells with both intracellular and extracellular bacteria.

The management of pneumonia is similar to the management of atelectasis, with the addition of parenteral antibiotics. The initial choice of parenteral antibiotics is usually based on the Gram stain and subsequently on sputum cultures. Most lung infections result when the contents of the mouth (mucus and bacteria that have a physiologic pH) are inhaled and subsequently produce bacterial pneumonia. A rare problem is pneumonitis produced by aspiration of gastric fluid (sterile and highly acidic), which produces a severe chemical pneumonitis. Women at high risk for aspiration pneumonia include the elderly, obese, and those with a hiatal hernia or emergency surgery associated with a full stomach. The latter condition does not usually involve bacterial infection. Acute respiratory distress syndrome is a complex, devastating clinical problem following acute lung injury. Recent clinical changes in mechanical ventilation using lower tidal volumes have reduced the mortality of this syndrome by 22%.

CARDIOVASCULAR PROBLEMS

Hemorrhagic Shock

Shock is defined as a condition in which circulatory insufficiency prevents adequate vascular perfusion of vital organs. Systemic hypotension results in poor tissue perfusion and reduced capillary filling. If this pathophysiologic state is neglected, prolonged hypotension results in oliguria, progressive metabolic acidosis, and multiple organ failure. Shock may be produced by hemorrhage, cardiac failure, sepsis, and anaphylactic reactions. Hypovolemic shock is by far the most common etiology of acute circulatory failure in gynecology. Cardiogenic and septic shock are rare. Shock from postoperative hemorrhage is usually seen in the first few hours following the operation. In the perioperative period, hypovolemia may be secondary to several factors, including the patient being volume deficient preoperatively, unreplaced blood loss during surgery, extracellular fluid loss during surgery, inadequate fluid replacement, and, most commonly, continued blood loss following the surgical procedure. Tachycardia is the classic cardiovascular physiologic response to hypotension. However, relative bradycardia in hypotensive women is also a common hemodynamic response.

The vast majority of perioperative cases of shock are related to hemorrhage secondary to inadequate hemostasis. The development of shock from acute blood loss depends on the rate of bleeding; for example, a slow venous ooze may produce a large amount of blood loss but not produce shock. Rapid loss of 20% of a woman's blood volume produces mild shock, whereas a loss of greater than 40% of blood volume results in severe shock. Actual measurement of intraoperative blood loss is imprecise even with extensive use of suction equipment. Studies have demonstrated that 15% to 45% of surgical blood loss is absorbed on the drapes, laparotomy pads, and other areas. Thus the level of blood in the suction bottle does not accurately represent the true loss from the procedure. Massive blood loss has been defined as hemorrhage that results in replacement of 50% of the circulating blood volume in less than 3 hours.

Hypotension in the immediate postoperative period may be secondary to the residual effects of anesthesia or oversedation. For example, elderly patients often experience prolonged vasodilation secondary to the sympathetic blockade produced by epidural or spinal anesthesia.

The most common cause of postoperative bleeding is either a less than ideal ligature or hemorrhage from a vessel that retracted during the operation. Bleeding may come from an isolated artery or vein or may be more generalized when the bleeding is secondary to a clotting diathesis. The differential diagnosis of postoperative hemorrhagic shock includes conditions such as pneumothorax, pulmonary embolus, massive pulmonary aspiration, myocardial infarction, and acute gastric dilation (see box on this page).

The differential diagnosis of ineffective coagulation includes sepsis, fibrinolysis, diffuse intravascular coagulation, and a previously unrecognized coagulation defect, such as von Willebrand's disease. Inadequate hemostasis sometimes develops from excessive transfusion. The progressive acidosis associated with shock increases hemostatic problems. Hypothermia further complicates hemostasis because it produces platelet dysfunction and coagulopathy secondary to decreased activity of thromboxanes. Thrombocytopenia, impaired platelet function, and a decrease in factors V, VIII, and XI occur with massive transfusions. Coagulopathy begins with the transfusion of greater than 5 units of blood. Hypofibrinogenemia is the first to develop followed by deficiencies of other coagulation factors. Thrombocytopenia is the last recognized defect in the coagulopathy cascade. However, the timing of its development varies from individual to individual. Thus transfusion of platelets should be determined by serial platelet counts.

Classification of Shock

I. Hypovolemic
   A. External loss (e.g., blood, plasma, water)
   B. Sequestration—distributive abnormality
      1. Intravascular
         a. Arteriolar resistance loss (e.g., spinal shock)
         b. Capacitance pooling, venous system (e.g., endotoxin)
      2. Extravascular
         a. Exudative (e.g., peritonitis)
         b. Traumatic (e.g., hematoma)
II. Cardiogenic
   A. Intrinsic power
      1. Focal (e.g., infarct or aneurysm)
      2. Generalized (e.g., drug effect or ischemia)
   B. Extrinsic factors
      1. Obstructive (e.g., pulmonary embolus)
      2. Compressive (e.g., cardiac tamponade)
III. Peripheral vascular
   A. Neural factors (e.g., neurogenic shock—fainting)
   B. Humoral factors (e.g., anaphylactic shock, histamine shock)

From Greenfield LJ: Shock. In Hardy JD, editor: Complications in surgery and their management, ed 4, Philadelphia, 1981, WB Saunders Co, p 34.

Tachycardia and decreased urine output are two early signs of hypovolemia caused by hidden internal bleeding. The body's adrenergic response to hemorrhage includes perspiration, tachycardia, and peripheral vasoconstriction. Urine output decreases to less than 25 ml per hour as a result of poor perfusion of the kidneys. Urine osmolality is an excellent test to help determine the etiology of the oliguria. With further loss of blood the woman becomes agitated, appears weak, and develops skin pallor with cold and clammy extremities. The systolic blood pressure drops below 80 mm Hg. Again, because of adaptive cardiovascular changes, it takes a rapid loss of approximately one third of the blood volume to produce significant hypotension.

After an operation both occult intraperitoneal and retroperitoneal bleeding often occur without significant local symptoms. Extraperitoneal bleeding may present as bleeding from the vaginal vault if the vaginal cuff was left open. There may be mild flank or back tenderness with rebound on abdominal palpation. However, abdominal distention, muscle rigidity, and shoulder pain are late signs of intraperitoneal hemorrhage. The diagnosis of clinically significant postoperative bleeding may be confirmed by serial changes in hematocrits and/or by paracentesis. However, it is important to caution that marked changes in hematocrit and hemoglobin require time to develop. Bimanual examination with the patient under anesthesia may help in the diagnosis of silent retroperitoneal bleeding immediately before reoperation. An intravenous pyelogram will sometimes demonstrate obliteration of the psoas shadow and deviation of the ureter by a large retroperitoneal hematoma.

To help gynecologists establish their priorities in treatment in an emergency situation, remembering the mnemonic ORDER may be helpful. The priorities are O for oxygenate, R for restore circulating volume, D for drug therapy, E for evaluation, and R for remedy the basic problem.

The goals of management of a woman who has developed postoperative shock are to replace, restore, and maintain the effective circulating blood volume and establish normal cellular perfusion and oxygenation (see the box below). To accomplish this goal, an adequate cardiac output and appropriate peripheral vascular resistance must be maintained. The first priority is to provide adequate ventilation because poor respiratory gas exchange is the most frequent cause of death in these patients. The second, almost simultaneous, priority is rapid fluid replacement with adequate amounts of blood and crystalloid solution (normal saline or lactated Ringer's solution). The three-to-one rule suggests a ratio of 3 ml of crystalloid solution for every 1 ml of blood loss. In a review of plasma expanders, Moss and Gould strongly expressed their opinion that there are no benefits to using colloid solutions rather than crystalloid solutions in the treatment of shock. The optimal fluid replacement is a fluid evenly distributed throughout multiple body compartments. They concluded that optimal replacement included packed red blood cells and a balanced electrolyte solution, such as lactated Ringer's solution or normal saline. In February 1995 the University Hospital Consortium developed guidelines for the use of albumin, nonprotein colloid, and crystalloid solutions. They recommended in hemorrhagic shock that crystalloids should be considered the initial resuscitation fluid of choice; colloids are appropriate for resuscitation in conjunction with crystalloids when blood products are not immediately available. A recent meta-analysis of patients with hypovolemia found an excess mortality of approximately 6% (1 excess death per 17 treated patients) in those who received albumin instead of or in addition to crystalloid solutions.

Management Priorities in Massive Transfusion (the Exact Priority Depends on the Circumstances)

Restore circulating blood volume
Maintain oxygenation
Correct coagulopathy
Maintain body temperature
Correct biochemical abnormalities
Prevent pulmonary and other organ dysfunction
Treat underlying cause of haemorrhage

From Donaldson MDJ, Seaman MJ, and Park GR: Br J Anaesth 69:621, 1992.

The goals of fluid replacement are to obtain and maintain a systolic blood pressure that is similar to preoperative readings, maintain urine output greater than 30 ml per hour, and maintain a pulmonary wedge pressure between 10 and 15 mm Hg. Table 25-2 lists types of blood components used for replacement therapy. To monitor the rapid replacement of large volumes of intravenous fluid, a Swan-Ganz catheter may be inserted to determine pulmonary artery pressure, pulmonary wedge pressure, central venous pressure, and cardiac output. These values allow adjustments in the rate of vascular volume replacement. A Foley catheter facilitates measurement of hourly urine outputs. We prefer a Swan-Ganz catheter over a traditional central venous pressure line. However, if one is using a central venous pressure line, it is important to measure the pressure with the patient at a 45-degree angle. Studies have demonstrated that a central venous pressure measurement in the supine position will severely underestimate the volume of intravascular depletion.

The gold standard of imaging studies to detect abdominal and pelvic hemorrhage is a CT scan performed without either oral or intravenous contrast. An unenhanced CT scan will determine rapidly the precise location of the hemorrhage. During the imaging studies, acute hemorrhage appears as a high attenuation area in contrast to the normal soft tissue. In an emergent situation, the use of a helical scanner allows for an even more rapid acquisition of images.

Returning a patient to the operating room to control hemorrhage is often a difficult decision. However, this decision should not be postponed, and the patient should have an exploratory operation as soon as possible after volume replacement. During this second operation excellent anesthesia, a full selection of surgical instruments, and the value of good assistance cannot be overemphasized. Proper exposure is paramount for the success of this operation. Initially the old clots are removed, and further bleeding is reduced by direct pressure over the pelvic vessels. A systematic search is conducted in an effort to identify the individual vessels that are bleeding. Often the offending artery or vein cannot be identified, or friability of the tissues results in further bleeding.

Bilateral ligation of the anterior divisions of the hypogastric arteries distal to the posterior parietal branch is an effective operation to control persistent postoperative pelvic hemorrhage. This procedure results in a reduction of pulse pressure, which allows a stable clot to form at the site where the pelvic vessels are injured. Classically, two ligatures are placed and tied around each hypogastric artery (Figure 25-2). The major potential complication of this procedure is injury to the hypogastric vein. If there is generalized oozing, thrombocytopenia, disseminated intravascular coagulation, or factor VIII deficiency should be suspected. If these conditions are excluded, venous oozing from small vessels in the pelvis may be controlled by local application of microfibrillar collagen (Avitene).

TABLE 25-2
Indications for Administration of Various Blood Products

Product	Content	Acceptable Indication	Unacceptable Indication
Red blood cells	Red cells	To increase oxygen-carrying capacity in anemic women For orthostatic hypotension secondary to blood loss	For volume expansion In place of a hematinic To enhance wound healing To improve general well-being
Platelet concentrates	Platelets	To control or prevent bleeding associated with deficiencies in platelet number or function	In patients with immune thrombocytopenic purpura (unless bleeding is life threatening) Prophylactically with massive blood transfusion
Fresh frozen plasma	Plasma, clotting factors	To increase the level of clotting factors in patients with demonstrated deficiency	For volume expansion As a nutritional supplement Prophylactically with massive blood transfusion
Cryoprecipitate	Factors I, V, VIII, XIII, von Willebrand factor, fibronectin	To increase the level of clotting factors in patients with demonstrated deficiency of fibrinogen, factor VIII, factor XIII, fibronectin, or von Willebrand factor	Prophylactically with massive blood transfusion

From ACOG Tech Bull 199:1, 1994.

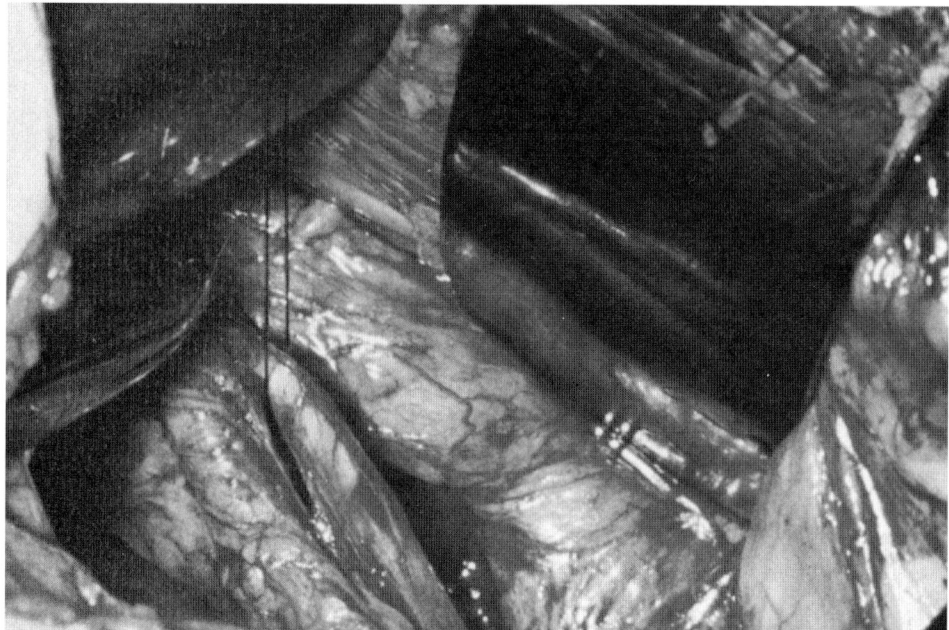

FIGURE 25-2   Ligation of internal iliac artery. Double loop is being directed toward bifurcation of common iliac artery. (From Breen JL, Gregori CA, and Kindzierski JA: Hemorrhage in gynecologic surgery. In Shaefer G and Graber EA, editors: Complications in obstetric and gynecologic surgery, Hagerstown, Md, 1981, Harper & Row, Publishers, Inc, p 439.)

Intraoperative rapid autologous blood transfusion is a commonly available technique that is used extensively in cardiovascular and trauma surgery. Regretfully, it is underused or rarely performed by gynecologists. Grimes has described a simple device that can adapt this technique for use in any operating room. The major complication of rapid autologous transfusion is a 10% hemolysis rate. The risks of air embolism or infusion of particulate matter have virtually been eliminated. Obviously, autologous blood does not contain platelets or clotting factors so that platelets and fresh frozen plasma will have to be given concurrently for severe hemorrhage. Rapid autologous transfusion is contraindicated in advanced pelvic infection or malignancy.

Most centers prefer using angiographic embolization instead of hypogastric artery ligation (Figure 25-3). To permit visualization of a bleeding vessel, a flow of 1 ml per minute is required. Recent introduction of digital road mapping technology has improved the rapid identification of bleeding vessels. Similarly, treatment of recurrent postoperative hemorrhage or hemorrhage late in the postoperative course (7 to 14 days), may be performed with angiographic arterial embolization. Either absorbable gelatin sponges, which produce vascular occlusion for 10 to 30 days, or metal coils with Dacron fibers, which produce permanent occlusion, may be used.

Hematomas

This section will describe the management of wounds or pelvic hematomas that develop slowly and are diagnosed after the first postoperative day. Proper management of postoperative hematomas is one of the most challenging and controversial subjects in operative gynecology. The incidence of hematomas is inversely related to the extent to which meticulous hemostasis is obtained intraoperatively. Women who are given low-dose heparin or chronically take aspirin are at a slightly higher risk of hematoma formation. Hematomas result from intermittent or slow, continuous venous bleeding and are almost always self-limiting. Eventually the pressure of the expanding hematoma will exceed the venous pressure, and a stable clot will form. The extent of the hematoma is determined partially by the potential size of the compartment into which the bleeding occurs. Retroperitoneal or broad ligament hematomas may contain several units of blood. The diagnosis of a wound or pelvic hematoma is usually suspected on the morning of the third postoperative day when the laboratory reports an unexpectedly low hematocrit. The patient may have mild to moderate tenderness over the affected area. By the fifth postoperative day the hematoma liquefies and is easier to outline during bimanual examination. Distinguishing between an uninfected hematoma and a hematoma that has become secondarily infected is difficult before incision and drainage. Both clinical situations produce tenderness and fever secondary to the inflammation surrounding the hematoma. The diagnosis of most retroperitoneal hematomas may be made by physical examination. Most important is a careful rectovaginal examination. Rarely, radiologic imaging studies are indicated when the hematoma cannot be palpated.

Hematomas less than 5 cm in diameter may be treated conservatively. Larger hematomas should be drained via an extraperitoneal approach as soon as they liquefy. If not treated by incision and drainage, most hematomas will become secondarily infected even when the patient is treated with parenteral antibiotics. Effective drainage of most pelvic and broad ligament hematomas usually can be

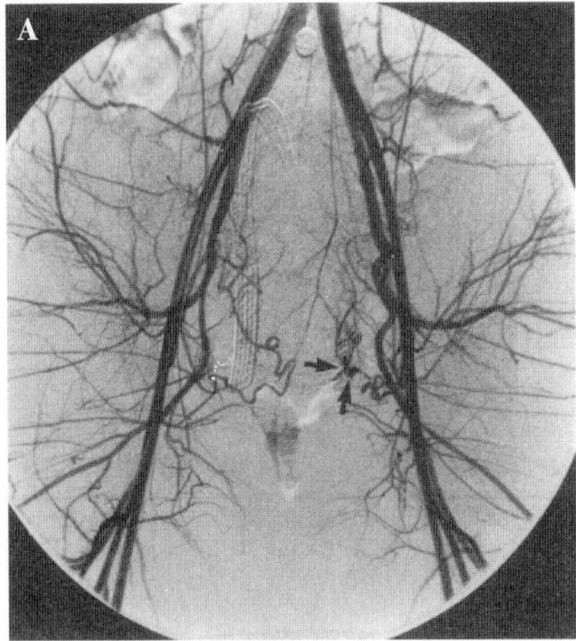
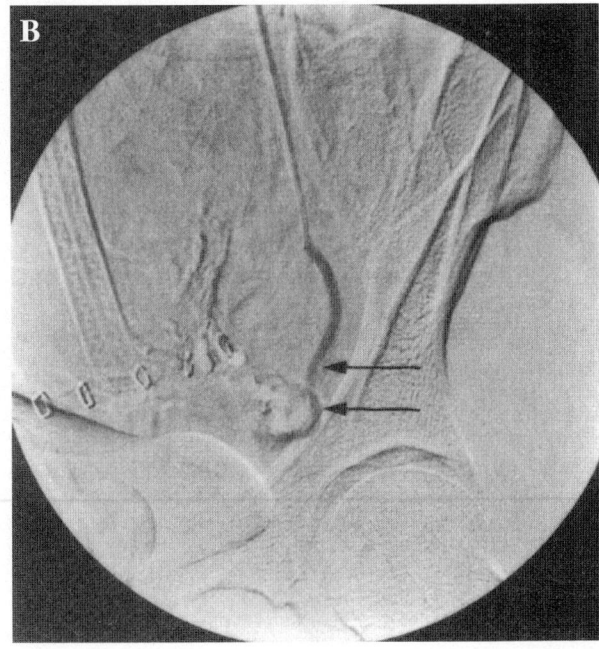

FIGURE 25-3   A, Anteroposterior digital subtraction pelvic angiogram in 37-year-old woman with persistent pelvic bleeding after surgical myomectomy for uterine leiomyomas demonstrates contrast pooling (*arrows*) from branches of left uterine artery, consistent with active hemorrhage. **B,** Postembolization left uterine arteriogram shows occluded left uterine artery (*long arrow*) with no evidence of active bleeding. (From Vedantham S, Goodwin SC, McLucas B, and Mohr G: Uterine artery embolization: an underused method of controlling pelvic hemorrhage, Am J Obstet Gynecol 176:938, 1997.)

accomplished vaginally. Small subcutaneous hematomas or fascial hematomas usually resolve. However, they are associated with an increased incidence of wound infection.

Any operation is accompanied by the potential risk of an unrecognized retained sponge or laparotomy pad. The exact incidence of this worrisome complication is difficult to establish but is estimated to be between 1 in 1200 and 1 in 1500 laparotomies. Most often the sponge counts at surgery have been correct. When this complication is discovered during the first postoperative week, the patient usually has a tender pelvic mass that is infected. When this mass is discovered after the immediate postoperative course, patients are often asymptomatic or exhibit minimal tenderness. The possibility of a retained foreign body should be considered in the differential diagnosis of pelvic hematomas and abscesses.

Thrombophlebitis and Pulmonary Embolus

Superficial Thrombophlebitis

Superficial thrombophlebitis is one of the most frequently occurring postoperative complications and is most commonly associated with intravenous catheters. Superficial thrombophlebitis is a benign disease. However, it is associated with deep vein thrombophlebitis in approximately 5% of cases. Superficial thrombophlebitis is frequently overlooked or disregarded as a cause of postoperative fever. However, this diagnosis should be suspected whenever an intravenous line with antibiotics or hypertonic solutions has been used. Superficial tenderness and erythema outline the course of the veins. Women with established superficial varicosities in the lower extremities are especially susceptible because of localized stasis or pressure during the operative procedure and inactivity during the first 24 hours after

operation. Patients with superficial thrombophlebitis of the legs also may have concomitant deep venous disease. Thus the finding of superficial thrombophlebitis does not eliminate the necessity to consider deep venous thrombosis as well. Recurrent, superficial phlebitis, in varying anatomic sites, may be a sign of occult malignant disease.

Detailed basic investigations have identified fibrin sheaths surrounding intravenous catheters in 60% to 100% of patients studied. The exact fate of the several inches of clot and fibrin sheath after the removal of the intravenous catheter is uncertain. Venography studies have found that these clots and fibrin sheaths do not break up on catheter removal but initially remain in situ. Intravenous catheters are an important source of nosocomial infections. Approximately 30% of all hospital-acquired bacteremias are secondary to intravenous lines. The most serious complication of intravenous catheter use is infection of the thrombus, producing suppurative phlebitis or catheter sepsis. The initial infection may occur via the bloodstream or via bacteria from the skin reaching the thrombus along the catheter line. When frank pus is expressed, the treatment of suppurative phlebitis includes excising the infected vein.

The natural history of intravenous catheter-associated phlebitis has been documented by Hershey et al. The classic symptom of phlebitis is inflammation of the subcutaneous tissue along the course of a vein or over the area of merging varicosities. The patient develops a painful, tender, erythematous induration (nodule or core). In the majority of severe cases there is associated fever. In studying 202 episodes of superficial phlebitis, Hershey et al. discovered that the disease develops relatively rapidly, giving few symptoms or signs that allow removal of the catheter to prevent the disease (Figures 25-4 and 25-5). After the process has begun, the inflammation does not

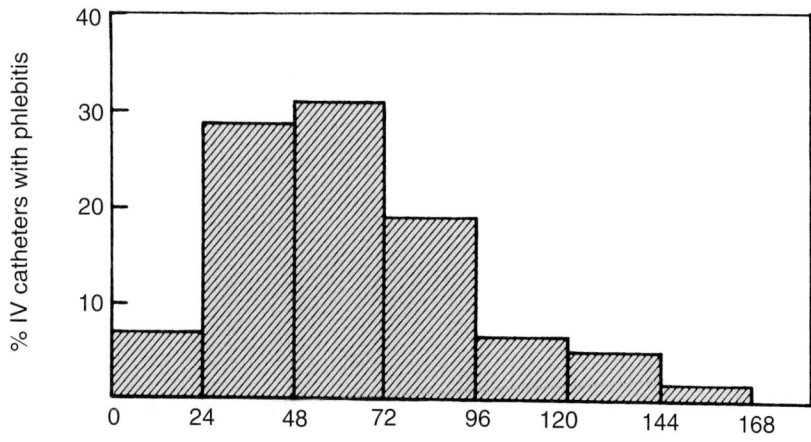

Hours after insertion that phlebitis was diagnosed

FIGURE 25-4 Hours after insertion that phlebitis was diagnosed. Time of diagnosis of phlebitis from time of intravenous catheter insertion. (From Hershey CO, Tomford JW, McLaren CE, et al: Arch Intern Med 144:1374, 1984, Copyright 1984, American Medical Association.)

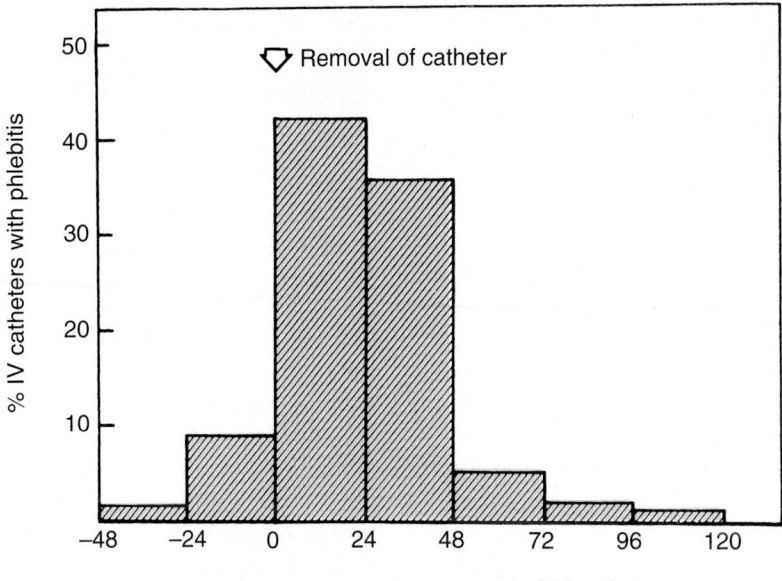

FIGURE 25-5 Distribution of intravenous catheter–induced phlebitis relative to interval between diagnosis of phlebitis and removal of catheter. (From Hershey CO, Tomford JW, McLaren CE, et al: Arch Intern Med 144:1374, 1984, Copyright 1984, American Medical Association.)

consistently terminate with removal of the catheter. In their study, more than 40% of cases occurred 24 hours or more after withdrawal of the intravenous line. Nevertheless, the duration of phlebitis is prolonged if the catheter is not immediately removed when the diagnosis of superficial phlebitis is made. The authors recommended that all intravenous catheters be removed and replaced at 48-hour intervals regardless of whether signs or symptoms of superficial phlebitis are present. In addition, the use of an intravenous team decreased the incidence of catheter-associated phlebitis from 32% to 15% in their series. Strict aseptic techniques should be used during catheter insertion. Catheters inserted into the hand or forearm, through which antibiotics are infused, should be changed at least every 36 hours. One recent observational study by Bregenzer et al. questions the concept of routine replacement of peripheral intravenous catheters. They believe that newer catheters made of fluorocarbon resins and polyurethane dramatically reduce catheter-related complications.

In summary, venous catheters should be removed at the first sign of induration, erythema, or edema. Superficial phlebitis is the leading cause of an enigmatic postoperative fever during the third, fourth, or fifth postoperative day.

The clinical management of mild superficial thrombophlebitis includes rest, elevation, and local heat. Moderate to severe superficial thrombophlebitis may be treated with a nonsteroidal antiinflammatory agent such as ibuprofen. The rare case of proximal progression of the inflammatory process should be treated with therapeutic doses of intravenous heparin and antibiotics.

Deep Vein Thrombophlebitis

Thrombophlebitis is a common postoperative complication in which the initial pathophysiology usually begins during the operation. It is the process of venous thrombosis formation occurring in any deep vein, secondary to coagulation of blood, and fibrin formation in the presence of venous stasis. Generally, thromboembolic complications occur early in the postoperative course—50% within the first 24 hours and 75% within 72 hours. Approximately 15% occur after the seventh postoperative day. Thus the potential threat is present even after the woman is discharged from the hospital. Diagnosis of deep vein thrombophlebitis by physical examination is very insensitive. Thus imaging studies are essential for establishing the correct diagnosis.

Venous thrombosis and pulmonary embolus are the direct causes of approximately 40% of deaths in gynecologic cases. The incidence of fatal pulmonary emboli following gynecologic operations is approximately 0.2%. Because women often die within a few hours of the appearance of initial symptoms, emphasis must be placed on prevention rather than treatment of this complication. (Refer to the discussion on thromboembolic disease in Chapter 24.) Pulmonary embolus is not the only major consequence of deep venous thrombophlebitis. Many women develop chronic venous insufficiency or "postphlebitic syndrome" of the legs as a major sequela following thrombophlebitis. The resulting damage to valves of the deep veins produces shunting of blood to superficial veins, chronic edema, pain on exercise, and skin ulceration.

The reported incidence of deep vein thrombosis with

gynecologic operations varies from 7% to 45%, with an average of approximately 15%. Walsh et al. found the incidence of deep venous thrombosis to be 7% following vaginal hysterectomy, 13% after abdominal hysterectomy for benign disease, 25% following Wertheim hysterectomy, and 45% following extensive gynecologic cancer operations. The incidence of thrombophlebitis is directly dependent on risk factors such as the type and duration of operation, the age of the woman, history of deep vein thrombophlebitis, peripheral edema, amount of blood lost at operation, restrictions in preoperative ambulation, obesity, immobility, malignancy, sepsis, diabetes, current oral contraceptive use, and conditions that produce venous stasis, such as ascites and heart failure (Table 25-3). Older and obese women have an increased incidence of thrombophlebitis because of dilation of their deep venous system. There is a two- to fourfold increased risk for venous thrombophlebitis in women taking postmenopausal estrogen therapy. The length of the surgical procedure also has an important influence on the development of thrombophlebitis. If the operation is 1 to 2 hours, approximately 15% of women develop the disease; if the surgery is longer than 3 hours, the risk is greater.

The process of thrombosis most often begins in the deep veins of the calf. It is estimated that 75% of pulmonary emboli originate from a thrombus that began in the leg veins. If one leg is involved, the other leg has thrombophlebitis in approximately 33% of women. Usually the thrombophlebitis remains localized and the clot lyses spontaneously, and the patient is free of symptoms. In approximately 1 in 20 cases the process extends centrally to the veins of the upper leg and pelvis. Involvement of the femoral vein often results in swelling caused by obstruction of this large vein. Pulmonary emboli from calf veins alone are rare, with only 4% to 10% of pulmonary emboli originating from this area. In contrast there is a 50% risk of a pulmonary embolus if thrombophlebitis of the femoral vein is not treated.

In 1854 Virchow described the three key predisposing or precipitating factors in the production of thrombi: an increase in coagulation factors, damage to the vessel wall, and venous stasis. Subsequent studies have documented that all three events occur with gynecologic operations. Blood flow in the iliac vein decreases by approximately 55% during an operation. During an operation there are several normal physiologic changes that produce hypercoagulability, including increases in the following: factors VIII, IX, and X, number of platelets, platelet aggregation and adherence, fibrinogen, and lastly, thromboplastin-like substance from tissue necrosis.

Kakkar has described the cascade of events leading to the development of thrombophlebitis. The initial event in the cascade is stasis. Stasis leads to localized anoxia with subsequent generation of thrombi at the anoxic site. This produces changes in the lining of the vessel with exposure of the basement membrane and platelet adhesion and local coagulation. Kakkar further postulated that the interaction of this process with activators of fibrinolysis and inhibitors of coagulation determines and regulates whether fibrin is deposited and a venous thrombus develops. Thus the most important event in thrombophlebitis is the generation of thrombi in the presence of venous stasis. A thrombus may generate in an area of stasis, or it may generate wherever a vessel wall is damaged with resultant exposure of the subendothelial collagen, to which platelets will adhere.

TABLE 25-3
Risk Categories of Thromboembolism in Gynecologic Operations

Risk Category	Low Risk	Medium Risk	High Risk
Age	40 years	40 years	50 years
Contributing factors			
Operation	Uncomplicated or minor	Major abdominal or pelvic	Major, extensive malignant disease
Weight		Moderately obese—75 to 90 kg or >20% above ideal weight	Morbidly obese—>115 kg or >30% above ideal weight
			Previous venous thrombosis
			Varicose veins
			Cardiac disease
			Diabetes (insulin dependent)
Calf vein thrombosis	2%	10%–35%	30%–60%
Iliofemoral vein thrombosis	0.4%	2%–8%	5%–10%
Fatal pulmonary emboli	0.2%	0.1%–0.5%	1%
Recommended prophylaxis	Early ambulation	Low-dose heparin or intermittent pneumatic compression	Low-dose heparin or intermittent pneumatic compression

From Mattingly RF and Thompson JD, editors: Te Linde's operative gynecology, ed 6, Philadelphia, 1985, LB Lippincott Co, p 106.

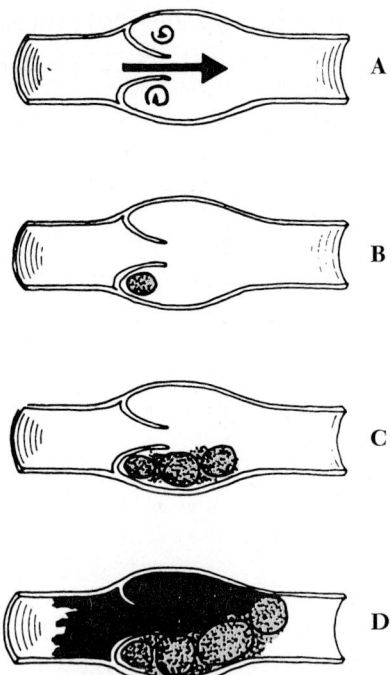

FIGURE 25-6 Stages in development of thrombus in valve pocket of deep veins of leg. **A,** Stasis in valve pocket results in thrombin generation. **B,** Platelet aggregation and fibrin formation. **C,** Propagation of platelet-fibrin nidus. **D,** Blockage of venous flow with resultant retrograde extension. (From Bloom AL and Thomas DP, editors: Haemostases and thrombosis, Edinburgh, 1981, Churchill Livingstone, Inc., p 684.)

The site of initial formation of the thrombus is most often near the base of a valve cusp in the calf of the leg (Figure 25-6). The thrombus propagates and grows by repetitive layers of platelet aggregation and deposition of fibrin from fibrinogen. The most recently formed portion of the propagating thrombi are free floating (not attached to the vein) and are most likely to become pulmonary emboli. The body attempts to repair the area of thrombosis through an invasion of fibroblasts from the vein wall to encompass the base of the thrombus. Eventually the thrombus is attached to the vein wall, the area is reepithelialized, organization occurs, and symptoms resolve.

The signs and symptoms of deep vein thrombophlebitis depend directly on the severity and extent of the process. Many localized cases of deep vein thrombophlebitis in the calf are asymptomatic and are only recognized by a screening procedure such as duplex ultrasonography. However, even extensive areas of deep vein thrombophlebitis may be asymptomatic, and the first sign may be the development of a pulmonary embolus. In a woman who is asymptomatic, the pathophysiologic process may not totally obstruct the individual vein and drainage is obtained via associated competent collateral circulation.

Studies using ^{125}I-labeled fibrinogen to screen the legs have documented that approximately one out of two women who develop deep vein thrombophlebitis follow-

ing gynecologic operation is totally free of symptoms. Among women who develop signs and symptoms, approximately 68% have induration of the calf muscles, 52% have minimum edema, 25% have calf tenderness, and 11% develop a difference of more than 1 cm in diameter of the leg. Homans' sign is present in 10%, and differential pain over the calf with a blood pressure cuff is present in approximately 40%. The clinical diagnosis of iliofemoral thrombosis is much easier, and the patient usually develops severe symptoms due to obstruction of venous return. Usually there is an acute onset of severe pain, swelling, and a sensation that the leg will "burst."

The clinician must have a high degree of suspicion to begin the diagnostic workup for deep vein thrombophlebitis. The clinical symptoms and signs of deep venous thrombosis are nonspecific. A clinical clue is the persistence of a low-grade fever with unexplained tachycardia. The tachycardia is often more rapid than one would expect with a low-grade fever. The finding of a definite difference in leg circumference is supportive evidence of deep venous thrombosis. However, physical examination of the legs produces false-positive findings in approximately 50% of cases. Thus, if the signs and symptoms are suspicious, or the woman is at high risk, the diagnosis should be confirmed by one of the imaging techniques currently available to detect deep vein thrombophlebitis (Table 25-4). One disturbing fact is that the more symptomatic the disease, the more adherent the thrombus. Relatively, patients with symptoms are less likely to develop pulmonary emboli.

Ascending contrast venography (phlebography) was the gold standard—the most accurate method—for detecting deep vein thrombophlebitis (Figure 25-7). However, duplex ultrasonography, the combination of Doppler and real-time B-mode ultrasound, and color Doppler have replaced venography as the preferred methods for diagnosis of deep vein thrombophlebitis. The diagnostic accuracy of venography is estimated to be 95% for peripheral disease and 90% for iliofemoral thrombophlebitis. The major drawback is that this invasive imaging procedure is quite painful when there is extravasation of the contrast material into the tissue. Contrast venography remains the most reliable means of detection of deep venous thrombosis isolated to the calf veins, the iliac veins, or the inferior vena cava. Contrast venography is superior to duplex ultrasonography for the diagnosis of deep venous thrombosis in asymptomatic women.

Scanning the leg with ^{125}I-labeled fibrinogen was an excellent method to screen women for occult thrombi. The test was not diagnostic above the midthigh because of the amount of radiation emanating from the femoral artery and urinary bladder. Recently, radioactive-labeled fibrinogen has been withdrawn from commercial use.

Duplex ultrasonography is a noninvasive screening test for deep vein thrombosis. This imaging modality has remarkably high sensitivity and specificity in sympto-

TABLE 25-4
Tests Used in the Diagnosis of Deep-Vein Thrombosis*

Test	Symptomatic Deep-Vein Thrombosis[†]		Asymptomatic Deep-Vein Thrombosis[‡]		Anatomic Area	Comment
	Sensitivity (%)	Specificity (%)	Sensitivity (%)	Specificity (%)		
Phlebography	Standard for comparison		Standard for comparison		Pelvis, thigh, popliteal area, calf	Invasive; provides equivocal results in cases of recurrent deep-vein thrombosis; not easily repeated
Inpedance plethysmography	92[§]	95	22	98	Thigh, popliteal area	For provisional diagnosis of primary or recurrent proximal deep-vein thrombosis; insensitive to calf thrombi and to nonocclusive proximal thrombi
Ultrasonography						
Real-time B-mode or duplex	97	97	59	98	Thigh, popliteal area	Most sensitive confirmatory test for symptomatic deep-vein thrombosis
Doppler flow velocity	88	88	—	—	Thigh, popliteal area	Can be used on limbs in traction or plaster; interpretation is subjective, requires skill
Magnetic resonance venography[¶]	96	100	—	—	Inferior, vena cava, pelvis, thigh	Can distinguish between acute and chronic occlusion; can identify associated abnormalities; noninvasive; expensive; limited availability

From Weinmann EE and Salzman EW: N Engl J Med 331:1630, 1994.

*No data on [¹²⁵I]-labeled fibrinogen scanning were included, since the test is no longer available.

†Testing is mostly used to verify clinical suspicion of deep-vein thrombosis.

‡Testing is mostly used to screen high-risk patients.

§Recent studies have reported lower sensitivity.

¶Magnetic resonance venography has only been evaluated in small clinical trials.

matic women. Real-time ultrasound imaging provides visualization of the larger veins, while sensitive Doppler ultrasound is focused simultaneously on the suspicious vessel. The technology depends on changes in venous flow for a positive diagnosis. In a recent meta-analysis of published studies, White et al. documented that the sensitivity of duplex ultrasonography to detect proximal thrombi is 95% (confidence intervals, 92% to 98%) and the specificity is 99% (confidence intervals, 98% to 100%). The advantages of this method are that it is noninvasive, easy to use, highly accurate, objective, simple, and reproducible. Color Doppler ultrasonography may improve the diagnostic accuracy in larger veins. The main disadvantage of duplex ultrasonography is its limited accuracy when investigating small vessels in the calf. The inability to compress the deep vein by moderate pressure with the ultrasound probe is the most widely used criteria for the positive diagnosis of deep venous thrombosis.

Lensing et al., in a prospective study of 220 patients, used compressibility of the vein as the sole criterion for diagnosis of deep vein thrombosis (Table 25-5). For all patients in their study, including both proximal vein and calf vein thrombosis, the sensitivity was 91% and the specificity was 99%.

Impedance plethysmography is another noninvasive screening method to detect deep vein thrombosis. A pneumatic cuff is applied around the thigh, and changes in blood volume are measured by changes in electrical resistance (impedance). Impedance is reduced with venous thrombi. This method has at least a 15% false-negative rate and a 20% false-positive rate. As with duplex ultrasonography, the accuracy of this method to detect thrombi of small vessels is limited.

Recently, magnetic resonance angiography (MRV) has been developed. Preliminary studies have found that MRV, which is noninvasive, is comparable diagnostically to contrast venography and duplex Doppler ultrasonography. Obviously the cost of MRV is 1.5 to 3 times greater than contrast or duplex scanning. However, there is the added benefit of soft tissue imaging, which may provide diagnostic information regarding the cause of the venous thrombosis.

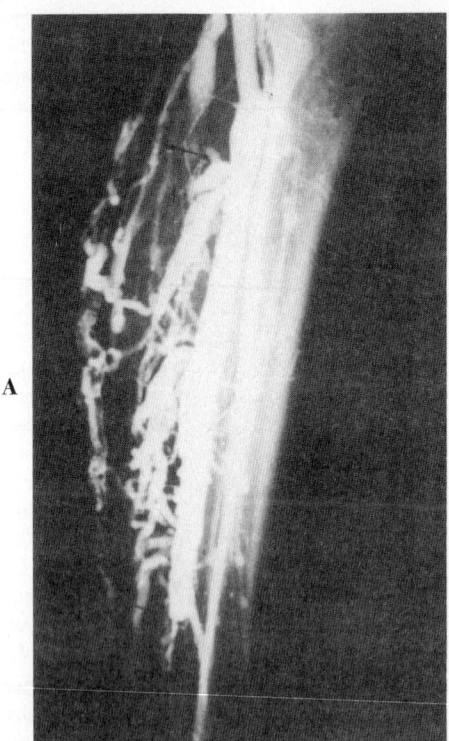 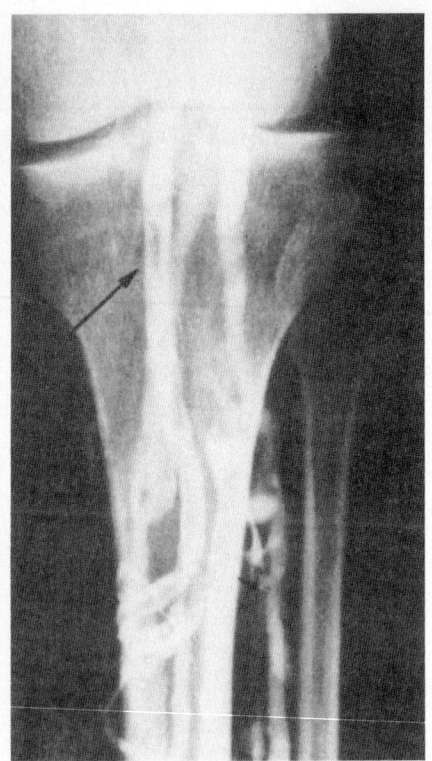

FIGURE 25-7 **A,** Phlebogram showing small thrombi in veins of calf, which are usually of no clinical significance. **B,** Thrombi in deep vein of calf showing extension into popliteal vein. (From Bonnar J: Clin Obstet Gynecol 28:439, 1985.)

TABLE 25-5

Comparison of Ultrasonographic and Venographic Results in 66 Patients with Proximal Vein Thrombosis and 143 Patients without Venous Thrombosis*

	Venogram	
Ultrasonographic Result	**Proximal Vein Thrombosis**	**Normal**
Noncompressible†	66	1
Compressible	0	142

From Lensing AWA, Prandoni P, Brandjes D, et al: N Engl J Med 320:342, 1989.

*The sensitivity of noncompressibility for the detection of proximal vein thrombosis was 100% (95% confidence interval, 95% to 100%); the specificity was 99% (95% confidence interval, 97% to 100%).

†Noncompressible denotes an inability to compress the common femoral vein, popliteal vein, or both with the transducer probe.

For years clinicians have sought to develop a blood test that would help in the differential diagnosis of deep vein thrombophlebitis. To date a reliable test that is positive when a woman has deep vein thrombophlebitis has not been found. However, plasma D-Dimer shows promise of identifying postoperative patients who have not developed deep vein thrombophlebitis. Clinical studies using a relatively low cut-off value for D-Dimer result in a sensitivity of approximately 100% (Table 25-6). Thus D-Dimer blood assay levels are helpful in excluding the diagnosis of deep vein thrombophlebitis in an individual woman when the clinical result is below the cut-off level. In women with suspected deep vein thrombosis in which the initial compression ultrasound test was normal, testing for the presence of D-Dimer helps to reduce the number of repeat ultrasound examinations.

The objectives of clinical management of deep vein thrombophlebitis associated with gynecologic operations are preventive medicine, early detection, and early therapy. In reality antithrombotic therapy, whether with heparin or warfarin sodium (Coumadin), is preventive medicine, since the therapeutic agent interrupts progression of the disease (thrombus formation) but does not actively resolve the disease process.

Anticoagulation with heparin is the drug of choice for the initial first-line treatment of deep vein thrombosis once the diagnosis is confirmed (Table 25-7). An initial loading dose of 5000 IU is given intravenously, followed by continuous infusion of 1000 to 1500 IU per hour. The dosage of unfractionated intravenous heparin should be adjusted to prolong the Lee-White clotting time to 2 to 3 times control

TABLE 25-6
Summary of Studies in the Evaluation of the Value of Plasma D-Dimer in the Diagnosis of DVT

Reference	No. of Patients	Cut Off (µg/L)	Sensitivity (%)	Specificity (%)
Rowbotham et al., 1987	104	250	100	36
Heaton et al., 1987	62	200	100	47
Bounameaux et al., 1989	53	200	100	31
Speiser et al., 1990	97	120	100	48
Boneu et al., 1991	116	500	94	51
Heyboer et al., 1992	309	300	100	29

From Koopman MMW, van Beek EJR, ten Cate JW: Prog Cardiovasc Dis 37:1, 1994.

TABLE 25-7
Treatment of Deep Vein Thrombosis

Superficial	Local measures, aspirin, nonsteroidal antiinflammatory drugs

Deep Vein Thrombosis

Proximal

Acute	Heparin
	Unfractionated intravenous—adjusted to a PTT 50–80 sec
	Porcine mucosal sodium subcutaneous—5000–7500 U q6h
	Calcium heparin subcutaneous—5000–7500 U q6h
	Low-molecular–weight subcutaneous—1 mg/kg q12h
Long-term	Heparin
	Calcium heparin subcutaneous—5000 U q8–12h
	Low-molecular–weight subcutaneous—0.8 mg/kg q24h
	Warfarin (Coumadin) titrated to INR 2.0 to 3.0
Duration	3 months and/or until predisposing factors alleviated

Calf

Acute	Heparin
	Unfractionated intravenous—adjusted to a PTT 50–80 sec
	Porcine mucosal sodium subcutaneous—5000–7500 U q6h
	Calcium heparin subcutaneous—5000–7500 U q6h
	Low-molecular–weight subcutaneous—1 mg/kg q12h
Long-term	Heparin
	Calcium heparin subcutaneous—5000 U q8–12h
	Low-molecular–weight subcutaneous—0.8 mg/kg q24h
	Coumadin titrated to INR 2.0 to 3.0
Duration	3–6 weeks Coumadin or heparin, then aspirin for 3 months or until predisposing factors alleviated

Modified from Baker WF Jr and Bick RL: Med Clin North Am 78:685, 1994.

values or, alternatively, to prolong an activated partial thromboplastin time to 1.5 to 2.5 times control values. Continuous heparin infusion is preferred over periodic bolus injections because there are fewer hemorrhagic complications (6% versus 14%). The half-life of heparin on the average is 1 to 2 hours after intravenous injection. Failure to achieve adequate anticoagulation in the first 24 hours of therapy increases the risk of recurrent venous thromboembolism fifteenfold. Heparin should be continued for 5 to 7 days. Oral warfarin (Coumadin), 15 mg daily, should be begun within the first 48 hours of heparin therapy. Following 2 to 3 days of 10 to 15 mg of Coumadin daily, the prothrombin time will usually be prolonged to 1.5 to 2 times the control value. This therapeutic level of 1.5 to 2 times normal control should be maintained by appropriate downward adjustment of the Coumadin dosage. The biologic half-life of Coumadin is 2 to 3 days. Anticoagulation with Coumadin should be continued for 3 months for adequate secondary prophylaxis.

In a double-blind, randomized trial, Hull et al. (1990) demonstrated that 5 days of heparin therapy was as effective as 10 days. Repeat venous thromboembolic events were similar in women receiving the shorter course of therapy. The authors believe that oral Coumadin may be started on the first day of heparin therapy, thus enabling patients to have a shorter hospital stay. The primary risk of chronic anticoagulation therapy is the potential for major bleeding complications. Major bleeding occurs in approximately 4% of woman-years of therapy. Thus it is important to carefully follow these women with serial coagulation studies. Approximately 1% of patients on full-dose heparin develop thrombocytopenia (platelet counts less than 100,000). If thrombocytopenia develops, heparin should be discontinued because of the potential risk of paradoxic thrombosis.

Low–molecular-weight heparin initially was reserved for the high-risk or difficult-to-manage patient because of its high cost. However, two recent large clinical trials assessed the advantages of outpatient treatment of deep vein thrombophlebitis with low molecular weight heparins. The medication is administered subcutaneously twice daily on a weight-adjusted basis without laboratory monitoring. This therapy is safe and effective for selective women and appreciably reduces inpatient costs.

The recent development and improvement of thrombolytic agents, such as plasminogen activators (streptokinase, urokinase, and recombinant tissue plasminogen activator), has offered an alternative medical therapy to heparin. The efficacy of these drugs in treating acute venous thrombosis has been established. For acute thrombi intravenous therapy is prescribed for 72 hours. It is important to underline that gynecologic surgery within the preceding 10 days is a relative contraindication to the use of these agents.

Pulmonary Embolus

The accurate diagnosis of pulmonary embolus is essential for the prevention of morbidity from lack of treatment or from unnecessary anticoagulation therapy. Autopsy studies have documented that pulmonary emboli are undiagnosed clinically in approximately 50% of women who experience this complication. Approximately 10% of women with a pulmonary embolus die within the first hour. The mortality of women with correctly diagnosed and treated pulmonary emboli is 8%, in contrast to approximately 30% if the disease is not treated. Most pulmonary emboli in gynecologic patients originate from thrombi in the pelvic and femoral veins. Predisposing risk factors are found in the majority of women with pulmonary embolus. Anticoagulation therapy is also dangerous, so there is the associated risk of heparin treatment if a false-positive diagnosis is made. Heparin is the leading cause of drug-related deaths in hospitalized patients.

No combination of symptoms or signs is pathognomonic for pulmonary embolus, and many patients are asymptomatic. The signs and symptoms of pulmonary embolus are nonspecific, and similar symptoms are caused by many other forms of cardiorespiratory disease. Common conditions considered in the differential diagnosis of pulmonary embolism include pneumonia, cardiac failure, atelectasis, aspiration, acute respiratory distress syndrome, and sepsis. However, they do alert the physician to the possibility of a pulmonary embolus, thus allowing a proper diagnostic workup to establish or rule out the disease. A national study of 327 patients with an angiographically proven pulmonary embolus found that chest pain, dyspnea, and apprehension are the most common symptoms. The dyspnea is often of abrupt onset. The classical triad of shortness of breath, chest pain, and hemoptysis is seen in less than 20% of women with proven pulmonary embolus. Tachypnea, rales, and an increase in the second heart sound over the pulmonic area are the most frequently found signs of pulmonary emboli (Table 25-8). Approximately 15% of women with pulmonary emboli have an unexplained low grade fever associated with a pulmonary embolus. A high fever is rarely associated with a pulmonary embolus but definitely may occur. The clinical manifestations of pulmonary embolus are produced primarily by occlusion of the large branches of the pulmonary arteries by embolic material. Pathophysiologically, associated reflex bronchial constriction and vasocon-

striction intensify the symptomatology. More than 50% of clinically recognized pulmonary emboli are multiple. The most frequent location of pulmonary emboli is in the lower lobes of the right lung. Shock and syncope are associated with massive pulmonary emboli.

Routine laboratory data, such as electrocardiograms (ECGs), chest x-ray films, and blood gas analyses, are important because they may contribute to the overall clinical impression, but individually or collectively they are not diagnostic. Less than 15% of ECGs demonstrate significant changes with a pulmonary embolus. Diminished pulmonary vascular markings may be a suspicious finding on a chest film. In the final analysis, imaging studies are of central importance in confirming the diagnosis of pulmonary embolus. However, the chest x-ray film may be helpful in the differential diagnosis by demonstrating other pulmonary complications, and the ECG helps to differentiate the symptom complex from myocardial infarction. The most common findings on chest x-ray examination with a pulmonary embolus are infiltrate, pleural effusion, atelectasis, and enlargement of the heart and/or descending pulmonary artery, although these findings are nonspecific. The majority of women with pulmonary emboli demonstrate hypoxemia on blood gas determinations, but as with other routine tests, these findings do not occur invariably. The rapid measurement of plasma D-Dimer levels is useful in screening women with a suspected pulmonary embolus. There is no need to perform pulmonary angiography when the concentration of D-Dimer is below the cut-off levels (less than 500 ng/ml) and the clinical suspicion is low. The

---

TABLE 25-8
Symptoms and Signs of Pulmonary Embolus

	Patients with Finding (%)
Symptoms	
Predisposing factors*	94
Dyspnea	84
Pleuritic chest pain	74
Apprehension	59
Cough	53
Hemoptysis	30
Syncope	14
Signs	
Tachypnea	92
Rales	58
Accentuation of pulmonic valve closure	53
Tachycardia	44
Cyanosis	20

From Blinder RA and Coleman RE: Radiol Clin North Am 23:392, 1985. Data from the Urokinase Pulmonary Embolism Trial—a national cooperative study, Circulation 47 (suppl II):1, 1973.

*Prolonged immobilization, postoperative state, congestive heart failure, carcinomatosis, and so on.

negative predictive value is 99% in women with a combination of a low pretest probability of pulmonary embolus and a normal D-Dimer. The clinician should appreciate that the units of value for the D-Dimer test have widely divergent sensitivities, specificities, and negative predictive values because many different D-Dimer tests are used. A negative D-Dimer test in women with cancer does not reliably exclude venous thrombosis and/or pulmonary embolus because the negative predictive value of the test is lower in women with cancer.

The first step in imaging techniques to establish or exclude the diagnosis of pulmonary embolus is a ventilation/perfusion lung scan. This test is safe and relatively easy to perform. The scan involves the injection of small radiocolloid particles into the circulation. They are trapped in small vessels, and their distribution depends on regional pulmonary blood flow. Ventilation scintigraphy uses radionuclides of technetium aerosol or xenon gas. The combination of lack of symmetry and a mismatch in the ventilation scan is the abnormality that leads to the diagnosis. The results of the ventilation/perfusion scan constitute the critical point in the differential diagnosis. However, the clinician should not place an overreliance on the ability of the ventilation/perfusion scan as a single test to diagnose a pulmonary embolus. In patients with a suspected pulmonary embolus, 40% will have a normal scan. A normal result effectively rules out the diagnosis of pulmonary embolus.

The results of 933 patients involved in the multicenter Prospective Investigation of Pulmonary Embolism Diagnosis (PIOPED) have been published. This report found that 4% of patients with normal or near-normal perfusion lung scans subsequently were discovered to have pulmonary emboli. This study emphasized a high sensitivity of 98% but a low specificity of 10% for ventilation/perfusion scans in the diagnosis of pulmonary embolus. The authors pointed out that almost all patients with acute pulmonary embolus had abnormal scans, but so did most patients without emboli. Therefore Bone has suggested the algorithm shown in Figure 25-8 for the diagnostic evaluation and management of a patient with pulmonary embolism.

Ventilation/perfusion scans have a high sensitivity but a variable specificity for the diagnosis of pulmonary embolism. For example, other cardiorespiratory diseases such as asthma may result in regional areas of decreased perfusion. If the scan documents multiple segments or lobar perfusion defects with a ventilation mismatch, the probability of pulmonary emboli is greater than 85%. Treatment is indicated without further imaging studies. However, ventilation/perfusion scans with less extensive perfusion abnormalities or matching ventilation defects do not reliably exclude the diagnosis of pulmonary embolus. McBride et al. studied 150 patients with clinically suspected pulmonary emboli, 56 of whom had pulmonary embolus documented by angiography. The presence or absence of pulmonary emboli could not be confidently predicted by ventilation/perfusion scans in the majority of patients (Table 25-9). Recently the Prospective Investigative Study of Acute Pulmonary Embolism Diagnosis reported angiography was required in only 21% of the patients when the perfusion scan was interpreted by the clinician in charge of the clinical assessment.

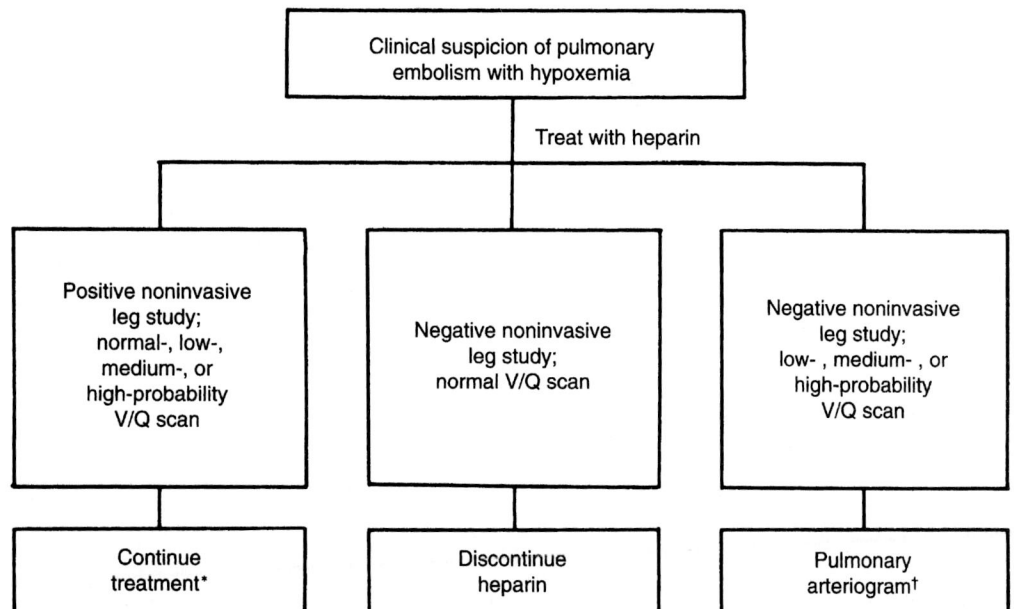

FIGURE 25-8 Algorithm for diagnostic evaluation of pulmonary embolus. Asterisk (*) indicates that treatment should be continued only if high-quality, noninvasive leg study can be performed. If one doubts quality of noninvasive study, venogram should be done. Dagger (†) indicates that, in selected patients with highly suspected pulmonary embolus (e.g., those with previously documented embolus), high-probability ventilation/perfusion (V/Q) scan might be accepted as proof of pulmonary embolus without angiogram. (Redrawn from Bone RC: JAMA 263:2794, 1990.)

TABLE 25-9
Ventilation/Perfusion Scans and Pulmonary Angiograms in the Diagnosis of Pulmonary Embolus

Ventilation/ Perfusion Scan Result	No. of Patients	Angiogram Result, No. of Patients (%)	
		Positive	Negative
Normal	7	0 (0)	7 (100)
Low probability	44	6 (13.6)	38 (86.4)
Indeterminate	38	7 (18.4)	31 (81.6)
Moderate probability	40	25 (62.5)	15 (37.5)
High probability	21	18 (85.7)	3 (14.3)
TOTAL	150	56	94

From McBride K, LaMorte, WW, and Menzoian JO: Arch Surg 121:755, 1986. Copyright 1986, American Medical Association.

Recently, radiologists have been enthusiastic about the use of helical computer tomography, sometimes called spiral computer tomography, as one of the initial screening tests for the diagnosis of a woman with a suspected pulmonary embolism. In helical CT scans, imaging of the pulmonary vessels is facilitated by the use of intravenous contrast media. The procedure is minimally invasive and provides a volumetric two-dimensional image of the lung by rotating the detector at a constant rate around the woman. A recent meta-analysis by Rathbun et al. concludes that to date the sensitivity and specificity of using helical computer tomography in the diagnosis of pulmonary embolism has not been adequately evaluated. Most importantly, the safety of withholding anticoagulation treatment in women with a negative study is controversial and uncertain.

Pulmonary angiography is the gold standard—the most definitive test presently available—to detect pulmonary emboli. This test is not ordered routinely because of the potential morbidity (hypotension and cardiac dysrhythmias) and risk of death associated with its use. Most deaths are directly related to pulmonary hypertension and right ventricular dysfunction. Approximately 5% of patients experience complications from this test, and the mortality is approximately 2 per 1000. The clinician must balance the risk of pulmonary angiography with the risk of anticoagulation in the individual patient. The significance of this imaging technique is unquestioned if one accepts intraluminal filling defects for the definitive diagnosis of pulmonary embolus. A series of 960 patients yielded only two false-positive tests. Digital subtraction pulmonary angiography and radiolabeled platelet scanning are promising but still experimental imaging techniques. Echocardiography, Doppler ultrasonography, and MRI are complementary diagnostic techniques that may identify differences in regional pulmonary blood flow.

The management of the vast majority of women with pulmonary emboli is by full-dose intravenous heparin therapy, similar to the management of deep vein thrombophlebitis (Figure 25-9). Prompt and early therapy with heparin provides anticoagulation and heparin also inhibits the release of serotonin from platelets. Potentially, this results in a decrease in the associated bronchoconstriction. Recently, more women are being treated with thrombolytic therapy (streptokinase-urokinase) or recombinant human tissue–type plasminogen activator. The time window for effective use of thrombolysis has been expanded with initiation of therapy as late as 14 days following the initial symptoms or signs of a pulmonary embolus. Thrombolytic therapy works by transforming plasminogen to plasmin. Use of thrombolytic therapy during the early postoperative period is a subject of great debate because of the increased risk of serious hemorrhage. Goldhaber et al. completed a randomized controlled study comparing urokinase and the new recombinant human tissue–type plasminogen activator. The latter was found to act more rapidly and to be safer than urokinase. Thrombolytic therapy is the method of choice in patients with massive pulmonary emboli (angiographically, greater than 50% obstruction of the pulmonary arterial bed) with associated moderate to severe hemodynamic embarrassment, lobular obstruction, or multiple segmental profusion defects. Random trials of heparin versus thrombolytic therapy have shown that emboli clear more rapidly with initial thrombolytic therapy. A thrombolytic agent is infused intravenously for the first 12 to 24 hours, and heparin therapy is continued for 7 to 10 days. The clinical assumption is that approximately 7 days are needed for the intravascular venous thrombus to become firmly attached to the vein's side wall. All patients with pulmonary emboli should have warfarin therapy after heparin treatment for 3 to 6 months. The risk of a woman developing a subsequent fatal pulmonary embolus during the 3 months of anticoagulation therapy is approximately 1 in 70 to 1 in 100. Recently, there has been increasing emphasis on treating pulmonary emboli with low-molecular–weight heparins. The most widely accepted indication for vena cava filters is failure of medical management or a contraindication to heparin therapy. Approximately 35% of vena cava filters are placed for prophylactic indications. A recent randomized trial reported by Decousos et al. compared vena cava filters to low-molecular–weight or unfractionated heparin. They concluded the initial beneficial effect of vena cava filters for the prevention of pulmonary embolus was counterbalanced by an excess of recurrent deep venous thrombosis without any difference in mortality rates. Treatment of a massive pulmonary embolus in an unstable patient involves a choice of thrombolytic therapy, pulmonary artery embolectomy, transvenous catheter embolectomy, and/or filter placement in the inferior vena cava.

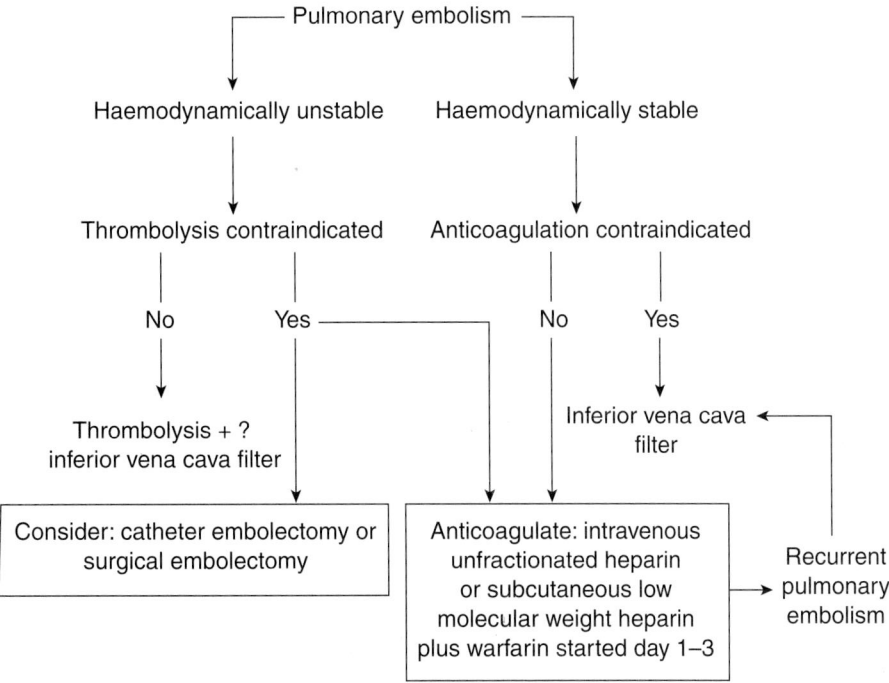

FIGURE 25-9 Treatment of pulmonary embolism. (From Tai MRM, Atwal AS, and Hamilton G: Modern management of pulmonary embolism, Br J Surg 86:853, 1999.)

URINARY TRACT PROBLEMS

Inability to Void

Many women experience an inability to void or an incomplete emptying of the bladder during the postoperative period. Inability to void is more frequent and lasts longer after an operation that involves the urethra or bladder neck. The etiology of postoperative voiding problems is complex. The major pathophysiologic change is the direct trauma and edema produced by the surgical procedure in the perivesical tissues. Other factors that contribute include the potential of overdistention from excessive hydration and dysynchronous contractions from the bladder neck. The differential diagnosis includes anxiety, mechanical interference, obstruction by swelling and edema, neurologic imbalance, and drug-associated detrusor hypotonia.

The woman's initial attempts at voiding should be made in a sitting position. Obviously, privacy is important to minimize performance anxiety. It is best not to remove the Foley catheter until the patient is ambulatory. Most women have difficulty in completely emptying their bladder either on a bedpan or in a semirecumbent position during the first 24 hours following abdominal hysterectomy. Catheter drainage keeps the bladder at rest and avoids acute bladder distention with resulting detrusor dysfunction and possibly retrograde reflux of urine. The age-old tradition of intermittent clamping and releasing of the Foley catheter to regain bladder tone is often counterproductive. We do not believe in this technique. It is not based on sound physiologic principles and overdistention is a possibility, which would compound voiding difficulties. There is no evidence to support the outdated practice of gradual emptying of the distended urinary bladder. The optimal management of urinary retention is quick, complete emptying.

Most problems with voiding resolve without medication and with time. If mechanical obstruction is not suspected to be a major factor, intermittent straight catheterization is indicated. This will result in a lower incidence of urinary tract infection and a more rapid return to normal function than periodic replacement and removal of a Foley catheter for the evaluation of residual urine volume. Although bacteriuria occurs secondary to intermittent catheterization, development of pyelonephritis is rare unless the patient has concomitant vesicoureteral reflux. Bacteriuria may occur with ever greater incidence with indwelling catheters. Most women prefer self-catheterization. They especially appreciate intermittent self-catheterization because it gives them control over a part of their postoperative care.

Rarely, medications may be given to patients who experience prolonged periods of inability to void. Reflex urethral spasm is common after plastic surgery to repair an enterocele or rectocele. Urethral spasm may be diminished by an alpha-adrenergic receptor blocking agent, phenoxybenzamine (Dibenzyline), in a dosage of 10 mg every

8 hours. However, hypotension is commonly associated with this drug. Bladder hypotonia may occur as a result of overdistention, prolonged inactivity, or use of medications such as beta-blockers. Bladder hypotonia may be treated with bethanechol (Urecholine) in a dosage of 25 to 50 mg every 8 hours. Urecholine effectively produces detrusor contractions. This medication is prescribed rarely. Recent studies have investigated the use of prostaglandins, both intravaginal and intravesical, to promote more rapid return to normal bladder function.

Infection

The most commonly acquired infection in the hospital and the most frequent cause of gram-negative bacteremia in hospitalized patients is catheter-associated urinary tract infection. Approximately 40% of nosocomial infections are urinary tract infections, and 60% of these are directly related to an indwelling urethral catheter. One percent of patients with infections from bladder catheters will develop bacteremia. However, patients without catheters may develop overdistention and bladder atony as a result of postoperative pain. Overdistention produces a temporary paralysis of the detrusor activity that may take several days to resolve. The atonic bladder is also prone to urinary tract infection. Thus, after a gynecologic operation, the patient is susceptible to urinary tract infection either with or without a catheter in place.

The normal uroepithelium inhibits adherence of surface bacteria to the walls of the urethra and bladder. A bladder catheter disrupts this property, and surface bacteria are able to colonize the lower urinary tract. Additionally, bacteria form a sheet or biofilm of microorganisms and bacterial bioproducts that adheres to the catheter. These biofilms protect bacteria from antibiotics. This characteristic of biofilms explains why antibiotic suppression is ineffective for patients with chronic catheterization and why replacement of a catheter is necessary in the treatment of systemic infection secondary to a colonized urinary tract. The incidence of a positive culture increases dramatically with

time. After a Foley catheter has been in place for 36 hours, approximately 20% of women have bacterial colonization, and after 72 hours, more than 75% have positive cultures. If the catheter drains into an open system for longer than 96 hours, 100% develop bacteriuria. Women with an indwelling catheter in place with a closed drainage system develop urinary tract infections at the rate of approximately 5% per 24 hours; this increases to 50% of women after 7 days of continuous catheterization.

Catheter-related urinary tract infections are related to the patient's age. In one study, 30% of women over age 50 developed an infection, compared with 16% of those postoperative women younger than age 50. Diabetes increased the incidence of catheter-related urinary tract infections threefold. The incidence of infection is directly related to the length of time the catheter is in place. Daifuku and Stamm performed a series of cultures and documented that rectal or urethral colonization precedes lower urinary tract infection by 24 to 48 hours (Table 25-10). The incidence of a positive urine culture after a single in-and-out catheterization is approximately 1%.

Sterile technique used during insertion, strict aseptic catheter care, and maintenance of a closed drainage system are all important steps to reduce the incidence of infection through reduced colonization. Bacteria ascend from the exterior to the bladder either via the lumen of the catheter or around the outside of the catheter. A recent meta-analysis by Saint et al. discovered that silver alloy–coated urinary catheters are significantly more effective in preventing urinary tract infection than are silver oxide catheters. The silver alloy–coated catheters cost approximately $6 more than standard Foley catheters. However, they reduce nosocomial urinary tract infection by approximately 50%. A sterile, closed drainage system is another prophylactic measure to reduce the incidence of urinary tract infections. In one study, strict closed drainage reduced the rate of infection from 80% to 23%. Studies have documented a lower risk of infection with a suprapubic, transabdominal urinary catheter. The latter technique also decreases patient discomfort and permits earlier spon-

TABLE 25-10
Occurrence of Antecedent Urethral or Rectal Bacterial Colonization in Patients with Catheter-Associated Urinary Tract Infections

	Women		Men	
	Urethral Colonization	Rectal Colonization	Urethral Colonization	Rectal Colonization
Gram-positive cocci	4/5	5/5	3/12	2/12
Gram-negative rods	6/9	7/9	1/4	3/4
Candida	2/4	2/4	1/1	0/1
All microorganisms	12/18	14/18	5/17	5/17

From Daifuku R and Stamm WE: JAMA 252:2029, 1984. Copyright 1984, American Medical Association.

taneous voiding. Systemic prophylactic antibiotics exert a short-term effect, decreasing the initial incidence of infection. However, the negative effect of prophylactic antibiotics is an increased emergence of antibiotic-resistant bacteria. Therefore prophylactic antibiotics are not used to "cover a catheter" except in immunocompromised patients. With catheterization for longer than 3 weeks, all patients have bacterial colonization regardless of the use of prophylactic antibiotics and a closed system.

The symptoms of urinary tract infection usually develop 24 to 48 hours after the Foley catheter is removed. Of interest, the signs and symptoms associated with a catheter-acquired lower urinary tract infection are not nearly as pronounced or as specific as those associated with cystitis unrelated to catheter use. Patients with lower urinary tract infections usually do not have fever but experience urinary frequency and mild dysuria, which are difficult to distinguish from normal postoperative discomfort. Women with upper urinary tract infections usually have a high fever, chills, and flank pain. If urinary tract symptoms persist after appropriate antibiotic therapy, one should obtain an intravenous pyelogram to evaluate the possibility of obstruction in the urinary tract. Obstruction of the ureter without associated infection may be asymptomatic or produce only mild flank tenderness. No appreciable change will be noted in urinary output with an isolated unilateral ureteral obstruction.

The diagnosis of urinary tract infection is established by urinalysis and urine culture. It is important to identify white blood cells and bacteria with the microscope. However, women with high-volume urine outputs may demonstrate minimal findings on urinalysis but have a positive urine culture. Stark and Maki have emphasized that a bacterial concentration of 10^2 organisms per milliliter in a catheterized specimen is significant. In their studies more than 95% of patients with 10^2 colony-forming units per milliliter subsequently developed the standard criterion of infection, which is 100,000 colonies per milliliter for a midstream culture.

We recommend a minimum of 3 days of antibiotic therapy for a woman who has developed cystitis after catheter use. One-day, single-dose antibiotic treatment is no longer considered an effective treatment for urinary tract infection.

To reduce the incidence of urinary tract infection, the Foley catheter should be used judiciously. When possible, use of a suprapubic catheter or intermittent in-and-out catheterization is preferable to continuous drainage with a Foley catheter. If a Foley catheter is used, retrograde flow of urine from the bag to the bladder during ambulation should be avoided. Preventive measures, such as aseptic care of the catheter and a closed, sterile drainage system, are also important. Modern practice is not to treat catheter-associated urinary tract infections unless the patient becomes febrile. If signs and symptoms of infection occur with a Foley in place, the woman should be

treated with systemic antibiotic therapy for 10 days. Prophylactic antibiotics are not used unless the patient is immunosuppressed, for they often result in a urinary tract infection with a *Proteus* or *Pseudomonas* species rather than the more common *Escherichia coli*.

Urinary Fistula

Vesicovaginal and ureterovaginal fistulas are infrequent yet troublesome complications of operations for benign gynecologic conditions. In the United States, gynecologic operations are found to be the cause of approximately 75% of urinary tract fistulas. Surprisingly, it is not the difficult cancer operation but rather the simple total abdominal hysterectomy for benign disease, such as myomas or abnormal bleeding, that is the most frequently associated with this complication. Fistulas following gynecologic operations are secondary to abdominal hysterectomy in 75% of cases and to vaginal operations in the remaining 25%. The exact incidence of injury to the ureter associated with gynecologic operations is unknown because many patients do not exhibit symptoms. However, it has been estimated that ureteral injury occurs as frequently as 1 per 200 abdominal hysterectomies. The ratio of injuries to the urinary bladder to ureteral injuries is approximately 5:1.

The classic clinical symptom of a urinary tract fistula is the painless and almost continuous loss of urine, usually from the vagina. On occasion the uncontrolled loss of urine is not continuous but may be related to change in position or posture. When urine loss is intermittent and related to position, one should suspect a ureterovaginal rather than vesicovaginal fistula. Urinary incontinence may be present within a few hours of the operative procedure. This symptom is secondary to a direct surgical injury to the bladder or ureter that was not appreciated during the operative procedure. The majority of fistulas become symptomatic 8 to 12 days and occasionally as late as 25 to 30 days after the operation. Occlusion of the blood supply from clamping or figure-of-8 sutures produces avascular necrosis and subsequent sloughing of the urogenital tissue. Pelvic examination often reveals a small reddened area of granulation tissue at the site of the fistula. In a review of unilateral ureteral obstruction secondary to gynecologic surgery, Stanhope et al. noted a mean increase of only 0.8 mg/dl in serum creatinine. The differential diagnosis of a ureterovaginal fistula includes spontaneous loss of peritoneal fluid or serosanguineous fluid from the retroperitoneal space.

A small fistula may be localized by placing a tampon in the vagina and instilling a dilute solution of methylene blue dye into the urinary bladder. This will also help differentiate between a vesicovaginal fistula and a ureterovaginal fistula. If the blue coloring is discovered on the tampon, then a defect in the bladder should be suspected. If the tampon is not colored, 3 to 5 ml of indigo carmine should be injected intravenously. The subsequent finding of blue coloring on the tampon is presumptive evidence of a ureterovaginal fistula. An intravenous pyelogram or enhanced CT scan should be obtained in either case to detect obstruction of the ureter and diagnose compound (ureter and bladder) fistulas.

As with most other postoperative complications, preventive medicine is paramount. Optimum operative technique should emphasize the standard axioms in the prevention of urinary tract injury. The patient should have an empty bladder, and the physician should obtain adequate exposure of the site. Sharp dissection should be made along tissue planes with proper traction and countertraction. When operating near the bladder or ureter, bleeding vessels should be ligated individually rather than with random clamping of tissue. If possible, the ureter should not be completely detached from the overlying peritonium. With extensive dissection of the periureteral tissue, care should be taken to avoid interference with the longitudinal vascular supply of the ureter. In the most difficult cases where anatomic landmarks are obscure, opening of the dome of the bladder and palpation with the index finger and thumb may help to identify the proper surgical plane. The urinary system, especially the bladder, is very "forgiving" if given a short period of rest to recover. If trauma to the bladder is suspected, continuous catheter drainage for 3 to 5 days usually results in spontaneous healing. A recent meta-analysis by Gilmore et al. reported the frequency of lower urinary tract injuries following gynecologic surgery. The overall frequency of ureteral and bladder injury was fourfold higher in the 8 studies that involved routine cystoscopy during major gynecologic operations than the 22 reports that did not involve the use of routine cystoscopy. The authors postulated that routine intraoperative cystoscopy would discover approximately 90% of unsuspected ureteral injuries and 85% of unsuspected bladder injuries. Obviously, a more conservative option is performing selective cystoscopy electively following complicated or difficult operative procedures when the gynecologist wonders whether or not the integrity of the lower urinary tract has been compromised.

When leakage from the urinary tract is first discovered, the bladder should be drained with a large-bore Foley catheter. Ureteral injuries should be treated with retrograde ureteral catheters. Approximately 20% of bladder injuries and 30% of ureteral injuries heal spontaneously without further operations. In these cases, splinting of the urinary tract facilitates healing of the defect before epithelization of the aberrant tract occurs, which would result in a true fistula. Spontaneous healing usually occurs within the first 4 weeks. With a ureteral fistula, follow-up intravenous pyelograms should be ordered at 3, 6, and 12 months to detect delayed ureteral strictures.

Unless the diagnosis is made in the immediate perioperative period, operative repair should usually be delayed 2 to 3 months after the initial injury to obtain optimum

results. The workup of a patient before operative repair of a vesicovaginal fistula includes intravenous pyelography, cystoscopy, and biopsy of the fistula's margins if carcinoma is suspected. Cystoscopy is mandatory and should be performed for two reasons: to establish that edema and inflammation have subsided around the fistulous tract and to establish the relationship of the fistulous tract to the trigone of the bladder, especially the ureteral orifices. Occasionally, repair of a fistula near the ureteral orifice compromises the ureter, and the ureter must be reimplanted into the bladder.

Operative repair of a vesicovaginal fistula is usually accomplished via a multilayered closure performed by the vaginal route. The principles for a successful operation include adequate exposure, dissection and mobilization of each tissue layer; excision of the fistulous tract; closure of each layer without tension on the suture line; and excellent hemostasis with closure of the dead space. Reliable bladder drainage is provided to avoid tension on the suture line for approximately 10 days. Latzko's operation is the simplest means of repairing a fistula at the vaginal apex. This technique of partial colpocleisis involves denudation of the vaginal mucosa surrounding the fistula and subsequent multilayer closure without entering the bladder. The primary disadvantage of the procedure is postoperative shortening of the vagina.

Many ureteral injuries discovered during the immediate postoperative period will heal when treated by percutaneous nephrostomy and ureteral catheters. Ureterovaginal fistulas that do not heal spontaneously are usually repaired 2 to 3 months after the original operation. The surgeon has several choices as to the operative technique. However, most persistent ureterovaginal fistulas involving the lower third of the ureter are repaired by reimplanting the ureter into the bladder.

GASTROINTESTINAL COMPLICATIONS

Nausea

Minor disturbances in gastrointestinal function are a normal consequence of anesthesia. The woman may experience nausea for approximately 12 hours, pass flatus some time during the first 48 hours, and have a spontaneous bowel movement by the third or fourth postoperative day.

Approximately 25% of adult women experience postoperative nausea and vomiting. Several factors affect the likelihood and severity of postoperative nausea, including preoperative anxiety, decreased threshold for nausea and vomiting, previous history of postoperative nausea and vomiting, duration of surgery, the type and drugs used for anesthesia, obesity, and postoperative pain medications. Certain preventive measures may be used to minimize postoperative nausea and vomiting including adequate hydration, minimizing use of narcotics and inhalation agents, avoiding nitrous oxide, the choice of regional anesthesia, and avoiding excessive movement in the immediate postoperative period. Many physicians, including anesthesiologists and gynecologists, selectively give medications prophylactically for women at high risk. Drugs commonly available for the prevention and treatment of postoperative nausea and vomiting include droperidol, metoclopramide, phenothiazines, and 5-HT$_3$ antagonists such as ondansedron and granisetron. The choice of the most appropriate drug depends on its cost and side effects.

Ileus

Ileus is an inhibition of the normal propulsive reflexes of the bowel that are regulated by the autonomic nervous system. Adynamic (paralytic) ileus is a normal event defined as an ileus of minor to moderate degree. It may be expected to follow any intraperitoneal or pelvic operation. An uncomplicated ileus may last 24 to 48 hours in the stomach, only a few hours in the small intestines, and 48 to 72 hours in the colon. The incidence and duration of adynamic ileus are less following vaginal hysterectomy than with abdominal hysterectomy. If adynamic ileus persists longer than 5 days, a diagnosis of mechanical bowel obstruction should be strongly considered. However, most gynecologists ignore the age-old surgical axiom of delaying postoperative oral feeding until spontaneous resolution of gastrointestinal dysfunction is demonstrated by the passage of flatus or a spontaneous bowel movement. Multiple recent articles reported that early postoperative oral feeding is safe and efficacious. This practice is preferred by women because it facilitates their recovery and shortens the hospital stay. The leading negative finding in randomized trials is an isolated increased incidence of nausea in the early postoperative feeding group. Obviously, the greatest risks associated with early feeding are vomiting and aspiration. Thus one should individualize postoperative orders depending on the woman's age and amount of sedation.

Adynamic ileus is believed to result from a lack of coordinated motor activity of the intestine, which results in disorganized, propulsive activity. Electrical activity is present, but the pathophysiologic problem is continuous activity of the intrinsic inhibitor neurons in the wall of the small intestine. Usually the process is generalized, but occasionally it may be localized, involving only an isolated loop of small intestine. The pathophysiology of severe postoperative ileus is a subject of great debate. Some speculate that the combination of abdominal and pelvic pain activates a reflex arc of the autonomic nervous system that inhibits motility of the intestines.

The classic symptoms of a prolonged ileus include absence of flatus, abdominal distention, and obstipation. Often these symptoms are associated with nausea and effortless vomiting. Bowel sounds may be hypoactive or absent. This condition may be associated with abdominal tenderness, and the abdomen is usually tympanic to percussion. Nausea and vomiting persisting longer than 24 hours after operation constitute cause for concern. The difference between small bowel obstruction and adynamic ileus is a subtle one, for adynamic ileus is normally associated with partial obstruction of the small intestine.

Diagnostic films of the abdomen (supine, erect, and lateral) help to establish the correct diagnosis (Table 25-11). In a woman with adynamic ileus, the intestinal gas is scattered throughout the gastrointestinal tract, including the small intestine and colon. Air-fluid levels, if present, tend to be at the same level. In a small series, Frager et al. found CT to be sensitive and specific in differentiating adynamic ileus from complete obstruction and helpful in differentiating ileus from partial obstruction.

Oral administration of radiocontrast material may be both a therapeutic and diagnostic test. The osmolality of the radiocontrast material is approximately 6 times greater than that of normal saline. Thus a large amount of fluid enters the small bowel and acts as a direct stimulant of peristalsis. In one study after preliminary abdominal films were obtained, 120 ml of 66% diatrizoate meglumine, 10% diatrizoate sodium (Gastrografin) was administered orally or via nasogastric tube. Passage of liquid stool occurred within a few hours in patients with adynamic ileus (Table 25-12). Gastrografin, unlike barium, is nontoxic if it accidentally contaminates the peritoneal cavity during an operation for bowel obstruction. In a different study, Finan et al. gave gastrografin on the third postoperative day to 57 women with ileus. These women were

---

TABLE 25-11

Differential Radiographic Findings in Ileus and Mechanical Obstruction

Adynamic Ileus	Mechanical Obstruction
Small and large bowel are distended in proportion to each other	In small-bowel obstruction there is dilated small bowel proximal to site of obstruction: in colonic obstruction the colon is distended and small-bowel distention is present with incompetent ileocecal valve
Air-fluid levels in small bowel are infrequent; when present, they are at the same levels	Air-fluid levels are common and at different levels in the bowel
Quantitative difference in small-bowel distention	Greater small-bowel distention than with ileus
Small-bowel distention in central part of abdomen with colon in periphery	Small-bowel distention present in central part of abdomen; no peripheral large-bowel distention

From Buchsbaum HJ and Mazer J: The gastrointestinal tract. In Buchsbaum HJ and Walton LA, editors: Strategies in gynecologic surgery, New York, 1986, Springer-Verlag New York, Inc, p 100.

TABLE 25-12
Study of 47 Cases of Adynamic Ileus Treated with Ingestion of Contrast Material

	Average	Range
Interim from operation to time of study	4.2 days	2–14 days
Approximate duration of ileus	35 hours	12–96 hours
Transit time from ingestion to large bowel	3 hours 20 minutes	25 minutes–6 hours
Transit time from ingestion to first stool	6 hours 20 minutes	1–18 hours
Duration of hospitalization after study	3.8 days	1–8 days
Obstetric-gynecologic patients	2.8 days	1–7 days

From Watkins DT and Robertson CL: Am J Obstet Gynecol 152:451, 1985.

compared with 58 women with ileus who received rectal suppositories. The investigators found no difference in the mean time of return of bowel function between the two groups of women.

Severe adynamic ileus is a self-limiting condition that responds to gastrointestinal rest and time. During the period of watchful expectancy, adequate fluid and electrolyte replacement is necessary. Patients experience mild cramping and passage of flatus and regain their appetite with the return of normal peristalsis. If adequate bowel sounds are present, a rectal tube, Fleet's enema, or rectal suppository may facilitate the initial passage of flatus. Some advocate the routine postoperative administration of a wetting agent, such as simethicone (Mylicon), to reduce surface tension of intestinal mucus and liberate entrapped gas. Opinions are mixed as to whether such an agent reduces the incidence or intensity of adynamic ileus.

Severe cases of adynamic ileus should be treated with intravenous fluids and, if they do not resolve, with nasogastric suctioning. Nasogastric suction prevents progression of the intestinal distention. During periods when nasogastric suctioning is used, special attention should be given to correct replacement of fluid and electrolytes (Tables 25-13 and 25-14). A rare but worrisome complication of prolonged ileus is massive dilation of the cecum. Massive dilatation of the colon related to a pseudo-obstruction produced by severe adynamic ileus in the absence of mechanical obstruction is known as Ogilive's syndrome. This condition may be treated medically by evacuating the air with colonoscopy. An alternative method of treating this condition was recently reported by Ponec et al. The authors demonstrated excellent decompression following 2.0 mg of neostigmine intravenously.

TABLE 25-13
Average Daily Volume and Electrolyte Concentrations of Gastrointestinal Secretions

	Volume (ml/day)	Electrolyte Concentrations (mEq/L)		
		Na+	K+	Cl−
Saliva	1000–1500	10–40	10–20	6–30
Gastric juice	2000–2500	60–120	10–20	10–30
Hepatic bile	600–800	130–155	2–12	80–100
Pancreatic juice	700–1000	150–155	5–10	30–50
Duodenal secretions	300–800	90–140	2–10	70–120
Jejunal and ileal secretions	2000–3000	125–140	5–10	100–130
Colonic mucosal secretions	200–500	140–148	5–10	60–90
TOTAL	8000–10,000			

From Buchsbaum HJ and Mazer J: The gastrointestinal tract. In Buchsbaum HJ and Walton LA, editors: Strategies in gynecologic surgery, New York, 1986, Springer-Verlag New York, Inc, p 103.

TABLE 25-14
Composition of Intravenous Solutions

Solutions	Glucose (g/L)	Na	Cl	HCO$_3$	K	Ca	Mg	HPO$_4$	NH$_4$
					(mEq/L)				
Extracellular fluid	1000	140	102	27	4.2	5	3	0.3	
5% Dextrose and water	50								
10% Dextrose and water	100								
0.9% Sodium chloride (normal saline)		154	154						
0.45% Sodium chloride (half-normal saline)		77	77						
0.21% Sodium chloride (1/4 normal saline)		34	34						
3% Sodium chloride (hypertonic saline)		513	513						
Lactated Ringer's solution		130	109	28*	4	2.7			
0.9% Ammonium chloride		168							168

From Miller TA and Duke JH: Fluid and electrolyte management. In Dudrick SJ, Baue AE, Eiseman B, et al, editors: Manual of preoperative and postoperative care, ed 3, Philadelphia, 1983, WB Saunders Co, p 47.

*Present in solution as lactate but is metabolized to bicarbonate.

Intestinal Obstruction

Adhesions are the most common etiology of intestinal obstruction postoperatively. During subsequent operations greater than 90% of women are found to have some adhesions following abdominal laparotomy. In a large retrospective cohort study covering a 10-year period following laparotomy for gynecologic conditions, approximately 1 in 3 women had adhesion-related readmissions to the hospital. Less common causes of intestinal obstruction are hernias, mesenteric defects, intussusception, volvulus, and neoplasm. Large raw areas of the pelvis with hypoxic tissue facilitate the attachment of small intestine following pelvic operations. Previous gynecologic operations are the most common cause of small-bowel obstruction in women. The incidence of operation for obstruction of the small intestine after an abdominal hysterectomy is estimated to be approximately 2%. Interestingly, in one series, adhesions involving the pelvic peritoneum were responsible for the intestinal obstruction in 85% of cases, and adhesions to the closure of the anterior abdominal wall accounted for the other 15%. Fortunately the fibrous adhesions that form during the first 2 to 3 weeks after an operation are soft and filmy. Thus intestinal strangulation during the postoperative period is extremely rare. Dense adhesions may develop several months after an operation. The incidence of intestinal obstruction depends on the type of gynecologic operation performed. Approximately two women in 1000 develop an obstruction after a benign gynecologic operation, whereas approximately 8% develop intestinal obstruction after radical cancer operations. Intestinal obstruction occurs in the small intestine in approximately 80% of cases and in the colon in the remaining 20%. As mentioned previously, the differential diagnosis between bowel obstruction and ileus is a difficult one (Table 25-15).

The acute symptoms of intestinal obstruction present most commonly between the fifth and seventh postoperative day. The majority of patients have a short period of normal intestinal function before the onset of symptoms. Women with bowel obstruction appear to have more toxicity and more acute distress than do women with ileus. The abdominal pain is intermittent, colicky, and sharp in nature. Episodes of colicky pain usually lasts from 1 to 3 minutes. Associated symptoms include vomiting, abdominal distention, and constipation. Bowel sounds are loud, high pitched, and metallic. Occasionally they may be heard without a stethoscope. Nasogastric drainage is more profuse than in patients with severe adynamic ileus. A patient with a complete small-bowel obstruction may have a bowel movement, eliminating fecal material that already existed in the colon.

Abdominal x-ray films demonstrate a stepladder appearance—multiple air-fluid levels throughout the small intestine with an absence of gas in the colon and rectum. Pneumoperitoneum from an exploratory celiotomy usually persists for 7 to 10 days. Thus, in the early postoperative period, free air under the diaphragm is not diagnostic of perforation of a hollow viscus. Obstruction of the colon may be diagnosed by retrograde infusion of contrast material or by flexible endoscopy.

The foundation of early treatment of postoperative intestinal obstruction is decompression of the small intestine and adequate replacement of fluids and electrolytes. Decompression may be accomplished by means of a nasogastric tube or, preferably, a long tube (Miller-Abbott or Cantor tube). Serial monitoring of white blood cell counts with differentials should be performed. Repeat abdominal

TABLE 25-15
Differential Diagnosis Between Postoperative Ileus and Postoperative Obstruction

Clinical Features	Postoperative Ileus	Postoperative Obstruction
Abdominal pain	Discomfort from distention but not cramping pains	Cramping, progressively severe
Relationship to previous operation	Usually within 48–72 hours of operation	Usually delayed; may be 5–7 days for remote onset
Nausea and vomiting	Present	Present
Distention	Present	Present
Bowel sounds	Absent or hypoactive	Borborygmi with peristaltic rushes and high-pitched tinkles
Fever	Only if related to associated peritonitis	Rarely present unless bowel becomes gangrenous
Abdominal x-ray film	Distended loops of small and large bowels; gas usually present in colon	Single or multiple loops of distended bowel, usually small bowel with air-fluid levels
Treatment	Conservative with nasogastric suction, enemas, cholinergic stimulation	Partial: conservative with nasogastric decompression; or Complete: surgical

From Mattingly RF and Thompson JD, editors: Te Linde's operative gynecology, ed 6, Philadelphia, 1985, JB Lippincott Co, p 102.

x-ray examinations at regular intervals are used to assess the degree of intestinal distention. Expectant management is successful in many patients. In the series by Wolfson et al., less than 40% of 112 patients with small-bowel obstruction due to adhesions required operation. Conservative therapy was most successful in those patients in whom the long intestinal drainage tube was successfully advanced from the stomach into the small intestine.

The major cause of morbidity and death with bowel obstruction is delay in diagnosis with resultant strangulation and secondary sepsis. Women who develop strangulation experience a dramatic increase in the intensity of abdominal pain, and the pain becomes continuous. Strangulation of the small bowel is associated with localized peritoneal irritation, increase in temperature, and marked leukocytosis. Bowel obstruction may also lead to translocation of intestinal bacteria across the bowel wall, promoting sepsis. A series by Sagar et al. found that the more distal the obstruction, the greater the incidence of anaerobic septicemia.

Fecal impaction is most often seen in elderly patients. It results from loss of peristalsis in the colon, with an impaired perception of rectal fullness. Fecal impaction is a humiliating experience for the woman. She may have either diarrhea around the impaction or obstipation. Treatment involves obtaining partial analgesia with lidocaine jelly and, subsequently, manually fragmenting and extracting the fecal mass.

Rectovaginal Fistula

Rectovaginal fistulas and fecal incontinence secondary to perineal tears are most commonly obstetric complications and are only rarely associated with gynecologic opera-

tions. In general, rectovaginal fistulas following hysterectomy or repair of an enterocele are usually located in the upper third of the vagina, while those secondary to a posterior colporrhaphy are in the lower third of the vagina. Other causes of rectovaginal fistula are carcinoma, radiation therapy, perirectal abscess, inflammatory bowel disease, lymphogranuloma venereum, and trauma.

The initial signs and symptoms associated with potential fistulous tracts between the rectum and vagina usually present 7 to 14 days after an operation. The first warning may be the rectal passage of several blood clots, indicating that a hematoma has ruptured into the rectum. Distressing symptoms include passage of gas from the vagina and, depending on the size of the opening, the passage of fecal material from the vagina. Associated with these classic symptoms and signs are chronic, foul-smelling vaginal discharge and subsequent dyspareunia. Aside from the physical symptoms of the anatomic defect, fistulas cause severe emotional distress because they affect almost every aspect of the patient's daily life.

The diagnosis is not difficult to establish, and only very small openings present a diagnostic problem. What appears to be granulation tissue in the posterior aspect of the vagina is the dark-red rectal mucosa, which stands out in contrast to the lighter vaginal mucosa. Usually the defect may be successfully defined with a small, malleable metal probe. If this is not successful, a Foley catheter should be placed in the rectum. Methylene blue dye or milk may then be instilled into the rectum with a tampon in the vagina, similar to the procedure establishing the diagnosis of a vesicovaginal fistula.

For initial treatment the woman should be obstipated with a low-residue diet and diphenoxylate hydrochloride (Lomotil). Approximately one in four anatomic defects heals spontaneously before epithelialization of the tract. A low residual diet or hyperalimentation may be helpful to facilitate spontaneous closure of some anatomic defects.

Timing of the operative repair is important. The gynecologist should inspect the area surrounding the fistula to make sure that the tissues are free of edema, induration, and infection. Preoperative evaluation includes visualization of the entire vagina and sigmoidoscopy of the rectal mucosa attempting to discover more than one opening. A barium enema or flexible endoscopy is important if there is any suspicion of coexistence of Crohn's disease.

The operative technique employed depends on the size and location of the fistula. Standard operative principles include removal of the entire fistulous tract and closure of tissue layers without tension on the suture line. In the repair of large rectovaginal fistulas in the lower part of the vagina, it is usually easier to convert the rectovaginal fistula into a fourth-degree laceration. Diverting colostomy should be used for all radiation-induced fistulas, the majority of fistulas associated with inflammatory bowel disease, and some large postoperative fistulas at the apex of the vagina. The woman may be discharged from the hospital after the first bowel movement. The stool should be kept soft with low-residue diets and stool softeners such as mineral oil for the first 2 weeks after the operation.

Antibiotic-Associated Diarrheas

Patients may develop diarrhea in the postoperative period after exposure to antibiotics. The antibiotic therapy, either for prophylaxis or for treatment, can disrupt the normal intestinal flora. If the patient is afebrile, the diarrhea is mild, and the abdominal examination is unremarkable, then stopping or changing antibiotics and providing supportive care are all that is necessary. If the patient has a temperature greater than 38° C, a leukocytosis, abdominal tenderness, severe abdominal distention, bloody diarrhea, or persistent diarrhea, then evaluation for *Clostridium difficile* infection is indicated.

Clostridium difficile is a species of spore-forming, gram-positive anaerobic bacteria found normally in 5% of healthy adults. However, after antibiotic treatment and disruption of normal enteric flora, up to 25% of hospitalized adults will become colonized with *C. difficile.* The organism is spread by nosocomial oral/fecal contamination. Persistence of the spores of *C. difficile* and contamination of the environment are primary factors in cross infection. The organism after colonizing the intestine may secrete two toxins, which produce a spectrum of clinical disease. Symptoms from the infection are varied and range from a mild diarrhea to colitis to a pseudomembranous colitis that in rare cases may be fatal. Nearly all antibiotics have been associated with the development of

TABLE 25-16
Antimicrobial Agents That Induce *C. difficile*–Associated Diarrhea and Colitis

Frequent Induction	Infrequent Induction	Rare or No Induction
Ampicillin and amoxicillin	Tetracyclines Sulfonamides	Parenteral aminoglycosides
Cephalosporins	Erythromycin	Bacitracin
Clindamycin	Chloramphenicol	Metronidazole
	Trimethoprim	Vancomycin
	Quinolones	

From Kelly CP, Pothoulakis C, LaMont JT: N Engl J Med 330:257, 1994.

C. difficile diarrhea (Table 25-16). Second- and third-generation cephalosporins, clindamycin, ampicillin, and amoxicillin are the antibiotics associated with the highest risk of developing *C. difficile* diarrhea. Symptoms usually appear 5 to 10 days after the initiation of antibiotic therapy. However, they may appear from a few days to a few weeks after antibiotic exposure. Diagnostic tests include culture for the organism; *C. difficile* cell cytotoxin B assay; ELISA kits for the *C. difficile* toxins A and B; stool leukocyte assay, which is nonspecific; colonoscopy for direct evaluation of pseudomembranes; abdominal x-rays; and CT. The test for *C. difficile* cell cytotoxin B in the stool is the gold standard for diagnosis as it is the most sensitive and specific. This test is also relatively inexpensive. The results are usually available within 24 hours. Discontinuing antibiotic therapy is the only treatment required in approximately 1 in 4 women. Use of drugs that slow intestinal transit time such as diphenoxylate atropine (Lomotil) or narcotics are definitely contraindicated because the toxins of *C. difficile* remain in the gastrointestinal tract for a longer period of time. The therapy for the infection is metronidazole, given 250 mg by mouth four times a day, or oral vancomycin, 125 mg four times a day. Gastrointestinal symptoms usually improve within the first 72 hours of therapy and complete resolution of symptoms occurs within 10 days. Host factors are involved in the pathogenesis of the disease; older and more chronically ill patients usually develop more severe symptoms. Up to 10% of women may develop a recurrence or relapse. Recent studies have confirmed that more than 50% of recurrence of symptoms after initial response to treatment are due to reinfection rather than due to a relapse. Recurrences usually can be successfully treated in the same manner as the initial therapy. Recently, Johnson et al. have reported a strain of *C. difficile* that is highly resistant to clindamycin and has been responsible for large outbreaks of diarrhea in several different hospitals.

WOUND COMPLICATIONS

Infection

A major wound infection prolongs the hospital stay approximately 2 to 6 days. In their extensive review of 23,649 operations, Cruse and Foord determined that the incidence of abdominal wound infection varied depending on risk factors; however, for abdominal hysterectomy the incidence was approximately 5%. In a population of women not at high risk, the incidence of infection should be 1% to 2%. Abdominal hysterectomy is classified as a clean-contaminated operative procedure because the bacterial flora of the vagina are in continuity with the operative site during the surgery. The Centers for Disease Control and Prevention has revised their nomenclature describing incisional infection. They subdivide incisional infections into superficial infections that involve only the skin and subcutaneous tissue and deep infections that involve the deep soft tissues including fascia and muscles.

The pathophysiology of wound infection depends on an interaction between the number and virulence of bacterial contamination and the resistance of the patient. Inoculation of bacteria into the wound occurs in the operating room during the surgical procedure. There is a wide spectrum of common, endogenous bacteria that produces wound infections, including most gram-positive cocci and both aerobic and anaerobic rods. Small numbers of bacteria are present in all surgical wounds; however, bacterial growth is facilitated by decreased tissue oxygen and excessive amounts of necrotic tissue. It takes between 100,000 and 1 million bacteria per gram of tissue to produce infection in a surgical wound of the skin and subcutaneous tissue. The incidence of superficial skin infection is directly related to the length of the operative procedure. Each additional hour of surgery results in a doubling of the incidence of superficial skin infections. The primary source of bacterial contamination of an abdominal wound may be exogenous to the patient, such as a break in sterile technique, or endogenous, such as purulent material from a pelvic abscess.

Both local and systemic factors contribute to the level of host resistance and thus to the incidence of wound infections. Local factors are more significant and include the presence of hematomas, necrotic tissue, foreign bodies, dead space, use of cautery, and decreased local tissue perfusion. Systemic factors include obesity, diabetes, liver disease, malnutrition, immunosuppression, defects in the reticuloendothelial system, age, and the duration of preoperative hospitalization. The incidence of postoperative wound infection is increased eightfold when the woman's preoperative weight exceeds 200 pounds. Soper et al. noted that the thickness of subcutaneous tissue is the greatest risk factor for wound infection in a series of women undergoing abdominal hysterectomy. If an abdominal incision is more than 4 cm in depth, the risk of a superficial skin infection is increased approximately threefold. Greer et al. have described a supraumbilical upper abdominal incision as a method to avoid cutting across a large, thick panniculus for pelvic surgery in the morbidly obese woman. Corticosteroid therapy may suppress the inflammatory phase of the healing process. However, after the first 5 days of wound healing, corticosteroid therapy has no effect on an uninfected wound.

The first symptom of most wound infections appears between the fifth and the tenth postoperative day. Wound infection may occur as late as several months following surgery, but more than 90% of cases present within the first 2 weeks of the postoperative period. The first sign is usually fever, followed by tachycardia and varying degrees of increased tenderness and pain. As the infection progresses, many wounds develop areas that are either fluctuant or firm, and some develop crepitus. The incision is swollen, erythematous, edematous, and tender. Occasionally, subcutaneous gas may be seen on radiographic examination. Later in the course of the infection there may be associated spontaneous purulent drainage from the wound.

Fever during the first 24 to 48 hours is usually secondary to atelectasis. However, two rare types of wound infections are so virulent that they produce toxicity within the first 48 hours. Classically, these early infections are those produced by *Clostridium* species and acute beta-hemolytic streptococcal infection. Clinically, wound infections secondary to beta-hemolytic streptococci appear swollen and red and have an odorless discharge. In contrast, infections secondary to *Clostridium* are boggy and edematous, and the discharge has a sweet odor.

Initial management of any wound infection consists of opening and drainage of the wound. The wound opens easily following removal of the skin sutures or clips. Purulent material exhibits a wide range of consistency from the thin watery discharge classical of a streptococcal infection to the thick pus associated with staphylococcal subcutaneous infections. Gram stain and both aerobic and anaerobic cultures of the wound should be obtained at this point. These initial cultures are most valuable if the patient does not respond to initial management. In such cases the differential diagnosis would be between infections involving deeper tissue planes and infection for which host resistance has failed even after drainage of the wound.

Once a wound infection has been opened and drained, care is directed toward initial packing of the wound with gauze to effect debridement and periodic irrigation. Rarely are antibiotics needed, unless there is a surrounding cellulitis. If there is a distinct zone of diffuse erythema surrounding a wound infection, the most likely organism is a streptococcal infection, and intravenous antibiotics are indicated. Systemic antibiotics are always indicated in women with immunosuppression or concomitant diseases with impaired defense mechanisms. Most women with a wound infection will become afebrile within 72 hours after the wound has been opened and debrided. When the woman becomes afebrile and granulation tissue begins to form, consideration may be given to delayed secondary closure.

Prevention is the foundation of any approach to the management of wound infections. Prevention involves consideration of both local and systemic factors, which if unattended, predispose to infection. Prophylactic antibiotics, especially in high-risk cases, definitely decrease the incidence of wound infection. If the wound is grossly contaminated, then delayed primary closure on the third or fourth postoperative day is appropriate. Women who should be considered as candidates for delayed primary closure include those who are immunosuppressed or malnourished, who have far-advanced malignancies, or who are markedly obese. Women having operative procedures that involve a simultaneous abdominal and vaginal approach and those with a surgical opening of unprepared large intestine are also candidates for delayed primary closure. In a small series, Brown et al. reported that the latter technique reduced the incidence of wound infection from 23% in a control group to 2% in the group having delayed closure. When delayed primary closure is planned, sutures may be placed at the time of surgery and secured, but not tied. The incision should be packed loosely with gauze. If the wound is dry and without evidence of infection on postoperative day 3, the edges may be approximated with the preplaced sutures.

Delayed secondary closure may be accomplished in previously infected wounds after several days of drainage and debridement. Delayed secondary closure markedly reduces the time necessary for eventual closure of the skin defect by secondary intention. Patient satisfaction is dramatically increased with delayed secondary closure.

A virulent, rapidly progressing form of soft tissue wound infection is necrotizing fasciitis. Often the diagnosis is not suspected during the early part of the infection because of the relative minor changes in the skin overlying the deeper infection. The early symptoms are local pain with systemic symptoms of tachycardia and fever, which are higher than would be expected with an uncomplicated wound infection. The woman experiences marked tenderness when the infected area is palpated. This classical sign should heighten the suspicion of the diagnosis of necrotizing fasciitis. As the disease progresses, the wound edges usually darken, with crepitance and bullae formation, and anesthetic areas adjacent to the wound develop. Necrotizing fasciitis involves the subcutaneous tissue and superficial fascia. The infection rapidly expands in the subcutaneous spaces and often tracks far beyond the superficial margins of the involved skin. If the diagnosis is questionable, a full-thickness core biopsy and frozen section of the tissue should be performed. This condition is a life-threatening surgical emergency, and patients should have debridement as soon as possible. It is most important for the gynecologist to have a high degree of suspicion for this condition because even with adequate surgical debridement, the mortality rate is 30% to 50%. This rare but potentially fatal condition necessitates wide debridement of all necrotic tissue, high levels of broad-spectrum antibiotics, and sometimes hyperbaric oxygen. Debridement to freely bleeding tissue helps determine the

surgical margin. It is not unusual for the patient to need repetitive debridements. Women with diabetes, malnutrition, immunosuppression, malignancy, obesity, and poor tissue perfusion are most susceptible to this complication.

Dehiscence and Evisceration

Dehiscence is a failure of normal healing and literally means disruption of any of the layers of a surgical incision. The physiologic, biochemical, and structural changes that characterize normal wound healing are complex and, at best, imperfectly understood. However, clinically the most important fact to the clinician is that the strength of the wound increases over time. The strength of a skin incision increases at a rapid and almost constant rate for the first 4 months and at a much slower rate for the first year. Clinically, dehiscence usually means that the previous incision of the skin, subcutaneous tissue, and fascia has separated, but not the peritoneum. This complication usually occurs during the first 2 postoperative weeks. Often dehiscence is recognized immediately or within the first 24 hours following the removal of skin clips. Evisceration is a complete breakdown of the healing process through all levels of the abdominal incision, with omentum or bowel presenting through the incision.

The incidence of wound dehiscence is approximately 1 in 200 gynecologic operations. The major short-term result of wound dehiscence is the prolongation of hospital stay. Over the long term, dehiscence predisposes to incisional hernias. Wound dehiscence is a rare cause of surgical mortality, especially in debilitated patients. Wound infection is present in approximately 50% of women with wound disruption. As with wound infections, preventive management is the most important therapeutic consideration. The incidence of dehiscence has decreased with the use of synthetic absorbable sutures, such as Dexon and Vicryl. They are superior to catgut in their more predictable absorption, reduction of tissue reaction, and greater tensile strength (Table 25-17).

TABLE 25-17
Qualities of Absorbable Sutures

Type	Knot Security	Tensile Strength	Wound Security
Gut	+	++	5–7 days (50%)
Chromic	++	++	10–14 days (50%)
Dexon*	++++	++++	25 days (50%)
Vicryl†	+++	++++	30 days (50%)

From Sanz L and Smith S: Mechanisms of wound healing, suture material, and wound closure. In Buchsbaum HJ and Walton LA, editors: Strategies in gynecologic surgery, New York, 1986, Springer-Verlag New York, Inc, p 63.

*Polyglycolic acid.

†Polyglactin.

Poole has reviewed the literature concerning prevention of disruption of fascial closure. The consensus of authorities is that local factors are much more important in the pathophysiology of wound disruption than are systemic factors, although both should be considered in preventive management. Important mechanical factors predisposing to disruption are conditions that increase the tension on the incision line, such as abdominal distention and chronic lung disease, or a technically inadequate closure of the wound. Other factors include obesity, advanced age, malignancy, uremia, liver failure, diabetes, hypoproteinemia, hematoma formation, sepsis, corticosteroids or chemotherapy, prior radiation therapy, and whether the incision is made through an area of a previous incision. Whether an incision is horizontal or vertical has little effect on the incidence of wound disruption. The pathophysiology of fascial dehiscence involves exaggerated collagen lysis in the wound. Clinically the sutures "tear through the fascia" rather than dissolving or becoming "untied." For example, approximating and tying sutures too vigorously, especially a figure-of-8 suture, may lead to strangulation and necrosis of the tissue and subsequent wound dehiscence. Some gynecologists are performing primary mass closure with a continuous monofilament, delayed absorbable suture to avoid this problem.

The classic symptom and sign of an impending wound disruption is the spontaneous passage of serosanguineous fluid from the abdominal incision. Most often this occurs between the fifth and eighth postoperative days. Patients with uninfected wounds generally have been asymptomatic. Patients who develop wound defects often lack the normal "healing ridge" of tissue that can be palpated in normal healing wounds.

Imperative for prevention of wound dehiscence is proper closure of the incision in a woman at high risk for less than optimum healing. Although there are many regional preferences for the choice of suture and method of closure, the most popular technique is some modification of the Smead-Jones closure with permanent suture (Figure 25-10). Closure with the Smead-Jones technique results in a dehiscence rate of approximately 1 in 1000 operations. With this technique it is important to place individual sutures at least 1 to 1.5 cm away from the adjacent sutures and include at least 2 cm of fascia on either side of the incision. The alternative technique is a mass closure using a monofilament permanent suture material such as nylon or polypropylene (Prolene). Delayed primary wound closure 3 to 5 days after the operation should be considered if the wound was contaminated during the procedure, such as with rupture of a tuboovarian abscess. Also, delayed closure should be considered for any patient already at high risk for wound complications, such as the malnourished patient, diabetic patient, markedly obese patient, or the woman who is immunosuppressed.

The treatment of wound disruption depends on the size

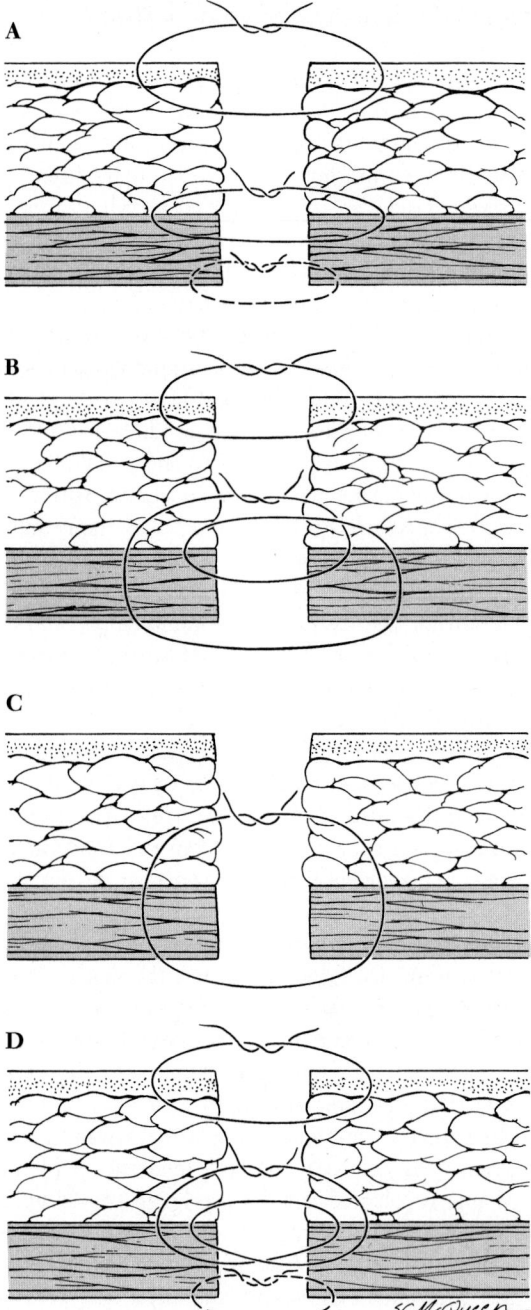

FIGURE 25-10 Types of abdominal incision closures. **A,** Layered. **B,** Smead-Jones. **C,** Through-and-through. **D,** Far-near. (From Braun TE: Wound dehiscence. In Schaefer G and Graber EA, editors: Complications in obstetric and gynecological surgery, Hagerstown, Md, 1981, Harper & Row, Publishers, Inc, p 159.)

and the depth of the defect. Similar to the management of wound infections, digital examination of the defect is important so that the full extent of the problem will be recognized. With larger defects the wound edges must be debrided and the wound closed with a modified Smead-Jones or mass closure technique.

OPERATIVE SITE COMPLICATIONS

Pelvic Cellulitis and Abscess

Infections of the contiguous retroperitoneal space immediately above the vaginal apex are common complications following abdominal or vaginal hysterectomy. However, the frequency of this postoperative complication has dramatically decreased in direct relation to the use of prophylactic antibiotics. These soft tissue infections range in severity from localized, minor cellulitis to large pelvic abscesses and have many names, from "cuff cellulitis" to "infected hematoma." Nevertheless, they are similar to soft tissue infections in other parts of the body and are either a cellulitis or an abscess. These infections prolong hospital stay and increase the cost of patient care. The bacterial spectrum that produces these infections includes aerobic and anaerobic bacteria from both exogenous and endogenous sources. Most postoperative pelvic infections are polymicrobial, usually from endogenous vaginal flora, and approximately 60% to 80% involve anaerobic organisms.

The pathophysiology of development of retroperitoneal infection is straightforward. The classic clamp-crush-cut-and-tie technique used in pelvic surgery produces an abundance of hypoxic and anoxic tissue that helps to establish an optimal environment for infection. This environment is further enhanced by the normal retroperitoneal hysterectomy site producing an average of 40 ml of serosanguineous fluid each day during the first 72 postoperative hours. The endogenous flora of the upper vagina colonize and multiply in this retroperitoneal serosanguineous fluid and in pelvic hematomas after the operation.

The major symptoms of an operative site infection are fever associated with lower quadrant abdominal and pelvic pain. The fever usually becomes prominent between the third and fifth postoperative days. As the infection becomes more severe, the fever becomes spiking in character, the pain intensifies, and the patient develops moderate leukocytosis.

The diagnosis of cuff cellulitis is confirmed by pelvic examination. Pelvic tenderness and induration are prominent during the bimanual examination. A subtle difference exists between normal postoperative pelvic tenderness and induration and the tenderness and induration produced by infection. Postoperative infection is accompanied by an increase in suprapubic pain and lateral parametrial tenderness. Cuff cellulitis sometimes responds to drainage by opening the vaginal cuff. Appropriate cultures of the site are difficult with cellulitis because of vaginal contamination. Both persistent cellulitis, or one encompassing a large area, and/or a pelvic abscess necessitate parenteral antibiotic therapy. Often the diagnosis of a retroperitoneal abscess is confirmed when the patient has ongoing fever and pelvic tenderness after 2 to 3 days of parenteral antibiotics for a suspected cuff cellulitis. Eason et al. reported that the volume of pelvic fluid 3 to 5 days postoperatively after a hysterectomy is a nonspecific finding and does not predict febrile morbidity or the need for drainage. They further commented that large or complex fluid collections may be present without adverse clinical consequences.

Because of their polymicrobial etiology, the infections are usually treated with an aminoglycoside (gentamicin) and an antibiotic specific for anaerobic infection (clindamycin). Metronidazole (Flagyl) may be substituted for clindamycin. An alternative therapy is substitution of a third-generation cephalosporin or the monobactam agent aztreonam (Azactam) for the aminoglycoside. Aztreonam has a similar spectrum of antibiotic coverage with much less renal toxicity; however, it is much more expensive. Intravenous antibiotics should be continued until the patient is afebrile for 24 hours. Recent studies have documented that oral antibiotic therapy is unnecessary following successful parenteral therapy. Alternatives to the aminoglycoside/clindamycin regimen include broad-spectrum antibiotics combined with betalactamase inhibitors such as ampicillin/sulbactam, amoxicillin/clavulanate, piperacillin/tazobactam, or ticarcillin/clavulanate. These drugs have better coverage of Enterobacteriaceae species and *Enterococcus*. Recently, increasing numbers of enterococci are resistant to both ampicillin and vancomycin.

Although many pelvic abscesses drain spontaneously, patients should have serial pelvic examinations and endovaginal ultrasound imaging to determine the most appropriate time to effect operative drainage. Appropriate cultures should be obtained from the center of an abscess cavity when the abscess is operatively incised. If a patient does not become afebrile within 48 hours of adequate drainage of a retroperitoneal abscess, a concomitant complication of pelvic thrombophlebitis should be suspected. If pelvic thrombophlebitis is suspected, a 72-hour trial of intravenous heparin therapy with concurrent antibiotics should be instituted.

Granulation Tissue

Granulation tissue at the apex of the vaginal vault is a frequent complication following hysterectomy. Small areas of friable, red granulation tissue are seen at the 6-week postoperative pelvic examination in more than 50% of women. Granulation tissue is more common following abdominal than vaginal hysterectomy. In a recent randomized study, Colombo et al. found that the incidence of both cuff cellulitis and formation of granulation tissue was no different between women with the vaginal cuff left open versus closed after abdominal hysterectomy.

Manyonda et al. conducted a prospective randomized trial of women with total abdominal hysterectomies and compared polygalactide (Vicryl) and chromic catgut. In this study 32% of the women had developed vault granulation tissue by their 6-week postoperative checkup. Of women who developed granulation tissue, chromic catgut was implicated twice as frequently as polygalactide suture, 68% versus 32%, respectively.

Excessive granulation tissue is the result of an exaggerated healing response of the vascular-rich pelvic tissues. One of the causes is believed to be inversion of the vaginal epithelium between the margins of the edges of the incision at the apex of the vaginal vault.

Some patients are asymptomatic, but many women experience spotting or a bloody discharge after intercourse. A rare patient may have mild pelvic discomfort. On speculum examination the granulation tissue appears as a polypoid projection hanging from the vaginal suture line. The differential diagnosis includes a prolapsed fallopian tube and recurrent carcinoma in a patient with a pelvic malignancy. The polypoid mass is easily avulsed from the vaginal apex. The remaining areas of granulation tissue should be treated with a chemical cautery (silver nitrate or Monsel's solution) or by cryocautery or electrocautery.

Prolapsed Fallopian Tube

Prolapse of the distal end of the fallopian tube is a rare complication of abdominal or vaginal hysterectomy. It is usually discovered during a routine visit during the first few months following the operation. Factors that may predispose a woman to develop prolapse of the fallopian tube include hematoma formation and postoperative pelvic infection.

Many women with this complication are free of symptoms, but others experience a watery discharge, postcoital spotting and pain, or moderate lower abdominal and pelvic pain. Differing from granulation tissue, the fallopian tube is not friable and is firmly attached. Grasping the fallopian tube with an instrument and applying traction produces much more pain than traction on granulation tissue. Treatment is the destruction of the segment of the fallopian tube protruding through the vaginal vault with cryocautery or the laser. The fallopian tube may be removed during a subsequent outpatient procedure using conduction anesthesia. Most clinicians opt for a vaginal approach with ligation of the fallopian tube as high as possible. The stump of the tube is buried retroperitoneally and the vaginal epithelium closed. Some difficult cases must be performed transabdominally via the laparoscope or minilaparotomy. An alternative treatment is coagulation of the segment of fallopian tube protruding through the vaginal apex with cryocautery. Often the vaginal wall reepithelializes over the area, thereby excluding the tube from any connection with the vaginal cavity.

MISCELLANEOUS COMPLICATIONS

Lymphocyst

A lymphocyst is a local collection of lymphatic fluid within the retroperitoneal spaces of the pelvis resulting from retrograde drainage of lymph. It is a rare complication, discovered most frequently after pelvic node dissections. In the past this complication occurred in approximately 20% of patients having undergone radical operations. However, with meticulous attention to ligation of distal lymphatic channels and abandonment of the practice of reperitonealization, this complication is reported in less than 5% of such cases. A peritoneal opening or "peritoneal window" allows flow of the lymphatic fluid into the peritoneal cavity with subsequent peritoneal resorption. The incidence is lower in series where palpation alone is used to identify the cysts. If ultrasound examination is used postoperatively to screen for lymphocysts, the incidence is 10-fold greater. Conditions that predispose the patient to formation of a lymphocyst are previous radiation and anticoagulation.

Lymphocysts usually present during the first 6 postoperative weeks. They vary greatly in size and seldom become infected. The cyst usually begins anterior and medial to the iliac vessels. As it expands, it may produce pelvic pain, leg pain, fever, obstruction or angulation of the ureter, pressure symptoms on the bladder, or partial venous obstruction. Small lymphocysts, less than 4 cm in diameter, are usually asymptomatic and regress spontaneously within 8 weeks. Larger cysts necessitate treatment either by intermittent aspiration followed by pressure dressings or insertion of an indwelling catheter under ultrasound guidance. Simple incision and drainage are usually unsuccessful because the condition often recurs. Injection of a sclerosing solution such as tetracycline is another therapeutic alternative. Traditional surgical management involves removing a large segment of the wall of the lymphocyst and placing a tongue of omentum in the cavity. Choo et al. have advised peritoneal marsupialization for lymphocysts that do not respond to traditional operative management.

Ovarian Abscess

Ovarian abscess is a rare but serious postoperative complication. This condition is potentially fatal because of intraperitoneal rupture of the abscess. Ovarian abscesses arise from bacterial colonization of the ovarian cortex without primary involvement of the fallopian tube. This may occur either via disruption of the ovarian capsule by the presence of a recently ruptured corpus luteum or via an operative disruption, such as cystectomy performed during vaginal hysterectomy.

The disease may follow either a slow, indolent course or a rapidly progressive one. Some patients with this complication present during the first postoperative week with high fever and severe pain, which are continuous until rupture occurs. Others become afebrile following the operation but return sometime during the first few months with a persistent low-grade fever and mild pain. Chronologically, most ovarian abscesses appear later in the postoperative course than other retroperitoneal abscesses.

Ovarian abscesses usually appear 2 to 3 weeks postoperatively, but cases have been reported as late as 3 to 4 months later. Willson and Black, in a classic work describing 28 patients with ovarian abscess, noted that the predominant symptom was abdominal pain associated with persistent tachycardia and high fever. This abscess is found higher in the pelvis than a retroperitoneal abscess at the apex of the vagina.

Initial treatment is medical therapy with intravenous antibiotics. However, most patients do not respond to medical therapy, and operative drainage of the abscess becomes a necessity. Surgical drainage often may not be accomplished transvaginally, and thus the abdominal approach is preferable. Percutaneous ultrasound or CT-directed drainage may also be an appropriate management strategy depending on location and clinical situation. This rare problem should be considered in any woman having a gynecologic operation, especially in women in which the integrity of the ovarian capsule is disrupted either physiologically or operatively.

Postoperative Neuropathy

The femoral nerve is the largest branch of the lumbar plexus and arises from the primary dorsal rami of L2, L3, and L4. It provides motor function to several leg muscles, including the quadriceps, and sensory fibers that innervate the anterior and medial surfaces of the thigh and leg. The vascular supply to the femoral nerve may be compromised during an abdominal or vaginal hysterectomy. Rosenblum et al. have described the pathophysiology of this complication as being secondary to continuous pressure, usually by a self-retaining retractor producing ischemic necrosis of the nerve. The vascular circulation of the nerve itself is compromised by diminished blood flow in the vasa nervorum. The most common site of nerve compression is 4 to 6 cm above the inguinal ligament where the nerve pierces the psoas muscle.

Factors that contribute to the development of this complication are thinness of the patient, long retractor blades, prolonged operative times, and systemic diseases such as diabetes mellitus, gout, alcoholism, and malnutrition. The classic patient who develops this complication is a short, thin, athletic woman who has a transverse incision in which a self-retaining retractor is used. A similar problem may develop after vaginal operations or laparoscopy in thin women who are placed into exaggerated hip flexion or abduction in the dorsal lithotomy position. Dunnihoo et al. reported on 33 cases of femoral neuropathy after vaginal hysterectomy. Femoral neuropathy following vaginal surgery is believed to be secondary to compromise of the nerve by severe angulation of the woman, not secondary to pressure injury from retractors.

Patients with this complication may experience numbness, paresthesias, and difficulty with their gait. Patients may have difficulty lifting the affected knee because of the involvement of the quadriceps. Symptoms may present with a spectrum of severity. Usually the neurologic symptoms develop within the first 24 to 72 hours following an operation. These symptoms are causes of great anxiety to the patient. Because of the inability to lift the leg, climbing stairs is a particular problem. The muscle and sensory function recovers spontaneously over several weeks to several months. The patient should be seen by a physical therapist to facilitate ambulation and prevent muscle atrophy.

To prevent this complication, it is important to palpate the lateral pelvic wall and femoral artery after placement of a self-retaining retractor. With the woman in the lithotomy position, one should check for pulsations in the popliteal or posterior tibial vessels. In a thin patient, placing folded towels between the skin surface and the self-retaining retractor helps to prevent this complication by decreasing the depth of penetration of the lateral retractor blades.

The ilioinguinal and iliohypogastric nerves pass in a transverse and diagonal course through the anterior lower abdominal musculature medial to the inguinal ligament and through the inguinal canal. The nerves supply sensory fibers to the labia, mons pubis, and medial thigh. The nerves may become injured during an operation with a Pfannenstiel incision or during urinary incontinence procedures (Figure 25-11). Pathophysiologically, the nerve may be transected or entrapped by suture or scar formation. Sharp or burning pain may develop immediately postoperatively or usually within a few days. The pain may radiate to the groin or vulva. Most symptoms will resolve spontaneously. Severe pain may necessitate nerve block or suture removal, or segmented removal of the involved nerve.

ESTROGEN REPLACEMENT

Bilateral salpingo-oophorectomy is sometimes performed on young women for conditions such as pelvic inflammatory disease. National surveys have documented that bilateral salpingo-oophorectomy concomitant with hysterectomy is performed in approximately 25% of premenopausal women. Removal of ovaries in a premenopausal woman reduces the serum estradiol concentrations by approximately 80% and serum testosterone concentrations by approximately 50%. The possible consequences of estrogen deprivation include vasomotor symptoms, urogenital tissue atrophy (atrophic vaginitis, dyspareunia, and urethral syndrome), and osteoporosis. For premenopausal women an additional risk is the development of atherosclerotic heart disease at an earlier age than for a woman with normal ovarian function. The pathophysiology of premature coronary vascular disease is complex and

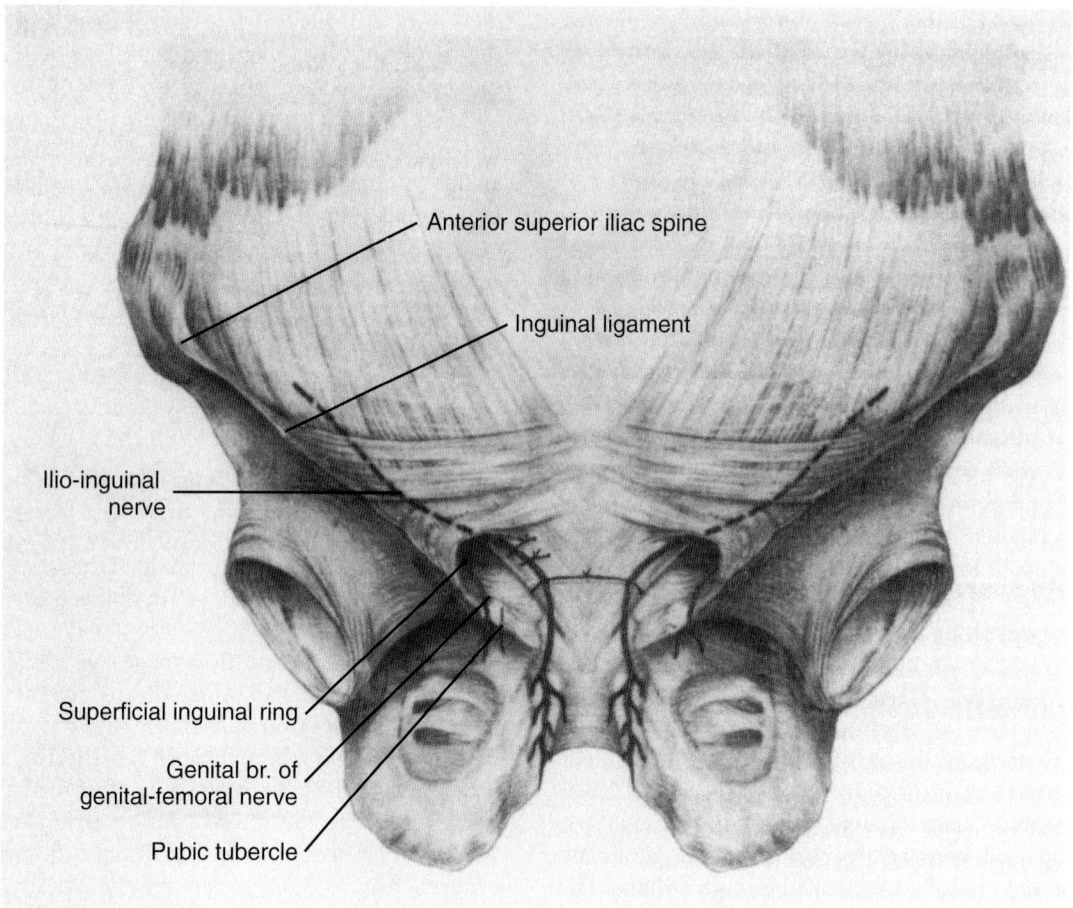

FIGURE 25-11 Ilioinguinal nerve entrapment during needle suspension for stress incontinence. (From Miyazaki F and Shook G: Obstet Gynecol 80:246, 1992.)

multifactorial, but the change in the ratio of high-density lipoproteins (HDLs) to low-density lipoproteins (LDLs) is an important factor. Removal of the ovaries in premenopausal women may lead to clinically significant sexual dysfunction.

Estrogen replacement is indicated in the vast majority of premenopausal women having bilateral oophorectomy. The increase in hypercoagulability produced by the doses of estrogen used for postmenopausal symptoms is negligible. Nevertheless, because of the physiologic hypercoagulability and injury to the intima of vessels associated with the operative procedure, oral estrogen therapy should not be started immediately after the procedure. Theoretically, estradiol given via a cutaneous patch is more acceptable in the immediate postoperative period than oral estrogen because of the difference in effect of the associated relative decrease in the liver's production of clotting factors. An oral tablet of 0.625 mg of conjugated estrogens daily is sufficient to protect from bone demineralization and osteoporosis. A higher dose may be required to alleviate hot flushes.

PSYCHOLOGIC SEQUELAE

Pain Relief

The proper management of pain during the postoperative period should be a primary goal of all gynecologists. Most women experience moderate to severe pain during the first 36 to 48 hours following a gynecologic operation. However, pain and suffering are personal, internal events, the extent and presence of which may best be measured by direct communication with the patient.

The current literature documents that pain relief is often treated inadequately in postoperative patients. For many women who undergo gynecologic operations, dosages of analgesics are prescribed that are less than adequate to relieve pain, and many nurses further reduce the amount of medication. The many misconceptions concerning postoperative pain include the dangers of addiction and the fear of respiratory depression. Kuhn et al. have emphasized that it is not only physicians and nurses who contribute to ineffective treatment. Patients also contribute by having a lower level of pain relief expectation.

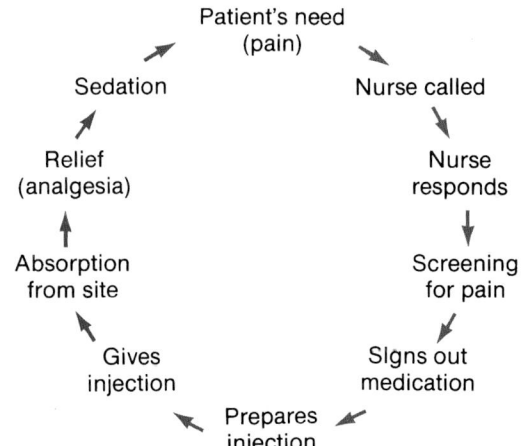

FIGURE 25-12   Pain cycle. (From White PF: Postgrad Med 80:8, 1986.)

These authors believe that pain relief is poor because of inadequate education of patients in what to expect from pain relief. Inadequate pain relief prolongs hospital stay and has adverse psychologic consequences.

White (1986) has presented a schematic diagram of the pain cycle and the potential delays in pain relief with traditional "prn" analgesic regimens (Figure 25-12). Many studies have confirmed that regular-interval preventive pain relief is superior to conventional "on demand" analgesic medication during the first 36 to 48 hours following the operation. Relative potencies of common analgesic medications are listed in Table 25-18. However, there is great variability in absorption. In addition, the therapeutic window (the range of effective blood concentration before undesired

side effects occur) is narrow. When 100 mg of meperidine hydrochloride (Demerol) is given every 4 hours intramuscularly, the concentration of the drug in the blood exceeds the minimum level necessary to produce adequate pain relief only 35% of the 4-hour period (Table 25-19).

TABLE 25-18
Relative* Potencies of Analgesics (mg/mg)

	Intramuscular	Oral
Alphaprodine	45	—
Buprenorphine	2.5–5	0.4 (sublingual)
Butorphanol	2–3	—
Codeine	130	200
Fentanyl	0.125	—
Heroin	4	—
Hydromorphone	1.5	7.5
Levorphanol	2	4
Meperidine	75	300
Methadone	10	20
Morphine	10	30–60
Nalbuphine	10	—
Oxycodone	10	30
Pentazocine	60	180
Propoxyphene	240	300
Sufentanil	0.0125	—

From Gorman ES and Warfield CA: Hosp Pract 21:48B, 1986.

*To 10 mg morphine, intramuscular.

TABLE 25-19
Blood Meperidine Concentrations After Intramuscular Administration of 100 mg Every 4 Hours in 10 Patients

	Peak Level (µg/ml)	Time to Peak Level (min)	Minimum Analgesic Concentration* (µg/ml)	Time Level Exceeded Minimum Analgesic Concentration* (min)
Initial postoperative injections				
Mean	0.51	57	0.43	43
Range	0.24–0.82	18–108	0.26–0.85	0–240
SD	0.14	27	0.14	57
Second postoperative day				
Mean	0.77	39	0.49	150
Range	0.51–1.21	18–108	0.28–0.66	54–240
SD	0.23	24	0.10	72

From White PF: Postgrad Med 80:9, 1986.

*Minimum analgesic concentration refers to the minimum level required to provide adequate pain relief.

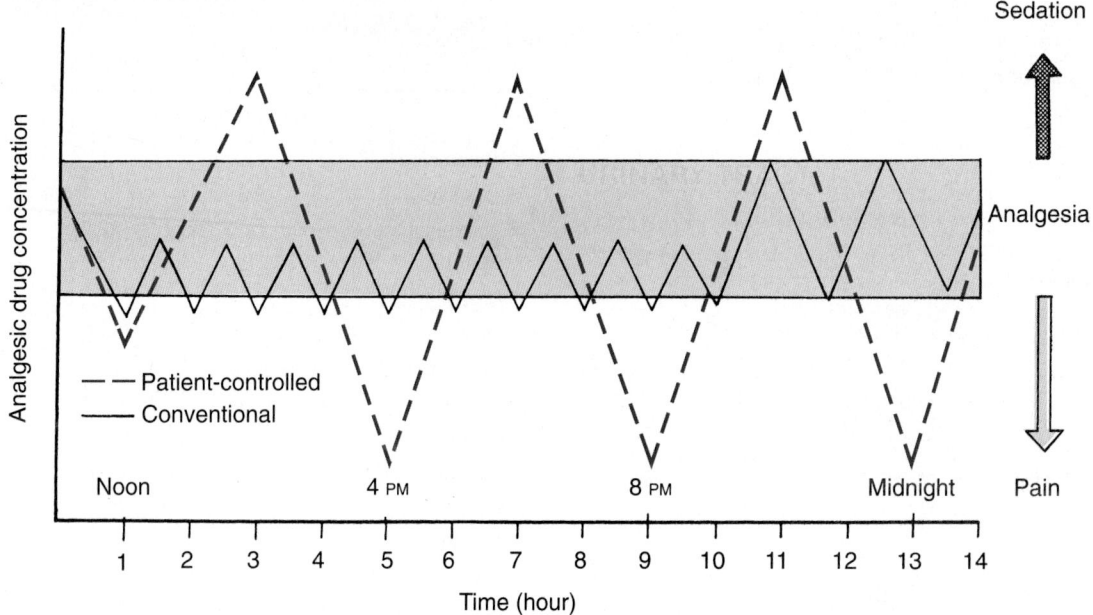

FIGURE 25-13 Theoretic relationships among dosing interval, analgesic drug concentration, and clinical effects when comparing patient-controlled analgesic (PCA) system *(solid lines)* with conventional intramuscular therapy *(dashed lines).* (Redrawn from White PF: Semin Anesthesiol 4:255, 1985.)

In White's study, peak concentrations varied as much as fivefold among the 10 different individuals, and the time to reach peak blood level varied as much as sevenfold. Thus patient-controlled analgesic (PCA) systems have become one of the preferred methods of pain relief during the immediate postoperative period (Figure 25-13). PCA systems dramatically decrease patients' anxiety because they are in control rather than the hospital staff. These systems are both safe and effective as long as there is a lockout period, and they help to minimize individual differences in pharmacokinetics. Modern PCA systems minimize the risk of drug overdose and allow the patient to titrate and therefore maximize analgesic effectiveness. In general, patients use the PCA system for approximately 12 to 36 hours until they are tolerating oral liquids. The suggested initial doses for PCA systems using meperidine and morphine are listed in Table 25-20. Women should be given instructions concerning PCA systems to alleviate inherent fears of addiction.

Perioperative injections of opioids intrathecal or epidural effectively relieve postoperative pelvic pain in most situations. Side effects are primarily itching and a small risk of hypotension. If severe pain is anticipated, continuous PCA epidurals may be used. The advantages and disadvantages of patient-controlled analgesia and epidural anesthesia are characterized in Table 25-21.

After the first 24 to 48 hours, pain relief may be successfully controlled with nonsteroidal antiinflammatory agents. Many of these agents are as effective as 10 mg intramuscular morphine for postoperative gynecologic pain. Advantages of prostaglandin synthetase inhibitors are a lack of effect on gastrointestinal motility and a much smaller effect on sensorium than narcotic

TABLE 25-20
Usual PCA Doses for Meperidine and Morphine*

Drug	Bolus Dose (mg)		Lockout Interval (min)		Basal Infusion (mg/hr)	
	Average	Range	Average	Range	Average	Range
Meperidine	10	5–30	6	5–15	5	5–20
Morphine	1	0.5–3	6	5–15	0.5	0.5–2

From Breslow MJ, Miller CF, and Rogers MC: Perioperative management, St Louis, 1990, Mosby–Year Book, Inc.

*These are suggested as starting doses only. After initiating therapy, titrate dose to analgesia versus sedation.

TABLE 25-21
Advantages and Disadvantages of Epidural Analgesia and Patient-Controlled Analgesia

	Epidural	Patient-Controlled
Advantages	Immediate pain relief May improve colon motility May improve postoperative pulmonary function after lower abdominal and pelvic surgery Less sedating than patient-controlled analgesia	Requires no special nursing or anesthesia support postoperatively Gives the patient "personal control" over administration of pain medication
Disadvantages	Requires a skilled anesthesiologist for correct placement May interfere with ambulation May delay removal of Foley catheter	Patient may experience pain in the recovery room until an adequate serum level of medication is achieved

From Baker VV: Principles of postoperative care. In Baker VV and Deppe G, editors: Management of perioperative complications in gynecology, Philadelphia, 1997, WB Saunders Co, p 141.

agents. Disadvantages include increased gastric acidity and potential compromise in patients with renal disease. Commonly used nonsteroidal agents for postoperative pain include ibuprofen, naproxen, and ketorolac (Toradol). Ketorolac may be given as an intramuscular or intravenous injection during the operative procedure. Intramuscular injections reach peak plasma levels in 40 to 50 minutes, with a half-life of 4 to 6 hours. The dose is an intramuscular loading dose of 30 to 60 mg followed with 15 to 30 mg every 6 hours during the first 24 to 36 hours. The drug works well when given concomitantly with narcotics. Toradol should not be used for more than 4 consecutive days because of gastrointestinal side effects.

Many surgeons and anesthesiologists believe that giving analgesics in the perioperative period prior to the patient's sensation of pain—giving them preemptively—leads to better pain control. Some physicians infiltrate the incision prior to closing with a local anesthetic such as lidocaine or bupivacaine. This effect is short lived and is more valuable in minor procedures with small incisions. Studies of this technique show effective pain relief with laparoscopy.

Psychosexual Problems and Depression

The time immediately before and after a surgical procedure is a stressful period for all women and their families. Anxiety and fear are normal responses and should be anticipated by health care providers. Any operation on the female reproductive organs stimulates questions and conflicts concerning body image, feminine identity, sexuality, and possibly future childbearing. The period following a gynecologic operation is one of transition and is a unique psychologic challenge to the woman. The reader should review Chapter 8 to emphasize the problems of loss and grief and the stages of depression. After gyneco-

logic operations, every patient needs support to overcome this challenge, and it is important to emphasize that it may take many months to complete the process. Personal issues that relate to a woman's body image and sexuality are particularly affected by hysterectomy. In premenopausal women who have undergone bilateral salpingo-oophorectomy, physiologic dosages of transdermal testosterone have been demonstrated to improve sexual function. The exogenous androgens also resulted in a beneficial effect on well-being and depression. Open discussions with the patient that allow her to discuss issues regarding sexuality are important during both preoperative and postoperative visits. Psychologic studies have confirmed that sexual function following a hysterectomy is related to a number of factors. Poor knowledge of reproductive anatomy, a negative expectation of sexual recovery following the operation, preoperative psychiatric morbidity, and a history of unsatisfactory sexual relations are all associated with a poor outcome. In summary the effect of hysterectomy on sexual function is an exceedingly complex topic with both physical and psychologic factors known to have varying and an almost unquantifiable influence.

Alcohol Withdrawal

A syndrome of nausea, sweating, tachycardia, tremors, delirium, and even grand mal seizures postoperatively is often misdiagnosed as a drug or anesthetic reaction. This constellation of signs and symptoms is usually alcohol withdrawal. The presence of a tremor should alert health care providers to the correct diagnosis. In the treatment of postalcohol withdrawal symptoms, benzodiazepines are the drug of choice. In elderly women especially after emergency surgery, postoperative confusion, anxiety, changes in personality, and memory impairment are frequent findings.

DISCHARGE INSTRUCTIONS

Simple but complete discharge instructions are an important component of postoperative care. The physician should anticipate the most common questions and give the woman explicit instructions. Particular attention should be given to limitations in physical activity, such as heavy lifting and resumption of sexual relations. Information should be given about vaginal spotting as sutures dissolve. Appropriate phone numbers should be provided in case of unanticipated complications and to schedule return appointments. One of the most accomplished clinicians of the previous generation was the internist Eugene A. Stead, Jr. He taught that discharge instructions should not be given on the morning of discharge. Rather, patients should receive these instructions the day before discharge; then a "posttest" is given on the morning of discharge to ensure that the patient understands. Instructions should be given in both verbal and written form. As an increasing number of procedures are performed as outpatient surgery or short stays, the physician must modify instructions to accommodate the gradual resumption of activity. The 24- to 48-hour postdischarge phone call to the recovering patient provides an excellent forum for answering questions and providing reassurance. Studies of outpatient surgeries have found this phone contact to be most important. Additionally, it is quite difficult for the patient and significant others to remember instructions received during the first 24 hours after surgery. Written guidelines are extremely valuable for outpatient procedures.

KEY POINTS

- Often, the woman and her family judge the competence of the gynecologist by the compassion displayed during the immediate postoperative period.

- Diurnal fluctuations are characteristic of the daily body temperature patterns of humans. A normal temperature is usually 37.2° C in the morning and 37.7° C overall.

- Postoperative febrile morbidity is related to infection in approximately 20% of cases and noninfectious causes in 80% of cases.

- The pathophysiology of postoperative fever is primarily related to the release of cytokines.

- Intraoperative factors that dramatically increase the risk of postoperative fever are an operative time longer than 2 hours and intraoperative transfusion.

- The proper workup of a postoperative fever involves three classic steps of history, physical examination, and laboratory evaluations, with the major emphasis placed on the physical examination.

- The findings of the history and especially the physical examination and considerations of cost containment all influence the extent of the laboratory tests ordered. Ordering a specific list of laboratory tests is unrewarding.

- Approximately 75% of patients develop a temperature greater than 37° C, which is usually not associated with an infectious process.

- Because of the shifts in water balance, the postoperative hematocrit at 72 hours is a more accurate measurement of operative and postoperative blood loss than a hematocrit at 24 hours.

- The normal physiologic response to the stress of an operation and tissue destruction is release of increased levels of antidiuretic hormone and aldosterone, producing both sodium and water retention.

- After subtracting the effects of the operative blood loss from the preoperative hematocrit, a further reduction in hematocrit of 3 to 5 points reflects a postoperative hemorrhage of approximately 500 ml.

- Women over the age of 60 should be transfused if their hematocrit falls below 28%.

- Microatelectasis is a common occurrence developing during almost all pelvic operations, and it is persistent 24 hours postoperatively in approximately 50% of women. Current studies have demonstrated that there is no association between fever and the amount of atelectasis diagnosed radiologically.

- Factors that predispose patients to atelectasis include supine position, obesity, smoking, age greater than 60 years, prolonged operative time, presence of nasogastric tube, and coexisting medical conditions such as cardiac disease or pulmonary infection.

- The clinical presentation of fever, tachypnea, and tachycardia within 72 hours of an operation is pathognomonic for atelectasis.

- Early mobilization and ambulation have been documented to be as effective as chest physical therapy in the prevention of pulmonary complications.

- Postoperative pneumonia is commonly associated with atelectasis, with predisposing factors including chronic pulmonary disease, heavy cigarette smoking, alcohol abuse, obesity, older age, nasogastric tubes, long procedures, gram-negative bacterial infections, postoperative peritonitis, and debilitating illnesses.

- Radiographic diagnoses are approximately 60% accurate for either bacterial or viral pneumonia in women with laboratory-proven pneumonia.

- In the perioperative period, hypovolemia may be secondary to several factors including preoperative volume deficit, unreplaced blood loss during surgery, extracellular fluid loss during surgery, inadequate fluid replacement, and, most commonly, continued blood loss after the surgical procedure.

- Tachycardia is the classic cardiovascular physiologic response of the body to hypotension. However, relative bradycardia in hypotensive women is also a common hemodynamic response.

- Rapid loss of 20% of a woman's blood volume produces mild shock, whereas a loss of greater than 40% of blood volume results in severe shock.

- From 15% to 45% of surgical blood loss is absorbed onto drapes, pads, and other areas. Thus blood levels in the suction bottle are inaccurate markers of total operative blood loss.

- Massive blood loss recently has been defined as hemorrhage that results in replacement of 50% of circulating blood volume in less than 3 hours.

- The differential diagnosis of hemorrhagic shock in the postoperative patient includes pneumothorax, pulmonary embolus, massive pulmonary aspiration, myocardial infarction, and acute gastric dilation.

- The goals of management of shock are to replace, restore, and maintain effective circulating blood volume and to establish normal cellular perfusion and oxygenation. To accomplish this goal, an adequate cardiac output and appropriate peripheral vascular resistance must be maintained.

- In hemorrhagic shock crystalloids should be considered the initial resuscitation fluid of choice; colloids are appropriate for resuscitation in conjunction with crystalloids when blood products are not immediately available.

- The gold standard of imaging studies to detect abdominal and pelvic hemorrhage is a CT scan performed without either oral or intravenous contrast.

- Returning a patient to the operating room to control hemorrhage is often a difficult decision. However, this decision should not be postponed, and the patient should have an exploratory operation as soon as possible after volume replacement.

- The extent of wound or pelvic hematomas is determined by the potential size of the compartment into which the bleeding occurs. Retroperitoneal or broad ligament hematomas may contain several units of blood.

- Superficial thrombophlebitis is frequently overlooked or disregarded as a cause of postoperative fever.

- Recurrent, superficial phlebitis, in varying anatomic sites, may be a sign of occult malignant disease.

- Approximately 30% of all hospital-acquired bacteremias are secondary to intravenous lines.

- Superficial phlebitis is the leading cause of an enigmatic postoperative fever during the third, fourth, or fifth postoperative day.

- The clinical management of mild superficial thrombophlebitis includes rest, elevation, and local heat. Moderate to severe superficial thrombophlebitis may be treated with nonsteroidal antiinflammatory agents.

- Generally, thromboembolic complications occur early in the postoperative course—50% within the first 24 hours and 75% within the first 72 hours. Approximately 15% occur after the seventh postoperative day.

- Diagnosis of deep vein thrombophlebitis by physical examination is very insensitive. Thus imaging studies are essential for establishing the correct diagnosis.

- Venous thrombosis and pulmonary embolus are the direct causes of approximately 40% of deaths in gynecologic cases.

- The reported incidence of deep vein thrombosis with gynecologic operations varies from 7% to 45%, with an average of approximately 15%.

- The incidence of thrombophlebitis is directly dependent on the risk factors of type and duration of operation, age of the woman, obesity, immobility, malignancy, sepsis, diabetes, current oral contraceptive use, and conditions producing venous stasis.

- Thrombophlebitis most often begins in the deep veins of the calf. Approximately 75% of pulmonary emboli originate from a thrombus that begins in the leg veins and extends to the femoral veins.

- The three precipitating factors that produce thrombi, as described by Virchow, are an increase in coagulability, damage to the vessel wall, and venous stasis.

- D-Dimer blood assay levels are helpful in excluding the diagnosis of deep vein thrombophlebitis in an individual woman when the clinical result is below the cut-off level.

- Heparin is the drug of choice for the initial treatment of thrombosis or pulmonary embolus once the diagnosis is confirmed.

- Failure to achieve adequate anticoagulation in the first 24 hours of therapy increases the risk of recurrent venous thromboembolism fifteenfold.

- The primary risk of chronic anticoagulation therapy is the potential for major bleeding complications. Major bleeding occurs in approximately 4% of woman-years of therapy.

- Autopsy studies have documented that pulmonary emboli are undiagnosed clinically in approximately 50% of women who experience this complication.

- Women with pulmonary emboli have a mortality rate of 30% in untreated cases versus 8% in treated cases.

- Signs and symptoms of pulmonary emboli are nonspecific; however, the most common symptoms are chest pain, dyspnea, apprehension, tachypnea, rales, and an increase in the second heart sound over the pulmonic area.

- Ventilation/perfusion scans are the first line in imaging techniques to rule out the diagnosis of pulmonary embolus. However, pulmonary angiography is the most definitive test in establishing the diagnosis. Five percent of patients experience complications from pulmonary angiography.

- The risk of a woman developing a subsequent fatal pulmonary embolus during the 3 months of anticoagulation therapy is approximately 1 in 70 to 1 in 100.

- The etiology of postoperative voiding problems includes anxiety, mechanical interference, obstruction by swelling and edema, overdistention from hydration, neurologic imbalance, drug-associated detrusor hypotonia, and dysynchronous bladder contractions.

- Intermittent in-and-out catheterization is preferable to continuous drainage with a Foley catheter. Women especially appreciate intermittent self-catheterization because it gives them control over a part of their postoperative care.

- The most commonly acquired infection in the hospital and most frequent cause of gram-negative bacteremia in hospitalized patients is catheter-associated urinary tract infection.

- Prophylactic antibiotics should not be used with a Foley catheter to cover for the possibility of urinary tract infection unless the patient is immunocompromised.

- In the United States, urinary fistulas following gynecologic operations are secondary to abdominal hysterectomy in 75% of cases and to vaginal procedures in the remaining 25%.

- The ratio of operative injuries to the urinary bladder compared to ureteral injuries is approximately 5:1.

- Although symptoms of urinary incontinence may present within a few hours of the operative procedure, the majority of fistulas usually present 8 to 12 days after operation, occasionally as late as 25 to 30 days after the operation.

- If there is a suspicion that trauma to the bladder has occurred during an operative procedure, continuous catheter drainage for 3 to 5 days usually results in spontaneous healing.

- Approximately 25% of adult women experience postoperative nausea and vomiting.

- An uncomplicated ileus may last 24 to 48 hours in the stomach, only a few hours in the small intestines, and 48 to 72 hours in the colon.

- If adynamic ileus persists for longer than 5 days, a diagnosis of mechanical bowel obstruction should be strongly considered.

- Multiple recent articles report early postoperative oral feeding is safe and efficacious. This practice is preferred by women because it facilitates their recovery and shortens hospital stay.

- The difference between small bowel obstruction and adynamic ileus is a subtle one, for adynamic ileus is normally associated with partial obstruction of the small intestine.

- Previous gynecologic operations are the most common cause of bowel obstruction in women.

- Pneumoperitoneum from an exploratory celiotomy usually persists for 7 to 10 days. Thus, in the early postoperative period, free air under the diaphragm is not diagnostic of perforation of a hollow viscus.

- After the diagnosis of a defect between the vagina and rectum has been made, the woman should be obstipated with a low-residue diet and diphenoxylate hydrochloride (Lomotil). Approximately one in four anatomic defects heals spontaneously before epithelialization of the tract occurs.

- *Clostridium difficile* is a species of spore-forming, gram-positive anaerobic bacteria found normally in 1% of healthy adults. However, after antibiotic treatment and disruption of normal enteric flora, up to 25% of hospitalized adults will become colonized with *C. difficile.*

- Second- and third-generation cephalosporins, clindamycin, ampicillin, and amoxicillin are the antibiotics associated with the highest risk of developing *C. difficile* diarrhea.

- The incidence of postoperative wound infection is increased eightfold when the woman's preoperative weight exceeds 200 pounds. The thickness of subcutaneous tissue is the greatest risk factor for wound infection in women undergoing abdominal hysterectomy.

- Symptoms of wound infections occur most commonly between the fifth and tenth postoperative day, with the patient usually exhibiting tachycardia and fever.

- Delayed secondary closure may be accomplished in previously infected wounds after several days of drainage and debridement. Delayed secondary closure markedly reduces the time necessary for eventual closure of the skin defect by secondary intention. Patient satisfaction dramatically increased with delayed secondary closure.

- Necrotizing fasciitis involves the subcutaneous tissue and superficial fascia. It rapidly expands in the subcutaneous spaces. If the diagnosis is questionable, a full-thickness core biopsy and frozen section of the tissue should be performed. This condition is a surgical emergency, and patients should have operative debridement as soon as possible.

- The incidence of wound dehiscence is approximately 1 in 200 gynecologic operations. Wound infection is found in approximately 50% of women with wound disruption.

- The classic symptom and sign of an impending wound disruption is the spontaneous passage of serosanguineous fluid from the abdominal incision.

- Most postoperative pelvic infections are polymicrobial, usually from endogenous vaginal flora, and approximately 60% to 80% involve anaerobic organisms.

- The volume of pelvic fluid 3 to 5 days postoperatively after a hysterectomy is a nonspecific finding and does not predict febrile morbidity or the need for drainage.

- If a patient does not become afebrile within 48 hours of adequate drainage of a retroperitoneal abscess, a concomitant complication of pelvic thrombophlebitis should be suspected. If pelvic thrombophlebitis is suspected, a 72-hour trial of intravenous heparin therapy with concurrent antibiotics should be instituted.

- Granulation tissue at the apex of the vaginal vault is a frequent complication following hysterectomy. Small areas of friable, red granulation tissue are seen at the 6-week postoperative pelvic examination in more than 50% of women.

- Ovarian abscesses arise from bacterial colonization of a disrupted ovarian capsule, usually by the presence of a recently ruptured corpus luteum or by operative disruption during a procedure.

- Ovarian abscesses usually present 2 to 3 weeks postoperatively, but cases have been reported as late as 3 to 4 months.

- Common causes of femoral neuropathy are continuous pressure from self-retaining retractors or exaggerated hip flexion or abduction in the dorsal lithotomy position in thin women.

- Patient-controlled analgesic (PCA) systems dramatically decrease patients' anxiety because they are in control rather than the hospital staff. These systems are both safe and effective as long as there is a lockout period, and they help to minimize individual differences in pharmacokinetics.

- Any operation on the female reproductive organs stimulates questions and conflicts concerning body image, feminine identity, sexuality, and possibly future childbearing.

- Discharge instructions should be given in both verbal and written forms, and the gynecologist should anticipate the most common questions.

BIBLIOGRAPHY

Acute Respiratory Distress Syndrome Network: Ventilation with lower tidal volumes as compared with traditional tidal volumes for acute lung injury and the acute respiratory distress syndrome, N Engl J Med 342:1301, 2000.

Allescia G, DiRicco G, Formichi B, et al: Invasive and noninvasive diagnosis of pulmonary embolism: preliminary results of the prospective investigative study of acute pulmonary embolism diagnosis, Chest 107:S33, 1995.

Al-Took S, Platt R, and Tulandi T: Adhesion-related small-bowel obstruction after gynecologic operations, Am J Obstet Gynecol 180:313, 1999.

Alvarez RD: Gastrointestinal complications in gynecologic surgery: a review for the general gynecologist, Obstet Gynecol 72:533, 1988.

American College of Obstetricians and Gynecologists: Blood component therapy, ACOG Tech Bull 199:1, 1994.

American College of Obstetricians and Gynecologists: Hemorrhagic shock, ACOG Educ Bull 235:1, 1997.

American College of Obstetricians and Gynecologists: Lower urinary tract operative injuries, ACOG Educ Bull 238:1, 1997.

Anand A and Feffer SE: Hematocrit and bleeding time: an update, South Med J 87:299, 1994.

Anderson CHM, Raju SK, Forsling ML, and Wheeler MJ: Oestrogen replacement after oophorectomy: comparison of patches and implants, BMJ 305:90, 1992.

Arcasoy SM and Kreit JW: Thrombolytic therapy of pulmonary embolism: a comprehensive review of current evidence, Chest 115:1695, 1999.

Atkinson TP and Kaliner MA: Anaphylaxis, Med Clin North Am 76:841, 1992.

AuBuchon JP and Birkmeyer JD: Controversies in transfusion medicine: is autologous blood transfusion worth the cost? Con Transfusion 34:79, 1994.

Baker WF Jr and Bick RL: Deep vein thrombosis, Med Clin North Am 78:685, 1994.

Baldo BA: Penicillins and cephalosporins as allergens—structural aspects of recognition and cross-reactions, Clin Exp Allergy 29:744, 1999.

Barnes J, Resch KL, and Ernst E: Homeopathy for postoperative ileus? A meta-analysis, J Clin Gastroenterol 25:628, 1997.

Barone JG and Cummings KB: Etiology of acute urinary retention following benign anorectal surgery, Am Surg 60:210, 1994.

Bates SM and Ginsberg JS: Helical computed tomography and the diagnosis of pulmonary embolism, Ann Intern Med 132:240, 2000.

Batres F and Barclay DL: Sciatic nerve injury during gynecologic procedures using the lithotomy position, Obstet Gynecol 62:92S, 1983.

Bates RD and Nahata MC: Once-daily administration of amnioglycosides, Ann Pharmacother 28:757, 1994.

Becker RC and Ansell J: Antithrombotic therapy: an abbreviated reference for clinicians, Arch Intern Med 155:149, 1995.

Bergman A, Mushket Y, Gordon D, and David MP: Prostaglandin prophylaxis and bladder function after vaginal hysterectomy: a prospective randomized study, Br J Obstet Gynaecol 100:69, 1993.

Bernardi E, Prandoni P, Lensing AWA, et al: D-dimer testing as an adjunct to ultrasonography in patients with clinically suspected deep vein thrombosis: prospective cohort study, BMJ 317:1037, 1998.

Birdwell BG, Raskob GE, Whitsett TL, et al: The clinical validity of normal compression ultrasonography in outpatients suspected of having deep venous thrombosis, Ann Intern Med 128:1, 1998.

Bloom SL, Ramin SM, and Gilstrap LC: Blood and blood component therapy, Prim Care Update Ob/Gyns 4:200, 1997.

Boardman A: Diagnosis and management of pseudomembranous colitis and Clostridium difficile-associated disease, Prim Care Update Ob/Gyns 5:219, 1998.

Bone RC: Ventilation/perfusion scan in pulmonary embolism: "The emperor is incompletely attired," JAMA 263:2794, 1990.

Bonnar J: Can more be done in obstetric and gynecologic practice to reduce morbidity and mortality associated with venous thromboembolism? Am J Obstet Gynecol 180:784, 1999.

Borstad E, Urdal K, Handeland G, and Abildgaard U: Comparison of low molecular weight heparin vs. unfractionated heparin in gynecological surgery: II. reduced dose of low molecular weight heparin, Acta Obstet Gynecol Scand 71:471, 1992.

Bounameaux H, Cirafici P, DeMoerloose P, et al: Measurement of D-dimer in plasma as diagnostic aid in suspected pulmonary embolism, Lancet 337:196, 1991.

Bounameaux H and Reber-Wasem MA: Superficial thrombophlebitis and deep vein thrombosis: a controversial association, Arch Intern Med 157:1822, 1997.

Bregenzer T, Conen D, Sakmann P, and Widmer AF: Is routine replacement of peripheral intravenous catheters necessary? Arch Intern Med 158:151, 1998.

Brenner DW, Fogle MA, and Schellhammer PF: Venous thromboembolism, J Urol 142:1403, 1989.

Breslow MJ, Miller CF, and Rogers MC, editors: Perioperative management, St Louis, 1990, Mosby–Year Book, Inc.

Broomhead CJ: Physiology of postoperative nausea and vomiting, Br J Hosp Med 53:327, 1995.

Cancio LC and Cohen DJ: Heparin-induced thrombocytopenia and thrombosis, J Am Coll Surg 186:76, 1998.

Carpenter JP, Holland GA, Baum RA, et al: Magnetic resonance venography for the detection of deep vein thrombosis: comparison with contrast venography and duplex Doppler ultrasonography, J Vasc Surg 18:734, 1993.

Carr JA and Silverman N: The heparin-protamine interaction: a review, J Cardiovasc Surg 40:659, 1999.

Carson JL and Willett LR: Is a hemoglobin of 10 g/dL required for surgery? Med Clin North Am 77:335, 1993.

Carter CJ: The natural history and epidemiology of venous thrombosis, Prog Cardiovasc Dis 36:423, 1994.

Castro CJ, Krammer J, and Drake J: Postoperative feeding: a clinical review, Obstet Gynecol Surv 55:571, 2000.

Cataldo PA, Senagore AJ, and Kilbride MJ: Ketorolac and patient controlled analgesia in the treatment of postoperative pain, Surg Obstet Gynecol 176:435, 1993.

Cercenado E, Ena J, Rodriguez-Creixems M, et al: A conservative procedure for the diagnosis of catheter-related infections, Arch Intern Med 150:1417, 1990.

Challis DE and Bennett MJ: Nerve entrapment—an important complication of transverse lower abdominal incisions, Aust N Z J Obstet Gynaecol 34:5, 1994.

Chassany O, Michaux A, and Bergmann JF: Drug-induced diarrhoea, Drug Safety 22:53, 2000.

Cholhan HJ and Kocur BA: Bladder care after gyn surgery, Contemp OB/GYN 39:35, 1994.

Chumbley GM, Hall GH, and Salmon P: Patient-controlled analgesia: an assessment by 200 patients, Anaesthesia 53:216, 1998.

Clagett GP, Anderson FA Jr, Heit J, et al: Prevention of venous thromboembolism, Chest 108:S312, 1995.

Clarke DB and Abrams LD: Pulmonary embolectomy: a 25 year experience, J Thorac Cardiovasc Surg 92:442, 1986.

Clarke-Pearson DL, Synan IS, Dodge R, et al: A randomized trial of low-dose heparin and intermittent pneumatic calf compression for the prevention of deep venous thrombosis after gynecologic oncology surgery, Am J Obstet Gynecol 168:1146, 1993.

Colombo M, Maggioni A, Zanini A, et al: A randomized trial of open versus closed vaginal vault in the prevention of postoperative morbidity after abdominal hysterectomy, Am J Obstet Gynecol 173:1807, 1995.

Cronan JJ: Venous thromboembolic disease: the role of US, Radiology 186:619, 1993.

Cruikshank MK, Levine MN, Hirsch J, et al: A standard heparin homogram for the management of heparin therapy, Arch Intern Med 151:333, 1991.

Cruse PJE and Foord R: A 5-year prospective study of 23,649 surgical wounds, Arch Surg 107:206, 1973.

Cumming PD, Wallace EL, Schorr JB, et al: Exposure of patients to human immunodeficiency virus through the transfusion of blood components that test antibody-negative, N Engl J Med 321:941, 1989.

Cuzen N, Haque R, and Timmis A: Applications of thrombolytic therapy, Intensive Care Med 24:756, 1998.

Dahl JB and Kehlet H: The value of pre-emptive analgesia in the treatment of postoperative pain, Br J Anaesth 70:434, 1993.

Dalen JE and Alpert JS: Thrombolytic therapy for pulmonary embolism: Is it effective? Is it safe? When is it indicated? Arch Intern Med 157:2550, 1997.

Darouiche RO, Raad II, Heard SO, et al: A comparison of two antimicrobial-impregnated central venous catheters, N Engl J Med 340:1, 1999.

Dauzat M, Laroche JP, Deklunder G, et al: Diagnosis of acute lower limb deep venous thrombosis with ultrasound: trends and controversies, J Clin Ultrasound 25:343, 1997.

Davis JH and Sheldon GF, editors: Surgery: a problem-solving approach, ed 2, St. Louis, 1995, Mosby–Year Book.

Decousus H, Leizorovica A, Parent F, et al: A clinical trial of vena cava filters in the prevention of pulmonary embolism in patients with proximal deep-vein thrombosis, N Engl J Med 338:409, 1998.

DeLancey JOL and Hartman RG: Operations on the abdominal wall. In Sciarra JJ, editor: Gynecology and Obstetrics, Philadelphia, 1992, JB Lippincott.

Demetriades D, Chan LS, Bhasin P, et al: Relative bradycardia in patients with traumatic hypotension, J Trauma Inj Infec Crit Care 45:534, 1998.

DeMoerloose P, Michiels JJ, and Bounameaux H: The place of D-Dimer testing in an integrated approach of patients suspected of pulmonary embolism, Semin Thromb Hemost 24:409, 1998.

Dodds C and Allison J: Postoperative cognitive deficit in the elderly surgical patient, Br J Anaesth 81:449, 1998.

Dodson MK, Magann EF, and Meeks GR: A randomized comparison of secondary closure and secondary intention in patients with superficial wound dehiscence, Obstet Gynecol 80:321, 1992.

Donaldson MDJ, Seaman MJ, and Park GR: Massive blood transfusion, Br J Anaesth 69:621, 1992.

Douketis JD, Kearon C, Bates S, et al: Risk of fatal pulmonary embolism in patients with treated venous thromboembolism, JAMA 279:458, 1998.

Duff GW: Is fever beneficial to the host? A clinical perspective, Yale J Biol Med 59:125, 1986.

Dunn LJ and Van Voorhis LW: Enigmatic fever and pelvic thrombophlebitis, N Engl J Med 276:265, 1967.

Dunnihoo DR, Huddleston HT, and North SC: Femoral nerve palsy as a complication of vaginal hysterectomy: review of the world literature, J Gynecol Surg 10:1, 1994.

Eason E, Aldis A, and Seymour RJ: Pelvic fluid collections by sonography and febrile morbidity after abdominal hysterectomy, Obstet Gynecol 90:58, 1997.

Ellis H, Niran BJ, Thompson JN, et al: Adhesion-related hospital readmissions after abdominal and pelvic surgery: a retrospective cohort study, Lancet 353:1476, 1999.

Engoren M: Lack of association between atelectasis and fever, Chest 107:81, 1995.

Fanning J, Neuhoff RA, Brewer JE, et al: Frequency and yield of postoperative fever evaluation, Infec Dis Obstet Gynecol 6:252, 1998.

Fejgin MD and Lourwood DL: Low molecular weight heparins and their use in obstetrics and gynecology, Obstet Gynecol Surv 49:424, 1994.

Fekety R and Shah AB: Diagnosis and treatment of *Clostridium difficile* colitis, JAMA 269:71, 1993.

Finan MA, Barton DPJ, Fiorica JV, et al: Ileus following gynecologic surgery: management with water-soluble hyperosmolar radiocontrast material, South Med J 88:539, 1995.

Fleenor-Ford A, Hayden MK, and Weinstein RA: Vancomycin-resistant enterococci: implications for surgeons, Surgery 125:121, 1999.

Frager DH, Baer JW, Rothpearl A, and Bossart PA: Distinction between postoperative ileus and mechanical small-bowel obstruction: value of CT compared with clinical and other radiographic findings, AJR 164:891, 1995.

Francis KR, Lamaute HR, Davis JM, and Pizzi WF: Implications of risk factors in necrotizing fasciitis, Am Surg 59:304, 1993.

Fraser JD and Anderson DR: Deep venous thrombosis: recent advances and optimal investigation with US, Radiology 211:9, 1999.

Fresh-Frozen Plasma, Cryoprecipitate, and Platelets Administration Practice Guidelines Development Task Force for the College of American Pathologists: Practice parameter for the use of fresh-frozen plasma, cryoprecipitate and platelets, JAMA 271:777, 1994.

Fujii Y, Tanaka H, and Somekawa Y: Granisetron, droperidol, and metoclopramide for the treatment of established postoperative nausea and vomiting in women undergoing gynecologic surgery, Am J Obstet Gynecol 182:13, 2000.

Gallup DG, Nolan TE, and Smith RP: Primary mass closure of midline incisions with a continuous polyglyconate monofilament absorbable suture, Obstet Gynecol 76:872, 1990.

Gefter WB, Hatabu H, Holland GA, et al: Pulmonary thromboembolism: recent developments in diagnosis with CT and MR imaging, Radiology 197:561, 1995.

Ghosh S and Sallam S: Patient satisfaction and postoperative demands on hospital and community services after day surgery, Br J Surg 81:1635, 1994.

Gilmour DT, Dwyer PL, and Carey MP: Lower urinary tract injury during gynecologic surgery and its detection by intraoperative cystoscopy, Obstet Gynecol 94:883, 1999.

Ginsberg JS, Wells PS, Kearson C, et al: Sensitivity and specificity in a rapid whole-blood assay for D-Dimer in the diagnosis of pulmonary embolism, Ann Intern Med 129:1006, 1998.

Giuntini C, Di Ricco G, Marini C, et al: Epidemiology, Chest 107:S3, 1995.

Goh JTW, Gregora MG, and Welch M: Lithotomy position-induced femoral neuropathy, Aust N Z J Obstet Gynaecol 34:596, 1994.

Goldhaber SZ: Contemporary pulmonary embolism thrombolysis, Chest 107:S45, 1995.

Goldhaber SZ, Kessler CM, Heit J, et al: Randomized controlled trial of recombinant tissue plasminogen activator versus urokinase in the treatment of acute pulmonary embolism, Lancet 8606:293, 1988.

Goldhaber SZ, Simons GR, Elliott CG, et al: Quantitative plasma D-dimer levels among patients undergoing pulmonary angiography for suspected pulmonary embolism, JAMA 270:2819, 1993.

Grady D and Sawaya G: Postmenopausal hormone therapy increases risk of deep vein thrombosis and pulmonary embolism, Am J Med 105:41, 1998.

Grimes DA: A simplified device for intraoperative autotransfusion, Obstet Gynecol 72:947, 1988.

Greer BE, Cain JM, Figge DC, et al: Supraumbilical upper abdominal midline incision for pelvic surgery in the morbidly obese patient, Obstet Gynecol 76:471, 1990.

Gunnarsson PS, Sawyer WT, Montague D, et al: Appropriate use of heparin: empiric vs nomogram-based dosing, Arch Intern Med 155:526, 1995.

Haire WD: Vena cava filters for the prevention of pulmonary embolism, N Engl J Med 338:463, 1998.

Hall JC, Heel KA, Papadimitriou JM, and Platell C: The pathobiology of peritonitis, Gastroenterology 114:185, 1998.

Harding GKM, Nicolle LE, Ronald AR, et al: How long should catheter-acquired urinary tract infection in women be treated? A randomized controlled study, Ann Intern Med 114:713, 1991.

Harrison L, McGinnis J, Crowther M, et al: Assessment of outpatient treatment of deep-vein thrombosis with low-molecular-weight heparin, Arch Intern Med 158:2001, 1998.

Heijboer H, Büller HR, Lensing AWA, et al: A comparison of real-time compression ultrasonography with impedance plethysmography for the diagnosis of deep-vein thrombosis in symptomatic outpatients, N Engl J Med 329:1365, 1993.

Hemsel DL: Post-hysterectomy cuff and pelvic cellulitis, Contemp Obstet Gynecol 32:39, 1990.

Hemsell DL: Infection after hysterectomy, Infec Dis Obstet Gynecol 5:52, 1997.

Hershey CO, Tomford JW, McLaren CE, et al: The natural history of intravenous catheter–associated phlebitis, Arch Intern Med 144:1373, 1984.

Hiippala S: Replacement of massive blood loss, Vox Sanguinis 74(S2):399, 1998.

Hirsh J, Raschke R, Warkentin TE, et al: Heparin: mechanism of action, pharmacokinetics, dosing considerations, monitoring, efficacy, and safety, Chest 108:S258, 1995.

Hohler A, Katz VL, Dotters DJ, and Rogers RG: *Clostridium difficile* infection in obstetric and gynecologic patients, SMJ 90:889, 1997.

Hopf HW and Weitz S: Postoperative pain management, Arch Surg 129:128, 1994.

Hull RD, Raskob GE, Pineo GF, and Brant RF: The low-probability lung scan: a need for change in nomenclature, Arch Intern Med 155:1845, 1995.

Hull RD, Raskob GE, Pineo GF, et al: Subcutaneous low-molecular–weight heparin compared with continuous intravenous heparin in the treatment of proximal-vein thrombosis, N Engl J Med 326:975, 1992.

Hull RD, Raskob GE, Pineo GF, et al: A comparison of subcutaneous low-molecular–weight heparin with warfarin sodium for prophylaxis against deep-vein thrombosis after hip or knee implantation, N Engl J Med 329:1370, 1993.

Hull RD, Raskob GE, Rosenbloom D, et al: Heparin for 5 days as compared with 10 days in the initial treatment of proximal venous thrombosis, N Engl J Med 322:1260, 1990.

Johnson S, Samore MH, Farrow KA, et al: Epidemics of diarrhea caused by a clindamycin-resistant strain of *Clostridium difficile* in four hospitals, N Engl J Med 341:1645, 1999.

Jones EM and MacGowan AP: Back to basics in management of *Clostridium difficile* infections, Lancet 352:505, 1998.

Kakkar VV: Pathophysiologic characteristics of venous thrombosis, Am J Surg 150:1, 1985.

Kakkar VV, Cohen AT, Edmonson RA, et al: Low molecular weight versus standard heparin for prevention of venous thromboembolism after major abdominal surgery, Lancet 341:259, 1993.

Katz DS, Lane MJ, and Mindelzun RE: Unenhanced CT of abdominal and pelvic hemorrhage, Semin Ultrasound CT MR 20:94, 1999.

Katz DS and Leung AN: Radiology of pneumonia, Clin Chest Med 20:549, 1999.

Keenan DL: The active management of postoperative pain. In Thompson JD and Rock JA, editors: TeLinde's Operative Gynecology Updates, ed 7, Philadelphia, 1992, JB Lippincott.

Kehlet H and Dahl JB: The value of multimodal or balanced analgesia in postoperative pain treatment, Anesth Analg 77:1048, 1993.

Kelly CP, Pothoulakis C, and LaMont JT: *Clostridium difficile* colitis, N Engl J Med 330:257, 1994.

Killewich LA, Sandager GP, Nguyen AH, et al: Venous hemodynamics during impulse foot pumping, J Vasc Surg 22:598, 1995.

Koopman MMW, van Beek EJR, and ten Cate JW: Diagnosis of deep vein thrombosis, Prog Cardiovasc Dis 37:1, 1994.

Kraus K and Fanning J: Prospective trial of early feeding and bowel stimulation after radical hysterectomy, Am J Obstet Gynecol 182:996, 2000.

Krebs HB: Intestinal injury in gynecologic surgery: a ten-year experience, Am J Obstet Gynecol 155:509, 1986.

Kuhn S, Cooke K, Collins M, et al: Perceptions of pain relief after surgery, Br Med J 300:1687, 1990.

Kuno K, Menzin A, Kauder HH, et al: Prophylactic ureteral catheterization in gynecologic surgery, Urology 52:1004, 1998.

Kyne L, Warny M, Qamar A, and Kelly CP: Asymptomatic carriage of *Clostridium difficile* and serum levels of IgG antibody against toxin A: N Engl J Med 342:390, 2000.

Kyrle PA, Minar E, Hirschl M, et al: High plasma levels of factor VIII and the risk of recurrent venous thromboembolism, N Engl J Med 343:457, 2000.

Landefeld CS and Beyth RJ: Anticoagulant-related bleeding: clinical epidemiology, prediction, and prevention, Am J Med 95:315, 1993.

Leith S, Wheatley RG, Jackson IJB, et al: Extradural infusion analgesia for postoperative pain relief, Br J Anaesth 73:552, 1994.

Leizorovicz A, Simonneau G, Decousus H, and Boissel JP: Comparison of efficacy and safety of low molecular weight heparins and unfractionated heparin in initial treatment of deep venous thrombosis: a meta-analysis, BMJ 309:299, 1994.

Lenhardt R, Negishi C, Sessler DI, et al: The effects of physical treatment on induced fever in humans, Am J Med 106:550, 1999.

Lensing AWA, Prandoni P, Brandjes D, et al: Detection of deep-vein thrombosis by real-time B-mode ultrasonography, N Engl J Med 320:342, 1989.

Liu S, Carpenter RL, and Neal JM: Epidural anesthesia and analgesia: their role in postoperative outcome, Anesthesiology 82:1474, 1995.

Lopes AD, Hall JR, and Monaghan JM: Drainage following radical hysterectomy and pelvic lymphadenectomy: dogma or need? Obstet Gynecol 86:960, 1995.

Lubin MF, Walker HK, and Smith RB, editors: Medical management of the surgical patient, ed 3, Philadelphia, 1995, JB Lippincott.

Lundberg GD: Practice parameter for the use of fresh-frozen plasma, cryoprecipitate, and platelets, JAMA 271:777, 1994.

MacFarland LV: Epidemiology, risk factors and treatments for antibiotic-associated diarrhea, Dig Dis 16:292, 1998.

Mackowiak PA, Wasserman SS, and Levine MM: A critical appraisal of 98.6° F, the upper limit of the normal body temperature, and other legacies of Carl Reinhold August Wunderlich, JAMA 268:1578, 1992.

Madan M, Alexander DJ, and McMahon MJ: Influence of catheter type on occurrence of thrombophlebitis during peripheral intravenous nutrition, Lancet 339:101, 1992.

Majeski J and Majeski E: Necrotizing fasciitis: improved survival with early recognition by tissue biopsy and aggressive surgical treatment, SMJ 90:1065, 1997.

Malins AF, Field JM, Nesling PM, and Cooper GM: Nausea and vomiting after gynaecological laparoscopy: comparison of premedication with oral ondansetron, metoclopramide and placebo, Br J Anaesth 72:231, 1994.

Manganelli D, Palla A, Donnamaria V, and Giuntini C: Clinical features of pulmonary embolism: doubts and certainties, Chest 107:S25, 1995.

Mann MC, Votto J, Kambe J, and McNamee MJ: Management of the severely anemic patient who refuses transfusion: lessons learned during the care of a Jehovah's Witness, Ann Intern Med 117:1042, 1992.

Mann WJ, Arato M, Patsner B, et al: Ureteral injuries in an obstetrics and gynecology training program: etiology and management, Obstet Gynecol 72:82, 1988.

Manyonda IT, Welch CR, McWhinney NA, et al: The influence of suture material on vaginal vault granulations following abdominal hysterectomy, Br J Obstet Gynaecol 97:608, 1990.

Matsumoto AH and Tegtmeyer CJ: Contemporary diagnostic approaches to acute pulmonary emboli, Radiol Clin North Am 33:167, 1995.

McBride K, LaMorte WW, and Menzoian JO: Can ventilation-perfusion scans accurately diagnose acute pulmonary embolism? Arch Surg 121:754, 1986.

McClean KL, Sheehan GJ, and Harding GKM: Intraabdominal infection: a review, Clin Infect Dis 19:100, 1994.

McIntosh DG and Rayburn WF: Patient-controlled analgesia in obstetrics and gynecology, Obstet Gynecol 78:1129, 1991.

McKenzie R, Kovac A, O'Connor T, et al: Comparison of ondansetron versus placebo to prevent postoperative nausea and vomiting in women undergoing ambulatory gynecologic surgery, Anesthesiology 78:21, 1993.

Meeks GR and Chez RA: Secondary closure, Contemp OB/GYN 38:35, 1993.

Meeks GR, Waller GA, Meydrech EF, and Flautt H Jr: Unscheduled hospital admission following ambulatory gynecologic surgery, Obstet Gynecol 80:446, 1992.

Mermel LA: Prevention of intravascular catheter-related infections, Ann Intern Med 132:391, 2000.

Meyer MA, Lalich RA, Meyer MM, and Widener J: Outpatient vaginal hysterectomy in a community hospital, Wis Med J 93:422, 1994.

Miyazaki F and Shook G: Ilioinguinal nerve entrapment during needle suspension for stress incontinence, Obstet Gynecol 80:246, 1992.

Moser KM, Fedullo PF, LitteJohn JK, and Crawford R: Frequent asymptomatic pulmonary embolism in patients with deep vein thrombosis, JAMA 271:223, 1994.

Moss GS and Gould SA: Plasma expanders: an update, Am J Surg 155:425, 1988.

Murry BE: Vancomycin-resistant enterococcal infections, N Engl J Med 342:710, 2000.

Neu HC: Emerging trends in antimicrobial resistance in surgical infections: a review, Eur J Surg S573:7, 1994.

Nyman MA, Schwenk NM, and Silverstein MD: Management of urinary retention: rapid versus gradual decompression and risk of complications, Mayo Clin Proc 72:951, 1997.

Palla S, Petruzzelli S, Donnamaria V, and Giuntini C: The role of suspicion in the diagnosis of pulmonary embolism, Chest 107:S21, 1995.

Patsner B: Closed-suction drainage versus no drainage following radical abdominal hysterectomy with pelvic lymphadenectomy for stage 1B cervical cancer, Gynecol Oncol 57:232, 1995.

Pearl ML, Valea VA, Fischer M, et al: A randomized controlled trial of early postoperative feeding in gynecologic oncology patients undergoing intra-abdominal surgery, Obstet Gynecol 92:94, 1998.

Perrier A: Noninvasive diagnosis of pulmonary embolism, Hosp Pract September 15, 1998, p 47.

Petty TL: The acute respiratory distress syndrome—historic perspective, Chest 105:S44, 1994.

PIOPED investigators: Value of the ventilation/perfusion scan in acute pulmonary embolism: results of the Prospective Investigation of Pulmonary Embolism Diagnosis, JAMA 263:2753, 1990.

Ponec RJ, Saunders MD, and Kimmey MB: Neostigmine for the treatment of acute colonic pseudo-obstruction, N Engl J Med 341:137, 1999.

Prandoni P, Lensing AWA, Büller HR, et al: Comparison of subcutaneous low-molecular–weight heparin with intravenous standard heparin in proximal deep-vein thrombosis, Lancet 339:441, 1992.

Ramin SM, Ramin KD, and Hemsell DL: Fallopian tube prolapse after hysterectomy, SMJ 92:963, 1999.

Rathbun SW, Raskob GE, and Whitsett TL: Sensitivity and specificity of helical computed tomography in the diagnosis of pulmonary embolism: a systematic review, Ann Intern Med 132:227, 2000.

Ripley DL: Necrotizing fasciitis, Prim Care Update Ob/Gyn 7:142, 2000.

Roberts HR and Lozier JN: New perspectives on the coagulation cascade, Hosp Pract 27:97, 1992.

Roberts JA, Fussell EN, and Kaack MB: Bacterial adherence to urethral catheters, J Urol 144:264, 1990.

Robertson PL, Goergen SK, Waugh JR, and Fabiny PJ: Colour-assisted compression ultrasound in the diagnosis of calf deep venous thrombosis, Med J Aust 163:515, 1995.

Sabiston DC Jr, editor: Textbook of surgery, ed 14, Philadelphia, 1991, WB Saunders Co.

Sagar PM, Sedman P, May J, et al: Intestinal obstruction promotes gut translocation of bacteria, Dis Colon Rectum 38:640, 1995.

Saint S, Elmore JG, Sullivan SD, et al: The efficacy of silver alloy-coated urinary catheters in preventing urinary tract infection: a meta-analysis, Am J Med 105:236, 1998.

Schulman S, Rhedin AS, Lindmarker P, et al: A comparison of six weeks with six months of oral anticoagulant therapy after a first episode of venous thromboembolism, N Engl J Med 322:1661, 1995.

Schwartz SI, editor: Principles of surgery, ed 7, New York, 1999, McGraw-Hill, Inc.

Shifren JL, Braunstein GD, Simon JA, et al: Transdermal testosterone treatment in women with impaired sexual function after oophorectomy, N Engl J Med 343:682, 2000.

Simonneau G, Sors H, Charbonnier B, et al: A comparison of low-molecular-weight heparin with unfractionated heparin for acute pulmonary embolism, N Engl J Med 337:663, 1997.

Soper DE, Bump RC, and Hurt WG: Wound infection after abdominal hysterectomy: effect of the depth of subcutaneous tissue, Am J Obstet Gynecol 173:465, 1995.

Spirt MJ: Antibiotics in inflammatory bowel disease: new choices for an old disease, Am J Gastroenterol 89:974, 1994.

Stamm WE and Hooten TM: Management of urinary tract infections in adults, N Engl J Med 329:1328, 1993.

Standards Care Committee of British Thoracic Society: Suspected acute pulmonary embolism: a practical approach, Thorax 52:S2, 1997.

Stanhope CR, Wilson TO, Utz WJ, et al: Suture entrapment and secondary ureteral obstruction, Am J Obstet Gynecol 164:1513, 1991.

Stark RP and Maki DG: Bacteriuria in the catheterized patient, N Engl J Med 311:560, 1984.

Stein PD, Afzal A, Henry JW, and Villareal CG: Fever in acute pulmonary embolism, Chest 117:39, 2000.

Stein PD, Hull RD, and Pineo G: Strategy that includes serial noninvasive leg tests for diagnosis of thromboembolic disease in patients with suspected acute pulmonary embolism based on data from PIOPED, Arch Intern Med 155:2101, 1995.

Stephenson H, Dotters DJ, Katz V, and Droegemueller W: Necrotizing fasciitis of the vulva, Am J Obstet Gynecol 166:1324, 1992.

Stovall TG, Summitt RL Jr., Bran DF, and Ling FW: Outpatient vaginal hysterectomy: a pilot study, Obstet Gynecol 80:145, 1992.

Strickler B, Blanco J, and Fox HE: The gynecologic contribution to intestinal obstruction in females, J Am Coll Surg 178:617, 1994.

Sutherland ME and Meyer AA: Necrotizing soft-tissue infections, Surg Clin North Am 74:591, 1994.

Suzuki M, Ohwada M, and Sato I: Pelvic lymphocysts following retroperitoneal lymphadenectomy: retroperitoneal partial "no-closure" for ovarian and endometrial cancers, J Surg Oncol 68:149, 1998.

Swisher ED, Kahleifeh B, and Polh JF: Blood cultures in febrile patients after hysterectomy: cost-effectiveness, J Reprod Med 42:547, 1997.

Symmonds RE: Ureteral injuries associated with gynecologic surgery: prevention and management, Clin Obstet Gynecol 19:623, 1976.

Symmonds RE: Prevention and management of genitourinary fistula, JCE Obstet Gynecol 21:13, 1979.

Tai NRM, Atwal AS, and Hamilton G: Modern management of pulmonary embolism, Br J Surg 86:853, 1999.

Tarkington MA, Dejter SW Jr, and Bresette JF: Early surgical management of extensive gynecologic ureteral injuries, Surg Gynecol Obstet 173:17, 1991.

Tewes PA, Taylor DR, and Bourke DL: Postoperative pain management. In Breslow MJ, Miller CF, and Rogers MC, editors: Perioperative management, St Louis, 1990, Mosby Year Book.

Thakar R and Clarkson P: Bladder, bowel and sexual function after hysterectomy for benign conditions, Br J Obstet Gynaecol 104:983, 1997.

Thomas JH: Pathogenesis, diagnosis, and treatment of thrombosis, Am J Surg 160:547, 1990.

Thompson CD, Brekken AL, and Kutteh WH: Necrotizing fasciitis: a review of management guidelines in a large obstetrics and gynecology teaching hospital, Infect Dis Obstet Gynecol 1:16, 1993.

Tobin MJ: Respiratory monitoring, JAMA 264:244, 1990.

Tønnesen H and Kehlet H: Preoperative alcoholism and postoperative morbidity, Br J Surg 83:869, 1999.

Traill ZC and Gleeson FV: Venous thromboembolic disease, Br J Radiol 71:129, 1998.

Vedantham S, Goodwin SC, McLucas B, and Mohr G: Uterine artery embolization: an underused method of controlling pelvic hemorrhage, Am J Obstet Gynecol 176:938, 1997.

Verma A, Mittal S, and Kumar S: Primary ovarian abscess, Int J Gynecol Obstet 68:263, 2000.

Vermeulen LC, Ratko TA, Erstat BL, et al: A paradigm for consensus: the University Hospital Consortium guidelines for the use of albumin, nonprotein colloid, and crystalloid solutions, Arch Intern Med 155:373, 1995.

von Gruenigen VE, Coleman RL, King MR, and Miller DS: Abdominal compartment syndrome in gynecologic surgery, Obstet Gynecol 994:830, 1999.

Wallace D, Hernandez W, Schlaerth JB, et al: Prevention of abdominal wound disruption utilizing the Smead-Jones closure technique, Obstet Gynecol 56:226, 1980.

Walsh JJ, Bomar J, and Wright FW: A study of pulmonary embolism and deep leg vein thrombosis after major gynaeco-logical surgery using labelled fibrinogen-phlebography and lung scanning, J Obstet Gynaecol Br Comm 81:311, 1974.

Walters MD, Dombroski RA, Davidson SA, et al: Reclosure of disrupted abdominal incisions, Obstet Gynecol 76:597, 1990.

Ware LB and Matthay MA: The acute respiratory distress syndrome, N Engl J Med 342:1334, 2000.

Warkentin TE, Levine MN, Hirsh J, et al: Heparin-induced thrombocytopenia in patients treated with low-molecular–weight heparin or unfractionated heparin, N Engl J Med 332:1330, 1995.

Watcha MF and White PF: Postoperative nausea and vomiting: its etiology, treatment, and prevention, Anesthesiology 77:162, 1992.

Watkins DT and Robertson CL: Water-soluble radiocontrast material in the treatment of postoperative ileus, Am J Obstet 152:450, 1985.

Weinmann EE and Salzman EW: Deep-vein thrombosis, N Engl J Med 331:1630, 1994.

Wells PS, Ginsberg JS, Anderson DR, et al: Use of a clinical model for safe management of patients with suspected pulmonary embolism, Ann Intern Med 129:997, 1998.

Wells PS, Hirsh J, Anderson DR, et al: Accuracy of clinical assessment of deep-vein thrombosis, Lancet 345:1326, 1995.

Wetchler SJ and Dunn LJ: Ovarian abscess, Obstet Gynecol Surv 40:476, 1985.

Wheeler AP and Bernard GR: Treating patients with severe sepsis, N Engl J Med 340:207, 1999.

White PF: Pain management (special report), Postgrad Med 80:7, 1986.

White RH, McGahan JP, Daschbach MM, et al: Diagnosis of deep-vein thrombosis using duplex ultrasound, Ann Intern Med 111:297, 1989.

Williams-Russo P, Charlson ME, MacKenzie R, et al: Predicting postoperative pulmonary complications: is it a real problem? Arch Intern Med 152:1209, 1992.

Willson JR and Black JR: Ovarian abscess, Am J Obstet Gynecol 90:34, 1964.

Wolfson PH, Bauer JJ, Gelernt IM, et al: Use of the long tube in the management of patients with small-intestine obstruction due to adhesions, Arch Surg 120:1001, 1985.

Wong HY, Carpenter RL, Kopacz DJ, et al: A randomized, double-blind evaluation of ketorolac tromethamine for postoperative analgesia in ambulatory surgery patients, Anesthesiology 78:6, 1993.

Wrenn K: Fecal impaction, N Engl J Med 321:658, 1989.

PART FOUR

Gynecologic Oncology

Principles of Radiation Therapy and Chemotherapy in Gynecologic Cancer

Basic Principles, Uses, and Complications

KEY TERMS AND DEFINITIONS

Alkylating Agent. A class of antineoplastic agents that covalently link (alkylation) with DNA, which inhibits the growth of dividing cells.

Alpha Particle. A type of particulate radiation that is the same as a helium nucleus.

Antimetabolites. Antineoplastic agents that resemble naturally occurring purines or pyrimidines and interfere with normal cell metabolism.

Antitumor Antibiotic. Antineoplastic agents derived from bacterial or fungal cultures.

Beta Rays. Low-energy electron radiation produced by radionuclide decay.

Betatron. A circular accelerator for electrons for production of high energy.

Brachytherapy. A form of radiation therapy in which the source is placed close to the tumor. The application may be in the form of needles implanted into the tumor (interstitial) or placed in the vagina or cervical canal (internal).

Centigray. One hundredth of a gray, a measure of radiation absorbed equal to 1 rad.

Complete Remission. Total disappearance of the tumor for at least 1 month.

Curie (Ci). A measure of the rate of disintegration of radioisotopes. One curie is equivalent to 3.7×10^{10} disintegrations per second.

Depth Dose. The specific dose of irradiation absorbed at a given distance beneath the surface.

Electron Volt (eV). A unit of measurement of electro-magnetic energy equivalent to 1.6×10^{-12} ergs. MeV = 1 million eV; keV = 1000 eV.

Erythropoietin (epo). A stimulator of bone marrow red cell production.

Fractionation. The practice of dividing radiation therapy treatments into numerous small doses to reduce damage to normal tissues.

Gamma Rays. A form of photon energy produced by the decay of radioactive isotopes.

Granulocyte cell stimulating factor (GCSF). An example of a growth factor.

Gray. A measurement of the dosage of radiation absorbed by tissue. 1 gray = 1 joule per kilogram (100 rads).

Growth Fraction. The proportion of tumor cells in a replicating phase.

Isodose Curve. A curve connecting points that receive equivalent doses of irradiation.

Linear Accelerator. A machine that accelerates electrons in a straight line to produce high energy.

Linear Energy Transfer (LET). The measurement of the amount of energy transferred by ionizing radiation per unit of distance traveled.

Log Cell Kill. The proportion of cells killed by a particular treatment: 90% equals a 1-log cell kill; 99% equals a 2-log cell kill.

Neutron. A subatomic particle with mass but no charge, making it a highly penetrating form of radiation.

Partial Objective Response. A more than 50% reduction in the greatest perpendicular dimension of the tumor for at least 1 month.

Photons. Quanta of radiation whose energy is proportional to their frequency and inversely proportional to their wavelength (gamma rays and x-rays).

Progression. Increase in size or spread of tumor in a patient receiving therapy.

Rad. A measurement of the dose of radiation absorbed in tissue equivalent to 100 ergs per gram or 1 centiGray (cGy).

Radiocurability. The ability to cure a malignant tumor with radiation.

Radiosensitivity. The relative response of tumor cells to radiation.

Source-to-Skin Distance (SSD). The distance from the external radiation source to the skin of the patient receiving external therapy.

Stabilization. A term occasionally used to indicate that a tumor has not changed in size while a patient has been receiving therapy.

Teletherapy. A form of radiation therapy with the placement of the radioactive source at a distance from the patient (external therapy).

Vinca Alkaloids. Antineoplastic agents derived from periwinkle plant *(Vinca rosea)* extracts.

X-ray. Electromagnetic radiation formed by accelerated electrons in a vacuum striking a target.

This chapter presents the general principles of radiation therapy and chemotherapy, with particular attention to those concepts that apply to the therapy of gynecologic cancers. The details of treatment of individual cancers are described separately in the various chapters dealing with specific gynecologic malignancies.

Included with the basic concepts of radiation physics are the types and measurements of radiation energy, the biologic effects of radiation on cells, and the factors that alter these effects. Common radiation sources and their properties are illustrated as they relate specifically to the treatment of gynecologic cancers. Risks and complications are also presented.

Cell growth and division are affected by cancerous processes and by chemotherapeutic treatments. The physician must know the various classes of chemotherapeutic agents, their actions in gynecologic malignancies, and their toxicities. There are also general approaches to be followed in administering chemotherapy, specifically including the monitoring of patients receiving these agents.

RADIATION THERAPY

Basic Radiation Physics

Radiation physics deals with the measurement of energy that is transferred from the source of the radiation to the tissues or cells being irradiated. One form of ionizing radiation is electromagnetic, which refers to x-rays or gamma rays. These sources of energy have no mass and no electrical charge. They are produced in discrete quanta or photons, and their energy is proportional to their frequency; that is, higher energies are transmitted at a higher frequency. Since the frequency of a photon is inversely pro-

portional to the wavelength, electromagnetic radiation with shorter wavelengths has a higher frequency and thus a higher energy. The energy that is produced is measured in electron volts (eV); 1 eV = 1.6×10^{-12} ergs. Various x-ray radiotherapy units can range from 50,000 eV (50 kV) to over 30 million eV (30 meV).

A second source of photon radiation comes from the production of gamma rays (similar to x-rays), which result from the decay of radioactive isotopes. Such decay or disintegration is measured in curies (Ci). One curie is defined as 3.7×10^{10} disintegrations per second, which is equivalent to the disintegration of 1 g of radium.

Regardless of the source of electromagnetic or photon radiation, the transmitted energy diverges as the distance it travels from the source increases. This divergence causes a decrease in energy, and the relationship is described by the inverse square law, which indicates that the energy dose of radiation per unit area decreases proportionately to the square of the distance from the site to the source ($1/d^2$). For example, the dose of radiation 2 cm from a point source is only one fourth of the value of the dose at 1 cm (Figure 26-1).

In general, x-rays or photons can be generated as a result of rapidly accelerated electrons in a vacuum striking a target. Modern generators that accelerate these elec-

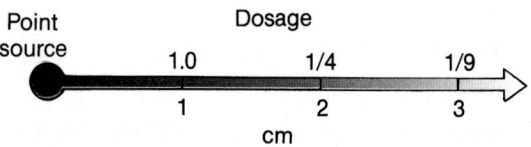

FIGURE 26-1 Radiation effects at various distances from point source of irradiation demonstrating the inverse square law.

trons at high speed may do so in a circular fashion (betatron) or linearly (linear accelerator). Another type of radiation energy is known as particulate radiation and is produced by subatomic particles with a discrete mass. These particles are usually released by the disintegration of radionuclides. Four common types are alpha particles (the same as a helium nucleus), neutrons, protons, and electrons. Alpha particles produce a large number of ions over a short distance. They currently have little use in radiation therapy because of their short range in tissue but are being investigated for intraperitoneal radiation application. Neutrons are usually machine produced and are highly penetrating with no charge but have a large mass. They cause high-energy collisions with atomic nuclei, principally of hydrogen, in the tissues. The resultant recoil proton loses energy to the surrounding tissue by ionization, which leads to cell death. Protons are positively charged particles, and generators are available for the direct production of protons to yield very high energy beams, which have specialized uses such as in the treatment of pituitary tumors.

Electrons may also be referred to as beta rays, produced by radionuclide disintegration. Electrons can be produced at different energies by machines for various therapeutic applications.

Radiation Biology

Photons (gamma rays or x-rays) act by dislodging orbital electrons from the atoms of the medium or tissue through which they pass. This collision produces a fast electron (Compton effect), which then ionizes molecules along its path, producing secondary electrons and free hydroxyl radicals. The process continues until the electromagnetic beam (photon) loses all of its energy. The cells are damaged by the free hydroxyl radicals and the negatively charged electrons that affect the DNA of the cell. This effect may be lethal and kill the cell, or it can be sublethal, in which case the cell will subsequently undergo repair of the DNA. In addition, free hydroxyl radicals may react with molecular oxygen to form peroxide in the tissues. This adds to the lethal effects of radiation on the cells. As shown by Gray et al., oxygen is important for the tissue effects of photon irradiation. This has practical implications in tumor therapy insofar as cancers tend to have poor blood supplies, which decreases the oxygenation, particularly at the center of large tumors. The effect of photon radiation in these hypoxic areas is therefore diminished.

The rate of loss of energy of an ionizing particle as it traverses a unit length of medium is known as linear energy transfer (LET). In the case of photon irradiation, the loss of energy per hit is small. This is described as low LET irradiation, which often causes a sublethal effect on a single cell and thus necessitates multiple hits to kill the cell, as well as to produce toxic hydroxyl radicals. In the case of particulate radiation with heavy particles, the ionization is known as high LET. Thus neutrons, with their large mass, produce high-energy recoil protons that kill the cell directly on impact, independent of oxygenation. For this reason research has been directed toward the development of neutron generators to try to improve tumor therapy by overcoming the limitation of poor oxygenation of cancer cells.

An important principle is that a given dose of radiation kills a constant fraction of the number of cells irradiated. For example, if 90% of the cells of a tumor are killed with each fraction of radiation delivered, then 10% of the cells would survive. Thus if one were to begin to irradiate a tumor with 10 million cells, there would be 1 million cells surviving after the first fraction, 100,000 cells after the second fraction, 10,000 cells after the third fraction, etc. By the seventh fraction all of the cells would be killed.

As shown in Figure 26-2 there are four phases of the cell cycle. Sinclair and Morton showed that during mitosis the cell is most sensitive to radiation. Thus rapidly dividing cells are the most radiosensitive. It has been demonstrated that dividing radiation treatment into a number of small doses (fractionation) allows for effective treatment of the tumor without increasing the complications of radiation to the normal tissues (bone marrow, intestine, and other rapidly dividing tissues) that would occur with single large doses. The more efficient repair of normal tissue occurring between treatment fractions affords a therapeutic advantage. The measurement of the amount of energy absorbed by tissue is the rad, which is defined as 100 ergs of energy absorbed per gram of tissue. The term *gray* (1 joule per kilogram) has been introduced; 1 gray is equivalent to 100 rads, and one rad to one centigray (cGy).

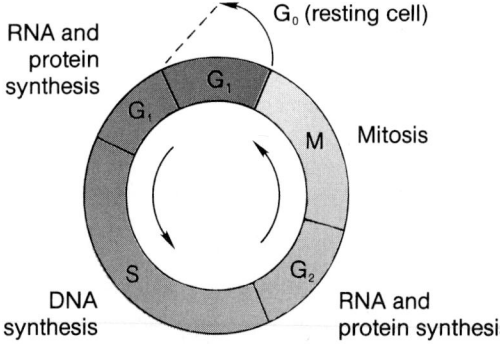

FIGURE 26-2 Phases of the cell. After mitosis *(M)* there is an interval of variable duration during which there is RNA and protein synthesis and a diploid DNA content (G_1 [gap$_1$]). The cell may also enter a prolonged or resting phase (G_0) and then reenter the cycle during DNA synthesis, the *(S)* phase, in which DNA is duplicated. During G_2 (gap$_2$) there again is protein and RNA synthesis. During the *M* phase the cell divides into two cells, each of which receives a diploid DNA content.

Radiation Sources— External and Internal Therapy

In general two techniques are utilized in radiation treatment: brachytherapy (internal) and teletherapy (external). Brachytherapy involves the placement of radioactive sources within an existing body cavity (e.g., the vagina) in close proximity to the tumor. In the treatment of gynecologic malignant tumors, radioactive needles may also be implanted directly into the tissue to be irradiated (interstitial implant), or a tandem containing radioactive sources may be placed within the cervix and uterus accompanied by two vaginal ovoids—one on each side of the tandem—that also contain radioactive sources (intracavitary therapy). Intracavitary brachytherapy is done with the aid of specialized applicators; the best known and most widely used is the Fletcher Suit applicator. Such an arrangement is useful for treatment of a cervical tumor or a tumor located near the cervix (Figure 26-3), and the dose delivered to the tissues is determined by the inverse square law. In practice the radioactive sources are placed in the devices after the apparatus has been properly placed within the endocervix and vagina. This "afterloading" technique reduces radiation exposure to the personnel treating the patient.

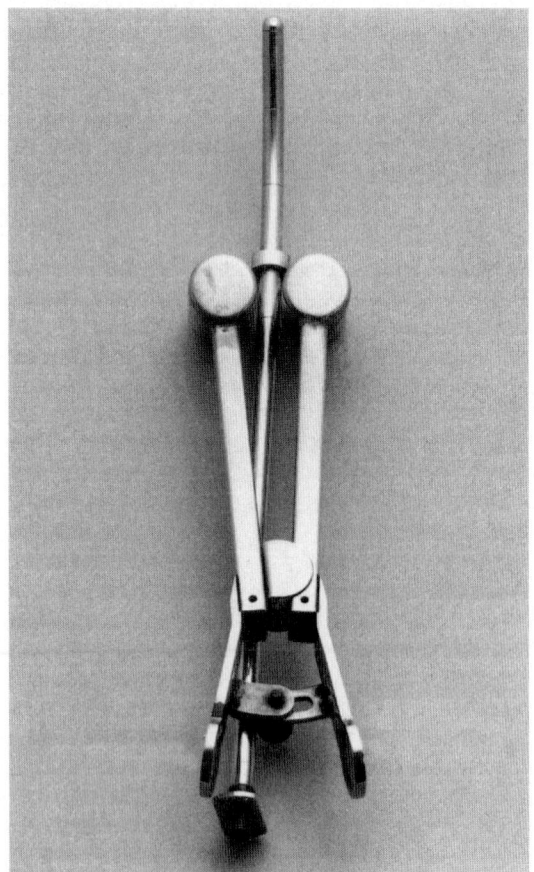

FIGURE 26-3 Fletcher-Suit applicator (tandem and ovoids) used for afterloading internal therapy.

Various radioisotopes are used in brachytherapy. In general those with a short half-life (such as gold 198) may be placed within the patient and left permanently, whereas those with a long half-life (cesium 137) are placed temporarily within the patient and then removed after a prescribed dose of irradiation has been administered. Brachytherapy has in the past been delivered over 3 to 4 days as an inpatient at a low-dose rate (LDR) (e.g., 40-70 cGy/hour). Recently high-dose rate (HDR) has been used in same settings using iridium at dose rates exceeding 200 cGy/min. Unlike LDR, HRD is an outpatient procedure requiring minimal anesthesia. Table 26-1 indicates the half-lives of some of the isotopes commonly used in treating gynecologic cancers. It is also important that a uniform distribution of radiation be achieved in the adjacent tissues to avoid "hot spots," which can damage normal tissue, as well as "cold spots," which can lead to undertreatment of the tumor.

Teletherapy refers to the placement of the radioactive source at a distance from the patient. With external therapy the source of radiation is located at a distance 5 to 10 times greater than the depth of the tumor being irradiated in order to deliver a uniform dose to the tumor and thus avoid the large dose changes that result because of the inverse square law. This distance is referred to as the source-to-skin distance (SSD).

With the utilization of different angles and ports of treatment, the concept of source axis distance (SAD) has been introduced; it denotes the distance from the radiation source to the central axis of machine rotation. The patient is positioned so that this axis passes through the center of the tumor, and treatment ports are arranged around this axis to optimize tumor dose and minimize the dose to vital structures.

Conventional external beam radiation is delivered with beams of uniform intensity. Recent advances have made the use of beams of varying intensity possible. This approach of planned dose intensification allows the high-dose region to be conformed precisely to the shape of the planned treatment volume. To focus the beam from the external source, a

TABLE 26-1
Half-Lives of Commonly Used Isotopes

Radionuclide	Half-Life
Gold 198	2.7 Days
Phosphorus 32	14.3 Days
Iodine 125	60 Days
Iridium 192	74.4 Days
Cobalt 60	5.3 Years
Cesium 137	30 Years
Radium 226	1620 Years

collimator is used. The collimator prevents scatter and allows for a directed beam for a given field size (10 cm × 10 cm, for example) to be applied to the tissue being irradiated (Figure 26-4). In general the higher the energy source of the radiation, the deeper the beam penetrates the tissue. Thus high-energy (short-wavelength) radiation has its predominant effect in deeper tissues and spares the surface or the skin of radiation effect. The term *orthovoltage* refers to machines in the 125,000 to 400,000 eV (125 to 400 keV) range, whereas supervoltage or megavoltage refers to machines with 2 to 35 million eV (megavolt) range. Cobalt machines (equivalent to 1.25 meV) and 4 to 6 meV machines have similar properties and achieve their maximum dosage at about 0.5 cm beneath the skin; higher energy machines such as the 22 meV have their maximum effect at a depth of about 5 cm beneath the skin.

An isodose curve is a line that connects points in the tissue that receive equivalent dosages of irradiation. Figure 26-5 contrasts the isodose curves for 6 and 22 meV machines. For the 6 meV machine the maximum dose is near the surface, with a more rapid falloff in the deeper tissues, in comparison to the 22 meV machine, which has its maximum dose well beneath the surface. Thus at a given depth the higher dose of radiation can be achieved with 22 meV, sparing the effects of radiation on the skin.

In addition to the energy of the beam, the energy of radiation absorbed at various depths is affected by the size of the field being treated. Larger fields contain more scattered radiation, which leads to a greater dose at a given depth. Figure 26-6 demonstrates the effect of increasing the size of the field with increasing dosage at a given depth for three different types of energy sources.

Thus the radiation dose delivered to the tumor is affected by the energy of the source, the depth of the tumor beneath the surface, and the size of the field undergoing irradiation. With external therapy, usually 160 to 200 cGy per day is given five times per week. Recently there has been experimental work evaluating hyperfractionation, which involves smaller multiple doses given more frequently (for example, 120 cGy three times a day or 160 cGy two times a day).

Multiple chemotherapeutic agents have been used to sensitize cells to radiation. These agents have included 5-fluorouracil, actinomycin-D, cisplatin, gemcitabine, paclitaxel (Taxol), doxorubicin, hydroxyurea, Mitomycin-C, topotecan, and vinorelbine (Navalbine). The mechanism of radiosensitization varies among agents. Cisplatin inhibits repair of lethal radiation damage. This inhibition of repair may also explain the radiosensitization effects of topotecan. Doxorubicin acts on cellular oxygen levels by inhibiting mitochondrial and tumor cell respiration. Paclitaxel synchronizes cells into G_2 and M of the cell cycle. Currently platinum is most commonly used in chemoradiation treatment. Hyperthermia has also been explored to potentiate the therapeutic effectiveness of radiation. It appears to offer the most promise for tumors localized in an area that can effectively and safely tolerate increased temperatures (42 degrees to 43 degrees C).

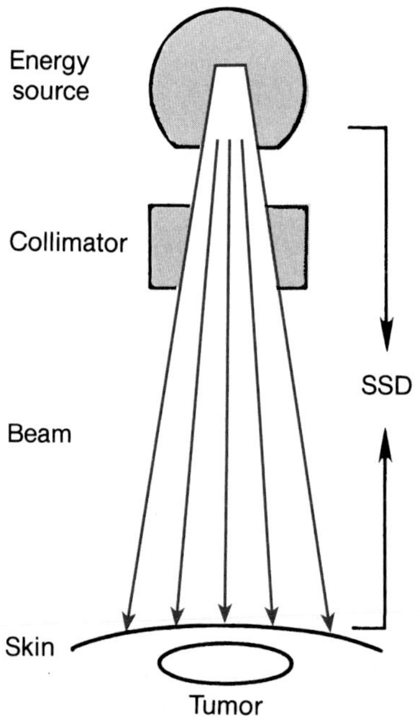

Tissue Tolerance and Radiation Complications

Radiation acutely affects tissues undergoing rapid cell division, such as the skin, the intestinal mucosa, and the mucosa of the vagina and bladder. Radiation given in the fractions noted previously reduces the untoward effects of cell damage on normal tissue and allows for normal healing to occur between treatment fractions. Systemic side effects of radiation include a decrease in circulating white cells, as well as gastrointestinal effects, such as nausea, anorexia, or diarrhea, which usually can be controlled with medication. The skin may be irritated with a "wet reaction," particularly if lower energy external sources are used; occasionally a treatment program may have to be temporarily discontinued.

Although the acute effects of radiation limit the rate at which the dosage is administered, late effects may occur many years later and can cause permanent damage. Late adverse effects include tissue necrosis and fibrosis, as well as fistula formation, ulceration, and bleeding. These late-stage complications depend on the total dose of the radiation administered, the volume of tissue treated, and the size of the radiation field. It is thought that these late effects are due to radiation damage to the vascular tissue and connective tissue. An alternate explanation is that the

FIGURE 26-4 External therapy unit. Divergence of beam increases with distance from source. (Redrawn from Kase NG and Weingold AB: Principles and practice of clinical gynecology, New York, 1983, John Wiley & Sons.)

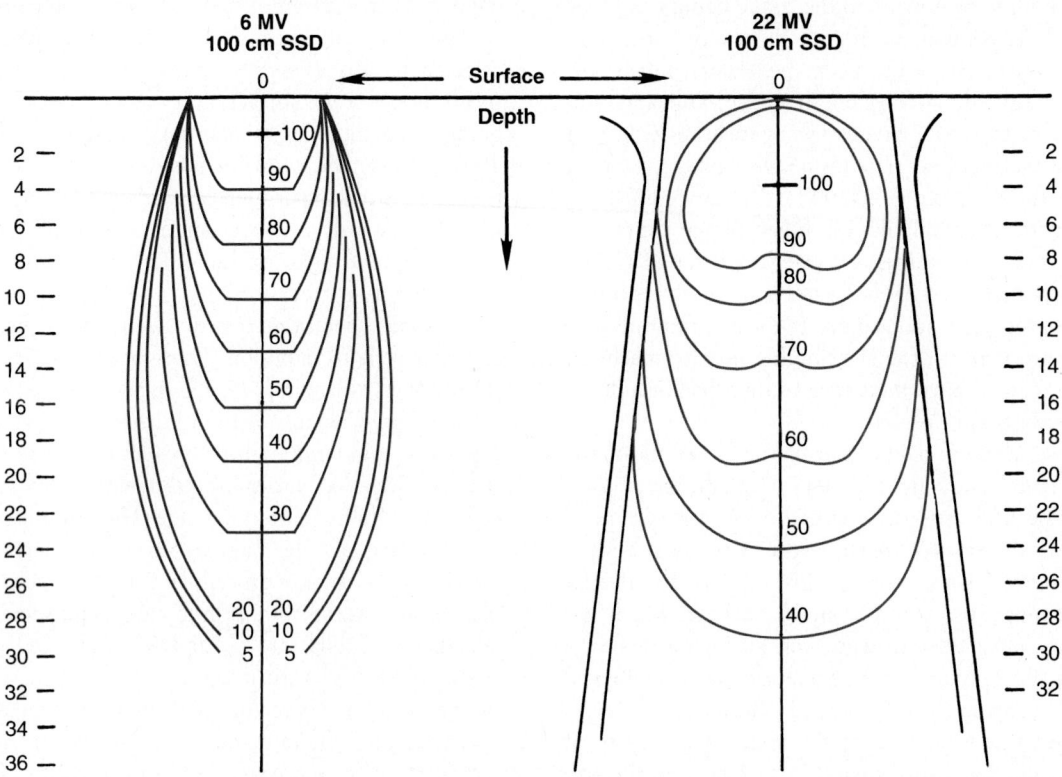

FIGURE 26-5   Comparison of isodose curves and depth-dose distribution for 6 MV and 22 MV betatrons. Note that the higher energy machine delivers radiation to greater depth for same surface dose, and there is considerable skin sparing. (Redrawn from DiSaia PJ and Creasman WT: Clinical gynecologic oncology, ed 4, St Louis, 1993, Mosby–Year Book, Inc.)

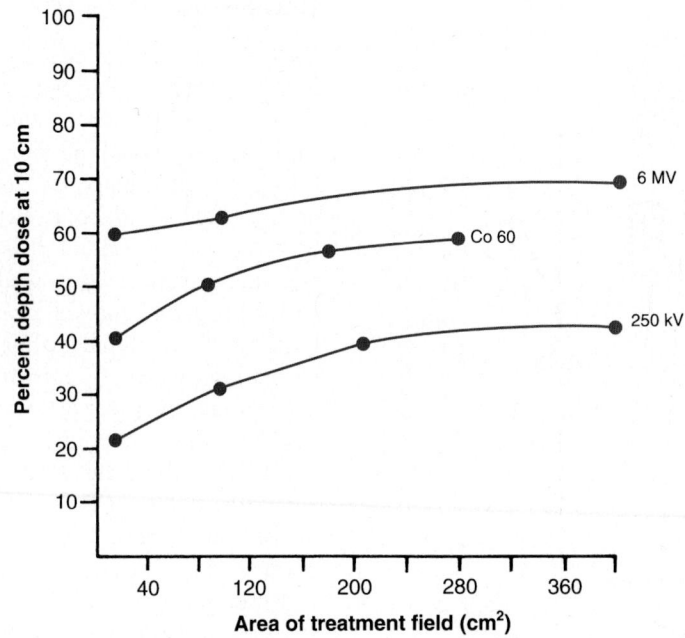

FIGURE 26-6   Variation of depth dose at 10 cm with energy and size of treatment field. (Redrawn from Joslin CAF: Basic parameters of radiotherapy. In Coppleson M, ed: Gynecologic oncology, Edinburgh, 1981, Churchill Livingstone.)

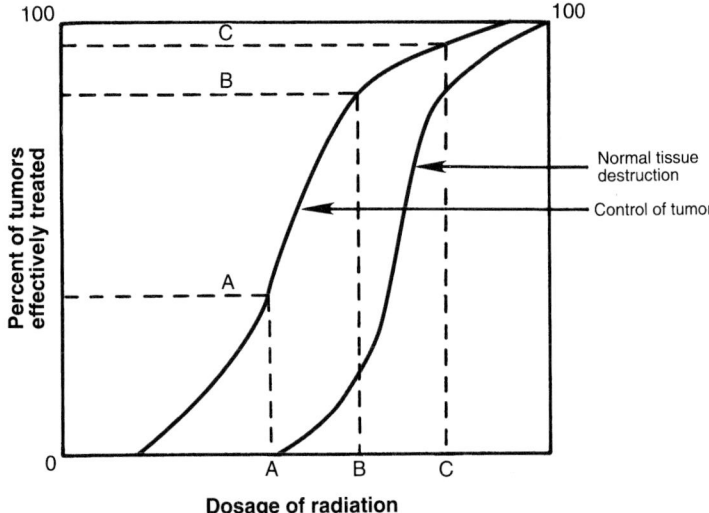

FIGURE 26-7   Concept of tumor control versus complications. At point *A* there are no complications but insufficient control. Point *C* has good control but excess complications. There is reasonable tumor control at *B* with a slight risk of complications.

radiation destroys the cells that are capable of regeneration, which eventually leads to tissue destruction. Second cancers induced after radiation are rare. Arai et al. noted an excess of rectal cancer, bladder cancer, and leukemia among patients with carcinoma of the cervix treated by radiation in comparison with those treated by operation.

It has been observed that the response of the tumor to radiation treatment follows a sigmoid curve, with increasingly effective tumor control associated with increasing dosage (Figure 26-7). A similar effect exists for normal tissues, and the ability of radiation therapy to control malignancy depends on the greater tolerance of normal tissues to radiation exposure. Thus if one were to use the level of radiation that causes no normal tissue damage, only a small proportion of cancers would be controlled. Conversely, if one were to use a dosage that could control almost all cancers, massive damage to normal tissue would occur and an unacceptable series of complications and even patient death could follow. The goal is to achieve maximum tumor control with as little risk of damage to normal tissues as possible.

In the treatment of gynecologic malignancies the main sites of radiation damage are the bladder, rectum, and large and small bowel. Complications of the bladder can occur in the form of radiation cystitis, which can lead to complaints of dysuria and frequency. Hematuria may also occur, and therapy with sclerosing solutions or fulguration through a cystoscope may be necessary. McIntyre et al. noted ureteral stricture after radiation for stage I carcinoma of the cervix was 1% at 5 years and 2.5% at 20 years, a rare but important complication. In rare instances urinary diversion may be required. Fistulas between the vagina and bladder or between the vagina and rectum may develop when there has been extensive radiation damage to the intervening tissues. This usually takes place during

therapy for large carcinomas of the cervix (see Chapter 29). As a general rule such complications will occur 6 months to 2 years after treatment, although they may occur many years after primary therapy. In addition, the bone marrow of the sacrum and lower vertebrae is compromised by pelvic irradiation, an important consideration if the patient is to receive subsequent chemotherapy.

Damage to the large bowel usually occurs in the form of inflammation (sigmoiditis), which may be associated with severe bleeding and pain. Less severe cases can often be controlled with a low-roughage diet and antispasmodic medication. Increase in bowel motility leading to diarrhea is common. More severe cases may require bowel resection or permanent bowel diversion through a colostomy. Covens et al. noted that those who required operation for radiation damage to the bowel had an approximately 25% risk of dying in 2 years, with ileal damage being the most risky. Those with complications not requiring operation frequently have decreased vitamin B_{12} and bile acid absorption. Recently, drugs have been used as radioprotectors to protect normal tissue from radiation damage while reportedly not affecting tumor radiosensitivity. The best known radioprotector is amifostine, a free radical scavenger. After administration this drug quickly penetrates into normal tissue, but only slowly into tumors, thereby protecting preferentially normal tissue.

Montana and Fowler showed that the risks of proctitis and cystitis are dose related. For example, severe proctitis and cystitis were noted at dosages of 6750 cGy and 6900 cGy respectively, while such complications were not observed in patients whose median dose was 6500 and 6300 cGy. The small bowel also receives irradiation during external therapy for pelvic tumors. In the acute phases of treatment this often leads to bowel irritability, and the patient complains of diarrhea. Long-term complications include

TABLE 26-2
Approximate Tolerance of Tissues
to Radiation Therapy

Tissue	Approximate Tolerance Dose (rads)
Bladder	6000–7000
Rectum	6000–7000
Vaginal mucosa	7000
Bowel	6000
Cervix	>12,000
Kidney	2000–2300
Liver	2500–3500

fibrosis of the wall of the intestine, which can lead to permanent narrowing and even obstruction. Occasionally enteric fistulas also develop and bowel perforation may occur. In the latter cases surgical therapy is required, usually to bypass the affected area of the intestine. As a general rule, extensive dissection of irradiated tissue is avoided. Small bowel injuries are more frequent in patients who have had a previous operation, particularly pelvic operations, which predispose to adhesions reducing bowel motility and increasing radiation damage. Table 26-2 presents the *approximate* tolerance of tissues to radiation therapy. Multiple factors, as already discussed, influence late effects of radiation on normal tissue, such as dose fractionation, field size, port arrangement, extent of tumor damage to normal tissues, previous operations, concurrent chemotherapy, and other less well-defined elements, including anemia, small vessel pathology, and the patient's nutritional status.

CHEMOTHERAPY

The use of drugs to treat disseminated cancer has developed into an extensive clinical discipline. Numerous compounds have been tested to treat human tumors, and the first successful effort in gynecologic cancer was the demonstration by Li et al. that the antimetabolite methotrexate could cause permanent remission in cases of metastatic trophoblastic disease (Chapter 35). A number of general principles have been developed that provide guidelines for the use of chemotherapeutic agents to treat malignant disease. Many of these principles were developed by Skipper, Bruce, and others and involve an understanding of the cell replication cycle.

Cell Kinetics

The cell replication cycle is demonstrated in Figure 26-2. After completion of mitosis, the cell usually enters the gap$_1$ (G$_1$) phase, during which there is a diploid content of DNA

and RNA and protein synthesis occurs. This phase is usually of variable length. The G$_1$ phase then leads into a phase of DNA synthesis (S), during which the DNA is duplicated. Then a second mitotic gap develops (G$_2$), during which DNA synthesis ceases and RNA and protein synthesis can again occur. During G$_2$ there is twice the DNA content of a normal cell. G$_2$ then leads into the mitosis (M) phase, during which the cell divides into two daughter cells, each of which contains a normal amount of DNA. Occasionally the cell enters a prolonged resting phase, termed the *G$_0$ phase*. During this phase the cell is not part of the active replication cycle and the cells are not generally sensitive at this time to chemotherapy or irradiation.

As has been noted previously, irradiation acts principally on the cell by attacking DNA and affecting the mitotic phase. Many chemotherapeutic drugs, such as alkylating agents, have actions similar to those of radiation. In many cases the specific site of action of a cytotoxic agent is unknown. However, in all cases these agents affect not only the tumor cells but also the normal tissues of the body, particularly those undergoing rapid cell replication, such as those of the hematopoietic system, mucosa of the gastrointestinal tract, the vagina, the bladder, germ cells, and skin. All these have relevance in patients with gynecologic malignancies.

As is the case in radiation, the proliferating cells are the most susceptible to chemotherapeutic agents. While normal tissues at steady state have cell growth occurring at a rate comparable to cell loss, malignant tumors have a rate of cell growth that greatly exceeds cell loss. The proportion of cells actively involved in proliferation of the tumor is known as the growth fraction (GF). The nondividing tumor cells may have reached a mature stage, may lack essential nutrition, may be anoxic, or may be inhibited by the host or other unknown influences. Different tumors require varying intervals for them to double in size (doubling time). In general, smaller tumors grow more rapidly than larger tumors, and it appears that metastases often grow more rapidly than the primary tumor, in part because they are smaller and in part because of the likelihood that more rapidly dividing cells will be the ones that tend to metastasize. This effect appears to be operative following the administration of cytotoxic agents, which reduce the mass of the tumor. But cell replication then appears to proceed at a faster rate. This has led to the assumption that chemotherapy not only reduces the number of cells but also leads to a smaller tumor mass, which allows the remaining cells to replicate faster. It is estimated that 1 g of tumor tissue is equal to 10^9 cells.

Apoptosis is a mode of cellular death that appears to be an energy-dependent programmed event. There are morphologic and biochemical changes that occur during apoptosis. These include nuclear condensation and fragmentation, cell shrinkage, relative sparing of cellular membrane and internal organelle, and DNA fragmentation. A variety of external stimuli such as irradiation, chemotherapy, viruses, hormones, and gene products, such as p53, can influence this death program.

Principles of Therapy

Some of the concepts used in antibiotic therapy of infections have been applied to cancer treatment. However, major differences exist. Infections are frequently caused by a single agent or even multiple types of bacteria with specific growth patterns and sensitivities to antibiotics. Although it is believed that a cancer can originate in a single (stem) cell, clinically evident disease is composed of a heterogeneous population of cells with different cell cycle durations and varying growth fractions. Larger tumors are more likely to contain cells resistant to a single cytotoxic agent.

An additional problem with larger tumors is their lower growth fraction, which is associated with a larger proportion of cells in the resting, or G_0 phase of the cell cycle. These cells are resistant to cytotoxic drugs and may become a source of future growth when they leave the G_0 phase to enter the cell replication cycle. Thus smaller tumors, those with a higher growth fraction, and those with a short doubling time are the most sensitive to cytotoxic agents.

Cytotoxic agents kill cancer cells according to first-order kinetics; that is, a given dose kills a constant fraction of malignant cells, similar in concept to that noted previously for radiation therapy. One of the reasons chemotherapy appears selectively to affect cancer tissue more than normal tissue is that malignant tumor cells have a higher growth fraction in comparison to normal cells and are thus more susceptible to the effects of the chemotherapeutic agent. The net effect of the agent depends on the proportion of the cells killed, as well as on the rapidity with which the surviving cells duplicate. The ability of a chemotherapeutic agent to destroy a greater proportion of cancer cells more effectively is enhanced if the agent can be given more frequently. The antitumor effect is also enhanced if a larger dose can be given, which will increase the proportion of the cells killed. However, the dose and frequency are both limited by the tolerance of normal tissues.

Figures 26-8 and 26-9 demonstrate these principles. Starting with a smaller tumor burden (Figure 26-8), and therefore fewer tumor cells, leads to a more rapid elimination of the entire tumor within fewer treatment cycles. This effect of shorter duration of treatment also provides for less time for the development of resistant cell strains. In addition, the selection of an agent that yields a greater cell kill leads to an increased net reduction in tumor mass between treatment cycles, which results in more effective control despite the tumor regeneration that occurs between cycles of chemotherapy. Figure 26-9 demonstrates the effects of frequency of therapy, illustrating that prolonging the interval between the cycles of treatment increases the risk of loss of tumor control and disease progression.

Since the risk of having multiple resistant cell lines increases as the tumor becomes larger, it is important to

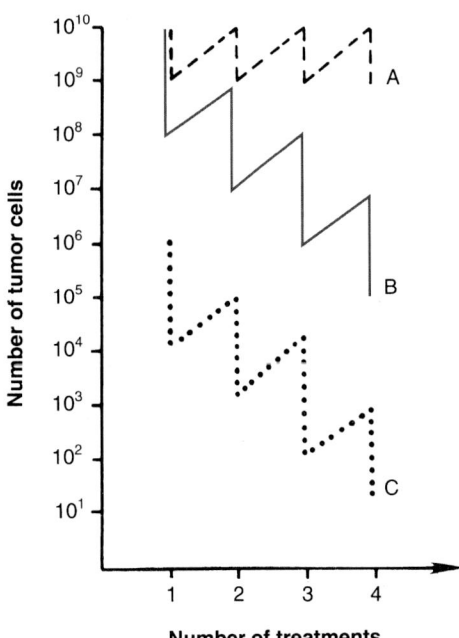

FIGURE 26-8 If treatment is initiated with lower tumor burden, fewer treatment courses are needed. *A,* One log cell kill (90% of cells) with smaller dose of drug. *B,* Two log cell kill (99% of cells) with larger dose of drug, leading to tumor regression. *C,* Two log cell kill (99% of cells) with larger dose of drug applied to smaller tumor burden, leading to more rapid tumor disappearance.

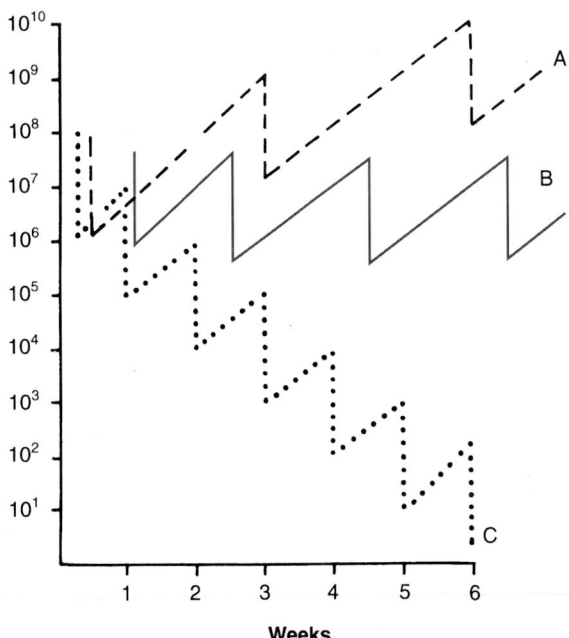

FIGURE 26-9 Importance of treatment frequency is illustrated in this example in which same drug is given at different intervals. *A,* Two log cell kill with recovery with therapy every 3 weeks (tumor progression). *B,* Two log cell kill with recovery with therapy every 2 weeks (no net change in tumor size). *C,* Two log cell kill with recovery with therapy weekly (tumor regression).

choose initially a therapeutic program that has the best chance of inducing tumor regression. The potential to treat simultaneously different cell lines within the tumor has led to the development of multiple-agent chemotherapy programs, which appear in many cases to be more effective than single agents. Such combination therapy appears to enhance the cell kill, provide broader coverage against multiple cell lines, and help prevent the emergence of resistant cells.

Approaches to Treatment

The dosage of an anticancer agent is usually calculated in body surface area (square meters), which provides a better measure of potential toxicity than body weight, in part because surface area more closely reflects cardiac output and blood flow. Chemotherapeutic agents have varying toxicities, which will be considered in the next section. A major problem with most agents is bone marrow toxicity, with the resultant necessity to monitor carefully the hemopoietic system. Most gynecologic chemotherapy protocols are administered in cycles with 3- to 4-week intervals. If the blood elements (white cells and platelets) have not recovered adequately by the time the next cycle of chemotherapy is due to be administered, the dosage of the agent or agents must be reduced or the time interval between treatments extended. Table 26-3 shows a schedule of approximate dosage reductions for myelosuppressive agents.

An additional consideration in toxicity of chemotherapeutic agents relates to hepatic metabolism and/or renal excretion. It may be necessary to modify the dosage of the drug administered when either renal or hepatic function is compromised. For example, doxorubicin (Adriamycin) and vincristine are metabolized in the liver, and dosage reductions must be made if the drug is administered to a patient with hepatic dysfunction; methotrexate and cisplatin effects are increased in patients with renal damage, necessitating dosage reduction in these patients; cisplatin not only has its effects

intensified in patients with renal damage but also is toxic to the kidney, requiring particular caution if it is administered to individuals with compromised renal function or patients receiving therapy with aminoglycosides, which are also toxic to the kidney. Methotrexate and cisplatin are also bound to albumin, and this binding is decreased in patients taking sulfonamides or salicylates, both of which increase the toxicity and effects of the chemotherapy. In general, low serum albumin leads to an increase in free circulating chemotherapeutic agent, one reason malnourished patients have heightened toxicity to chemotherapy.

Various chemotherapeutic agents can be differentially toxic to other organ systems of the body, including the intestine, nervous system, and lungs. Cessation of menstrual function occurs in women receiving chemotherapy but in most cases it returns in a few months. In addition, subsequent successful pregnancies do occur with no evidence at present of an increased risk of congenital anomalies in those who have had chemotherapy. The therapist must be aware of the individual adverse affects when administering these agents. The goal of treatment is to provide as high a dosage of the chemotherapeutic agent as possible to produce maximum therapeutic effectiveness without causing unacceptable toxicity and side effects.

These are four ways chemotherapy is generally used. Chemotherapy can be used (1) as an induction treatment for advanced disease, (2) as an adjunct to local methods of treatment, (3) as primary treatment for localized cancer, and (4) by direct instillation into specific regions of the body (i.e., intraperitoneal chemotherapy).

Adjunctive therapy describes therapy given as primary treatment for patients with advanced cancer for which there is no alternative therapy. Adjunctive therapy can be used as systemic therapy after the cancer has been controlled by an alternative therapy.

Primary (neoadjunctive) therapy is the use of chemotherapy as the initial therapy for which there is an alternative, but less than completely effective therapy, in order to try to improve overall therapeutic results.

In assessment of the effect of chemotherapeutic agents, a number of definitions are used to describe the response of the tumor being treated. A *complete remission* or *response* is total disappearance of the tumor for at least 1 month. A partial *objective response* is the reduction in the size of the tumor greater than 50% in its greatest perpendicular diameter for at least 1 month. *Progression* indicates an increase in tumor size or the appearance of new lesions. Occasionally the term *stabilization* is used to indicate that the disease has not changed in size and no new lesions have appeared. However, clinically the possibility of confusion exists, insofar as stabilization of the disease may be assumed to be due to chemotherapy when the lack of observed increase in size may be related in part to a prolonged doubling time of the tumor.

TABLE 26-3
A Schedule of Approximate Dosage Reductions for Myelosuppressive Agents

Dose	White blood count
Total dose	>4000/mm³
½ dose	≥3000–4000 mm³
¼ dose	≥1500–3000 mm³
Withhold dose	<1000/mm³

Dose	Platelet count
Total dose	>100,000/mm³
½ dose	50,000–100,000/mm³
Withhold dose	< 50,000/mm³

Evaluation of New Agents

In the development of new drugs, serial evaluations are necessary to assess the effectiveness of the drug as well as to ascertain its toxicity. A number of trials are necessary to move a new agent from the point of evaluation to allow it to be used in regular medical practice. Such "phase trials" are defined as follows:

PHASE I TRIAL. An initial trial to test new drugs at various doses to evaluate toxicity and determine tolerance to the drug. At the various doses tested some therapeutic effects may be observed.

PHASE II TRIAL. Tests to determine the therapeutic effectiveness and extent of the toxicity of the drug at doses expected to be effective against a specific tumor type.

PHASE III TRIAL. Trials to compare the drug therapy to treatment currently in use to ascertain if the new therapy is superior.

A standard method frequently used to measure the patient's status in chemotherapy trials is the Karnofsky Performance Status (Table 26-4). In general, patients are not accepted to trials of new agents if their Karnofsky status is 50 or less.

Chemotherapeutic Agents Commonly Used in Gynecologic Cancer

A large number of drugs have been used in the therapy of cancer. In general the agents used in gynecologic oncology can be classified into alkylating agents, antitumor antibiotics, antimetabolites, vinca (plant) alkaloids, synthetic and miscellaneous compounds, and hormones.

TABLE 26-4
Karnofsky Performance Status

100 =	Normal, no complaints; no evidence of disease
90 =	Able to carry on normal activity; minor signs or symptoms of disease
80 =	Normal activity with effort; some signs or symptoms of disease
70 =	Cares for self but unable to carry on normal activity or do active work
60 =	Requires occasional assistance but is able to care for most personal needs
50 =	Requires considerable assistance and frequent medical care
40 =	Disabled; requires special care and assistance
30 =	Severely disabled; hospitalization indicated, although death not imminent
20 =	Very sick; hospitalization necessary; active support treatment necessary
10 =	Moribund; fatal process progressing rapidly
0 =	Death

Alkylating Agents

The primary action of these chemicals appears to be via direct interaction with DNA. The process of alkylation leads to the development of positively charged alkyl groups, which react with the negatively charged portion of DNA, leading to interference with DNA function. Cross-linking of DNA also occurs. The alkylating agents affect rapidly dividing cells and are particularly toxic to the bone marrow, leading to severe myelosuppression. They may be administered intravenously or orally and have been used extensively in gynecologic malignancies, particularly in ovarian cancers. The most commonly used agents are cyclophosphamide (Cytoxan), chlorambucil (Leukeran), phenylalanine mustard (melphalan or Alkeran), and ifosfamide. In general the effectiveness of these agents appears similar, but there are some variations in toxicity. Phenylalanine mustard not only is acutely toxic to the bone marrow, but also appears to have a cumulative effect on the marrow that may compromise marrow function after its use has been discontinued.

Cyclophosphamide is associated with hemorrhagic cystitis. A urinary metabolite, acrolein, causes urothelial damage. A structural analog of cyclophosphamide, Ifosfamide, has been evaluated for its marked antitumor effects, which are similar to those of other alkylating agents. However, it is highly toxic to the bladder and urothelium, and severe hemorrhagic cystitis can be prevented by the prophylactic administration of 2-mercaptoethane sulfonate (MESNA), which binds to acrolein and prevents urotoxicity. In addition, it has been noted that therapy with alkylating agents is associated with the subsequent risk of the patient's developing acute leukemia. This risk may range from 2% to 10% and appears to be related to the dose and the duration of treatment.

Antitumor Antibiotics

Antitumor antibiotics are derived from products of bacterial or fungal cultures. Their mechanism of action is not clearly delineated, but it is thought that they directly attack DNA and appear to be able to produce DNA breaks and also interfere with DNA synthesis and transcription. The ones most commonly used in gynecologic cancer are actinomycin D (Dactinomycin), doxorubicin (Adriamycin), and bleomycin (Blenoxane).

Actinomycin-D intercalates between adjacent guanine-cytosine base pairs resulting in blockage of DNA transcription by RNA polymerase. Actinomycin D is usually given intravenously often in 5-day courses every 4 weeks. The drug causes severe myelosuppression and can affect the gastrointestinal mucosa, leading to diarrhea and ulcers in the mouth. Alopecia and skin toxicity may also occur. The drug has a potentiating effect with radiation therapy, and this increased activity may be observed even when the drug is given after radiation treatment is completed. The drug is widely used to treat trophoblastic disease. It is also sclerosing and has been used to treat malignant pleural effusions.

Doxorubicin (Adriamycin) is an anthracyclin that intercalates with DNA preventing DNA and RNA synthesis. Other anthracyclines are epirubicin and idarubicin. Adriamycin must be carefully administered intravenously, since extravasation leads to soft tissue and skin necrosis and ulceration. It is metabolized in the liver, and dosages must be reduced in patients with compromised hepatic function. Myelosuppression occurs regularly with therapeutic doses. Complete alopecia is a constant side effect. The alopecia is reversible after cessation of the use of the drug, but it tends to be one of the greatest causes of patient distress. The drug also causes cardiomyopathy, which leads to congestive heart failure and can be life threatening. In general, doses are kept below 550 mg/m², and cardiac function is often monitored by ultrasound evaluation or radionuclide scans. Clinical resistance is thought to be caused by the overexpression of MDR1 gene (p-glycoprotein).

Bleomycin's action results from single strand scission of DNA. Bleomycin may be administered intravenously, intramuscularly, or subcutaneously. It is excreted via the kidney, and some dosage reduction is made if renal function is compromised. The drug does *not* have significant myelosuppressant properties, in contrast to most of the other cytotoxic agents. It is, however, highly toxic to the lungs, and pneumonitis and pulmonary fibrosis may occur. Thus particular care must be used in persons with compromised lung function. The drug is also toxic to skin and can produce erythema, peeling, and pigmentation. It has been used as part of combination therapy with particular effectiveness against ovarian germ cell tumors, and it has been tried for a variety of other gynecologic malignancies, particularly carcinoma of the cervix.

Antimetabolites

Antimetabolites interfere with cell metabolism by competing with naturally occurring purines or pyrimidines, whose chemical structure they resemble. In this way they interfere or prevent vital biochemical reactions.

5-Fluorouracil (5-FU) is a pyrimidine analogue with the capacity to inhibit the biosynthesis of pyrimidine nucleotides. It is usually given intravenously and is also active orally. It is myelosuppressive, although less so than many other cytotoxic agents used in gynecologic cancer treatment. It causes gastrointestinal side effects (diarrhea) and ulceration of the oral mucosa. Other toxicities may include alopecia, nail changes, dermatitis, acute cerebellar syndrome, cardiac toxicity, hyperpigmentation over the vein used for infusion, and hand-foot syndrome, especially with continuous infusion. It is effectively metabolized in the liver, which has led to its use in hepatic artery infusions for liver metastasis. The

clearing of 5-FU from the blood by the liver markedly reduces systemic toxicity in patients receiving these infusions. The drug is extensively used in gynecologic cancer, including ovarian carcinomas, endometrial adenocarcinomas, and some cases of cervical squamous cell carcinomas. It has also been used topically to treat intraepithelial neoplasia of the lower genital tract. Newer oral analogues are being investigated. These include doxifluridine and capecitabine.

Methotrexate (MTX) is a folic acid analogue that is a specific inhibitor of the enzyme dihydrofolate reductase (DHFR), which plays a critical role in intracellular folate metabolism. This prevents metabolic transfer of one carbon unit and inhibits the synthesis of thymidylic acid as well as different purine nucleotides. RNA and DNA syntheses are inhibited, and the drug works primarily in the S phase. Nondividing or resting cells are resistant. The effects of methotrexate can be overcome by the administration of folinic acid (citrovorum factor) 24 hours after methotrexate, which replenishes the tetrahydrofolate. Some chemotherapy protocols have used very high doses of methotrexate to treat the tumor, followed by citrovorum rescue to avoid severe toxic side effects. Methotrexate is administered intravenously, intramuscularly, or orally. It is excreted in the urine, and dosage adjustments must be made if there is decreased renal function. There are recognized mechanisms for intrinsic and acquired resistance to MTX in tumors. These mechanisms generally involve increased levels of DHFR due to gene amplification. Methotrexate is severely myelosuppressive and causes toxicity to the oral mucosa and intestines, as well as the liver, and an increase in liver enzymes is seen after treatment. The serum levels are also prolonged in patients with ascites or pleural effusion, since these act as a reservoir for the drug. Blood levels of methotrexate can be monitored with radioimmunoassay. The predominant use of the drug in gynecologic cancer has been the effective treatment of trophoblastic disease.

Gemcitibine is a newer antimetabolite under investigation for many gynecologic tumors. It is a deoxycytidine (nucleoside) analogue. The treatment toxicities include myelosuppression, transient elevation of liver enzymes, nausea, vomiting, flulike symptoms, and fatigue.

Antimicrotubular (Antimitotic) Drugs

A number of cytotoxic drugs have been isolated from plant extracts. Most of the antimitotics are plant alkaloids. These include naturally occurring vinca alkaloids, such as vincristine, vinblastine, and their semisynthetic analogues, and the taxanes (Taxol). The vinca alkaloids bind to the β-tubulin subunits, blocking polymerization of the microtubules in mitosis. Taxanes, on the other hand, bind to the β-tubulin of microtubules preventing depolymerization preventing chromosomes from moving to the metaphase plate.

TABLE 26-5
Side Effects of Drugs Often Used in Gynecologic Oncology

	Bone Marrow	Phlebitis Sclerosant	Neurologic	Skin	Pulm.	Renal	Hepatic	Cardiac	Endo.	Bladder	Gut Mucositis	Allergic	Alopecia	Metabolic	Nausea Vomiting
Antimetabolites															
Methotrexate	***		*	*	*	*	**				***		*		*
5-Fluorouracil	***		*	*							**		*		*
Alkylating agents															
Cyclophosphamide	***			*			*	*	*	**	**		**	*	**
Ifosfamide	**		**							**			**		*
Antitumor antibiotics															
Actinomycin D	***	*	*	*							**		**	*	**
Mitoxantrone	***							**			**		*		*
Adriamycin	***	**	*					**			**		**		**
Bleomycin	*			***	***							*			**
Mitomycin C	***	*	**				*				*				**
Vinca alkaloids															
Vinblastine	***	*	*										*		
Vincristine	*	*	***										*		
Etoposide (VP-16)	***						*	*			*		**	*	*
Miscellaneous compounds															
Hexamethylmelamine	*		*								***				**
Cisplatin	*		*			***									**
Carboplatin	**					*					*				*
Taxol	***	*	**	*				*			*	**	**		
Hydroxyurea	***		*	*							*	*	*		

Modified from Tattersall MHN: Pharmacology and selection of cytotoxic drugs. In Coppleson M, ed: Gynecologic oncology, ed 2, Edinburgh, 1992, Churchill-Livingstone, p 180.

***indicates dose limiting; **indicates common; *indicates rare.

Vinca (Plant) Alkaloids

Those in current use in gynecologic oncology include vinblastine, vincristine, and VP-16 (etoposide). These drugs are cell cycle dependent and arrest cells at metaphase by blocking the assembly of tubulin, and cause toxic destruction of the mitotic spindle and thus arrest mitosis. This can result in synchronization of the cell cycle for those cells surviving therapy. The drugs are given intravenously and have different side effects. Vincristine is severely neurotoxic and can produce numbness, motor weakness, and constipation as a result of its autonomic effects. There is little myelosuppression. Vinblastine is myelotoxic, and this tends to be a dose-limiting factor. However, it has less neurotoxicity than vincristine. VP-16 (etoposide) is a plant-derived drug that is a topoisomerase-II (enzyme) inhibitor, which is involved in DNA synthesis. It appears to have fewer toxic side effects but is myelotoxic. These drugs are used to treat ovarian germ cell tumors, as well as in trophoblastic disease.

Taxanes

Paclitaxel (Taxol) is derived from the bark of the Western yew and is used in the treatment of ovarian carcinoma. Its use has been markedly increased since the drug has been successfully synthesized. It disrupts the function of microtubules and thereby inhibits cell division. It is a potent agent whose administration can be accompanied by severe hypersensitivity reactions and hypotension. Premedication with antihistamines and steroids are recommended to minimize hypersensitivity reactions. Neutropenia is the major toxic side effect, but sensory peripheral neuropathy is also a serious problem. As noted by Warner, the distribution of neurotoxicity of Taxol is similar to that of platinum, *but* they do not appear to be synergistic, which fortunately allows them to be used together effectively. Bradycardia can also occur. Although severe cardiac problems have been reported with the administration of Taxol, they are rare. In addition to its use in the treatment of ovarian cancer, Taxol is being evaluated in a number of other gynecologic malignancies. A rare complication has been the report of bowel perforation in a few individuals while on Taxol therapy, as noted by Rose and Piver. Table 26-5 summarizes the major side effects of many of the drugs currently used in gynecologic oncology.

Semisynthetic analogues of paclitaxel are being investigated. Their mechanism of tumor cell kill and spectrum of clinical activity are similar to that of paclitaxel. They act as a spindle poison stabilizing the microtubule assembly. Dose-limiting toxicities include myelosuppression with platelet sparing, cutaneous toxicity, edema, pleural effusions, alopecia, and severe myalgias.

Topoisomerase Inhibitors

Topoisomerases are DNA enzymes that control the topology of DNA double-helix cellular functions (i.e., transcription and replication of genetic material). There are two classes of topoisomerases, I and II. Drugs that prevent these functions are referred to as inhibitors. Two newer drugs being investigated for the treatment of gynecologic malignancies are topotecan and CPT-11. Both of these drugs are topoisomerase I inhibitors.

CPT 11 is a semisynthetic analogue of camptothecin. It is given intravenously and is metabolized by the liver. It is being investigated for therapy against cervical cancers. Dose-limiting toxicity is myelosuppression and diarrhea.

Topotecan is also a semisynthetic analogue of camptothecin. It is used for cisplatin refractory ovarian cancer. Topotecan is administered intravenously or orally and is excreted by the renal route. Toxicity includes granulocytopenia, nausea and vomiting, dermatitis, neuropathy, conjunctivitis, headache, and occasionally psychiatric symptoms.

Synthetic and Miscellaneous Compounds

A number of drugs have been introduced that have antitumor activity. Many are synthetically produced. They do not have any single mode of action, and in some instances their mechanism of antitumor activity is uncertain.

Cisplatin (cis-diamminedichloroplatinum, cis-DDP) has been found to have wide antitumor activity. It appears to bind to DNA and interfere with DNA synthesis, but its cell cycle specificity has not been clearly defined. It is administered intravenously and is very toxic to the kidney. A high urine output must be maintained during administration to try to reduce kidney toxicity, since the drug is excreted in the urine in its active form. It induces myelosuppression and also causes high-frequency ototoxicity, so that renal and auditory function must be monitored during treatment in addition to peripheral blood counts. Cisplatin induces severe peripheral neuropathy, which may improve somewhat after cessation of therapy but tends to be permanent. Metabolic changes including hypomagnesemia and hypokalemia occur, and seizures have been reported in severe cases. One of the side effects most annoying to the patient is the production of severe nausea with vomiting, which may be controlled in part by antiemetic medication. The drug is widely used in the treatment of ovarian epithelial and germ cell tumors and many types of gynecologic cancers.

New analogues have been introduced, such as carboplatinum, which appear to have comparable activity in ovarian epithelial carcinoma as cisplatin. Its mechanism of action and antitumor activity is similar to cisplatin, yet it is less potent in producing DNA interstrand cross-links compared to cisplatin. Carboplatinum is not toxic to the kidneys but appears more suppressive to the bone marrow, especially to platelets. Rare toxicities include rash, alopecia, and hepatotoxicity. Dose is usually based on the area under the curve (AUC). The preferred dose in an AUC = 5-7 mg/mL. The dose (mg) = AUC X (creatinine clearance + 25). It is readily administered on an outpatient basis.

Hexamethylmelamine is orally active, but its mechanism of antitumor activity is unclear. It is thought to act somewhat similarly to alkylating agents, but it is structurally different from that class of compounds. It is myelosuppressive and causes nausea and vomiting. It is active in ovarian epithelial carcinomas and frequently is used as part of combination chemotherapy in the treatment of these tumors.

Hormones

Hormone therapy has been effectively developed in the treatment of breast cancer. Estrogen and progesterone receptors have been clearly identified in endometrial carcinomas and have been recently found in other types of gynecologic cancers, particularly ovarian epithelial carcinomas. Progestins such as megestrol (Megace), depo-medroxyprogesterone (Depo-Provera), and 17-OH progesterone caproate (Delalutin), as well as antiestrogens such as tamoxifen and raloxifene, have been used in the treatment of endometrial carcinomas and seem to have their best effects against well-differentiated tumors. Hormonal therapy is also being evaluated in the treatment of some well-differentiated ovarian epithelial carcinomas.

Alternative Modes of Therapy

Many new modes of therapy are being tried, particularly those that are being adapted from trials of nongynecologic tumors; this includes high-dose chemotherapy as well as concomitant chemoradiation. Concurrent administration of chemotherapy and radiation may improve local cancer control particularly with squamous cell cancer. Several phase II trials have been conducted showing improved survival in advanced stage cervical carcinoma (Chapter 29).

Stimulators of the hematopoietic system are also being used to diminish the toxicity of chemotherapeutic agents; this includes the use of erythropoietin (epo) to overcome the chronic anemia that often occurs with chemotherapy. In addition, granulocyte-monocyte colony stimulating factor (GM-CSF) and granulocyte colony stimulating factor (G-CSF) stimulate white cell proliferation to allow higher doses of myelosuppressive chemotherapy to be administered. As noted by Vose and Armitage, these agents have been used successfully to diminish the risk of infection and reduce morbidity associated with neutropenia. Newer agents are being developed, including stem cell factor and the number of the interleukins that act earlier in the hematopoetic cycle.

KEY POINTS

- Electromagnetic radiation is a form of energy that has no mass or charge and travels at the speed of light.

- Particulate energy is a form of ionizing radiation consisting of subatomic particles (electrons, neutrons, and protons) whose energy is in part related to their mass and velocity.

- Inverse square law states that the energy measured from a radiation source is inversely proportional to the distance from the source.

- A given dose of radiation kills a constant fraction of tumor cells radiated. The tissue effects of electromagnetic radiation (x-rays and gamma rays) are dependent on oxygenation.

- The effect of photon radiation (low LET) on tissues is altered by tissue oxygenation, while neutron (high LET) radiation is independent of oxygenation.

- The cell replication cycle consists of M (mitosis), G_1 (Gap$_1$ = RNA and protein synthesis), S (DNA synthesis), and G_2 (Gap$_2$ = RNA and protein synthesis). When the cell is not in the replication cycle, it is in the G_0 phase.

- The dose of radiation delivered to a tumor depends on the energy of the source, the size of the treatment field, and the depth of the tumor beneath the surface. Increasing the dosage increases the depth of maximum dose beneath the skin surface.

- Radiation acts on cells primarily in the M phase, making rapidly proliferating cells the most radiosensitive. Normal tissues recover from the effects of radiation therapy more efficiently than tumor tissue does.

- Multiple chemotherapeutic agents have been used to sensitize cells to radiation, and such chemoradiation appears to give improved results particularly with squamous cell cancers.

- Ureteral stricture occurs after radiation for stage I carcinoma of the cervix and is estimated to be 1% at 5 years and 2.5% at 20 years, a rare but important complication.

- Cytotoxic chemotherapeutic agents act on various phases of the cell cycle, primarily affecting rapidly proliferating cells, and at a given dose destroy a constant fraction of tumor cells.

- Most chemotherapeutic drugs are severely myelosuppressive, with the exception of bleomycin and vincristine.

- In general, low serum albumin leads to an increase in free circulating chemotherapeutic agent, one reason malnourished patients have heightened toxicity to chemotherapy.

- Methotrexate and cisplatin are excreted by the kidney, and their effects are increased in patients with diminished renal function. Because of displacement from serum albumin, both salicylates and sulfa drugs increase toxicity of these agents.

- Vincristine and cisplatin cause severe peripheral neurotoxicity.

- Bleomycin is associated with severe pulmonary toxicity.

- Doxorubicin is associated with severe cardiomyopathy.

- Cisplatin is nephrotoxic and myelosuppressive. Its analogue, carboplatin, is also excreted by the kidney but is not nephrotoxic.

- Taxol is a powerful antineoplastic agent that disrupts the function of microtubules. It is effective particularly in cases of ovarian cancer. It can cause severe neutropenia and neurotoxicity.

- Alopecia can occur with any chemotherapy, but it is total and severe with doxorubicin, actinomycin, and paclitaxel. Hair growth resumes after cessation of treatment.

- Large tumors tend to have smaller growth fractions and a higher proportion of cells in the resting phase (G_0) of the cycle than small tumors. Tumors consist of a heterogeneous population of cells and have variable growth fractions.

- The major classes of cytotoxic chemotherapeutic agents used in gynecologic oncology are alkylating agents, antitumor antibiotics, antimetabolites, vinca (plant) alkaloids, topoisomerase inhibitors, and specially synthesized compounds.

- Topoisomerase inhibitors are drugs that prevent transcription and replication. Examples are topotecan and CPT-11.

- Growth factors or granulocyte colony stimulating factor (G-CSF) are used to limit hematologic toxicity of chemotherapy.

BIBLIOGRAPHY

Arai A, Nakano T, Fukuhisa K, et al: Second cancer after radiation therapy for cancer of the uterine cervix, Cancer 67:398, 1991.

Asco Ad Hoc Colony-Stimulating Factor Guidelines Expert Panel: American Society of Clinical Oncologists recommendation for use of hematopoietic colony-stimulating factors: evidence based, clinical practical guidelines. J Clin Oncol 12:2471, 1994.

Bellin SL and Selin M: Cisplatin-induced hypomagnesemia with seizures: a case report and review of the literature, Gynecol Oncol 30:104, 1988.

Bruce WR, Meeker RE, and Valeriote FA: Comparison of the sensitivity of normal hematopoietic and transplanted lymphoma colony-forming cells to chemotherapeutic agents administered in vivo, J Natl Cancer Inst 37:233, 1966.

Bunn HF: Recombinant erythropoietin therapy in cancer patients, J Clin Oncol 6:949, 1990.

Buntzel J, Kuttner K, Frahlich D, and Glatzel M: Selective cytoprotection with amifostene in concurrent radiochemistry, Ann Oncol 9:505, 1998.

Byrne A, Mulvihill JJ, Myers MH, et al: Effects of treatment on fertility in long-term survivals of childhood or adolescent cancer, N Engl J Med 317:1315, 1987.

Calvert AH, Newell DR, Grumbell LA, et al: Carboplatin dosage: prospective evaluation of a simple formula based on renal function, J Clin Oncol 7:1748, 1989.

Canman C, Gilmer T, Coutts S, et al: Growth factor modulation of p53-mediated growth arrest versus apoptosis, Genes Dev 9:600, 1995.

Chambers SK, Chopyk RL, Chambers JT, et al: Development of leukemia after doxorubicin and cisplatin treatment for ovarian cancer, Cancer 64:2459, 1989.

Covens A, Thomas G, DePetrillo A, et al: The prognostic importance of site and type of radiation-induced bowel injury in patients requiring surgical management, Gynecol Oncol 43:270, 1991.

Dauplat J, Legros M, Condat P, et al: High-dose melphalan and autologous bone marrow support for treatment of ovarian carcinoma with positive second-look operation, Gynecol Oncol 34:294, 1989.

DeVita VT: On the value of response criteria in therapeutic research. Le Bulletin du Cancer. Collogue Inserm—John Library Series. Proc 2nd International Congress of Neoadjuvant Chemotherapy, 75:863, 1998.

DiSaia PJ and Creasman W: Clinical gynecologic oncology, ed 4, St. Louis, 1993, Mosby.

Erslev AJ: Erythropoietin, N Engl J Med 324:1339, 1991.

Gray LH, Coger AD, Ebert M, et al: The concentration of oxygen dissolved in tissues at the time of radiation as a factor in radiotherapy, Br J Radiol 26:638, 1953.

Joslin CAF: Basic parameters of radiotherapy. In Coppleson M, ed: Gynecologic oncology, ed 2, Edinburgh, 1992, Churchill Livingstone.

Lederer CM, Hollander J, and Perlman I: Table of isotopes, New York, 1967, John Wiley & Sons.

Li MC, Hertz R, and Spencer DB: Effect of methotrexate therapy upon choriocarcinoma and chorioadenoma, Proc Soc Exp Biol Med 93:361, 1956.

Ling V: Multidrug resistance: molecular mechanisms and clinical relevance, Cancer Chemother Pharmacol 40 (suppl 1):53, 1997.

Lucerno MA and McCloskey WW: Alternatives to estrogen for the treatment of hot flashes, Ann Pharmaco Ther 31:915, 1997.

Lund B, Hansen OP, Theilade K, et al: Phase II Study of gemcitibine (2^1 2^1-difluoro-deoxycytidine) in previously treated ovarian cancer patients, J Natl Cancer Inst 86:1530, 1994.

Mangioni C, Bolis G, Pecorelli K, et al: Randomized trial in advanced ovarian cancer comparing cisplatin and carboplatin, J Natl Cancer Inst 81:1464, 1989.

McIntyre JF, Eifel PJ, Levenback C, and Oswald MJ: Ureteral stricture as a late complication of radiotherapy for stage Ib carcinoma of the uterine cervix, Cancer 75:836, 1995.

Montana GS and Fowler WC: Carcinoma of the cervix: analysis of bladder and rectal radiation dose and complications, Int J Radiat Oncol Biol Phys 16:95, 1989.

Ringel I and Horowitz SB: Studies with RP 56976 (taxotere): a semisynthetic analogue of Taxol, J Natl Cancer Inst 83:288, 1991.

Rose PG and Piver MS: Case report: intestinal perforation secondary to paclitaxel, Gynecol Oncol 57:270, 1995.

Rowinsky EK and Donehower RC: Paclitaxel (Taxol), N Engl J Med 332:1004, 1995.

Sinclair WK and Morton RA: X-ray sensitivity during cell generation cycle of cultured Chinese hamster cells, Radiat Res 29:450, 1966.

Sitt JA, Fowler JF, Thomadsen BR, Buchler DA, Paliwal BP, and Kinsella TJ: High dose rate intracavitary brachytherapy for carcinoma of the cervix: The Madison System: I. Clinical and biological considerations, Int J Radiat Oncol Phys 24:335, 1992.

Skipper HE: Biochemical, pharmacologic, toxicological, kinetic, and chemical (subhuman and human) relationships, Cancer 21:600, 1968.

Stillwell TJ and Benson RC: Cyclophosphamide-induced hemorrhagic cystitis: a review of 100 patients, Cancer 61:451, 1988.

Tattersall MHN: Pharmacology and selection of cytotoxic drugs. In Coppleson M, ed: Gynecologic oncology, ed 2, Edinburgh, 1992, Churchill-Livingstone.

Tucker MA and Fraumeni JF Jr: Treatment-related cancers after gynecologic malignancy, Cancer 60:2117, 1987.

Vose JM and Armitage JO: Clinical applications of hematopoietic growth factors, J Clin Oncol 13:1023, 1995.

Warner E: Neurotoxicity of cisplatin and taxol, Int J Gynecol Cancer 5:161, 1995.

Weiss RB, Donehower RC, Wiernik PH, et al: Hypersensitivity reactions from Taxol, J Clin Oncol 8:1263, 1990.

Yeoh E, Horowitz M, Russo A, et al: A retrospective study of the effects of pelvic irradiation for carcinoma of the cervix on gastrointestinal function, Int J Radiat Biol Phys 26:229, 1993.

Yves P: Eukaryotic DNA isomerase I: genome gatekeeper and its intruders, camptothecins, Semin Oncol 23 (suppl 3):3, 1996.

Immunology and Molecular Oncology in Gynecologic Cancer

Immunologic Response, Cytokines, Tumor Cell Killing and Immunotherapy

KEY TERMS AND DEFINITIONS

Adoptive Immunotherapy. The use of extracts derived from sensitized lymphocytes to transfer "immunologic memory" and induce an antitumor response.

Adenovirus. An RNA virus that can be used as a vector in gene therapy.

Allele. Abbreviation for "allelomorph." The form of DNA sequences in a gene on a given locus. If the genes are identical the individual is homozygous. Different genes result in heterozygosity.

Amplification. Increase in the number of copies of a DNA sequence in a cell.

Antigen Presenting Cell. A cell, often a macrophage, that digests the antigen involved in cellular immunity and then displays the foreign antigen on its surface, which reacts with the T cell.

Angiogenesis. The formation of new capillary blood vessels. A critical process in neoplasia whereby malignant cells release substances that eventually lead to the activation and reproduction of normal endothelial cells and the establishment of new capillary blood supply to a growing tumor.

Antibody. A molecule produced by a plasma cell that binds to foreign antigens.

Apoptosis. The process of programmed cell death leading to degradation of DNA, fragmentation of the cell, and phagocytosis by macrophages.

B Lymphocyte. A lymphocyte that leads to antibody synthesis in response to an antigenic stimulus and is responsible for humoral immunity. It differentiates into a plasma cell, which secretes the antibody.

BRCA1, BRCA2. BReast CAncer and ovarian suscepti-

bility genes. Thought to function primarily as DNA repair genes. Mutation of BRCA1 or 2 confers a high lifetime risk of breast or ovarian cancer.

Cellular Immunity. Cell-mediated immunity in which lymphoid cells, usually T cells or NK cells, directly react with foreign cells or antigens.

Cluster of Differentiation (CD). Cell surface markers on the surface of T cells that recognize antibodies which allow characterization of specific T cells.

Complement. A component of the immune system consisting of interacting proteins and nine parts (C1-9) that play a role in the inflammatory response to destroy invading organisms and can also lead to cytotoxicity.

Cytokines. Modulators of the immune system that are secreted into the circulation which affect cellular proliferation.

Fab. The variable portion of the immunoglobulin molecule that binds to the antigen.

Fc. The "constant" region of the immunoglobulin molecule that is responsible for biologic activity. It allows for antibody binding to a phagocyte.

Helper T Cells. A T cell lymphocyte that is differentiated to stimulate immune response as well as B cell immunoglobulin production.

Humoral Immunity. Antibody-mediated immunity resulting from antibodies secreted into the circulation that are produced in response to a variety of foreign antigens.

Immunoglobulin. The basic structure of antibodies that are secreted on the surface of plasma cells. Five types are recognized (IgG, IgM, IgA, IgD, IgE).

Interferon (IFN). A cytokine produced by lymphocytes or fibroblasts in response to viral infection. There are three types: alpha, beta, and gamma, and they may have an antiproliferative effect on tumor cells.

Interleukin (IL). A class of cytokines secreted by monocytes, lymphocytes, and macrophages. They are numerically designated.

Lymphokine. See cytokine.

MHC—Major Histocompatibility Complex. A cluster of genes that include human leukocyte antigens (HLA). The gene complex is found in nearly all nucleated cells of the body of chromosome 6 and have been termed "transplantation" antigens in the past.

Mutation. An alteration of normal genetic composition that leads to a change in the DNA sequence that is perpetuated in subsequent cell divisions.

Mutator Gene. A set of cancer-causing genes that prevents the cell from repairing DNA mismatches during replication, which in turn can lead to malignant development.

Natural Killer (NK) Cells. A type of mononuclear cell (null cell) that mediates the killing of tumor cells by the immune system. They can react without antigenic stimulation.

Oncogene. A class of genes governing cellular processes that were mutated, overexpressed, or amplified and are associated with the development of malignant growth.

Overexpression. Increase in the amount of protein products secreted by a gene.

Passive Immunity. The transfer of specific antibodies to try to enhance the immune response.

Proto-oncogene. A normal gene component in cells that plays a role in physiologic growth and development. When abnormally activated they become oncogenes and lead to malignant cell growth.

Retrovirus. An RNA tumor virus that when integrated into certain animal cells leads to oncogene development. It has an RNA genome and can propagate by reverse transcription of its RNA into DNA.

Suppressor T Cells. A differentiated T cell lymphocyte that functions to suppress B cell production and T cell cytotoxicity.

Systemic-Active Nonspecific Immunotherapy. Use of adjuvant agents, usually of microbiologic origin, to increase cellular and humoral immunity. Examples are Bacillus Calmette-Guerin (BCG) and *Corynebacterium parvum (C. Parvum)*.

T Cell Lymphocyte. Lymphocytes that exhibit cell surface antigenicity via the T cell receptor (TcR) and mediate cellular immunity.

Transfection. The transfer of DNA sequences (genetic material) into a cell.

Translocation. The transfer or exchange of genetic material between two nonhomologous chromosomes.

Transcription. Transcription is a process by which messenger RNA is synthesized from a DNA template in the nucleus, then RNA enters the cytoplasm and serves as a template for protein synthesis.

Tumor Necrosis Factor (TNF). A cytokine that mediates endotoxic shock and is capable of inhibiting tumor cell growth.

Tumor Suppressor Gene. A normal genetic component of the cell that controls cell growth and proliferation. Mutations in the gene can lead to malignancy.

This chapter will summarize general principles of tumor immunology followed by a description of molecular genetics and angiogenesis that apply to gynecologic tumors. These are rapidly expanding fields and it is not possible in this text to explore them in detail. However, in the following sections some basic immunologic mechanisms will be reviewed and the possible application of this information to gynecologic tumor therapy will be explored. This will be followed by a summary of the molecular and genetic changes associated with malignant cellular growth and a consideration of the application of this knowledge to tumor therapy.

THE IMMUNOLOGIC RESPONSE

Immune responses are usually characterized as cellular or humoral. These responses occur as a result of specific antigenic determinants often referred to as *epitopes*. These distinctions refer to whether the response is mediated primarily by T cells (cellular) or through antibody responses by B cells (humoral). The components of each system interact, but for simplicity each will be considered separately. A cellular immune response occurs as a result of a direct interaction between the T-cell receptor (TcR) and a foreign antigen presented by an HLA (MHC) molecule on an antigen presenting cell (such as a macrophage). Cellular responses by cytotoxic T cells (Tc) lead to the direct lysis of infected cells harboring the antigen determinant or to signaling of B cells to produce antibodies. The latter is mediated through the production of cytokines. Humoral or antibody responses occur from antigen stimulation that leads to antibody (immunoglobulin) production. Antibodies are synthesized from B-lymphocytes, which differentiate into plasma cells that secrete large quantities of antibodies in response to the antigenic stimulant. In humans B cells are derived from hematapoetic stem cells and aggregate in lymph nodes, the spleen, or the gastrointestinal tract. T-helper (Th) cells regulate this function by producing cytokines that stimulate B cell differentiation into plasma cells, thus "helping" with antibody production. Other types of T-suppressor (Ts) cells act in opposite fashion and in this way "suppress" antibody production.

Humoral Immunity: B Cells and Immunoglobulins

Immunoglobulins are the basic structure of antibodies and are produced by plasma cells. Most antibodies are capable of exerting a physiologic response remote from the site of production. Figure 27-1, *A*, illustrates the B-lymphocyte, which differentiates into a plasma cell that secretes large quantities of immunoglobulin (antibody). Five types of related immunoglobulin molecules are recognized (IgG, IgM, IgA, IgD, IgE [see box below]). The immunoglobulin molecule has a fixed constant region that directs the biologic activity of the antibody (Fc region) and a unique variable (Fab) region that is formed in a response to the antigenic stimulus. The Fc region thus carries the biologic activity that can then allow the antibody to bind to a phagocyte leading to phagocytosis, and elimination of the cell expressing the antigens.

Classes of Immunoglobulins

IgG, the major class of immunoglobulin, comprises approximately 70% of total serum immunoglobulin and is the predominant form of antibody. Only IgG crosses the placenta and is important for the transfer of passive immunity to the newborn.

IgA comprises about 20% of total serum immunoglobulin. It is found in saliva, milk colostrum, and genitourinary secretions.

IgM represents about 10% of total serum immunoglobulin. It is the predominant antibody produced early in the humoral immune responses and is the most efficient in activating complement.

IgD accounts for less than 1% of total serum immunoglobulin, and it is found on the surface of B cells. The precise role of IgD is not understood but presumably plays a role in B lymphocyte activation.

IgE is associated with hypersensitivity and also infection with parasites.

Some understanding of the details of immunoglobulin structure is important. There are four polypeptide chains connected by a disulfide bond near the center. Two of these chains are termed heavy and the other two, light. There are variable regions (V) and constant regions (C) on each chain (Figure 27-1, *B*). There are five types of heavy chains and two types of light chains, each of which has specific domains. Differences in the variable region of the immunoglobulin account for its specificity. Thus the B cell is programmed to secrete a specific type of antibody, and it is estimated that more than 10^7 different antibodies are capable of being produced in response to the presence of foreign antigens. Without the specific antigenic stimulants, antibody production by the given B cell will not occur. The repeated specificity of given antibody production by the B cell results in a process known as *clonal selection*.

In addition to phagocytosis, there can be an immune response by the activation of complement. This is a complicated system that consists of a large group of interacting proteins. It is believed that there are nine serum components that participate in the complement destruction of cells expressing foreign antigens, including, in some cases, tumor cells. Essentially there are two overlapping pathways in the complement cascade. In the first case the antigen-antibody complex leads to activation of complement beginning with the C1 component and proceeding to C3. In the alternative pathway, C3 is activated directly with Factor B (polysaccharides) or similar external stimuli. The first pathway can also be activated by aggregated immunoglobulins of the IgG or IgM types. The alternative pathway, as is already mentioned, can react to polysaccharides, dextran or also to IgA complexes. The alternative pathway thus can be activated in the absence of antibody. Powerful biologic substances can be released during the complement cascade, including those involved in the inflammatory response with polymorphonuclear leukocytes and the process of opsonization and phagocytosis. In addition the activation of C9 leads to complement-dependent cytotoxicity that attacks the membrane and can lyse the cell. Unfortunately, many tumor cells are resistant to this complement-dependent cytotoxicity and other cytotoxic mechanisms described below need to be applied.

Cellular Immunity: T Cells

Cell-mediated immunity occurs in response to antigens, which cause activation of "T" lymphocytes as a consequence of cell-cell interaction, in contrast to B cells that can recognize antigens in fluids. T cells originate in the bone marrow and then differentiate in the thymus. They may be found in the blood or areas such as lymph nodes, the spleen, or the intestine (Peyer's patches). The cellular response is recognized on the surface of the T cell by the T-cell receptor (TcR) having been processed in the context

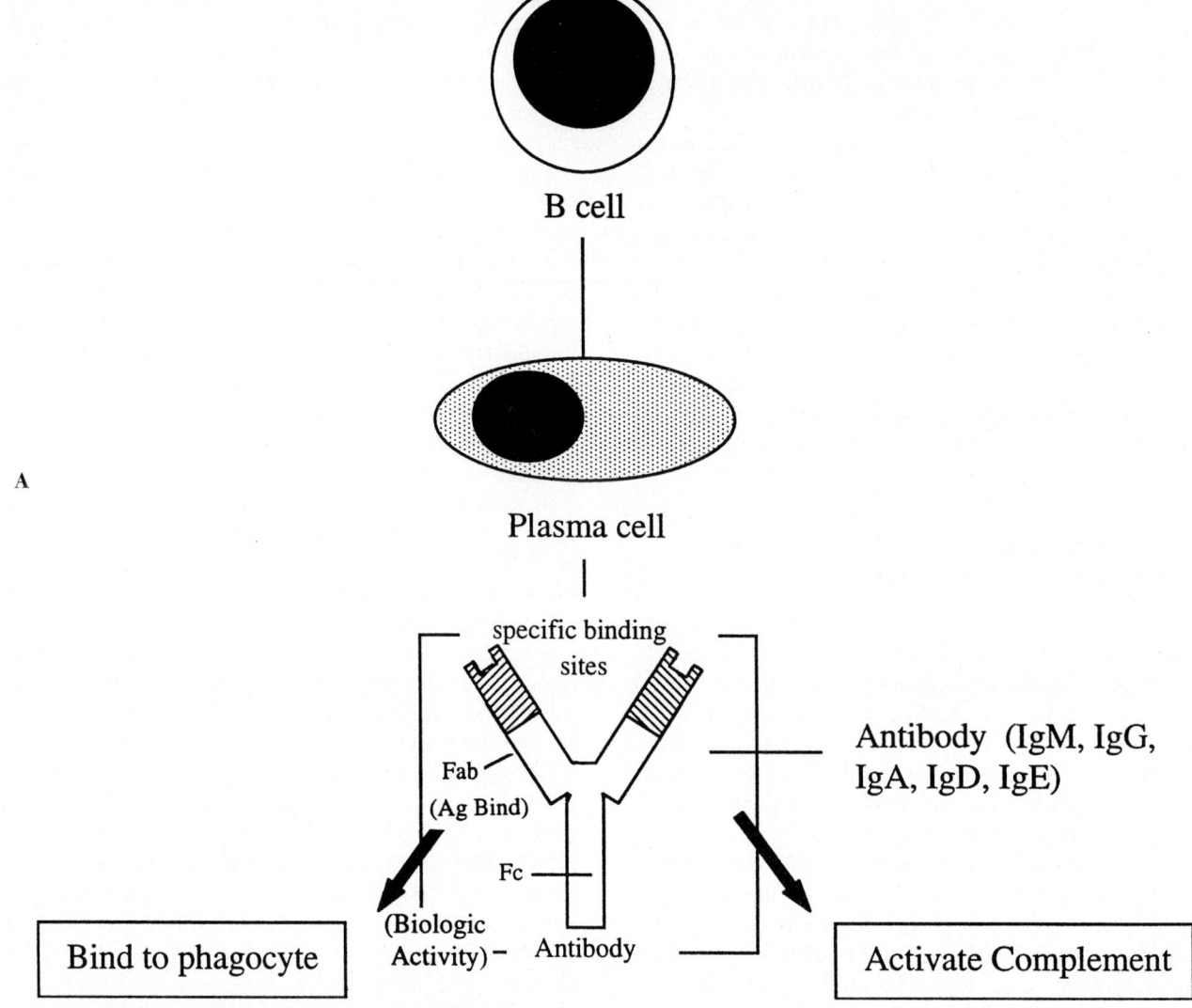

A

FIGURE 27-1 **A,** B cell response leading to antibody production. The B cell is stimulated to differentiate into a plasma cell, which produces specific antibodies that then lead either to phagocytes or activation of complement. **B,** Structure of an immunoglobulin monomer. V_{LH}, variable light and heavy chain regions; C_H 1, 2, 3, constant heavy chain regions; V_L, light chain variable region; V_H, heavy chain variable region; C_L, light chain constant region; C_H, heavy chain constant region. (Modified from Claman HN: The immunology of human pregnancy, Totowa, NJ, 1993, The Humana Press.)

of major compatibility molecules (MHC), or HLA (Figure 27-2) by an antigen presenting cell (APC), often a macrophage or dendritic cell. Specific reactivity of the T cell depends on the structure of the T-cell receptor and those with similar receptors form a "clone" of comparable T cells similar to the clonality of B cells described earlier. Thus the antigen presenting cell (APC) processes the antigen and in conjunction with HLA molecules presents a processed antigen on the surface of the cell. The specific T-cell receptor (TcR) and the processed antigen-HLA complex lead to a cellular response. Two classes of MHC molecules are recognized (Class I and II), which contribute to specific TcR response. Thus the recognition of the antigen-HLA complex is an integral part of the cellular immune process. Unfortunately, not all

cancers express Class I or Class II MHC antigens and are therefore capable of evading the cellular immune response.

T cells can be characterized by their cell surface lymphocyte markers, which are termed *clusters of differentiation*, or CD groups. T cells, in general, have the CD 2 surface marker while CD 3 is linked to the T-cell receptor; Th (helper/inducer) cells have a CD 4 surface marker; and Ts (suppressor/cytotoxic) cells have CD 8 surface markers. The CD 4 surface markers are on T cells that recognize antigens that are presented by HLA (MHC) Class II molecules (Th cell), and the CD 8 surface markers are on T cells that recognize antigens presented by HLA (MHC) Class I (suppressor/cytotoxic) cells. In both of these situations the CD 2 surface marker is present and interactions between

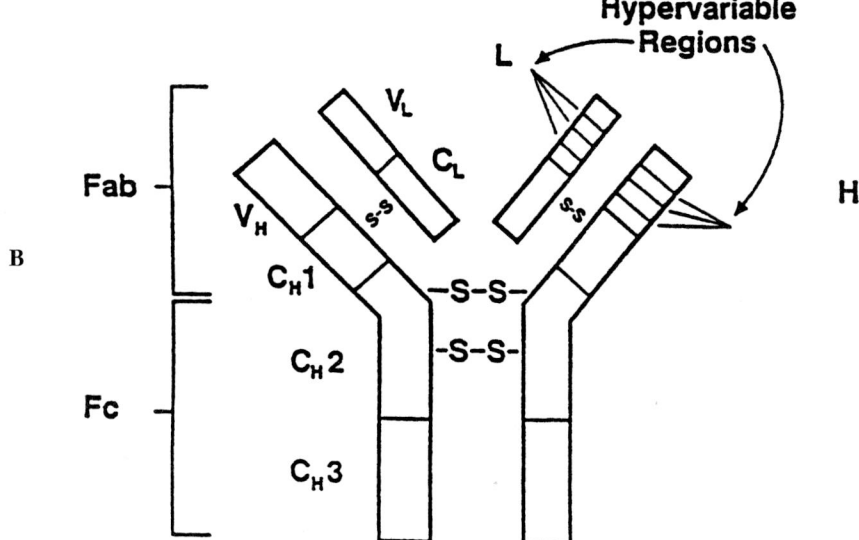

FIGURE 27-1 cont'd For legend see opposite page.

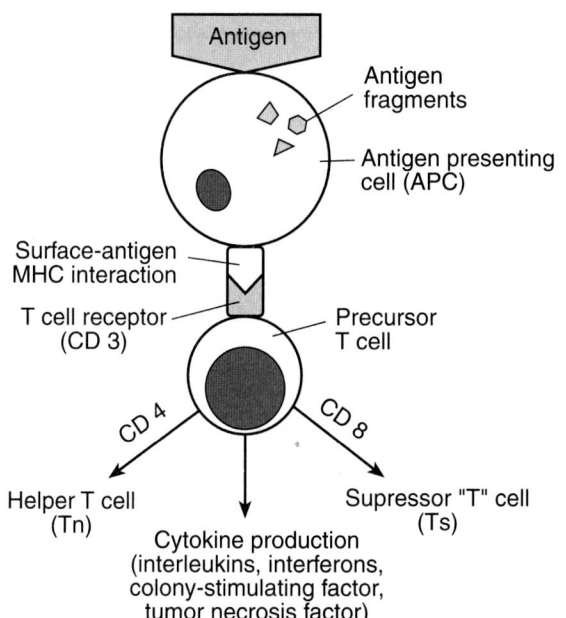

FIGURE 27-2 The antigen is processed by the antigen-presenting cell and broken into smaller fragments. These fragments and major histocompatability complex (MHC) or HLA molecules (Class I or II) then interact with the receptor on the surface of the "T" cell (TcR) to produce the immune response.

the TcR and antigen-HLA complex are "stabilized" by the CD 3 surface marker.

Activated T cells, as well as monocytes, produce a number of regulatory substances (cytokines) that can affect both arms of the immune system (see Figure 27-2). Examples of such cytokines are interleukins, interferons, colony-stimulating factors, and tumor necrosis factor,

which are subsequently summarized. In addition, in 1986 Townsend et al. noted that cytotoxic T cells (CTLs) could recognize viral antigens that were expressed inside an infected cell rather than on the surface. This raised the possibility of CTLs being able to recognize small changes in the cell that could lead to cytotoxicity (see discussion on ras oncogenes later in this chapter).

As previously noted, there are two classes of T cells: helper/inducer cells, which activate monocytes, stimulate cytotoxic T cells, and help immunoglobulin production by B cells; and suppressor/cytotoxic cells, which inhibit the function of other T cells, as well as B cells. There is a third type of cell, known as a *null cell* or *natural killer (NK) lymphocyte*, that is effective in nonspecific cytotoxicity. NK cells do not require antigen stimulation, but their activity can be enhanced by exposure to interferons.

An additional type of cytotoxic cell can be derived by culturing mononuclear cells in vitro with IL2. This results in production of lymphokine-activated (LAK) cells. Most of these are believed to be derived from NK cells. Activated macrophages can also occur in response to gamma interferon and to bacterial stimulation via BCG and *C. parvum* (see following discussion) and these activated macrophages can also be destructive to tumor cells.

CYTOKINES

Interleukins

Interleukins (IL) are potent cytokines that are designated numerically.

IL-1 is released in response to cell damage. Macrophages and monocytes release IL-1 in response to antigens leading to a number of immune messages, including stimulation of T cells and IL-2 production, hematopoietic factors, and glucocorticoid release.

IL-2 is produced by T cells and has a primary role of cell-mediated immunity. It is being evaluated as an antitumor agent in gynecologic and other malignancies, particularly ovarian carcinomas. IL-2 stimulates T lymphocytes, natural killer (NK) cells, and lymphokine-activated killer cells (LAK cells) and leads to the secretion of other lymphokines, including tumor necrosis factor (see following discussion). In addition, IL-2 is being used to promote thrombocytosis in patients with chemotherapy-induced thrombocytopenia.

Other interleukins include the following: IL-3 stimulates differentiation of myeloid stem cells; IL-4, formerly called B cell stimulating factor-1, stimulates the proliferation of B cells; IL-5 also stimulates B cells and has been termed B cell stimulating factor 2; IL-6 is a B cell stimulant as well. Additional interleukins have been described (IL 7-16) that affect the immune response, and new ones are being discovered.

Interferon

Interferons (IFNs) are produced in response to viral infection and act to inhibit viral replication. Three major types of these lymphokines have been described: alpha, beta, and gamma. IFN-alpha is secreted by leukocytes and macrophages and may enhance the antiviral response by stimulating cell surface antigens (major histocompatability complex [MHC]). It has antiproliferative activity; IFN-beta is produced by fibroblasts and epithelial cells and also acts to stimulate MHC antigens and has antiviral and antiproliferative activity; IFN-gamma is produced by activated T cells. It appears to have a wide-ranging set of actions, including enhancing MHC expression and inducing cytotoxic T cell maturation. The interferons have also been observed in vitro to inhibit tumor cell proliferation. Interferons bind to cell surface receptors and become biologically active, which can result both in antiviral and antiproliferative effects. Their precise mechanism of action is not known, but they appear to interact with T and B cells to augment cellular and humoral immunity. Interferon is being used clinically for treatment of some hematologic malignancies and has shown efficacy in some studies of cervical cancer and lower genital tract condylomas.

Tumor Necrosis Factor

Tumor necrosis factor (TNF) induces necrosis of tumor cells in vitro and also appears to act synergistically with interferons. It is a mediator of endotoxic shock and can stimulate hematopoietic cells. Furthermore, it can induce production of other cytokines, including GM-CSF. TNF cytotoxicity appears to be selective for tumor cells. This characteristic provides a theoretical advantage over classical chemotherapeutic agents inasmuch as approximately 100 to 10,000 × concentration of TNF is needed to affect normal cells in comparison with malignant cells in vitro. Moreover, TNF can act synergistically with IFN-gamma as well as chemotherapeutic agents such as 5-FU, alkylating agents, and etoposide. However, its administration has also been accompanied by severe toxicity, including shock-like symptoms, fever, and hypotension.

Colony-Stimulating Factors

Granulocyte colony-stimulating factor (G-CSF), a cytokine, promotes growth of granulocytes and is secreted by lymphocytes, as well as macrophages. It is used primarily in patients receiving cytotoxic chemotherapy to stimulate neutrophil production and thus shorten the duration of the myelosuppressive response. Granulocyte-macrophage colony-stimulating factor (GM-CSF) stimulates neutrophils and other granulocytes, monocytes, and early erythroid cells.

Erythropoetin, although not involved in the immune response, is a potent stimulatory factor of the erythroid system and can also stimulate megakaryocytes. It is secreted by peritubal renal cells and Kupffer cells in the human and serves as an important stimulus of red cell production. As with G-CSF and GM-CSF, the gene for erythropoetin has been cloned and the protein can now be mass produced. Erythropoetin is indicated for the treatment of chemotherapy-induced anemia, and its use in oncology patients alleviates the need for red cell transfusion in many cases.

TUMOR CELL KILLING AND IMMUNOTHERAPY

Active Immunotherapy

Various approaches have been evaluated in an attempt to use the immune system to eradicate cancer cells. Nonspecific active immunotherapy classically involved bacterial immunostimulants such as Bacillus Calmette-Guerin (BCG) and *Corynebacterium parvum (C. parvum)* to stimulate the system leading to tumor cell destruction. Chemicals such as levamisole, an anthelmintic agent used in veterinary work, also have immunomodulator action by restoring cell-mediated immune mechanisms and stimulating precursor T lymphocytes to differentiate into mature T cells. Interferons and cytokines such as IL-2 and TNF have had success in animal models, though efforts to replicate these responses in humans with cancer have been unrewarding. In many instances these substances have been combined with chemotherapy in order to enhance their effectiveness, often at the expense of increased toxicity.

In summary active, nonspecific immunotherapy can consist of a number of different approaches, including bacterial preparations and chemicals, both of which are immunostimulants, as well as the use of cytokines. More recently, experimental work has been directed toward development of tumor vaccines that in theory would inhibit tumor growth. Such efforts are in early development. A vaccine, designed to stimulate the immune system against oncoproteins produced by tumorigenic human papillomavirus, is presently undergoing early human trials in patients with advanced cervical cancer.

Passive Adoptive Immunotherapy

Passive adoptive immunotherapy involves the transfer of specialized cells that have the capacity to mediate directly an anti-tumor response. A well-known example is the use of LAK cells with IL-2, which in trials in the 1980s caused regressions of some instances of metastatic disease, mostly in melanomas and hypernephromas. Presumably IL-2–activated lymphocytes resulted in lymphokine-activated killer cells and these attached to tumor cells nonspecifically without disturbing normal cells. In these trials toxicity was a dose limiting problem. Such strategies have been investigated by Rosenberg et al., with some success reported. In general it is believed that large quantities of immune-lymphoid cells are required to be effective even against micrometastases. Canevari et al. recently reported on the use of retargeted T lymphocytes prepared using FAB fragments of a bispecific monoclonal antibody directed to the CD 3 molecule on T lymphocytes and the folate receptor on ovarian carcinoma. In a phase II trial 28 patients were treated intraperitoneally with these lymphocytes plus IL-2. Nineteen patients improved clinically and 3 had a complete response, lasting 26, 23, and 18 months, and the remainder either partial response or progression. While this is a low rate of response, it could provide the basis for further development of this approach.

MOLECULAR ONCOLOGY

There are three categories of genes that are associated with the development or prevention of malignancy: oncogenes, tumor suppressor genes, and DNA mismatch repair genes. Knowledge regarding these gene functions is rapidly expanding, and each category will be separately considered. Alterations in one or more of these genes may lead to disturbances in apoptosis, the complex, multistep process of programmed cell death. Apoptosis typically occurs as a result of accumulated genetic damage and is a key means of preventing an organism from passing on genetic injury during cell replication.

The term *oncogene* has been applied to one set of genes that when altered are associated with the development of a malignant cell. Most studies describing oncogenes were done in animals such as chickens, mice, and rats. Many of the oncogenes described in the literature probably do not play a role in human disease. A detailed discussion of this complicated subject is well beyond the scope of this text, but a general overview is provided.

The ability of certain genes to transform animals cells was identified through the study of RNA-tumor viruses (retroviruses). An interesting observation was that the sequences identified in the oncogene region of the virus were present in normal host cells. These normal sequences are called *proto-oncogenes.* Oncogenes carried by viruses are designated as *v-onc* while those that are in the cell are termed *c-onc.* More than 20 viral oncogenes have been identified, and these all have counterparts (proto-oncogenes) in normal cells. Usually viral oncogenes are slightly altered from their normal cellular counterparts; therefore these gene components in normal cells do not lead to malignant growth. Viral oncogenes may also exert their transforming effect by loss of their relationship with genes involved in regulating their expression. Proto-oncogenes play a role in normal cellular growth and development. When the proto-oncogenes become activated as a result of external stimuli, such as irradiation, chemical, or aging, malignant cell growth can result.

Proto-oncogenes are involved in cell division and as a group are generally placed into six classes: (1) growth factors, (2) receptors with protein kinase activity, (3) nonreceptor kinases, (4) signal transducers, (5) transcription factors, and (6) nuclear proteins.

The alterations that can lead to malignancy occur either by point mutations, amplification (increase in numbers of copies of genes in the cell), or chromosomal disturbances that free the oncogene from normal suppressive effects of regulatory genes. Transcription is the process whereby mRNA is transcribed from a DNA template in the nucleus, which leads to protein expression as a result of the mRNA serving as a template in the cytoplasm. The abnormal protein derived from oncogene RNA can lead to uncontrolled cellular growth. The term *overexpression* refers to excessive and abnormal protein production. Thus proto-oncogenes are normal cellular components that become altered in a way that permits transformed cell growth. Figure 27-3, *A,* shows the theoretic mechanisms of viral oncogene transformation; Figure 27-3, *B,* depicts a cellular oncogene model.

Cellular genes that code for growth factors or hormone receptors can be altered to become virally transduced oncogenes. Examples of some genes that code for hormone receptors are erb-B, which codes for epidermal growth factor (EGF); c-fms, which codes for the CSF-1 receptor, an important stimulator of the hemopoetic system; c-erb-A, which codes for thyroid hormone receptor; and c-erb-B, which also plays a role in erythrocyte differentiation. The c-erb-B2 gene, also termed *HER-2/neu gene,* is an example of a receptor gene (tyrosine kinase) that may be activated as a result of point mutation or gene amplification. HER-2/*neu* overexpression has been associated with poor prognosis in breast and ovarian cancers. The effect of this

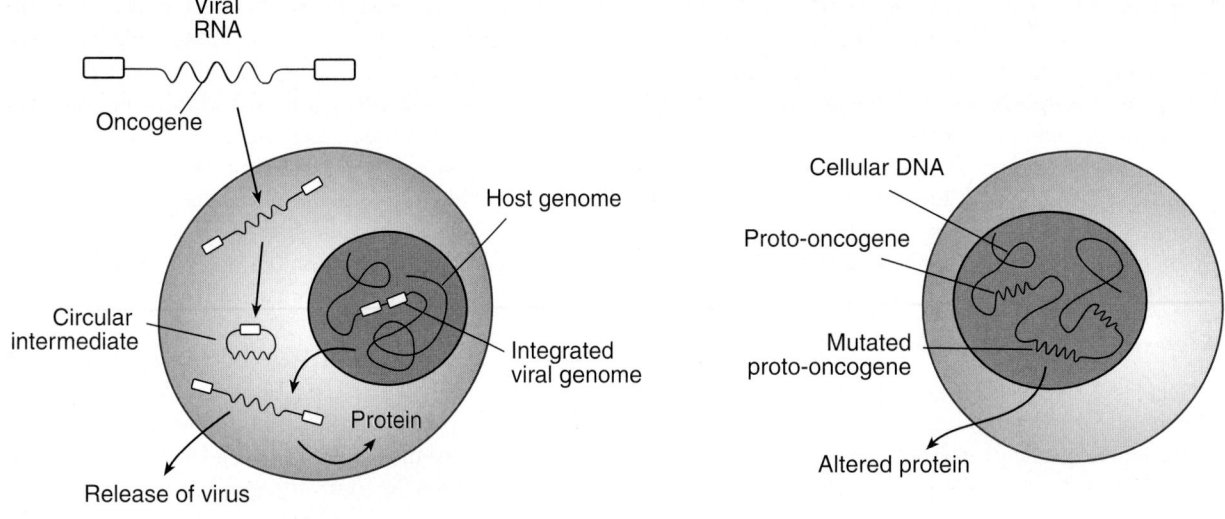

FIGURE 27-3 **A,** In the viral oncogene model, an RNA virus carrying an oncogene enters a cell. Double-stranded DNA is made from viral RNA, using the viral enzyme reverse transcriptase. The double-stranded DNA may integrate into the host genome. This genetic information may be transcribed to produce an mRNA, which is packaged as a mature virus or is translated into a protein that leads to malignant transformation. **B,** In the cellular-oncogene model, proto-oncogenes are genes in mammalian cells that regulate normal cell growth and differentiation. Alterations by mutation, amplification, or translocation may lead to gene products that cause malignant transformation. (Modified from Minden MD: Oncogenes. In Tannok IF and Hill RP, editors: The basic science of oncology, New York, 1987, Pergamon Press.)

cell membrane growth factor receptor is believed to be due to the level of stimulation of tyrosine phosphorylation. Recently, a humanized monoclonal antibody directed against the HER-2/*neu* receptor has been cloned and can now be produced in large quantities for clinical use. This product, approved for patients with breast cancer overexpressing HER-2/*neu* protein (approximately 15% of tumors), has been associated with an improved antitumor response, as summarized by Shak. Epithelial ovarian cancers overexpress HER-2/*neu* in about 10% of tumors, and phase II clinical trials are presently testing the efficacy of anti HER-2/*neu* receptor therapy in this group of patients.

Signal transducers are an important group of oncogenes represented by the ras genes. These resemble G-proteins and participate in signal transduction from the cell membrane to the interior of the cell. Ras oncogenes have been designated as H-ras, N-ras, and K-ras. Generally these are dormant but when stimulated, protein encoded by these genes causes GTP (guanisine triphosphate) to be formed from GDP (guanisine diphosphate), presumably leading to signal transduction followed by alteration to the ras genes. The signaling leads to an activated state that can provide messages to lead to other activations or deactivations of processes within the cell. It appears, as noted by Berchuck et al., that ras is a final common pathway that becomes activated following binding of growth factors previously described to receptor tyrosine kinases. Ras genes acquire the ability to transform as a consequence of point mutations or overexpression, either

of which can lead to malignant change. As noted previously, cytotoxic T lymphocytes (CTLs) can recognize intracellular alterations as well as surface antigens. In 1991 Jung and Schluesener reported that T lymphocytes could recognize point mutations of the ras oncogene. This raises the possibility of using CTLs targeted against ras mutations as a mechanism of tumor cytotoxicity. The mutant ras gene is thought to be more effective in causing malignant change than overexpression of the gene. Ras genes are referred to as *transforming genes* for their ability in some systems to alter cell-to-cell relationships.

Transcription factors are important in controlling gene expression, as explained previously. Activation of the gene alters its normal regulatory function and allows carcinogenesis to develop as a result of aberrant protein secretion that occurs abnormally during the cell cycle.

There are a number of nuclear oncogenes, including myc, myb, fos, etc. They can transactivate other genes and stimulate DNA replication. The cellular myc proto-oncogene can be activated by retrovirus insertion or by translocation to a highly active chromosomal region such as the immunoglobulin locus in B cells. With elevated c-myc expression the growth factor requirements of normal cells are altered. For example, hemopoetic cells dependent on IL-2 or IL-3 are able to grow independently of these factors when retrovirus-infected myc is introduced. The cells may become tumorogenic in mice, as noted by Klein. The c-myc gene is in the category that can be amplified as one way to contribute to tumor growth. Growth factors can stimulate its overexpression, that is, abnormal increased production of its protein products. The overexpression of myc can lead to cell proliferation independent of normal growth factor activity that is seen, for example, in leukemias and neuroblastomas. This has led to the categorization of myc genes as "immortalizing genes" in comparison to ras genes, which as previously noted are termed "transforming genes," although under some circumstances these categories may be interchangeable.

Tumor Suppressor Genes

Tumor suppressor genes restrain cellular proliferation. In this capacity they serve vital functions in normal cell regulation. The retinoblastoma gene (rb) was the first tumor suppressor gene that was characterized. In this hereditary disease two gene copies are inherited. In the inherited form of retinoblastoma, affected individuals inherit one defective copy of the rb gene but since there is a normal intact copy a malignancy does not develop until the second copy of the gene is inactivated, presumably as a result of mutation. Thus there is a "two-hit" theory of the action of the tumor suppressor gene, with the first hit being present in the inherited abnormal gene and the second as a consequence of somatic effects that occur later. These two hits are necessary in order for tumor to develop.

Mutant alleles from constitutional cells of individuals with inherited retinoblastoma, as well as from those from the "sporadic" type, have been recently sequenced. These analyses have provided molecular evidence that supports the two-hit model. As was predicted, those patients with retinoblastoma had one mutated and one normal allele in their blood cells. As described later in this chapter, the "two-hit" theory is also proposed to explain the substantially increased risk of breast cancer and ovarian cancer in women born with a germ line BRCA1 or BRCA2 mutation.

The most widely known tumor suppressor gene in gynecologic oncology is the p53 gene, which is located on the short arm of human chromosome 17. P53 normally suppresses the activity of oncogenes and plays a role in apoptosis. Loss of tumor suppressor function can occur due to deletion of the gene (both copies), gene mutation, or by partial deletion and other changes that inactivate the protein product of the gene. When p53 undergoes mutation, it loses its normal suppressive cellular function and then it can become associated with cell transformation and the development of neoplasia.

As noted by Berchuck et al., loss of p53 tumor suppressor gene function is a common event described in human cancers. It is important to recognize that p53 protein inhibits cellular proliferation, and binding of p53 to DNA results in the expression of several genes that are growth inhibitory. Thus normal p53 plays an important and active role in preventing malignancy. It functions as a surveillance mechanism by which cells that have undergone genetic damage are arrested in the G_1 phase of the cell

cycle, and this then allows DNA repair. If for some reason the DNA repair is not adequate, then p53 triggers programmed cell death through the process of apoptosis.

As in the case of retinoblastoma gene, it is generally believed that both alleles of p53 have to be altered in order for the p53 gene to be inactivated so that it cannot bind to DNA. However, mutation of one copy of the p53 gene is frequently accompanied by deletion of the other copy. Thus the cancer cell has only mutant p53 protein, which is not effective in inhibiting cellular proliferation. Furthermore, mutant p53 protein can form a complex with normal p53 protein and also prevent it from interacting with DNA. The E6 gene of certain oncogenic HPV types codes for a protein that complexes with wild-type p53 and facilitates its degradation and functionally deactivates the gene, in the absence of mutation. Thus inactivation of both p53 alleles is *not required* in order for p53 cellular growth inhibition to occur. Furthermore, mutant p53 proteins are resistant to degradation and will accumulate in the nucleus and this overexpression of mutant p53 leads to abnormal cell growth.

It is interesting, as noted by Fearon and Vogelstein, that wild-type p53 genes can inhibit the transforming ability of mutant p53 genes as well as other oncogenes. For example, it has been shown that the wild-type p53 gene suppresses the growth of human colorectal carcinoma cells with p53 mutations and that mutations in the p53 gene itself will abrogate its suppressor function. On the other hand, the growth suppressor effect of wild-type p53 gene can be observed even though the cells may have other genetic alterations. All of this highlights the role of wild-type p53 in normal regulation of cell growth, as noted by Baker et al.

BRCA1 and BRCA2

Genetic mutations have been identified as the cause of breast and ovarian cancer in many cancer-prone families; these mutations are rare and are estimated to account for no more than 5% to 10% of breast and ovarian cancer cases overall. The pattern of inheritance is autosomal dominant in nearly all families studied. In 1990 King and associates localized the first major susceptibility gene for breast and ovarian cancer on chromosome 17 and referred to it as BRCA1 (BR = Breast and CA = Cancer). Since that time BRCA2, localized to the long arm of chromosome 13, has also been isolated. BRCA2 mutations predispose their carriers predominately to breast cancer and are responsible for only a small proportion of hereditary ovarian cancers.

BRCA1 mutations appear to be responsible for about 45% of hereditary breast cancers in families without a history of ovarian cancer, BRCA2 are responsible for about 40%, and the remaining are due to other less common genetic causes. In families with both breast and ovarian cancer, BRCA1 mutations account for about 90% of these malignancies and BRCA2 mutations are much less common. Over 600 mutations and sequence variations in BRCA1 have been described for this large gene. A large percentage of these mutations leads to frameshifts resulting in a missing or nonfunctional protein. While a small number of these mutations have been found repeatedly in unrelated families, the majority are sporadic and have not been reported in more than a few families. Although fewer total mutations have been described in BRCA2 compared to BRCA1 (approximately 450), this gene was cloned later than BRCA1, is larger, and is more difficult to screen.

BRCA1 and 2 are thought to be tumor suppressor genes that code for a protein which regulates transcription of genes involved in DNA repair and cellular proliferation. The "two-hit" model, as described earlier, assumes that a carrier inherits a single mutated BRCA gene from one of her parents, but that the second, normal BRCA gene imparts its protective effects until such time that the normal gene undergoes a mutation. At that point, a functional tumor suppressor protein is no longer present, and a cancer develops. The cause or causes of the second "hit" are unknown, as are the reasons the ovary and breast are most susceptible to these malignant transformations.

It is suspected that as many as a million (about 0.5% to 0.6%) U.S. women are carriers of an altered BRCA1 or BRCA2 gene. Ashkenazi Jewish women are at particularly high risk with over 1% carrying the gene. It is estimated that for carriers of BRCA1 and BRCA2 mutations, breast cancer will develop by age 70 in 36% to 85% of women and ovarian cancer in 16% to 60%. Unfortunately, these women often develop breast cancer at a younger age than is typically seen with sporadic carcinomas and 60% will be diagnosed before the age of 50. BRCA mutation–associated ovarian cancer before the age of 50, however, is uncommon.

Personal characteristics associated with an increased likelihood of a BRCA1 or BRCA2 mutation include breast cancer diagnosed at an early age, bilateral breast cancer, or a history of both breast and ovarian cancer. Family history characteristics associated with an increased likelihood of carrying a BRCA1 or BRCA2 mutation include multiple cases of breast cancer in the family, both breast and ovarian cancer in the family, or one or more family members with two primary cancers.

The guidelines for screening cancer patients or their unaffected family members for BRCA gene mutations are evolving. As epidemiologic research progresses, more accurate information will become available on risks of BRCA1 and 2 mutation in a given family.

Mismatch Repair Genes

Mutator genes are the most recently described of the three types of cancer-causing genes. These genes have been characterized in bacteria by Fishel et al., and they noted that a gene in humans (designated MSH) is analogous to a bacterial gene. Mutation of this gene leads to the

inability of the bacteria to proceed with DNA mismatch repair. This human gene has been studied in a type of hereditary colon cancer known as hereditary nonpolyposis colon cancer (HNPCC—Lynch type II). It has been found on chromosome 2 and in this condition there are mutations in the MSH2 gene, and this gene is involved in DNA mismatch repair. Papadopoulos et al. have described another gene, MLH1, on chromosome 3P. MLH1 is important in correcting DNA mismatch repair and is mutated in some patients with HNPCC. The inability to provide effective DNA mismatch repair during replication leads to the accumulation of genetically altered material in the genome. If these mutations occur in the oncogenes or tumor suppressor genes, aberrant cell growth will result.

Multiple gene abnormalities are usually present in a single tumor and in general no single genetic change leads to malignant transformation. Nonetheless, major research efforts are under way to develop delivery systems to reverse the malignant process and thus induce remission of the cancer. In general these approaches involve the use of vectors (frequently adenoviruses or plasmid DNA), which are used to transfect the genetic material into the target cell. The system could be utilized to inhibit cell growth as was done by Ohno et al. in experiments with smooth muscle cells, which are normally stimulated after arterial injury. An adenoviral vector-encoding herpes virus thymidine kinase (tk) infected the smooth muscle cells and produced a toxic product resulting in cell death. As mentioned earlier, antibodies to HER-2/*neu* have been developed and are being used with some success in breast cancer patients. In a recent review Stauss summarized the work that was previously noted, namely that there is now evidence that cytotoxic T cells could recognize point mutations of the ras oncogene. Fenton et al. reported that CTLs that were developed as a result of immunization of mice with mutant ras protein could provide protection for mice against a tumor challenge. This approach raises the possibility of vaccines against ras proteins. Other potential applications include the use of genes that stimulate the immune response as a way of enhancing immunotherapeutic systems.

Angiogenesis

Angiogenesis, the formation of new capillary blood vessels, plays a crucial role in the pathogenesis of benign and malignant neoplasia. Under normal conditions, capillaries do not increase in size or number because the endothelial cells lining these small vessels do not reproduce. Tumor cells, however, are capable of reactivating the process of angiogenesis. This complex, multistep process appears to be triggered by growth factors secreted by tumor cells in the vicinity of the capillaries or by macrophages attracted to the site of developing neoplasia. One or more of these factors activates the normally quiescent endothelial cell, which then secretes enzymes that degrade the extracellular

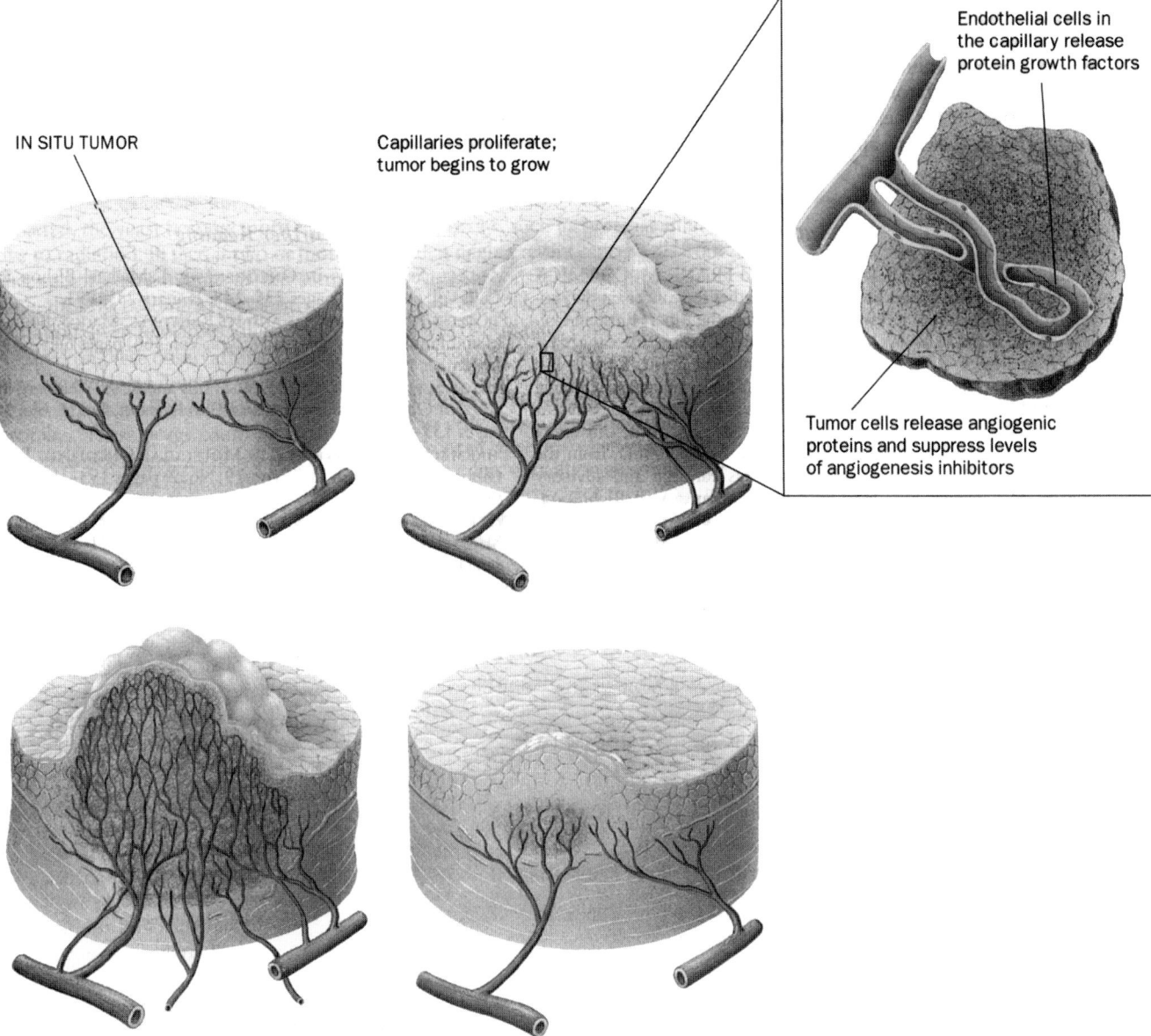

IN SITU TUMOR

Capillaries proliferate;
tumor begins to grow

Endothelial cells in
the capillary release
protein growth factors

Tumor cells release angiogenic
proteins and suppress levels
of angiogenesis inhibitors

FIGURE 27-4 Angiogenesis, or neovascularization, involves the proliferation of new blood vessels. The process transforms a small, usually harmless cluster of abnormal cells (known as an in situ tumor) into a large mass that can spread to other organs. Drugs that aim to interfere with angiogenesis, for example by halting the action of angiogenic proteins, can reduce the size of tumors and potentially maintain them in a dormant state. (From Folkman J: Fighting cancer by attacking its blood supply, Scientific American, September 1996, pp. 116-117).

matrix. The endothelial cells then invade the matrix and begin dividing. Eventually, the new cells organize into hollow tubes, and reestablish communication with preexisting capillary channels. This process is one of the integral steps in a tumor's transition from a minute, harmless cluster of cells to a large, malignant growth, capable of metastasizing to other organs throughout the body (Figure 27-4).

At present over 15 proteins are known to activate endothelial cell growth and movement, including angiogenin, epidermal growth factor, estrogen, fibroblast growth factors, interleukin 8, prostaglandin E1 and E2, tumor necrosis factor, vascular endothelial growth factor (VEGF), and granulocyte colony-stimulating factor. Some of the known inhibitors of angiogenesis include angiostatin, endostatin, interferon, retinoid acid, and tissue inhibitors of metalloproteinase.

In laboratory animals, it is possible to shrink tumors and prevent metastasis following treatment with one or more antiangiogenic compounds. These drugs prevent tumors from establishing new capillaries, and in many cases established capillaries within tumors are disrupted, essentially starving the tumor from essential nutrients.

About 20 angiogenesis inhibitors are currently being tested in human trials. Most are in early phase I or II clinical (human) studies. Because these drugs are designed to target normal endothelial cells, it is generally felt that these agents will have fewer side effects than cytotoxic chemotherapy agents and will not be as likely to induce resistance in malignant cells themselves. Antiangiogenic therapy may ultimately prove most useful when combined with standard chemotherapy because each therapy is aimed at a different cellular target.

KEY POINTS

- The cellular immune response occurs as a result of T lymphocytes reacting via a surface T cell receptor (TcR) that processes antigens presented to it by an antigen presenting cell (APC) in conjunction with HLA (MHC) molecules.

- T cell activation can result in helper/inducer (Th) cells, cytotoxic/suppressor (Ts) cells, or cytokine production.

- Cytotoxic T cells have the ability to recognize intracellularly expressed viral antigens and oncogene mutations.

- Humoral immunity results from antigen stimulation of a B lymphocyte, which differentiates into a plasma cell and secretes antibody (immunoglobulin).

- There are five types of immunoglobulins (IgG, IgM, IgD, IgA, and IgE). The immunoglobulin molecule consists of a fixed region (Fc), which carries the biologic activity, and a variable region (Fab), which reacts to a specific antigen.

- The complement cascade provides a basis for the inflammatory response and can also mediate cytotoxicity.

- T cells are characterized by cell surface markers, which are termed clusters of differentiation, and are numbered CD1 to CD80.

- Cytokines (lymphokines) are regulatory substances of the immune system produced as a result of T cell activation, cell damage by a virus, or other cells, such as macrophages and monocytes, involved in the immune response.

- Interferons are a group of cytokines produced in response to viral infections. They also have antiproliferative effects and can enhance the antitumor immune response as well as interact with other cytokines and chemotherapeutic agents.

- Colony-stimulating factors are a group of cytokines that can stimulate various parts of the bone marrow and can help to overcome the suppressive effects of chemotherapy.

- Systemic-active nonspecific immunotherapy results from the injection of agents derived from bacteriologic sources mixed with an adjuvant that causes a proliferation of lymphocytes leading to cellular and humoral immunity.

- Active specific immunotherapy is the use of tumor cells and their surface antigens to produce tumor immunity.

- There are three types of genes associated with malignant development: oncogenes, tumor suppressor genes, and mutator genes.

- Proto-oncogenes are protein sequences of oncogenes that occur in normal cells and regulate physiologic growth and development. When activated they can lead to malignant change.

- Malignant change is seen with point mutations, chromosomal aberration, gene amplification (increase in number of copies), or chromosomal translocation.

- Overexpression is excessive protein production in the cytoplasm, a result of gene alterations that can lead to abnormal cell growth.

- Retroviruses are RNA tumor viruses that identified animal cellular oncogenes. Many animal oncogenes do not lead to human tumor development.

- Ras oncogenes are part of a group of signal transducer oncogenes that relay messages from the membrane to the cell interior. They are activated generally by point mutations.

- Growth factor genes include C-erb-B2 (HER-2/*neu*), whose overexpression has been associated with poor prognosis in some human tumors.

- Nuclear oncogenes include myc and fos and can activate other genes as well as stimulate DNA replication.

- Tumor suppressor genes restrain cell growth. They have two copies and, in general, alteration of both copies leads to a mutant expression, which allows malignant growth to occur.

- Rb (retinoblastoma) and p53 are two widely studied tumor suppressor genes. Mutations of either allele of p53, as well as both alleles, can lead to malignant development. Wild-type p53 produces normal development and leads to apoptosis.

- Mutant p53 prevents normal p53 from interacting with DNA, which prevents cellular growth inhibition.

- BRCA1 and BRCA2 mutation confer an extremely high lifetime risk of breast and/or ovarian cancer. Mutation screening may be appropriate for women with family histories suggesting a hereditary predisposition to breast or ovarian cancer.

- Mutator genes act by preventing DNA mismatch repair during replication, which allows genetically damaged material to accumulate in the cell.

- Angiogenesis is the formation of new capillary blood vessels. This is considered an integral process in the progression of tumor from tiny in situ lesions to large malignant tumors capable of metastasizing to distant organs.

BIBLIOGRAPHY

Arbuck SG, Christian MC, Fisherman JS, et al: Clinical development of taxol, J NCI Monograph No. 15, 11, 1993.

Baker SJ, Markowitz S, Fearon ER, et al: Suppression of human colorectal carcinoma cell growth by wild-type p53, Science 249:912, 1990.

Bast RC Jr and Boyer CM: Tumor immunology. In Holland JF, Frei E III, Bast RC Jr, et al, editors: Cancer medicine, ed 3, Philadelphia, 1993, Lea & Febiger.

Berchuck A, Elbendary A, Havrilseky L, et al: Pathogenesis of ovarian cancers, J Soc Gynecol Invest 1:181, 1994.

Berek JS, Martinez-Maza O, and Montz FJ: The immune system and gynecologic cancer. In Coppleson M, editor: Gynecologic oncology, ed 2, London, 1992, Churchill Livingstone.

Canevari S, Stoter G, Arienti F, et al: Regression of advanced ovarian carcinoma by intraperitoneal treatment with autologous T lymphocytes retargeted by a bispecific monoclonal antibody, J Natl Cancer Inst 87:1463, 1995.

Claman HN: The immunology of human pregnancy. Totowa, NJ, 1993, The Humana Press.

Covens A, Thomas G, DePetrillo A, et al: The prognostic importance of site and type of radiation-induced bowel injury in patients requiring surgical management, Gynecol Oncol 43:270, 1991.

Deshane J, Cabrera G, Grim JE, et al: Targeted eradication of ovarian cancer mediated by intracellular expression of anti-erbB-2 single-chain antibody, Gynecol Oncol 59:8, 1995.

Druker BJ, Mamon HJ, and Roberts TM: Oncogenes, growth factors, and signal transduction, Semin Med Beth Israel Hospital, 321:1383, 1989.

Fearon ER and Vogelstein B: Tumor suppressor genes and cancer. In Holland JF, Frei E III, Bast RC Jr, et al, editors: Cancer medicine, Philadelphia, 1993, Lea & Febiger.

Fenton RG, Keller CJ, Hanna N, and Taub DD: Induction of T-cell immunity against ras oncoproteins by soluble protein or ras-expressing *Escherichia coli*, J Natl Cancer Inst 87:1853, 1995.

Ferrara N, Alitalo K: Clinical applications of angiogenic growth factors and their inhibitors, Nat Med 5:1359, 1999.

Fishel R, Lescoe MK, Rao MRS, et al: The human mutator gene homolog *MSH2* and its association with hereditary nonpolyposis colon cancer, Cell 75:1027, 1993.

Folkman J: Tumor angiogenesis. In Mendelsohn J, Howley PM, Israel MA, and Liotta LA, editors: The molecular basis of cancer, Philadelphia, 1995, WB Saunders Co.

Folkman J: Fighting cancer by attacking its blood supply, Scientific American, September, 1996.

Frank TS, Mankley SA, Olopade OI, et al: Sequence analysis of BRCA1 and BRCA2: correlation of mutations with family history and ovarian cancer risk, J Clin Oncol 16:2417, 1998.

Hall JM, Lee MK, Newman B, et al: Linkage of early-onset familial breast cancer to chromosome 17q21, Science 250:1684, 1990.

Jorde LB, Carey JC, and White RL: Medical genetics, St. Louis, 1995, Mosby–Year Book, Inc.

Jung S and Schluesener HJ: Human T lymphocytes recognize a peptide of single point-mutated, oncogenic ras proteins, J Exp Med 173:273, 1991.

Klein G: Oncogenes. In Holland JF, Frei E III, Bast RC Jr, et al, editors: Cancer medicine, ed 3, Philadelphia, 1993, Lea & Febiger.

Krontiris TG: Molecular medicine—oncogenes, N Engl J Med 333:303, 1995.

Leach FS, Nicolaides NC, Papadopoulos NC, et al: Mutations of a *mutS* homolog in hereditary nonpolyposis colorectal cancer, Cell 75:1215, 1993.

Minden MD: Oncogenes. In Tannock IF and Hill RP, editors: The basic science of oncology, New York, 1987, Pergamon Press.

Ohno T, Gordon D, San H, et al: Gene therapy for vascular smooth muscle cell proliferation after arterial injury, Science 265:781, 1994.

O'Reilly MS, Holmgren L, Chen C, and Folkman J: Angiostatin induces and sustains dormancy of human primary tumors in mice, Nat Med 2:689, 1996.

Papadopoulos N, Nicolaides NC, Wei YF, et al: Mutation of a *mutL* homolog in hereditary colon cancer, Science 263:1625, 1994.

Rosenberg S, Abersold P, Kenneth C, et al: Gene transfer in humans: immunotherapy of patients with advanced melanoma using tumor infiltrating lymphocytes modified by retroviral transduction, N Engl J Med 323:570, 1990.

Rosenberg SA, Lotz MT, Yang JC, et al: Experience with the use of high dose interleukin-2 in the treatment of 652 cancer patients, Ann Surg 210:474, 1989.

Shank S: Overview of the trastuzumab (Herceptin) anti-HER2 monoclonal antibody clinical program in HER2-overexpressing metastatic breast cancer. Herceptin Multinational Investigator Study Group, Semin Oncol 26:4 (Suppl 12), 1999.

Shattuck-Eidens D, Oliphant A, McClure M, et al: BRCA1 sequence analysis in women at high risk for susceptibility mutations: risk factor analysis and implications for genetic testing, JAMA 278:1242, 1997.

Smith SA, Easton DF, Evans DG, et al: Allele losses in the region 12q12-21 in familial breast and ovarian cancer involve the wild-type chromosome, Nat Genet 2:128, 1992.

Stauss HJ: Mutant ras proteins and peptides: bad news for tumors, J Natl Cancer Inst 87:1820, 1995.

Teicher BA, Holden SA, Ara G, et al: Potentiation of cytotoxic cancer therapies by TNP-470 alone and with other anti-angiogenic agents, Int J Cancer 57:920, 1994.

Thompson MW, McInnes RR, and Willard HF: Genetics in medicine, Philadelphia, 1991, WB Saunders Co.

Townsend AR, Rothbard J, Gotch FM, et al: The epitopes of influenza nucleoprotein recognized by cytotoxic T lymphocytes can be defined with short synthetic peptides, Cell 44:959, 1986.

Vose JM and Armitage JO: Clinical applications of hematopoietic growth factors, J Clin Oncol 13:1023, 1995.

Wooster R, Neuhausen SL, Mangion J, et al: Localization of the breast cancer susceptibility gene, BRCA2, to chromosome 13q12-13, Science 265:2088, 1994.

Intraepithelial Neoplasia of the Cervix
Etiology, Screening, Diagnostic Techniques, Management

KEY TERMS AND DEFINITIONS

Abnormal Transformation Zone. Area on the cervix or vagina that may contain columnar epithelium and squamous metaplasia and that often contains intraepithelial neoplasia with an abnormal colposcopic pattern.

Acetowhite Epithelium. A colposcopic term to describe epithelium that initially looks normal but appears white after acetic acid application. The area is frequently found to have histologic evidence of intraepithelial neoplasia or human papillomavirus (HPV) infection, in which case the term *subclinical papilloma infection (SPI)* is used.

AGCUS. Atypical Glandular Cells of Undetermined Significance. A term in the Bethesda cytologic classification used to indicate abnormal glandular cells that are not sufficiently abnormal to allow a definite diagnosis of neoplasia.

ASCUS. Atypical Squamous Cells of Undetermined Significance. A term in the Bethesda cytologic classification used to indicate abnormal squamous cells that are not sufficiently abnormal to allow a specific diagnosis of neoplasia.

Bethesda Classification. A cytologic classification developed in the United States in 1988, which defines two levels of squamous neoplasia (low-grade or high-grade squamous intraepithelial neoplasia).

Carcinoma in Situ. A morphologic alteration of the epithelium that usually precedes, occasionally gives rise to, and is usually present in the vicinity of invasive carcinoma. The full thickness of the epithelium is replaced with neoplastic cells.

Cervical Intraepithelial Neoplasia (CIN). A premalignant change in the cervical epithelium that can progress to the development of cervical carcinoma. The degree of change from mild to severe is described as CIN I, CIN II, or CIN III.

Colposcope. An instrument used to magnify and examine the epithelium of the transformation zone to identify abnormal areas in the lower genital tract that warrant biopsy.

Conization. An excisional technique to remove a cone-shaped central core of the cervix for diagnosis or treatment of intraepithelial neoplasia.

Cryotherapy. Freezing of the cervix to abate abnormal epithelium.

Dysplasia. A traditional term used to describe varying degrees of cervical intraepithelial neoplasia. It may be mild, involving approximately one third of the epithelium (CIN I); moderate, approximately two thirds of the epithelium (CIN II); or severe, full thickness of the epithelium (CIN III).

Endocervical Curettage (ECC). A biopsy procedure used to obtain endocervical tissue for histologic diagnosis.

Flat Wart. An alternate term to describe subclinical human papillomavirus (HPV) infection.

Human Papillomavirus (HPV) Types. A numeric designation given to varying types of HPVs, as determined by their DNA sequence. New types are being continuously described.

Koilocytosis. A cellular change associated with papillomavirus infection, which includes perinuclear cavitation and nuclear atypicality.

Leukoplakia. A colposcopic term to describe an area that appears white to the naked eye even before application of 3% acetic acid.

Loop Electrosurgical Excision Procedure (LEEP). An excisional procedure utilizing a thin electric wire loop to excise a cone of cervical tissue, usually utilized on an outpatient basis.

Mosaic Pattern. A colposcopic term to describe the rosette appearance of capillary vessels in an abnormal transformation zone.

Native Squamous Epithelium. The normal original squamous epithelium found in the vagina and on the portio of the cervix.

Normal Transformation Zone. Area of columnar epithelium and squamous metaplasia that has a normal colposcopic pattern.

Punctation. A colposcopic term to describe the stippled appearance of capillary vessels in the abnormal transformation zone.

Radiation Dysplasia. A term to describe abnormal cells in the cytologic smear of patients who have been treated by ionizing irradiation for lower genital tract malignancies. These patients are at increased risk for recurrent disease.

Satisfactory Colposcopy. A colposcopic examination in which the entire transformation zone, including the squamocolumnar junction, is adequately visualized. If not visualized, it is termed unsatisfactory colposcopy.

Squamocolumnar Junction. The junction of the squamous epithelium and columnar (glandular) epithelium, usually located near the external cervical os.

Squamous Intraepithelial Lesion (SIL). A cytologic term used to describe abnormal squamous cells according to the Bethesda Classification. Low grade (LGSIL) corresponds to koilocytosis and CIN I. High grade (HGSIL) corresponds to CIN II and III.

Squamous Metaplasia. A physiologic process whereby squamous tissue replaces columnar tissue.

Subclinical Papilloma Infection (SPI). Colposcopically evident papilloma infection not clinically visible. An area that looks normal to the naked eye but colposcopically appears white after acetic acid application. It usually contains papillomavirus infection.

Because of the accessible location of the cervix and the upper vagina, intraepithelial neoplasia of the cervix has been investigated more than any other premalignant lesion of the female genital tract, and this process has resulted in improved detection and treatment. The development of cytology to aid in the detection of neoplasia of the cervix and the colposcope as an instrument to localize the site of the most severe change and allow directed biopsy has contributed to improvement of the management of these disorders. This chapter reviews the morphologic changes that characterize the intraepithelial neoplastic lesions of the cervix. The current concepts of the factors thought to lead to the development of cervical neoplasia, including a detailed consideration of human papillomavirus infection (HPV), are reviewed and the methods of diagnosis and treatment described.

DEFINITIONS AND MORPHOLOGY

The squamocolumnar junction is an important landmark where neoplastic change develops in the cervix. In young adults this intersection between the cervical glandular (columnar) epithelium and the native squamous epithelium is usually located on the exocervix just distal to the external os. During pregnancy and after childbirth this area may enlarge and become more distally located on the portio of the cervix away from the os. After menopause the junction usually recedes and is frequently located in the endocervical canal. Thus in the normal adult female of reproductive age, there are usually areas of columnar epithelium surrounding the exocervix. During puberty and throughout reproductive life, especially during pregnancy, this exposed columnar epithelium undergoes gradual replacement by squamous epithelium (squamous metaplasia), and the areas of columnar epithelium and squamous metaplasia constitute the normal transformation zone. In contrast, abnormal or neoplastic squamous epithelium can also be found in the transformation zone, which leads to abnormal colposcopic patterns and characterizes the abnormal transformation zone (see colposcopy section).

Three terminologies have been used in recent years to describe premalignant conditions of the cervix (Figure 28-1). One relies on the term *dysplasia* (mild, moderate, or severe) to describe the early premalignant changes in the epithelium and *carcinoma in situ* to describe the most advanced premalignant change. A second nomenclature that describes the same histologic features utilizes the terminology of *cervical intraepithelial neoplasia (CIN):* CIN I (mild dysplasia), CIN II (moderate dysplasia), and CIN III (severe dysplasia to carcinoma in situ). The Bethesda System is a two-tier system that combines koilocytosis and mild dysplasia into Low-Grade Squamous Intraepithelial Lesion (LGSIL) and moderate and

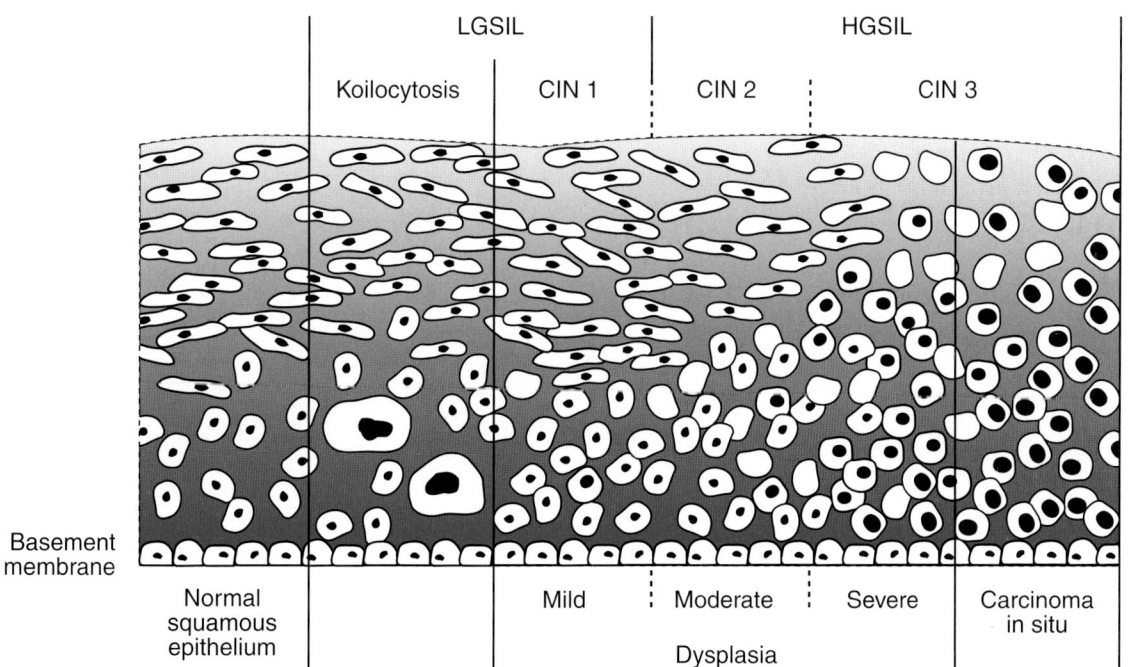

FIGURE 28-1 Diagram of cervical epithelium showing various terminologies used to characterize progressive degrees of cervical neoplasia.

severe dysplasia and carcinoma in situ into High-Grade Squamous Intraepithelial Lesion (HGSIL).

The cytologic and histologic features of mild, moderate, and severe dysplasia and carcinoma in situ are illustrated in Figures 28-2 to 28-5. Further progression leads to invasive carcinoma (Figures 28-6 and 28-7). The diagnosis of koilocytosis is discussed separately in the section on human papillomavirus and is illustrated in Figures 28-8 to 28-10. Unfortunately, there is a lack of agreement regarding the precise definition of each category of intraepithelial neoplasia, and there is no sharp morphologic boundary between them, a problem that often leads to disagreements in the diagnosis of the degree of severity. In general for dysplasia, if up to one third of the basal epithelium is abnormal, the term "mild" is applied; up to two thirds, "moderate"; more than two thirds, "severe"; and full thickness, "carcinoma in situ." In addition, carcinoma in situ may develop in the crypts of the glands of the cervix as well as in the surface epithelium. Involvement of the glands leads to a diagnosis of "carcinoma in situ with gland involvement." For purposes of patient management, this entity is the same as carcinoma in situ without gland involvement.

EPIDEMIOLOGY

Potential Factors in Carcinogenesis

Intraepithelial neoplasia of the cervix occurs mainly in young women. The incidence is approximately twice as high in black women as in white in the United States. The peak in the age incidence of the disease is in those in their 20s and 30s, and occasionally younger. Furthermore, it appears that the frequency of the diagnosis of carcinoma in situ has increased in the past 25 years, in part because of the effectiveness of cytologic screening (Pap smear). This has been accompanied by a concomitant decrease in the frequency of invasive carcinoma, with a drop of approximately 50% in the frequency of cervical carcinoma in the United States in the latter part of the 20th century. The low-grade lesions (LGSIL) are the most common and these frequently will spontaneously regress. On the other hand, even a few low-grade abnormalities can progress to cancer, and the risk of such progression increases with more severe lesions, such as carcinoma in situ.

The precise cause of cervical neoplasia is not known. The box on p. 864 outlines the major factors believed to be related to its development. Many have a venereal association. It is generally agreed that the atypical epithelium develops in the transformation zone of the cervix during the process of squamous metaplasia. Viruses, particularly HPV, have a major role in the genesis of premalignant lesions. In addition to this pathway of cervical carcinogenesis, it is recognized that some squamous cell cancers can arise de novo in areas outside the transformation zone.

Women who have multiple sex partners are at increased risk, and the disease is more frequent in young prostitutes. The age at first intercourse appears particularly important. Herrero et al. noted a greater than twofold risk of cervical cancer for those starting intercourse at ages 14 to 15 years

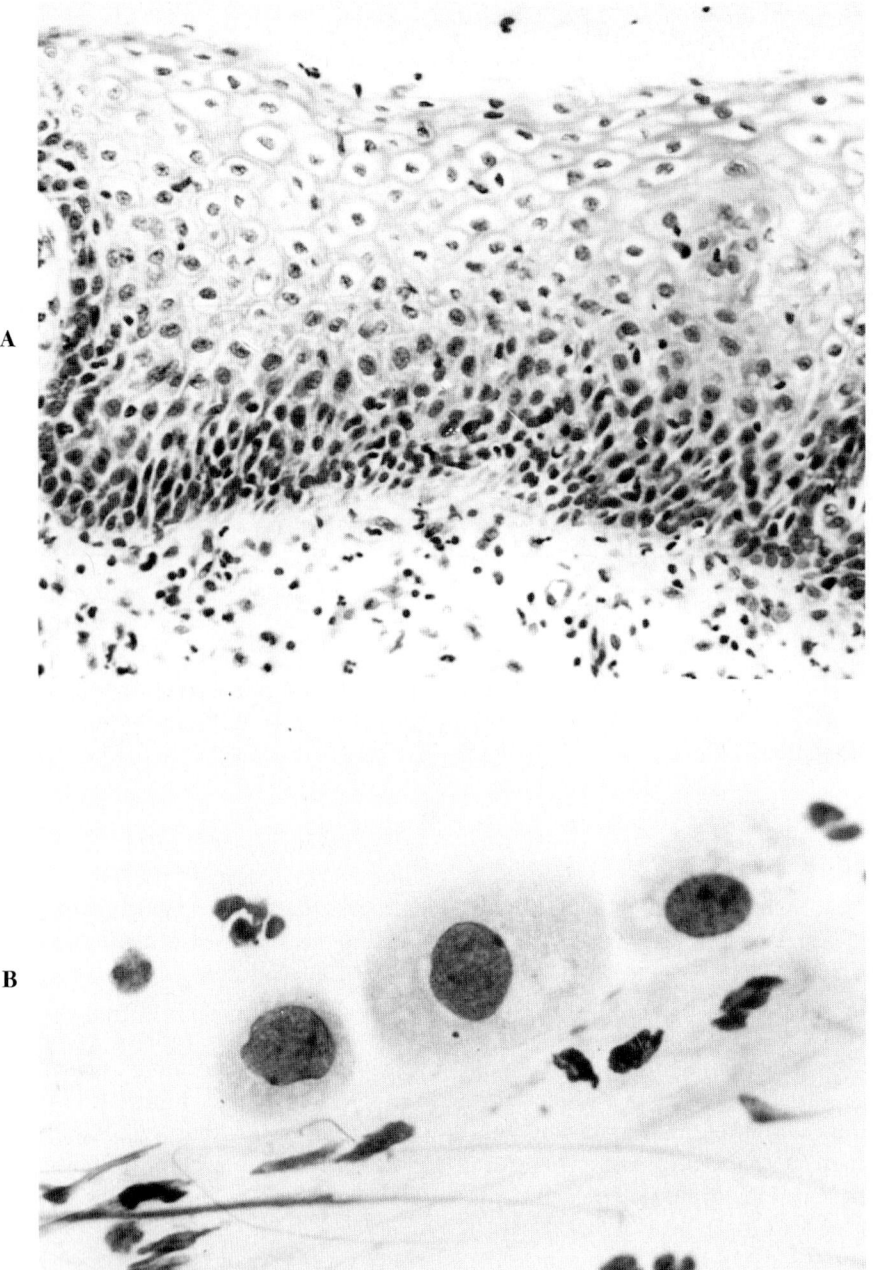

FIGURE 28-2   **A,** Mild dysplasia (histology) (CIN-I), (LGSIL). Undifferentiated cells are confined to lower two to four layers of epithelium. Cells of middle and upper third show nuclear enlargement and irregular nuclei. (H&E stain; ×250.) **B,** Mild dysplasia (cytology). Dysplastic cells have altered nuclear-cytoplasmic ratio, exhibit nuclear enlargement, and have finely granular chromatin structure. (Papanicolaou stain; ×800.)

compared with those over 20 years, suggesting that the younger patients may be more susceptible to carcinogenic influences. In contrast, squamous cell carcinoma of the cervix is almost unknown in nuns.

The male consort can also be important in the development of the disease. For example, Kessler studied women married to men whose previous wives had developed cervical cancer. This cohort was compared with women married to men whose previous wives had not had cervical cancer. A threefold increased frequency of cervical cancer occurred among the former group.

The occurrence of diseases such as gonorrhea has also been shown to be associated with the frequency of cervical carcinoma. Beral and colleagues noted that an increase in the frequency of gonorrhea in a given group was accompanied by a subsequent increase in cervical carcinoma. However, current data do not indicate a direct role for venereal diseases such as gonorrhea, *Trichomonas vagi-*

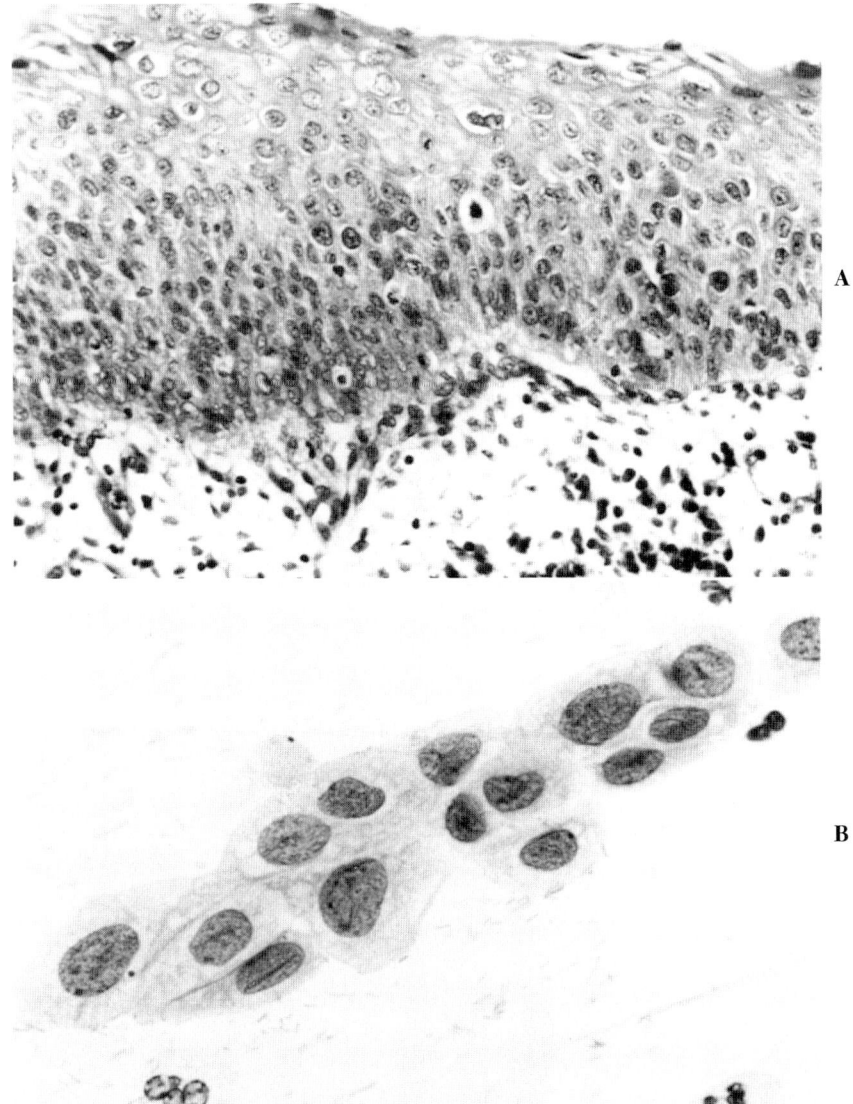

FIGURE 28-3   A, Moderate dysplasia (histology) (CIN-II) (HGSIL). Immature cells are confined to lower half of epithelium. Cells of upper half show well-defined cell borders and enlarged, pleomorphic nuclei. (H&E stain; ×300.) **B,** Moderate dysplasia (cytology). Cells derived from moderate dysplasia exhibit altered nuclear-cytoplasmic ratio with less cytoplasm than in cells of mild dysplasia. There may be a uniformly finely granular chromatin pattern, with occasional chromocenter and (as cell at right) irregular nuclear envelope. (Papanicolaou stain; ×800.)

nalis, or syphilis in the genesis of cervical carcinoma but suggest that the causative agent or agents may be transmitted as a result of sexual activity, during which these diseases are also transmitted.

Alteration in immune function increases the risk of neoplasia. For example, transplant patients receiving immunosuppressive therapy have been noted to be at increased risk for recurrent HPV infection (see following). In addition, HIV-infected women not only have increased frequency of HPV infection and CIN but also the frequency of these problems correlates with the CD4 counts. Wright et al. noted a frequency of CIN of 30% in HIV-positive women compared with 4% in those who are HIV-negative. A low

CD4+ lymphocyte count increased the risk. Fink et al. reported a prevalence of CIN of 35% in HIV-seropositive females with CD counts over 400 in contrast to 56% in those with counts under 200. Ellerbrock et al. noted 1 in 5 HIV-infected women with no evidence of cervical disease developed biopsy-proven SIL within 3 years.

Other Potential Factors

In studies of women ingesting oral contraceptives, Vessey et al. suggested an increased risk of CIN in comparison to controls with comparable sexual histories who used an IUD. Beral et al. studied 47,000 women and showed that

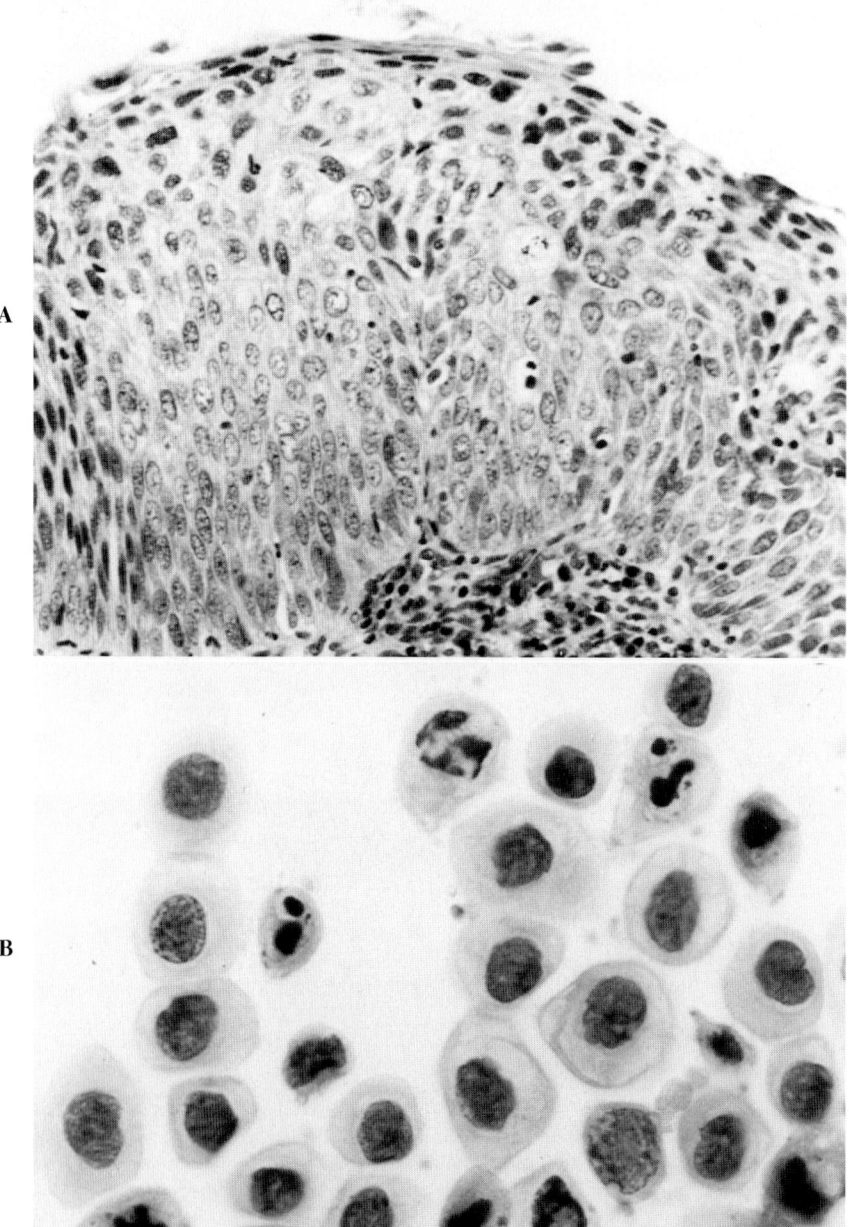

FIGURE 28-4   **A,** Severe dysplasia (histology) (CIN-III) (HGSIL). In this lesion, immature cells with spindle-shaped nuclei replace more than two thirds of the mucosal thickness. Upper layers show evidence of squamous cell differentiation (H&E stain; ×300.) **B,** Severe dysplasia (cytology). Cells derived from a severe dysplasia may exhibit enlarged hyperchromatic nuclei, an irregular nuclear envelope, a coarse chromatin structure, and less cytoplasm than less severe dysplastic reactions. (Papanicolaou stain, ×1000.)

oral contraceptive users were at increased risk for CIN. The increase in cervical neoplasia was most prominent in those who used oral contraceptives for more than 5 to 10 years. These results may be affected by other confounding factors, and other studies have not shown a relationship between oral contraceptives and CIN. Moreover, Ursin et al. suggested an association between oral contraceptives and cervical adenocarcinomas. Despite conflicting data patients taking oral contraceptives should have at least

annual cytologic screening, since they appear to have 2 to 4 times the risk of developing neoplasia. As noted in a review by Grimes and Economy, a number of studies suggest a protective effect for barrier contraceptives (condom and diaphragm and spermcides) but not all studies are consistent on this point. Cigarette smoking has also been implicated as a factor. Brinton et al. found a relative risk of 1.5 for the development of cervical neoplasia among women who smoke. Schiffman and Brinton noted in their

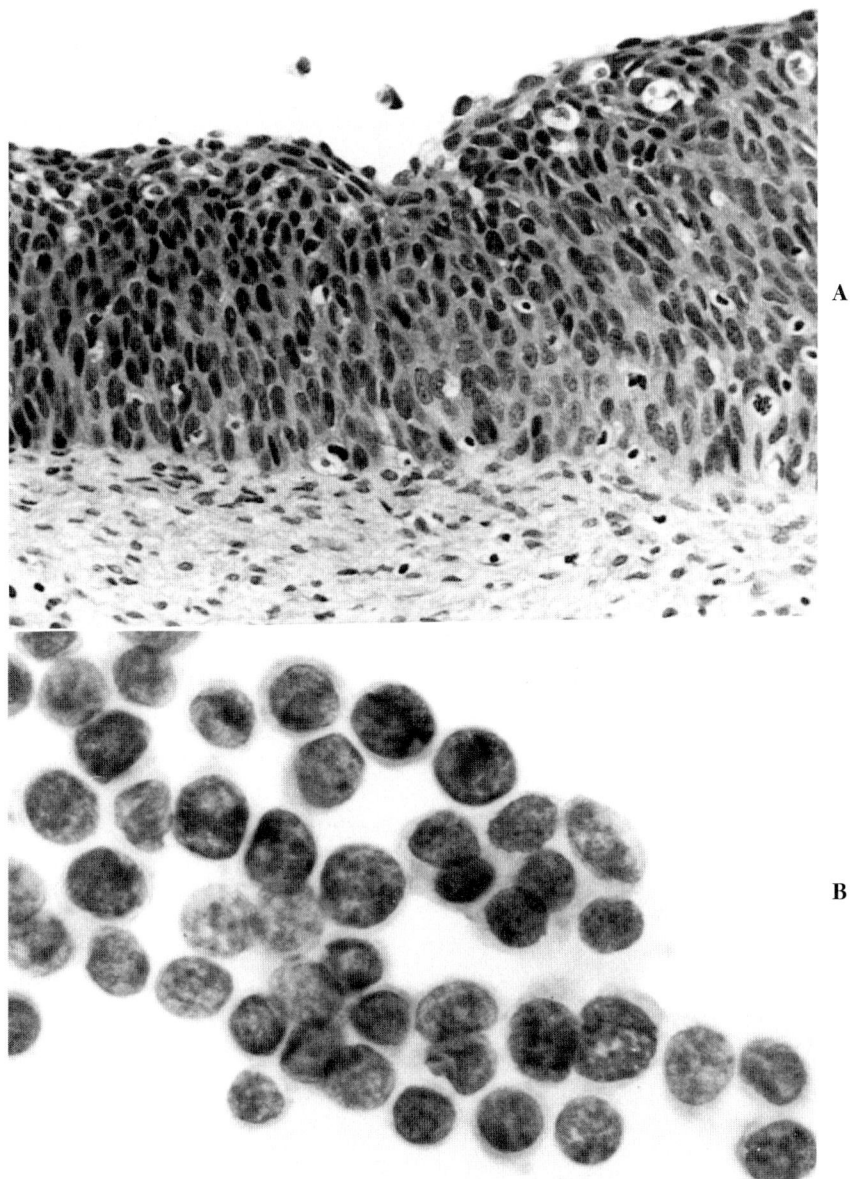

FIGURE 28-5 **A,** Carcinoma in situ (CIS) (histology) (CIN III, HGSIL). Basal-type cells with elongated nuclei and indistinct cytoplasmic boundaries occupy full thickness of mucosa. No maturation is present. (H&E stain; ×300.) **B,** CIS (cytology). CIS in cytologic sample may reveal groups of primitive cells with scant, ill-defined cytoplasm, nuclei that are round or oval, and a coarsely granular chromatin pattern with distinct chromocenters. Nucleoli are usually absent. (Papanicolaou stain; ×800.)

1995 review, the association of cervical dysplasia with smoking is weak and may, in part, be related to the association of HPV infection in smokers.

Vitamins have also been evaluated as potential risk factors. Animal studies have suggested that deficiencies in vitamin A can promote neoplasia. Vitamin A deficiencies in humans have been associated with dysplastic-type changes in cytologic smears of the cervix, and these changes have been reversed by vitamin A administration. Romney et al. noted a deficiency of vitamin C in patients who had an abnormal Pap smear in comparison to those who had normal smears, and they suggested that vitamin C deficiency might also be a factor. There are also theories that other nutrients, such as vitamin E and folate, may be protective, but such studies are difficult to control and may be confounded by the fact that smoking lowers some vitamin serum levels.

Radiation has also been considered as a potential factor in CIN. Cervical dysplasia has been reported in cytologic (Pap) smears in patients after irradiation therapy for carci-

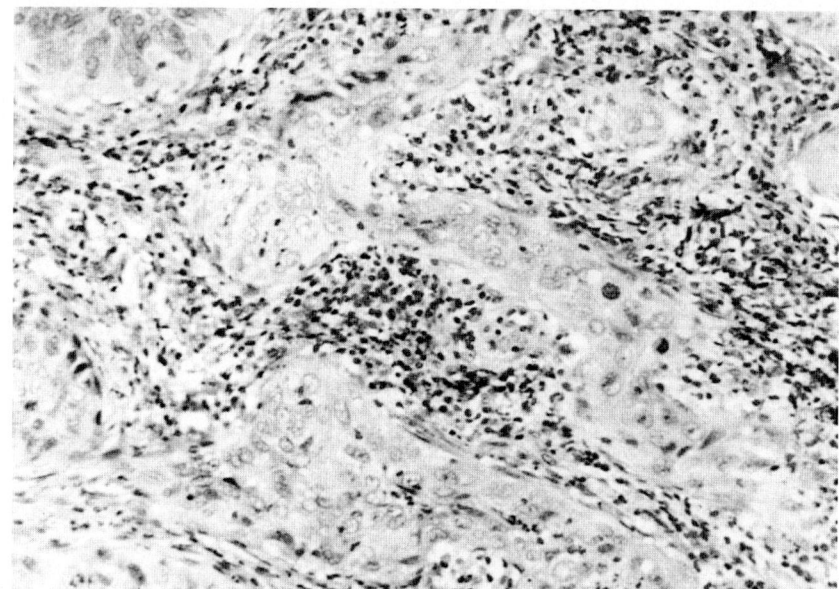

FIGURE 28-6   Invasive squamous carcinoma (histology). Irregular tumor nests infiltrate a stroma rich in inflammatory cells. Tumor cells are pleomorphic. A mitotic figure is seen at left. (H&E stain; ×200.)

noma of the cervix. If these patients with so-called radiation dysplasia are carefully followed, they are found to be at increased risk for the development of recurrent disease compared with those who do not show radiation dysplasia changes. However, it is not clear if this radiation dysplasia is a result of the radiation or is an early morphologic cellular change that precedes the development of recurrence.

> ### Potential Risk Factors for Cervical Neoplasia
>
> **Epidemiologic Characteristics**
>   Early intercourse
>   Multiple sex partners
>   Early marriage
>   Early childbearing
>   Prostitution
>   Male factors –"high-risk" consort
>   Socioeconomic status, race
>   STD infection
>   Immune status, including HIV infection
>
> **Other Potential Factors**
>   Oral contraceptives
>   Cigarette smoking
>   Vitamin C
>   Prior radiation
>   Intrauterine DES exposure
>   Lupus erythematosus
>   Vitamins A and E, folates
>
> **Viral Relations**
>   Papillomavirus
>   Herpesvirus
>   Cytomegalovirus

Intrauterine diethylstilbestrol (DES) exposure is discussed in detail in Chapter 15. Because of the enlarged transformation zone that occurs in the cervix and occasionally the vagina of these females with concomitant larger areas of squamous metaplasia, there is concern that such patients may be at increased risk for squamous neoplasia. Although such patients require regular medical surveillance for the development of squamous neoplasia, current evidence has not established that DES exposure is a risk factor for squamous neoplasia.

Viral Hypothesis

Human Papillomavirus

Papillomaviruses belong to the Papovaviridae family. They are double-stranded deoxyribonucleic acid (DNA) viruses that replicate within epithelial cells. They are commonly associated with genital warts and have been extensively studied in the past few years for their potential role in the genesis of CIN. Human papillomavirus (HPV) does not cause systemic infection. Like HSV II (see following section), papillomaviruses are sexually transmitted, and infections have been identified in the asymptomatic male partners of infected females. Moreover, women having sexual relations with these male partners appear to be at increased risk for CIN.

In recent years extensive evidence has accumulated linking HPV to CIN. HPV causes distinct cellular changes, the most common of which is koilocytosis (perinuclear cavitation with nuclear abnormalities) (Figure 28-8). These cells are found in genital warts and are frequently identified in areas of intraepithelial neoplasia.

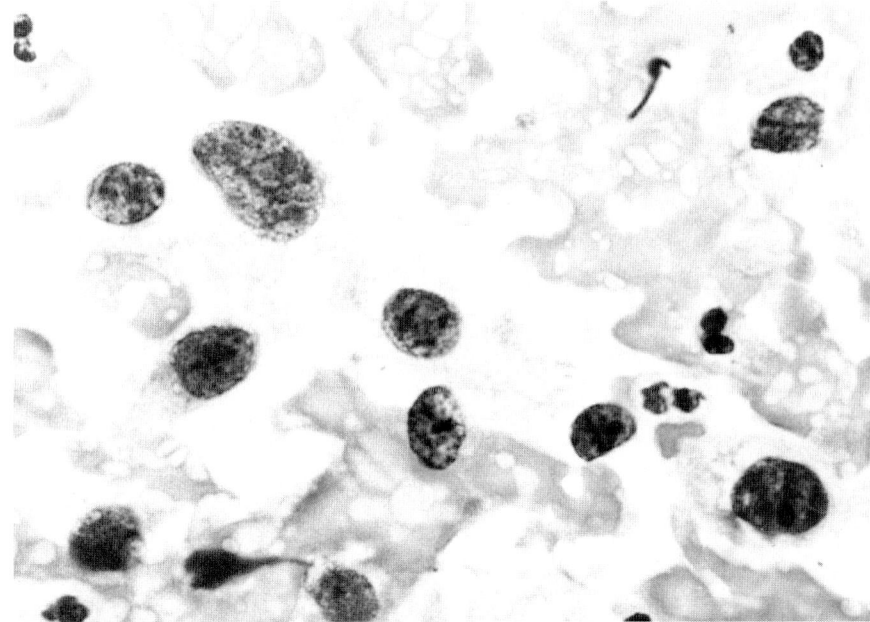

FIGURE 28-7 Invasive squamous cell carcinoma (cytology). Poorly differentiated squamous cell carcinoma may exhibit in the cytologic sample isolated malignant tumor cells with marked variation in nuclear size and shape. Because of the coarse and irregular chromatin pattern, nucleoli are not easily discerned here but are usually evident on direct microscopic examination. Background shows degenerated red blood cells and a few polymorphonuclear leukocytes. (Papanicolaou stain; ×1000.)

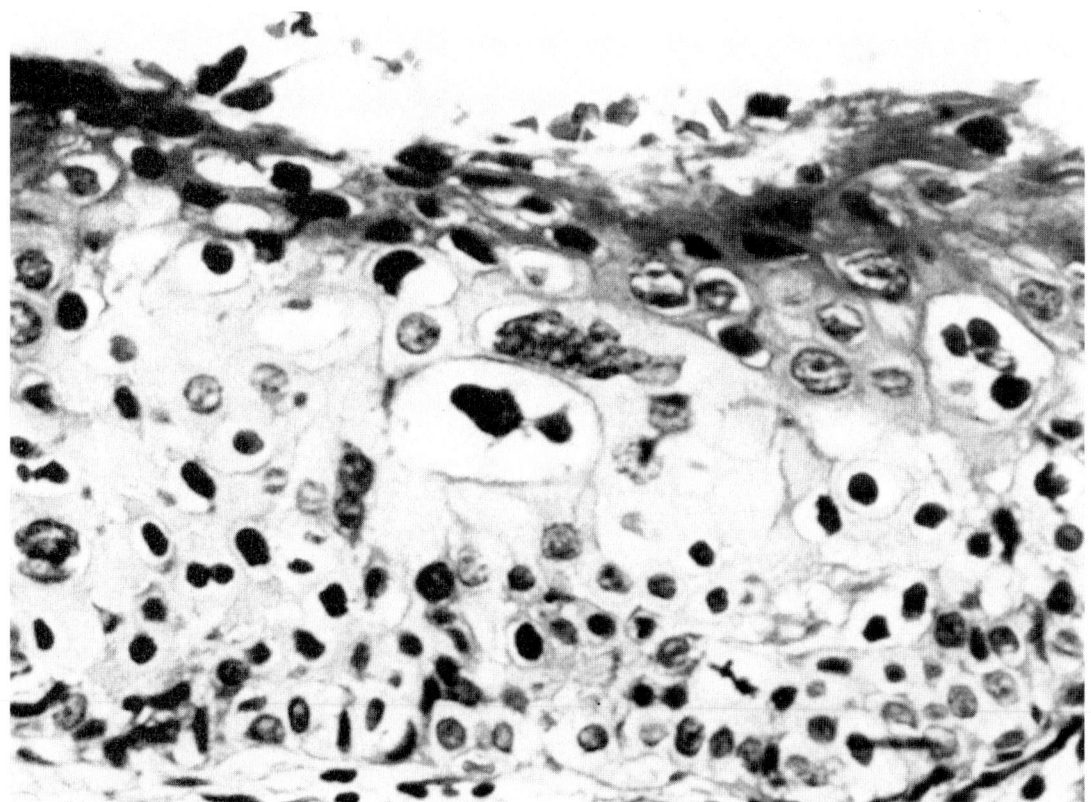

FIGURE 28-8 Human papillomavirus changes: koilocytosis, multinucleation, parakeratosis, and dyskeratosis. (Light microscopy: H&E stain.) (From Grunebaum AN, Sedlis A, Sillman F, et al: Obstet Gynecol 62:448, 1983. Reprinted with permission from The American College of Obstetricians and Gynecologists.)

Some of the morphologic changes of HPV infection mimic the changes of mild dysplasia (CIN I), which is one basis of the Bethesda Cytology Classification (see following). The rapid increase in knowledge regarding HPV has affected both the diagnosis and management of atypias of the cervix. The cytologic and histologic features of HPV infection of the lower female genital tract are illustrated in Figure 28-9. One problem is that the diagnosis of koilocytosis has been made erroneously on the basis of perinuclear cavitation only. Nuclear atypia is mandatory. In addition, Jovanovic et al. recently reported "pseudokoilocytotic" cells in postmenopausal women (Figure 28-10).

HPVs are classified by DNA-hybridization techniques, which differentiate the major DNA composition of the viruses. Each type is designated by a number, depending upon the order in which the type is discovered. More than 100 human types have been described, and new ones can be anticipated to be discovered.

Several DNA-hybridization techniques have been used to study and characterize HPVs. One must have a general understanding of these techniques to interpret the varying results of the many studies published. The *Southern blot technique* has been frequently used and was the basis of the characterization of HPV-DNA in vulvar warts and vulvar neoplasia by zur Hausen and other researchers. Regardless of the technique, the identification depends on the hybridization between a specific DNA or ribonucleic acid (RNA) probe and the target HPV in the cell. Some studies have used a *dot-blot procedure*, which depends on HPV-DNA hybridization but eliminates the electrophoretic

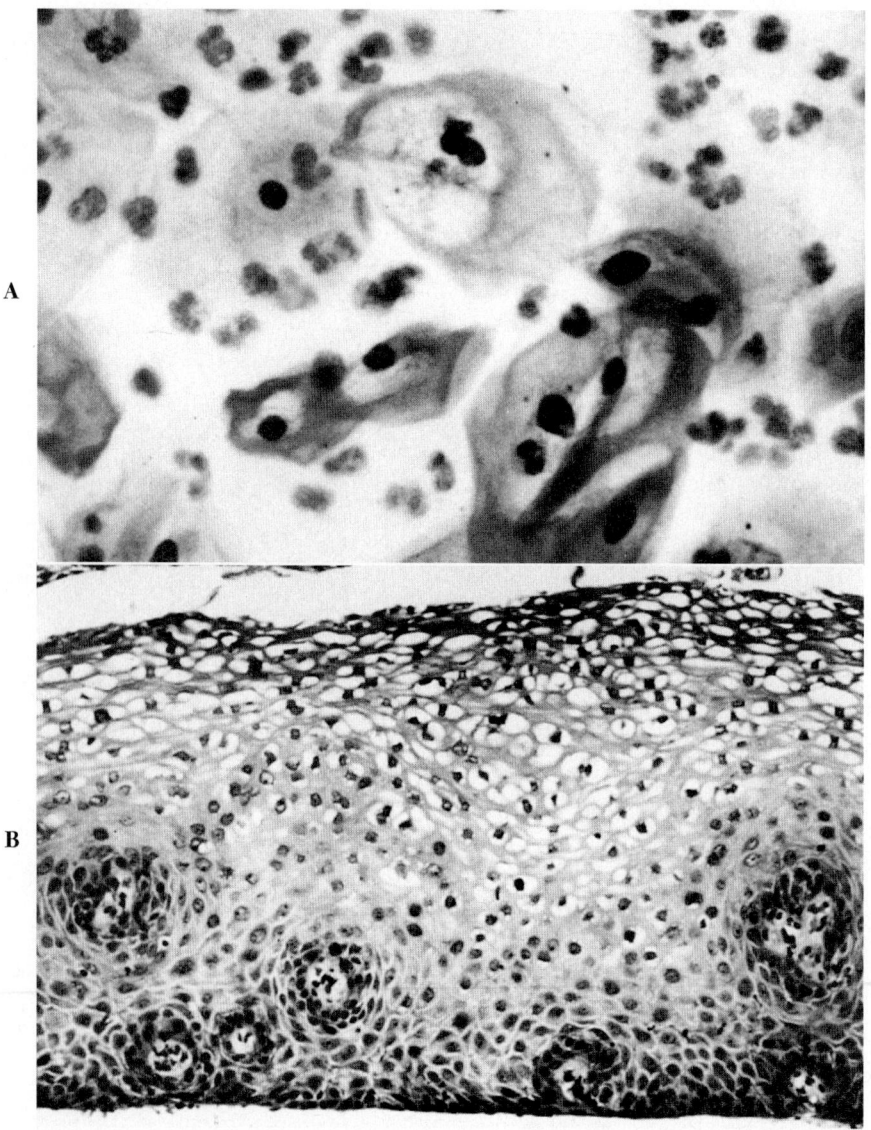

FIGURE 28-9 **A,** Typical koilocytic cells in HPV infection of uterine cervix. Note cavitation of cytoplasm, binucleation, and pyknotic nuclei. (Papanicolaou stain; ×400.) **B,** Condyloma of uterine cervix. Note koilocytes in superficial layers of epithelium and many binucleated cells. (H&E stain; ×240.) (Courtesy Marluce Bibbo, M.D.)

step needed with the Southern blot technique. Both are sensitive but time consuming. Techniques are also available to study formalin-processed tissue sections already fixed in paraffin, called *in situ hybridization*. These can be performed without radioactive probes. However, the technique is much less sensitive than the Southern or the dot-blot procedure. A much more sensitive technique is known as the *polymerase chain reaction* (PCR). It involves the enzymatic amplification of DNA sequences and is reported to be capable of detecting a single HPV molecule in a million cells, compared with the Southern blot technique, which is reported to require about one copy per hundred cells. PCR is used commonly today in research studies.

Hybrid capture is a recently introduced technique that has been evaluated in a number of trials. The test depends on the collection of a specimen from the cervix. HPV-DNA, if present, is hybridized with varying nonradioactive HPV-derived RNA probes. The resulting DNA-RNA hybrid is reacted against specific antibodies resulting in varying degrees of luminescence, which is compared with controls. RNA probes from a number of different HPV types are usually combined in a single "cocktail." The degree of light emitted from the antibody DNA-RNA complex is read by a machine that provides a measure of the amount of HPV-DNA detected. A recent development is an HPV test (Hybrid Capture II) that has a sensitivity of detecting HPV-DNA of 1 pg/ml. A cocktail of oncogenic types (Table 28-1) is combined and is being evaluated as a potential future clinical tool (see later).

The association of HPV infection with cervical neoplasia is very strong. Most women with cervical intraepithelial neoplasia and carcinoma are infected with HPV-DNA. However, most women with HPV infection do not develop cervical neoplasia. Moreover, 10% to 15% of cervical cancers appear to arise in the absence of detectable HPV-DNA. The prevalence of HPV infection is related both to sexual practices and patient age. The highest rates of detection are among those with increased sexually transmitted disease and multiple partners. Thus young individuals in a sexually active population have the highest HPV prevalence rates, and these women are usually in their late teens and early twenties. The prevalence drops among older women, with a sharp drop after age 30, presumably in part due to host response and immunologic clearance of HPV. In addition, Moscicki et al., in a study of 300 HPV-positive women, noted that approximately two thirds of them had cleared the infection spontaneously within 2 years. DeVilliers et al. estimated that females in Germany with detectable HPV-DNA by in-situ hybridization and normal cytology had a lifetime cumulative risk of developing either CIN or invasive cancer of 3.7%.

Recent studies by Josefsson et al. and Ylitalo et al. suggest that those with persistent high viral loads of HPV-16 have an increased risk for developing carcinoma in situ. An important observation by Wallin et al. was that the finding of oncogenic HPV-DNA in a Pap smear increased the risk of future development of invasive cervical cancer with the same HPV type.

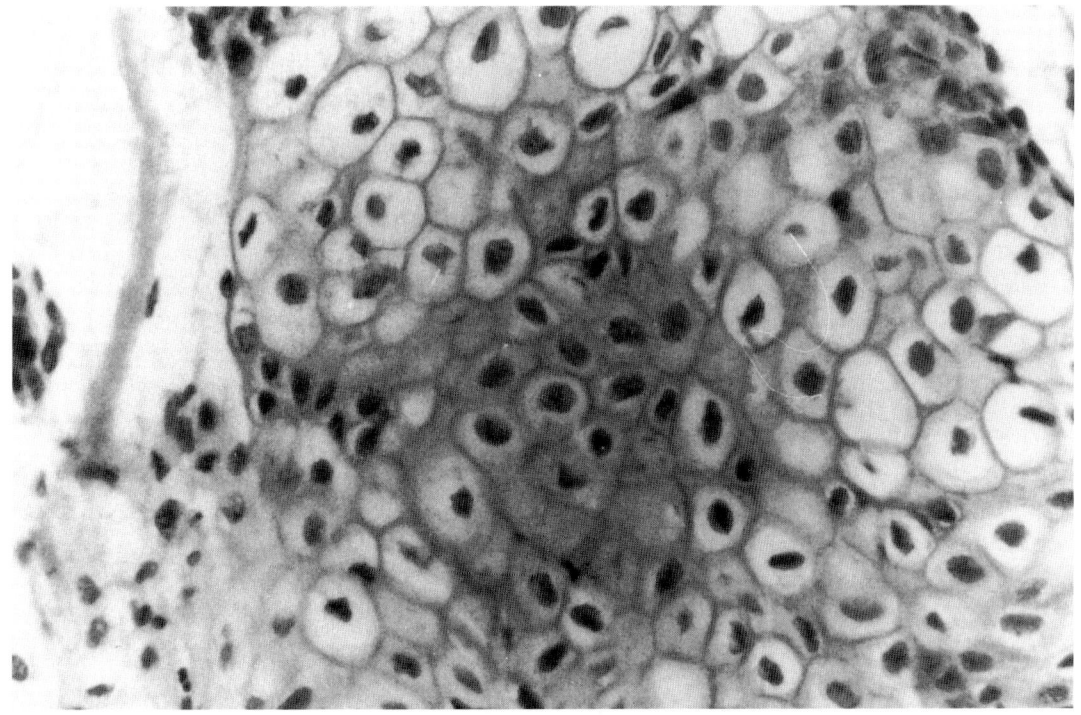

FIGURE 28-10 Postmenopausal squamous mucosa with moderate nuclear enlargement and moderate differences in nuclear staining intensity mimicking koilocytosis. (From Jovanovic AS, McLachlin CM, Shen L, et al: Mod Pathol 8:408, 1995.)

TABLE 28-1
Oncogenic Potential of HPV Types

Potential	HPV Types
Nononcogenic	6, 11, 42, 43, 44
Oncogenic	16, 18, 31, 33, 35, 39, 45, 51, 52, 56, 58, 59, 68

The strong associations between HPV and CIN suggest a causative role for the virus. As noted by Koss, HPV is a prime candidate for transforming the cervical epithelial cell. Repeated infections or perhaps other viral infections are needed to promote the change, and environmental or hormonal factors previously discussed may also play a role. These various factors could then combine to lead to genetic changes, producing neoplasia. Such events are supported by the studies of protooncogenes by Riou et al., who noted deletion and mutation in the C-ha-*ras* gene in cervical cancers and amplification of C-*myc* gene. Oncogene amplification (ha-*ras* and c-*myc*) have been reported in CIN III and invasive carcinoma in comparison to normal cervix and CIN I by Pinion et al.

A possible molecular mechanism explaining the potential role of HPV in cervical neoplasia has been proposed and reviewed by Park et al. and Schiffman and Brinton. In brief, oncogenic HPV infects the cervical epithelium and initially is in an episomal (nonintegrated) form. It then becomes integrated into the host genome. Two viral open reading frames from the genome designated E6 and E7 are then able to encode for oncoproteins that are important for cell transformation as well as viral replication. The E6 protein appears to affect tumor suppressor gene p53, leading to a loss of wild-type and a loss therefore of the normal tumor suppressor function. As noted in Chapter 27, this impairment of p53 and the concomitant loss of tumor suppressor function leads to oncogenic activity and malignant cell growth. A similar type of mechanism appears to be exerted by E7 protein on the retinoblastoma (Rb) tumor suppressor gene. Thus genomic instability arising from loss of normal tumor suppressor gene function appears to contribute to the development of cervical neoplasia.

Herpesvirus

Various studies have related genital tract infections with herpes simplex virus II (HSV II) to cervical carcinoma. The herpesvirus elicits antibody responses in humans, and elevated serum antibody titers to HSV II have been found more frequently among women with premalignant and malignant cervical lesions. The virus has been detected in tissues from cervical carcinoma, and viral antigens have also been detected in carcinoma tissues. Cervical carcinoma has also been found to contain antibodies to HSV II antigens. The virus has been found to be capable of transform-ing mammalian cells in vitro and of producing tumors in experimental animals. Although HSV II is suspect in the etiology of cervical cancer, a definitive cause-and-effect relationship has not been established.

Cytomegalovirus

The cytomegalovirus is the largest member of the Herpetoviridae family and also has been studied for its potential role in cervical carcinogenesis. It is transmitted by sexual contact. Viral particles have been uncovered in cervical carcinoma biopsies, and in vitro malignant cellular transformation has been observed. However, cytomegalovirus has not been extensively studied and is not currently thought to have a major role in cervical carcinogenesis.

DIAGNOSIS AND MANAGEMENT

The term *subclinical papillomavirus infection* (SPI) has been used to describe an entity that is not clinically visible to the naked eye but that can be recognized utilizing the colposcope and staining the vagina and cervix with acetic acid (see colposcopy section). Subclinical HPV infection and clinically evident condyloma constitute important manifestations of HPV infection of the lower genital tract. The morphologic manifestations of HPV infection (koilocytosis) is most prominent in the early premalignant lesions, such as mild dysplasia (CIN I), and decrease as the more severe alterations of the cervical epithelium occur. Moreover, it appears that some diagnoses reported as dysplasia in the past may in fact have been HPV infection. Therapy should be limited to women who have clinically evident or symptomatic condyloma or morphologic evidence of neoplasia.

Risks of Progression and Natural History

What are the rates of progression of premalignant lesions of the cervix? Precise data are not available. In cytologic studies of mild and moderate cervical dysplasia, Nasiell et al. used cervical cytology or biopsy to follow women in 1962 to 1983. Regression to normal from mild dysplasia occurred in 62% of the cases, while progression to more severe lesions of carcinoma in situ or severe dysplasia occurred in 16%. The remaining 22% had persistence of mild dysplasia. In a similar study of moderate dysplasia, the same authors noted that regression occurred in 54% over 6 years, progression to severe dysplasia or carcinoma in situ in 30%, and persistence of severe dysplasia in 16%. Two patients lost to follow-up from the study eventually developed invasive cancer.

While some have concern in regard to these studies, particularly with diagnoses based only on cytology findings, the results are consistent with the concept that the risk of progression of CIN is higher for those with high-grade lesions but that spontaneous regression can also occur. Current evidence suggests a slow progression to

TABLE 28-2
Natural History CIN: A Critical Review

Citat. (N)	Subjects (N)		Regress	Persist	Prog. CIN III	Prog. Invasive
17	4504	CIN I	57%	32%	11%	1%
12	2247	CIN II	43%	35%	22%	5%
21	767	CIN III	32%	?<56%*	–	12%*

From Östor AJ: Int J Gynecol Pathol 12:186, 1993.

*Limited follow-up in some series.

Limit to report of Cytol. and/or Bx alone. Exclude cone and destructive Rx.

invasive cancer from CIN, but the risk of such progression is small and usually takes many months or years to occur. The studies of McIndoe et al. from the early 1980s indicate the risk is greatly elevated in patients with persistent abnormal cytology after treatment for carcinoma in situ. In their series, 29 of 131 patients (22%) subsequently developed invasive carcinoma. Östor reviewed the world literature on premalignant cervical lesions, and Table 28-2 summarizes data from the article and gives approximate rates of progression, regression, and persistence for CIN I, II, and III. Thus the risk for the development of invasive disease from carcinoma in situ is high, and all of these latter lesions require therapy, and CIN II is usually treated as well. The recent study of Holowaty et al. confirms that moderate dysplasia (CIN II) has a risk of progression intermediate between mild dysplasia (CIN I) and CIN III.

Methods of Detection and Diagnosis

The Papanicolaou (Pap) smear has been used widely for about 50 years to screen women for malignant and premalignant cervical disease. It has been effective to reduce the frequency of invasive carcinoma of the cervix. It is essential to realize that cervical cytology is useful only for screening, and its results do not establish definitive diagnosis. False-negative and false-positive results can also occur. For example, in the detection of cervical carcinoma it is estimated that some cases will be missed by routine cytologic screening because of sampling variation or other interpretive difficulties that may contribute to false-negative rates of 5% to 20% (false negatives/true positives plus false negatives). In addition, some cells appear atypical and mimic neoplastic changes. Examples are severe cervical infection, *Trichomonas vaginalis* infection, herpesvirus infection (which can cause cellular nuclear change), as well as erroneous diagnoses of koilocytosis discussed previously (see Figures 28-9 and 28-10). Abnormal-appearing cells on the cytologic smear have also been reported in patients who have received chemotherapy. In addition, abnormal cervical cellular changes are reported with increasing frequency in those with lupus erythematosus and these latter patients deserve close follow-up at least annually.

Cytology

TECHNIQUE. The Pap smear is best obtained by taking a direct scrape (sample) from the tissue being studied. This is usually accomplished by exposing the cervix. A sample is taken from the endocervix using a brush and rotating it 90 to 180 degrees (Figure 28-11). A wood or plastic spatula

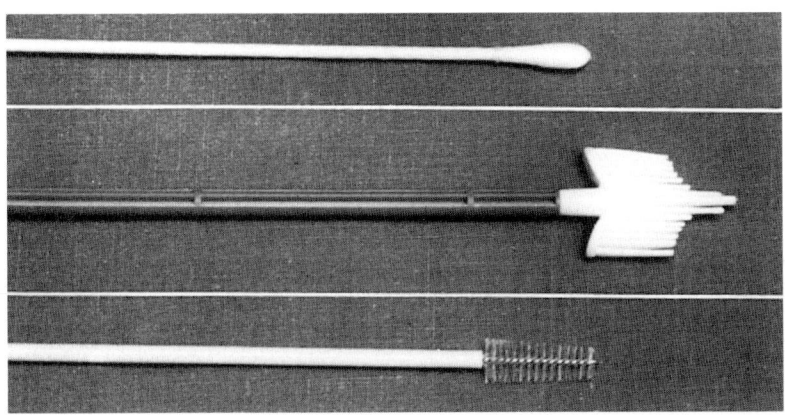

FIGURE 28-11 Narrow brushes for endocervical sampling. *Top,* Q-Tip; *middle,* Cervix Brush (Unimar); *bottom,* Cytobrush (Medscand).

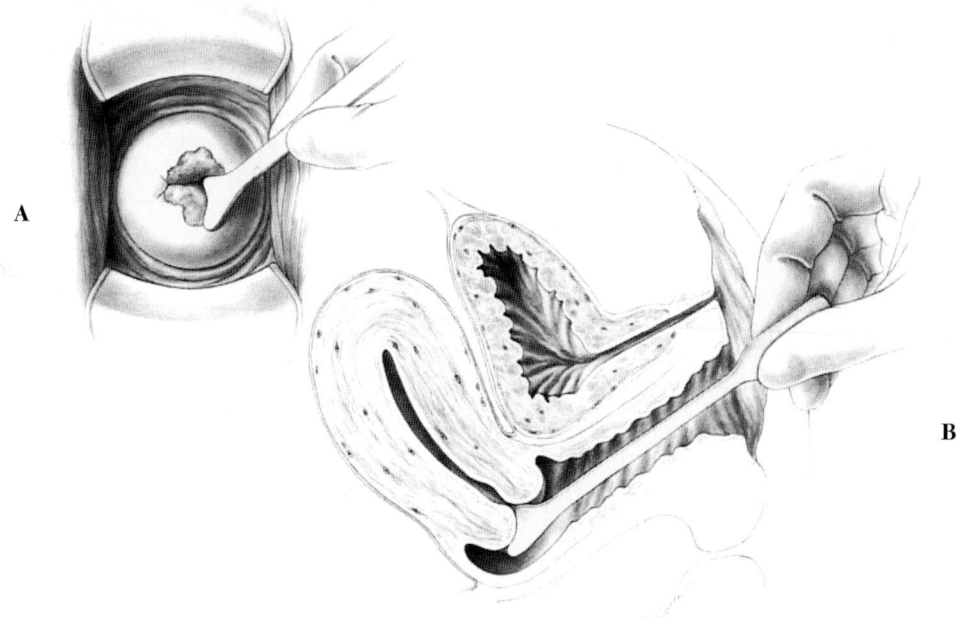

FIGURE 28-12   **A,** Scrape of endocervix. **B,** Scrape of exocervix.

is used to scrape the exocervix separately so as to include the entire transformation zone (Figure 28-12). Some centers obtain a separate smear from the vagina and from the cervix and endocervix (V, vaginal; C, cervical; E, endocervical), and these are placed separately on a single glass slide. The cellular specimen is immediately fixed, either in 90% alcohol or sprayed with fixative. It is important to hold the fixative spray more than 12 inches (30 cm) from the smear and not to allow the smear to air dry before fixing in order to preserve the cellular architecture and not introduce artifacts.

INTERPRETATION OF THE SMEAR.   Numerous classifications have been used to describe the Pap smear results. The most useful information is conveyed by describing the type of cellular changes observed by the cytologist. It is very important that the smear be interpreted by laboratories with adequate volumes to maintain diagnostic skills. It is recommended that a cytopathologist annually supervise at least 25,000 cervical smears to achieve this. Cytologists also frequently indicate the type of inflammation or infection that may exist if morphologic changes that allow infectious agents, such as herpesvirus, HPV, *Chlamydia,* or *Trichomonas vaginalis,* to be identified. Figures 28-2 to 28-7 illustrate the various cytologic changes that correspond to the various types of cervical neoplasia that are also demonstrated histologically. One classification used for many years is demonstrated in the upper part of the box on this page. It has been replaced by the Bethesda System in the United States as well as in some other countries.

The Bethesda System is based on a conference sponsored by the National Institutes of Health (NIH) in 1988. It is summarized in the lower part of the box on this page.

Traditional Classification and Bethesda Classification (Modified) of Papanicolaou Smear

Traditional Classification of Papanicolaou Smear
Normal
Metaplasia
Inflammation
Minimal atypia—koilocytosis
Mild dysplasia (CIN I)
Moderate dysplasia (CIN II)
Severe dysplasia—carcinoma in situ (CIN III)
Invasive carcinoma

Bethesda Classification (Modified)
Adequacy of smear
Infection type
Squamous abnormalities
    Reactive (inflammatory change)
    Epithelial cell abnormalities
        Atypical type, undetermined
        Squamous intraepithelial lesions (SILs)
    Low grade: HPV or mild dysplasia (CIN I)
    High grade: moderate to severe dysplasia– carcinoma in situ (CIN II-III)
Glandular cells
    Atypical and source
    Adenocarcinoma and source

There has been controversy among gynecologists and cytologists regarding this terminology, which lumps koilocytosis and CIN I into LGSIL and combines CIN II and III into the category of HGSIL. In this system koilocytosis and mild dysplasia are considered low-grade squamous intraepithelial lesions. However, based on the descriptions in the bottom of the box on p. 870, the clinician can request the descriptive terms of CIN or dysplasia–CIS, which are allowed as part of the Bethesda System reporting mechanism. The category of LGSIL (koilocytosis and CIN I) encompasses a large and less severely atypical category than CIN I alone. As noted by Syrjanen et al., the reduction of two grades of cytologic abnormality (LGSIL and HGSIL) leads to a loss of useful diagnostic information and can increase the risk of overtreatment for these conditions. The recent studies of Abadi et al. demonstrate that even using stringent morphologic criteria for koilocytosis, many smears did not in fact have evidence of HPV infection, which would lead to overdiagnosis of LGSIL.

The terms *atypical squamous cells of undetermined significance (ASCUS)* and *atypical glandular cells of undetermined significance (AGUS or AGCUS)* are controversial and cause diagnostic and management confusion. The categories were intended to indicate minor cytologic abnormalities not sufficiently severe to diagnose neoplasia. Despite over a decade of use of the Bethesda System in the United States, the interpretation and management of these categories is not clarified. Most patients with ASCUS smears will have spontaneous regression, as shown by the studies of Montz et al. Current guidelines with the Bethesda System indicate that the ASCUS reading should comprise no more than 3% to 5% of smears, but many centers experience higher numbers. As noted subsequently, those with an ASCUS diagnosis who are reliable for follow-up may have the smear repeated in 4 to 6 months. Some centers qualify the ASCUS diagnosis with a "rule out" modifier—that is, R/O HGSIL. In this case the patient usually undergoes triage by colposcopic evaluation. This was confirmed in the recent studies of Vlahos et al. who noted a higher percentage of biopsy-positive cases among those over age 35 years with ASCUS. Unfortunately the recent review of Smith et al. indicates that the diagnosis of ASCUS does not appear to be reproducible or accurate between observers. However, a new finding of ASCUS in a menopausal patient should lead to a consideration of a trial of vaginal estrogen therapy prior to repeating the smear. This topic is considered in detail further under "Management."

The category of AGUS or AGCUS is even less well defined. Some studies have shown that many patients with this diagnosis have inflammatory or other innocent cells that appear atypical but appear to have been detected because of the increased efficiency of the sampling of small brushes that are used in the endocervical canal (Figure 28-12). The rate of AGCUS has been reported to be from 0.2% to 0.46% in large studies by Kennedy et al. and Goff et al. comprising more than 80,000 smears from the referral centers of the Cleveland Clinic and Massachusetts General Hospital. Among these cases were 12 instances of invasive and/or in situ adenocarcinoma. Interestingly, squamous intraepithelial lesions were much more frequently noted in these patients. Recent efforts by Raab

et al. and Doss et al. have been directed to subdividing the AGCUS smears into categories of reactive or "favor benign" categories as opposed to those that "suggest neoplasia." These modifiers aid in the clinical management of ACGUS, as was also shown in the study of Veljovich et al. Once these divisions are made, premalignant or invasive lesions have been observed in about one third of the neoplastic category. A repeat of an AGCUS smear is appropriate particularly if a reactive process is favored. However, in the absence of extensive data, those with AGCUS favoring a neoplastic or high-grade lesion should have endocervical biopsy and colposcopy. Endometrial biopsy should also be done in older menopause patients. A conization may be needed to evaluate endocervical disease.

A particular problem in cytologic screening is the issue of false negatives. This area has been recently studied extensively by Schwartz et al. and Sherman et al. under the category of "rapidly progressing" cervical carcinoma. The cases studied by these authors and others are those in which invasive carcinoma or a high-grade lesion has been diagnosed in a patient who previously had a number of normal smears. Careful evaluation of these prior "negative" smears indicates that they most likely were false negative, that is, abnormal cells were present that were not detected. When one considers there are 300,000 to 500,000 cells on a normal smear and some slides contain fewer than 100 abnormal cells, it is perhaps not surprising that some false negatives do occur. An additional problem is inflammation obscuring the abnormal cells as well as the occasional problem of inadequate sampling. A technique of placing the cytologic sample in fluid and passing it through a millipore filter to produce a clear monolayer cellular preparation (ThinPrep, Cytyc Corp., Marlboro, Mass.) has also been introduced to try to facilitate more accurate readings and reduce unsatisfactory smears. New techniques, including molecular studies of probes that react with neoplastic cells, are being investigated as tools to improve morphologic diagnosis as well as computers using neural networks to automate the identification of abnormal cells.

CYTOLOGIC SCREENING GUIDELINES. The American College of Obstetricians and Gynecologists (ACOG) and the International Academy of Cytology recommend that cytologic screening start at age 18 or when the individual becomes sexually active and continue annually indefinitely. In addition, the development of cervical cancer has been reported to occur within 3 to 4 years after a negative Pap smear (see false-negative discussion above). Even after hysterectomy some risk for neoplasia remains. Stuart et al., in a study of 29 cases of vaginal cancer, noted a 5.7-year interval for diagnosis of cancer after hysterectomy when the operation was performed for CIN. When hysterectomy was performed for benign disease, the interval was 13.1 years. A retrospective study of women with cervical cancer by Shy et al. suggested an increased risk of cervical cancer if the screening interval exceeds 2 years. Conversely, Sawaya et al. studied a cohort of 128,805

TABLE 28-3
Recommendations on the Frequency of Pap Testing

	ACOG (1993)	American Cancer Society (1980)	Canadian Task Force (1982)	International Academy of Cytology (1980)	National Cancer Institute (1980)
Start	Age 18 or when sexually active	Age 20 or when sexually active	When sexually active	Age 18 or when sexually active	When sexually active
Age 18–35	Annually	Annually until two negative tests; then continue every 3 years	Annually if sexually active	—	After two negative tests, continue every 1–3 years
Age 36–60	Annually	At least every 3 years; more frequently if high risk; pelvic examination should be done annually after age 40	After two negative tests, continue every 5 years	Annually	Every 1–3 years
Over age 60	Annually	At least every 3 years; more frequently if high risk; pelvic examination should be done annually	After two negative tests, testing may be stopped	Annually	After two negative tests, testing may be stopped

women and found that following a normal smear result, the frequency of a future abnormal smear did not change if the screening interval was 1 or 2 or 3 years. Table 28-3 shows a composite of recommended intervals for Pap smear screening from various organizations. Patients treated for CIN should have annual cytology indefinitely.

An additional factor for the physician to consider is the importance of an annual pelvic examination, particularly for women over age 40, which allows for evaluation of ovarian size as well as breast examination and scheduling of mammography. In general, for women interested in an effective health maintenance program, an annual Pap smear and pelvic and physical examinations are indicated. For those who have had a hysterectomy for benign disease and in whom the ovaries remain, an annual pelvic examination should be done and some recommend vaginal cytology also be performed periodically, although the recent review by Fetters et al. suggests that such a policy will rarely yield a positive result.

A flowchart showing a scheme for evaluating the abnormal Pap smear is shown in the box on the opposite page. The techniques of colposcopy and biopsy are discussed subsequently.

Biopsy

Instruments useful for biopsy of the cervix are shown in Figure 28-13. The punch biopsy is capable of removing a small tissue sample 2 to 3 mm in size from the cervix. The colposcopically directed biopsy can easily be obtained in the office without anesthesia. An endocervical

curette is used to obtain an endocervical curettage (ECC) specimen. To obtain an adequate sample, the curette is introduced into the endocervix approximately 1 to 2 cm, and firm pressure is applied to obtain a sample from the four quadrants of the endocervix. This part of the procedure often causes discomfort to the patient, and the administration of an oral analgesic is occasionally helpful. Usually the examination can be completed without analgesia. The ECC specimens are grouped together in one container and submitted to pathology, since it is important to only ascertain whether neoplasia exists in the cervical canal. It is not feasible to identify which portion of the canal contains abnormal epithelium. Endocervical cytology with one of the previously described brushes appears to provide information that is equivalent to an ECC.

Colposcopy

The colposcope is a magnifying instrument used to identify those abnormal cervical areas that require biopsy. The pertinent area is the transformation zone, which may be either normal or abnormal. A normal transformation zone, as previously noted, is the junction of normal columnar epithelium and physiologic squamous metaplasia, while the abnormal transformation zone contains patterns that may indicate the presence of neoplastic tissue or a premalignant process.

Colposcopic examination is usually performed at a magnification of 10 to 16. After excess mucus is gently wiped away from the cervix and the Pap smear has

Evaluation of Abnormal Pap Smear

Reliable patient

ASCUS*   LGSIL*

Not reliable patient or HGSIL

Repeat smear in 4-6 months or triage (see text)   Repeat smear in 4-6 months or triage (see text)

Regress to normal   Progress   Regress to normal   Persist   Progress   Colpo.

Repeat yearly   Same as LGSIL or triage   Repeat yearly   Colpo.   Colpo.

Colposcopy

Colposcopic examination with
3% acetic acid and green filter

Satisfactory colposcopy
Limits of lesion seen and biopsied

and

ECC or cytology of endocervix negative

Therapy or follow-up as indicated

Unsatisfactory colposcopy
Limits of lesion not seen

or

ECC or cytology of endocervix positive

Conization or LEEP

*Possible alternative techniques being evaluated are HPV testing, cervicography, and others.
ECC, endocervical curettage.

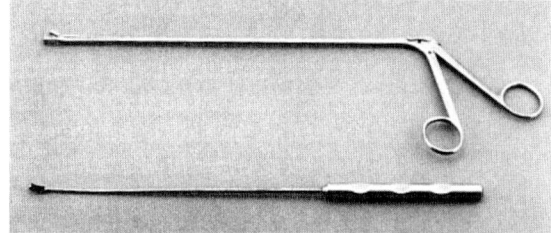

FIGURE 28-13 Cervical biopsy instruments. *Above,* Punch biopsy; *below,* endocervical curette.

been taken, 3% acetic acid is applied and the examination is often performed using a green filter. Normal columnar epithelium will often produce a grapelike pattern, while squamous metaplasia appears as a smooth, gray-white epithelium after the application of acetic acid (Figure 28-14). The native squamous epithelium outside the transformation zone has a smooth, red-tan appearance.

An abnormal transformation zone may be marked by white areas with red stippling (punctation), sharp-bordered lesions with vessels in a mosaic pattern (mosaic), white tissue with sharp borders (white epithelium), or atypical vessels. The white epithelium is seen best after acetic acid application and results from the piling up of cells with an increased nuclear-cytoplasmic ratio. A mosaic pattern results from neovascularization with capillaries running just beneath the surface epithelium, whereas punctation results from capillaries growing perpendicular to the surface. In addition, some areas may appear white before the application of acetic acid (leukoplakia).

High-grade intraepithelial lesions are usually found in large abnormal transformation zones, whereas small abnormal transformation zones are associated with low-grade lesions. A large abnormal transformation zone should heighten the examiner's suspicion of a high-grade lesion and possibly an invasive carcinoma. Similarly, atypical vessels usually indicate a high-grade intraepithelial lesion or invasive cancer.

An additional diagnostic criterion is the presence of *aceto-white epithelium.* This is tissue that initially looks normal but takes a white color after acetic acid is applied. Areas found outside the transformation zone frequently contain HPV infection (SPI, "flat warts," or "flat condyloma"). An example of intraepithelial neoplasia is shown

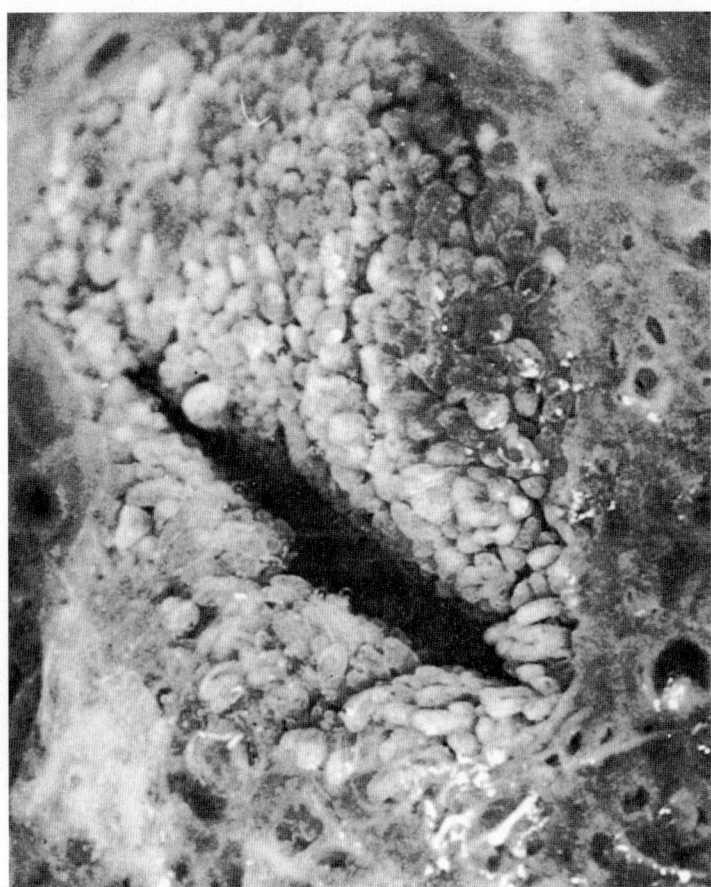

FIGURE 28-14 Typical transformation zone. The distal portion of columnar (grapelike) epithelium is replaced by a crescentic sheet of white metaplastic epithelium. At its inner edge it adjoins columnar epithelium. (From Coppleson M, Pixley E, and Reid B: Colposcopy—a scientific and practical approach to the cervix in health and disease, Springfield, Ill, 1971, Charles C Thomas, Publisher.)

in Figure 28-15, which demonstrates punctation and variably sized mosaic structures in the abnormal transformation zone. For a detailed description of the important colposcopic changes of the abnormal transformation zone and their interpretation, the reader should consult an atlas of colposcopy.

Only if the entire transformation zone can be seen colposcopically and if biopsies are obtained from the most abnormal areas is the examination considered technically satisfactory. If the transformation zone extends into the endocervical canal above the examiner's vision, the colposcopic examination is termed unsatisfactory, and diagnostic conization or Loop ElectroExcision Procedure (LEEP [see later discussion]) is performed. If the colposcopic examination is technically satisfactory, biopsy specimens are taken of the most abnormal areas. Before initiating outpatient therapy, an ECC is usually performed, even though the entire transformation zone can be seen. As already noted some consider a normal endocervical brush cytologic sample to indicate outpatient therapy may be undertaken. Others have advocated immediate LEEP to evaluate an abnormal smear. Such a "See and Treat"

approach is appropriate for women only who are multiparous and have cytologic evidence of a high-grade CIN III lesion. Holschneider et al. noted this technique was cost effective for those with HGSIL. The approach may also be appropriate for women who are in markedly underserved areas and are not likely to return for a follow-up evaluation or treatment, as was noted by Spitzer et al. The technique is also useful to consider for those with HIV infection and an abnormal smear, as noted in the studies of Del Priore et al. and Wright et al., particularly if the patient has a low CD4+ lymphocyte count. However, the widespread use of the procedure in low-risk patients to evaluate abnormal smears can lead both to complications and also to increased cost, as noted by Roland et al.

A scheme for the colposcopic evaluation of the abnormal Pap smear is shown in the box on p. 873. The biopsy results of the abnormal areas are compared with the results of the cytologic examination to verify that the tissue samples appear to be representative of the abnormal cells identified cytologically. Precise agreement between the cytologic and histologic diagnoses is not necessary and often does not occur. However, it is vital that an invasive

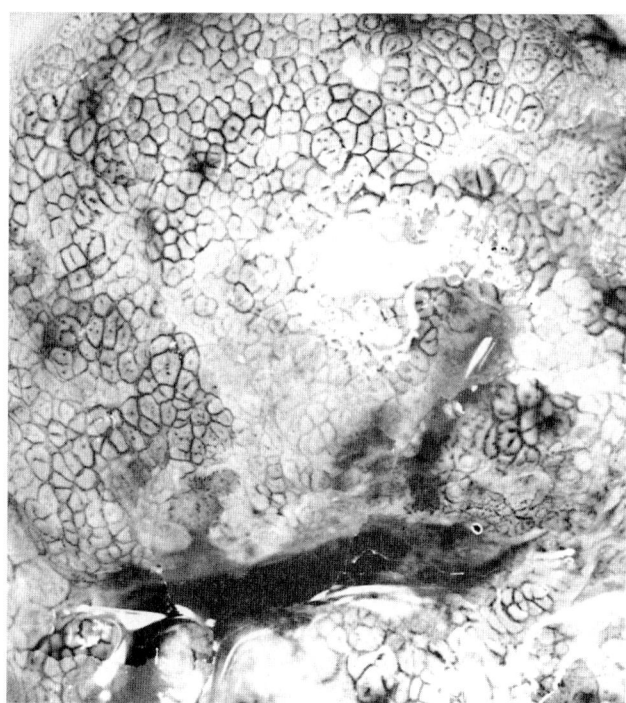

FIGURE 28-15 Extensive in situ carcinoma almost completely covers the visible part of ectocervix. The picture is dominated by coarse but regular mosaic vascular figures with greatly increased intercapillary distance. Atypical vessels are not to be seen. (×8.) (From Kolstad P and Stafl A: Atlas of colposcopy, Baltimore, 1972, University Park Press.)

carcinoma not be missed, and the degree of atypicality found cytologically must be adequately explained by the tissue obtained on biopsy.

MANAGEMENT

General Principles

If severe inflammation or infection is present, it should be treated as outlined in Chapter 22. If atypical squamous cells of undetermined significance (ASCUS) are diagnosed, it is often only necessary in a reliable patient to repeat the smear in 4 to 6 months unless a modifier of rule out HGSIL is present, which would lead to more immediate triage. Follow-up is appropriate for women who have koilocytosis and mild dysplasia (LGSIL). However, these "follow-up" guidelines, which are incorporated into the Interim Guidelines for the Bethesda System, are appropriate only for patients who are reliable. For those who are at high risk, such as patients with HIV infection or patients who will not adhere to a close follow-up protocol, colposcopy and biopsy are indicated (see subsequent discussion). The category of AGCUS is even less well understood. In reactive cases a repeat smear is indicated. If the cytologist indicates the likely presence of neoplasia, then further histologic evaluation is usually performed.

Papillomavirus Infection

If clinically evident condyloma are identified, therapy of the affected area is usually undertaken. It is clear most HPV infections regress spontaneously. If all women with HPV infection were treated to prevent neoplasia, most patients would be treated unnecessarily. Many have suggested that the male sexual partner should be evaluated and treated if condylomas are found. Krebs noted that two thirds of male partners of females with dysplasia or condyloma have HPV genital warts, which he treated with cryotherapy, laser, or 5-FU. However, in a follow-up study he noted that therapy of the male did not affect the rate of subsequent development of dysplasia in the female partner. Hippelainen et al., in extensive studies from Finland, noted a marked lack of concordance of HPV types between male and female partners and the finding in the female did not predict results in the male. Furthermore, only men with exophytic warts or clinical symptoms had any benefit from therapy. Those with asymptomatic HPV infection had a benign course. Their study suggested that condom use was protective only for those men who initially were HPV-negative. The futility of trying to treat subclinical papillomavirus infection (SPI) in the female was emphasized by the studies of Riva et al., who performed extensive CO_2 laser vaporization of the lower female genital tract in 25 women with confirmed SPI. Significant febrile and pain morbidity resulted, and 88% of the patients still had evidence of SPI at follow-up examination.

For condylomata involving the cervix and vagina, the laser is often employed. For those only on the cervix, either the laser or cryotherapy is used. Cautery with anesthesia can also be used for isolated vaginal or cervical condylomata. Local application of trichloroacetic acid has been tried (Chapter 22) but occasionally can cause excess tissue slough. It is important that the patient wash or douche 1 to 2 hours after its application to reduce normal tissue destruction. Therapy with interferon has also been utilized with some success reported (see Chapter 22).

Much research is in progress to stimulate the immunologic system in order to treat or prevent HPV infections. Two strategies being investigated include stimulating the immune system through the use of cytokines or adoptive immunotherapy by transferring sensitized cytotoxic T cells to the host (see Chapter 27). If successful, such therapy might prevent or possibly even treat malignant transformation resulting from HPV infection. As noted in a review by Hines et al., vaccination directed against HPV infection offers a different approach by providing a strategy to deal with the widespread population-based problem of HPV infection. In these cases, papillomavirus subunits and virions (a central nucleic acid core surrounded by a protein [capsid] envelope) are used to raise antibodies against HPV infection. The neutralizing antibodies are produced by B cells, and these have been produced in animal models by injection of papillomavirus subunits (conformational epitopes) that are found on the surface of virions (Figure 28-16). Using recombinant DNA technology, HPV-type specific antibodies have been developed. These vaccines would not lead to HPV infection in humans but would result in antibodies that theoretically offer a promising preventive tool.

HPV-DNA testing has been extensively studied as a tool for triaging women with abnormal Pap smears to try to decide which lesions are at higher risk for progression. A large-scale NIH trial—ASCUS/LGSIL Triage Study (ALTS Trial)—was set up to test the optimal method to manage these lesions. Over 5000 women were studied and were randomized to immediate colposcopy and biopsy if indicated, repeat Pap smear, and HPV testing with colposcopy for those who were positive for HPV oncogene types as measured in the Hybrid Capture II assay (Digene, Silver Springs, Md.). The first publication analyzed those with LGSIL and showed that almost 85% of these patients were positive for HPV, which meant that it could not separate those who needed immediate triage from those who could be followed.

The previously mentioned ALTS Trial also evaluated those with an ASCUS smear. Over 3500 women with an ASCUS smear were studied and randomized as noted above. Definitive results have not been published, but preliminary reports have indicated a higher sensitivity with over 95% of those found to have ASCUS and positive HPV are found on biopsy to have CIN II or III. However, there appears to be a high false-positive rate insofar as many patients with ASCUS and positive HPV tests did not have CIN II or III. ASCUS and HPV testing has also been studied by Manos et al. who evaluated 973 women with ASCUS. The sensitivity to detect a high-grade lesion was excellent (90%), but there were many false positives with a specificity of only 64%. HPV testing appears to be more accurate for those over age 30 years but as noted by Follen and Richards-Kortum, and Kaufman et al. there remain questions both regarding the specificity and technique and its cost effectiveness. Bergeron et al. also noted HPV testing for triage of ASCUS was compromised by low specificity. It does appear, however, that those who are HPV negative are at very low risk for cervical neoplasia, a potential useful aspect of this test, since as noted by Johnston, there is a strong long-term correlation between initial HPV infection and the eventual development of cervical neoplasia.

The general principle for treatment of cervical premalignant lesions is the eradication of the abnormal epithelium. In most instances, this can be accomplished by procedures completed in the physician's office. A number of modalities are available to destroy the abnormal tissue, which is usually a few millimeters thick. Deeper destruction is required if the crypt of the glands is involved, since the glands usually lie approximately 5 mm below the surface. The size and extent of the lesion are also factors influencing therapy. As previously noted, high-grade lesions are more extensive than low-grade lesions. Boonstra et al. studied the depth and extent of CIN III lesions in conization specimens. Of the lesions, 97.7% (mean, 2 standard deviation) had depth of crypt involvement less than 3.6 mm and extended linearly to the proximal border less than 19.3 mm from the cervical os. Moreover, similar to previous reports, younger patients had smaller transformation zones with a more ectocervical location. Also, in women over age 50, the depth of the crypt involvement increased significantly, indicating more extensive tissue destruction (if needed) for therapy of older patients.

Prior to performing outpatient ablative therapy (laser, cautery, cryotherapy), a colposcopic examination must be satisfactory and the entire transformation zone visualized and the endocervix by biopsy or brush technique found to be free of neoplastic cells. The biopsy results should provide appropriate consistency with the abnormal cells seen cytologically, as well as with the colposcopic appearance of the transformation zone. If the colposcopic examination is technically unsatisfactory, that is, the entire transformation zone cannot be seen, or if there is marked disparity

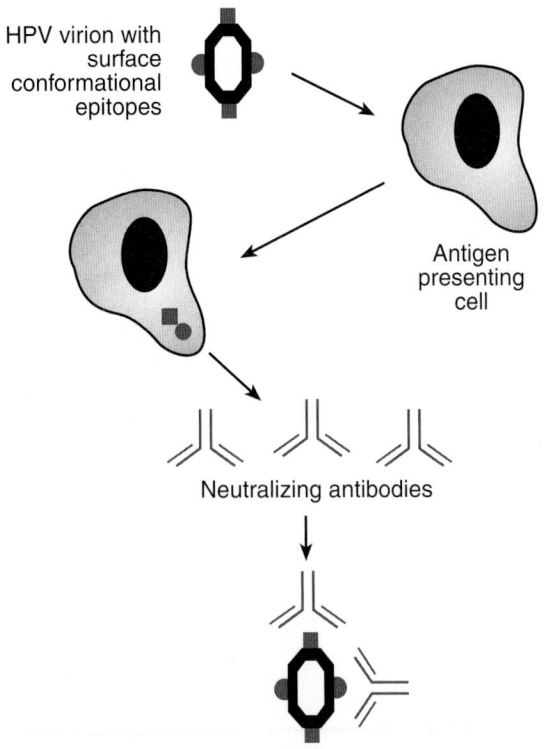

FIGURE 28-16 Antibody-mediated viral neutralization. Neutralizing, conformational isotopes are expressed on the surface of human papillomavirus (HPV) virions. The epitopes (antigens) are recognized by lymphocytes, and specific neutralizing antibodies are generated. These neutralizing antibodies bind specifically to surface epitopes and inhibit viral infection. (From Hines JF et al: Obstet Gynecol 86:860, 1995.)

between the cytology and biopsy results, excisional therapy (conization or LEEP) is indicated. Hysterectomy is considered only after it is ascertained that the patient does not have invasive cancer and no longer wishes to maintain childbearing function.

Therapy of Intraepithelial Neoplasia— Ablative Treatment

Cryotherapy

Cryotherapy is accomplished by a freezing process that results from rapid expansion of fluid, usually carbon dioxide or nitrous oxide, into a probe (Figure 28-17), which is placed against the cervix. The probe chosen depends on the size of the lesion to be treated, but the flat probes are most commonly used, particularly since probes with long endocervical nipples can cause extensive destruction of the endocervix with resulting cervical stenosis. The contact with the cervix is enhanced by putting water-soluble lubricating jelly on the tip of the probe. While cryotherapy can be used in other areas, such as the vulva, local anesthesia is usually required, but no anesthesia is required for cervical treatment. It is important that the ice ball extend 4 to 5 mm beyond the edge of the lesion to ensure adequate freezing and destruction of abnormal epithelium. Usually a second freeze is carried out, particularly with large lesions and when more extensive tissue necrosis is desired (double-freeze technique). It is sometimes necessary to reapply the probe to a different area to treat larger areas of CIN adequately. For CIN III lesions, Boonstra et al. noted failures at the 3 and 9 o'clock positions, presumably because of increased vascularity from cervical vessels, if the freeze lasted less than 5 minutes. Initial cure rates approximate 90% and averaged 89% for 4549 patients summarized from the literature in a review by Charles and Savage. Andersen and Husth noted a 91% cure with CIN II but only 78% for CIN III.

After initial cryotherapy a follow-up examination is carried out in 4 months. Further evaluation is in accordance with the guidelines discussed for all cervical neoplasia. It is recommended that ECC or endocervical brush cytology be performed at least once after freezing to be certain there is no disease in the canal.

Possible complications in addition to recurrence of neoplasia include infertility and cervical stenosis. Although both have been reported, there is no clear evidence of an increased risk of these adverse outcomes in patients treated with cryotherapy. Recurrent treatments or extensive therapy of the endocervical canal does appear to increase the risk because of the more extensive destruction of the normal endocervix.

Laser Therapy

The laser has been widely used in conjunction with the colposcope. The energy from the laser beam is absorbed by water with resultant vaporization of the target tissue. The laser beam is controlled by a small "joystick," and the spot size of the laser can be varied but is usually less than 1 mm. Different degrees of power are available, and for therapy of intraepithelial neoplasia approximately 25 to 35 watts are utilized. Most reports express the treatment mode as a power density, that is, watts per square centimeter. Because therapy results in tissue vaporization, the resultant smoke must be evacuated with vacuum suction; thus a speculum with a smoke evacuator is used. Graduated millimeter probes can be used to gauge the depth of the laser crater.

Usually therapy is carried to a depth of 5 to 7 mm and a power density of over 600 W/cm^2. The treatment is more effective at higher power densities. However, the complications of pain and bleeding are also related to the power density and depth of treatment. If bleeding occurs during therapy, it can easily be controlled by coagulating the site by defocusing the laser beam and using a lower power density. Healing in the laser crater is usually complete in 4 to 6 weeks, and an advantage of the laser is that the transformation zone is likely to remain visible colposcopically. However, the technique is used less frequently than other ablative and excisional techniques in part due to the cost of laser equipment in comparison to other modalities.

Cautery

Electrocautery was the mainstay of outpatient therapy of CIN before the advent of cryosurgery, laser therapy, and the LEEP procedure (see subsequent discussion). The treatment can be accomplished with a hot wire unit generating heat to the cervix or an electrodiathermy unit, which requires current to be passed through the tissues and electrical grounding of the patient. The treatment is carried out with sufficient depth to destroy cervical glands. An electrocautery unit is less expensive than the laser and appears able to yield comparable therapy results to cryosurgery but is infrequently used today.

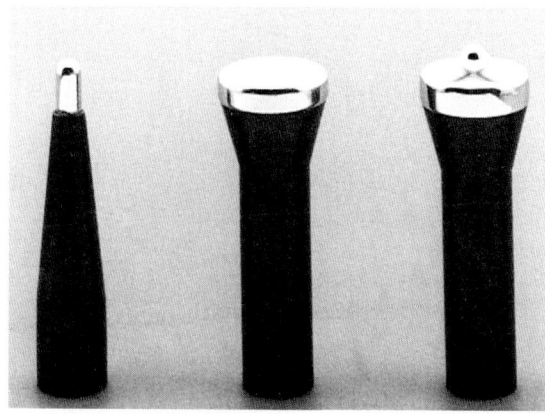

FIGURE 28-17 Three varieties of cryotherapy probes.

Summary of Ablative Management

Ablative therapy of intraepithelial neoplasia depends on adequate destruction of all abnormal tissues. The transformation zone should be completely visualized colposcopically with no neoplasia in the endocervical canal, and the treatment should be carried out to a depth to reach the cervical crypts. It should also extend a few millimeters beyond the transformation zone to include normal-appearing tissue. Many authors have reported increased failure rates with high-grade lesions and carcinoma in situ with cryotherapy, but this is partly because these high-grade lesions cover larger areas of the cervix and extend more deeply into the cervical crypts. Overall success rates approximate 90%. Ferenczy noted that lesions smaller than 3 cm could be equivalently treated by cryosurgery or laser but that larger lesions or those that extended up to 5 mm into the cervical canal fared better with laser treatment. Larger lesions, particularly those that extend onto the vagina, are treated usually with the laser or by operative excision.

Mitchell et al. did a randomized trial of cryotherapy, laser vaporization, and loop electrosurgical excision (LEEP—see next section) for treatment of SIL (CIN). In the trial 390 patients were studied and all three modalities were comparably effective in successful treatment. Patients over age 30 years and those with larger transformation zones or history of prior therapy were more likely to have a recurrence.

Excisional Therapy

Conization

Conization of the cervix is performed if the colposcopic examination is unsatisfactory, if there is uncertainty regarding the presence of invasive disease, if there is neoplasm in the endocervix, or if the cells seen on cytologic examination are not adequately explained by the biopsy specimens. If the biopsy suggests the possibility of microinvasion or if invasion is suspected but cannot be confirmed, conization is mandatory because the proper diagnosis of microinvasion cannot be made from a biopsy specimen. Excisional therapy is also carried out when childbearing function is to be maintained or when a patient prefers therapy less extensive than hysterectomy and is willing to adhere to a strict protocol for follow-up.

Conization may also be needed to evaluate abnormal endocervical glandular cells. Widrich et al. noted that cold knife conization is superior to LEEP in terms of improved negative margins. In addition there was less recurrence of adenocarcinoma in situ with cold knife conization. In evaluating adenocarcinoma in situ, the risk of residual disease and/or invasion is high if the margins of the cone are positive, as noted by Wolf et al.

TECHNIQUE—COLD KNIFE CONE.   The extent of the transformation zone on the exocervix is outlined by use of the colposcope. In addition, it is advisable to stain the cervix with iodine (Lugol's or Schiller's solution) to outline the limits of the resection margin of the cone. The degree to

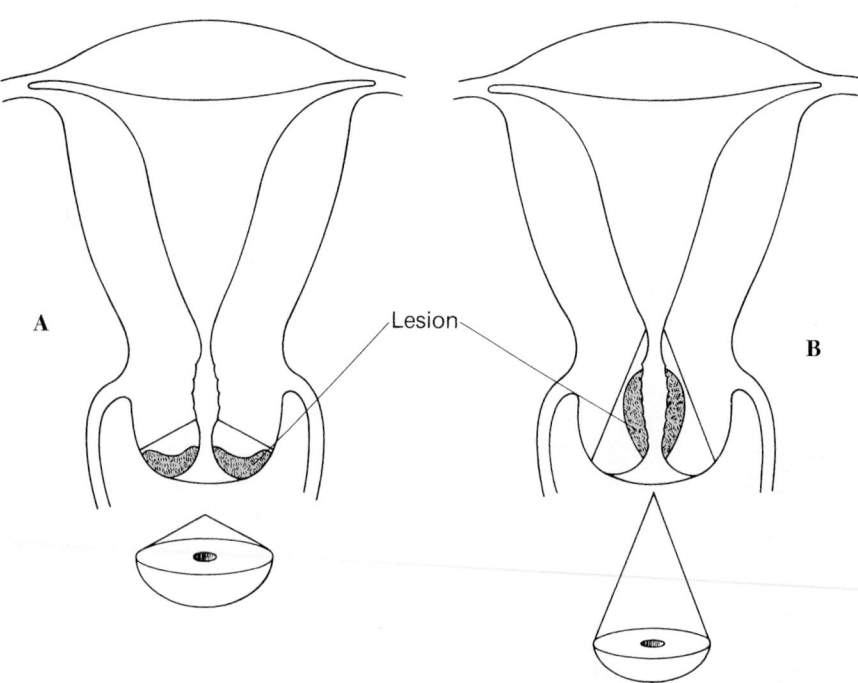

FIGURE 28-18   **A,** Cone biopsy for CIN of exocervix. Limits of lesion were identified colposcopically. **B,** Cone biopsy for endocervical disease. Limits of lesions were not seen colposcopically. (Redrawn from DiSaia PJ and Creasman WT: Clinical gynecologic oncology, St Louis, 1984, Mosby–Year Book, Inc.)

which the cone extends into the endocervical canal depends on the extent of the transformation zone. If the upper limits cannot be seen in the endocervical canal or the ECC results are positive, the operation is adjusted so as to place the apex of the cone higher in the canal than in instances where the upper part of the transformation zone can be visualized, as illustrated in Figure 28-18.

The procedure can be done with a scalpel (cold knife cone). One useful technique uses dilute vasopressin (10 IU in 100 ml sterile saline), which is injected into the stroma of the cervix to reduce bleeding. The endocervical canal is sounded and the cone cut so as to keep the apex below the internal os. The posterior part of the cone (3 to 9 o'clock) is usually cut first so any bleeding does not obscure the operative field. The upper margin of the cone is usually dissected free with scissors, and the 12 o'clock position of the cone identified for the pathologists with a suture. An ECC is performed after the completion of the conization, and, if indicated, uterine curettage is done. If the postconization ECC is positive, residual disease is likely to be present. Usually the cone bed is repaired with a running or running-locked vicryl suture, and in the experience of the author blood loss is negligible with this technique. Cauterization of the bed is undertaken by many therapists, but this adds to destruction of the endocervical glands and possibly increases the risk of subsequent infertility. The author prefers to utilize Surgicel in the cone bed after the vicryl suture is completed. So-called Sturmdorf hemostatic sutures turn the edge of the cervix into the canal. They should never be used as they may bury abnormal cervical epithelium and also interfere with future colposcopic follow-up examination. It is advisable to sound the cervix a few weeks after the procedure to help avoid stenosis.

LASER CONIZATION. The laser has also been used frequently to perform conization. However, excessive burn artifacts have been reported, and the use of loop diatheramy (see subsequent discussion) has become much more common. Thus laser cones are not usually performed.

LOOP ELECTROEXCISION PROCEDURE (LEEP). This technique involves the use of an electrosurgical unit with both cutting and coagulation currents. It has been termed LEEP (loop electrosurgical excision procedure) or LLETZ (large loop excision of the transformation zone). Various-sized loops and cautery tips (Figure 28-19) can be used to excise the abnormal epithelium after colposcopy is completed. The cervix is usually infiltrated with dilute vasopressin and local anesthetic at a location "every two hours" around the os. A combination loop is used that blends both cutting and cautery energies. The depth of the excision is regulated with some loops (Figure 28-19) by setting the crossbar at the base of the electrode. The loop is gently passed across the cervix, excising the transformation zone. A smaller biopsy can be taken with a small loop if desired. The entire excision procedure can be accomplished in a few minutes, and any bleeding from the cervical base is usually coagulated or treated with Monsel's (ferrous subsulfate) solution.

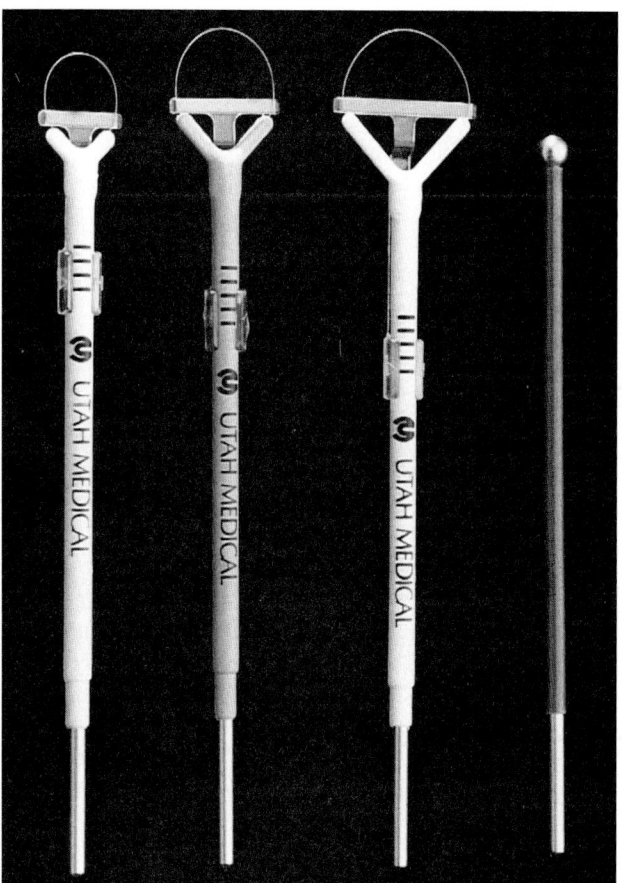

FIGURE 28-19 Examples of electrodes (Utah Medical Corp., Midvale, Utah) used for a LEEP procedure. The width of the excised tissue specimens can range from 1.0 to 2.0 cm, and the specimen depth can be adjusted by sliding the guard attached to the electrode shaft. Following excision the base of the cervix is often gently cauterized with a ball electrode. (Courtesy Steven E. Waggoner, M.D., The University of Chicago.)

COMPLICATIONS AND COMPARISON OF EXCISIONAL THERAPY. Bleeding is the major short-term complication of conization and LEEP. Long-term complications that have been of concern include cervical stenosis, infertility, loss of cervical mucus, and an increase in adverse pregnancy outcome (incompetent cervix). Definitive data are not available concerning the degree of risk of these adverse outcomes, but they are thought to be related in part to the degree to which the endocervical glands are removed. Buller and Jones evaluated infertility and pregnancy outcome in 166 patients following conization and found no evidence of an increased rate of infertility or alteration of pregnancy outcome as a complication of the operation. In contrast, a case-control study from England of 66 matched patients found a statistically significant association between conization and preterm delivery (17% versus 3%) and the risk of pregnancy loss was even more frequent among their patients with second pregnancies. Bigrigg et al. evaluated LLETZ in 330 women with 3 to 4 years follow-up and found their rates of fertility and menstrual patterns were not significantly different from a group of matched controls. Unfortunately, their study size was such that it was only possible to detect a threefold difference in infertility rates. Similar results were shown by Ferenczy et al., who noted no effects, and they advise limiting the cone to a maximum depth of 1.5 cm and a diameter of 1.8 cm. Kristensen et al. evaluated 170 Danish women who had been treated with conization and found the procedure significantly increased the risk of subsequent preterm birth and this increase in prematurity post cone was also noted in the study of El-Bastawissi et al. It appears excisional procedures may lead to infertility and preterm delivery but the risks are small, particularly in patients with excisional specimens that do not remove large portions of the cervix. It is, however, a cost-effective technique for the management of CIN.

FOLLOW-UP. If the margin of the excision specimen is free of neoplastic epithelium, the patient still requires long-term follow-up, since new lesions can develop. If the margins of the cone specimen are involved with neoplasia, the patient can be considered for further treatment with hysterectomy, since there is an increased risk of failure in these cases. However, many patients with "positive" margins are found to have no residual disease at subsequent hysterectomy.

At the time of 5-year follow-up examination, Ahlgren et al. noted 98% cure rates if the margin of the cervical conization was free, while the rate fell to 70% for those with positive margins. Kolstad and Klem followed 1128 patients for 15 to 25 years. Twenty-five of their patients had conization margins involved with neoplastic disease, and four of them eventually developed recurrence, some as long as 6 years after therapy. However, the remaining 21 were free of disease up to 15 years. These data emphasize that it is *not* always mandatory to perform hysterectomy if the margins of the cone are involved with CIN. This is particularly true if the ectocervical margins are involved, since subsequent outpatient ablative therapy can usually eradicate any residual CIN at this site. In the patient desiring to preserve childbearing function, careful cytologic and colposcopic follow-up are reasonable options.

It has been customary to perform the hysterectomy within 48 hours of conization or to wait more than 6 weeks to reduce the risk of postoperative infection at the time of the hysterectomy. Webb and Symmonds, as well as others, suggest that it is not always necessary to operate within these intervals. It is thought to be advisable to prescribe prophylactic antibiotics, such as a cephalosporin, during the hysterectomy to reduce infections. However, in most cases a 6-week delay is reasonable.

Kolstad and Klem also noted that conization and hysterectomy were approximately equivalent in their effectiveness in treating carcinoma in situ. Conization was done in 795 patients, and with 5 to 25 years of follow-up, recurrences of carcinoma in situ occurred in 2.3%, whereas invasive cancer occurred in 0.9% (seven patients). For the 238 patients treated by hysterectomy, recurrence of carcinoma in situ occurred in 1.2% and invasive cancer in 2.1%. The recurrent carcinoma in situ or invasive cancer developed up to 10 years after primary treatment. These data indicate that conization is approximately as effective as hysterectomy for treatment of carcinoma in situ, particularly if the surgical margins are free. However, long-term follow-up is mandatory because of the risk of subsequent development of neoplasia. It should be emphasized that good results presented for conization are partly due to adequate pretherapy colposcopic evaluation.

Because of the apparent increased risk of invasive disease in older patients, Killackey et al. recommend that all patients over age 50 with a biopsy diagnosis of carcinoma in situ undergo conization to rule out invasive disease. In their series, 3 of 16 patients (19%) so treated were found to have unsuspected invasive carcinoma despite adequate colposcopic evaluation with cytology and negative ECC results.

Hysterectomy

Simple total hysterectomy is performed for treatment of CIN if childbearing function is not to be preserved and if there is no evidence of invasive disease (Chapter 29 discusses invasive carcinoma). The need to perform hysterectomy following excision therapy must be individualized depending on the clinicopathologic circumstances, including the patient's willingness to be followed and desire to preserve childbearing function. A vaginal hysterectomy is usually performed, or if the abdominal route is chosen, a class I hysterectomy (as described in Chapter 29) is done. Many patients, particularly those with normal-sized uteri in whom ovarian removal is desired, are candidates for laparoscopically assisted vaginal hysterectomy (LAVH). If the vagina is involved with neoplasia, it is important to extend the surgical margins to include the abnormal vaginal tissue. Follow-up is required after hysterectomy, since the patient is at risk for the development of lower genital tract intraepithelial neoplasia years later.

ABNORMAL PAP SMEAR IN PREGNANCY

When an abnormal Pap smear is discovered initially in a pregnant patient, evaluation is more complicated than in the nonpregnant patient because of the increased vascularity of the cervix, the presence of the fetus, and morphologic changes (edema, decidual reaction, etc.) in the cervix that develop as pregnancy progresses. Evaluation in the pregnant patient is best performed by physicians with extensive colposcopic experience. CIN is not treated during pregnancy; therapy is postponed until the postpartum period. The prime objective in the pregnant patient with an abnormal Pap smear is to rule out invasive carcinoma.

Years ago DePetrillo et al. introduced a scheme for the evaluation of the abnormal Pap smear during pregnancy utilizing colposcopy. A modified plan is shown in Figure 28-20. Insofar as the cervix everts during pregnancy, the squamocolumnar junction is more easily visible for evaluation. This circumstance also lessens the need for an ECC, which increases the risk of interrupting the pregnancy. A gentle brush sampling of the endocervix for cytologic evaluation is preferable, with care taken not to go high into the canal. When a patient has abnormal cytologic findings during pregnancy and the colposcopic examination is within normal limits, these examinations are periodically repeated, usually every trimester depend-

ing upon the severity of the lesion. If there is neither evidence of neoplasia nor indication of a lesion requiring biopsy, the patient is followed and evaluated postpartum. If the colposcopic examination is abnormal, a biopsy is usually taken of the most abnormal area to confirm the cytologic and colposcopic findings, and the examination (including Pap smear) and colposcopy are repeated periodically until the patient delivers. Then definitive evaluation is performed in the postpartum period. A major problem arises if the patient has an undetected invasive lesion. In all circumstances a directed biopsy is needed, and then the management is carried out as outlined in Figure 28-20, B.

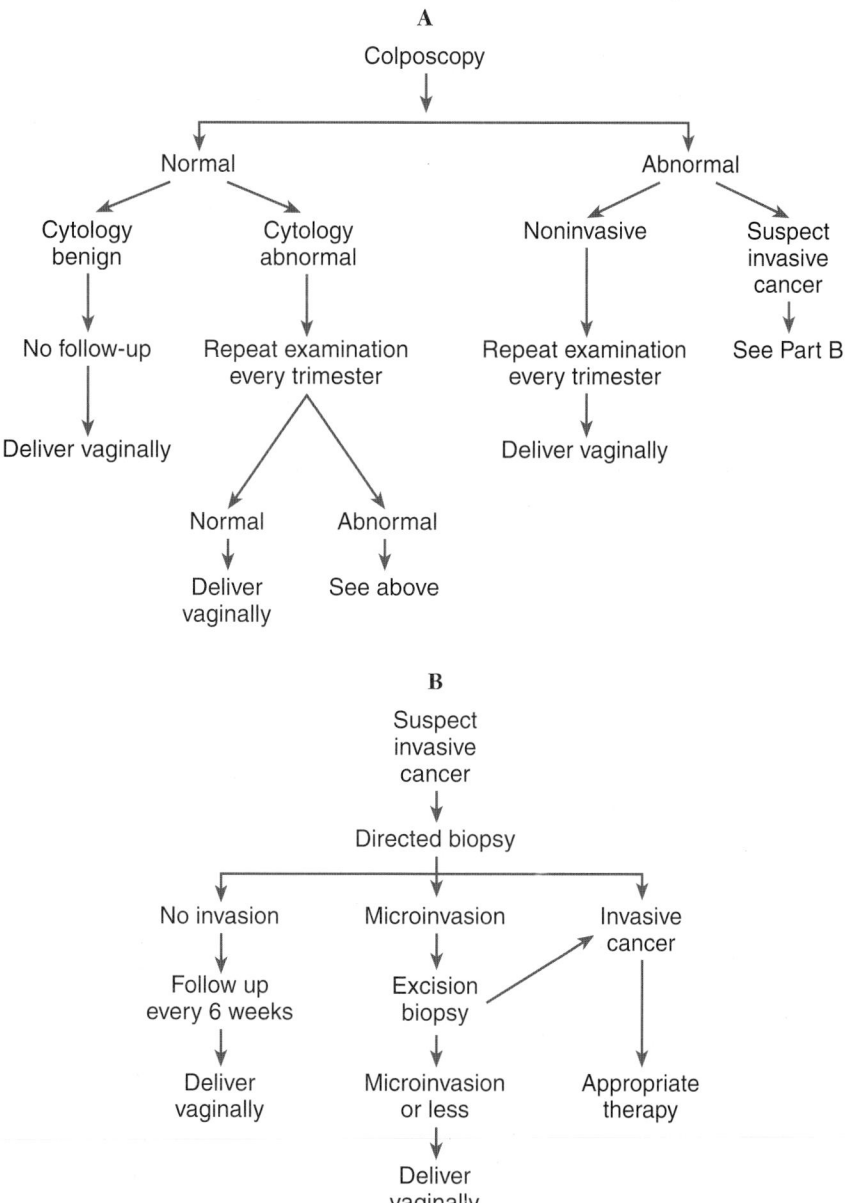

FIGURE 28-20   Scheme for evaluation of abnormal Pap smear during pregnancy utilizing colposcopy. **A,** Screening evaluation of abnormal Pap smear in pregnancy. **B,** Schematic of evaluation when an invasive lesion is suspected. (Modified from DePetrillo AD, Townsend DE, Morrow CP, et al: Am J Obstet Gynecol 121:441, 1975.)

In a study of 401 pregnant patients, Benedet et al. noted that the antepartum colposcopic impression was within one degree of the postpartum diagnosis in 87% of the women. Of the nine invasive cancers, five were found in 83 patients over age 30 (6%), in contrast to 3 of 318 patients (1%) under age 30, indicating a greater risk in older patients.

If microinvasion is suspected, either conization or excision of the abnormal area may be carried out but only to rule out invasive carcinoma. It is preferable to evaluate the patient in the postpartum period unless invasive cancer is present. If invasive cancer is discovered, management is carried out in accordance with the guidelines in Chapter 29. Wedge resection or conization is needed if there is cytologic suspicion of invasion not explained by colposcopically directed biopsy or if the colposcopic pattern suggests invasion but the biopsy did not confirm its presence. The conization (or wedge resection of the poorly visualized or colposcopically abnormal area) in the pregnant patient is usually less extensive than that in the nonpregnant patient. Conization should be avoided because of the risk of blood loss and the potential of disturbing the pregnancy.

DePetrillo et al. evaluated 300 pregnant patients with abnormal cytologic smears and found it necessary to perform conization only on three. Hannigan et al. summarized the literature on the treatment of 448 patients by conization during pregnancy and noted that approximately 9% had serious blood loss (more than 500 ml) and required blood transfusion. In their summary pregnancy losses did not appear to be increased for women who underwent conization. The authors noted that their data did not substantiate the need to perform conization in the second trimester, as generally practiced.

There are studies to suggest that CIN has higher regression rates when detected in pregnant women than in nonpregnant individuals. The precise reason for this is not known, but two explanations are generally offered: (1) the low-grade intraepithelial changes, particularly those with mild dysplasia recorded during pregnancy, may represent cytologic changes that occur as a consequence of pregnancy itself, and (2) intraepithelial lesions may be removed during the trauma of vaginal delivery. Ahdoot et al. reported higher CIN regression rates for women delivered vaginally. Yost et al. showed that most lesions in their study regressed postpartum but the regression was not affected by the method of delivery.

LONG-TERM FOLLOW-UP

After treatment for CIN a patient requires long-term follow-up. As has been previously discussed, the recurrence of intraepithelial neoplasia in the cervix, vagina, or vulva can take place many years after treatment. The risk of development of neoplasia is also small (about 3%) but is ever present. Generally the initial screening examination is performed in 3 to 4 months and usually repeated in 6 months. For low-grade lesions, two negative consecutive examinations are sufficient and such a patient is then placed on a schedule of annual follow-up. For those treated for a high-grade lesion, three negative follow-up smears are often advised before returning to annual follow-up. Hatch et al., in a follow-up study of intraepithelial neoplasia with cryotherapy, noted that 90% of their failures were detected in the first two examinations. In their study the failure rate was highest in the CIN III group, emphasizing the importance of more intensive and prolonged follow-up for high-grade lesions. Chew et al., in a study of 2130 patients, noted lesions detected even after 10 years of follow-up after initial therapy.

The posttherapy evaluation includes both cytology and colposcopy. If the initial lesion occupied the endocervical canal, many therapists advise a routine ECC as part of the initial posttherapy evaluation. The use of an endocervical brush improves the detection of abnormal endocervical cells. However, biopsies are usually performed only when indicated as a result of the cytologic and colposcopic examinations, and after initial posttherapy evaluation cytologic follow-up is sufficient with colposcopic evaluation if an abnormal smear develops.

KEY POINTS

- Intraepithelial neoplasia is a spectrum of premalignant changes in the epithelium of the cervix that histologically show varying degrees of cellular atypia. Numerous terms are used to describe the severity of the atypias, but there is no clearly defined boundary between them.

- During reproductive life the squamocolumnar junction is usually on the portio of the cervix near the external os. It may be found farther away from the os during and after pregnancy and usually recedes into the endocervical canal after menopause.

- Pap smear (cytology) screening appears to have decreased the frequency of invasive carcinoma of the cervix by 50% in the past 25 years.

- Many cases of cervical intraepithelial neoplasia (CIN) do not progress. Some particularly low-grade lesions spontaneously regress, but all have the potential for progression to malignancy.

- The risk of progression for CIN I (mild dysplasia—LGSIL) to a higher grade lesion is approximately 16%.

- High-grade lesions (carcinoma in situ [CIN III]—HGSIL) are at greater risk for malignant progression and usually are found in larger abnormal transformation zones.

- Malignant progression risk is greatest for CIN III, least for CIN I, and intermediate for CIN II.

- Carcinoma in situ with gland involvement is treated the same as carcinoma in situ without gland involvement.

- The precise cause of CIN is not known but appears to be associated with sexual activity and HPV infection.

- Females with multiple sex partners are at increased risk for CIN, and males with multiple sex partners increase the risk of neoplasia for a female sex partner.

- Cigarette smoking increases the risk of CIN. Increased levels of vitamins A and E may decrease the risk.

- Prolonged oral contraceptive use (more than 5 years) is associated with an increased frequency of cervical neoplasia.

- Human papillomavirus (HPV) infection is associated with an increased risk of CIN. HPV types 16, 18, 31, 33, 35, 39, 45, 51, 52, 56, 58, 59, and 68 are considered oncogenic.

- Immunosuppressed patients are at an increased risk for genital HPV infection and CIN. HIV-infected individuals have the highest risk when CD4 counts drop below 200.

- HPV infection can progress to CIN. However, HPV infections also spontaneously regress, usually within 2 years. The prevalence drops among older patients, with a sharp drop after age 30, presumably in part due to host response and immunologic clearance of HPV.

- Patients without HPV infection usually do not develop CIN.

- The false negative rate for properly performed cytology smears is approximately 5% to 20%.

- "Rapidly progressing" cervical carcinoma appears primarily due to false-negative smears rather than to a true rapid progression from normal to malignant epithelium.

- Abnormal cells on Pap smears occur with increasing frequency in those receiving chemotherapy and in patients with lupus erythematosus.

- The colposcope is used to evaluate the cervix if an abnormal Pap smear is present. Usually multiple biopsy specimens of an abnormal transformation zone are needed for an adequate evaluation.

- Colposcopic and cytologic findings do not establish a diagnosis; biopsy is necessary.

- The endocervix should be free of neoplastic cells prior to undertaking outpatient ablative therapy for CIN. In addition, the entire transformation zone must be seen, and the evaluation must be adequate to rule out the presence of invasive carcinoma.

- The crypts of the endocervical glands are located as deep as 5 mm beneath the surface.

- Atypical cells seen on the biopsy specimen should be of similar magnitude (within one degree) of abnormality as those seen on cytologic smears before therapy is begun. If there is a major discrepancy, a conization should be performed.

- Therapy of all HPV infections would result in treatment of many women to try to prevent a few cases of invasive carcinoma of the cervix.

- An excisional procedure (LEEP or cone) of the cervix should be performed if colposcopy is unsatisfactory, if the biopsy results do not explain the cytologic findings, if the ECC sample has neoplastic cells, or if there is suspicion of invasive or microinvasive disease.

- The diagnosis of microinvasion requires a conization specimen.

- Conization is usually performed for therapy of carcinoma in situ if childbearing function is to be preserved.

- Cold knife conization is preferable to LEEP in evaluation of endocervical adenocarcinoma in situ. If the cone margins are positive in this disease, the risk of recurrence and possibly invasive adenocarcinoma markedly increases.

- Young patients with CIN tend to have smaller transformation zones with an ectocervical location when compared with older patients, who have larger areas of neoplasia and more cervical crypt involvement.

- The goal of treatment in CIN is eradication of all abnormal tissue.

- Laser therapy, cryotherapy, and electrocautery have been reported to have equivalent results and lead to eradication of the lesions in about 90% of the patients with carcinoma in situ after initial therapy.

- Cervical stenosis, infertility, and premature birth may result from excisional therapy of CIN if large areas of the endocervix are destroyed. Limiting the cone or LEEP height to less than 1.5 to 2.0 cm decreases this risk.

- Conization for the therapy of CIN is as effective as hysterectomy, especially if the margins are free of disease.

- Immediate LEEP is an effective method to triage and treat HGSIL, particularly in a parous patient and in those with reduced access to health care.

- Simple total hysterectomy is not always necessary if the margins of the conization specimen contain neoplastic tissue, especially low-grade lesions.

- Hysterectomy may be performed for therapy of CIN if childbearing function is not to be preserved and there is no evidence of invasive disease.

- Evaluation of the abnormal Pap smear in pregnancy is conducted primarily to rule out the presence of invasive carcinoma. CIN is evaluated and treated in the postpartum period.

- Some CIN lesions discovered during pregnancy spontaneously regress postpartum.

- When two consecutive examinations on patients with low-grade lesions or three consecutive examinations on patients with high-grade lesions are negative, annual follow-up is instituted and continued indefinitely.

- The risk of long-term development (up to 10 years) of intraepithelial neoplasia following initial therapy is about 3%.

- Most short-term recurrences of intraepithelial neoplasia occur within 1 to 2 years after initial treatment.

- Patients treated for CIN should have annual cytology indefinitely.

BIBLIOGRAPHY

Abadi MA, Ho GYF, Burk RD, et al: Stringent criteria for histological diagnosis of koilocytosis fail to eliminate overdiagnosis of human papillomavirus infection and cervical intraepithelial neoplasia grade 1, Human Pathol 29:54, 1998.

Ahdoot D, van Nostrand KM, Nguyen NJ, et al: The effect of route of delivery on regression of abnormal cervical findings in the postpartum period, Am J Obstet Gynecol 178:1116, 1998.

Ahlgren M, Ingemarsson I, Lindberg LG, et al: Conization as treatment of carcinoma in situ of the uterine cervix, Obstet Gynecol 46:135, 1975.

Andersen ES and Husth M: Cryosurgery for cervical intraepithelial neoplasia: 10-year follow-up, Gynecol Oncol 40:240, 1992.

Benedet JL, Selke PA, and Nickerson KG: Colposcopic evaluation of abnormal Papanicolaou smears in pregnancy, Am J Obstet Gynecol 157:932, 1987.

Beral V, Hannaford P, and Kay C: Oral contraceptive use and malignancies of the genital tract, Lancet 2(8624):1331, 1988.

Bergeron C, Jeannel D, Poveda J-D, et al: Human papillomavirus testing in women with mild cytologic atypia, Obstet Gynecol 95:821, 2000.

Bigrigg A, Haffenden DK, Sheehan AL, et al: Efficacy and safety of large-loop excision of the transformation zone, Lancet 343:32, 1994.

Blumenfield Z, Lorber M, Yoffe N, and Scharf Y: Systemic lupus erythematosus: predisposition for uterine cervical dysplasia, Lupus 3:59, 1994.

Boonstra H, Aalders JG, Koudstaal J, et al: Minimum extension and appropriate topographic position of tissue destruction for treatment of cervical intraepithelial neoplasia, Obstet Gynecol 75:227, 1990.

Boonstra H, Koudstaal J, Oosterhuis JW, et al: Analysis of cryolesions in the uterine cervix: application techniques, extension, and failures, Obstet Gynecol 75:232, 1990.

Bosch FX, Manos MM, Munoz N, et al: Prevalence of human

papillomavirus in cervical cancer, J Natl Cancer Inst 87:796, 1995.

Buller RE and Jones HW: Pregnancy following cervical conization, Am J Obstet Gynecol 142:506, 1982.

Burghardt E and Ostor AG: Site and origin of squamous cervical cancer: a histomorphologic study, Obstet Gynecol 62:117, 1983.

Chew GK, Jandial L, Paraskevaidis E, et al: Pattern of CIN recurrence following laser ablation treatment: long-term follow-up, Int J Gynecol Cancer 9:487, 1999.

Cox JT, Lorincz AT, Schiffman MH, et al: Human papillomavirus testing by hybrid capture appears to be useful in triaging women with a cytologic diagnosis of atypical squamous cells of undetermined significance, Am J Obstet Gynecol 172:946, 1995.

Cramer DW: The role of cervical cytology in declining morbidity and mortality of cervical cancer, Cancer 34:2018, 1974.

Del Priore GD, Maag T, Bhattacharya M, et al: The value of cervical cytology in HIV-infected women, Gynecol Oncol 56:395, 1995.

DeMay RM: The pap smear. In The art and science of cytopathology, Chicago, 1996, ASCP Press.

DePetrillo AD, Townsend DE, Morrow CP, et al: Colposcopic evaluation of the abnormal Papanicolaou test in pregnancy, Am J Obstet Gynecol 121:441, 1975.

DeVilliers EM, Wagner D, Schneider A, et al: Human papillomavirus DNA in women without and with cytological abnormalities: results of a 5-year follow-up study, Gynecol Oncol 44:33, 1992.

Doss BJ, Montag AG, Schrader T, and DeMay RM: The significance of atypical glandular cells of undetermined significance, Mod Pathol, 1996. In press.

El-Bastawissi AY, Becker TM, Daling JR: Effect of cervical carcinoma in situ and its management on pregnancy outcome, Obstet Gynecol 93:207, 1999.

Ellerbrock TV, Chaisson MA, Bush TJ, et al: Incidence of cervical squamous intraepithelial lesions in HIV-infected women, JAMA 283:1031, 2000.

Ferenczy A: Comparison of cryo- and carbon dioxide laser therapy for cervical intraepithelial neoplasia, Obstet Gynecol 66:793, 1985.

Ferenczy A, Choukroun D, Falcone T, and Franco E: The effect of cervical loop electrosurgical excision on subsequent pregnancy outcome: North American experience, Am J Obstet Gynecol 172:1246, 1995.

Fetters MD, Fischer G, and Reed BD: Effectiveness of vaginal Papanicolaou smear screening after total hysterectomy for benign disease, JAMA 275:940, 1996.

Fink MJ, Fruchter RG, Maiman M, et al: The adequacy of cytology and colposcopy in diagnosing cervical neoplasia in HIV-seropositive women, Gynecol Oncol 55:133, 1994.

Follen M and Richards-Kortum R: Emerging technologies and cervical cancer, J Natl Cancer Inst 92:363, 2000.

Goff BA, Atanasoff P, Brown E, et al: Endocervical glandular atypia in Papanicolaou smears, Obstet Gynecol 79:101, 1992.

Grimes DA and Economy KD: Primary prevention of gynecologic cancers, Am J Obstet Gynecol 172:227, 1995.

Hatch KD, Shingleton HM, Orr JW, et al: Role of endocervical curettage in colposcopy, Obstet Gynecol 65:403, 1985.

Hellberg D, Valentin J, and Nilsson S: Smoking and cervical intraepithelial neoplasia—an association independent of sexual and other risk factors? Acta Obstet Gynecol Scand 65:625, 1986.

Herbst AL: The Bethesda System for cervical/vaginal cytologic diagnoses: a note of caution, Obstet Gynecol 76:449, 1990.

Herrero R, Brinton LA, Reeves WC, et al: Sexual behavior, venereal diseases, hygiene practices, and invasive cervical cancer in a high-risk population, Cancer 65:380, 1990.

Hines JF, Ghim S, Schlegel R, et al: Prospects for a vaccine against human papillomavirus, Obstet Gynecol 86:860, 1995.

Hippelainen MI, Hippelainen M, Saarikoski S, et al: Clinical course and prognostic factors of human papillomavirus infections in men, Sex Trans Dis 21:272, 1994.

Hippelainen MI, Yliskoski M, Syrjanen S, et al: Low concordance of genital human papillomavirus (HPV) lesions and viral types in HPV-infected women and their male sexual partner, Sex Trans Dis 21:76, 1994.

Hollyhock VE, Chanen W, and Wein R: Cervical function following treatment of intraepithelial neoplasia by electrocoagulation diathermy, Obstet Gynecol 61:79, 1983.

Holowaty P, Miller AB, Rohan T, et al: Natural history of dysplasia and the uterine cervix, J Natl Cancer Inst 91:252, 1999.

Holschneider CH, Ghosh K, Montz FJ: See-and-treat in the management of high-grade squamous intraepithelial lesions of the cervix: a resource utilization analysis, Obstet Gynecol 94:377, 1999.

Johnston C: Quantitative tests for human papillomavirus, Lancet 355:2179, 2000.

Jones JM, Sweetnam P, and Hibbard BM: The outcome of pregnancy after cone biopsy of the cervix: a case-control study, Br J Obstet Gynaecol 86:913, 1979.

Josefsson AM, Magnusson PK, Ylitalo N, et al: Viral load of human papillomavirus 16 as a determinant for development of cervical carcinoma in situ: a nested case-control study, Lancet 355:2189, 2000.

Jovanovic AS, McLachlin CM, Shen L, et al: Postmenopausal squamous atypia: a spectrum including "pseudo-koilocytosis," Mod Pathol 8:408, 1995.

Kaufman RH, Adam E, Icenogle J, et al: Relevance of HPV screening in management of cervical intraepithelial neoplasia, Am J Obstet Gynecol 176:87, 1997.

Kennedy AW, Salmieri SS, Wirth SL, et al: Results of the Clinical Evaluation of Atypical Glandular Cells of Undertermined Significance (AGCUS) On Routine Cervical Cytology Screening, Gynecol Oncol, In press.

Killackey MA, Jones WB, and Lewis JL Jr: Diagnostic conization of the cervix: review of 460 consecutive cases, Obstet Gynecol 67:766, 1986.

Kobak WH, Roman LD, Felix JC, et al: The role of endocervical curettage at cervical conization for high-grade dysplasia, Obstet Gynecol 85:197, 1995.

Kolstad P and Klem V: Long-term follow-up of 1121 cases of carcinoma in situ, Obstet Gynecol 48:125, 1976.

Kolstad P and Stafl A: Atlas of colposcopy, Baltimore, 1972, University Park Press, p 91.

Koss LG: Dysplasia: a real concept or misnomer? Obstet Gynecol 51:374, 1978.

Koss LG, Stewart FW, Foote FW, et al: Some histological aspects of behavior of epidermoid carcinoma in situ and related lesions of the uterine cervix: a long-term prospective study, Cancer 16:1160, 1963.

Koutsky LA, et al: Human papillomavirus testing for triage of women with cytologic evidence of low-grade squamous intraepithelial lesions: baseline data from a randomized trial. The Atypical Squamous Cells of Undetermined Significance/Low-Grade Squamous Intraepithelial Lesions Triage Study (ALTS) Group, J Natl Cancer Inst 92:397, 2000.

Krebs HB and Helmkamp BF: Does the treatment of genital condyloma in men decrease the treatment failure rate of cervical dysplasia in the female sexual partner? Obstet Gynecol 76:660, 1990.

Kristensen J, Langhoff-Roos J, and Kristensen FB: Increased risk of pre-term birth in women with cervical conization, Obstet Gynecol 81:1005, 1993.

Manos MM, Kinney WK, Hurley LB, et al: Identifying women with cervical neoplasia. Using human papillomavirus DNA testing for equivocal Papanicolaou results, JAMA 281:1605, 1999.

Mathevet P, Dargent D, Roy M, and Beau G: A randomized prospective study comparing three techniques of conization: cold knife, laser, and LEEP, Gynecol Oncol 54:175, 1994.

McIndoe WA, McLean MR, Jones RW, and Mullins PR: The invasive potential of carcinoma in situ of the cervix, Obstet Gynecol 64:451, 1984.

Mitchell MF, Tortolero-Luna G, Cook E, et al: A radomized clinical trial of cryotherapy, laser vaporization, and LEEP electrosurgical excision for treatment of squamous intraepithelial lesions of the cervix, Obstet Gynecol 92:737, 1998.

Montz FJ, Holschneider CH, and Thompson LDR: Large-loop excision of the transformation zone: effect on the pathologic interpretation of resection margins, Obstet Gynecol 81:976, 1993.

Montz FJ, Monk BJ, Fowler JM, et al: Natural history of the minimally abnormal Papanicolaou smear, Obstet Gynecol 80:385, 1992.

Moscicki AB, Palefsky J, Smith G, et al: Variability of human papillomavirus DNA testing in a longitudinal cohort of young women, Obstet Gynecol 82:578, 1993.

Nasiell K, Nasiell M, and Vaclavinkova V: Behavior of moderate cervical dysplasia during long-term follow-up, Obstet Gynecol 61:609, 1983.

Nasiell K, Roger V, and Nasiell M: Behavior of mild cervical dysplasia during long-term follow-up, Obstet Gynecol 67:665, 1986.

Östor AG: Natural history of cervical intraepithelial neoplasia: a critical review, Int J Gynecol Pathol 12:186, 1993.

Park TW, Fujiwara H, and Wright TC: Molecular biology of cervical cancer and its precursors, Cancer 76:1902, 1995.

Pinion SB, Kennedy JH, Miller RW, et al: Oncogene expression in cervical intraepithelial neoplasia and invasive cancer of the cervix, Lancet 337:819, 1991.

Porreco R, Penn I, Droegemueller W, et al: Gynecologic malignancies in immunosuppressed organ transplant recipients, Obstet Gynecol 45:359, 1975.

Raab SS, Isacson C, Layfield JF, et al: Atypical glandular cells of undetermined significance, Am J Clin Pathol 104:574, 1995.

Rader AE, Rose PG, Rodriguez M, et al: Atypical squamous cells of undetermined significance in women over 55, ACTA Cytol 43:357, 1999.

Richart RM and Barron BA: A follow-up study of patients with cervical dysplasia, Am J Obstet Gynecol 105:386, 1969.

Riou G, Barrois M, Sheng ZM, et al: Somatic deletions and mutations of c-Ha-*ras* gene in human cervical cancers, Oncogene 2:329, 1988.

Riva JM, Sedlacek TV, Cunnane MF, and Mangan CE: Extended carbon dioxide laser vaporization in the treatment of subclinical papillomavirus infection of the lower genital tract, Obstet Gynecol 73:25, 1989.

Roland PY, Naumann RW, Alvarez RD, et al: A decision analysis of practice patterns used in evaluating and treating abnormal Pap smears, Gynecol Oncol 59:75, 1995.

Santos C, Galdos R, Alvarez M, et al: One-session management of cervical intraepithelial neoplasia: a solution for developing countries, Gynecol Oncol 61:11, 1996.

Sawaya GF, Kerlikowske K, Lee NC, et al: Frequency of cervical smear abnormalities within 3 years of normal cytology, Obstet Gynecol 96:219, 2000.

Schiffman MH and Brinton LA: The epidemiology of cervical carcinogenesis, Cancer 76:1888, 1995.

Sherman ME and Kelly D: High-grade squamous intraepithelial lesions and invasive carcinoma following the report of three negative papanicolaou smears: screening failures or rapid progression? Mod Pathol 5:337, 1992.

Shy K, Chu J, Mandelson M, et al: Papanicolaou smear screening interval and risk of cervical cancer, Obstet Gynecol 74:838, 1989.

Smith AE, Sherman ME, Scott DR, et al: Review of the Bethesda System atlas does not improve reproducibility or accuracy in the classification of atypical squamous cells of undetermined significance smears, Cancer (Cancer Cytopathol) 90:201, 2000.

Solomon D: The 1988 Bethesda System for reporting cervical/vaginal diagnoses: a National Cancer Institute Workshop, JAMA 262:931, 1989.

Spitzer M, Chernys AE, and Seltzer VL, The use of large-loop excision of the transformation zone in an inner-city population, Obstet Gynecol 82:731, 1993.

Stuart GCE, Allen HH, and Anderson RJ: Squamous cell carcinoma of the vagina following hysterectomy, Am J Obstet Gynecol 139:311, 1981.

Syrjanen K: Cervical papillomavirus infection progressing to invasive cancer in less than three years, Lancet 1:510, 1985.

Syrjanen K, Kataja V, Yliskoski M, et al: Natural history of cervical human papillomavirus lesions does not substantiate the biologic relevance of the Bethesda System, Obstet Gynecol 79:675, 1992.

Ursin G, Peters RK, Henderson BE, et al: Oral contraceptive use and adenocarcinoma of cervix, Lancet 344:1390, 1994.

Veljovich DS, Stoler MH, Andersen WA, et al: Atypical glandular cells of undetermined significance: a five-year retrospective histopathologic study, Am J Obstet Gynecol 179:38, 1998.

Vessey MP, McPherson K, Lawless M, et al: Neoplasia of the cervix uteri and contraception: a possible adverse effect of the pill, Lancet 2:930, 1983.

Vlahos NP, Dragisic KG, Wallach EE, et al: Clinical significance of the qualification of atypical squamous cells of undetermined significance: an analysis on the basis of histologic diagnoses, Am J Obstet Gynecol 182:885, 2000.

Wallin K-L, Wiklund F, Angstrom T, et al: Type-specific persistence of human papillomavirus DNA before the development of invasive cervical cancer, N Engl J Med 341:1633, 1999.

Whiteley PF and Olah KS: Treatment of cervical intraepithelial neoplasia: experience with the low-voltage diathermy loop, Am J Obstet Gynecol 162:127, 1990.

Widrich T, Kennedy AW, Myers TM, et al: Adenocarcinoma in

situ of the uterine cervix: management and outcome, Gynecol Oncol 61:304, 1996.

Wolf JK, Levenback C, Malpica A, et al: Adenocarcinoma in situ of the cervix: significance of cone biopsy margins, Obstet Gynecol 88:82, 1996.

Wright TC Jr, Ellerbrock TV, Chiasson MA, et al: Cervical intraepithelial neoplasia in women infected with human immunodeficiency virus: prevalence, risk factors, and validity of Papanicolaou smears, Obstet Gynecol 84:591, 1994.

Wright TC, Koulos J, Schnoll F, et al: Cervical intraepithelial neoplasia in women infected with the human immunodeficiency virus: outcome after loop electrosurgical excision, Gynecol Oncol 55:253, 1994.

Wright TC and Richart RM: Review: role of human papillomavirus in the pathogenesis of genital tract warts and cancer, Gynecol Oncol 37:151, 1990.

Ylitalo N, Sorensen P, Josefsson AM, et al: Consistent high viral load of human papillomavirus 16 and risk of cervical carcinoma in situ: a nested case-control study, Lancet 355:2194, 2000.

Yost NP, Santoso JT, McIntire DD, et al: Postpartum regression rates of antepartum cervical intraepithelial neoplasia II and III lesions, Obstet Gynecol 93:3559, 1999.

zur Hausen H: Human papillomavirus and their possible role in squamous cell carcinoma, Can Top Microbiol Immunol 78:1, 1977.

Malignant Diseases of the Cervix

Microinvasive and Invasive Carcinoma: Diagnosis and Management

KEY TERMS AND DEFINITIONS

Adenoma Malignum. A virulent adenocarcinoma of the cervix that histologically consists of glands that appear well differentiated (minimal deviation adenocarcinoma).

Barrel-Shaped Cervix. A cervix containing a large carcinoma, *generally* of endocervical origin, that has replaced much of the cervix, causing its diameter to widen (usually more than 4 cm).

Brachytherapy. A form of radiation therapy in which the source is placed close to the tumor. The application may be in the form of needles implanted into the tumor (interstitial therapy) or into the vagina or cervical canal (internal therapy). For cervical tumors an intracervical tandem and vaginal ovoids (colpostats) are usually used.

Endophytic. A term used to describe a tumor that begins in the endocervical canal.

Exophytic. A term used to describe a cervical tumor that grows on the outside surface primarily of the cervix (portio).

Extrafascial Hysterectomy. An operation that develops the pubocervical fascia to allow total removal of the cervix and uterus (class I hysterectomy).

Fletcher-Suit Applicator. A system that delivers brachytherapy to cervical carcinomas by use of a tandem in the cervical canal and ovoids (colpostats) in the vagina.

Glassy Cell Carcinoma. A virulent adenosquamous carcinoma that occurs in the cervix and metastasizes early in the course of the disease.

Microinvasive Carcinoma. A small (stage IA) carcinoma detected by microscopic examination with little or no risk of spread to regional lymph nodes (see text for detailed discussion).

Modified Radical Hysterectomy. An operation that removes the uterus and cervix and some paracervical tissues but does not dissect the ureters distal to the uterine artery (class II hysterectomy).

Pelvic Exenteration. An extensive pelvic operation usually employed to treat a central pelvic recurrence of cervical carcinoma after radiation. A total exenteration involves removal of the bladder, uterus, cervix, and rectum. An anterior exenteration spares the rectum, while a posterior exenteration spares the bladder.

Persistent Tumor. The identification of invasive disease at the site of primary therapy less than 6 months after therapy.

Point A. A term used in radiation therapy of carcinoma of the cervix to identify a point 2 cm above the external os of the cervix and 2 cm lateral to the cervical canal.

Point B. A term used in the radiation treatment of carcinoma of the cervix to identify a point 3 cm lateral to point A or 5 cm from the cervical canal.

Radical Hysterectomy. An operation that removes the uterus, upper third of the vagina, cervix, and paracervical-parametrial tissues. The pelvic ureters are dissected to the uterovesical junction. It is usually combined with a pelvic lymph node dissection (class III hysterectomy).

Recurrent Tumor. The identification of invasive disease 6 months or more after therapy.

Summary of Stages of Carcinoma:
  I: Tumor confined to the cervix
  IA: Microinvasion (preclinical)
  IB: All other cases confined to cervix
  IIA: Tumor spread to the vagina—upper two thirds

IIB: Tumor spread to paracervical tissue but not to pelvic walls

IIIA: Tumor spread to lower third of vagina

IIIB: Tumor spread to pelvic wall or obstruction of either ureter by tumor

IV: Tumor spread to mucosa of bladder or rectum or outside the pelvis.

Teletherapy. A form of radiation with placement of the radioactive source at a distance from the patient (external therapy). It is usually used to treat the pelvis and occasionally the paraaortic nodes in patients with cervical carcinoma.

Verrucous Carcinoma. A warty appearing, well-differentiated squamous malignancy that rarely metastasizes.

Malignancies of the cervix are almost always carcinomas, and a summary of the more common histologic types are shown in the box to the right. Approximately 85% to 90% of these tumors are squamous cell carcinomas, and from 10% to 15% are adenocarcinomas. The proportion of adenocarcinomas has increased in the United States, partly because of a decrease in the frequency of occurrence of squamous cell carcinomas. Squamous cell carcinoma of the cervix is closely associated with early and frequent sexual contact and cervical viral infection, particularly human papillomavirus (HPV), as detailed in Chapter 28. According to the American Cancer Society, the frequency of cervical cancer has been steadily decreasing, in part because of the effect of widespread screening for premalignant cervical changes by cervical cytology (Pap smear). Approximately 12,400 cases of cervical cancer occur in the United States annually, making it the third most frequent malignancy of the lower female genital tract after endometrial and ovarian carcinomas.

Summary of Major Categories of Cervical Carcinoma

Squamous Cell Carcinomas
Large cell (keratinizing or nonkeratinizing)
Small cell
Verrucous

Adenocarcinomas
Typical (endocervical)
Endometrioid
Clear cell
Adenoid cystic (basaloid cylindroma)
Adenoma malignum (Minimal deviation adenocarcinoma)

Mixed Carcinomas
Adenosquamous
Glassy cell

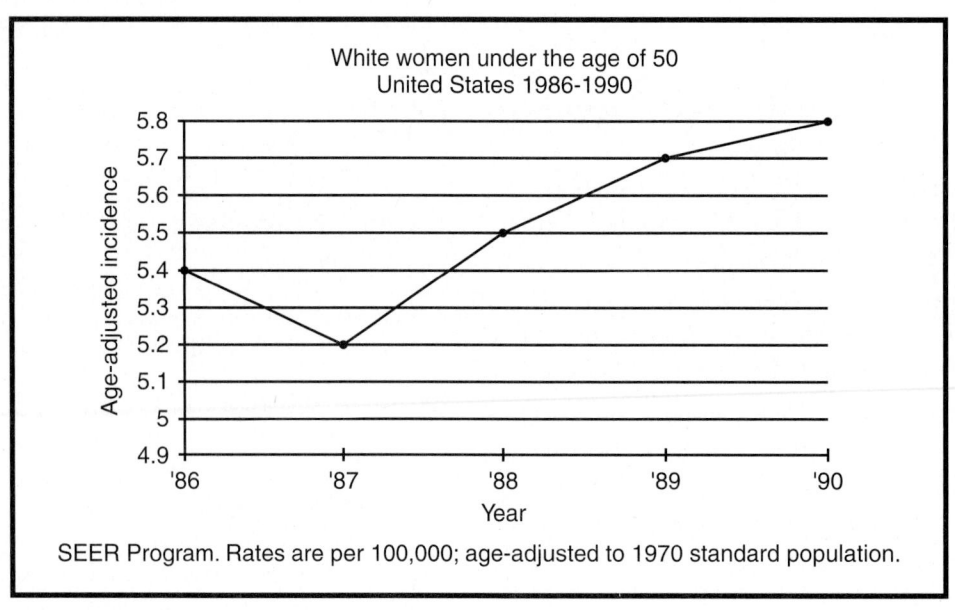

FIGURE 29-1 Incidence rates of invasive carcinoma. (From U.S. Department of Health and Human Services. Ries LAG et al, editors: SEER Cancer Statistics Review, 1973-1991, 136-144, 1994.)

Approximately 4600 deaths annually result from cervical cancer, which is less than the approximately 14,000 for ovarian cancer. Unfortunately SEER data has shown an increase in invasive cancer for women under age 50 starting in 1987 (Figure 29-1).

This chapter will detail the various types of cervical carcinomas and consider their natural history, methods of diagnosis and evaluation, and the details of therapy. Primary sarcomas and melanomas of the cervix are extremely rare and are not considered separately.

HISTOLOGIC TYPES

Varieties of squamous cell carcinoma of the cervix are illustrated in Figure 29-2. An early form, microinvasive carcinoma, is considered separately in the next section. Most squamous cell carcinomas of the cervix are reported to be of the large cell, nonkeratinizing type, but many are keratinized, and squamous pearls may be seen. About 2% to 5% are small cell carcinomas, and these tend to be more virulent than the other types. They resemble small (OAT)

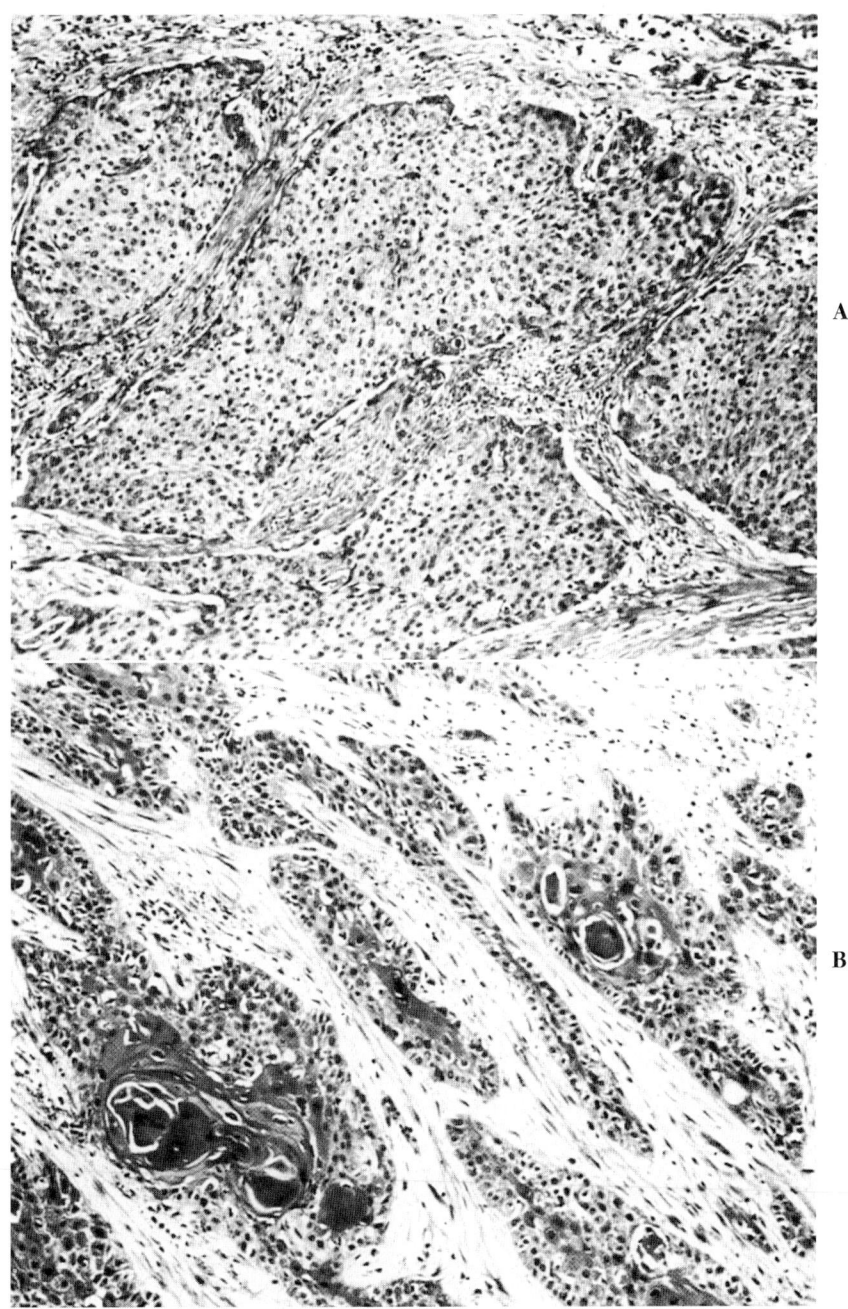

FIGURE 29-2 **A,** Large cell, nonkeratinizing squamous cell carcinoma. Discrete islands of uniform, large cells with abundant cytoplasm are separated by fibrous stroma. (×160.) **B,** Keratinizing squamous cell carcinoma. Irregular nests of squamous cells forming several pearls are separated by fibrous stroma. The nests have pointed projections. (×160.)

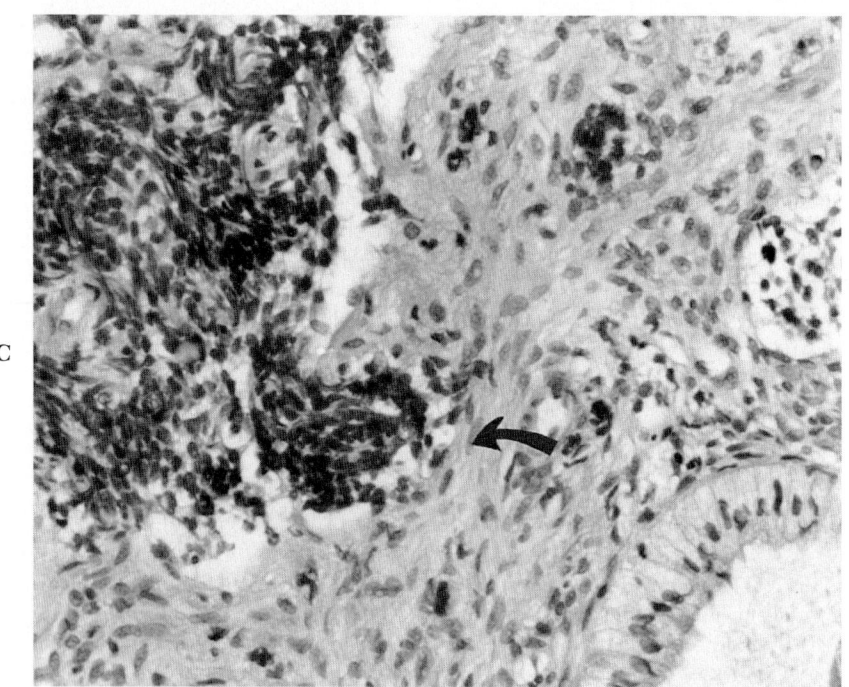

FIGURE 29-2, cont'd. **C,** Small cell neuroendocrine carcinoma of the cervix *(arrow)* infiltrating between normal endocervical glands (H&E; ×240.) (A and B from Clement PB and Scully RE: Semin Oncol 9:251, 1982. C courtesy of Anthony Montag, M.D., Department of Pathology, the University of Chicago.)

cell carcinomas of the lung, often containing neuroendocrine granules. They frequently occur in younger women. Van Nagell et al. noted that small cell carcinomas tend to have higher recurrence rates and more distant spread than squamous cell carcinomas, with poorer patient survival rates. Adjuvant chemotherapy (see subsequent section) has been used before radical operation or radiation with apparent improvement in results. The degree of differentiation of tumors is usually designated by three grades: G1, well differentiated; G2, intermediate; and G3, undifferentiated. However, there is no consensus on the value of tumor grade as a major prognostic factor for squamous cell carcinoma of the cervix.

A rare variety of squamous cell carcinoma is the so-called verrucous carcinoma, which is morphologically similar to those found in the vulva (Chapter 32). These warty tumors appear as large, bulbous masses (Figure 29-3). They rarely metastasize but unfortunately may be admixed with the more virulent, typical squamous cell carcinomas, in which case metastatic spread is more likely.

Adenocarcinomas may have a number of histologic varieties. As noted by Brinton et al., adenocarcinomas do not appear to be affected by the usual sexual factors associated with squamous carcinomas. However, HPV-DNA, oral contraceptive use, and lack of cervical cytologic screening heightened the risk of developing these tumors. The typical variant often contains intracytoplasmic mucin

and is related to the mucinous cells of the endocervix (endocervical pattern) (Figure 29-4). However, on occasion the cells contain little or no mucin, and then the tumor may resemble an endometrial carcinoma (endometrioid pattern). It may be difficult histologically to ascertain if these carcinomas arise in the cervix or endometrium. Endocervical tumors more frequently stain positive for carcinoembryonic antigen (CEA) than do endometrial tumors, and this histochemical observation has been used to try to distinguish the tumors microscopically by an immunoperoxidase reaction.

A rare but important virulent variety of adenocarcinoma is the adenoma malignum. These microscopically innocuous-appearing tumors consist of well-differentiated mucinous glands (Figure 29-5) that vary in size and shape and infiltrate the stroma. Despite their bland histologic appearance, they tend to be deeply invasive and metastasize early. The term *minimal deviation adenocarcinoma* is applied to these tumors. According to McGowan et al., patients with Peutz-Jeghers syndrome are at increased risk for development of these tumors.

Clear cell adenocarcinomas of the cervix are histologically identical to those of the ovary (Chapter 31) and vagina (Chapter 33). They are uncommon in the cervix and can also be associated with intrauterine diethylstilbestrol (DES) exposure (Chapter 15), although they also often develop spontaneously in the absence of DES exposure.

Adenoid cystic carcinomas are rare. Berchuk and

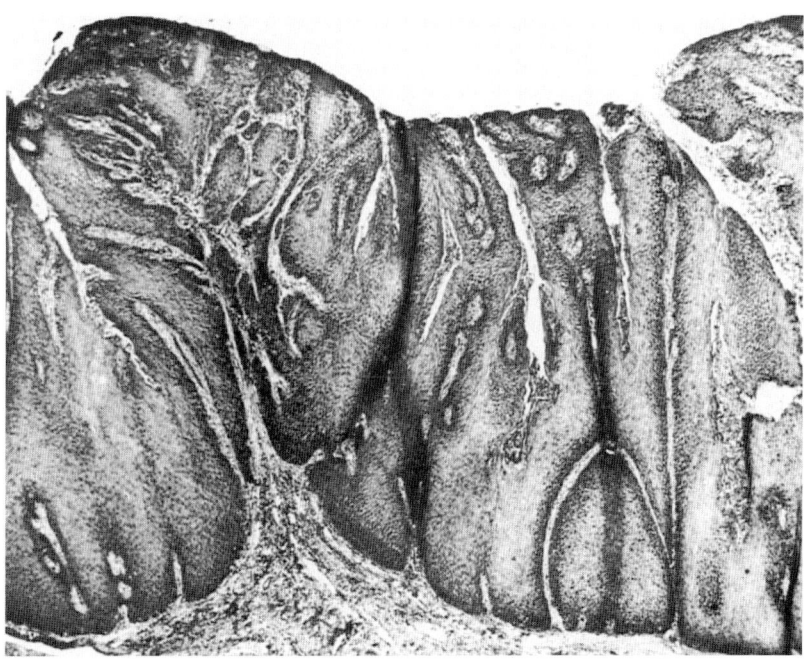

FIGURE 29-3 Verrucous carcinoma. Downgrowns of papillae have broad bases. Tumor cells are well differentiated. (×34.) (From Clement PB and Scully RE: Semin Oncol 9:251, 1982.)

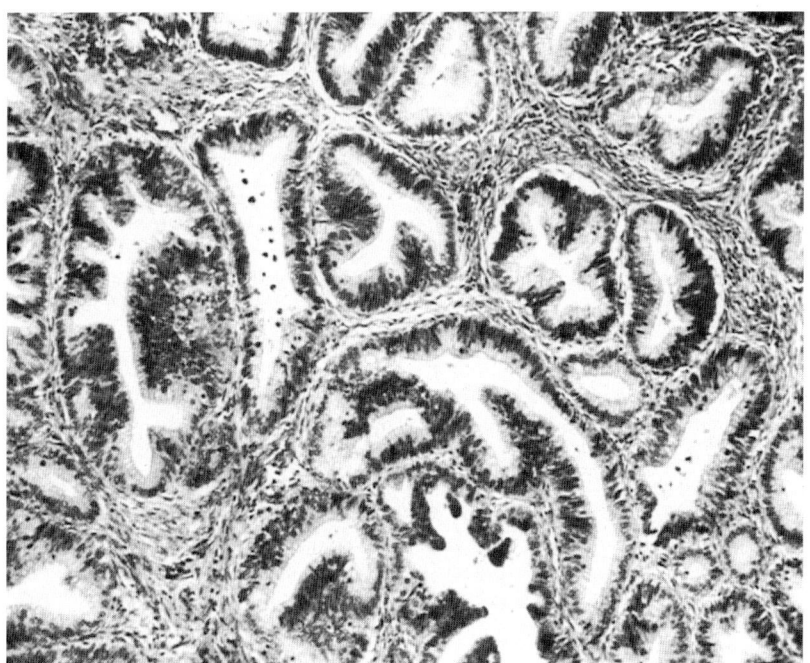

FIGURE 29-4 Typical adenocarcinoma. Irregular glands are lined by stratified mucin-containing epithelium. Mitotic figures are numerous. (×160.) (From Clement PB and Scully RE: Semin Oncol 9:251, 1982.)

Mullin summarized 88 cases reported in the literature. These tumors are aggressive and may resemble cylindromas of salivary gland or breast origin and histologically may resemble basal cell carcinomas of the skin (adenoid basal, or basaloid, carcinomas). Most patients with these tumors are over age 60 years. The basaloid variety appears to be less aggressive. King et al. reported four unusual cases in women under age 40. One patient was noted to survive more than 5 years.

Adenosquamous carcinomas, as the name implies, consist of both squamous carcinoma and adenocarcinoma elements in varying proportions (Figure 29-6). They occur

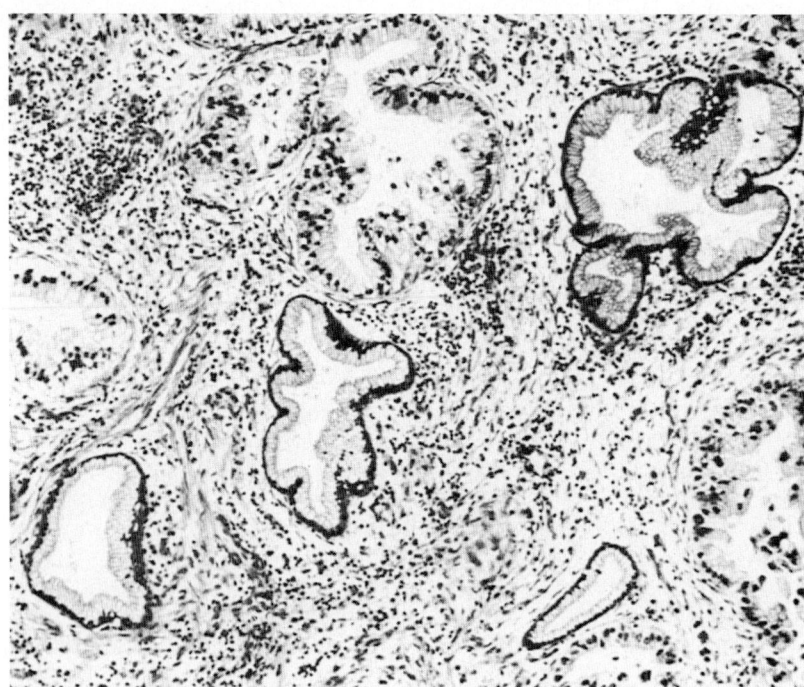

FIGURE 29-5 Adenoma malignum. Glands are mostly well differentiated, appearing normal except for their irregular shapes. A few obviously malignant glands are also present. (×160.) (From Clement PB and Scully RE: Semin Oncol 9:251, 1982.)

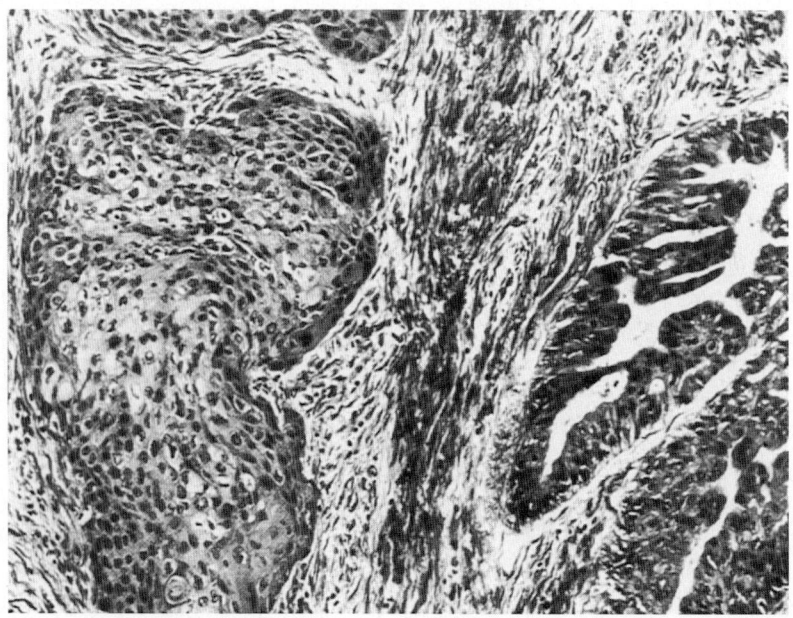

FIGURE 29-6 Well-differentiated adenosquamous carcinoma. Glandular structure lies adjacent to nest of nonkeratinizing, large squamous cells. (×400.) (From Clement PB and Scully RE: Semin Oncol 9:251, 1982.)

frequently in pregnant women. A particularly virulent variety is termed *glassy cell carcinoma* (Figure 29-7). This is an undifferentiated tumor consisting of large cells containing cytoplasm with a ground-glass appearance. Glassy cell carcinomas tend to metastasize early to lymph nodes as well as to distant sites, and usually have a fatal outcome.

MICROINVASIVE CARCINOMA OF THE CERVIX

Microinvasive carcinoma of the cervix is part of the spectrum of cervical neoplasia between intraepithelial carcinoma (Chapter 28) and frankly invasive carcinoma. These are tiny lesions that have begun to invade the cervical

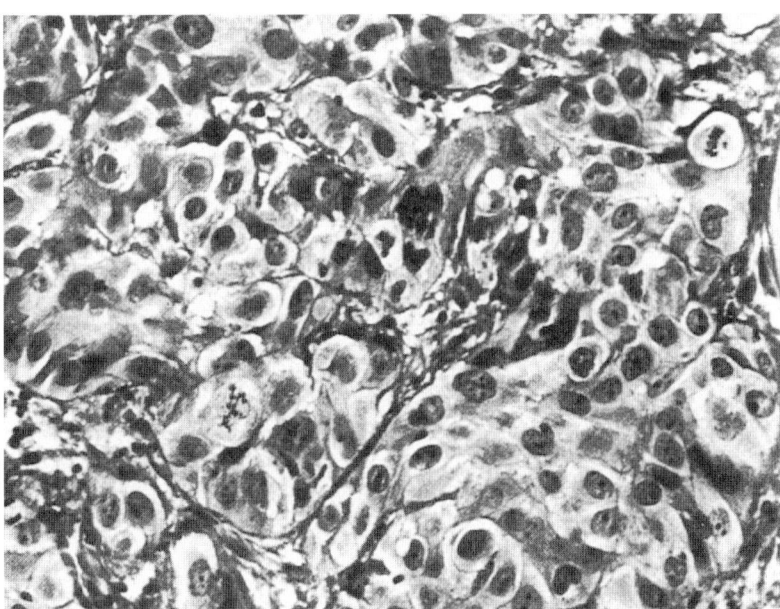

FIGURE 29-7   Glassy cell carcinoma. Cells have sharp borders, ground-glass–type cytoplasm, and nuclei containing prominent nucleoli. (×1000.) (From Clement PB and Scully RE: Semin Oncol 9:251, 1982.)

stroma (Figure 29-8), but can often be treated by less extensive measures than those required for larger invasive cancers. In the International Federation of Gynecology and Obstetrics (FIGO) staging classification, these preclinical carcinomas are designated as stage IA.

A major problem in gynecologic oncology is that there is no uniform agreement on the appropriate definition of microinvasive carcinoma. The ideal definition is one that would have widespread clinicopathologic applicability and describe an early invasive lesion that has little or no risk of spread beyond the cervix, such as to regional pelvic lymph nodes. It is important to consider some of the definitions that have been used to describe this entity and also to consider the results of therapy that have been obtained. The important factors are the depth of stromal invasion, the presence or absence of vascular or lymphatic space involvement (capillary-like spaces), the presence or absence of tumor confluence, and the lateral extent (width) of the lesion.

FIGO (1994) defines a stage IA lesion as a preclinical cervical carcinoma and divides microinvasion into two categories: stages IA1 and IA2. Stage IA1 is minimal stromal invasion that most authorities believe can be treated as a carcinoma in situ. Stage IA1 is a microinvasive tumor whose dimensions are less than 3 mm depth of invasion and 7 mm width. It is not clear whether this definition provides reliable criteria for lack of risk of tumor spread to regional nodes. Stage IA2 is microscopic tumor that is 3 to 5 mm in depth and less than 7 mm in width (Table 29-1). Kolstad summarized 411 patients with stage IA2, 245 of whom were treated by hysterectomy and 166 by more radical therapy. Two patients had node metastases, and four died. The poor outcome occurred primarily in those with vascu-

lar space involvement. Kolstad recommends conservative therapy if the margins of the cone are clearly negative and there is no lymphatic or vascular space involvement.

The Society of Gynecologic Oncologists in 1974 described microinvasive carcinoma of the cervix as "a lesion in which the neoplastic epithelium invades the stroma in one or more places to a depth of 3 mm or less below the basement membrane of the epithelium and in which lymphatic or vascular involvement is not demonstrated." Currently available studies indicate that almost all lesions meeting the latter definition will not have spread beyond the cervix, but the definition, while widely used, does not provide sufficient precision for many clinical situations. As pointed out by Burghardt et al. these 0 to 3 mm cases include very early cases of "early stromal invasion." For these tumors a small band of eosinophilic neoplastic tissue invades overlying carcinoma in situ (Figure 29-9). These cases are virtually 100% curable, and if they are removed from the analysis of the 0 to 3 mm invasive category, the stage IA1 and IA2 appear to have a similar prognosis (see therapy discussion later).

A further refinement has been reported by investigators from Western Europe, who used a meticulous and time-consuming three-dimensional microscopic study to calculate the *volume* of neoplastic tissue. Using a 50 mm^2 two-dimensional criterion, Lohe et al. reported no positive nodes in 134 cases studied in numerous centers in Western Europe. This two-dimensional definition has the advantage of considering both the depth of invasion and the width of tumor and provides a general guide that is used by many pathologists for determination of microinvasive disease. The current stage IA1 definition allows for an area of 21 mm^2, and 35 mm^2 for IA2.

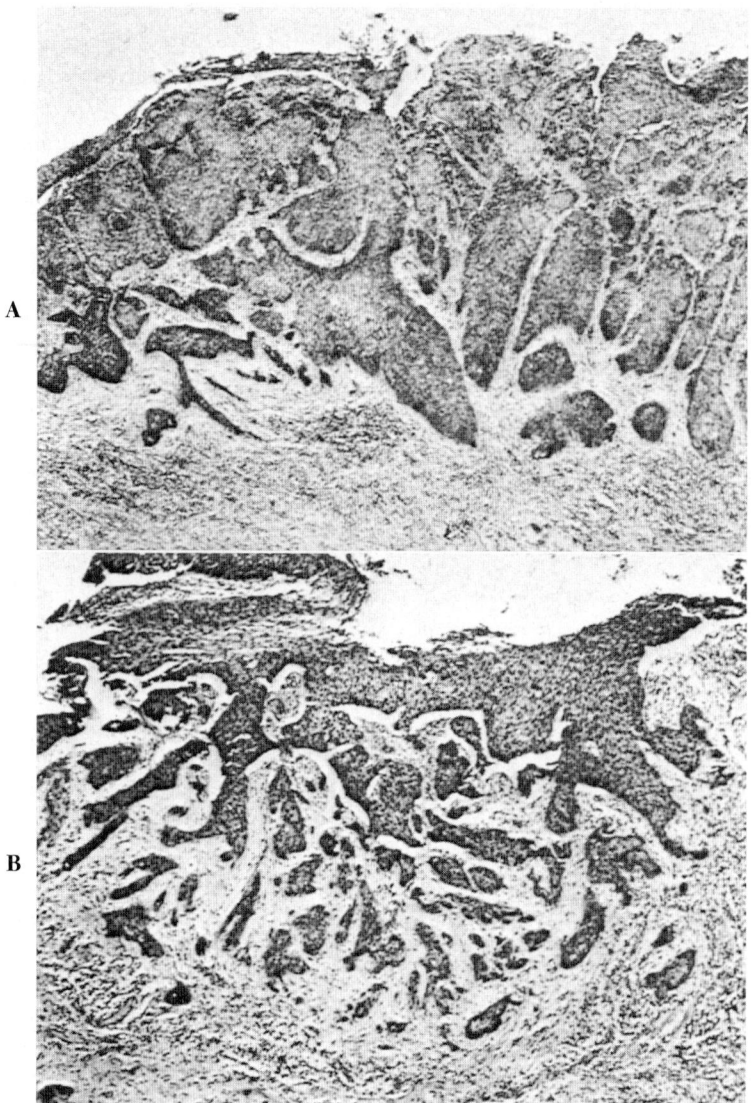

FIGURE 29-8   **A,** Tumor with only 0.5 mm of invasion. (×40.) **B,** Example of so-called spray pattern with multiple invasive nodules in stroma. Invasion is only 1 mm. (×50.) (From Creasman WT, Fetter BF, Clarke-Pearson DL, et al: Am J Obstet Gynecol 153:164, 1985.)

These area measurements provide the general guidelines but there are other factors to consider when undertaking conservative treatment for suspected microinvasive tumors. First, the diagnosis of microinvasive tumor cannot be made on the basis of a biopsy specimen alone and a cervical conization must be performed. Second, if the margin of the cervical cone specimen contains neoplastic epithelium, the risk of invasive tumor in the remaining uterus is increased. Third, endocervical tumors have an increased risk of being associated with invasion, and this may occur when the exocervix is covered with normal squamous epithelium. Östor and Rome evaluated 200 patients from Australia with microinvasive tumors, 91 of which invaded less than 5 mm and were less than 7 mm in width. Four of the latter recurred in the vagina, and one patient has died. Twenty-three patients had conization as the sole treat-

ment. None of these have recurred, but none had more than 3 mm of invasion. Morris et al. studied 14 patients treated by conization and followed for a mean of 26.5 months. All had lesions with less than 3 mm of invasion without capillary-lymphatic space involvement. One patient had a hysterectomy that showed mild dysplasia in the specimen. The remaining 13 were free of disease at the time of the report. A study of 51 patients with 3 to 5 mm invasion by Creasman et al. indicated that if the tumor had these dimensions, subsequent radical hysterectomy and node dissection showed no cases of lymph node metastases. Impressively, no patients died of cancer at 5 years and none recurred in spite of the fact that one quarter of the cases showed vascular invasion. Thus, truly negative margins which existed in these cases is an excellent prognostic sign in spite of the fact that these cases belong to stage IA2.

TABLE 29-1
Clinical Stages of Carcinoma of the Cervix Uteri (FIGO, Revised 1994)

Stage			Characteristics
I			Carcinoma is strictly confined to cervix (extension to corpus should be disregarded)
	IA		Invasive cancer identified only microscopically. All gross lesions, even with superficial invasion, are stage IB cancers. Invasion is limited to measured stromal invasion with a maximum depth of 5 mm and no wider than 7 mm.*
		IA1	Measured invasion of stroma no greater than 3 mm in depth and no wider than 7 mm
		IA2	Measured invasion of stroma greater than 3 mm and no greater than 5 mm in depth and no wider than 7 mm
	IB		Clinical lesions confined to the cervix or preclinical lesions greater than IA
		IB1	Clinical lesions no greater than 4 cm in size
		IB2	Clinical lesions greater than 4 cm in size
II			Carcinoma extends beyond cervix but has not extended to pelvic wall; it involves vagina, but not as far as lower third
	IIA		No obvious parametrial involvement
	IIB		Obvious parametrial involvement
III			Carcinoma has extended to pelvic wall; on rectal examination there is no cancer-free space between tumor and pelvic wall; tumor involves lower third of vagina; all cases with hydronephrosis or nonfunctioning kidney should be included, unless they are known to be due to another cause
	IIIA		No extension to pelvic wall, but involvement of lower third of vagina
	IIIB		Extension to pelvic wall, or hydronephrosis or nonfunctioning kidney due to tumor
IV			Carcinoma has extended beyond true pelvis or has clinically involved mucosa of bladder or rectum
	IVA		Spread of growth to adjacent pelvic organs
	IVB		Spread to distant organs

*The depth of invasion should not be more than 5 mm taken from the base of the epithelium, either surface or glandular, from which it originates. Vascular space involvement, either venous or lymphatic, should not alter the staging.

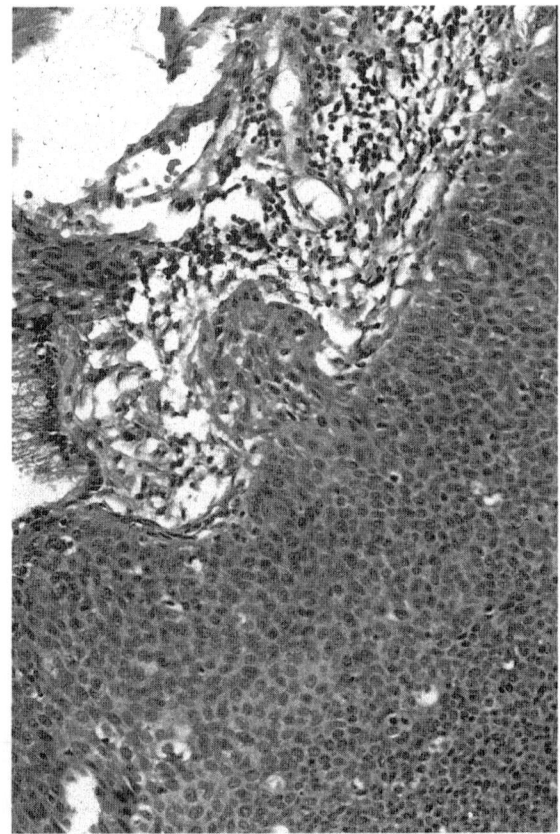

FIGURE 29-9 Photomicrograph showing early stromal invasion. (Courtesy of Dr. Anthony Montag, University of Chicago, Department of Pathology.)

In considering the therapy of microinvasive carcinoma of the cervix, the clinician must weigh the risk that an invasive lesion may be mistakenly treated by conservative means. If an early invasive carcinoma is present, it can usually be successfully treated by means of a radical or modified radical hysterectomy (see later discussion). The risk of death or serious morbidity from such operation is probably on the order of 1%, and the risk of error or misdiagnosis of a lesion should be comparably small.

At present a patient suspected of having microinvasive carcinoma of the cervix should first have conization of the cervix. If the lesion is less than 21 to 35 mm^2, the patient can often be treated by conservative means, which is usually a simple hysterectomy, particularly if invasion from the basement membrane is less than 3 mm. If the lesion is less than 21 mm^2 and there is only infrequent capillary-like space involvement, such conservative treatment is usually adequate. Conization may be used as sole therapy in carefully selected cases in which the cone margins are free of tumor and accurate measurements of the tumor dimensions are available. The presence of capillary-like space involvement does not preclude conservative therapy, but the risk of invasive disease or future recurrence increases with capillary-like space involvement and larger lesions. Conservative therapy should not be attempted if the conization margins are involved with neoplasia. It is usually wise to do an endocervical curettage after the conization to be sure neoplastic epithelium is not higher in the canal. All patients must be followed with periodic physical and cytologic (Pap smear) examinations, since recurrences may develop late and have been noted more than 15 years after primary therapy. The 5-year survival rate following appropriately chosen therapy of microinvasive carcinoma of the cervix should approach 100%.

CARCINOMA OF THE CERVIX

Clinical Considerations

Patients with carcinoma of the cervix characteristically present with abnormal bleeding or brownish discharge, frequently noted following douching or intercourse and also occurring spontaneously between menstrual periods. The patients often have a history of not having had a cytologic (Pap) smear for many years. Other symptoms, such as back pain, loss of appetite, and weight loss, are late manifestations and occur when there is extensive spread of cervical carcinoma. The patients tend to be in their 40s to 60s, with a median age of 52 years noted worldwide by Pecorelli et al. It is more frequent in blacks than whites in the United States. Preinvasive intraepithelial carcinoma of the cervix (Chapter 28) occurs primarily in women in their 20s and 30s and has become more common among those in their 20s, leading to a gradual increase in the incidence of invasive carcinoma in younger patients.

The diagnosis is established by biopsy of the tumor; a specimen can be easily obtained at office examination. A Kevorkian, Eppendorf, Tishler, or similar punch biopsy instrument (see Chapters 28 and 33) is convenient to use. Occasionally it is necessary to biopsy nodularity or induration in the vagina near the cervix to ascertain the limit of tumor spread and to define a correct tumor stage. If the patient's cytologic smear is suggestive of invasive carcinoma with no gross lesion visible and endocervical curettage does not demonstrate carcinoma, or if an adequate biopsy specimen to establish carcinoma cannot be obtained, then cervical conization should be performed.

Staging

The staging of carcinoma of the cervix depends primarily on the pelvic examination, and the designation may be modified by general physical examination, by chest x-ray examination, by intravenous pyelogram, or CT scan and is not changed based on operative findings. Table 29-1 shows the definition of the four stages of cervical carcinoma according to FIGO (revised in 1994), and the various types of tumor distribution that may be observed in the various stages are illustrated in Figure 29-10.

Natural History and Spread

Carcinoma of the cervix is initially a locally infiltrating cancer that spreads from the cervix to the vagina and paracervical and parametrial areas. Grossly the tumors may be ulcerated (Figure 29-11), similar to carcinomas occurring elsewhere in the female genital tract, and may have an exophytic growth pattern or cauliflower-like appearance extruding from the cervix, usually producing abnormal bleeding and staining. Alternatively, they may be endophytic, in which case they are asymptomatic, particularly in the early stage of development, and tend to be deeply invasive when diagnosed. These usually start initially from an endocervical location and often fill the cervix and lower uterine segment, resulting in a "barrel-shaped" cervix. The latter tumors tend to metastasize to regional pelvic nodes, and because of the tendency of late diagnosis, they are often more advanced than the exophytic variety. The primary path for distant spread is through lymphatics to the regional pelvic nodes. Blood-borne metastases from cervical carcinomas do occur, but they are less frequent and usually are seen late in the course of the disease.

Initially, cervical carcinoma spreads to the primary pelvic nodes, which include the pericervical (ureteral) node, which lies near the intersection of the uterine artery and ureter; the hypogastric (internal iliac) and external iliac nodes, which lie along their respective vessels; and the nodes in the obturator fossa near the vessels and nerve. From this primary group, tumor spread proceeds secondarily to the common iliac and paraaortic nodes. Rarely the inguinal nodes or the presacral nodes may be involved; the latter are particularly at risk for tumors that grow into the area of the rectum. The distribution of lymph node involvement was studied in detail in 26 cases of untreated carcinoma of the cervix by Henriksen (Figure 29-12) (five stage I, six stage II, eight stage III, and seven stage IV). All were examined at autopsy, and the primary pelvic group had the highest frequency of metastases with distal sites also involved, but less frequently. An important distal node that becomes involved after the paraaortic group is the left scalene node, that is the left supraclavicular node. A clinical correlation is that biopsy of this node is frequently performed in the assessment of advanced cervical carcinoma to clarify whether the tumor has spread outside the abdomen. In addition to nodal spread, hematogenous spread of cervical carcinoma occurs primarily to the lung, liver, and, less frequently, bone (see recurrence section).

Prognostic Factors

Clinical stage is the most important determinant of prognosis for carcinoma of the cervix. Table 29-2 demonstrates the collated results for 11,945 cases treated worldwide between 1990 and 1992. Approximately 75% of the tumors are in stage I or II, about 21% in stage III, and

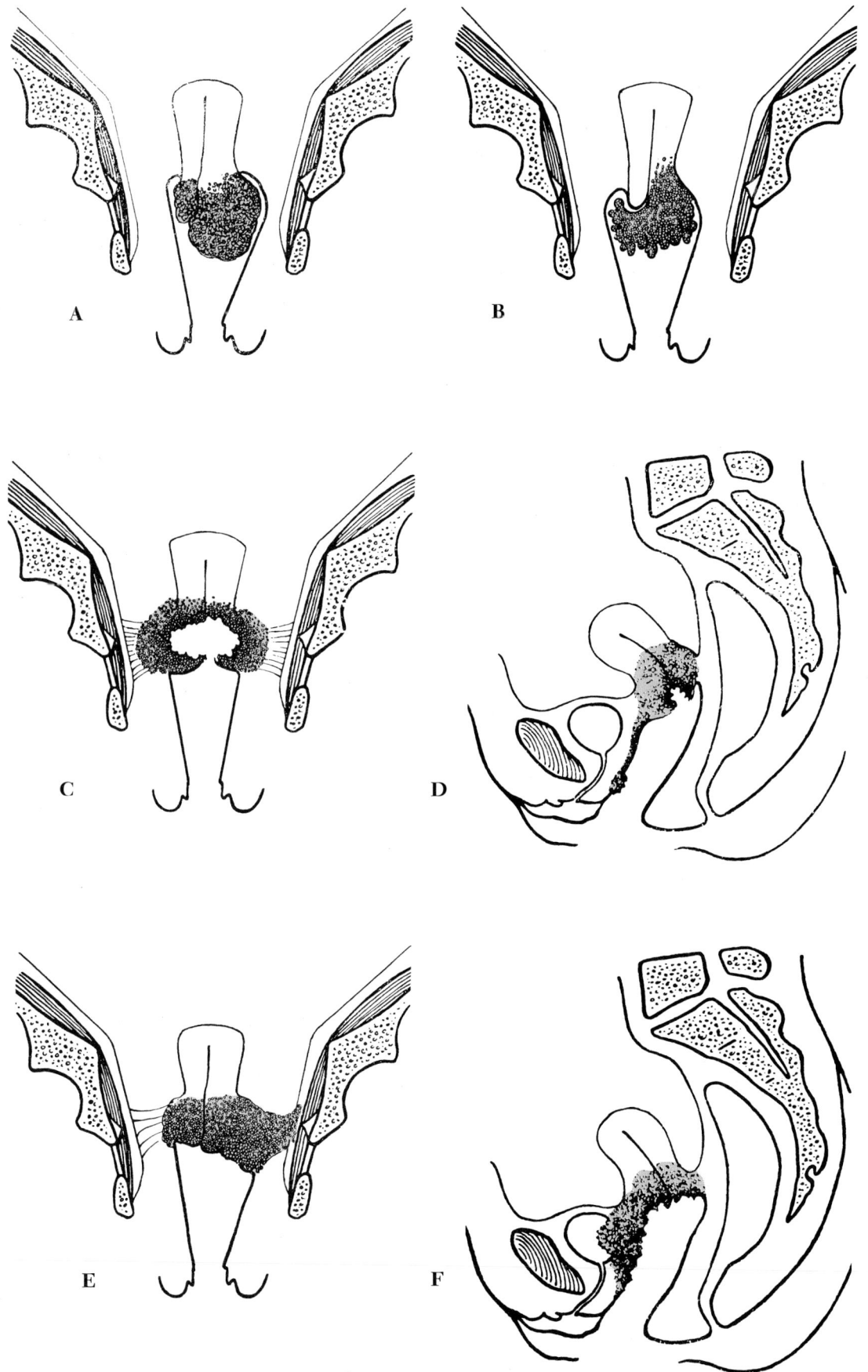

FIGURE 29-10 Staging of cervical carcinoma. **A,** Stage IB: nodular cervix. **B,** Stage IIA: carcinoma extending into left vault. **C,** Stage IIB: parametrium involved on both sides, but carcinoma has not invaded pelvic wall; endocervical crater. **D,** Stage IIIA: submucosal involvement of anterior vaginal wall and small, papillomatous nodule in its lower third. **E,** Stage IIIB: parametrium involved on both sides; at left, carcinoma has invaded pelvic wall. **F,** Stage IVA: involvement of bladder. (From Pettersson F and Bjorkholm E: Semin Oncol 9:289, 1982.)

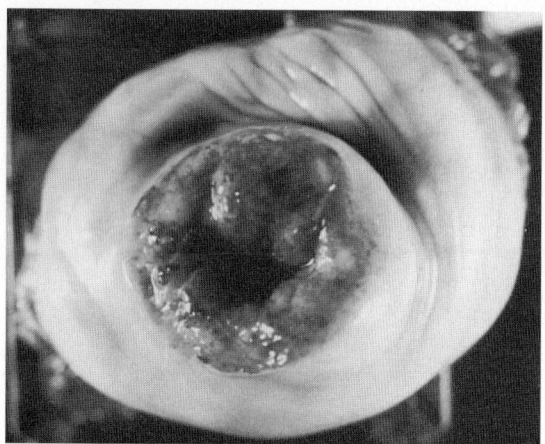

FIGURE 29-11 Carcinoma of cervix (gross specimen).

fewer than 5% in stage IV. Age appears to be a factor, insofar as those under age 40 have a lower rate of survival than those between ages 40 and 69. This was emphasized by the studies of Dattoli et al., who noted a 5-year survival of 54% for those with stage IB who were younger than age 40, compared with 91% for older patients. As noted in Chapter 28, HPV is strongly associated with cervical neoplasia. Molecular studies by DeBritton et al. and Higgins et al. have shown that HPV tends to occur in cervical carcinomas in younger women and these tumors have a better prognosis than the HPV-negative tumors.

Numerous other factors have been evaluated to ascertain their importance in predicting the behavior of cervical carcinoma. These include tumor grade, lesion size, depth of invasion, histologic type, presence of lymph-vascular (capillary-like) space involvement, and status of regional pelvic nodes. Many of these factors, however, are interrelated; that is, the stage of the tumor closely correlates with the status of the regional pelvic nodes. For example, in a summary of 6560 cases, Plentl and Friedman noted a frequency of 15% positive pelvic nodes in 3391 cases of stage I, 29% in 2952 cases of stage II, and 47% in 217 cases of stage III. Percentages based on a single series of patients are not available for paraaortic node involvement, but in a multiinstitutional review of 290 patients by Lagasse et al., the proportion was 6% in stage I, 19% in stage IIA, and 33% in stages IIB and III; overall, 29% of the patients in stage II and higher had positive paraaortic nodes.

Within stage IB, lesion size has proved to be a very effective predictor of tumor behavior, as has the depth of tumor invasion into the stroma. In three-dimensional studies Burghardt et al. correlated tumor volume with patient survival, emphasizing the effect of lesion size on prognosis. The importance of lymph-vascular (capillary-like) space involvement in the prognosis of cervical carcinoma is not clear. Delgado et al., in a cooperative Gyneco-

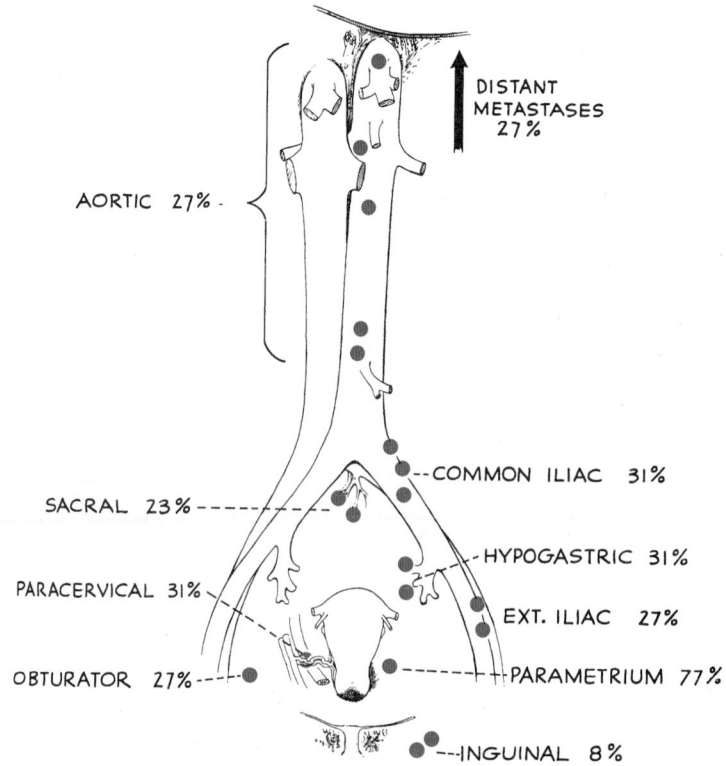

FIGURE 29-12 Frequency of lymph node metastases in cervical carcinoma. Incidence of node group involvement in 26 non-treated cases of cervical carcinoma. (From Henriksen E: Am J Obstet Gynecol 58:924, 1949.)

TABLE 29-2

TABLE 29-2
Carcinoma of the Uterine Cervix: Distribution by Stage and 5-Year Survival Rates for Patients Treated in 1990–1992 ($n = 11,945$)

Stage	Patients (n)	5-Year Survival
Stage Ia	902	95.01%
Stage Ib	4657	80.1%
Stage II	3364	64.2%
Stage III	2530	38.31%
Stage IV	492	14%

Modified from Pecorelli et al: Annual report on the Results of Treatment in Gynaecological Cancer, XXIII Volume, Milan, 1998. Federation Internationale de Gynecologie et d'Obstetrique.

logic Oncology Group study, analyzed 645 patients with stage I disease who had radical hysterectomy and node dissections at 33 institutions. The presence of pelvic node metastases independently correlated with lymphvascular space involvement, depth of invasion, parametrial involvement, and patient age. In a follow-up GOG study the authors noted disease-free interval following therapy also correlated with lesion size, capillary-lymphatic space involvement, and depth of tumor invasion. Similar correlations for lesion size, capillary-like space involvement, and depth of invasion were noted by Gauthier et al. Involvement of the endometrium by tumor does not change the stage but does appear to predispose to distant metastases, as noted by Fagundes et al. Molecular studies indicate that overexpression of the C-*myc* and *ras* oncogenes are also associated with a poor prognosis.

ADENOCARCINOMAS OF THE CERVIX

Cervical adenocarcinomas occur in women of all ages, but the typical mucinous variety occurs primarily in women in their 50s. These tumors appear to have a different etiology than squamous cell carcinomas of the cervix insofar as there does not appear to be a clear relationship to sexual transmission or a viral infection. HPV studies by a number of investigators, including Bosch et al., indicate that HPV-18 is predominant in adenocarcinomas while HPV-16 is most common in squamous cell carcinomas. Patients with clear cell adenocarcinoma of the cervix are often younger, particularly individuals who are exposed to DES in utero (Chapter 15). The prognosis of adenocarcinoma may be worse within comparable stages than for squamous cell carcinoma, but this is debatable. Kleine et al., in a study of 145 patients with adenocarcinoma, noted poorer survival rates, particularly in patients with stage I or II disease. However, Leminen

et al., in a study of 106, observed no difference. Anton-Culver et al. studied 152 cases of adenocarcinoma and 456 squamous cell carcinomas from Southern California. Their results indicated the prevalence for adenocarcinomas was 22%, which is higher than reported in earlier studies. However, the authors did not note a survival difference between the squamous cell carcinoma and the adenocarcinoma groups. Hirai et al. reported 5-year cures of the rare and virulent adenoma malignum. In 4 cases of stage I treated by radical hysterectomy the 5-year survival was a surprising 100% indicating that cure is possible in these tumors.

Prognosis is related not only to the stage of the tumor but also to tumor grade and size and depth of stromal invasion. Berek et al. reported that the size of the adenocarcinoma, its degree of differentiation, and the depth of stromal invasion all correlated with the frequency of metastases to lymph nodes and thus patient survival. For adenocarcinomas with less than 2 mm of invasion, there was no lymph node metastases, while the frequency was greater than 50% for tumors that invaded more than 10 mm. Similarly, among stage I tumors less than 2 cm in diameter, all pelvic lymph node studies were negative for tumor, while larger tumors had an increasing proportion of positive nodes as tumor size or dedifferentiation increased. In a recent literature review, Ostor noted that cold knife cone is preferred for the proper diagnosis of margins and the depth of invasion in cases of early adenocarcinoma. Invasion was limited to 5 mm or less. Of 219 patients whose pelvic nodes were removed, 2% had positive nodes. A small group of 21 patients had only conization as treatment, and none recurred. This latter treatment is acceptable for early lesions with negative margins in reliable patients who wish to preserve fertility. Covens et al. reviewed 16 cases of early stage I adenocarcinoma of the cervix with tumor thickness <10 mm and patients whose tumor volumes were <600 mm^2. None had tumor recurrence in pelvic nodes or elsewhere. Many of these patients had a depth of invasion <2 mm. Therapy is considered in subsequent discussions.

MANAGEMENT

Pretherapy Evaluation

Once the patient has been diagnosed as having an invasive carcinoma, pretreatment evaluation is conducted to determine the extent of disease, to arrive at an accurate clinical staging, and to plan the program of therapy. The usual evaluation consists of a thorough history and physical examination, routine blood studies, an intravenous pyelogram (IVP) or computed tomography (CT) scan, and chest x-ray. Demonstration of an obstructed ureter or nonfunctioning kidney caused by tumor automatically assigns the case at least to stage III (see Table 29-1). A barium enema test or flexible sigmoidoscopy is sometimes performed, in the case of large tumors, or for those who will be receiving radiation treatment.

The CT scan is more expensive than IVP but has the advantage of being able to provide greater information concerning tumor spread to lymph nodes, particularly in cases of higher-stage disease. CT scan and IVP provide approximately equivalent information for most cases of stages I and IIA but CT allows detection of enlarged pelvic and paraaortic nodes that were suspicious for involvement of tumor. However, the CT scan is not particularly useful to detect the parametrial extent of cervical carcinoma, which is evaluated more reliably by pelvic examination. Magnetic resonance imaging (MRI) (Chapter 10) has also been used to evaluate local spread, but the test is not used routinely. The suggestion of tumor in retroperitoneal nodes by CT scan does not affect stage, which relies primarily on clinical examination and the status of the ureters.

A pelvic examination for determining tumor stage is often performed with anesthesia to assess accurately the extent of disease. Cystoscopy may be performed at this time to rule out extension of tumor to the bladder. The results are usually normal for tumors of low stage (i.e., I or IIA) and this test can be omitted for these cases as shown in the studies of Liang et al.

If a pelvic or paraaortic node appears to be involved with tumor by CT scan, further evaluation is indicated. If possible, fine-needle aspiration (FNA) of the suspicious node should be performed under CT guidance. Nash et al. utilized FNA with cytologic analysis of 177 aspirations, with a reported sensitivity of 68%; since there were no false positive results, their specificity and positive predictive value were 100%. If the fine-needle aspiration does not yield a positive diagnosis of a suspicious node, particularly those in the paraaortic area, many therapists will proceed with open biopsy removal of the node through a retroperitoneal approach (see the discussions of therapy of high-stage tumors). The advantage of the retroperitoneal approach is that subsequent radiation therapy results in less bowel injury than a transperitoneal approach.

A scalene node biopsy of the left supraclavicular area is sometimes performed for evaluation of tumor spread. Vasilev and Schlaerth used the procedure before paraaortic irradiation for positive nodes and found 4 of 17 patients had a positive scalene evaluation indicative of systemic disease. The diagnostic step is particularly useful in high-stage disease or in cases of patients with pelvic tumor recurrence who are being considered for exenterative therapy.

Low-Stage (IB-IIA) Disease

Radical hysterectomy and radiation therapy are equally effective as treatments for low-stage disease, and comparable survival statistics have been reported for stage IB and early stage IIA (i.e., minimal spread to the vagina). Numerous studies have been conducted to try to ascertain which tumors will respond preferentially either to radiation or to operation, but no reliable method of predicting which modality is optimum for a given tumor has been developed. Five-year survival rates from some centers of approximately 80% to 90% have been reported for stage IB and 70% to 80% for stage IIA with either radiation or radical hysterectomy; these statistics are somewhat better than most recently published, collated worldwide percentages (Table 29-2).

Both modalities have advantages and disadvantages. Operation allows preservation of ovarian function and completion of therapy in one hospitalization and causes less vaginal radiation fibrosis and compromise of sexual function. It also permits a thorough exploration of the abdomen. Chambers et al. reported on 38 patients whose ovaries were transposed laterally and superiorly. This procedure often preserves ovarian function in patients who are subsequently radiated, but ovarian cyst development can be a troublesome postoperative problem. The best results are obtained when operation is performed on small tumors, particularly those that are exophytic. Short-term complications such as infection, thromboembolic disease, and rarely fistula formation may occur, but there are few long-term complications (see later discussion). Short-term serious complications will occur in 1% to 2% of cases. Patients selected for radical hysterectomy are usually younger and in general in better health and thus are better able to tolerate a major surgical procedure. Patients who have had salpingitis or inflammatory bowel disease or who have unexplained pelvic masses are also treated by operation because of the increased risk of complications with radiation. Radiation therapy is also effective to treat low-stage carcinomas of the cervix. Attempts have been made to combine full radiation treatment with radical hysterectomy, but this leads to frequent severe complications, including lack of healing and fistula formation. Einhorn et al. have reported promising effective combined results by using preliminary brachytherapy alone followed by radical hysterectomy, primarily for stage IB disease (see next section).

Operative Therapy: Radical Hysterectomy, Pelvic Node Dissection

Radical hysterectomy and bilateral pelvic lymphadenectomy are effective for treatment of many stage IB and some early stage IIA cancers. It is important that the operation remove the same volume of tissues that receive cancerocidal doses of radiation in cases for which radiation is the sole therapy. The amount of tissue removed, particularly in the paracervical and parametrial areas near the ureter, depends on the extent and location of the tumor. Piver et al. defined five classes to describe the extent of the operation. Class I guarantees the removal of the entire

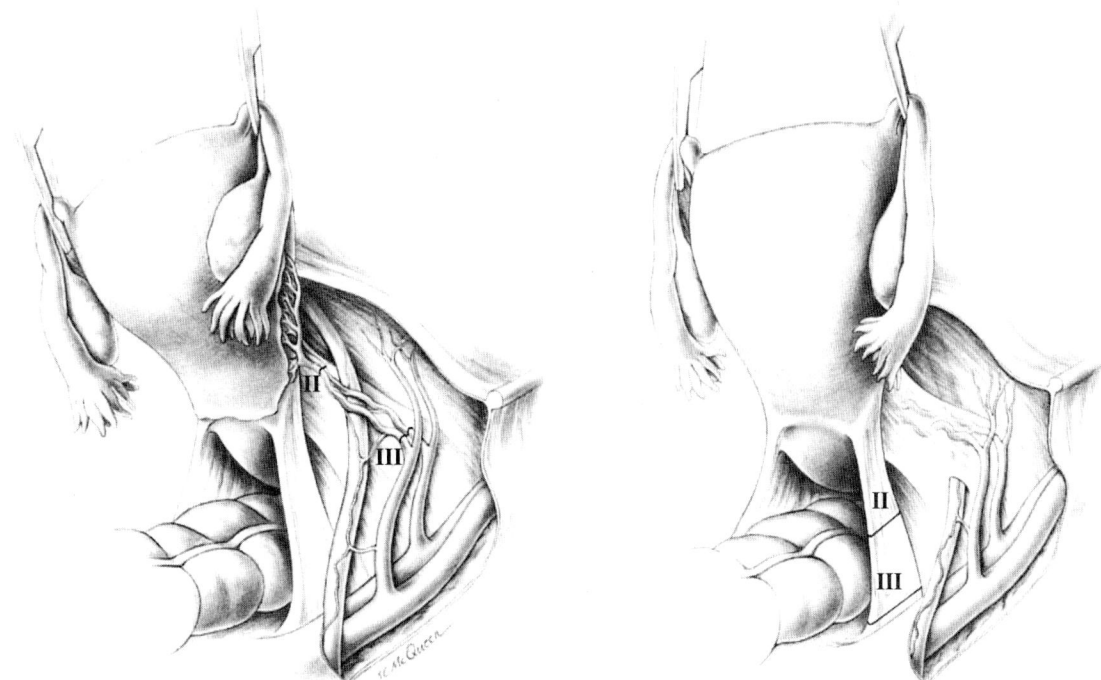

FIGURE 29-13 Classes II and III radical hysterectomy with points of dissection shown (see text).

cervix and uterus. The ureter is not disturbed from its bed. In many instances this is described as an *extrafascial hysterectomy*, the type used after preoperative radiation for treatment of a barrel-shaped cervix (see later discussion). A class II operation (Figure 29-13) removes more paracervical tissue than class I, but the ureters are retracted laterally yet are not dissected from their attachments distal to the uterine artery, and the uterosacral ligaments are ligated approximately halfway between the uterus and rectum. The operation is usually performed with pelvic lymphadenectomy and is often termed a *modified radical hysterectomy*. The operation is useful to treat small microscopic carcinomas of the cervix. Magrina et al. utilized modified radical hysterectomy primarily for tumors <2 cm (median 1.1 cm) with 5-year survival of 96%. This procedure may occasionally be used to treat small, central cervical recurrences of carcinoma that are diagnosed following radiation therapy of the primary tumor. For a class III operation, the uterine artery is ligated at its origin from the anterior division of the hypogastric artery, and the uterosacrals are ligated deep in the pelvis near the rectum (Figure 29-12). This operation is usually termed a *radical hysterectomy* (Meigs-Wertheim hysterectomy) and is performed for stage IB and rarely for stage IIA carcinomas of the cervix.

Class IV and V operations are infrequently performed. The former involves a complete dissection of the ureter from its bed and sacrifice of the superior vesical artery. A class V operation involves resection of the distal ureter or bladder or both with reimplantation of the ureter into the

bladder (ureteroneocystotomy). Both operations are designed to remove small, central recurrent disease and would be attempted to avoid an anterior exenteration (see following discussion). Extensive data are not available but the latter two procedures appear to have high complication rates.

Preoperative preparation for a patient who is to undergo radical hysterectomy includes the same basic considerations for anyone undergoing a major operative procedure. Graduated-compression below-the-knee leg stockings are utilized to reduce the risk of thromboembolism. Prophylactic antibiotics are also frequently prescribed (see Chapter 24). During the course of the operation care is taken not to grasp the ureters with instruments such as forceps to avoid damaging the periureteral capillary blood supply. In addition, following removal of the pelvic nodes, suction catheters may be left in the retroperitoneal space, and the upper and lower margins of the excised lymphatic tissue (near the femoral vessels inferiorly and the common iliac vessels superiorly) are ligated to reduce the risk of lymphocyst formation. Some therapists leave the pelvic peritoneum open, and with free drainage into the peritoneal cavity, suction catheters are not used. Ovarian function may be preserved in younger patients if there is little likelihood of postoperative radiation. Many surgeons prefer a suprapubic cystotomy, which is more convenient for the patient and less likely to be accompanied by postoperative infection than a transurethral catheter. If a pelvic node dissection is not performed, particularly in an obese patient, a radical hysterectomy can also be accomplished vaginally

(Shauta-Aumreich procedure). This operation has been more widely practiced in Europe than in the United States.

In stage I cases treated by radical hysterectomy and node dissection, the results obtained are related primarily to the status of the pelvic nodes, as well as the surgical resection margins around the primary tumor (ideally more than 1 cm). If the pelvic nodes are free of tumor, the 5-year survival rate can be expected to exceed 90%, whereas if the nodes are found to contain tumor, the 5-year survival rate drops to 45% to 50%. Lerner et al. reported a 5-year survival rate (life table technique) of 93.4% for 108 patients using class III hysterectomy for stage IB carcinomas of the cervix. All but five of these tumors were less than 5 cm in diameter. Six patients experienced prolonged bladder dysfunction after operation. Only one postoperative ureterovaginal fistula developed, and there were no postoperative deaths, indicating that excellent results can be obtained with operation, particularly if the patients are carefully selected. If the patient is found to have extensive spread of gross disease to pelvic nodes, the studies of Potter et al. suggest it is preferable to cease the operation and complete radiation therapy to improve pelvic control of tumor. However, Hacker et al. reported an estimated 5-year survival of 80% for 34 patients whose tumor-positive pelvic or paraaortic nodes were resected and the areas subsequently radiated. In a recent Gynecologic Oncology Group Study, Sedlis et al. evaluated disease-free survival for patients treated with radical hysterectomy with adverse prognostic factors including more than one third stromal invasion, capillary lymphatic space involvement, and large tumor diameter. Survival was improved in those who received postoperative pelvic radiation.

Numerous studies have been published evaluating low-dose preoperative radiation followed by radical hysterectomy and pelvic node dissection. The technique has been particularly widely used in Western Europe, and Einhorn et al. evaluated the Swedish experience comparing complete treatment with full radiation therapy alone, or preoperative partial radiation (two intracavitary radiums) and radical hysterectomy for patients under age 41 with stage IB or IIA carcinoma of the cervix. A significant ($P < 0.004$) improvement was noted in stage IB for the combined-therapy group as compared with radiation alone (5-year survival rate: 96% versus 81%). No significant difference was noted in stage IIA. Calais et al. used combined therapy for tumors less than 4 cm in diameter in 70 patients and reported a 10-year survival of 96%, an excellent result. However, definitive trials have not proven the superiority of this technique.

Postoperative Therapy and Care

If the pelvic nodes are found to contain metastatic tumor following radical hysterectomy, it is current practice at most centers to add external pelvic radiation (teletherapy). Usually, approximately 50 Gy (5000 rads) are delivered by megavoltage radiation. Unfortunately, current data do not establish that this practice improves patient survival. Kinney et al. performed a matched retrospective analysis of adjuvant radiotherapy in 185 patients and noted no differences in survival. Soisson et al. also noted no improved survival with fewer pelvic recurrences in their series of 72 patients who tended to fail with distant metastases, indicating the need for effective systemic therapy. The number of positive nodes appears to have prognostic importance. Inoue and Morita noted decreasing 5-year survival in patients with stage IB cervical carcinoma as follows: no nodes, 92%; one node, 91%; two to three nodes, 71%; and four or more nodes, 50%. Survival appeared to improve in patients with one node who had postoperative radiotherapy, but a control group was not available for comparison.

Following radical hysterectomy many patients experience long-term complications. Montz et al. noted a 5% frequency of small bowel obstruction, which rose to 20% if radiation was used postoperatively. Fistulas from the urinary tract, particularly ureterovaginal fistulas, have been reported to occur in about 1% of cases. The low rate appears to result from administration of antibiotics, the prevention of retroperitoneal serosanguineous collections, and avoidance of direct manipulation of the ureter to avoid injury to the periureteral blood supply. Some therapists do not reperitonealize the pelvis, which causes drainage directly to the peritoneal cavity, in which case suction catheters are not usually used.

Many patients suffer postoperative bladder dysfunction. In part this appears to be due to disruption of the sympathetic nerve supply to the bladder. However, the dysfunction may be temporary. Low et al. noted an increase in bladder pressure with a decrease in urethral pressure (see Chapter 21) following radical hysterectomy. There was reduced bladder compliance with detrusor instability. The bladder can develop hypotonicity, and overdistention can then become a problem. If overdistention of the bladder and infection are avoided, progressive improvement of bladder function usually occurs. Forney correlated the degree of bladder dysfunction after radical hysterectomy with the extent of resection of the cardinal ligament. Those who had a complete resection of cardinal ligaments could void satisfactorily in an average of 51 days, in comparison to 20 days for those with only partial resection of the ligaments. All the patients experienced a decrease in bladder sensation. In a few patients the decrease in bladder sensation can be permanent. For patients in whom it is temporary, recovery usually occurs after continuous drainage of the bladder with an indwelling catheter. Westby and Asmussen observed that by 1 year after operation, a slight decrease in urethral pressure persists but that the decrease is not as great as that noted immediately after operation. After 1 year the postoperative changes and bladder function usually recover. In a recent study from Sweden, Bergmark et al. noted compromised sexual activity, decreased lubrication, and shortened vagina in women treated for cervical cancer both by operation and/or radiation.

TABLE 29-3
Approximate Radiation Therapy Dosages for Carcinoma of the Cervix*

Stage	External Therapy	Local Implant† Dosage to Pt A (Gy)
IB (small, 1 cm)	45 Gy	35
IB (bulky, 3 cm)	45 Gy	40
IB (barrel, 4 cm)	Combination radiation and operation (see text)	
IIA	Similar to IB (bulky)	
IIB	45 Gy, may have additional boost to parametrial disease up to 6 Gy	40
III	45 Gy, may have additional boost to parametrial disease up to 10 Gy	40
IVA	Individualized or similar to stage III	

*Average dosages will vary among patients and treatment centers.

†Usually done in two applications.

Radiation Treatment

The majority of patients with carcinoma of the cervix are treated by radiation. The principles of external megavoltage treatment (teletherapy) and local implants (brachytherapy) are reviewed in Chapter 26. External beam radiation is administered in fractions, usually 180 cGy daily 5 days per week, so as to destroy the tumor without causing permanent damage to normal tissues. This delivers uniform dosages to the entire pelvis, including the regional pelvic nodes. The local implant delivers its highest energy locally to the cervix and surface of the vagina, and paravaginal and paracervical tissues. The radiation from the implant diminishes according to the inverse square law, and the uterus and cervix serve as a receptacle for arranging and holding the intracavitary applicator stem (tandem) and accompanying vaginal applicators (ovoids) in a fixed and optimum position for delivering the desired radiation dosimetry (Fletcher-Suit applicator, see Figure 26-3). Results appear to be improved if hemoglobin levels are at 12 gm/dL or higher as shown by the study of Grogan et al. Mundt et al. noted that African Americans from lower socioeconomic groups tended to have more anemia and more medical problems, compromising the success of radiation treatment. The analysis showed that socioeconomic status, not race, was the contributing factor.

Current technique delivers about 40 cGy per hour to point A with shielding on the posterior ovoids to protect the rectum. The tandem and ovoids are inserted with the patient anesthetized, and a pack is placed in the vagina to stabilize the apparatus and increase the distance from the mucosa of the bladder and rectum. After the position of the applicator has been confirmed to be satisfactory by x-ray films, the radioactive sources, such as cesium 137, are inserted (afterloading technique). Other types of applicators are available, but the principle of delivering intense radiation to the cervix and paracervical areas is the same.

The goal is to increase the total dosage of radiation to the maximum allowable to achieve tumor control without introducing a major risk of complications and injury to adjacent normal tissue. The specific protocols followed in various treatment centers differ, and individualization for specific patients is often needed depending on the stage and size of the cervical tumor as well as the patient's local anatomy. In general, external therapy is given first both to treat the regional pelvic nodes and to shrink the central tumor mass, which then is more amenable for a local implant (Table 29-3). In some patients external therapy can lead to excessive shrinkage of the vaginal apex, making safe, effective implantation of local radiation sources difficult. This can be a problem particularly in older or postmenopausal patients. Occasionally in those patients, the implant is done first, especially for smaller stage I tumors. Rotmensch et al. also used intraoperative ultrasound to provide optimal implant positioning in these difficult patients. In some instances the central pelvis is shielded during external radiation therapy to allow for subsequent higher dosages from the implant. Occasionally, interstitial therapy in the form of needles implanted into the area of the tumor is needed to achieve effective local tumor control. Recently, high dose rate (HDR) brachytherapy given on an outpatient basis has been introduced. Preliminary data by Sarkaria et al. are encouraging for this modality, which eliminates the need for patient hospitalization for brachytherapy. Clark et al. used HDR with concomitant cisplatin chemotherapy and noted increasing complications if the rectal dose exceeded 7600 cGy. (See section on radiation complications.)

In calculating the dosages of radiation, two reference points, A and B, are used (Figure 29-14). Point A is 2 cm above the external os and 2 cm lateral to the cervical canal. Point B is 5 cm lateral to the cervical canal and 3 cm lateral to point A which places point B in the vicinity of the lateral pelvic wall. The total dosage administered depends on tumor stage, but in general at the pelvic wall it is in the

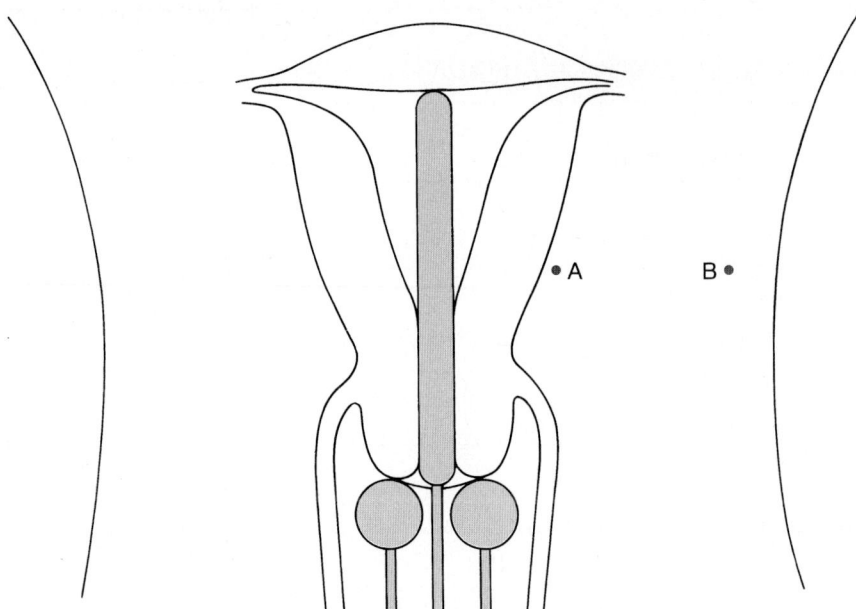

FIGURE 29-14 Points A and B with central stem (tandem) and two ovoids in place.

range of 50 to 65 Gy, with the higher dosages used for high-stage disease. At point A it varies but approximates 85 Gy. The normal cervix is particularly resistant to radiation and can tolerate doses as high as 200 to 250 Gy over 2 months, whereas the adjacent bladder and in particular the rectum are much more sensitive, and their exposure in general should be limited at the point of maximum radiation to 80 Gy, with overall average dosages in the range of 65 to 70 Gy. The small bowel can be damaged at dosages above 45 to 50 Gy, especially if adhesions limit intestinal mobility and a large volume is treated.

A general scheme for treating the various stages of carcinoma of the cervix by radiation is summarized in Table 29-3. The sum of external radiation therapy (Gy/10) plus the implant dose (mg hr/1000) equals approximately 10. At many treatment centers this sum varies from 9.0 to 10.0, and in general as the sum increases, the risk of complications from radiation therapy increases (see following discussion). In addition, as the volume of tissue that receives high doses of radiation increases, the risk of complications also increases. Therapeutic results with radiation therapy in the past have been generally similar to those with surgery for low-stage disease, and representative values are shown in Table 29-2.

CHEMORADIATION

The general approach to radiation has just been summarized. However, the overall approach for treatment of carcinoma of the cervix has been greatly modified by the recent reported success of chemoradiation. Runowicz et

al., in 1989, reported 32 evaluable patients with tumors greater than 4 cm in diameter. They administered cisplatin (20 mg/m²) continuously for 5 days every 3 weeks during radiation treatment. Twenty had high-stage tumors (IIB, III, or IV). There were 29 complete responses with a 28-month survival rate of over 80%. Most patients received four courses of cisplatin with future courses prevented by bone marrow depression. In addition, chemotherapy-radiation treatments have also been tried to improve results in patients with paraaortic node involvement, but long-term results are not available. Podczaski et al. noted two late bowel injuries in patients receiving extended-field irradiation with 5-fluorouracil (5-FU) and cisplatin. Radiation myelitis has also been reported.

The results of subsequent chemoradiation trials sponsored by the National Cancer Institute Gynecologic Oncology Group (GOG) were published in 1999. The preliminary results from these trials showed such improved survival that the trials were preliminarily halted in order to release the results, which changed clinical practice.

Rose et al. treated patients with advanced squamous cell, adenosquamous, or adenocarcinoma of the cervix (stages IIB, III, and/or IVA) in a recent GOG study. The patients received external radiation therapy (40.8-51 Gy) followed by 1 or 2 brachytherapy implants. Total dosages to point B were 55 Gy for stage IIB cases and 60 Gy for stages III and IVA. The patients were randomized to receive 1 of 3 concomitant chemotherapy regimens (hydroxyurea; cisplatin, 5-FU, and hydroxyurea; or cisplatin alone). The best results were obtained with the cisplatin-containing regimens with the least complications that with weekly cisplatin (40 mg/m²) alone. Progression-free survival at 24 months was an impressive 67% for this very high-risk group of patients.

Keys et al., in a further collaborative trial, studied 369 women with bulky stage Ib carcinoma (> 4 cm) in diameter. They were randomized to receive radiation alone or with concomitant weekly cisplatin (40 mg/m²). Total dose to point B was 55 Gy. Patients with radiographic evidence of hydronephrosis or lympadenopathy were excluded. Adjuvant extrafascial hysterectomy was performed in 3 to 6 weeks after conclusion of the chemoradiation treatments. Acute severe toxicity, especially hematologic but also gastrointestinal, was noted. However, the therapeutic results were markedly better in the chemoradiation group with a 3-year 83% disease-free survival compared to 74% in the radiation group alone (*P* = .008). Recurrences and death were higher in the radiation-alone group.

Chemoradiation has also proven superior for treating both paraaortic and pelvic nodes. Morris et al., also in a GOG trial, studied 403 women with advanced cervical cancer (stages IIB-IVA) or stages IB-IIA with tumor diameter >5 cm or biopsy-proven metastases to pelvic nodes. Four field external beam therapy was used. Dosage to the pelvis and paraaortic nodes was 45 Gy. In most cases, brachytherapy followed external treatment. The patients were randomized to receive radiation alone or chemoradiation (5-FU plus platinum days 1-5, 22-26, and during brachytherapy). More hematologic toxicity was noted in the combined group but late term side effects in the 2 groups were comparable. A marked improvement in the chemoradiation arm was noted with overall survival in the chemoradiation group 73% versus 58% in the radiation group alone.

In another trial of biopsy-proven paraaortic node metastases, Varia et al. treated 95 patients with extended field radiation including the paraaortic nodes (45 Gy) with concomitant 5-FU and cisplatin weeks 1 and 5. The trial showed chemoradiation was feasible in this group and a progression-free survival at 3 years of 33% was obtained.

In view of the studies of Rose et al. cited earlier showing comparable chemoradiation results but less toxicity with weekly cisplatin, most therapists now utilize that protocol for chemoradiation (i.e., weekly cisplatin 40 mg/m²).

PARAAORTIC RADIATION. The field of external radiation is often extended from the pelvis to the paraaortic nodes, particularly for high-stage disease (IIB or greater). The risk of paraaortic metastases in these cases is approximately 30%. Most therapists prefer to treat individuals in whom there is evidence of spread to paraaortic nodes. As noted previously, a CT scan is often obtained to evaluate advanced cervical carcinoma. In cases that appear to have suspected paraaortic node involvement by tumor, a CT scan–directed, fine-needle aspiration biopsy is performed to document tumor spread. However, a negative test result does not guarantee lack of tumor spread. Therefore, to provide more precise information, some therapists have evaluated the paraaortic node by performing a pretherapy laparotomy. Unfortunately, a transperitoneal approach lends to a high rate of intestinal complications if subsequent paraaortic irradiation is given. In some series severe complications have been noted in a majority of the patients treated, particularly if the dose of radiation exceeded 5000 cGy. Lagasse et al. suggested a retroperitoneal approach to evaluate the paraaortic nodes, which reduced the risk of intraperitoneal adhesions and provided a basis for selection of patients for paraaortic irradiation. Vigliotti et al. noted that complication rates were related to dose and operative approach, that is, 8% following retroperitoneal lymphadenectomy and 8% with dosages ranging from 40 to 45 Gy, rising to 10% with 50 Gy, and rising dramatically to 32% for dosages around 55 Gy. As noted previously, chemoradiation with cisplatin is the preferred approach.

RADIATION COMPLICATIONS. Complications following radiation therapy are related to dosage, volume treated, and sensitivity of the various tissues receiving radiation. The patient's habitus and presence of diseases that affect circulation, such as diabetes and high blood pressure, increase the risk, as does prior intraabdominal operation. Acute minor complications, such as diarrhea and nausea, subside after radiation therapy is completed. Complications usually arise in 1 to 2 years but can occur as early as 6 months or as late as many years after radiation therapy is completed. Scarring of normal tissues can lead to severe radiation fibrosis. The rare development of a second primary cancer after radiation for cervical cancer was reported by Kleinerman et al. from 13 population-based European registries. With 30 years of survival, there was approximately a doubling of risk of a new primary in an irradiated pelvic organ, including ovary and bladder, as well as the vagina and vulva.

The treatment of radiation complications depends on the symptoms and site of the complication. Vaginal or cervical ulcerations occasionally occur, and local treatment with topical antibiotics and estrogen creams is usually satisfactory. Postradiation cystitis may manifest itself as urinary frequency or dysuria. After infection has been ruled out, symptomatic treatment is undertaken with drugs such as antispasmodics or urinary analgesics (e.g., phenazopyridine [Pyridium], 100 mg three times daily), and these are prescribed until the symptoms clear. Occasionally hemorrhagic cystitis develops and this may require hospitalization for continuous bladder irrigation or instillation of agents to control bleeding, such as silver nitrate or sometimes fulguration of the bleeding points. In cases of hematuria, recurrent tumor should first be ruled out. Periureteral fibrosis can lead to ureteral obstruction and loss of kidney function. McIntyre et al. studied 1784 patients with stage IB carcinomas who were treated by radiation therapy, and found 29 cases of ureteral stenoses, which rose from a frequency of 1% at 5 years to 2.5% at 20 years. While tumor recurrence was the most common cause of early ureteral obstruction, radiation fibrosis can be a rare but occasionally fatal late complication.

Bowel complications tend to be more frequent than urinary complications. Proctosigmoiditis can lead to diarrhea, severe pain on defecation, or gastrointestinal bleeding. Conservative therapy with stool softeners and a low-roughage diet may suffice; occasionally local corticosteroids (Cort enema) are of assistance. Fistulas or rectal ulcerations are occasionally seen in the area adjacent to the tip of the cervix, which is also the area maximally radiated during the local vaginocervical implant. If a fistula develops, or in cases of ulceration or severe bleeding and pain, a diverting colostomy is required. Serious small bowel complications may occur, leading to obstruction, fistula formation, or necrosis. The use of parenteral nutrition and intravenous hyperalimentation has provided an excellent mechanism to help deal with these problems. Follow-up studies by Klee et al. show bladder and bowel symptoms tend to be chronic in some patients but long-term fatigue was also reported. In most patients it regressed in a few months.

The rate of complications also is related to the frequency of cure, especially for high-stage disease. Montana et al. noted a 19.5% complication rate in the therapy of 251 patients with stage II disease, and the risk of complications increased with radiation dose. For example, patients with complications had a mean dose of 7877 cGy to point A, in comparison to 7593 cGy for those without complications. In a follow-up study, the risk of proctitis was also related to increasing doses of external beam treatment. The balancing of the risk of complication with increasing radiation dosage to improve cure rates was further demonstrated by Orton and Wolf-Rosenblum, who studied patients with stages IIB and III carcinoma of the cervix. Higher dosages had been used in persons who survived 5 years, and their complication rate was 21%, in comparison to only 6% for those who did not survive 5 years. Compromise of sexual function due to inelastic vagina and decreased utilization was noted in the studies of Bergmark et al. In a randomized trial of experimental psycho-educational intervention, involving regular vaginal dilation, Robinson et. al. noted reduced fear of sexual activity post treatment in the experimental group.

Adenocarcinomas

The appropriate therapy of adenocarcinoma of the cervix has been debated, and many therapists use the same approaches as have been described for squamous cell carcinoma. Some have suggested that these tumors may be more resistant to radiation than comparable squamous cell carcinomas of the cervix. There are no data from randomized studies, but some data support the impression of a worse prognosis, stage for stage, for adenocarcinoma of the cervix as does the report of Hopkins and Morley. Furthermore, these results suggest that, particularly for low-stage tumor, the combination of operation and radiation is preferable to radiation alone. Patients who are able to receive only radiation do worse, in part because the larger and more extensive tumors are chosen to be radiated. As shown by Weiss and Lucas, larger tumors tend to be poorly differentiated and have a higher frequency of node metastases. Duk et al. reported the tumor marker CA-125, usually used for ovarian carcinoma (Chapter 31), may predict prognosis in cervical adenocarcinoma, since patients with elevated levels had a worse prognosis. Cohn et al. evaluated retrospectively 40 cases of cervical adenocarcinoma. The median survival with stage I disease was 69 months. For patients with positive nodes in this study, chemoradiation (platinum and bleomycin) appeared to improve the results.

Although many authors have reported comparable survival statistics for adenocarcinoma of the cervix following operation alone or radiation alone, the desirability of utilizing a combined modality has been supported in a study of 211 cases of pure or typical adenocarcinoma of the cervix by Moberg et al. in which stage IB or IIA cases were treated by either full radiation alone or partial radiation (two local implants into the cervix and vagina) followed by radical hysterectomy within 3 months. The overall 5-year survival rates for patients with stage IB were 79% and 92%, respectively, and stage IIA, 46% and 67%, respectively, suggesting that a combined radiation and surgical approach may give superior results. For higher stage tumors, the results presented in the prior section for chemoradiation indicate that radiation plus weekly cisplatin is the preferred treatment.

Bulky Stage IB Carcinomas

Bulky tumors of the cervix over 4 to 6 cm in diameter, particularly those of an endocervical location, give rise to a barrel-shaped cervix. Because of the large volume of hypoxic tumor, such lesions are believed to be more resistant to conventional ionizing radiation, which requires oxygen (Chapter 26). This leads to an increased risk of radiation failure and local tumor recurrence. To avoid those risks a combined radiation and surgical approach has been used. Usually 4000 rads at approximately 180 rads per day external therapy is given, followed by an intracavitary implant and in 4 to 6 weeks an extrafascial (class I) hysterectomy is performed. Gallion et al. compared such combined therapy with radiation treatment alone for stage IB barrel-shaped cervical lesions and noted improved results with the combined approach (16% recurrence rate versus 47% for radiation alone). The results of the Gynecologic Oncology Group Study by Keys et al., cited earlier, demonstrated that weekly cisplatin 40 mg/m^2 (6 doses) with external radiation and a single implant to give 55 Gy at point B, followed by extrafascial hysterectomy, gave the best outcome.

Cervical Stump Tumors

Some patients undergo supracervical hysterectomy for nonmalignant disease. Carcinomas that subsequently develop in the cervical stump pose special problems because of the shortness of the cervical canal and absence of the uterus, both of which curtail the effective use of brachytherapy, especially insertion of an intracervical tandem. There is also the risk that bowel adhesions to the apex of the vagina and cervix will increase the chances of radiation complications, and a pretherapy barium study of the small and large bowel may be helpful to identify loops that adhere to the cervical apex. For patients with small stage IB tumors, an operative approach similar to radical hysterectomy can be considered. However, most patients are treated with radiation. External treatment is emphasized because of the difficulty of an optimum intracavitary implant. A transvaginal cone may also be used to supplement external pelvic therapy. Effective treatment of cervical stump carcinoma can be achieved, and an overall 5-year survival rate of 45% in 173 patients was reported by Wolff et al., and 60% for 70 patients reported by Kovalic et al. Stage for stage, the survival rates are comparable to those achieved for invasive carcinoma of the cervix, but because of the prior supracervical hysterectomy, there is an increased risk of complications. Chemoradiation studies of these tumors are not currently available, but based on data already presented, radiation combined with weekly cisplatin appears to be optimal.

Carcinoma of the Cervix Inadvertently Removed at Simple Hysterectomy

Unfortunately the situation occasionally arises in which a patient undergoes simple total hysterectomy and an invasive carcinoma of the cervix is found after operation. Optimum radiation treatment of the cancer is not possible, since the uterus and cervix are no longer present and the receptacle for a tandem for brachytherapy has been removed. The therapist can subsequently perform a radical operation, removing the tissues that would normally be removed at radical hysterectomy, including the regional pelvic nodes. Such an approach has been utilized particularly in younger patients, particularly those with small tumors. A 5-year survival of 89% for 18 patients was reported by Chapman et al. More commonly, however, the patient is treated with radiation therapy. Usually external therapy is initiated and supplemented with local brachytherapy with vaginal colpostats. Heller et al. reported a 5-year survival rate of 70% for 25 patients. Crane and Schneider reported on 18 patients followed for a median of 42 months (2 to 102) with 5-year survival of 93% and local control of 88%. External therapy alone and/or brachytherapy was used. Four patients had gross disease postoperatively. In general, this complication is best treated by chemoradiation, which would be accomplished by previously described cisplatin chemotherapy weekly to give optimal results.

Carcinoma of the Cervix in Pregnancy

Rarely an invasive carcinoma of the cervix is discovered in a pregnant patient. Within each stage, survival statistics are similar in pregnant and nonpregnant women. A concern has been that the delivery of a fetus through a cervix replaced by carcinoma might worsen the prognosis due to tumor dissemination, but there is no clear evidence to indicate that tumor dissemination is caused by the birth process. However, tumor recurrence in episiotomy sites following vaginal delivery has been reported by Cliby et al. The major risk to the patient of delivery through a cervix containing invasive carcinoma is the risk of hemorrhage as a result of tearing of the tumor during cervical dilation and delivery.

A problem arising in pregnancy is whether a patient with an abnormal cytologic smear has intraepithelial neoplasia or invasive cancer. In general, if the cytologic and histologic findings of colposcopically directed biopsies are comparable and suggest intraepithelial neoplasia or carcinoma in situ, the patient is observed and delivered, with final evaluation and therapy completed approximately 6 weeks after delivery, as outlined in Chapter 28. Even if there is a question of microinvasion, a patient so diagnosed in the last trimester of pregnancy is usually followed and evaluated further after delivery. Cervical conization during pregnancy can lead to severe complications, particularly hemorrhage and also loss of the fetus. If it is necessary to perform a conization or preferably a wedge resection of the cervix during pregnancy, it is probably best to perform this during the second trimester, when the risks of fetal loss and hemorrhage are minimal. For patients in whom invasive cancer is diagnosed, a therapeutic plan must be developed to deliver appropriate care, with regard also for the outcome of the pregnancy.

The therapy of carcinoma during pregnancy is influenced by the stage of the disease, the time in pregnancy the cancer is diagnosed, and the beliefs and desires of the patient in terms of initiating therapy that can terminate the pregnancy as opposed to postponing the therapy until fetal viability is achieved. If carcinoma is diagnosed in the first trimester or early in the second trimester (before 20 weeks), treatment may be undertaken immediately because of the concern that a delay could lead to tumor progression or spread. However, Duggan et al. had delays of 2 to 7 months in 8 pregnant patients with stage I disease and demonstrated no adverse effects from the delay. If the patient has resectable tumor (stage IB or early IIA), then effective treatment consists of radical hysterectomy and node dissection (class III). This procedure can usually be carried out without difficulty on a pregnant woman. Increased uterine motility and edema of the pelvic tissue planes help to simplify the procedure for the experienced surgeon, but pregnancy does increase the risk of blood loss. For higher stage tumors therapy is begun with external beam radiation (teletherapy), and usually in 4 to 6 weeks this leads to spontaneous abortion. The dosage of external therapy prescribed varies depending on the stage of the tumor, but approximately 40 to 50 Gy is given. Although the results of a published series are not available, it would appear preferable to augment the radiation with weekly cisplatin, since the pregnancy in this instance would be terminated. Following abortion the uterus involutes, and an implant (brachytherapy) is performed. If the pregnancy does not spontaneously abort, dilation and curettage, prostaglandin-assisted delivery, or rarely hysterotomy may be necessary to empty the uterus before brachytherapy. Alternatively, if the initial tumor was small and has completely regressed, an extrafascial hysterectomy or modified radical hysterectomy may be performed.

For patients beyond the twentieth week of gestation, therapy is often delayed until fetal viability. The health and maturity of the fetus are determined by appropriate ultrasound studies and amniotic fluid analysis to ensure fetal lung maturity. Delivery is usually accomplished by cesarean section, and after this, therapy is completed by operation or radiation with the usual considerations of tumor stage and size. Overall, treatment results in pregnant patients are similar to those in nonpregnant patients, stage for stage, as recently confirmed by van der Vange et al. The reader should be aware that many published studies dealing with carcinoma of the cervix in pregnancy include cases treated as long as 1 year postpartum, which assumes the carcinoma was present during pregnancy. Hacker et al. summarized the results of 1249 cases reported in various series in the literature. Overall, a 5-year survival rate of 49.2% was recorded for pregnant patients, in comparison to 51% for nonpregnant patients treated during the same period of time. Their statistics included not only patients treated during pregnancy but also those treated up to 6 months after delivery, and the postpartum group had the poorest survival statistics. Survival was most closely related to stage, as expected, and persons diagnosed during the first trimester had a better prognosis than those diagnosed during the third trimester.

RECURRENCES

Approximately one third of patients treated for cancer of the cervix will experience tumor recurrence, which is defined as the reappearance of tumor 6 months or more after therapy. Metastases can occur anywhere, but most are in the pelvis (centrally in the vagina or cervix or laterally near the pelvic walls) or less frequently distally in the periaortic nodes, lung, liver, or bone. It should be noted that liver, lung, and distal bone metastases outside the pelvis likely result from hematogenous tumor spread.

The symptoms caused by recurrence depend on the site and extent of metastatic disease. Vaginal discharge and abnormal bleeding are often symptoms of an early central pelvic recurrence. Malaise, loss of appetite, and general symptoms associated with widespread metastatic disease are late manifestations of recurrence. Lateral pelvic recurrences often have a retroperitoneal component, which can lead to sciatic nerve irritation and cause severe pain around the distribution of the sciatic nerve in back of the leg as well as loss of muscle strength causing the patient to walk with a limp. Unilateral leg edema frequently accompanies such metastases, or leg swelling may occur from fibrosis of lymphatics following operation or radiation. In addition, tumor recurrence can also cause ureteral obstruction, leading to unilateral or bilateral compromise of kidney function. Low back pain frequently occurs.

Patients treated for carcinoma of the cervix are examined according to the same schedule as patients with other malignancies: every 3 months the first year, every 4 months the second year, every 6 months from years 3 to 5, and yearly thereafter. More frequent examinations are done if abnormal symptoms or signs develop. Examination consists of vaginal and cervical cytology (Pap smear), as well as complete physical and pelvic examinations. Generally, chest x-ray films are obtained annually, and an IVP or abdominal pelvic CT is also performed annually, particularly during the first 2 years after treatment, when the majority of recurrences will develop. Renal function tests may be indicated, since ureteral fibrosis can occur more than 5 years after the completion of radiation therapy. A blood test for squamous cell carcinoma (SCC) antigen has been studied as a modality to follow patients who have detectable levels of the antigen in their blood. Holloway et al. noted elevated levels in 72 of 153 patients (53%) and found the test useful for following patients who initially had elevated levels. Once recurrent disease is suspected, verification is usually obtained by biopsy of an accessible mass or CT-directed thin-needle aspiration, depending on the location of the tumor recurrence.

Pelvic Recurrences

Approximately half of the recurrences will develop in the pelvis. In addition to clinical assessment and CT, vaginal ultrasound is often useful to document pelvic recurrence. Recurrences of adenocarcinoma are less frequent in the pelvis and are more likely to be at distant sites, such as the lung or supraclavicular areas. For patients who were initially treated by operation, radiation is usually prescribed for pelvic recurrences, and approximately 50 Gy whole pelvic irradiation is given. Supplemental interstitial or intracavitary radiation is also prescribed, depending on the size and location of recurrence in the pelvis. As described previously, chemoradiation is preferably utilized. For patients who were initially treated with radiation who have developed a localized pelvic recurrence, surgical eradication of the tumor should be considered, since further effective radiation is not possible and limited surgical resection of the pelvic recurrence will not lead to a cure but will often cause severe complications of wound healing and intestinal and urinary fistulas. If neither operation nor radiation are feasible alternatives, palliative chemotherapy is considered.

Pelvic Exenteration

Exenterative therapy for central pelvic tumor recurrence is an extensive operative procedure used only if preoperative evaluation suggests that the patient's condition can be cured by this procedure. Exenteration is not performed for palliation. Three types of operation may be used. *Anterior pelvic exenteration* is the removal of the bladder, uterus, cervix, and part or all of the vagina. *Posterior pelvic exenteration* is the removal of the anus and rectum and resection of the uterus, cervix, and all or part of the vagina. *Total exenteration* is combined anteroposterior exenteration to remove all the pelvic contents. Shepherd et al. noted that patients over age 69, those who recurred within 3 years, or who had persistent disease or positive resection margins, had a poorer prognosis for the procedure.

Before an exenterative operation is undertaken, the patient is thoroughly evaluated for any evidence of disease spread outside the pelvis, and if there is any evidence of disease spread, the procedure is not performed. At operation abdominal exploration is carried out to be sure the tumor is resectable. Biopsy specimens of any enlarged lymph nodes or suspicious areas outside the pelvis are taken, and frozen-section studies are performed, including evaluation of the operative margins. Usually total exenteration is performed. The recent introduction of a continent urinary pouch has contributed to patient comfort; the operation is well described by Penalver et al. Generally the urinary stoma is located in the abdomen on the right side and the intestinal stoma on the left side. However, 3 of 39 patients (7%) died of operative complications. The use of intestinal stapling devices sometimes allows preservation of the rectal sphincter and anal function, and avoids a permanent colostomy. Long-term complications are usually ureteral stricture and/or difficulty catheterizing the intestinal reservoir.

Severe postoperative and intraoperative complications can occur with this extensive procedure, and perioperative mortalities as high as 10% to 20% have been reported in the past. Infection and bowel obstruction are the major risks. However, current surgical techniques of preoperative bowel preparation, use of antibiotics, careful intraoperative fluid and volume monitoring, and the use

of parenteral nutrition have reduced the immediate postoperative mortality to less than 5%. The use of a peritoneal graft or an omental flap, created from the right or left side of the omentum and placed in the pelvis to protect the denuded pelvic floor, can help to avoid bowel obstruction, and reduce postoperative morbidity, as noted by Miller et al. Occasionally, gracilis myocutaneous grafts are used both to create a new vagina and to bring a new blood supply to the previously irradiated pelvis, which aids in wound healing. Morley et al. reported a 5-year survival of 61% in 100 patients ages 21 to 74 years. No patients with positive nodes in the operative specimen survived.

Nonpelvic Recurrences

Recurrences outside of the pelvis can be treated with radiation, operation, or chemotherapy. Localized recurrences in areas not previously irradiated are occasionally treated by means of radiation. Resection of the metastasis is rarely done, and it is usually restricted to a localized lesion that occurs 3 to 4 years after primary therapy on the assumption that such a solitary metastasis can be effectively treated with local resection. However, in general, distant metastases are usually manifestations of systemic disease and are not cured with local therapy.

Chemotherapy

Chemotherapy is used as adjuvant treatment for poor-prognosis tumors. For example, to treat small cell carcinoma of the cervix, Morris et al. used cisplatin, doxorubicin, and etoposide in 10 patients, with a median survival of 28 months in 4 of 6 patients who had stage IB disease. The patients survived free of disease for 7 to 60 months after primary chemotherapy followed by radical hysterectomy. A similar approach was also reported with some success by Lewandowski and Copeland. Chemoradiation for this disease has been reported by Hoskins et al. with a 28% 3-year survival in 11 patients. They also used prophylactic cranial irradiation for those patients with small cell carcinoma whose tumors locally responded to treatment.

Chemotherapy is usually prescribed for patients with unresectable pelvic recurrences following radiation therapy or for patients with disseminated metastatic disease. A variety of chemotherapeutic agents, either singly or in combination, have been used to treat recurrent squamous cell carcinoma of the vagina with generally poor results. Part of the problem is that in many of the cases there is often compromise of renal function due to ureteral obstruction or loss of bone marrow due to prior pelvic irradiation that reduces the dosage of chemotherapeutic agent that can be administered. In addition, squamous cell carcinomas in general have proven to be resistant to many chemotherapy programs.

A study by Rose et al. demonstrated partial activity

(12% complete response and 34% partial response) with Taxol 135 to 170 mg/m^2 with cisplatin 75 mg/m^2. The best responses were in tumors that recurred in nonradiated sites. Unfortunately, no truly effective regimen has been reported for this disease.

Advanced Disease

As noted previously, pelvic pain can be a severe problem in patients with recurrent carcinoma of the cervix, especially when there is irritation or invasion of nerve trunks by tumor. This often becomes a particularly serious problem in patients with pelvic recurrence, where back pain and lower limb pain are often severe. Analgesics, including narcotics, are used as needed to control pain. Continuous intravenous infusion of narcotics, such as morphine, is occasionally very helpful. Local nerve blocks are also used, and in selected cases neurosurgical procedures, such as cordotomy (interruption of the lateral spinothalamic tract), provide the patient with excellent pain relief. Unfortunately, the operation also has potential severe side effects, such as bladder atony.

In addition to pain, urinary or intestinal fistulas or obstruction may develop. In certain selected cases this is relieved with an operation to divert the feces or urine, although if possible an operation is avoided in patients with advanced disease. Urinary diversion is generally avoided, since persons who undergo such a diversion frequently have prolonged periods of severe pain from metastatic disease in comparison to patients who do not have diversion and who succumb to uremia. The decision to use an operative approach to provide palliation to these patients depends on their activity status and near-term prognosis. The appropriate management of these difficult therapeutic problems requires sensitive and close interaction among the physician, allied health workers, and the patient and her family.

Sarcomas

Very rare sarcomas of the cervix have been reported. Brand et al. summarized 21 cases of sarcoma botryoides with encouraging results using multiagent chemotherapy followed by operation. A report by Daya and Scully suggests that patients with these tumors may have a better prognosis than those with tumors of similar histology arising in the vagina (Chapter 33).

KEY POINTS

- Carcinomas of the cervix are predominantly squamous cell carcinomas (85% to 90%), and about 10% to 15% are adenocarcinomas.

- Squamous cell carcinomas appear to have a viral and venereal association, particularly with HPV. In the United States squamous cell carcinoma is more frequent in blacks than in whites.

- Cervical carcinoma is the third most frequent malignancy of the lower female genital tract, after endometrial and ovarian cancer, and the second most frequent cause of death, after ovarian cancer.

- The definitive diagnosis of microinvasive carcinoma is established only by means of cervical conization, not biopsy. The margins of the cone should be free of neoplastic epithelium before conservative therapy is undertaken

- Microinvasive carcinoma of the cervix can be effectively treated by total hysterectomy, with a 5-year survival rate of almost 100%, but recurrent neoplasia can develop after 5 years. However, a precise and reliable definition of microinvasion is controversial.

- Prognosis in squamous cell cancer of the cervix is related to tumor stage and lesion volume (size), depth of invasion, and spread to lymph nodes. Older patients tend to have a worse prognosis, and HPV-positive younger patients have a better prognosis.

- The prognosis of adenocarcinoma of the cervix is related to tumor stage, size, grade, and depth of invasion. Large adenocarcinomas tend to be poorly differentiated.

- Metastases to regional pelvic nodes in stage I squamous carcinomas correlate with lesion size, depth of invasion, presence of capillary lymphatic space involvement, and correlate inversely with patient age.

- Cervical carcinomas are locally invasive tumors that spread primarily to the pelvic tissues and then to the pelvic and paraaortic lymph nodes. Less frequently, hematogenous spread to the liver, lung, and bone occurs.

- The risk of the spread of cervical carcinoma to pelvic nodes is about 15% for stage I, 29% for stage II, and 47% for stage III. For the paraaortic nodes, percentages are 6% for stage I, 19% for stage II, and 33% for stage III.

- Stage IB carcinomas of the cervix may be treated equally effectively by radical hysterectomy and pelvic node dissection or radiation. The 5-year survival rate is approximately 80%. If lymph nodes are free of tumor, the 5-year survival rate is approximately 90%, and if the nodes contain metastatic tumor, 50%. Improved overall survival rates have been reported for patients with tumors less than 4 cm in diameter treated by preliminary brachytherapy followed by radical hysterectomy.

- During radical hysterectomy the ureter should never be grasped with surgical instruments so as to avoid damaging the periureteral blood supply.

- Operation is often used for treating stage IB and early stage IIA carcinomas of the cervix, particularly for smaller tumors and for younger patients to preserve their ovarian function. Operation produces less scarring and vaginal fibrosis than does irradiation. Operation is preferred for women with pelvic mass, pelvic infection, or history of conditions such as inflammatory bowel disease, which increase the risk for radiation complications.

- High-stage tumors are treated by chemo-irradiation. Current programs usually utilize cisplatin 40 mg/m^2 weekly during external treatment and with brachytherapy.

- Urinary fistulas follow radical hysterectomy in approximately 1% of cases.

- Most cancers of the cervix are treated by irradiation (teletherapy and brachytherapy). Radiation dosages vary with tumor size and stage but approximate 50 to 65 Gy at point B and 85 Gy at point A. Current practice is to combine radiation with simultaneous chemotherapy to optimize the results.

- Improved cure rates of cervical cancers are obtained with increased dosages, which also lead to an increased frequency of complications. Large increments in dosage may increase complications without increasing cure rates.

- Complications following radiation are related to dosage and volume of tissue treated and include radiation inflammation of the bladder or bowel, which may lead to pain, bleeding, or, infrequently, fistula formation. The normal cervix is resistant to radiation, and the dose can be as high as 200 to 250 Gy over 2 months. The bladder and rectum can be injured at average dosages in the range of 65 to 70 Gy. Overall moderate to severe radiation complications for treatment of all stages approximate 10%.

- Radiation complications of the intestine are more frequent than bladder complications. Both tend to occur more than 1 year after therapy.

- Worldwide 5-year survival rates reported for patients with carcinomas of the cervix are as follows: stage Ia, 95%; stage Ib, 80%; stage II, 64%; stage III, 38%; and stage IV, 14%.

- Pregnancy does not adversely affect the survival rate for women with carcinoma of the cervix, stage for stage.

- Approximately one third of patients treated for cervical carcinoma develop tumor recurrence, and about half of these recurrences are located in the pelvis and most occur within 2 years.

- Patients whose recurrences occur more than 3 years after primary therapy have a better prognosis than those with earlier recurrence.

- Pelvic exenteration in carefully selected patients with central pelvic recurrence can lead to a 5-year survival of 50% or better.

- Chemotherapy of recurrent squamous cell carcinoma of the cervix does not produce long-term cures, but response rates of approximately 50% (partial and complete) have been obtained with multiple-agent regimens that contain cisplatin.

- Leg pain following the distribution of the sciatic nerve or unilateral leg swelling is often an indication of pelvic recurrence of carcinoma of the cervix.

BIBLIOGRAPHY

Abell MR and Ramirez JA: Sarcomas and carcinosarcomas of the uterine cervix, Cancer 31:1176, 1973.

Alvarez RD, Soong S-J, Kinney WK, et al: Identification of prognostic factors and risk groups in patients found to have nodal metastasis at the time of radical hysterectomy for early-stage squamous cell carcinoma of the cervix, Gynecol Oncol 35:130, 1989.

Angioli R, Estape R, Cantuaria G, et al: Urinary complications of Miami pouch: trend of conservative management, Am J Obstet Gynecol 179:343, 1998.

Anton-Culver H, Bloss JD, Bringman D, et al: Comparison of adenocarcinoma and squamous cell carcinoma of the uterine cervix: a population-based epidemiologic study, Am J Obstet Gynecol 166:1507, 1992.

Balderson K, Tewari K, Gregory WT, et al: Neuroendocrine small cell uterine cervix cancer in pregnancy: long-term survival following combined therapy, Gynecol Oncol 71:128, 1998.

Berchuk A and Mullin TJ: Cervical adenoid cystic carcinoma associated with ascites, Gynecol Oncol 22:201, 1985.

Berek JS, Hacker NF, Fu YS, et al: Adenocarcinoma of the uterine cervix: histologic variables associated with lymph node metastasis and spread, Obstet Gynecol 65:46, 1985.

Bergmark K, Avall-Lundqvist E, Dickman PW, et al: Vaginal changes and sexuality in women with a history of cervical cancer, N Engl J Med 340:1383, 1999.

Berman ML, Keys H, and Creasman W: Survival and patterns of recurrence in cervical cancer metastatic to periaortic lymph nodes, Gynecol Oncol 19:8, 1984.

Bloss JD, DiSaiia PJ, Mannel RS, et al: Radiation myelitis: a complication of concurrent cisplatin and 5-fluorouracil chemotherapy with extended field radiotherapy for carcinoma of the uterine cervix, Gynecol Oncol 43:305, 1991.

Bosch FX, Manos MM, Munoz N, et al: Prevalence of human papillomavirus in cervical cancer: a worldwide perspective, J Natl Cancer Inst 87:796, 1995.

Brand E, Berek JS, and Hacker N: Controversies in the management of cervical adenocarcinoma, Obstet Gynecol 71:261, 1988.

Brand E, Berek JS, Nieberg RK, and Hacker NF: Rhabdomyosarcoma of the uterine cervix, Cancer 60:1552, 1987.

Brinton LA, Herrero R, Reeves WC, et al: Risk factors for cervical cancer by histology, Gynecol Oncol 51:301, 1993.

Burghardt E, Baltzer J, Tulusan H, et al: Results of surgical treatment of 1028 cervical cancers studied with volumetry, Cancer 70:648, 1992.

Burghardt E, Ostor A, and Fox H: The new FIGO definition of cervical cancer stage IA: a critique (Editorial), Gynecol Oncol 65:1, 1997.

Calais G, Le Floch O, Chauvet B, et al: Carcinoma of the uterine cervix stage Ib and early stage II: prognostic value of the histological tumor regression after initial brachytherapy, Int J Radiat Oncol Biol Phys 17:1231, 1989.

Chambers SK, Chambers JT, Kier R, et al: Sequelae of lateral ovarian transposition in irradiated cervical cancer patients, Int J Radiat Oncol Biol Phys 20:1305, 1991.

Chapman JA, Mannel RS, Disala PJ, et al: Surgical treatment of unexpected invasive cervical cancer found at total hysterectomy, Obstet Gynecol 80:931, 1992.

Clark BG, Souhami L, Roman TN, et al: Rectal complications in patients with carcinoma of the cervix treated with concomitant cisplatin and external beam irradiation with high dose rate brachytherapy: a dosimetric analysis, Int J Radiat Oncol Biol Phys 28(5):1243, 1994.

Clement PB and Scully RE: Carcinoma of the cervix: histologic types, Semin Oncol 9:251, 1982.

Cliby WA, Dodson MK, and Podratz KC: Cervical cancer complicated by pregnancy: episiotomy site recurrences following vaginal delivery, Obstet Gynecol 84:179, 1994.

Cohn DE, Peters WA III, Muntz HG, et al: Adenocarcinoma of the uterine cervix metastatic to lymph nodes, Am J Obstet Gynecol 178:1131, 1998.

Covens A, Kirby J, Shaw P, et al: Prognostic factors for relapse and pelvic lymph node metastases in early stage I adenocarcinoma of the cervix, Gynecol Oncol 74:423, 1999.

Covens A, Shaw P, Murphy J, et al: Is radical trachelectomy a safe alternative to radical hysterectomy for patients with Stage IA-B carcinoma of the cervix? Cancer 86:2273, 1999.

Crane CH and Schneider BF: Occult carcinoma discovered after simple hysterectomy treated with postoperative radiotherapy, Int J Radiation Oncol Biol 43:1049, 1999.

Creasman WT: New gynecologic cancer staging, Gynecol Oncol 58:157, 1995.

Creasman WT, Zaino RJ, Major FJ, et al: Early invasive carcinoma of the cervix (3 to 5 mm invasion): risk factors and prognosis, Am J Obstet Gynecol 178:62, 1998.

Dattoli MJ, Gretz HF III, Beller U, et al: Analysis of multiple prognostic factors in patients with stage Ib cervical cancer: age as a major determinant, Int J Radiat Oncol Biol Phys 17:41, 1989.

Davidson SE, Symonds RP, Lamont D, and Watson ER: Does adenocarcinoma of uterine cervix have a worse prognosis than squamous carcinoma when treated by radiotherapy? Gynecol Oncol 33:23, 1989.

Daya DA and Scully RE: Sarcoma botryoides of the uterine cervix in young women: a clinicopathological study of 13 cases, Gynecol Oncol 29:290, 1988.

DeBritton RC, Hildesheim A, DeLao SL, et al: Human papillomaviruses and other influences on survival from cervical cancer in Panama, Obstet Gynecol 81:19, 1993.

Delgado G, Bundy BN, Fowler WC, et al: A prospective surgical pathological study of stage I squamous carcinoma of the cervix: a gynecologic oncology group study, Gynecol Oncol 35:314, 1989.

Delgado G, Bundy B, Zaino R, et al: Prospective surgical-pathologic study of disease-free interval in patients with stage IB squamous cell carcinoma of the cervix: a Gynecologic Oncology Group study, Gynecol Oncol 38:352, 1990.

Duggan B, Muderspach LI, Roman LD, et al: Cervical cancer in pregnancy: reporting on planned delay in therapy, Obstet Gynecol 82:598, 1993.

Eifel PJ, Morris M, Wharton JT, and Oswald MJ: The influence of tumor size and morphology on the outcome of patients with FIGO stage IB squamous cell carcinoma of the uterine cervix, Int J Radiation Oncol Biol Phys 29:9, 1994.

Einhorn N, Patek E, and Sjoberg B: Outcome of different treatment modalities in cervix carcinoma stages Ib and IIa: observations in a well-defined Swedish population, Cancer 55:949, 1985.

Fagundes H, Perez CA, Grigsby PW, et al: Distant metastases after irradiation alone in carcinoma of the uterine cervix, Int J Radiat Oncol Biol Phys 24:197, 1992.

Forney JP: The effect of radical hysterectomy on bladder physiology, Am J Obstet Gynecol 138:374, 1980.

Gallion HH, van Nagell JR, Donaldson ES, et al: Combined radiation therapy and extrafascial hysterectomy in the treatment of stage Ib barrel-shaped cervical cancer, Cancer 56:262, 1985.

Greenlee RT, Murray T, Bolen S, and Wingo PA: Cancer Statistics, 2000, CA Cancer J Clin 50:7, 2000.

Greer BE, Koh W, Stelzer KJ, et al: Expanded pelvic radiotherapy fields for treatment of local-regionally advanced carcinoma of the cervix, Am J Obstet Gynecol 174:1141, 1996.

Grigsby PW: Rectal complications in patients with carcinoma of the cervix: the concept of a rectal reference dose, Int J Radiat Oncol Biol Phys 28:1271, 1994.

Grogan M, Thomas GM, Melamed I, et al: The importance of hemoglobin levels during radiotherapy for carcinoma of the cervix, Cancer 86:1528, 1999.

Heller PB, Barnhill DR, Mayer AR, et al: Cervical carcinoma found incidentally in a uterus removed for benign indications, Obstet Gynecol 67:187, 1986.

Henriksen E: The lymphatic spread of carcinoma of the cervix and of the body of the uterus, Am J Obstet Gynecol 58:924, 1949.

Higgins GD, Davy M, Roder D, et al: Increased age and mortality associated with cervical carcinomas negative for human papillomavirus RNA, Lancet 338:910, 1991.

Hirai Y, Takeshima N, Haga A, et al: A clinicopathologic study of adenoma malignum of the uterine cervix, Gynecol Oncol 70:219, 1998.

Holloway RW, To A, Moradi M, et al: Monitoring the course of cervical carcinoma with the squamous cell carcinoma serum radioimmunoassay, Obstet Gynecol 74:944, 1989.

Hoskins PJ, Wong F, Swenerton KD, et al: Small cell carcinoma of the cervix treated with concurrent radiotherapy, cisplatin, and etoposide, Gynecol Oncol 56:218, 1995.

Inoue T and Morita K: Long-term observation of patients treated by postoperative extended-field irradiation for nodal metastases from cervical carcinoma stages IB, IIA, and IIB, Gynecol Oncol 58:4, 1995.

Inoue T and Morita K: The prognostic significance of number of positive nodes in cervical carcinoma stages Ib, IIa, and IIb, Cancer 65:1923, 1990.

Kaspar HG, Dinh TV, Doherty MG, et al: Clinical implication of tumor volume measurement in stage I adenocarcinoma of the cervix, Obstet Gynecol 81:296, 1993.

Keys HM, Bundy BN, Stehman FB, et al: Cisplatin, radiation, and adjuvant hysterectomy compared with radiation and adjuvant hysterectomy for bulky stage IB cervical carcinoma, N Engl J Med 340:1154, 1999.

King LA, Talledo OE, Gallup DG, et al: Adenoid cystic carcinoma of the cervix in women under age 40, Gynecol Oncol 32:26, 1989.

Kinney WK, Alvarez RD, Reid GC, et al: Value of adjuvant whole-pelvis irradiation after Wertheim hysterectomy for early-stage squamous carcinoma of the cervix with pelvic nodal metastasis: a matched-control study, Gynecol Oncol 34:258, 1989.

Klee M, Thranov I, and Machin D: The patients' perspective on physical symptoms after radiotherapy for cervical cancer, Gynecol Oncol 76:14, 2000.

Kleine W, Rau K, Schwoeorer D, et al: Prognosis of the adenocarcinoma of the cervix uteri: a comparative study, Gynecol Oncol 35:145, 1989.

Kleinerman RA, Boice JD, Storm HH, et al: Second primary cancer after treatment for cervical cancer, Cancer 76:442, 1995.

Kolstad P: Follow-up study of 232 patients with stage Ia1 and 411 patients with stage Ia2 squamous cell carcinoma of the cervix (microinvasive carcinoma), Gynecol Oncol 33:265, 1989.

Kovalic JJ, Grigsby PW, Perez CA, et al: Cervical stump carcinoma, Int J Radiat Oncol Biol Phys 20:933, 1991.

Lagasse LD, Creasman WT, and Shingleton HM: Results and complications of operative staging in cervical cancer: experience of the Gynecologic Oncology Group, Gynecol Oncol 9:90, 1980.

Larsen NS: Invasive cancer rising in young white females, J Natl Cancer Inst 86:6, 1994.

Leminen A, Paavonen J, Forss M, et al: Adenocarcinoma of the uterine cervix, Cancer 65:53, 1990.

Lewandowski GS and Copeland LJ: A potential role for intensive chemotherapy in the treatment of small cell neuroendocrine tumors of the cervix, Gynecol Oncol 48:127, 1993.

Liang C-C, Tseng C-J, and Soong Y-K: The usefulness of cystoscopy in the staging of cervical cancer, Gynecol Oncol 76:200, 2000.

Lohe KJ, Burghardt E, Hillemanns HG, et al: Early squamous cell carcinoma of the uterine cervix. II. Clinical results of a cooperative study in the management of 419 patients with early stromal invasion and microcarcinoma, Gynecol Oncol 6:31, 1978.

Low JA, Mauger GM, and Carmichael JA: The effect of Wertheim hysterectomy on bladder and urethral function, Am J Obstet Gynecol 139:826, 1981.

Magrina JF, Goodrich MA, Lidner TK, et al: Modified radical hysterectomy in the treatment of early squamous cervical cancer, Gynecol Oncol 72:183, 1999.

McGowan L, Young RH, and Scully RE: Peutz-Jeghers syndrome with "adenoma malignum" of the cervix, Gynecol Oncol 10:125, 1980.

McIntyre JF, Eifel PJ, Levenback C, et al: Ureteral stricture as a late complication of radiotherapy for stage Ib carcinoma of the uterine cervix, Cancer 75:836, 1995.

McKelvey JL and Goodlin RR: Adenoma malignum of the cervix: a cancer of deceptively innocent histological pattern, Cancer 16:549, 1963.

Miller B, Morris M, Gershenson DM, et al: Intestinal fistulae formation following pelvic exenteration: a review of the University of Texas MD Anderson Cancer Center experience, 1957-1990, Gynecol Oncol 56:207, 1995.

Monk BJ, Cha DS, Walker JL, et al: Extent of disease as an indication for pelvic radiation following radical hysterectomy and bilateral pelvic lymph node dissection in the treatment of stage Ib and IIa cervical carcinoma, Gynecol Oncol 54:4, 1994.

Montana GS and Fowler WC: Carcinoma of the cervix: analysis of bladder and rectal radiation dose and complications, Int J Radiat Oncol Biol Phys 16:95, 1989.

Montz FJ, Holschneider CH, Solh S, et al: Small bowel obstruction following radical hysterectomy: risk factors, incidence, and operative findings, Gynecol Oncol 53:114, 1994.

Morley GW, Hopkins MP, Lindenauer SM, and Roberts JA: Pelvic exenteration, University of Michigan: 100 patients at 5 years, Obstet Gynecol 74:934, 1989.

Morris M, Eifel P, Lu J, et al: Pelvic radiation with concurrent chemotherapy compared with pelvic and para-aortic radiation for high risk cervical cancer, N Engl J Med 340:1137, 1999.

Morris M, Gershenson DM, Eifel P, et al: Treatment of small cell carcinoma of the cervix with cisplatin, doxorubicin, and etoposide, Gynecol Oncol 47:62, 1992.

Morris M, Mitchell MF, Silva EG, et al: Cervical conization as definitive therapy for early invasive squamous carcinoma of the cervix, Gynecol Oncol 51:193, 1993.

Mundt AJ, Connel PP, Campbell T, et al: Race and clinical outcome in patients with carcinoma of the uterine cervix treated with radiation therapy, Gynecol Oncol 71:151, 1998.

Nash JD, Burke TW, Woodward JE, et al: Diagnosis of recurrent gynecologic malignancy with fine-needle aspiration cytology, Obstet Gynecol 71:333, 1988.

Orton CG and Wolf-Rosenblum S: Dose dependence of complication rates in cervix cancer radiotherapy, Int J Radiat Oncol Biol Phys 12:37, 1986.

Östor AG: Studies on 200 cases of early squamous cell carcinoma of the cervix, Int J Gynecol Pathol 12:193, 1993.

Östor AG: Early invasive adenocarcinoma of the uterine cervix, Int J Gynecol Pathol 19:29, 2000.

Östor AG and Rome RM: Micro-invasive squamous cell carcinoma of the cervix: a clinico-pathologic study of 200 cases with long-term follow-up, Int J Gynecol Cancer 4:257, 1994.

Pecorelli S, Creasman WT, Pettersson F, et al: FIGO annual report on the results of treatment in gynaecological cancer, vol. 23. Milano, Italy, International Federation of Gynecology and Obstetrics, J Epidemiol Biostatistics, 3(1), 1998.

Penalver MA, Bejany DE, Averette HE, et al: Continent urinary diversion in gynecologic oncology, Gynecol Oncol 34:274, 1989.

Penalver M, Donato D, Sevin B, et al: Complications of the Ileocolonic Continent Urinary Reservoir (Miami Pouch), Gynecol Oncol 52:360, 1994.

Piver MS, Rutledge F, and Smith JR: Five classes of extended hysterectomy for women with cervical cancer, Obstet Gynecol 44:265, 1974.

Plentl AA and Friedman EA: Lymphatic system of the female genitalia, Philadelphia, 1971, WB Saunders Co.

Potter ME, Alvarez RD, Shingleton HM, et al: Early invasive cervical cancer with pelvic lymph node involvement: to complete or not to complete radical hysterectomy? Gynecol Oncol 37:78, 1990.

Reich O, Tamussino K, Lahousen M, et al: Clear cell carcinoma of the uterine cervix: pathology and prognosis in surgically treated stage IB-IIB disease in women not exposed in utero to diethylstilbestrol, Gynecol Oncol 76:331, 2000.

Riou G, Barrois M, Le MG, et al: C-*myc* proto-oncogene expression and prognosis in early carcinoma of the uterine cervix, Lancet April 1987, p 761.

Robinson JW, Faris PD, and Scott CB: Psychoeducational group increases vaginal dilation for younger women and reduces sexual fears for women of all ages with gynecologic carcinoma treated with radiotherapy, Int J Radiat Oncol Biol Phys 44:497, 1999.

Rose PG, Blessing JA, Gershenson DM, and McGehee R: Paclitaxel and cisplatin as first-line therapy in recurrent or advanced squamous cell carcinoma of the cervix: a Gynecologic Oncology Group Study, J Clin Oncol 17:2676, 1999.

Rose PG, Bundy BN, Watkins EB, et al: Concurrent cisplatin-based radiotherapy and chemotherapy for locally advanced cervical cancer, N Engl J Med 340:1144, 1999.

Rotman M, Pajak TF, Choi K, et al: Prophylactic extended-field irradiation of para-aortic lymph nodes in stages IIb and bulky Ib and IIa cervical carcinoma, JAMA 274:387, 1995.

Rotmensch J, Rosenshein NB, and Woodruff JD: Cervical sarcoma: a review, Obstet Gynecol Surv 38:456, 1983.

Rotmensch J, Waggoner SE, and Quiet C: Ultrasound guidance for placement of difficult intracavitary implants, Gynecol Oncology 54:159, 1994.

Runowicz CD, Wadler S, Rodriguez-Rodriguez L, et al: Concomitant cisplatin and radiotherapy in locally advanced cervical carcinoma, Gynecol Oncol 34:395, 1989.

Sagal S, Kuzumaki N, Hisada T, et al: Ras oncogene expression and prognosis of invasive squamous cell carcinoma of the uterine cervix, Cancer 63:1577, 1989.

Sardi J, Sananes C, Giaroli A, et al: Results of a prospective randomized trial with neoadjuvant chemotherapy in stage Ib bulky, squamous carcinoma of the cervix, Gynecol Oncol 49:156, 1993.

Sarkaria JN, Petereit DG, Stitt JA, et al: A comparison of the efficacy and complication rates of low dose-rate versus high dose-rate brachytherapy in the treatment of uterine cervical carcinoma, Int J Radiat Oncol Biol Phys 30:75, 1994.

Sedlis A, Bundy BN, Rotman MZ, et al: A randomized trial of pelvic radiation therapy versus no further therapy in selected patients with stage IB carcinoma of the cervix after radical hysterectomy and pelvic lymphadenectomy: a Gynecologic Oncology Group Study, Gynecol Oncol 73:177, 1999.

Shepherd JH, Ngan HYS, Neven P, et al: Multivariate analysis of factors affecting survival in pelvic exenteration, Int J Gynecol Cancer 4:361, 1994.

Shepherd JH: Staging announcement FIGO staging of gynecologic cancers: cervical and vulva, Int J Gynecol Cancer 5:319, 1995.

Soisson AP, Soper JT, Clarke-Pearson DL, et al: Adjuvant radiotherapy following radical hysterectomy for patients with stage Ib and IIa cervical cancer, Gynecol Oncol 37:390, 1990.

Sorosky JI, Squatrito R, Ndubisi BU, et al: Stage 1 squamous cell cervical carcinoma in pregnancy: planned delay in therapy awaiting fetal maturity, Gynecol Oncol 59:207, 1995.

Spirtos NM, Schlaerth JB, Kimball RE, et al: Laparoscopic radical hysterectomy (type III) with aortic and pelvic lymphadenectomy, Am J Obstet Gynecol 174:1763, 1996.

Stock RG, Chen ASJ, Flickinger JC, et al: Node-positive cervical cancer: impact of pelvic irradiation and patterns of failure, Int J Radiat Oncol Biol Phys 31:31, 1995.

U.S. Department of Health and Human Services. Ries ALG, Miller BA, Hankey BF, et al: SEER Cancer Statistics Review, 1973-1991, 136-144, 1994.

Van der Vange N, Weverling GJ, Ketting BW, et al: The prognosis of cervical cancer associated with pregnancy: a matched cohort study, Obstet Gynecol 85:1022, 1995.

van Nagell JR, Maruyama Y, Donaldson ES, et al: Phase II clinical trial using californium 252 fast neutron brachytherapy, external pelvic radiation and extrafascial hysterectomy in the treatment of bulky, barrel-shaped stage Ib cervical cancer, Cancer 57:1918, 1986.

van Nagell JR, Powell DE, Gallion HH, et al: Small cell carcinoma of the uterine cervix, Cancer 62:1586, 1988.

Varia MA, Bundy BN, Deppe G, et al: Cervical carcinoma metastatic to para-aortic nodes: extended field radiation therapy with concomitant 5-fluorouracil and cisplatin chemotherapy: a Gynecologic Oncology Group Study, Int J Radiat Oncol Biol Phys 42:1015, 1998.

Vasilev SA and Schlaerth JB: Scalene lymph node sampling in cervical carcinoma: a reappraisal, Gynecol Oncol 37:120, 1990.

Vigliotti AP, Wen B, Hussey DH, et al: Extended field irradiation for carcinoma of the uterine cervix with positive periaortic nodes, Int J Radiat Oncol Biol Phys 23:501, 1992.

Westby M and Asmussen M: Anatomical and functional changes in the lower urinary tract after radical hysterectomy with lymph node dissection as studied by dynamic urethrocystography in simultaneous urethrocystometrics, Gynecol Oncol 21:261, 1985.

Wolff JP, Lacour J, Chassagne D, et al: Cancer of the cervical stump: a study of 173 patients, Obstet Gynecol 39:10, 1972.

CHAPTER

30

Neoplastic Diseases of the Uterus

Endometrial Hyperplasia, Endometrial Carcinoma, Sarcoma: Diagnosis and Management

KEY TERMS AND DEFINITIONS

Carcinosarcoma. A term used to describe uterine cancers that contain adenocarcinoma and sarcoma components; also termed malignant mixed müllerian tumor (MMMT). The tumor consists of both adenocarcinoma and sarcomatous elements. Depending on the appearance of the sarcomatous elements, it is designated as a homologous or a heterologous (MMMT).

Clear Cell Endometrial Carcinoma. A virulent form of endometrial carcinoma that histologically is similar to clear cell adenocarcinomas that arise in the ovary, cervix, and vagina.

Endolymphatic Stromal Myosis (ESM). A term that describes a low-grade (<10 mitoses/10 hpf) endometrial stromal sarcoma.

Endometrial Carcinoma Grade. A pathologic classification that describes the degree of differentiation of endometrial carcinoma. G1, well differentiated; G2, intermediate; G3, poorly differentiated.

Endometrial Carcinoma Stage. A classification that describes the extent of spread of endometrial carcinoma:
Stage I: Tumor confined to the uterine corpus.
Stage II: Tumor involving the corpus and cervix.
Stage III: Tumor spreading outside the uterus but confined in the pelvis.
Stage IV: Tumor spreading outside the pelvis or into the mucosa of the bladder or rectum.

Endometrial Hyperplasia. A general term that encompasses a variety of proliferative endometrial patterns. Hyperplasia often occurs with abnormal bleeding during times of anovulation. Unless there is cellular atypia, the hyperplasias are not generally considered to have marked premalignant potential.

Atypical hyperplasia. A variant of endometrial hyperplasia that is premalignant. The glands are often severely crowded and have abnormal outpouchings and there is an abnormal appearance to the epithelial cells of the glands (cytologic atypia). The degree of atypia is occasionally further described as mild, moderate, or severe.

Complex Hyperplasia. A type of endometrial hyperplasia in which the glands are irregular in shape and often close together. Its premalignant potential is low.

Cystic Endometrial Hyperplasia. An older term to describe hyperplasia in which the glands are markedly dilated and lined by relatively uniform epithelial cells without cytologic atypia. It frequently occurs in the perimenopausal period. When many glands are greatly dilated, the term *Swiss-cheese hyperplasia* is sometimes used.

Simple Hyperplasia. A type of endometrial hyperplasia consisting of a proliferation of glands, some of which are dilated, and with abundant stroma.

Heterologous Uterine Sarcoma. A sarcoma consisting of mesenchymal elements foreign to the uterus, that is, chondrosarcoma, osteosarcoma, liposarcoma, and rhabdomyosarcoma.

Homologous Uterine Sarcoma. A sarcoma consisting of mesenchymal elements normally found in the uterus, that is, leiomyosarcoma and endometrial stromal sarcoma.

Leiomyosarcoma. A smooth muscle malignancy with >5 mitoses/10 hpf and bizarre cells with nuclear atypia.

Malignant Mixed Müllerian Tumor (MMMT). (see *carcinosarcoma*)

Serous Endometrial Carcinoma. A virulent form of endometrial carcinoma that histologically resembles papillary serous adenocarcinoma of the ovary.

Endometrial carcinoma is the most common malignancy of the lower female genital tract in the United States. Approximately 36,100 new cases develop in the United States each year, according to recent figures (2000) from the American Cancer Society. This is about 1.3 times the frequency of ovarian cancer and approximately twice the number of new cases of cervical cancer. However, 6500 deaths occurred annually from uterine cancer, slightly more than for cervical cancer and much less than the approximately 14,000 for ovarian cancer. Overall, about 1 woman in 50 in the United States will develop this disease during her life.

This chapter reviews the clinical and pathologic features of endometrial hyperplasias and carcinomas. The factors that contribute to the development of these diseases and the appropriate methods of management are discussed separately. Sarcomas of the uterus and their clinical behavior and therapy are also presented.

EPIDEMIOLOGY

Adenocarcinoma of the endometrium affects women primarily in the perimenopausal and postmenopausal years and is most frequently diagnosed in those between the ages of 50 and 65. However, these cancers can also develop in young women during their reproductive years, and about 5% of the cases are diagnosed in women under 40. Figure 30-1 plots a typical age-incidence curve for cancers of the endometrium according to age. The curve rises sharply after age 45 and peaks between 55 and 69; then there is a gradual decrease.

Atypical endometrial hyperplasia may develop into endometrial carcinoma after unopposed estrogen stimulation of the endometrium. However, there is a second pathway insofar as some endometrial cancers develop without prior hyperplasia and these non–estrogen-related carcinomas tend to be poorly differentiated and are aggressive tumors (see later discussion).

Multiple factors increase the risk of developing endometrial carcinoma (and hyperplasia). Unopposed estrogen stimulation appears to be a primary factor, increasing the risk 4 to 8 times for a woman using estrogens alone for menopausal replacement therapy. The risk increases with higher doses of estrogen (greater than 0.625 mg conjugated estrogens) and more prolonged use but can be markedly reduced with the use of progestin (see Chapter 42). Similarly, combination (progestin-containing) oral contraceptives decrease the risk. As noted by Grimes and Economy, combination oral contraceptives protect against endometrial cancer, with most studies showing a relative risk reduction to about 0.5. The protection begins after 1 year of use and lasts about 15 years after discontinuation. Schlesselman estimates that 8 years of oral contraceptive use in 100,000 women decreases the number of endometrial cancer for those ages 20 to 54 by about 200 cases. However, other conditions leading to long-term estrogen stimulation,

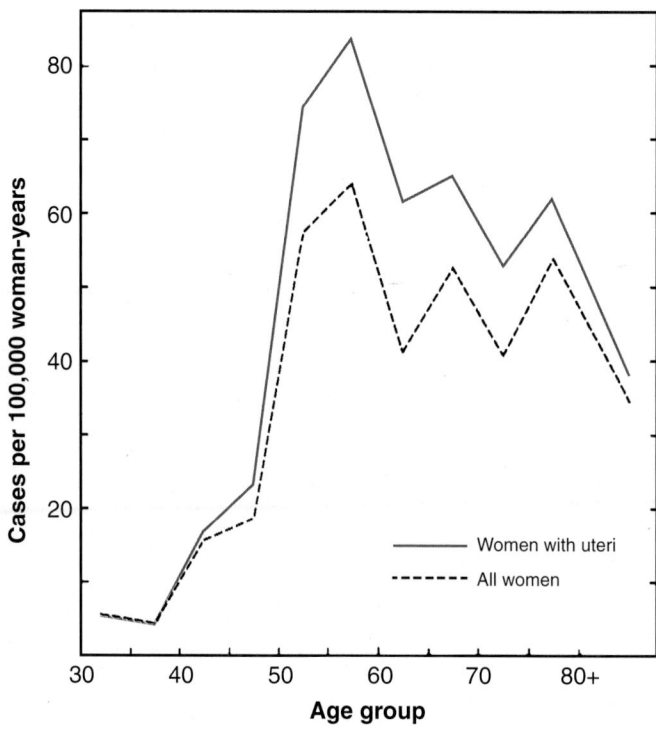

FIGURE 30-1 Incidence curve for carcinoma of the endometrium by age. (From Elwood JM, Cole P, Rothman KJ, and Kaplan SD: J Natl Cancer Inst 59:1055, 1977.)

including the polycystic ovary syndrome (Stein-Leventhal syndrome) and the much more rare feminizing ovarian tumors, are also associated with increased risk of endometrial carcinoma.

Patients with breast cancer who receive the anti-estrogen tamoxifen are also at increased risk of developing endometrial carcinoma. The risk may go up by as much as 6 times, as noted by the population-based study of Rutqvist et al. after 10 years of follow-up. However, Cook et al. did not note any increase in risk for patients who used tamoxifen for less than 2 years. Endometrial hyperplasia and high-grade and well-differentiated tumors have been reported in long-term tamoxifen patients. A recent French case-control study noted a significant increase in risk for those who used tamoxifen for 3 or more years. Bernstein et al. noted those using tamoxifen who are obese and have a history of estrogen replacement therapy warrant close surveillance for endometrial neoplasia.

MacMahon defines three important factors as obesity, nulliparity, and late menopause (over the age of 52 years). The risk for endometrial carcinoma increased 3 times for those overweight by 21 to 50 pounds and 10 times for those more than 50 pounds. Nulliparous women have twice the risk in comparison with those with one child and 3 times in comparison with those with five or more children. Elwood et al. noted that the risk for women whose menopause occurred after age 52 was 2.4 times that for women whose menopause occurred before age 49.

Various other factors have been found or postulated. Diabetes increases the risk by 2.8. Hypertension has frequently been reported to be a risk factor, and many obese patients do have hypertension. Hypertension has not been established as an independent risk factor, nor has prior pelvic irradiation. Regarding racial factors, the incidence of endometrial cancer among white women is approximately twice the rate in black women. Studies of Hill et al. demonstrated that black women tend to develop a much higher percentage of poorly differentiated tumors. The National Cancer Database report by Partridge et al. confirms that patients who are black and have a low income do present at an advanced stage and have a poor survival compared with non-Hispanic whites. The box below summarizes the risk factors for endometrial carcinoma with estimates of the increased relative risk.

Berchuck et al. noted that HER-2/neu oncogene over-expression occurs in about 10% of endometrial carcinomas and correlates with poor survival. In other molecular studies, Pisani et al. noted that overexpression of mutant p53 tumor suppressor gene was a significant independent prognostic factor for poor survival. As noted by Braly, DNA ploidy may also be a useful prognostic marker. Mariani et al. also noted that p53 overexpression predicted advanced disease and poor survival. In addition two other markers, overexpression of M1B and non-diploid DNA content, also predicted poor survival. In this study, overexpression of HER-2/neu did not predict poor survival. Although numerous alterations have been studied, the molecular basis of endometrial carcinoma is not yet defined.

ENDOMETRIAL HYPERPLASIA

The normal morphologic changes that occur in the endometrium during the menstrual cycle are reviewed in Chapter 4. Endometrial hyperplasia occurs during periods of long-term unopposed estrogen stimulation, such as anovulation, particularly around the time of menopause. Normally, perimenopausal bleeding is characterized by "skips and delays." Marked increases in the quantity of menstrual flow or more frequent bleeding can have multiple causes (Chapter 7), including endometrial hyperplasia and occasionally endometrial carcinoma.

Kurman and Norris introduced and studied a new terminology that has been adopted by the World Health Organization to describe endometrial hyperplasias and their premalignant potential. There are two important separate categories: atypical hyperplasia and hyperplasia without atypia. Within these categories, two types are recognized: simple hyperplasia and complex hyperplasia (Table 30-1).

Endometrial Carcinoma Risk Factors

Increases the Risk	Diminishes the Risk
Unopposed estrogen stimulation	Ovulation
Unopposed menopausal estrogen (4–8×) replacement therapy	Progestin therapy
Menopause after 52 years (2.4×)	Combination oral contraceptives
Obesity (3*, 21–50 lb; 10*, over 50 lb)	Menopause prior to 49 years
Nulliparity (2–3×)	Normal weight
Diabetes (2.8×)	Multiparity
Feminizing ovarian tumors	
Polycystic ovarian syndrome	
Tamoxifen therapy for breast cancer (more than 2 years)	

Simple Hyperplasia

This term defines an endometrium with dilated glands that may contain some outpouching and abundant endometrial stroma (Figure 30-2). The term *cystic hyperplasia* has been used to describe dilation of the endometrial glands (Figure 30-3), which often occurs in a hyperplastic endometrium in a menopausal or postmenopausal woman (cystic atrophy). It is also referred to as *Swiss-cheese hyperplasia* and is considered to be weakly premalignant.

Complex Hyperplasia

In this condition, glands are crowded with very little endometrial stroma, and a very complex gland pattern and outpouching formations (Figure 30-4). In traditional terminology this is a variant of adenomatous hyperplasia with moderate to severe degrees of architectural atypia but with no cytologic atypia. These hyperplasias have a low premalignant potential.

Atypical Hyperplasia

This term refers to hyperplasias that contain glands with cytologic atypia, and the degree of cytologic atypia is a major determinant of their premalignant potential. There is an increase in the nuclear/cytoplasmic ratio with irregularity in the size and shape of the nuclei (see Figure 30-5). Atypicality may occur in either simple (atypical simple hyperplasia) or in complex hyperplasia (complex atypical hyperplasia). Complex atypical hyperplasia has the greatest premalignant potential.

The term *carcinoma in situ* may be applied by some when the cytologic atypia is most severe. In addition, eosinophilia of the cytoplasm and intraglandular epithelial bridges are present, but there is insufficient abnormal tissue to warrant the diagnosis of invasive adenocarcinoma. No uniformly accepted criteria exist to distinguish small, well-differentiated endometrial adenocarcinomas from adenocarcinoma in situ, but they usually require similar therapy (see discussion of management). Because there is no uniformly applicable definition for in situ lesions, many pathologists do not apply the term *adenocarcinoma*

TABLE 30-1
Classifications of Endometrial Hyperplasias

World Health Organization

Simple hyperplasia

Complex hyperplasia

Atypical simple hyperplasia

Atypical complex hyperplasia

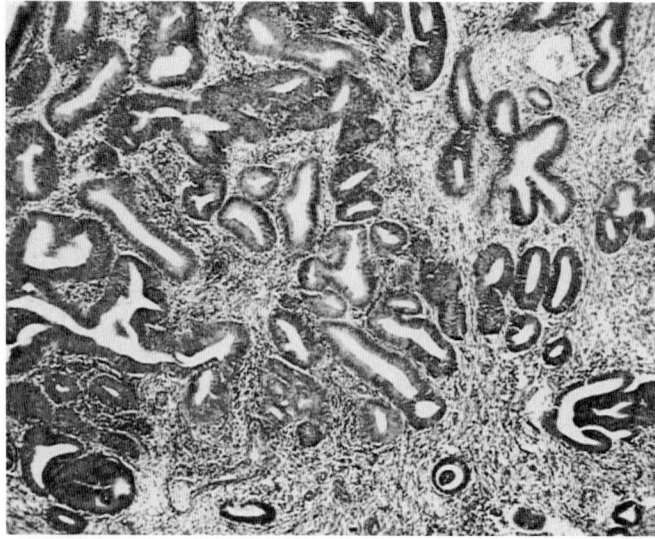

FIGURE 30-2 Benign simple hyperplasia. (From Kurman RJ, Kaminski PF, and Norris HJ: Cancer 56:403, 1985.)

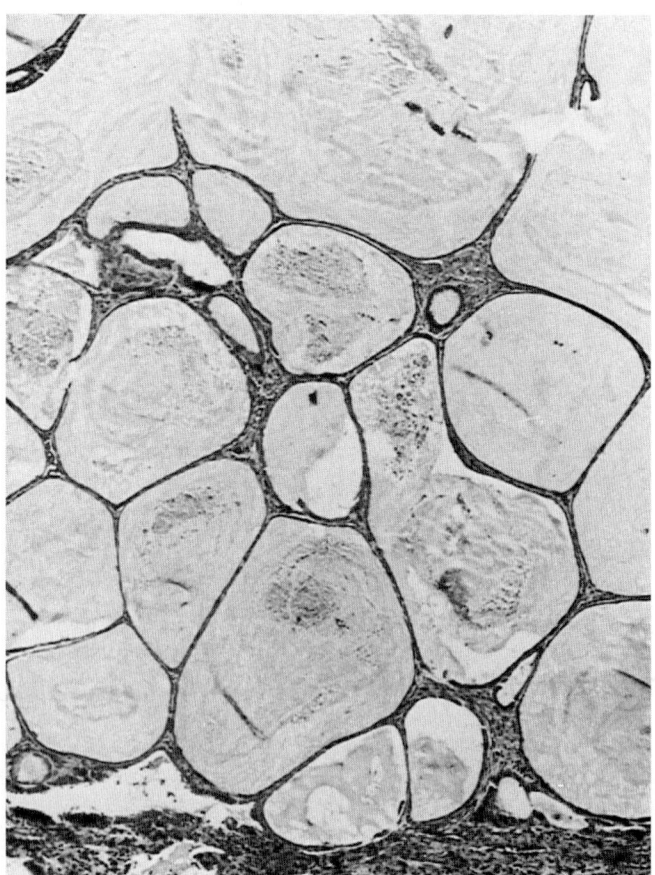

FIGURE 30-3 Cystic (swiss cheese) hyperplasia. (×79.) (From Christopherson WM and Gray LA: Premalignant lesions of the endometrium: endometrial hyperplasia and adenocarcinoma in situ. In Coppleson M, editor: Gynecologic oncology, Edinburgh, 1981, Churchill-Livingstone. Reprinted by permission.)

in situ to endometrial disease but restrict their microscopic diagnosis to hyperplasia or invasive carcinoma.

Other Endometrial Changes

All endometrial hyperplasias may be accompanied by squamous metaplasia, and squamous epithelium can also be seen with endometrial carcinomas. Squamous epithelium is more likely to be seen with the more severely atypical hyperplasias. Occasionally secretory changes are seen with endometrial hyperplasias, usually as a result of progestin therapy or superimposed ovulation. Occasion-

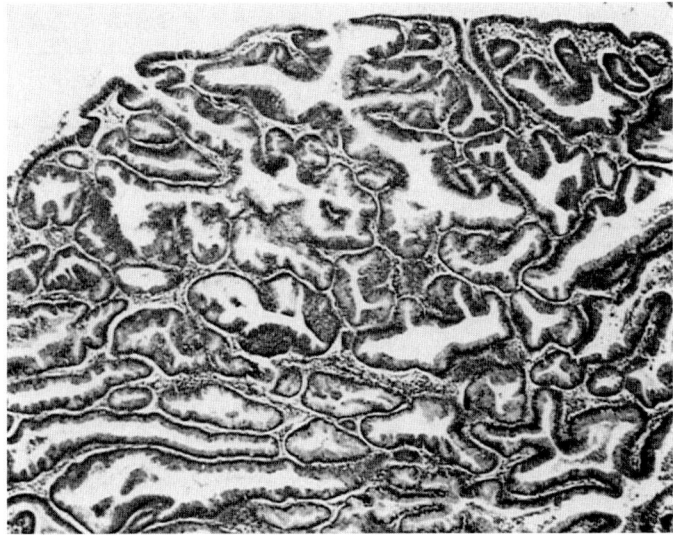

FIGURE 30-4 Complex hyperplasia characterized by crowded back-to-back glands with complex outlines. (From Kurman RJ, Kaminski PF, and Norris HJ: Cancer 56:403, 1985.)

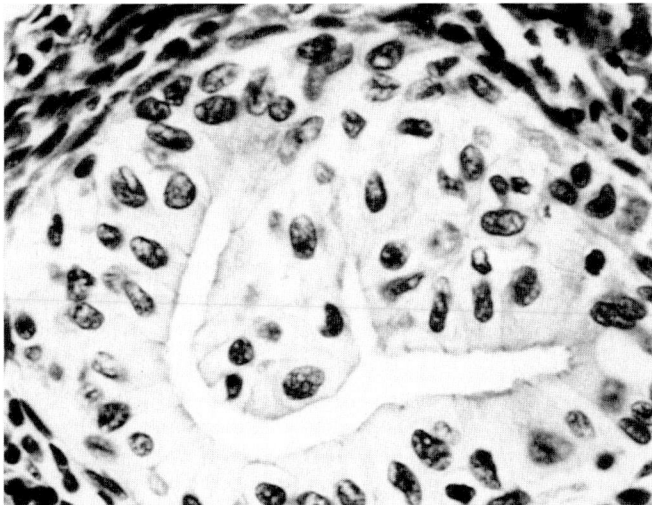

FIGURE 30-5 Severely atypical hyperplasia (complex) of the endometrium with marked irregularity of nuclei. (×720.) (From Welch WR and Scully RE: Hum Pathol 8:503, 1977. Reprinted with permission from WB Saunders Co.)

ally ciliated cells are present resembling the epithelium of the fallopian tube, in which case the term *tubal* or *ciliated metaplasia* is applied. These usually occur in the less severe forms of hyperplasia.

Polyps may also develop in the endometrium and may contain areas of hyperplasia or occasionally even carcinoma. Although polyps frequently coexist with carcinoma, they do not appear to be precursors of endometrial carcinoma. The atypical hyperplasia found in a polyp may appear histologically more severe than that found in nonpolypoid areas of the endometrium.

The clinician must consult directly with the pathologist interpreting the endometrial histologic picture to be certain of the terminology used. The lack of uniform terminology, the fact that the demarcations between various diagnostic categories are not sharply defined, and the presence of multiple patterns in the same endometrial tissue make this communication important.

Natural History

The rate at which endometrial hyperplasia progresses to endometrial carcinoma has not been accurately determined. Studies addressing this area have been retrospective, based on samples obtained from dilation-and-curettage (D&C) specimens at a single institution, and are therefore not necessarily generalizable. Kurman et al. studied 170 patients with endometrial hyperplasia diagnosed by D&C at least 1 year before hysterectomy. Table 30-2 shows the results of their study. Overall, most of the hyperplasias regressed, whereas the atypical hyperplasias had the highest risk for progression to carcinoma. A few patients in each category became pregnant after medical therapy. The atypical endometrial hyperplasias regressed in 15 patients after withdrawal of estrogen therapy. This study provides excellent evidence that many endometrial hyperplasias spontaneously regress and that progression to cancer from atypical lesions may take years.

Diagnosis and Endometrial Sampling

Abnormal vaginal bleeding is the most frequent symptom of endometrial hyperplasia. In younger patients, hyperplasia may develop during anovulatory bleeding and may even be detected after prolonged periods of oligomenorrhea or amenorrhea. It can occur at any time during the reproductive years but is most common with abnormal bleeding in the perimenopausal period, although it also occurs in women taking menopausal estrogen replacement therapy without an accompanying progestin.

Diagnosis may be made from tissue samples obtained during office endometrial sampling or at D&C, usually with hysteroscopy. The office sampling instruments, such as a thin, plastic pipelle, which can provide very accurate information (see Chapter 10), are introduced through the cervical os into the endometrial cavity. Many patients tolerate

TABLE 30-2
Endometrial Hyperplasia Follow-up

Type	Number	Age	(Mean)	Regressed*	Progressed to Carcinoma No. of Cases	Progressed to Carcinoma Mean (Years)	Follow-up (Years)
Simple hyperplasia†	93	17–71	(42)	74 (80%)	1	11	1–26.7 10 pregnancies
Complex hyperplasia‡	29	20–67	(39)	23 (79%)	1	8.3	2–26 3 pregnancies
Atypical hyperplasia	48	20–70	(40)	28 (58%)	11	4.1	1–25 3 pregnancies
Atypical simple hyperplasia	13			9	1		
Atypical complex hyperplasia	35			20	10		

Adapted from Kurman RJ, Kaminski PF, and Norris HJ: Cancer 56:403, 1985, and Kurman RJ and Norris HJ: Endometrial hyperplasia and related cellular changes. In Blaustein's pathology of the female genital tract, ed 4, New York, 1994, Springer-Verlag.

*A total of 34 patients with simple hyperplasia, 7 with complex hyperplasia, and 15 with atypical hyperplasia had no further therapy.

†Benign proliferation of the glands.

‡Greater crowding of glands—no cytologic atypia present.

office endometrial sampling without an analgesic agent, but paracervical block can be an effective anesthetic aid, particularly in nulliparous women or at the time of D&C. Some patients benefit from an oral nonsteroidal antiinflammatory drug (NSAID) taken about 30 minutes before biopsy.

Studies with transvaginal ultrasound suggest that this modality may be of use to detect endometrial abnormalities. Kurjak et al. studied 750 postmenopausal women prior to hysterectomy. None of 35 women with carcinoma had endometrial thickness <5 mm, and 90% had an endometrial thickness >10 mm. Moreover, blood flow studies showed a resistance index of about 0.4 or less for cancer cases but no flow in atrophic cases, as well as in more than 90% of those with hyperplasia. One must be cautious in interpreting endometrial thickness in patients on tamoxifen. Langer et al., in a study of 448 women, found a threshold of 5 mm endometrial thickness had only a 9% predictive value for detecting endometrial abnormalities. Its greater use was eliminating the diagnosis of neoplasia for those with thickness < 5 mm (negative predictive value of 99%). These findings were confirmed in a literature review by Smith-Bindman et al. who found 96% of women with carcinoma had an abnormal ultrasound (endometrial thickness > 5 mm). Conversely 8% of postmenopausal women with an abnormal scan had no histologic abnormality and the percentage grew to 23% for those on hormone replacement therapy.

It would appear that a finding of endometrial thickness < 5 mm is a reasonable predictor of lack of endometrial pathology even in a patient with bleeding. However, persistent bleeding should lead to endometrial sampling regardless of the ultrasound findings. Gull et al. found no cancers or hyperplasias by limiting the thickness of the endometrium to < 4 mm, and this appears to be a useful guideline.

Cecchini et al. biopsied 108 patients on long-term tamoxifen with endometrial thickness >6 mm. One case of hyperplasia and one of carcinoma were found, and most patients had atrophic endometrium. Franchi et al. reported that women taking tamoxifen longer than 27 months with vaginal bleeding and an endometrial thickness over 9 mm were at greater risk for endometrial neoplasia. Among 46 patients who bled, there were 18 cases of polyps, 6 of hyperplasia, and 2 carcinomas. Endometrial thickness is not necessarily a useful guide for biopsy in tamoxifen patients as noted by Love et al., but sampling should be done if the patient experiences bleeding.

As noted, many recent studies on ultrasound evaluation of endometrial thickness in various clinical situations have been published, including a recent study by Omodei et al. Endometrial thickness values for various clinical situations are shown in the box on page 925. These are not rigid values but provide the reader with guidelines as to what may be normal or abnormal. Generally, if the thickness is less than the values shown in the "preferred upper limit" column, the patient will not have endometrial pathology. However, as already noted, abnormal bleeding does require investigation even if the findings are within the upper limits.

Koss et al. studied the endometria of 2586 asymptomatic women, 98% of whom were older than 45 years. Only 16 carcinomas and 17 cases of hyperplasia were detected. They concluded that the endometrial sampling procedure was not cost-effective in asymptomatic women.

Ultrasound Criteria for Endometrial Thickness			
	Thickness Measurement (mm)		
Clinical Status	Mean	Normal Range	Preferred Upper Limit
Premenopause			
Proliferative Phase		4–8	
Secretory Phase		7–14	
Postmenopause			
No HRT		4–8	4–5
HRT, unopposed, sequential	3.6	6–10	8
HRT, combined	3.2	4–8	6
Tamoxifen	7.3	6–10	10

Courtesy Professor Jacque Abramowicz, Department of Obstetrics and Gynecology, University of Chicago.

However a most important conclusion from their study was that endometrial hyperplasia did *not* always precede endometrial carcinoma, indicating two different pathways for carcinoma development. These are, first, endometrial hyperplasia occurring after unopposed estrogen stimulation leading to carcinoma, and second, endometrial adenocarcinoma developing without prior endometrial hyperplasia. These non–estrogen-stimulated cancers tend to be less well differentiated and to have a poorer prognosis.

Endometrial ablation is sometimes undertaken to control severe uterine bleeding (see Chapter 37). However recent reports of endometrial carcinoma developing after this procedure provide evidence that ablation should not be attempted in those with hyperplasia or at high risk for its development.

Management

The therapy employed for endometrial hyperplasia depends on the degree of atypicality of the hyperplasia and the patient's age. In addition, the risk of carcinoma development without atypia from the studies of Kurman is about 2%. Therapy for young women in their 20s and 30s is usually conservative and directed toward preservation of childbearing function. After a D&C, providing no further symptoms develop, a patient with hyperplasia without atypia can simply be managed by long-term follow-up. Kurman's studies showed that most endometrial hyperplasias without cytologic atypia regress. Such lesions include simple and complex hyperplasias and these are frequently removed by D&C alone. Endometrial sampling should be repeated if abnormal bleeding occurs. Usually progestin (Provera), 10 mg daily for 10 days, or an estrogen-progestin combination (oral contraceptives) will induce monthly withdrawal bleeding in young women who are having anovulatory and irregular menstrual bleeding (Figure 30-6, *A*).

Patients with atypical hyperplasia require therapy

even though about half can regress spontaneously. Mild atypia can be treated with a progestin (Provera), 10 mg bid continuously or for 10 to 14 days monthly, or an estrogen-progestin combination oral contraceptive if contraception is desired. Women who desire preservation of childbearing function are treated with high-dose progestin therapy. The patient should remain amenorrheic and should have long-term follow-up and periodic sampling, at least every 6 months (Figure 30-6, *A*). If continuous therapy is stopped, it is advisable in these anovulatory patients to continue at least intermittent progestin to induce endometrial sloughing. Recently Perez-Medina et al. reported regression of atypical endometrial hyperplasia giving continuous progestogen (5 years) with gonadotrophin releasing analog (6 months) in patients desiring to preserve fertility.

Younger patients with chronic anovulation and hyperplasia who desire children may be treated by induction of ovulation with clomiphene citrate (Clomid) (see Chapter 41), especially if the hyperplasia is mildly atypical. Weight reduction for very obese patients is also advised.

For older patients the risk of carcinoma increases. For example, Kurman et al. studied the uterus of patients after curettage had been performed, and atypical hyperplasia was found in the curettings. In their study, 11% of those under age 35, 12% of those 36 to 54, and 28% of those over age 55 with atypical hyperplasia were found to have carcinoma in their uterus. Thus older patients with moderate or severe atypical hyperplasia generally require hysterectomy. In addition, those who fail progestin therapy and especially those with severe cytologic atypia should also be considered for hysterectomy (Figure 30-6, *B*). If hysterectomy is not medically advisable, long-term high-dose progestin therapy can be used (megestrol acetate 40 to 160 mg/day or its equivalent depending on the endometrial response). Periodic sampling (every 6 months) of the endometrium is also performed. High-dose progestin therapy does carry the risk of thrombophlebitis.

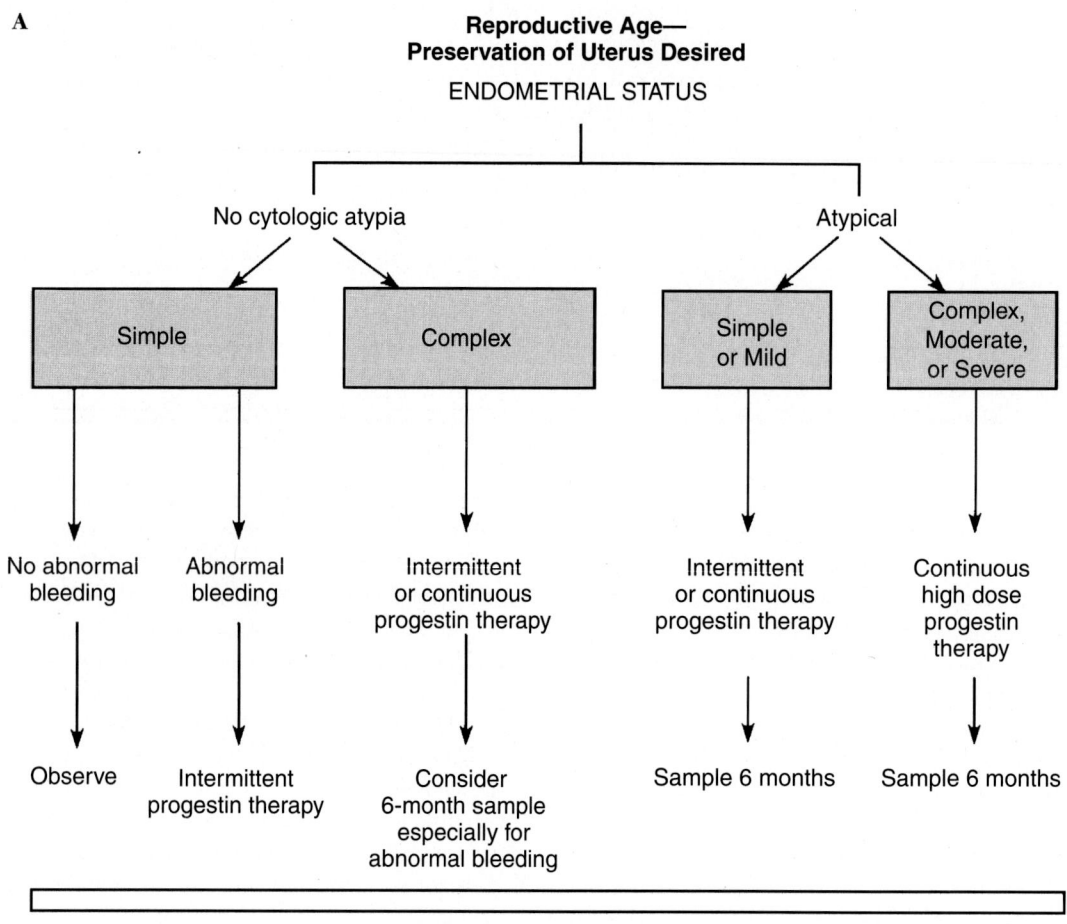

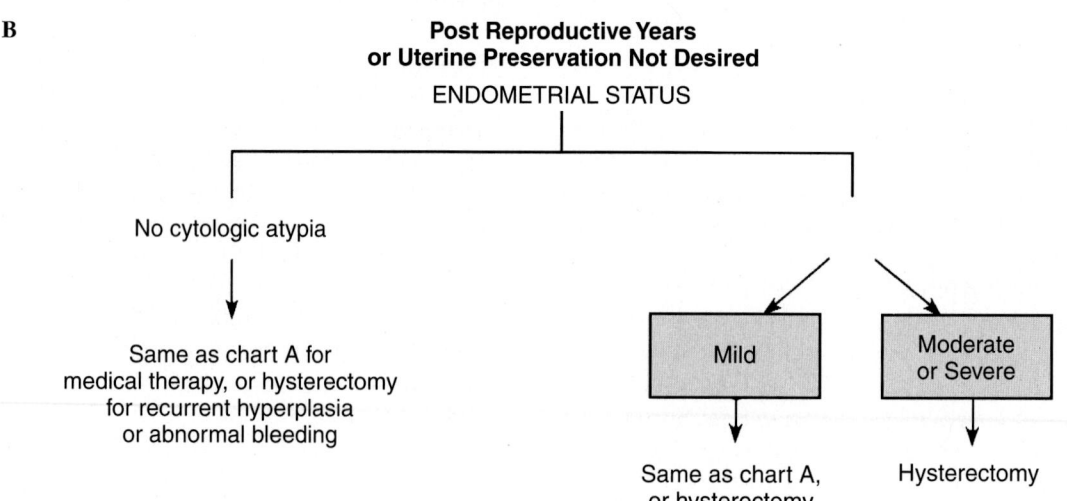

FIGURE 30-6 Schematic diagram for endometrial hyperplasia management for **A,** reproductive and **B,** postreproductive patients.

An alternative approach is depo Provera (depo medroxy-progesterone acetate) 200 mg IM initially followed by 100 mg IM every 2 weeks two times, and 100 mg IM monthly for 6 months. The patient will remain amenorrheic after therapy, but sampling of the endometrium should be performed at 6-month intervals.

Figure 30-6, *A* and *B* displays a flow chart as a guide to the management of endometrial hyperplasia. It is important to emphasize that the diagnoses are not precisely defined, and these proliferative disorders are a continuum from mild abnormalities to malignant change.

Endometrial Primary Adenocarcinomas

Typical endometrioid adenocarcinoma
    Adenocarcinoma with squamous elements*
Clear cell carcinoma
Serous carcinoma
Secretory carcinoma
Mucinous carcinoma
Squamous carcinoma

*Previously termed adenoacanthoma or adenosquamous carcinoma

ENDOMETRIAL CARCINOMA

Symptoms, Signs, and Diagnosis

Postmenopausal bleeding and abnormal perimenopausal bleeding are the primary symptoms of endometrial carcinoma. A routine cytologic examination (Papanicolaou smear) from the exocervix, which screens for cervical neoplasia, detects endometrial carcinoma in only about 50% of the cases.

The diagnosis of endometrial carcinoma is established by histologic examination of the endometrium. Initial diagnosis can frequently be made on an outpatient basis, with an endometrial biopsy. If endometrial carcinoma is found, endocervical curettage is performed to rule out invasion of the endocervix.

If adequate outpatient evaluation cannot be obtained or if the diagnosis or cause of the abnormal bleeding is not clear from the tissue obtained, a fractional D&C, usually with hysteroscopy, or vaginal ultrasound with saline instillation should be performed to rule out intrauterine pathology. The endocervix is first sampled to rule out cervical involvement by endometrial cancer (invasion of the cervical stroma by tumor should be demonstrated), and then a sound is used to determine uterine depth. A complete uterine curettage is then performed.

Histologic Types

Almost all endometrial carcinomas are adenocarcinomas. The various types are listed in the box at the right.

Figure 30-7 illustrates typical adenocarcinomas of the endometrium and demonstrates varying degrees of differentiation (G1, well differentiated; G2, intermediate differentiation; G3, poorly differentiated).

Squamous epithelium commonly coexists with the glandular elements of endometrial carcinoma. Previously the term *adenoacanthoma* was used to describe a well-differentiated tumor and *adenosquamous carcinoma* to describe a poorly differentiated carcinoma with squamous elements. More recently the term *adenocarcinoma with squamous elements* has been used with a description of the degree of differentiation of both the glandular and squa-

mous components. Zaino et al., in a Gynecologic Oncology Group (GOG) study of 456 cases with squamous elements, showed prognosis was related to the grade of the glandular component and the degree of myometrial invasion. They suggested the term *adenocarcinoma with squamous differentiation,* and this has been generally adopted.

Clear cell adenocarcinomas of the endometrium are less common. Histologically they resemble clear cell adenocarcinomas of the ovary, cervix, and vagina. Clear cell tumors tend to develop in postmenopausal women and carry a prognosis much worse than typical endometrial adenocarcinomas. Survival rates of 39% to 55% have been reported, much less than the 65% or better usually recorded for endometrial carcinoma. Abeler and Kjorstad reviewed 97 cases and noted the best prognosis (90%) for those without myometrial invasion. Patients whose tumors had blood vessel invasion experienced a 15% 5-year survival. Carcangiu and Chambers reviewed 29 cases and found 5-year survivals for stages I and II of 72% and 59%, respectively.

Serous carcinomas are also highly virulent and uncommon endometrial carcinomas. Because of a frequent papillary pattern, they are at times termed *uterine papillary serous carcinoma* (UPSC). Histologically they demonstrate epithelial anaplasia and papillary growth (Figure 30-8). These tumors histologically resemble papillary serous carcinomas of the ovary. Goff et al. studied 50 patients with UPSC and found a high rate of extrauterine disease even in cases without myometrial invasion. They recommend a thorough operative staging (see following discussion) in all cases of these tumors because of the high risk of extrauterine disease even in cases admixed with other histologic types. The necessity of a thorough staging laparotomy similar to the operation for ovarian carcinoma (Chapter 31) was emphasized by the recent study of Cirisano et al. both for papillary serous and clear cell endometrial carcinomas. The report of Gitsch et al. suggests supplemental chemotherapy may be effective.

Secretory carcinomas are extremely rare, occurring primarily in premenopausal patients. They are diagnosed in the presence of progestational stimulation, and corpus luteum is frequently detected in the ovary of patients with this tumor. The prognosis is good.

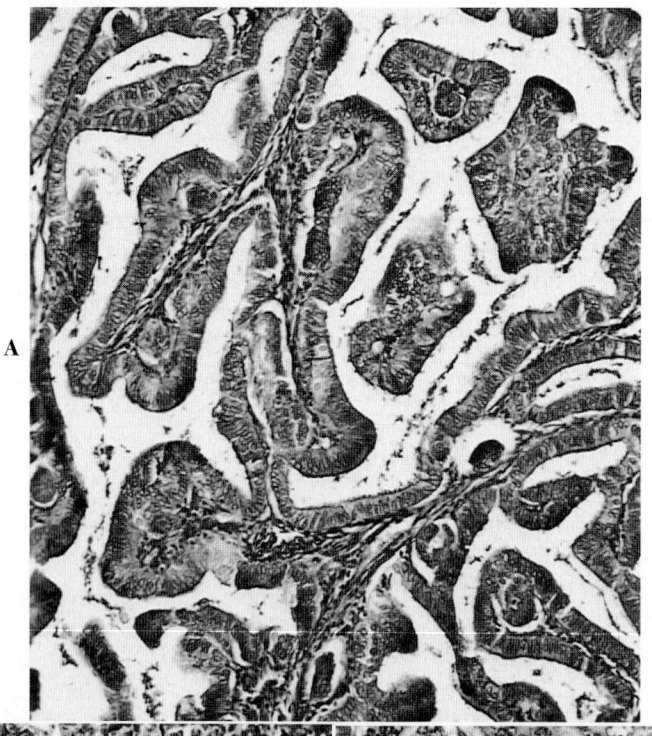

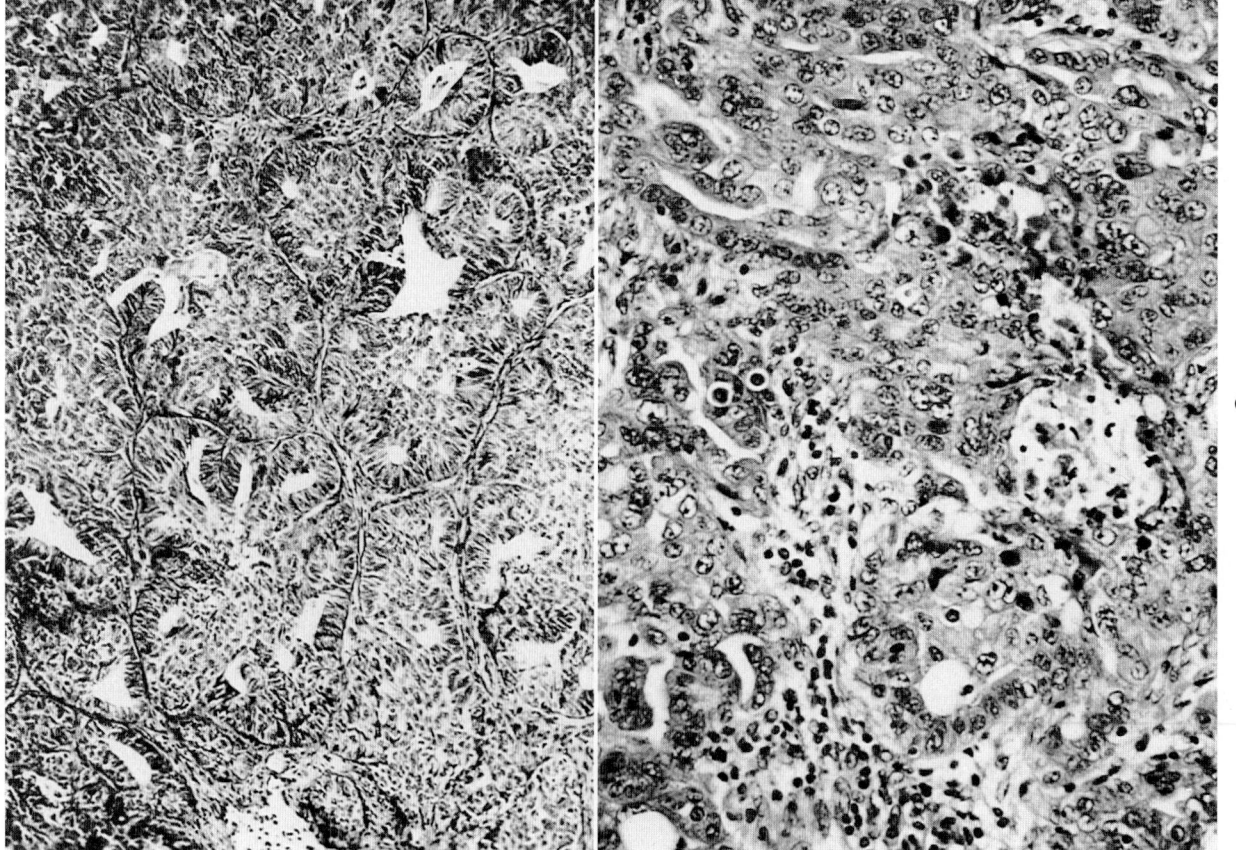

FIGURE 30-7   **A,** Well-differentiated adenocarcinoma of endometrium. The glands are confluent. (×130.) **B,** Moderately differentiated adenocarcinoma of endometrium. The glands are more solid, but some lumens remain. (×100.) **C,** Poorly differentiated adenocarcinoma of endometrium. The epithelium shows solid proliferation with only a rare lumen. (×100.) (From Kurman RJ and Norris HJ: Endometrial neoplasia: hyperplasia and carcinoma. In Blaustein A, editor: Pathology of the female genital tract, ed 2, New York, 1982, Springer-Verlag.)

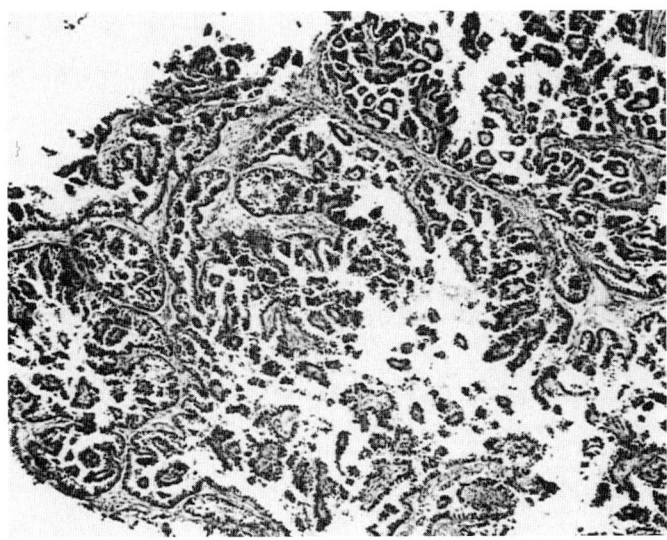

FIGURE 30-8 Serous carcinoma characterized by a complex papillary architecture resembling serous carcinoma of the ovary. (From Kurman RJ: Blaustein's pathology of the female genital tract, ed 3, New York, 1987, Springer-Verlag.)

TABLE 30-3
FIGO Staging Classification of Endometrial Carcinoma (1971–1988)

Stage	Characteristic
I	Confined to corpus
IA	Uterine cavity ≤8 cm
	G1: Well-differentiated tumor
	G2: Moderately differentiated tumor
	G3: Poorly differentiated tumor
IB	Uterine cavity >8 cmG1, G2, or G3
II	Involvement of corpus and cervix
III	Extension outside uterus but not outside true pelvis; may involve bladder or parametrium but not mucosa of bladder or rectum
IV	Extends outside true pelvis or involves mucosa of bladder or rectum

TABLE 30-4
Corpus Cancer Staging (Adopted 1988)

Stages	Characteristic
IA G123	Tumor limited to endometrium
IB G123	Invasion to <½ myometrium
IC G123	Invasion to >½ myometrium
IIA G123	Endocervical glandular involvement only
IIB G123	Cervical stromal invasion
IIIA G123	Tumor invades serosa and/or adnexae, and/or positive peritoneal cytology
IIIB G123	Vaginal metastases
IIIC G123	Metastases to pelvic and/or paraaortic lymph nodes
IVA G123	Tumor invasion of bladder and/or bowel mucosa
IVB	Distant metastases including intraabdominal and/or inguinal lymph node

Mucinous carcinomas are also extremely rare; only a few cases have been reported, primarily in postmenopausal women. They can be confused with primary mucinous carcinomas of the ovary, cervix, or bowel. They appear to have a good prognosis.

Primary squamous cell carcinoma of the endometrium usually occurs in postmenopausal women. Approximately 50 cases have been reported. As noted in the review by Kennedy et al. radiation, chemotherapy, and operation are used in individual cases.

Staging

Tables 30-3 and 30-4 demonstrate the staging classifications of the International Federation of Gynecology and Obstetrics (FIGO) for endometrial carcinoma. Table 30-3 shows the classification in use from 1971 to 1988. In 1988 a new classification was introduced (Table 30-4) that relies on an operative evaluation with particular emphasis on myometrial invasion in stage I. Figure 30-9 displays the various stages of endometrial carcinoma based on the varying degrees of uterine involvement according to the new FIGO system. For patients who are treated primarily with radiation, the older staging system is applied.

Prognostic Factors

Many variables affect the behavior of endometrial adenocarcinomas. These variables can be conveniently divided into clinical and pathologic factors. The clinical determinants are patient age at diagnosis, race, and clinical tumor stage. The pathologic determinants are tumor grade, histologic type, uterine size, depth of myometrial invasion, microscopic involvement of vascular spaces in the uterus by tumor, and spread of tumor outside the uterus to the retroperitoneal lymph nodes, peritoneal cavity, or uterine adnexa. In addition, steroid receptor hormone content affects prognosis, although this is not usually measured clinically.

Clinical Factors

A number of studies have shown that younger women with endometrial carcinoma have an improved prognosis. Older patients have tumors of a higher stage and grade than younger patients. The finding of malignant endometrial cells in routine cervical-vaginal cytology (Pap smear) is a poor prognostic factor. DuBeshter et al. noted that

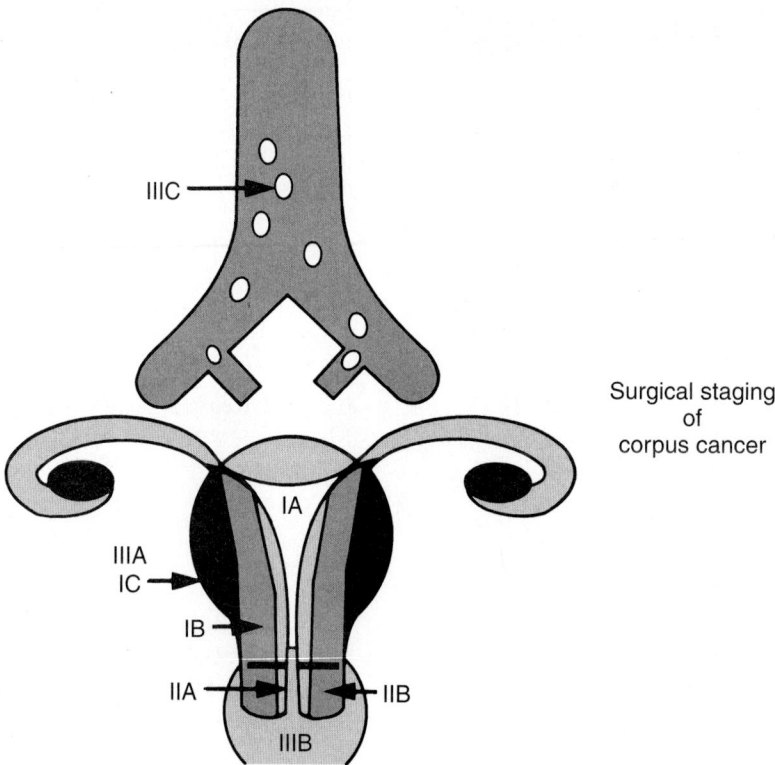

Surgical staging
of
corpus cancer

FIGURE 30-9 Schematic for surgical staging for endometrial carcinoma according to 1988 FIGO definitions (Table 30-4). Courtesy of Dr. James Orr, Watson Clinic, Lakeland, Florida.

among 66 women with suspicious or malignant endometrial cells in their cervical smears, only 2 were stage IA while 24 had a stage III-IV disease (1988 revised FIGO staging). These findings were confirmed in a recent study by Fukada et al., who noted more extensive endometrial carcinomas in those with positive or suspicious cytology. In addition, the findings of histiocytes or lipid-laden cells in a cervical cytologic smear suggest the possibility of endometrial neoplasia.

White patients have a higher survival rate than black patients, a finding partially explained by higher-stage and higher-grade tumors among black women. The 10-year survival of 136 black patients in the series of Aziz et al. was 40%, in comparison with 72% for 135 white patients.

Tumor stage is a well-recognized prognostic factor for endometrial carcinoma (Table 30-5), and the results reflect a combination of clinical and operative staging, since the latter was introduced in 1988, which was the midpoint of the reporting period. Fortunately, most cases are diagnosed in stage I, which provides a favorable prognosis.

Pathologic Factors

The histologic grade of the tumor is a major determinant of prognosis. Endometrial carcinomas are divided into three grades: grade 1, well differentiated; grade 2, intermediate differentiation; and grade 3, poorly differentiated. Figure 30-10 shows the survival of 895 patients studied by

TABLE 30-5
Carcinoma of the Corpus Uteri: Patients Treated in 1990–1992. Survival by FIGO Surgical Stage, n = 5562

Stage	5-Year Survival
IA	90.9%
IB	88.2%
IC	81.0%
II	71.6%
III	51.4%
IV	8.9%

Modified from Pecorelli S, Creasman WT, Pettersson F, et al: FIGO annual report on the results of treatment in gynaecological cancer. Twenty-third volume, Milano, Italy. J Epidemiol Biostat, 1998.

the GOG which relates endometrial carcinoma survival to tumor grade and demonstrates the worsening of prognosis with advancing grade.

The histologic type of the endometrial carcinoma is also related to prognosis, with the best prognosis associated with typical adenocarcinomas, as well as better-differentiated tumors with or without squamous elements, and secretory carcinomas. Approximately 80% of all endome-

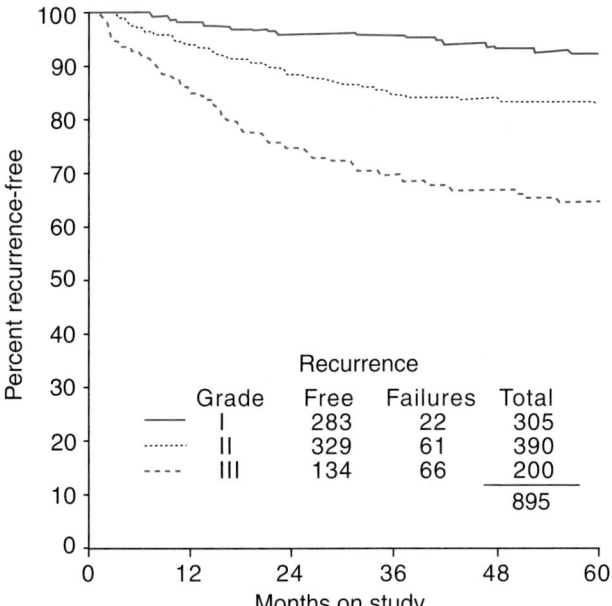

Grade	Recurrence		
	Free	Failures	Total
—— I	283	22	305
······· II	329	61	390
---- III	134	66	200
			895

FIGURE 30-10 Recurrence-free interval by histologic grade. (Redrawn from Morrow CP, Bundy BN, Kurman RJ, et al: Relationship between surgical-pathologic risk factors and outcome in clinical stage I and II carcinoma of the endometrium: a Gynecologic Oncology Group study, Gynecol Oncol 40:55, 1991.)

trial carcinomas fall into the favorable category. Poor prognostic histologic types are papillary serous carcinomas, clear cell carcinomas, and poorly differentiated carcinomas with or without squamous elements, as previously noted.

The degree of myometrial invasion correlates with the risk of tumor spread outside the uterus, but the higher grade and higher stage tumors in general have the deepest myometrial penetration. The importance of tumor grade and myometrial invasion is also illustrated by a study of their relationship to their spread to the retroperitoneal pelvic and paraaortic lymph nodes. Studies of 142 patients by Schink et al. indicate that tumor size is also prognostic. Only 4% of those with tumors ≤2 cm in size had lymph node metastases. The rate increased to 15% for those with tumors >2 cm to 35% when the entire endometrial cavity was involved.

Peritoneal cytology has been studied as a prognostic factor, and the results are conflicting. In a study of 567 surgical stage I cases, Turner et al. found that positive peritoneal cytology was an independent prognostic factor. In contrast, Grimshaw et al. evaluated 322 clinical stage I cases and found that positive peritoneal cytology was an adverse prognostic factor, but they did not find it to be an independent risk factor when other variables were considered. More recently Kadar et al. and Lurain noted that positive peritoneal cytology was associated primarily with adverse features such as extrauterine disease, and that therapy (see following discussion) for positive peritoneal cytology as an isolated finding did not appear to improve survival.

A GOG study of 597 patients with stages I or II disease provides useful information to predict survival. Both clinical and operative stages were analyzed. Table 30-6 and Figure 30-11 demonstrate the results. For example, the values for operative staging from Table 30-6 for a grade 3 serous carcinoma (4.4) with middle one-third myometrial invasion (3.3) gives a total value of 4.4 × 3.3 = 14.52. Figure 30-11 indicates the value of 15 leads to a 5-year survival of approximately 90%. The study confirmed the importance of older age and deeper myometrial invasion and to a lesser extent higher grade and adverse histologic types (serous and clear cell) as worsening the prognosis. However, it provides no information on the effects of therapy insofar as the patients were presumably treated on a number of different protocols at various institutions. Nonetheless the apparent good result for serous tumors in this example is due to the fact that the data are based on operative staging.

PATTERNS OF SPREAD OF ENDOMETRIAL CARCINOMA. Plentl and Friedman noted four major channels of lymphatic drainage from the uterus that serve as sites for extrauterine spread of tumor: (1) a small lymphatic branch along the round ligament that runs to the inguinal femoral nodes, (2) branches from the tubal and (3) ovarian pedicles (infundibulopelvic ligaments), which are large lymphatics that drain into the paraaortic nodes, and (4) the broad ligament lymphatics that drain directly to the pelvic nodes. The pelvic and paraaortic node drainage sites (2, 3, and 4) are the most important clinically. In addition, direct peritoneal spread of tumor can occur through the uterine wall or via the lumen of the fallopian tube. Clinically, therefore, the clinician must assess the retroperitoneal nodes, the peritoneal cavity, and the uterine adnexa for the spread of endometrial carcinoma (Figure 30-12).

Extensive studies by the GOG have elucidated both the frequency of lymph node metastases in endometrial carcinoma and the pathologic factors that modify this risk in stage I disease. Tumor grade, size of the uterus, and degree of myometrial invasion were studied. Table 30-7 illustrates the frequency of lymph node metastases according to uterine size and tumor grade. There are differences in the proportion of positive nodes between stage IB and IA (pre-1988 staging) cases, as well as tumor grade. Table 30-8 shows the effects of tumor grade and depth of myometrial invasion. The frequency of nodal involvement becomes much greater with higher-grade tumors and with greater depth of myometrial invasion. The risk of lymph node involvement appears to be negligible for endometrial carcinoma involving only the endometrium. With invasion of the inner third of the myometrium there is negligible risk of node involvement for grade 1 and grade 2 cases. If the outer third of the myometrium is involved, the risk of nodal metastases is greatly increased. These data emphasize the importance of myometrial invasion and tumor spread providing the basis for FIGO Operative

TABLE 30-6
Surgical Stage I and II Tumors: The Proportional Hazards Modeling of Relative Survival Time

Variable	Regression Coefficient	Relative Risk	Significance Test* (*P* value)
Endometrioid			—
Grade 1	—	1.0	
Grade 2	0.28	1.3	2.7 (0.1)
Grade 3	0.56	1.8	
Clear cell			2.5 (0.1)
Grade 1	1.62	5.1	
Grade 2	1.26	3.5	0.3 (0.6)
Grade 3	0.91	2.5	1.7 (0.2)
Serous			
Grade 1	0.80	2.2	
Grade 2	1.15	3.1	0.7 (0.4)
Grade 3	1.49	4.4	
Endometrioid with squamous differentiation			0.1 (0.7)
Grade 1	0.20	1.2	
Grade 2	−0.01	1.0	0.3 (0.6)
Grade 3	0.22	0.8	
Villoglandular			2.2 (0.1)
Grade 1	−4.91	0.01	
Grade 2	−0.59	0.5	10.4 (0.001)
Grade 3	3.73	41.9	
Myometrial invasion			
Endometrium only	—	1.0	
Superficial	0.39	0.5	
Middle	1.20	3.3	19.6 (0.0002)
Deep	1.53	4.6	
Age	0.17	—	
Age^2	−0.000837	—	20.7 (0.0001)
45 (arbitrary reference)	—	1.0	
55	0.85	2.3	
65	1.52	4.6	
75	2.03	7.6	
Vascular space involvement	0.32	1.4	1.2 (0.3)

Modified from Zaino RJ, Kurman RJ, Diana KL, and Morrow CP: Cancer 77:1115, 1996.

*Wald chi-square test.

P value for grading is for overall grade within cell type.

Staging System. Table 30-9 summarizes the risk of nodal metastases based on the GOG studies published by Creasman et al. In a more recent GOG study cited previously, Morrow et al. noted that for patients without metastases at operation, the greatest risk of future recurrence was grade 3 histology. Furthermore, among 48 patients with histologically documented aortic node metastases, 47 were found to have positive pelvic nodes, adnexal metastases, or tumor invasion to the outer one third of the myometrium, emphasizing the poor prognostic aspects of these three findings.

STEROID HORMONE RECEPTORS. Steroid hormones affect the growth of target cells by binding with steroid receptors in the cell. The receptor steroid complex then interacts with DNA in the cell nucleus, stimulating the synthesis of messenger RNA (mRNA), which acts in the cytoplasm to stimulate protein synthesis.

The steroid receptor level in endometrial carcinoma is lower than in normal endometrium. The highest levels of estrogen and progesterone receptors in tumors have been found in the well-differentiated (grade 1) tumors and the lowest in grade 3 tumors. Vihko et al. noted a correlation between tumor stage and receptor status, with 65% of stage I tumors "receptor positive" and the proportion decreasing for stages II, III, and IV to 50%, 17%, and 0%, respectively. The survival rate within each stage was also better for women with receptor-rich tumors than for those with receptor-negative tumors. Palmer et al. noticed that ER values over 70 fmol/mg and PR values greater than 30 fmol/mg were associated with improved survival.

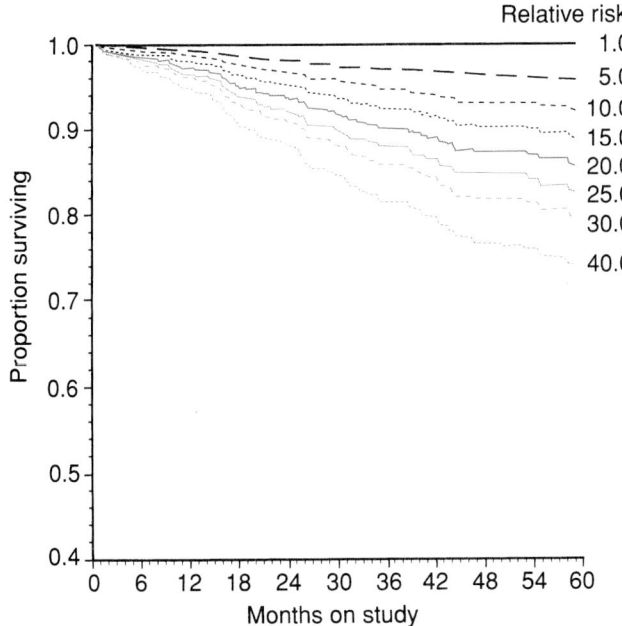

FIGURE 30-11 Predicted survival time by initial tumor relative risk surgical stage I and II patients. (Modified from Zaino RJ et al: Cancer 77:1115, 1996.)

These levels are 2 to 3 times higher than cutoffs used in other studies, some of which have not demonstrated a receptor-survival association. However, Palmer's data and those of others suggest receptor status is an important prognostic parameter. In a study of 309 tumors, Kleine et al. performed a multivariate analysis of survival and found progesterone receptor status, not estrogen receptor status, the most significant prognostic factor after clinical stage. Receptor status appears to influence tumor response to progestational therapy. Despite extensive research in this area, receptor status in endometrial carcinoma does not appear to have the same clinically relevant role as it does in cases of breast carcinoma.

Evaluation

When the patient's disease is diagnosed as adenocarcinoma of the endometrium, fractional D&C or endometrial biopsy and endocervical curettage are usually performed to ascertain tumor grade, uterine size, and cervical involvement and the depth of the uterus is determined.

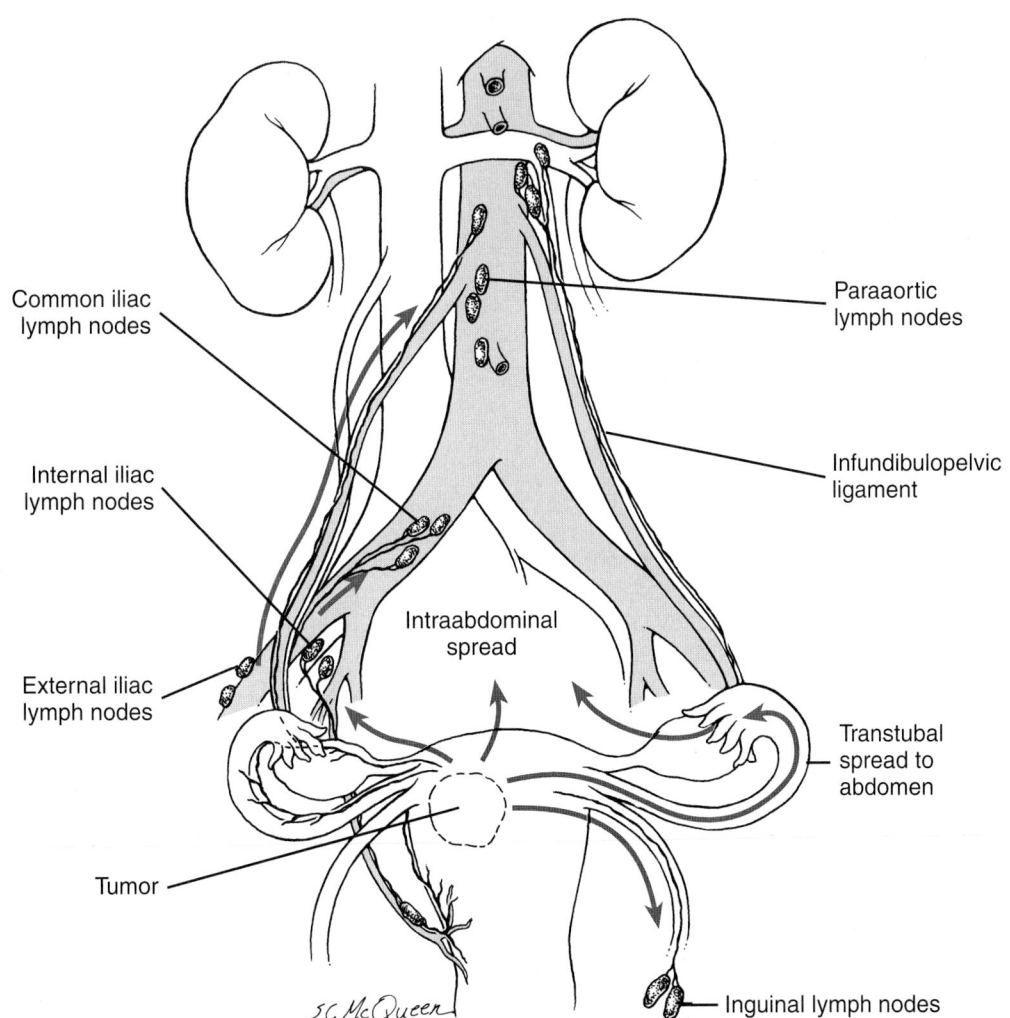

FIGURE 30-12 Spread of endometrial carcinoma. The major pathways of tumor spread are illustrated (see text).

TABLE 30-7
Grade, Depth of Myometrial Invasion, and Node Metastasis—Stage I

| Depth of Invasion | Pelvic | | |
	G1 n = 180	G2 n = 288	G3 n = 153
Endomet. only (n = 86)	0 (0%)	1 (3%)	0 (0%)
Inner (n = 281)	3 (3%)	7 (5%)	5 (9%)
Middle (n = 115)	0 (0%)	6 (9%)	1 (4%)
Deep (n = 139)	2 (11%)	11 (19%)	23 (34%)

| Depth of Invasion | Aortic | | |
	G1 n = 180	G2 n = 288	G3 n = 153
Endomet. only (n = 86)	0 (0%)	1 (3%)	0 (0%)
Inner (n = 281)	1 (1%)	5 (4%)	2 (4%)
Middle (n = 115)	1 (5%)	0 (0%)	0 (0%)
Deep (n = 139)	1 (6%)	8 (14%)	15 (23%)

Adapted from Creasman WT et al: Cancer 60:2035, 1987.

TABLE 30-8
FIGO Staging and Nodal Metastasis

| Staging | Metastasis | |
	Pelvic	Aortic
IA G1 (n = 101)	2 (2%)	0 (0%)
G2 (n = 169)	13 (8%)	6 (4%)
G3 (n = 76)	8 (11%)	5 (7%)
IB G1 (n = 79)	3 (4%)	3 (4%)
G2 (n = 119)	12 (10%)	8 (7%)
G3 (n = 77)	20 (26%)	12 (16%)

From Creasman WT et al: Cancer 60:2035, 1987. Reprinted with permission.

TABLE 30-9
Risk Factors for Nodal Metastases—Stage I

Factor	Pelvic	Aortic

Low Risk
  Grade 1
  Endometrium only
  No intraperitoneal spread
	0/44 (0%)	0/44 (0%)

Moderate Risk
  Grade 2 or 3
  Invasion to middle ⅓
	15/268 (6%)	6/268 (2%)

High Risk Invasion to outer ⅓	21/116 (18%)	17/118 (15%)

Adapted from Creasman WT, Morrow CP, Bundy BN, et al: Cancer 60:2035, 1987.

However, a recent GOG study by Creasman et al. showed that almost one half of those classified as stage II did not have tumor in the cervix, but rather in the lower uterine segment and these thus were in fact stage I. In addition, extrauterine disease was found in about 50% of those with cervical involvement. The risk of extrauterine disease is particularly great for high-grade tumors. In some cases conization may be necessary to define accurately cervical involvement when planning treatment, since microscopic tumor found on endocervical curettage without invasion of the cervical stroma is not conclusive evidence of cervical involvement.

In addition to the usual routine preoperative evaluation, the patient should have a chest x-ray examination, intravenous pyelogram, and/or a chest and abdominal pelvic CT scan. However, a recent study by Connor et al. noted that preoperative CT scan had only a 50% positive predictive value for nodal disease. Furthermore, postoperative CT monitoring did not appear to improve survival. The measurement of antigen CA-125, usually used in cases of ovarian carcinoma, may occasionally be useful. If elevated preoperatively, it usually indicates extrauterine disease. It may be a particularly useful marker for those with serous carcinoma of the endometrium (see recurrences). Cervical cytology may also be helpful, as noted previously. A positive or suspicious smear markedly increases the likelihood of extrauterine disease, and these patients should have a full operative staging procedure (see later). However, as noted recently by DuBeshter, those with a negative Pap smear result are least likely to benefit from a full staging procedure and this test may be as useful as more expensive CT scan in helping to make therapeutic decisions.

Management

Stage I

Both operation and irradiation have been used effectively to treat carcinoma of the endometrium. For patients in satisfactory physical condition, a surgical procedure is the primary treatment modality, with irradiation used as an adjunct. For patients who cannot medically tolerate an operation, irradiation alone can be used. However, irradiation as the sole method of therapy yields inferior results, as Bickenbach et al. noted, with an 87% 5-year survival rate for patients with stage I carcinoma treated by an operation alone, in comparison with a 69% survival rate for those treated with irradiation alone. For those who cannot tolerate operation or external beam therapy, treatment by intracavitary radiation alone offers some benefit. Lehoczky et al. reported on 170 elderly patients treated with brachytherapy alone with uncorrected 5-year survival for stages IA and IB of 46% and 30%, respectively. Sometimes very obese patients are encountered for whom an abdominal operation is very risky. Sood et al. noted that for stage I patients with a preoperative CA-125, < 20 U/ml, the risk of extrauterine disease was only 3%, making vaginal hysterectomy a therapeutic option. Dotters reported CA-125 > 35 U/ml usually predicted extrauterine disease, although about one third of patients needing full operative staging were not identified by an elevated CA-125 for grade 1 or 2 cases while for grade 3, the sensitivity increased to 88%. However, a few false-positive cases were noted, making the results a useful guide but not sufficiently precise to be the sole criterion for performing lymphadenectomy.

Initial operation followed by irradiation, when needed, allows accurate surgical and histologic assessment of (1) tumor spread in the uterus, (2) degree of penetration into the myometrium, and (3) extrauterine spread to retroperitoneal nodes, adnexa, and/or the peritoneal cavity. This is the approach used for cases that are staged according to the 1988 FIGO system (see Table 30-4). Laparoscopic node sampling can be used particularly for patients who are incompletely staged at the time of initial operation.

The operation performed for stage I carcinoma depends on tumor grade determined preoperatively, intraoperative findings, and results of pathologic examination of the removed hysterectomy specimen. The extent of the operative approach is based on the relative risk of disease outside the uterus.

STAGE I, GRADE 1.   The risk of spread of grade 1 tumor to pelvic nodes is extremely small (see Table 30-8). Operatively the abdomen is explored, and peritoneal cytology is obtained, and an extrafascial total abdominal hysterectomy with bilateral salpingo-oophorectomy is performed. Before the hysterectomy, clamps are placed across both fallopian tubes to obtain traction on the uterus and allow its manipulation during surgery. In theory this reduces the risk of dissemination of endometrial tumor cells. Routine sampling of retroperitoneal nodes is not performed in these cases, but any clinically enlarged pelvic or paraaortic lymph nodes are removed for histologic evaluation. The surgical specimen should be opened and a frozen section performed if there is evidence of deep myometrial penetration. Doering et al. have shown that visual inspection of the opened uterus in the operating room accurately determines the depth of invasion confirmed microscopically in 91% of 148 cases. The technique of opening and sampling the uterus with demonstration of the depth of tumor invasion is shown in Figure 30-13, *A* and *B*. If deep penetration is present or if there is a well-differentiated tumor penetrating into the outer one third of the uterus, the tumor could have microscopic areas advanced beyond grade 1, in which case lymph node dissection would be indicated. In contrast, Shim et al. found a good correlation separating depth of myometrial invasion into inner one third and outer two thirds and did not note any difference for tumor grade and similar results were reported by Franchi et al. If the patient has only grade 1 tumor and

the pathologic evaluation shows no deep penetration of the myometrium, the operation is concluded for grade 1 cases.

If peritoneal cytologic sampling shows tumor cells and there is no indication for external irradiation or brachytherapy, 15 mCi of ^{32}P may be given intraperitoneally 2 to 3 weeks postoperatively (Chapter 31). However, the efficacy of ^{32}P in endometrial carcinoma has not been established. If there is deep myometrial invasion to the outer one third, postoperative irradiation delivered via vaginal implant provides a surface dose to the vagina of approximately 5000 to 6000 cGy (50 to 60 Gy) or external pelvic irradiation should be considered particularly if there is tumor penetration close to the peritoneal surface (see later discussion). The combination of external therapy and 15 mCi of ^{32}P can result in serious bowel complications, as noted by Heath et al. It should be noted that laparoscopic-assisted vaginal hysterectomy (LAVH) and pretreatment hysteroscopy both appear to increase the frequency of positive peritoneal cytology according to the recent studies of Sonoda et al. and Zerbe et al.

STAGE I, GRADES 2 AND 3.   Insofar as there is a definite risk of nodal tumor spread for grade 2 and particularly grade 3, the operative approach often includes sampling of the paraaortic and pelvic nodes. This is usually done for grade 3 cases with any invasion of the myometrium and grade 2 cases with invasion of one third to half or more of the myometrium. These are only rough guidelines, and the decision to do a pelvic and paraaortic node sampling is also affected by the degree of operative risk, including the patient's obesity and medical risk factors. Node sampling is usually performed in patients with poor prognostic cell types (clear cell, papillary serous tumors, and undifferentiated tumors). For node sampling, the aorta and iliac vessels are identified and palpated, and any enlarged nodes up to the level of the third portion of the duodenum as it crosses the aorta are identified and removed. If no enlarged nodes are encountered, the retroperitoneal space along the pelvic wall is opened, and the ureters are retracted medially. Usually lymph node tissue over the external iliac vessels and obturator spaces is removed, with particular emphasis on any enlarged nodes identified in this area or along the common iliac artery. The peritoneum over the aorta is incised. The ureter is retracted laterally, as is the inferior mesenteric artery; the lymph node tissue over the anterior part of the aorta and vena cava is removed up to the level of the duodenum (Figure 30-14). However, Chuang et al. in a study of 295 cases from MD Anderson Hospital noted that selective sampling to include biopsy of the paraaortic nodes and also bilateral pelvic nodes were effective in detecting most cases of nodal disease. Mariani et al. reported improved survival in patients at high risk for nodal disease who underwent paraaortic lymphadenectomy in comparison to those who did not have this procedure.

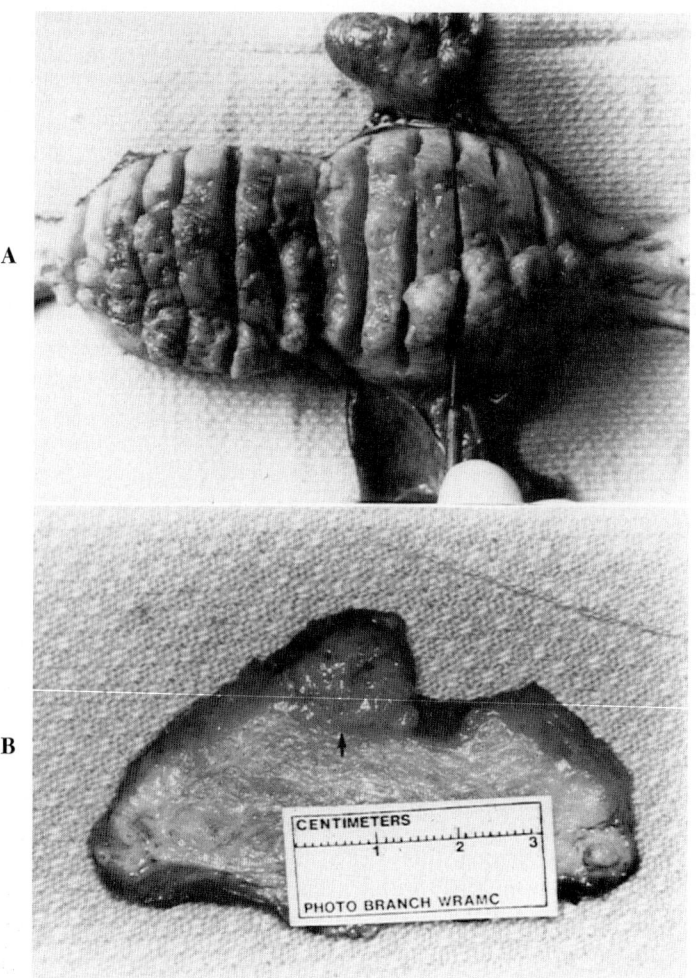

FIGURE 30-13   **A,** Technique for intraoperative assessment of the depth of myometrial invasion. **B,** Cross section of uterine wall demonstrating superficial myometrial invasion. Arrow shows tumor-myometrial junction. (From Doering DL, Barnhill DR, Weiser EB, et al: Obstet Gynecol 74:930, 1989.)

Use of postoperative irradiation depends on the pathologic findings. For grade 2 tumors that invade the myometrium to the middle third or beyond or for grade 3 tumors that invade the myometrium, full pelvic irradiation is usually given in view of the risk of pelvic recurrence. However, if the pelvic nodes are free of tumor, local vaginal irradiation alone may be sufficient. For grade 2 tumors confined to the inner third of the myometrium or grade 3 tumors only in the endometrium, vaginal irradiation is often prescribed. If the nodes are found to contain tumor, external irradiation encompasses the area from which the tumor-bearing node was removed. Recently Mariani et al. noted that for grade 1 or grade 2 cases with surface diameter < 2 cm, myometrial invasion < 50%, and no macroscopic evidence of extrauterine tumor, hysterectomy alone was adequate treatment .

Adnexal spread of tumor is usually managed by external pelvic irradiation, usually extended to include the entire abdomen, since transperitoneal seeding is likely. Some therapists advocate[32]P for cases with positive peritoneal cytology who do not require pelvic irradiation, but the efficacy of such therapy is not proven.

PAPILLARY SEROUS AND CLEAR CELL ENDOMETRIAL ADENOCARCINOMAS   Endometrial carcinomas with a clear cell or papillary serous histology have a poor prognosis and deserve careful and unique therapeutic management. Cirisano et al. showed both of these tumors had more frequent extrauterine disease than poorly differentiated (grade 3) endometrial carcinomas. In addition, there was a lack of correlation with extrauterine disease and myometrial invasion for these histologies leading to the recommendation that all patients with these histologic types have a full staging operation including dissection of retroperitoneal nodes. Geisler et al. further noted that the risk for extensive intraperitoneal spread for papillary serous endometrial carcinoma should lead to the same staging procedure as is done for ovarian carcinoma (Chapter 31). However, Aquino-Parsons et al. noted that if clear cell or papillary features are only noted in the curettage specimen but not in the hysterectomy speci-

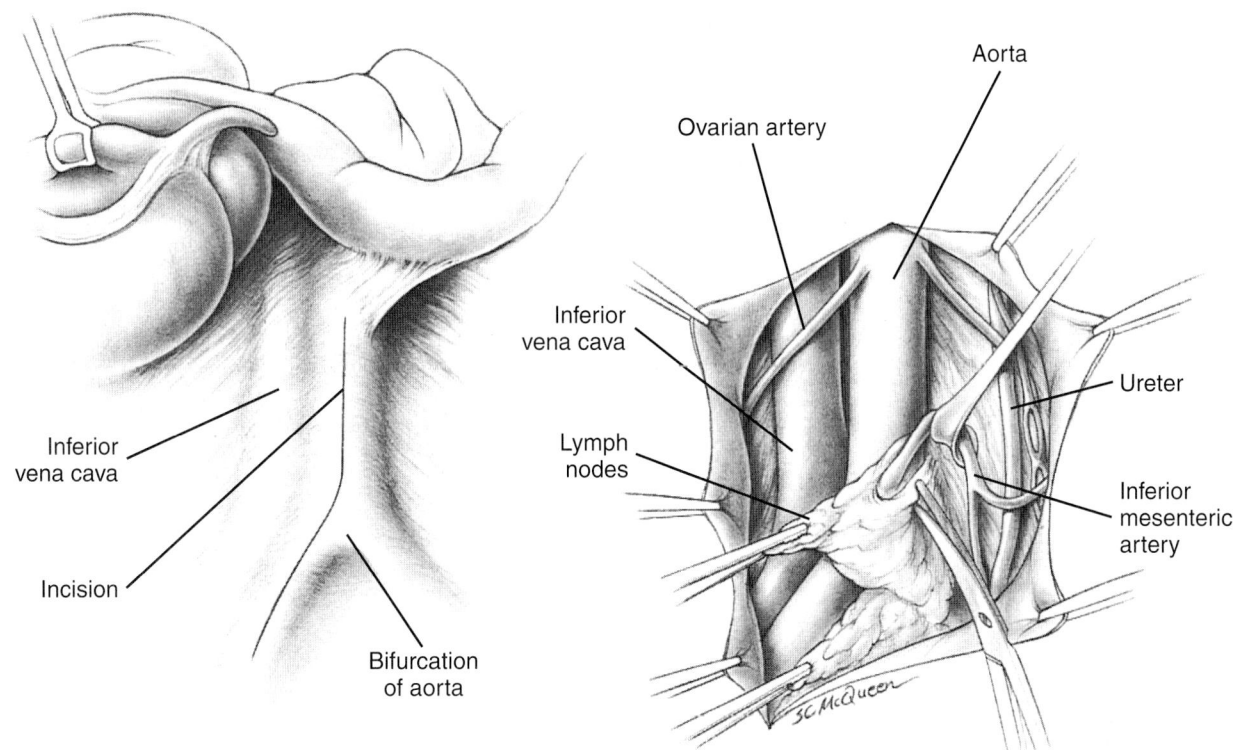

FIGURE 30-14 Removal of lymph node tissue. The technique of removal of retroperitoneal paraaortic nodes is demonstrated with the important anatomic landmarks.

men, then the usual therapy for adenocarcinoma of the endometrial carcinoma may be undertaken. In spite of the general poor prognosis for papillary serous tumors, patients who are surgically staged completely and have findings consistent with stage I/II have an excellent prognosis with 12 of 14 such patients free of disease with a median follow-up of 50 months as noted by Grice et al.

RADIATION THERAPY CONSIDERATIONS. As previously discussed, radiation therapy may be prescribed for stage I endometrial carcinomas preoperatively, postoperatively, or as the sole therapy for patients unable to undergo surgery. Deep penetration of the myometrium is also associated with increased spread of tumor to retroperitoneal nodes. Lower uterine segment involvement by tumor is also an indication for postoperative radiation, according to the studies of Mayr et al., insofar as 5 of their 68 patients with this finding had pelvic recurrence compared with only 1 of 136 without lower segment involvement.

A study of 605 patients by Kucera et al. demonstrated the efficacy of postoperative irradiation in improving survival in stage I patients and also provided useful guidelines for therapy. They administered vaginal irradiation only (3200 cGy) to the vaginal surface to 376 patients with inner one-third myometrial involvement regardless of grade or for middle one-third involvement for grade 1 cases. No pelvic irradiation was given to these patients with a good prognosis, and the 5-year survival was 91.8%.

External pelvic irradiation to give a total dose of 5400 to 5600 cGy was prescribed for patients with grade 2 or 3 tumors that penetrated to the middle one third of the myometrium or for all grades that penetrated to the outer one third. The overall 5-year survival for these 229 high-risk patients was 87.8%, almost as good as the 91.8% for those with good prognostic factors. A study of 86 patients by Stryker et al. suggests 4250 cGy whole-pelvis radiotherapy may be adequate following total abdominal hysterectomy and bilateral salpingo-oophorectomy for patients with disease confined to the uterus or occultly extending to the cervix. Carey et al. defined low-risk patients as stage I, grades 1 or 2 with less than half myometrial invasion. No further therapy was given to these patients, and a 95% 5-year survival was observed. These findings were also demonstrated in a study of Poulsen et al., who defined low risk as stage I, grades 1 or 2, with less than half myometrial invasion, while high risk was defined as stage I, grades 1 or 2, with more than half myometrial invasion, or any grade 3. No further therapy was given to 641 low-risk cases and only 45 recurred and 4 died (Table 30-10). Fifteen of the 72 patients with vaginal recurrence were subsequently salvaged with pelvic irradiation. It appears that patients who do not need additional irradiation therapy after operation for endometrial carcinoma are those with grade 1 or 2 endometrial tumor with less than half myometrial invasion.

TABLE 30-10
Adjuvant Radiation Therapy

	Follow-up Radiotherapy	No. of Cases	68–72 Month Follow-up Recurrence	Death
Low risk	None	641*	45† (7%)	4
Stage I Grade 1–2 ≤50% myometrial invasion	None			
High risk				
Stage I Grade 1–2, >50% myometrial invasion or Grade 3	External radiotherapy, whole pelvis 4500 cGy	235	36 (15%)	11

Modified from Poulsen HK, Jacobsen M, Bertelsen K, et al: Int J Gynecol Cancer 6:38, 1996.

*Clear cell and serous cases included.

†15 of 17 vaginal recurrences salvaged with radiotherapy.

The uncertain area is grade 3 with any myometrial invasion and grade 2 cases with invasion between one third and half of the myometrium. It is important to try to start irradiation therapy within 6 weeks of operation, since a longer delay increases the risk of treatment failure, as noted in a study of 195 cases by Ahmad et al. However, as noted by Bruner et al., a disadvantage of combined external beam and brachytherapy is an association with a decrease in vaginal length and an apparent decrease in sexual activity. Furthermore Greven et al. noted the addition of vaginal cuff brachytherapy with pelvic irradiation did not enhance survival or pelvic disease control. A recent randomized trial from the Netherlands by Creutzberg et al. reported on 714 patients with stage I disease and grade 1 with more than 50% myometrial invasion or grade 2 with any invasion or grade 3 with < 50% invasion. They received full pelvic irradiation or no further treatment. Local regional control was better in the radiation group but complications (some mild) from radiation (4600 cGy) were seen in one quarter of the patients. No survival advantage was demonstrated in the radiation group. Nonetheless, increased death was noted in the grade 3 patients. The study indicates a large group of patients do exist who do not gain a survival advantage with postop irradiation.

Paraaortic irradiation is also used. It carries with it an increased risk of bowel complications, particularly if the patient has undergone prior transperitoneal exploration or removal of the paraaortic nodes. Such complications are dose related and usually become most severe above dosages of 5000 cGy. Potish et al. treated 48 women with 4500 to 5075 cGy to the paraaortic areas; 22 had had nodal metastases established at operation, and the remainder had suspected nodal disease documented on lymphangiogram. Overall, a salvage rate of 47% was achieved in patients with metastatic tumor. Only one patient (2%) experienced a small bowel complication. Further efficacy of paraaortic node therapy was reported by Feuer and Calanog, who salvaged 10 of 15 patients with microscopic tumor in paraaortic nodes. Corn et al. reported 26 patients with paraaortic disease and found the probability of cure was enhanced if grossly abnormal paraaortic nodes were removed. In addition, chemoradiation, as indicated elsewhere, has produced markedly improved results with cervical carcinomas (Chapter 29). Radiation accompanied by weekly cisplatin (50 mg/m²) is the current standard utilized. No large similar studies are reported with this technique for endometrial carcinoma but it is being tried by some therapists to enhance treatment effectiveness, particularly when treating known disease.

Stage II

Three therapeutic options have been employed for the treatment of stage II carcinoma of the endometrium that also involves the endocervix: (1) primary operation (radical hysterectomy and pelvic node dissection), (2) primary irradiation (intrauterine and vaginal implant and external irradiation) followed by an operation (extrafascial hysterectomy), and (3) irradiation as the sole method of management. Because tumor involves the cervix, as well as the endometrium, in stage II carcinoma, dissemination of malignancy from both the uterus and cervix must be considered.

Radical hysterectomy and pelvic node dissection have been used as effective therapy and have resulted in a 75% 5-year survival for the 26 patients treated by Homesley et al. and 65% for the 20 patients reported by Wallin et al. External irradiation is usually added if the pelvic nodes are involved with tumor. For grade 1 tumors, particularly those with less than one-third myometrial invasion, no postoperative irradiation is used.

Most patients with stage II carcinoma of the endometrium are treated with a combination of radiation and extrafascial hysterectomy. A widely used protocol includes external radiation (45 Gy) and a single brachytherapy implant usually followed in 4 to 6 weeks by extrafascial total abdominal hysterectomy, bilateral salpingo-oophorectomy, and paraaortic node sampling. Podczaski et al. noted that those with gross cervical tumor had a poor prognosis and were likely to have extrauterine disease at operation. For patients with cervical involvement on biopsy but no gross tumor, Trimble and Jones found radiation treatment by a single implant alone followed by a hysterectomy to be effective, and they added external therapy depending on the nodal findings and myometrial invasion. Andersen reported on 54 patients with stage II tumors and found a 70.6% survival in patients treated by abdominal hysterectomy followed by radiation.

If the patient is able to tolerate an operation, removal of the uterus appears to improve prognosis and survival. If the patient is unable to tolerate an operation, irradiation alone (combined uterine and vaginal local irradiation and external therapy) is utilized (see later discussion). Most patients with stage II adenocarcinoma of the endometrium are elderly and obese and thus are not good candidates for radical hysterectomy, and are treated by preoperative external irradiation, an implant, and then extrafascial hysterectomy. However, for good operative candidates, especially younger, thin patients and those with "occult" cervical involvement rather than gross clinical disease, radical hysterectomy and pelvic node dissection can be effective. Radiation therapy may be added for higher grade lesions, patients with deep myometrial invasion (beyond the inner third), lymphvascular space involvement or those with evidence of spread of tumor to regional pelvic nodes. For well-differentiated tumors or only microscopic involvement of the cervix, an extrafascial hysterectomy with selective lymph node sampling can be performed after intrauterine irradiation. External irradiation is added postoperatively, depending on the pathologic findings. Recent reports by Feltmate et al. and Eltabbakh and Moore indicate 5-year survivals of over 90% can be achieved for stage II cases treated by operation and radiation.

Radiation Therapy as the Sole Treatment of Stage I or II

Occasionally irradiation is used alone to treat stage I or II adenocarcinoma of the endometrium. Landgren et al. used Heyman packing with vaginal ovoids and two or three applications to treat stage I carcinomas. Either a dosage of 6000 mg-hours of radium was given to the uterus, or this dosage was reduced to 2500 mg-hours and supplemented later with 4000 cGy of external radiation therapy. The best results were obtained with radium packing alone. This older series was not randomized, but an improved result with the added external therapy was not demonstrated. The 5-year survival for stage I patients was approximately 75% in comparison with 55% for stage II patients. Later the same authors noted that treatment by uterine packing (6000 mg-hours) provided greater pelvic control of stage I disease than did 4000 cGy of external irradiation in combination with only 2500 mg-hours of uterine packing. Lehoczky et al., as previously noted, used intracavitary radiation alone to salvage stage I patients. The results, however, were not as good as full external radiation supplemented by an implant.

As previously noted, patients unable to undergo surgery can be treated with radiation therapy alone. Traditionally, low-dose-rate approaches have been used that utilize Heyman-Simon capsules. The uterus is packed with multiple capsules that are afterloaded with cesium-137, and the myometrial wall is distended, as shown in Figure 30-16. Intrauterine packing with multiple capsules is preferable to a single linear intracavitary source because multiple sources deliver more effective doses of radiation to the uterus. In more recent years, high-dose-rate approaches have been developed that utilize iridium-192. High-dose-rate brachytherapy is particularly appealing in elderly patients with multiple comorbid conditions who are poor candidates for general anesthesia and prolonged hospitalizations. It can be administered on an outpatient basis. Anderson et al. utilized three brachytherapy HDR insertions of 1500 cGy each weekly as sole therapy for stages Ib and Ic in 102 patients. A 5-year disease-free survival of 93% was obtained. Moreover, 97% of the patients were disease-free at 5 years with only three pelvic failures occurring in high-risk patients (grade 3 outer one third, or lymph-vascular space involvement, or lower uterine segment involvement).

Comparable outcomes have recently been reported using high-dose-rate brachytherapy approaches in stage I-II patients unable to undergo surgery. Nguygen et al. reported a 3-year disease-free survival rate of 85% in 36 stage I patients treated with definitive radiation therapy. Nineteen patients were considered inoperable due to morbid obesity, and the remainder had significant medical problems precluding anesthesia. All patients were treated as outpatients with five weekly brachytherapy applications performed under conscious sedation. At a median follow-up of 32 months, the 3-year actuarial uterine-control rate was 88%.

Stage III

In stage III carcinoma the disease has spread outside the uterus but remains confined to the pelvis with the exception of stage IIIc, which involves the retroperitoneal nodes. These tumors do not involve the mucosa of the rectum or bladder. They account for approximately 7% of all endometrial carcinomas and occur in patients who are older than those with lower stage tumors and often medically less able to undergo an operation. Aalders et al. reported on the results of 175 patients with stage III tumor, 52% of whom were over 60 years of age. These patients were divided into two groups: those with clinical evidence of extrauterine spread before therapy (usually to the vagina or parametrium, 108 cases) and those with subclinical evidence of spread to the adnexa (fallopian tube or ovary) discovered at the time of operation in a patient believed to have stage I or II carcinoma initially (but IIIA by the operative classification, 67 cases). Operative eradication of microscopic tumor was of major prognostic importance in these cases; eradication was usually possible if the tumor involved only the uterine adnexa. The optimal therapy, when possible, was a total abdominal hysterectomy and bilateral salpingo-oophorectomy followed by external irradiation (40 to 50 Gy). If there was vaginal extension of cervical disease, the cervical field was shielded at 20 Gy and subsequent brachytherapy was administered to the vagina, bringing the vaginal surface dose to 60 Gy. For patients who could not undergo surgery, packing of the uterus was done as described (see Figure 30-15), followed by external irradia-

tion therapy. Those with subclinical spread of tumor had a much better 5-year survival (40%) than those with overt clinical stage III disease (16%). Pliskow et al. noted a 5-year survival of 27% for 22 patients with stage III disease with the best results for those treated by operation and irradiation. Gerszten et al. used radiation after hysterectomy for those who at operation were discovered to have stage III disease, excluding clear cell and papillary serous histologies. Extended field radiation was given for those with positive nodes. For stage IIIa cases, 2 of 19 developed recurrence compared to 5 of 8 for stage IIIc. The addition of radiation appears to have enhanced salvage in many of these cases and, as mentioned previously, the possibility of chemoradiation improving results is being considered at various treatment centers.

For intraperitoneal metastatic disease, Greer and Hamburger used whole abdominal irradiation in 31 patients. In 27 of the patients with residual tumor less than 2 cm, a 5-year survival of 63% was noted. These authors recommend that such salvage therapy could be effective for individuals with endometrial carcinoma, particularly stage III disease, providing tumor reduction surgery results in residual tumor under 2 cm in diameter, as shown in the data for ovarian epithelial carcinoma.

The patients with stage III endometrial carcinoma with the best prognosis have tumor spread only to the fallopian tubes or ovaries or both (stage IIIA). Greven et al. noted a 60% 5-year survival for those with adnexal involvement and only 45% for those with parametrial or pelvic peritoneal involvement. If possible, therapy should include operative eradication of macroscopic tumor. This is combined with radiotherapy. The previously cited study of Gerszten et al. reported that 24 of 32 patients with stage III carcinomas were disease-free with a mean follow-up of 68 months following operation and radiation. If there is no extensive involvement of the cervix and paracervical areas, initial Heyman packing can be done before hysterectomy and external beam therapy. For tumor that extends into the vagina and paravaginal tissues, intracavitary irradiation is combined with external therapy, followed by hysterectomy if technically feasible. For tumor extending to the pelvic wall or patients in poor medical condition, usually only irradiation therapy is possible.

Stage IV

Approximately 3% of endometrial carcinomas are at stage IV, and many of these patients have tumor metastases outside the pelvis. In a series of 83 patients from the Norwegian Radium Hospital, Aalders et al. reported that the lung was the main site of extrauterine spread (36% of the cases), which is consistent with the generalized pattern of recurrent adenocarcinoma of the endometrium. They utilized hysterectomy to achieve local control of stage IV disease, usually followed by postoperative external irradiation ther-

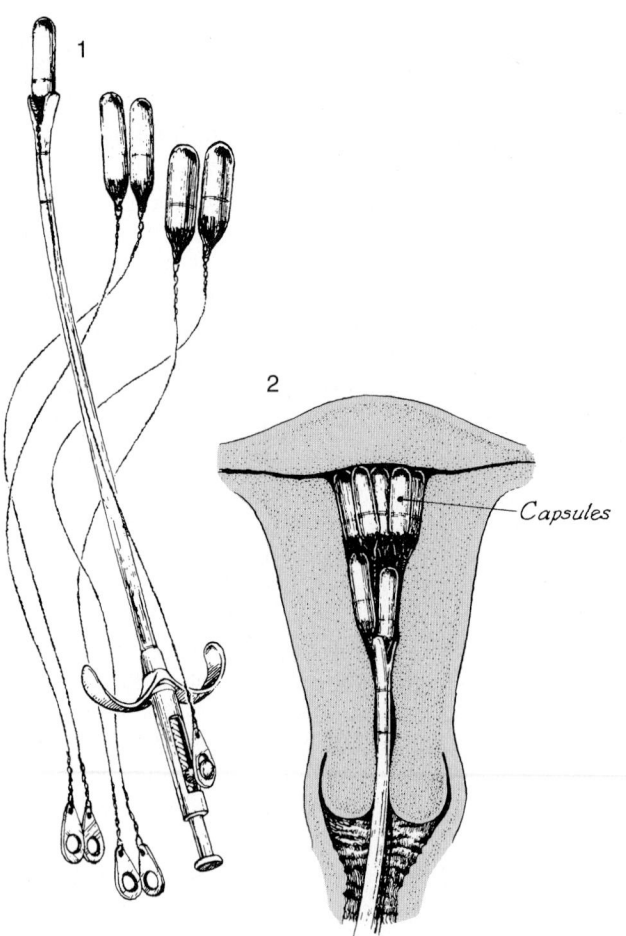

FIGURE 30-15 Heyman's capsules used to pack and distend the endometrial cavity. (From Wheeless CR: Atlas of pelvic surgery, Philadelphia, 1981, Lea & Febiger.)

apy. Progestational therapy (17 α-hydroxyprogesterone caproate, 1000 mg intramuscularly daily for 1 week, weekly for 3 months, and every other week for at least 1 year) was also prescribed for 17 patients, two of whom survived 3 and 13 years, respectively. Progestins were also used in 30 patients with pulmonary metastases, and 8 had a complete remission (disappearance) of metastatic tumor. The 5-year survival was 10% for all 83 cases, similar to the general experience (see Table 30-5).

Individualization of therapy is necessary for the patient with stage IV endometrial carcinoma. If feasible, the uterus, tubes, and ovaries are removed to achieve local control. Irradiation therapy is administered as an adjunct or, if necessary, as the sole therapy for palliation to achieve pelvic control of disease. Progestational agents and/or combination chemotherapy are usually added. A collaborative group from the United Kingdom-Australia and New Zealand (COSA-NZ-UK) randomized patients with high-risk endometrial carcinoma who had been treated with operation and radiation. They received medroxyprogesterone 200 mg twice daily or no further therapy. Fewer recurrences were observed in the treated group, suggesting a possible beneficial effect, but no survival advantage was noted.

Recurrent Adenocarcinoma of the Endometrium

Most recurrences of adenocarcinoma of the endometrium occur within 3 years of diagnosis, and 90% occur within 5 years of diagnosis. Rose et al. used CA-125, a more common marker for ovarian carcinoma, to follow patients with endometrial carcinoma whose pretreatment CA-125 levels were elevated. It was a useful marker for recurrence in about 60% of cases but was falsely elevated (40 to 605 IU) in 11 patients who received radiation, particularly outside of the pelvis.

Since 10% of recurrences will occur more than 5 years after initial diagnosis, patients with adenocarcinoma of the endometrium need prolonged follow-up. In the series of Aalders et al. involving 379 patients, half of the recurrences were in the pelvis and vagina; the most frequent sites of nonpelvic metastases were lung (17%), upper portion of the abdomen (10%), and bone (6%). Irradiation was the primary treatment of localized recurrent disease in patients who had an operation alone as the initial treatment, but operative excision of resectable nodules was also done when feasible. The 5-year survival rate for those patients who received progestins with other forms of treatment for grade 1 and grade 2 recurrences was 26%, in comparison with 14% for those who did not. For undifferentiated tumors the comparable survival was 9%.

Radiotherapy can be useful to salvage patients with pelvic recurrence who had only operation for primary therapy. Ackerman et al. treated 21 patients with pelvic relapse and found radiation achieved pelvic control of dis-

ease in 14 (67%). The best results were with recurrences in the vaginal mucosa. Similarly, Sears et al. treated 45 patients with vaginal recurrence of endometrial cancer with irradiation and achieved a 44% 5-year survival. As noted earlier, Carey salvaged 15 of 17 patients with vaginal recurrence initially treated by operation alone. Trials of chemoradiation with cisplatin are being tried, as noted previously.

CHEMOTHERAPY. Chemotherapy for endometrial carcinoma has primarily involved the use of progestins and cytotoxic agents. Unfortunately, no clearly effective program has emerged. Progestins have been used frequently, and responses of 10% to 20% have been reported.

Steroid hormone receptor content of tumor has been studied in relation to chemotherapeutic response. It has been shown that the well-differentiated tumors also have the highest content of estrogen and progestin steroid hormone receptors. Numerous and various dosage schedules have been employed, including 17 α-hydroxyprogesterone (Delalutin), discussed earlier; medroxyprogesterone (Depo-Provera), 400 mg intramuscularly weekly for 3 months, and then every 2 weeks; and oral megestrol acetate (Megace), 160 to 320 mg daily. Recent data from the Gynecologic Oncology Group (GOG) reported by Thigpen et al. indicate a dose of oral medroxyprogesterone of 200 mg/day is adequate and effective, particularly in well-differentiated tumors, which have the best response. The results do not appear to depend on the type of progestin administered. Antiestrogens, such as tamoxifen, have been added to treat recurrent endometrial carcinoma. Well-differentiated tumors respond better than poorly differentiated tumors. A regimen of 5 days of therapy (10 mg orally twice daily) was associated with increased receptor content of endometrial carcinoma in the patients studied. Carlson et al. noted that only 13 of 25 tumors were progesterone receptor positive before tamoxifen therapy, whereas 21 of 25 tumors became positive after tamoxifen.

Cytotoxic chemotherapy.
A number of cytotoxic agents have been used to treat endometrial carcinoma. No effective therapy has emerged.

There is some evidence that combined chemohormonal therapy provides better results. Ayoub et al. showed that 3 weeks of tamoxifen 20 mg PO daily alternating with 3 weeks of Provera 200 mg daily plus Cytoxan 400 mg/m^2 IV on days 1 and 8, Adriamycin 30 mg/m^2 IV day 1 and 5-fluorouracil 400/m^2 IV days 1 and 8 (CAF) gave significantly better results in a randomized trial than CAF alone. The combined chemohormonal therapy was also effective in reducing the frequency of relapses when used adjuvantly in high-risk cases (ER-negative, grade 3 tumors). Effective chemohormonal results were also reported by Hoffman et al. using Cytoxan (250 to 500 mg/m^2), Adriamycin (30 mg/m^2), and platinum (50 mg/m^2) (CAP) with megestrol acetate (40 to 160 mg PO daily). Of 15 patients, 4 had complete responses in their studies. Pinelli et al. utilized Megace alternating with tamoxifen combined with carboplatin (300 mg/m^2) and noted a 33-month survival for 4 of 13 patients who had a complete response. An ideal regimen for recurrent endometrial carcinoma has yet to be identified. One protocol currently being evaluated compares Adriamycin 60 mg/m^2 (45 mg/m^2 for those with prior radiation therapy or over age 65 years) with cisplatinum 50 mg/m^2 every 3 weeks (AP) or Adriamycin 45 mg/m^2 and cisplatin 50 mg/m^2 day 1 and taxol 160 mg/m^2 day 2 supplemented by GCSF days 3-12 (TAP). Definitive results are not currently available.

Post Treatment Estrogen Replacement Therapy

Since estrogens have been implicated in the genesis of many endometrial carcinomas, it has usually been advised to avoid estrogen replacement therapy (ERT) (see Chapter 42) in these patients. However, a retrospective nonrandomized study by Creasman et al. suggested that those receiving ERT may not have an increased risk of tumor recurrence and are also protected against the complications of estrogen lack, i.e., osteoporosis, coronary artery disease, etc. In a nonrandomized study of 221 patients with stage I disease, 47 received ERT and 174 did not. Recurrence occurred in 26 (14.7%) of the non-ERT group and in 1 (2.1%) of the ERT group. Moreover, in a 5-year follow-up, 26 of the non-ERT group had died in comparison with only 1 of the ERT group, suggesting the ERT group was protected. Further studies are needed, but these data suggest that ERT may be administered to those treated for stage I endometrial carcinoma without increased risk of tumor recurrence and with likely health benefits. The patient needs to be informed of the various risks and benefits.

SARCOMAS

Sarcomas comprise less than 5% of uterine malignancies and are much less frequent than endometrial carcinomas, particularly in Western countries. Numerous terms have been used to describe the many histologic types. One useful classification is based on determination of the resemblance of the sarcomatous elements to mesenchymal tissue normally found in the uterus (homologous sarcomas) in contrast to tissues foreign to the uterus (heterologous sarcomas). Homologous types include leiomyosarcomas, endometrial stromal sarcomas, and rarely angiosarcomas. Heterologous types include rhabdomyosarcomas, chondrosarcomas, osteosarcomas, and liposarcomas. These sarcomas may exist exclusively or may be admixed with epithelial adenocarcinoma, in which case the term *carcinosarcoma* (*malignant mixed müllerian tumor* [MMMT]) is applied. The box at right shows a morphologic classification for uterine sarcomas.

A recent study by Zelmanowicz et al. suggests risk factors for these tumors are similar to those of endometrial carcinoma, that is, estrogens and obesity increase the risk and oral contraceptive use decreases the risk. No uniformly defined staging criteria exist for these tumors, and the most widely used definitions are similar to those for endometrial carcinoma, that is, stage I, confined to the corpus; stage II, corpus and cervix involved; stage III, spread outside the uterus but confined to the pelvis; and stage IV, spread outside the true pelvis or into the mucosa of the bladder or rectum. Wolfson et al. conducted a study of 62 patients with a variety of uterine sarcomas and found operative stage to be the most important predictor of survival. Yamada et al. noted a high rate (over one half) of occult metastases, including nodal and intraperitoneal disease, in these patients, suggesting an operative staging similar to endometrial carcinoma should be used, particularly to evaluate the results of various therapeutic regimens.

Modified Classification of Uterine Sarcomas

I. Pure sarcoma
  A. Homologous
    1. Smooth muscle tumors
      a. Leiomyosarcoma
      b. Leiomyoblastoma
      c. Metastasizing tumors with benign histologic appearance
        (1) Intravenous leiomyomatosis
        (2) Metastasizing uterine leiomyoma
        (3) Leiomyomatosis peritonealis disseminata
    2. Endometrial stromal sarcomas
      a. Low grade: endolymphatic stromal myosis (ESM)
      b. High grade: endometrial stromal sarcoma (ESS)
  B. Heterologous
    1. Rhabdomyosarcoma
    2. Chondrosarcoma
    3. Osteosarcoma
    4. Liposarcoma
  C. Other sarcomas
II. Carcinosarcoma—Malignant mixed müllerian tumors (MMMT)
  A. Homologous (carcinosarcoma): Carcinoma + Homologous sarcoma
  B. Heterologous: Carcinoma + Heterologous sarcoma
III. Müllerian adenosarcoma
IV. Lymphoma

Modified from Clement P and Scully RE: Pathology of uterine sarcomas. In Coppleson M, editor: Gynecologic oncology, New York, 1981, Churchill Livingstone, p 591. Reprinted by permission.

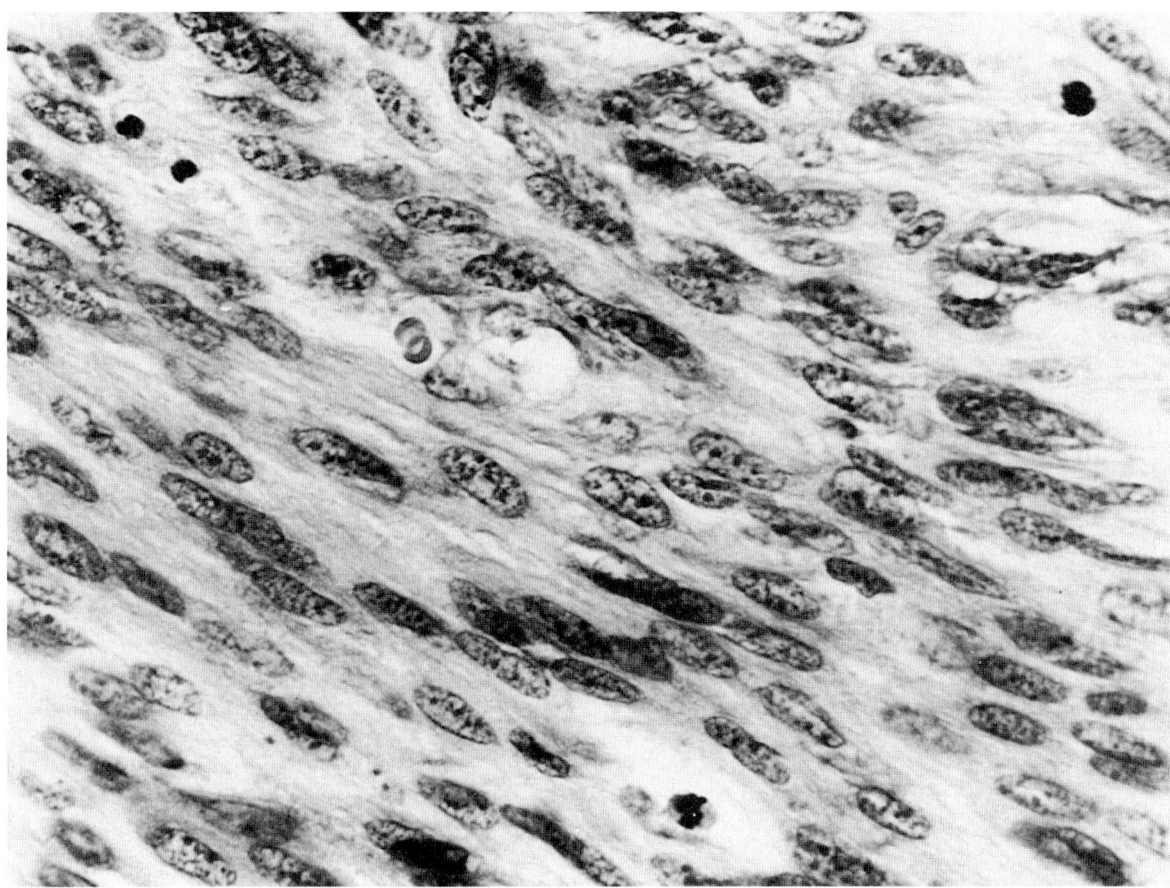

FIGURE 30-16 Leiomyosarcoma. Nuclear hyperchromatism and mitotic figures are present. (×660.) (From Clement PB and Scully RE: Pathology of uterine sarcomas. In Coppleson M, editor: Gynecologic oncology, Edinburgh, 1981, Churchill-Livingstone. Reprinted by permission.)

Homologous Sarcoma

Leiomyosarcoma

Among the uterine sarcomas, leiomyosarcomas are the most common, occurring somewhat more frequently than carcinosarcomas. In summarizing 1089 uterine sarcomas from the literature, Lurain and Piver noted that leiomyosarcomas comprised 45% of the group. The determination of malignancy is made in part by ascertaining the number of mitoses in 10 high-power fields (hpf), as well as the presence of cytologic atypia, abnormal mitotic figures, and nuclear pleomorphism (Figure 30-16). Vascular invasion and extrauterine spread of tumor are associated with worse prognoses. A finding of more than 5 mitoses/10 hpf with cytologic atypia leads to a diagnosis of leiomyosarcoma; when there are 4 mitoses/10 hpf or less, the tumors usually have a more benign clinical course. The prognosis worsens for tumors with over 10 mitoses/10 hpf. The presence of bizarre cells may not necessarily establish the diagnosis (Figure 30-17) because they can occasionally be seen in benign leiomyomas and in patients receiving progestational agents. Furthermore, it is important to note that an increase in mitotic count in leiomyomas occurs in pregnancy as well as during oral contraceptive use. This can occasionally cause confusion in the histologic diagnosis. Leiomyosarcomas tend to occur in patients in their 50s and occasionally in conjunction with leiomyomas, although leiomyosarcomas usually infiltrate diffusely into the myometrium.

The development of leiomyosarcoma from leiomyoma is rare. Leibsohn and co-workers noted that among 1423 patients who had hysterectomies for presumed leiomyomas with a uterine size comparable with a 12-week pregnancy or larger, the risk of sarcoma increased with age, from 0.4% for those in their 30s to 1.4% for those in their 50s. Premenopausal patients have been reported to have a better prognosis than postmenopausal patients. Usually the patient has an enlarged pelvic mass, occasionally accompanied by pain or vaginal bleeding. Leiomyosarcomas are suspected if the uterus undergoes rapid enlargement, particularly in patients in the perimenopausal or postmenopausal age group. However, Parker et al. noted a frequency of only 0.27% among 371 women ages 22 to 68.

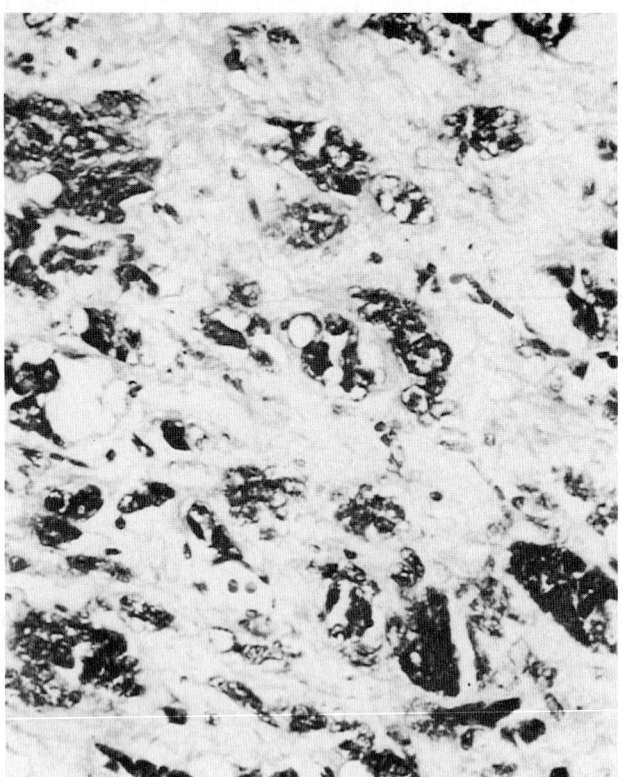

FIGURE 30-17 Leiomyoma with bizarre nuclei. No mitoses are present. (×256.) (From Clement PB and Scully RE: Pathology of uterine sarcomas. In Coppleson M, editor: Gynecologic oncology, Edinburgh, 1981, Churchill-Livingstone. Reprinted by permission.)

It is also occasionally possible to detect uterine sarcomas with ultrasound using a vaginal probe, because of the enhancement of the sarcoma image as a consequence of increased vascularity as illustrated in Figure 30-18, *A*. In addition, with a leiomyoma, there is acoustic shadowing as shown in Figure 30-18, *B*. The increased vascularity, irregularity, and random distribution of vessels can also be demonstrated with color imaging or power Doppler, although differentiating with this modality between simple leiomyoma and one with sarcomatous changes is not always feasible. Kurjak et al. examined a group of more than 2000 women 1 day before hysterectomy with transvaginal ultrasonography using color Doppler. There were 10 cases of uterine sarcoma compared with 1850 cases of uterine leiomyomata and 150 controls. All 10 cases of sarcoma demonstrated abnormal vascularization and lower Doppler indices than normal or myomatous uteri. Sensitivity and specificity were 90.9% and 99.8%, respectively.

Treatment consists of surgical removal of all disease if possible. Mitotic rate is important in determining prognosis. With increasing mitotic rate the prognosis becomes worse. For patients with well-documented leiomyosarcoma the overall 5-year survival rate is about 20%; for those with stage I and II tumors it is approximately 40%.

The most important aspect of treatment is removal of the tumor, usually by total abdominal hysterectomy with bilateral salpingo-oophorectomy (TAH-BSO). Irradiation therapy has been used to treat residual pelvic disease but is of unproved value. Salazar et al. noted that irradiation therapy appeared to decrease the risk of pelvic recurrence of tumor but did not significantly improve survival rates. Radiation is usually not prescribed except to control pelvic disease. Chemotherapy with Adriamycin and/or platinum, often in combination with other agents, is usually tried with fair results (see below). Berchuck et al. reported responses of only 16% to chemotherapy for these tumors.

In addition to local pelvic recurrences, distant metastases are frequent and most often occur in the lungs or intraabdominally. These are preferably treated by multiple-agent chemotherapy. Occasionally a patient of reproductive age has an unsuspected leiomyosarcoma diagnosed in a leiomyoma removed at myomectomy. Usually in such cases, hysterectomy is subsequently performed, but a few cures have been reported in individuals who have had no further treatment beyond myomectomy; a complete, accurate histologic assessment is vital to ascertain the risk. As previously noted, pregnancy can increase the mitotic rate in smooth muscle tumors, which should be remembered when myomas are removed from pregnant or recently pregnant patients.

The clinician should be aware of variations of smooth muscle tumors that are not leiomyosarcomas or benign leiomyomas. These tumors include leiomyoblastoma, intravenous leiomyomatosis, metastasizing uterine leiomyoma, and leiomyomatosis peritonealis disseminata. Leiomyoblastomas are very rare smooth muscle tumors that grossly resemble leiomyomas. They contain epithelial-like cells with spindle-shaped cells characteristic of smooth muscle tumors. Usually the mitotic rate is less than 5/10 hpf, and these tumors should be regarded as low-grade sarcomas for which operative removal is the preferred therapy. Intravenous leiomyomatosis is also rare and is usually a condition characterized by intravenous extension of smooth muscle tissue outside the uterus (Figure 30-19). Wormlike projections of the tumor may be found in vascular spaces in the broad ligament or extending even into the vena cava. Occasionally smooth muscle nodules are found outside the pelvis either in lymph nodes or in the lungs, in which case the term *metastasizing leiomyoma* is used. Removal of the uterus and the extrauterine lesion, if possible, is the treatment of choice, although leaving some tissue in cases of intravenous leiomyomatosis does not appear to lead to spread of the disease. Very rarely, small nodes of leiomyoma are found in the peritoneal cavity (leiomyomatosis peritonealis disseminata). The condition is usually found during pregnancy and regresses after delivery. However, it can exist in the absence of pregnancy, in which case it may require operative removal.

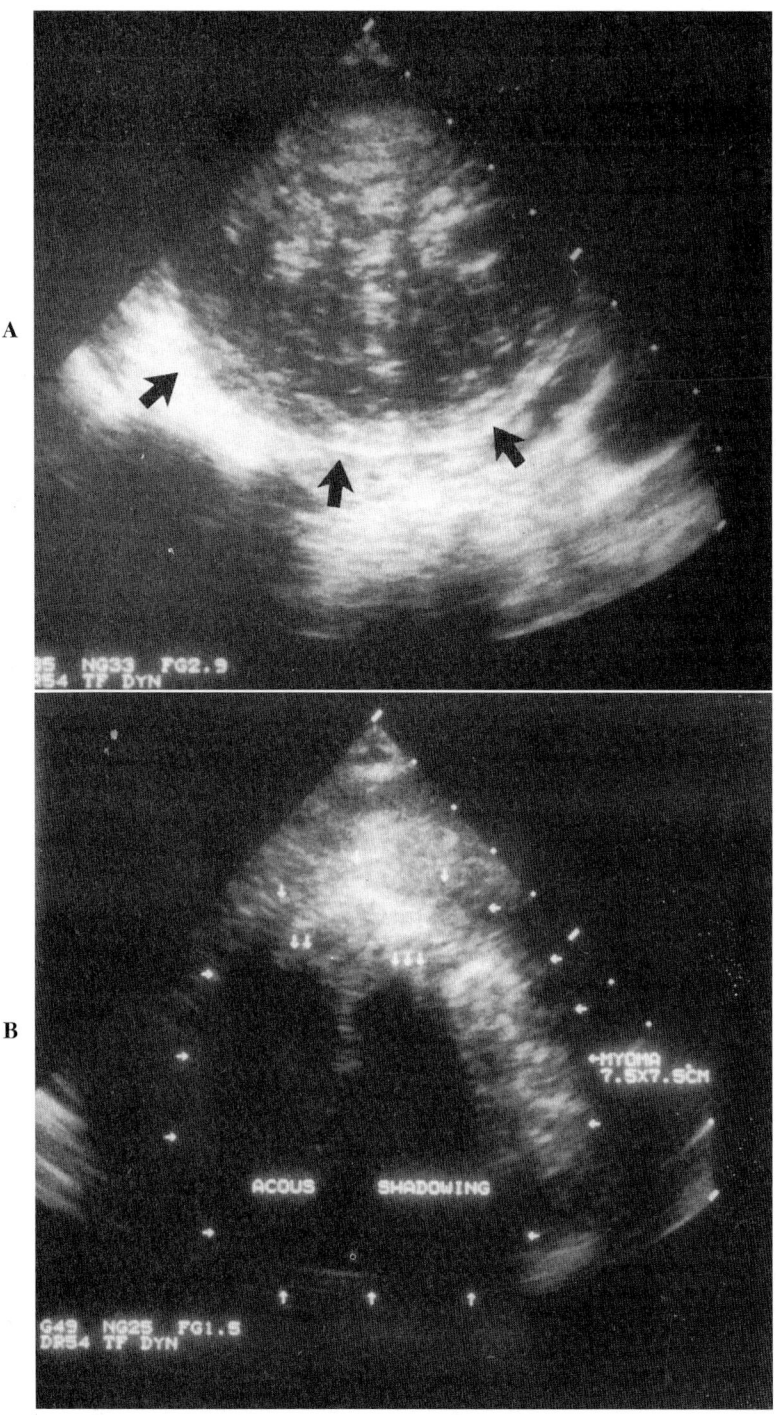

FIGURE 30-18   **A,** Transvaginal ultrasound image of uterine sarcoma; posterior wall enhancement *(arrows);* no acoustic shadowing. **B,** Transvaginal ultrasound depicting a myoma (fibroid) between the arrows. The arrows at the top point to acoustic shadowing, which is a typical characteristic of a fibroid. (Courtesy Dr. Zubie Sheikh, Department of Obstetrics & Gynecology, The University of Chicago.)

ENDOMETRIAL STROMAL SARCOMA

Overall, stromal tumors comprise about 10% of uterine sarcomas. Their behavior correlates primarily with mitotic rate, and they usually are divided into low-grade and high-grade tumors.

LOW GRADE—ENDOLYMPHATIC STROMAL MYOSIS. Endolymphatic stromal myosis is the least frequent among the uterine sarcomas, leiomyosarcomas, and malignant mixed müllerian tumors. The tumor consists of cells that resemble those of the uterine stroma, with a spindle-like appearance somewhat resembling fibrous sarcoma.

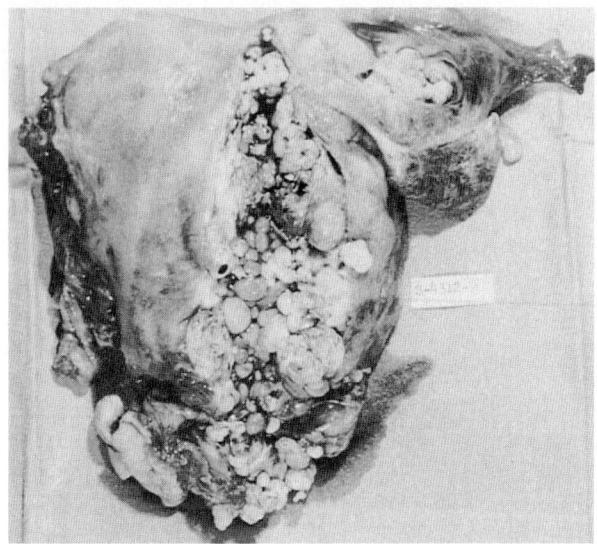

FIGURE 30-19 Intravenous leiomyomatosis replacing most of the uterus and extending into the broad ligaments and adjacent veins. (From Norris HJ and Zaloudek CJ: Mesenchymal tumors of the uterus. In Blaustein A, editor: Pathology of the female genital tract, ed 2, New York, 1982, Springer-Verlag.)

Endolymphatic stromal myosis is diagnosed if the mitotic rate in the tumor is less than 5/10 hpf. Occasionally these tumors have 10 mitoses/10 hpf. Despite the comparatively innocuous appearance and prolonged clinical course, these tumors can be fatal.

Piver et al. summarized a comparative study of 152 cases of endolymphatic stromal myosis. The patients with this tumor were 20 to 70 years of age, but almost three fourths were under age 50. Most had abnormal vaginal bleeding, and pelvic examination frequently revealed a large, irregularly shaped uterus. Occasionally the diagnosis is made on tissue obtained at diagnostic D&C. Press and Scully reported six cases associated with chronic estrogen stimulation and suggested that unopposed estrogen stimulation might increase the risk of these tumors.

The predominant mode of treatment is surgical and usually consists of total abdominal hysterectomy and bilateral salpingo-oophorectomy. Occasionally for tumors that spread to the cervix or paracervical areas a more radical procedure is performed, and a major effort is made to remove all gross disease. Long-term survivors are common, and 5-year survival of 100% was reported for the 15 patients originally described by Norris and Taylor; it was 88% in the collaborative series collected by Piver et al. for patients with tumors confined to the uterus.

Recurrence. Endolymphatic stromal myosis tends to recur locally in the pelvis or peritoneal cavity and frequently spreads to the lungs. In treating metastatic disease it should be remembered that these tumors contain estrogen and progestin steroid hormone receptors and are sensitive to progestational therapy. Megestrol acetate (Megace), medroxyprogesterone (Provera), and 17α-hydroxyprogesterone caproate (Delalutin) have been used. Complete resolution of the pulmonary lesions has been reported, and dosages of progestational drugs used are comparable to those for endometrial carcinoma. Nine patients reported by Thatcher and Woodruff were all living without evidence of disease 2 to 8 years after treatment, even though five had disease beyond the uterus at the time of initial operation. In view of the potential reappearance of disease, it is advisable to continue progestational therapy indefinitely after successful initial treatment of metastatic disease.

Irradiation has also been used to treat recurrences of these tumors, especially in the pelvis, with resolution of all residual tumor, but extensive experience with irradiation treatment is not available. Systemic chemotherapy with cytotoxic agents has not been reported generally to be effective, although complete response to doxorubicin (Adriamycin) has been reported.

HIGH GRADE—ENDOMETRIAL STROMAL SARCOMA. Endometrial stromal sarcomas are high-grade stromal tumors that behave aggressively and have a poor prognosis; microscopically more than 10 mitoses/10 hpf are present, and frequently 20 or more mitoses/10 hpf are present. Some series have reported 100% fatalities, although Vongtama et al. reported survival of over 60% for 24 patients with stage I and 1 patient with stage II disease. All cases of endolymphatic stromal myosis were eliminated, and treatment consisted of either operation alone or operation plus irradiation.

Patients with endometrial stromal sarcoma have abnormal bleeding or a pelvic mass. The tumor can occur at any age during reproductive life but tends to be primarily diagnosed in women under age 50 years. Operative removal of the tumor is the treatment of choice, but in view of the frequently poor survival rate, adjuvant therapy is occasionally considered. Unfortunately current data do not show a beneficial effect of adjuvant therapy in uterine sarcomas. A randomized trial using Adriamycin for stage I or II uterine sarcomas was reported for the GOG by Omura et al. and showed no benefit to the adjuvant group.

Recurrence. Recurrences are common in the pelvis, lung, and abdomen. If there has not been prior irradiation and the recurrence is confined to the pelvis, usually pelvic irradiation is prescribed. If there is disseminated disease, multiple-agent chemotherapy is used.

Carcinosarcoma (Malignant Mixed Müllerian Tumors)

Carcinosarcomas are aggressive malignancies that comprise about 40% of uterine sarcomas. As shown in the box on p. 942, these tumors consist of carcinomatous and sarcomatous elements native to the uterus that may resemble the endometrial stroma of smooth muscle (homologous) or of sarcomatous tissues foreign to the uterus (heterologous). Spanos et al. reviewed 188 patients with mixed mesodermal tumor and found both the prognosis and the pattern of survival similar for both homologous and heterologous tumors. The study of George et al. showed that patients with these tumors had a markedly worse prognosis than patients with high-grade endometrial carcinomas. Unlike patients with endometrial stromal sarcoma or leiomyosarcoma, those with carcinosarcoma tend to be older and primarily postmenopausal, usually beyond the age of 62 years. Prior pelvic irradiation has been identified as an occasional predisposing factor and was experienced by 17 of the 136 patients reviewed by Norris and Taylor. The heterologous and homologous tumors occur with approximately equivalent frequency. These tumors spread into the myometrium and then to the pelvis, to the abdomen including the peritoneum, and frequently to the lungs and pleura, a pattern similar to the spread of endometrial carcinoma.

A common symptom is postmenopausal bleeding, often accompanied by a large uterus. Occasionally the diagnosis is made in tissue removed with D&C, and the tumor may appear to be a polypoid excrescence from the cervix; diagnosis may be made also by vaginal ultrasound examination.

As is true for other sarcomas, the primary treatment is operative removal of the uterus. An additional problem is the older age of these patients. The extent of the tumor and the depth of myometrial invasion are important prognostic factors. Those with deep myometrial invasion are more likely to have spread to pelvic or paraaortic nodes, as in endometrial carcinomas. Patients with tumors confined to the uterus and little or no myometrial spread have the best prognosis. TAH and BSO are completed with stage I tumors; more extensive procedures are occasionally attempted for stage II tumors, as well as for those with early extrauterine spread. Nielsen et al. reported a 5-year survival of 58% for these tumors when the disease was confined to the uterus.

Because of the poor results with operation alone, supplemental treatment with irradiation or chemotherapy has been advocated. Perez et al. used preoperative intracavitary irradiation (5000 mg-hours) followed by TAH and BSO and then supplemented with full pelvic irradiation for stage I and stage II. The pelvic disease was eradicated, but distant metastases were common. Although irradiation may augment the beneficial effects of operation, particularly for the carcinomatous elements, systemic dissemination of disease is common. Current evidence fails to support a survival advantage for those receiving pelvic irradiation, although the frequency of pelvic recurrence is thought to be reduced. Full control depends on the identification of an effective program of chemotherapy to control systemic disease, particularly because lung metastases are so common in uterine sarcomas.

Müllerian Adenosarcoma

Müllerian adenosarcoma is a rare low-grade malignancy composed of both a sarcomatous stroma (homologous) and a proliferation of benign glandular elements that are intimately associated. It occurs predominantly in women older than 60 years. Ten cases were described initially by Clement and Scully. TAH with BSO is the treatment of choice, but Kaku et al. reported on the GOG experience and found a few cases behave aggressively and these authors recommend a staging laparotomy for apparent stage I and II cases. Mitotic index was related to prognosis.

Lymphoma

On rare occasions the uterus can be the original site for lymphoma, or, more commonly, involvement of the uterus may be the initial presentation of disseminated lymphoma. About 40 cases of primary lymphoma of the uterus have been reported. They are usually treated by irradiation.

Chemotherapy

It is evident from available data that treatment beyond operative resection and irradiation therapy is needed to achieve control of uterine sarcomas. Once resection has been accomplished, cytotoxic chemotherapy has been considered as an adjuvant to improve survival, particularly with high-grade tumors. Unfortunately, few data are available, and conflicting results have been reported. Marchese et al. studied 38 patients with sarcomas. Six with complete resection received adjuvant chemotherapy, primarily with vincristine, actinomycin D, and cyclophosphamide, and had a 5-year survival of 61%; survival was 15% for 23 patients with complete resections who did not receive chemotherapy. Confounding factors, such as tumor histologic findings and stage, were not controlled. A recent meta-analysis from the United Kingdom indicates that regimens containing doxorubicin (Adriamycin) improve both recurrence and survival-free time as well as time to develop a recurrence.

No single program has proved superior for the treatment of endometrial stromal sarcoma, leiomyosarcoma, or mixed müllerian malignant tumor, with the exception of progestin therapy to treat low-grade endometrial stromal sarcoma (endolymphatic stromal myosis). Thus chemotherapy programs for these sarcomas can be considered together.

Aziz et al. treated six cases of metastatic leiomyosarcoma with vincristine, 1.2 mg/m² weekly for 7 to 8 weeks; doxorubicin, 20 to 25 mg/m² intravenously for 3 days; and dacarbazine (DTIC), 250 mg/m² for 5 days every 3 weeks. Three complete responses lasting up to 2 years and one partial response were observed. Hannigan et al. used vincristine, actinomycin D, and cyclophosphamide (Cytoxan) (VAC protocol, Chapter 31) and noted a 13% complete response rate and 16% partial response rate in 74 patients with advanced metastatic uterine sarcomas. A large collaborative trial was conducted by the Gynecologic Oncology Group and reported by Omura et al. The best responses were obtained for patients with lung metastases who received doxorubicin and DTIC. Current evidence suggests that a multidrug program offers the greatest potential for inducing remission of uterine sarcomas. Cisplatin, Adriamycin, Taxol, ifosfamide, and VP 16 all appear to have some effectiveness. Peters et al. reported response in 8 of 11 patients treated with cisplatin (100 mg/m^2) and Adriamycin (40 to 60 mg/m^2) every 3 weeks. Current trials are directed toward finding an effective regimen for these aggressive tumors.

KEY POINTS

- Endometrial carcinoma is the most common malignancy of the lower female genital tract. In the United States about 1 woman in 50 will develop the disease.

- More deaths occur from ovarian and cervical cancer than from endometrial cancer.

- Most women who develop endometrial cancer are between 50 and 65 years of age.

- The primary symptom of endometrial carcinoma is postmenopausal bleeding.

- Chronic unopposed estrogen stimulation of the endometrium leads to endometrial hyperplasia and in some cases adenocarcinoma. Other important predisposing factors include obesity, nulliparity, late menopause, and diabetes.

- The risk of a woman developing endometrial carcinoma is increased 3 times if she is 21 to 50 pounds overweight and 10 times if she is more than 50 pounds overweight. Nulliparous women have twice the risk of those with one child and 3 times the risk of those with five or more children. Menopause after 52 years of age increases the risk by 2.4 times in comparison with menopause before age 49 years. Diabetes raises the risk by a factor of 2.8.

- Tamoxifen use in breast cancer patients increases the risk of endometrial neoplasia predominantly after 2 years of use.

- Prognosis in endometrial carcinoma is related to tumor grade, tumor stage, histologic type, and degree of myometrial invasion.

- Endometrial carcinoma can develop without preexisting endometrial hyperplasia, particularly in older patients and those with less well-differentiated tumors.

- Younger women with endometrial cancer have a better prognosis than older women.

- Most endometrial hyperplasias regress without treatment.

- Cytologic atypia in endometrial hyperplasia is the most important factor in determining premalignant potential.

- Older patients with atypical hyperplasia are at increased risk for malignant progression in comparison with younger patients.

- Adenocarcinoma of the endometrium is detected only in about 50% of the cases by routine cervical-vaginal cytologic study (Papanicolaou smear).

- Patients with adenocarcinoma of the endometrium and positive pretherapy Pap smears are likely to have extrauterine spread.

- Endometrial carcinoma spreads outside the uterus, to the retroperitoneal, pelvic, and paraaortic lymph nodes, to the adnexa, and then to the peritoneal cavity.

- CT scans may miss up to 50% of patients with nodal disease.

- A key determinant of risk of nodal spread of endometrial carcinoma is depth of myometrial invasion, which is often related to tumor grade.

- Well-differentiated (grade 1) endometrial carcinomas usually contain measurable levels of steroid hormone receptors, whereas poorly differentiated (grade 3) tumors usually do not contain measurable levels of receptors.

- Receptor-positive endometrial carcinomas have a better prognosis than do those that are receptor negative.

- Ninety percent of recurrences of adenocarcinoma of the endometrium occur within 5 years.

- Overall survival rates for patients with adenocarcinoma of the endometrium by stage are as follows: stage I, 86%; stage II, 66%; stage III, 44%; stage IV, 16% (overall 72.7% 5-year survival combining clinical and operative staging systems).

- Histologic variants of endometrial carcinoma with a poor prognosis include serous carcinoma and clear cell carcinoma.

- Patients with clear cell or papillary serous carcinoma of the endometrium should have a full staging laparotomy similar to that for ovarian carcinoma.

- The most frequent sites of distant metastasis of adenocarcinoma of the endometrium are the lung, retroperitoneal nodes, and abdomen. CA-125 can be used to follow patients with elevated pretreatment values, but many may be falsely elevated particularly in patients who received irradiation therapy.

- Progestin therapy results in responses of 10% to 20% in recurrent endometrial carcinoma. The highest response rates are in tumors with elevated sex steroid receptor levels, well-differentiated tumors, and recurrences at sites not previously irradiated. A dosage of medroxyprogesterone of 200 mg/day is effective.

- The optimal treatment of resectable endometrial carcinoma is by operation that includes total abdominal hysterectomy and bilateral salpingo-oophorectomy. Supplemental irradiation is prescribed depending on the extent of the disease and the histologic features of the tumor.

- Patients with grade 1 and possibly grade 2 endometrial carcinomas that penetrate to one third of the myometrium (stage IB) do not require supplemental irradiation, and 5-year survivals in excess of 90% can be expected postoperatively.

- Irradiation can be used effectively to cure endometrial carcinoma in patients who are a poor risk for operation.

- CA-125 can be falsely elevated in patients who receive radiation therapy. A pretherapy CA-125 > 35 U/ml usually suggests extrauterine disease.

- Vaginal cuff brachytherapy with pelvic irradiation postoperatively increases complications and does not enhance survival or pelvic disease control.

- Uterine sarcomas comprise less than 5% of uterine malignancies.

- Uterine sarcomas are treated primarily by operation including removal of the uterus, tubes, and ovaries.

- Mitotic rate is an important prognostic factor in uterine leiomyosarcomas and is worse for those with more than 10 mitoses/10 hpf. Tumors with 5 to 9 mitoses/10 hpf have a low malignant potential.

- Endometrial stromal sarcomas are virulent sarcomas with 10 or more mitoses/10 hpf. For tumors with less than 10 mitoses/10 hpf, the prognosis is improved, and a diagnosis of endolymphatic stromal myosis or low-grade stromal sarcoma is made if there are less than 5 mitoses/10 hpf.

- Recurrences of uterine sarcomas are most frequent locally in the pelvis, the abdomen, and the lungs.

- Metastatic endolymphatic stromal myosis (low-grade stromal sarcoma) is treated with progestin therapy initially. More than half will resolve.

- Multiagent chemotherapeutic regimens are usually prescribed for metastatic sarcomas; complete responses are rare and usually temporary.

BIBLIOGRAPHY

Aalders JG, Abeler V, and Kolstad P: Clinical (stage III) as compared to subclinical intrapelvic extrauterine tumor spread in endometrial carcinoma: a clinical and histopathological study of 175 patients, Gynecol Oncol 17:64, 1984.

Aalders JG, Abeler V, and Kolstad P: Stage IV endometrial carcinoma: a clinical and histopathological study of 83 patients, Gynecol Oncol 17:75, 1984.

Aalders JG, Abelar V, and Kolstad P: Recurrent adenocarcinoma of the endometrium: a clinical and histopathological study of 379 patients, Gynecol Oncol 17:85, 1984.

Abeler VM and Kjorstad KE: Clear cell carcinoma of the endometrium: a histopathological and clinical study of 97 cases, Gynecol Oncol 40:207, 1991.

Ackerman I, Malone S, Thomas G, et al: Endometrial carcinoma: relative effectiveness of adjuvant irradiation vs therapy reserved for relapse, Gynecol Oncol 60:177, 1996.

Ahmad NR, Lanciano RM, Corn BW, et al: Postoperative radiation therapy for surgically staged endometrial cancer: impact of time factors (overall treatment time and surgery-to-radiation interval) on outcome, Int J Radiat Oncol Biol Phys 33:837, 1995.

Andersen ES: Stage II endometrial carcinoma: prognostic factors and the results of treatment, Gynecol Oncol 38:220, 1990.

Anderson JM, Baldassarre S, Hallum AV, et al: High-dose-rate postoperative vaginal cuff irradiation alone for stage IB and IC endometrial cancer, Int J Radiat Oncol Biol Phys 46:417, 2000.

Aquino-Parsons C, Lim P, Wong F, et al: Papillary serous and clear cell carcinoma limited to endometrial curettings in FIGO stage 1a and 1b endometrial adenocarcinoma: treatment implications, Gynecol Oncol 71:83, 1998.

Ahmad K, Kim YH, Deppe G, et al: Radiation therapy in stage II carcinoma of the endometrium, Cancer 63:854, 1989.

Ayoub J, Audet-Lapointe P, Methot Y, et al: Efficacy of sequential cyclical hormone therapy in endometrial cancer and its correlation with steroid hormone receptor status, Gynecol Oncol 31:327, 1988.

Aziz H, Rotman M, Hussain F, et al: Poor survival of black patients in carcinoma of the endometrium, Int J Radiat Oncol Biol Phys 27:293, 1993.

Barakat RR, Wong G, Curtain JP, et al: Tamoxifen use in breast cancer patients who subsequently develop corpus cancer is not associated with a higher incidence of adverse histologic features, Gynecol Oncol 55:164, 1994.

Barter JF, Smith EB, Szpak CA, et al: Leiomyosarcoma of the uterus: clinicopathologic study of 21 cases, Gynecol Oncol 21:220, 1985.

Berchuck A, Anspach C, Evans A, et al: Postsurgical surveillance of patients with FIGO stage I/II endometrial carcinoma, Gynecol Oncol 59:20, 1995.

Berchuck A and Boyd J: Molecular basis of endometrial cancer, Cancer 76:2034, 1995.

Berchuck A, Rodriguez G, Kinney RB, et al: Overexpression of HER-2/*neu* in endometrial cancer is associated with advanced stage disease, Am J Obstet Gynecol 164:15, 1991.

Berchuck A, Rubin SC, Hoskins WJ, et al: Treatment of uterine leiomyosarcoma, Obstet Gynecol 71:845, 1988.

Bernstein L, Deapen D, Cerhan JR, et al: Tamoxifen therapy for breast cancer and endometrial cancer risk, JNCI 91:1654, 1999.

Braly PS: Flow cytometry as a prognostic factor in endometrial cancer: what does it add? Gynecol Oncol 58:145, 1995.

Bruckman JE, Bloomer WD, Marck A, et al: Stage III adenocarcinoma of the endometrium: two prognostic groups, Gynecol Oncol 9:12, 1980.

Bruner DW, Lanciano R, Keegan M, et al: Vaginal stenosis and sexual function following intracavitary radiation for the treatment of cervical and endometrial carcinoma, Int J Radiat Oncol Biol Phys 27:825, 1993.

Carcangiu ML and Chambers JT: Early pathologic stage clear cell carcinoma and uterine papillary serous carcinoma of the endometrium: comparison of clinicopathologic features and survival, Int J Gynecol Pathol 14:30, 1995.

Carey MS, O'Connell GJ, Johanson CR, et al: Good outcome associated with a standardized treatment protocol using selective postoperative radiation in patients with clinical stage I adenocarcinoma of the endometrium, Gynecol Oncol 57:138, 1995.

Cecchini S, Ciatto S, Bonardi R, et al: Screening by ultrasonography for endometrial carcinoma in postmenopausal breast cancer patients under adjuvant tamoxifen, Gynecol Oncol 60:409, 1996.

Childers JM, Spirtos NM, Brainard P, et al: Laparoscopic staging of the patient with incompletely staged early adenocarcinoma of the endometrium, Obstet Gynecol 83:597, 1994.

Chuang L, Burke TW, Tornos C, et al: Staging laparotomy for endometrial carcinoma: assessment of retroperitoneal lymph nodes, Gynecol Oncol 58:189, 1995.

Cirisano FD, Robboy SJ, Dodge RK, et al: Epidemiology and surgicopathologic findings of papillary serous and clear cell endometrial cancers when compared to endometrioid carcinoma, Gynecol Oncol 74:385, 1999.

Clement PB and Scully RE: Müllerian adenosarcoma of the uterus, Cancer 34:1138, 1974.

Clement PB and Scully RE: Pathology of uterine sarcomas. In Coppleson M, editor: Gynecologic oncology, ed 2, Edinburgh, 1992, Churchill Livingstone.

Connor JP, Andrews JI, Anderson B, and Buller RE: Computed tomography in endometrial carcinoma, Obstet Gynecol 95:692, 2000.

Cook LS, Weiss NS, Schwartz SM, et al: Population-based study of tamoxifen therapy and subsequent ovarian, endometrial, and breast cancers, J Natl Cancer Inst 87:1359, 1995.

Connelly PJ, Alberhasky RC, and Christopherson WM: Carcinoma of the endometrium. III. Analysis of 865 cases of adenocarcinoma and adenoacanthoma, Obstet Gynecol 59:569, 1982.

Corn BW, Lanciano RM, Greven KM, et al: Endometrial cancer with para-aortic adenopathy: patterns of failure and opportunities for cure, Int J Radiat Oncol Biol Phys 24:223, 1992.

COSA-NZ-UK Endometrial Cancer Study Groups: Adjuvant medroxyprogesterone acetate in high-risk endometrial cancer, Int J Gynecol Cancer 8:387, 1998.

Cramer DW, Cutler SJ, and Christine B: Trends in the incidence of endometrial cancer in the United States, Gynecol Oncol 2:130, 1974.

Creasman WT: New gynecologic cancer staging, Obstet Gynecol 75:287, 1990.

Creasman WT: Estrogen replacement therapy: is previously treated cancer a contraindication? Obstet Gynecol 77:308, 1991.

Creasman WT, DeGeest K, DiSaia PJ, et al: Significance of true surgical pathologic staging: a Gynecologic Group Study, Am J Obstet Gynecol 181:31, 1999.

Creasman WT, Henderson D, Hinshaw W, et al: Estrogen replacement therapy in the patient treated for endometrial cancer, Obstet Gynecol 67:326, 1986.

Creasman WT, Morrow CP, Bundy BN, et al: Surgical pathologic spread patterns of endometrial cancer, Cancer 60:2035, 1987.

Creutzberg CL, van Putten WLJ, Kiper PCM, et al: Surgery and postoperative radiotherapy versus surgery alone for patients with stage-1 endometrial carcinoma: multicentre randomised trial, Lancet 355:1404, 2000.

Currie JL, Blessing JA, Muss HB, et al: Combination chemotherapy with hydroxyurea, dacarbazine (DTIC), and etoposide in the treatment of uterine leiomyosarcoma: a Gynecologic Oncology Group study, Gynecol Oncol 61:27, 1996.

Doering DL, Barnhill DR, Weiser EB, et al: Intraoperative evaluation of depth of superficial invasion in stage I endometrial carcinoma, Obstet Gynecol 74:930, 1989.

Dotters DJ: Preoperative CA 125 in endometrial cancer: is it useful? Obstet Gynecol 182:1328, 2000.

DuBeshter B: Endometrial cancer: predictive value of cervical cytology (editorial), Gynecol Oncol 72:271, 1999.

Eifel PJ, Ross J, Hendrickson M, et al: Adenocarcinoma of the endometrium: analysis of 256 cases with disease limited to the uterine corpus: treatment comparison, Cancer 52:1026, 1983.

Eltabbakh GH and Moore AD: Survival of women with surgical stage II endometrial cancer, Gynecol Oncol 74:80, 1999.

Feltmate CM, Duska LR, Change Y, et al: Predictors of recurrence in surgical stage II endometrial adenocarcinoma, Gynecol Oncol 73:407, 1999.

Feuer GA and Calanog A: Endometrial carcinoma: treatment of positive paraaortic nodes, Gynecol Oncol 27:104, 1987.

Fornander T, Cedermark B, Mattsson A, et al: Adjuvant tamoxifen in early breast cancer: occurrence of new primary cancers, Lancet 1(8630):117, 1989.

Franchi M, Ghezzi F, Donadello N, et al: Endometrial thickness in tamoxifen-treated patients: an independent predictor of endometrial disease, Obstet Gynecol 93:1004, 1999.

Franchi M, Ghezzi F, Melpignano M, et al: Clinical value of intraoperative gross examination in endometrial cancer, Gynecol Oncol 76:357, 2000.

Fukuda K, Mori M, Uchiyama M, et al: Preoperative cervical cytology in endometrial carcinoma and its clinicopathologic relevance, Gynecol Oncol 72:273, 1999.

Gallion HH, van Nagell JR, Powell DF, et al: Stage I serous papillary carcinoma of the endometrium, Cancer 63:2224, 1989.

Geisler JP, Geisler HE, Melton ME, and Wiemann MC: What staging surgery should be performed on patients with uterine papillary serous carcinoma? Gynecol Oncol 74:465, 1999.

George E, Lillemoe TJ, Twiggs LB, et al: Malignant mixed müllerian tumor versus high-grade endometrial carcinoma and aggressive variants of endometrial carcinoma: a comparative analysis of survival, Int J Gynecol Pathol 14:39, 1995.

Gerszten K, Faul C, and Huang Q: Pathologic stage III endometrial cancer treated with adjuvant radiation therapy, Int J Gynecol Cancer 9:243, 1999.

Gitsch G, Friedlander ML, Wain GV, et al: Uterine papillary serous carcinoma: a clinical study, Cancer 75:2239, 1995.

Goff BA, Kato D, Schmidt RA, et al: Uterine papillary serous carcinoma: patterns of metastatic spread, Gynecol Oncol 54:264, 1994.

Goldschmidt R, Katz Z, Blickstein I, et al: The accuracy of endometrial pipelle sampling with and without sonographic measurement of endometrial thickness, Obstet Gynecol 82:727, 1993.

Goodman A, Zukerberg LR, Rice LW, et al: Squamous cell carcinoma of the endometrium: a report of eight cases and a review of the literature, Gynecol Oncol 61:54, 1996.

Granberg S, Wikland M, Karlsson B, et al: Endometrial thickness as measured by endovaginal ultrasonography for identifying endometrial abnormality, Am J Obstet Gynecol 164:47, 1991.

Greven KM, Curran WJ, Whittington R, et al: Analysis of failure patterns in stage III endometrial carcinoma and therapeutic implications, Int J Radiat Oncol Biol Phys 17:35, 1989.

Greven KM, D'Agostino RB, Lanciano RM, and Corn BW: Is there a role for a brachytherapy vaginal cuff boost in the adjuvant management of patients with uterine-confined endometrial cancer? Int J Radiat Oncol Biol Phys 42:101, 1998.

Grice J, Ek M, Greer B, et al: Uterine papillary serous carcinoma: evaluation of long-term survival in surgically staged patients, Gynecol Oncol 69:69, 1998.

Grimes DA and Economy KE: Primary prevention of gynecologic cancers, Am J Obstet Gynecol 172:227, 1995.

Grimshaw RN, Tupper WC, Fraser RC, et al: Prognostic value of peritoneal cytology in endometrial carcinoma, Gynecol Oncol 36:97, 1990.

Gull B, Carlsson SA, Karlsson B, et al: Transvaginal ultrasonography of the endometrium in women with postmenopausal bleeding: is it always necessary to perform an endometrial biopsy? Am J Obstet Gynecol 182:509, 2000.

Hill HA, Coates RJ, Austin H, et al: Racial differences in tumor grade among women with endometrial cancer, Gynecol Oncol 56:154, 1995.

Hoffman MS, Roberts WS, Cavanagh D, et al: Treatment of recurrent and metastatic endometrial cancer and cisplatin, doxorubicin, cyclophosphamide, and megestrol acetate, Gynecol Oncol 35:75, 1989.

Homesley HD, Boronow RC, and Lewis JL: Stage II endometrial adenocarcinoma, Obstet Gynecol 49:604, 1977.

Kadar N, Homesley HD, and Malfetano JH: Positive peritoneal cytology is an adverse factor in endometrial carcinoma only if there is other evidence of extrauterine disease, Gynecol Oncol 46:145, 1992.

Kaku T, Silverberg SG, Major FJ, et al: Adenosarcoma of the uterus: a Gynecologic Oncology Group clinicopathologic study of 31 cases, Int J Gynecol Pathol 11:75, 1992.

Kato DT, Ferry JA, Goodman A, et al: Uterine papillary serous carcinoma (UPSC): a clinicopathologic study of 30 cases, Gynecol Oncol 59:384, 195.

Kendall BS, Ronnett BM, Isacson C, et al: Reproducibility of the diagnosis of endometrial hyperplasia, atypical hyperplasia, and well-differentiated carcinoma, Am J Surg Pathol 22:1012, 1998.

Kennedy AS, DeMars LR, Flannagan LM, et al: Primary squamous cell carcinoma of the endometrium: a first report of adjuvant chemoradiation, Gynecol Oncol 59:117, 1995.

Koss LG, Schreiber K, Oberlander SG, et al: Detection of endometrial carcinoma and hyperplasia in asymptomatic women, Obstet Gynecol 64:1, 1984.

Kucera H, Vavra N, and Weghaupt K: Benefit of external irradiation in pathologic stage I endometrial carcinoma: a prospective clinical trial of 605 patients who received postoperative vaginal irradiation and additional pelvic irradiation in the presence of unfavorable prognostic factors, Gynecol Oncol 38:99, 1990.

Kurjak A, Kupesic S, Shalan H, et al: Uterine sarcoma: a report of 10 cases studied by transvaginal color and pulsed Doppler sonography, Gynecol Oncol 59:342, 1995.

Kurjak A, Shalan H, Sosic A, et al: Endometrial carcinoma in postmenopausal women: evaluation by transvaginal color doppler ultrasonography, Am J Obstet Gynecol 169:1597, 1993.

Kurman RJ, Kaminski PF, and Norris HJ: Behavior of endometrial hyperplasia: a long-term study of "untreated" hyperplasias in 170 patients, Cancer 56:403, 1985.

Kurman RJ and Norris HJ: Endometrial hyperplasia and related cellular changes. In Blaustein's pathology of the female genital tract, ed 4, New York, 1994, Springer-Verlag.

Kurman RJ and Scully RE: Clear cell carcinoma of the endometrium, Cancer 37:872, 1976.

Lanciano RM and Greven KM: Adjuvant treatment for endometrial cancer: who needs it? Gynecol Oncol 57:135, 1995 (editorial).

Langer RD, Pierce JJ, O'Hanlan KA, et al: Transvaginal ultrasonography compared with endometrial biopsy for the detection of endometrial disease, N Engl J Med 337:1792, 1997.

Lee RB, Burke TW, and Park RC: Estrogen replacement therapy following treatment for stage I endometrial carcinoma, Gynecol Oncol 36:189, 1990.

Lehoczky O, Bosze P, Ungar L, et al: Stage I endometrial carcinoma: treatment of nonoperable patients with intracavitary radiation therapy alone, Gynecol Oncol 43:211, 1991.

Leibsohn S, Mishell DR, d'Ablaing G, and Schlaerth JB: Leiomyosarcomas in a series of hysterectomies performed for presumed uterine leiomyomata, Am J Obstet Gynecol 162:968, 1990.

Love CDB, Muir BB, Scrimgeour JB, et al: Investigation of endometrial abnormalities in asymptomatic women treated with tamoxifen and an evaluation of the role of endometrial screening, J Clin Oncol 17:2050, 1999.

Lurain JR and Piver MS: Uterine sarcomas: clinical features and management. In Coppleson M, editor: Gynecologic oncology, ed 2, Edinburgh, 1992, Churchill Livingstone, p 827.

MacMahon B: Risk factors for endometrial cancer, Gynecol Oncol 2:122, 1974.

Magriples U, Naftolin F, Schwartz PE, et al: High-grade endometrial carcinoma in tamoxifen-treated breast cancer patients, J Clin Oncol 11:485, 1993.

Malfetano JH: Tamoxifen-associated endometrial carcinoma in postmenopausal breast cancer patients, Gynecol Oncol 39:82, 1990.

Mariani A, Sebo TJ, Katzmann JA, et al: Pretreatment assessment of prognostic indicators in endometrial cancer, Am J Obstet Gynecol 182:1535, 2000.

Mariani A, Webb MJ, Galli L, and Podratz KC: Potential therapeutic role of para-aortic lymphadenectomy in node-positive endometrial cancer, Gynecol Oncol 76:348, 2000.

Mariani A, Webb MJ, Kenney GL, et al: Low-risk corpus cancer: is lymphadenectomy or radiotherapy necessary? Am J Obstet Gynecol 182:1506, 2000.

Mayr NA, Wen BC, Benda J, et al: Postoperative radiation therapy in clinical stage I endometrial cancer: corpus, cervical, and lower uterine segment involvement—patterns of failure, Radiology 196:323, 1995.

Melhem MF and Tobon H: Mucinous adenocarcinoma of the endometrium: a clinico-pathological review of 18 cases, Int J Gynecol Pathol 6:347, 1987.

Mignotte H, Lasset C, Bonadana V, et al: Iatrogenic risks of endometrial carcinoma after treatment for breast cancer in large French case-control study, Int J Cancer 76:325, 1998.

Miller B, Umpierre S, Tornas C, and Burke T: Histologic characterization of uterine papillary serous adenocarcinoma, Gynecol Oncol 56:425, 1995.

Moore DH, Fowler WC, Walton LA, and Droegemueller W: Morbidity of lymph node sampling in cancers of the uterine corpus and cervix, Obstet Gynecol 74:180, 1989.

Morrow CP, Bundy BN, Kurman RJ, et al: Relationship between surgical-pathological risk factors and outcome in clinical stage I and II carcinoma of the endometrium: a Gynecologic Oncology Group study, Gynecol Oncol 40:55, 1991.

Nguyen T-V and Petereit DG: High-dose-rate brachytherapy for medically inoperable stage I endometrial cancer, Gynecol Oncol 71:196, 1998.

Nielsen SN, Podratz KC, Scheithauer BW, and O'Brien PC: Clinicopathologic analysis of uterine malignant mixed müllerian tumors, Gynecol Oncol 34:372, 1989.

Norris HJ and Taylor HB: Mesenchymal tumors of the uterus. I. A clinical and pathologic study of 53 endometrial stromal tumors, Cancer 19:755, 1966.

Omodei U, Ferrazzia E, Ruggeri C, et al: Endometrial thickness and histological abnormalities in women on hormonal replacement therapy: a transvaginal ultrasound/hysteroscopic study, Ultrasound Obstet Gynecol 15:317, 2000.

Omura GA, Blessing JA, Major FJ, et al: A randomized clinical trial of adjuvant Adriamycin in uterine sarcomas: a Gynecologic Oncology Group study, J Clin Oncol 3:1240, 1985.

Omura GA, Major FJ, Blessing JA, et al: A randomized study of Adriamycin with and without dimethyl-triazeno-imidazole-carboxamide in advanced uterine sarcomas, Cancer 52:626, 1983.

Onsrud M, Kolstad P, and Normann T: Postoperative external pelvic irradiation in carcinoma of the corpus, stage I: a controlled clinical trial, Gynecol Oncol 4:222, 1976.

Parker SL, Tong T, Bolden S, and Wingo PA: Cancer statistics, 1996, CA Cancer J Clin 46:5, 1996.

Parker WH, Fu YS, and Berek JS: Uterine sarcoma in patients operated on for presumed leiomyoma and rapidly growing leiomyoma, Obstet Gynecol 83:414, 1994.

Partridge EE, Shingleton HM, and Menck HR: The national cancer data base report on endometrial cancer, J Surg Oncol 61:111, 1996.

Patsner B, Mann WJ, Cohen H, and Loesch M: Predictive value of preoperative serum CA-125 levels in clinically localized and advanced endometrial carcinoma, Am J Obstet Gynecol 158:399, 1988.

Pecorelli S, Creasman WT, Pettersson F, et al: FIGO annual report on the results of treatment in gynaecological cancer. Twenty-third volume, Milano, Italy. J Epidemiol Biostatistics, 1998.

Perez CA, Grigsby PW, Castro-Vita H, and Lockett MA: Carcinoma of the uterine cervix. I. Impact of prolongation of overall treatment time and timing of brachytherapy on outcome of radiation therapy, Int J Radiat Oncol Biol Phys 31:1275, 1995.

Perez-Medina T, Bajo J, Folgueira G, et al: Atypical endometrial hyperplasia treatment with progestogens and gonadotropin-releasing hormone analogues: long-term follow-up, Gynecol Oncol 73:299, 1999.

Petereit DG, Tannehill SP, Grosen EA, et al: Outpatient vaginal cuff brachytherapy for endometrial cancer, Int J Gynecol Cancer 9:456, 1999.

Peters WA, Rivkin SE, Smith MR, and Tesh DE: Cisplatin and Adriamycin combination chemotherapy for uterine stromal sarcomas and mixed mesodermal tumors, Gynecol Oncol 34:323, 1989.

Pinelli DM, Fiorica JV, Roberts WS, et al: Chemotherapy plus sequential hormonal therapy for advanced and recurrent endometrial carcinoma: a phase II study, Gynecol Oncol 60:462, 1996.

Pisani AL, Barbuto DA, Chen D, et al: Her-2/*neu*, p53, and DNA analyses as prognosticators for survival in endometrial carcinoma, Obstet Gynecol 85:729, 1995.

Piver MS, Rutledge FN, Copeland L, et al: Uterine endolymphatic stromal myosis: a collaborative study, Obstet Gynecol 64:173, 1984.

Plentl AA and Friedman EA: Lymphatic system of the female genitalia, Philadelphia, 1971, WB Saunders Co.

Pliskow S, Penalver M, and Averette H: Stage III and stage IV endometrial carcinoma: a review of 41 cases, Gynecol Oncol 38:210, 1990.

Podczaski ES, Kaminski P, Manetta A, et al: Stage II endometrial carcinoma treated with external-beam radiotherapy, intracavitary application of cesium, and surgery, Gynecol Oncol 35:251, 1989.

Potish RA, Twiggs LB, Adcock LL, et al: Paraaortic lymph node radiotherapy in cancer of the uterine corpus, Obstet Gynecol 65:251, 1985.

Poulsen HK, Jacobsen M, Bertelsen K, et al: Adjuvant radiation therapy is not necessary in the management of endometrial carcinoma stage I, low-risk cases, Int J Gynecol Cancer 6:38, 1996.

Press MF and Scully RE: Endometrial "sarcomas" complicating ovarian thecoma, polycystic ovarian disease and estrogen therapy, Gynecol Oncol 21:135, 1985.

Rose PG, Sommers RM, Reale FR, et al: Serial serum CA 125 measurements for evaluation of recurrence in patients with endometrial carcinoma, Obstet Gynecol 84:12, 1994.

Rutqvist LE, Johansson H, Signomklao T, et al: Adjuvant tamoxifen therapy for early stage breast cancer and second primary malignancies, J Natl Cancer Inst 87:645, 1995.

Sarcoma Meta-Analysis Collaboration: Adjuvant chemotherapy for localised resectable soft-tissue sarcoma of adults: meta-analysis of individual data, Lancet 350:1647, 1997.

Schink JC, Rademaker AW, Miller DS, et al: Tumor size in endometrial cancer, Cancer 67:2791, 1991.

Schlesselman JJ: Net effect of oral contraceptive use on the risk of cancer in women in the United States, Obstet Gynecol 85:793, 1995.

Sears JD, Greven KM, Hoen HM, et al: Prognostic factors and treatment outcome for patients with locally recurrent endometrial cancer, Cancer 74:1303, 1994.

Shim JU, Rose PG, Reale FR, et al: Accuracy of frozen-section diagnosis at surgery in clinical stage I and II endometrial carcinoma, Am J Obstet Gynecol 166:1335, 1992.

Smith-Bindman R, Kerlikowske K, Feldstein VA, et al: Endovaginal ultrasound to exclude endometrial cancer and other endometrial abnormalities, JAMA 280:1510, 1998.

Sonoda Y, Zerbe M, Barakat RR, et al: High incidence of positive peritoneal cytology in low-risk endometrial cancer treated by laparoscopically assisted vaginal hysterectomy (LAVH), SGO Abstracts 19, 2000.

Sood AK, Buller RE, Burger RA, et al: Value of preoperative CA 125 level in the management of uterine cancer and prediction of clinical outcome, Obstet Gynecol 90:441, 1997.

Thatcher SS and Woodruff JD: Uterine stromatosis: a report of 33 cases, Obstet Gynecol 59:428, 1982.

Thigpen JT, Brady MF, Alvarez RD, et al: Oral medroxyprogesterone acetate in the treatment of advance or recurrence endometrial carcinoma: a dose-response study by the Gynecology Oncology Group, J Clin Oncol 17:1736, 1999.

Thoms WM, Eifel PJ, Smith TL, et al: Bulky endocervical carcinoma: a 23-year experience, Int J Radiat Oncol Biol Phys 23:491, 1992.

Tiltman AJ: Mucinous carcinoma of the endometrium, Obstet Gynecol 55:244, 1980.

Turner DA, Gershenson DM, Atkinson N, et al: The prognostic significance of peritoneal cytology for stage I endometrial cancer, Obstet Gynecol 74:775, 1989.

Valle RF and Baggish MS: Endometrial carcinoma after endometrial ablation: high-risk factors predicting its occurrence, Am J Obstet Gynecol 179:569, 1998.

Vergote I, Kjorstad K, Abeler V, et al: A randomized trial of adjuvant progestagen in early endometrial cancer, Cancer 64:1011, 1989.

Wilson TO, Podratz KC, Gaffey TA, et al: Evaluation of unfavorable histologic subtypes in endometrial adenocarcinoma, Am J Obstet Gynecol 162:418, 1990.

Wolfson AH, Wolfson DJ, Sittler SY, et al: A multivariate analysis of clinicopathologic factors for predicting outcome in uterine sarcomas, Gynecol Oncol 52:56, 1994.

Yamada SD, Burger RA, Brewster WR, et al: Pathologic variables and adjuvant therapy as predictors of recurrence and survival for patients with surgically evaluated carcinosarcoma of the uterus, Cancer 88:2782, 2000.

Zaino RJ, Kurman RJ, Diana KL, and Morrow CP: Pathologic models to predict outcome for women with endometrial adenocarcinoma, Cancer 77:1115, 1996.

Zaino RJ, Kurman R, Herbold D, et al: The significance of squamous differentiation in endometrial carcinoma: data from a Gynecologic Oncology Group study, Cancer 68:2293, 1991.

Zelmanowicz A, Hildescheim A, Sherman ME, et al: Evidence for a common etiology for endometrial carcinomas and malignant mixed mullerian tumors, Gynecol Oncol 69:253, 1998.

Zerbe MJ, Zhang J, Bristow RE, et al: Retrograde seeding of malignant cells during hysteroscopy in endometrial cancer, SGO Abstracts 20, 2000.

Neoplastic Diseases of the Ovary

Screening, Benign and Malignant Epithelial and Germ Cell Neoplasms, Sex-Cord Stromal Tumors

Adenofibroma. An epithelial tumor that consists of glandular elements and large amounts of ovarian stromal (fibroblast) elements.

Adenoma. A benign ovarian epithelial tumor consisting of glandular (adenomatous) elements.

Alpha-fetoprotein. A secretory product from endodermal sinus tumors that can be measured in serum and serves as a specific tumor marker.

Borderline Tumors. A term used to describe an epithelial carcinoma of low malignant potential (grade 0). The malignant cells do not invade the stroma.

Brenner Tumor. An epithelial neoplasm that consists of cells resembling urothelium and so-called Walthard nests of the ovary. These are mixed with ovarian stroma.

Carcinoid. A rare type of teratoma that histologically resembles the carcinoid tumors that arise in the gastrointestinal tract.

Clear Cell Tumor (Mesonephroma). An ovarian neoplasm that consists of clear cells (containing glycogen) or "hobnail" cells. Histologically they resemble clear cell tumors that arise in the endocervix, endometrium, and vagina.

Cyst. A descriptive term added as a prefix to the designation of epithelial tumors to indicate the presence of cystlike spaces, for example, cystadenoma.

Cytoreductive Surgery. The practice of reducing the bulk of malignant tissue and removing, if possible, all gross disease.

Dermoid. A benign cystic germ cell tumor (cystic teratoma) that may contain elements of all three germ cell layers. It is the most common ovarian neoplasm in those under 30 years of age.

Dysgerminoma. The most common of ovarian malignant germ cell tumors. It consists of primitive germ cells.

Endodermal Sinus Tumor. A malignant germ cell tumor. It recapitulates extraembryonic tissue and may resemble the yolk sac of the rodent placenta.

Endometrioid Tumor. An ovarian epithelial tumor whose cells resemble those of the uterine endometrial adenocarcinoma.

Epithelial Stromal Tumors. The most common type of ovarian neoplasms. They are derived from the surface (coelomic) epithelium and ovarian stroma. Have previously been termed *common epithelial tumors*. The most common cell types are serous, mucinous, and endometroid.

Fibroma. The most common benign ovarian solid tumor. It is composed of stromal cells (fibroblasts) and in some cases is associated with benign ascites and hydrothorax (Meigs' syndrome).

Germ Cell Tumor. The second most common type of ovarian neoplasm after epithelial tumors. Germ cell tumors contain cells that recapitulate embryonic tissues (ectoderm, mesoderm, or endoderm) or extraembryonic elements.

Gonadoblastoma. A rare tumor that arises in abnormal (dysgenetic) gonads and consists of sex-cord stromal elements and germ cells.

Granulosa-Thecal Cell Tumor. A sex-cord stromal tumor that often secretes estrogens and consists of granulosa cells (sex cord) and ovarian stromal cells (thecal cells or fibroblasts).

Immature Teratoma. A teratoma with malignant (immature) embryonic elements (ectoderm, mesoderm, or endoderm).

955

Krukenberg Tumor. A tumor metastatic to the ovary, usually bilateral, consisting of signet-ring cells that usually originate from the gastrointestinal tract, most frequently the stomach, and then from the large intestine.

Mucinous Tumor. An ovarian epithelial tumor whose cells contain mucin and resemble those of the endocervix.

Ovarian Neoplasm. An ovarian tumor that is not physiologic and will not regress with time. It may be benign or malignant.

Papillary. A descriptive term added to the designation of epithelial tumors if papillary-like projections are present, for example, papillary cystadenocarcinoma.

Papillary Serous Carcinoma of the Ovary. A variant of carcinoma leading to widespread peritoneal carcinomatosis. It has microscopically a papillary serous appearance and usually small (<4 cm) ovaries. A tumor of similar histology may arise from the peritoneum in which case it is termed *primary peritoneal carcinoma.*

Primary Peritoneal Carcinoma. A malignant process predominantly involving the peritoneum and histologically resembling serous carcinoma. The ovaries are usually of normal size with surface metastatic deposits (up to 5 mm).

Pseudomyxoma Peritonei. Intraperitoneal spread of mucin-secreting cells that originate from ovarian mucinous cystadenoma or cystadenocarcinoma or frequently from the appendix that may lead to recurrent abdominal masses and bowel obstruction.

Second-Look Operation. A procedure with extensive biopsy sampling and cytologic sampling of the peritoneal cavity, as well as evaluation of the retroperitoneal nodes. It is usually performed after chemotherapy in a patient who is clinically in complete remission.

Serous Tumor. An ovarian epithelial tumor whose cells resemble those of the fallopian tube.

Sertoli-Leydig Cell Tumor. A rare sex cord–stromal tumor with male elements. It often causes virilization.

Sex Cord–Stromal Tumors. A class of ovarian tumors in which the constituents of the ovary or testes are recapitulated.

Small Cell Carcinoma. A highly virulent, usually fatal ovarian malignancy occurring in young women, often accompanied by hypercalcemia.

Stages of Ovarian Cancer:

Stage I: Confined to one or both ovaries.

Stage II: Extension to pelvic structures.

Stage III: Extension outside of pelvis or to retroperitoneal or inguinal nodes.

Stage IV: Extension outside of peritoneal cavity or to liver parenchyma—pleural effusion with malignant cells.

Struma Ovarii. A specialized ovarian teratoma that consists of thyroid tissue as a major or exclusive component. It may rarely produce sufficient thyroid hormone to induce hyperthyroidism.

Teratoma. An ovarian germ cell tumor that recapitulates any one or all of tissues of the ectoderm, mesoderm, or endoderm. The tissues can be benign (mature) or malignant (immature).

Thecoma. A benign ovarian stromal tumor consisting of thecal cells.

Ovarian cancer is the second most common malignancy of the lower part of the female genital tract, occurring less frequently than cancers of the endometrium but more frequently than cancers of the cervix. However, it is the most frequent cause of death from gynecologic neoplasms in the United States. Cancer Statistics 2000 reports that approximately 23,100 new cases of ovarian cancer will be diagnosed yearly in the United States, and there will be 14,000 deaths. A major contributing factor to the high death rate from relatively few cases is the detection of the disease in advanced stages because of the intraabdominal location of the ovary and the fact that these cancers often do not cause symptoms until the malignancy is widespread. The incidence of ovarian cancer (Figure 31-1) rises with age, becoming most marked beyond 50 years, with a gradual increase continuing to age 70 years followed by a decrease for those over age 80.

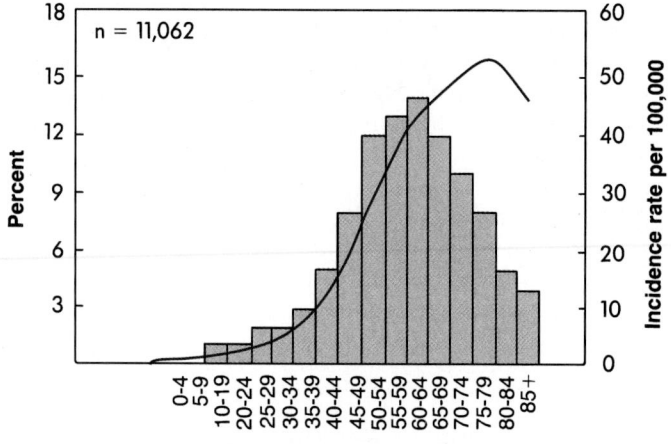

FIGURE 31-1 Ovarian cancer incidence rates by age, 1973 to 1982. (From Yancik R, Ries LG, and Yates JW: Am J Obstet Gynecol 154:639, 1986.)

Moreover, Yancik et al. noted that those over 65 were more likely to have their cancers diagnosed at an advanced stage, leading to a worse prognosis and poorer survival compared to those under age 65 years.

Despite numerous epidemiologic investigations, a clear-cut cause of ovarian cancer has not been defined. A number of theories have been advanced. It is thought that these malignancies are related to frequent ovulation, and therefore women who ovulate regularly appear to be at higher risk. Included are those with a late menopause, a history of nulliparity, or late childbearing. Conversely, women who have had several pregnancies or who have used oral contraceptives appear to have some protection against ovarian cancer. Casagrande et al. related the development of ovarian cancer to "ovulatory age," that is, the number of years during which the patient has ovulated. This number would be reduced by pregnancy, breast-feeding, or oral contraceptive use. Schildkraut et al. correlated overexpression of mutant p53 protein in ovarian cancers with reproductive histories and found that overexpression was more likely in those who had high ovulatory cycle histories. In addition, talcum powder used on the perineum has been postulated to increase the risk, but as noted by Cramer et al. it is a weak association. The use of oral contraceptives decreases the risk by about 50% after 5 years of use (about 10% to 12% per year). The protection increases with duration of use to 10 years and appears to last for about 15 years after discontinuation of use. Schlesselman calculated a decrease of 369 ovarian cancer cases per 100,000 women for 8 years of use. Given that the approximate occurrence of ovarian cancer cases in this group would be expected to be 1400, such a decrease approximates 25%. Breast-feeding and pregnancy also are protective and perhaps, surprisingly, tubal ligation and to a lesser extent hysterectomy with ovarian preservation also lower the risk of ovarian cancer. It has been suggested that ovulation-inducing drugs such as Clomid increase the risk of ovarian cancer, as noted by Whittemore et al. Rossing et al. reported an increase in risk from a population-based study that suggested that the risk was associated with prolonged use of clomiphene insofar as no association was noted with less than 1 year of use. The study was significant but with wide 95% confidence limits, and only 11 cancer cases occurred in the clomiphene group among 3837 women studied in the Infertility Clinic. However, the recent study of Venn et al. from Australia did not demonstrate an increase in ovarian cancer for those using fertility drugs for in vitro fertilization. Cramer et al. found women with ovarian cancer to have a diet high in animal fat in comparison with control subjects, and studies of Risch et al. suggest that saturated fat increases the risk of ovarian cancer while vegetable fiber may reduce it. Table 31-1 shows the various factors that alter the risk of ovarian cancer. The familial or inherited aspects of the disease are considered subsequently.

There are geographic and racial differences in the distribution of ovarian cancers. These cancers occur most fre-

TABLE 31-1
Putative Associations of Increasing and Decreasing Risks of Ovarian Epithelial Carcinoma

Increases	Decreases
Age	Breast-feeding
Diet	Oral contraceptives
Family history	Pregnancy
Industrialized country	Tubal ligation and hysterectomy with ovarian conservation
Infertility	
Nulliparity	
Ovulation	
Ovulatory drugs	
Talc?	

From Herbst AL: Am J Obstet Gynecol 170:1099, 1994.

quently in industrialized and affluent countries such as the United States and Western Europe, and less frequently in Asia and Africa. The disease is more frequent among white than black women. Finally, patients with ovarian carcinoma have an increased risk of developing breast and endometrial cancer. The major factors, however, appear to be related to the frequency of ovulation and residence in an industrialized country.

In a case-control study Hartge et al. showed a familial history of breast cancer and a personal history of breast cancer were risk factors. Lynch et al. have reported on families with these hereditary ovarian cancers and noted that they tend to occur at a younger age than in the general population. It appears that germline mutations of the BRCA tumor suppressor gene on chromosome 17q are responsible for a large proportion of hereditary cancers (see later discussion). However, these are a small proportion of all ovarian carcinomas. A recent study by Narod et al. suggests it may be possible to reduce ovarian cancer risk in these patients with BRCA mutation by oral contraceptive use, but the data are not definitive.

Hereditary ovarian cancers are rare, occur in a few families, and are usually lethal. The term *familial ovarian cancer* denotes an inherited trait that predisposes to ovarian cancer development. It has been widely studied and two definitions are important: A first-degree relative is a mother, sister, or daughter of an affected individual; a second-degree relative is a maternal or paternal aunt or grandmother. As noted in the review by Kerlikowske et al., prior literature studies suggest an increase from about 1.5% to 5% in the lifetime risk of ovarian cancer with one first-degree relative; with two or more the risk reaches about 7%. Unfortunately, many of the studies showing statistical significance were based on self-reporting of family history rather than documentation by medical records. Thus the increase in risk may well be less. Current information suggests that about 90% of ovarian cancers develop sporadically. For the woman with a familial history of ovarian cancer (not the dominant genetic hereditary type), periodic surveillance with transvaginal ultrasound every 6 months beyond the age of 35 has been suggested (see ultrasound discussion later in this chapter). Unfortunately, such a strategy has not been shown to be worthwhile or cost effective in disease prevention and may on occasion lead to additional tests or unnecessary procedures when a questionable ultrasound result is obtained (see subsequent discussion on ultrasound screening and natural history of ovarian cancer). The use of prophylactic oophorectomy in patients whose mothers had ovarian cancer has been a controversial topic. Kerlikowske et al. and Herbst provided reasons against the widespread use of such a practice. However, if a patient with a positive family history requires operation such as hysterectomy, removal of both ovaries at the time of operation is appropriate. The patient must be aware that peritoneal carcinomatosis, a process resembling serous carcinoma of the ovary, can rarely develop despite the removal of both ovaries.

The following describes the classification and histology of the major ovarian neoplasms. Pertinent microscopic findings, clinical behavior, and appropriate therapy are presented.

CLASSIFICATION OF OVARIAN NEOPLASMS

The most widely used classification of ovarian neoplasms is that of the World Health Organization. This classification, along with frequency of occurrence of the primary ovarian neoplasms, is shown in Table 31-2.

The epithelial stromal (common epithelial) tumors are the most frequent ovarian neoplasms. They are believed to arise from the surface (coelomic) epithelium. Germ cell tumors are the second most frequent and are the most common among young women. Histologically they may be composed of extraembryonic elements or may have features that resemble any or all of the three embryonic layers (ectoderm, mesoderm, or endoderm). Germ cell tumors are the main cause of ovarian malignancy in young women, particularly those in their teens and early 20s. Sex cord–stromal tumors are the third most frequent and contain elements that recapitulate the constituents of the ovary or testis. These tumors may secrete sex steroid hormones or may be hormonally inactive. Lipid (lipoid) cell tumors are extremely rare and histologically resemble the adrenal gland. Gonadoblastomas consist of germ cells and sex cord–stromal elements. They occur in individuals with dysgenetic gonads, particularly when a Y chromosome is present. All these ovarian neoplasms are discussed later in this chapter.

Soft tissue tumors not specific to the ovary, such as hemangioma or lipoma, are extremely rare and are categorized according to the criteria for soft tissue tumors arising elsewhere in the body. Unclassified tumors, as the name implies, cannot be placed in any of the preceding categories. One example is small cell carcinoma, which is a highly virulent cancer affecting primarily young women (see discussion later in chapter). Metastatic tumors to the ovary may arise elsewhere in the reproductive tract, or from distant sites such as the bowel or stomach (Krukenberg tumors). Tumorlike conditions refer to enlargements of the ovary, such as extensive edema, pregnancy luteoma, endometriomas, and follicular or luteal cysts, none of which are true neoplasms. With the exceptions of metastatic tumors and small cell carcinoma of the ovary, none of these are considered further in this chapter.

EPITHELIAL STROMAL OVARIAN NEOPLASMS

According to Scully, two thirds of ovarian neoplasms are epithelial tumors; malignant epithelial tumors account for about 85% of ovarian cancers, probably arising from the surface (coelomic) epithelium and adjacent ovarian stroma. Table 31-3 summarizes the five cell types that most commonly comprise epithelial ovarian tumors, indicating their relative frequency.

TABLE 31-2
Frequency of Ovarian Neoplasms
(WHO Classification)

Class	Approximate Frequency (%)
Epithelial stromal (common epithelial) tumors	65
Germ cell tumors	20–25
Sex–cord stromal tumors	6
Lipid (lipoid) cell tumors	<0.1
Gonadoblastoma	<0.1
Soft tissue tumors (not specific to ovary)	
Unclassified tumors	
Secondary (metastatic) tumors	
Tumorlike conditions (not true neoplasm)	

TABLE 31-3
Epithelial Ovarian Tumor Cell Types

	Approximate Frequency (%)	
	All Ovarian Neoplasms	**Ovarian Cancers**
Serous	20–50	35–40
Mucinous	15–25	6–10
Endometrioid	5	15–25
Clear cell (mesonephroid)	<5	5
Brenner	2–3	Rare

Modified from Scully RE: Tumors of the ovary and maldeveloped gonads. In Atlas of tumor pathology, fascicle 16, series 2, Washington, DC, 1979, Armed Forces Institute of Pathology.

Epithelial tumors can be categorized as benign (adenoma), malignant (adenocarcinoma), or of an intermediate form, known as *borderline malignant adenocarcinoma* or *tumors of low malignant potential.* The term *papillary* or the prefix *cyst* (as in cystadenoma) is used when the tumor has, respectively, papillae or cystic structures. The suffix *fibroma* (as in adenofibroma) is added when the ovarian stroma predominates, with the exception of a Brenner tumor, which normally contains a large amount of ovarian stroma.

Well-differentiated serous tumors (Figure 31-2, *A* and *B*) consist of ciliated epithelial cells that resemble those of the fallopian tube. Serous tumors (Figure 31-2, *C*) are the most frequent ovarian epithelial tumors. The malignant forms account for up to 40% of ovarian cancers; the benign forms (serous cystadenomas) occur primarily during the reproductive years; the borderline tumors occur in women 30 to 50 years of age; the carcinomas typically occur in women over 40 years of age.

Two histologically similar variants of serous tumors occur. One is an aggressive tumor with small ovaries that are usually less than 4 to 5 cm in diameter, with extensive disease on the ovarian surface and metastatic disease in the abdomen. The process is termed *serous surface papillary carcinoma of the ovary.* The other type presents in a clinically similar fashion as a primary peritoneal serous adenocarcinoma. It is often difficult histologically to distinguish these entities.

Mucinous tumors (Figure 31-3, *A* and *B*) consist of epithelial cells filled with mucin; most are benign. These cells resemble cells of the endocervix or may mimic intestinal cells, which can pose a problem in the differential diagnosis of tumors that appear to originate from the ovary or intestine. Benign mucinous tumors are found primarily during the reproductive years, and mucinous carcinomas (Figure 31-3, *C*) usually occur among those in the 30- to 60-year age range. Overall they can account for about one fourth of ovarian tumors and up to 10% of ovarian cancers.

Endometrioid tumors (Figure 31-4), as the name implies, consist of epithelial cells resembling those of the endometrium. In the ovary these neoplasms are less frequent (approximately 5%) than either the serous or mucinous tumors, but the malignant variety accounts for about 20% of ovarian carcinomas. Endometrioid carcinomas usually occur in women in their 40s and 50s. They may be seen in conjunction with endometriosis and ovarian endometriomas, although an origin from endometriosis is rarely demonstrated. Most endometrioid carcinomas arise directly from the surface epithelium of the ovary, as do the other epithelial tumors.

Clear cell (mesonephroid) tumors contain cells with abundant glycogen (Figure 31-5, *A*) and so-called *hobnail* cells (Figure 31-5, *B*), in which the nuclei of the cells protrude into the glandular lumen. Tumors with identical histologic features are found in the endometrium, cervix, and

vagina, the latter two often associated with intrauterine diethylstilbestrol (DES) exposure. Clear cell ovarian tumors are not related to DES exposure and comprise about 5% of ovarian cancers. They occur primarily in women 40 to 70 years of age and are highly aggressive.

The major cell types of ovarian epithelial tumors recapitulate the müllerian-derived epithelium of the female reproductive system (serous—endosalpinx; mucinous—endocervix; endometrioid—endometrium). This differentiation occurs even though the ovary is not derived directly from the müllerian ducts (Chapter 2). The clear cell tumors also mimic this müllerian tendency, frequently being admixed with endometrioid carcinomas, as well as with ovarian endometriomas.

Brenner tumors (Figure 31-6) consist of cells that resemble the transitional epithelium of the bladder and Walthard nests of the ovary. There is abundant stroma. These tumors constitute only 2% to 3% of all ovarian tumors.

In addition to the cell types shown in Table 31-3, epithelial tumors may be classified as undifferentiated if the tumor consists of poorly differentiated epithelial cells not characteristic of any particular cell type. They may be considered unclassifiable if they cannot be placed in any of the categories shown in Table 31-3.

Many epithelial ovarian tumors can be bilateral, and the risk of bilaterality is an important consideration in therapy, particularly when an ovarian tumor is discovered in a young woman of reproductive age. Widely varying percentages have been reported for bilaterality in ovarian tumors, and the most widely quoted are summarized in Table 31-4. Malignant epithelial tumors tend to involve both ovaries more frequently than do benign epithelial tumors. Serous tumors also tend to be bilateral more frequently than do mucinous tumors.

Benign Epithelial Ovarian Tumors— The Adnexal Mass

As noted in Chapter 7, enlargement of the ovary beyond 5 cm is considered abnormal. However, age and menstrual status must also be considered before the appropriate course of action is chosen. A 5- to 8-cm ovarian mass in a woman with regular menses, even if she is in her 40s, is frequently a functioning ovarian cyst, such as a follicular or corpus luteum cyst. It will usually regress spontaneously during a subsequent menstrual cycle. Enlargements of this type in young patients in their 20s or early 30s do not automatically require immediate operative intervention and can be observed for two menstrual cycles. An exception would be a mass in a patient who is taking oral contraceptives, in which case a neoplastic mass is most likely. Shushan et al. reported ovarian cysts detected by ultrasound in pre- and postmenopausal patients taking tamoxifen for breast cancer. Unilocular 5- to 8-cm cysts are likely to be functional (Chapter 17),

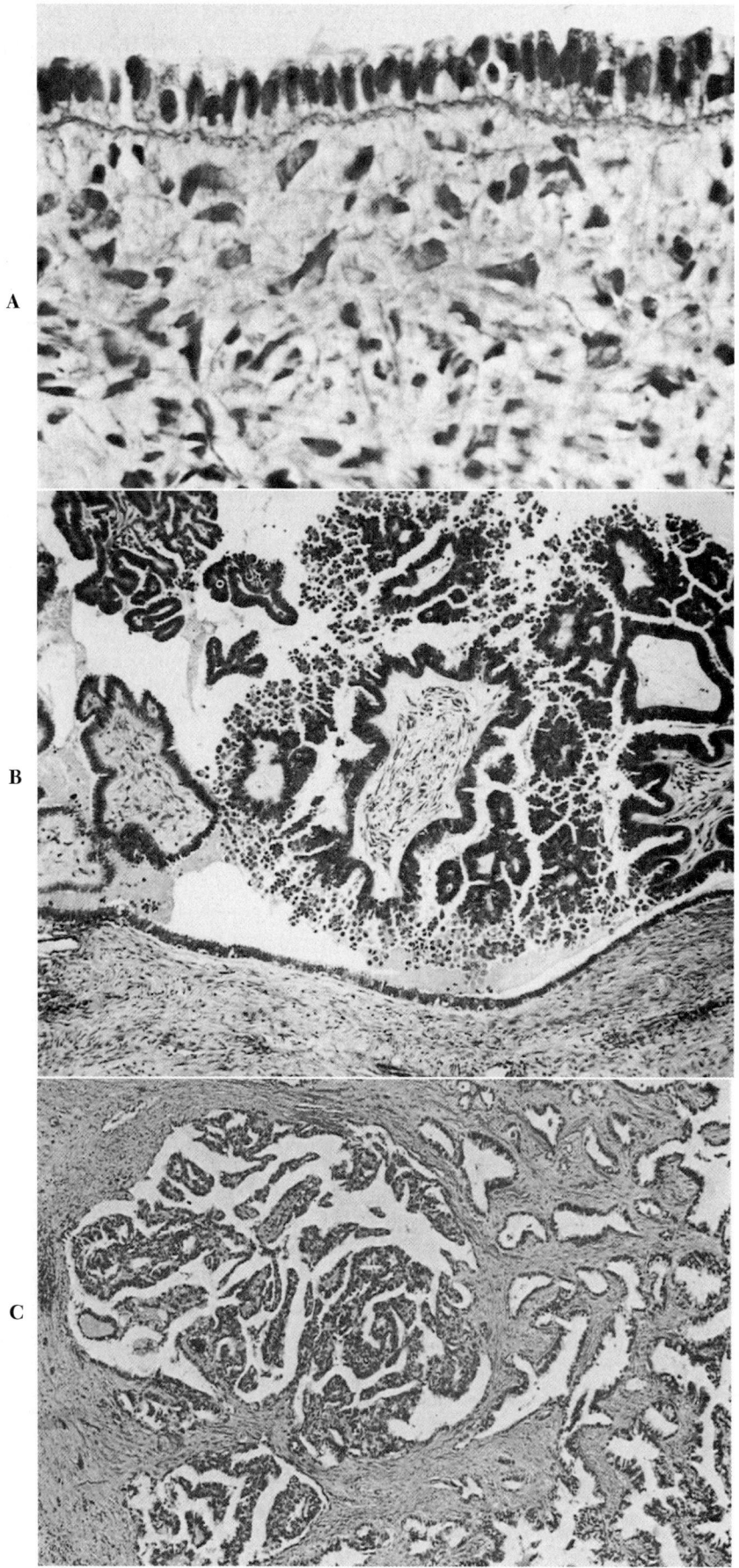

FIGURE 31-2   **A,** Ciliated epithelium of a well-differentiated serous tumor. (×800.) **B,** Serous papillary cystadenoma of borderline malignancy. The epithelium resembles that of the fallopian tube, and a well-developed papillary pattern is present. (×80.) **C,** Serous papillary adenocarcinoma. (×50.) The neoplastic epithelium invades the stroma. (**A** and **C** from Serov SF, Scully RE, and Sobin LH: Histologic typing of ovarian tumors, Geneva, 1973, World Health Organization. **B,** Courtesy Dr. R.E. Scully.)

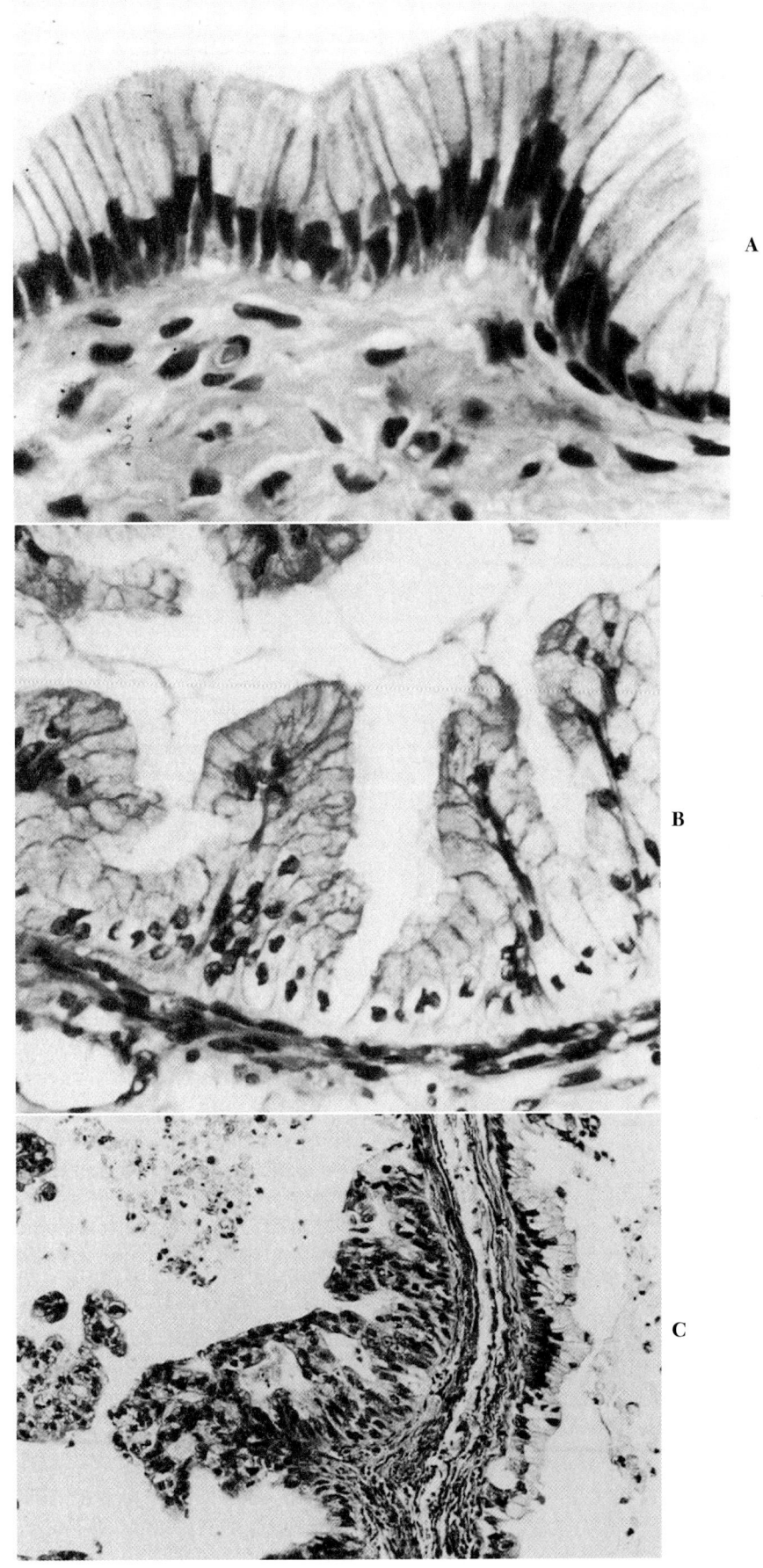

FIGURE 31-3 **A,** Mucinous cystadenoma. (×800.) **B,** Mucinous borderline tumor. Epithelium resembles that of the endocervix. **C,** Mucinous carcinoma. (×120.) Incomplete stratification of cells and atypicality is present. (**A** and **C** from Serov SF, Scully RE, and Sobin LH: Histologic typing of ovarian tumors, Geneva, 1973, World Health Organization. **B,** Courtesy Dr. R.E. Scully.)

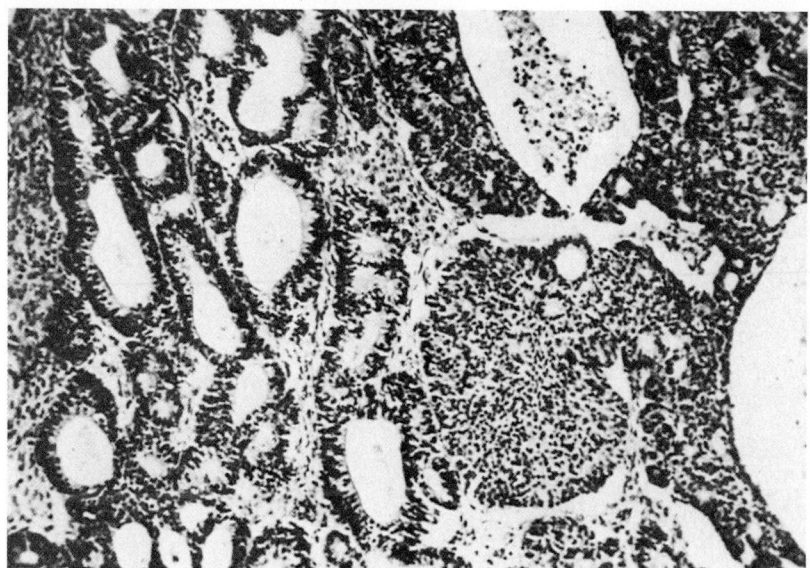

FIGURE 31-4 Endometrioid carcinoma. Tubular glands are lined by stratified endometrium. (×80.) (From Meadowbrook Staff Journal 1:148, 1968. Courtesy Dr. R.E. Scully.)

whereas multilocular or partially solid tumors are more likely to be neoplastic. Beyond the age of 40 the risk of malignancy rises. The ovary shrinks during menopause and normally is about 1.5 to 2.0 cm in size. Transvaginal ultrasound can reliably detect an ovary greater than 1.0 to 1.5 cm in diameter. Higgins et al. estimated the upper limit of the volume of a postmenopausal ovary was about 8 cm^3 in comparison with 18 cm^3 for the premenopausal ovary. Ten of their patients who exceeded these criteria and had solid or complex echo patterns all had neoplastic tumors, and one carcinoma was discovered. An ultrasound examination, preferably with a vaginal probe, helps to differentiate these adnexal masses (see following discussion).

Occasionally it is discovered that the adnexal mass is paraovarian. In a study of 168 paraovarian tumors, Stein et al. noted that only 3 (2%) were malignant. The 3 cysts all had solid components, and the cysts were 8 to 12 cm size in patients 19 to 48 years of age.

Adnexal Mass and Ovarian Cancer Ultrasound Screening and CA-125

CA-125 was described by Bast et al. in the 1980s. It is expressed by approximately 80% of ovarian epithelial carcinomas but less frequently by mucinous tumors. The marker is elevated in endometrial and tubal carcinoma, in addition to ovarian carcinoma, and in other malignancies, including those originating in the lung, breast, and pancreas. A level >35 U/ml is generally considered elevated. The box at right lists some of the benign conditions for which CA-125 also has frequently been found to be elevated. As can be seen, many of these are frequently found in women of childbearing age. This lack of specificity must

---

Benign Conditions in Which CA-125 Has Been Found to Be Elevated

Endometriosis
Peritoneal inflammation, including pelvic inflammatory disease
Leiomyoma
Pregnancy
Hemorrhagic ovarian cysts
Liver disease

---

be remembered when one is interpreting elevated CA-125 values in younger women with adnexal masses or when screening is being considered (see following discussion). In addition (Bast RC, personal communication), there are rare individuals who have no disease but are found to have levels of CA-125 as high as 200 to 300 U/ml, as a consequence of developing idiopathic antibodies to mouse IgG.

One must also be cautious in the interpretation of an elevated CA-125, particularly in a premenopausal patient with an adnexal mass. The specificity appears to be better for elevated values in the postmenopausal patient. In a study of 182 patients Vasilev et al. noted CA-125 was elevated in 22% of cases of benign masses but for postmenopausal patients an elevated value usually indicated malignancy as was also shown in the CA-125–vaginal ultrasound study of 290 postmenopausal patients by Maggino et al.

Ultrasound has helped to define criteria to allow conservative follow-up and the risk of malignancy of some adnexal masses. Goldstein et al. studied 42 postmenopausal patients whose ultrasound scans showed unilocular cysts less than 5 cm in diameter. Twenty-eight were explored,

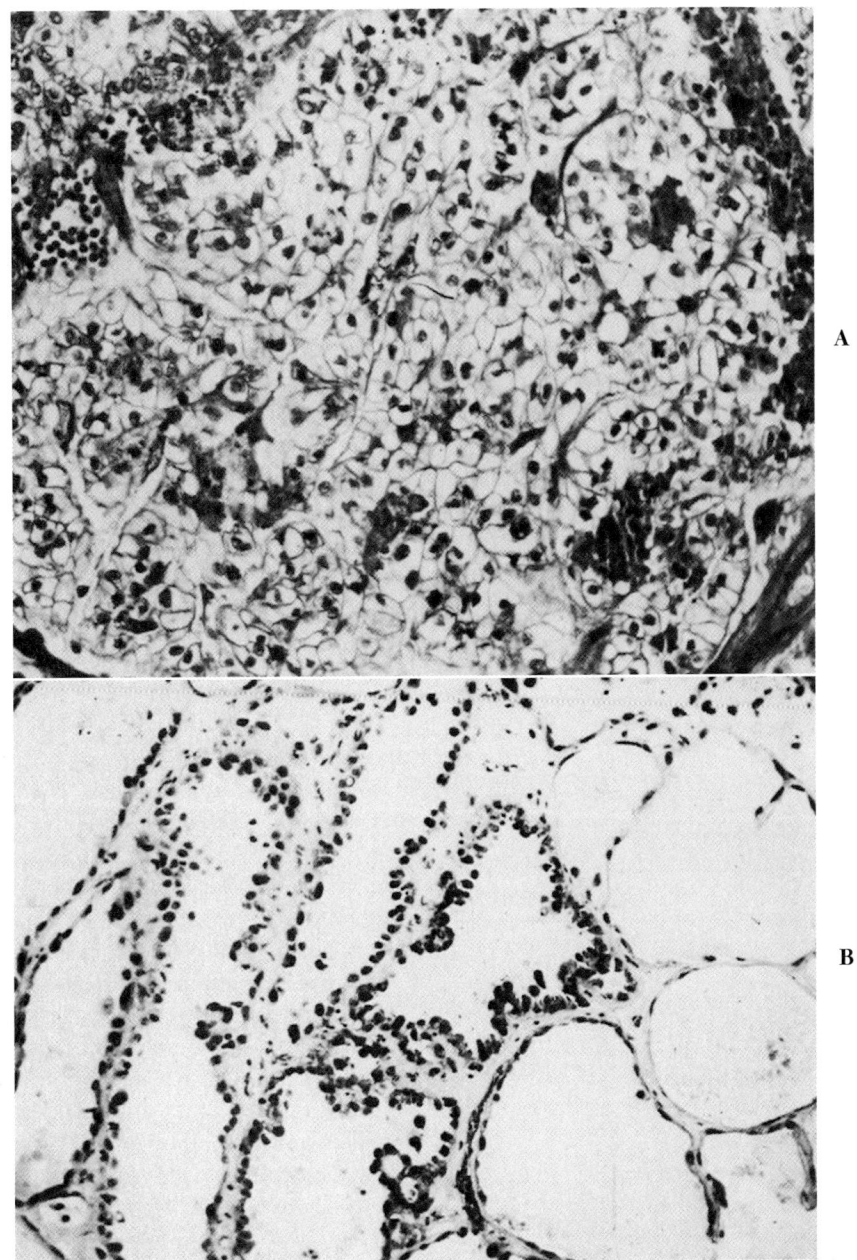

FIGURE 31-5 **A,** Clear cell adenocarcinoma. (×200.) Solid pattern of abundant polyhedral tumor cells containing abundant clear cytoplasm is present. **B,** Clear cell adenocarcinoma. (×200.) *Left:* Hobnail cells with scant cytoplasm: protruding nuclei line shows tubules. *Right:* Cysts lined by flattened tumor cells. (**A** from Barlow JF and Scully RE: Cancer 20:1405, 1967. **B** from Meadowbrook Staff Journal 1:148, 1968. Courtesy Dr. R.E. Scully.)

and none had malignancy. Fourteen were followed for up to 6 years with no change in ultrasound appearance. Finkler et al. noted that the addition of CA-125 serum assay to their ultrasound criteria in postmenopausal women increased the accuracy of preoperative evaluation. In a clinical pathologic study to define ultrasound criteria of malignancy, Granberg et al. studied the ovarian tumors in 1017 women. Of 296 with unilocular cysts, only 1 was malignant, this had visible papillary formations on the cyst wall, and 60% of these women were over age 40. In contrast, malignancy rates were 8% (20 of 229) for multilocular

cysts, 65% (147 of 201) for multilocular-solid tumors, and 39% (31 of 80) for solid ovarian masses. In a follow-up study of 180 women, the authors noted that 45 of 45 unilocular cysts were benign. In a recent ultrasound study of cystic ovarian masses in women over age 50 years, Bailey et al. noted unilocular cysts <10 cm in diameter are rarely malignant, whereas complex cysts or those with solid areas are at high risk for malignancy.

Several scoring systems have been proposed to try to determine the risk of an ovarian mass being malignant. They usually include (1) Is the finding a simple cyst

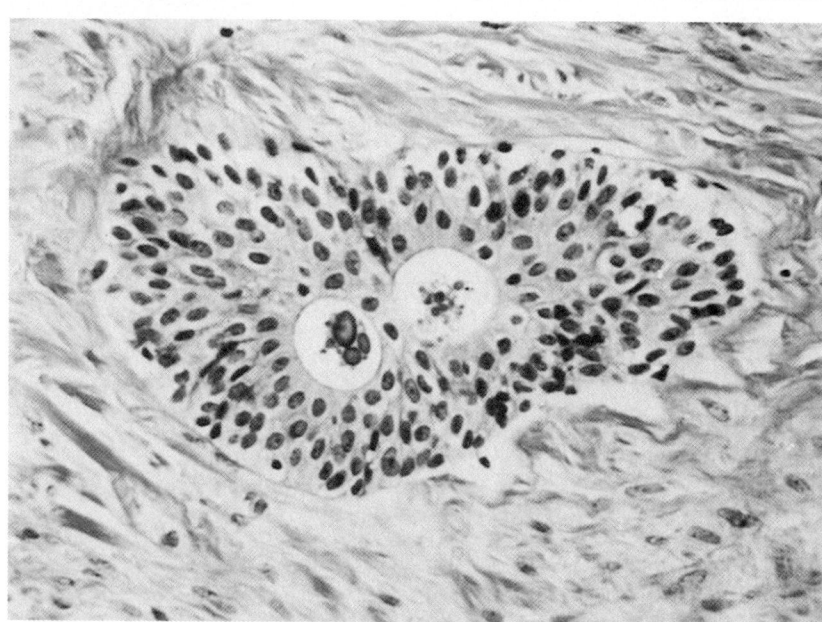

FIGURE 31-6 Brenner tumor. (×350.) Note nest of transition-like epithelium containing spaces with eosinophilic material. (From Atlas of tumor pathology, fascicle 16, series 2, Washington DC, 1979, Armed Forces Institute of Pathology.)

TABLE 31-4
Bilaterality of Ovarian Tumors

Type of Tumor	Occurrence (%)
Epithelial tumors	
Serous cystadenoma	10
Serous cystadenocarcinoma	33–66
Mucinous cystadenoma	5
Mucinous cystadenocarcinoma	10–20
Endometrioid carcinoma	13–30
Benign Brenner tumor	6
Germ cell tumors	
Benign cystic teratoma (dermoid)	12
Immature teratoma (malignant)	2–5
Dysgerminoma	5–10
Other malignant germ cell tumors	Rare
Sex cord–stromal tumors	
Thecoma	Rare
Sertoli-Leydig cell tumor	Rare
Granulosa-theca cell tumor	Rare

(unilocular) or complex (multicystic/multilocular with solid components)?; (2) Are there papillary projections?; (3) Are the cystic walls and/or septa regular and smooth?; (4) What is the echogenicity (tissue characterization)? These components help to refine the likelihood of malignancy.

A number of studies have been undertaken using transvaginal ultrasound to detect ovarian cancers early, particularly in high-risk women. Bourne et al. screened 775 women who had at least one first-degree (677) or second-degree (98) relative with ovarian cancer. Overall 43 women were referred for operation with abnormal-appearing ovaries and 39 underwent surgery, with 3 stage IA ovarian carcinomas discovered (3.9/1000 screened); one of these was a borderline tumor. One screened patient was found to have peritoneal carcinomatosis 11 months after a normal screening study. The remainder had nonmalignant findings. DePriest et al. screened 6470 asymptomatic postmenopausal women and defined abnormality as an ovary with volume >10 cm³ and/or papillary projections in a cystic ovarian tumor. Ninety patients who had persistent findings by repeat ultrasound at 4 to 6 weeks had an operation, with the finding of five early (stage IA—see subsequent discussion) and one advanced (stage IIIB) carcinomas. There were 37 serous cystadenomas and 20 assorted benign ovarian conditions. One patient with a normal scan was found to have peritoneal carcinomatosis 11 months later. These investigators noted that normal ovarian volume in a postmenopausal woman is <10 cm³ and in a premenopausal woman it is up to 20 cm³ as reported by Pavlik et al.

In addition, Creasman and DiSaia et al. estimated that if a vaginal ultrasound and CA-125 were performed annually on all women over the age of 45 in the United States, the cost would exceed $10 billion per year. Shalev et al. combined transvaginal ultrasound and normal CA-125 values in 55 postmenopausal women with simple cystic or septate cystic ovarian masses, and all 55 had benign disease. Although this is a small study, it suggests the potential of applying stringent ultrasound criteria with CA-125 evaluation of ovarian masses in postmenopausal women.

Recent clinicopathologic studies of Bell and Scully, as well as ultrasound screening trials by Crayford et al., provide an explanation for the lack of success with ultrasound screening in detecting low-stage ovarian carcinomas. Bell and Scully proposed the term *early de novo carcinoma* to explain their findings of 14 carefully studied cases. None of these patients at the time of operation had clinical evidence of ovarian carcinoma. All cases had microscopic foci of carcinoma in their ovaries and 3 cases were detected only years postoperatively when the patients were discovered to have widespread carcinoma consistent with what was found in their ovaries on retrospective study. Crayford et al. screened 5479 self-referred asymptomatic women by vaginal ultrasound and removed all persistent ovarian cysts in an attempt to reduce the frequency of ovarian cancer. Eighty-eight patients had cysts removed. Twelve years after the conclusion of the study showed a slight nonsignificant increase in ovarian cancer deaths for this group. Therefore it appears that the majority of ovarian carcinomas (particularly serous) arise from a tiny cancer of the surface of the ovary from which it can spread rapidly before the ovary enlarges. Some ovarian tumors such as endometrioid carcinoma may have an origin from endometriosis. These carcinomas, as well as mucinous, tend to be detected more frequently in lower stages. Therefore they appear more likely to have a cystic rather than a "de novo" origin. These observations strongly suggest that current strategies to use vaginal ultrasound screening to detect early ovarian carcinoma will have only limited success as recently noted by Herbst.

Some have advocated using transvaginal pulsed Doppler color-enhanced flow studies to identify benign from malignant masses. The resistance index has been employed, which measures resistance to flow in the vessels and presumably is low in the presence of neovascularization that is seen with malignant tumors. The vessels of neoangiogenesis are abnormal in their distribution with disorganized branching and a loss of the muscularis layer, all of which contribute to the decreased resistance to flow. A resistance of 0.40 or less was found useful by Kurjak et al. in a study of 254 women. In contrast, Bromley et al., in a study of 33 postmenopausal women, used a cutoff of 0.6, which did not greatly add to their specificities, and these authors rely on morphologic criteria, that is, solid elements, papillary projections, etc., to diagnose malignancy.

It should be noted there is a difference in using ultrasound to screen for ovarian cancer as opposed to using different modalities of ultrasound to characterize an ovarian mass as benign or malignant. For example, the addition of color Doppler, which measures blood flow and direction of flow, and power Doppler, which can detect slow flow in small vessels, can add useful information. These permit visualization of flow location (peripheral, central, or within a septum). Most malignant tumors have a central flow (75% to 100%) in comparison to only 5% to 40% of benign ovarian tumors. Schelling et al. studied transvaginal B-mode and color Doppler sonography for diagnosis of malignancy in 257 adnexal masses with unclear malignant

status. They achieved 92% sensitivity and 94% specificity. The recent development of three-dimensional (3-D) ultrasound may allow more accurate volume assessments. In addition, color Doppler with 3-D may permit better detection of vessel irregularity, coiling, and branching. A future possibility is the use of contrast media to quantify and permit earlier detection of abnormal angiogenesis as noted by Abramowicz.

Nonmalignant Neoplasms

Most nonmalignant epithelial ovarian tumors are asymptomatic unilateral adnexal masses that can be treated by oophorectomy or occasionally cystectomy (see section on benign cystic teratomas later in this chapter). In the past some have recommended bisecting the opposite ovary to rule out bilaterality in the case of benign epithelial ovarian tumors (see Table 31-4), but in view of the risk of adhesions and infertility as well as the availability of vaginal ultrasound, this is no longer done. In a woman beyond her reproductive years, especially in the presence of a serous cystadenoma, which tends to be bilateral, hysterectomy and bilateral salpingo-oophorectomy are usually performed.

Mucinous tumors can become particularly large and reach sizes up to 30 cm. Possible complications of mucinous cystadenoma are perforation and rupture, which can lead to the deposit and growth of mucin-secreting epithelium in the peritoneal cavity (pseudomyxoma peritonei, discussed later under borderline mucinous tumors).

Adenofibromas consist of fibrous and epithelial elements. The epithelial component may be serous, mucinous, clear cell, or endometrioid—the architectural subtypes of these benign ovarian tumors. Their appearance will depend on the predominant histologic features—epithelial or fibrous. These tumors are also managed by simple excision. Endometriomas are considered in Chapter 19.

Brenner tumors (see Figure 31-6) are rare and often incidental findings when oophorectomy is performed for an indication other than ovarian enlargement. Most often, these tumors occur in women in their 40s and 50s, but both younger and older patients have been found to have them. Brenner tumors are almost always benign and can usually be managed by oophorectomy. When the ovary is palpably enlarged, approximately 5% of Brenner tumors will prove to be malignant. These tumors often occur in perimenopausal and postmenopausal women, in which case hysterectomy and bilateral salpingo-oophorectomy are indicated. Unfortunately, malignant Brenner tumors appear to have a poor prognosis despite this operative therapy, and an effective program of chemotherapy has not been developed.

The differential diagnosis for and approach to an adnexal mass in female patients of various ages are discussed in Chapter 7. Ovarian enlargement in the premenarchal female is usually the result of a germ cell tumor, which may be malignant but is usually benign (see later discussion of germ cell tumors). During the reproductive years ovarian neoplasms are usually benign. For the patient in her 20s or 30s most ovarian enlargements can be approached operatively through a lower abdominal transverse (Pfannenstiel) incision or by laparoscope, unless there is a likelihood of malignancy, such as a solid tumor or one with papillae viewed on ultrasound examination. However, the risk of laparoscopic excision was emphasized in a report by Maiman et al. They conducted a national survey and discovered 42 cases of ovarian malignancy in patients who had laparoscopic aspiration and/or excision of an adnexal mass that subsequently proved to be malignant. More recently, Lehner et al. and Leminen and Lehtovirta reported early spread of malignancy after laparoscopic removal of ovarian masses that were found postoperatively to be malignant. In these cases, as well as in women over age 40 or those with a large mass extending out of the pelvis and into the abdomen, a vertical incision is indicated. The tumor should be removed intact, and if malignancy is present, as is more likely in older patients, a thorough surgical evaluation is indicated (outlined in the section on epithelial carcinoma).

A frozen section should be obtained if gross examination of the ovarian tumor is at all suspicious for malignancy. For women of reproductive age, if the diagnosis of malignancy is suspected but uncertain even after a frozen section is obtained, the operation should be terminated after removal of the ovarian tumor. A second procedure can be performed if malignancy is confirmed after detailed histologic study of the permanent sections. This is preferable to risking an unnecessary hysterectomy or bilateral salpingo-oophorectomy in a patient who desires to preserve childbearing function.

Epithelial Carcinomas

Diagnosis, Staging, Spread, and Preoperative Evaluation

Ovarian carcinomas are usually diagnosed by detection of an adnexal mass on pelvic examination. Unfortunately the diagnosis is frequently made only after the disease has spread beyond the ovary, as noted in the prior section describing the "de novo" origin of these tumors. Scully estimates that the risk of malignancy in a primary ovarian tumor rises to about 33% in a woman over the age of 45, whereas it is less than 1 in 15 for women who are 20 to 45 years of age. In general, over half of ovarian carcinomas occur in women beyond the age of 50. In a hospital-based study of ovarian neoplasms in 861 women, Koonings et al. noted the risk of malignancy was 13% in premenopausal women but rose to 45% in postmenopausal women. In their study, benign ovarian neoplasms were most common among those 20 to 29 years of age.

Patients with ovarian carcinoma frequently develop ascites, and a swollen abdomen may be the first sign of disease. Vague lower abdominal discomfort is a frequent complaint, but severe pain is not a prominent symptom. Vaginal cytologic testing can detect ovarian carcinoma cells because of their transmigration through the tubes, uterus, and cervix into the vagina. However, an ovarian carcinoma is rarely initially detected from vaginal cytologic smears. The diagnosis is established by histologic examination of tumor tissue removed at operation. Occasionally the initial diagnosis is suggested by malignant cells found in ascitic fluid obtained at paracentesis.

The staging of ovarian cancer (Table 31-5) is designed according to the criteria of the International Federation of Gynecology and Obstetrics (FIGO) and is based on the results of operative exploration.

TABLE 31-5
Staging of Ovarian Carcinomas (FIGO)
Modified 1985

Stage	Characteristics
I	Growth limited to the ovaries.
IA	Growth limited to one ovary; no ascites present containing malignant cells. No tumor on the external surface; capsule intact.
IB	Growth limited to both ovaries; no ascites present containing malignant cells. No tumor on the external surfaces; capsules intact.
IC	Tumor either stage IA or IB but with tumor on surface of one or both ovaries; or with capsule ruptured; or with ascites present containing malignant cells; or with positive peritoneal washings.
II	Growth involving one or both ovaries with pelvic extension.
IIA	Extension and/or metastases to the uterus and/or tubes.
IIB	Extension to other pelvic tissues.
IIC	Tumor either stage IIA or IIB, but with tumor on surface of one or both ovaries; or with capsule(s) ruptured; or with ascites present containing malignant cells; or with positive peritoneal washings.
III	Tumor involving one or both ovaries with peritoneal implants outside the pelvis and/or positive retroperitoneal or inguinal nodes. Superficial liver metastasis equals stage III. Tumor is limited to the true pelvis but with histologically proven malignant extension to small bowel or omentum.
IIIA	Tumor grossly limited to the true pelvis with negative nodes but with histologically confirmed microscopic seeding of abdominal peritoneal surfaces.
IIIB	Tumor of one or both ovaries with histologically confirmed implants of abdominal peritoneal surfaces, none exceeding 2 cm in diameter. Nodes are negative.
IIIC	Abdominal implants greater than 2 cm in diameter and/or positive retroperitoneal or inguinal nodes.
IV	Growth involving one or both ovaries with distant metastases. If pleural effusion is present, there must be positive cytology to allot a case to stage IV.
IVA	Parenchymal liver metastasis equals stage IV

Before operative exploration for suspected ovarian carcinoma, the patient has the preoperative workup usual for a major abdominal operation (Chapter 24). Additional diagnostic studies may include a CT scan of the abdomen to search for retroperitoneal node enlargement or parenchymal liver masses and often a barium enema or colonoscopy. The latter is of particular importance for the potential of a primary colon carcinoma, which may present initially as an adnexal mass in the older patient. An endoscopic or gastrointestinal radiographic examination is performed if there is evidence of gastrointestinal bleeding or the suggestion of any GI pathology. A CA-125 is obtained and if elevated at the time of operation, it is useful for following the progress of the patient during and after treatment, and demonstrating the response to therapy or detecting tumor progression. Buller et al. studied the regression slope for CA-125 during chemotherapy and found the slope of the regression curve to be predictive of therapeutic outcome. Other investigators have shown that patients whose CA-125 values drop from elevated to normal rapidly while undergoing primary chemotherapy have an improved prognosis over those whose values regress more slowly. Serum inhibin has been reported to

be elevated in mucinous carcinomas and may serve as a marker, according to the studies of Henley et al. Frias et al. reported pretreatment levels of inhibin A to be a prognostic factor for survival in postmenopausal women with ovarian cancer.

Preoperatively a program to cleanse the bowel is instituted in case intestinal resection is required. One widely used program utilizes 4 L of GoLYTELY given over 3 to 4 hours the evening before operation. Neomycin sulfate 1 g, with 1 g erythromycin base, may be given 3 times (3 PM, 7 PM, and 11 PM) on the day before surgery or intravenous broad-spectrum antibiotics prophylactically IV just prior to operation. Alternatively, 60 cc castor oil may be used with a sweetening vehicle such as orange juice at approximately 4 PM the day prior to surgery. However, the important principle is mechanical cleansing of the bowel (see Chapter 24). Treatment with variable compression leg support stockings appears to reduce the risk of thromboembolism.

Ovarian carcinomas infiltrate the peritoneal surfaces of both the parietal and intestinal areas, as well as the undersurface of the diaphragm, particularly on the right side (Figure 31-7). This is particularly important because tumors that appear at operation to be confined to the ovary may

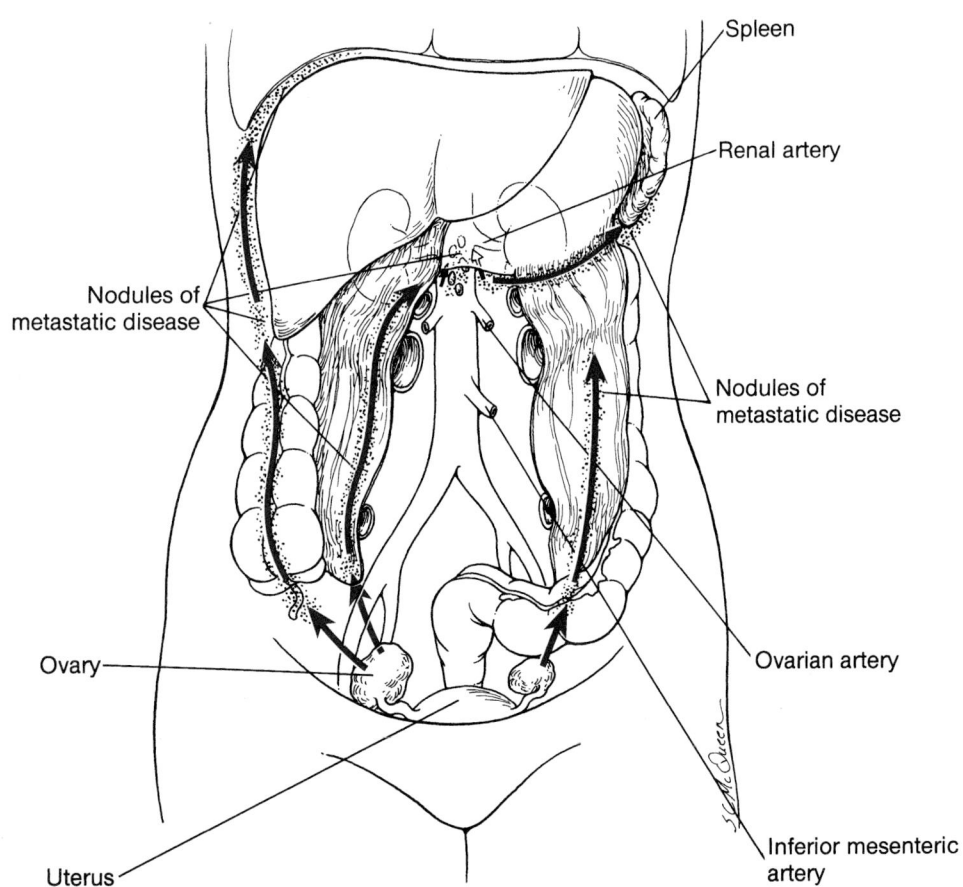

FIGURE 31-7 Peritoneal spread of ovarian cancer. Portions of omentum, small intestine, and transverse colon have been resected. (From Knapp RC, Berkowitz RS, and Leavitt T Jr: Natural history and detection of ovarian cancer. In Gynecology and obstetrics, vol 4, Philadelphia, 1986, JB Lippincott Co.)

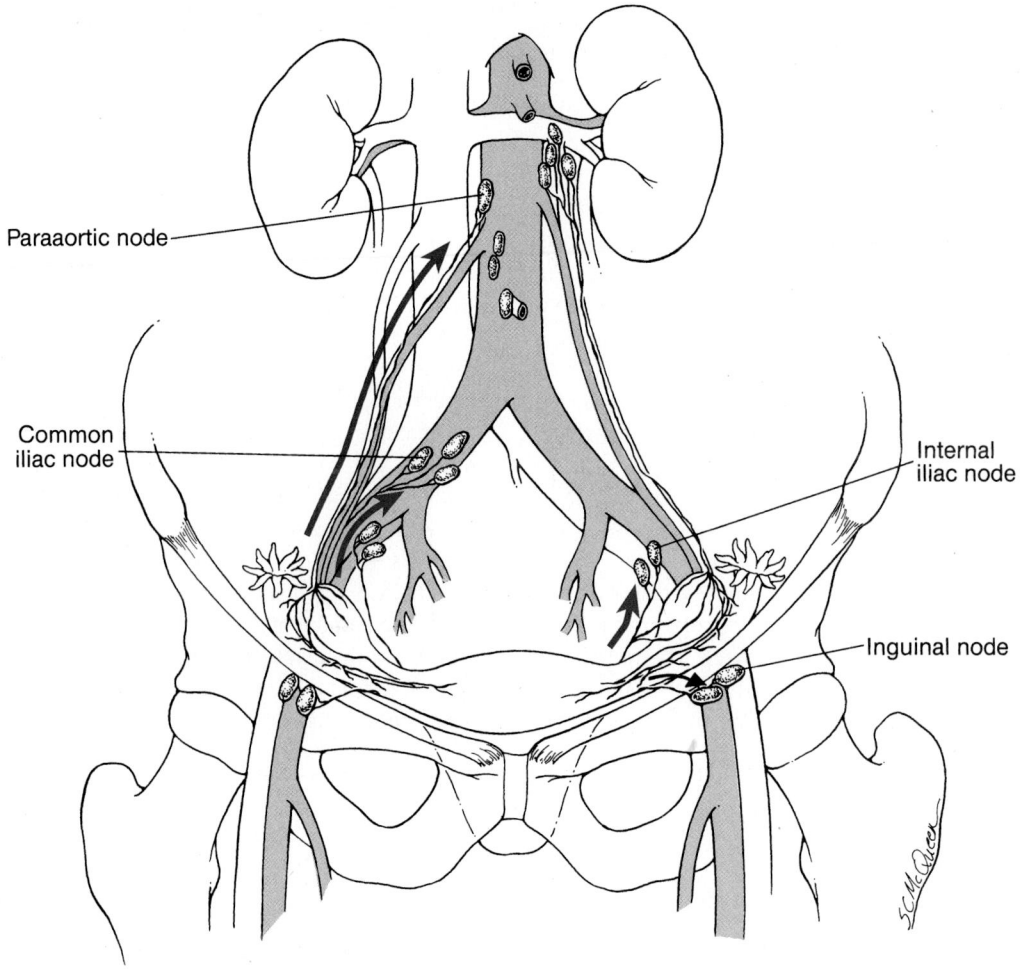

Paraaortic node

Common iliac node

Internal iliac node

Inguinal node

FIGURE 31-8 Lymph nodes draining ovaries. Primary routes of spread to the pelvic and paraaortic nodes are illustrated. (Redrawn from Musumeci R: Cancer 40:1444, 1977.)

have small areas of diaphragmatic involvement as the sole site of extraovarian spread. As noted earlier most ovarian carcinomas, particularly the serous type, appear to arise from microscopic ovarian sites and do not become clinically evident until there is widespread metastatic disease. Lymphatic dissemination is also a prominent part of disease spread (Figure 31-8), and it is particularly important to note that the paraaortic nodes are at risk through lymphatics that run parallel to the ovarian vessels. Knapp and Friedman noted that, of 26 patients with ovarian cancer apparently limited to the ovary, 19% had paraaortic involvement and all had poorly differentiated tumors. In a study of 180 patients, Burghardt et al. observed that the proportion of positive nodes rose with higher stage tumors: 24% in stage I, 50% in stage II, and 73.5% in stages III and IV.

The prognosis for patients with ovarian carcinoma is related to tumor stage, tumor grade, cell type, and the amount of residual tumor after resection. Worldwide results for patients treated from 1990 to 1992 are summarized in Table 31-6.

TABLE 31-6

Carcinoma of the Ovary: Survival by FIGO Stage for Patients Treated 1990–92

Stage	Number	5-year Survival %
IA	342	86.9
IB	49	71.3
IC	352	79.2
IIA	64	66.6
IIB	92	55.1
IIC	136	57.0
IIIA	129	41.1
IIIB	137	24.9
IIIC	1193	23.4
IV	360	11.1

Modified from Pecorelli S, Creasman WT, Pettersson F, et al: FIGO annual report on the results of treatment in gynaecological cancer, vol 23, Milano, Italy, J Epidemiol Biostat, 1998.

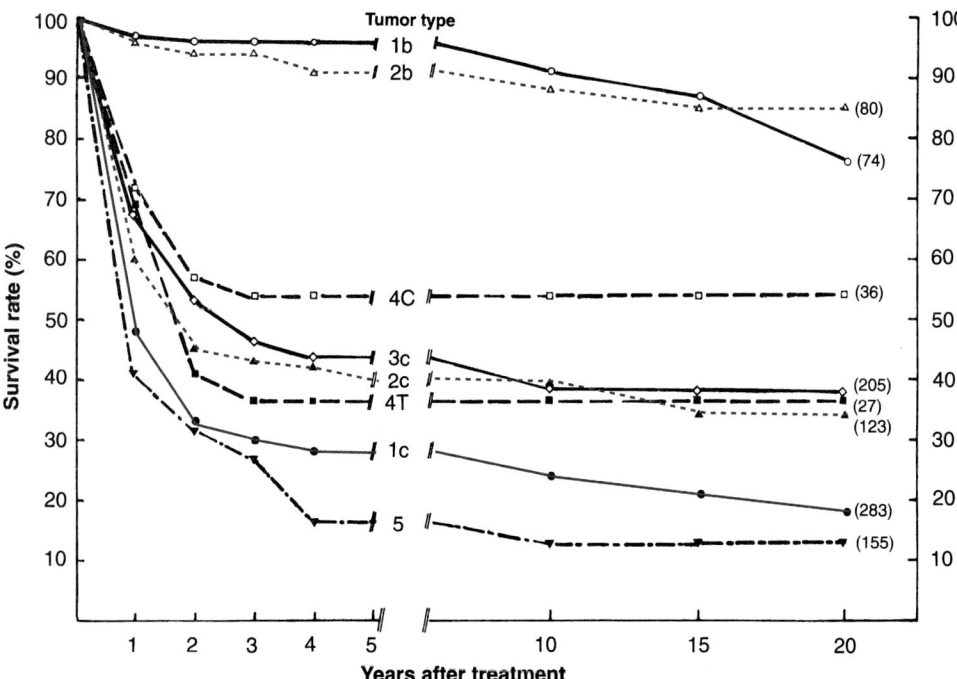

FIGURE 31-9 Survival rates for 983 patients with all stages of ovarian cancer by histologic type. *1b*, Serous, low malignant potential (74 cases); *2b*, Mucinous, low malignant potential (80 cases); *1c*, Serous carcinoma (283 cases); *2c*, Mucinous carcinoma (123 cases); *3c*, Endometrioid carcinoma (205 cases); *4c*, Clear cell (36 cases); *4T*, Tubulocystic pattern of clear cell (27 cases); *5*, Undifferentiated (155 cases). (Redrawn from Aure JC, Hoeg K, and Kolstad P: Obstet Gynecol 37:1, 1971. Reprinted with permission from The American College of Obstetricians and Gynecologists.)

Cell type has been reported to be an important factor in prognosis, as shown in Figure 31-9, which summarizes the 20-year survival rate of a group of patients. The most common invasive epithelial cancers, serous carcinomas, have the worst prognosis; prognosis is better for mucinous, endometrioid, and clear cell tumors, although clear cell carcinomas do have a poor prognosis. A variant of papillary serous carcinoma termed *transitional cell carcinoma* is thought by some to be a rare but more chemosensitive tumor. However, this has not been established in multi-institutional studies. Endometrioid carcinoma is rarely associated with endometriosis and according to McMeekin et al. such cases more commonly occur in younger women and have a better prognosis than typical endometrioid carcinomas of the ovary. Clear cell cancers have a worse prognosis, but Kennedy et al. noted that mitotic activity and tumor stage were important prognostic features of this tumor in their series. Tubulocystic pattern did not appear to affect prognosis, as was suggested by the earlier studies of Aure et al., depicted in Figure 31-9. Nonetheless these are aggressive tumors with a propensity for recurrence even in stage I. In a follow-up analysis Kennedy et al. noted a survival probability of only 50% for stage I-II, which was similar to that of high-grade epithelial cancers of comparable stage. It should be noted that both stage and grade affect these observations. Serous tumors tend to be more poorly differentiated and discovered at a higher stage than are mucinous tumors.

In some cases patients are found to have small ovaries (less than 4 cm in diameter) and widespread papillary serous carcinoma in the abdomen. In such cases the term *serous surface papillary carcinoma of the ovary* is applied. Fromm et al. reported on 74 patients and found survival improved if the patients were treated postoperatively with combination chemotherapy (see later discussion for therapy of high stage carcinoma of the ovary). Another variety of serous carcinoma is "primary peritoneal carcinoma." In these cases the ovaries may be of normal size with surface metastatic tumor deposits. There is widespread intraabdominal spread of carcinoma of serous histology. These cases are associated with BRCA1 and BRCA2 mutations as shown by the studies of Karlan et al.

The cloning of the BRCA1 gene has advanced our knowledge of the molecular genetics of ovarian cancer, but the role of this gene that resides on chromosome 17q21 is not clear. It appears to be a tumor suppressor gene that is highly expressed in ovarian borderline carcinoma. Mutations in BRCA1 are strongly associated with increased risk of breast and ovarian cancer, and a similar increase in risks occurs with mutations in BRCA2 (see Table 31-7). These mutations are seen in approximately 2% to 2.5% of Ashkenazi Jewish women, who appear to be an appropriate target group for testing if breast cancer is diagnosed prior to age 50 in the patient or a close relative according to the analysis of Warner et al. Prophylactic oophorectomy reduces the risk of ovarian cancer in those with a mutation, but does not eliminate the problem because of the potential for primary peritoneal carcinoma. The study of Rebbeck et al. of BRCA1 mutation carriers suggests prophylactic oophorectomy may also reduce the subsequent risk of breast cancer. Boyd et al. reported that stage for stage, the hereditary ovarian cancer group may have a better prognosis than the spontaneously occurring tumors. Lu et al. noted a high proportion of microscopic carcinomas in apparently normal ovaries removed from patients with BRCA mutations, an observation consistent with the "de novo" origin of serous and poorly differentiated carcinomas.

In addition to stage, the grade of the tumor is a major determinant of patient prognosis. Figure 31-10 demonstrates the survival of 442 patients with ovarian carcinoma by grade, with a markedly worse prognosis for poorly differentiated tumors (grade 3). The relationship between grade and survival also exists when the results are examined separately for each stage of disease. Grade 0 (borderline) tumors have the best prognosis (see Figure 31-9).

Studies of flow cytometry indicate that the ploidy of the tumor is prognostic with aneuploidy being a negative prognostic factor. Klemi et al. noted an independent prognostic association with the DNA index and S phase fraction. A better prognosis was observed if the proportion of S phase cells was less than 11% or if the DNA index (the relative DNA content of aneuploid cells compared with diploid) was less than 1.3. Genetic studies by Slamon et al. have shown that the HER-2/*neu* oncogene is found to be amplified in ovarian and breast cancers. As noted in a review by Berchuck et al. the overexpression of HER-2/*neu* occurs in about 30% of epithelial ovarian cancers and appears associated with a worse prognosis. The p53 tumor suppressor gene is mutated in about half of ovarian epithelial cancers studied while the C-myc oncogene is overexpressed more commonly in serous cases and the K-ras oncogene has been identified more frequently in borderline ovarian cancers. The molecular genetic events surrounding ovarian carcinoma development and biologic behavior are incompletely understood.

TABLE 31-7
Cancer Risk Estimates for BRCA1 or BRCA2 Carriers

Genetic Alteration	Ovarian Cancer Risk	Breast Cancer Risk	Other Considerations
BRCA1	40–60%	80–90%	Colon cancer—8%
BRCA2	20%	80–90%	Increased risk for colon cancer
None	1–2%	10–12%	Colon cancer—2%

The size of residual nodules and the presence or absence of tumor after operation have been shown to be related to the survival of patients treated for ovarian carcinoma. Aure et al., in their classic studies, noted a 5-year survival of over 30% for stage III tumors that were completely resected, in comparison with 10% when resection was incomplete. The 5-year survival of incompletely resected stage II tumors was approximately 18%. Patients with small postoperative residual tumors have a better prognosis than those with larger diameter residual tumors. Frequently used categories are microscopic (present on biopsy, but not grossly), less than 1.0 cm, or greater than 1.0 cm.

Management

BORDERLINE OVARIAN TUMORS (OVARIAN CARCINOMAS OF LOW MALIGNANT POTENTIAL). Approximately 20% of ovarian epithelial cancers are of tumors of low malignant potential (grade 0) and usually have an excellent prognosis regardless of stage. Most studies have been confined to borderline tumors of the serous (see Figure 31-2, *B*) and mucinous (see Figure 31-3, *B*) varieties, which are the most common of borderline tumors, but other epithelial types (see Table 31-3) can occur. The cells of these epithelial tumors do not invade the stroma of the ovary. It is extremely important that the ovarian tumor be thoroughly sampled by the pathologist to be certain that a borderline tumor is not mixed with invasive elements. Numerous studies have confirmed that borderline tumors have a slower growth rate than do invasive ovarian carcinomas, and the patients have a prolonged survival time (see Figure 31-9).

Since these tumors tend to occur in young women during the reproductive years, it is desirable to ascertain the safety of conservative therapy for patients with borderline stage 1A tumors (confined to one ovary). Leake et al. reported on 200 patients with borderline serous tumors. With a median follow-up of 11.2 years, the 5-year survival for *all* stages was 97% and for 20 years, 89%.

Recurrences in stages I and II were very rare and despite recurrences, the 20-year survival in stage III was approximately 40%. Patients with stage I disease can be treated by unilateral adnexectomy and if the opposite ovary is normal, it need not be biopsied. Lim-Tan et al. reported on 33 cases of stage I serous borderline tumors initially treated by cystectomy. Only 3 of 33 patients undergoing cystectomy had recurrence or persistence, and these 3 patients had positive resection margins and/or multiple cysts present in the ovary, emphasizing the effectiveness of conservative operation. However, for most stage IA cases, unilateral adnexectomy is performed, and if the opposite ovary looks normal, no biopsy or wedge resection is done.

Mucinous borderline tumors also are associated with an excellent prognosis. Hart and Norris reviewed 97

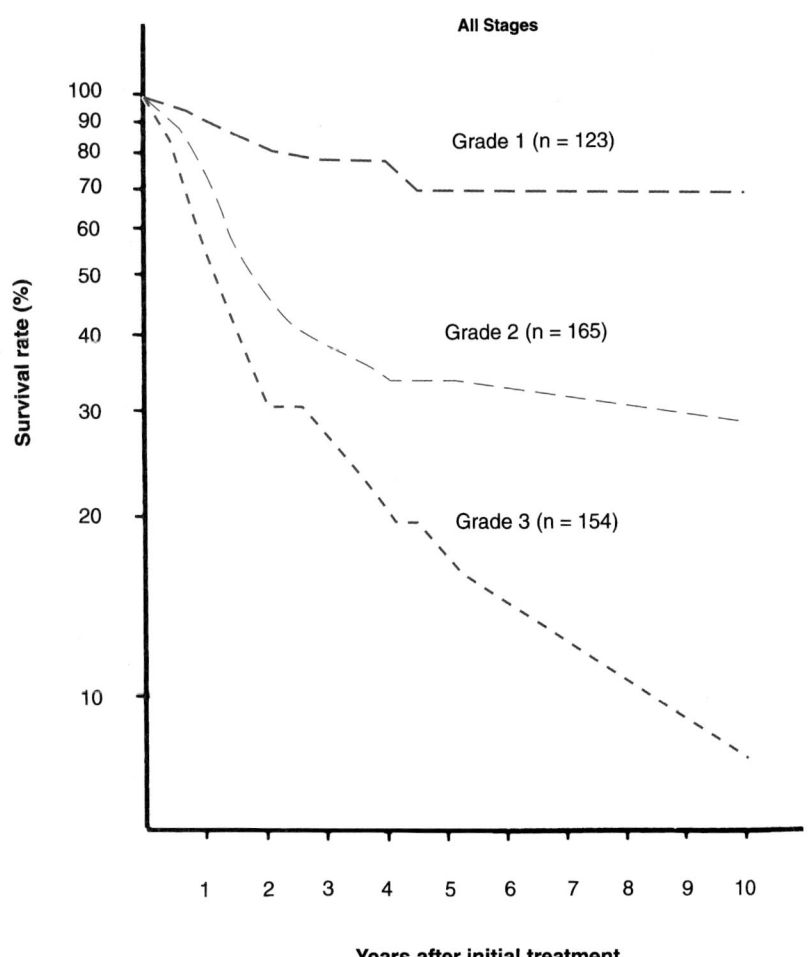

FIGURE 31-10 Survival rates for patients with ovarian cancer by tumor grade. Survival curves for the complete series according to the histologic degree of differentiation. All differences between curves are highly significant. (From Sorbe B, Frankendal B, and Veress B: Obstet Gynecol 59:576, 1982. Reprinted with permission from the American College of Obstetricians and Gynecologists.)

patients with stage I tumors who were 9 to 70 years of age with a median of 35 years. Over 10% of the tumors were discovered during pregnancy or in the immediate postpartum period. Follow-up data were available on 87 of the patients, and there were only three tumor-related deaths during the 5- to 10-year follow-up. The actuarial survival was 98% at 5 years and 96% at 10 years. This was also noted by Bostwick et al., who reported on 109 borderline tumors, 33 of which were mucinous, and all of which were stage I, contributing to the good prognosis.

Borderline mucinous tumors have also been associated with widespread growth of mucin-producing cells in the peritoneum (pseudomyxoma peritonei). The result may be the accumulation of large amounts of mucinous material, which is sometimes associated with recurrent bouts of bowel obstruction. Studies by Young et al. suggest pseudomyxoma peritonei usually arise in the appendix. The review of Ronnett et al. supports a primary appendicial origin for these tumors, and therefore appendectomy is indicated in these cases. Those associated with appendi-

cial adenoma have a better prognosis than those associated with appendicial carcinoma and the same is true of ovarian tumors, as noted by Wertheim et al. The disease tends to recur and to require repeated laparotomy to relieve bowel obstruction. Chemotherapy and mucolytic agents have been tried but are usually not successful. However, Jones and Homesley reported a single case with a complete remission following eight courses of cyclophosphamide (Cytoxan), 500 mg/m^2; doxorubicin (Adriamycin), 50 mg/m^2; and cisplatin, 50 mg/m^2.

Conservative therapy of borderline ovarian tumors with preservation of childbearing function may be carried out by unilateral oophorectomy if the following criteria are met: the tumor is confirmed to be at stage IA; extensive histologic sampling of the tumor confirms it to be grade 0 (borderline); the contralateral ovary appears normal; biopsy specimens of areas of omental or peritoneal nodularity are negative; and results of peritoneal cytologic tests are negative for tumor cells. Retroperitoneal nodes are rarely involved and are not routinely sampled. No recurrences were noted in 156 stage I patients in a Gynecologic Oncology Group (GOG) study treated by operation alone, as reported by Barnhill et al.

For borderline tumors beyond stage I, both irradiation therapy and chemotherapy have been prescribed to attempt to improve survival. However, as noted in Figure 31-9, the 5-year survival of patients with all stages of borderline tumors is high (over 90%) after resection alone. Operative removal of all gross disease remains the most important factor in primary treatment, with extensive biopsy of any peritoneal or omental implants. As emphasized by Prat, peritoneal implants should be meticulously sampled to determine if they are noninvasive or invasive. Bell et al. studied peritoneal implants (Figures 31-11 and 31-12) in 56 patients with 368 person-years of follow-up. Patients with benign implants, that is, endometriosis or endosalpingosis (benign tubal-appearing epithelium), were eliminated because they require no therapy. Three adverse histologic features were identified in the implants: invasiveness, cytologic atypia, and mitotic count. Gross residual disease after primary operation was also a factor. A group of 27 patients without adverse features had a 100% survival. The risk of death was least (4%) for those whose invasive implants were confined to the pelvis, but rose to 20% for stage III cases. *Additional therapy should be reserved for those with implants with adverse features, primarily invasiveness and cytologic atypia.* Recently Mooney et al. noted spontaneous regression of invasive implants postpartum in patients whose borderline tumors were diagnosed during pregnancy. Gershenson and Silva recommend six cycles of chemotherapy (see later discussion) for patients with invasive implants. Histologic examination of the implants may provide a basis to choose patients who might potentially benefit from therapy. However, definite evidence of a survival benefit by treating these cases is lacking. Based on current evidence, operative removal offers the best treatment for borderline tumors.

INVASIVE EPITHELIAL CARCINOMAS. The primary treatment of ovarian epithelial carcinoma is removal of all resectable gross disease. The patient's abdomen is explored through a vertical incision. If ascitic fluid is present, it is sent for cytologic evaluation; if ascites is not present, 200 to 400 ml of normal saline solution is used to obtain cytologic samples from the peritoneum by irrigating at least the pelvis, upper abdomen, and right and left paracolic gutters before any resection is done. The diaphragm can be cytologically sampled by scraping the undersurface with a sterile tongue depressor and sample placed on a glass slide and sprayed with a fixative. Biopsy or, preferably, excision of any suspicious nodules are taken. A total abdominal hysterectomy, bilateral salpingo-oophorectomy, and appendectomy as well as infracolic omentectomy, are performed if technically possible. When there is no gross disease outside the pelvis, paraaortic and pelvic lymph node sampling is recommended, with care taken to remove enlarged nodes. Current evidence suggests that if all gross disease can be resected, duration of patient survival is enhanced.

It may occasionally be necessary to resect bowel to relieve impending obstruction or to remove a tumor nodule and thereby eliminate all gross disease from the peritoneal cavity. Heintz et al. noted prognosis was improved for younger patients (age ≤50 years), those with good initial performance status (Karnofsky >80, Table 26-4), as well as those whose disease could be cytoreduced to less than 1.5 cm. Adverse factors were large metastases before initial operation, ascites, and peritoneal carcinomatosis. In a small collaborative GOG study, Hoskins et al. found that those who started with large-volume disease did worse than those who initially had small-volume disease and no survival advantage could be demonstrated for the debulking operation in the large-volume disease group. Chi et al. noted that those with advanced disease and a preoperative CA-125 > 500 U/ml had less than a 20% chance of an optimal operative debulking (see later).

One exception to the required removal of the uterus and opposite ovary occurs in the case of well-differentiated (grade 1) ovarian tumors confined to one ovary (stage IA). DiSaia et al. outlined criteria for preserving childbearing function in a young woman with stage IA, grade 1 ovarian epithelial carcinoma, as follows:

1. Tumor confined to one ovary
2. Tumor well differentiated (grade 1) with no invasion of capsule, lymphatics, or mesovarium
3. Peritoneal washings negative
4. Omental biopsy specimen negative
5. Young woman of childbearing years with strong desire to preserve reproductive function

These criteria can be applied to all types of epithelial ovarian tumors but are more likely to be satisfied in the case of mucinous tumors, which are more frequently well differentiated and unilateral than serous carcinomas. Wedge resection of a normal-appearing contralateral ovary is unlikely to uncover an occult tumor. It is reasonable to follow the patient closely for any evidence of future ovarian enlargement with vaginal ultrasound in these cases.

LOW-STAGE OVARIAN CARCINOMAS

Stage I. Operative exploration is performed. It is important to emphasize that careful assessment of the subdiaphragmatic areas and inspection of the entire peritoneum and the retroperitoneal paraaortic and pelvic nodes are important, particularly in view of the risk of diaphragmatic and nodal spread in higher-grade tumors that initially appear to be at stage I, particularly those on frozen section that appear to be less well differentiated than grade 1. In addition, the omentum, uterus, tubes, and contralateral ovary are removed.

Rupture of ovary. Occasionally during removal a stage I ovarian carcinoma is inadvertently ruptured (stage IC,

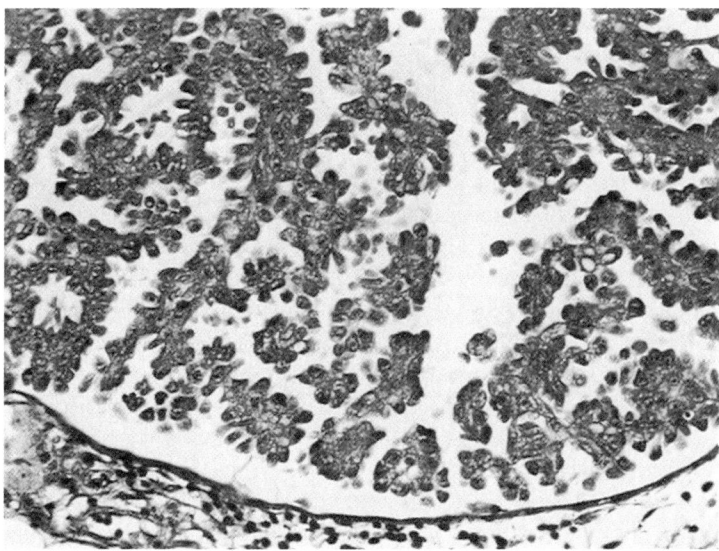

FIGURE 31-11 Noninvasive implant of epithelial type. Branching papillae and detached clusters of polygonal cells showing moderate cytologic atypicality are present (H&E; ×313). (From Bell DA, Weinstock MA, and Scully RE: Cancer 62:2212, 1988.)

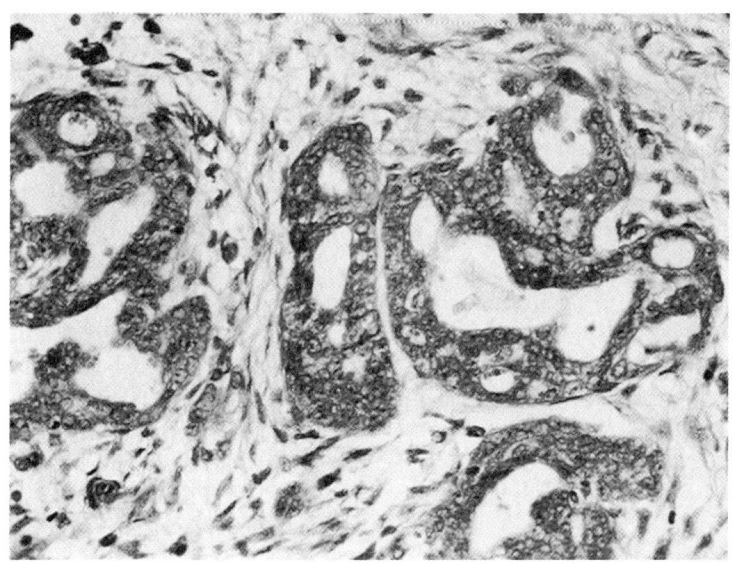

FIGURE 31-12 Invasive implant. Glands with an irregular contour lined by severely atypical epithelial cells with extensive intraglandular bridging are present (H&E, ×313). (From Bell DA, Weinstock MA, and Scully RE: Cancer 62:2212, 1988.)

Table 31-6). There are conflicting opinions as to the potential adverse effects on patient prognosis. Sjövall, in an analysis of 394 patients, found that rupture during surgery did not affect survival, while there was marked reduction in survival in that study among those whose ovarian rupture occurred *before* operation. In general the spilled fluid and all residual tumor should be removed promptly from the operative field following rupture (see later discussion). Presumably higher-grade and larger tumors are most prone to rupture.

A study by Dembo et al. of 519 stage I patients found that adverse factors were grade of tumor, dense pelvic adherence (no invasion but adhesion), or over 250 ml of ascites. Patients without these features had a 98% 5-year survival. It appears that patients with stage I grade 3 tumors should have postoperative therapy, but data are unclear for stage I grade 2 patients.

Stage II. Stage II ovarian cancer is initially treated by removal of all gross disease, including the uterus, tubes, and ovaries, and an omentectomy (infracolic) is performed. The pelvic and paraaortic nodes are sampled.

Postoperative management for stages I-II. After operative therapy is completed, the patient may receive additional treatment with irradiation or chemotherapy. It is not clearly defined which patients will benefit from adjuvant therapy. Guthrie et al. evaluated 656 patients treated for epithelial ovarian carcinomas that had been totally excised. Most carcinomas were at stage I or II, and patients were randomly assigned to receive postoperative treatment of radiation therapy alone, chemotherapy alone, radiation therapy and chemotherapy, or no postoperative therapy. Follow-up was for at least 2 years. Approximately 20% of the tumors were borderline malignancies, and the rest were invasive carcinomas. Perhaps surprisingly, the lowest frequency of death or recurrence was noted in the group receiving no postoperative therapy (2%), whereas in the other groups the death or recurrence incidence was 14% to 17%. Thus this study showed no benefit for adjuvant therapy in completely excised stage I and II carcinomas, emphasizing the importance of a control-nontreatment group in adjuvant therapy trials.

Radioactive colloids and adjuvant chemotherapy have been used postoperatively in an attempt to improve survival rates in patients with stage I and II disease or with no gross residual tumor after operation. ^{32}P, a primary beta emitter, has been used. Usually 15 mCi of ^{32}P in 500 ml of saline solution is injected intraperitoneally and distributed widely throughout the peritoneal cavity. Radioactive gold (^{198}Au) had also been used in the past but because of gamma ray emission (see Chapter 26) it is associated with more post-therapy complications and is not used.

Young et al. conducted two randomized studies for adjuvant therapy of stage I disease. The first showed those with stage IA grades 1 and 2 had 5-year survivals of greater than 90% and did not benefit from adjuvant alkylating agent chemotherapy. The second study showed comparable results both for adjuvant ^{32}P and alkylating agent therapy for stage I grade 3, as well as completely resected stage II cases. The latter had no "control group." Piver et al. reported 93% 5-year survival for stage IC or stage I grade 3 patients who received multiagent chemotherapy containing cisplatinum. Vergote et al. analyzed 313 patients treated with ^{32}P either after primary operation or second-look (see discussion later in chapter) operation. Bowel complications occurred in 22 (7%), and 13 required operation. Bolis et al. reported two randomized trials comparing ^{32}P versus chemotherapy with cisplatinum at 50 mg/m^2 for six cycles. Both for stages IA and IB grades 2 to 3 and stages IC showed significantly reduced relapse rates in the cisplatinum arms. Unfortunately a survival advantage was not demonstrated, and those who recurred after receiving chemotherapy did worse than those who received ^{32}P. The optimal treatment is not known, but those requiring adjuvant therapy for low-stage disease are usually treated with multiagent chemotherapy with Taxol and carboplatin (see following discussion).

Unfortunately, chemotherapy administration, particularly with alkylating agents, is associated with an increased risk of subsequently developing leukemia, which is related to the dose and duration of treatment. This risk increases from about 2% within 4 years of therapy to as great as 10% 8 years after treatment. Kaldor et al. reported that alkylating agents, as well as cisplatin and doxorubicin, used for ovarian cancer were all associated with an increased risk of leukemia that was not seen after radiotherapy. This risk must be balanced against the potential benefits of improved survival when adjuvant therapy is prescribed for patients with completely resected disease. A recent study by Travis et al. showed a significant increase in relative risk of secondary leukemia for both cisplatin and carboplatin, which was dose related. However, the total number of excess cases did not negate the substantially better survivals in ovarian cancer patients treated with platinum compounds.

External irradiation has been used as treatment for ovarian carcinoma, particularly stage II disease. Dembo and Bush used pelvic irradiation (4500 cGy to the midpoint of the pelvis) plus upper abdominal radiation, including the liver and diaphragm (2250 cGy), to treat stage IB, stage II, and asymptomatic stage III ovarian cancer. They reported abdominopelvic irradiation to be superior to pelvic irradiation alone or pelvic irradiation plus adjuvant chemotherapy only with an alkylating agent. Over 78% of their patients treated with abdominopelvic irradiation survived at least 5 years, in comparison with 50% of those in the other treatment group, but this was a nonrandomized study.

The results with postoperative irradiation have not been confirmed, and a randomized trial of radiation therapy versus chemotherapy for low-stage ovarian cancer has not been conducted. An additional concern regarding the use of external therapy is that the therapy compromises bone marrow function because wide areas of pelvic bone marrow are irradiated, necessitating dosage reduction in subsequent chemotherapy, and there is an increased risk of bowel complications if subsequent surgery is required.

ADVANCED EPITHELIAL CARCINOMAS (STAGES III AND IV). A maximal surgical resection is completed to minimize the amount of residual disease in the case of advanced ovarian cancer. Heintz et al. also reported that diffuse peritoneal carcinomatosis and the presence of ascites worsen the prognosis. As previously noted, bowel resection may be needed to complete effective removal of tumor, but this procedure is not advisable if large residual tumors would be left after intestinal resection is completed. Bristow et al. reported improved survival in optimally debulked stage IV ovarian cancer (<1 cm residual nodules). These patients also had a better performance status and may have had cancers more amenable to resection. However, it is believed that optimal surgical debulking confers a survival advantage in advanced ovarian carcinoma.

For patients who are cachectic or those who are undergoing extensive operative procedures leading to prolonged periods of compromised bowel function, total parenteral nutrition (hyperalimentation) via a centrally placed intravenous catheter that will allow delivery of 2000 to 3000 calories daily (20% dextrose, amino acids, and lipid for essential nutrients) is advised. For short-term therapy, a peripheral vein may be used and hyperalimentation accomplished with 10% dextrose and lipids, but phlebitis will eventually develop, and only about half as many calories can be administered. Patients treated with hyperalimentation are better able to tolerate intestinal resection and also appear to be more resistant to the adverse effects of subsequent chemotherapy.

As noted previously (see p. 969), the term *serous surface papillary carcinoma of the ovary* is applied to cases of small (<4 cm) ovaries and widespread peritoneal tumor. These tumors, as noted by Altaras et al., often elaborate CA-125 and appear to respond best to multiagent chemotherapy following maximal surgical debulking.

Chemotherapy for ovarian carcinoma. Until the late 1970s, chemotherapy for ovarian carcinoma was usually in the form of a single alkylating agent (melphalan, cyclophosphamide [Cytoxan], or chlorambucil) (see Chapter 26), and complete response rates of 10% to 20% were reported, with overall responses (complete plus partial) on the order of 50%.

In the 1980s platinum-based regimens were commonly used with apparent improvement in response rates. Usually cisplatin and an alkylating agent were prescribed. Other drugs were occasionally added, including Adriamycin and hexamethylmelamine, and the toxicity of these various agents is discussed in Chapter 26. Venesmaa reported on 523 women with stage III ovarian cancer treated in Finland between 1977 and 1990 and showed a statistically significant improvement in 5-year survival from the preplatinum era of 10% to 27% among those who received a platinum protocol. Although this was an impressive improvement, it still clearly resulted in failure for most patients.

Current therapy has been developed to include the drug paclitaxel (Taxol). McGuire et al. conducted a randomized trial comparing cisplatinum 75 mg/m^2 with either cyclophosphamide 750 mg/m^2 or paclitaxel 135 mg/m^2 over 24 hours and demonstrated a survival advantage in the Taxol arm. All patients had residual disease >1 cm after primary operation so that they were in a somewhat unfavorable category. However, the median progression-free survival was only 18 months in the paclitaxel arm compared with 13 months in the platinum arm. This protocol has generally been adopted in the United States as first-line therapy for ovarian cancer. Because the analog carboplatin is readily administered on an outpatient basis, most therapists have substituted it for cisplatinum and have shortened the Taxol infusion to 3 hours (175 mg/m^2). A recent phase III trial by Neijt et al. showed paclitaxel and carboplatin is a feasible outpatient regimen with less toxicity than paclitaxel-cisplatin. It should be noted that carboplatin is quantitatively secreted by the kidney and its effective serum concentration can be calculated from a formula based on the patient's size and the drug's renal clearance. The formula gives a dosage expression as "the area under curve (AUC)," which provides a measure of the drug's concentration and is a preferable means of calculating carboplatin dosage than dosage expressed as mg/m^2. A usual dose for carboplatin is calculated for AUC values of 5 to 7.5. Both Taxol and platinum compounds are neurotoxic, as noted by Warner, and this is often the dose-limiting toxicity. G-CSF (granulocyte colony stimulating factor) is occasionally needed to reduce the duration of significant neutropenia in these programs. A commonly used program is Taxol 175 mg/m^2 over 3 hours and carboplatin (AUC = 5) given in a 1 to 2 hour infusion every 3 weeks.

A'Hern and Gore conducted a meta-analysis and suggested improved results for the addition of Adriamycin to platinum and alkylating chemotherapy regimens and indicated that these agents should be compared to the efficacy of paclitaxel and platinum. An ideal first-line effective treatment for advanced ovarian cancer has not yet been identified.

Evaluation of Chemotherapy Results

Chemotherapy is usually administered every 3 weeks. The patient is monitored with careful physical examination; blood tests to measure hematologic, liver, and kidney functions; and radiologic studies, such as chest x-ray examinations, ultrasound tests, or (usually) computed tomography (CT) scans of the abdomen and the pelvis. G-CSF is added as needed to combat neutropenia. Mild neutropenia following chemotherapy can be managed expectantly but for the patient who develops severe neutropenia with fever and an absolute neutrophil count (ANC) of <500 cells/μl, antibiotics are prescribed to prevent septic complications.

If tumor is suspected on CT scan, fine-needle biopsy can frequently document the presence of persistent or recurrent disease. A negative CT scan, however, does not guarantee complete clinical response. Goldhirsch et al. noted that 5 of 26 patients with tumor nodules larger than 1 cm had negative CT scans, and the examination was most effective (80%) for detecting metastasis in retroperitoneal nodes. In 1989 Reuter et al. reported improved results of 8% false negatives using newer equipment with CT slices at 10- to 15-mm intervals. Patsner reported that 24 of 60 patients with negative CT scans had positive second-look operations, calling into question the value of this imaging study. Vaginal ultrasound is particularly useful to assess the pelvis. CA-125 levels are used to monitor the course of the patient with carcinoma. Buller et al., as noted previously, calculated that CA-125 followed an exponential regression curve in successfully treated patients. This provides the possibility of mathematically estimating early in treatment the patient's response to chemotherapy. Bridgewater et al. reported a greater than 50% drop in CA-125 was a good sign of clinical response.

Occasionally the problem arises of a patient whose tumor was incompletely resected at initial operation, usually because an ovarian cancer was not suspected preoperatively. Some therapists advocate reexploration to achieve maximum debulking. An alternative approach was suggested by Lawton et al., who administered 3 cycles of platinum-based multiagent chemotherapy to 36 incompletely resected ovarian cancer patients. They concluded such neoadjuvant therapy improved the likelihood of subsequent successful resection and subsequent effectiveness of chemotherapy. Van der Burg et al., in a collaborative effort, studied patients with residual nodules >1 cm after primary operation. They gave three cycles of chemotherapy and then randomized the patients to a second operation or no operation followed by additional chemotherapy. There was a slight survival advantage (56% versus 46%) in the group receiving interval debulking, which was statistically significant and suggests a possible benefit to this approach in some patients. A recent retrospective analysis by Vergote et al. also suggests an advantage for neoadjuvant chemotherapy before complete debulking. Chi et al. noted previously that those with preoperative CA-125 > 500 were less likely to be optimally debulked. They suggest these patients might benefit from laparoscopic confirmation of the diagnosis. They could then be followed by neoadjuvant chemotherapy and then debulking. However, there are no data currently to indicate the superiority of this approach.

Second-Look Procedures

Some therapists perform a laparoscopy before second-look laparotomy. If a second-look laparotomy is performed, it is important to extensively sample the peritoneal surfaces and lymph nodes. Particular attention is paid to areas that contained residual disease at the conclusion of the initial surgical procedure.

There are conflicting opinions regarding the value and indications of a second-look procedure in the therapy of ovarian cancer and these are mostly done by major centers as part of large-scale protocol studies. Many patients with negative second-look operation eventually develop recurrent disease. Early studies of second-look laparotomy showed about half (25% to 75%) of the patients thought clinically and radiologically to be free of disease actually had persistent disease at second-look operation. Walton et al. showed that patients who initially have stage I or II disease rarely have positive second-look procedures, and they recommend the operation not be done for those with low-stage tumors, a result confirmed by Sonnendecker. Favorable factors for negative second-look are low tumor grade, no residual disease after primary operation, young age (<55 years), and rapid regression to normal of elevated CA-125 values during chemotherapy.

Unfortunately, many patients develop recurrent disease, even after negative second-look operation. Rubin et al. noted a high (45%) rate of recurrence in patients with negative second-look laparotomy. Those initially with higher-stage and higher-grade tumors are more likely to recur after negative second-look operation. However, those who were disease free at 5 years were likely to remain disease free at subsequent follow-up.

It is controversial whether additional debulking at the time of second-look operation helps improve survival rates. Some patients are discovered to have recurrent ovarian carcinoma years after primary therapy. Recent studies by Markman et al. and others indicate that secondary regimens are more likely to produce a response if the patient initially responded and was at least 2 years from the completion of initial therapy. The likelihood of response increases the longer the interval since primary treatment.

A randomized clinical trial is needed to demonstrate the optimal management of patients after second-look operation and also to determine the potential value of the procedure. Intraperitoneal chemotherapy and whole abdominal radiation (WAR) are considered later in this section.

INTRAPERITONEAL THERAPY. Intraperitoneal instillation of chemotherapeutic agents has been tried to increase the effect of cytotoxic drugs on the tumor within the abdominal cavity. High intraperitoneal concentrations are achieved with instillation of the drug into the peritoneal cavity. Eventually serum levels comparable to those seen after intravenous therapy are obtained. The drug can be instilled with a catheter similar to that used for peritoneal dialysis. One modification is shown in Figure 31-13, in which a needle is allowed subcutaneous access through the skin into the port to administer the chemotherapy intraperitoneally through the catheter.

The effectiveness of the drug is increased by higher intraperitoneal concentrations and longer residence within the peritoneal cavity before escaping into the systemic circulation. The ideal agent would be one that slowly leaves the peritoneal cavity but then is rapidly metabolized once it reaches the systemic circulation, thus reducing side effects of the agent. In general, peritoneal absorption is decreased as molecular weight increases and lipid solubility decreases. In addition, drugs that are highly ionized at physiologic pH absorb more slowly from the peritoneal cavity than un-ionized agents.

In another GOG study Braly et al. used cisplatinum and 5-FU in 45 patients with <1 cm residual disease. Pathologic complete responses were documented in 3 of 15 patients who had third-look laparotomy, and the best results were in the platinum-sensitive patients. Platinum refractory patients did poorly as also noted in the study of Morgan et al. Barakat et al. report improved 3-year survivals in those receiving intraperitoneal therapy after negative second-look operation in comparison to those not treated (54% versus 39%). Despite great initial enthusiasm for intraperitoneal treatment, its efficacy and use in the treatment of ovarian carcinoma has yet to be defini-

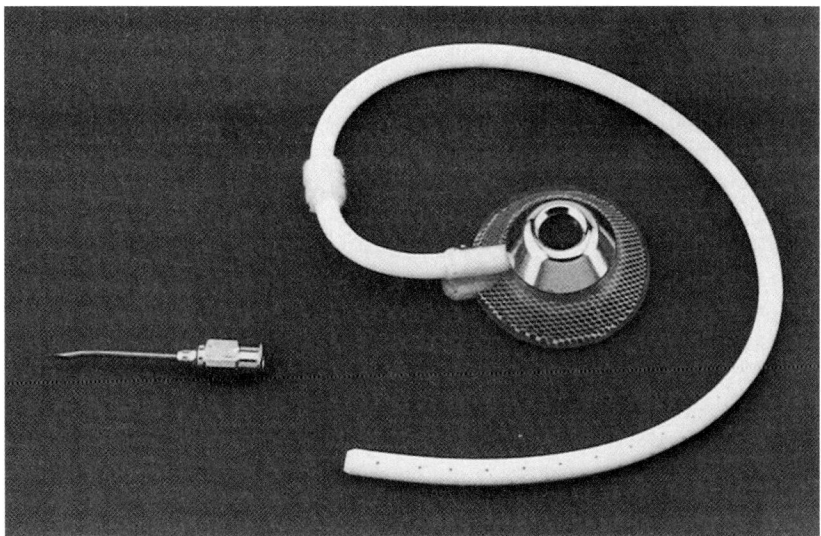

FIGURE 31-13   Peritoneal catheter with access port for infusion of drugs. (Port-A-Cath, Pharmacia Deltec, Inc.)

tively established. Cooperative trials are ongoing to find the optimal use of this modality.

IRRADIATION THERAPY.   Whole abdominal radiation (WAR) has been studied to improve salvage, with varying results and a high frequency of bowel complications, often serious, requiring operative intervention. Goldhirsch et al. studied whole abdominal radiation in 45 patients who had documented pathologic complete responses. A group of 24 received whole abdominal radiation and the remainder no therapy. The addition of irradiation did not improve the results. Menczer et al. compared intraperitoneal cisplatin with abdominal pelvic irradiation in individuals who were in complete clinical remission with minimal or no residual disease at second-look laparotomy. Eighteen patients received irradiation therapy to the abdomen and pelvis, and 19 received three courses of intraperitoneal cisplatin with systemic thiosulfate protection. A statistically significant difference in overall survival was observed at 36 months (76.6% versus 44.4%), suggesting an advantage to intraperitoneal cisplatin treatment in these patients in comparison with irradiation. Because of the risk of complications and the lack of extensive data regarding its effectiveness, whole abdominal radiation has generally not been used in these cases. Such radiation should not be used in patients who have received intraperitoneal P^{32} because of the risk of bowel complications.

Recently, Cmelak and Kapp treated 41 patients with platinum refractory ovarian cancer who had undergone operation. They treated the whole abdomen with 28 Gy and a pelvic boost to 48 Gy. For 28 patients with residual disease less than 1.5 cm the 5-year survival was 53%, which is better than would be expected with chemotherapy. However, no large-scale trial data are available for this technique.

Complications and Alternative Considerations

MALIGNANT EFFUSIONS.   Patients with ovarian cancer frequently develop ascites or hydrothorax or both, requiring repeated drainage by paracentesis or thoracentesis. Occasionally sclerosing solutions are used in the thoracic cavity to prevent reaccumulation of fluid, with resultant adherence of the pleural surfaces. Nitrogen mustard, tetracycline, and quinacrine have all been used successfully for this purpose.

IMMUNOTHERAPY AND GENE THERAPY.   Immunotherapy agents, such as *Corynebacterium parvum (C. parvum)*, and bacille Calmette-Guerin (BCG) have been administered to try to augment the immunologic response and promote tumor resistance in the host. These agents have also been used in combination with cytotoxic chemotherapy, and preliminary improved results have been reported. Intraperitoneal immunotherapy approaches have been evaluated with such agents as interferon, lymphokine-activated killer (LAK) cells, interleukin-2, and tumor necrosis factor (TNF). Berek et al. conducted a phase I-II trial of IP cisplatinum (60 mg/m^2) and α-Interferon (25 $\times$ 10^6 IV) given every 4 weeks. Among 18 patients there were 3 complete and 4 partial responses.

The use of monoclonal antibodies as a form of site-directed therapy has been investigated. Epenetos et al. have used tumor-associated antigens linked to ^{131}I to treat recurrent ovarian carcinoma. After intraperitoneal administration to 24 patients, responses were noted primarily in those with small-volume disease, with some responses evaluated by follow-up laparoscopy lasting up to 3 years. Canevari et al. noted responses in 3 of 26 patients treated with autologous T-lymphocytes targeted with a bispecific monoclonal antibody. Although these techniques hold promise, they have not yet proven to be of great clinical value.

The potential of gene therapy is also under active investigation. Santoso et al. reported that transfection of a wild-type p53 into ovarian cancer cells in vitro inhibited cellular proliferation. As noted by Berchuck and Bast, there are a number of hurdles to developing this type of therapy to clinical usefulness.

HUMAN TUMOR STEM CELL ASSAY.   The in vitro method of human tumor stem cell assay was developed by Slamon et al. The test is based on the growth of cultured cells in vitro, which are then tested against a variety of chemotherapeutic agents. Such clonogenic assays may potentially provide useful clinical information regarding drug selection for chemotherapy in gynecologic malignancies, primarily for drug resistance, but at present they are not reliable for regular clinical use.

SUMMARY

Therapy for epithelial ovarian carcinoma is based on removal of all gross disease and sampling of areas at high risk for spread in the peritoneal cavity and retroperitoneal nodes. Postoperative therapy is employed depending on the stage and grade of the primary tumor. For accurately staged cases, postoperative ^{32}P may be used in low-stage tumors, such as stage IC carcinomas where there is a risk of intraperitoneal tumor seeding but no residual disease. Multiagent chemotherapy with carboplatin and Taxol is frequently employed as adjunctive treatment for poorly differentiated tumors, such as stage I, grade 3, or for stage II cases without residual tumor, but such treatment carries with it a risk of subsequent development of leukemia. External irradiation has been used, but its use usually compromises bone marrow function and interferes with the future use of chemotherapy.

For high-stage tumors and for patients with residual disease after initial operation, multiple-agent chemotherapy, usually Taxol and carboplatin, is used. It is accompanied by multiple short- and long-term toxic side effects, but results in initial response rates in stage III cases may exceed 90%. Five-year survival rates drop to 30% or less. Long-term randomized trials and the development of new agents will be needed to improve rates of salvage and to optimize therapy for epithelial ovarian carcinomas. Currently second-line chemotherapy offers remission to some patients, but the best response rates are achieved with initial chemotherapy.

SMALL CELL CARCINOMA

Dickerson et al. described a new and virulent type of ovarian malignancy that occurs in young women, usually between the ages of 15 and 30 years. Because of its histologic appearance, it has been designated a small cell carcinoma. The tumor is often but not always accompa-

nied by hypercalcemia as noted by Young et al. in an analysis of 150 cases. Most patients have died, although a few stage I survivors have been reported, some of whom have been treated with adjuvant multiagent chemotherapy. Reed reported a patient with stage IC disease treated with cisplatinum, etoposide, and bleomycin who survived 5 years. Benrubi et al. treated a patient with stage II small cell carcinoma with debulking and multiagent chemotherapy followed by radiation, and the patient was 4 years disease-free at the time of the report. Other isolated stage I 5-year survivals have been reported with multiagent chemotherapy programs augmented with subsequent pelvic radiation. However, for advanced-stage disease, and even in most stage I cases, the course of the tumor has been fatal.

MALIGNANT MIXED MÜLLERIAN TUMORS (CARCINOSARCOMAS)

These are extremely rare ovarian malignancies that histologically resemble comparable tumors in the uterus. Treatment involves operation for cytoreduction, as noted by Muntz et al., with added therapy usually in the form of multiagent chemotherapy. Stage is prognostic, and those with advanced stages usually do not survive.

As noted by Hellstrom et al., about 500 of these rare tumors have been reported. In their series of 36 such cases over 20 years the median survival was 16.6 months with a 5-year actuarial survival of only 18%. Low-stage tumors and those treated with multiagent chemotherapy (cytoxan, Adriamycin, cisplatin) had an improved survival.

GERM CELL TUMORS

These tumors are derived from the germ cells of the ovary. As a group they are the second most frequent of ovarian neoplasms, and they account for about 20% to 25% of all ovarian tumors. The classification of germ cell tumors according to the World Health Organization (WHO) designation is shown in the box on the opposite page.

The most frequent germ cell tumor is the benign cystic teratoma (dermoid); overall, only 2% to 3% of germ cell tumors are malignant. Among the malignant germ cell tumors, the most frequent is the dysgerminoma, which accounts for about 45% of malignant germ cell tumors. Next in frequency are the immature teratomas and then endodermal sinus tumors. In female patients under age 30, germ cell tumors are the most frequent ovarian neoplasm, and about one third of the germ cell tumors encountered in those under age 21 are malignant.

The histogenesis of germ cell tumors has been extensively studied and summarized by Talerman. Figure 31-14 shows the theory of the histogenesis of these tumors—

WHO Classification of Germ Cell Tumors

Dysgerminoma
    Endodermal sinus tumor
    Embryonal carcinoma
    Polyembryoma
    Choriocarcinoma
    Teratomas
    Immature
    Mature
        Solid
        Cystic
Dermoid cyst (mature cystic teratoma)
Dermoid cyst with malignant transformation
    Monodermal and highly specialized
        Struma ovarii
        Carcinoid
        Struma ovarii and carcinoid
        Others
    Mixed forms

that they originate from the primitive germ cell and then gradually differentiate to mimic the developmental tissues of embryonic origin (ectoderm, mesoderm, or endoderm) and the extraembryonic tissues (yolk sac and trophoblast). Germ cell tumors that originate in the ovary have homologous counterparts in the testes, that is, dysgerminoma and seminoma. Germ cell tumors are usually unilateral, with the exception of teratomas and dysgerminomas (see Table 31-4). The morphologic and clinical aspects of each of the various types of germ cell tumors will be separately considered.

Teratomas

Teratomas consist of tissues that recapitulate the three layers of the developing embryo (ectoderm, mesoderm, and endoderm). One or more of the layers may be represented, and the tissues can be mature (benign) or immature (malignant). Chromosomal studies indicate that teratomas appear to arise from a single germ and have an XX karyotype. In the older literature, terms such as *malignant teratoma* and *teratocarcinoma* were used to denote the malignant variety of these tumors, but these terms have been replaced by the nomenclature shown in the box at left.

Benign Cystic Teratomas (Dermoids)

Benign cystic teratomas are the most common germ cell tumors and account for 25% of all ovarian neoplasms. They primarily occur during the reproductive years but may occur in postmenopausal women and in children. The risk of malignant transformation (see later discussion) is markedly increased if these tumors are found in postmenopausal women. One of the interesting facets of teratomas is their ability to produce adult tissue, including skin, bone, teeth, hair, and dermal tissue. The presence of calcified bone or teeth allows the tumor to be diagnosed preoperatively with ultrasound or radiography (Figure 31-15).

Dermoids are usually unilateral, but 10% to 15% are bilateral. The outside wall of the tumor tends to be smooth with a yellowish appearance caused by the sebaceous fatty material that fills the tumor. Hair is also a prominent fea-

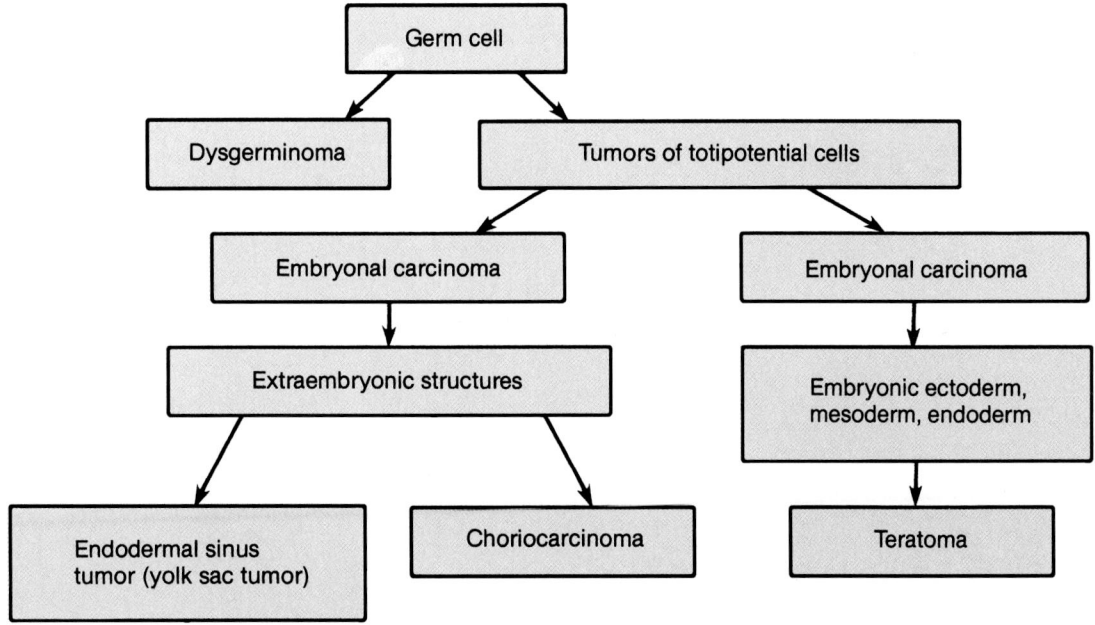

FIGURE 31-14 Histogenesis of germ cell tumors. (Modified from Talerman A: Germ cell tumors of the ovary. In Blaustein A, editor: Pathology of the female genital tract, New York, 1982, Springer-Verlag.)

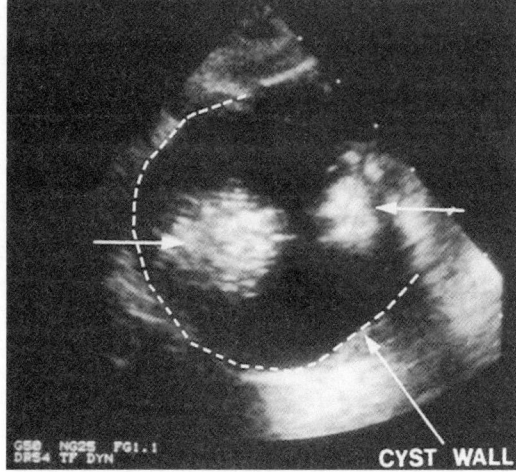

FIGURE 31-15 Transvaginal ultrasound image of an ovarian dermoid cyst. The arrows indicate balls of hair. (Courtesy Dr. Zubie Sheikh, The University of Chicago, Department of Obstetrics & Gynecology.)

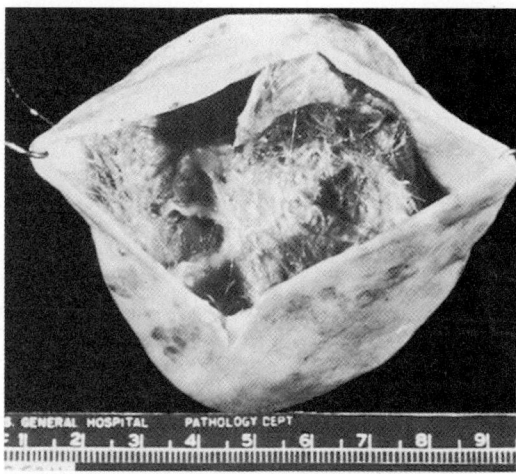

FIGURE 31-16 Gross specimen of a dermoid cyst that was filled with sebaceous material and hair. (Courtesy Dr. R.E. Scully.)

ture once the cyst is opened (Figure 31-16). Usually the tumors are asymptomatic, but they can cause severe pain if there is torsion or if the sebaceous material perforates the cyst wall, leading to a reactive peritonitis. This rare complication is severe and can occur during pregnancy. Microscopically a number of adult tissues are seen (Figure 31-17).

Treatment of the reproductive-age female patient or of the child consists of either cystectomy or unilateral oophorectomy. In most cases it should be possible to remove only the cyst and preserve normal ovarian tissue.

The technique at open laparotomy is demonstrated in Figure 31-18. The opposite ovary should be inspected. If it is grossly normal, nothing further need be done. Some therapists remove the mass laparoscopically, but rupture can result in local chemical peritonitis unless all irritating substances are completely removed with saline lavage. Current treatment involves preservation of the contralateral ovary without any biopsy if it grossly appears normal. In women beyond childbearing years, therapy for a dermoid usually consists of removal of the uterus, both tubes, and the ovaries.

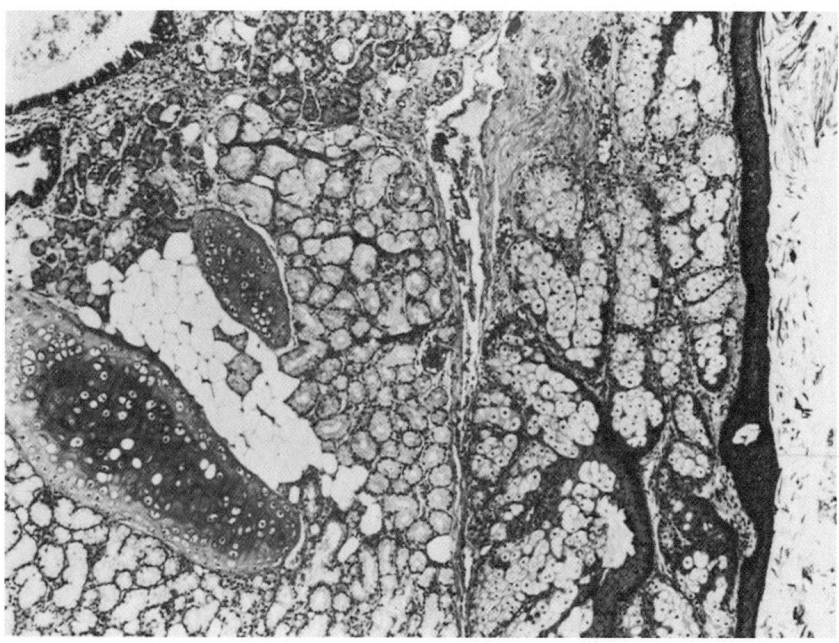

FIGURE 31-17 Photomicrograph of dermoid. Cartilage is shown *(right)* lined by epidermis and accompanying appendages *(left).* (×50.) (From Serov SF, Scully RE, and Sobin LH: Histologic typing of ovarian tumors, Geneva, 1973, World Health Organization.)

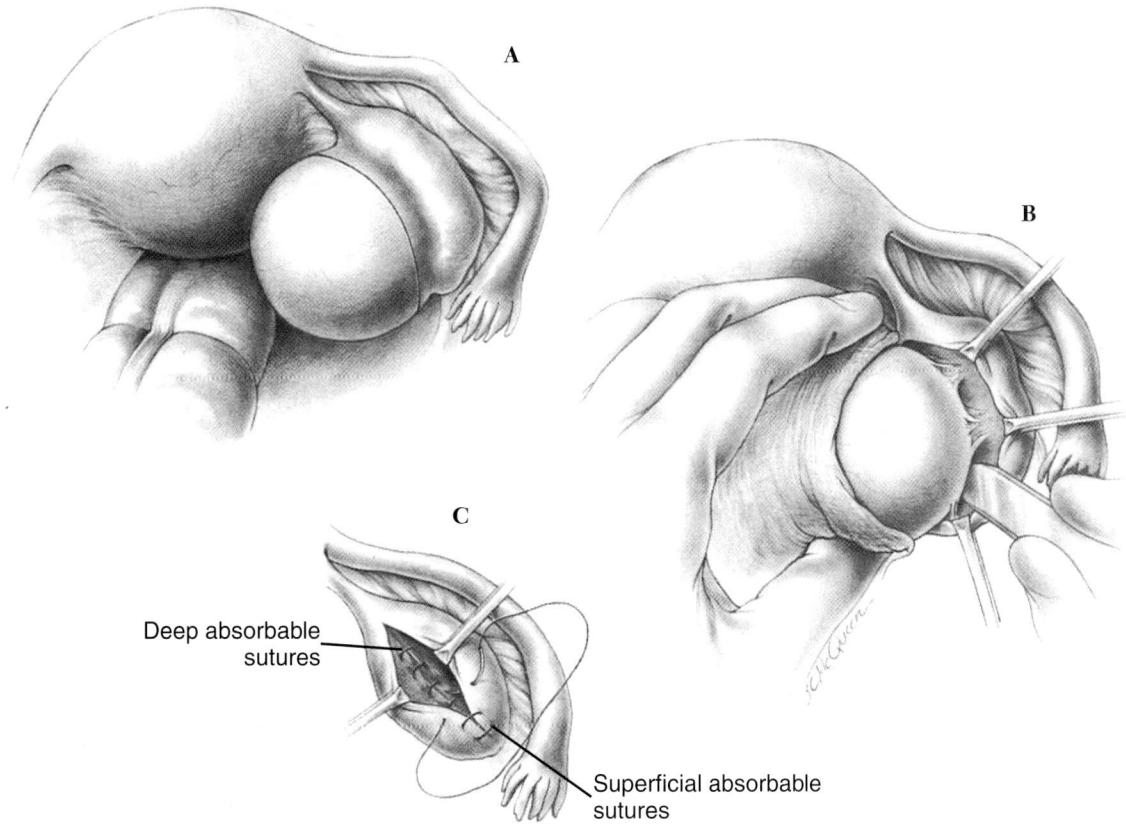

Deep absorbable
sutures

Superficial absorbable
sutures

FIGURE 31-18 Shelling out of teratoma. **A,** Scalpel incision in ovary at intersection of dermoid and normal ovary. **B,** Dermoid being separated. Note how upper part peels away. **C,** Reconstruction of normal ovary.

Occasionally teratomas may be solid and may consist only of adult tissues, leading to the diagnosis of solid, mature teratoma. These benign germ cell tumors are rare.

A cystic teratoma can undergo malignant degeneration, usually after menopause. Generally it occurs in the squamous epithelial elements of the dermoid, producing a squamous cell carcinoma. It is a rare complication estimated to occur in fewer than 2% of these tumors. If the malignant tissue has spread beyond the confines of the ovary, the prognosis is poor. In such cases additional therapy for squamous cell carcinoma with irradiation or chemotherapy or both are utilized.

Immature Teratomas

Immature teratomas are malignant and account for up to 20% of the malignant ovarian tumors found in women under the age of 20 but less than 1% of all ovarian cancers. They do not occur in women after menopause. They consist of immature embryonic structures that can be admixed with mature elements.

The prognosis for patients with immature teratomas is related to the stage (FIGO) and grade of the tumor. The grade of the tumor is based on the degree of immaturity of the various tissues. Grade 3 tumors consist of the most

immature tissues and often have a high proportion of immature neuroepithelium. Figure 31-19 shows the survival of patients with immature teratomas by stage and grade before the advent of modern chemotherapy. Because these tumors occur in young women, preservation of childbearing function is an important consideration. Kurman and Norris reported that patients with stage IA immature teratoma had a 10-year actuarial survival of 70% after unilateral salpingo-oophorectomy; this rate is comparable to that recorded after bilateral salpingo-oophorectomy. The opposite ovary is rarely involved by immature teratoma, although a benign cystic teratoma (dermoid) is present in about 10% of cases. If the opposite ovary appears grossly normal, unilateral salpingo-oophorectomy alone is adequate. If there is extension of tumor outside the ovary, implants and metastases should be extensively sampled and graded histologically to decide on therapy. The retroperitoneal nodes also should be evaluated and sampled, especially for grades 2 and 3 cases.

Multiple-agent chemotherapy has greatly improved the outlook for patients with immature teratoma. One protocol is the so-called VAC regimen (vincristine, 1.5 mg/m^2 given intravenously weekly for 12 weeks and actinomycin D, 0.5 mg, with cyclophosphamide [Cytoxan] 5 to 7 mg/kg/day given intravenously daily for 5 days every 4 weeks).

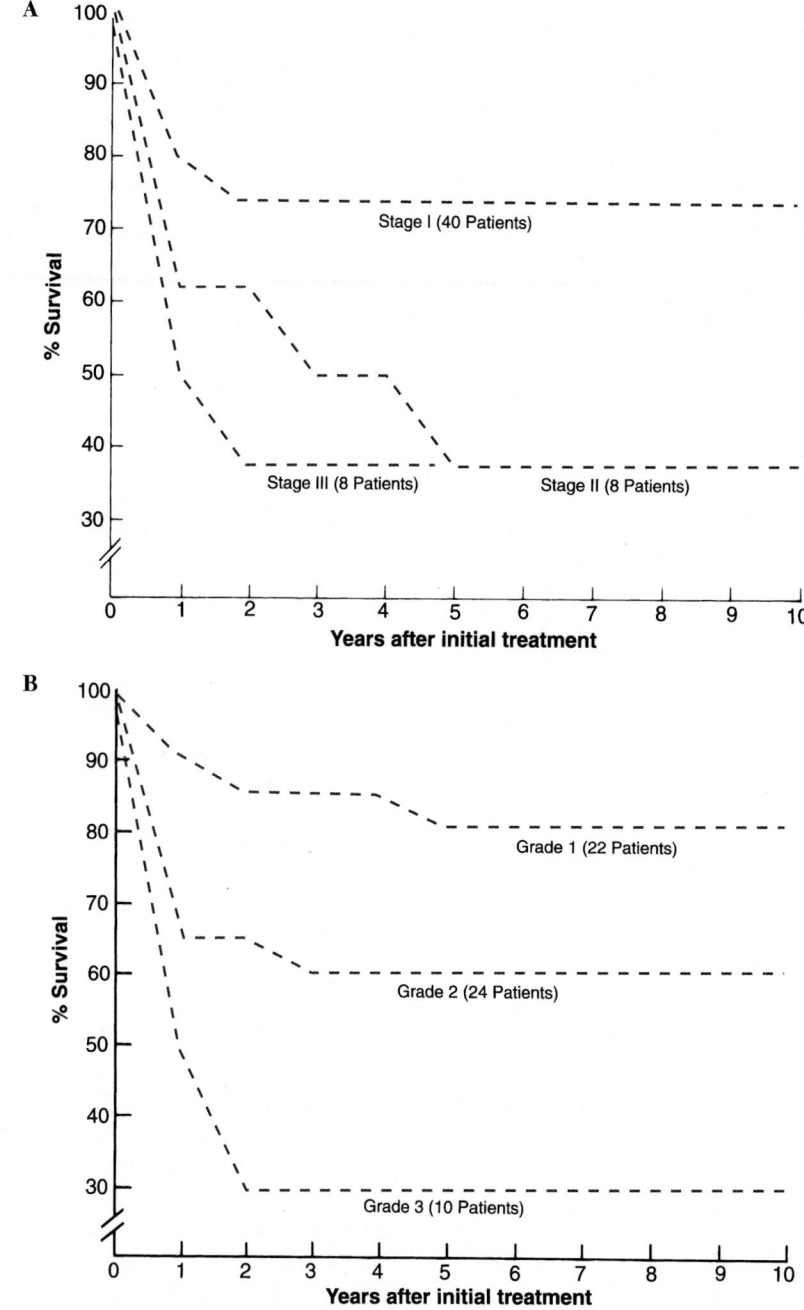

FIGURE 31-19 **A,** Actuarial survival of 56 patients with malignant teratoma by neoplasm stage. **B,** By neoplasm grade. (From Norris HJ, Zirkin JH, and Benson WL: Cancer 37:2359, 1976.)

Gershenson et al. noted excellent chemotherapy results with immature teratoma. Of 21 patients stages I to III treated with VAC, 18 survived. The progression-free survival rate was significantly better for those who received postoperative chemotherapy in comparison with those who did not (approximately 90% versus 10%). All 22 patients who underwent second-look laparotomy were free of disease. Conversion of metastatic immature teratoma (grades 2 and 3) after chemotherapy to mature elements (grade 0) has been reported by DiSaia et al. Mature elements require

no further therapy. Currently vinblastine, bleomycin, and cisplatin (VBP) (see "Endodermal Sinus Tumors") or etoposide and platinum are employed initially and are frequently effective. Bonazzi et al. treated 32 patients with operation alone for stage I to II tumors, grades 1 to 2. All patients with grade 3 tumors or stage III tumors, or those with tumor recurrence, received cisplatin, etoposide, and bleomycin. Most patients underwent fertility-sparing operation. Ten received chemotherapy. All patients were free of disease with a median follow-up of 47 months, and

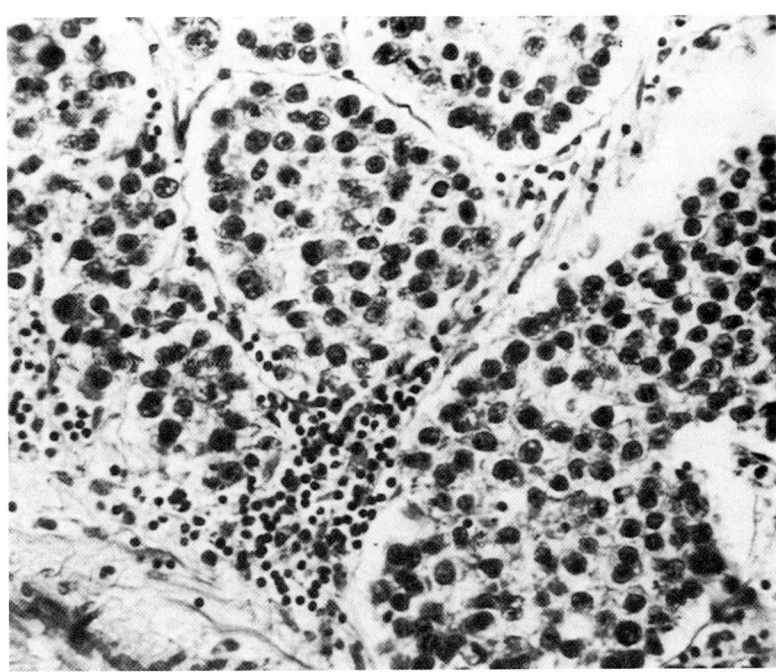

FIGURE 31-20   Dysgerminoma. (×300.) Dysgerminoma cells are demonstrated, as well as infiltration of stroma by lymphocytes. (From Scully RE: Germ cell tumors of the ovary and fallopian tube. In Meigs JV and Sturgis SH, editors: Progress in gynecology, vol 4, New York, 1963, Grune & Stratton.)

5 had delivered healthy infants. A recent Pediatric Oncology Group Study reported by Cushing et al. indicated that patients under age 15 with pure immature teratoma could be followed without chemotherapy; however over 90% of the tumors in their series were grade 1 or 2.

Chemotherapy is indicated for metastatic immature teratoma (other than grade 0). For stage IA tumors that are composed of grade 2 or 3 elements, adjunctive chemotherapy is indicated for most patients because of the associated poor prognosis (see Figure 31-19).

Specialized Germ Cell Tumors—Struma Ovarii and Carcinoids

Specialized ovarian germ cell tumors are rare; two types are commonly recognized (see box on p. 979): the struma ovarii and carcinoids. Struma ovarii are dermoids with thyroid tissue exclusively or as a major component. The thyroid tissue can be functional, leading to clinical hyperthyroidism. Most of these tumors are benign, but malignant changes are possible. Metastatic disease, if present, has been reported to be effectively treated with ^{131}I, as in the case of primary thyroid carcinoma.

Carcinoids are ovarian teratomas that histologically resemble similar tumors in the gastrointestinal tract. Carcinoids are rare and are unilateral in the ovary. In about 30% of cases a true carcinoid syndrome will develop, and 5-hydroxyindoleacetic acid (5-HIAA) can be detected and used to monitor the tumor postoperatively. These tumors occur primarily in older women and tend to grow slowly;

the prognosis after hysterectomy and bilateral salpingo-oophorectomy is excellent. For a young woman desiring preservation of childbearing function, a stage IA carcinoid can be treated by unilateral salpingo-oophorectomy.

Dysgerminomas

Dysgerminomas are the most common type of malignant germ cell tumors. They consist of primitive germ cells with stroma infiltrated by lymphocytes (Figure 31-20). They are analogous to seminoma in the male testis, and they comprise about 1% of ovarian malignancies. Dysgerminomas occur primarily in women under the age of 30. The tumor can be discovered during pregnancy. Some arise in dysgenetic gonads (see later discussion of gonadoblastomas). Unlike other malignant germ cell tumors, dysgerminomas are bilateral in about 10% of cases (see Table 31-4). The prognosis is related to tumor size (improved if less than 15 cm), unilaterality, encapsulation (not ruptured), lack of spread to retroperitoneal nodes, and lack of ascites. If all these criteria are present, the prognosis in stage IA cases is excellent (greater than 90% 5-year survival). Fortunately about two thirds of the cases present as stage IA. Sampling of a normal-appearing contralateral ovary is not necessary, particularly with the availability of vaginal ultrasound to follow ovarian size.

Insofar as patients with dysgerminoma are young, preservation of childbearing function is desirable. The tumor can spread within the peritoneal cavity and to retroperitoneal nodes, a more likely occurrence with larger dysgerminomas. If the tumor is confined to one ovary, a unilateral salpingo-oophorectomy should be performed and the abdomen thoroughly explored to determine the presence of intraperitoneal and retroperitoneal spread. Any enlarged pelvic or paraaortic nodes should be excised. If frozen section indicates pure dysgerminoma and there is no evidence of spread outside the primary tumor, only a unilateral salpingo-oophorectomy is indicated. Patients so treated have a 5-year survival in excess of 90%. Assadourian and Taylor noted that unilateral salpingo-oophorectomy was as effective as more radical treatment for unilateral dysgerminoma. There can be a recurrence in as many as 20% of cases, primarily in tumors over 15 cm, but most of these tumors can be effectively treated by an additional operative procedure or chemotherapy or irradiation. These tumors are extremely radiosensitive and can be cured with less than 3000 cGy, a dosage used to treat extraovarian residual tumor after primary surgery or for recurrence, but multiagent chemotherapy is effective with fewer side effects in these young patients and is generally preferred.

Patients treated conservatively should be closely followed with periodic pelvic ultrasound and/or CT imaging evaluations. Occasionally the serum lactic dehydrogenase (LDH) is elevated as a nonspecific tumor marker as summarized by Schwartz and Morris. Vaginal ultrasound is used if the contralateral ovary is preserved.

The successful therapy of germ cell tumors has improved the prognosis and results of all germ cell tumors. Effective regressions have been accomplished and menstrual and childbearing function have been preserved in many of these patients after successful chemotherapy. Wu et al. reported 6 normal pregnancies among 12 married women previously treated successfully by chemotherapy for malignant germ cell tumors. Williams et al. reported the GOG experience for 20 patients with dysgerminoma treated with platinum and bleomycin plus etoposide or vinblastine and a few subsequently received VAC. Nineteen of 20 patients were disease-free with median follow-up of 26 months, emphasizing the effectiveness of multiagent chemotherapy in this disease. Recently Brewer et al. reported on 26 patients treated with bleomycin, etoposide, and cisplatin with 25 alive and disease free with median follow-up of 89 months. They reported 71% resumed normal menstrual function and 6 patients conceived. Blumenfeld et al. administered gonadotrophin-releasing hormone agnoist (GnRHa) during chemotherapy for nongynecologic tumors to women of reproductive age and 15 of 16 surviving patients (93.7%) resumed menses and ovulation. This suggests such GnRHa prophylaxis may be worthwhile for young patients needing chemotherapy in order to preserve future ovarian function.

Other germ cell elements may coexist with these tumors (mixed germ cell tumor), in which case the prognosis is markedly worse. Some of the reports in the earlier literature of poor prognosis with unilateral dysgerminoma were probably unrecognized cases of mixed germ cell tumors, such as would be suggested if alpha-fetoprotein is found elevated in a case thought to be dysgerminoma (see later discussion). However, minor elevations of hCG have been reported in pure dysgerminoma. If the levels exceed 100 mIU/ml, the tumor probably contains choriocarcinoma elements and should be considered a mixed germ cell tumor.

Endodermal Sinus Tumors (Yolk Sac Tumors)

The endodermal sinus tumor, which comprises 10% of malignant germ cell tumors, in part resembles the yolk sac of the rodent placenta, thus recapitulating extraembryonic tissues (see Figure 31-14). One typical histologic pattern is shown in Figure 31-21. The tumor secretes alpha-fetoprotein, which is a specific marker that is useful in identifying and following these tumors clinically.

These rapidly growing tumors occur in females between 13 months and 45 years of age. A median age of 19 years at diagnosis was noted by Kurman and Norris. Stage IA cases can be treated by unilateral adnexectomy. Before modern chemotherapy, the tumor was usually fatal, even if it was confined to one ovary. Therefore all patients with endodermal sinus tumor should undergo chemotherapy postoperatively. The VAC protocol (see previous section on immature teratoma) has been widely used. Another effective regimen has been a 5-day program: actinomycin D, 10 g/kg/day; 5-fluorouracil (5-FU), 8 mg/kg/day up to 500 mg; and cyclophosphamide (Cytoxan), 7 mg/kg/day up to 450 mg (Act-FU-Cy). Forney noted regression of endodermal sinus tumor with this program and also reported subsequent pregnancy in a patient so treated. Einhorn and Donahue initially reported a potent combination of vinblastine, 12 mg/m² intravenously every 3 weeks for four doses; bleomycin, 20 units/m² (maximum dose, 30 units/m²) intravenously given weekly for seven doses and an eighth course on week 10; and cisplatin (cis-platinum), 20 mg/m² daily for 5 days given every 3 weeks for up to four courses (VBP). This regimen has been found to be effective in treating patients with metastatic germ cell tumors of the testis and in inducing remissions in endodermal sinus tumors. Multiple-agent chemotherapy is needed, and of the 41 patients reported by Gershenson et al., all of the 21 who survived had received multiple-agent chemotherapy with one of these protocols. Bleomycin, etoposide, and platinum are probably used most frequently.

Choriocarcinomas

Nongestational choriocarcinoma is a highly malignant rare germ cell tumor resembling extraembryonic tissues. Like gestational choriocarcinoma (see Chapter 35), it consists of malignant cytotrophoblasts and syncytio-

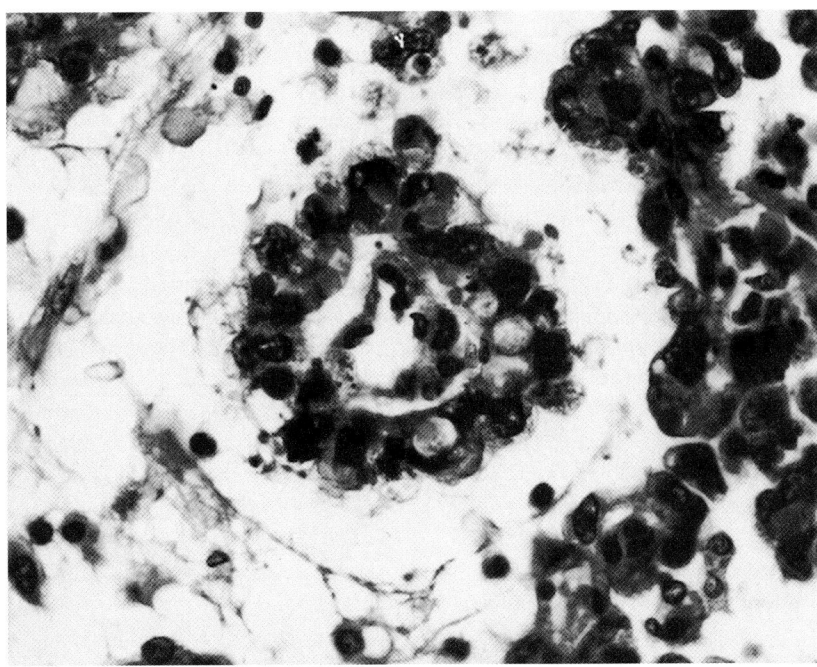

FIGURE 31-21 Schiller-Duvall body associated with numerous hyaline droplets in an endodermal sinus tumor. (×350.) (From Kurman RJ and Norris HJ: Hum Pathol 8:551, 1977. Reprinted with permission from WB Saunders Co, Philadelphia, 1977.)

trophoblasts; human chorionic gonadotrophin (hCG) is a useful tumor marker. Most patients developing this tumor primarily in the ovary are under the age of 20. The disease was usually fatal in the past and does not appear to respond to single-agent chemotherapy, such as methotrexate or actinomycin D, with the same frequency as gestational trophoblastic disease. This lack of response may be due in part to the occurrence of these tumors in combination with other malignant germ cell tumors (mixed germ cell tumor), and on occasion the other germ cell elements may not be histologically recognized. Multiple-agent chemotherapy is advisable.

Embryonal Carcinomas

An embryonal carcinoma is a rare malignant germ cell tumor composed of primitive embryonal cells. It occurs in young females between the ages of 4 and 28 years. Kurman and Norris summarized 15 cases. Trophoblastic elements may be present, and both hCG and alpha-fetoprotein have been reported to be present.

Polyembryomas

Polyembryomas are exceedingly rare tumors that are usually found in the testes. They can occur in the ovary and consist of embryonal bodies that resemble early embryos. Trophoblastic elements with hCG and placental lactogen secretion have been reported.

Mixed Germ Cell Tumors

Mixed germ cell tumors are combinations of any of the previously described germ cell tumors of the ovary. They can be bilateral if dysgerminoma elements are involved; otherwise they are unilateral. Treatment of apparent stage IA mixed germ cell tumors consists of unilateral adnexectomy. Multiple-agent chemotherapy is recommended. The most frequently found elements in mixed germ cell tumors are dysgerminomas and teratomas. Survival of patients with mixed germ cell tumors is related primarily to the immaturity of the constituent tissues; it can reach 100% for small mixed germ cell tumors. It is diminished for women with large tumors or with a predominance of endodermal sinus elements, choriocarcinoma, or grade 3 immature teratoma.

SUMMARY AND CONSIDERATIONS OF CHEMOTHERAPY FOR MALIGNANT GERM CELL TUMORS

As noted, the advent of modern multiagent chemotherapy has vastly improved the prognosis of these tumors. Frequent regimens are VBP (see previous section on endodermal sinus tumor) or EP (etoposide 100 mg/m^2 per day IV for 5 days and cisplatin 20 mg/m^2 per day for 5 days every 3 weeks). Although the optimal approach for these tumors is not certain, those cases that require adjuvant treatment usually receive three to six cycles. For cases in which a tumor marker is present and elevated, chemotherapy is usually prescribed for 2 cycles after the tumor marker becomes negative. Childbearing potential can be preserved in these individuals. In a report of 40 patients Gershenson et al. noted 27 had normal menses after multiagent chemotherapy for germ cell tumors, and 11 of 16 patients who attempted pregnancy were successful in bearing 22 children. Peccatori et al. reported on 139 patients with malignant germ cell tumors, 108 of whom had fertility-sparing operations. Multiagent platinum-containing chemotherapy was used with a 96% survival with a mean follow-up of 55 months. In a GOG study, Williams et al. reported on 93 patients treated adjuvantly with cisplatinum, etoposide, and bleomycin for three cycles. Ninety-one of 93 patients were free of disease 4 to 90 months posttreatment, although leukemia developed in one patient and lymphoma in a second patient. Excellent results are obtained with these multiagent regimens and fertility-sparing surgery should be undertaken. Postchemotherapy ovarian function may possibly be enhanced with simultaneous administration of gonadotrophin-releasing hormone agonist (GnRHa).

The role of second-look operation in these tumors has been controversial. Gershenson advised that in the high proportion of negative second-look procedures, the operation was not needed, particularly if a tumor marker is elevated prior to therapy and reverts to a normal value. In addition, a recurrence, if it develops, can usually be effectively treated with chemotherapy. The procedure does appear to have potential value in patients with immature teratoma, as noted by Culine et al. Although second-look operation would appear to be most useful for patients whose germ cell tumors do not have a tumor marker, the need for second-look operation in most patients with germ cell tumors will rarely arise.

GONADOBLASTOMAS (GERM CELL SEX CORD–STROMAL TUMORS)

The term *gonadoblastoma* was introduced by Scully in 1953 to describe a tumor that consists of germ cell and sex cord–stromal elements. Approximately 100 cases have been reported. The germ cells usually resemble dysgerminoma, whereas the sex cord–stromal elements may consist of immature granulosa and Sertoli cells. Leydig cells and luteinized cells may be present. The tumor usually occurs in patients with abnormal (dysgenetic) gonads. Most patients have a female phenotype but may be virilized. These patients have a Y chromosome detected in their karyotype, and patients with gonadal dysgenesis and a Y chromosome are at risk for the development of gonadoblastoma or malignant germ cell tumors, predominantly dysgerminoma, which may occur in an individual as young as 6 months of age. Removal of these gonads is indicated when they are discovered. Both gonads should be removed, and if the presence of pure gonadoblastoma is confirmed, the prognosis is excellent, since these tumors have not been reported to metastasize.

SEX CORD–STROMAL TUMORS

The sex cord–stromal tumors are derived from the sex cords of the ovary and the specialized stroma of the developing gonad. The elements can have a male or female differentiation, and some of these tumors are hormonally active. The group accounts for about 6% of ovarian neoplasms and the majority of hormonally functioning ovarian tumors. For the female derivatives the sex cord component is the granulosa cell, and the stromal component is the theca cell or fibroblast. For the male counterpart the similar components are the Sertoli cell and the Leydig cell. Granulosa-theca cell tumors and Sertoli-Leydig cell tumors tend to behave as low-grade malignancies. Their clinical and morphologic aspects will be separately considered.

Granulosa-Theca Cell Tumors

Granulosa cell tumors consist primarily of granulosa cells and a varying proportion of theca cells or fibroblasts or both. One characteristic microscopic pattern is shown in Figure 31-22, which demonstrates the so-called *Call Exner bodies,* eosinophilic bodies surrounded by granulosa cells. Functional granulosa cell tumors are primarily estrogenic. About 5% occur before puberty, and they can be one of the causes of precocious puberty, but the tumors have been described in women of all ages. In postmenopausal women these tumors can produce elevated levels of blood estrogens, uterine bleeding, and occasionally endometrial carcinoma. It is estimated that about 5% of the granulosa cell tumors in adults are associated with endometrial carcinoma. In menstruating women the functional granulosa cell tumor can produce abnormal menstrual patterns, menorrhagia, and even amenorrhea.

These tumors can become large and may present as a ruptured mass, leading to laparotomy for an acute abdomen with hemoperitoneum. Because of the low-grade malignant character of these tumors, recurrences are frequently more than 5 years after primary therapy. In general, prognosis does not correlate with the histologic pattern of the tumor. A total of 90% of granulosa cell tumors present as stage I. Advanced clinical stage, the presence of tumor rupture, a large primary tumor (greater than 15 cm), and a high mitotic rate have been associated with a poorer prognosis. Overall 10-year survival rates of 90% have been reported. Studies by Klemi et al. and others suggest that most granulosa cell tumors have a diploid pattern and a low (<60%) S phase fraction when analyzed by flow cytometry. Those with an aneuploid pattern had a worse prognosis in the study of Klemi et al. However, it is important to recognize that granulosa cell tumors can be confused histologically with poorly

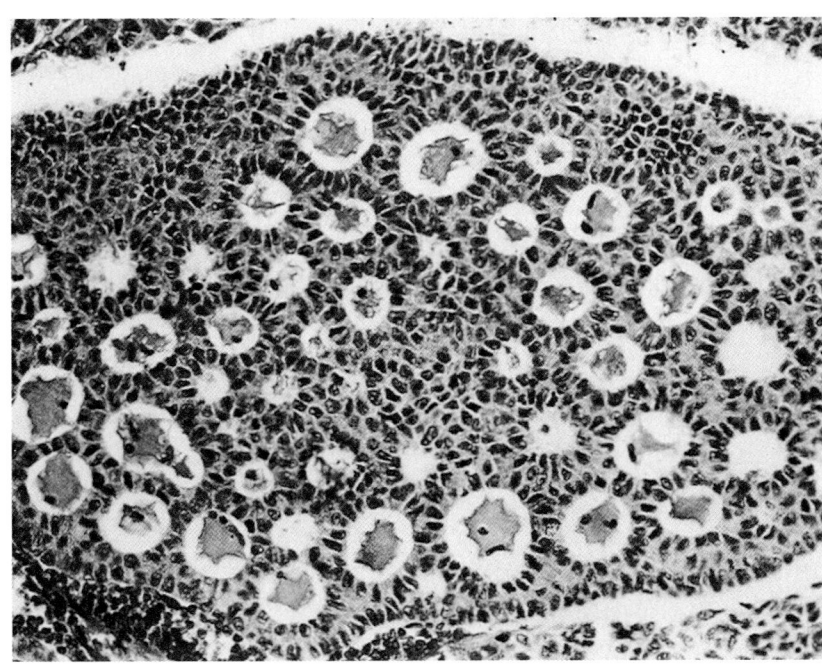

FIGURE 31-22 Granulosa cell tumor. (×460.) (From Scully RE and Morris J: Functioning ovarian tumors. In Meigs JV and Sturgis SH, editors: Progress in gynecology, vol 3, New York, 1957, Grune & Stratton.)

differentiated adenocarcinomas, and the latter would also have an aneuploid pattern, as well as a poor prognosis. A variant found predominantly in females under age 20 years is known as juvenile granulosa cell tumor. It was described by Young, Dickersen, and Scully and has an excellent prognosis, particularly if the tumor is confined to one ovary.

The primary therapeutic approach is the operative removal of the tumor. Since these tumors are rarely bilateral (less than 5%), stage IA tumors can be treated by unilateral adnexectomy. Lack et al. reported 10 cases of granulosa cell tumors in premenarchal female patients, all of whom were treated by unilateral salpingo-oophorectomy. Two tumors were ruptured. All 10 of the patients were alive with no evidence of disease 2 to 33 years after therapy. Evans et al. did note a higher recurrence rate among women who were treated by unilateral salpingo-oophorectomy for stage IA cases in comparison with those treated with bilateral salpingo-oophorectomy. This finding has led to the recommendation that women of reproductive age treated for granulosa cell tumor by unilateral salpingo-oophorectomy have close follow-up. The removal of the contralateral ovary is considered after reproductive function is completed or if there is evidence of ovarian enlargement. Recent studies by Lappohn et al. suggest that the peptide hormone, inhibin, is secreted by some granulosa cell tumors and serum measurements could serve as a tumor marker.

Although radiation and chemotherapy have been employed for the treatment of recurrent or metastatic granulosa cell tumors, there is insufficient experience to warrant conclusions regarding their effectiveness. Complete responses to chemotherapy have been reported in patients using multiple-agent protocols, including cisplatin, 50 mg/m^2, and doxorubicin (Adriamycin), 50 mg/m^2, as well as in patients receiving Act-FU-Cy or vinblastine, bleomycin, and cisplatin (see previous section on endodermal sinus tumor). Many such patients will develop recurrent disease following initial response to chemotherapy, however. Segal et al. noted there is little evidence to support the use of adjuvant therapy in patients with granulosa cell tumors. Responses to chemotherapy have been identified with vinblastine, cisplatinum, and bleomycin, with response rates as high as 90% reported. Homesley et al. in a GOG study of these agents reported 11 of 16 primary cases and 21 of 41 recurrent cases were disease free at second-look operation. However, toxicity was severe in addition to 2 bleomycin-related deaths. Responses to Taxol have also been reported.

Thecomas and Fibromas

Thecomas are benign tumors that consist entirely of stroma (theca) cells. They occur in women predominantly in the perimenopausal and menopausal years. These tumors can be associated with estrogen production but not as frequently as are granulosa cell tumors. Removal of the tumor alone is adequate treatment in women in the reproductive years. For older women, total abdominal hysterectomy and bilateral salpingo-oophorectomy are performed. Rarely, thecomas have

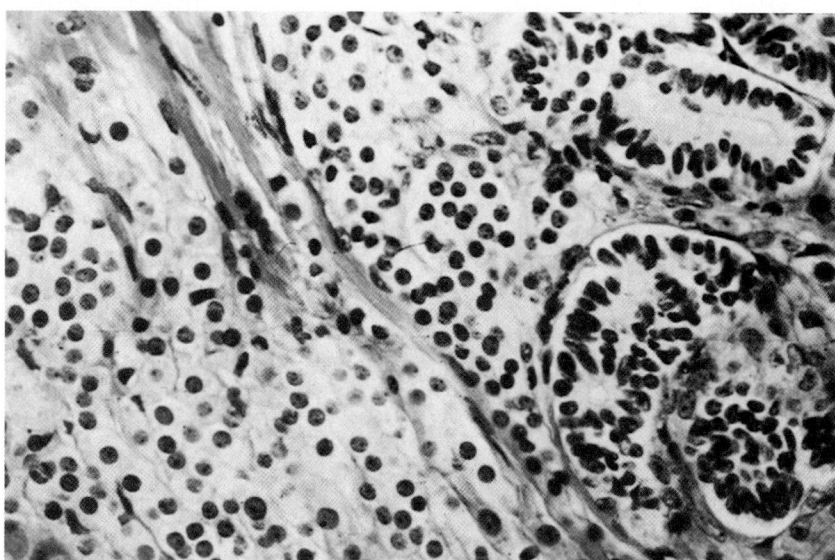

FIGURE 31-23 Sertoli-Leydig cell tumor. Tubules of Sertoli cells *(right)* and Leydig cells *(left)* are shown. (×250.) (Courtesy Dr. R.E. Scully.)

been reported to be malignant, and these are most likely fibrosarcomas. A closely related tumor is the fibroma, which is the most common benign solid ovarian tumor and accounts for 4% of all ovarian tumors. Like the thecoma, it can occur at any age but is more common in older women; it does not secrete hormones. These tumors contain spindle cells, and the tumors can grow to a large size. They are benign, and excision is adequate treatment. These tumors are associated with ascites in about 40% of cases if the tumor exceeds 10 cm, according to Samanth and Black. They can also be responsible for hydrothorax with a benign ascites (Meigs' syndrome), which regresses following tumor removal.

Sertoli-Leydig Cell Tumors (Androblastomas)

Sertoli-Leydig cell tumors are very rare. Sertoli (sex cord) and Leydig (stromal) cells are present in varying amounts, and the tumor may consist almost entirely of either Sertoli or Leydig cells (Figure 31-23). These tumors tend to occur in young women of reproductive age and frequently are the cause of masculinization and hirsutism. The symptoms of virilization usually regress after tumor removal, but temporal hair recession and a deeper voice tend to remain. Rarely they have been reported also to have estrogenic activity, leading to the same symptoms and signs as granulosa cell tumors. The tumors tend to behave as low-grade malignancies, and 5-year survival is reported to vary from 70% to 90%. Poorly differentiated types tend to have a poor prognosis, as do higher stage tumors. Young and Scully reviewed 207 cases. Seventy-five percent were 30 years of age or younger, and fewer than 10% were over 50 years old. One third had evidence of androgen excess.

Both ovaries were involved in only three cases. The well-differentiated tumors behaved clinically as benign tumors, whereas recurrence or extrauterine spread was noted occasionally in women with intermediate differentiation (11%) and frequently in those with poor differentiation (59%). Of 164 patients available for follow-up, 18% had metastasis or recurrence. There is insufficient experience to provide guidelines for therapy. Irradiation for localized pelvic disease has been beneficial, and chemotherapy with agents such as VAC (see previous section on immature teratoma) would be considered for disseminated disease or in the case of undifferentiated tumors.

Gynandroblastomas

Gynandroblastomas are rare sex cord–stromal tumors consisting of both female and male cell types.

Sex Cord Tumors with Annular Tubules

Sex cord tumors with annular tubules (SCTAT) are unusual. As suggested by the name, there is a prominent tubular pattern. Features of both Sertoli and granulosa cell tumors are present. Seventy-four cases were reviewed by Young et al., and 27 were associated with mucocutaneous pigmentation and gastrointestinal tract polyposis (Peutz-Jeghers syndrome). The tumors may have estrogenic manifestations. Those associated with Peutz-Jeghers syndrome are benign, and those not associated with this syndrome can be malignant. It is of interest that 4 of the 74 cases reported by Young et al. were associated with a virulent form of cervical adenocarcinoma (adenoma malignum).

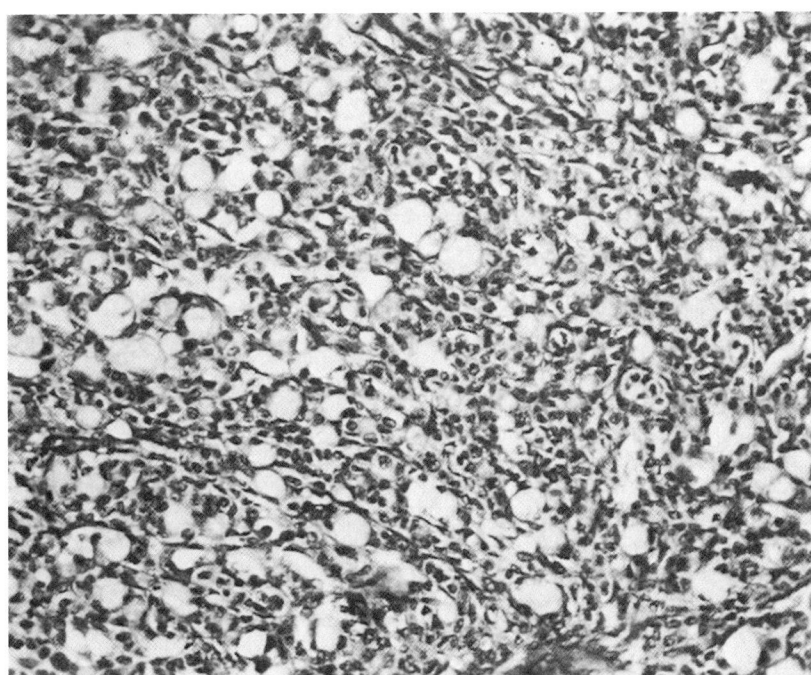

FIGURE 31-24   Krukenberg tumor. (×256.) Mucin-filled signet-ring cells are present. (Courtesy Dr. R.E. Scully.)

Leydig Cell and Hilus Cell Tumors

Leydig cell and hilus cell tumors are rare and are composed of Leydig cells or cells of the ovarian hilus. Their cytoplasm contains hyaline bodies known as *crystalloids of Reinke*. They usually cause virilization and are benign. They tend to be small (under 6 cm) and develop primarily in perimenopausal women.

LIPID (LIPOID) TUMORS

Lipid tumors are infrequently occurring ovarian tumors composed of large cells that resemble Leydig cells, luteinized cells, or cells that arise in the adrenal cortex. About 100 tumors have been reported. These tumors usually cause virilization but have also been associated with excess cortisol production. There is not enough experience with them to delineate an effective form of treatment. However, metastases of lipid cell tumors have been reported.

METASTATIC OVARIAN TUMORS

Tumors from distant primary sites can metastasize to the ovary. Frequently metastases are from primary tumors that originate elsewhere in the female repro-ductive tract, particularly from the endometrium and fallopian tube. Distant sites of origin occur most frequently from the breast and gastrointestinal tract. Metastatic tumors from the gastrointestinal tract to the ovary can be associated with sex hormone production, which usually leads to estrogenic manifestations. One special type of metastatic ovarian tumor is known as *Krukenberg's tumor,* which histologically consists of nests of mucin-filled signet-ring cells in a cellular stroma (Figure 31-24). The most common gastrointestinal tract origin for these tumors is the stomach, and the next frequent is the large intestine. However, breast metastases to the ovary can on occasion give the same histologic picture. A few cases of Krukenberg's tumors have been described with no apparent distant primary malignancy, suggesting the rare possibility of a primary ovarian tumor with the histologic features of a Krukenberg's tumor. A primary gastrointestinal tract malignancy should be considered in older women with an adnexal mass, particularly if it is bilateral and solid. Pretherapy evaluation to rule out a gastrointestinal tract or breast primary tumor is indicated. The tumor should be removed when discovered, and the primary site should be treated. The prognosis is poor, and it is rare for a patient to survive for 5 or more years after treatment.

KEY POINTS

- Ovarian cancer is the leading cause of death from gynecologic cancer, but it occurs less frequently than endometrial cancers.

- Ovarian cancers of women older than age 50 are diagnosed at a more advanced stage, leading to a worse prognosis than for younger women.

- The risk of ovarian cancer is decreased by oral contraceptive use. Tubal ligation and hysterectomy also appear to decrease the risk.

- Most ovarian carcinomas are diagnosed in stage III or IV.

- Ovarian cancer risk rises from about 1.4% in general to 5%–7% with one to two first- or second-degree relatives with ovarian cancer.

- Patients with ovarian cancer are at increased risk of developing breast cancer and endometrial cancer. It is important that the follow-up of ovarian cancer patients include monitoring for breast cancer.

- Epithelial tumors are the most frequent ovarian neoplasm. They account for two thirds of all ovarian neoplasms and 85% of ovarian cancers.

- The major ovarian epithelial tumor cell types recapitulate müllerian-type epithelium (serous-endosalpinx, mucinous-endocervix, and endometrioid-endometrium).

- Serous ovarian neoplasms are the most common type of epithelial tumors. Serous adenocarcinomas tend to be high grade, are the most virulent, and have the worst prognosis of epithelial adenocarcinomas. They are bilateral in 33% to 66% of cases.

- A cystic adnexal mass less than 8 cm in diameter in a menstruating female is most frequently functional.

- The normal postmenopausal ovary is approximately 1.5 to 2 cm in diameter.

- The risk of an ovarian tumor being malignant is about 33% in a woman over age 45, whereas it is less than 1 in 15 for those 20 to 45 years of age. More than half of ovarian cancers occur in women beyond the age of 50.

- There are three types of ovarian tumors with a serous histology: traditional serous adenocarcinoma; surface papillary tumors (ovary <4 cm); and primary peritoneal carcinomas (serous carcinoma metastatic to the ovary with normal ovarian size).

- Most ovarian carcinomas start from small microscopic foci and spread throughout the peritoneum before becoming clinically evident (de novo origin), particularly serous and poorly differentiated tumors.

- Ovarian carcinomas having a cystic origin are primary mucinous or endometrioid and these are more likely to be discovered at a low stage.

- A vaginal ultrasound finding of a unilocular cyst of 5 cm or less in a perimenopausal woman can usually be followed without operative intervention.

- Vaginal ultrasound may detect early ovarian carcinoma but has not been proven to be a cost-effective screening technique.

- The primary distribution spread of epithelial carcinoma is transcoelomic to the visceral and parietal peritoneum and diaphragm and to the retroperitoneal nodes.

- The risk of retroperitoneal node spread of epithelial carcinoma in apparent stage I cases is greatest for poorly differentiated tumors, for which the risk can reach 10% to 20%. The risk of retroperitoneal node spread increases in higher-stage cases.

- The prognosis of a patient with ovarian epithelial carcinoma is related primarily to tumor stage and tumor grade, as well as to the amount of residual tumor remaining after primary resection.

- The 5-year survival rate for patients with borderline epithelial ovarian carcinoma (grade 0) is close to 100% for stage I cases and over 90% for all stages.

- The overall 5-year survival rate for patients with stage I ovarian carcinoma is 65%. For stage I, grade 1, survival is reported to be over 80%.

- Optimal surgical debulking (<1 cm residual nodules) appears to confer a survival advantage in cases of stage III-IV ovarian carcinoma.

- Alkylating agent chemotherapy administration is accompanied by an increased risk of subsequent development of leukemia, which can reach almost 10% 8 years after therapy.

- Platinum-based chemotherapy increases the risk of secondary leukemia 4-7X, which is dose related. However, the small total number of patients developing leukemia does not overcome the greatly improved survivals for platinum-based ovarian cancer therapy.

- Computed tomographic scan for patients with ovarian cancer can be approximately 80% to 90% effective for detecting tumor in retroperitoneal nodes. The test is much less successful for detecting intraabdominal disease.

- The ovarian antigen CA-125 is useful in helping to monitor patients with ovarian carcinoma. Reaction to the antigen is positive in about 80% of cases.

- A rapid decrease in CA-125 values after treatment indicates a more favorable prognosis.

- The initial response rate of ovarian epithelial carcinomas multiple-agent chemotherapy is over 90%, but the proportion of patients who survive drops to around 30% in 4 years. Initial treatment is usually with carboplatin and Taxol.

- Approximately half of patients thought initially to be clinically free of disease are found at second-look laparotomy to have gross or microscopic tumor.

- The 5-year survival rate after negative second-look operation is about 50%.

- Germ cell tumors are the second most common type of ovarian neoplasms and account for about 20% to 25% of all ovarian tumors.

- In young women under age 30 the most frequent ovarian neoplasm is a germ cell tumor, and about one third of these germ cell tumors are malignant under age 21.

- The most common germ cell tumor is the benign cystic teratoma (dermoid). It is bilateral in 10% to 15% of the cases. Approximately 30% are calcified.

- For women under age 30 the most common ovarian neoplasm is the dermoid.

- Malignant germ cell tumors are usually unilateral except dysgerminomas, which are bilateral in about 10% of the cases.

- Dysgerminomas are the most common malignant germ cell tumors and account for 1% to 2% of ovarian cancers.

- The prognosis for a patient with immature teratoma is related to tumor grade and tumor stage. These tumors are the second most common type of malignant germ cell tumor.

- The 5-year survival of stage IA pure dysgerminoma treated by unilateral salpingo-oophorectomy is over 90%.

- Pure dysgerminomas are radiocurable. However, multiagent chemotherapy, particularly with etoposide and platinum with or without bleomycin, will frequently result in complete remission. Favorable prognostic factors include size under 15 cm, encapsulation without rupture, lack of ascites, and no spread to retroperitoneal nodes. About two thirds of cases present as stage IA.

- Patients with immature teratoma stage IA grade 3 should receive postoperative adjuvant chemotherapy.

- Patients with endodermal sinus tumors have a median age of 19. These tumors can be followed by measuring serum levels of alpha-fetoprotein. They should be treated with adjuvant multiagent chemotherapy even in stage IA.

- Multiple-agent chemotherapy has improved the survival in patients with malignant germ cell tumors, preserving child-bearing function in most cases. Commonly used protocols include VAC (vincristine, actinomycin D, and Cytoxan), VBP (vinblastine, bleomycin, and platinum), and EP (etoposide and platinum).

- Gonadoblastomas are sex cord–stromal germ cell tumors that arise in dysgenetic gonads in patients with a Y chromosome. They are cured by removal.

- Granulosa cell tumors and Sertoli-Leydig tumors usually behave as low-grade malignancies, but there may be late recurrences. Responses have been observed with vinblastine, cisplatin, and bleomycin for granulosa cell tumors.

- Fibroma is the most common benign solid ovarian tumor.

- The most frequent sites of origin of tumors metastatic to the ovary are the lower reproductive tract, the gastrointestinal tract, and the breast.

BIBLIOGRAPHY

Abramowicz JS: Ultrasound contrast media and their use in obstetrics and gynecology, Ultrasound Med Biol, 23:1287, 1997.

A'Hern RP and Gore ME: Impact of doxorubicin on survival in advanced ovarian cancer, J Clin Oncol 13:726, 1995.

Altaras MM, Aviram R, Cohen I, et al: Primary peritoneal papillary serous adenocarcinoma: clinical and management aspects, Gynecol Oncol 40:230, 1991.

Assadourian LA and Taylor HB: Dysgerminoma: an analysis of 105 cases, Obstet Gynecol 33:370, 1969.

Aure JC, Hoeg K, and Kolstad P: The clinical and histologic studies of ovarian carcinoma: long-term follow-up of 990 cases, Obstet Gynecol 37:1, 1971.

Bailey CL, Ueland FR, Land GL, et al: The malignant potential of small cystic ovarian tumors in women over 50 years of age, Gynecol Oncol 69:3, 1998.

Barakat RR, Almadrones L, Venkatramman ES, et al: A phase II trial of intraperitoneal cisplatin and estoposide as consolidation therapy in patients with stage II-IV epithelial ovarian cancer following negative surgical assessment, Gynecol Oncol 69:17, 1998.

Bast RC, Feene M, Lazarus H, et al: Reactivity of a monoclonal antibody with human ovarian carcinoma, J Clin Invest 68:1331, 1981.

Behbakht K, Randall TC, Benjamin I, et al: Clinical characteristics of clear cell carcinoma of the ovary, Gynecol Oncol 70:255, 1998.

Bell DA, Weinstock MA, and Scully RE: Peritoneal implants of ovarian serous borderline tumors: histologic features and prognosis, Cancer 62:2212, 1988.

Bell DA and Scully RE: Early de novo ovarian carcinoma, Cancer 73:1859, 1994.

Ben-Baruch G, Siven E, Moran O, et al: Primary peritoneal serous papillary carcinoma: a study of 25 cases and comparison with stage III-IV ovarian papillary serous carcinoma, Gynecol Oncol 60:393, 1996.

Benrubi GI, Pitel P, and Lammert N: Small cell carcinoma of the ovary with hypercalcemia responsive to sequencing chemotherapy, South Med J 86:247, 1993.

Berchuck A and Bast RC: P53-based gene therapy of ovarian cancer: magic bullet? Gynecol Oncol 59:169, 1995.

Berchuck A, Elbendary A, Havrilesky L, et al: Pathogenesis of ovarian cancers, J Soc Gynecol Invest 1:181, 1994.

Berek JS, Knapp RC, Malkasian GD, et al: CA-125 serum levels correlated with second-look operations among ovarian cancer patients, Obstet Gynecol 67:685, 1986.

Bjorkholm E and Silfversward C: Prognostic factors in granulosa cell tumor, Gynecol Oncol 11:261, 1981.

Blumfeld Z, Aviv I, Linn S, et al: Prevention of irreversible chemotherapy-induced ovarian damage in young women with lymphoma by a gonadotrophin-releasing hormone agonist in parallel to chemotherapy, Hum Reprod 11:1620, 1996.

Bolis G, Colombo N, Pecorelli S, et al: Adjuvant treatment for early epithelial ovarian cancer: results of two randomised clinical trials comparing cisplatin to no further treatment or chromic phosphate (^{32}P), Ann Oncol 6:887, 1995.

Bonazzi C, Peccatori F, Colombo N, et al: Pure ovarian immature teratoma, a unique and curable disease: 10 years' experience of 32 prospectively treated patients, Obstet Gynecol 84:598, 1994.

Bostwick DG, Tazelaar HD, Ballon SC, et al: Ovarian epithelial tumors of borderline malignancy: clinical and pathologic study of 109 cases, Cancer 58:2052, 1986.

Bourne TH, Whitehead MI, Campbell S, et al: Ultrasound screening for familial ovarian cancer, Gynecol Oncol 43:92, 1991.

Boyd J, Sonoda Y, Frederici MG, et al: Clinicopathologic features of BRCA-linked and sporadic ovarian cancer, JAMA 283:2260, 2000.

Braly PS, Berek JS, Blessing JA, et al: Intraperitoneal administration of cisplatin and 5-fluorouracil in residual ovarian cancer: a phase II Gynecologic Oncology Group trial, Gynecol Oncol 56:164, 1995.

Brewer M, Gershenson DM, Herzog CE, et al: Outcome and reproductive function after chemotherapy for ovarian dysgerminoma, J Clin Oncol 17:2670, 1999.

Bridgewater JA, Nelstrop AE, Rustin GJS, et al: Comparison of standard and CA-125 response criteria in patients with epithelial ovarian cancer treated with platinum and paclitaxel, J Clin Oncol 17:501, 1999.

Bristow RE, Montz FJ, Lagasse LD, et al: Survival impact of surgical cytoreduction in stage IV epithelial ovarian cancer, Gynecol Oncol 72:278, 1999.

Buller RE: BRCA1:What do we know? What do we think we know? What do we really need to know? (Editorial) Gynecol Oncol 76:291, 2000.

Buller RE, Berman ML, Bloss JD, et al: CA-125 regression: a model for epithelial ovarian cancer response, Am J Obstet Gynecol 165:360, 1991.

Buller RE, Vasilev S, and DiSaia PJ: CA 125 kinetics: a cost effective clinical tool to evaluate clinical trial outcomes in the 1990s, Am J Obstet Gynecol 174:1241, 1996.

Burghardt E, Girardi F, Lahousen M, et al: Patterns of pelvic and paraaortic lymph node involvement in ovarian cancer, Gynecol Oncol 40:103, 1991.

Canevari S, Stoter G, Arienti F, et al: Regression of advanced ovarian carcinoma by intraperitoneal treatment with autologous T lymphocytes retargeted by bispecific monoclonal antibody, J Natl Cancer Inst 87:1463, 1995.

Casagrande JT, Louie EW, Pike MC, et al: "Incessant ovulation" and ovarian cancer, Lancet 2:170, 1979.

Chadha S, Cornelisse CJ, and Schaberg A: Flow cytometry DNA ploidy analysis of ovarian granulosa cell tumor, Gynecol Oncol 36:240, 1990.

Chi DS, Venkatraman ES, Masson V, and Hoskins WJ: Ability of preoperative serum CA-125 to predict optimal primary tumor cytoreduction in stage III epithelial ovarian carcinoma, Gynecol Oncol 77:237, 2000.

Childers JM, Lang J, Surwit EA, and Hatch KD: Laparoscopic surgical staging of ovarian cancer, Gynecol Oncol 59:25, 1995.

Cmelak AJ and Kapp DS: Long-term survival with whole abdominal irradiation in platinum-refractory persistent or recurrent ovarian cancer, Gynecol Oncol 65:453, 1997.

Colditz GA, Hankinson SE, Hunter DJ, et al: The use of estrogens and progestins and the risk of breast cancer in postmenopausal women, N Engl J Med 332:1589, 1995.

Columbo N, Sessa C, Landoni F, et al: Cisplatin, vinblastine and bleomycin, combination chemotherapy in metastatic granulosa cell tumor of the ovary, Obstet Gynecol 67:265, 1986.

Cramer DW, Liberman RF, Titus-Ersntoff L, et al: Genital talc exposure and risk of ovarian cancer, Int J Cancer 81:351, 1999.

Cramer DW, Welch WR, Hutchinson GB, et al: Dietary animal fat in relation to ovarian cancer risk, Obstet Gynecol 63:833, 1984.

Crayford TJB, Campbell S, Bourne TH, et al: Benign ovarian cysts and ovarian cancer: a cohort study with implications for screening, Lancet 355:1060, 2000.

Creasman WT: New gynecologic cancer staging, Obstet Gynecol 75:287, 1990.

Creasman WT and DiSaia PJ: Screening in ovarian cancer, Am J Obstet Gynecol 165:7, 1991.

Creasman WT and Soper JT: Assessment of the contemporary management of germ cell malignancies of the ovary, Am J Obstet Gynecol 153:828, 1985.

Culine S, Lhomme C, Kattan J, et al: Pure malignant immature teratoma of the ovary: the role of chemotherapy and second-look surgery, Int J Gynecol Cancer 5:432, 1995.

Curry SL, Smith JP, and Gallagher HS: Malignant teratoma of the ovary: prognostic factors and treatment, Am J Obstet Gynecol 131:845, 1978.

Cushing B, Giller R, Ablin A, et al: Surgical resection alone is effective treatment for ovarian immature teratoma in children and adolescents: a report of the Pediatric Oncology Group and the Children's Cancer Group, Am J Obstet Gynecol 181: 353, 1999.

Dembo AJ, Bush RS, Beale FA, et al: Ovarian carcinoma: improved survival following abdominopelvic irradiation in patients with a completed pelvic operation, Am J Obstet Gynecol 134:793, 1979.

Dembo AJ, Davy M, Stenwig AE, et al: Prognostic factors in patients with stage I epithelial ovarian cancer, Obstet Gynecol 75:263, 1990.

DePriest PD, Gallion HH, Pavlik EJ, et al: Transvaginal sonography as a screening method for the detection of early ovarian cancer, Gynecol Oncol 65:408, 1997.

Dickersin GR, Kline IW, and Scully RE: Small cell carcinoma of the ovary with hypercalcemia: a report of 11 cases, Cancer 49:188, 1982.

DiSaia PJ, Saltz A, Kagan AR, et al: Chemotherapeutic retroconversion of immature teratoma of the ovary, Obstet Gynecol 49:347, 1977.

Einhorn LH and Donahue J: Cis-diamminedichloroplatinum, vinblastine, and bleomycin combination chemotherapy in disseminated testicular cancer, Ann Intern Med 87:87, 1977.

Epenetos AA, Munro AJ, Stewart S, et al: Antibody guided irradiation of advanced ovarian cancer with intraperitoneally administered radiolabeled monoclonal antibodies, J Clin Oncol 5:1890, 1987.

Evans AT, Gaffey TA, and Malkasian GD: Clinical pathologic review of 118 granulosa and 82 theca cell tumors, Obstet Gynecol 55:231, 1980.

Finkler NJ, Benacerraf B, Lavin PT, et al: Comparison of serum CA-125, clinical impression, and ultrasound in the preoperative evaluation of ovarian masses, Obstet Gynecol 72:659, 1988.

Ford D, Easton DF, Bishop DT, et al: Risks of cancer in BRCA1-mutation carriers, Lancet 343:692, 1994.

Forney JP: Pregnancy following removal and chemotherapy of ovarian endodermal sinus tumor, Obstet Gynecol 52:360, 1978.

Fox H: Primary neoplasia of the female peritoneum, Histopathology 23:103, 1993.

Frias AE, Li H, Keeney GL, et al: Preoperative serum level of inhibin A is an independent prognostic factor for the survival of postmenopausal women with epithelial ovarian carcinoma, Cancer 85:465, 1999.

Frasci G, Conforti S, Zullo F, et al: A risk model for ovarian carcinoma patients using CA 125, Cancer 77:1122, 1996.

Fromm GL, Gershenson DM, and Silva EG: Papillary serous carcinoma of the peritoneum, Obstet Gynecol 75:89, 1990.

Gershenson DM: Menstrual and reproductive function after treatment with combination chemotherapy for malignant ovarian germ cell tumors, J Clin Oncol 6:270, 1988.

Gershenson DM: The obsolescence of second-look laparotomy in the management of malignant ovarian germ cell tumors, Gynecol Oncol 52:283, 1994 (letter to the editor).

Gershenson DM, Copeland LJ, Kavanagh JJ, et al: Treatment of metastatic stromal tumors of the ovary with cisplatin, doxorubicin, and cyclophosphamide, Obstet Gynecol 70:765, 1987.

Gershenson DM, Del Junco G, Herson J, et al: Endodermal sinus tumor of the ovary: the MD Anderson experience, Obstet Gynecol 61:194, 1983.

Gershenson DM, Del Junco G, Silva EG, et al: Immature teratoma of the ovary, Obstet Gynecol 68:624, 1986.

Gershenson DM and Silva EG: Metastatic serous ovarian tumors of low malignant potential, Cancer 65:578, 1990.

Gershenson DM, Silva EG, Levy L, et al: Ovarian serous tumors with invasive peritoneal implants, Cancer 82:1096, 1998.

Gershenson DM, Silva EG, Mitchell MF, et al: Transitional cell carcinoma of the ovary: a matched control study of advanced-stage patients treated with cisplatin-based chemotherapy, Am J Obstet Gynecol 168:1178, 1993.

Gershenson DM, Silva EG, Tortolero-Luna G, et al: Serous borderline tumors of the ovary with noninvasive peritoneal implants, Cancer 83:2157, 1998.

Gloeckler LA, Hankey BF, and Edwards BK, editors: Cancer statistics review 1973-87. Prepared by the Surveillance Program, division of Cancer Prevention and Control, National Cancer Institute, Besthesda, Md, 1992. Available from U.S. Department of Health and Human Services, National Institutes of Health (NIH), National Cancer Institute, PB90-2789.

Goldhirsch A, Greiner R, Dreher E, et al: Treatment of advanced ovarian cancer with surgery, chemotherapy, and consolidation of response by whole-abdominal radiotherapy, Cancer 62:40, 1988.

Goldhirsch A, Triller JF, Greiner R, et al: Computed tomography prior to second-look operation in advanced ovarian cancer, Obstet Gynecol 62:630, 1983.

Greenlee RT, Murray T, Bolden S, et al: Cancer Statistics, 2000. CA Cancer J Clin, 50:7, 2000.

Grimes DA and Economy KE: Primary prevention of gynecologic cancers, Am J Obstet Gynecol 172:227, 1995.

Gross TP and Schlesselman JJ: The estimated effect of oral contraceptive use on the cumulative risk of epithelial ovarian cancer, Obstet Gynecol 83:419, 1994.

Guthrie D, Davy MLJ, and Philips PR: A study of 656 patients with "early" ovarian cancer, Gynecol Oncol 17:363, 1984.

Hacker NF: Systematic pelvic and paraaortic lymphadenectomy for advanced ovarian cancer: therapeutic advance or surgical folly? Gynecol Oncol 56:325, 1995.

Hankinson SE, Colditz GA, Hunter DJ, et al: A quantitative assessment of oral contraceptive use and risk of ovarian cancer, Obstet Gynecol 80:708, 1992.

Hankinson SE, Hunter DJ, Colditz GA, et al: Tubal ligation, hysterectomy, and risk of ovarian cancer: a prospective study, JAMA 270:2813, 1993.

Hart WR and Norris HJ: Borderline and malignant mucinous tumors of the ovary: histologic criteria and clinical behavior, Cancer 31:1031, 1973.

Hartge P, Schiffman MH, Hoover R, et al: A case-control study of epithelial ovarian cancer, Am J Obstet Gynecol 161:10, 1989.

Healy DL, Burger HG, Mamers P, et al: Elevated serum inhibin concentrations in postmenopausal women with ovarian tumors, N Engl J Med 329:1539, 1993.

Hellstrom A-C, Tegerstedt G, Silfversward C, and Pettersson F: Malignant mixed mullerian tumors of the ovary: histopathologic and clinical review of 36 cases, Int J Gynecol Cancer 9:312, 1999.

Herbst AL: The epidemiology of ovarian carcinoma and the current status of tumor markers to detect disease, Am J Obstet Gynecol 170:1099, 1994.

Herbst AL: Letter to the editor: Efficacy of transvaginal sonographic screening, Gynecol Oncol (in press).

Higgins RV, van Nagell JR, Donaldson ES, et al: Transvaginal sonography as a screening method for ovarian cancer, Gynecol Oncol 34:402, 1989.

Hoerl HD and Hart WR: Primary ovarian mucinous cystadenocarcinomas, Am J Surg Pathol 22:1449, 1998.

Homesley HD, Bundy BN, Hurteau JA, et al: Bleomycin, etoposide, and cisplatin combination therapy of ovarian granulosa cell tumors and other stromal malignancies: a Gynecologic Oncology Group Study, Gynecol Oncol 72:131, 1999.

Hoskins WJ, Bundy BN, Thigpen JT, and Omura GA: The influence of cytoreductive surgery on recurrence-free interval and survival in small-volume stage III epithelial ovarian cancer: a Gynecologic Oncology Group study, Gynecol Oncol 47:159, 1992.

Hunter VJ, Daly L, Helms M, et al: The prognostic significance of CA-125 half-life in patients with ovarian cancer who have received primary chemotherapy after surgical cytoreduction, Am J Obstet Gynecol 163:1164, 1990.

Iversen O-E and Skaarland E: Ploidy assessment of benign and malignant ovarian tumors by flow cytometry, Cancer 60:82, 1987.

Jacobs A, Deppe G, and Cohen CJ: Combination chemotherapy of ovarian granulosa cell tumor with cis-platinum and doxorubicin, Gynecol Oncol 14:294, 1982.

Jacobs I and Lancaster J: The molecular genetics of sporadic and familial epithelial ovarian cancer, Int J Gynecol Cancer 6:337, 1996.

Jones HW III and Homesley HD: Successful treatment of pseudo-myxoma peritonei of ovarian origin with cis-platinum, doxorubicin, and cyclophosphamide, Gynecol Oncol 22:257, 1985.

Julian CG, Barrett JM, Richardson RC, et al: Bleomycin, vinblastine, and cis-platinum in the treatment of advanced endodermal sinus tumors, Obstet Gynecol 56:396, 1980.

Kaldor JM, Day NE, Pettersson F, et al: Leukemia following chemotherapy for ovarian cancer, N Engl J Med 322:1, 1990.

Kamiya N, Mizuno K, Kawai M, et al: Simultaneous measurement of CA 125, CA 19-9, tissue polypeptide antigen, and immunosuppressive acidic protein to predict recurrence of ovarian cancer, Obstet Gynecol 76:417, 1990.

Karlan BY, Baldwin RL, Lopez-Luevanos E, et al: Peritoneal serous papillary carcinoma, a phenotypic variant of familial ovarian cancer: implications for ovarian cancer screening, Am J Obstet Gynecol 180:917, 1999.

Kennedy AW, Biscotti CV, Hart WR, et al: Histologic correlates of progression-free interval and survival in ovarian clear cell adenocarcinoma, Gynecol Oncol 50:334, 1993.

Kennedy AW, Markman M, Biscotti CV, et al: Survival probability in ovarian clear cell adenocarcinoma, Gynecol Oncol 74:108, 1999.

Kerlikowske K, Brown JS, and Grady DG: Should women with familial ovarian cancer undergo prophylactic oophorectomy? Obstet Gynecol 80:700, 1992.

Kim DS and Park MI: Maternal and fetal survival following surgery and chemotherapy of endodermal sinus tumor of the ovary during pregnancy: a case report, Obstet Gynecol 73:503, 1989.

Kirmani S, Lucas WE, Kim S, et al: A phase II trial of intraperitoneal cisplatin and etoposide as salvage treatment for minimal residual ovarian carcinoma, J Clin Oncol 9:649, 1991.

Klemi PJ, Joensuu H, and Salmi T: Prognostic value of flow cytometric DNA content analysis in granulosa cell tumor of the ovary, Cancer 65:1189, 1990.

Koonings PP, Campbell K, Mishell DR, and Grimes DA: Relative frequency of primary ovarian neoplasms: a 10-year review, Obstet Gynecol 74:921, 1989.

Kurjak A, Kupesic S, Breye B, et al: The assessment of ovarian tumor angiogenesis: what does three-dimensional power Doppler add? Ultrasound Obstet Gynecol 12:136, 1998.

Kurman RJ and Norris HJ: Embryonal carcinoma of the ovary: a clinical pathogenic entity distinct from endodermal sinus tumor resembling embryonal carcinoma of the adult testes, Cancer 38:2420, 1976.

Kurman RJ and Norris HJ: Malignant germ cell tumors of the ovary, Hum Pathol 8:551, 1977.

Lack EE, Perez-Atayde AR, Murthy ASK, et al: Granulosa theca cell tumors in premenarcheal girls: a clinical and pathologic study of 10 cases, Cancer 48:1846, 1981.

Lappohn RE, Burger HG, Bouma J, et al: Inhibin as a marker for granulosa-cell tumors, N Engl J Med 321:790, 1989.

Leake JF, Currie JL, Rosenshein NB, and Woodruff D: Long-term follow-up of serous ovarian tumors of low malignant potential, Gynecol Oncol 47:150, 1992.

Lehner R, Wenzl R, Heinzl H, et al: Influence of delayed staging laparotomy after laparoscopic removal of ovarian masses later found malignant, Obstet Gynecol 92:967, 1998.

Leminen A and Lehtovirta P: Spread of ovarian cancer after laparoscopic surgery: report of eight cases, Gynecol Oncol 75:387, 1999.

Lenhard RE Jr: Cancer statistics: a measure of progress, CA Cancer J Clin 46:3, 1996.

Lim-Tan SK, Cajigas HE, and Scully RE: Ovarian cystectomy for serous borderline tumors: a follow-up of 35 cases, Obstet Gynecol 72:775, 1988.

Linder D et al: Pathogenetic origin of benign ovarian teratomas, N Engl J Med 292:63, 1975.

Lu KH, Garber JE, Cramer DW, et al: Occult ovarian tumors in women with *BRCA1* or *BRCA2* mutations undergoing prophylactic oophorectomy, J Clin Oncol 18:2728, 2000.

Lund B and Williamson P: Prognostic factors for outcome of and survival after second-look laparotomy in patients with advanced ovarian carcinoma, Obstet Gynecol 76:617, 1990.

Lynch HT, Watson P, Bewtra C, et al: Hereditary ovarian cancer: heterogeneity in age at diagnosis, Cancer 67:1460, 1991.

Maggino T, Gadducci A, D'Addario V, et al: Prospective multicenter study on CA 125 in postmenopausal pelvic masses, Gynecol Oncol 54:117, 1994.

Maiman M, Seltzer V, and Boyce J: Laparoscopic excision of ovarian neoplasms subsequently found to be malignant, Obstet Gynecol 77:563, 1991.

Malfetano JH: The appendix and its metastatic potential in epithelial ovarian cancer, Obstet Gynecol 69:396, 1987.

Markman M: CA-125: an evolving role in the management of ovarian cancer, J Clin Oncol 14:1411, 1996.

Markman M, Berek JS, Blessing JA, et al: Characteristics of patients with small-volume residual ovarian cancer unresponsive to cisplatin-based ip chemotherapy: lessons learned from a Gynecologic Oncology Group phase II trial of ip cisplatin and recombinant α-interferon, Gynecol Oncol 45:3, 1992.

Markman M, Lewis JL Jr, Saigo P, et al: Impact of age on survival of patients with ovarian cancer, Gynecol Oncol 49:236, 1993.

McGuire WP, Hoskins W, Brady MF, et al: Cyclophosphamide and cisplatin compared with paclitaxel and cisplatin in patients with stage III and stage IV ovarian cancer, N Engl J Med 334:1, 1996.

McMeekin DS, Burger RA, Manetta A, et al: Endometrioid adenocarcinoma of the ovary and its relationship to endometriosis, Gynecol Oncol 59:81, 1995.

Menczer J, Ben-Baruch G, Modan M, and Brenner H: Intraperitoneal cisplatin chemotherapy versus abdominopelvic irradiation in ovarian carcinoma patients after second-look laparotomy, Cancer 63:1509, 1989.

Menczer M, Modan M, Brenner J, et al: Abdominal pelvic irradiation for stage II-IV ovarian carcinoma patients with limited or no residual disease at second-look laparotomy after completion of *cis*-platinum-based combination chemotherapy, Gynecol Oncol 24:149, 1986.

Mishell DR: Contraception, N Engl J Med 320:777, 1989.

Mooney J, Silva E, Tornos C, et al: Unusual features of serous neoplasms of low malignant potential during pregnancy, Gynecol Oncol 65:830, 1997.

Morgan RJ, Braly P, Leong L, et al: Phase II trial of combination intraperitoneal cisplatin and 5-fluorouracil in previously treated patients with advanced ovarian cancer: long-term follow-up, Gynecol Oncol 77:433, 2000.

Mulhollan TJ, Silva EG, Tornos C, et al: Ovarian involvement by serous surface papillary carcinoma, Int J Gynecol Pathol 13:120, 1994.

Munkarah A, Gershenson DM, Levenback C, et al: Salvage surgery for chemorefractory ovarian germ cell tumors, Gynecol Oncol 55:217, 1994.

Muntz HG, Jones MA, Godd BA, et al: Malignant mixed müllerian tumors of the ovary, Cancer 76:1209, 1995.

Narod SA, Risch H, Moslehi R, et al: Oral contraceptives and the risk of hereditary ovarian cancer, N Engl J Med 339:424, 1998.

Neijt JP, Engelholm SA, Tuxen MK, et al: Exploratory phase III study of paclitaxel and cisplatin versus paclitaxel and carboplatin in advanced ovarian cancer, J Clin Oncol 18:3084, 2000.

Nichols CR, Tricot G, Williams SD, et al: Dose-intensive chemotherapy in refractory germ cell cancer: a phase I/II trial of high-dose carboplatin and etoposide with autologous bone marrow transplant, J Clin Oncol 7:932, 1989.

Norris HJ, Zirkin HJ, and Benson WL: Immature (malignant) teratoma of the ovary: a clinical and pathologic study of 58 cases, Cancer 37:2359, 1976.

Ozols RF: Intraperitoneal therapy in ovarian cancer: time's up, J Clin Oncol 9:197, 1991.

Patsner B: Is there a role for CT scanning to monitor therapy of optimally debulked patients with advanced ovarian epithelial cancer? Int J Gynecol Cancer 4:19, 1994.

Pavlik EJ, DePriest PD, Gallion HH, et al: Ovarian volume related to age, Gynecol Oncol 77:410, 2000.

Peccatori F, Bonazzi C, Chiari S, et al: Surgical management of malignant ovarian germ-cell tumors: 10 years' experience of 129 patients, Obstet Gynecol 86:367, 1995.

Pecorelli S, Creasman WT, Pettersson F, et al: FIGO annual report on the results of treatment in gynaecological cancer, vol 23, Milano, Italy. J Epidemiol Biostat, 1998.

Piver MS, Malfetano J, Baker TR, and Hempling RE: Five-year survival for stage Ic or stage I grade 3 epithelial ovarian cancer treated with cisplatin-based chemotherapy, Gynecol Oncol 46:35, 1992.

Prat J: Ovarian tumors of borderline malignancy (tumors of low malignant potential): a critical appraisal, Adv Anat Pathol 6:247, 1999.

Pujade-Lauraine E, Guastalla JP, Colombo N, et al: Intraperitoneal recombinant interferon gamma in ovarian cancer patients with residual disease at second-look laparotomy, J Clin Oncol 14:343, 1996.

Randall ME, Barrett RJ, Spirtos NM, et al: Chemotherapy, early surgical reassessment and hyperfractionated abdominal radiotherapy in stage III ovarian cancer: results of a Gynecologic Oncology Group study, Int J Radiat Oncol Biol Phys 34:139, 1996.

Rebbeck TR, Levin AM, Eisen A, et al: Breast cancer risk after bilateral prophylactic oophorectomy in BRCA1 mutation carriers, J Natl Cancer Inst 91:1475, 1999.

Reed WC: Small cell carcinoma of the ovary with hypercalcemia: report of a case of survival without recurrence 5 years after surgery and chemotherapy, Gynecol Oncol 56:452, 1995.

Reimer RR, Hoover R, Fraumeini JF, et al: Acute leukemia after alkylating-agent therapy of ovarian cancer, N Engl J Med 297:177, 1977.

Risch HA, Jain M, Marrett LD, et al: Dietary fat intake and risk of epithelial ovarian cancer, J Natl Cancer Inst 86:1409, 1994.

Robey SS, Silva EG, Gershenson DM, et al: Transitional cell carcinoma in high-grade high-stage ovarian carcinoma, Cancer 63:839, 1989.

Ronnett BM, Kurman RJ, Zahn CM, et al: Pseudomyxoma peritonei in women: a clinicopathologic analysis of 30 cases with emphasis on site of origin, prognosis, and relationship to ovarian mucinous tumors of low malignant potential, Hum Pathol 26:509, 1990.

Rossing MA, Daling JR, Weiss NS, et al: Ovarian tumors in a cohort of infertile women, N Engl J Med 331:771, 1994.

Rota SM, Zanetta G, Ieda N, et al: Clinical relevance of retroperitoneal involvement from epithelial ovarian tumors of borderline malignancy, Int J Gynecol Cancer 9:477, 1999.

Rubin SC, Randall TC, Armstrong KA, et al: Ten-year follow-up of ovarian cancer patients after second-look laparotomy with negative findings, Obstet Gynecol 93:21, 1999.

Rustin G, Nelstrop AE, McClean P, et al: Defining response of ovarian carcinoma to initial chemotherapy according to serum CA-125, J Clin Oncol 14:1545, 1996.

Samanth KK and Black WC: Benign ovarian stromal tumors associated with free peritoneal fluid, Am J Obstet Gynecol 197:538, 1970.

Santoso JT, Tang D, Lane SB, et al: Adenovirus-based p53 gene therapy in ovarian cancer, Gynecol Oncol 59:171, 1995.

Schelling M, Braun M, Kuhn W, et al: Combined transvaginal B-mode and color Doppler sonography for differential diagnosis of ovarian tumors: results of a multivariate logistic regression analysis, Gynecol Oncol 77:78, 2000.

Schildkraut JM, Bastos E, and Berchuck A: Relationship between lifetime ovulatory cycles and overexpression of mutant p[53] in epithelial ovarian cancer, J Natl Cancer Inst 89:932, 1997.

Schlesselman JJ: Net effect of oral contraceptive use on the risk of cancer in women in the United States, Obstet Gynecol 85:793, 1995.

Schneider J, Erasun F, Hervas JL, et al: Normal pregnancy and delivery 2 years after adjuvant chemotherapy for grade III immature ovarian teratoma, Gynecol Oncol 29:245, 1988.

Schwartz PE and Morris JM: Serum lactic dehydrogenase: a tumor marker for dysgerminoma, Obstet Gynecol 72:511, 1988.

Schwartz PE and Smith JP: Treatment of ovarian stromal tumors, Am J Obstet Gynecol 125:402, 1976.

Scully RE: Gonadoblastoma: a gonadal tumor related to dysgerminoma (seminoma) and capable of sex hormone production, Cancer 6:455, 1953.

Scully RE: Sex cord–stromal tumors. In Blaustein A, editor: Pathology of the female genital tract, ed 4, New York, 1994, Springer-Verlag.

Scully RE: Influence of origin of ovarian cancer on efficacy of screening [Commentary], Lancet 355:1028, 2000.

Scully RE, Young RH, and Clement PB: Tumors of the ovary, maldeveloped gonads, fallopian tube, and broad ligament. In Atlas of tumor pathology, fascicle 23, series 3, Washington, DC, Armed Forces Institute of Pathology, 1998.

Segal R, DePetrillo AD, and Thomas G: Clinical review of adult granulosa cell tumors of the ovary, Gynecol Oncol 56:338, 1995.

Serov SF, Scully RE, and Sobin LH: Histological typing of ovarian tumors, Geneva, 1973, World Health Organization.

Sevinc A, Buyukberber S, Sari R, et al: Elevated serum CA-125 levels in hemodialysis patients with peritoneal, pleural, or pericardial fluids, Gynecol Oncol 77:254, 2000.

Shakfeh AM and Woodruff JD: Primary ovarian sarcomas: report of 46 cases and review of literature, Obstet Gynecol Surv 42:331, 1987.

Shalev E, Eliyahu S, Peleg D, and Tsabari A: Laparoscopic management of adnexal cystic masses in postmenopausal women, Obstet Gynecol 83:594, 1994.

Sharp F, Blackett AD, Leake RE, and Berek JS: Conclusions and recommendations from the Helene Harris memorial trust fund biennial international forum on ovarian cancer, May 4-7, 1995, Glasgow, UK, Int J Gynecol Cancer 5:449, 1995.

Shushan A, Peretz T, Uziely B, et al: Ovarian cysts in premenopausal and postmenopausal tamoxifen-treated women with breast cancer, Am J Obstet Gynecol 174:141, 1996.

Sjöval K, Nilsson B, and Einhorn N: Different types of rupture of the tumor capsule and the impact on survival in early ovarian carcinoma, Int J Gynecol Cancer 4:333, 1994.

Slamon DJ, Godolophin W, Jones LA, et al: Studies of the HER-2/*neu* protooncogene in human breast and ovarian cancer, Science 244:707, 1989.

Sorbe B, Frankendal B, and Veress B: Importance of histologic grading in the prognosis of epithelial cancer, Obstet Gynecol 59:576, 1982.

Stein AL, Koonings PP, Schlaerth JB, et al: Relative frequency of malignant paraovarian tumors: should paraovarian tumors be aspirated? Obstet Gynecol 75:1029, 1990.

Swanson SA, Norris HJ, Kelsten ML, and Wheeler JE: DNA content of juvenile granulosa tumors determined by flow cytometry, Int J Gynecol Pathol 9:101, 1990.

Talerman A: Germ cell tumors of the ovary. In Blaustein A, editor: Pathology of the female genital tract, ed 4, New York, 1994, Springer-Verlag.

Travis LB, Holowaty EJ, Bergfelt K, et al: Risk of leukemia after platinum-based chemotherapy for ovarian cancer, N Engl J Med 340:351, 1999.

Tresukosol D, Kudelka AP, Edwards CL, et al: Recurrent ovarian granulosa cell tumor: a case report of a dramatic response to taxol, Int J Gynecol Cancer 5:156, 1995.

Thigpen JT, Blessing JA, Ball H, et al: Phase II trial of paclitaxel in patients with progressive ovarian carcinoma after platinum-based chemotherapy: a Gynecologic Oncology Group study, J Clin Oncol 12:1748, 1994.

Troche V and Hernandez E: Neoplasia arising in dysgenetic gonads, Obstet Gynecol Surv 41:74, 1986.

Trope C, Kaern J, Vergote IB, et al: Are borderline tumors of the ovary overtreated both surgically and systemically?: a review of four prospective randomized trials including 253 patients with borderline tumors, Gynecol Oncol 51:236, 1993.

Vaccarello L, Rubin SC, Vlamis V, et al: Cytoreductive surgery in ovarian carcinoma patients with a documented previously complete surgical response, Gynecol Oncol 57:61, 1995.

van der Burg MEL, van Lent M, Buyse M, et al: The effect of debulking surgery after induction chemotherapy on the prognosis in advanced epithelial ovarian cancer, N Engl J Med 332:629, 1995.

Venesmaa P: Epithelial ovarian cancer: impact of surgery and chemotherapy on survival during 1977-1990, Obstet Gynecol 84:8, 1994.

Vergote I, De Wever I, Tjalma W, et al: Neoadjuvant chemotherapy or primary debulking surgery in advanced ovarian carcinoma: a retrospective analysis of 285 patients, Gynecol Oncol 71:431, 1998.

Vergote IB, Winderen M, De Vos LN, and Trope CG: Intraperitoneal radioactive phosphorus therapy in ovarian cancer, Cancer 71:2250, 1993.

Von Hoff DD, Kronmal R, Salmon SE, et al: A Southwest Oncology Group study for the use of a human tumor cloning assay for predicting response in patients with ovarian cancer, Cancer 67:20, 1991.

Warner E: Neurotoxicity of cisplatin and taxol, Int J Gynecol Cancer 5:161, 1995.

Warner E, Foulkes W, Goodwin P, et al: Prevalence and penetrance of BRCA1 and BRCA2 gene mutations in unselected Ashkenazi Jewish women with breast cancer, J Natl Cancer Inst 91:1241, 1999.

Wertheim I, Fleischhacker D, McLachlin CM, et al: Pseudomyxoma peritonei: a review of 23 cases, Obstet Gynecol 84:17, 1994.

Westhoff C and Randall MC: Ovarian cancer screening: potential effect on mortality, Am J Obstet Gynecol 165:502, 1991.

Whittemore AS, Harris R, Itnyre J, et al: Characteristics relating to ovarian cancer risk: collaborative analysis of 12 U.S. case-control studies, Am J Epidemiol 136:1184, 1992.

Wick MR, Mills SE, Dehner LP, et al: Serous papillary carcinomas arising from the peritoneum and ovaries, Int J Gynecol Pathol 8:179, 1989.

Willemse PHB, Aalders JG, Bouma J, et al: Long-term survival after vinblastine, bleomycin, and cisplatin treatment in patients with germ cell tumors of the ovary: an update, Gynecol Oncol 28:268, 1987.

Willemse PHB, Oosterhuis JW, Aalders JG, et al: Malignant struma ovarii by ovariectomy, thyroidectomy, and ^{131}I administration, Cancer 60:182, 1987.

Williams SD, Blessing JA, DiSaia PJ, et al: Second-look laparotomy in ovarian germ cell tumors: the Gynecologic Oncology Group experience, Gynecol Oncol 52:287, 1994.

Williams SD, Blessing JA, Hatch KD, and Homesley HD: Chemotherapy of advanced dysgerminoma: trials of the Gynecologic Oncology Group, J Clin Oncol 9:1950, 1991.

Williams S, Blessing JA, Liao SY, et al: Adjuvant therapy of ovarian germ cell tumors with cisplatin, etoposide, and bleomycin: a trial of the Gynecologic Oncology Group, J Clin Oncol 12:701, 1994.

Wingo PA, Tong T, and Bolden S: Cancer statistics, 1995, CA Cancer J Clin 45:8, 1995.

Wu PC, Huang RL, Lang JH, et al: Treatment of malignant ovarian germ cell tumors with preservation of fertility: a report of 28 cases, Gynecol Oncol 40:2, 1991.

Yancik R, Ries LG, and Yates JW: An analysis of surveillance, epidemiology, and end results program data, Am J Obstet Gynecol 154:639, 1986.

Young RH, Dickersin GR, and Scully RE: Juvenile granulosa cell tumor of the ovary, Am J Surg Pathol 8:575, 1984.

Young RH, Gilks CB, and Scully RE: Mucinous tumors of the appendix associated with mucinous tumors of the ovary and pseudomyxoma peritonei, Am J Surg Pathol 15(5):415, 1991.

Young RH, Olivia E, and Scully RE: Small cell carcinoma of the ovary, hypercalcemia type, Am J Surg Pathol 18:1102, 1994.

Young RH, Welch WR, Dickersin GR, et al: Ovarian sex cord tumor with annular tubules, Cancer 50:1384, 1982.

Young RH and Scully RE: Ovarian Sertoli-Leydig cell tumors: a clinicopathological analysis of 207 cases, Am J Surg Pathol 9:543, 1985.

Young RC, Walton LA, Ellenberg SS, et al: Adjuvant therapy in stage I and stage II epithelial ovarian cancer: results of two prospective randomized trials, N Engl J Med 332:1021, 1990.

Zambetti M, Escobedo A, Pilotti S, and De Palo G: Cis-platinum/vinblastine/bleomycin combination chemotherapy in advanced or recurrent granulosa cell tumors of the ovary, Gynecol Oncol 36:317, 1990.

CHAPTER
32

Neoplastic Diseases of the Vulva
Lichen Sclerosus, Intraepithelial Neoplasia, Paget's Disease, Carcinoma

KEY TERMS AND DEFINITIONS

Carcinoma in Situ. Premalignant epithelial change throughout the full thickness of the vulvar epithelium. It is also comparable to vulvar intraepithelial neoplasia (VIN) III.

Keyes Punch. An instrument used to biopsy the vulva.

Lichen Sclerosus. A vulvar abnormality usually characterized by thinning of the epithelium with a loss of subcutaneous adnexal structures, hyalinization of the superficial dermis, and lymphocytic infiltrates below the zone of dermal homogenization.

Melanoma Level. A system (I to V) used to define the depth or level to which a malignant melanoma invades the epithelium.

Microinvasive Vulvar Carcinoma. A controversial term used to describe a superficially invasive carcinoma of the vulva that is not expected to be associated with lymph node metastasis. The lesion is ≤2 cm in diameter; the invasion is less than 1 mm into the stroma (stage IA).

Paget's Disease of the Vulva. An itchy, usually erythematous, lesion microscopically containing large cells similar to Paget cells seen in the breast. The squamous epithelium is studded with large cells containing clear cytoplasm and pleomorphic nuclei with prominent nucleoli.

Radical Vulvectomy. An operation that removes the entire vulva, including subcutaneous and fatty tissue, the labia minora and majora, perineal skin, and clitoris, to treat cancer.

Simple Vulvectomy. An operation that removes the skin of the vulva, including the labia majora and minora, the clitoris, and perineal skin.

Stages of Vulvar Cancer:
  Stage I: Less than 2 cm in diameter and confined to the vulva and/or perineum.
  Stage II: Over 2 cm in diameter and confined to the vulva and/or perineum.
  Stage III: Extends to the anus and/or lower urethra, and/or unilateral regional node metastasis.
  Stage IV: Spreads to the bladder or rectum or pelvic bone or upper urethra or nonvulvar sites, or bilateral regional node metastases.

TNM System. A system used to describe the extent of tumor (T), node status (N), and presence of metastatic disease (M) (see box on p. 000).

Verrucous Carcinoma. An uncommon well-differentiated squamous carcinoma with a gross wartlike appearance that is curable with a local excision.

Vulvar Atypia. A mild, moderate, or severe neoplastic or dysplastic change in the vulvar squamous epithelium. It may also be termed *vulvar intraepithelial neoplasia (VIN I, II, or III)*.

Cancer of the vulva accounts for about 4% of malignancies of the lower female genital tract, which ranks it fourth in frequency among these malignancies, after cancers of the endometrium, ovary, and cervix.

Well-defined predisposing factors for the development of vulvar carcinoma have not been identified. In general, premalignant and malignant changes frequently arise at multifocal points on the vulva. Occasionally invasive carcinoma arises from areas of carcinoma in situ, similar to the mechanism in cervical squamous cell carcinoma (Chapter 29). However, many cases of squamous cell carcinoma of the vulva appear to develop in the absence of premalignant changes in the vulvar epithelium. Human papillomavirus (HPV) has been noted in many patients with carcinoma of the vulva. Other factors, such as granulomatous disease of the vulva, diabetes, hypertension, smoking, and obesity, have all been suggested as etiologic factors, but current data do not provide consistent evidence regarding their association with vulvar carcinoma. Carcinoma of the vulva does occur with increasing frequency in those who have been treated for squamous cell carcinoma of the cervix or vagina, presumably as a result of the increased risk of carcinogenesis in the squamous epithelium of the lower genital tract in these patients. It appears HPV DNA is involved in the development of a subset of vulvar carcinomas that tend to occur in younger patients, as noted by Crum et al. Monk et al. demonstrated that not only were the HPV-DNA–associated carcinomas found in younger patients but also the HPV-negative patients appear to have a poor prognosis with tumors that were more likely to recur and lead to patient death. As demonstrated by Hording et al. HPV-positive tumors tend to have a warty or basiloid appearance while HPV-negative tumors tend to be keratinized. The former tend to be associated with premalignant vulvar changes (vulvar intraepithelial neoplasia).

Most vulvar malignancies are squamous cell carcinomas. Although this is a disease of older women, Franklin and Rutledge noted that 15% of cancers of the vulva in their series occurred in women under the age of 40. The incidence of squamous cell carcinoma of the vulva in the United States increases progressively with age (Figure 32-1). More than half of patients with carcinoma of the vulva are 60 to 79 years of age at the time of diagnosis. While most patients with carcinoma of the vulva are older than 60, those with carcinoma in situ of the vulva are usually 10 to 15 years younger, that is, 40 to 55 years of age. In recent years premalignant changes of the vulva are being seen with increasing frequency among younger patients, often in their 20s and 20s, possibly as a result of an increasing rate of multiple sexual contacts and increased venereal-viral, particularly HPV, infections in the population. An increase in the frequency of invasive carcinoma of the vulva, however, has not yet been detected, but it may well develop in future years.

This chapter reviews the clinical and pathologic aspects of premalignant vulvar lesions and vulvar atypias. This is followed by consideration of the diagnosis, natural history,

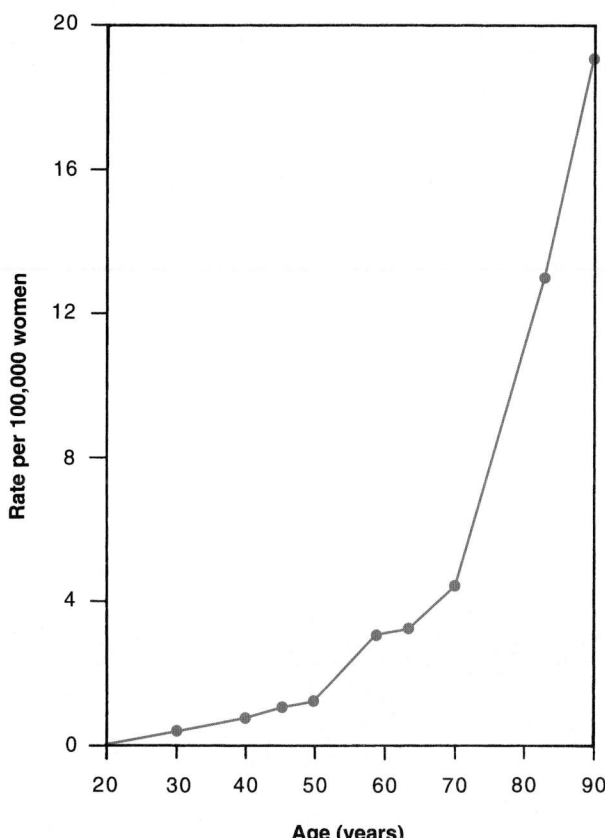

FIGURE 32-1 Age incidence curve for carcinoma of vulva in white women in the United States. (Adapted from Menczer J, Voliovitch Y, Modan B, et al: Am J Obstet Gynecol 143:893, 1982.)

and management of invasive cancers of the vulva, which includes not only the squamous cell carcinomas but also the rarer melanomas and sarcomas.

VULVAR ATYPIAS

Specific Conditions

The diagnosis and treatment of premalignant conditions of the vulva have been confusing in the past because of the lack of a uniform definition of the various lesions encountered. The current definition of vulvar atypias is shown in the box on the facing page. A number of ambiguous terms have been eliminated. For example, terms such as *leukoplakia* and *leukoplakic vulvitis* have been discarded, and terms such as *Bowen's disease, erythroplasia of Queyrat*, and *carcinoma simplex* are all grouped under the term *carcinoma in situ* or *vulvar intraepithelial neoplasia (VIN)*.

Vulvar Atypias—Intraepithelial Neoplasia

Lichen sclerosus (Figure 32-2) is a change in the vulvar skin that often appears whitish. Microscopically the epithelium becomes markedly thinned with a loss or

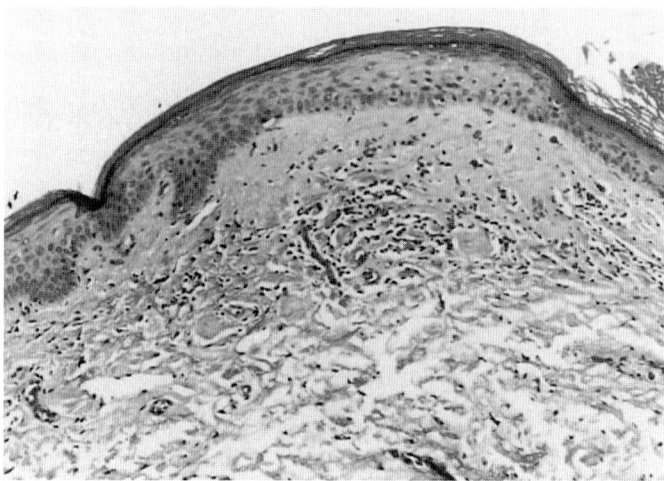

FIGURE 32-2 Lichen sclerosus et atrophicus. Homogenous collagen in the papillary dermis is accompanied by a scattered lymphocytic infiltrate and atrophy of the epithelium. (H&E; ×80.) (Courtesy Dr. Anthony Montag, The University of Chicago.)

Classification of Vulvar Atypias

Squamous cell hyperplasia (formerly hyperplastic dystrophy)
Lichen sclerosus
Intraepithelial neoplasia
    VIN I   Mild dysplasia
    VIN II Moderate dysplasia
    VIN III Severe dysplasia—carcinoma in situ
Others:
    Paget's disease
    Melanoma in situ (level 1)

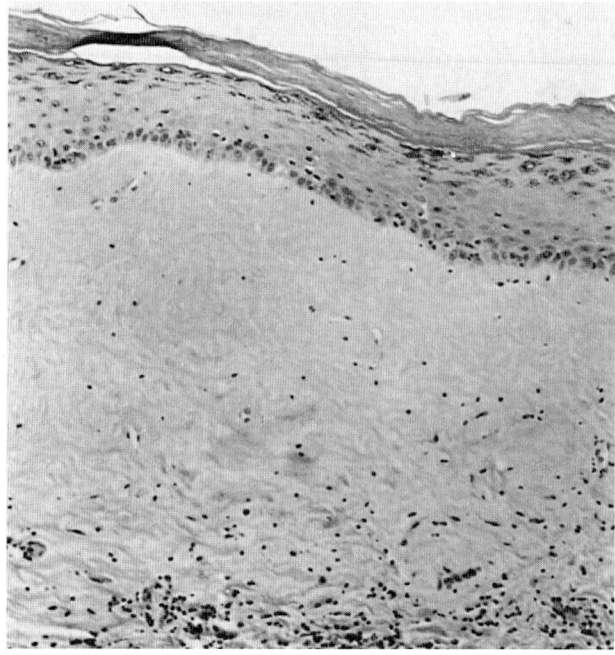

FIGURE 32-3 Lichen sclerosus. Hyperkeratosis is occasionally present. (From Friedrich EG and Wilkinson EJ: The vulva. In Blaustein A, ed: Pathology of the female genital tract, New York, 1982, Springer-Verlag.)

blunting of the rete ridges. In some cases there is also a thickening or hyperkeratosis of the surface layers (Figure 32-3). Inflammation is usually present. Hart et al. studied 107 patients with lichen sclerosus, and only one followed for 12 years eventually developed vulvar carcinoma. Five patients had vulvar carcinoma at the time lichen sclerosus was diagnosed. Twelve other patients subsequently developed malignancies at other sites, such as the cervix, colon, breast, ovary, and endometrium. Patients with lichen sclerosus in the past were deemed not to be at increased risk for the development of vulvar carcinoma. A recent study by Carlson et al. supports a small premalignant potential of lichen sclerosus. Their study and a literature review showed a risk of lichen sclerosus (LS) and squamous cell carcinoma (SCC) was 4.5% with an average of 4 years latency between symptomatic LS and SCC. The tumors that developed tended to be clitoral in location.

Squamous hyperplasia (formerly hyperplastic dystrophy) changes involve elongation and widening of the rete ridges, which may be confluent (Figure 32-4). There may also be hyperkeratotic surface layers, and the tissue grossly often is whitish or reddish.

Atypical changes may appear in the vulvar epithelium.

These changes are usually marked by a loss of maturation process usually seen in squamous epithelium as well as an increase in mitotic activity and in the nuclear-cytoplasmic ratio (Figure 32-5). Mild dysplasia (atypia) is diagnosed if these changes involve the lower third of the epithelium; moderate dysplasia (atypia) if half to two thirds of the epithelium is involved; and severe dysplasia (atypia) if over two thirds of the epithelium is affected. Carcinoma in situ involves full thickness of the epithelium. The term *VIN I* is used for mild atypia, *VIN II* for moderate atypia,

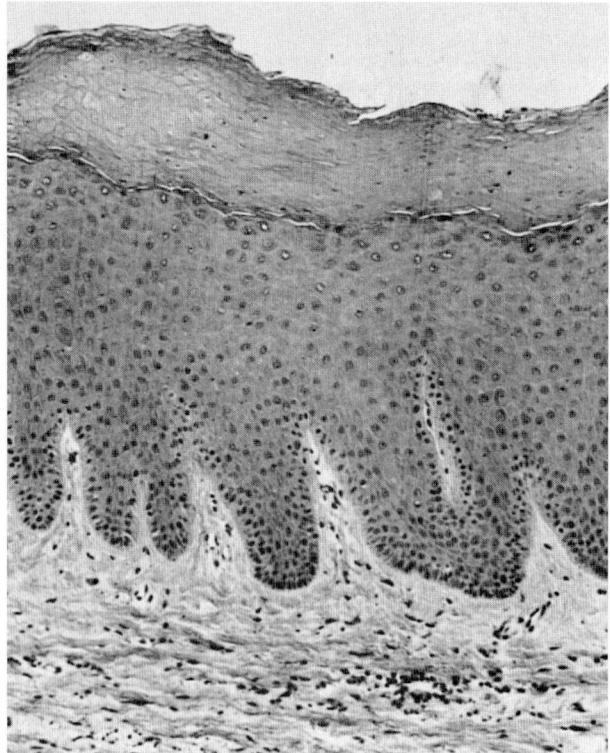

FIGURE 32-4 Squamous hyperplasia (formerly hyperplastic dystrophy), benign. Hyperkeratosis, acanthosis, and mild inflammation are present. (From Friedrich EG and Wilkinson EJ: The vulva. In Blaustein A, ed: Pathology of the female genital tract, New York, 1982, Springer-Verlag.)

and *VIN III* for severe atypia, as well as carcinoma in situ. It is sometimes difficult to distinguish between squamous hyperplasia and intraepithelial neoplasia. Crum has suggested that intraepithelial neoplasia of the vulva almost always contains nuclei which are fourfold or greater different in size, while differences in the size of nuclei in condyloma or nonneoplastic epithelia are threefold or less. Furthermore, abnormal mitoses are usually observed in vulvar intraepithelial neoplasia.

Carcinoma in Situ (VIN III)

Carcinoma in situ is diagnosed if the full thickness of the epithelium is abnormal (Figure 32-6, *A*). Occasionally the process may histologically resemble carcinoma in situ of the cervix, and in many lesions there are multinucleated cells, abnormal mitoses, an increased density in cells, and an increase in the nuclear-cytoplasmic ratio.

Paget's Disease

Paget's disease is a rare intraepithelial disorder that occurs in the vulvar skin and histologically resembles Paget's disease in the breast. Paget cells are large pale cells (Figure 32-7). The cells often occur in nests and infiltrate

upward through the epithelium. Frequently, histologic abnormalities of the apocrine glands of the skin may be noted in these lesions. There is an increased association of Paget's disease of the vulva with invasive GI and breast carcinomas. Paget's disease of the vulva tends to spread, often in an occult fashion, and recurrences are frequent after treatment.

Diagnosis

Clinical Presentation

Atypias of the vulva present with a variety of symptoms and signs. Irritation or itching is common, although some patients frequently do not complain of these symptoms. The vulva often has a whitish change due to a thickened keratin layer. In the past the term *leukoplakia* was used. This term has been discarded in part because abnormal lesions of the vulva require biopsy to establish a correct diagnosis. When lichen sclerosus is present, there is usually a diffuse whitish change to the vulvar skin (Figure 32-8). The vulvar skin often appears thin, and there may be scarring and contracture. In addition, fissuring of the skin is often present, accompanied by excoriation secondary to itching. Areas of squamous hyperplasias (formerly called *hyperplastic dystrophy without atypia*) also appear as whitish lesions in general, but the tissues of the vulva usually appear thickened and the process tends to be more focal or multifocal than diffuse (Figure 32-9).

Abnormal areas of vulvar atypia or intraepithelial neoplasia may also appear as white, red, or pigmented areas on the vulva. However, the clinical appearance of vulvar intraepithelial neoplasia is variable. Wilkinson and Friedrich estimate that about one third of patients with carcinoma in situ will present with pigmented lesions, emphasizing the importance of a biopsy to establish the diagnosis. The lesions tend to be discrete and multifocal, and they occur more frequently in those who have had squamous cell neoplasia of the cervix. In addition, reddish nodules may also be foci of Paget's disease, as well as carcinoma in situ. Paget's disease often has a reddish, eczematoid appearance. It should be reemphasized that these conditions cannot be accurately diagnosed from their clinical appearance, and biopsies are needed.

Diagnostic Methods

In general, the cytologic evaluation (Pap smear) of the vulva has often not been helpful, in part because the vulvar skin is thick and keratinized and does not shed cells as readily as the epithelium of the vagina and cervix. However, in some cases, particularly if there is ulceration of the vulva, a cytologic smear can be helpful diagnostically (Figure 32-6, *B*). A tongue depressor moistened with normal saline or tap water is scraped over the surface portion of

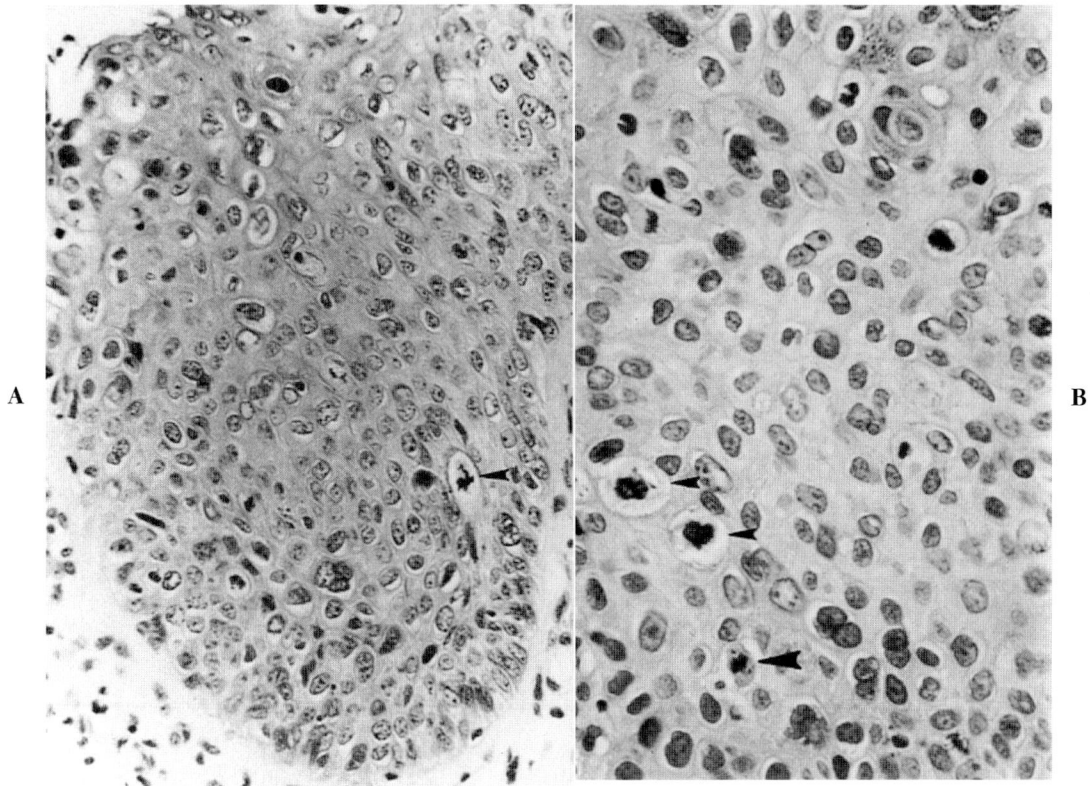

FIGURE 32-5   A, Vulvar intraepithelial neoplasia from which HPV type 16 was isolated. Characteristic features displayed here include abnormal mitoses (a two-group metaphase is denoted by the arrow), a full-thickness population of abnormal cells and abnormal differentiation. Superficial cells contain perinuclear halos, which in contrast to condylomata are small and concentric. **B,** The higher power photomicrograph of vulvar intraepithelial neoplasia illustrates the marked variability in nuclear size and staining with both enlarged nuclei and multinucleated cells. Coarsely clumped mitoses *(small arrows)* and a three-group metaphase *(large arrow)* are present. (From Crum CP: Pathology of the vulva and vagina, New York, 1987, Churchill-Livingstone.)

the vulva to be sampled, and the specimen is placed on a glass slide and then fixed.

The toluidine blue test (1% toluidine blue applied for 1 minute followed by 1% acetic acid) with biopsy of the retained blue staining areas has generally been discarded, since it appears to be so nonspecific.

Colposcopy of the vulva is difficult because the characteristic changes in vascular appearance and tissue patterns that are seen in the cervix are not present (Chapter 28). Nevertheless, the magnification of the colposcope may be used to help follow patients with intraepithelial neoplasia of the vulva, as well as to identify the discrete whitish or pigmented areas that warrant biopsy. The colposcope is not used for routine vulvar examination but is primarily employed for those who are being evaluated or followed for vulvar atypia or intraepithelial neoplasia. However, the addition of 3% acetic acid highlights whitish areas for biopsy.

Biopsy of the vulva can be conveniently accomplished with a Keyes dermal punch (Figure 32-10). Usually a 3 to 5 mm diameter punch is used. Each area to be biopsied is usually is infiltrated with local anesthesia using a fine 25-gauge needle. The punch is then rotated and a downward

pressure applied so that a disc of tissue is circumscribed. When the entire thickness of the skin has been incised, the specimen is elevated with forceps and then removed with a sharp scissors. Occasionally a larger biopsy is needed, in which case a larger field is anesthetized and a small scalpel or cervical punch biopsy (see Figure 28-14) is used to obtain the specimen. Usually little bleeding is encountered, and it can generally be controlled by applying silver nitrate or ferrous subsulfate (Monsel's solution). Depending on the size of the atypical area and the variety of atypical appearing areas, one or multiple biopsies may be needed.

Management

Vulvar Atypias

Most vulvar atypias have pruritus as the major symptom, so the relief of itching is often the main concern of the patient. Once the correct diagnosis has been established by biopsy, appropriate therapy can be undertaken. Most whitish lesions will be benign, as lichen sclerosus is the most common condition encountered.

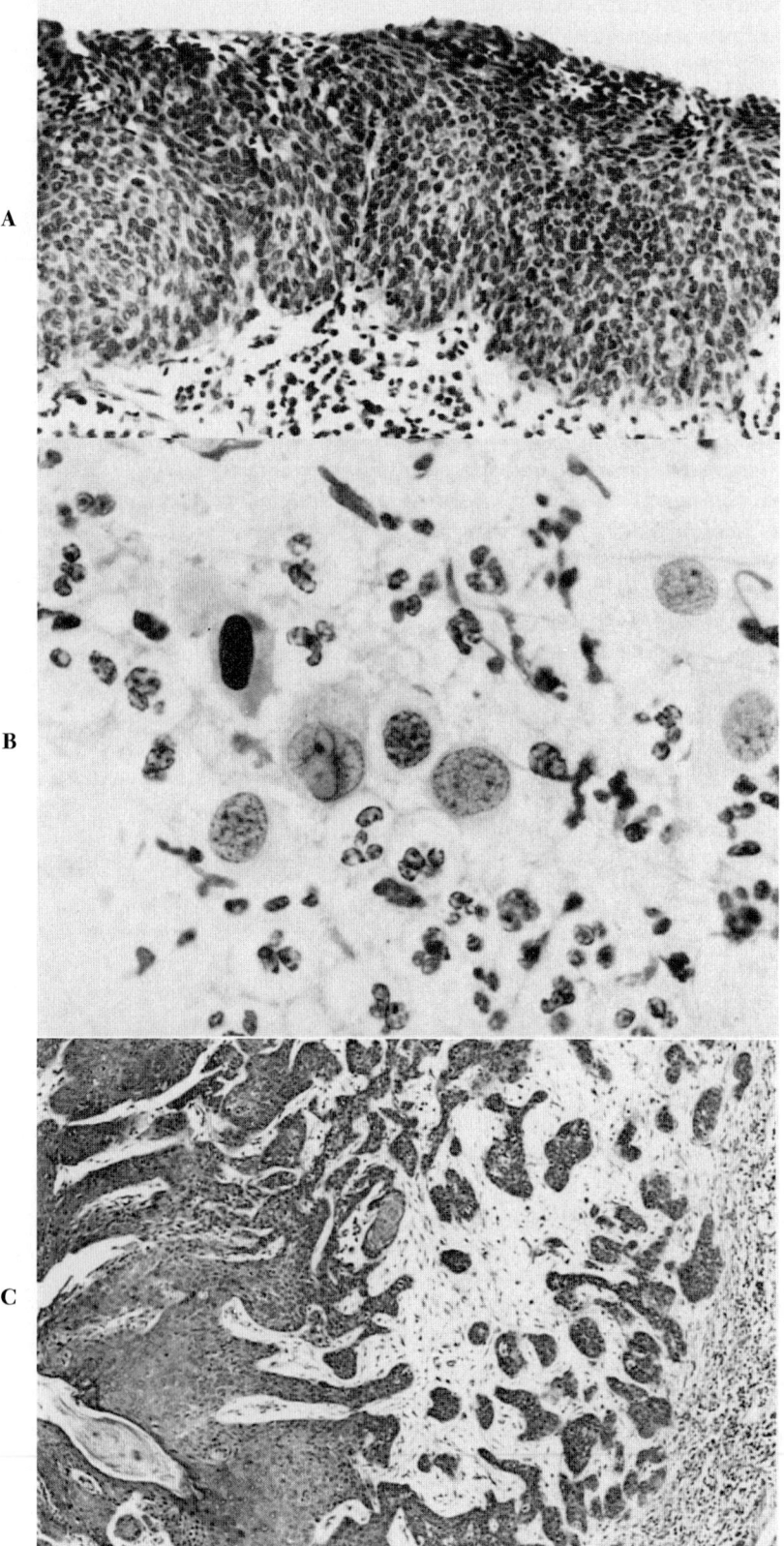

FIGURE 32-6 A, Carcinoma in situ, histology. Full thickness of epithelium is replaced by hyperchromatic cells with poorly defined cellular borders. (×80.) **B,** Carcinoma in situ, cytology. Cells derived from carcinoma in situ of vulva may exhibit varying sizes and shapes as depicted in this photomicrograph. Note variation in nuclear pattern from one nucleus to another. Degenerated polymorphonuclear leukocytes are present in background. (×800.) **C,** Invasive squamous carcinoma, histology. Tumor nests and cords infiltrate stroma. The squamous nature of tumor is more apparent on surface *(left),* where cells have abundant dense cytoplasm. Keratin is also seen. (×80.)

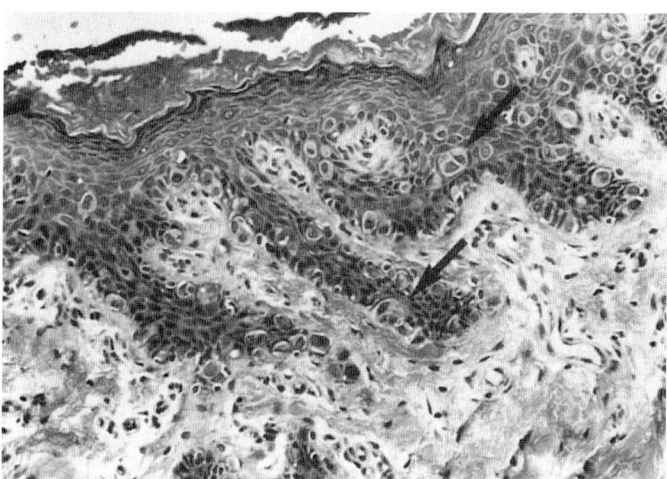

FIGURE 32-7 Vulvar epidermis with Paget's disease. Malignant cells *(arrows)* are seen infiltrating the epidermis and spreading along the dermal-epidermal junction. (H&E; ×160.) (Courtesy Dr. Anthony Montag, The University of Chicago.)

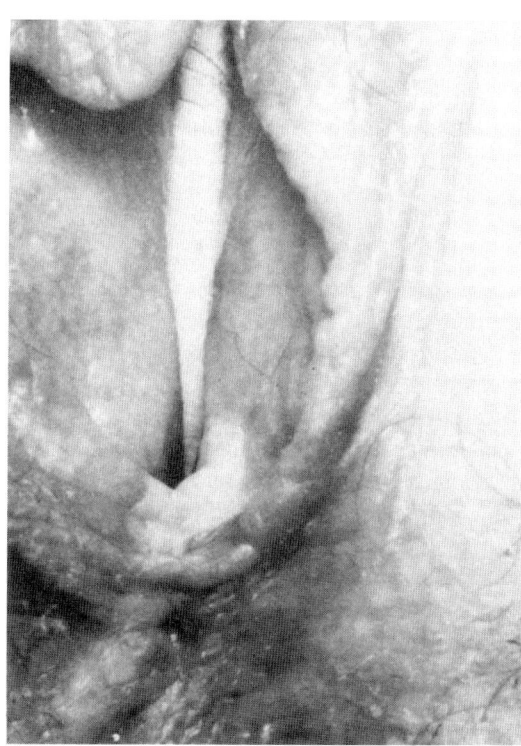

FIGURE 32-9 Vulva, hyperplastic dystrophy. Sharply demarcated, raised, white area is noted at lower tip of white pointer. (From Kaufman RH, Gardner HL, and Merrill JA: Diseases of the vulva and vagina. In Romney SL et al, eds: Gynecology and obstetrics. New York, 1980, McGraw-Hill Book Co.)

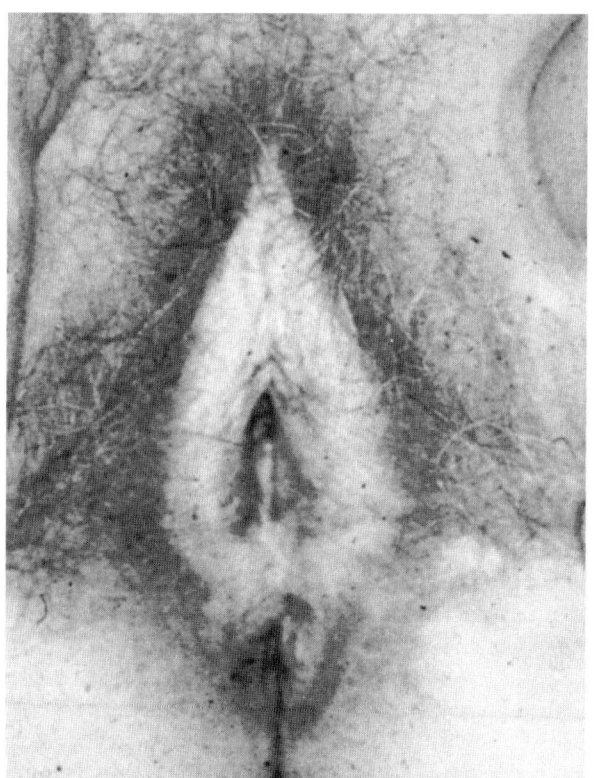

FIGURE 32-8 Vulva, lichen sclerosus. Tissue of labia minora and perineum has white, brittle "cigarette paper" appearance. (From Kaufman RH, Gardner HL, and Merrill JA: Diseases of the vulva and vagina. In Romney SL et al, eds: Gynecology and obstetrics, New York, 1980, McGraw-Hill Book Co.)

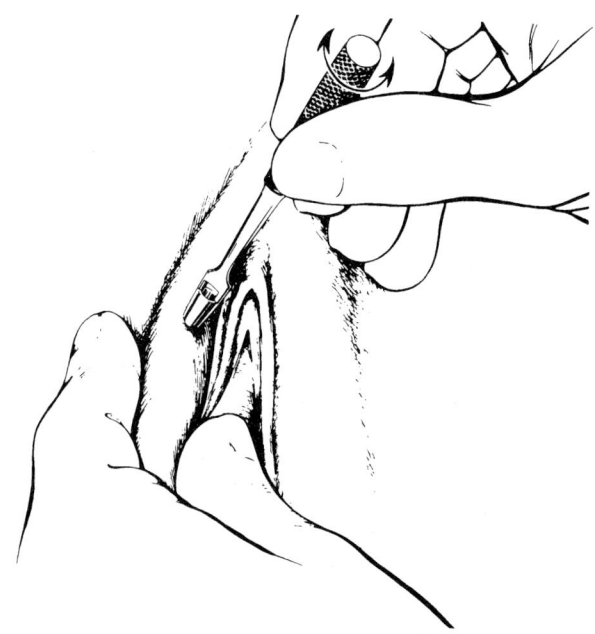

FIGURE 32-10 Diagnostic Keyes punch biopsy. (From Friedrich EG: Vulvar disease, ed 2, Philadelphia, 1983, WB Saunders Co.)

Topical testosterone is employed for atrophic conditions of the vulva, particularly lichen sclerosus. An effective preparation is 2% testosterone proprionate in petrolatum, which is used twice daily. Once daily is often sufficient maintenance after the first week. Side effects, such as clitoral hypertrophy and increased hair growth, can occur. If there are undesirable side effects with testosterone, then local progesterone cream is sometimes tried, with variable success. Those who have a beneficial response to testosterone should be continued on the medication indefinitely. Often testosterone cream twice weekly is a sufficient maintenance dose.

The control of local irritation of the vulva is discussed in Chapter 18. In addition to local measures to diminish irritation (cotton underclothes, avoidance of strong soaps and detergents, and avoidance of synthetic undergarments), topical fluorinated corticosteroids are helpful to control itching. Frequently used preparations are 0.025% or 0.1% triamcinolone acetonide (Aristocort, Kenalog), fluorocinolone acetonide (Synalar), or 0.01% or 0.1% betamethasone valerate. These are usually applied twice daily to control the itching, which is often relieved in 1 to 2 weeks. Unfortunately the prolonged use of fluorinated topical steroids can lead to vulvar atrophy and contraction. Thus once the symptoms of itching are controlled, the dosage of topical corticosteroids is tapered off, or if long-term therapy is needed, a nonfluorinated compound such as 1.0% hydrocortisone is used to avoid vulvar contraction. Occasionally 1% hydrocortisone is sufficient for initial therapy. In some cases the corticosteroids are not successful, and numerous types of topical therapy need to be tried to control symptoms. Gentle soaps such as Basis are helpful. Burow's solution (5% solution of aluminum acetate) is frequently used as a wet dressing to help control irritation and itching. Three percent Doak's Tar in petrolatum (USP) or in 1% hydrocortisone ointment is useful for severe cases.

In some patients with lichen sclerosus, severe contracture of the vulva, particularly in the area of the posterior fourchette, will occur with concomitant scarring and tenderness. Intercourse may then become painful in these patients. Woodruff et al. have described a useful surgical technique to treat these vaginal outlet disorders by plastic repair of the perineum. The contractured and fissured area in the posterior fourchette is excised, which results in an elliptical defect. This defect is then closed by undermining the distal 3 to 4 cm of the posterior vaginal mucosa and suturing the freed mucosa to the perineal skin (Figure 32-11).

Vulvar Intraepithelial Neoplasia

Once the diagnosis of VIN has been established by biopsy, therapy is performed to eradicate the area containing the neoplasia. The clinician must be aware that the progress of vulvar atypia (mild dysplasia—VIN I) to moderate dysplasia (VIN II) to severe dysplasia and carcinoma in situ (VIN III) and then to invasive carcinoma is not as well documented for vulvar neoplasia as it is for squamous cell neoplasia of the cervix. Moreover, vulvar neoplasia is frequently multifocal, requiring treatment of several areas. An additional complication is that some cases originally diagnosed as intraepithelial neoplasia have been reported to regress spontaneously.

In 1972 Friedrich reported Bowenoid atypia (histologically similar to carcinoma in situ) in a pregnant patient that regressed spontaneously postpartum. Others also reported spontaneous regression of this lesion. These spontaneously regressing lesions tend to be discrete elevations in young women. Some may be explained by studies of nuclear DNA content of vulvar atypias that suggest not all lesions with this designation are premalignant. Fu et al. noted that only four of eight cases of vulvar atypia had an aneuploid (neoplastic) distribution. A polyploid distribution was noted in four of the cases, which is consistent with a benign process, whereas aneuploidy is consistent with intraepithelial neoplasia.

Although VIN is being diagnosed more commonly in younger women, the risk of progression to invasive cancer is higher for those who are older as well as for those who are immunosuppressed, such as transplant recipients. Chafe et al. studied 69 patients with a diagnosis of VIN treated by surgical excision. Unsuspected invasion was found in 13 patients. The median age was 36 years for those without invasive carcinoma, whereas the median age was 58 years ($p = .003$) for those with invasion found in the excision specimen, emphasizing the increased risk of invasion in the older patients. *Furthermore, the risk of invasion was higher in those who had raised lesions with irregular surface patterns.* Thus patients who were older and those with irregular raised lesions had the greatest risk of unrecognized invasive carcinoma. A recent study by Modesitt et al. of 73 patients of mean age 45 years found an invasive carcinoma in 22% of VIN III excision specimens. Not surprisingly the risk of recurrence was almost 50% if the margins were positive and only 17% if they were negative. A frequency of 20% invasive disease in 78 patients was also reported by Husseinzadeh and Recinto. Twelve of the 16 malignancies occurred in patients over age 40 years. The risk of progression from intraepithelial disease to invasive carcinoma appears to be less for vulvar cases than for cervical disease (Chapter 28).

Current evidence suggests that the potential of VIN to develop into invasive cancer is low. Buscema et al. followed 102 patients with vulvar carcinoma in situ for 1 to 15 years without treatment, and four patients developed invasive disease, two of whom were immunosuppressed. Unfortunately, current techniques do not allow precise prediction of which lesions of VIN are at the greatest risk for progression to invasive disease. A recent population-based study from Norway confirms an increasing frequency of VIN III that nearly tripled in frequency in that country from the mid-1970s to 1988-91. However, during the same period

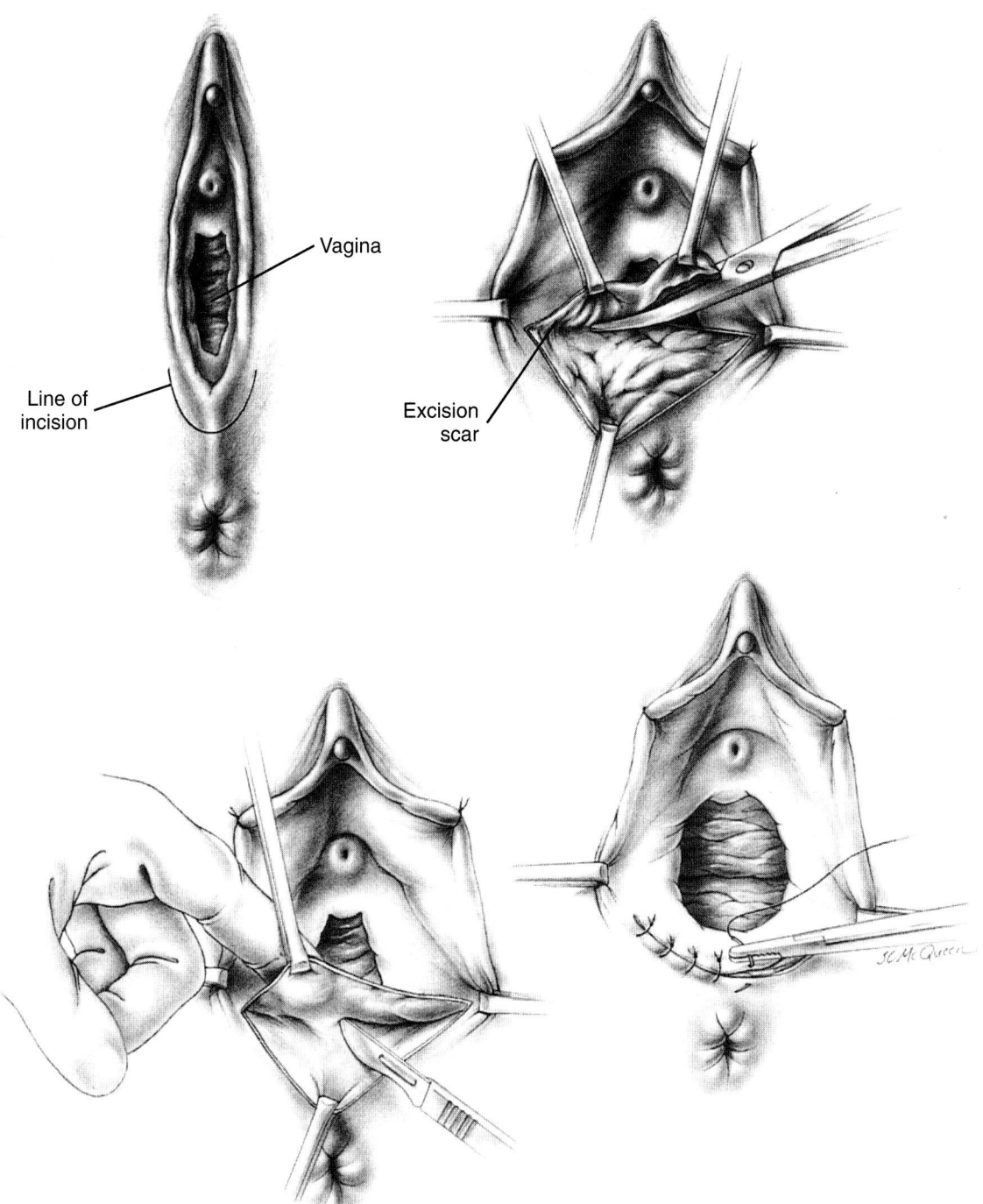

Vagina

Line of
incision

Excision
scar

FIGURE 32-11 Surgical correction of perineal scars. (From Woodruff JD and Julian CJ: Surgery of the vulva. In Ridley JH, ed: Gynecologic surgery: errors, safeguards, salvage, Baltimore, 1974, Williams & Wilkins Co.)

the age-adjusted frequency of invasive vulvar carcinomas remained virtually constant. Iversen and Tretli further noted an estimated conversion of VIN III to invasive carcinoma of about 3.4% for these in situ lesions. Jones et al. recently noted spontaneous regression of VIN 2-3 pigmented lesions in young women under age 30 years.

Currently HPV types 6 and 11 are generally recognized as being found most frequently in benign vulvar warts, whereas primarily HPV types 16, 18, 31, 33, and 35 are more frequently associated with intraepithelial neoplasia or invasive carcinoma (see Chapter 28). Crum has estimated that perineal warts develop in more than 1 million women per year in the United States, and perhaps as many as 10% of all women harbor HPV infection. An additional complication is that HPV type 16 infection is not always accompanied by histologic evidence of VIN.

Moreover, HPV types 6, 11, and 16 can be recovered from a single site, including those that show only condyloma, as well as those that show carcinoma. Thus a unique role for HPV types in VIN has not been elucidated. At the current state of our knowledge, therapy should be based on histologic findings and not on the presence or absence of HPV infection or specific HPV types. Studies by Buscema et al. suggest that HPV type 16 is frequently found in vulvar neoplasia, and as noted previously HPV 16 has been frequently associated with some vulvar carcinomas.

THERAPY. The problem of the management of vulvar HPV infection is particularly complicated, since it is extremely prevalent and the risk of progression from HPV infection to VIN is small. Planner et al. evaluated 148 women with cytologic evidence of vulvar HPV infection and found that two thirds of them had pruritus and dyspareunia. Results of the biopsy revealed that 11 of the 148 women had VIN. Follow-up showed spontaneous regression of HPV infection in 56 patients, whereas VIN III developed in 2 and invasive cancer eventually developed in 1. It appears that the best approach is to restrict therapy to individuals with clinically bothersome symptoms such as warts or to eradicate lesions with VIN, particularly VIN II and III. Cytologic or histologic evidence of an asymptomatic HPV infection, such as koilocytosis, is not an indication for therapy. Riva et al. treated lower genital tract HPV infection with laser to include the cervix, vagina, and vulva. Twenty-five patients had proven subclinical HPV infection, and the male partners were also evaluated and treated. All 25 patients suffered severe pain, and many required hospitalization. At 3 months after therapy, 24 of the 25 had evidence again of subclinical HPV infection and 22 had persistent histologic evidence of koilocytosis, indicating the futility of trying to eradicate HPV infection by this method.

Many lesions of intraepithelial neoplasia of the vulva tend to be posterior, predominantly in the perineal area. Surgical removal has been effectively used but the type of operation has changed in recent years. In the past, simple vulvectomy was widely practiced to treat carcinoma in situ of the vulva, but this disfiguring operation is now infrequently used, particularly since the disease is occurring in younger women. To improve the cosmetic result and sexual function, Rutledge and Sinclair introduced the method of "skinning vulvectomy." This removes the superficial vulvar skin, preserving the clitoris, and replaces the removed skin with a split-thickness vulvar graft. In many cases, however, such extensive surgery is not needed. Often the abnormal area of the vulva can be removed only with wide local excision. Sixty-two of the patients in the series reported by Buscema et al. were treated with local excision; 68% showed no recurrence. For comparison, in 28 patients treated by vulvectomy, 70% showed no recurrence. The risk of recurrence is higher if neoplastic epithelium is found at the resection margin. Friedrich noted a 10% risk of recurrence if the surgical margins were free of disease in comparison to a 50% risk if the surgical margins were involved with neoplasia. However, since recurrence may develop even if the resection margins are negative, long-term follow-up is mandatory.

The carbon dioxide laser has been utilized to treat VIN, usually to a depth of 1 to 3 mm, with deeper depth being used for areas that contain hair. This results in eradication of the abnormal vulvar tissue and healing without scarring. Most patients require a single treatment, but some patients require more, particularly those with large or multiple lesions. Usually patients can be treated on an outpatient basis with local, general, or regional anesthesia. The laser is particularly useful for younger patients. It is essential to be certain that the patient does not have invasive disease before utilizing the laser. Therefore the therapist should be experienced in the diagnosis and treatment of vulvar disease before utilizing laser ablation. Older patients or those with raised lesions should be treated by surgical excision. Treatment is usually carried out to a depth of 3 to 4 mm, and healing is usually complete within 2 to 3 weeks. Leuchter et al. treated 142 patients with carcinoma in situ of the vulva. Of the 42 treated by laser, 17% had recurrence; 4 (25%) of the 16 treated with vulvectomy and 15 (33%) of 45 treated by local excision also had recurrence. In view of the risk of unsuspected carcinoma in older patients as noted by the studies of Chafe et al., those over the age of 45 and those with raised or irregular lesions should have an excision performed and have the entire tissue submitted for histologic evaluation. Posterior lesions near the anus require particular attention, since often the anal canal is involved and this abnormal tissue also needs to be removed.

5-Fluorouracil (5-FU) cream has been tried to treat carcinoma in situ of the vulva, but it causes severe burning and is generally not utilized.

Paget's Disease of the Vulva

Paget's disease is generally seen in postmenopausal women and usually appears grossly as a diffuse erythematous eczematoid lesion that has usually been present for a prolonged time. Itching is a common problem. The disease is primarily seen in whites, and the average age of the patient is approximately 65 years. The major importance of Paget's disease of the vulva is the frequent association with other invasive carcinomas. Squamous carcinoma of the vulva or cervix or an adenocarcinoma of the sweat glands of the vulva or Bartholin's gland carcinoma may be present. Cases of adenocarcinoma of the gastrointestinal tract and breast accompanying Paget's disease have also been reported. Once a diagnosis of Paget's disease of the vulva is made, it is important for the gynecologist to rule out the presence of breast and GI malignancy. In a review by Lee et al. a total of 75 cases of Paget's disease of the vulva were identified, and an underlying invasive carcinoma of the adnexal structures of the skin was reported in only 16 (22%) and a carcinoma in situ in 7 (9%). Twenty-two of the patients (29%) had cancer at distant sites, including adenocarcinoma of the rectum, carcinoma of the breast, carcinoma of the urethra, basal cell carcinoma of the skin, and carcinoma of the cervix.

If no local or distant primary malignancy is uncovered, a wide excision of the affected area can be performed. It is important to remove the full thickness of the skin to the subcutaneous fat to be certain that all the skin adnexal structures are excised, as they may have a subclinical malignancy. Bergen et al. evaluated 14 patients with Paget's disease of the vulva treated by operation, usually vulvectomy, skinning vulvectomy with graft, or hemivulvectomy. With a median follow-up of 50 months, all patients were free of disease, although two with positive margins and one with negative margins required treatment for recurrence. Fishman et al. studied 14 patients treated by various surgical procedures for Paget's disease. Either frozen section or gross visual inspection was utilized to judge the operative margins. In this series, visual estimation was as useful as frozen section insofar as the error rate for judging margins by the final pathology report was approximately 35%. In addition, two of five patients with positive margins recurred after initial operation compared with three of nine with negative margins. This small series, therefore, suggests that gross visual inspection may be as useful as frozen section when judg-

ing the extent of surgical operation. A conservative approach involving removal of gross Paget's disease with approximately a 1-cm margin appears to be most appropriate, with the understanding that re-excision may be required for recurrence in the future. The full thickness of the vulvar skin to the adipose layer should be removed.

Even if resection margins are free of Paget's disease at the time of surgical excision, local recurrence remains a risk. Women who have been treated for Paget's disease of the vulva should have as part of their routine follow-up annual examination of the breast, cytologic evaluation of the cervix and vulva, and screening for gastrointestinal disease at least by testing for occult blood in the stool. Progression of Paget's disease of the vulva to invasive adenocarcinoma has been rarely reported.

MALIGNANT CONDITIONS

Squamous Cell Carcinoma

Squamous cell carcinomas comprise approximately 90% of primary vulvar malignancies, but a variety of other vulvar cancers are encountered; the primary ones are listed in the box on this page. Melanomas account for about 4% to 5% and the other types for the remainder.

TNM* and Staging Classifications of Carcinoma of the Vulva

TNM

T primary tumor

Tis	Preinvasive carcinoma (carcinoma in situ)
T 1	Tumor confined to the vulva and/or perineum—2 cm or less in diameter
T 2	Tumor confined to the vulva and/or perineum—more than 2 cm in diameter
T 3	Tumor of any size with adjacent spread to the urethra, vagina, anus or all of these
T 4	Tumor of any size infiltrating the bladder mucosa or the rectal mucosa or both, including the upper part of the urethral mucosa or fixed to the anus

N regional lymph nodes

N 0	No nodes palpable
N 1	Unilateral regional lymph node metastases
N 2	Bilateral regional lymph node metastases

M distant metastases

M 0	No clinical metastases
M 1	Distant metastases (including pelvic lymph node metastases)

Staging (FIGO)† Modified 1994

Stage 0	Tis	Carcinoma in situ; intraepithelial carcinoma
Stage I	T1 N0 M0	Tumor confined to the vulva and/or perineum—2 cm or less in greatest dimension. No nodal metastases.
	IA invasion 1 mm or less	
	IB invasion >1 mm	
Stage II	T2 N0 M0	Tumor confined to the vulva and/or perineum—more than 2 cm in greatest dimension. No nodal metastases.
Stage III	T3 N0 M0	Tumor of any size with the following:
	T3 N1 M0 (1)	Adjacent spread to the lower urethra, the vagina, the anus, and/or the following:
	T1 N1 M0 (2)	
	T2 N1 M0	Unilateral regional lymph node metastases
Stage IVA	T1 N2 M0	Tumor invades any of the following:
	T2 N2 M0	
	T3 N2 M0	
	T4 any N M0	Upper urethra, bladder mucosa, rectal mucosa, pelvic bone, and/or bilateral regional node metastases
Stage IVB any T, any N, M1		Any distant metastases, including pelvic lymph nodes.

Modified from Shepherd JH: Int J Gynecol Cancer 5:319, 1995.
*TNM = Tumor—Nodes—Metastases.
†FIGO = International Federation of Gynecology and Obstetrics.

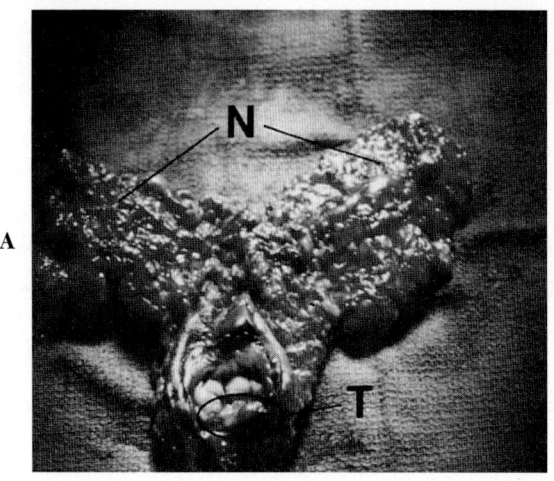

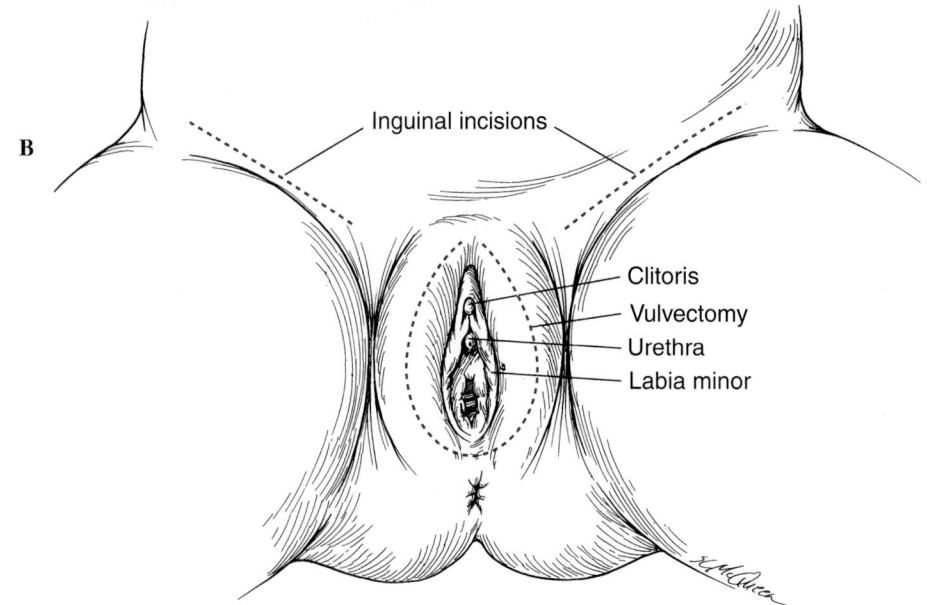

FIGURE 32-12   **A,** Radical vulvectomy specimen. **B,** Vulvectomy with operative incision lines shown. Note groin incisions.

Primary Vulvar Malignancies

Squamous cell carcinoma
Adenocarcinoma (including Bartholin's gland)
Verrucous carcinoma
Basal cell carcinoma
Melanoma
Sarcoma

Morphology and Staging

Grossly, vulvar carcinomas usually appear as polypoid masses on the vulva (Figure 32-12, *A*). Biopsy of the lesion reveals the characteristic histologic appearance of squamous cell carcinoma (Figure 32-6, *C*).

Four clinical stages are defined for carcinoma of the vulva according to the International Federation of Gyne-

cology and Obstetrics (FIGO), similar to the system used for other gynecologic malignancies. In addition, many centers use the T (tumor), N (nodes), M (metastases) classification; T denotes the size and extent of the tumor, N the clinical status of the nodes, and M the presence or absence of metastatic disease.

In 1988 the FIGO staging was modified to reflect lymph node status, as well as location of the tumor on the vulva. A location on the perineum is no longer allotted to stage III. This system with the modifications introduced in 1994 for stages IA and IB is shown in the box on p. 1009.

Natural History, Spread, and Prognostic Factors

The vulvar area is rich in lymphatics with numerous cross connections. The main lymphatic pathways are illustrated in Figure 32-13. Tumors located in the mid-

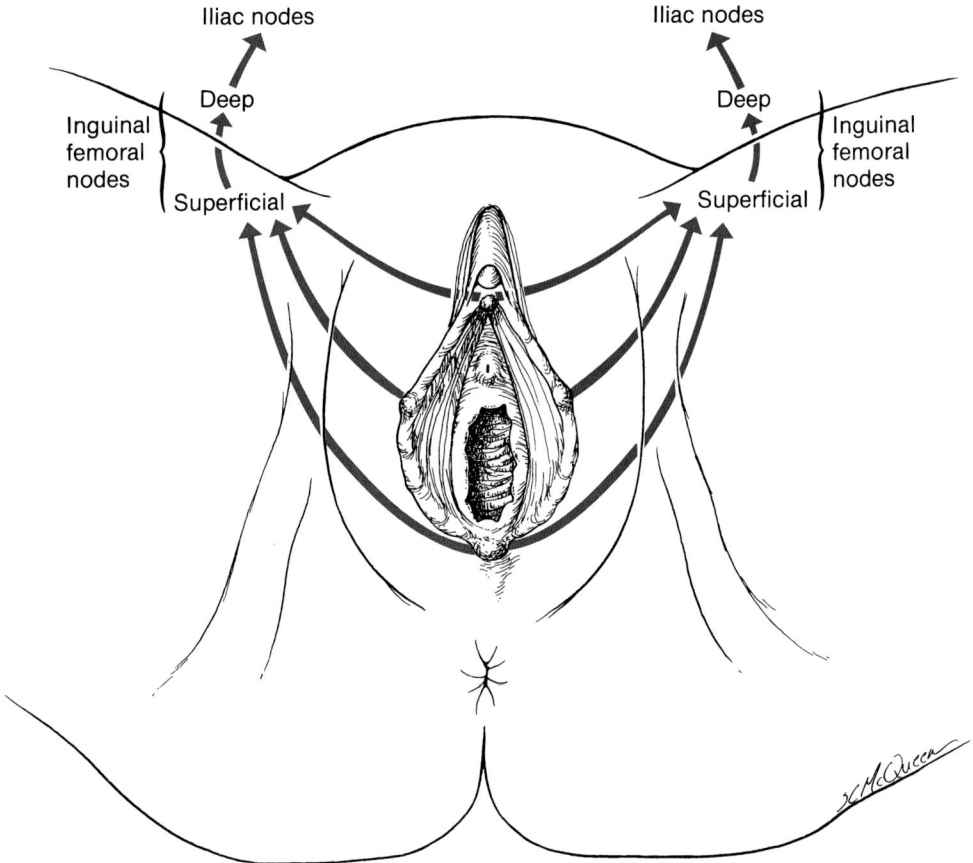

FIGURE 32-13   Vulva lymph drainage. General schematic representation of major drainage channels of vulva.

dle of either labium tend to drain initially to the ipsilateral femoral-inguinal nodes, whereas perineal tumors can spread to either the left or the right side. Tumors in the clitoral or urethral areas can also spread to either side. From the inguinal-femoral nodes, the lymphatic spread of tumor is cephalad to the deep pelvic iliac and obturator nodes. Although there has been concern in the past that tumors in the clitoral-urethral area would spread directly to the deep pelvic nodes, this rarely, if ever, occurs. The characteristics of lymph drainage of the vulva were evaluated by Iverson and Aas, who injected ^{99m}Tc-colloid subcutaneously into the anterior and posterior labia majora, anterior and posterior labia minora, clitoral area, and perineum. They then measured the radioactivity in the pelvic lymph nodes, which were surgically removed 5 hours later. Over 98% of the radioactivity was found in the ipsilateral node and less than 2% on the contralateral side. The anterior labial injections resulted in 92% concentration of radioactivity in the ipsilateral side with 8% on the contralateral side. The clitoral and perineal injections developed a bilateral nodal distribution of radioactivity in all the patients. It is of interest that two thirds of the patients with labial injections had a small amount of detectable radioactivity in the contralateral nodes. Thus anastomoses of the lymphatics do exist,

but a direct connection from the clitoris to the deep nodes was not demonstrated.

The prognosis of a patient with vulvar carcinoma is related to the stage of the disease (Figure 32-14), lesion size, as well as the presence or absence of cancer in regional nodes. The worldwide actuarial 5-year survival results from the *23rd FIGO Annual Report on the Results of Treatment of Gynaecologic Cancer* are stage I, 71.4%; stage II, 61.3%; stage III, 43.8%; and stage IV, 8.3%. The presence of carcinoma in regional lymph nodes correlates with the size of the primary lesion, the degree of tumor differentiation, and the extent of involvement of vascular spaces by tumor. Tumor size is usually estimated by the greatest tumor diameter; for example, ≤2 cm or >2 cm separates stage I from stage II disease.

The status of the regional lymph nodes is important prognostically, as well as therapeutically. Numerous studies, including a multicenter collaborative investigation from the Gynecologic Oncology Group (GOG), indicate that tumor stage, location on the vulva, microscopic differentiation, presence or absence of vascular space involvement, and tumor thickness are all important prognostic factors. In a GOG study of 588 patients reported by Homesley et al., the risk of lymph node metastases was

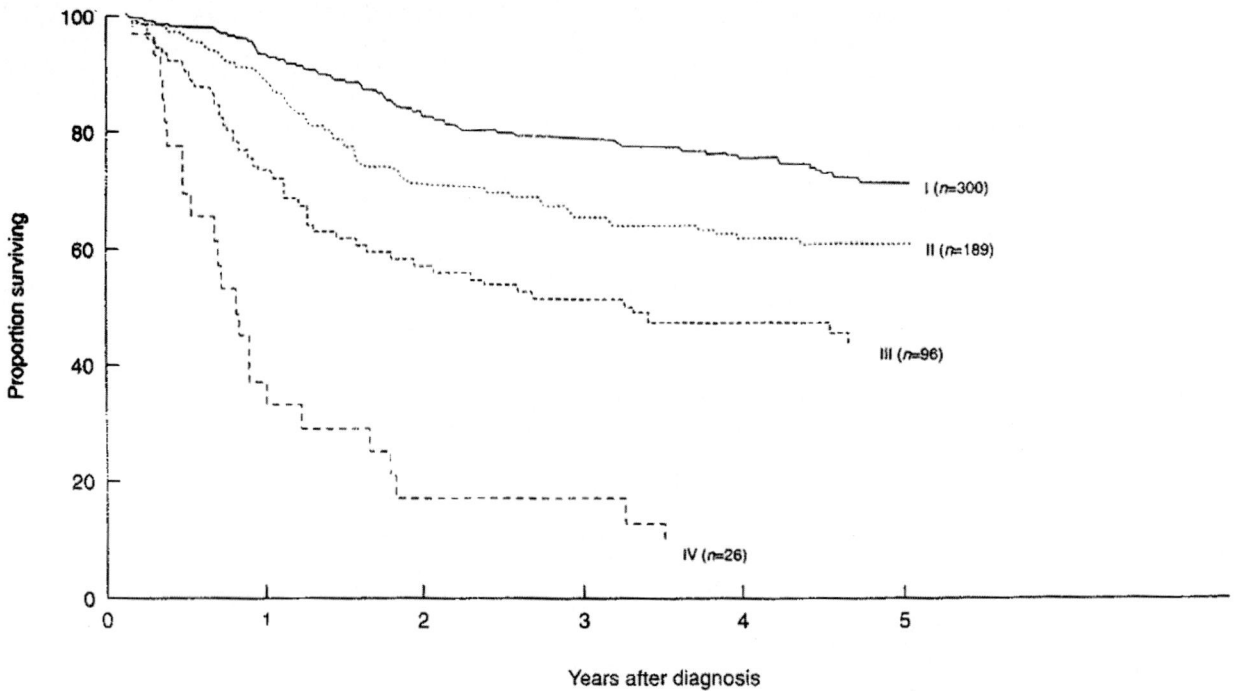

Strata	Patients (n)	Mean age (years)	Overall survival at					Hazards ratio[a] (95% Confidence Intervals)
			1 year	2 years	3 years	4 years	5 years	
I	300	64.7	92.3%	82.3%	78.7%	75.7%	71.4%	Reference
II	189	67.4	86.5%	71.0%	65.8%	62.2%	61.3%	1.94 (1.36–2.75)
III	96	69.4	72.0%	57.2%	51.3%	47.5%	43.8%	3.84 (2.55–5.78)
IV	26	72.8	33.3%	16.7%	16.7%	8.3%	8.3%	12.2 (7.08–21.2)

[a]Hazards ratio and 95% Confidence Intervals obtained from a Cox model adjusted for country.

FIGURE 32-14 Carcinoma of the vulva: Patients treated in 1990-92. Survival by FIGO stage (epidermoid invasive cancer only) n = 611. (From Pecorelli S, Creasman WT, Pettersson F, et al: FIGO annual report on the results of treatment in gynaecological cancer, vol 23, Milano, Italy. Epidemiol Biostat, 1998.)

related to lesion size (19% ≤ 2 cm and 42% > 2 cm). Additional independent predictors of positive nodes were (1) tumor de-differentiation; (2) suspicious, fixed, or ulcerated lymph nodes; (3) capillary-lymphatic space involvement; (4) older age of the patient; and (5) tumor thickness. Table 32-1 summarizes these factors.

Perineural invasion also appears to be a factor in vulvar tumors as it is in cervical carcinoma (Chapter 28). In a small study of 22 patients Rowley et al. noted no metastases in 20 patients without perineural invasion and in 2 of 2 patients with perineural invasion.

In assessing the patient, the clinician's evaluation of the regional nodes can be a factor in the choice of therapy. In the GOG study, if the nodes were not palpable and were considered normal by the clinician, 23.9% of cases were found to have positive nodes, whereas the figure rose to 76% for those with suspicious nodes and 92.6% for clini-

cally fixed or ulcerated nodes. Because the FIGO staging system of carcinoma of the vulva (see box on p. 000) includes the morphologic status of the regional nodes, it is helpful in treatment planning to confirm the status of the nodes with fine-needle aspiration. Using this technique, Crosby et al. found no false positive and only two false negative results among 34 patients evaluated, 19 of whom had positive and 15 negative cytologic fine-needle aspirations, indicating that the technique can be highly useful.

Stage IA: Carcinoma of the Vulva (Early or Microinvasive Carcinoma)

DEFINITION AND CLINICAL-PATHOLOGIC RELATIONSHIPS. The term *microinvasive carcinoma of the vulva* has no uniformly accepted definition. Most therapists would use the stage IA definition, that is, <2 cm with ≤1 mm invasion to

TABLE 32-1
Factors Related to Positive Inguinal Nodes (588 Cases)

GOG Grade	% Positive Nodes	Tumor Thick (mm)	% Positive Nodes	Age (Yrs)	% Positive Nodes	C-L Space Involve	% Positive Nodes
1	2.8	≤1	2.6	<55	25.2	+	75
2	15.1	2	8.9	55–64	25.4	−	27
3	41.2	3	18.6	65–74	36.4		
4	59.7	4	30.9	>75	46		
		≥5	43				

Modified from Homesley H, Bundy BN, Sedlis A, et al: Gynecol Oncol 49:279, 1993.

identify early tumors unlikely to spread to regional nodes. However, varying clinico-pathologic results are reported when this definition is used.

Part of the confusion is due to different reference points from which the depth of invasion is measured, that is, from the surface or basement membrane. Dvoretsky et al. carefully analyzed the microscopic aspects of 36 cases of superficial vulvar carcinoma. Tumor penetration into the stroma was measured from the surface of the squamous epithelium (neoplastic thickness) (Figure 32-15, *A*) and also from the tip of the adjacent epithelial ridge (stromal invasion) (Figure 32-15, *B*). Six of the 36 cases had spread to regional nodes, and all had invaded over 3 mm from the surface. Kneale et al. have pointed out that although there is almost no risk of metastases to regional nodes in stage IA lesions, late recurrence of these tumors can develop years after primary therapy, and in a literature review, eight instances of recurrence were reported in 88 cases of superficial vulvar carcinoma. All tumors were less than 2 cm diameter and invaded less than 1 mm into the stroma measured from the adjacent rete peg, which would approximately correspond to 3 mm measured from the surface, since the vulvar epithelium is about 2 mm thick.

The presence of carcinoma in situ in the primary lesion decreases the risk of node involvement in these cases. Ross and Ehrman noted only 1 of 35 cases with adjacent CIS had nodal metastases, and this tumor penetrated into the stroma 1.7 mm. In contrast, 5 of 27 cases of superficial stage I cases (2.1 to 5.0 mm penetration) without adjacent CIS had positive nodes. Thus spread to regional nodes is unlikely, particularly if the tumor is well differentiated (grade 1), invades less than 3 mm measured from the surface or has a depth of invasion measured from the adjacent rete pegs of less than 1 mm, and is without vascular space involvement. The presence of carcinoma in situ is a favorable factor. Less well-differentiated tumors or those with vascular involvement or confluence and with greater depths of invasion have an increased risk of lymph node involvement by cancer.

MANAGEMENT. Based on available evidence, it would appear prudent that most patients with stage IA carcinoma of the vulva by the criteria previously described should be treated at least with a wide excision to give a margin of 1 to 2 cm. Depending on the location of the tumor, a hemivulvectomy may be needed. The lymph node dissection may be omitted or deferred depending on the final pathologic evaluation of the tumor in the surgical specimen. For younger patients, especially with tumors that involve either the labia or the perineum at a distance from the clitoris, an operation that spares the clitoris should be utilized. Even if the criteria for stage IA is rigorously applied, a rare nodal metastasis may occur, as reported by Van der Velden. However, a recent report by Magrina et al. on 40 patients with T1 lesions (less than 2 cm in diameter) and less than 1 mm invasion could be effectively treated with wide excision. No nodal metastases were noted in this small group, and excision appeared to be as effective as more radical operation in preventing recurrent disease.

Invasive Carcinoma of the Vulva

Figure 32-12, *A* shows a typical carcinoma of the vulva, which usually appears as a polyploid mass. The patient frequently complains of a "sore" that has not healed. The patient may also complain of bleeding, but this does not usually occur early in the course of the disease. Unfortunately, the delay in diagnosis is common because older patients frequently fail to seek prompt medical attention, and often, when they do, a biopsy is not initially performed. For example, some patients have their symptoms of irritation or itching treated with various medications to eradicate the symptoms. It is vital that a biopsy be taken of any vulvar lesion before undertaking therapy, as was emphasized earlier. A biopsy of a tumor like that shown in Figure 32-12, *A* can easily be obtained on an outpatient basis utilizing local anesthesia and biopsy forceps, for example, a Kevorkian punch as illustrated in Chapter 28.

Effective therapy of stage I or II and early stage III vulvar carcinoma can be accomplished with a radical vulvec-

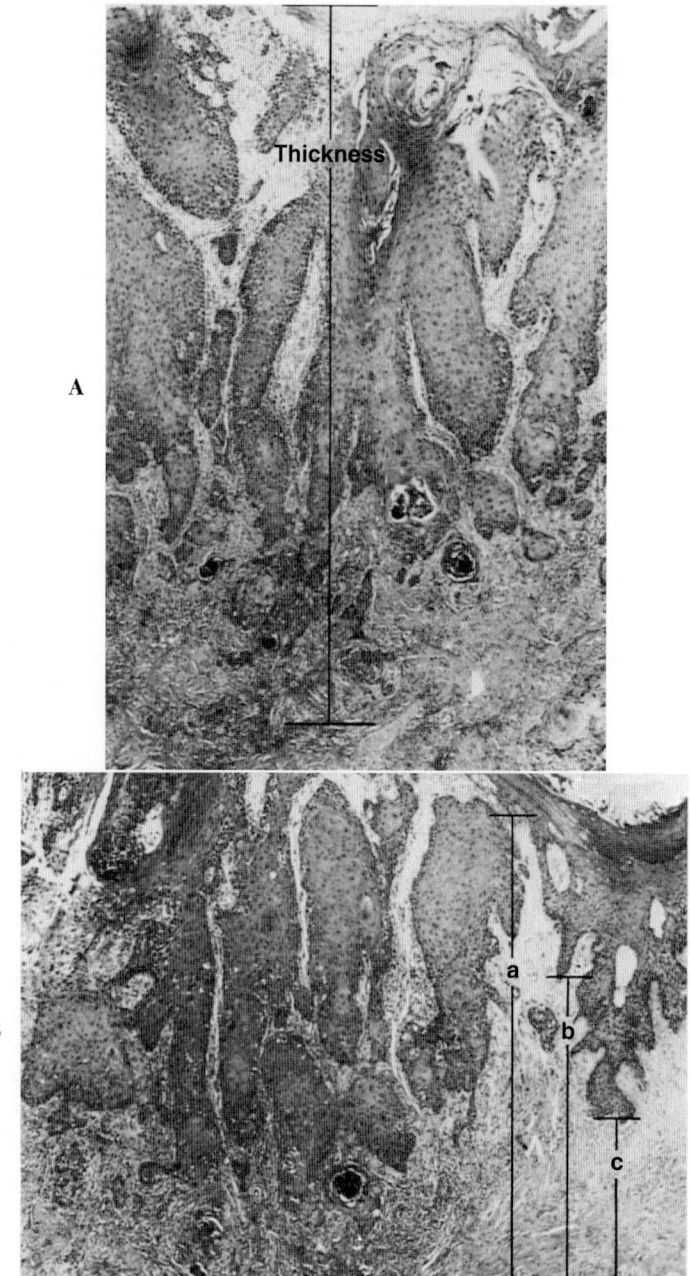

FIGURE 32-15   A, Measurement of neoplastic thickness in squamous cell carcinoma. (×35.) **B,** Superficially invasive squamous cell carcinoma. Reference point used to measure depth of stromal invasion is demonstrated by line *b*. Note striking variation in measurement of stromal invasion, depending on which reference point is chosen (line *a, b,* or *c*). (×35.) (From Dvoretsky PM, Bonfiglio TA, Helkamp BF, et al: The pathology of superficially invasive thin vulva squamous cell carcinoma, Int J Gynecol Pathol 3:331, 1984.)

tomy and bilateral inguinal-femoral node dissection. Because the deep pelvic nodes are virtually never involved unless the inguinal nodes are also involved, only the inguinal femoral nodes are removed at the time of primary operation and the deep pelvic nodes subsequently treated with external radiation if the superficial nodes are involved with tumor. The radical vulvectomy is usually tailored to remove the affected area. For example, in the case of a mid-labial lesion, a hemivulvectomy is often sufficient, while for a lesion away from the clitoris, the operation usually can spare that organ, particularly in younger patients.

Usually the inguinal-femoral node dissection is performed through separate inguinal incisions followed by the vulvectomy portion. Figure 32-12, *A* shows the type of specimen that can be obtained through separate groin

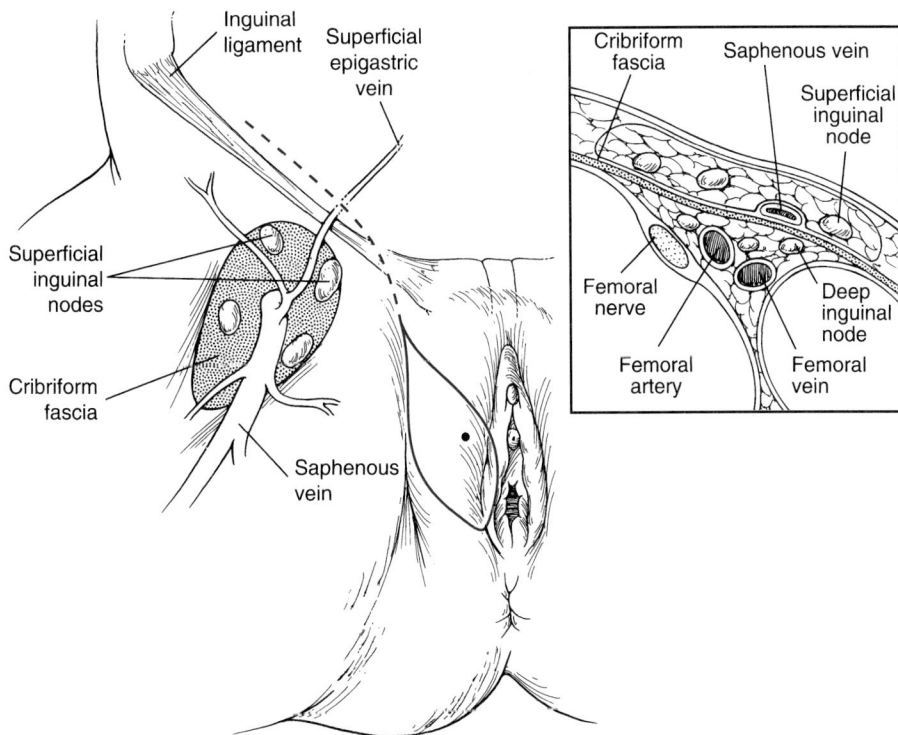

FIGURE 32-16 Early vulvar cancer. Wide local excision with ipsilateral superficial lymph node dissection. Lymph nodes removed are above cribriform fascia. (From Rowley KC, Gallion HH, Donaldson ES, et al: Gynecol Oncol 31:43, 1988.)

incisions. The operative incisions are shown in Figure 32-12, *B*. It appears that an adequate surgical dissection with decreased wound complications can be accomplished by this technique. It is advisable to use suction drainage in the inguinal area until all drainage is complete, which usually takes 7 to 10 days, and drains are frequently also used in the vulvar area. It is important that an adequate margin, usually 2 to 3 cm, be obtained around the primary tumor at the time of surgery. Grimshaw et al. reported on 100 cases operated through separate incisions and noted superb results with a corrected 5-year survival in stage I of 96.7% and stage II of 85%. Similar excellent results for separate skin incisions were reported by Farias-Eisner et al. on 74 patients with 5-year survivals of 97% and 90% for stages I and II, respectively. Tumor recurrence has occurred rarely in the skin bridge over the symphysis when separate groin incisions are used, without an en bloc dissection of the vulva and intervening lymph tissue. Magrina et al. noted comparable survivals with fewer complications in those undergoing modified radical vulvectomy with inguinal incisions done separately.

To lessen extensive and mutilating procedures, particularly in stage I cases, modifications have been introduced in recent years. Rowley et al. performed wide local excision and superficial inguinal dissection for 20 patients with stage I lesions and a depth of invasion less than 5 mm. The operative technique is illustrated in Figure 32-16. The deep inguinal nodes are removed only if the superficial nodes contain tumor, and in this case the contralateral inguinal-femoral nodes are also dissected. The unilateral approach is most appropriate for labial lesions, but bilateral inguinal node dissections must be performed for lesions near the midline. The approach appears effective and is accompanied by less morbidity than radical vulvectomy. Stehman et al. reported a GOG study of 121 stage I evaluable patients with tumor invasion less than 5 mm. The patients were treated by modified radical vulvectomy and ipsilateral node dissection. In this group there were 19 recurrences and 7 deaths, with 5 of the 7 deaths among those whose initial recurrence was in the groin nodes.

In treating stage I and stage II tumors of the vulva, the results of histologic evaluation of the inguinal-femoral nodes are important. Many therapists initially treat the superficial nodes above the cribriform fascia (Figure 32-17). If these nodes are negative, the deep nodes are spared. The procedure can be accomplished even occasionally with preservation of the saphenous vein, which has traditionally been sacrificed. However, while these modifications reduce the risk of leg edema, long-term follow-up regarding recurrences currently is not available. If the lymph nodes, particularly the upper femoral group, are involved with tumor, the deep pelvic nodes require treatment. Homesley et al. reported improved survival for those who received radiation (4500 to 5000 rads) to the deep pelvic nodes in comparison with those who had a pelvic node dissection.

The results of therapy in stage I and II disease relate not only to the stage of the disease but also to the status of the regional pelvic nodes. If the nodes do not contain metastatic tumor and the patient can be successfully treated by radical vulvectomy and bilateral node dissection, 5-year survivals of about 95% are reported. Iverson et al. in a series of 424 patients noted lymph node metastasis in 10.5% of stage I cases, 30% of stage II, 66% of stage III, and 100% of stage IV. The number of positive nodes in the radical vulvectomy specimen correlates with the size of the primary tumor and also with the patient's survival. Andrews et al. noted in a study of T_1 and T_2 tumors that only unilateral inguinal node metastases occurred, and furthermore, the deep nodes were involved only if the superficial nodes were positive. However, there is a small (2% to 3%) risk of contralateral node involvement for the larger T_2 lesions. In a study of 113 patients, Hacker et al. noted an actuarial 5-year survival of 96% for those with negative nodes, but there was a progressive fall in survival to 94% for those having one positive node; 80% for two positive nodes; and 12% for three or more positive nodes. In various cases that have been studied, the deep pelvic nodes do not contain tumor unless the upper inguinal-femoral nodes contain metastatic disease. The number of nodes involved as well as the size of the metastasis are both important. Hoffman et al. noted that 14 of 15 patients with inguinal lymph node metastasis measuring less than 36 mm^2 survived free of disease 5 years in comparison to 12 of 29 whose lymph node metastases measured more than 100 mm^2. These results should be taken into consideration when planning additional therapy for patients with positive nodes.

If tumor spread to the regional inguinal-femoral nodes is identified, further treatment should be considered. If only one node is microscopically involved with tumor, usually no further therapy is needed particularly if only a small volume is present. However, if three or more nodes are involved, pelvic radiation as outlined is usually prescribed. For patients with only two nodes involved, the decision for further therapy will depend on the location of the nodes and the size of the metastatic deposit of tumor, although many therapists would opt for radiotherapy in such cases.

Advanced Vulvar Tumors

Large tumors of the vulva, particularly those that encroach on the anal-rectal area or the urethra, require more extensive treatment than radical vulvectomy to achieve effective tumor control. In such instances, removal of the anus or urethra is necessary as part of a primary operative procedure, in which case diversion of the urinary or fecal stream is required (see discussion of exenterative surgery for carcinoma of the cervix, Chapter 29).

A useful therapeutic approach has been to treat large vulvar tumors with external radiation and then after the tumor has been reduced in size, remove the residual tumor surgically, usually by radical vulvectomy. External radiation is used to deliver approximately 4000 cGy to the tumor and 4500 cGy to the pelvis and inguinal nodes. Operation is usually performed about 5 weeks after the completion of radiation therapy. Although a large series of patients has not been treated by this technique, a sufficient number have been treated to demonstrate that marked tumor regression does occur. The primary cancer can be eradicated by an operation that does not require diversion of the urine or feces. Boronow initially summarized the treatment of 26 patients with primary carcinoma of the vaginal vulvar area with this technique and noted a 5-year survival of 80%. Rotmensch et al. reported on 16 patients, 13 stage III and 3 stage IV, and achieved an overall 5-year survival of 45% with this technique, somewhat better than might be expected with stage III-IV (see Figure 32-14). Recurrences are more likely if the resection margins were within 1 cm of the tumor. The introduction of chemotherapy with radiation appears to offer therapeutic advantage. Koh et al. studied 20 patients with stages III to IV disease, and 3 with recurrence, utilizing 5-FU with radiation. In addition, some patients also received cisplatin with concurrent radiotherapy. Actuarial 3- and 5-year survival rates in this small group were 59% and 49%, respectively. Similar results with 5-FU and radiation, occasionally with the addition of cisplatinum, in 25 patients was also reported by Russell et al. Moore et al. reported on a phase II GOG study and noted the need for less extensive operation when chemotherapy with cisplatin and 5-FU were combined with preoperative radiation. Multiple chemoradiation programs are available, but a convenient outpatient regimen consists of weekly cisplatin 50 mg/m^2 IV with radiation usually to 4500 cGy. Other complications reported include stenosis of the introitus, urethral stenosis, and rectovaginal fistula, but this technique is an effective alternative to primary exenteration for large vulvar vaginal carcinomas and is preferred in most treatment centers although success with exenteration can occasionally be achieved, as noted by Miller et al.

Radiation Therapy and Recurrences

In a few instances the medical condition of the patient precludes operation, and radiation therapy may be employed as the sole treatment. However, the vulvar skin is prone to radiation dermatitis fibrosis and ulceration, making irradiation, as the sole form of therapy, a less desirable treatment. Therefore irradiation is seldom used as the sole treatment of carcinoma of the vulva. To manage recurrences, reoperation is often tried. Piura et al. analyzed 73 patients whose disease recurred only on the vulva. Salvage was achieved with wide radical local excision, which appeared to be successful in 30 of the patients who recurred only on the vulva.

As may be expected, the risk of recurring carcinoma rises as the stage of the disease increases. Podratz et al. in an analysis of 224 patients with vulvar carcinoma noted a recurrence rate of 14% in stage I and 71% in stage IV. Local vulvar recurrences were the most common and occurred in 40 of 74 cases of recurrence (54%). The remaining recurrences were in the groin, pelvis, or distant sites. Radiation therapy or additional operations for local vulvar recurrences usually provide effective control and 5-year survivals of approximately 50%. The risk of recurrence of the disease in the vulva requires careful attention to the surgical resection margins at the time of initial operation.

Combined use of chemotherapy and radiation has been utilized for primary treatment of late-stage advanced vulvar tumors as previously described. It has also been applied to recurrences, especially those near the anus and/or urethra. Radiation alone may also be used for vulvar recurrences as reported by Perez et al., although chemoradiation would appear to be a more effective choice.

Treatment of patients with disseminated disease requires chemotherapy but, unfortunately, no chemotherapeutic regimen has been very successful in this disease. Squamous cell carcinomas of the female genital tract have generally not been responsive to cytotoxic chemotherapy, and the protocols followed are similar to those described for recurrent squamous cell carcinomas of the cervix (Chapter 29).

Other Vulvar Malignancies

Bartholin's Gland Carcinoma

These are adenocarcinomas which comprise about 1% to 2% of vulvar carcinomas. An enlargement of Bartholin's gland in a postmenopausal patient should raise suspicion for this malignancy. These tumors are treated similarly to primary squamous cell carcinoma of the vulva, and radical vulvectomy with bilateral inguinal-femoral lymphadenectomy is the treatment of choice. If the regional lymph nodes are free of tumor, the prognosis is good. Rosenberg has reported on five cases of adenoid cystic carcinoma of Bartholin's gland treated by operation (usually hemivulvectomy) and postoperative irradiation. Four of the five patients were living and free of disease 28 to 57 months after treatment.

Basal Cell Carcinoma

Basal cell carcinomas can arise in the vulva as they can arise in the skin elsewhere in the body. They are rare and comprise about 2% of vulvar carcinomas. Therapy consists of wide local excision of the lesion, which is generally ulcerated. If the surgical resection margins are free of tumor, the disease is cured.

Verrucous Carcinoma

Verrucous carcinomas of the vulva are also rare. They are a special variant of squamous cell cancer with distinctive histologic features. Clinically they appear as a large condylomatous mass on the vulva. Histologically they consist of mature squamous cells and extensive keratinization with nests that invade the underlying vulvar tissue. It is often necessary to perform multiple biopsies of the condylomatous lesion to establish a diagnosis of malignancy. Radiation therapy is ineffective and can worsen the prognosis by causing anaplastic change in the tumor and is therefore contraindicated. The treatment of an authentic verrucous carcinoma is wide excision.

In 24 cases of verrucous carcinoma Japaze et al. noted no lymph node metastases. Some of the primary tumors were as large as 10 cm in diameter. Recurrences developed in nine of the patients, five of whom had prior irradiation. Wide local excision is effective therapy. Depending on the size and location of the tumor, simple vulvectomy may be needed, but a radical vulvectomy or inguinal node dissection is not indicated. The 17 cases treated surgically and reported by Japaze et al. had a 5-year survival of 94%. As noted by Crowther et al., it is important to take a large biopsy specimen to establish the diagnosis. This is particularly important when dealing with a malignant-appearing tumor from a biopsy specimen that has been reported as benign. This can lead to incorrect therapy for "condyloma acuminatum." Conversely, too shallow a biopsy may fail to show areas of squamous cell carcinoma that can coexist with verrucous carcinoma. However, in the presence of areas of squamous cell carcinoma, local excision is inadequate therapy. Verrucous tumors with squamous cell carcinoma elements can metastasize to regional nodes, and such tumors should not be treated as true verrucous carcinomas.

Melanoma

Melanoma is the most frequent nonsquamous cell malignancy of the vulva. It comprises about 5% of primary cancers of this area. As is true elsewhere in the body, melanomas arise from junctional or compound nevi. Pigmented lesions of the vulva are usually junctional nevi, and all such lesions should be removed by excision.

Patients with malignant melanoma of the vulva vary widely in age from the late teens to women in their 80s. The average age is approximately 50 years. Clinically, melanomas appear as brown, black, or blue-black masses on the vulva. The lesion can be flat or ulcerated. Occasionally it is nodular, and small, darkly pigmented areas (satellite nodules) may surround the primary lesion. Some melanomas may be without pigment and can grossly resemble squamous cell carcinoma of the vulva. Most melanomas of the vulva occur on the labia minora or the clitoris (Figure 32-17).

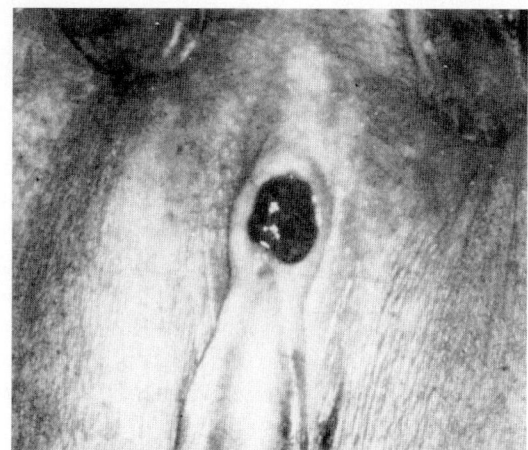

FIGURE 32-17 Nodular melanoma arising directly from glans clitoris. (Courtesy J McL. Morris, M.D., deceased, Yale University School of Medicine, New Haven, Conn.)

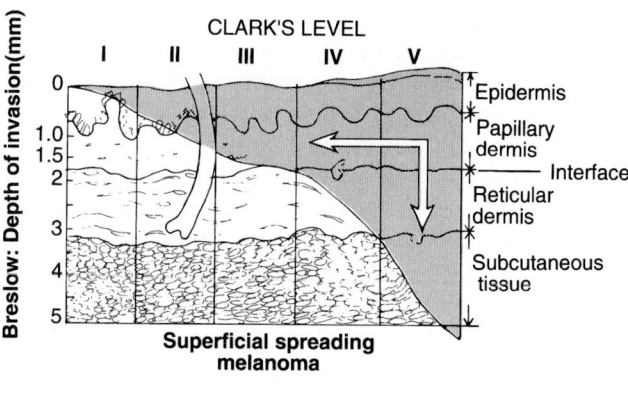

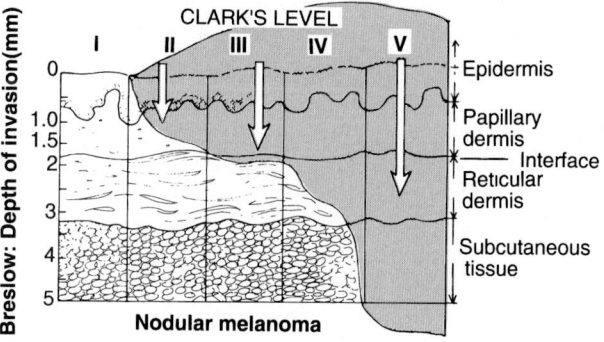

FIGURE 32-18 Level of invasion for superficial spreading melanoma and nodular melanoma. (From Podratz KC, Gaffey TA, Symmonds RE, et al: Gynecol Oncol 16:153, 1983.)

Vulvar melanomas if staged, use the same FIGO classification employed for squamous carcinomas (see box, p. 1009). However, staging is not as useful a prognostic indicator as is the depth of invasion. A system for vulvar melanoma analogous to that used by Clark for cutaneous melanomas has been adopted. Five levels (I to V) have been defined based on the Clark classification. Figure 32-18 shows the depth of invasion for each level of superficial spreading melanoma and nodular melanoma, the two most common varieties of melanomas that occur on the vulva. Superficial spreading melanoma is more common and fortunately has a better prognosis, with a 5-year survival of 71% reported in the series by Podratz et al. The 5-year survival for nodular melanoma, which is more invasive, was only 38%. The level of invasion correlates with survival, which varies from 100% for level II, to 83% for level IV, to 28% for level V.

Tumor thickness is also useful to evaluate the tumor. Breslow reported that overall prognosis is excellent, and spread to regional node is not likely for melanomas whose thickness measured from the surface epithelium to the deepest point of penetration is less than 0.76 mm. Most of these lesions would correspond to level I or level II penetration by the modified Clark system. Stefanon et al., in a study of 28 patients, noted no lymph node metastasis if melanoma thickness was less than 3 mm and the 5-year survival in this group was 50% in comparison with 25% for those whose melanomas were more than 3 mm thick. In a comprehensive long-term study of 219 Swedish females, Ragnarsson-Olding et al. noted that tumor thickness and ulceration were prognostic factors. In addition, gross amelanosis and advanced age worsened the prognosis. The authors further noted that amelanotic tumors were seen in about one fourth of the patients and that overall the

vulvar melanomas were about 2.5 times more frequent than cutaneous melanomas. A preexisting nevus was not necessary and de novo melanoma development does appear to occur on the vulva, particularly in the glabrous (hairless) skin.

The standard therapy for vulvar melanoma is a wide excision of the primary tumor. Because the tumors are rare, a large clinical experience is not available. It was believed that melanoma of the vulva could metastasize to pelvic nodes, bypassing the inguinal femoral nodes; current evidence indicates that there is no pelvic node involvement without prior inguinal node involvement. A further therapeutic consideration is that patients with melanoma whose pelvic nodes are involved with tumor usually do not survive the disease.

Excision margins have been extensively studied for cutaneous melanomas. Veronesi et al. found that cutaneous melanomas less than 2 mm thick could be adequately treated with a 1 cm margin, which was as effective as a 3 cm margin for these thin lesions. Although comparable data do not exist for vulvar melanomas, the data from cutaneous melanomas suggest that a 1 cm margin could be used for very thin vulvar melanomas. In a report of 36 melanoma cases, Rose et al. noted that wide excision was as effective as radical vulvectomy. They noted that the prognosis was improved in younger patients, presumably because most of them had superficial spreading (good prognosis) rather than nodular (poor prognosis) melanomas. Although firm recommendations from available data are not possible, a reasonable approach would be to excise a melanoma with a 2 cm margin without node dissection for tumors that are less than 0.76 mm thick. An excision with a 2 to 3 cm margin combined with node dissection would be carried out for more advanced melanomas.

For lesions that correspond to Clark level 1 or 2, that is, less than 0.76 mm thick, a wide local excision results in 5-year survivals in the vicinity of 100%. The prognosis is poor for patients with melanomas more than 3 mm thick. If the regional nodes are negative, survival is greater than 60%, but survival drops to less than 30% if the regional nodes are involved with tumor. Most series of malignant melanoma report overall survivals of approximately 50%. Although metastases of melanoma to regional inguinal nodes are usually fatal, isolated prolonged survivals have been observed as was reported by Trimble et al. and also by Tasseron et al., who noted in a series of 30 patients, 6 had positive nodes and 2 survived for more than 5 years.

Distant metastases are frequently noted, and no effective program of chemotherapy has been described. Regressions (but not cures) have been reported with various multiagent cytotoxic programs. Current efforts are devoted to developing an effective program of immunotherapy.

Sarcoma

Sarcomas of the vulva are extremely rare. Twelve cases were reported by DiSaia et al., and surgical removal of the primary tumor is the treatment of choice. Chemotherapeutic considerations are the same as those for sarcomas of other sites in the female genital tract.

Granular Cell Myoblastomas

Granular cell myoblastoma is also an extremely rare tumor that is almost invariably benign but does morphologically show pleomorphism. Local excision is generally sufficient therapy. The tumor appears as a solitary, firm, nontender, slowly growing nodule in the subcutaneous tissue of the vulva.

KEY POINTS

- Squamous cell carcinomas comprise 90% of primary vulvar malignancies. More than half the patients are over 60 years of age at the time of diagnosis.

- Cancer of the vulva accounts for about 4% of malignancies of the lower female genital tract and is less frequent than uterine, ovarian, and cervical cancers.

- Paget's disease generally occurs in postmenopausal women and is usually treated by wide excision. Invasive carcinomas at other sites should be ruled out.

- Prolonged use of fluorinated corticosteroids to treat itching accompanying vulvar dystrophy can lead to vulvar contraction.

- Topical testosterone is often beneficial to treat lichen sclerosus but is absorbed systemically and occasionally can produce masculinizing symptoms.

- Recent studies indicate symptomatic lichen sclerosus is a premalignant condition preceding carcinoma by a mean of 4.0 years. The tumors that do develop tend to be clitoral in location and are in patients over age 40 years.

- HPV vulvar infection is common. Intraepithelial neoplasia occurs much less frequently.

- HPV-positive tumors tend to occur in younger patients, and these tumors tend to have a better prognosis than HPV-negative tumors.

- A clear progression of dysplasia-CIS (VIN I, II, and III) to invasive carcinoma in the vulva has not been clearly established. Intraepithelial neoplasia in the vulva may spontaneously regress. VIN III has an approximate 3.4% risk of progression to invasive carcinoma.

- Intraepithelial neoplasia of the vulva is usually treated by local excision. Laser therapy of the atypical area may be utilized in younger patients who do not have raised lesions.

- Vulvar carcinomas less than 2 cm in diameter and depth of invasion less than 1 mm (3 mm thickness) rarely metastasize to regional nodes.

- Unilateral vulvar tumors metastasize to ipsilateral inguinal-femoral nodes.

- Prognosis in vulvar carcinoma is primarily related to lesion size, stage, and lymph node status, which determines stage.

- The risk of lymph node groin metastases is related to tumor differentiation, lesion thickness, capillary-lymphatic space involvement, older age of patient, and tumor size.

- The deep pelvic nodes do not become involved with metastatic vulvar cancer unless the inguinal-femoral nodes are affected.

- The 5-year survival of vulvar carcinoma with negative nodes is over 95%. With one positive node the 5-year survival is approximately the same, that is, 94%; with two nodes it decreases to 80%; with three or more, to 12%.

- The worldwide 5-year survival for carcinoma of the vulva by stage is I, 71.4%; II, 61.3%; III, 43.8%; and IV, 8.3%.

- Advanced vulvar tumors encroaching on the urethra and/or anus may be treated by preliminary radiation followed by radical vulvectomy rather than exenteration. Enhanced results have also been reported with the combined use of chemotherapy and radiation.

- Verrucous carcinomas are a variant of squamous cancer that do not metastasize to regional nodes. Radiation therapy is contraindicated, and local surgical excision is the treatment of choice.

- Melanomas comprise 5% of vulvar cancers and are the most frequent non–squamous cell malignancies.

- The overall 5-year survival of patients with vulvar melanoma is about 50%.

- Superficial spreading melanomas tend to occur in younger patients and have a better prognosis than nodular melanomas.

- Prognosis of vulvar melanoma is related to tumor invasion (level) and to tumor thickness.

- Basal cell carcinoma of the vulva is treated by wide local excision.

BIBLIOGRAPHY

Andrews SJ, Williams BT, DePriest PD, et al: Therapeutic implications of lymph nodal spread in lateral T_1 and T_2 squamous cell carcinoma of the vulva, Gynecol Oncol 55:41, 1994.

Baehrendtz H, Einhorn N, Pettersson F, and Silfersward C: Paget's disease of the vulva: the Radiumhemmet series 1975-1990, Int J Gynecol Cancer 4:1, 1994.

Bergen S, DiSaia PJ, Liao SY, et al: Conservative management of extramammary Paget's disease of the vulva, Gynecol Oncol 33:151, 1989.

Berman ML, Soper JT, Creasman WT, et al: Conservative surgical management in superficially invasive stage I vulvar carcinoma, Gynecol Oncol 35:352, 1989.

Boronow RC, Hickman BT, Reagan MT, et al: Combined therapy as an alternative to exenteration for locally advanced vulvovaginal cancer, Am J Clin Oncol 10(2):1711, 1987.

Breslow A: Thickness, cross-sectional areas, and depth of invasion in the prognosis of cutaneous melanoma, Ann Surg 172:908, 1970.

Buscema J, Woodruff JD, Parmley TH, et al: Carcinoma in situ of the vulva, Obstet Gynecol 55:225, 1980.

Carlson JA, Ambros R, Malfetano J, et al: Vulvar lichen sclerosus and squamous cell carcinoma: a cohort, case control, and investigational study with historical perspective; implications for chronic inflammation and sclerosis in the development of neoplasia, Hum Pathol 29:932, 1998.

Christopherson W, Buchsbaum HJ, Vort R, et al: Radical vulvectomy and bilateral groin lymphadenectomy utilizing separate groin incisions: report of a case with recurrence in the intervening skin bridge, Gynecol Oncol 21:247, 1985.

Creasman WT: New gynecologic cancer staging, Gynecol Oncol 58:157, 1995.

Crosby JH, Bryan AB, Gallup D, et al: Fine-needle aspiration of inguinal lymph nodes in gynecologic practice, Obstet Gynecol 73:281, 1989.

Crowther ME, Lowe DG, and Shepherd JH: Verrucous carcinoma of the female genital tract: a review, Obstet Gynecol Surv 43:263, 1988.

Crum CP: Vulvar intraepithelial neoplasia: histology and associated viral changes. In Wilkinson EJ, ed: Pathology of the vulva and vagina, New York, 1987, Churchill Livingstone.

Crum CP: Carcinoma of the vulva: epidemiology and pathogenesis, Obstet Gynecol 79:448, 1992.

Curtin JP, Rubey SR, Jones WB, et al: Paget's disease of the vulva, Gynecol Oncol 39:374, 1990.

DiSaia PJ, Rutledge F, and Smith JP: Sarcoma of the vulva—report of 12 patients, Obstet Gynecol 38:180, 1971.

Dvoretsky PM, Bonfiglio TA, Helkamp BF, et al: The pathology of superficially invasive thin vulva squamous cell carcinoma, Int J Gynecol Pathol 3:331, 1984.

Farias-Eisner R, Cirisano FD, Grouse D, et al: Conservative and individualized surgery for early squamous carcinoma of the vulva: the treatment of choice for stage I and II (T_{1-2} N_{0-1} M_0) disease, Gynecol Oncol 53:55, 1994.

Fishman DA, Chambers SK, Schwartz PE, et al: Extramammary Paget's disease of the vulva, Gynecol Oncol 56:266, 1995.

Friedrich EG: Reversible vulvar atypia: a case report, Obstet Gynecol 39:173, 1972.

Greenlee RT, Murray T, Bolden S, and Wingo PA: Cancer Statistics, 2000, CA Cancer J Clin 50:7-33, 2000.

Grimshaw RN, Murdoch JB, and Monaghan JM: Radical vulvectomy and bilateral inguinal-femoral lymphadenectomy through separate incisions: experience with 100 cases, Int J Gynecol Cancer 3:18, 1993.

Hacker NF, Berek JS, Lagasse LD, et al: Management of regional lymph nodes and their prognostic influence in vulvar cancer, Obstet Gynecol 61:408, 1983.

Hart WR, Norris HJ, and Helwig ED: Relation of lichen sclerosus et atrophicus of the vulva to development of carcinoma, Obstet Gynecol 45:369, 1975.

Hoffman JS, Kumar NB, and Morley GW: Prognostic significance of groin lymph node metastases of squamous carcinoma of the vulva, Obstet Gynecol 66:402, 1985.

Homesley HD, Bundy BN, Sedlis A, and Adcock L: A randomized study of radiation therapy versus pelvic node resection for patients with invasive squamous cell carcinoma of the vulva having positive groin nodes (a Gynecologic Oncology Group Study), Obstet Gynecol 68:733, 1986.

Homesley HD, Bundy BN, Sedlis A, et al: Assessment of current International Federation of Gynecology and Obstetrics staging of vulvar carcinoma relative to prognostic factors for survival (a Gynecologic Oncology Group study), Am J Obstet Gynecol 164:997, 1991.

Homesley HD, Bundy BN, Sedlis A, et al: Prognostic factors for groin node metastasis in squamous cell carcinoma of the vulva (a Gynecologic Oncology Group study), Gynecol Oncol 49:279, 1993.

Hording U, Junge J, Daugaard S, et al: Vulvar squamous cell carcinoma and papillomaviruses: indications for two different etiologies, Gynecol Oncol 52:241, 1994.

Husseinzadeh N and Recinto C: Frequency of invasive cancer in surgically excised vulvar lesions with intraepithelial neoplasia (VIN 3), Gynecol Oncol 73:119, 1999.

Iversen T and Aas M: Lymph drainage from the vulva, Gynecol Oncol 16:179, 1983.

Iversen T, Abler V, and Aalder J: Individual treatment of stage I carcinoma of the vulva, Obstet Gynecol 57:85, 1981.

Iversen T, Elders JG, Christensen A, et al: Squamous cell carcinoma of the vulva: review of 424 patients, 1957-1974, Gynecol Oncol 9:271, 1980.

Iversen T and Tretli S: Intraepithelial and invasive squamous cell neoplasia of the vulva: trends in incidence, recurrence, and survival rate in Norway, Obstet Gynecol 91:969, 1998.

Japaze H, Dinh TV, and Woodruff JD: Verrucous carcinoma of the vulva: study of 24 cases, Obstet Gynecol 60:462, 1982.

Jones RW and Rowan DM: Spontaneous regression of vulvar intraepithelial neoplasia 2-3, Obstet Gynecol 96:470, 2000.

Kaufman RH: Distinguished professor series. Intraepithelial neoplasia of the vulva, Gynecol Oncol 56:8, 1995.

Koh WJ, Wallace HJ, Greer BE, et al: Combined radiotherapy and chemotherapy in the management of local-regionally advanced vulvar cancer, Int J Radiat Oncol Biol Phys 26:809, 1993.

Leuchter RS, Hacker NF, Voet RL, et al: Primary carcinoma of the Bartholin gland: a report of 14 cases and review of the literature, Obstet Gynecol 60:361, 1982.

Lieb SM, Gallousis S, and Freedman H: Granular cell myoblastoma of the vulva, Gynecol Oncol 8:12, 1979.

Magrina JF, Gonzalez-Bosquet J, Weaver AL, et al: Primary squamous cell cancer of the vulva: radical versus modified radical vulvar surgery, Gynecol Oncol 71:116, 1998.

Magrina JF, Gonzalez-Bosquet J, Weaver AL, et al: Squamous cell carcinoma of the vulva Stage IA: long-term results, Gynecol Oncol 76:24, 2000.

Messing MJ and Gallup DG: Carcinoma of the vulva in young women, Obstet Gynecol 86:51, 1995.

Miller B, Morris M, Levenback C, et al: Pelvic exenteration for primary and recurrent vulvar cancer, Gynecol Oncol 58:202, 1995.

Modesitt SC, Waters AB, Walton L, et al: Vulvar intraepithelial neoplasia III: occult cancer and the impact of margin status on recurrence, Obstet Gynecol 92:962, 1998.

Monk BJ, Burger RA, Lin F, et al: Prognostic significance of human papillomavirus DNA in vulvar carcinoma, Obstet Gynecol 85:709, 1995.

Pecorelli S, Creasman WT, Pettersson F, et al: FIGO annual report on the results of treatment in gynaecological cancer, vol 23, Milano, Italy, Epidemiol Biostat, 1998.

Piura B, Masotina A, Murdoch J, et al: Recurrent squamous cell carcinoma of the vulva: a study of 73 cases, Gynecol Oncol 48:189, 1993.

Podratz KC, Gaffey TA, Symmonds RE, et al: Melanoma of the vulva: an update, Gynecol Oncol 16:153, 1983.

Ragnarsson-Olding BK, Kanter-Lewensohn LR, Lagerlof B, et al: Malignant melanoma of the vulva in a nationwide, 25-year study of 219 Swedish females. Clinical observations and histopathologic features, Cancer 86:1273, 1999.

Ragnarsson-Olding BK, Nilsson BR, Kanter-Lewensohn LR, et al: Malignant melanoma of the vulva in a nationwide, 25-year study of 219 Swedish females. Predictors of survival, Cancer 86:1285, 1999.

Riva JM, Sedlacek TV, Cunnane MF, and Mangan CE: Extended carbon dioxide laser vaporization in the treatment of subclinical papillomavirus infection of the lower genital tract, Obstet Gynecol 73:25, 1989.

Rose PG, Piver S, Tsukada Y, et al: Conservative therapy for melanoma of the vulva, Am J Obstet Gynecol 159:57, 1988.

Rosenberg P, Simonsen E, and Risberg B: Adenoid cystic carcinoma of Bartholin's gland: a report of 5 new cases treated with surgery and radiotherapy, Gynecol Oncol 34:145, 1989.

Rotmensch J, Rubin SJ, Sutton HG, et al: Preoperative radiotherapy followed by radical vulvectomy with inguinal lymphadenectomy for advanced vulvar cancer, Gynecol Oncol 36:181, 1990.

Rowley KC, Gallion IIII, Donaldson ES, et al: Prognostic factors in early vulvar cancer, Gynecol Oncol 31:43, 1988.

Russell AH, Mesic JB, Scudder SA, et al: Synchronous radiation and cytotoxic chemotherapy for locally advanced or recurrent squamous cancer of the vulva, Gynecol Oncol 47:14, 1992.

Sedlis A, Homesley H, Bundy BN, et al: Positive groin lymph nodes in superficial squamous vulvar cancer, Am J Obstet Gynecol 156:1159, 1987.

Shepherd JH: Staging announcement: FIGO staging of gynecologic cancers: cervix and vulva, Int J Gynecol Cancer 5:319, 1995.

Siller BS: Vulvar cancer: a case-control study of triple incision vs. en bloc radical vulvectomy and inguinal lymphadenectomy, Gynecol Oncol 57:335, 1995.

Skinner MS, Sternberg WH, Ichinose H, et al: Spontaneous regression of Bowenoid atypia of the vulva, Obstet Gynecol 42:40, 1973.

Stefanon B, Clemente C, Lupi G, et al: Malignant melanoma of the vulva: a clinicopathologic study of 28 cases, Cervix & IFGT 5:223, 1987.

Stehman FB and Bundy BN: Sites of failure and times to failure in carcinoma of the vulva treated conservatively: a Gynecologic Oncology Group report, Am J Obstet Gynecol 174:1128, 1996.

Stehman FB, Bundy BN, Dvoretsky PM, and Creasman WT: Early stage I carcinoma of the vulva treated with ipsilateral superficial inguinal lymphadenectomy and modified radical hemivulvectomy: a prospective study of the Gynecology Oncology Group, Obstet Gynecol 79:490, 1992.

Tasseron EWK, Van der Esch EP, Hart AAM, et al: A clinicopathological study of 30 melanomas of the vulva, Gynecol Oncol 46:170, 1992.

Thomas G, Dembo A, and DePetrillo A: Concurrent radiation and chemotherapy in vulvar carcinoma, Gynecol Oncol 34:263, 1989.

Trimble EL, Lewis JL, Williams LL, et al: Management of vulvar melanomas, Gynecol Oncol 45:254, 1992.

Van der Velden J, Kooyman CD, Van Lindert ACM, and Heintz APM: A stage Ia vulvar carcinoma with an inguinal lymph node recurrence after local excision: a case report and literature review, Int J Gynecol Cancer 2:157, 1992.

Veronesi V, Cascinelli N, Adams J, et al: Thin stage I primary cutaneous malignant melanomas: comparison of excision with margins of 1 or 3 cm, N Engl J Med 318:1159, 1988.

Woodruff JD, Genadry R, and Poliakoff S: Treatment of dyspareunia and vaginal outlet distortions by perineoplasty, Obstet Gynecol 57:750, 1981.

Neoplastic Diseases of the Vagina

Intraepithelial Neoplasia, Carcinoma, Sarcoma

Clear Cell Adenocarcinoma. A vaginal or cervical malignancy occurring primarily after 14 years of age. It is often associated with prenatal exposure to diethylstilbestrol (DES).

Endodermal Sinus Tumor. A rare adenocarcinoma of the vagina occurring in infants less than 2 years of age.

Field Defect. The propensity of squamous epithelium of the lower genital tract (cervix, vagina, and vulva) to undergo premalignant change.

Laser (*Light Amplification by Stimulated Emission of Radiation*). An energized source of light that can be used to vaporize tissue and to treat intraepithelial neoplasia.

Pelvic Exenteration. An extensive pelvic operation usually employed to treat a central pelvic recurrence of cervical carcinoma after radiation. A total exenteration involves removal of the bladder, uterus, cervix, and rectum. An anterior exenteration spares the rectum, while a posterior exenteration spares the bladder.

Pseudosarcoma Botryoides. A benign tumor occurring in the vagina of infants and pregnant women that has a polyploid shape. Microscopically it may be confused with sarcoma botryoides.

Sarcoma Botryoides (Embryonal Rhabdomyosarcoma). A rare, often fatal, malignancy of the vagina that occurs in infants and children.

Vaginal Tumor Stage. A clinical classification that describes the extent of spread of vaginal carcinoma.
  Stage I: Limited to vaginal wall
  Stage II: Extends to subvaginal tissue
  Stage III: Reaches the pelvic wall
  Stage IV: Extends beyond the true pelvis or into mucosa of the bladder or rectum

VAIN-1. Vaginal intraepithelial neoplasia of the least severe type (comparable to mild dysplasia), usually occupying the lower one third of the epithelium. Also termed low grade squamous intraepithelial lesion (LGSIL).

VAIN-2. Vaginal intraepithelial neoplasia of intermediate severity (comparable to moderate dysplasia), usually occupying the lower two thirds of the epithelium.

VAIN-3. Vaginal intraepithelial neoplasia of the most severe type (comparable to severe dysplasia and carcinoma in situ), usually replacing the full thickness of the epithelium. VAIN 2 and 3 are also combined into high grade squamous intraepithelial lesion (HGSIL).

Premalignant changes in the vagina occur less frequently than comparable lesions in the cervix and vulva. However, the histologic appearance of intraepithelial neoplasia of the vagina is similar to that described for the cervix (Chapter 28). These changes are also similarly designated as dysplasia (mild, moderate, or severe) and carcinoma in situ. The term *VAIN* (vaginal, *VA;* intraepithelial, *I;* neoplasia, *N*) has been used to describe these histologic changes; the comparable categories are VAIN-1 (mild dysplasia), VAIN-2 (moderate dysplasia), and VAIN-3 (severe dysplasia to carcinoma in situ). With the recent Bethesda terminology (see Chapter 28), VAIN 1 is classified as a low grade squamous intraepithelial lesion (LGSIL) while VAIN 2 and 3 are grouped as high grade squamous intraepithelial lesions (HGSIL). The cytologic and histologic features of these changes are illustrated in Figure 33-1.

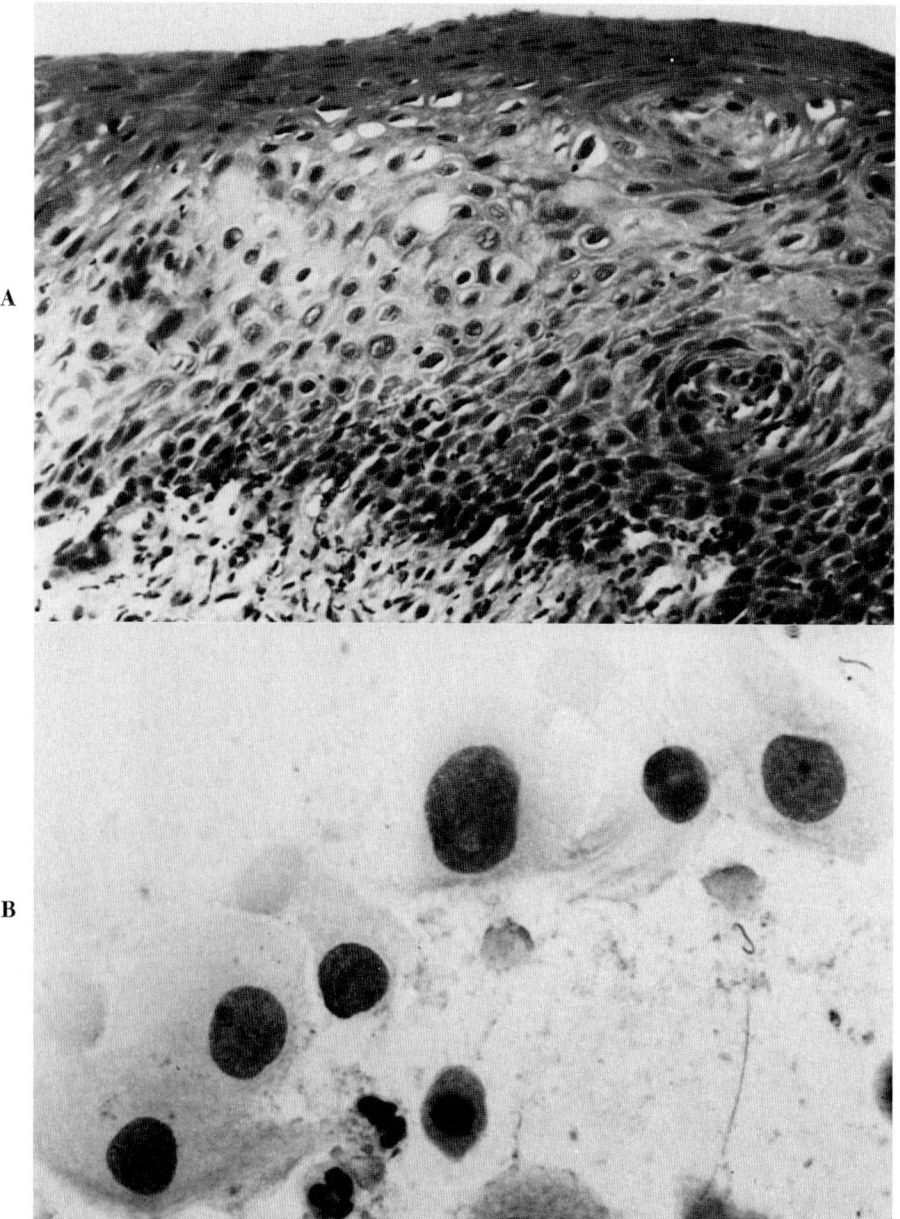

FIGURE 33-1 **A,** Section of vagina showing dysplasia. Epithelium appears thickened and shows abnormal maturation. Immature, hyperchromatic cells occupy lower two to four layers. Middle and upper third of mucosa show evidence of cytoplasmic differentiation with well-defined cellular borders. Nuclei in these areas are enlarged and pleomorphic. Parakeratosis is apparent on surface. Because immature cells are confined to lower third of mucosa, dysplasia is classified as mild. (H&E stain; ×250.) **B,** Cytologic specimen showing mild dysplasia. Note sheet of dysplastic cells. Cells show well-defined cytoplasmic borders. Nuclei are enlarged, and nuclear contour is smooth. Chromatin is uniformly, finely granular. Focal condensations of chromatin (chromocenters) are present in some nuclei. Nucleoli are not present. (Papanicolaou stain; ×1000.)

(continued)

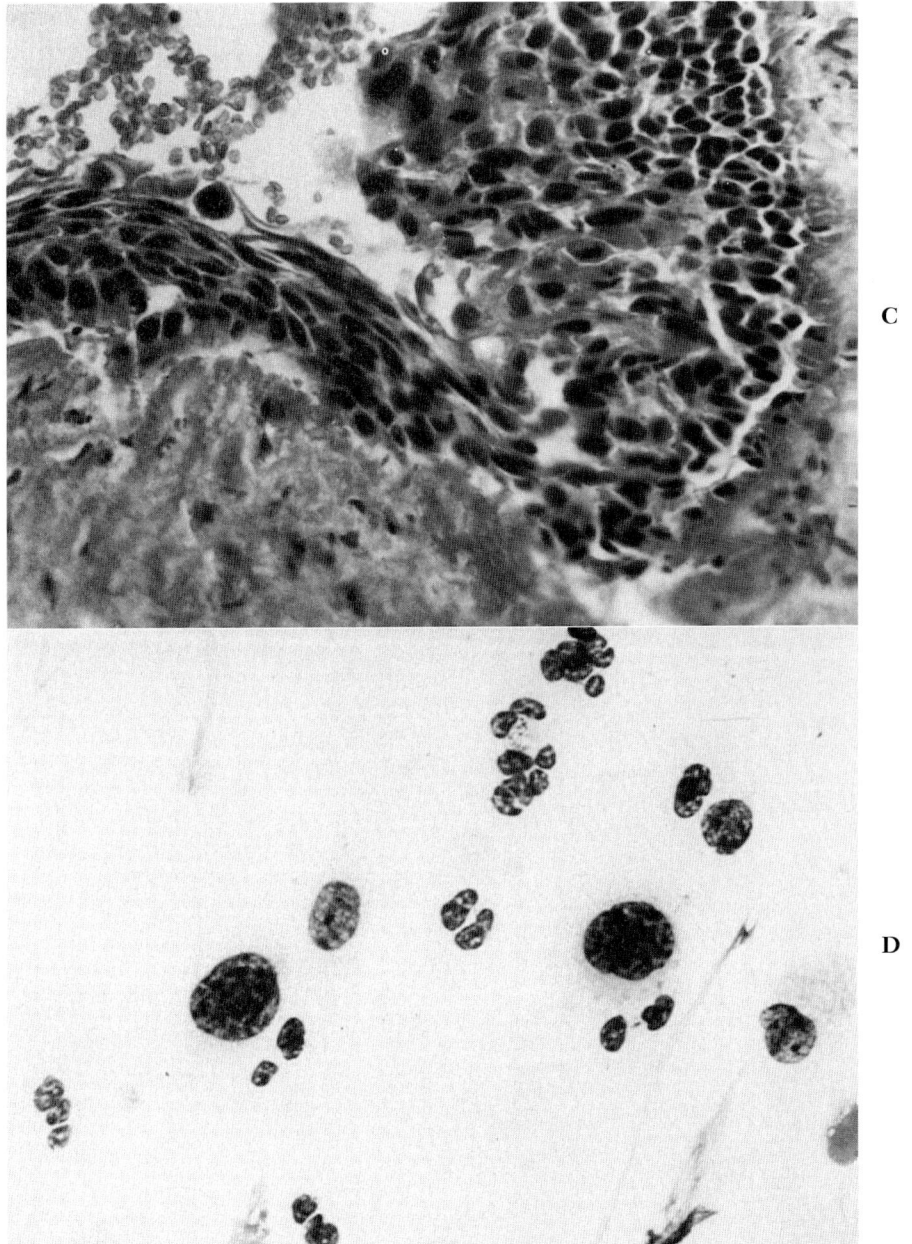

C

D

FIGURE 33-1 cont'd.   C, Section showing severe dysplasia to carcinoma in situ. Entire epithelial thickness is occupied by hyperchromatic, dysplastic cells. Marked nuclear variation and mitoses are seen. Because of occasional cells with squamous differentiation (spindle-shaped cells, cells with well-defined cytoplasmic borders) in superficial layers, this lesion is sometimes classified as severe dysplasia. In carcinoma in situ immature cells replace the full thickness, and there is no evidence of squamous differentiation on the surface. (H&E stain; ×400.) **D,** Cytologic specimen showing carcinoma in situ. Several isolated immature cells with high nuclear-cytoplasmic ratio and poorly defined cytoplasmic borders can be seen. Chromatin is coarsely granular, and no nucleoli are present. In background are several polymorphonuclear leukocytes and strings of mucus. (Papanicolaou stain; ×1000.)   *(continued)*

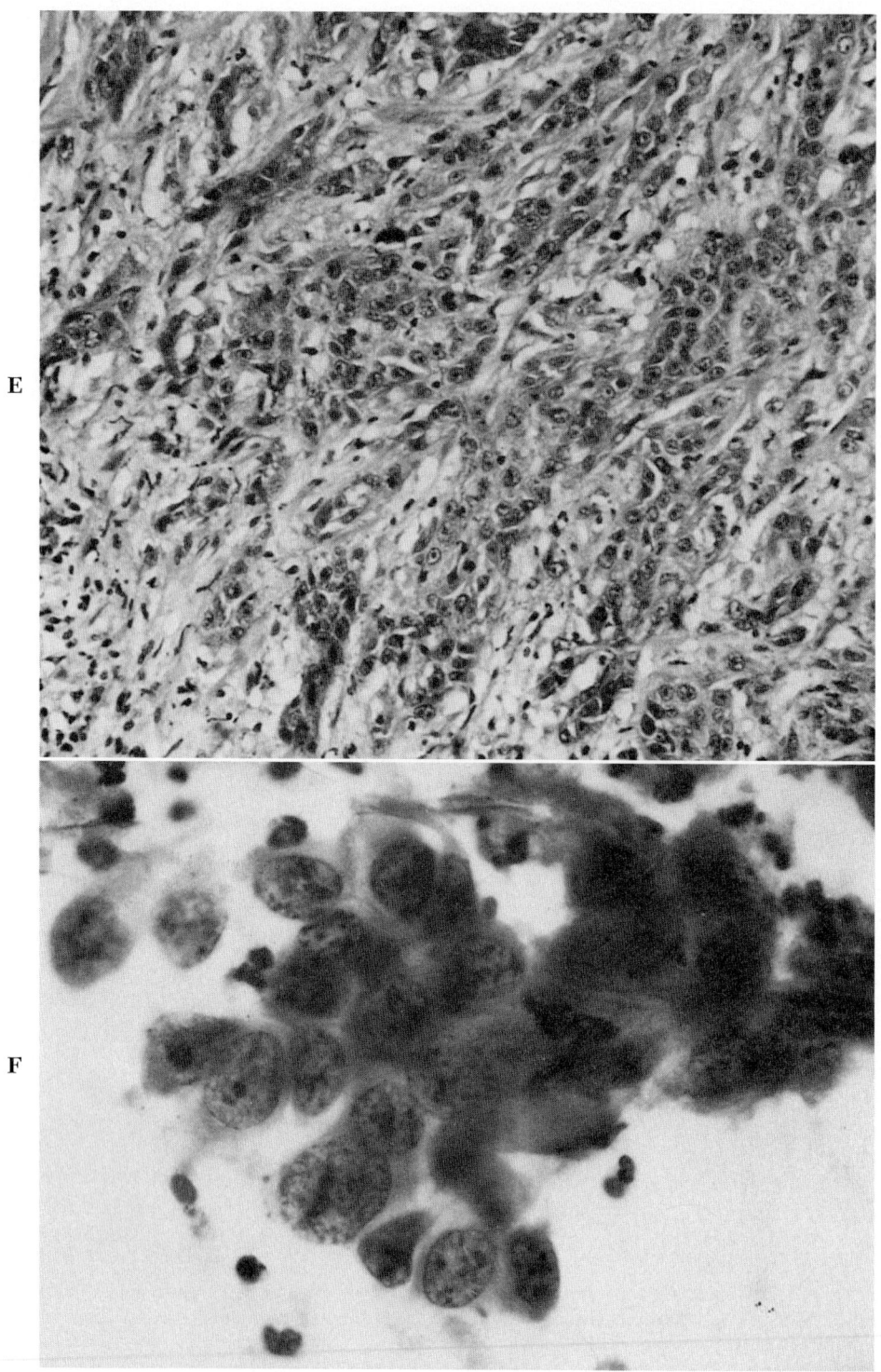

FIGURE 33-1 cont'd. **E,** Section showing invasive squamous carcinoma. Cords and sheets of poorly differentiated tumor cells infiltrate stroma. Nuclei are pleomorphic, and nucleoli are distinct. Mitotic rate is high. Squamous differentiation (keratin pearl formation, single-cell keratinization) was present in other areas of tumor. (H&E stain; ×200.) **F,** Cytologic specimen showing invasive squamous cell carcinoma. Note aggregate of tumor cells. Cellular boundaries are poorly defined, and nuclear orientation is lacking. Chromatin is irregularly distributed and has areas of clumping and clearing. Note nucleoli in some cells, which were absent in cells of patient with dysplasia and carcinoma in situ. (Papanicolaou stain; ×800.)

VAIN occurs more commonly in patients previously treated for cervical intraepithelial neoplasia. The frequency of vaginal premalignancy in these patients is about 1% to 3%. Similarly, there is an increased risk for VAIN in those previously treated for squamous cell neoplasia of the vulva. The tendency to develop premalignant changes in the lower genital tract has been termed a *field defect* and denotes the increased risk of squamous cell neoplasia arising anywhere in the lower genital tract in such individuals. As with the cervix, predisposing factors associated with these changes may include venereal diseases, herpes virus type II infection, and human papillomavirus infection as well as HIV infection. Additional risk factors include prior radiation therapy of the genital tract, immunosuppressive therapy in transplant patients, and chemotherapy in patients undergoing treatment for malignant disease.

Primary cancer of the vagina is rare and constitutes less than 2% of gynecologic malignancies. Most vaginal malignancies are metastatic, primarily from the cervix and endometrium. Less commonly, ovarian and rectosigmoid carcinomas, as well as choriocarcinoma, metastasize to the vagina. The most common histologic type of primary vaginal cancer is squamous cell carcinoma, but numerous other types of carcinomas, as well as primary sarcomas, occur. Table 33-1 summarizes the major primary malignancies of the vagina arranged according to the age of occurrence.

PREMALIGNANT DISEASE OF THE VAGINA

Detection and Diagnosis

Since premalignant disease of the vagina is generally asymptomatic, detection depends primarily on cytologic screening (Figure 33-1, *B* and *D*). Most commonly the changes will be observed in patients who have undergone prior therapy for intraepithelial disease of the cervix. Once an abnormal smear from vaginal epithelium is identified, a biopsy is required for histologic identification (Figure 33-1, *A* and *C*). A colposcopic examination is usually performed to identify the areas requiring biopsy. As in the case of cervical neoplasia, a repeat Pap smear is often taken prior to the colposcopic examination. Vaginal colposcopic techniques are similar to those described for the cervix. A large speculum is used to aid in visualizing the entire vaginal wall. While the abnormal colposcopic findings resemble those of the cervix (Chapter 28), full visualization of the entire vaginal wall is often difficult and time consuming.

A biopsy is performed with small instruments, such as the Kevorkian or Eppendorf punch biopsy forceps (Figure 33-2), or similar instruments also used for the cervix. Occasionally it is necessary to use a fine instrument, such as a nerve hook, to provide traction on the vaginal epithelium to obtain a biopsy. Most patients experience some discomfort during the biopsy, but usually local anesthesia is not needed, since injection of the anesthetic is often as uncomfortable as the biopsy itself. A less precise but useful method for identifying an area for biopsy is to stain the vaginal epithelium with half-strength Lugol's solution and to take a biopsy specimen from the nonstaining areas. The vaginal epithelium must be adequately estrogenized so that sufficient epithelial glycogen is present for the normal tissue to stain dark brown. Local estrogen cream used for 1 to 2 weeks before examination is frequently helpful in postmenopausal patients and in patients with severe atrophic vaginitis in which atypical cells are first detected on cytologic (Pap) smear. The estrogen cream should not be used for 2 days prior to the examination in order to avoid excess buildup of superficial vaginal cells.

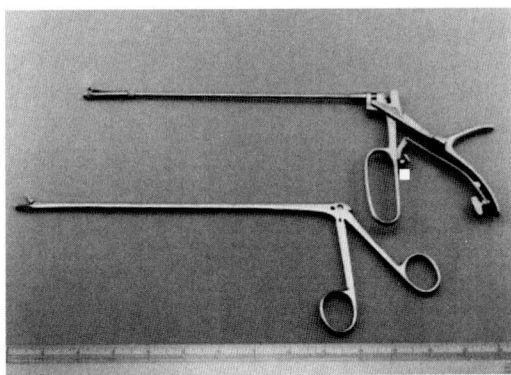

FIGURE 33-2 Eppendorf (upper) and Kevorkian (lower) punch biopsy instruments.

TABLE 33-1
Common Primary Vaginal Cancers

Tumor Type	Predominant Age (years)	Clinical Correlations
Endodermal sinus tumor (adenocarcinoma)	<2	Extremely rare, alpha-fetoprotein secretion, often fatal, multimodality therapy
Sarcoma botryoides	<8	Aggressive malignancy, multimodality therapy
Clear cell adenocarcinoma	>14	Associated with intrauterine exposure to DES
Melanoma	>50	Very rare, poor survival
Squamous cell carcinoma	>50	Most common primary vaginal cancer

It is important for the examiner to realize that vaginal neoplasia is often multifocal. While the process is frequently located in the vaginal apex, it can occur anywhere along the vaginal tube, necessitating examination of the vagina in its entirety.

Management

As is true for cervical intraepithelial neoplasia, the abnormal vaginal epithelium must be completely eradicated. Small lesions, particularly those at the vaginal apex in patients who have undergone hysterectomy, usually are excised. However, excision of large areas may require skin grafting, and for that reason, other therapeutic modalities are often chosen.

Alternate nonsurgical treatment modalities are also directed toward destruction of all the abnormal epithelium. Radiation therapy, although used in the past, often leads to scarring and fibrosis and is generally not recommended for treatment of noninvasive disease. Because of the proximity of the bladder and rectum, cryotherapy is usually not used. Widely used nonsurgical approaches include the laser, which is most commonly employed, or 5-fluorouracil (5-FU) cream for widespread multicentric lesions, particularly those with papillomavirus infection.

The carbon dioxide laser allows vaporization of the abnormal tissue. The beam is directed colposcopically. Iodine staining of the vagina can also outline those areas requiring therapy. Treatment is occasionally performed on an outpatient basis with a local anesthetic and an analgesic. More frequently, general or regional anesthesia is required. The intensity of therapy is regulated by adjusting the wattage of the laser, most commonly 15 to 20 watts if carried to a depth of 2 to 4 mm. The patient will experience a discharge for a few days after therapy. Healing usually requires a few weeks. Although long-term experience and follow-up with laser treatment of vaginal neoplasia is not available, results reported by Petrilli et al. show success rates on the order of 90%. Regular follow-up every 4 months, including a Pap smear and colposcopy, is required during the first year and usually 6 to 12 months thereafter.

Five percent 5-FU cream is often used for approximately 7 days. One half of a vaginal applicator (approximately 5 g) is inserted into the vagina nightly. Because the cream is irritating, some protective ointment such as zinc oxide should be applied to the vulva. If excess leakage occurs, less than half of an applicator should be used. In addition, the treatment should be discontinued before 7 days if the patient notes excessive irritation. A cycle of therapy should be repeated in 3 to 4 weeks if intraepithelial neoplasia persists. In some cases the application of 5-FU is continued for 10 to 14 days, in which case the nontherapy interval is increased to 2 or 3 months. Lesions with a thickened white crust (hyper-

keratosis) appear to be less sensitive to this treatment. In contrast, postmenopausal women tolerate only small doses of 5-FU, presumably because of the comparative thinness of the vaginal epithelium. Krebs used one third of an applicator of 5% 5-FU weekly for 10 weeks and noted that 17 of 20 patients with vaginal condyloma were free of disease at 3 months. Three patients received a second cycle, and 16 of 18 were free of disease at 10 to 20 months. Ballon et al. and Petrilli et al. reported success rates of 80% to 90% for patients with vaginal intraepithelial neoplasia after multiple treatment cycles; the method appears particularly useful for patients with multifocal diffuse lesions.

Audet-Lapointe et al. noted that 61 of 66 cases of VAIN occurred in the upper one third of the vagina. For apical lesions, especially after hysterectomy, excision is advisable; for multifocal lesions and condyloma, they used 5-FU. The laser was used to eradicate discrete lesions.

MALIGNANT DISEASE OF THE VAGINA

Symptoms and Diagnosis

Primary vaginal cancers usually occur as squamous cell carcinomas in women over age 50. To be considered a primary vaginal tumor, the malignancy must arise in the vagina and not involve the external os of the cervix superiorly or the vulva inferiorly. Otherwise the tumor is classified as cervical or vulvar. This is also an important therapeutic consideration, insofar as the same management techniques apply to small tumors of the upper one third of the vagina and cervical carcinomas. Tumors of the lower one third of the vagina are treated similarly to vulvar cancers (Chapter 32). Table 33-2 lists the staging criteria for vaginal cancers according to the International Federation of Gynecology and Obstetrics, which are illustrated in Figure 33-3.

TABLE 33-2

International Federation of Gynecology and Obstetrics (FIGO) Staging Classification for Vaginal Cancer

Stage	Characteristics
0	Carcinoma in situ
I	Carcinoma limited to vaginal wall
II	Carcinoma involves subvaginal tissue but has not extended to pelvic wall
III	Carcinoma extends to pelvic wall
IV	Carcinoma extends beyond true pelvis or involves mucosa of bladder or rectum (bullous edema as such does not assign a patient to stage IV)

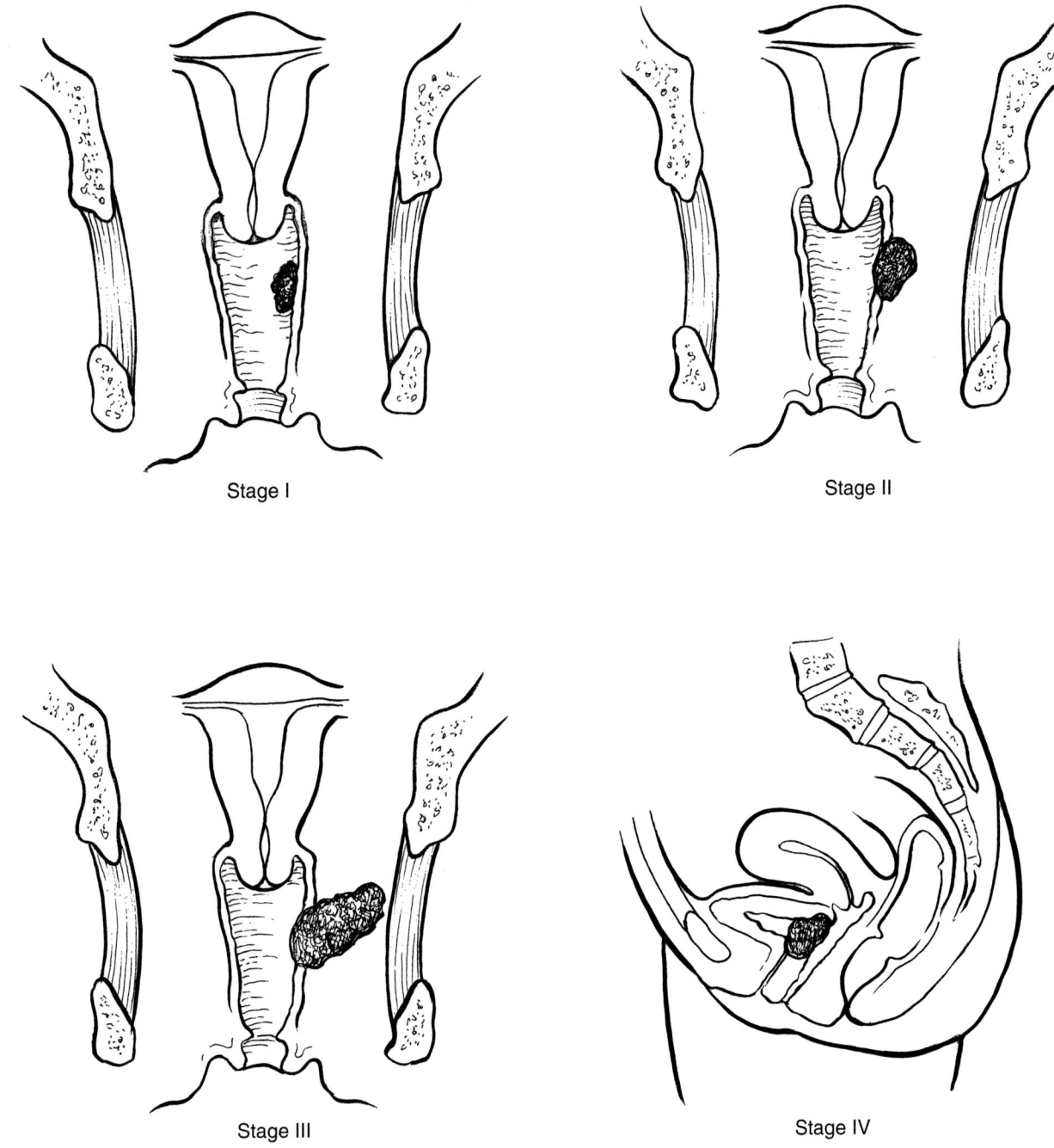

Stage I

Stage II

Stage III

Stage IV

FIGURE 33-3 Staging of vaginal cancer.

Delay in the diagnosis of these cancers frequently occurs, in part because of their rarity as well as because of a lack of recognition that the abnormal symptoms may be due to a malignancy. The most common symptom of vaginal cancer is abnormal bleeding or discharge. Pain is usually a symptom of an advanced tumor. Urinary frequency is also reported occasionally, particularly in the case of anterior wall tumors, whereas constipation or tenesmus may be reported when the tumors involve the posterior vaginal wall. In general, the longer the delay in diagnosis,

the worse the prognosis and the more difficult the therapy. Vaginal cancer is usually diagnosed by direct biopsy of the tumor mass (Figure 33-1, *E*). Abnormal cytologic findings (Figure 33-1, *F*) may prompt a thorough pelvic examination that will lead to diagnosis of vaginal cancer. It is important during the course of the pelvic examination to inspect and palpate the entire vaginal tube and to rotate the speculum carefully to visualize the entire vagina, since often a small tumor may occupy the anterior or posterior vaginal wall.

Tumors of Adult Vagina

Squamous Cell Carcinoma

Squamous cell carcinoma is the most common of the vaginal malignancies and accounts for 90% of primary vaginal cancers. Although reported in women in their 30s, the disease occurs primarily in those over age 50. Most squamous cell carcinomas occur in the upper third of the vagina, but primary tumors in the middle third and lower third are also common. Grossly the tumor appears as a fungating, ulcerating mass, often accompanied by a foul smell and discharge related to a secondary infection. Microscopically (Figure 33-1, *E*) the tumor demonstrates the classic findings of an invasive squamous cell carcinoma infiltrating the vaginal epithelium.

Treatment of these tumors is based on the size, stage, and location. Therapy is limited by the proximity of the bladder anteriorly and the rectum posteriorly. It is also influenced by the location of the tumor in the vagina, which determines the area of lymphatic spread (Figure 33-4).

The lymphatics of the vagina envelop the mucosa and anastomose with lymphatic vessels in the muscularis. Those of the middle to upper vagina communicate superiorly with the lymphatics of the cervix and drain into the pelvic nodes of the obturator and internal and external iliac chains. In contrast, the lymphatics of the distal third of the vagina drain to both the inguinal nodes as well as to the pelvic nodes, similar to the drainage of the vulva. The posterior wall lymphatics anastomose with the rectal lymphatic system and then to the nodes that drain the rectum, such as the inferior gluteal, sacral, and rectal nodes.

MANAGEMENT. Both operation and irradiation therapy have been effective, considering the limits imposed by the proximity to the bladder and rectum and the risk of fistula formation from these organs to the vagina. Radiation therapy has been the most frequent mode of treatment. External radiation therapy with megavoltage equipment is initially utilized to shrink the tumor. This is then followed by a local cesium or radium implant placed interstitially with needles or by intracavitary radiation using a tandem

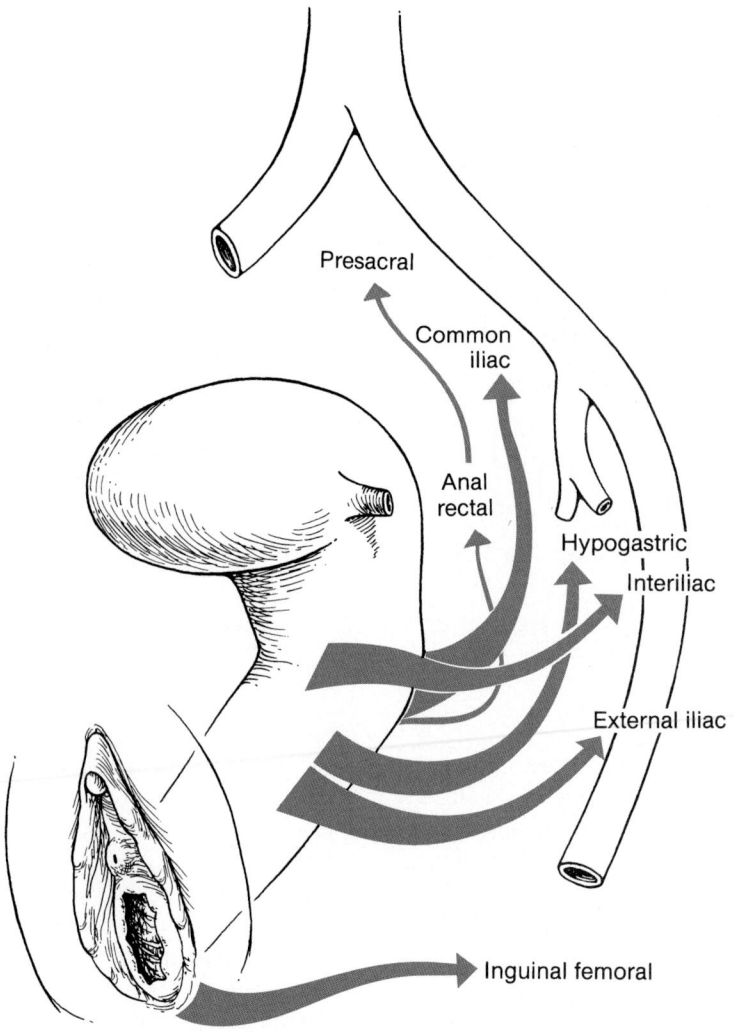

FIGURE 33-4 Lymphatic drainage of vagina. Predominant pathways from various parts of vagina are shown.

TABLE 33-3
Summary of Average Dosages* for Treatment of Vaginal Carcinoma

	External Therapy	Implant (Interstitial)
Stage I		
Small tumors (<2 cm)	May omit	6000–7000 cGy, 6–7 days
All others	4000 cGy, whole pelvis	3000–4000 cGy, 3–4 days
Stage II	4000–5000 cGy, whole pelvis	3000–4000 cGy, 3–4 days
Stages III and IV	5000 cGy, whole pelvis; an additional 1000–2000 cGy through reduced field if implant not possible	2000 cGy, by implant if possible

Modified from Nori D, Hilaris BS, Stanimir G, et al: Int J Radiat Oncol Biol Phys 9:1471, 1983.

*1 cGy = 1 rad.

or ovoids, similar to the delivery systems used for cervical carcinoma (particularly in the case of a tumor in the upper one third of the vagina if the cervix is present) (Chapter 29). Prognosis appears to improve if the interval from the end of external therapy to the initiation of brachytherapy is less than 28 days.

DiSaia et al. have reported using a fixed perineal template (Syed/Neblett applicator) to achieve reproducible isodose delivery to a large vaginal tumor volume. For lesions of the upper vagina after hysterectomy, a laparotomy is done to remove any bowel loops from the vaginal apex and in some instances omentum is used to provide additional separation of the bowel from the vaginal apex. Paley et al. reported using a retropubic approach in a small series of six patients to achieve direct visualization of needle placement. The treatment is individualized depending on tumor size and stage. Some therapists have advocated using only local sources of radiation if the primary carcinoma is small (under 2 cm) and accessible to needle implantation. For larger lesions the dosage of the external component of radiation therapy is increased, with a concomitant reduction in the local vaginal component of treatment of the primary tumor. Usually a total tumor dose of approximately 7500 cGy is administered. Implants cannot be done in some patients with stage III or IV carcinoma; in such cases only external therapy can be used, and a central "boost" is given after an initial 5000 cGy whole-pelvic treatment (Table 33-3). Spirtos et al., in a study of 23 stage I patients, noted only two local recurrences, and both patients had tumor dosages less than 7500 cGy. However, Perez et al. noted increasingly severe complications if the vaginal dose exceeded 9800 cGy. Kucera and Vavra, in a series of 434 patients treated with irradiation, noted results were best for low stage tumors, those in the upper one third of the vagina and if the tumor was well differentiated. Kirkbride et al. reported that stage and tumor size and tumor grade were prognostic and that the tumor dose must reach at least 7000 cGy, consistent with other studies. Treatment time is also important, and it is preferable as noted by Lee et al. to complete the radiation within 9

TABLE 33-4
Stage and Survival—Carcinoma of the Vagina: Patients Treated in 1990–92

	Patient (no.)	5-Year Survival (%)
Stage I	69	62.7
Stage II	78	45.0
Stage III	50	21.8
Stage IVA	16	—
Stage IVB	6	50.0

Modified from Pecorelli S, Creasman WT, Pettersson F, et al: FIGO annual report on the results of treatment in gynaecological cancer. Twenty-third volume, Milano, Italy. J Epidemiol Biostat, 1998.

weeks. For advanced lesions, chemoradiation with sensitizers, such as cisplatin, are being tried similar to protocols followed for carcinoma of the cervix (see Chapter 29).

For localized tumors in the upper one third of the vagina, radical hysterectomy and vaginectomy can be effective, especially in younger patients. In most instances, radical pelvic surgery, including removal of the bladder (anterior exenteration) or removal of the rectum (posterior exenteration), or both (total exenteration), is necessary only in patients with localized recurrence after radiation therapy. Initially the tumors usually recur locally, as in squamous cell carcinoma of the cervix and vulva, but distant metastases also occur, as in vulvar and cervical cancers. An effective chemotherapy program for recurrent squamous cell vaginal carcinoma has not been developed. A variety of regimens for squamous cell carcinoma utilizing multiple-agent chemotherapy is usually employed, similar to those for squamous cell carcinoma of the cervix (Chapter 29).

SURVIVAL. Overall 5-year survival rates for patients with primary carcinoma of the vagina have been reported to be approximately 45%. Table 33-4 demonstrates that survival is related to stage. However, as noted by Davis et al. stage is a vital prognostic factor. In their series of 89 patients treated with operation and/or irradiation, the 5-year survival for stage I was 82% and for stage II, 53%.

Clear Cell Adenocarcinoma

Clear cell adenocarcinomas in young women have been seen more frequently since 1970 as a result of the association of many of these cancers with intrauterine exposure to diethylstilbestrol (DES). The nonmalignant manifestations of this exposure are discussed in Chapter 15.

MANAGEMENT. Therapeutic considerations are similar to those for squamous cell carcinoma, taking into account the young age of the patients undergoing therapy. Cervical clear cell adenocarcinomas are treated like primary cervical carcinomas (Chapter 29). The results of therapy for both vaginal and cervical clear cell adenocarcinoma in young women will be discussed together in this section. These tumors are also staged according to the FIGO classification (see Tables 29-2 and 33-2). The majority (80%) have been diagnosed as stage I or II. The overall results of therapy, based on the stage of the tumor at the time of treatment, are shown in Table 33-5. As can be seen, the survival rate is related directly to the stage of the tumor, similar to other gynecologic malignancies at these sites.

In general, operation is the primary treatment modality because of the young age of the patients. For stage I and early stage II tumors, radical hysterectomy with partial or complete vaginectomy, pelvic lymphadenectomy, and replacement of the vagina with split-thickness skin grafts has been the most common approach. In most cases, ovarian function is preserved. In addition, efforts have been made to preserve fertility in patients who have small tumors of the vagina by the use of local irradiation of the primary tumor and immediate adjacent tissues to spare the ovaries. Since metastases to regional pelvic nodes can occur even with small stage I tumors, retroperitoneal lymph node dissections are usually performed before local therapy.

Usually local excision of the tumor has been performed before irradiation to facilitate local application. Senekjian et al. in 1987 have noted that the survival of patients with small vaginal tumors treated by local excision and then local irradiation is comparable to those with conventional extensive therapy. The best candidates are those with tumors less than 2 cm in diameter, a predominant tubulocystic pattern (Figure 33-5, A) and depth of invasion less than 3 mm. After wide local excision, the pelvic nodes are sampled to rule out tumor spread. If these are negative, local irradiation can then be given. Pregnancies have occurred in patients so treated. Larger tumors, however, are treated with full pelvic irradiation, in addition to an intracavitary implant. In a few instances exenterative surgery has been successfully performed, but as noted in 1989 by Senekjian et al., this procedure is preferably applied to central recurrences after primary irradiation. Local vaginal excision as the sole therapy is not usually adequate for small tumors, since the tumor frequently recurs.

SURVIVAL. Three predominant histologic patterns are found in patients with clear cell adenocarcinoma (Figure 33-5). In addition, a number of prognostic factors have been identified. The older patients (over 19 years of age) have been found to have a more favorable prognosis in comparison to younger subjects (under 15 years of age). This difference is associated with a more favorable outcome for those with the tubulocystic pattern of clear cell adenocarcinoma, which is the most frequent histologic pattern found in older patients. In addition, smaller tumor diameter and superficial depth of invasion correlate with improved patient survival. Recently Waggoner et al. showed that patients with clear cell adenocarcinoma and a positive maternal DES history do better than those with a negative maternal DES history. If the regional pelvic nodes are free of tumor, the prognosis is also more favorable. It is more likely that the regional pelvic lymph nodes will be free of tumor if other factors are favorable (see box below).

Clear cell adenocarcinomas can spread locally as well as by lymphatics and blood vessels. Metastases to regional pelvic nodes are found in about one sixth of stage I cases. The spread to regional pelvic nodes becomes more frequent in higher stage tumors. Depending on the

---

TABLE 33-5

5- and 10-Year Survival Rates for 588 Patients with Clear Cell Adenocarcinoma of the Vagina and Cervix

Stage	5-Year Survival (%)	10-Year Survival (%)
Stage I	91	85
Stage IIA	80	67
Stage IIB	56	47
Stage II (vagina)	82	67
Stage III	37	25
Stage IV	0	0

Modified from unpublished Registry Data, The University of Chicago.

Favorable Factors in Survival of Patients with Clear Cell Adenocarcinoma

Low stage
Older age
Tubulocystic histologic pattern
Small tumor diameter
Reduced depth of invasion
Regional lymph nodes free of tumor
Positive DES history

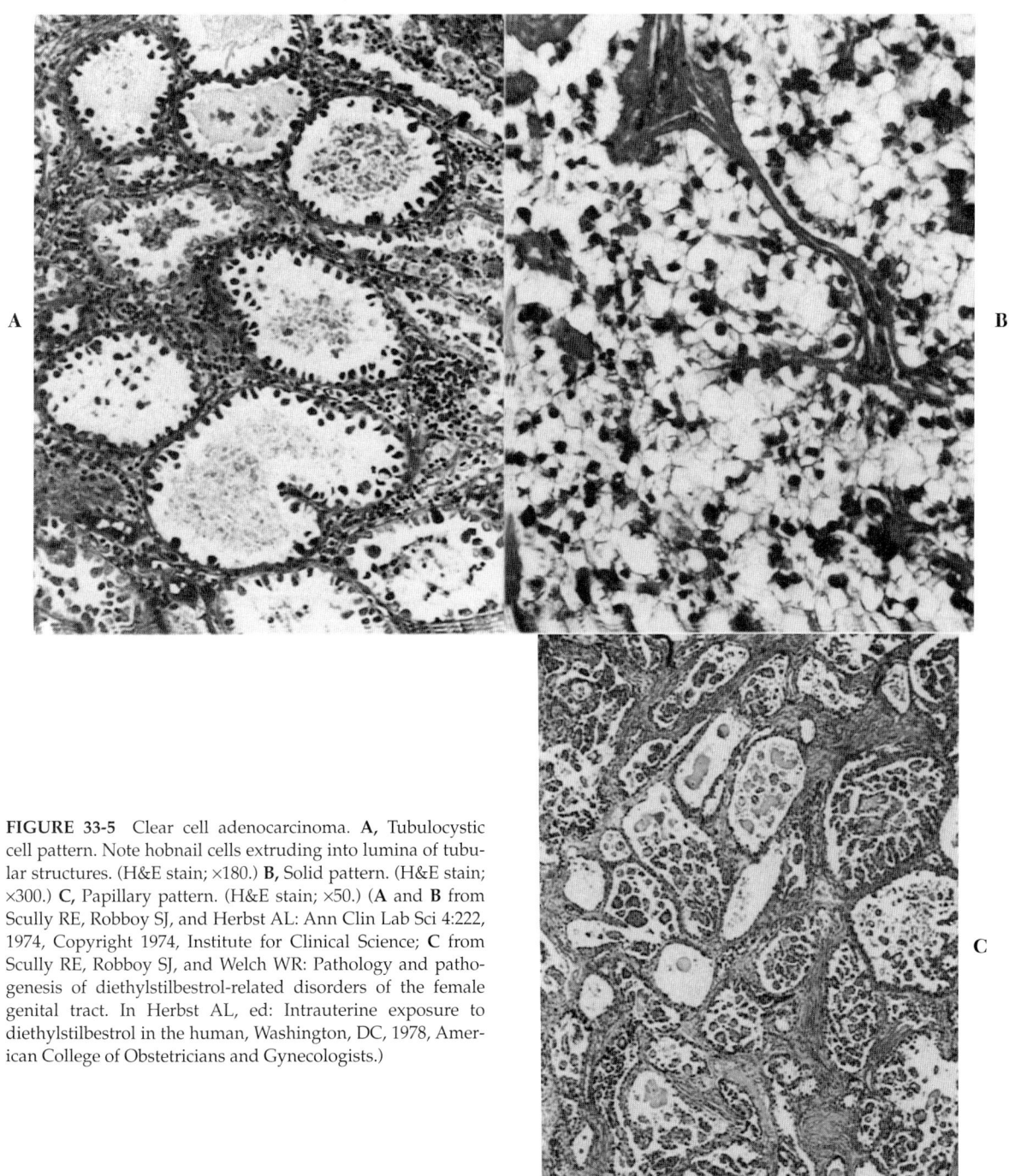

FIGURE 33-5 Clear cell adenocarcinoma. **A,** Tubulocystic cell pattern. Note hobnail cells extruding into lumina of tubular structures. (H&E stain; ×180.) **B,** Solid pattern. (H&E stain; ×300.) **C,** Papillary pattern. (H&E stain; ×50.) (**A** and **B** from Scully RE, Robboy SJ, and Herbst AL: Ann Clin Lab Sci 4:222, 1974, Copyright 1974, Institute for Clinical Science; **C** from Scully RE, Robboy SJ, and Welch WR: Pathology and pathogenesis of diethylstilbestrol-related disorders of the female genital tract. In Herbst AL, ed: Intrauterine exposure to diethylstilbestrol in the human, Washington, DC, 1978, American College of Obstetricians and Gynecologists.)

location of the tumor recurrence, therapy has consisted of additional radical surgery or extensive radiation in localized pelvic disease and systemic chemotherapy in cases of metastatic disease. Unfortunately, no single agent or combination of chemotherapeutic agents has currently emerged as an effective therapy. Prolonged follow-up is necessary for these patients, since recurrences have been reported as long as 20 years after primary therapy, particularly in the lungs and supraclavicular areas.

Data from the Registry on Hormonal Transplacental Carcinogenesis indicate that ovarian preservation with concomitant estrogen stimulation does not adversely affect survival in clear cell adenocarcinoma (see box on page 1034).

Stage I Cases Clear Cell Adenocarcinoma	
Ovarian function preserved	228/244 = 92% 5-year survival
Ovarian function *not* preserved*	98/107 = 90% 5-year survival
*Some may have received hormone replacement therapy.	

Malignant Melanoma

Vaginal melanomas are rare. The tumors occur in adult patients predominantly (average age 60 years). They tend to be deeply invasive in the vagina, although histologically they may resemble other melanomas, such as those of the vulva. However, patients with vaginal melanoma have a worse prognosis than those with vulvar melanoma, in part probably due to delay in diagnosis in comparison to vulvar carcinomas, which are more accessible.

MANAGEMENT. Treatment usually consists of operation with wide excision of the vagina and often dissection of the regional nodes (pelvic or inguinal-femoral, or both), depending on the location of the lesion. However, these very rare lesions are often advanced and have not been eradicated with conventional radiation or chemotherapy. The goal is operative removal with clear surgical margins as noted by Buchanan et al.

SURVIVAL. Local recurrence is common, and the disease is usually fatal. Chung et al. reported a 5-year survival of only 21% in a series of 19 patients. Reid et al. noted 17.4% 5-year survival in 15 patients, but the prognosis improved for those with tumors less than 3 cm in diameter. More recently, Borazjani et al. noted improved survival for patients whose tumors had less than six mitoses per 10 hpf. Van Nostrand et al. reported a 2-year survival for 3 of 4 patients with tumors <10 cm², that is, approximately 3.0 cm in diameter. However, Neven et al. noted that among 9 patients, all those with melanomas >2 mm thick either died or recurred regardless of therapy, emphasizing the importance of tumor thickness on melanoma prognosis (see Chapter 32).

Vaginal Tumors of Infants and Children

Endodermal Sinus Tumor (Yolk-Sac Tumor)

This type of adenocarcinoma is a rare germ cell tumor that usually occurs in the ovary (Chapter 31). The tumor secretes alpha-fetoprotein (AFP), which provides a useful tumor marker to monitor patients treated for these neoplasms. Approximately 20 cases of this unusual malignancy originating in the vagina of infants, predominantly those under 2 years of age, have been reported. The tumor is aggressive, and most patients have died.

Young and Scully reported six patients who were free of disease 2 to 9 years after operation or irradiation, or both, with vincristine, actinomycin D, and cyclophosphamide (VAC; Chapter 31) chemotherapy. Copeland et al. reported similar good results with combination chemotherapy and excision. Collins et al. noted tumor regression in a 5-month-old patient after VAC therapy alone.

Sarcoma Botryoides (Embryonal Rhabdomyosarcoma)

This rare sarcoma is usually diagnosed in the vagina of a young female. Rarely does it occur in a young child over 8 years of age, although cases in adolescents have been reported. The most common symptom is abnormal vaginal bleeding, with an occasional mass at the introitus (Figure 33-6). The tumor grossly will resemble a cluster of grapes forming multiple polypoid masses.

The tumors are believed to begin in the subepithelial layers of the vagina and expand rapidly to fill the vagina. These sarcomas often are multicentric. Histologically, they have a loose myxomatous stroma with malignant pleomorphic cells and occasional eosinophilic rhabdomyoblasts that often contain characteristic cross-striations (strap cells) (Figure 33-7).

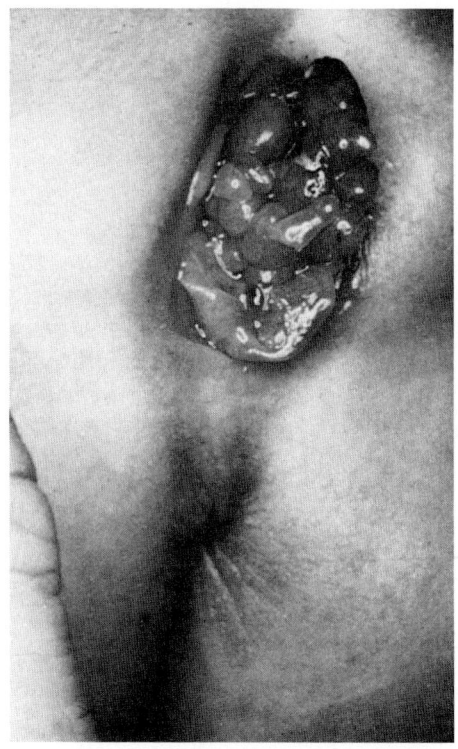

FIGURE 33-6 Sarcoma botryoides protruding through vaginal introitus. (From Herbst AL: Cancer of the vagina. In Gusberg SB and Frick HC, eds: Gynecologic cancer, ed 5, Baltimore, 1978, Williams & Wilkins. Copyright 1978 by Williams & Wilkins Co.)

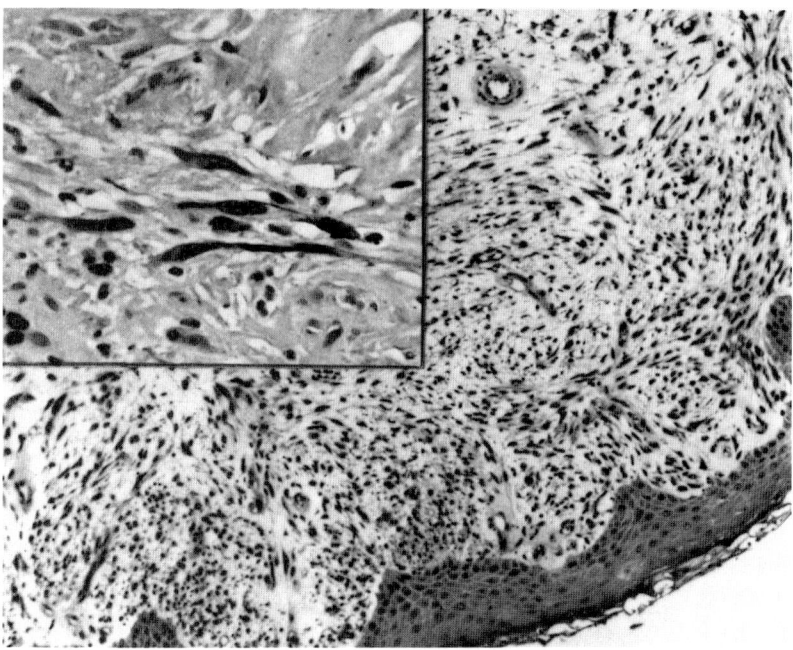

FIGURE 33-7   Vaginal mucosa with sarcoma botryoides showing condensation of malignant cells under epithelium (H&E, ×100). Insert: Immunohistochemical stain for desmin illustrating strap cells (×240). Courtesy of A. Montag, M.D., University of Chicago.

These virulent tumors have been treated in the past by radical surgery, such as pelvic exenteration. However, effective control with less radical surgery has been achieved with a multimodality approach consisting of multiagent chemotherapy (VAC), usually combined with operation. Radiation therapy has also been used. Hays et al. reported recently on 21 patients with vaginal rhabdomyosarcomas who received chemotherapy. Seven relapsed, five of whom had residual disease after incomplete resection. One had disseminated disease. In 17 patients who received chemotherapy for 8 to 48 weeks, a delayed excision could be performed. Long-term survival data for a large number of patients are not available, but such a combined approach appears to result in effective treatment with less mutilating surgery. A multimodality approach including chemotherapy was used by Flamant et al. in 17 females with rhabdomyosarcoma of the vagina or vulva. At the time of their 1990 report 15 appeared cured and 11 of 12 pubescent females have had menses, while 2 have successfully conceived and delivered healthy children. This was emphasized in a report from the Intergroup Rhabdomyosarcoma Study (IRS) by Maurer et al. They found VAC to be effective for disease confined to the vagina without nodal spread. Therapy was effective without irradiation for disease that was locally resected, suggesting for these patients chemotherapy plus operation can be effective therapy.

Pseudosarcoma Botryoides

A rare, benign vaginal polyp that resembles sarcoma botryoides is found in the vagina of infants or pregnant women. Although large atypical cells may be present microscopically, strap cells are absent. Grossly these polyps do not resemble the grapelike appearance of sarcoma botryoides. They are called *pseudosarcoma* botryoides. Treatment by local excision is effective.

KEY POINTS

- Predisposing factors associated with the development of vaginal intraepithelial neoplasia include infection with papillomavirus and herpesvirus II, prior radiation therapy to the vagina, and immunosuppression in patients receiving transplants and those with HIV infection.

- The tendency of intraepithelial squamous neoplasia to develop anywhere in the lower female genital tract is termed *field defect* and describes the increased risk of premalignant changes occurring in the cervix, vagina, or vulva.

- Most cases of vaginal intraepithelial neoplasia (VAIN) occur in the upper one third of the vagina.

- VAIN can be treated by excision, laser, or 5-fluorouracil (5-FU). Excision is often used if the apex is involved, particularly after hysterectomy; laser is generally used for discreet lesions; and 5-FU cream for diffuse multicentric disease.

- The most common primary vaginal malignancy is squamous cell carcinoma (90%).

- Most cancers occurring in the vagina are metastatic.

- Vaginal cancers constitute less than 2% of gynecologic malignancies.

- Tumors of the upper vagina have a lymphatic drainage to the pelvis similar to cervical tumors while those of the lower one third of the vagina go to the pelvic nodes and also the inguinal nodes similar to vulvar tumors.

- Operation is used to treat low-stage tumors primarily of the upper vagina in younger patients.

- Radiation therapy is the most frequently used modality for treatment of squamous cell carcinoma of the vagina. Ideally at least 7000 to 7500 cGy is administered in less than 9 weeks.

- Overall 5-year survival of patients treated for squamous cell carcinoma of the vagina is approximately 45%.

- Clear cell adenocarcinoma is often associated with prenatal DES exposure and has an improved prognosis if the patient is over age 19 years, has a predominant tubulocystic tumor pattern, and has low-stage disease. Those with a positive DES maternal history have a better prognosis.

- Local therapy for small stage I clear cell adenocarcinomas of the vagina is best considered if the tumor is less than 2 cm in diameter, invades less than 3 mm, and is predominantly of the tubulocystic histologic type. Pelvic nodes should be sampled and be free of tumor.

- The overall 5-year survival of patients treated for clear cell adenocarcinoma is approximately 80%, in part due to the high proportion of low-stage cases.

- Vaginal melanomas are usually fatal. They occur primarily in patients over age 50 years.

- Endodermal sinus tumors occur in infants under age 2 years. They secrete alpha-fetoprotein and are usually treated by multiagent chemotherapy followed by operative excision.

- Sarcoma botryoides occurs primarily in children under age 8 years. It is treated by a multimodality approach using multiagent chemotherapy with operative removal and occasionally irradiation.

BIBLIOGRAPHY

Andersen ES: Primary carcinoma of the vagina: a study of 29 cases, Gynecol Oncol 33:317, 1989.

Andersen WA, Sabio H, Durso N, et al: Endodermal sinus tumor of the vagina, Cancer 56:1025, 1985.

Audet-Lapointe P, Body G, Vauclair R, et al: Vaginal intraepithelial neoplasia, Gynecol Oncol 36:232, 1990.

Ballon SC, Roberts JA, and Lagasse LD: Topical 5-fluorouracil in the treatment of intraepithelial neoplasia of the vagina, Obstet Gynecol 54:163, 1979.

Borazjani G, Prem KA, Okagaki T, et al: Primary malignant melanoma of the vagina: a clinicopathological analysis of 10 cases, Gynecol Oncol 37:264, 1990.

Buchanan DJ, Schlaerth J, and Kurosaki T: Primary vaginal melanoma: thirteen-year disease-free survival after wide local excision and review of recent literature, Am J Obstet Gynecol 178:1177, 1998.

Collins HS, Burke TW, Heller PB, et al: Endodermal sinus tumor of the infant vagina treated exclusively by chemotherapy, Obstet Gynecol 73:507, 1989.

Copeland LJ, Gershenson DM, Saul PB, et al: Sarcoma botryoides of the female genital tract, Obstet Gynecol 66:262, 1985.

Creasman WT, Phillips JL, and Menck HR: The national cancer data base report on cancer of the vagina, Cancer 83:1033, 1998.

Davis KP, Stanhope CR, Garton GR, et al: Invasive vaginal carcinoma: analysis of early-stage disease, Gynecol Oncol 42:131, 1991.

DiSaia PJ, Syed AMN, and Puthawala AA: Malignant neoplasia of the upper vagina, Endocrine/Hypertherm Oncol 6:251, 1990.

Elliott GB, Reynolds HA, and Fidler HK: Pseudosarcoma botryoides of cervix and vagina in pregnancy, J Obstet Gynaecol Br Comm 74:728, 1967.

Flamant F, Gerbaulet A, Nihoul-Fekete C, et al: Long-term sequelae of conservative treatment by surgery, brachytherapy, and chemotherapy for vulval and vaginal rhabdomyosarcoma in children, J Clin Oncol 8:1847, 1990.

Herbst AL and Anderson D: Recent advances in clear cell adenocarcinoma of the vagina and cervix secondary to intrauterine exposure to DES, Semin Surg Oncol 6:343, 1990.

Herbst AL, Ulfelder H, and Poskanzer DC: Adenocarcinoma of the vagina, N Engl J Med 284:878, 1971.

Kirkbride P, Fyles A, Rawlings GA, et al: Carcinoma of the vagina—experience at the Princess Margaret Hospital (1974-1989), Gynecol Oncol 56:435, 1995.

Krebs HB: Treatment of vaginal condylomata acuminata by weekly topical application of 5-fluorouracil, Obstet Gynecol 70:68, 1987.

Kucera H and Vavra N: Radiation management of primary carcinoma of the vagina: clinical and histopathological variables associated with survival, Gynecol Oncol 40:12, 1991.

Lee WR, Marcus RB, Sombeck MD, et al: Radiotherapy alone for carcinoma of the vagina: the importance of overall treatment time, Int J Radiat Oncol Biol Phys 29:983, 1994.

Miettinen M, Wahlstrom T, Vesterinen E, et al: Vaginal polyps with pseudosarcomatous features: a clinicopathologic study of seven cases, Cancer 51:1148, 1983.

Mittendorf R and Herbst AL: Diethylstilbestrol: an update, Cancer Prevention, 1-12, August, 1992.

Neven P, Shepherd JH, Masotina A, et al: Malignant melanoma of the vulva and vagina: a report of 23 cases presenting in a 10-year period, Int J Gynecol Cancer 4:383, 1994.

Nori D, Hilaris BS, Stanimir G, et al: Radiation therapy of primary vaginal carcinoma, Int J Radiat Oncol Biol Phys 9:1471, 1983.

Paley PJ, Koh W-J, Stelzer KJ, et al: A new technique for performing Syed template interstitial implants for anterior vaginal tumors using an open retropubic approach, Gynecol Oncol 73:121, 1998.

Pecorelli S, Creasman WT, Pettersson F, et al: FIGO annual report on the results of treatment in gynaecological cancer, vol 23, Milano, Italy. Epidemiol Biostat, 1998.

Perez CA, Camel HM, Galakatos AE, et al: Definitive irradiation in carcinoma of the vagina: long-term evaluation of results, Int J Radiat Oncol Biol Phys 15:1283, 1988.

Petrilli ES, Townsend DE, Morrow CP, et al: Vaginal intraepithelial neoplasm: biologic aspects and treatment with topical 5-fluorouracil and the carbon dioxide laser, Am J Obstet Gynecol 38:321, 1980.

Pingley S, Shrivastava SK, Sarin R, et al: Primary carcinoma of the vagina: Tata Memorial Hospital experience, Int J Radiat Oncol Biol Phys 46:101, 2000.

Piver MS and Rose PG: Long-term follow-up and complications of infants with vulvovaginal embryonal rhabdomyosarcoma treated with surgery, radiation therapy, and chemotherapy, Obstet Gynecol 71:435, 1988.

Plentl AA and Friedman EA: Lymphatic system of the female genitalia, Philadelphia, 1971, WB Saunders Co.

Reid GC, Schmidt RW, Roberts JA, et al: Primary melanoma of the vagina: a clinicopathologic analysis, Obstet Gynecol 74:190, 1989.

Scully RE and Welch WR: Pathology of the female genital tract after prenatal exposure to diethylstilbestrol. In Herbst AL and Bern HA, eds: Developmental effects of diethylstilbestrol (DES) in pregnancy, New York, 1981, Thieme-Stratton.

Senekjian EK, Frey KW, Anderson D, and Herbst AL: Local therapy in stage I clear cell adenocarcinoma of the vagina, Cancer 60:1319, 1987.

Senekjian EK, Frey KW, and Herbst AL: Pelvic exenteration in clear cell adenocarcinoma of the vagina and cervix, Gynecol Oncol 34:413, 1989.

Senekjian EK, Frey KW, Stone C, and Herbst AL: An evaluation of stage II vaginal clear cell adenocarcinoma according to substages, Gynecol Oncol 31:56, 1988.

Spirtos NM, Doshi BP, Kapp DS, and Teng N: Radiation therapy for primary squamous cell carcinoma of the vagina: Stanford University experience, Gynecol Oncol 35:20, 1989.

Sulak P, Barnhill D, Heller P, et al: Nonsquamous cancer of the vagina, Gynecol Oncol 29:309, 1988.

Van Nostrand KM, Lucci III JA, Schell M, et al: Primary vaginal melanoma: improved survival with radical pelvic surgery, Gynecol Oncol 55:234, 1994.

Waggoner SE, Mittendorf R, Biney N, et al: Influence of *in utero* diethylstilbestrol exposure on the prognosis and biologic behavior of vaginal clear cell adenocarcinoma, Gynecol Oncol 55:238, 1994.

Wharton JT, Fletcher GH, and Delclos L: Invasive tumors of the vagina. In Coppleson M, ed: Gynecologic oncology, New York, 1981, Churchill Livingstone, Inc.

Young RH and Scully RE: Endodermal sinus tumor of the vagina: a report of nine cases and review of the literature, Gynecol Oncol 18:380, 1984.

Malignant Disease of the Fallopian Tube
Diagnosis, Management

Hydrops Tubae Profluens. A symptom complex of abnormal vaginal discharge preceded by pain and a mass that may disappear after the discharge is noted. This complex occasionally occurs in patients with tubal carcinoma, but most do not have this complex.

Primary Tubal Carcinoma. An adenocarcinoma usually of papillary or medullary variety arising within the lumen of the oviduct. A transition can often be demon-

strated between nonneoplastic and malignant tubal epithelium.

Tubal carcinoma staging (summary).
  Stage I: Confined to the tubes
  Stage II: Spread to ovaries or pelvic tissues
  Stage III: Intraperitoneal spread or involvement of retroperitoneal nodes
  Stage IV: Metastases to liver parenchyma, outside the peritoneum, or malignant cells in pleural fluid

Primary cancers of the fallopian tube are the rarest of female genital tract malignancies, and almost all are adenocarcinomas. This malignancy comprises approximately 0.3% to 1.1% of all gynecologic cancers. Approximately 80% to 90% of fallopian tube malignancies are metastatic from other sites, usually arising in the ovary or uterus and occasionally in the gastrointestinal tract. Metastatic carcinomas are approximately 10 times as frequent as primary tumors. This chapter reviews current information, with particular emphasis on diagnosis, natural history, and management.

ETIOLOGY AND AGE DISTRIBUTION

The etiology of adenocarcinoma of the fallopian tube is unclear. It has been postulated that chronic salpingitis and prior pelvic inflammatory disease are associated factors. However, pelvic inflammatory disease is common, and the carcinomas rare, suggesting that other factors are involved.

The disease primarily affects older women, the average

age being in the 50s, with a range from 18 to 80 years. Podczaski and Herbst summarized the age distribution of 188 cases reported in the literature since 1970 (Figure 34-1) and noted an average age of 54.9 years. In a recent review of 105 cases, Alvarado-Cabrero et al. noted an age range of 26 to 85 years with an average of 58.5 years. These findings were confirmed in a review by Baekelandt et al., who also noted a history of infertility, low parity, and pelvic infection as possible predisposing factors. In a molecular genetic study, abnormalities of p53 and c-erbB-2 protooncogenes were observed similar to those noted in ovarian carcinoma, suggesting a possible similar biologic behavior between fallopian tube and ovarian carcinoma. A recent epidemiologic study by Rosen et al. indicates that oral contraceptives and pregnancy may reduce the risk of these cancers similar to the effect on ovarian carcinoma. In addition there may be a genetic effect insofar as these investigators found a hereditary association with ovarian carcinoma increase in BRCA1 and 2 mutations in these patients. The increase in fallopian tube carcinoma in patients with BRCA1 mutations was additionally demonstrated by Zweemer et al.

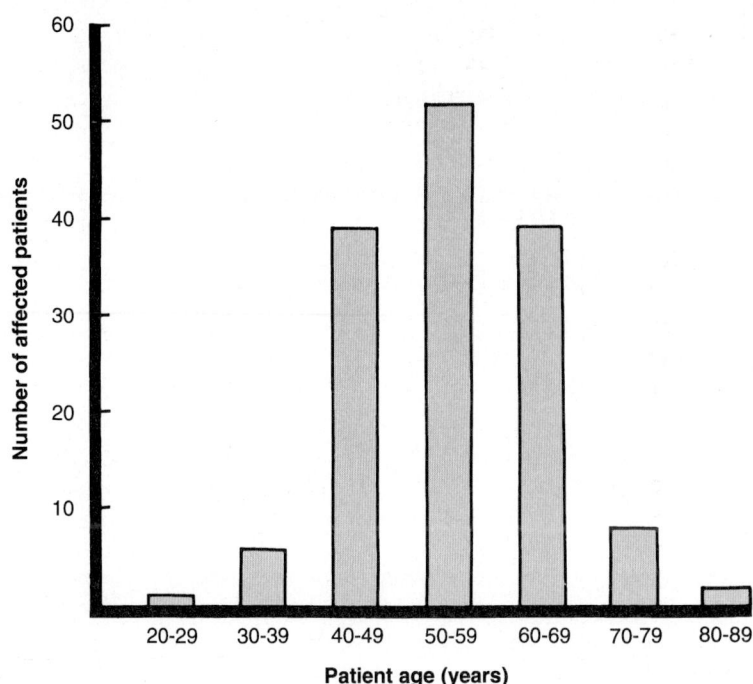

FIGURE 34-1   Histogram illustrating age distribution of patients with tubal carcinomas. (From Podczaski E and Herbst AL: Cancer of the vagina and fallopian tube. In Knapp RC and Berkowitz RS, eds: Gynecologic oncology, New York, 1983, Macmillan Publishing Co.)

DIAGNOSIS

These tumors are usually asymptomatic, and the diagnosis is most frequently made only after the patient has undergone surgical exploration. The most commonly reported sign is abnormal or excessive vaginal bleeding or discharge, which occurs in about 50% of the patients. Pain is less frequently reported. Occasionally an adnexal mass is noted. Abnormal vaginal discharge and bleeding, combined with lower abdominal pain and an adnexal mass in the postmenopausal woman, are considered pathognomonic for the diagnosis of tubal malignancy. Unfortunately, these three conditions rarely exist together, which is why the diagnosis is frequently made postoperatively. The term *hydrops tubae profluens* has been used to describe the abnormal discharge and pain that presumably result from blockage of the distal part of the fallopian tube. Subsequent peristalsis produces the discharge, occasionally accompanied by the disappearance of the mass secondary to the expulsion of fluid from the dilated tube. The disease should be strongly suspected in anyone with these findings, which rarely occurs. Vaginal cytology may show malignant adenocarcinoma cells. However, vaginal cytology is usually negative; Benedet et al. found it to be positive in only 10% of their 40 patients, although Hirai et al. reported preoperative cytology was positive in 6 (40%) of their 15 cases.

The diagnosis of tubal carcinoma should be considered in any patient with vaginal cytology positive for adenocarcinoma in whom the diagnosis of endometrial carcinoma has been excluded, although ovarian and endocervical adenocarcinomas are other possibilities. The diagnosis should also be suspected in patients with postmenopausal uterine bleeding for whom dilation and curettage and hysteroscopy fail to reveal the cause. Transvaginal ultrasound can be of aid in diagnosing abnormal adnexal masses. Laparoscopy can be of benefit in establishing the diagnosis for patients, particularly those with questionable or abnormal ultrasound appearances.

PATHOLOGY

On gross examination the fallopian tube containing primary adenocarcinoma often appears dilated and may resemble a hydrosalpinx until the tube is opened, revealing an infiltrating tumor (Figures 34-2 and 34-3). Sometimes it is difficult to be certain that the tumor is of tubal origin, and confusion with metastatic carcinoma, particularly from the ovary, can be a diagnostic problem. In 1950 Hu, Taymor, and Hertig suggested the following criteria to allow the diagnosis of primary tubal carcinoma:

1. The primary tumor is grossly within the lumen of the tube.
2. The mucosa of the tube is involved with the tumor, which displays a papillary (or medullary) pattern.
3. A transition can be demonstrated between the malignant and nonmalignant tubal epithelium (if the tubal wall is involved to a great extent).

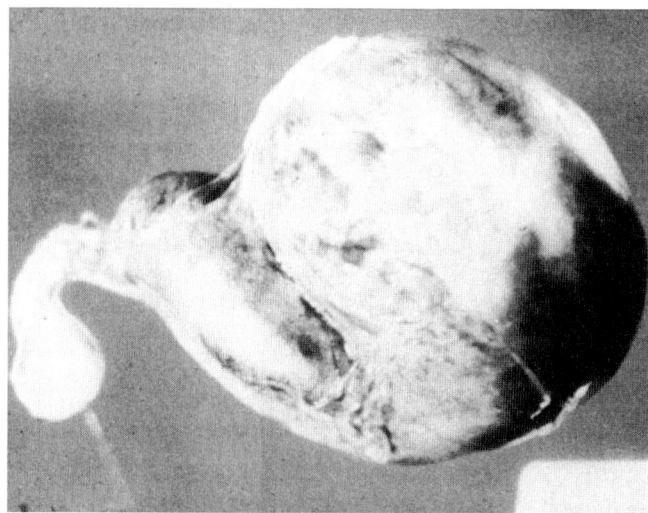

FIGURE 34-2 External appearance of fallopian tube with primary adenocarcinoma. (From Podczaski E and Herbst AL: Cancer of the vagina and fallopian tube. In Knapp RC and Berkowitz RS, eds: Gynecologic oncology, New York, 1983, Macmillan Publishing Co. [Courtesy Freidoon Azizi, M.D.])

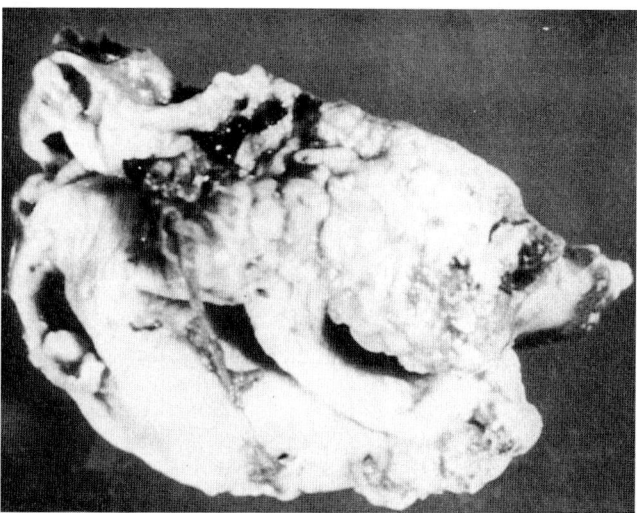

FIGURE 34-3 Cross section through fallopian tube demonstrating primary adenocarcinoma. (From Podczaski E and Herbst AL: Cancer of the vagina and fallopian tube. In Knapp RC and Berkowitz RS, eds: Gynecologic oncology, New York, 1983, Macmillan Publishing Co. [Courtesy Freidoon Azizi, M.D.])

Figures 34-4 and 34-5 demonstrate a primary tubal carcinoma showing a papillary-alveolar pattern. Serous histology resembling ovarian carcinoma is most common, but endometrioid, clear cell, and other rare patterns have been reported. These tumors can arise in either tube with approximately equal frequency and occasionally may be bilateral.

CLINICAL STAGING AND NATURAL HISTORY

The 1991 FIGO staging system for fallopian tube carcinoma is shown in Table 34-1. The tumor spreads in a manner similar to epithelial carcinoma of the ovary.

The carcinoma is initially confined to the lumen of the tube but can penetrate to the serosa and then spread intraperitoneally to involve the surface of the bowel, the omentum, and the parietal peritoneum, similar to ovarian carcinoma. The peritoneum is the most frequent site of metastatic spread of tubal carcinoma. In addition, lymphatic spread occurs, particularly to the paraaortic nodes. Tamini and Figge noted metastases to the paraaortic nodes in 5 of 15 patients, and these nodes were the only site of metastatic disease in two patients. Thus the retroperitoneal nodes must also be considered as sites of common spread in the management of these cancers, similar to considerations for ovarian epithelial carcinomas.

Prognosis in tubal carcinoma is related to the extent ("stage") of disease (see Table 34-1). In addition, Asmussen et al. noted in a study of 33 cases that vessel invasion was a poor prognostic factor. In a study of 115 patients,

Peters et al. noted that depth of invasion of the tubal wall was also a factor for those with disease confined to the tube. A comprehensive review of 128 cases from the Radiumhemmet, by Hellström et al., confirmed stage to be the primary prognostic factor. Additionally the degree of differentiation of the tumor affected prognosis. The study of Alvarado-Cabrero et al. confirmed higher stage tumors and age greater than 66 years as well as absence of closure of the fimbriated end of the tube worsened the prognosis. They also correlated prognosis with the depth of invasion of the tumor into the tubal wall and noted a markedly worse prognosis for tumors that had a fimbrial location. Recently Hefler et al. noted CA 125 levels were also prognostic with elevated values associated with a worse prognosis. Chemotherapy with cisplatin (see following discussion) also prolonged survival.

MANAGEMENT

As noted previously, the diagnosis of primary tubal carcinoma is most frequently made at the time of surgical exploration. Once the diagnosis is established, frequently by frozen section, a thorough operative staging procedure is carried out, including a total abdominal hysterectomy and bilateral salpingo-oophorectomy. Peritoneal cytology testing is performed using 200 to 300 ml of normal saline solution mixed with 0.5 ml (5000 IU) of heparin to prevent clotting of any blood present in the fluid. If there is no evidence of intraperitoneal spread, a paraaortic node sampling should be performed to rule out extrapelvic spread. This is particularly important in cases of large or

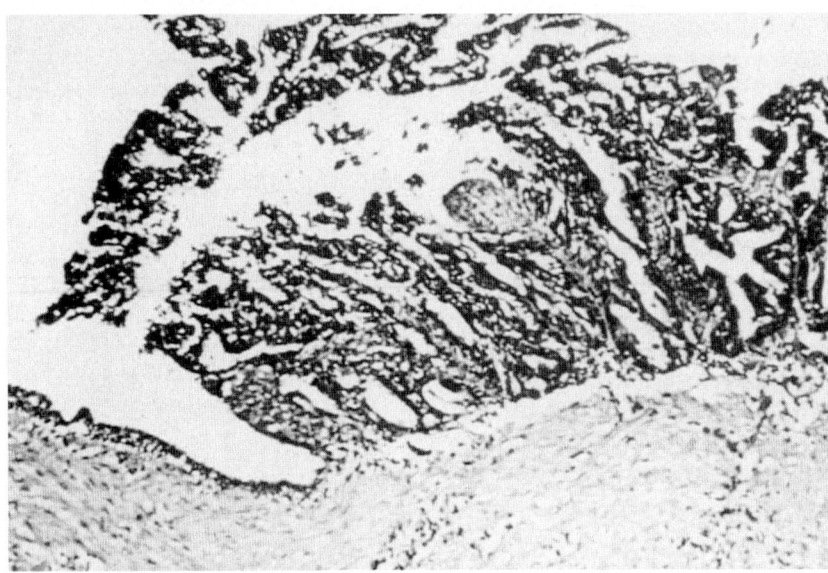

FIGURE 34-4 Microscopic appearance of well-differentiated papillary adenocarcinoma of fallopian tube. (From Podczaski E and Herbst AL: Cancer of the vagina and fallopian tube. In Knapp RC and Berkowitz RS, eds: Gynecologic oncology, New York, 1983, Macmillan Publishing Co. [Courtesy Elizabeth Alenghat, M.D.])

poorly differentiated tumors, in view of the fact that these carcinomas often metastasize to the paraaortic nodes. An omentectomy should also be performed and an attempt made to remove all gross disease. As emphasized by Podratz et al., meticulous staging is important both for optimal effective treatment and to help decide if additional postoperative therapy is advisable.

Because of the varied experience in the treatment of these malignancies, a number of therapeutic approaches have been suggested. The value of postoperative radiation therapy or chemotherapy is not established, although those modalities have been reported to be effective. In the case of a stage I carcinoma, in which the cancer is confined to the tubal lumen and peritoneal cytology is negative, therapy usually consists only of primary operation. If there is positive peritoneal cytology (stage IC), postoperative intraperitoneal ^{32}P is often advised or whole-abdominal radiation may be used. However, successful remissions have also been reported with platinum-containing chemotherapy regimens. If there is spread of tumor outside of the tube to the pelvis, postoperative radiation including the paraaortic nodes has also been considered, depending on the extent of disease discovered at surgery. Brown et al. recommend abdominopelvic radiation postoperatively providing there is no residual disease greater than 2 cm^2 after operation.

For intraperitoneal disease or for recurrent metastatic carcinoma, chemotherapy usually is prescribed. Deppe et al. reported two patients with widespread disseminated fallopian tube carcinoma who were treated with *cis*-diamminedichloroplatinum (cisplatin, 50 mg/m^2)

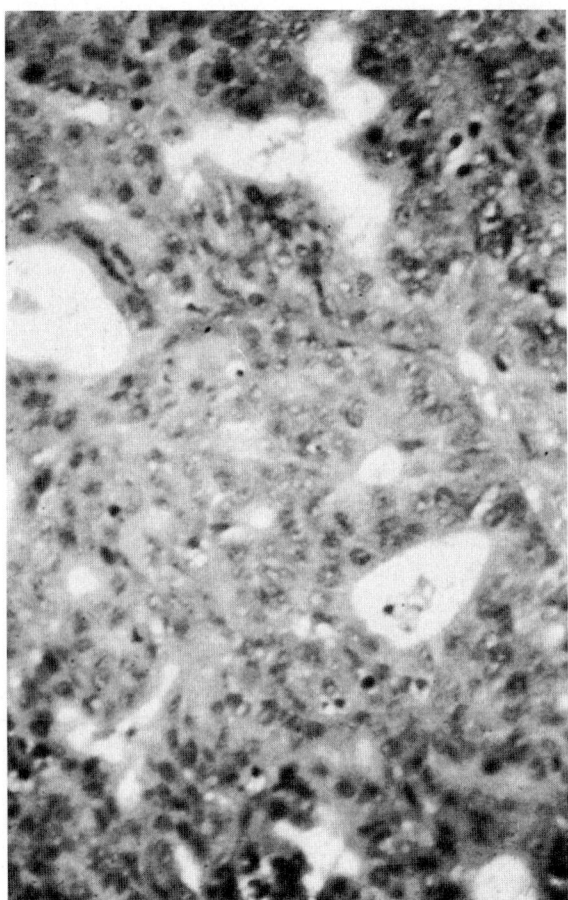

FIGURE 34-5 Poorly differentiated tubal carcinoma with a predominantly solid growth pattern. (From Azizi F and Johnston GA: Female Patient 7:42, 1982.)

TABLE 34-1
FIGO Staging System for Tubal Carcinoma

Stage	Characteristics
Stage 0	Carcinoma in situ (limited to tubal mucosa)
Stage I	Growth limited to the fallopian tube
Stage IA	Growth is limited to one tube with extension into the submucosa and/or muscularis, but not penetrating the serosal surface; no ascites
Stage IB	Growth is limited to both tubes with extension into the submucosa and/or muscularis, but not penetrating the serosal surface; no ascites
Stage IC	Tumor either stage IA or IB, but with tumor extension through or onto the tubal serosa; or with ascites present containing malignant cells or with positive peritoneal washings
Stage II	Growth involving one or both fallopian tubes with pelvic extension
Stage IIA	Extension and/or metastasis to the uterus and/or ovaries
Stage IIB	Extension to other pelvic tissues
Stage IIC	Tumor either stage IIA or IIB and with ascites present containing malignant cells or with positive peritoneal washings
Stage III	Tumor involves one or both fallopian tubes with peritoneal implants outside of the pelvis and/or positive retroperitoneal or inguinal nodes. Superficial liver metastasis equals stage III. Tumor appears limited to the true pelvis, but with histologically proven malignant extension to the small bowel or omentum
Stage IIIA	Tumor is grossly limited to the true pelvis with negative nodes, but with histologically confirmed microscopic seeding of abdominal peritoneal surfaces
Stage IIIB	Tumor involving one or both tubes with histologically confirmed implants of abdominal peritoneal surfaces none exceeding 2 cm in diameter. Lymph nodes are negative
Stage IIIC	Abdominal implants greater than 2 cm in diameter and/or positive retroperitoneal or inguinal nodes
Stage IV	Growth involving one or both fallopian tubes with distant metastases. If pleural effusion is present, there must be positive cytology to be stage IV. Parenchymal liver metastases equals stage IV

Note: Staging for fallopian tube is by the surgical-pathologic system. Operative findings designating stage are determined prior to tumor debulking.

and doxorubicin (Adriamycin, 37.5 mg/m^2) as well as a progestin, megestrol acetate (Megace, 160 mg daily). One patient also received cyclophosphamide (Cytoxan, 400 mg/m^2). At a second-look procedure 10 to 13 months later, both patients showed no evidence of disease. In a multicenter analysis, Peters et al. noted a significant improvement in patient survival for "stage III" disease with combination chemotherapy, primarily platinum,

Cytoxan, and Adriamycin, as reported by Morris et al., from MD Anderson Cancer Center. The effectiveness of platinum chemotherapy for tubal carcinoma was confirmed in the multivariant analysis of 128 cases by Hellström et al. Barakat et al. also confirmed a favorable response to cisplatinum. They also utilized a second-look procedure and found an 80% survival for those with a negative second-look, and in this small series of 35 cases stage was not a predictor of a negative second-look operation but lack of residual disease after primary operation was. In view of the resemblance of the behavior of fallopian tube carcinoma to ovarian carcinoma, Taxol (see Chapter 31) is also being tried.

Definitive conclusions cannot be drawn regarding the results of therapy. Sedlis noted a 5-year survival of 38% for all stages of tubal carcinoma. Patients with tubal carcinoma confined to the tube have the best prognosis, expecting a 70% to 80% 5-year survival. High-grade tumors behave more aggressively, and platinum therapy appears to enhance survival. A complete response of fallopian tube carcinoma to paclitaxel (Taxol) has been reported. In a selected literature review of 409 patients, Baekelandt et al. noted an overall survival of approximately 40% for all stages.

In summary, operation by TAH-BSO is adequate for stages IA and IB. For stage IC, either P32 or adjuvant chemotherapy with platinum-containing regimens are appropriate. For stages II and III, chemotherapy would be chosen by most therapists after operation, although some centers might advocate whole-abdominal radiation with a pelvic boost for stage II disease. Chemotherapy would be most likely used for stage IV disease.

OTHER TUMORS

Sarcomas of the fallopian tube are extremely rare. They may be mixed, containing carcinomatous elements (carcinosarcoma), or may have heterologous sarcomatous tissue, and the term *mixed mesodermal tumors* has also been used. These tumors' behavior is similar to that of other sarcomas and carcinosarcomas within the uterus (Chapter 30). Treatment consists of surgery, with removal of the uterus and tube, and follow-up chemotherapy, usually with a regimen including doxorubicin (Adriamycin). Paclitaxel (Taxol) and platinum have also been used as described in Chapter 31 (ovarian carcinoma). Choriocarcinoma of the tube has also been reported and is believed to result from trophoblastic disease associated with ectopic pregnancy. The same considerations of therapy apply to these lesions as for trophoblastic disease elsewhere (Chapter 35).

- Ninety percent of tubal cancers are metastatic, mostly from the ovary, uterus, or gastrointestinal tract.

- Only 10% of patients with fallopian tube carcinoma have positive vaginal cytology.

- Primary tubal carcinoma is the rarest gynecologic malignancy (0.3% to 1.1%).

- The diagnosis of tubal carcinoma is usually made at operation.

- The average age of patients with tubal carcinoma is 55 years.

- Predisposing factors for primary tubal carcinoma appear to be infertility, nulliparity or low parity, pelvic infection, and a family history of ovarian cancer.

- Oral contraceptives and pregnancy may decrease the risk.

- The most common site of spread of tubal carcinoma is to the peritoneum and retroperitoneal lymph nodes.

- Overall 5-year survival for all stages of primary tubal carcinoma is approximately 40%.

- The diagnosis of tubal carcinoma should be considered for anyone with vaginal cytology positive for adenocarcinoma in whom the diagnosis of endometrial carcinoma has been excluded. It should also be considered for anyone with postmenopausal uterine bleeding in whom a D&C and hysteroscopy fail to reveal the cause. Ultrasound can aid in the preoperative diagnosis.

- The triad of abnormal bleeding, adnexal mass, and watery discharge in a postmenopausal woman is suggestive of tubal carcinoma, although most fallopian tube carcinomas present without the triad.

- Prognosis in tubal carcinoma is related to stage of disease, tumor differentiation, vascular invasion histologically, and, for tumors confined to the tube, depth of invasion of the muscularis and pretreatment CA 125 levels.

- Combination chemotherapy using cisplatin improves survival in disseminated or recurrent fallopian tube carcinoma.

BIBLIOGRAPHY

Alvarado-Cabrero I, Young RH, Vamvakas EC, et al: Carcinoma of the fallopian tube: a clinicopathologic study of 105 cases with observations on staging and prognostic factors, Gynecol Oncol 72:367, 1999.

Asmussen M, Kaern J, Kjoerstad K, et al: Primary adenocarcinoma localized to the fallopian tubes: report on 33 cases, Gynecol Oncol 30:183, 1988.

Baekelandt M, Kock M, Wesling F, and Gerris J: Primary adenocarcinoma of the fallopian tube: review of the literature, Int J Gynecol Cancer 3:65, 1993.

Barakat RR, Rubin SC, Saigo PE, et al: Cisplatin-based combination chemotherapy in carcinoma of the fallopian tube, Gynecol Oncol 42:156, 1991.

Barakat R, Rubin SC, Saigo PE, et al: Second-look laparotomy in carcinoma of the fallopian tube, Obstet Gynecol 82:748, 1993.

Benedet JL, White GW, Fairey RN, and Boyes DA: Adenocarcinoma of the fallopian tube, Obstet Gynecol 50:654, 1977.

Brown MD, Kohorn EI, Kapp DS, et al: Fallopian tube carcinoma, Int J Radiat Oncol Biol Phys 11:583, 1985.

Daya D, Young RH, and Scully RE: Endometrioid carcinoma of the fallopian tube resembling an adnexal tumor of probable wolffian origin: a report of six cases, Int J Gynecol Pathol 11:122, 1992.

Deppe G, Bruckner HW, and Cohen CJ: Combination chemotherapy for advanced carcinoma of the fallopian tube, Obstet Gynecol 56:530, 1980.

Hefler LA, Rosen AC, Graf AH, et al: The clinical value of serum concentrations of cancer antigen 125 in patients with primary fallopian tube carcinoma, Cancer 89:1555, 2000.

Hellström AC, Silfversward C, Nillson B, and Petterson F: Carcinoma of the fallopian tube: a clinical and histopathologic review. The Radiumhemmet series, Int J Gynecol Cancer 4:395, 1994.

Hershey DW, Fennell RH, and Major FJ: Primary carcinoma of the fallopian tube, Obstet Gynecol 57:367, 1981.

Hirai Y, Kaku S, Teshima H, et al: Clinical study of primary carcinoma of the fallopian tube: experience with 15 cases, Gynecol Oncol 34:20, 1989.

Hu CY, Taymor ML, and Hertig AT: Primary carcinoma of the fallopian tube, Am J Obstet Gynecol 59:58, 1950.

Lacy MQ, Hartmann CL, Kenney GL, et al: c-erbB-2 and p53 expression in fallopian tube carcinoma, Cancer 75:2891, 1995.

Morris M, Gershenson DM, Burke TW, et al: Treatment of fallopian tube carcinoma with cisplatin, doxorubicin, and cyclophosphamide, Obstet Gynecol 76:1020, 1990.

Peters WA, Andersen WA, Hopkins MP, et al: Prognostic features of carcinoma of the fallopian tube, Obstet Gynecol 71:757, 1988.

Phelps HM and Chapman KE: Role of radiation therapy in treatment of primary carcinoma of the uterine tube, Obstet Gynecol 43:669, 1974.

Podczaski E and Herbst AL: Cancer of the vagina and fallopian tube. In Knapp RC and Berkowitz RS, eds: Gynecologic oncology, ed 2, New York, 1990, Macmillan Publishing Co.

Podratz KC, Podczaski ES, Gaffey TA, et al: Primary carcinoma of the fallopian tube, Am J Obstet Gynecol 154:1319, 1986.

Puls LE, Davey DD, DePriest D, et al: Immunohistochemical staining for CA-125 in fallopian tube carcinomas, Gynecol Oncol 48:360, 1993.

Rose PG, Piver MS, and Tsukada Y: Fallopian tube cancer: the Roswell Park experience, Cancer 66:2661, 1990.

Rosen B, Aziz S, Narod S, et al: Hereditary and reproductive influences on fallopian tube carcinoma (abstract), Gynecol Oncol 76:231, 2000.

Schiller HM and Silverberg SG: Staging and prognosis in primary carcinoma of the fallopian tube, Cancer 28:389, 1971.

Sedlis A: Carcinoma of the fallopian tube, Surg Clin North Am 58:121, 1978.

Tamini HK and Figge DC: Adenocarcinoma of the uterine tube: potential for lymph node metastases, Am J Obstet Gynecol 141:132, 1981.

Tresukosol D, Kudelka AP, Edwards CL, et al: Primary fallopian tube adenocarcinoma: clinical complete response after salvage treatment with high-dose paclitaxel, Gynecol Oncol 58:258, 1995.

Wu JP, Tanner WS, and Fardal PM: Malignant mixed müllerian tumor of the uterine tube, Obstet Gynecol 41:707, 1981.

Yoonessi M: Carcinoma of the fallopian tube, Obstet Gynecol Surv 34:257, 1979.

Zweemer RP, van Diest PJ, Verheijen RHM, et al: Molecular evidence linking primary cancer of the fallopian tube to BRCA1 mutations, Gynecol Oncol 76:45, 2000.

Gestational Trophoblastic Disease

Hydatidiform Mole, Nonmetastatic and Metastatic Gestational Trophoblastic Tumor: Diagnosis and Management

KEY TERMS AND DEFINITIONS

Androgenesis. Impregnation of an inactive egg by a paternal haploid sperm that duplicates its chromosomes to provide a diploid complement. This results in a complete mole.

Choriocarcinoma. A morphologic term applied to a highly malignant type of trophoblastic neoplasia in which both the cytotrophoblast and syncytiotrophoblast grow in a malignant fashion.

Complete Mole. A molar pregnancy with swelling of all placental villi. Fetal tissues are absent.

Gestational Trophoblastic Disease (GTD). The spectrum of diseases resulting from the abnormal proliferation of trophoblast associated with pregnancy.

Gestational Trophoblastic Tumor (GTT). A term applied to gestational diseases that have neoplastic malignant potential, including invasive mole, choriocarcinoma, and placental-site trophoblastic tumor. It can be either nonmetastatic or metastatic. It is occasionally termed gestational trophoblastic neoplasia (GTN).

High Risk Metastatic Gestational Trophoblastic Disease (GTD [GTT]). Patient with pretreatment serum β-hCG greater than 40,000 mIU/ml; or more than 4 months' duration of disease; or previous chemotherapy failure; and brain or liver metastases (vagina and lung excluded).

Hydatidiform Mole. A placental abnormality involving swollen placental villi and trophoblastic hyperplasia with loss of fetal blood vessels. There are two types: partial and complete.

Invasive Mole. A variant of hydatidiform mole in which the hydropic villi invade into the myometrium or blood vessels. It may spread to extrauterine sites.

Low Risk Metastatic GTD (GTT). Patients with metastatic disease outside the uterus, excluding the brain or liver; serum β-hCG less than 40,000 mIU/ml; duration of disease less than 4 months; and no prior chemotherapy.

Partial Mole. A molar pregnancy with some normal and some swollen villi plus fetal, cord, and/or amniotic membrane elements.

Placental-Site Trophoblastic Tumor. A rare type of GTT arising in the uterus that secretes human placental lactogen (HPL) and human chorionic gonadotrophin (hCG) and is often resistant to chemotherapy.

Stages of GTT:
I: Confined to corpus uteri
II: Metastases to the pelvis and vagina
III: Metastases to the lungs
IV: Distant metastases (liver, brain, etc.) In each stage subsets are:
   A. No risk factor
   B. One risk factor
   C. 2 risk factors
Risk factor definitions:
   1. Pretherapy serum hCG > 100,000 mIU/ml
   2. Disease duration > 6 months

Theca Lutein Cysts. Enlargements of the ovary occurring with hydatidiform moles and consisting of theca lutein cells. Usually they regress after treatment of the mole.

Gestational trophoblastic disease (GTD) refers to the spectrum of abnormalities of the trophoblastic associated with pregnancy. These neoplasias have been known for hundreds of years, and they specifically secrete human chorionic gonadotrophin (hCG). The availability of extremely sensitive and specific assays to measure hCG allows prediction of the clinical status of the disease, as well as monitoring of treatment. The initial use of methotrexate in 1956 by Li, Hertz, and Spencer to successfully treat malignant trophoblastic disease completely altered the prognosis of patients with these tumors and represented a milestone in the cure of human tumors by chemotherapeutic agents.

This chapter presents the current classification of GTDs and the factors that appear to be associated with their development. The methods of diagnosis, therapy, and follow-up of these patients are reviewed.

CHARACTERISTICS

Trophoblastic tissue normally shares certain characteristics with malignancies, such as the ability to divide rapidly, to invade locally, and occasionally to metastasize to distant sites such as the lung, yet these activities usually cease at the end of pregnancy, and the trophoblast disappears. However, in GTD, abnormal growth and development continue beyond the end of pregnancy.

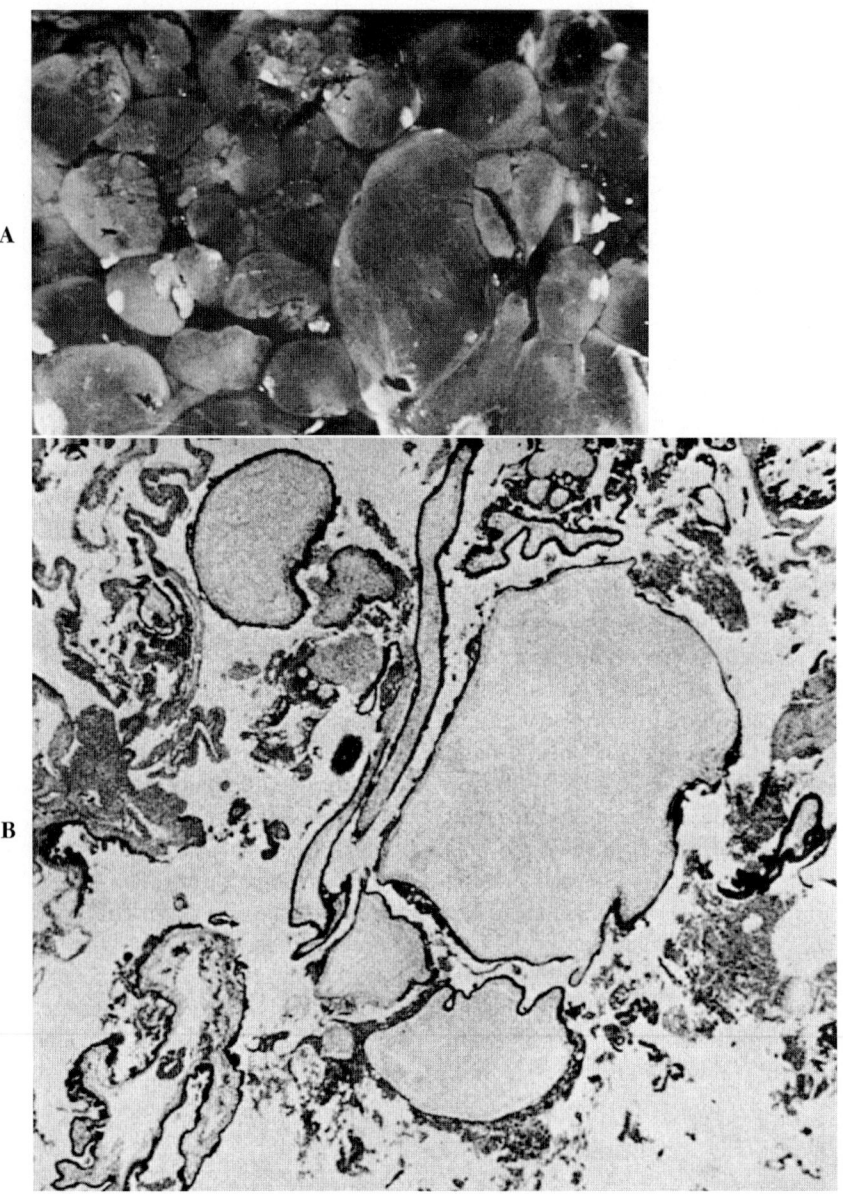

FIGURE 35-1 **A,** Hydatidiform mole. A few vesicles approach 1 cm in diameter. The background is formed by smaller vesicles. **B,** Hydatidiform mole aborted by suction curettage. A large intact vesicle is near the center. Many vesicles, however, have been ruptured and have collapsed. (From Bigelow B: Gestational trophoblast disease. In Blaustein A, editor: Pathology of the female genital tract, ed 2, New York, 1982, Springer-Verlag New York, Inc.)

MORPHOLOGY

Hydatidiform Mole

A hydatidiform mole has three morphologic characteristics: (1) a mass of vesicles (distended villi) that appear as large, grapelike dilations (Figure 35-1); (2) a loss of fetal blood vessels, which are either diminished or absent from the villi; and (3) hyperplasia of the syncytiotrophoblast and cytotrophoblast.

The terms *complete mole* and *partial mole* have been used to describe the variations of molar pregnancies. With a complete mole, all placental villi are swollen and the fetus, cord, and amniotic membrane are absent. In partial molar pregnancy, only some chorionic villi are swollen, and fetal tissues are present, such as amniotic membrane, cord, or even rarely a full-term fetus, although the fetus is usually chromosomally abnormal (see following discussion). With a partial mole the trophoblastic hyperplasia is limited to the syncytiotrophoblast.

The genetics of molar pregnancy has been extensively studied. In normal pregnancy, half the chromosomes of the conceptus are paternal and the other half maternal, resulting in a diploid content. In complete mole, only paternal chromosomes are believed to be present; there are 46 chromosomes and nearly always 46, XX, although a few moles with 46, XY karyotype have been reported. The development of complete mole appears to result from the fertilization of an "empty egg," one with an absent or inactive nucleus. The haploid paternal set of chromosomes from the sperm impregnate the inactive egg. These paternal chromosomes then duplicate to give the diploid number, a process known as *androgenesis,* the development of an "embryo" due only to chromosomes from an X-bearing sperm (Figure 35-2). In the rare case of complete mole with an XY chromosomal content, the "empty egg" appears to be fertilized by two haploid sperm, one X and one Y.

Incomplete, or partial, moles are usually triploid and have 69 chromosomes of both maternal and paternal origin. The most common mechanism for the origin of partial mole (Figure 35-3) is a haploid egg being fertilized by two sperm, resulting in three sets of chromosomes. Alternatively, triploidy could result when an abnormal diploid sperm fertilizes the haploid egg. It is also possible for an abnormal diploid egg to be fertilized by a haploid sperm, but this latter mechanism usually results in an abnormal conceptus with congenital abnormalities rather than a partial mole. Partial mole is often difficult to diagnose and may present as a missed abortion in the second trimester. Although these fetuses are usually abnormal, Watson et al. noted that some partial moles have occurred with phenotypically normal fetuses. In such cases the uterus is small for dates. As noted by Lage et al., a few partial moles are diploid, and these very rare cases may be less sensitive to chemotherapy than triploid moles if subsequent GTT develops (see following discussion).

Partial moles are rarely associated with the subsequent development of GTT. Bagshawe et al. reported that neoplasia requiring chemotherapy occurs in approximately 1 in 200 cases of partial mole, compared with 1 in 12 with complete mole. However, Rice et al. noted 16 of 240 partial moles (6.6%) had malignant *sequelae,* all of which responded to chemotherapy. Goldstein et al. summarized a number of published reports that indicated that GTT followed partial mole in 39 of 1125 (3.5%) cases. Despite rare subsequent malignancy, patients with partial moles need the same follow-up as those with complete mole.

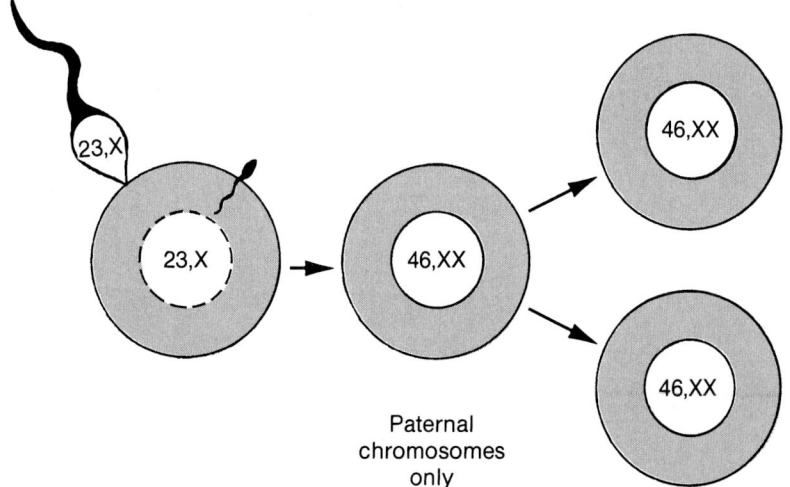

FIGURE 35-2 Paternal chromosomal origin of a complete classic mode (46,XX). *Left to right,* entry of normal sperm with haploid set of 23,X into egg whose 23,X haploid set is lost; egg is "taken over" by paternal chromosomes, which duplicate (without cell's division) to reach requisite complement of 46. Observe that virtually the same result can be obtained through a fertilization by two sperm gaining entry into an "empty egg" (dispermy). (From Szulman AE and Surti U: Clin Obstet Gynecol 27:172, 1984.)

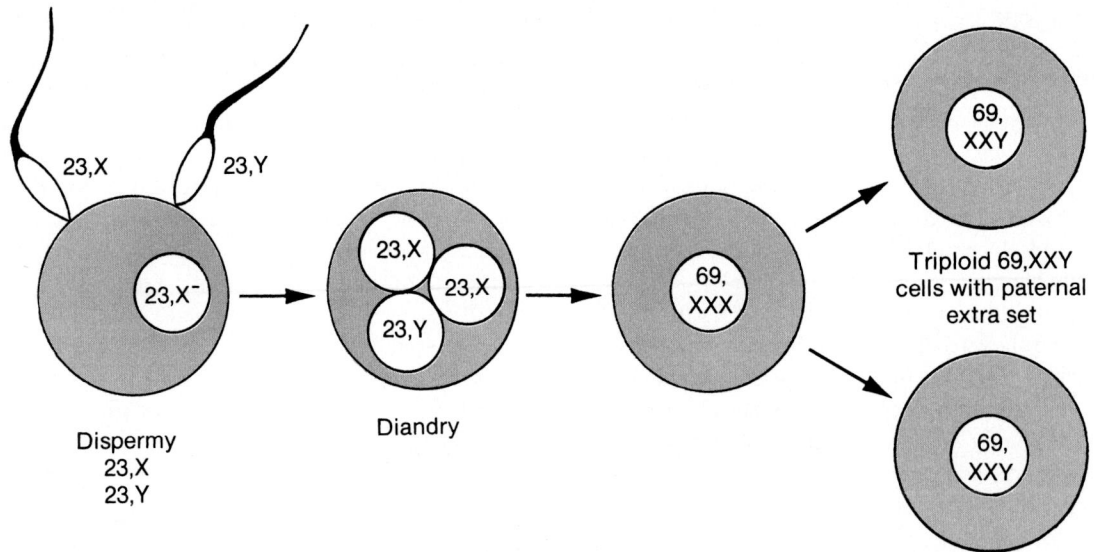

FIGURE 35-3   Triploid chromosomal origin of partial mole (69,XXY—dispermy). Fertilization of an egg equipped with a normal 23,X complement by two independently produced sperm (dispermy) to give total of 69 chromosomes. Observe that triploidy can also result through fertilization by sperm carrying father's total complement of 46,XY. (From Szulman AE and Surti U: Clin Obstet Gynecol 27:172, 1984.)

Choriocarcinoma

Choriocarcinomas are malignancies that occur after or in association with pregnancy, although the same histologic tumor can develop without pregnancy as a primary neoplasm in the ovaries. The prognosis for primary gonadal choriocarcinomas, which also occur in testes, is worse than for those associated with gestation.

The diagnosis is made histologically, and the term is applied to the finding of malignant cytotrophoblast and syncytiotrophoblast. Chorionic villi are absent. These tumors (Figure 35-4) tend to be hemorrhagic and necrotic. The latter is common because these tumors frequently outgrow their blood supply. Metastases are common.

Most but not all gestational choriocarcinomas develop after molar pregnancies. Trophoblastic tissue normally regresses within 2 to 3 weeks after delivery, including cells that may have spread to the lung. The normal processes leading to this regression are unknown, but the finding of trophoblastic cells in the uterus more than 3 weeks after delivery should lead one to consider the possibility of choriocarcinoma.

Placental-Site Trophoblastic Tumor

The term *placental-site trophoblastic tumor* (trophoblastic pseudotumor) was introduced by Young and Scully to describe a rare tumor that consists of excessive groups of mononucleate and multinucleate trophoblastic cells at the implantation site accompanied by an inflammatory cell reaction. Histocytochemical studies have shown that the cells of these tumors tend to stain more for human placental lactogen (HPL) than for hCG, and both hCG

and HPL should be monitored. The tumor can lead to hemorrhage and uterine perforation. It tends to be locally invasive and most patients do not develop metastases. Hysterectomy is the treatment of choice. How et al. noted 77 patients reported as of 1995, with 62 of them alive.

Chemotherapy is usually administered for metastatic disease when it occurs, but is less effective with these tumors than with other gestational trophoblastic tumors, which is another reason for prompt operative treatment. The EMA/CO regimen (see following discussion) has been reported by Dessau et al. to produce long-term survival.

EPIDEMIOLOGY AND INCIDENCE

Extensive investigation has been performed to ascertain the factors that enhance the occurrence of trophoblastic disease. The major areas that have been evaluated are maternal age, history of fetal wastage or prior hydatidiform mole, geographic and racial distribution, and ABO blood groupings.

Hydatidiform Mole

There is wide variation in the reported incidence of hydatidiform mole. The rates are usually expressed in terms of molar gestations per numbers of pregnancies. In the United States the rate is estimated to be approximately 0.75 to 1.0 per 1000. The rates from Southeast Asia are 1.5 to 2.5 times higher with much larger variations, and rates up to 8 per 1000 have been reported. The high rates

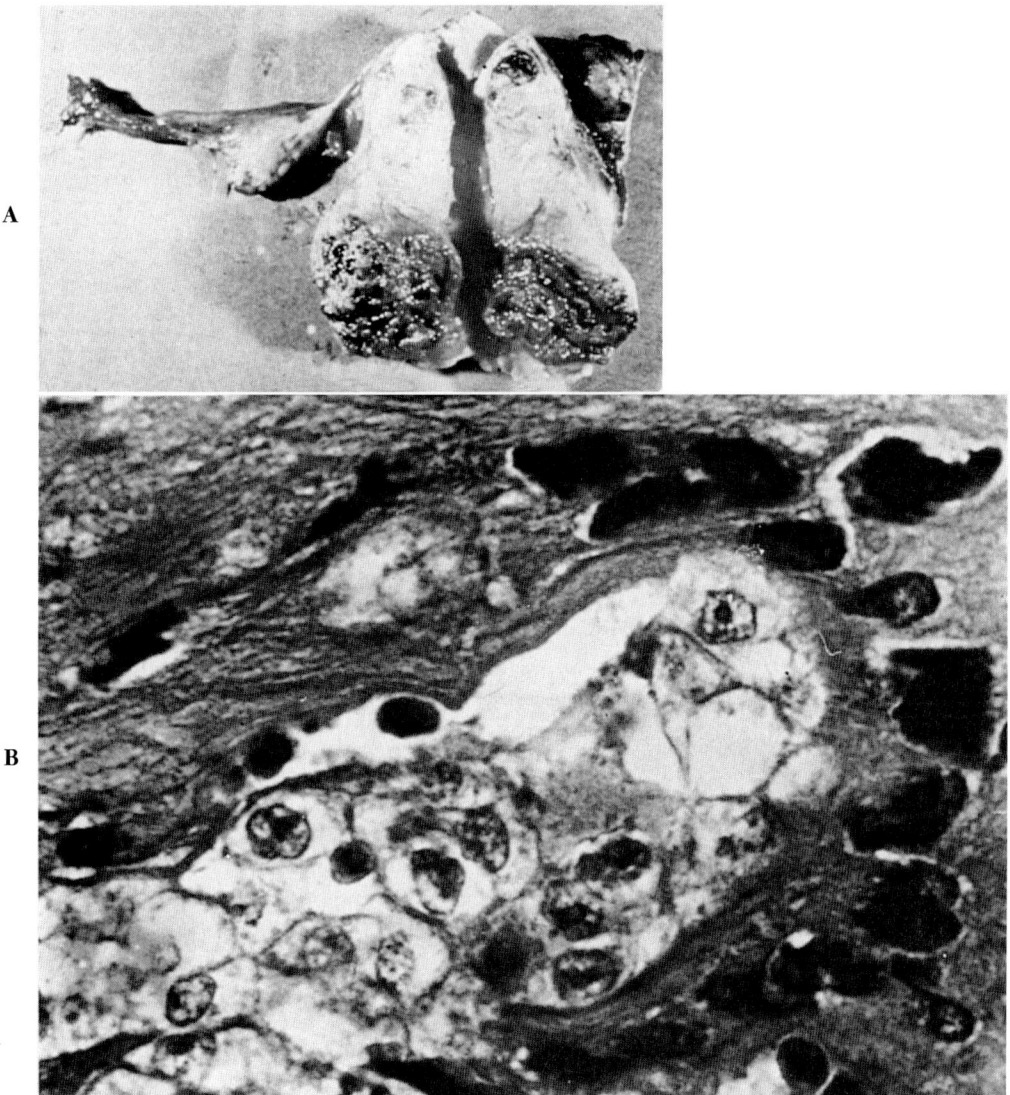

FIGURE 35-4 **A,** Choriocarcinoma. Hemorrhagic tumor occupies lower uterine segment and cervix. Smaller foci of choriocarcinoma can be seen in left and right fundal walls. **B,** Choriocarcinoma, high-power view. Central pale cytotrophoblast is surrounded by syncytiotrophoblasts. Nuclei are pleomorphic. (From Bigelow B: Gestational trophoblast disease. In Blaustein A, editor: Pathology of the female genital tract, ed 2, New York, 1982, Springer-Verlag New York, Inc.)

reported in some studies result from hospital-based rather than population-based statistics. As already noted, hydatidiform mole develops because of abnormal fertilization.

Maternal age is an extremely important risk factor. The lowest rates are among those in their 20s and 30s, with a great increase in those over age 40, after which the risk progressively increases with age. There is also an increase in risk among those under age 20, but the magnitude is not nearly so great as it is among older women. A summary of age-related risks for hydatidiform mole is shown in Table 35-1. An additional risk factor is a history of prior hydatidiform mole, which increases the risk of subsequent mole by 20 to 40 times. Prior recurrent spontaneous abortion is also a risk factor.

The increased frequency among those with lower socioeconomic status, as well as in underdeveloped areas, particularly in Southeast Asia, has led to the suggestion that poor nutrition is a factor in the development of this disease. However, evidence is conflicting, and as noted by Grimes, a dietary etiology for hydatidiform mole has not been supported. A recent report by Palmer et al. suggests a slight increase in risk for GTT (but not hydatidiform mole) with oral contraceptive use, particularly if conception occurs while using oral contraceptives.

The risk appears to vary with race and ethnic origin. In Southeast Asia the rates are double for Eurasians as compared to those of Chinese, Malaysian, or Indian origin. A decreased rate has also been reported among blacks in the United States in comparison to whites, and rates are higher among those of Latin American origin. Mexicans and Filipinos appear to have elevated rates in comparison to Japanese and Chinese.

TABLE 35-1
Relationship of Age to Risk of Hydatidiform Mole

Age	Risk
Less than 20	1.53
20–24	1.17
25–29	1
30–34	1.04
35–39	1.33
40–44	2.66
45–49	24.89
Over 50	80.76

Adapted from Buckley JD: Clin Obstet Gynecol 27:153, 1984.

Classification of Gestational Trophoblastic Disease (GTD)

Hydatidiform mole
1. Complete
2. Incomplete (Partial)

Gestational trophoblastic tumor (GTT); (Malignant GTD)
3. Nonmetastatic
4. Metastatic
   a. Low risk
   b. High risk

Choriocarcinoma

Choriocarcinoma primarily occurs in about 3% to 5% of those who have had a prior complete hydatidiform mole and a prior hydatidiform mole is the major risk factor for the development of gestational choriocarcinoma. However, Secki et al. recently reported choriocarcinoma after partial mole. In Western countries choriocarcinomas are reported at rates between 0.014 and 0.2 per 1000 pregnancies. The rate in the United States is about 1 per 20,000 pregnancies. Rare choriocarcinomas have developed after normal pregnancy (1 per 40,000 term pregnancies). The disease also follows incomplete abortion and ectopic pregnancy. The risk factors for complete mole, particularly maternal age and pregnancy loss, are indirectly associated with choriocarcinoma. An additional factor for choriocarcinoma has been described among ABO blood groups. Some studies, including those of Bagshawe, have shown that women with type A blood married to men with type O, and vice versa, are at higher risk for choriocarcinoma in comparison to matings of other blood groups. No differential in the risk for hydatidiform mole for ABO blood groups has been demonstrated.

CLINICAL CLASSIFICATION OF GTD

The histologic terminology used to describe GTD may be confusing, since the prior terms were based on the morphologic appearance of the abnormal tissue. With the use of sensitive and specific assays for hCG, clinical terminology is more useful in describing GTD, as shown in the box on this page. This offers an effective way of analyzing the treatment and the biologic behavior of these abnormal trophoblastic conditions.

CLINICAL ASPECTS OF GTD

Hydatidiform Mole

Symptoms and Signs

The most common presenting symptom is abnormal bleeding in a patient who has experienced delayed menses and seems to be pregnant. Abnormal bleeding is present in almost all patients, and associated symptoms often mimic an incomplete or threatened abortion. Occasionally the patient notices a swollen villus that has been passed from the uterus. The uterus is frequently large for dates; Curry et al. noted this change in about half of their patients with molar pregnancy. However, as many as one fourth of the patients may have a uterus small for dates. Sequelae appear to be more common among those with an enlarged uterus. In about 20% of the patients, an additional physical finding is enlargement of the ovaries (theca lutein cysts), which is associated with a higher frequency of future sequelae (approximately 50%) as compared to less than 15% for those without ovarian enlargement. The development of these theca lutein cysts is believed to be secondary to the luteinizing hormone-like effect of excessive hCG stimulation. However, in a study of 102 patients with theca lutein cysts, Montz et al. noted that cyst growth did not correlate with changes in hCG concentrations and that some persisted after hCG disappeared from the circulation. Three of the cysts ruptured; the remaining spontaneously regressed.

Nausea and vomiting are common complaints, as is true in normal pregnancy, and hyperemesis gravidarum has been reported. Additionally, preeclamptic toxemia may occur in as many as one fourth of the patients, although its frequency has been reported to be less in many series.

Insofar as molar pregnancies are frequently diagnosed in the latter part of the first trimester of pregnancy, GTD should be considered in any patient with signs of toxemia during this time or during the early part of the second trimester. In addition, laboratory manifestations of hyperthyroidism have been reported, but clinical manifestations of hyperthyroidism are rare. The changes are in part due to the production of thyrotrophin-like hormone by the abnormal trophoblastic tissue, although a weak thyroid-

TABLE 35-2
Complete Versus Partial Hydatidiform Moles

	Complete Mole		Partial Mole	
Clinical presentation and average gestational age	Molar pregnancy 16 weeks	48%	Molar pregnancy 19.7 weeks 8	%
	Spontaneous abortion 13.7 weeks	40%	Spontaneous abortion 14.4 weeks	49%
	Missed abortion 19.5 weeks	6%	Missed abortion 24.8 weeks	43%
Preeclampsia		6%		8%
Uterus large for dates		33%		11%

Adapted from Szulman AE and Surti U: Clin Obstet Gynecol 27:172, 1984.

Symptoms and Signs of Hydatidiform Mole

Abnormal bleeding in early pregnancy
Lower abdominal pain
Toxemia before 24 weeks of gestation
Hyperemesis gravidarum
Hyperthyroidism (rare)
Uterus large for dates (50%)
Enlargement of ovaries (20%)
Absent fetal heart tones and fetal parts
Expulsion of swollen villi

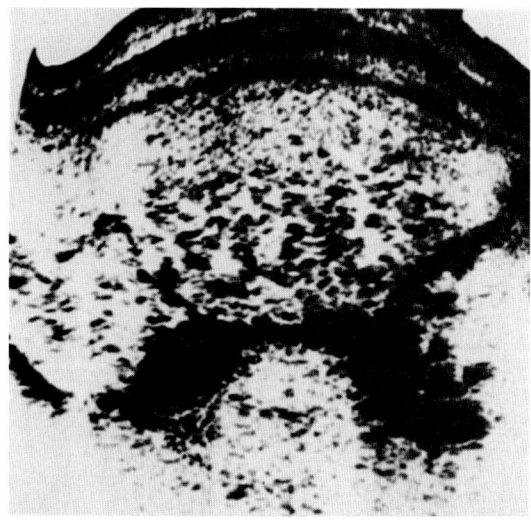

FIGURE 35-5 Ultrasound of uterus demonstrating "snowstorm" appearance of hydatidiform mole.

stimulating hormone action for hCG has also been hypothesized. These changes are reversible and usually abate after treatment of trophoblastic disease. The signs and symptoms of hydatidiform moles are summarized in the box above.

Clinically the behaviors of partial and complete moles differ. Complete mole is the more common and also has a more serious prognosis, with increased risk for the subsequent development of a GTT. Partial moles usually present as an incomplete or missed abortion. Szulman and Surti analyzed the characteristics of 200 moles, both complete and partial; their results are summarized in Table 35-2. HCG levels tend to be lower in partial moles.

Diagnosis

In a patient suspected of having a molar pregnancy, the most valuable diagnostic aid is ultrasound (Figure 35-5). The examination usually reveals absence of a fetus (in the case of a complete mole) and characteristic swollen villi that produce a snowstorm-like pattern or multicystic appearance. The examination may also demonstrate ovarian enlargement secondary to the development of a theca lutein cyst. If a fetal sac is detected, the possibility of a partial mole still exists. However, beyond the seventh week a fetal heart should be detected by ultrasound; its absence may suggest a missed abortion. If hydropic villi are present, it is possible that a blood clot in the uterus has been mistaken for a fetal sac. If there is doubt con-

cerning the presence of fetal tissue and the existence of a partial mole, follow-up sonographic examinations are indicated.

The measurement of hCG is an integral part of the diagnosis and evaluation of the patient suspected of having GTD. Immunoassays allow the measurement of extremely small amounts of hCG in blood and urine. The levels in normal pregnancy reach a peak at about 10 to 14 weeks and rarely exceed levels of 100,000 mIU/ml. They can be higher in twin gestation, are frequently elevated in GTD, and may appear elevated in patients whose dates are not accurate. With molar pregnancy it is possible that the level of hCG may not be elevated, so that a single determination is not diagnostic and will not necessarily differentiate normal pregnancy, multiple pregnancy, and GTD. However, a level in excess of 100,000 mIU/ml suggests GTD. The hCG levels tend to be elevated above normal pregnancy values in complete mole, whereas partial mole tends to produce lower levels.

Management

Once the diagnosis of molar pregnancy is made, the uterus should be evacuated. Medical problems, such as anemia due to blood loss, pregnancy-induced hypertension, pulmonary insufficiency, and hyperthyroidism, should be evaluated and, when necessary, corrected. Hyperemesis gravidarum may develop, necessitating antiemetic and intravenous therapy. Occasionally, disseminated intravascular coagulation (DIC) occurs, leading to a consumptive coagulopathy that requires correction, as well as prompt uterine evacuation. Preevacuation chest x-ray examination is performed to rule out the spread of GTD to the lungs and also for comparison in future follow-up. Unless a viable fetus is found, the pregnancy should be promptly terminated. If hyperthyroidism is present, it should be treated before operative removal of the molar tissue. Theca-lutein cysts usually regress spontaneously and do not require operative intervention unless an acute episode (e.g., rupture) occurs. In general, they regress spontaneously in about 2 months.

Pulmonary insufficiency may also occur following evacuation of a molar pregnancy. Acute dyspnea and cyanosis may develop, usually within 4 hours of evacuation. As noted by Cotton et al., this risk is greatest in patients whose uterus is more than 16 weeks' gestation size. Trophoblastic embolization and fluid overload with blood volume expansion contribute to cardiac decompensation and pulmonary edema. If there are signs of pulmonary distress, arterial PO_2 should be monitored. In severely compromised patients ventilatory assistance, monitoring of pulmonary arterial pressure, and management in an intensive care unit may be needed. Respiratory failure can occur.

Goldstein et al. have advocated the use of prophylactic cytotoxic chemotherapy to prevent the neoplastic sequelae of molar pregnancy. However, this practice has not gained widespread acceptance because giving chemotherapy at the time of evacuation of the mole exposes the patient to toxic drugs, even though most patients with hydatidiform mole do not require further treatment. Approximately 80% of the patients require only uterine evacuation as definitive therapy. If sequelae do develop, which is a risk for the remaining 20%, chemotherapy can then be used. Chemotherapy in young females does increase the risk of ovarian failure and menopause. Byrne et al. studied 1067 females treated with chemotherapy prior to age 19 and noted a markedly increased risk of menopause for these women once they reached their 20s.

The most effective and widely used method of emptying the uterus of a molar pregnancy is suction curettage. In many instances the molar pregnancy will have already begun to abort, and suction can complete the process. The level of hCG is determined prior to evacuation. Intravenous oxytocic agents are used during the evacuation and immediately postoperatively to aid in uterine contraction and to help reduce blood loss, unless the uterus is only minimally enlarged. However, it is not advisable to use oxytocic drugs before evacuation of the molar pregnancy because of the risk of disseminating abnormal trophoblastic cells. If possible, a large suction curette (12 mm) should be used to aid in evacuation. The operator should begin the evacuation in the lower part of the uterus near the cervix and gradually extend it toward the fundus. After evacuation by suction curettage is complete, a gentle sharp curettage should be performed to ensure completion of the procedure. Intravenous oxytocin is continued post evacuation to ensure uterine contraction.

If the patient has completed childbearing, hysterectomy may be considered as primary therapy for molar pregnancy. This is particularly desirable treatment in patients at greater risk for GTT following the molar pregnancy, especially older patients with ovarian lutein cysts or a greatly enlarged uterus. Since the ovarian lutein cysts regress after termination, it is not necessary to remove them, although older patients or those with risk factors for ovarian carcinoma may wish to consider elective removal. In an analysis of 358 patients with hydatidiform mole, Schlaerth et al. primarily used suction evacuation followed by gentle curettage in 88% of their patients. Major complications included infection, toxemia, anemia, and postevacuation respiratory insufficiency.

Follow-up

After evacuation of the uterus (or in the rare case of therapy by hysterectomy), the patient should be carefully monitored for the potential development of malignant sequelae, specifically gestational trophoblastic tumor (GTT). The key is the serial determination of β-hCG in the patient's serum. Abnormal regression of the hCG levels following evacuation of a hydatidiform mole is an indication of GTT.

Evaluation of the patient treated for a molar pregnancy should include the data summarized in the box on page 1055, which also allow identification of those at higher risk for GTT. The risk of GTT is increased in those with a large uterus, high hCG level, lutein cysts, and a history of molar pregnancy and toxemia, as well as in older exposed patients, particularly individuals over 40. The risk of sequelae is less in the absence of these factors and also if fetal tissue is present (partial mole).

To follow the course of the disease after evacuation of a molar pregnancy, the physician must carefully monitor the hCG levels. A normal regression curve is shown in Figure 35-6. Following evacuation of hydatidiform mole, a normal range is usually reached by the fourteenth week. However, in some instances the level returns to normal after a longer interval. Weekly hCGs are measured until the level reaches normal values. The patient must not become pregnant, and usually oral contraceptives are prescribed. There has been a controversial sug-

Baseline Data for Patient with Molar Pregnancy

HCG serum level (preevacuation)
Chest x-ray
Age
Uterine size
Presence or absence of ovarian theca-lutein cysts
Presence or absence of fetal tissue
History of prior molar pregnancy
Assessment for medical complications
  Anemia
  Toxemia
  Hyperemesis
  Hyperthyroidism
  Pulmonary compromise

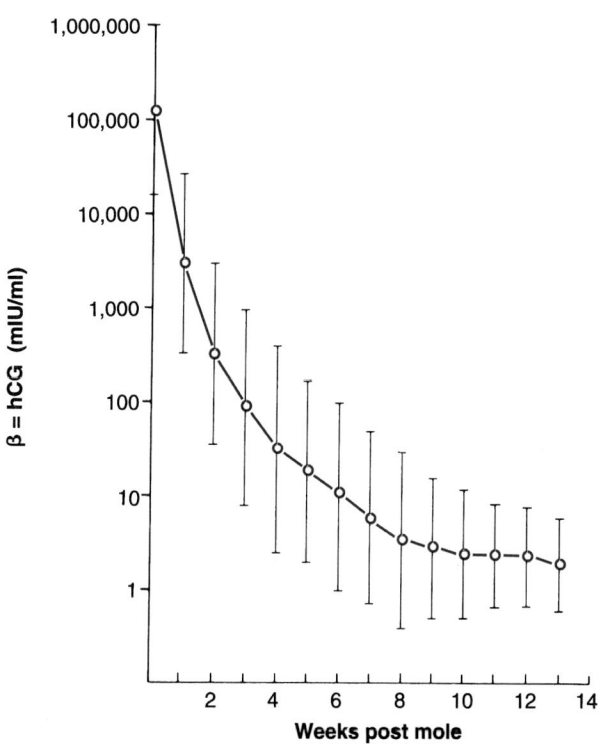

FIGURE 35-6 Mean value and 95% confidence limits describing normal postmolar β-hCG regression curve. (From Schlaerth JB, Morrow CP, Kletzky OA, et al: Obstet Gynecol 58:478, 1981. Reprinted with permission from The American College of Obstetricians and Gynecologists.)

gestion in the literature that birth control pills might increase the risk of GTT, but data from Morrow et al. suggest that birth control pills are safe and effective in this situation. A study by Deicas et al. indicates that oral contraceptives actually offer a therapeutic advantage with fewer patients developing GTT who used birth control pills.

After the initial pelvic examination a repeat periodic evaluation is performed, usually every 2 weeks until the uterus and ovaries have returned to normal size. Theca-lutein cysts characteristically resolve within 2 months, but Montz et al. showed they may last as long as 4 months. However, patients with the high-risk factors listed earlier are approximately 10 times more likely to develop the sequelae of neoplasia in comparison to those without these factors. Once the hCG reaches undetectable levels, it is preferable to monitor them monthly for 6 to 12 months, after which the patient may be advised that she can safely attempt another pregnancy. For partial moles, 6 months of follow-up is probably sufficient. However, the isolated recurrence of trophoblastic disease 16 months after complete molar evacuation in a patient on oral contraceptives has been reported.

There may be an abnormal regression curve after evacuation (Figure 35-7), and in such instances the patient requires therapy for GTT. A rise in hCG (a doubling over a 2-week period) or a plateau in hCG (failure to fall by at least 10% per week) indicates the presence of postmolar trophoblastic tumor. As noted by Kohorn, a higher plateau of hCG values is a stronger indication for chemotherapy. He suggests a level of 10^5 or greater over 2 values required treatment, while at 10^4 to 10^5 3 values are appropriate over 2 weeks, with a range up to a month of follow-up for values that appear to plateau under 100 mIU/ml. A general rule suggested by Berkowitz et al. is a level of >20,000 mIU/ml more than 4 months post mole evacuation is an indication for initiation of chemotherapy. The box at right out-

lines the management of hydatidiform mole, including the indications for chemotherapy. Thus either an abnormal regression curve or the finding of choriocarcinoma in uterine curettings is an indication for the initiation of chemotherapy (see following discussion). The finding of placental site trophoblast tumor would be an indication for hysterectomy if the disease is confined to the uterus.

Management of Hydatidiform Mole

HCG weekly serum determination until normal for two values, then monthly for 6 to 12 months
Chest x-ray examination initially and repeat if abnormal or if hCG plateaus or rises
Contraception for 1 year
Pelvic examination every 2 weeks until normal, then every 3 months
Initiate chemotherapy if:
  HCG level increases or plateaus Metastatic disease is present Choriocarcinoma is diagnosed on tissue
  HCG level still elevated 6 months after molar evacuation
Elevated hCG is detected after normal levels are reached

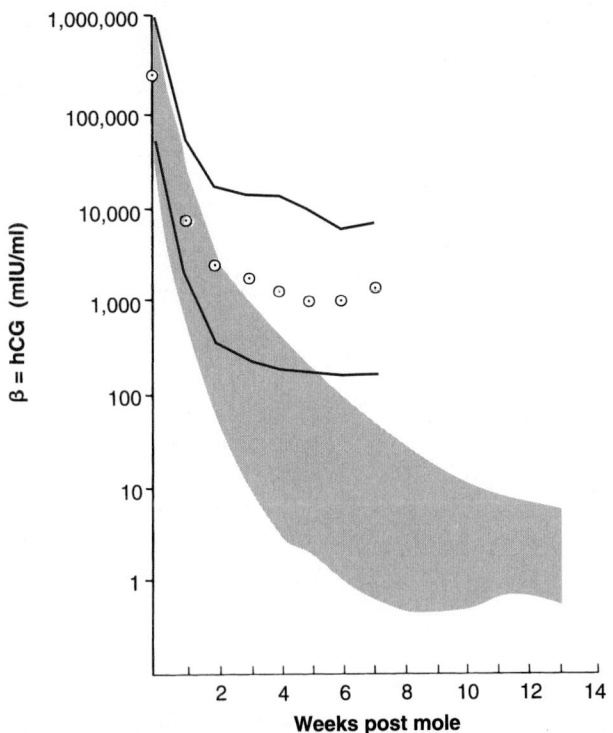

FIGURE 35-7 Mean value and 95% confidence limits for serum β-hCG titers obtained weekly after molar pregnancy in 38 patients whose regression curve deviated early in follow-up from normal regression curve, represented by stippled area. (From Schlaerth JB, Morrow CP, Kletzky OA, et al: Obstet Gynecol 58:478, 1981. Reprinted with permission from The American College of Obstetricians and Gynecologists.)

Gestational Trophoblastic Neoplasia

Incidence and Diagnosis

As has been noted, malignancy (gestational trophoblastic tumor, GTT) develops after approximately 20% of complete hydatidiform moles. Conversely, about half the cases of GTT arise after molar pregnancy, while one fourth occur after normal pregnancy and one fourth after abortion or ectopic pregnancy. Therefore patients who continue to have abnormal bleeding after any pregnancy should have a β-hCG assay performed. Once GTT is diagnosed, chemotherapy is initiated unless complications, such as uterine hemorrhage or perforation, arise that require hysterectomy.

First, a thorough evaluation must be done, including a complete physical examination, measurement of β-hCG level, and diagnostic tests to rule out metastatic disease. The physical examination includes pelvic and neurologic evaluations. These patients may have symptoms of metastatic disease, such as hemoptysis (due to pulmonary lesions), or neurologic signs (secondary to brain metastases). Because of the fatal ramifications of brain and liver metastases, these areas are usually assessed with a computed tomography (CT) scan or radionuclide brain scan. Some therapists omit a brain scan unless neurologic examination or fundoscopic eye examination suggests a brain metastasis. In the absence of liver and/or lung metastases and a negative neurologic examination, a head CT is probably not necessary.

CT is usually preferred for evaluating both the brain and the liver. A pelvic ultrasound examination should be combined with the abdominal CT scan to complete the evaluation of the pelvis. In addition, MRI evaluation has been used and occasionally reported to be helpful. The most frequent site of metastatic GTT is the lungs (80% to 90% of cases), and less frequently the liver, brain, ovary, and vagina are involved. Chest CT will be more sensitive in detecting chest metastases than a chest x-ray. In addition, metastatic disease can occur at any site but false positive results are more frequent with chest CT. Tests of renal and liver chemistries should also be performed, in addition to a hematologic profile. Depending on the location of the disease, the duration of symptoms, the level of hCG, and a history of prior chemotherapy, it is possible to categorize the patient as having low-risk or high-risk GTT, as outlined in the box on the facing page. This terminology is commonly used in the United States and adopted by the National Institutes of Health. It has been stated that associated term pregnancy results in high-risk GTT, but evidence by Olive et al. from the Brewer Trophoblastic Disease Center indicates that GTT after term pregnancy may be considered as low risk unless one of the poor prognosis factors listed is also present.

In addition, two other methods have been used to classify GTT: clinical staging and prognostic scoring, as suggested by Bagshawe, which has been adopted by the World Health Organization. The International Federation of Gynecology and Obstetrics (FIGO) anatomic staging system is shown in Table 35-3 and allows a comparison of treatment results from various centers but is rarely used in the United States. The prognostic scoring system is shown in Table 35-4. It provides a useful mechanism to evaluate GTT and then summing the scores assigned to the various risk factors, a total score is provided that predicts chemotherapy resistance.

Gordon et al. noted that patients with a score of 8 or higher required multiagent chemotherapy. In 1989 Bagshawe et al. summarized results on 487 patients. In this report a score of 5 or less was considered low risk, and 347 of 348 patients survived. Those authors advise that those with medium- and high-risk disease should begin with multiagent chemotherapy. In a multivariate analysis, Soper et al. noted that the clinical classification (see the box on p. 1057) provided the best method of identifying patient prognosis and the indication for single or multiple-agent initial chemotherapy (see following discussion). It is important to emphasize that regardless of the classification system, the most important factor for following the patient is the level of hCG.

TABLE 35-3
FIGO Classification System of GTT

Stage	Anatomic Location
I	Confined to corpus uteri
II	Metastases outside uterus limited to vagina or pelvic structures
III	Metastases to lungs
IV	Distant metastases to other sites

Substages for each stage as follows:

  A. No risk factors
  B. One risk factor
  C. Two risk factors

Definition of risk factors
  1. Pretherapy serum hCG:100,000 mIU/ml
  2. Disease duration > 6 months

Prognostic Classification of GTT (Malignant GTD)

  I. Nonmetastatic GTT
  II. Metastatic GTT: disease outside the uterus
    A. Good prognosis
      1. Disease present less than 4 months (short duration)
      2. Pretreatment b-hCG less than 40,000 mIU/ml
      3. No prior chemotherapy
    B. Poor prognosis
      1. Disease present more than 4 months (long duration), or
      2. Pretreatment b-hCG greater than 40,000 mIU/ml, or
      3. Presence of metastases to sites other than lungs or vagina, i.e., liver or brain, or
      4. Failure of prior chemotherapy

Management

NONMETASTATIC AND GOOD-PROGNOSIS METASTATIC GTT.
Single-agent chemotherapy is started for nonmetastatic GTT and good-prognosis (low-risk) metastatic GTT. Many programs of single-agent chemotherapy have been used, including methotrexate, 0.4 mg/kg body weight (maximum, 25 mg) intravenously or intramuscularly daily for 5 days every 2 weeks; actinomycin D, 10 to 12 μg/kg intravenously daily for 5 days every 2 weeks; or methotrexate, 1 to 1.5 mg/kg intramuscularly or intravenously on days 1, 3, 5, and 7, followed by citrovorum factor rescue (leucovorin), 0.1 to 0.15 μg/kg intramuscularly on days 2, 4, 6, and 8. Pulse actinomycin D, 1.25 mg/m^2 intravenously once every 2 weeks, has also been used. The latter regimen was introduced by Morrow et al. to treat low-risk nonmetastatic disease and has the advantage of being able to be given conveniently on an outpatient basis. It is used for low-risk postmolar trophoblastic neoplasia. It appears to be a cost-effective regimen, although it may require a longer treatment time to attain regression of hCG to normal values.

Petrilli et al. reported on single-dose actinomycin D for 31 patients in a cooperative Gynecologic Oncology Group (GOG) study. Twenty-nine (94%) achieved remission after a median of four courses of therapy. Another alternative was reported by Homesley et al., who summarized a GOG study of 63 patients with nonmetastatic GTD. Fifty-one responded completely to weekly intramuscular methotrexate, initially 30 mg/m^2 and increased as tolerated 5 mg/m^2/week to 50 mg/m^2. However, 11 patients failed and subsequently required 5-day actinomycin D therapy.

The 5-day actinomycin D and methotrexate courses have been found to be equally effective, but methotrexate appears to have more toxicity, particularly for the oral mucosa, and the severity of its toxicity increases with liver

TABLE 35-4
Prognostic Scoring System for GTT

Factor	Score*			
	0	1	2	4
Age (years)	≥39	>39		
Antecedent pregnancy	H. Mole	Abortion	Term	
Interval between end of antecedent pregnancy and start of chemotherapy (months)	<4	4–6	7–12	>12
HCG (IU/L)	<10^3	10^3–10^4	10^4–10^5	>10^5
Largest tumor, including uterine (cm)	<3	3–4 cm	≥5 cm	
Site of metastases		Spleen, kidney	GI tract	Brain, liver
Number of metastases		1–3	4–8	>8
Prior chemotherapy			1 drug	≥2 drugs

Modified from Kohorn EI, Goldstein DP, Hancock BW, et al: Int J Gynecol Cancer 10:84, 2000.

*Low risk, ≤4; middle risk, 5–7; high risk ≥8.

or renal compromise (Chapter 26). High-dose methotrexate with citrovorum rescue has not proven to be more effective than the other single agents given alone. Some investigators have alternated the 5-day actinomycin D and methotrexate courses in the belief that this results in reduced toxicity and more rapid resolution of the disease. VP-16 (etoposide) has also been effectively used as single-agent therapy given for 5 days 200 mg/m^2 repeated about every 2 weeks. The single-dose weekly methotrexate regimen at 30 mg/m^2 intramuscularly or actinomycin D 1.25 mg/m^2 every 2 weeks provide a cost-effective advantage in terms of outpatient therapy. As noted by Homesley, however, weekly methotrexate has less gastrointestinal toxicity. Oral etoposide is expensive and causes total alopecia, with gastrointestinal and hematologic toxicity.

Patients are treated until a normal β-hCG level has been obtained; then one to two additional courses of chemotherapy are usually given. Although recurrence rates of approximately 5% may be expected after therapy, recurrence more than 6 to 12 months after treatment is extremely unusual. Weekly serum hCG determinations are made until three negative β-hCG levels are obtained. Then monthly levels are taken for at least 6 to 12 months, after which pregnancy may be attempted. Even with recurrence, chemotherapy can be expected to cure 100% of patients with low-risk nonmetastatic trophoblastic disease. Hysterectomy may be performed in good operative candidates with nonmetastatic GTT who desire no further children or who have uterine disease resistant to chemotherapy.

HIGH-RISK METASTATIC GTT. The treatment of poor-prognosis GTT requires multiple-agent chemotherapy. One protocol was designated MAC, consisting of methotrexate (0.3 mg/kg), actinomycin D (8 to 10 μg/kg), and chlorambucil (oral, 0.2 mg/kg) or cyclophosphamide (3 to 5 mg/kg) given intravenously daily for 5 days. The cycle is repeated in 9 to 14 days as toxicity permits. In a cooperative, randomized GOG study, Curry et al. reported good results for MAC therapy. The chemotherapy of poor-prognosis GTT

is continued for two courses after levels become negative, a practice that appears to decrease the rate of relapse.

In recent years effective protocols have been introduced using etoposide (VP-16). This drug is usually reserved for high-risk and/or drug-resistant cases, since secondary malignancies have been reported following its use (see Chapter 26). A widely used protocol uses etoposide, high-dose methotrexate with citrovorin rescue, actinomycin D, cyclophosphamide, and vincristine (Oncovin) (EMA/CO) (Table 35-5). Bolis et al., in a study of 36 high-risk patients, noted EMA/CO to be effective, including a 64% response rate when used as second-line therapy, which was higher than MAC or other multiagent protocols. Schink et al. reported a complete response in 10 of 12 patients when used as primary therapy for high-risk disease. EMA/CO is widely used for poor-prognosis GTT. Using this protocol in 272 high-risk patients, Bower et al. reported 112 subsequent live births but also 5 subsequent secondary malignancies. The use of granulocyte colony stimulating factor (G-CSF) can reduce neutropenic toxicity. Some therapists have used platinum and etoposide (EP) for high-risk disease. Soper et al. reported six of seven chemorefractory GTD patients had a complete response but with serious side effects, including grade IV neutropenia and severe renal toxicity. Recently Newlands et al. reported a multiagent regimen of etoposide/platinum (EP) alternating weekly with etoposide, methotrexate, and actinomycin D (EMA) to treat EMA/CO failures and rare metastatic placental site trophoblastic (PSTT) tumors, which are usually resistant to chemotherapy. Thirty of 34 patients with GTT and 4 of 8 with PSTT survived. Operation was used in some cases. This appears to be an effective regimen with frequent severe toxicity especially hematologic.

If brain metastases are diagnosed, 2000 to 3000 rads are often given immediately along with systemic chemotherapy. Bakri et al. reported responses of brain metastases to chemotherapy without radiation. Liver metastases are

---

TABLE 35-5
EMA/CO Regimen*

Day	Drug/Dosage	Abbreviation
1	Etoposide; 100 mg/m^2 IV over 30 minutes Actinomycin D: 0.5 mg IV push Methotrexate: 100 mg/m^2 IV push Methotrexate: 200 mg/m^2 IV infusion in 1000 ml D5W over 12 hours	E (etoposide) M (methotrexate) A (actinomycin D)
2	Etoposide: 100 mg/m^2 IV infusion in 250 ml NS over 30 minutes Actinomycin D: 0.5 mg IV push Folinic acid: 15 mg IM every 12 hours for 4 doses beginning 24 hours after starting methotrexate	
8	Cyclophosphamide: 600 mg/m^2 IV Vincristine: 1.0 mg/m^2 IV push	C (cyclophosphamide) O (Oncovin)

*Repeat cycle on days 15, 16, and 22 (every 2 weeks).

usually treated by systemic chemotherapy, and intraarterial chemotherapy infusion has been tried.

Occasionally, operation will benefit those with localized chemorefractory GTD. Lehman et al. reported 33 patients from M.D. Anderson Hospital who had hysterectomy (29), thoracotomy (4), and 1 nephrectomy. Fourteen (42%) of the patients had postoperative complete responses, while 8 of the 19 remaining had a complete response to subsequent chemotherapy.

As many as 20% of patients with poor-prognosis GTT who attain a negative hCG level have a recurrence. In comparison, the recurrence rate for those with good-prognosis GTT is 5%, while those with nonmetastatic GTT have recurrence rates of 1% to 2%. High-dose salvage therapy has resulted in remission. Giacalone et al. used high-dose chemotherapy with autologous bone marrow transplantation in a patient who is free of disease 3 years after such treatment.

After a negative hCG level is achieved for three cycles in patients with high-risk GTT, hCG measurements are repeated every 2 weeks for 3 months and then monthly for 1 year. Some therapists continue the measurement of hCG levels every 6 months for as long as 5 years because of the slight risk of late recurrence of the disease. Chest x-ray examinations are also usually repeated every 3 months during the first year of follow-up, but the hCG level is the crucial element in following the patient. A few isolated cases of choriocarcinomas have been reported in the absence of elevated levels of hCG. After 1 year of negative follow-up, the patient may again attempt pregnancy.

Fertility After Treatment for GTT

There is concern, particularly among patients who have been treated for GTD, that a subsequent pregnancy will lead to repeat GTD or recrudescence of the disease. While repeat molar pregnancy is an increased risk, current evidence suggests that normal pregnancy usually results. Data from Rustin et al. indicate no increased frequency of congenital anomalies among infants whose mothers received chemotherapy. Goldstein et al. reported that 67.4% of 929 individuals treated at various centers for GTD subsequently had a normal term delivery, while only 1.4% experienced a recurrent molar pregnancy. Green et al. reported that those treated with chemotherapy for a variety of tumors are not at increased risk for having offspring with congenital anomalies. However, the patients receiving actinomycin D 2-16 mg/m^2 had the greatest frequency of congenital anomalies suggesting further study is indicated for this drug. If pregnancy occurs following GTD, it is important to perform an ultrasound examination early to identify a gestational sac in the uterus, as well as a fetal heart, which should be evident by the seventh week of pregnancy. hCG levels should be obtained after delivery to rule out any recurrence of GTD. Products of conception or placentas should be examined histopathologically.

KEY POINTS

- The monitoring of trophoblastic disease and its follow-up is accomplished by the measurement of the beta-subunit of hCG (β-hCG).

- The risk of hydatidiform mole is about 0.75 to 1.0 per 1000 pregnancies in the United States.

- Choriocarcinomas follow 1 in 40,000 term pregnancies and 3% to 5% of complete molar pregnancies.

- The major risk factors for molar pregnancy include maternal age (over 40 and under 20 years), and a history of prior molar pregnancy. Choriocarcinoma risk factors are similar. There appears to be an increased frequency of these diseases in Southeast Asia and Mexico.

- The risk of developing a second molar pregnancy after a primary mole is about 20 to 40 times greater than the initial risk.

- Trophoblastic cells normally regress within 3 weeks following delivery.

- The finding of trophoblast cells in the uterus more than 3 weeks after delivery should lead to the consideration of the diagnosis of choriocarcinoma.

- About half the cases of gestational trophoblastic tumor (GTT) follow molar pregnancy, one fourth follow normal pregnancy, and one fourth follow abortion or ectopic pregnancy.

- Persistent abnormal bleeding following normal pregnancy, abortion, or ectopic pregnancy should lead to a consideration of the diagnosis of GTT. The finding of pulmonary nodules on chest x-ray after normal pregnancy suggests GTT.

- Complete moles are of paternal origin, are diploid, and carry a 20% risk of GTT sequelae.

- Partial moles are of maternal and paternal origin, are triploid, and rarely are followed by GTT, but these require the same follow-up for potential malignant sequelae as a complete mole.

- Hydatidiform molar pregnancy should be suspected in a woman with persistent bleeding in the first half of pregnancy, toxemia before 24 weeks' gestation, or hyperemesis. The uterus is large for gestational dates in about half the cases, and ovarian enlargement occurs in about 20%.

- An elevated serum level of hCG is not diagnostic of molar pregnancy but may indicate a multiple gestation or a normal pregnancy with incorrect gestational dates.

- The diagnosis of a molar pregnancy (complete mole) can be established with ultrasound, which displays a "snowstorm" pattern.

- Hydatidiform moles are effectively and safely evacuated from the uterus using suction curettage.

- Medical complications of hydatidiform mole include anemia from blood loss, toxemia, hyperthyroidism, hyperemesis gravidarum, and rarely pulmonary insufficiency.

- In low-risk GTT, the initial serum hCG level is less than 40,000 mIU/ml; the disease is present less than 4 months; metastases, if present, involve the lung and vagina only; and there has been no prior chemotherapy. It is usually treated by single-agent chemotherapy.

- In high-risk metastatic GTT, one or more of the following are present: the initial serum hCG level is greater than 40,000 mIU/ml, the disease has been present more than 4 months; metastases beyond the lung and vagina are present; and there is failure of prior chemotherapy. It is treated with multiple-agent chemotherapy.

- Recurrence rate for patients treated for GTT whose hCG level reached normal is 5% for good-prognosis metastatic GTT and 1% to 2% for nonmetastatic GTT. However, nonmetastatic GTT and low-risk GTT are 100% curable by repeated courses of chemotherapy.

- Patients with high-risk metastatic GTT are successfully treated with chemotherapy in more than 70% of the cases.

- Patients treated for GTT should not become pregnant for 6 to 12 months after treatment to allow accurate assessment of β-hCG levels.

- Chemotherapy administration to young females increases the risk of early menopause.

- Infants born to mothers treated for GTD do not appear to have an increased frequency of congenital anomalies.

BIBLIOGRAPHY

Acaia B, Parazzini F, La Vecchia C, et al: Increased frequency of complete hydatidiform mole in women with repeated abortion, Gynecol Oncol 31:310, 1988.

Atrash HK, Hogue CJR, and Grimes DA: Epidemiology of hydatidiform mole during early gestation, Am J Obstet Gynecol 154:906, 1986.

Bagshawe KD: Treatment of high-risk choriocarcinoma, J Reprod Med 29:813, 1984.

Bagshawe KD, Lawler SD, Paradinas FJ, et al: Gestational trophoblastic tumours following initial diagnosis of partial hydatidiform mole, Lancet 335:1074, 1990.

Bagshawe KD, Rawlings G, Pike MC, et al: The ABO blood groups in trophoblastic neoplasia, Lancet 1:553, 1971.

Bakri Y, Berkowitz RS, Goldstein DP, et al: Brain metastases of gestational trophoblastic tumor, J Reprod Med 39:179, 1994.

Bandy LC, Clarke-Pearson DL, and Hammond C: Malignant potential of gestational trophoblastic disease at the extreme ages of reproductive life, Obstet Gynecol 64:395, 1984.

Berkowitz RS, Bernstein MR, Laborde O, and Goldstein DP: Subsequent pregnancy experience in patients with gestational trophoblastic disease: New England Trophoblastic Disease Center, 1965-1992, J Reprod Med 39:228, 1994.

Berkowitz RS, Goldstein DP, DuBeshter B, et al: Management of complete molar pregnancy, J Reprod Med 32:634, 1987.

Bigelow B: Gestational trophoblast disease. In Blaustein A, editor: Pathology of the female genital tract, ed 2, New York, 1982, Springer-Verlag New York Inc.

Bolis G, Bonazzi C, Landoni F, et al: EMA/CO regimen in high-risk gestational trophoblastic tumor (GTT), Gynecol Oncol 31:439, 1988.

Bower M, Newlands ES, Holden D, et al: EMA/CO for high-risk gestational trophoblastic tumors: results from a cohort of 272 patients. J Clin Oncol 15:2636, 1997.

Buckley JD: The epidemiology of molar pregnancy and choriocarcinoma, Clin Obstet Gynecol 27:153, 1984.

Byrne J, Fears TR, Gail MH, et al: Early menopause in long-term survivors of cancer during adolescence, Am J Obstet Gynecol 166:788, 1992.

Chang Y-L, Chang T-C, Hsueh S, et al: Prognostic factors and treatment for placental site trophoblastic tumor—report of 3 cases and analysis of 88 cases, Gynecol Oncol 73:216, 1999.

Cotton DB, Bernstein SG, Read SA, et al: Hemodynamic observations in evacuation of molar pregnancy, Am J Obstet Gynecol 138:6, 1980.

Curry SL, Blessing J, DiSaia P, et al: A prospective randomized comparison of methotrexate, dactinomycin, and chlorambucil versus methotrexate, dactinomycin, cyclophosphamide, doxorubicin, melphalan, hydroxyurea, and vincristine in "poor prognosis" metastatic gestational trophoblastic disease: a Gynecologic Oncology Group study, Obstet Gynecol 73:357, 1989.

Deicas RE, Miller DS, Rademaker AW, et al: The role of contraception in the development of postmolar gestational trophoblastic disease, Obstet Gynecol 78:221, 1991.

Dessau R, Rustin GJS, Paradinas FJ, et al: Surgery and chemotherapy in the management of placental site tumor, Gynecol Oncol 39:56, 1990.

Elmer DB, Granai CO, Ball HG, and Curry SL: Persistence of gestational trophoblastic disease for longer than 1 year following evacuation of hydatidiform mole, Obstet Gynecol 81:888, 1993.

Giacalone PL, Benos P, Donnadio D, and Laffargue F: High-dose chemotherapy with autologous bone marrow transplantation for refractory metastatic gestational trophoblastic disease, Gynecol Oncol 58:383, 1995.

Goldstein DP, Berkowitz RS, and Bernstein MR: Reproductive performance after molar pregnancy and gestational trophoblastic tumor, Clin Obstet Gynecol 27:221, 1984.

Gordon AN, Gershenson DM, Copeland LJ, et al: High-risk metastatic gestational trophoblastic disease: further stratification into two clinical entities, Gynecol Oncol 34:54, 1989.

Green DM, Zevon MA, Lowrie G, et al: Congenital anomalies in children of patients who received chemotherapy for cancer in childhood and adolescence, N Engl J Med 325:141, 1991.

Grimes DA: Epidemiology of gestational trophoblastic disease, Am J Obstet Gynecol 150:309, 1984.

Hammond CB and Soper JT: Poor-prognostic metastatic gestational trophoblastic neoplasia, Clin Obstet Gynecol 27:228, 1984.

Homesley HD: Development of single-agent chemotherapy regimens for gestational trophoblastic disease, J Reprod Med 39:185, 1994.

Homesley HD, Blessing JA, Rettenmaier M, et al: Weekly intramuscular methotrexate for nonmetastatic gestational trophoblastic disease, Obstet Gynecol 72:413, 1988.

How J, Scurry J, Grant P, et al: Placental site trophoblastic tumor: report of three cases and review of the literature, Int J Gynecol Cancer 5:241, 1995.

Kelly MP, Rustin GJS, Ivory C, et al: Respiratory failure due to choriocarcinoma: a study of 103 dyspneic patients, Gynecol Oncol 38:149, 1990.

Kim JH, Park DC, Bae SN, et al: Subsequent reproductive experience after treatment for gestational trophoblastic disease, Gynecol Oncol 71:108, 1998.

Kohorn EI: Evaluation of the criteria used to make the diagnosis of nonmetastatic gestational trophoblastic neoplasia, Gynecol Oncol 48:139, 1993.

Kohorn EI, Goldstein DP, Hancock BW, et al: Combining the staging system of the International Federation of Gynecology and Obstetrics with the scoring system of the World Health Organization for Trophoblastic Neoplasia. Report of the Working Committee of the International Society for the Study of Trophoblastic Disease and the International Gynecologic Cancer Society, Int J Gynecol Cancer 10:84, 2000.

Lage JM, Berkowitz, RS, Rice LW, et al: Flow cytometric analysis of DNA content in partial hydatidiform moles with persistent gestational trophoblastic tumor, Obstet Gynecol 77:111, 1991.

Lathrop JC, Lauchlan S, Nayaf R, et al: Clinical characteristics of placental site trophoblastic tumor (PSTT), Gynecol Oncol 31:32, 1988.

Lehman E, Gershenson DM, Burke TW, et al: Salvage surgery for chemorefractory gestational trophoblastic disease, J Clin Oncol 12:2737, 1994.

Lemonnier M-C, Glezerman V, Auclair R, et al: Choriocarcinoma associated with undetectable levels of human chorionic gonadotropin, Gynecol Oncol 25:48, 1986.

Li MC, Hertz R, and Spencer DB: Effect of methotrexate therapy upon choriocarcinoma and chorioadenoma, Proc Soc Exp Biol Med 93:36, 1956.

Lurain JR: High-risk metastatic gestational trophoblastic tumors: current management, J Reprod Med 39:217, 1994.

Lurain JR and Elfstrand EP: Single-agent methotrexate chemotherapy for the treatment of nonmetastatic gestational trophoblastic tumors, Am J Obstet Gynecol 172:574, 1995.

Montz FJ, Schlaerth JB, and Morrow CP: The natural history of theca lutein cysts, Obstet Gynecol 72:247, 1988.

Morrow P, Nakamura R, Schlaerth JB, et al: The influence of oral contraceptives on the post molar HCG regression curve, Am J Obstet Gynecol 151:906, 1985.

Mortakis AE and Braga CA: "Poor prognosis" metastatic gestational trophoblastic disease: the prognostic significance of the scoring system in predicting chemotherapy failures, Obstet Gynecol 76:272, 1990.

Newlands ES, Mulholland PJ, Holden L, et al: Estoposide and cis-platin/estoposide, methotrexate, and actinomycin D (EMA) chemotherapy for patients with high-risk gestational trophoblastic tumors refractory to EMA/cyclophosphamide and vincristine chemotherapy and patients presenting with metastatic placental site trophoblastic tumors, J Clin Oncol 18:854, 2000.

Olive DL, Lurain JR, and Brewer JI: Choriocarcinoma associated with term gestation, Am J Obstet Gynecol 148:711, 1984.

Palmer JR: Advances in the epidemiology of gestational trophoblastic disease, J Reprod Med 39:155, 1994.

Palmer JR, Driscoll SG, Rosenberg L, et al: Oral contraceptive use and risk of gestational trophoblastic tumors, J Natl Cancer Inst 91:635, 1999.

Petrilli ES, Twiggs LB, Blessing JA, et al: Single-dose actinomycin D treatment for nonmetastatic gestational trophoblastic disease: a prospective phase II trial of the gynecologic oncology group, Cancer 60:2173, 1987.

Rice LW, Berkowitz RS, Lage JM, et al: Persistent gestational trophoblastic tumor after partial hydatidiform mole, Gynecol Oncol 36:358, 1990.

Rustin GJS, Booth M, Dent J, et al: Pregnancy after cytotoxic chemotherapy for gestational trophoblastic tumors, Br Med J 288:103, 1984.

Schink JC, Singh DK, Rademaker AW, et al: Etoposide, methotrexate, actinomycin D, cyclophosphamide, and vincristine for the treatment of metastatic, high-risk gestational trophoblastic disease, Obstet Gynecol 80:817, 1992.

Schlaerth JB, Morrow CR, Kletzky OA, et al: Prognostic characteristics of serum human chorionic gonadotropin titer regression following molar pregnancy, Obstet Gynecol 58:478, 1981.

Schlaerth JB, Morrow CP, Montz FJ, and d'Ablaing G: Initial management of hydatidiform mole, Am J Obstet Gynecol 158:1299, 1988.

Schlaerth JB, Morrow CP, Nalick RH, et al: Single-dose actinomycin D in the treatment of post molar trophoblastic disease, Gynecol Oncol 19:53, 1984.

Secki MJ, Fisher RA, Salerno G, et al: Choriocarcinoma and partial hydatidiform moles, Lancet 356:36, 2000.

Smith EB, Szulman AE, Hinshaw W, et al: Human chorionic gonadotropin levels in complete and partial hydatidiform moles and in nonmolar abortuses, Am J Obstet Gynecol 149:129, 1984.

Soper JT: Surgical therapy for gestational trophoblastic disease, J Reprod Med 39:168, 1994.

Soper JT, Clarke-Pearson DL, Berchuck A, et al: 5-day methotrexate for women with metastatic gestational trophoblastic disease, Gynecol Oncol 54:76, 1994.

Soper JT, Evans AC, Conaway MR, et al: Evaluation of prognostic factors and staging in gestational trophoblastic tumor, Obstet Gynecol 84:969, 1994.

Soper JT, Evans AC, Rodriguez G, et al: Etoposide-platin combination therapy for chemorefractory gestational trophoblastic disease, Gynecol Oncol 56:421, 1995.

Szulman AE and Surti U: The syndromes of partial and complete molar gestation, Clin Obstet Gynecol 27:172, 1984.

Watson EJ, Hernandez E, and Miyazawa K: Partial hydatidiform moles: a review, Obstet Gynecol Surv 42:540, 1987.

Wren BG: Hormonal therapy following female genital tract cancer, Int J Gynecol Cancer 4:217, 1994.

Young RH and Scully RE: Placental-site trophoblastic tumor: current status, Clin Obstet Gynecol 27:248, 1984.

PART FIVE

Reproductive Endocrinology and Infertility

Primary and Secondary Dysmenorrhea and Premenstrual Syndrome

Etiology, Diagnosis, Management

Cervical Stenosis. Narrowing of the cervical canal, often at the level of the internal os, in such a way that menstrual flow is impeded and intrauterine pressure is increased at the time of menses.

Dysmenorrhea. Painful cramping sensation in the lower abdomen often accompanied by other symptoms such as sweating, tachycardia, headaches, nausea, vomiting, diarrhea, and tremulousness. These all occur just before or during the menses. Primary dysmenorrhea begins at or shortly after menarche and is usually not accompanied by pelvic pathologic conditions. Secondary dysmenorrhea arises later and usually is associated with other pelvic conditions.

Mittelschmerz. Midcycle pelvic pain usually related to ovulation. The actual mechanism is not clearly understood.

Nonsteroidal Antiinflammatory Drugs (NSAIDs). Also known as *prostaglandin synthetase inhibitors.* Substances that block the activity of prostaglandin synthetase, thereby preventing the effect of prostaglandins on tissue. These basically consist of two chemical groups: the arylcarboxylic acids and the arylalkanoic acids.

Pelvic Congestion Syndrome. Vascular engorgement of the uterus and the vessels of the broad ligament and lateral pelvic walls, which may lead to chronic pelvic pain.

Premenstrual Syndrome (PMS). A group of symptoms, both physical and behavioral, that occur in the second half of the menstrual cycle and often interfere with work and personal relationships. They are followed by a period entirely free of symptoms.

Dysmenorrhea and premenstrual syndrome afflict a large percentage of women in the reproductive years. These conditions have a negative effect on the quality of the patients' lives and on the lives of their families, and they are also responsible for a huge economic loss as a result of the cost of medications, medical care, and decreased productivity. This chapter will discuss current thinking with respect to the etiology, pathophysiology, and management of these two conditions, which are not always related.

DYSMENORRHEA

Dysmenorrhea is defined as a severe, painful cramping sensation in the lower abdomen often accompanied by other biologic symptoms, including sweating, tachycardia, headaches, nausea, vomiting, diarrhea, and tremulousness, all occurring just before or during the menses. In the past the definition has been subdivided into primary and secondary dysmenorrhea. The term *primary dysmenorrhea* was reserved for women who had no obvious pathologic condition. We currently recognize that these patients are suffering from the effects of endogenous prostaglandins. *Secondary dysmenorrhea,* on the other hand, is associated with pelvic conditions or pathology that causes pelvic pain in conjunction with the menses. Primary dysmenorrhea almost always first occurs in women younger than 20. Indeed, the patient will report pain as soon as she establishes ovulatory cycles. Secondary dysmenorrhea may, of course, occur in women under 20, but it is most often seen in women over 20.

Incidence

A number of studies have attempted to determine the prevalence of dysmenorrhea; a wide range (3% to 90%) has been reported. These studies have been performed on students, teenagers and their mothers, and individuals from various specific populations, such as industrial workers or college students. The best estimate of the prevalence of primary dysmenorrhea is about 75%. Andersch and Milsom surveyed all the 19-year-old women in the city of Gothenburg, Sweden. A total of 90.9% of such women responded to a randomly distributed questionnaire, and 72.4% of these stated that they suffered from dysmenorrhea. In addition, 34.3% of the total population reported mild menstrual symptoms, 22.7% cited moderate symptoms that required analgesia, and 15.4% stated that they had severe dysmenorrhea that clearly inhibited their working ability and that could not be adequately assuaged by general analgesia (Table 36-1). This study verified the work of others who found that women who had vaginally delivered a child, who took birth control pills, or who were smokers were less likely to have dysmenorrhea. Pregnancy itself without actual birth did not seem to alleviate dysmenorrhea, as women who had ectopic pregnancies or spontaneous or voluntary terminations of pregnancy were not relieved of their symptoms, whereas women who delivered babies were.

TABLE 36-1
Severity of Primary Dysmenorrhea in a Population of 586 Swedish, 19-year-old Women

Severity	Number	Percent
None	162	27.6
Mild*	201	34.3
Moderate†	133	22.7
Severe‡	90	15.4

Data from Andersch B and Milsom I: Am J Obstet Gynecol 144:655, 1982.

*No systemic symptoms, medication rarely required, work rarely affected.

†Few systemic symptoms, medication required, work moderately affected.

‡Multiple symptoms, poor medication response, work inhibited.

Oral contraceptive use was noted by these investigators to reduce the prevalence and severity of dysmenorrhea significantly ($P \leq 0.01$). IUD use did not affect prevalence or severity in any measurable way.

Relationship to Menstruation and the Menstrual Cycle

Andersch and Milsom demonstrated a significant positive correlation between the severity of dysmenorrhea and the duration of menstrual flow, amount of menstrual flow, and early menarche. They showed no relationship with the actual duration of the menstrual cycle.

In their series, 38.3% of the patients reported that they had experienced dysmenorrhea for the first time during the first year after menarche, and only 20.8% reported that dysmenorrhea had not occurred until 4 years after menarche.

Family History

Dysmenorrhea has been reported to be significantly increased among mothers and sisters of women with dysmenorrhea.

Pathogenesis of Primary Dysmenorrhea

Although the pathogenesis of dysmenorrhea is still unknown, the fact that there is a close association between an elevated prostaglandin $F_{2\alpha}$ level in the secretory endometrium and the symptoms of dysmenorrhea, including uterine hypercontractility, complaints of severe cramping, and other prostaglandin-induced symptoms, has led to the theory that prostaglandin $F_{2\alpha}$ is associated with the pathogenesis of dysmenorrhea. Nonsteroidal antiinflammatory drugs (NSAIDs) are prostaglandin synthetase inhibitors and have been demonstrated to alleviate these symptoms. These substances are nonsteroidal and antiinflammatory. They have been used as analgesics for a number of conditions, including arthritis, and generally are divided into two chemical groups—the arylcarboxylic acids, which include acetylsalicylic acid (aspirin) and fenamates, and the arylalkanoic acids, including the arylpropionic acids (ibuprofen, naproxen, and ketoprofen), as well as the indoleacetic acids (indomethacin). The specific effect of these agents on the uterine musculature is reduction of contractility as measured by reduction of intrauterine pressure.

In 1984 Owen reviewed the effectiveness of NSAIDs in the treatment of primary dysmenorrhea. She reviewed 51 trials carried out in 1649 women. More than 72% of the women suffering from dysmenorrhea reported significant pain relief with NSAIDs, 18% reported minimal or no pain relief, and 15% showed a placebo response. Owen concluded that PGSI compounds were effective and safe for the majority of women with primary dysmenorrhea.

The fenamates seemed to be more effective in providing pain relief than ibuprofen, indomethacin, or naproxen. All the compounds demonstrated minimal NSAID-associated side effects with the exception of indomethacin. In trials with indomethacin the dropout rate was higher primarily because of symptoms involving the central nervous system and gastrointestinal tract.

Smith has demonstrated that the effectiveness of NSAIDs is related to tissue concentration. Using meclofenamate in 18 subjects who participated in a double-blind, placebo-controlled, cross-over study, he was able to show a parallel in time response curves between the plasma levels of the drug and decrease in uterine contractility. Figure 36-1 demonstrates the average intrauterine pressure relationships between placebo-treated and drug-treated patients over time. Intrauterine pressure declined 20% to 56% in these patients during meclofenamate therapy.

NSAIDs should not be given to patients who have shown previous hypersensitivity to such drugs. It is also contraindicated for individuals who have had nasal polyps, angioedema, and bronchospasm related to aspirin or nonsteroidal antiinflammatory agents. In addition, these agents are contraindicated for individuals with a history of chronic

ulceration or inflammatory reaction of the upper or lower gastrointestinal tract and for those with preexisting chronic renal disease. During the use of such agents, autoimmune hemolytic anemia, rash, edema and fluid retention, and central nervous system symptoms, such as dizziness, headache, nervousness, and blurred vision, can occur. In up to 15% of users slight elevation of hepatic enzymes may also be found. Table 36-2 lists some of the NSAIDs in common use for the treatment of dysmenorrhea.

Other Therapy

Although NSAIDs are the standard therapy available for primary dysmenorrhea, other approaches are possible. Oral contraceptives will relieve the symptoms of primary dysmenorrhea in about 90% of patients treated. This may be because of either a modulating effect on the hypothalamus or a direct reduction in the amount of endometrium present in women on oral contraceptive therapy. If the patient also requires contraception, oral contraceptive therapy may prove to be the treatment of choice.

Analgesics may be necessary in treating patients with primary dysmenorrhea but should be used as back-up drugs when the desired therapeutic effect is not achieved with NSAID medication or oral contraceptives.

Kaplan et al. reported on the use of transcutaneous electrical nerve stimulation (TENS) for 2 menstrual cycles in 61 Israeli women suffering from primary dysmenorrhea. Thirty percent reported marked pain relief, 60% moderate relief, and 10% no change in symptoms. They suggested that this method could be considered as primary therapy or in conjunction with pharmacologic therapy. Milsom et al. in Sweden, and Smith and Heltzel in the United States noted that TENS relieved menstrual pain without reducing intrauterine pressure, suggesting that its mode of action may be in the central nervous system.

TABLE 36-2
Commonly Used Nonsteroidal Antiinflammatory Drugs (NSAIDs)

Brand Name	Generic Name	Usual Regimen (mg q6h)
Motrin	Ibuprofen	400–800
Naprosyn	Naproxen	250–500
Anaprox	Naproxen sodium	275–550
Ponstel	Mefenamic acid	250–500

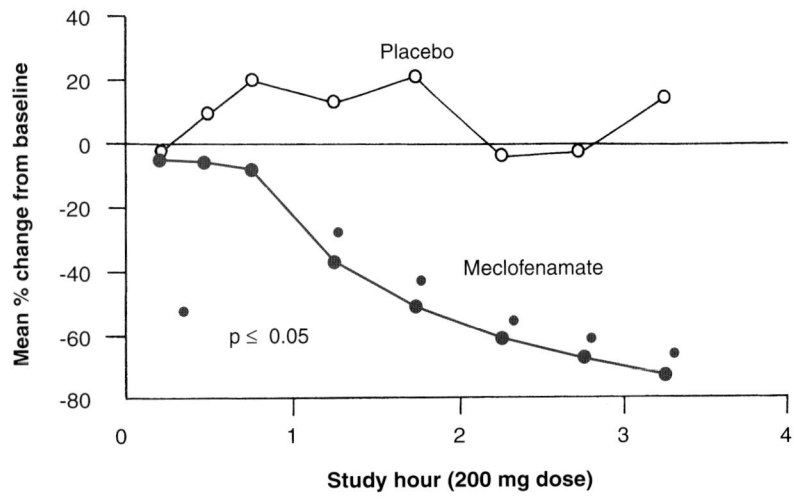

FIGURE 36-1   Average pressure: meclofenamate versus placebo. (Redrawn from Smith RP: Obstet Gynecol 70:785, 1987.)

Etiology and Management of Secondary Dysmenorrhea

A variety of other conditions cause or are associated with dysmenorrhea. These conditions may occur at any age, and in most cases the pain experienced is either secondary to the pathologic process of the condition or a specific result of the condition. These constitute the so-called secondary dysmenorrhea group of problems and include cervical stenosis, ectopic endometrial tissue, pelvic inflammation, pelvic congestion, conditioned behavior, and stress and tension (see box above).

Cervical Stenosis

Severe narrowing of the cervical canal, particularly at the level of the internal os, may impede menstrual flow, causing an increase in intrauterine pressure at the time of menses. In addition, retrograde menstrual flow through the fallopian tubes into the peritoneal cavity may take place. Thus severe cervical stenosis may eventually be associated with pelvic endometriosis as well. The etiology of cervical stenosis may be congenital or may be secondary to cervical injury, such as with electrocautery, cryocautery, or operative trauma (i.e., conization). The condition may also result from an inflammatory process caused by infection or by the application of caustic substances. After any of these conditions the cervical canal may narrow because of the formation of scar tissue.

The possibility of cervical stenosis should be considered if there is a history of scant menstrual flow and if severe cramping continues throughout the menstrual period.

The diagnosis is suspected when the external os appears scarred or when it is impossible to pass a uterine sound through the internal os during the proliferative stage of the menstrual cycle. Diagnosis is generally documented by the inability to pass a thin probe of a few millimeters' diameter through the internal os or by hysterosalpingogram, which demonstrates a thin, stringy-appearing canal. If dilation and curettage (D&C) are performed, finding the passage through the internal os with a thin probe is often difficult but can frequently be accomplished with patience. The patient should be anesthetized.

Treatment consists of dilating the cervix; this may be accomplished by D&C with progressive dilators or by the use of progressive *laminaria* tents. In the past the insertion of stem pessaries has been noted to be of some value in such cases. Unfortunately, cervical stenosis often recurs after therapy, necessitating repeat procedures. Pregnancy and vaginal delivery often afford more lasting cure.

Often other problems obstructing the cervix can have a similar presentation. Figure 36-2 shows anteroposterior and lateral views of a hysterogram in an 18-year-old nulliparous woman who had a 2-year history of severe, disabling dysmenorrhea that usually required morphine therapy with each menstrual period. At hysteroscopy she was found to have a tissue band across her internal os, at which site a large endocervical polyp had formed. Transecting the band and removing the polyp completely relieved the dysmenorrhea, and she had no further symptoms after 3 years.

Ectopic Endometrial Tissue (Endometriosis)

Ectopic endometrial tissue or endometriosis (including endometriosis and adenomyosis) should be considered when there is a history of pain becoming more severe during menses. Frequently dyspareunia and infertility are accompanying symptoms. Pertinent physical findings may include uterosacral ligament nodules or evidence for endometriosis in the vagina or cervix.

In a study from Japan, Koike et al., in an in vitro experiment using tissue slices, found that prostaglandin in endometriosis implants was significantly higher than in normal endometrium, myometrium, leiomyomata, and normal ovarian tissue and that adenomyosis implants produced larger amounts of 6-keto PGF when the dysmenorrhea had been severe. They believed that prostaglandins in endometriosis increased painful menstruation.

Specific diagnosis of endometriosis is made by direct visualization via laparoscopy or laparotomy or by direct biopsy of vaginal or cervical lesions.

Treatment of endometriosis is discussed in Chapter 19. Management should be designed for the patient's specific needs.

Pelvic Inflammation

Pelvic infections secondary to gonorrhea, chlamydia, or other infectious agents may cause pelvic inflammation or pelvic abscess and with healing may be associated with pelvic adhesions that may cause pelvic pain. Often this may be aggravated at menses, causing dysmenorrhea. Infections secondary to other conditions, such as appendicitis or IUD use, may also create a similar response. The pain may be secondary to the congestion and edema that occur normally at menses, which may subsequently be aggravated by the healed inflammatory areas and adhesions.

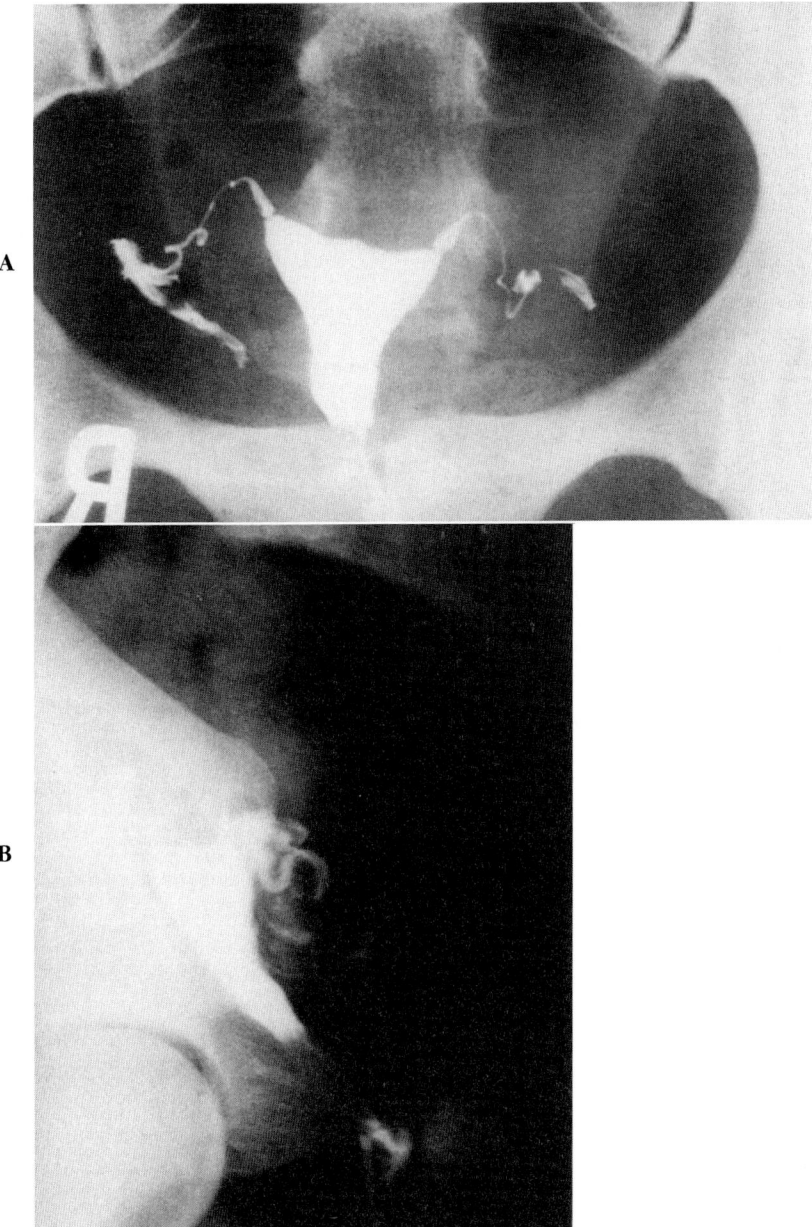

FIGURE 36-2   Hysterogram. **A,** Anteroposterior view and **B,** lateral view of an 18-year-old patient with severe disabling dysmenorrhea. At hysteroscopy she was found to have a tissue band across the internal os and an endocervical polyp at this site. Removal of the polyp and transection of the band completely relieved the dysmenorrhea.

Pelvic Congestion Syndrome

Pelvic congestion syndrome, which was first described by Taylor in 1949, results from engorgement of pelvic vasculature. The pain is usually burning or throbbing in nature, worse at night, and worse after standing. Physical examination of the vagina and cervix usually reveals vasocongestion with evidence of some uterine enlargement and tenderness. Diagnosis is made by observation of the features noted and by laparoscopy, which not only rules out other causes of pelvic pain but also demonstrates congestion of the uterus and engorgement or varicosities of the broad ligament and pelvic side wall veins. If laparoscopy is used for diagnosis, it is important to observe the broad ligament vasculature as the pressure of the carbon dioxide or nitrous oxide is released. At full pressure during the procedure these vessels may be obliterated but will reappear as pressure is reduced.

The pathophysiology of pelvic congestion syndrome is probably related to tension and psychosomatic problems. Consequently, management relates to careful history of the patient's past and present social situation and, where appropriate, the use of counseling.

Severe cases of pelvic congestion syndrome associated

with dysmenorrhea that do not respond to counseling or other medical types of pain management may respond to hysterectomy, although such management should be considered a last resort (see Chapter 7).

Conditioned Behavior

In individuals with strong family histories of dysmenorrhea or in situations where a careful history demonstrates a possibility for societal reward or control because of the symptoms of pain, a conditioned behavior should be considered. It is important to obtain a careful medical and social history and to rule out all other causes of acquired dysmenorrhea.

Diagnosis can often be verified by the use of a personality profile test, such as the Minnesota Multiphasic Personality Index. This test has been used clinically on many different groups of patients and is well standardized. It is frequently necessary to use such a test to demonstrate to the patient that she does indeed fit into such a category.

Treatment of patients with conditioned behavior dysmenorrhea includes reeducation so that the pain is not looked on as a rewarding experience. Teaching the patient an understanding of the pathophysiology of the problem and applying reconditioning techniques are useful. Psychologists or other similarly trained mental health workers can be consulted for this purpose.

Stress and Tension

Dysmenorrhea resulting from stress and tension usually is accompanied by a history of gradual onset, and the pain is generally worse at times, particularly when stress is severe and when there may be a possibility for secondary gain. The pathophysiology is difficult to define; it may be a combination of prostaglandin activity and engorgement.

The treatment is centered on finding the means to relieve stress, which may include education, the teaching of relaxation techniques, counseling, and, on rare occasions, antidepression or tranquilizing medications for short periods of time.

Relation to Functional Bowel Disease

Crowell et al. studied 383 women ages 20 to 40 using a NEO Personality Inventory on entry into the program and a Moos' Menstrual Distress Questionnaire and a bowel symptom inventory every 3 months for 12 months. Dysmenorrhea was diagnosed in 19.8% of the 383 women. Functional bowel disorder, defined as abdominal pain with altered bowel function, occurred in 61% of the women with dysmenorrhea but in only 20% of the others ($P < 0.05$). Although neuroticism was significantly more often diagnosed in patients with functional bowel disorder with or without dysmenorrhea, bowel symptoms were significantly correlated with dysmenorrhea even after controlling for the effects of neuroticism. Prostaglandin levels in vaginal fluid were elevated in patients with dysmenorrhea but did not consistently differentiate the diagnostic groups. These authors concluded that there was a strong covariance of menstrual and bowel symptoms, along with an overlap in their diagnosis suggesting a common physiologic basis.

Other Causes

At times dysmenorrhea may be related to unusual pathologic findings. These include small leiomyomas or polyps at the junction of the internal os and lower uterine segment. Such a condition may produce a valvelike effect at the os at the time of menses. Frequently myomas or polyps become engorged or edematous at the time of menses, accentuating the problem. Diagnosis is generally made by history and by hysterosalpingography, hysteroscopy, or D&C. Therapy consists of excising the pathologic tissue. In the case of a myoma a hysterectomy may be necessary.

PREMENSTRUAL SYNDROME

Premenstrual syndrome (PMS) is defined as a group of symptoms, both physical and behavioral, that occur in the second half of the menstrual cycle and that often interfere with work and personal relationships. These are followed by a period entirely free of symptoms. The condition was first described by Frank in 1931. That author attempted to relate symptoms of then so-called *premenstrual tension* with hormonal changes of the menstrual cycle. The term *premenstrual syndrome* was first used by Dalton in 1953. The symptoms do vary from woman to woman, and more than 150 symptoms have been linked with the disorder.

Incidence

Although various reports place the prevalence of PMS at 5% to 95% of menstruating women, it is generally agreed that about 40% of women are significantly affected at one time or another. Severe symptoms occur in only 2% or 3% of women between the ages of 18 and 48.

Symptoms

In a review by O'Brien a number of common somatic and psychologic symptoms were enumerated. These are summarized in the box (see facing page). In general, somatic symptoms relate to presumed fluid retention, breast tenderness, and various pain constellations, such as headache or pelvic pain. Psychologic symptoms vary from irritability and tension to anxiety, aggression, and depression. The personality changes that occur in the second half of the

Symptoms of Premenstrual Syndrome
Somatic Symptoms
Bloated feeling
Feeling of weight increase
Breast pain or tenderness
Skin disorders
Hot flushes
Headache
Pelvic pain
Change in bowel habits
Psychologic Symptoms
Irritability
Aggression
Tension
Anxiety
Depression
Lethargy
Insomnia
Change in appetite
Crying
Change in libido
Thirst
Loss of concentration
Poor coordination, clumsiness, accidents
From O'Brien PM: Drugs 24:140, 1982.

menstrual cycle are so severe in some patients that the term *Dr. Jekyl and Mr. Hyde* is frequently used. In a few instances PMS has been used as a defense in murder trials.

Freeman et al. in a study of 60 women ages 18 to 45 who were newly enrolled in a PMS program at the University of Pennsylvania found that four major history variables explained 34% of the variance of symptom severity using step regression analysis. These were PMS in the patient's mother, low level of exercise, younger age, and more children. These relationships suggested to the authors that familial and stress factors had a role in the syndrome.

Depression is a common complaint in the population in general and also in PMS sufferers during the luteal phase. Mortola et al. have recently shown that 16 PMS patients had marked worsening of scores on the Profile of Mood States and Beck Depression Inventory during the luteal phase compared with 16 controls. However, six patients suffering from endogenous depression had scores three-fold higher on both indices than PMS patients who were in the luteal phase. Also, the amplitude of cortisol secretion pulses was higher in the depressed patients than either PMS patients or control patients. The data of this study demonstrate that PMS patients do have more episodes of depression during the luteal phase compared with controls, but these episodes are distinctly different from those suffered by patients with endogenous depression.

In addition, Rapkin et al. have demonstrated that PMS patients show no deficit in cognitive processing and performance, as well as no loss in ability to concentrate and

sustain attention and motivation. No such alterations were seen in 10 PMS patients during the luteal phase. Their performance was similar to nine controls when tested in these areas. In a later study, this group studied 30 patients with PMS and 31 controls during the follicular and luteal phases. Despite feelings of inadequacy, patients showed no statistically significant differences from controls in tests for attention, memory, cognitive flexibility, and overall mental agility.

Etiology

When Frank first described the syndrome, he attributed it to estrogen excess. Israel theorized 7 years later that it resulted from an imbalance of estrogen and progesterone. Others have offered theories that the disorder is related to endogenous hormone allergy, hypoglycemia, vitamin B_6 deficiency, prolactin excess, fluid retention, inappropriate prostaglandin activity, elevated monoamine oxidase (MAO), endorphin malfunction, and multiple psychologic disturbances. In 1981, Reid and Yen reviewed the subject and concluded that PMS was a multifactorial psychoendocrine disorder. Recent studies indicate that alterations in serotoninergic neuronal mechanisms in the central nervous system may have a major involvement. Evidence for this is indirect but includes successful clinical trials with selective serotonin reuptake inhibitors (SSRIs) and other neurotropic agents thought to affect the serotonin pump mechanism between CNS neurons. Other indirect evidence includes the fact that platelet tritium-labeled, imipramine-binding sites that are felt to be reduced in patients suffering from depression and are believed to represent receptor sites that label for presynaptic serotonin transporter on the presynaptic nerve terminal, in some studies, have returned to normal several months after clinical remission of depression or during the response to psychotropic medications or electroconvulsive therapy. These platelet-binding sites therefore have been used as an indirect measure of the neuron receptor site. Recently, Steege et al. demonstrated lower platelet tritium-labeled imipramine binding in women with late luteal phase dysphoric disorder (PMS) and felt this supported the hypothesis that such patients suffered from alterations of the central serotonergic systems.

That ovulation and therefore progesterone production is important in this syndrome has been known for some time, but studies related to the relationship of progesterone in the circulation and the severity of the symptoms have not been fruitful. In fact, some have demonstrated an increased level of progesterone in the circulation in PMS sufferers, while others have demonstrated a decrease or no change at all. Although symptom relief has been noted in several studies using GnRH agonists to block ovulation completely, no relief was found in a study by Chan et al. who blocked progesterone receptors with the progesterone antagonist RU 486. Rapkin et al. evaluated the anxiolytic $3-\alpha-5-\alpha$ reduced progesterone metabolite allopregnanediol during the luteal phase of 35 women with PMS and 36 controls. Serum progesterone and allopregnanediol levels were measured on days 19 and 26 of the cycles as determined by LH kits. Allopregnanediol levels were significantly lower in the PMS patients than controls on day 26, but there were not significant differences with respect to progesterone itself. They concluded that since PMS patients had lower levels of this anxiolytic metabolite during the luteal phase, they could be at greater susceptability for various mood symptoms such as anxiety, tension, and depression. Chuong et al. have recently demonstrated that beta endorphin levels throughout the periovulatory phase were lower in PMS patients than in controls, especially in postovulatory days 0 to 4. Likewise, Halbreich et al. demonstrated that PMS patients treated with 200 mg per day of danazol for 90 days demonstrated a complete relief of symptoms in 23 anovulatory cycles but relief of symptoms occurred in only 6 of 32 ovulatory cycles. They concluded that the beneficial effect of danazol in the treatment of PMS was achieved only when the anovulatory state eliminated the hormonal cyclicity of the normal cycle and not because of action of drug per se. Further evidence for this was advanced by O'Brien and Abukhalil. They studied 100 women with premenstrual syndrome and premenstrual breast pain using a randomized double-masked placebo-controlled study of 3 menstrual cycles, using danazol 20 mg qd as the active drug. Treatment was given only during the luteal phase. Danazol did not effectively reduce the general symptoms of PMS, but did relieve mastalgia. Severe PMS has been shown to be relieved by total abdominal hysterectomy and bilateral salpingo-oophorectomy even with hormone replacement therapy using an estrogen, but some women on cyclic estrogen and progesterone therapy postmenopausally continue to complain of PMS symptoms.

The theory that steroid allergy might be the basis of PMS symptomatology was advanced by several many years ago, but none held the test of a carefully controlled study. Likewise, dietary and vitamin deficiency theories have been difficult to prove and have not been found to be a major cause of this syndrome. Several have looked for prolactin excess since some of the patients complain of breast tenderness, but no positive findings have been found. Although some of the symptomatology seems to relate to prostaglandin activity and these symptoms are often reduced with treatment with nonsteroidal antiinflammatory drugs, a direct cause and effect has not been established.

Diagnosis

Because the etiology of PMS is still unknown, the diagnosis is made by history. The facts given by the patient may allow the physician to construct a specific treatment regimen for that patient. It is important that the physician have a clear understanding of the patient's symptoms before undertaking therapy. After a complete history and physical examination, the physician should rule out any medical problems that could be influencing the symptomatology. The physician should then ask the patient to keep a diary of her symptoms throughout two menstrual cycles. Although the patient and the physician may focus on the second half of the menstrual cycle, the patient should be encouraged to keep track of all symptoms regardless of the stage of the menstrual cycle. A number of commercial diary sheets and symptom checkoff lists are available, but it is probably better to have the patient write the symptoms she perceives in her own words rather than clue her to specific response patterns. At the end of two cycles the physician should review the symptom diary with the patient and discuss carefully those symptoms that seem to be causing her the most difficulty.

It is important to differentiate PMS from other illnesses with similar symptomatology. Patients with psychiatric disorders, such as different types of depression, anxiety reactions, and psychosis, may present believing that they have PMS. A differentiating aspect is that PMS patients suffer their symptoms *only* during the luteal phase.

That many women who do not actually have PMS may be self-referred to a facility that treats this condition is well appreciated. In one study, Plouffe et al. carefully analyzed 100 consecutive women prospectively entering the Uniform Diagnostic and Treatment Protocol for PMS and found that 38 women had premenstrual syndrome; 24 had premenstrual magnification syndrome, that is, other conditions that were magnified during the luteal phase, and 13 had affective or other psychiatric disorders. Only 44% of the women previously given a diagnosis of premenstrual syndrome were found to have this syndrome. Overall, in this study, 84% of the women with premenstrual syndrome and premenstrual magnification syndrome responded to treatment. A variety of currently accepted therapies were used.

No laboratory tests are available to make the diagnosis. Although it has been reported that many patients with PMS suffer thyroid hypofunction, a study by Nikolai et al. demonstrated that there was no significant thyroid disease in 44 carefully studied PMS patients compared with 15 normal controls. In addition, treating 22 with L-thyroxine and 22 with placebo led to no differences in relief of symptoms.

The diagnosis of PMS is therefore made by symptom diary and by the elimination of other diagnoses.

Management

Diet and Exercise

Although many individuals will suffer from symptomatology related to premenstrual syndrome, only about 2% to 3% are seriously affected. Thus the selection of medications and other regimens should be tailored to the symptomatic needs of the patient. In 1953 Morton et al. observed that glucose tolerance tests were occasionally flattened prior to menses and restored to normal thereafter. Individuals demonstrating this often crave sweets and complain of headaches. He therefore treated 249 volunteers in a New York state prison with a high-protein diet, placebo, other medications consisting of diuretic, caffeine, and vitamin B complex or combinations thereof. He demonstrated that 15% of those treated with placebo noted an improvement in symptoms, 39% treated with placebo and high-protein diet noted improvement, 61% of those treated with a drug regimen reported improvement, and 79% of those treated with a drug regimen plus a high-protein diet showed improvement. The greatest improvement was in symptoms that were related to nervousness and emotional dysfunction. Vitamin B_6 deficiency in PMS patients has been suggested because B_6 is a coenzyme in the biosynthesis of dopamine and serotonin and the possibility that this agent may be involved in the etiology of PMS has been raised. In 1973 Adams et al. noted that vitamin B_6 therapy seemed to be associated with improvement of depression in women taking oral contraceptives in a double-blind trial. It was believed that the oral contraceptives cause an abnormal tryptophan metabolism and that B_6, to some extent, reversed this. One double-blind study by Abraham and Hargrove demonstrated that vitamin B_6 administered at 200- to 800-mg doses daily prevented some of the symptoms of PMS in women with this affliction, significantly better than placebo. They theorized that deficiencies of vitamin B_6 and magnesium could result in lower thresholds to stress and to potential hormone imbalance. They also noted that giving vitamin B_6 to a patient raised serum progesterone levels at mid-luteal cycle. They felt that eventually the vitamin B_6 activity might lower brain serotonin levels. Doll et al. studied 32 women ages 18 to 49 with a double-blind, placebo-controlled, cross-over protocol utilizing 200 mg of pyridoxine daily. They noted a significant beneficial effect on emotional symptoms (depression, irritability, and tiredness) but on no other PMS symptoms. Higher doses of pyridoxine should be administered with caution since neuropathy occurred in several patients treated with as little as 100 to 200 mg daily. Such symptoms as sensory deficit, paresthesia, numbness, ataxia, and muscle weakness may occur. The physician therefore should review the patient's diet and initially suggest a high-protein, well-balanced diet. Supplemental vitamins may be used, and the physician may elect to suggest that the patient use a vitamin B_6 (pyridoxine) supplement at the rate of 50 mg per day. It is appropriate to begin with this therapy and add other medications if necessary. The patient should be encouraged to exercise at least 3 to 4 times per week, particularly during the luteal phase.

Diuretics

The physician may elect to add a diuretic to the regimen if the patient complaints involve bloating and perceived change in body habitus during the luteal phase of the cycle.

A potassium-saving diuretic should be selected, and the lowest dose possible to achieve symptomatic relief should be used. Although many patients do report a feeling of fluid retention during the luteal phase, this has been difficult to demonstrate. Perceived swelling of the body is difficult to prove unless actual careful weight analysis is utilized. Faratian et al. evaluated 148 menstrual cycles in 52 women and in each cycle various parameters were measured to determine an objective means of assessing the syndrome. These included daily mood assessment, measurement of body weight, plasma 17 β-estradiol levels, and plasma progesterone levels. The abdominal girth was measured carefully in two dimensions: at the level of the umbilicus and then 10 cm below the umbilicus. At the same time the dimensions were subjectively judged by the patient. Mood scores showed a marked shifting during the premenstrual phase of each cycle. The symptoms of bloatedness were most marked during the premenstrual phase of the cycle. Despite these elevated scores for bloatedness, there was no increase in body weight or measured body dimension changes in any plane during this period. The patient's perception of body size did increase and a discrepancy between the perceived body size and actual body size was noted. The authors divided their patients into those with predominantly somatic symptoms and those with predominantly psychologic symptoms and also studied a control group. No hormonal differences were noted in the three groups. Freeman et al. studied transcapillary fluid balance in 10 women with well-defined PMS. The capillary filtration coefficient was measured by string gauge plethysmography. They noted that from the follicular to the luteal phase, interstitial colloid osmotic pressure on the leg was significantly reduced (mean of 3.6 mm Hg), whereas the interstitial colloid osmotic pressure on the thorax remained constant. The capillary filtration coefficient increased 30% from the follicular to the luteal phase. No change was observed in body weight. The authors felt that these changes represented an instability of vascular regulation in women with PMS and that this led support to the hypothesis that redistribution of fluid rather than water retention is responsible for the subjective symptom of bloatedness in premenstrual syndrome. This would explain why diuretics might appear beneficial to the patient. They should be avoided in patients with chronic renal disease or in those who are suffering from diarrhea or other fluid loss.

Progesterone

Although Dalton advocates the use of naturally occurring progesterone, the fact that progesterone receptors will respond to both synthetic progestins and progesterone implies that any reasonable progestational agent would be appropriate. However, in all double-blind studies to date, progesterone has not been shown to be effective. In the rare patient in whom progesterone is to be tried, a regimen of 10 to 20 mg per day of medroxyprogesterone acetate (Provera) or 50 to 100 mg twice a day of progesterone vaginal suppositories can be tried.

Some relief of symptoms was noted in a double-blind, placebo-controlled, cross-over study using estradiol patches (200 μg every 3 days) and norethisterone 5 mg (days 19 to 26 of each cycle) when compared with placebo by Watson et al. The authors realized they were suppressing ovulation and that this may have been the mechanism for obtaining symptom relief.

Psychotherapy

Studies in the 1950s showed that 50% of patients improved with psychotherapy alone. However, this is similar to the response rate of many placebo therapies. Certainly if patients have obvious psychiatric problems as detected by history, psychotherapy should be added. It is less effective as a primary therapy.

Psychoactive Drugs

Although continuous use of psychoactive drugs, such as tricyclics and lithium, has not yielded good PMS symptom relief, Smith et al. noted in a carefully performed double-blind, placebo-controlled, cross-over study of 19 patients suffering from PMS using alprazolam (Xanax) that the drug significantly relieved the severity of premenstrual nervous tension, mood swings, irritability, anxiety, depression, fatigue, forgetfulness, crying, cravings for sweets, abdominal bloating, cramps, and headaches, compared with the placebo. These investigators prescribed 0.25 mg tid days 20 to 28 of each cycle, tapering to 0.25 mg bid on day 1 and 0.25 mg on day 2. On this regimen in my hands, many patients complain of sleepiness, but 0.25 mg bid and even 0.125 mg bid has proved to be equally effective in many cases. In fact, I usually use 0.25 mg bid days 20 to 28 with one 0.25-mg dose on day 1. Patients with strong tendencies to habituation should not be treated with this regimen. Berger and Presser studied two groups of patients with alprazolam therapy. The first group was diagnosed as having late luteal phase dysphoric disorder (PMS); the second group experienced this disorder, as well as symptoms of mild anxiety or depression during the follicular phase. Although alprazolam definitely reduced symptoms of PMS compared with placebo in the pure PMS group, no difference was noted in symptoms in the patients with PMS plus mild anxiety or depression during the follicular phase. Also, in 22 patients with confirmed premenstrual syndrome studied by Schmidt et al., no significant differences were noted in symptoms between the drug and placebo cycles except for an alleviation of depression. Certainly, symptom differences noted in various studies may relate to the selection of patients.

Other antianxiety drugs seem to have value in the control of PMS symptoms. One such drug, fluoxetine hydrochloride (Prozac), has been effectively used in several clinics, including mine. Fluoxetine hydrochloride has been utilized in continuous therapy with doses of 5 to 20 mg per day and in regimens of therapy from day 20 to 28 of the menstrual cycle and seems to have efficacy in both types of regimens. Since the medication is an SSRI, it may turn out to be one of the more specific agents for this condition. Many other SSRI drugs are also effective.

Before using psychoactive drugs, it is extremely important to be sure of the diagnosis as the drugs may not be effective and may actually be contraindicated in other psychiatric conditions that mimic PMS.

Danazol

Sarno et al. reported on the apparent effectiveness of danazol in doses of 200 mg qd, days 20 to 28 of each menstrual cycle, in relieving PMS symptoms. Studying 14 patients in a double-blind, placebo-controlled protocol, they found significant relief of symptoms in 11 of the 14 patients, compared with placebo. Because such a small dose given during only the luteal phase will not prevent pregnancy, patients should be cautioned to avoid this agent if pregnancy is contemplated, to avoid the potential of masculinizing a female fetus. As noted previously, danazol may be effective because it causes anovulation in some subjects at this dose level.

Bromocriptine

Bromocriptine may be used in patients with breast tenderness and may be helpful for some of the other symptoms of PMS, although its use in any individual case will need to be evaluated. A dose of 5 mg per day during the luteal phase is appropriate.

Nonsteroidal Antiinflammatory Drugs

For patients who complain of cramping or other systemic symptoms, such as diarrhea or heat intolerance, a trial with a nonsteroidal antiinflammatory drug (NSAID) may be useful. It should be noted, however, that a toxic complication of NSAID use is nonoliguric renal failure. Because it is more likely to occur with NSAID use associated with severe dehydration, the agent should be discontinued if severe diarrhea is present and should not be used with diuretics.

Hysterectomy and Bilateral Oophorectomy

Casper and Hearn reported complete relief of symptoms in 14 women with severe debilitating symptoms of PMS who had completed their families, had been demonstrated to have relief of symptoms with ovarian-suppressing doses of danazol, and now were treated with total hysterectomy and bilateral oophorectomy followed by continuous low-dose estrogen replacement therapy. Casson et al. have noted similar results. Although this approach is not offered as standard therapy for severe PMS, it may be a reasonable alternative for selective cases. The use of a GnRH analog for short periods of time with or without estrogen add back may be useful as therapy in severe cases or at least helpful in deciding who may benefit from surgical treatment.

The physician should be cautious in building a treatment regimen for any individual patient and should attempt to verify the patient's symptoms and to add medications only when relief has not been achieved. Medications that do not seem to be helping should be stopped. Because most agents when scrutinized by double-blind control methods are less than utopian in the treatment of this condition, it is not surprising that individualization of treatment is essential. Many of the therapies just mentioned, however, do offer relief of most symptoms and hope for many sufferers.

KEY POINTS

- Primary dysmenorrhea almost always occurs before the age of 20. Secondary dysmenorrhea may occur at any time during the menstrual years.

- Approximately 75% of all women complain of primary dysmenorrhea. Roughly 15% have severe symptoms.

- Pregnancy without vaginal birth does not seem to alleviate primary dysmenorrhea, whereas childbirth does.

- Oral contraceptives reduce the prevalence and severity of dysmenorrhea.

- IUD use does not affect the prevalence or severity of primary dysmenorrhea.

- The severity of primary dysmenorrhea correlates directly with the duration of menstrual flow, amount of menstrual flow, and age at menarche but does not correlate with the duration of the menstrual cycle.

- Among patients who had primary dysmenorrhea, 38% reported onset of symptoms within the first year after menarche.

- Nonsteroidal antiinflammatory drugs (NSAIDs) are the treatment of choice in primary dysmenorrhea, with 72% of women suffering from dysmenorrhea reporting significant pain relief.

- NSAIDs reduced intrauterine pressure 20% to 56% during treatment of patients with dysmenorrhea in one study.

- Approximately 40% of all women suffer considerably from premenstrual syndrome (PMS), with 2% to 3% demonstrating severe symptoms.

- Common historical findings in PMS patients are (1) a history of maternal PMS, (2) low levels of exercise, (3) younger age, and (4) higher parity.

- PMS patients often suffer depression during the luteal phase but not as severe as depression noted by endogenous depression patients when measured by standard depression scales or the amplitude of cortisol secretion pulses.

- PMS patients show no deficit in cognitive function during the luteal phase.

- Bromocriptine is effective primarily in relieving breast tenderness in PMS.

- Although fluid retention–related symptoms are prevalent in patients with PMS, it is difficult to document such retention. Redistribution of fluid may occur.

- There is no evidence that women with symptoms of PMS have impaired corpus luteal function.

- The most useful diagnostic tool in caring for PMS patients is a symptom diary.

- There is little objective data to support the concept that vitamin B_6 therapy relieves PMS symptoms.

- There is little objective data to support the concept that progesterone relieves PMS symptoms in most women.

- Therapy with psychoactive drugs, such as alprazolam (Xanax) and fluoxetine hydrochloride (Prozac), in relatively small doses given during the luteal phase may be helpful in relieving PMS symptoms. Specific cautions for the use of these agents must be followed.

- In severe cases of PMS involving older women who have completed their families, hysterectomy and bilateral oophorectomy can give symptom relief. Small, daily dosage of estrogen may then be given.

BIBLIOGRAPHY

Abraham GE and Hargrove JT: Effect of vitamin B_6 on premenstrual symptomatology in women with premenstrual tension syndrome: a double blind crossover study, Infertility 3:155, 1980.

Abramson M and Torghele JR: Weight, temperature changes and psychosomatic symptomatology in relation to the menstrual cycle, Am J Obstet Gynecol 81:223, 1961.

Adams PW, Rose DP, Folkard J, et al: Effect of pyridoxine hydrochloride (vitamin B_6) upon depression associated with oral contraception, Lancet 1:897, 1973.

Andersch B: Bromocriptine and premenstrual symptoms: a survey of double blind trials, Obstet Gynecol Surv 38:643, 1983.

Andersch B and Hahn L: Bromocriptine and premenstrual tension: a clinical and hormonal study, Pharmatherapeutica 3:107, 1982.

Andersch B and Milsom I: An epidemiologic study of young women with dysmenorrhea, Am J Obstet Gynecol 144:655, 1982.

Berger CP and Presser B: Alprazolam in the treatment of two subsamples of patients with late luteal phase dysphoric disorder: a double-blind, placebo-controlled crossover study, Obstet Gynecol 84:379, 1994.

Brown CS, Ling FW, Andersen RN, et al: Efficacy of depot leuprolide in premenstrual syndrome: effect of symptom severity and type in a controlled trial, Obstet Gynecol 84:779, 1994.

Bruce J and Russell GFM: Premenstrual tension: a study of weight changes and balances of water, sodium and potassium, Lancet 2:267, 1962.

Budoff PW: Zomepirac sodium in the treatment of primary dysmenorrhea syndrome, N Engl J Med 307:714, 1982.

Casper RF and Hearn MT: The effect of hysterectomy and bilateral oophorectomy in women with severe premenstrual syndrome, Am J Obstet Gynecol 162:105, 1990.

Casson P, Hahn PM, Van Vugt DA, and Reid RL: Lasting response to ovariectomy in severe intractable premenstrual syndrome, Am J Obstet Gynecol 162:99, 1990.

Chan AF, Mortola JF, Wood SH, and Yen SSC: Persistence of premenstrual syndrome during low-dose administration of the progesterone antagonist RU 486, Obstet Gynecol 84:1001, 1994.

Chuong CJ, Hsi BP, and Gibbons WE: Periovulatory b-endorphin levels in premenstrual syndrome, Obstet Gynecol 83:755, 1994.

Cohen MR, Cohen RM, Pickar D, et al: Behavioral effect of high dose naloxone administration in normal volunteers, Lancet 1:1110, 1981.

Crowell MD, Dubin NH, Robinson JC, et al. Functional bowel disorders in women with dysmenorrhea, Am J Gastroenterol 89:1973, 1994.

Dalton K: The premenstrual syndrome and progesterone therapy, London, 1977, William Heinemann Medical Books.

Doll H, Brown S, Thurston A, and Vessey M: Pyridoxine (vitamin B_6) and the premenstrual syndrome: a randomized crossover trial, J R Coll Gen Pract 39:364, 1989.

Facchinetti F, Fioroni L, Sances G, et al: Naproxen sodium in the treatment of premenstrual symptoms: a placebo-controlled study, Gynecol Obstet Invest 28:205, 1989.

Faratian B, Gaspar A, O'Brien PM, et al: Premenstrual syndrome, weight, abdominal swelling and perceived body image, Am J Obstet Gynecol 150:200, 1984.

Frank RT: The hormonal causes of premenstrual tension, Arch Neurol Psychol 126:1052, 1931.

Freeman E, Rickels K, Sondheimer SJ, and Polansky M: Ineffectiveness of progesterone suppository treatment for premenstrual syndrome, JAMA 264:349, 1990.

Freeman EW, Sondheimer SJ, and Rickels K: Effects of medical history factors on symptoms severity in women meeting criteria for premenstrual syndrome, Obstet Gynecol 72:236, 1988.

Green R and Dalton K: The premenstrual syndrome, Br Med J 1:1007, 1953.

Halbreich U, Assael M, Ben-David M, et al: Serum prolactin in women with premenstrual syndrome, Lancet 2:654, 1976.

Halbreich U, Rojansky N, and Palter S: Elimination of ovulation and menstrual cyclicity (with danazol) improves dysphoric premenstrual syndromes, Fertil Steril 56:1066, 1991.

Henzl MR, Ortega-Herrera E, Rodriguez C, and Izu A: Anaprox in dysmenorrhea: reduction of pain in intrauterine pressure, Am J Obstet Gynecol 135:455, 1979.

Kaplan B, Peled Y, Pardo J, et al: Transcutaneous electrical nerve stimulation (TENS) as a relief for dysmenorrhea, Clin Exp Obstet Gynecol 21:87, 1994.

Koike H, Ikenoue T, and Mori N: Studies on prostaglandin production relating to the mechanism of dysmenorrhea in endometriosis, Nippon Naibunpi Gakkai Zasshi. Folia Endocrinologica Japonica 20:43, 1994.

Korzekwa MI and Steiner M: Assessment and treatment of premenstrual syndrome, Prim Care Update OB/GYN 6:153, 1999.

Kullander S and Svanberg L: Bromocriptine treatment of the premenstrual syndrome, Acta Obstet Gynecol Scand 58:375, 1979.

Mattes JA and Martin D: Pyridoxine in premenstrual depression, Hum Nutr Appl Nutr 36(2):131, 1982.

Menkes DB, Taghavi E, Mason PA, and Howard RC: Fluoxetine's spectrum of action in premenstrual syndrome, Int Clin Psychopharmacol 8:95, 1993.

Metz A: Fluoxetine treatment of premenstrual syndrome, J Clin Psychiatry 51:260, 1990.

Mezrow G, Shoupe D, Spicer D, et al: Depot leuprolide acetate with estrogen and progestin add-back for long-term treatment of premenstrual syndrome, Fertil Steril 62:932, 1994.

Milsom I, Hedner N, and Mannheimer C: A comparative study of the effect of high-intensity transcutaneous nerve stimulation and oral naproxen on intrauterine pressure and menstrual pain in patients with primary dysmenorrhea, Am J Obstet Gynecol 170:123, 1994.

Morgan M, Rapkin AJ, D'Ella I, et al: Cognitive functioning in premenstrual syndrome, Obstet Gynecol 88:961, 1996.

Mortola JF, Girton L, and Fischer U: Successful treatment of severe premenstrual syndrome by combined use of gonadotropin-releasing hormone agonist and estrogen/progestin, J Clin Endocrinol Metab 71:252A, 1991.

Mortola JF, Girton L, and Yen SSC: Depressive episodes in premenstrual syndrome, Am J Obstet Gynecol 161:1682, 1989.

Morton JH, Additon H, Addison RG, et al: A clinical study of premenstrual tension, Am J Obstet Gynecol 65:1182, 1953.

Nikolai TF, Mulligan GM, Gribble RK, et al: Thyroid function and treatment in premenstrual syndrome, J Clin Endocrinol Metab 70:1108, 1990.

O'Brien PM: The premenstrual syndrome: a review of the present status of therapy, Drugs 24:140, 1982.

O'Brien PM and Abukhalil IEH: Randomized controlled trial of the management of premenstrual syndrome and premenstrual mastalgia using luteal phase–only danazol, Am J Obstet Gynecol 180:18, 1999.

Owen PR: Prostaglandin synthetase inhibitors in the treatment of primary dysmenorrhea: outcome trials reviewed, Am J Obstet Gynecol 148:96, 1984.

Pearlstein TB and Stone AB: Long-term fluoxetine treatment of late luteal phase dysphoric disorder, J Clin Psychiatry 55:332, 1994.

Plouffe L Jr, Stewart K, Craft KS, et al: Diagnostic and treatment results from a southeastern academic center-based premenstrual syndrome clinic: the first year, Am J Obstet Gynecol 169:295, 1993.

Rapkin AJ, Chang LI, and Reading AE: Mood and cognitive style in premenstrual syndrome, Obstet Gynecol 74:644, 1989.

Rapkin AJ, Morgan M, Goldman L, et al: Progesterone metabolite allopregnanediol in women with premenstrual syndrome. Obstet Gynecol 90:709, 1997.

Reid RL and Yen SSC: Premenstrual syndrome, Am J Obstet Gynecol 139:85, 1981.

Rogers WC: The role of endocrine allergy in the production of premenstrual tension, West J Surg Obstet Gynecol 70:100, 1962.

Sampson GA: Premenstrual syndrome: a double blind control trial of progesterone and placebo, Br J Psychiatry 135:209, 1979.

Sarno AP Jr, Miller EJ, and Lundblad EG: Premenstrual syndrome: beneficial effects of periodic, low-dose danazol, Obstet Gynecol 70:33, 1987.

Schmidt PJ, Grover GN, and Rubinow DR: Alprazolam in the treatment of premenstrual syndrome: a double-blind, placebo-controlled trial, Arch Gen Psychiatry 50:467, 1993.

Smith RP: The dynamics of nonsteroidal antiinflammatory therapy for primary dysmenorrhea, Obstet Gynecol 70:785, 1987.

Smith RP and Heltzel JA: Interrelation of analgesia and uterine activity in women with primary dysmenorrhea: a preliminary report, J Reprod Med 36:260, 1991.

Smith S, Rinehart JS, Ruddock VE, and Schiff I: Treatment of premenstrual syndrome with alprazolam: results of a double-blind, placebo-controlled, randomized crossover clinical trial, Obstet Gynecol 70:37, 1987.

Smith S and Schiff I: The premenstrual syndrome: diagnosis and management, Fertil Steril 52:527, 1989.

Smith SL: Mood and the menstrual cycle. In Sacher EJ, editor: Topics in cycle endocrinology, New York, 1975, Grune & Stratton.

Speroff L and Ramwell P: Prostaglandins in reproductive physiology, Am J Obstet Gynecol 107:1111, 1970.

Steege JR, Stout AL, Knight DL, and Nemeroff CB: Reduced platelet tritium-labeled imipramine binding sites in women with premenstrual syndrome, Am J Obstet Gynecol 167:168, 1992.

Steiner M, Steinberg S, Stewart D, et al: Fluoxetine in the treatment of premenstrual syndrome. N Engl J Med 332:1529, 1995.

Stokes J and Mendels J: Pyridoxine and premenstrual tension, Lancet 1:1177, 1972.

Stone AB, Pearlstein TB, and Brown WA: Fluoxetine in the treatment of late luteal phase dysphoric disorder, J Clin Psychiatry 52:290, 1991.

Taylor HC: Vascular congestion and hyperemia, their effect on the structure and function in the female reproductive system, Am J Obstet Gynecol 57:211, 1949.

Taylor JW: The timing of menstruation-related symptoms assessed by a daily symptom rating scale, Acta Psychiatr Scand 60:87, 1979.

Tollan A, Oian P, Fadness HO, and Maltau JM: Evidence for altered transcapillary fluid balance in women with the premenstrual syndrome, Acta Obstet Gynecol Scand 72:238, 1993.

Watson NR, Studd JWW, Savvas M, et al: Treatment of severe premenstrual syndrome with oestradiol patches and cyclical oral norethisterone, Lancet 2:730, 1989.

Ylikorkala O and Dawood MY: New concepts in dysmenorrhea, Am J Obstet Gynecol 130:833, 1978.

Ylöstalo P, Kauppila A, Puolakka J, et al: Bromocriptine and norethisterone in the treatment of premenstrual syndrome, Obstet Gynecol 58:292, 1982.

Abnormal Uterine Bleeding

Ovulatory and Anovulatory Dysfunctional Uterine Bleeding, Management of Acute and Chronic Excessive Bleeding

KEY TERMS AND DEFINITIONS

Dysfunctional Uterine Bleeding (DUB). Excessive uterine bleeding with no demonstrable organic cause (genital or extragenital). It is most frequently due to abnormalities of endocrine origin, particularly anovulation.

Endometrial Ablation. Destruction of the endometrium by laser or electrocoagulation with instruments placed through a hysteroscope.

Intermenstrual Bleeding. Bleeding of variable amounts occurring between regular menstrual periods.

Menometrorrhagia. Prolonged uterine bleeding occurring at irregular intervals.

Menorrhagia. Prolonged (more than 7 days) or excessive (greater than 80 ml) uterine bleeding occurring at regular intervals. The term *hypermenorrhea* is synonymous.

Metrorrhagia. Uterine bleeding occurring at irregular but frequent intervals, the amount being variable.

Nonsteroidal Antiinflammatory Drugs (NSAIDs). Drugs that inhibit the synthesis of prostaglandins.

Polymenorrhea. Uterine bleeding occurring at regular intervals of less than 21 days.

Sonohysterography. Sonographic imaging of the endometrial cavity after installation of 10 to 15 ml of saline to improve contrast and facilitate diagnosis of endometrial lesions.

Abnormal uterine bleeding can take many forms: infrequent episodes, excessive flow, or prolonged duration of menses and intermenstrual bleeding. Alterations in the pattern or volume of blood flow of menses are among the most common health concerns of women. Infrequent uterine bleeding, defined as *oligomenorrhea* if the intervals between bleeding episodes vary from 35 days to 6 months, and *amenorrhea*, defined as no menses for at least 6 months, are discussed fully in Chapter 38. Excessive or prolonged bleeding will be discussed in this chapter. Recently several new therapeutic modalities have been successfully utilized to treat excessive uterine bleeding, and they will also be discussed in this chapter.

To define excessive abnormal uterine bleeding it is necessary to define normal menstrual flow. The mean interval between menses is 28 days (±7 days). Thus if bleeding occurs at intervals of 21 days or less, it is abnormal. The mean duration of menstrual flow is 4 days. Since few women with normal menses bleed more than 7 days, bleeding more than 7 days is considered to be abnormally prolonged (menorrhagia). It is useful to document the duration and frequency of menstrual flow with the use of menstrual diary cards; however, it is difficult to determine the amount of menstrual blood loss (MBL) by subjective means. Several studies have shown that there is poor correlation between subjective judgment and objective measurement of MBL. Hallberg et al. found that 40% of women with blood loss greater than 80 ml considered their menstrual flow to be small or moderate in amount (Figure 37-1), whereas 14% of women with blood loss less than 20 ml thought their menses were heavy. In a study by Chimbira et al., there was also poor correlation between a woman's perception of menstrual blood loss and the actual amount lost. These investigators reported that

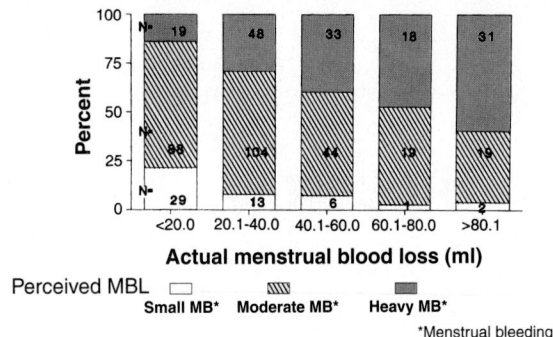

FIGURE 37-1 Subjective judgments of menstrual blood loss. (From Hallberg L, Högdahl AM, Nilsson L, and Rybo G: Acta Obstet Gynecol Scand 45:320, 1966.)

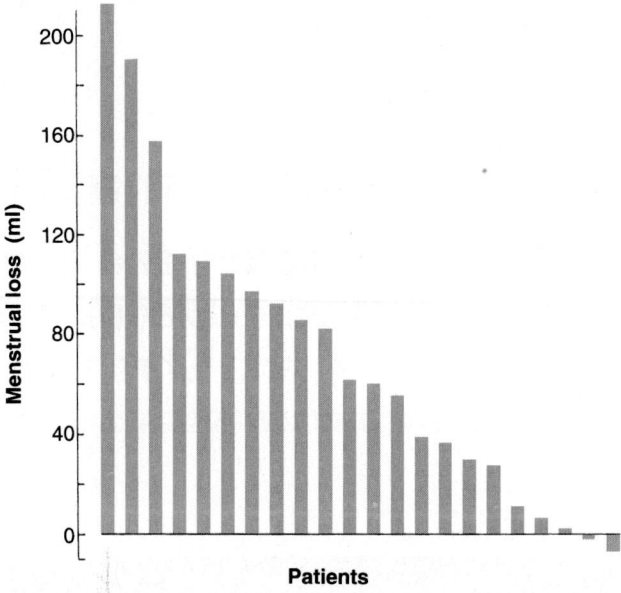

FIGURE 37-2 Distribution of menstrual blood loss in population sample from women living in Göteborg. (From Hallberg L, Högdahl AM, Nilsson L, and Rybo G: Acta Obstet Gynecol Scand 45:320, 1966.)

one third of the menses described as light were more than 80 ml and that about half of those believed to be heavy were less than 80 ml. Determining the number of sanitary pads used is also an unreliable indication of MBL. Grimes found that there is great variability of absorption among different types of sanitary products as well as among different devices in the same package. Fraser et al. reported that the percentage contribution of blood to the total fluid volume of the menstrual discharge varied extensively among different women, from 1.6% to 81% with a mean of 36%. Thus the majority of fluid volume in menstrual discharge is probably derived from endometrial tissue exudate. These investigators also reported that there was a very significant correlation between the total fluid loss and blood loss. Women differ markedly in their fastidiousness in changing sanitary products. Thus queries about the passage of blood clots or the degree of inconvenience caused by the bleeding are more helpful than counting the number of pads used in order to ascertain whether menorrhagia exists.

Because of the unreliability of subjective assessment, objective methods have been developed to quantify MBL. One method involves radioisotopic labeling of the woman's red blood cells. The other, which is the most widely used technique, involves photometric measurement to quantify hematin collected onto sanitary napkins. This alkaline hematin method, originated by Hallberg and Nilsson, has been refined by Newton et al. and van Eijkeren et al. and is very accurate. Nevertheless the accuracy depends on complete collection of the sanitary napkins used by the woman. With this technique it has been found in several studies published in the 1960s and 1970s that the mean amount of MBL in normal women (women with normal hemoglobin, hematocrit, and plasma iron) is about 35 ml, with the mean in various studies ranging from 31 to 44 ml. About 95% of normal women lose less than an average of 60 ml of blood during each menses. In several recent studies in the 1990s one laboratory in Sweden has reported that the mean MBL in normal women is between 55 and 60 ml. In contrast to the earlier studies in which

the extraction of the blood from the sanitary napkins was performed manually, in this laboratory a machine was used to press out the hematin and the women were instructed to meticulously collect all menstrual blood. Thus it is possible that the mean amount of MBL in normal women is greater than previously reported.

In each of the studies of populations of normal women, there was a wide range of menstrual blood loss with a marked positive skewness of the distribution of different volumes (Figure 37-2). In the study by Cole et al. of 280 women using neither oral contraceptives nor an IUD, about one third of women lost less than 20 ml (light) during each menstrual episode, one third lost 20 to 44 ml (medium), and one third lost more than 45 ml (heavy). These investigators also reported that there was a significant increase in menstrual blood loss with increasing parity, but not with age, and that short women lost less blood than women of normal or tall height.

Hallberg and Nilsson reported that in normal women there is little variation in volume of menstrual blood loss in successive menses of the same individual (standard deviation [SD], 1.9 ml) during a 1-year period, whereas the variation between women is great (SD, 15.3 ml) (Figure 37-3). In this study the average loss of iron in each menses was 13.0 mg. In normal women about 70% of the total blood loss occurs during the first 2 days of menses.

Hallberg et al. found that individuals with blood loss greater than 80 ml have significantly lower mean hemoglobin, hematocrit, and serum iron levels than do women with less MBL (Figure 37-4). Therefore an MBL greater than 80 ml should be regarded as hypermenorrhea. For practical pur-

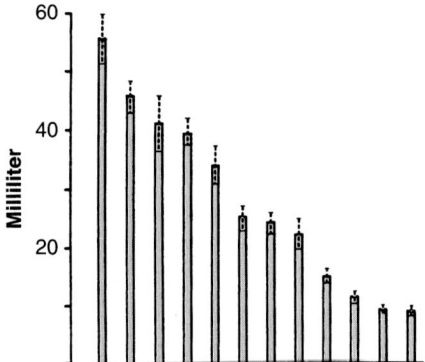

FIGURE 37-3 Menstrual blood loss in 12 subjects. Mean values of 12 periods and standard error of means. (From Hallberg L and Nilsson L: Acta Obstet Gynecol Scand 43:352, 1964.)

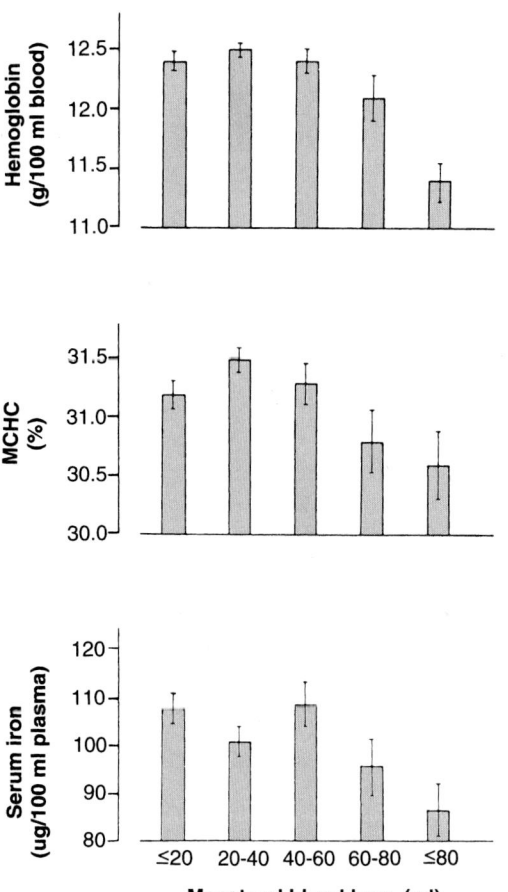

FIGURE 37-4 Mean values (±SEM) of hemoglobin concentration, menstrual cycle hematocrit *(MCHC)*, and plasma iron concentration in different ranges of menstrual blood loss. (From Hallberg L, Högdahl AM, Nilsson L, and Rybo G: Acta Obstet Gynecol Scand 45:320, 1966.)

poses, if a woman experiences a change in duration of flow (e.g., from 3 to 6 days), it must be considered abnormal, even though by definition she does not have menorrhagia.

Menorrhagia has been reported to occur in 9% to 14% of healthy women who participated in the various studies of measurement of MBL. In women complaining of menorrhagia, Haynes et al. reported that, as with women with normal menses, 70% of the blood was lost within the first 2 days of menses and 92% by the end of the third day. Also, there was no relation between the number of days of menstrual bleeding and the total MBL. The majority of these women with menorrhagia did not have increased duration of menses but rather had a markedly increased amount of menstrual flow for the first few days of menses. Thus the mechanisms responsible for control of menses are as effective in these women as in women with normal menses. The mechanisms responsible for the increased menstrual flow are unclear but may result from alterations in prostaglandin metabolism, as discussed later.

ETIOLOGY

The etiology of abnormal uterine bleeding is usually divided into two major categories—organic and dysfunctional (or endocrinologic). The organic causes of abnormal uterine bleeding are discussed in detail in other chapters of this book and will only be briefly outlined here.

Organic Causes

The organic causes can be subdivided into systemic disease and reproductive tract disease.

Systemic Disease

Systemic diseases, particularly disorders of blood coagulation such as von Willebrand's disease and prothrombin deficiency, may initially present as abnormal uterine bleeding.

Other disorders that produce platelet deficiency, such as leukemia, severe sepsis, idiopathic thrombocytopenic purpura, and hypersplenism, can also cause excessive bleeding. Routine screening for coagulation defects is mainly indicated in the adolescent who has prolonged heavy menses beginning at menarche, unless otherwise indicated by clinical signs such as petechiae or ecchymosis. Claessens and Cowell reported that coagulation disorders are found in about 20% of adolescent females who require hospitalization for abnormal uterine bleeding. Coagulation defects are present in about one fourth of those whose hemoglobin levels fall below 10 g/100 ml, in one third of those who require transfusions, and in half of those whose severe menorrhagia occurred at the time of the first menstrual period. A more recent study by Falcone et al. indicated that a coagulation disorder was found in only 5% of adolescents hospitalized for heavy bleeding. Both studies indicate that the likelihood of a blood disorder in adolescents with heavy menses is sufficiently high so that they should all be evaluated to determine if a coagulopathy is present.

Hypothyroidism is frequently associated with menorrhagia as well as intermenstrual bleeding. Thyroid-stimulating hormone (TSH) should be measured in women with menorrhagia of undetermined etiology. When standard tests of thyroid function are used to diagnose hypothyroidism, the incidence of this disorder among women with menorrhagia has been estimated to range between 0.3% and 2.5%. Wilansky and Greisman studied 67 clinically euthyroid women with normal serum thyroxine and triiodothyronine levels who had symptoms of severe menorrhagia with a thyrotropin-releasing hormone (TRH) stimulation test. They found that 15 of these women had small but significantly elevated baseline TSH levels as well as significantly elevated TSH responses (>30 mU/L) 30 minutes after TRH infusion. They characterized those women as having early or potential hypothyroidism instead of subclinical hypothyroidism. Treatment of these women with 50 to 200 mg of L-thyroxine daily resulted in normalization of their TSH levels and disappearance of the menorrhagia within 3 to 6 months in all the women treated. If these results are confirmed elsewhere, a sensitive TSH assay and/or a TRH stimulation test should be performed in all women with unexplained menorrhagia. If the test is abnormal, thyroxine therapy is indicated. Although hyperthyroidism is usually not associated with menstrual abnormalities, hypomenorrhea, oligomenorrhea, and amenorrhea have been reported.

Cirrhosis is associated with excessive bleeding secondary to the reduced capacity of the liver to metabolize estrogens. If hypoprothrombinemia is present, the incidence of abnormal bleeding will be increased.

Reproductive Tract Disease

The most common causes of abnormal uterine bleeding during reproductive age are accidents of pregnancy such as threatened, incomplete, or missed abortion and ectopic pregnancy. In addition, trophoblastic disease must be considered in the differential diagnosis of abnormal bleeding in any woman who has had a recent pregnancy, so a sensitive beta–human chorionic gonadotrophin (b-hCG) assay should be performed as part of the diagnostic evaluation.

Malignancies of any portion of the genital tract may present as abnormal bleeding, particularly endometrial and cervical cancer. Less commonly, vaginal, vulvar, and oviductal cancer may produce abnormal bleeding. In addition, estrogen-producing ovarian tumors may become manifest by abnormal uterine bleeding. Thus granulosa-theca cell tumors may present with excessive uterine bleeding. Infection of the upper genital tract, particularly endometritis, may present as prolonged menses, although episodic intermenstrual spotting is a more common symptom.

Anatomic uterine abnormalities such as submucous myomas, endometrial polyps, and adenomyosis frequently produce symptoms of prolonged and excessive regular uterine bleeding. The mechanisms whereby these lesions

cause menorrhagia are unclear. Makarainen and Ylikorkala reported that release of thromboxane and prostacycline from endometrial specimens of normal women and women with menorrhagia associated with leiomyomas was similar. Cervical lesions such as erosions, polyps, and cervicitis may cause irregular bleeding, particularly postcoital spotting. These lesions can usually be diagnosed by visualization of the cervix. In addition, traumatic vaginal lesions, severe vaginal infections, and foreign bodies have been associated with abnormal bleeding.

Foreign bodies in the uterus, such as the IUD, frequently produce abnormal uterine bleeding. Other iatrogenic causes include oral and injectable steroids such as those used for contraception and hormonal replacement or for the management of dysmenorrhea, hirsutism, acne, or endometriosis. Tranquilizers and other psychotropic drugs may interfere with the neurotransmitters responsible for releasing and inhibiting hypothalamic hormones, thus causing anovulation and abnormal bleeding.

Dysfunctional Causes

After organic, systemic, and iatrogenic causes for the abnormal bleeding are ruled out, the diagnosis of dysfunctional uterine bleeding (DUB) can be made. There are two types of DUB, anovulatory and ovulatory. The predominant cause of DUB in the postmenarcheal and premenopausal years is anovulation secondary to alterations in neuroendocrinologic function. In women with anovulatory DUB there is continuous estradiol production without corpus luteum formation and progesterone production. The steady state of estrogen stimulation leads to a continuously proliferating endometrium, which may outgrow its blood supply or lose nutrients with varying degrees of necrosis. In contrast to normal menstruation, uniform slough to the basalis layer does not occur, which produces excessive uterine blood flow. Ovulatory DUB occurs most commonly after the adolescent years and before the perimenopausal years. The incidence of this disorder has been reported to occur in as many as 10% of ovulatory women.

In the past, prolonged life of the corpus luteum was reported to be a cause of abnormal bleeding (Halban's syndrome). This disorder is associated with a normal-appearing secretory endometrium. A sensitive serum hCG assay should be performed to differentiate this disorder from early pregnancy loss. Irregular shedding of the endometrium has also been reported to produce menorrhagia. The diagnosis of this disorder is made if an endometrial biopsy obtained during the fourth day of the flow reveals both proliferative and secretory endometrium. No recent studies have documented the presence of these two conditions. Thus the prevalence of these disorders, if they actually exist, is uncertain.

In most tissues, following blood vessel damage, the process of hemostasis consists of five actions, some of which occur concomitantly: (1) localized vasoconstriction, (2) platelet adhesion, (3) formation of a platelet plug, (4) reinforcement of the platelet plug with fibrin, and (5) removal of the coagulated material by fibrinolytic mechanisms. The process of hemostasis in the endometrial vessels differs somewhat from the response to vessel damage elsewhere in the body. Morphologic studies by Christiaens et al. have revealed that hemostatic plugs in the endometrium are smaller, have a different morphology, and persist for a shorter time than those in other tissues.

These investigators found that there are two main mechanisms for hemostasis during menstruation. The first, hemostatic plug formation, is the most important mechanism in the functional endometrium. The second, vasoconstriction, is more important in the basalis layer. Since vascular occlusion by both mechanisms is never total, blood leakage continues for several days until endometrial regeneration is completed.

Sheppard et al. performed ultrastructural studies of samples of menstrual fluid obtained from the uterine cavity and vagina of 10 women with normal menses and 10 women with DUB. Fibrin and platelets were found in nearly all samples. No differences were found in the morphology of fibrin and platelets in the samples collected from the two groups of women. Rees et al. reported that there was no significant difference in amounts of coagulation factors or fibrinolytic proteins in the menstrual fluid of women with normal blood loss compared with those with menorrhagia.

Hahn and Rybo reported that there was no difference in the concentrations of fibrinogen-fibrin degradation products in menstrual blood samples obtained from normal women and those with menorrhagia. Rees et al. reported no difference in clotting factors in menstrual fluid between the two groups of women.

Rees et al. performed a histologic study of the endometrium and myometrium in uteri removed by hysterectomy from women with normal and excessive amounts of uterine bleeding. No pathologic findings were found in the specimens. These investigators found no correlation between menstrual blood loss and endometrial and myometrial arterial density and endometrial glandular density. Thus menorrhagia in the absence of pathologic findings does not result from an excessive number of arteries or abnormal distribution of the endometrial glands.

With the discovery that prostaglandins are involved with the regulation of vasodilation and vasoconstriction, as well as the clotting process, numerous studies were conducted in the 1980s in which various prostaglandins and their metabolites were measured in endometrial and myometrial samples obtained from normal women and women with menorrhagia. The majority of the studies were performed by two groups in Britain, one in Oxford and the other in Edinburgh, and sometimes the results were contradictory because of differences in methodology.

Since PGE_2 produces vasodilation while $PGF_{2\alpha}$ increases vasoconstriction, and thromboxane promotes platelet aggregation while prostacycline inhibits this process, most of the studies measured these prostaglandins or their metabolites. In women with regular ovulatory cycles with normal menstrual blood loss, there was an increase in the amount of both $PGF_{2\alpha}$ and PGE_2 found in the endometrium in the late secretory phase and during menses, with the endometrial $PGF_{2\alpha}/PGE_2$ ratio steadily increasing from midcycle to menses.

Smith et al. found that the levels of $PGF_{2\alpha}$ in persistently proliferative endometria obtained from women with anovulatory DUB were lower than the levels in women with normal secretory endometria. They theorized that progesterone was necessary to increase levels of arachidonic acid, the precursor of $PGF_{2\alpha}$, while estradiol stimulates synthesis of prostaglandins from arachidonic acid by cyclic endoperoxides. With the absence of progesterone in anovulatory cycles, there are reduced levels of $PGF_{2\alpha}$ with normal levels of PGE_2, resulting in a decreased $PGF_{2\alpha}/PGE_2$ ratio. Since $PGF_{2\alpha}$ binds to receptors in the spiral arteries in the late secretory phase to cause vasoconstriction and control menstrual flow, decreased levels of $PGF_{2\alpha}$ could cause heavier and/or more prolonged bleeding.

These investigators found there was an inverse correlation between the endometrial $PGF_{2\alpha}/PGE$ ratio and the amount of menstrual blood loss (Figure 37-5). PGE_2 also stimulates contraction of the smooth muscle cells in the myometrium, and elevated levels of $PGF_{2\alpha}$ are found in the menstrual blood of women with dysmenorrhea. Anovulatory cycles are usually not associated with dysmenorrhea, probably because of the reduced levels of $PGF_{2\alpha}$. Progesterone treatment of women with anovulatory DUB rapidly reduces the amount of menstrual blood loss, probably by stimulating production of arachidonic acid, the precursor of $PGF_{2\alpha}$.

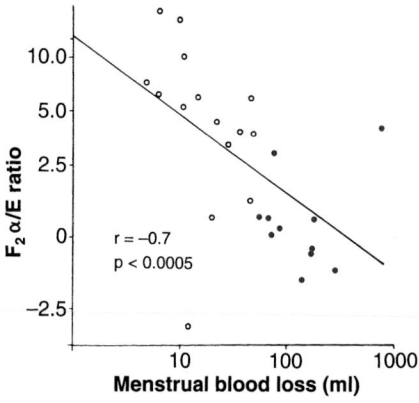

FIGURE 37-5 Correlation between ratio of endogenous concentrations of $PGF_{2\alpha}$ and PGE and menstrual blood loss (MBL). Normal secretory endometrium; persistent proliferative endometrium. (From Smith SK, Abel MH, Kelly RW, and Baird DT: J Clin Endocrinol Metab 55:284, 1982.)

Circulating levels of reproductive hormones are not different in women with ovulatory DUB and those with normal cycles. Various investigators have shown that the increased MBL in women with ovulatory DUB is also associated with reduced uterine synthesis of $PGF_{2\alpha}$ and an increase in synthesis of PGE_2 and prostacycline.

Furthermore, Adelantado et al. reported that PGE receptor concentrations in the myometrium of hysterectomy specimens were significantly greater in women with unexplained ovulatory menorrhagia than in women with normal MBL. Also, there was a direct correlation between the concentration of myometrial PGE receptor concentration and MBL.

Makarainen and Ylikorkala reported that the ratio of release of thromboxane to prostacycline in endometrial biopsy specimens was inversely related to the amount of MBL in a group of women with menorrhagia. They concluded that the menorrhagia could be due in part to a relative deficiency of thromboxane in the endometrium.

Bonney et al. reported that there was a significantly greater amount of phospholipase C, but not phospholipase A_2 types 1 and 2, in the endometrium of women with ovulatory menorrhagia. Phospholipases release arachidonic acid from cell membrane phospholipids. Several investigators have reported that there is an increased availability of arachidonic acid in the endometrium of women with ovulatory menorrhagia, in contrast to the decreased amount of this substance in the endometrium of women with anovulatory DUB.

Thus alterations in prostaglandin synthesis and release appear to occur in women with both anovulatory as well as ovulatory DUB. The reasons why these changes occur and their exact causal relation with menorrhagia have not yet been determined.

DIAGNOSIS

When a woman presents with a complaint of abnormal bleeding, it is essential to take a thorough history regarding the frequency, duration, and amount of bleeding, as well as to inquire whether and when the menstrual pattern has changed. This history is extremely important to determine whether the menstrual abnormality is polymenorrhea, menorrhagia (hypermenorrhea), metrorrhagia, menometrorrhagia, or intermenstrual bleeding. Providing the woman with a calendar to record her bleeding episodes is a very helpful way to characterize definitively the bleeding episodes. Since there is a poor correlation between a woman's estimate of the amount of blood flow and the measured loss, as well as great variation in the amount of blood and fluid absorbed by different types of sanitary napkins and in the same type of napkin in different individuals, objective criteria should be used to determine if menorrhagia (blood loss more than 80 ml) is present.

Since direct measurement of MBL is not generally available, indirect assessment by measurement of hemoglobin concentration, serum iron levels, and serum ferritin levels is useful. Serum ferritin provides a valid indirect assessment of iron stores in the bone marrow. Additional useful laboratory tests include a sensitive hCG determination and a sensitive TSH assay. For adolescent women, as well as older women with systemic disease, a coagulation profile should be performed to rule out a coagulation defect. If the woman has regular cycles, it is important to determine whether she is ovulating by obtaining a luteal phase serum progesterone measurement, a daily basal body temperature, or a premenstrual sampling of the endometrium.

If a woman is ovulating and has menorrhagia, it is important to rule out the presence of a uterine lesion such as an endometrial polyp, submucous leiomyoma, or carcinoma by performing an endocervical curettage, pelvic sonography with a vaginal probe (which also permits measurement of the endometrial thickness), and hysterosalpingography or hysteroscopy. Hysteroscopy, which can be performed in the office or clinic setting with local anesthesia even when the patient is bleeding, is a more accurate diagnostic procedure than a dilation and curettage (D&C). Therefore hysteroscopy should be utilized in all women who have ovulatory menorrhagia to determine if endometrial pathology exists. D&C is a blind technique and does not always detect focal lesions. It has been estimated that D&C misses the diagnosis in 10% to 25% of women. In a comparison of panoramic hysteroscopy with endometrial biopsy and D&C in a group of 342 women, Gimpelson and Rappold found that hysteroscopy permitted the accurate diagnosis in 60 women in whom the diagnosis was not made by D&C. Most of these individuals had the diagnosis of submucous myomas and endometrial polyps made by hysteroscopy and missed by D&C. March reported that one fourth of women with a presumptive diagnosis of DUB were found to have uterine lesions at the time of hysteroscopy. Following the diagnosis of a uterine lesion, it is then usually possible to resect the polyp or submucous leiomyoma by operative hysteroscopy. Recently it has been suggested that pelvic sonography with a vaginal transducer be utilized as a screening procedure in women with ovulatory menorrhagia to determine if a lesion is present in the endometrial cavity prior to performing hysteroscopy. With routine sonographic imaging of the endometrial cavity, it is usually possible to detect the presence of an endometrial polyp or submucous leiomyoma. However, the likelihood of visualizing these lesions sonographically is markedly enhanced if fluid is placed into the endometrial cavity prior to the sonographic examination. Placement of 10 to 15 ml of saline into the endometrial cavity can be easily accomplished through a small insemination catheter. Visualization of the endometrial cavity with this technique, called *sonohysterography*, or saline infusion sonography, is sufficiently sensitive so that if no lesion is visualized it is unnecessary to perform a hysteroscopy as it is very unlikely that an anatomic lesion is present.

MANAGEMENT

In the absence of an organic cause for excessive uterine bleeding, it is preferable to use medical instead of surgical treatment, especially if the woman desires to retain her uterus for future childbearing or will be undergoing natural menopause within a short time. There are several effective medical methods for treatment of DUB. These include estrogens, progestins (delivered systemically or locally), nonsteroidal antiinflammatory agents, antifibrinolytic agents, danazol, and gonadotrophin-releasing hormone (GnRH) agonists. The type of treatment utilized depends on whether it is used to stop an acute heavy bleeding episode or whether it is given to reduce the amount of MBL in subsequent menstrual cycles. Before instituting long-term treatment, definitive diagnosis is required and should be made on the basis of hysteroscopy or sonohysterography and directed endometrial biopsies, with definitive treatment determined by the diagnosis.

Estrogens

The rationale for the therapeutic use of estrogen for the treatment of DUB is based on the fact that estrogen in pharmacologic doses causes rapid growth of the endometrium. The bleeding that results from most causes of DUB will respond to such therapy because a rapid growth of endometrial tissue occurs over the denuded and raw epithelial surfaces. To control an acute bleeding episode, the use of oral conjugated estrogen (CE) in a dose of 10 mg a day, administered in four divided doses, is a therapeutic regimen that has been found to be clinically useful. Acute bleeding from most causes is usually controlled by this method. If bleeding is not controlled within the first 24 hours with this dose of estrogen, higher doses of CE (20 mg) may be effective; however, consideration must be given to the fact that an organic cause, such as an accident of pregnancy, may be the cause of the bleeding, and curettage should usually be performed.

Intravenous administration of estrogen is also effective in the acute treatment of menorrhagia. DeVore et al. reported that, compared with women given a placebo, a significantly greater percentage of women had cessation of bleeding 2 hours after the second of two 25-mg doses of conjugated equine estrogens (CEE) were administered intravenously 3 hours apart. There was no significant difference in cessation of bleeding between women administered estrogen and those given a placebo 3 hours after the first infusion. This study indicates that at least several hours are required to induce mitotic activity and growth of the endometrium, whether the estrogen is administered orally or parenterally. Thus intravenous estrogen therapy

accompanied by its rapid metabolic clearance does not appear to offer a significant advantage compared with the same dose of estrogen given orally.

Livio et al. reported that 6 hours after infusion of an average dose of 30 mg of CEE to individuals with a prolonged bleeding time due to renal failure, the bleeding time was significantly shortened. In this study, measurements of various clotting factors were unchanged after CEE infusion. Therefore the mechanism whereby intravenous CEE controls bleeding is unknown. No studies indicate that intravenous estrogen acts quicker or is more effective than high doses of oral estrogen. The latter route of administration is less costly, is easier to administer, and therefore is preferred.

Usually estrogen therapy reduces the amount of uterine bleeding within the first 24 hours after treatment is initiated. However, because most women with an acute heavy bleeding episode bleed because of anovulation, progestin treatment is also required. Therefore, after bleeding has ceased, oral estrogen therapy is continued at the same dosage, and a progestin, usually medroxyprogesterone acetate (MPA) 10 mg once a day, is added. Both hormones are administered for another 7 to 10 days, after which treatment is stopped to allow withdrawal bleeding, which may have an increased amount of flow but is rarely prolonged. Following the withdrawal bleeding episode, one of several alternate treatment modalities should be used. Before instituting long-term treatment, a definite diagnosis should be made after reviewing the endometrial histology. Definitive treatment should be based on these findings. Oral contraceptives are usually the best long-term treatment.

A more convenient regimen to stop acute bleeding than the sequential high-dose estrogen-progestin regimen is the use of a combination oral contraceptive containing both estrogen and progestin. Four tablets of an oral contraceptive containing 50 μg of estrogen taken every 24 hours in divided doses will usually provide sufficient estrogen to stop acute bleeding and simultaneously provide progestin. Treatment is continued for at least 1 week after the bleeding stops. This regimen is successful and convenient and is thus the preferred method of some clinicians. However, in one study it was found not to be as effective as the use of high doses of CE. A theoretic reason for this difference might be the fact that the combined use of estrogen and progestin does not afford as rapid endometrial growth as estrogen alone, because the progestin decreases the synthesis of estrogen receptors and increases estradiol dehydrogenase in the endometrial cell, thus inhibiting the growth-promoting action of estrogen.

Progestins

Progestins not only stop endometrial growth but also support and organize the endometrium in such a way that an organized slough occurs after their withdrawal. In the absence of progesterone, erratic unorganized breakdown of the endometrium occurs. With progesterone or progestin treatment, an organized slough to the basalis layer allows a rapid cessation of bleeding. In addition, progestins stimulate arachidonic acid formation in the endometrium, increasing the $PGF_{2\alpha}/PGE$ ratio. Progestins usually do not stop the acute bleeding episode and should not be used for this purpose. However, after the acute bleeding has ceased, progestins should be added to the estrogen therapy to produce a normal bleeding episode following their withdrawal.

Progestin therapy is ultimately the treatment of choice for the majority of women with anovulatory DUB, as already mentioned. However, progestin therapy usually does not stop the acute bleeding episode as effectively as estrogen and is warranted only for long-term treatment after the acute episode of bleeding has been controlled by other means.

MPA in a dose of 10 mg daily for 10 days each month is a successful therapeutic regimen that produces regular withdrawal bleeding in women with adequate amounts of endogenous estrogen to cause endometrial growth. Although other progestins have been used, MPA does not adversely alter serum lipids as much as the 19-nortestosterone derivatives and thus may have fewer adverse long-term effects. Progestins are beneficial, since in pharmacologic doses they act as antiestrogens. They diminish the effect of estrogen on target cells by inhibiting estrogen receptor replenishment in the cell and induce the activation of 17-hydroxysteroid dehydrogenase, which converts estradiol to the less active estrone. These findings account for the antimitotic, antigrowth effect of the progestins and support the rationale for their use in the treatment of unopposed estrogen and endometrial hyperplasia.

Adolescent anovulatory women represent an ideal model for the use of progestins in the treatment of DUB. These women have immaturity of the hypothalamic-pituitary axis, and progestin therapy for 10 days every month is a reasonable mode of treatment that is highly successful and produces regular cyclic withdrawal bleeding until maturity of the positive feedback system is achieved. This therapy does not interfere with the normal resumption of ovulatory cycles. Theoretically it may be better for these women not to use oral contraceptives, since this therapy inhibits hypothalamic-pituitary gonadotrophin synthesis and may delay the maturation of the hypothalamic-pituitary axis. However, there are no data to support this belief. In women of reproductive age who have anovulatory DUB, long-term use of oral contraceptives is useful after the acute bleeding episode is controlled unless the woman wishes to conceive, in which case cyclic treatment with clomiphene citrate should be used.

The major therapeutic use of progestins is to treat anovulatory women for 10 to 14 days each month. However, because progestins have a profound effect on inhibiting endometrial growth and inducing atrophic changes, a therapeutic trial with these agents may be useful in women with menorrhagia who also ovulate.

For women with ovulatory DUB and mean MBL more than 80 ml, administration of high doses of progestin for only 1 week each month from cycle day 19 to 26 does not reduce MBL. When norethindrone was given for 1 week at doses of either 5 mg twice or 3 times a day in 2 recent British studies, MBL was not reduced. However, Fraser reported that administration of two oral progestins, norethindrone and MPA, in high doses of 5 to 10 mg 3 times a day for 2 to 3 weeks each month, significantly reduced MBL by 40% to 50% in women with both ovulatory and anovulatory DUB. In women with anovulatory DUB the progestins were given from cycle days 12 to 25, whereas the ovulatory women received progestins from days 5 to 25. Prolonged use of these high doses of progestins may cause unpleasant adverse effects, including tiredness, mood changes, and weight gain, as well as unfavorably alter the lipid profile. To eliminate these effects, local administration of progestins can be utilized.

The progesterone-releasing IUD has been found to be effective in the treatment of women with ovulatory DUB. Bergqvist and Rybo inserted this device into 12 women with ovulatory DUB and found their MBL declined from an average of 138 ml to 49 ml in 1 year, a 65% reduction in MBL (Figure 37-6). This device needs to be reinserted annually because of the rapid diffusion of progesterone through polysiloxone.

A levonorgestrol-releasing intrauterine system (IUS) has been developed that has an effective duration of action of more than 5 years. Milson et al. studied use of this IUS as treatment for menorrhagia and found that at the end of 3 months it caused an average 80% reduction in MBL, which increased to 100% at the end of 1 year. This reduction in MBL was significantly greater than that achieved with either an antifibrinolytic agent or a prostaglandin synthetase inhibitor in studies by the same investigators (Figure 37-7).

Nonsteroidal Antiinflammatory Drugs

Nonsteroidal antiinflammatory drugs (NSAIDs) are prostaglandin synthetase inhibitors that inhibit the biosynthesis of the cyclic endoperoxides, which convert arachidonic acid to prostaglandins. In addition, these agents block the action of prostaglandins by interfering directly at their receptor sites.

To decrease bleeding of the endometrium, it would be ideal to block selectively the synthesis of prostacyclin alone, without decreasing thromboxane formation, as the latter increases platelet aggregation. Presently there are no NSAIDs that possess this ability. All NSAIDs are cyclooxygenase inhibitors and thus block the formation of both thromboxane and the prostacyclin pathway. Nevertheless, NSAIDs have been shown to reduce MBL, primarily in women who ovulate. However, a complete understanding

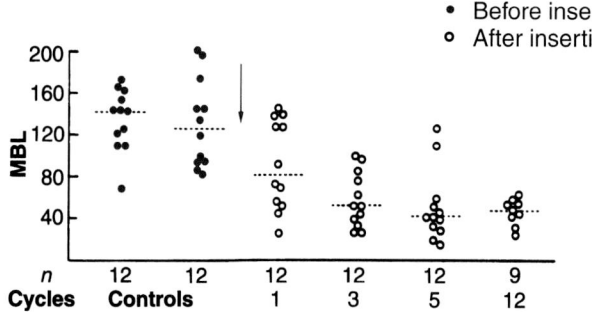

FIGURE 37-6 Menstrual blood loss (MBL) before and after insertion of Progestasert *(arrow)* in menorrhagic women. (Each dot marks a separate patient, and the median value is marked with a line.) (From Bergqvist A and Rybo G: Br J Obstet Gynaecol 90:255, 1983.)

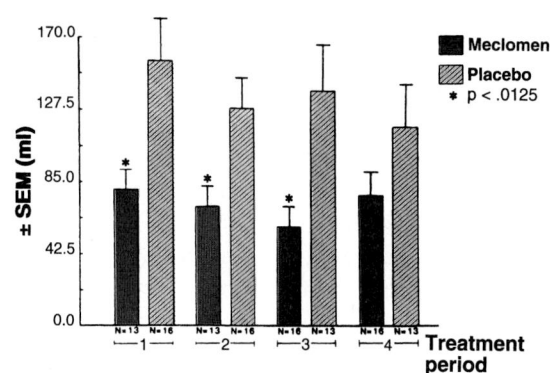

FIGURE 37-8 Menstrual blood loss (MBL) by treatment period and drug. (From Vargyas JM, Campeau JD, and Mishell DA: Am J Obstet Gynecol 157:944, 1987.)

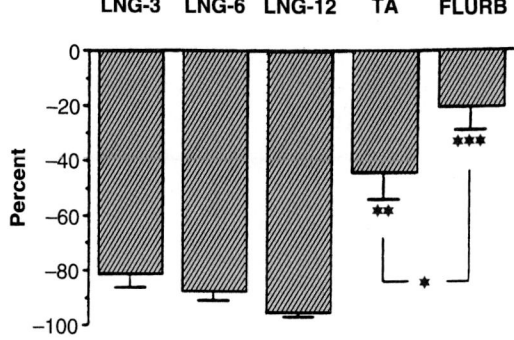

FIGURE 37-7 Reduction in menstrual blood loss (MBL) expressed as percentage of mean of two control cycles for each form of treatment. Significance of difference between treatment with levonorgestrel-releasing IUD *(LNG)* and tranexamic acid *(TA)* and flurbiprofen *(FLURB)* indicated by double asterisks ($P < 0.01$) and triple asterisks ($P < 0.001$) and between treatment with tranexamic acid and flurbiprofen indicated by asterisk ($P < 0.05$). (From Milson I, Andersson K, Andersch B, and Rybo G: Am J Obstet Gynecol 164:879, 1991.)

of the mechanisms whereby prostaglandin inhibitors reduce MBL is still undetermined, and their therapeutic action may take place through some as yet undiscovered mechanism. Several NSAIDs have been administered during menses to groups of women with menorrhagia and ovulatory DUB and have been found to reduce mean MBL by about 20% to 50% (Figure 37-8). Irvine et al. performed a randomized trial comparing the use of the levonorgestrel IUS and oral norethindrone for the treatment of idiopathic menorrhagia. The IUS caused a 94% reduction in MBL, similar to 5 mg norethindrone three times a day. However the IUS was better tolerated and had a higher continuation rate than oral norethindrone.

Drugs used in studies include mefenamic acid, 500 mg 3 times a day; ibuprofen, 400 mg 3 times a day; meclofenamate sodium, 100 mg 3 times a day; and naproxen sodium, 275 mg every 6 hours after a loading dose of 550

mg, as well as other NSAIDs. These drugs are usually given for the first 3 days of menses or throughout the bleeding episode, and they appear to have a similar level of effectiveness.

Not all women treated with these agents have reduction in blood flow, but those without a decrease usually had only a mildly increased amount of MBL. The greatest amount of MBL reduction occurs in the women with the greatest pretreatment blood loss. Fraser et al. reported that treatment of menorrhagia with mefenamic acid in 36 women for more than 1 year resulted in a significantly sustained reduction in amounts of MBL and a significant increase in serum ferritin. Thus this therapy can be used for long-term treatment because side effects, mainly gastrointestinal, are mild with this intermittent therapy.

To date, there have been very few studies comparing NSAIDs with other treatment modalities. It appears, however, that the beneficial reduction in MBL with NSAIDs occurs primarily in women who ovulate. Furthermore the degree of reduction of MBL with NSAIDs in noncomparative studies is similar to that reported for the use of either antifibrinolytic agents or oral contraceptives alone.

Although NSAIDs are used by themselves to treat women with MBL who ovulate, they can also be given in combination with oral contraceptives or progestins. With this combined approach, reduction in MBL can be achieved more effectively than with use of any of these agents by themselves.

Antifibrinolytic Agents

Epsilon-aminocaproic acid (EACA), tranexamic acid (AMCA), and para-aminomethylbenzoic acid (PAMBA) are potent inhibitors of fibrinolysis and have, therefore, been used in the treatment of various hemorrhagic conditions. Nilsson and Rybo compared the effect on blood loss of EACA, AMCA, and oral contraceptives in 215 women with menorrhagia. EACA was given in a dose of 18 g per day for 3 days and then 12, 9, 6, and 3 g daily on successive days. The total dose was always at least 48 g. AMCA was administered in a dose of 6 g per day for 3 days followed by 4, 3, 2, and 1 g daily on successive days. The total dose of AMCA was at least 22 g. There was a significant reduction in blood loss after treatment with EACA, AMCA, and oral contraceptives, and use of each of these agents resulted in about a 50% reduction in MBL (Table 37-1). Of interest was the finding that the greatest reduction in blood loss with antifibrinolytic therapy occurred in women who exhibited the greatest MBL. Preston et al. compared the effects of 4 g of AMCA daily for 4 days each cycle with 10 mg of norethindrone for 7 days each cycle in a group of women with ovulatory menorrhagia with a mean MBL of 175 ml. AMCA reduced MBL by 45%, while there was a 20% increase with norethindrone. The side effects of this class of drugs in decreasing order of frequency are nausea, dizziness, diarrhea, headaches, abdominal pain, and allergic manifestations. These side effects are much more common with EACA than with AMCA. Other investigators have compared use of AMCA to placebo in double-blind studies and have found no significant differences in the occurrence of side effects. Renal failure and pregnancy are contraindications to the use of antifibrinolytic agents.

Antifibrinolytic agents clearly produce a reduction in blood loss and may be used as therapy for women with menorrhagia who ovulate. However, their use is somewhat limited by the side effects. Furthermore, as with NSAIDs, they are best combined with another agent, such as oral contraceptives, for a greater effect on MBL reduction.

Ergot

Ergot derivatives are not recommended for therapy because they are rarely effective and have a high incidence of side effects (nausea, vertigo, abdominal cramps). Nilsson and Rybo demonstrated no reduction in blood loss among 82 women with menorrhagia who were treated with methylergobaseimmaleate (Table 37-1).

TABLE 37-1

Mean Menstrual Blood Loss and Reduction with Treatment with EACA, AMCA, Oral Contraceptives, and Methylergobaseimmaleate

	Mean Blood Loss (ml)		
	Before Treatment	After Treatment	% Decrease
EACA	164	87	47
AMCA	182	84	54
Oral contraceptives	158	75	52
Methylergobaseimmaleate	164	164	0

Adapted from Nilsson L and Rybo G: Am J Obstet Gynecol 110:713, 1971.

Androgenic Steroids (Danazol)

Danazol has been used by several investigators for the treatment of menorrhagia. Doses of 200 and 400 mg daily have been given over 12 weeks after careful pretreatment observation and evaluation. MBL was markedly reduced in these studies from more than 200 ml to less than 25 ml. Also, there was an increased interval between bleeding episodes (Figure 37-9). The most common side effects of danazol treatment are weight gain and acne. Reduction of dosage from 400 to 200 mg daily decreased the side effects but did not alter the reduction in blood loss (Figure 37-10). Some women may ovulate when receiving this dose of danazol. Further reduction to 100 mg daily did not effectively reduce MBL in most women. Although danazol is effective, it is also expensive and has moderate side effects.

Dockeray et al. treated 40 women with DUB, half with mefenamic acid, 500 mg three times a day for 3 to 5 days of menses, and half with danazol, 100 mg twice a day for 60 days. Danazol was more effective in reducing MBL, 60% compared with 20% for mefenamic acid (Figure 37-11). However, adverse side effects were more severe with danazol and occurred in 75% of patients, compared with side effects in only 30% of patients treated with mefenamic acid.

GnRH Agonists

Although no large-scale studies have been performed, it is possible to inhibit ovarian steroid production with GnRH agonists. In a small study of four women, daily administration of a GnRH agonist for 3 months markedly reduced MBL from 100 to 200 ml per cycle to 0 to 30 ml per cycle. Unfortunately, after therapy was discontinued, blood loss returned to pretreatment levels (Figure 37-12). Because of the expense and side effects of these agents, their use for menorrhagia caused by ovulatory DUB is limited to women with severe MBL who fail to respond to other methods of medical management and wish to retain their childbearing capacity. Use of an estrogen and/or progestin ("add back" therapy) together with the agonist will help prevent bone loss.

Surgical Therapy

Dilation and Curettage

The performance of a D&C can be both diagnostic and therapeutic. For women with markedly excessive uterine bleeding who may be hypovolemic, the D&C is the quickest way to stop acute bleeding. Therefore it is the treatment of choice in women with DUB who suffer from hypovolemia. A D&C may also be utilized to stop an acute bleeding episode in women over the age of 35 when the incidence of pathologic findings increases.

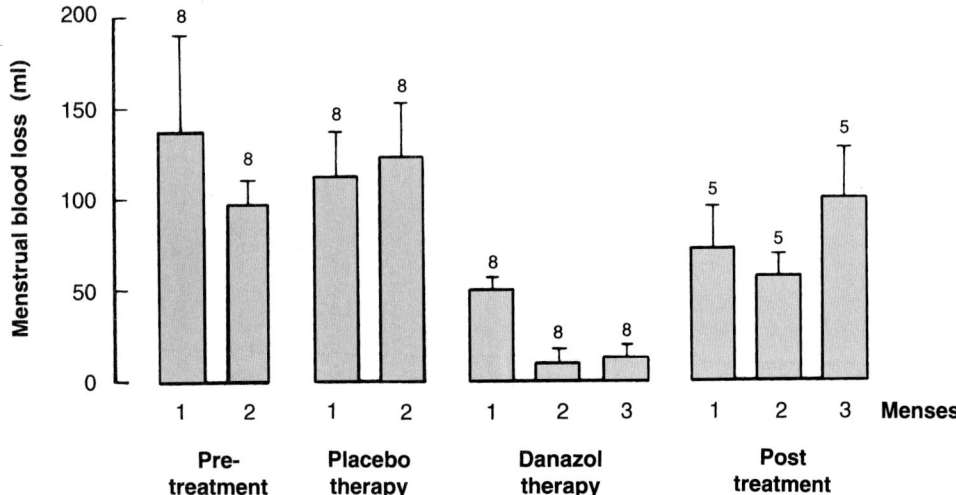

FIGURE 37-9   Mean (±SEM) menstrual blood loss in eight patients with menorrhagia before treatment, with placebo therapy, with 200 mg danazol daily, and after treatment. Number of patients is shown above each histogram. (From Chimbria TH, Anderson ABM, Naish C, et al: Br J Obstet Gynaecol 87:1152, 1980.)

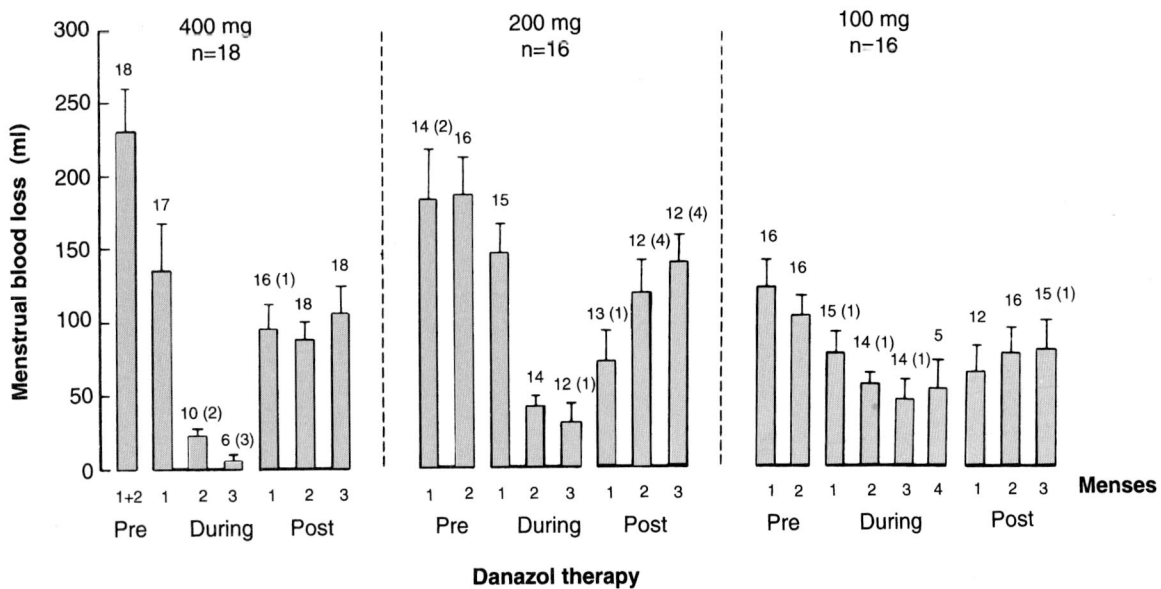

FIGURE 37-10   Mean (±SEM) menstrual blood loss in three groups of patients with menorrhagia treated with 400, 200, or 100 mg danazol daily for 12 weeks. Menstrual blood loss measurements are shown for each group before, during, and after danazol therapy. Number of patients menstruating is shown above each histogram, with number of missing menstrual loss collections in parentheses. (Adapted from Chimbria TH, Anderson ABM, Naish C, et al: Br J Obstet Gynaecol 87:1152, 1980.)

The use of D&C for the treatment of DUB has been reported to be curative in only a minority of women. Temporary cure of the problem may occur in some women with chronic anovulation, since the curettage removes much of the hyperplastic endometrium; however, the underlying pathophysiologic cause is unchanged. A D&C has not proved useful for treatment of women who ovulate and have menorrhagia. More than 1 month after the D&C, Nilsson and Rybo have shown that there was either no difference or an increase in MBL in women with menorrhagia who ovulate.

Therefore D&C is only indicated for women with acute bleeding resulting in hypovolemia, and for older women who are at higher risk of having endometrial neoplasia. All other women, after having an endometrial biopsy, sonohysteroscopy, or diagnostic hysteroscopy to rule out organic disease, are best managed by medical therapy, as outlined earlier, without a D&C.

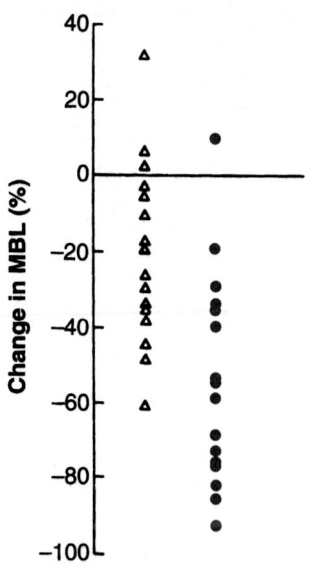

FIGURE 37-11 Percentage change in menstrual blood loss (MBL) between pretreatment cycles 1 and 2 and treatment cycles 3 and 4 shown for individual women treated with (Δ) mefenamic acid or (●) danazol. Mean % change is –22.3% in the mefenamic acid group and –56.0% in the danazol-treated group. (From Dockeray CJ, Sheppard BL, and Bonnard J: Br J Obstet Gynaecol 96:840, 1989.)

Endometrial Ablation

Laser photovaporization of the endometrium for treatment of menorrhagia was originally reported by Goldrath et al. in 1981. Photovaporization of the endometrium was performed by use of a neodymium-YAG laser with hysteroscopic visualization and fluid distention of the uterine cavity. Danazol 800 mg per day was ingested for 2 to 3 weeks before the procedure, and an additional 2 weeks of danazol treatment was given afterward. This procedure was curative in 160 of 180 women, and follow-up biopsies showed no evidence of inflammation other than foreign body giant cells secondary to the carbon particles left after laser treatment. There was minimum endometrial regeneration. Photovaporization causes varying degrees of uterine contraction, scarring, and adhesion formation, as demonstrated by follow-up hysterosalpingograms and hysteroscopy.

Subsequently a large, prospective, 5-year, multicenter study with this technique was reported by Erian. A total of 2342 women with menorrhagia, most with ovulatory DUB, were enrolled. After producing endometrial atrophy with at least 1 month of 600 mg danazol daily, progestins, or a

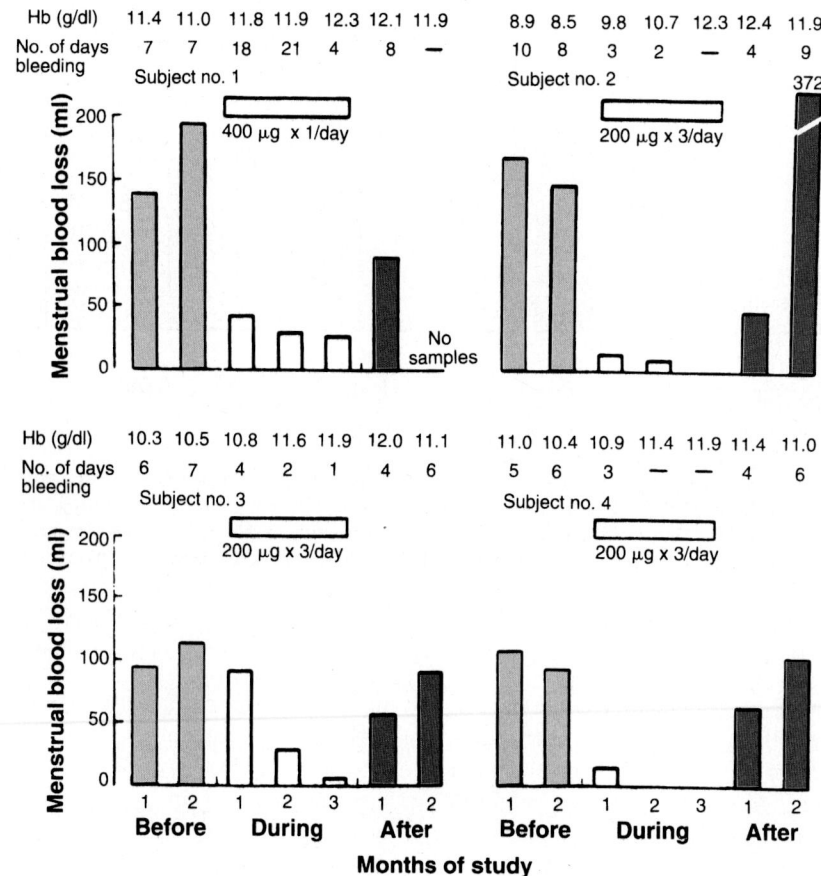

FIGURE 37-12 Alterations in measured monthly menstrual blood losses, number of days of menstrual bleeding, and hemoglobin estimates before, during, and after therapy with intranasal luteinizing hormone–releasing hormone (LHRH) agonist. (From Shaw RW and Fraser HM: Br J Obstet Gynaecol 9:913, 1984.)

TABLE 37-2
Menstrual Bleeding at Different Ages Following Hysteroscopic Endometrial Laser Ablation of Patients with Disabling Menorrhagia Resistant to Other Treatment

Age (years)	No. of Patients	Amenorrhea	Reduced Menses	Normal Period	No Improvement
14–19	4	0	3	1	0
20–29	35	2	11	4	18
30–34	96	18	32	20	26
35–39	242	64	55	96	27
40–44	867	502	135	194	36
45–49	510	352	112	32	14
50–56	112	105	5	1	1
TOTAL (%)	1866	1043 (56)	353 (19)	348 (19)	122 (7)

From Erian J: Br J Obstet Gynaecol 101(suppl 11):19, 1994.

GnRH agonist, the endometrium was ablated with an Nd-YAG laser inserted through a hysteroscope. Complications were uncommon and minor: 0.4% fluid overload, 0.5% infection, and 0.29% uterine perforation. No major hemorrhage requiring a transfusion or laparotomy occurred. The mean duration of the procedure was 24 minutes. Of the 1866 women followed for 1 year, 56% had amenorrhea, 38% had a satisfactorily reduced amount of menses, and 7% had no reduction, requiring a second treatment (Table 37-2). Most of the latter responded to a second treatment, and only 2% required a hysterectomy.

Because the Nd-YAG laser is expensive, others have ablated the endometrium with electrocautery delivered by a urologic resectoscope placed through a hysteroscope. Magos et al. utilized this technique, termed *transcervical resection of the endometrium*, in 234 women with menorrhagia and produced amenorrhea in about 30%; 1 of the treatment groups (overall 90%) had improvement in the symptoms of heavy bleeding (Figure 37-13).

In 1989 Vancaillie reported that thermal destruction of the endometrium could be accomplished easily and rapidly with electrocautery applied through a ball-end electrode attached to a urologic resectoscope. The ball-end electrode has several advantages compared with the loop electrode. These include a larger contact area, better fit into the cornual area, and because of the rotation, easier contact with the tissue as the ball-end electrode moves (Figure 37-14). Paskowitz reported that in a study of 200 women treated with this technique, amenorrhea occurred in 40% and the remainder reported decreased bleeding. The procedure was performed on an outpatient basis with general anesthesia. Preoperative endometrial suppression was accompanied with at least 1 month of danazol, GnRH analogues, or progestin. Of the 200 women, 10 (15%) had hysterectomies following the ablation.

The time to learn the roller-ball technique is shorter than for the laser, and the equipment is less expensive.

However, both techniques require preoperative medications for several weeks, training and experience with operative hysteroscopy, and the use of general anesthesia. Another technique to cause endometrial ablation is to insert a latex balloon into the endometrial cavity, inject 5% dextrose in water into the balloon, heat the fluid to 87° C, and leave the heated filled balloon in the cavity for 8 minutes. This procedure does not require pretreatment regimens to the endometrium, does not require hysteroscopy training, and can be performed with local anesthesia. A randomized trial comparing the thermal balloon with rollerball ablating by Meyer et al. found that both techniques result in about an 80% return to normal bleeding. The long-term effects of all techniques of endometrial ablation are not yet known. After ablation, the rates of amenorrhea in large studies vary between 25% and 60%, with most of the remainder having a decrease in the amount of menstrual bleeding. In one follow-up study in Britain 4 years after ablation, 24% of the women had a hysterectomy but most series report lower rates. The three techniques of endometrial ablation are being used with increasing frequency for the treatment of women with menorrhagia without uterine lesions who are unresponsive to medical therapy, since the cost, mortality, and length of hospitalization is less than with hysterectomy. Endometrial ablation may therefore be used as an alternative to hysterectomy when other medical modalities fail or when there are contraindications to their use. Ablation is also useful in treating women with severe menorrhagia who have medical contraindications against performing a hysterectomy or for treating women with ovulatory DUB who do not wish to take medications. Obviously, ablation should not be used in women who wish to maintain their reproductive capacity. Complications of hysteroscopic endometrial ablation include fluid overload, uterine hemorrhage, uterine perforation, thermal damage to adjacent organs, and hematometra. Most of

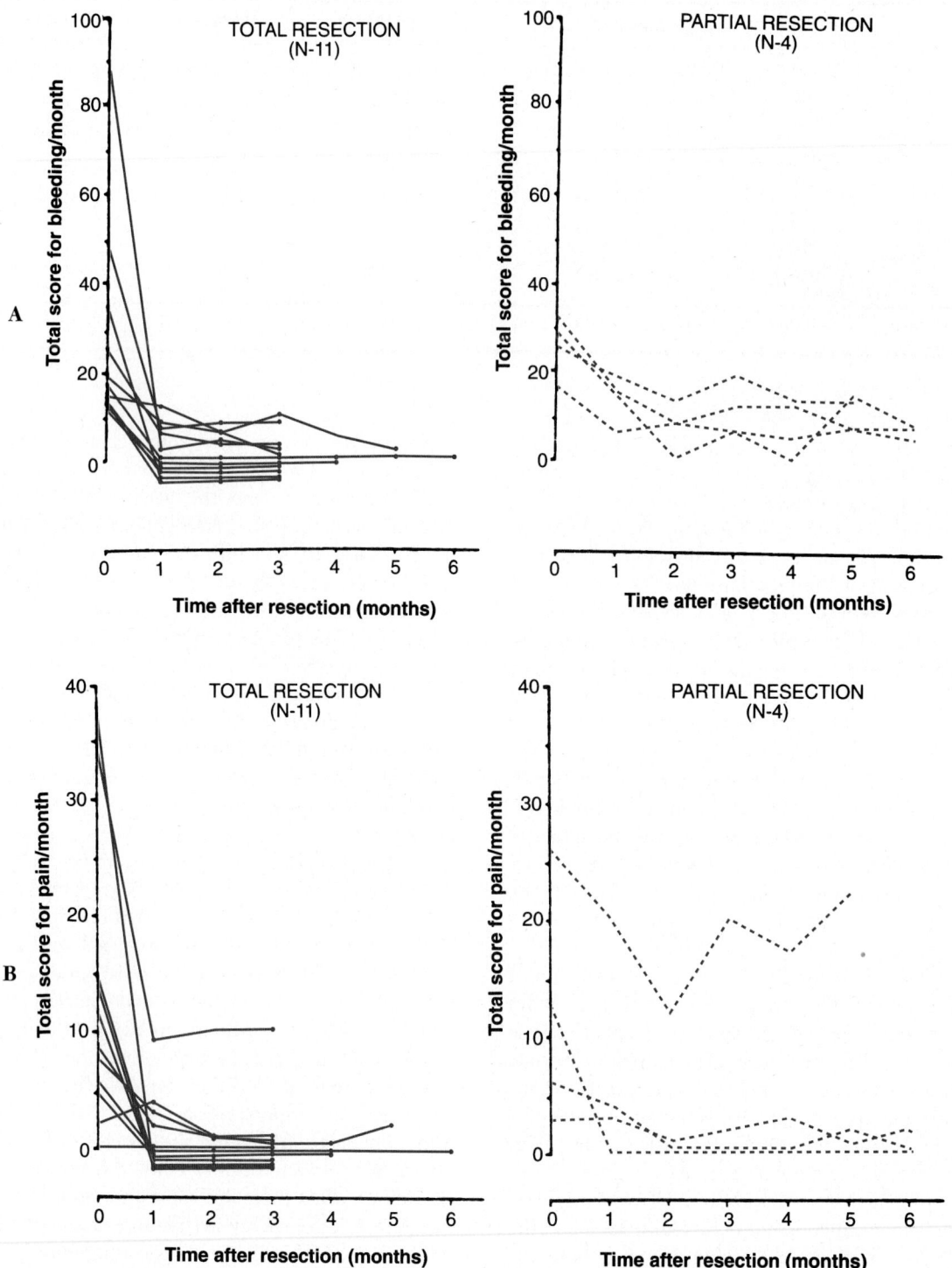

FIGURE 37-13 **A,** Effect of total and partial endometrial resection on total amount of menstrual bleeding each month. Blood loss was scored daily on scale of 0 to 3 (none to heavy). **B,** Effect of total and partial endometrial resection on total amount of menstrual pain each month. Pain was scored daily on score of 0 to 3 (none to severe). (From Magos AL, Baumann R, and Turnbull AC: Br Med J 298:1209, 1989.)

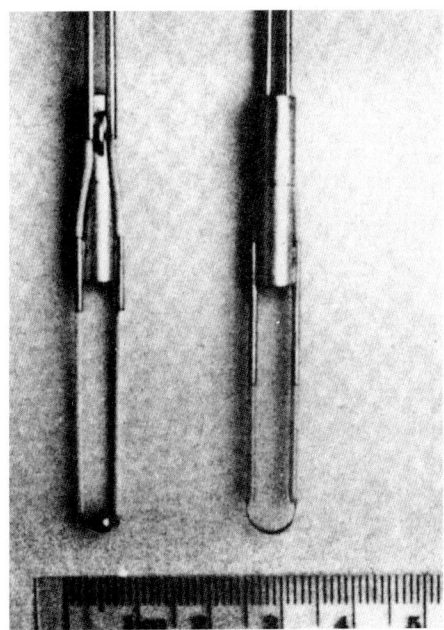

FIGURE 37-14 Ball-end and loop electrodes, side by side. Ball-end electrode is 2 mm in diameter and the loop, 7 mm. (From Vancaillie TG: Obstet Gynecol 74:425, 1989.)

these complications occur because the ablation extends too deeply into the endometrium, opening up uterine vessels and exposing adjacent tissues to thermal injury. Guidelines for the safe and effective practice of endometrial ablation, including correct patient selection, were recently summarized by Garry after a meeting of a group of experts from several countries. They concluded that correct patient selection should be restricted to women with heavy menstrual blood loss in the absence of organic distress. Ablation can be performed with either general or local anesthesia. The ablation should destroy all of the endometrium but only the superficial myometrium to reduce the rate of posttreatment problems. Similar guidelines by a British group were summarized by Lewis, who suggested that the operating surgeon perform at least 15 supervised procedures before being credentialed.

Hysterectomy

The decision to remove the uterus should be made on an individual basis and should usually be reserved for the woman with other indications for hysterectomy, such as leiomyomas or uterine prolapse. Hysterectomy should only be used to treat persistent ovulatory DUB after all medical therapy has failed and the amount of MBL has

been documented to be excessive by direct measurement or by abnormally low serum ferritin levels. With increasing use of endometrial ablation to treat this problem, the incidence of hysterectomy as therapy for ovulatory DUB should decrease. It has been estimated that as many as half the women over 40 years of age with menorrhagia without uterine lesions are now being treated by hysterectomy and that 20% of all hysterectomies in women of reproductive age are performed for excessive uterine bleeding.

Short- and Long-Term Treatment

Women who are treated for menorrhagia should be divided into those with acute symptoms and signs and those with chronic problems.

Acute bleeding is best controlled with the use of estrogen. A curettage or thorough endometrial aspiration is indicated for women over the age of 35 who have persistent abnormal bleeding or for women with bleeding that is sufficiently severe to produce anemia.

After the diagnosis of anovulation is confirmed, long-term therapy should be directed by individual needs in the majority of women. In the adolescent, 10 mg of MPA for 10 days each month for at least 3 months should be prescribed, and the woman should be observed carefully thereafter. In this group of women additional diagnostic studies should be performed to detect possible defects in the coagulation process, particularly if bleeding is severe. For the woman of reproductive age, long-term therapy depends on whether she requires contraception, induction of ovulation, or treatment of DUB alone. In the last circumstance oral contraceptive or MPA can be administered, as stated above, monthly for at least 6 months, while oral contraceptives and clomiphene citrate are used for the other indications. For the perimenopausal woman who characteristically has lower amounts of circulating estrogen, use of cyclic MPA alone is frequently not curative. In these women abnormal bleeding is best treated by low-dose oral contraceptives. The cyclic use of CE (0.625 to 1.25 mg) given for 25 days, with 10 mg of MPA added to the CE from days 15 to 25 can also be used after abnormal endometrial histologic findings have been ruled out.

The most difficult management of DUB is chronic treatment of ovulatory women with menorrhagia. If anatomic abnormalities are not present, long-term treatment is necessary to reduce MBL. For these women NSAIDs, progestins, oral contraceptives, danazol, and GnRH analogues are all useful therapeutic modalities. A combination of two or more of these agents is often required to obviate the need for endometrial ablation or hysterectomy.

KEY POINTS

- The percentage of blood to total fluid volume of menstrual discharge averages 36%.

- The most precise method to measure menstrual blood loss (MBL) is the alkaline hematin method.

- Average loss of iron in each menses is 13 mg.

- The mean amount of MBL in one cycle in normal women was previously reported to be about 35 ml but may be as much as 60 ml.

- About 70% of total MBL occurs in the first 2 days of menses.

- Menorrhagia occurs in 9% to 14% of healthy women, and most have normal duration of menses.

- The predominant cause of dysfunctional uterine bleeding (DUB) in the postmenstrual and premenopausal years is anovulation. During the rest of the reproductive years, most DUB is associated with ovulation.

- Hemostatic plugs in the endometrium are smaller, have different morphology, and persist for a shorter time than when vessel damage occurs in other tissue.

- Following the treatment of menorrhagia in women with a normal uterus by endometrial ablation with laser or electrocoagulation, amenorrhea occurs in about half the women. About 40% have decreased bleeding, and 10% have no improvement.

- Within four years after endometrial ablation about 25% of women so treated will have a hysterectomy.

- There is an increase in the amount of both PGE_2 and $PGF_{2\alpha}$ in the endometrium in the late secretory phase and during menses, with the $PGF_{2\alpha}/PGE_2$ ratio steadily increasing from midcycle to menses.

- There is an inverse correlation between endometrial $PGF_{2\alpha}/PGE_2$ ratio and MBL.

- Anovulatory cycles are usually not associated with dysmenorrhea because of reduced levels of $PGF_{2\alpha}$ in the endometrium.

- Alterations in prostaglandin synthesis and release occur in women with both ovulatory and anovulatory DUB.

- Endometrial ablation by the thermal balloon technique yields similar results as electrocoagulation without the need to perform hysteroscopy.

- Diagnostic tests in women with menorrhagia include measurement of hemoglobin, serum iron, serum ferritin, hCG, TSH, endometrial biopsy, and hysteroscopy or hysterosalpingography.

- High doses of oral or intravenous estrogen will usually stop acute bleeding episodes caused by anovulatory DUB. Oral estrogen is less expensive and easier to administer than the intravenous form.

- Ergot derivatives do not reduce MBL and should not be used as therapy.

- Anovulatory DUB can be treated by cyclic use of progestins, oral contraceptives, or intermittent clomiphene citrate.

- Patients with ovulatory DUB are best treated with oral contraceptives, NSAIDs (antiprostaglandins), danazol, or progestins during the luteal phase or progesterone or progestins released locally from an IUD.

- NSAIDs administered during menses reduce MBL by 20% to 50% in women with ovulatory DUB.

- The blind technique of dilation and curettage (D&C) misses the diagnosis of uterine lesions in 10% to 25% of women.

- A D&C should be used to stop the acute bleeding episode in patients with hypovolemia or those over age 35. A D&C only treats the acute episode of excess uterine bleeding, not subsequent episodes.

- Endometrial ablation with laser or electrocautery is a useful technique to control ovulatory DUB in women who do not respond to medical management, have excessive side effects with medical therapy, or have no other indications for hysterectomy.

- Hysterectomy should be used to treat women with ovulatory DUB only after medical therapy has failed and excessive MBL has been documented by objective measurement.

BIBLIOGRAPHY

Adelantado JM, Rees CP, Bernal AL, and Turnbull AC: Increased uterine prostaglandin E receptors in menorrhagic women, Br J Obstet Gynaecol 95:162, 1988.

Amso NN, for the International Collaborative Uterine Thermal Balloon Working Group: Uterine thermal balloon therapy for the treatment of menorrhagia: the first 300 patients from a multi-centre study, Br J Obstet Gynaecol 105:517, 1998.

Bergqvist A and Rybo G: Treatment of menorrhagia with intrauterine release of progesterone, Br J Obstet Gynaecol 90:255, 1983.

Bonney RC, Higham JM, Watson H, et al: Phospholipase activity in the endometrium of women with normal menstrual blood loss and women with proven ovulatory menorrhagia, Br J Obstet Gynaecol 98:363, 1991.

Chimbria TH, Anderson ABM, Naish C, et al: Reduction of menstrual blood loss by danazol in unexplained menorrhagia: lack of effect of placebo, Br J Obstet Gynaecol 87:1152, 1980.

Chimbira TH, Anderson AC, and Turnbull AC: Relation between measured menstrual blood loss and patients' subjective assessment of loss, duration of bleeding, number of sanitary towels used, uterine weight and endometrial surface area, Br J Obstet Gynaecol 87:603, 1980.

Chimbria TH, Cope E, Anderson ABM, et al: The effect of danazol on menorrhagia, coagulation mechanisms, haematological indices and body weight, Br J Obstet Gynaecol 86:46, 1979.

Christiaens GC, Sixma JJ, and Haspels AA: Morphology of haemostasis in menstrual endometrium, Br J Obstet Gynaecol 87:425, 1980.

Cicinelli E, Romano F, Anastasio PS, et al: Transabdominal sonohysterography, transvaginal sonography, and hysteroscopy in the evaluation of submucous myomas, Obstet Gynecol 85:42, 1995.

Claessens EA and Cowell CL: Acute adolescent menorrhagia, Am J Obstet Gynecol 139:277, 1981.

Cole SK, Billwicz WZ, and Thomson AM: Sources of variation in menstrual blood Loss, J Obstet Gynaecol Br Commonwlth 78:933, 1971.

DeVore GR, Owens O, and Kase N: Use of intravenous Premarin in the treatment of dysfunctional uterine bleeding: a double-blind randomized control study, Obstet Gynecol 59:285, 1982.

Dockeray CJ, Sheppard BL, and Bonnard J: Comparison between mefenamic acid and danazol in the treatment of established menorrhagia, Br J Obstet Gynaecol 96:840, 1989.

Erian J: Endometrial ablation in the treatment of menorrhagia, Br J Obstet Gynaecol 101:19, 1994.

Falcone T, Desjardins C, Bourque J, et al: Dysfunctional uterine bleeding in adolescents, J Reprod Med 39:761, 1994.

Fraser IS; Menorrhagia due to myometrial hypertrophy: treatment with tamoxifen, Obstet Gynecol 70:505, 1987.

Fraser IS: Treatment of ovulatory and anovulatory dysfunctional uterine bleeding with oral progestogens, Aust N Z J Obstet Gynecol 30:353, 1990.

Fraser IS, McCarron G, and Markham R: A preliminary study of factors influencing perception of menstrual blood loss volume, Am J Obstet Gynecol 149:788, 1984.

Fraser IS, McCarron G, Markham R, and Resta T: Blood and total fluid content of menstrual discharge, Obstet Gynecol 65:194, 1985.

Fraser IS, McCarron G, Markham R, et al: Long-term treatment of menorrhagia with mefenamic acid, Obstet Gynecol 61:109, 1983.

Fraser IS, McCarron G, Markham R, et al: Measured menstrual blood loss in women with menorrhagia associated with pelvic disease or coagulation disorder, Obstet Gynecol 68:630, 1986.

Garry R: Good practice with endometrial ablation, Obstet Gynecol 85:144, 1995.

Garry R, Erian J, and Grochmal SA: A multi-centre collaborative study into the treatment of menorrhagia by Nd-YAG laser ablation of the endometrium, Br J Obstet Gynaecol 98:357, 1991.

Garry R, Shelley-Jones D, Mooney P, and Phillips G: Six hundred endometrial laser ablations, Obstet Gynecol 85:24, 1995.

Gimpelson RJ and Rappold HO: A comparative study between panoramic hysteroscopy with directed biopsies and dilatation and curettage, Am J Obstet Gynecol 158:489, 1988.

Goldrath MH, Fuller TA, and Segal S: Laser photovaporization of endometrium for the treatment of menorrhagia, Am J Obstet Gynecol 140:14, 1981.

Goldstein SR: Use of ultrasonohysterography for triage of perimenopausal patients with unexplained uterine bleeding, Am J Obstet Gynecol 170:565, 1994.

Granstrom E, Swahn ML, and Lundstrom V: The possible roles of prostaglandins and related compounds in endometrial bleeding, Acta Obstet Gynecol Scand Suppl 113:91, 1983.

Grant AM for the Aberdeen Endometrial Ablation Trials Group: A randomised trial of endometrial ablation versus hysterectomy for the treatment of dysfunctional uterine bleeding: outcome at four years, Br J Obstet Gynaecol 106:360, 1999.

Hallberg L, Högdahl AM, Nilsson L, and Rybo G: Menstrual blood loss—a population study: variation at different ages and attempts to define normality, Acta Obstet Gynecol Scand 45:320, 1966.

Hallberg L and Nilsson L: Constancy of individual menstrual blood loss, Acta Obstet Gynecol Scand 43:352, 1964.

Hammond RH, Oppenheimer LW, and Saunders PG: Diagnostic role of dilatation and curettage in the management of abnormal premenopausal bleeding, Br J Obstet Gynaecol 96:496, 1989.

Haynes PJ, Hodgson H, Anderson ABM, and Turnbull AC: Measurement of menstrual blood loss in patients complaining of menorrhagia, Br J Obstet Gynaecol 84:763, 1977.

Higham JM and Shaw RW: A comparative study of danazol, a regimen of decreasing doses of danazol, and norethindrone in the treatment of objectively proven unexplained menorrhagia, Am J Obstet Gynecol 169:1134, 1993.

Irvine GA, Campbell-Brolwn MB, Lumsden MA, et al: Randomised comparative trial of levonorgestrel intrauterine system and norethisterone for treatment of idiopathic menorrhagia, Br J Obstet Gynaecol 105:592, 1998.

LaLonde A: Evaluation of surgical options in menorrhagia, Br J Obstet Gynaecol 101:8, 1994.

Lewis BV: Guidelines for endometrial ablation, Br J Obstet Gynaecol 101:470, 1994.

Loffer FD: Hysteroscopy with selective endometrial sampling compared with D&C for abnormal uterine bleeding: the value of a negative hysteroscopic view, Obstet Gynecol 73:16, 1989.

Magos AL, Baumann R, Lockwood GM, and Turnbull AC: Experience with the first 250 endometrial resections for menorrhagia, Lancet 337:1074, 1991.

Makarainen L and Ylikorkala O: Primary and myoma-associated menorrhagia: role of prostaglandins and effects of ibuprofen, Br J Obstet Gynaecol 93:974, 1986.

Meyer WR, Walsh BW, Grainger DA, et al: Thermal balloon and rollerball ablation to treat menorrhagia: a multicenter comparison, Obstet Gynecol 92:98, 1998.

Milson I, Andersson K, Andersch B, and Rybo G: A comparison of flurbiprofen, tranexamic acid, and a levonorgestrel-releasing intrauterine contraceptive device in the treatment of idiopathic menorrhagia, Am J Obstet Gynecol 164:879, 1991.

Newton J, Barnard G, and Collins W: A rapid method for measuring menstrual blood loss using automatic extraction, Contraception 16:269, 1977.

Nilsson L and Rybo G: Treatment of menorrhagia with an antifibrinolytic agent, tranexamic acid (AMCA): a double-blind investigation, Acta Obstet Gynecol Scand 46:572, 1967.

Nilsson L and Rybo G: Treatment of menorrhagia, Am J Obstet Gynecol 110:713, 1971.

Parmer J: Long-term suppression of hypermenorrhea by progesterone intrauterine contraceptive devices, Am J Obstet Gynecol 149:578, 1984.

Paskowitz RA: "Rollerball" ablation of the endometrium, J Reprod Med 40:333, 1995.

Preston JT, Cameron IT, Adams EJ, and Smith SK: Comparative study of tranexamic acid and norethisterone in the treatment of ovulatory menorrhagia, Br J Obstet Gynaecol 102:401, 1995.

Rees MCP, Cederholm-Williams SA, and Turnbull AC: Coagulation factors and fibrinolytic proteins in menstrual fluid collected from normal and menorrhagic women, Br J Obstet Gynaecol 92:1164, 1985.

Rees MCP, Dunnill MS, Anderson ABM, and Turnbull AC: Quantitative uterine histology during the menstrual cycle in relation to measured menstrual blood loss, Br J Obstet Gynaecol 91:662, 1984.

Ross D, Cooper AJ, Pryse-Davies J, et al: Randomized, double-blind, dose-ranging study of the endometrial effects of a vaginal progesterone gel in estrogen-treated postmenopausal women, Obstet Gynecol 1777:937, 1997.

Rybo G: Plasminogen activators in the endometrium, Acta Obstet Gynecol Scand 45:411, 1966.

Scottish Hysteroscopy Audit Group: A Scottish audit of hysteroscopic surgery for menorrhagia: complications and follow up, Br J Obstet Gynaecol 102:249, 1995.

Shaw RW and Fraser HM: Use of a superactive luteinizing hormone releasing hormone (LHRH) agonist in the treatment of menorrhagia, Br J Obstet Gynaecol 9:913, 1984.

Sheppard BL, Dockeray CJ, and Bonnar J: An ultrastructural study of menstrual blood in normal menstruation and dysfunctional uterine bleeding, Br J Obstet Gynaecol 90:259, 1983.

Smith SK, Abel MH, Kelly RW, and Baird DT: Prostaglandin synthesis in the endometrium of women with ovular dysfunctional uterine bleeding, Br J Obstet Gynaecol 88:434, 1981.

Smith SK, Abel MH, Kelly RW, and Baird DT: The synthesis of prostaglandins from persistent proliferative endometrium, J Clin Endocrinol Metab 55:284, 1982.

Smith SK, Kelly RW, Abel MH, and Baird DT: A role for prostacyclin (PGI2) in excessive menstrual bleeding, Lancet, March 1981, p 522.

Syrop CH and Sahakian V: Transvaginal sonographic detection of endometrial polyps with fluid contrast augmentation, Obstet Gynecol 79:1041, 1992.

Vancaillie TG: Electrocoagulation of the endometrium with the ball-end resectoscope, Obstet Gynecol 74:425, 1989.

van Eijkeren MA, Christiaens GC, Sixma JJ, and Haspels AA: Menorrhagia: a review, Obstet Gynecol Surv 44:421, 1989.

van Eijkeren MA, Scholten PC, Christiaens GC, et al: The alkaline hematin method for measuring menstrual blood loss—a modification and its clinical use in menorrhagia, Eur J Obstet Gynecol Reprod Biol 22:345, 1986.

Vargyas JM, Campeau JD, and Mishell DA: Treatment of menorrhagia with meclofenamate sodium, Am J Obstet Gynecol 157:944, 1987.

Wilansky DL and Greisman B: Early hypothyroidism in patients with menorrhagia, Am J Obstet Gynecol 160:673, 1989.

CHAPTER 38

Primary and Secondary Amenorrhea
Etiology, Diagnostic Evaluation, Management

KEY TERMS AND DEFINITIONS

Amenorrhea. Absence of menses during the reproductive years. It can be either physiologic (pregnancy) or pathologic.

Androgen Resistance Syndrome (Testicular Feminization). A genetically transmitted androgen receptor defect in a 46,XY individual with testes and normal male testosterone levels. These individuals have normal female phenotype, absent uterus, and scant body hair.

Anorexia Nervosa. A psychiatric disease associated with a fear of weight gain or obesity, food aversion, and a distorted body image in which the individual limits caloric intake to starvation levels. In addition to severe weight loss, there is a decreased metabolic rate and amenorrhea.

Chromophobe Adenoma. A non–hormone-secreting pituitary tumor that can disrupt normal pituitary function and thus produce low gonadotrophin levels.

Congenital Absence of Uterus and Vagina. A malformation in a 46,XX individual with normal ovarian function resulting in failure of the uterus and vagina to form. It is also called *uterovaginal agenesis* and *Rokitansky-Kuster-Hauser syndrome*.

Cryptomenorrhea. Menstruation without egress of menses through the introitus.

Delayed Menarche. Onset of menses in women older than 16.5 years who have no reproductive abnormalities.

Functional Hypothalamic Amenorrhea. Amenorrhea caused by nonorganic impairment of normal hypothalamic function with slowing of normal gonadotrophin-releasing hormone (GnRH) pulsatility.

Gonadal Failure. Failure of the gonads to develop. It is also called *gonadal dysgenesis* if the karyotype is abnormal and *gonadal agenesis* if the karyotype is normal.

Gonadal Streaks. Streaks of fibrous tissue in the normal position of the ovaries.

Gonadotrophin-Resistant Ovary Syndrome. Premature ovarian failure in which the ovary contains normal-appearing primordial follicles but no follicular development. It is also called *ovarian hypofolliculogenesis*.

Hypogonadotrophic Hypogonadism. Failure of the ovaries to develop as a result of low amounts of circulatory gonadotrophins. When anosmia is present, the term *Kallmann syndrome* is used.

Hypothalamic Dysfunction. Secondary amenorrhea caused by an abnormal pattern of GnRH pulsatility and circulatory estradiol levels above 40 pg/ml.

Hypothalamic Failure. Secondary amenorrhea caused by an abnormal pattern of GnRH pulsatility and estradiol levels below 40 pg/ml.

Insulin Tolerance Test. A test of adrenocorticotropic hormone function in which hypoglycemia is produced and cortisol measured.

Intrauterine Adhesions or Synechiae. A condition in which fibrous tissue partially or completely obliterates the uterine cavity. It is also called *Asherman syndrome*.

Isolated Gonadotrophin Deficiency. The presence of hypogonadotrophic hypogonadism in individuals who do not produce gonadotrophins after prolonged administration of GnRH.

Pituitary Destruction. Damage or necrosis of the pituitary gland caused by anoxia, thrombosis, or hemorrhage. It is called *Sheehan syndrome* when related to pregnancy and *Simmond disease* when unrelated to pregnancy.

Polycystic Ovary Syndrome. An endocrinologic disorder characterized by excessive androgen production, inappropriate gonadotrophin secretion, and chronic anovulation. It begins perimenarcheally, and its clinical manifestations include signs of hyperandrogenism (hirsutism) and menstrual irregularity (oligomenorrhea or amenorrhea).

Premature Ovarian Failure. Cessation of menstruation caused by depletion of ovarian follicles or failure of primordial follicles to respond to gonadotrophin before

the age of 40. It is also called *hypergonadotrophic hypogonadism.*

Primary Amenorrhea. Absence of any spontaneous menses in an individual older than 16.5 years of age.

Pure Gonadal Dysgenesis. Absence of the gonads in an individual with a normal 46,XX or 46,XY karyotype. It is also called *gonadal agenesis.*

Secondary Amenorrhea. Absence of menses for a variable period of time (for at least 3 to 12 months, usually 6 months or longer) in an individual who has previously had spontaneous menstrual periods.

Amenorrhea can be either physiologic, when it occurs during pregnancy and the postpartum period (particularly when nursing), or pathologic, when it is produced by a variety of endocrinologic and anatomic disorders. In the latter circumstance the failure to menstruate is a symptom of these various pathologic conditions. Thus amenorrhea itself is not a pathologic entity and should not be used as a final diagnosis.

Although the absence of menses causes no harm to the body, in a woman who is not pregnant or postpartum it is abnormal and thus is a source of concern. For this reason women usually seek medical assistance when the condition occurs. Therefore the clinician needs to know the various etiologies of amenorrhea, how to diagnose the etiology, and how to treat the underlying pathologic condition. This chapter will present the etiology, diagnostic evaluation, and treatment of the various causes of both primary and secondary amenorrhea.

Many individuals with ambiguous external genitalia resulting from various intersex problems are raised as females and never menstruate. The etiology of the intersex problem is usually determined at birth or soon thereafter. Since such disorders are discussed in Chapter 11, they will not be discussed in this chapter. Although women with cryptomenorrhea caused by anatomic disorders interfering with the outflow of menses, such as an imperforate hymen or transverse vaginal septum, have the symptom of amenorrhea, they are actually menstruating. These conditions are discussed in Chapter 11. Severe systemic diseases such as metastatic carcinoma and chronic renal failure can also cause amenorrhea; however, since amenorrhea is not the presenting symp-

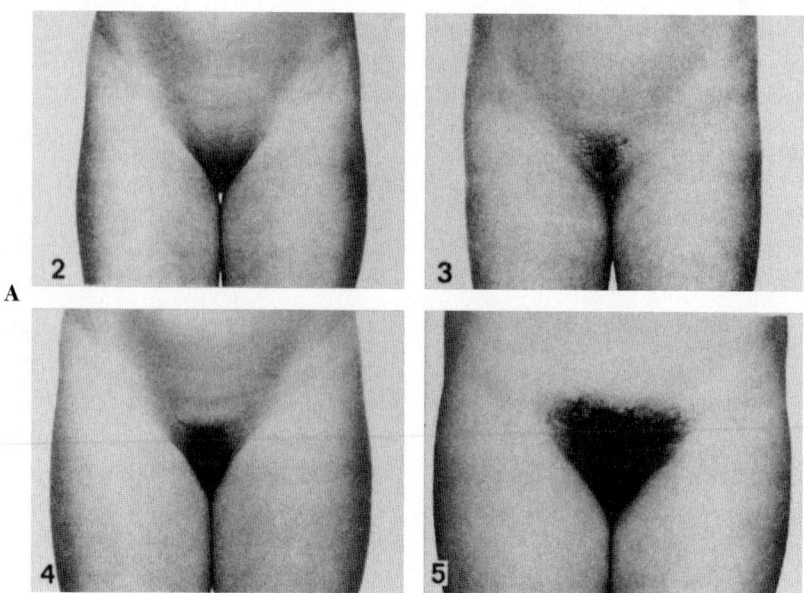

FIGURE 38-1 Standards for **(A)** pubic hair and **(B)** breast ratings. (Modified from Tanner JM: Growth and endocrinology of the adolescent. In Gardner L, editor: Endocrine and genetic diseases of childhood, ed 2, Philadelphia, 1975, WB Saunders Co.)

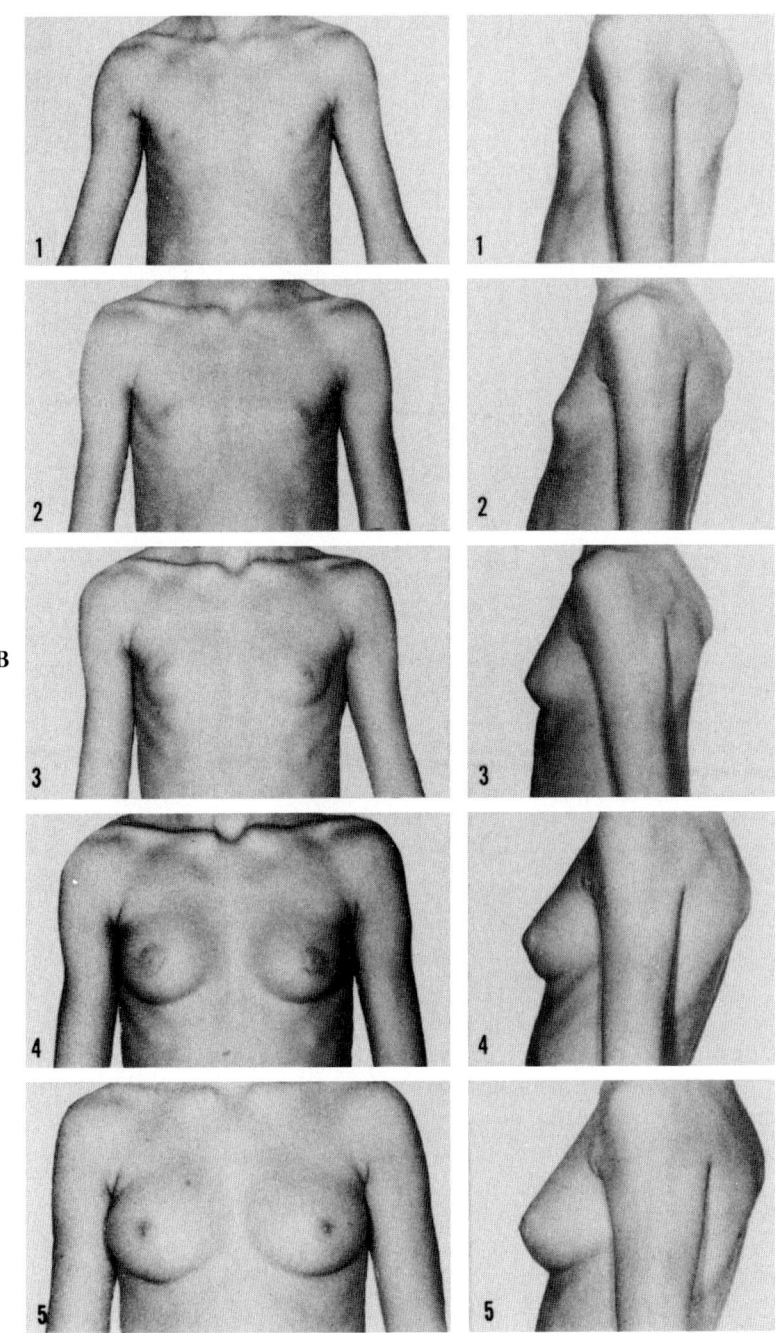

FIGURE 38-1, cont'd. For legend see opposite page.

tom of these disorders, they will not be discussed in this chapter.

Primary amenorrhea is defined as the absence of menses in a woman who has never menstruated by the age of 16½ years. The incidence of primary amenorrhea is less than 0.1%. Secondary amenorrhea is defined as the absence of menses for an arbitrary time period, usually longer than 6 to 12 months. The incidence of secondary amenorrhea of more than 6 months' duration in a survey of a general population of Swedish women of reproductive age was found to be 0.7%. The incidence was significantly higher in women younger than 25 years of age and those with a prior history of menstrual irregularity.

DELAYED MENARCHE

Before the onset of menses the normal female goes through a progressive series of morphologic changes produced by the pubertal increase in estrogen and androgen production. In 1969 Marshall and Tanner defined five stages of breast development and pubic hair development (Figure 38-1,

TABLE 38-1
Classifications of Breast Growth
and Pubic Hair Growth

Classification	Description
Breast Growth	
B1	Prepubertal: elevation of papilla only
B2	Breast budding
B3	Enlargement of breasts with glandular tissue, without separation of breast contours
B4	Secondary mound formed by areola
B5	Single contour of breast and areola
Pubic hair growth	
PH1	Prepubertal: no pubic hair
PH2	Labial hair present
PH3	Labial hair spreads over mons pubis
PH4	Slight lateral spread
PH5	Further lateral spread to form inverse triangle and reach medial thighs

Adapted from Roy S: Puberty. Reproduced with permission from Infertility, contraception and reproductive endocrinology, ed 4, by Daniel R. Mishell, Jr., M.D., and Val Davajan, M.D. Copyright 1997 by Blackwell Scientific Publications, Malden, Mass. All rights reserved.

TABLE 38-2
Mean Ages of Girls at the Onset of Pubertal
Events (United States)

Event	Mean Age ± SD (Years)
Initiation of breast development (B2)	10.8 ± 1.10
Appearance of pubic hair (PH2)	11.0 ± 1.21
Menarche	12.9 ± 1.20

Adapted from Frisch RE and Revelle R: Arch Dis Child 46:695, 1971.

TABLE 38-3
Pubertal Intervals

Interval	Mean Age ± SD (Years)
B2-peak height velocity	1.0 ± 0.77
B2-menarche	2.3 ± 1.03
B2-PH5	3.1 ± 1.04
B2-B5 (average duration of puberty)	4.5 ± 2.04

Adapted from Frisch RE and Revelle R: Arch Dis Child 46:695, 1971.

Table 38-1). These changes sometimes are combined and called *Tanner* or *pubertal stages 1 through 5*. The first sign of puberty is usually the appearance of breast budding followed within a few months by the appearance of pubic hair.

Thereafter the breasts enlarge, the external pelvic contour becomes rounder, and the most rapid rate of growth occurs (peak height velocity). These changes precede menarche. Thus breast budding is the earliest sign of puberty and menarche the latest. The mean ages of occurrence of these events in American women are shown in Table 38-2, and the mean intervals (with standard deviation) between initiation of breast budding and other pubertal events are shown in Table 38-3. The mean interval between breast budding and menarche is 2.3 years, with a standard deviation of about 1 year. Some individuals can progress from breast budding to menarche in 18 months, while others may take 5 years. Thus although the arbitrary age of primary amenorrhea is 16½ years, if a woman 14 years of age or older presents to the clinician with absence of breast budding, a diagnostic evaluation should be performed at this time. The absence of breast development is indicative of a lack of estradiol synthesis. The cause of this abnormality should be determined; then estrogen replacement can be initiated to cause breast development.

The mean time of onset of menarche was previously thought to occur when a critical body weight of about 48 kg, or 106 lb, was reached. However, it is now believed that body composition is more important than total body weight in determining the time of onset of puberty and menstruation. Thus the ratio of fat to both total body weight and lean body weight is probably the most relevant factor that determines the time of onset of puberty and menstruation. Individuals who are moderately obese, between 20% and 30% above the ideal body weight, have an earlier onset of menarche than nonobese women. Malnutrition, such as occurs with anorexia nervosa or starvation, is known to delay the onset of puberty. Well-nourished individuals with prepubertal strenuous exercise programs resulting in less total body fat have also been shown to have a delayed onset of puberty. Warren et al. reported that ballet dancers, swimmers, and runners had menarche delayed to about age 15 if they began exercising strenuously before menarche (Figure 38-2). These investigators also determined that stress is not the cause of the delayed menarche in these exercising girls, as girls of the same age with stressful musical careers did not have a delayed onset of menarche. Young women with strenuous exercise programs have sufficient estrogen to produce some breast development and thus do not need extensive endocrinologic evaluation if concern arises about lack of onset of menses. Frisch et al. reported that for girls engaged in premenarcheal athletic training, menarche was delayed 0.4 years for each year of training. Individuals

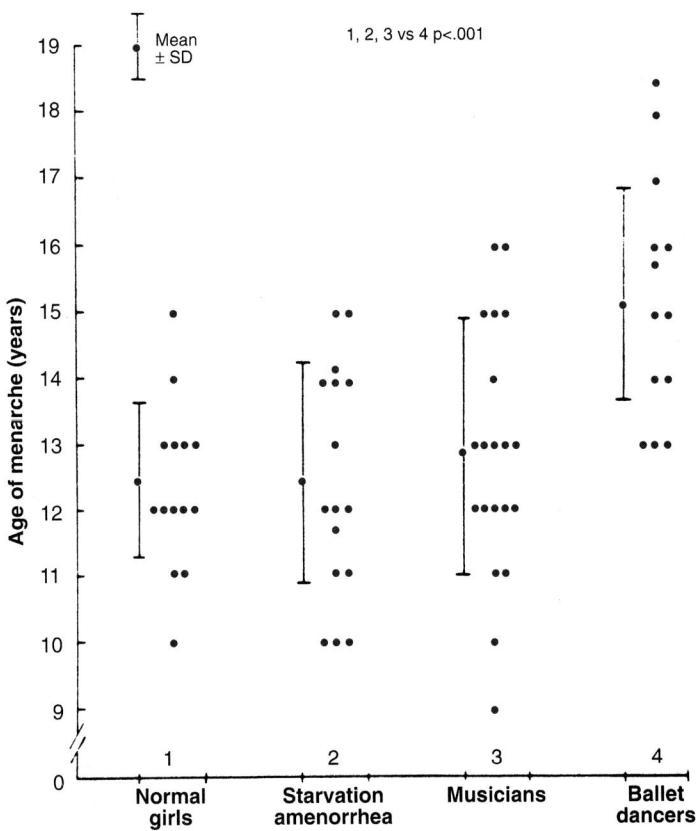

FIGURE 38-2 Ages of menarche in ballet dancers compared with those of three other groups. (From Warren MP: J Clin Endocrinol Metab 51:1150, 1980. Copyright 1980 by The Endocrine Society.)

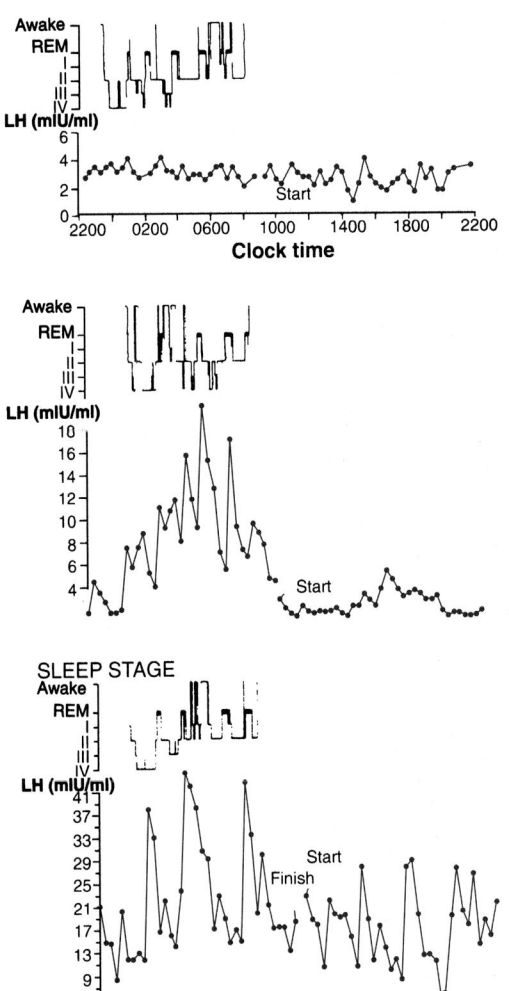

FIGURE 38-3 Plasma LH concentration measured every 20 minutes for 24 hours in normal prepubertal girl *(upper panel),* early pubertal girl *(center panel),* and normal late pubertal girl *(lower panel).* In top and center panels sleep histogram is shown above period of nocturnal sleep. Sleep stages are awake, rapid eye movement (REM), and stages I to IV by depth of line graph. Plasma LH concentrations are expressed as milli–international units per milliliter of Second International Reference Preparation of Human Menopausal Gonadotropin. (Modified from Boyar RM, Katz J, Finkelstein JW, et al: N Engl J Med 291:861, 1974. Reprinted by permission of The New England Journal of Medicine.)

who exercise strenuously should be counseled that they will usually have a delayed onset of menses, but it is not a health problem. They should be told that they will most likely have regular ovulatory cycles when they either stop exercising or become older.

Before puberty, circulating levels of luteinizing hormone (LH) and follicle-stimulating hormone (FSH) are low (FSH/LH ratio being greater than 1) because the central nervous system (CNS)-hypothalamic axis is extremely sensitive to the negative feedback effects of low levels of circulating estrogen. As the critical weight or body composition is approached, the CNS-hypothalamic axis becomes less sensitive to the negative effect of estrogen, and gonadotrophin-releasing hormone (GnRH) is secreted in greater amounts, causing an increase in both LH and to a lesser extent FSH. The initial endocrinologic change associated with the onset of puberty is the occurrence of episodic pulses of LH occurring during sleep (Figure 38-3). These pulses are absent before the onset of puberty. After menarche the episodic secretions of LH occur both during sleep and while awake. The last endocrinologic event of puberty is activation of the positive gonadotrophin response to increasing levels of estradiol, which results in the midcycle gonadotrophic surge and ovulation.

PRIMARY AMENORRHEA

It is important that the clinician understand both the sequential endocrinologic and the morphologic chronologic changes taking place during normal puberty in order to make the differential diagnosis between delayed menarche and primary amenorrhea. Although the former condition requires only reassurance, the latter requires an endocrinologic evaluation to establish the etiology of this symptom.

Classification of Disorders with Primary Amenorrhea and Normal Female External Genitalia

I. Absent breast development; uterus present
  A. Gonadal failure
    1. a. 45,X (Turner syndrome)
       b. 46,X, abnormal X (e.g., short- or long-arm deletion)
       c. Mosaicism (e.g., X/XX, X/XX/XXX)
       d. 46,XX or 46,XY pure gonadal dysgenesis
       e. 17α-hydroxylase deficiency with 46,XX
  B. Hypothalamic failure secondary to inadequate GnRH release
    1. Insufficient GnRH secretion due to neurotransmitter defect
    2. Inadequate GnRH synthesis (Kallman syndrome)
    3. Congenital anatomic defect in central nervous system
    4. CNS neoplasm (craniopharyngioma)
  C. Pituitary failure
    1. Isolated gonadotrophin insufficiency (thalassemia major, retinitis pigmentosa)
    2. Pituitary neoplasia (chromophobe adenoma)
    3. Mumps, encephalitis
    4. Newborn kernicterus
    5. Prepubertal hypothyroidism
II. Breast development; uterus absent
  A. Androgen resistance (testicular feminization)
  B. Congenital absence of uterus (utero-vaginal agenesis)
III. Absent breast development; uterus absent
  A. 17,20-desmolase deficiency
  B. Agonadism
  C. 17α-hydroxylase deficiency with 46,XY karyotype
IV. Breast development; uterus present
  A. Hypothalamic etiology
  B. Pituitary etiology
  C. Ovarian etiology
  D. Uterine etiology

Etiology

Although numerous classifications have been used for the various etiologies of primary amenorrhea, it has been found most clinically useful to group them on the basis of whether secondary sexual characteristics (breasts) and female internal genitalia (uterus) are present or absent (see the box above). Thus the findings of a physical examination can alert the clinician to possible causes and indicate which laboratory tests should be performed. In a series of 62 individuals reported by Maschchak et al. the largest subgroup with primary amenorrhea (29) were those with absent breasts and a uterus present; the second largest subgroup (22) had both breasts and uterus; an absent uterus together with breast development accounted for the third largest category (9); and absent breasts and uterus were the least common (2).

Breasts Absent and Uterus Present

All individuals with no breast development and a uterus present have no ovarian estrogen production as a result of either a gonadal disorder or a CNS hypothalamic-pituitary abnormality. The phenotype of individuals with either of these causes of low estrogen synthesis is similar. However, since the etiology and prognosis for fertility differs, it is important to establish the specific diagnosis.

GONADAL FAILURE (HYPERGONADOTROPHIC HYPOGONADISM). Failure of gonadal development is the most common cause of primary amenorrhea, occurring in almost half the individuals with this symptom. Gonadal failure is most frequently due to a chromosomal disorder or deletion of all or part of an X chromosome, but it is sometimes due to a genetic defect and rarely 17α-hydroxylase deficiencies. The chromosome disorders are usually due to a random meiotic or mitotic abnormality (e.g., nondisjunction or anaphase lag) and thus are not inherited. However, if absent gonadal development occurs in the presence of a 46,XX or 46,XY karyotype, called *pure gonadal dysgenesis,* a gene disorder may be present, as it has been reported to occur in siblings. Reindollar et al., in the largest single series of patients with primary amenorrhea, reported that all individuals with gonadal failure and an X chromosome abnormality were less than 63 inches in height. About one third had major cardiovascular or renal anomalies.

Since at least two X chromosomes are necessary for normal ovarian development, individuals with a 45,X karyotype, mosaicism involving a single X chromosome, or abnormalities of the X chromosome usually do not develop ovaries. In place of the ovary a band of fibrous tissue called a *gonadal streak* is present (Figure 38-4). Streaks are also present in individuals with absent gonads and pure gonadal dysgenesis. With the absence of ovarian follicles, synthesis of ovarian steroids and inhibin does not occur. Breast development does not occur because of the very low circulating estradiol levels. Because the negative hypothalamic-pituitary action of estrogen and inhibin is not present, gonadotrophin levels are markedly elevated. Since estrogen is not necessary for müllerian duct development or wolffian duct regression, the internal and external genitalia are phenotypically normal female. Individuals with 17α-hydroxylase deficiency do have primordial follicles but cannot synthesize sex steroids. An occasional individual with mosaicism, an abnormal X, or pure gonadal dysgenesis (46,XX) may have a few follicles that develop under endogenous gonadotrophin stimulation early in puberty and may synthesize enough estrogen to induce breast development and a few episodes of uterine bleeding. Rarely, ovulation and pregnancy can occur. However, nearly all individuals with hypergonadotrophic hypogonadism have primary amenorrhea and no breast development.

Goldenberg et al. reported that all individuals with pri-

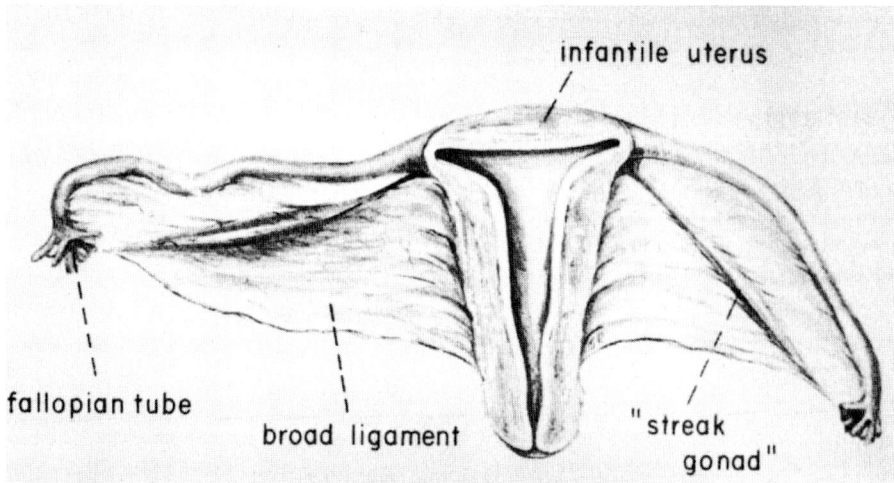

FIGURE 38-4 Internal genitalia of patient with gonadal dysgenesis (Turner syndrome), featuring normal but infantile uterus, normal fallopian tubes, and pale, glistening "streak" gonads in both broad ligaments. (From Federman DD, editor: Disorders of gonadal development: gonadal dysgenesis [Turner syndrome]. In Abnormal sexual development, Philadelphia, 1967, WB Saunders Co.)

mary amenorrhea and plasma FSH levels greater than 40 mIU/ml had no functioning ovarian follicles in the gonadal tissue. Thus, in women with primary amenorrhea, the diagnosis of gonadal failure can be established if the FSH levels are abnormally elevated.

45,X anomalies. *Turner syndrome* occurs in about 1 per 2000 to 1 per 3000 live births but is much more frequent in abortuses. In addition to primary amenorrhea and absent breast development, these individuals have other somatic abnormalities, the most prevalent being short stature (less than 60 inches in height), webbing of the neck, a short fourth metacarpal, and cubitus valgus. Thus the diagnosis is usually made before puberty (Chapter 2).

A wide variety of chromosomal mosaics are associated with primary amenorrhea and normal female external genitalia, the most common being X/XX. In addition, individuals with X/XXX and X/XX/XXX mosaicism have primary amenorrhea. These individuals are generally taller and have fewer anatomic abnormalities than individuals with a 45,X karyotype. In addition, some of them may have a few gonadal follicles, and about 20% have sufficient estrogen production to menstruate. Occasionally ovulation may occur.

Structurally abnormal X chromosome. Although individuals with this disorder have a 46,XX karyotype, part of one X chromosome is structurally abnormal. If there is deletion of the long arm of the X chromosome (Xq), normal height has been reported to occur, but in Reindollar's series such individuals were all short. These individuals have no somatic abnormalities. However, if there is deletion of the short arm of the X chromosome (Xp), the individual phenotypically resembles those with a 45,X karyotype (Turner syndrome). A similar phenotype occurs in

persons with isochrome of the long arm of the X chromosome. Other X chromosome abnormalities include a ring X and minute fragmentation of the X chromosome.

Pure gonadal dysgenesis (46,XX and 46,XY with gonad streaks; gonadal agenesis). As already mentioned, this abnormality is probably a genetic disorder, as it has been reported in siblings. These individuals have normal stature and phenotype, absence of secondary sexual characteristics, and primary amenorrhea. Some of these individuals have a few ovarian follicles, develop breasts, and may even menstruate spontaneously for a few years. In Reindollar's series nearly all such individuals were taller than 63 inches.

17α-hydroxylase deficiency with 46,XX karyotype. A rare gonadal cause of primary amenorrhea without breast development and normal female internal genitalia is deficiency of the enzyme 17α-hydroxylase in an individual with a 46,XX karyotype. Only a few such individuals have been described in the literature, but it is important for the clinician to be aware of this entity because these individuals, in contrast to those described earlier, have hypernatremia and hypokalemia. Because of decreased cortisol, adrenocorticotropic hormone (ACTH) levels are elevated. The mineralocorticoid levels are also elevated, as 17α-hydroxylase is not necessary for the conversion of progesterone to deoxycortisol or corticosterone. Thus there is excessive sodium retention and potassium excretion, leading to hypertension and hypokalemia. Serum progesterone levels are also elevated because progesterone is not converted to cortisol. In addition to sex steroid replacement, these individuals need cortisol administration.

GENETIC DISORDERS WITH HYPERANDROGENISM. Hyperandrogenism occurs in about 10% of women with gonadal dysgenesis. Most have a Y chromosome or fragment of a Y chromosome, but some may only have a DNA fragment that contains the testes-determining gene (probably SRY) without a full Y chromosome. Individuals with hypergonadotrophic hypogonadism and a female phenotype who have any clinical manifestation of hyperandrogenism, such as hirsutism, should have a gonadectomy even if a Y chromosome is not present because gonadal neoplasms are frequent. Although not yet considered routine, in the future all individuals with gonadal dysgenesis will be screened for the presence of SRY or even more specific testis-determining regions.

CNS-HYPOTHALAMIC-PITUITARY DISORDERS. With CNS-hypothalamic-pituitary disorders the low estrogen levels are due to very low gonadotrophin release. The etiology of low gonadotrophin production can be morphologic or endocrinologic.

Lesions. Any anatomic lesion of the hypothalamus or pituitary can be a cause of low gonadotrophin production. These lesions can be congenital (stenosis of aqueduct or absence of sellar floor) or acquired (tumors). Many of these lesions, particularly pituitary adenomas, result in elevated prolactin levels (Chapter 39).

However, non–prolactin-secreting pituitary tumors (chromophobe adenomas) as well as craniopharyngiomas may not be associated with hyperprolactinemia and can rarely be the cause of primary amenorrhea with low gonadotrophin levels. Thus all individuals with primary amenorrhea and low gonadotrophin levels, with or without an elevated prolactin, should have computed tomography (CT) scanning or magnetic resonance imaging (MRI) of the hypothalamic-pituitary region to rule out the presence of a lesion.

Inadequate GnRH release (hypogonadotrophic hypogonadism). Individuals without a demonstrable lesion and a low gonadotrophin level were previously thought to have primary pituitary failure (hypogonadotrophic hypogonadism). However, when they are stimulated with GnRH, there is an increase in FSH and LH, indicating that the basic defect is either hypothalamic with insufficient GnRH synthesis or a CNS neurotransmitter defect resulting in inadequate GnRH synthesis or release or both. Although a single bolus of GnRH may not initially cause a rise in gonadotrophin level in these individuals, after 4 days of GnRH administration they will have a rise in gonadotrophins after a single GnRH bolus. Some of these individuals also have anosmia (Kallman syndrome), and they should be tested for olfaction with coffee, orange, and cocoa. Kallman syndrome is a genetically transmitted disorder and is frequently associated with other anatomic and functional abnormalities.

Isolated gonadotrophin deficiency. Rarely, individuals with primary amenorrhea and low gonadotrophin levels do not respond to GnRH even after 4 days of administration. These individuals nearly always have an associated disorder such as thalassemia major or retinitis pigmentosa. Occasionally this pituitary abnormality had been associated with prepubertal hypothyroidism, kernicterus, or mumps encephalitis.

Breast Development Present and Uterus Absent

Two etiologies cause primary amenorrhea associated with normal breast development and an absent uterus: androgen resistance and congenital absence of the uterus. The former is a genetically inherited disorder, whereas the latter is an accident of development and is only rarely genetically inherited.

ANDROGEN RESISTANCE. Androgen resistance, originally termed *testicular feminization*, is a genetically transmitted disorder in which there is an absence of androgen receptor synthesis or action. The syndrome is due to absence of an X-chromosomal gene responsible for the cytoplasmic or nuclear testosterone receptor. It is either an X-linked recessive or sex-limited autosomal dominant disorder with transmission through the mother. These individuals have an XY karyotype and normally functioning male gonads that produce normal male levels of testosterone and dihydrotestosterone. However, because of a lack of receptors in the target organs, there is a lack of male differentiation of the external and internal genitalia. The external genitalia remain feminine, as occurs in the absence of sex steroids. Wolffian duct development, which normally occurs as a result of testosterone stimulation, fails to take place. Since müllerian duct regression is induced by anti-müllerian hormone (AMH), a glycoprotein synthesized by the Sertoli cells of the fetal testes, this process occurs normally in these individuals as steroid receptors are unnecessary for the action of glycoproteins. Thus individuals with this condition have no female or male internal genitalia, normal female external genitalia, and either a short or absent vagina. Pubic and axillary hair is absent or scanty as a result of a lack of androgenic receptors, but breast development is normal or enhanced due to the fact that there is no androgenic opposition to the stimulation of breast tissue by the small circulating levels of estrogen secreted by the gonads and adrenals, as well as the estrogen produced by peripheral conversion of androstenedione. The abnormal gonads have an increased risk of developing a malignancy (gonadoblastoma or dysgerminoma), with an incidence reported to be about 20%. However, these malignancies rarely occur before age 20. Therefore it is usually recommended that the gonads be left in place until after puberty is completed to allow full breast development and epiphyseal closure to occur. After these events occur, usually about age 18, the gonads should be removed. It is recommended that individuals with androgen resistance syndrome be informed that they have an abnormal sex chromosome, without specifically mentioning a Y chromosome, because it is well known that an XY karyotype indicates maleness. In addition, because psychologically and phenotypically these individuals are female and have been raised as such, the term *gonads* should be used instead of testes. These individuals should also be informed that they can never become pregnant because they do not have a uterus and that their gonads (not testes) need to be removed after age 18 because of their high malignant potential.

CONGENITAL ABSENCE OF THE UTERUS (UTERINE AGENESIS; UTEROVAGINAL AGENESIS; ROKI-TANSKY-KUSTER-HAUSER SYNDROME). This disorder is the second most frequent cause of primary amenorrhea. It occurs in 1 in 4000 to 5000 female births and accounts for about 15% of individuals with primary amenorrhea. Individuals with complete uterine agenesis have normal ovaries with regular cyclic ovulation and normal endocrine function. Women with this disorder have normal breast and pubic and axillary hair development but have a shortened or absent vagina in addition to absence of the uterus (Figure 38-5). Congenital renal abnormalities occur in about one third of these individuals and skeletal abnormalities in about 12%. Cardiac and other congenital abnormalities also occur with increased frequency. The overwhelming majority of these disorders are due to an isolated developmental defect, but on occasion the condition is genetically inherited. It is usually easy to differentiate these individuals from those with androgen resistance by the presence of normal pubic hair, but some individuals with incomplete androgen resis-

tance have some pubic hair. Since women with congenital absence of the uterus are endocrinologically normal females, whereas those with androgen resistance are endocrinologically male with male testosterone levels and an XY karyotype, the differential diagnosis is easily made.

Absent Breast and Uterine Development

Individuals with no breast or uterine development are rare and have a male karyotype, elevated gonadotrophin levels, and testosterone levels in the normal or below normal female range. Etiologies for this phenotype include 17α-hydroxylase deficiency, 17,20-desmolase deficiency, and agonadism. Individuals with the first disorder have testes present but lack the enzyme necessary to synthesize sex steroids and thus have female external genitalia. Because they have testes, AMH is produced and the female internal genitalia regress; with low testosterone levels the male internal genitalia do not develop. Insufficient estrogen is synthesized to develop breasts. A similar lack of sex steroid synthesis occurs in males with a 17,20-desmolase deficiency. Individuals with agonadism, sometimes called the *vanishing testes syndrome*, have no gonads present, but since the female internal genitalia are also absent it has been postulated that testicular AMH production occurred during fetal life, but the gonadal tissue subsequently regressed.

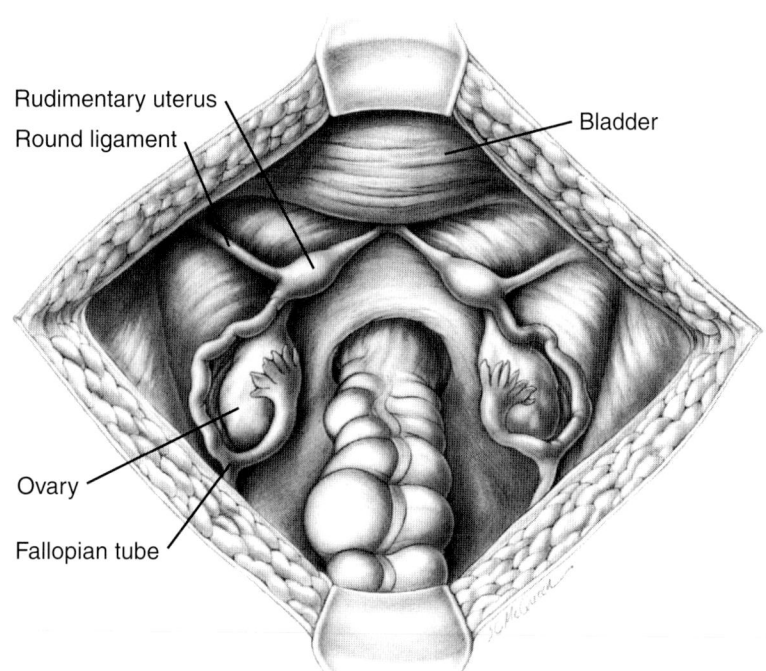

Rudimentary uterus

Round ligament

Bladder

Ovary

Fallopian tube

FIGURE 38-5 Congenital absence of vagina. Laparotomy revealed rudimentary uterus that showed evidence of failure of fusion of müllerian ducts. This is a common finding in this condition and indicates that disorder is more extensive than simple anomaly of vagina. (Redrawn from Jones HW Jr and Scott WW, editors: Hermaphroditism, genital anomalies and related endocrine disorders, ed 2, Baltimore, 1971, Williams & Wilkins Co.)

Secondary Sex Characteristics and Female Internal Genitalia Present

This is the second largest category of individuals with primary amenorrhea, accounting for about one third of them. In the series reported by Maschchak et al., about 25% of these individuals had hyperprolactinemia and prolactinomas. The remaining women had etiologies similar to those with secondary amenorrhea and thus should be subcategorized and treated similarly to women with secondary amenorrhea. Secondary amenorrhea is discussed in the latter half of this chapter.

Differential Diagnosis and Management

After a history is obtained and a physical examination performed, including measurement of height, span, and weight, individuals with primary amenorrhea can be grouped into one of the four general categories listed in the box on p. 1104 depending on the presence or absence of breasts and a uterus.

If breast development is absent and a uterus is present, the diagnostic evaluation should differentiate between CNS-hypothalamic-pituitary disorders and failure of normal gonadal development. Although individuals with both these disorders have similar phenotypes because of low estradiol levels, a single serum FSH assay can differentiate between these two major etiologic categories (Figure 38-6). Women with hypergonadotrophic hypogo-

nadism (FSH >30 mIU/ml), not those with hypogonadotrophic hypogonadism, should have a peripheral white blood cell karyotype performed to determine if a Y chromosome is present. If a Y chromosome is present, the streak gonads should be excised, as the incidence of malignancy occurring subsequently, mainly gonadoblastomas, is relatively high. If a Y chromosome is absent, it is unnecessary to remove the gonads unless there are signs of hyperandrogenism. It is also unnecessary to perform a karyotype on the gonadal tissue to detect possible mosaicism with a Y chromosome in the gonad unless hyperandrogenism is present.

All women with an elevated FSH level and an XX karyotype should have electrolyte and serum progesterone levels measured to rule out 17α-hydroxylase deficiency. In addition to hypernatremia and hypokalemia, individuals with 17α-hydroxylase deficiency have an elevated serum progesterone level (>3 ng/ml), a low 17α-hydroxyprogesterone level (<0.2 ng/ml), and an elevated serum deoxycorticosterone level (>17 ng/100 ml), so the diagnosis is easily established.

All individuals in this category need estrogen-progestin replacement therapy to develop breast tissue and prevent osteoporosis. The progestin is necessary to decrease the risk of endometrial carcinoma, which is increased by long-term unopposed estrogen administration. Ingestion of 0.625 mg conjugated estrogen or 1 mg estradiol daily and 2.5 mg medroxyprogesterone acetate daily or 5 mg for the first 12 days of the month is sufficient to achieve maximal breast growth, and prevent osteoporosis and endometrial

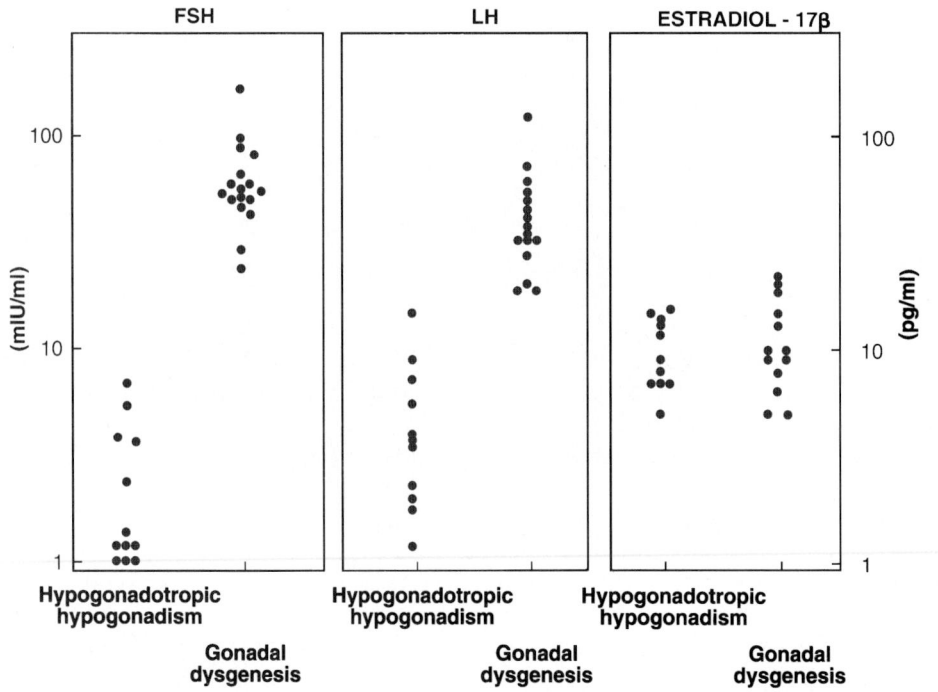

FIGURE 38-6 Levels of serum FSH, LH, and estradiol in patients with primary amenorrhea who have an intact uterus and no breast development. (From Maschchak CA, Kletzky OA, Davajan V, et al: Obstet Gynecol 57:715, 1981. Reprinted with permission from The American College of Obstetricians and Gynecologists.)

hyperplasia. Larger doses of estrogen will not result in larger breasts. Those rare individuals with 17α-hydroxylase deficiency need to have adequate cortisol replacement in addition to sex steroid treatment. It is possible for women with hypergonadotrophic hypogonadism to become pregnant with appropriate endometrial stimulation with exogenous steroids and transfer of embryos following fertilization of donor eggs.

If the FSH level is low, the underlying disorder is in the CNS-hypothalamic-pituitary region, and a serum prolactin measurement should be obtained. Even if the prolactin level is not elevated, all women with hypogonadotrophic hypogonadism should have a cranial CT scan or MRI obtained to rule out a lesion. It is unnecessary to perform a karyotype, as all individuals with hypogonadotrophic hypogonadism are 46,XX. The use of GnRH testing is optional but is expensive and is clinically unnecessary unless GnRH is going to be used for ovulation induction. Ovulation can usually be induced in women with this disorder because their ovaries are normal. Initially they should receive estrogen-progestogen treatment to induce breast development and cause epiphyseal closure. When fertility is desired, human menopausal gonadotrophins or pulsatile GnRH should be administered to induce ovulation. Clomiphene citrate will be ineffective because of the low endogenous estradiol levels.

The differential diagnosis of androgen resistance from uterine agenesis can easily be made by the presence in the latter condition of normal body hair, ovulatory and premenstrual-type symptoms, a biphasic basal temperature, and a normal female testosterone level. Since women with uterine agenesis have normal female endocrine function, they do not need hormonal therapy. An intravenous urogram or some type of scanning should be performed because of the high incidence of renal abnormalities. They may need surgical reconstruction of an absent vagina (McIndoe procedure), but progressive mechanical dilation with plastic dilators as described by Frank should be tried first. These women can now have their own genetic children. After ovarian stimulation and follicle aspiration, their ova can be fertilized and placed in the uterus of a surrogate recipient.

Individuals with androgen resistance have an XY karyotype and male levels of testosterone. After full breast development is obtained and epiphyseal closure occurs, the gonads should be removed because of their malignant potential. Thereafter estrogen-replacement therapy should be administered. These individuals do not need progestin therapy as they do not have endometrial tissue. To prevent constant breast stimulation the estrogen is best administered 5 days out of each week.

The rare individuals with absent breast development and absent internal genitalia should be referred to an endocrine center for the extensive evaluation necessary to establish the diagnosis. If gonads are present, they should be removed, because a Y chromosome is present. Steroid

hormonal replacement therapy should be administered to individuals with this disorder.

SECONDARY AMENORRHEA

Etiology

The symptom of amenorrhea associated with hyperprolactinemia or excessive androgen or cortisol production will not be considered in this chapter as these disorders are discussed in Chapters 39 and 40. If amenorrhea is present without galactorrhea, hyperprolactinemia, or hirsutism, the symptom can result from disorders in the CNS-hypothalamic-pituitary axis, ovary, or uterus. In a review of 262 patients presenting with secondary amenorrhea during a 20-year period at a tertiary medical center, Reindollar et al. (1986) reported that 12% of cases resulted from a primary ovarian problem, 62% from a hypothalamic disorder, 16% from a pituitary problem (including prolactinomas), and 7% from a uterine disorder. The uterine cause of secondary amenorrhea is the only one in which normal endocrinologic function is present and will be discussed first.

Uterine Cause

Intrauterine adhesions (IUAs) or synechiae (Asherman syndrome) can obliterate the endometrial cavity and produce secondary amenorrhea. Rarely, a missed abortion or endometrial tuberculosis can also cause endometrial destruction. The most frequent antecedent factor of IUAs is endometrial curettage associated with pregnancy: either evacuation of a live or dead fetus by mechanical means or postpartum or postabortal curettage. Curettage for a missed abortion results in a high (30%) incidence of IUA formation. IUAs may also occur after diagnostic dilation and curettage (D&C) in a nonpregnant individual, so this procedure should be performed only when indicated and not routinely at the time of other surgical procedures such as diagnostic laparoscopy. A less common cause of IUA is severe endometritis or fibrosis following a myomectomy, metroplasty, or cesarean delivery. This etiology of amenorrhea should be considered to be most likely if a temporal relation exists between the onset of symptoms and a uterine curettage. The likelihood of the diagnosis is strengthened if there is difficulty or inability to pass a sound into the uterine cavity.

Confirmation of the diagnosis is usually made by hysterography (Figure 38-7) or hysteroscopy. Although it has been suggested that sequential administration of estrogen-progestogen be used as the initial diagnostic procedure when IUA is suspected, withdrawal bleeding occurs following administration of the steroids in most women with IUA. Because of the lack of specificity of this test, steroid administration should not be performed prior to indirect or direct visualization of the uterine cavity.

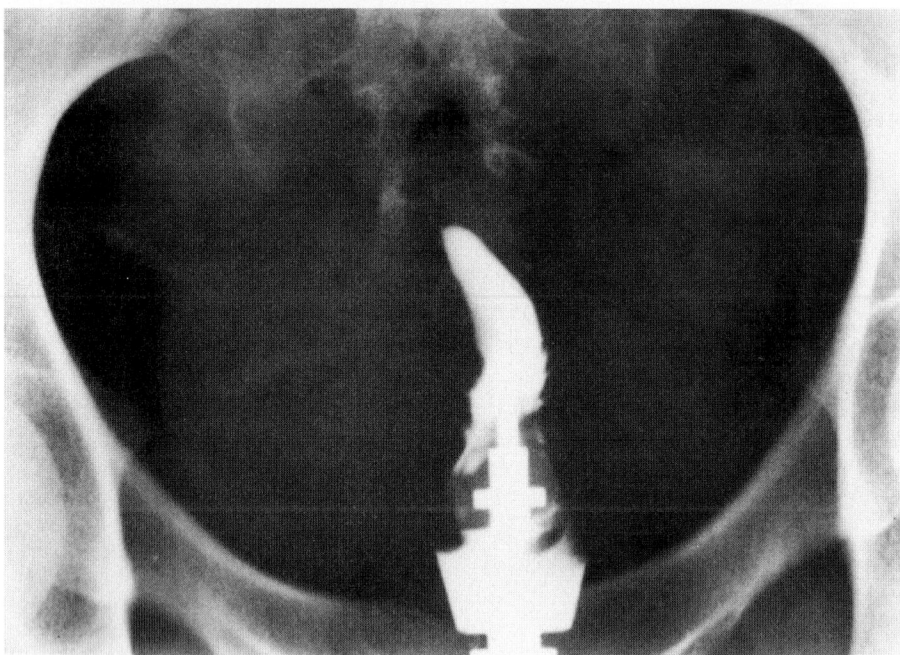

FIGURE 38-7   X-ray film of patient with Asherman syndrome. Patient (33 years, gravida 3, para O, abortus 3) had been amenorrheic for 6 months after D&C for most recent therapeutic abortion (TAB). Filling of endocervical canal and nonvisualization of endometrial cavity are consistent with complete obliteration of cavity by adhesions or with obstruction at internal os level by adhesions in lower endometrial cavity. This appearance may also be seen with advanced endometrial tuberculosis. (From Richmond JA: Hysterosalpingography. Reproduced with permission from Infertility, contraception and reproductive endocrinology, ed 4, by Daniel R. Mishell, Jr., M.D., and Val Davajan, M.D. Copyright 1997 by Blackwell Scientific Publications, Malden, Mass. All rights reserved.)

CNS-Hypothalamic Causes

LESIONS.   The same anatomic lesions in the brainstem or hypothalamus that can produce primary amenorrhea by interfering with GnRH release can also cause secondary amenorrhea. Hypothalamic lesions include craniopharyngiomas, granulomatous disease (tuberculosis and sarcoidosis), and sequelae of encephalitis. When such uncommon lesions are present, circulating gonadotrophin levels and estradiol levels are low, and withdrawal uterine bleeding will not occur after progesterone administration.

DRUGS.   Phenothiazine derivatives, certain antihypertensive agents, and other drugs listed in Chapter 39 can also produce amenorrhea without hyperprolactinemia, although usually the prolactin levels are elevated. Therefore, every individual with secondary amenorrhea should have a detailed medication history obtained even if galactorrhea is not present. Oral contraceptive steroids inhibit ovulation by acting both on the hypothalamus to suppress GnRH and directly on the pituitary to suppress FSH and LH. Occasionally this hypothalamic-pituitary suppression persists for several months after oral contraceptives are discontinued, producing the syndrome termed *postpill amenorrhea.* This oral contraceptive-induced suppression does not last more than 6 months. It has been reported that the incidence of amenorrhea persisting more than 6 months after discontinuation of high-dose oral contraceptives (0.8%) is about the same as the incidence of secondary amenorrhea in the general population (0.7%). Thus the etiology of amenorrhea persisting more than 6 months after discontinuation of oral contraceptives is unrelated to their use, except that the regular withdrawal bleeding produced by oral contraceptives masks the development of this symptom. With use of lower-dose contraception steroids, ovulation usually resumes promptly after their discontinuation, and the syndrome of postpill amenorrhea is an uncommon occurrence.

STRESS AND EXERCISE.   Stressful situations including a sudden change in environment (e.g., going away to school), a death in the family, or divorce can produce amenorrhea. A high percentage of women who had been placed in concentration camps or those sentenced for execution also became amenorrheic as a result of stress.

It is also now believed that the amenorrhea associated with strenuous exercise is also related to stress. Feicht et al. reported that the incidence of secondary amenorrhea in runners had a positive correlation with the number of miles run per week (Figure 38-8). In a comparison of amenorrheic and eumenorrheic athletes, they reported that physical parameters such as age, weight, lean body mass, and body fat were similar. The only significant difference between the two groups was the fact that the amenorrheic athletes ran more miles per week. McArthur et al. also reported there was no significant difference in the percent-

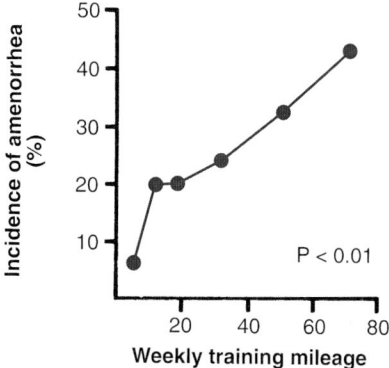

FIGURE 38-8 Correlation between training mileage and amenorrhea. Each point represents average of 21 respondents. Statistical significance of relationship was obtained from point-biserial correlation (1 mile [1.6 km]). (From Feicht CB, Johnson TS, and Matrin BJ: Lancet 2:1145, 1978.)

age of body fat in amenorrheic runners compared with runners who were menstruating. In a longitudinal study of competitive swimmers, Russell et al. found that when the training became more strenuous, their LH and FSH levels fell significantly, while levels of beta-endorphin and catechol estrogens rose significantly as compared with levels of these hormones when the swimmers were exercising to a moderate degree (Tables 38-4 and 38-5). Individuals with a low percentage of adipose tissue have a shift in the pathway of estrogen metabolism from 16-hydroxylation, which forms estriol, to 2-hydroxylation, which forms catechol estrogens. It has been postulated that the decreased fatty tissue in individuals who exercise is the reason for the increased levels of catechol estrogens. However, when the swimmers were exercising only moderately, levels of catechol estrogens as well as beta-endorphin were not significantly different from those of a control group of similar body weight and percentage body fat who were not participating in organized physical activity. This group of investigators also reported that another group of swimmers and runners had significantly higher levels of catechol estrogens than a control group of normally menstruating women with a similar weight and low percentage of body fat. Whether catechol estrogens are increased as a result of less fatty tissue, the stress of training, or a combination of both, the increase may be the cause of the amenorrhea. The competition between catecholamine and catechol estrogens for catechol-O-methyltransferase may result in increased levels of dopamine, which in turn suppresses the release of GnRH and thus LH. Adashi et al. showed that infusion or injection of catechol estrogens decreased LH levels in humans.

Carr et al. also reported that physical conditioning facilitates the exercise-induced secretion of beta-endorphin and its precursor beta-lipoprotein in women. Reid et al. showed that infusion of beta-endorphin into women caused a significant decrease in LH. Beta-endorphin and its analogues inhibit GnRH release, possibly by inhibiting the stimulating effect of norepinephrine on GnRH. Russell et al. (1989) administered the opioid antagonist naloxone to a group of oligomenorrheic and eumenorrheic competitive swimmers and noted an increase in baseline LH only in the former group.

Nappi et al. measured both pulsatile cortisol secretion and plasma cortisol response to naloxone and corticotropin-releasing hormone in a group of women with stress-related amenorrhea. There was a lack of naloxone-stimulated adrenal release of cortisol and a blunted response to corticotropin-releasing hormone in these women. As a result it was concluded that the stress caused impaired activity of the opioid and serotonin neurotransmitters, resulting in

TABLE 38-4

Analysis* of Protein Hormones for Swimmers During Moderate and Strenuous Exercise and for Nonexercising Control Subjects

	Swimmers			Group Comparison (Median Values)		
Hormone	Control Subjects	Moderate (60,000 yards)	Strenuous (100,000 yards)	C vs. 60	C vs. 100	100 vs. 60
No.	6	5	5			
LH (mIU/ml)	23.1[21.4] ± 10.5 (12.3–13.3)	22.9[22.2] ± 5.7 (15.9–30.7)	10.9[11.3] ± 2.8 (7.4–13.6)	$P = 0.66$	$P = 0.02$	$P = 0.02$
FSH (mIU/ml)	10.9[9.6] ± 3.5 (7.1–15.7)	20.2[18.2] ± 5.1 (15.3–27.7)	6.54[6.8] ± 2.1 (4.0–9.5)	$P = 0.05$	$P = 0.04$	$P \leq 0.001$
Prolactin (ng/ml)	20.8[13.5] ± 15.0 (9.0–47.2)	10.6[10.5] ± 3.6 (5.9–16.1)	1.36[1.0] ± 0.9 (0.7–3.0)	$P = 0.18$	$P = 0.004$	$P = 0.006$

Adapted from Russel JB, Mitchell DE, Musey PI, et al: Fertil Steril 42:690, 1984. Reproduced with permission of the publisher, The American Fertility Society.

*Mean (median) value ± SD with range in parentheses.

TABLE 38-5
Analysis* of Beta-Endorphin Immunoreactivity, Estradiol, and Catechol Estrogens for Swimmers During Moderate and Strenuous Exercise and for Nonexercising Control Subjects

| Hormone | Swimmers | | | Group Comparison | | |
	Control Subjects	Moderate (60,000 yards)	Strenuous (100,000 yards)	C vs. 60	C vs. 100	100 vs. 60
No.	6	5	5			
Estradiol (pg/ml)	264[193] ± 253 (78–759)	61.8[65] ± 16.8 (36–79)	76.8[52] ± 61.9 (36–185)	$P = 0.009$	$P = 0.003$	$P = 0.68$
Catechol estrogens (pg/ml)	35.3[35] ± 7.5 (25–46)	28.6[28] ± 1.2 (26–29)	92.4[88] ± 12.8 (83–115)	$P = 0.08$	$P \leq 0.001$	$P \leq 0.001$
Beta-endorphin immuno-reactivity (pmol/L)	8.50[2] ± 15.4 (2–40)	4.40[4] ± 2.2 (2–8)	31.2[24] ± 14.3 (18–52)	$P = 0.25$	$P = 0.03$	$P = 0.01$

Adapted from Russel JB, Mitchell DE, Musey PI, et al: Fertil Steril 42:690, 1984. Reproduced with permission of the publisher, The American Fertility Society.

*Mean (median) value ± SD with range in parentheses.

multiple alterations in the hypothalamic control of the pituitary gland. Thus the increase in both catechol estrogens and beta-endorphins associated with strenuous exercise appears to be the mechanism whereby LH and probably FSH release is inhibited, most likely by acting on the neurotransmitters responsible for release of GnRH. The decreased gonadotrophin levels produce amenorrhea by failing to stimulate sex steroid production.

It is probable that emotionally stressful situations such as divorce or a sudden change in environment can also cause alterations in beta-endorphin and catechol estrogens. When the stressful situation (whether emotional in origin or related to strenuous exercise) abates, normal cyclic ovarian function and regular menses usually resume in a few months.

WEIGHT LOSS. Both male and female animals who are malnourished have decreased reproductive capacity. Weight loss is also associated with amenorrhea in women and has been classified into two groups: the moderately underweight group includes individuals whose weight is 15% to 25% below ideal body weight; severely underweight women are those whose weight loss is greater than 25% of ideal body weight. Weight loss can occur from excessive dietary restrictions as well as malnutrition. Vigersky et al. have demonstrated that women with amenorrhea associated with simple weight loss have both direct and indirect evidence of hypothalamic dysfunction, while pituitary and end-organ function is normal. Mason and Sagle showed that in contrast to women with normal cycles, a group of women with weight loss amenorrhea had similar mean levels of LH as well as LH pulse amplitude but decreased frequency of LH pulses. Warren et al. however, showed that when women were severely underweight, in addition to hypothalamic dysfunction, pituitary gonadotrophin function was also altered because

there was no increase in LH and a decreased response of FSH following GnRH administration. However, these responses could be due to a lack of prolonged GnRH secretion, because the studies were not performed after several days of GnRH priming. Thus the amenorrhea associated with weight loss appears to be due mainly to failure of normal GnRH release, with a possible pituitary disorder also occurring when the weight loss is severe.

Criteria for Diagnosis of Anorexia Nervosa

Onset before 25 years of age
Anorexia with accompanying weight loss of at least 25% of original body weight
Distorted, implacable attitude toward eating, food, or weight that overrides hunger, admonitions, reassurance, and threats; for example:
Denial of illness
Failure to recognize nutritional needs
Apparent enjoyment in losing weight
Desired body image of extreme thinness
Unusual hoarding or handling of food
No known medical illness that could account for the anorexia and weight loss
No other known psychiatric disorder
At least two of the following manifestations:
Amenorrhea
Lanugo
Bradycardia (persistent resting pulse of 60 bpm or less)
Periods of overactivity
Episodes of bulimia
Vomiting (may be self-induced)

From Sherman BM, Halmi KA, and Zamudio R: J Clin Endocrinol Metab 41:135, 1975. Copyright 1975 by the Endocrine Society.

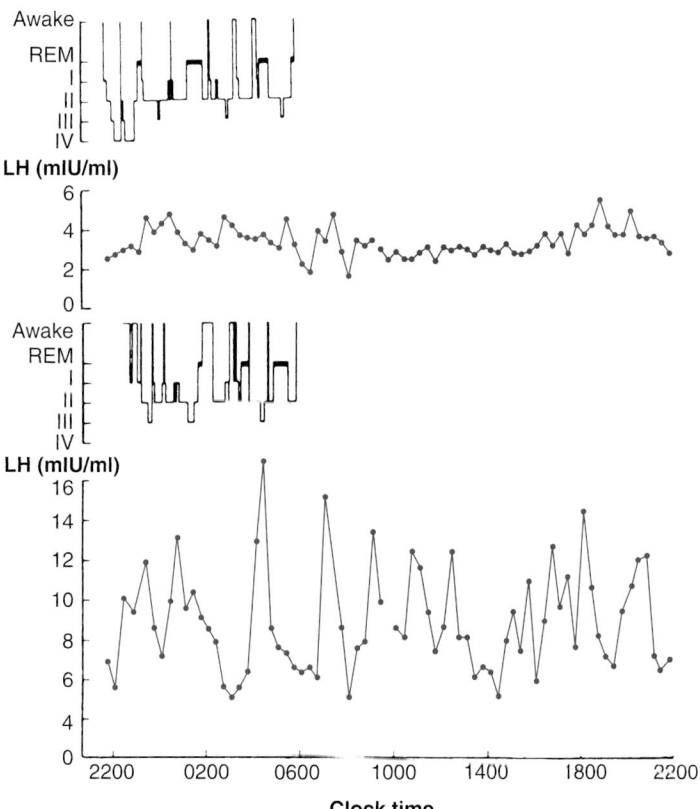

FIGURE 38-9 Plasma LH concentrations every 20 minutes for 24 hours during acute exacerbation of anorexia nervosa *(upper panel)* and after clinical remission with return of body weight to normal *(lower panel)*. (From Boyar RM, Katz J, Finkelstein JW, et al: N Engl J Med 291:861, 1974. Reprinted by permission of The New England Journal of Medicine.)

A severe psychiatric disorder called *anorexia nervosa* is also associated with severe weight loss and amenorrhea. Anorexia nervosa is not rare; it is estimated to occur in about 1 in 1000 white women in the United States. It is uncommon in men and rare in blacks and Asians. This disorder is most frequent in teenagers and is uncommon after the age of 25. It is one of the most important and probably the most common causes of secondary amenorrhea in adolescent women. This disorder is associated with other physical changes, including dry skin, bradycardia, hypotension, constipation, and hypothermia (see box at left). Individuals with anorexia nervosa usually have a normal thyroxine (T_4) level and an abnormally low serum triiodothyronine (T_3) level. If the clinician cannot make the differential diagnosis between amenorrhea caused by simple weight loss and that caused by anorexia nervosa on clinical findings alone, measurement of the serum T_3 level is most helpful, as individuals with simple weight loss usually have normal T_3 levels. In women with anorexia nervosa T_4 levels are normal, T_3 levels are low, and reverse T_3 (an inactive metabolite) levels are increased, indicating that peripheral conversion of T_4 to T_3 is impaired. Women with anorexia nervosa have a hypothalamic disorder interfering with normal GnRH release, and their amenorrhea frequently occurs at the time of initiation of food restric-

tion before they lose weight. However, after severe weight loss occurs in these individuals and they are less than 25% of ideal body weight, an abnormal gonadotrophin response to GnRH takes place similar to that seen in individuals with severe weight loss caused by dieting. This indicates that pituitary dysfunction also occurs in persons with anorexia nervosa when the weight loss becomes severe. Boyar et al. have shown that women with anorexia nervosa have an LH secretion pattern similar to that observed in prepubertal children (absent LH pulses) (Figure 38-9) or pubertal premenarcheal girls (nocturnal LH pulses only). When these individuals gain weight, the normal 24-hour LH pulsatile patterns return. Weight gain in either individuals with anorexia nervosa or those with severe simple weight loss results in their gonadotrophin response to GnRH infusion becoming normal or even exaggerated, with the FSH response resuming in proportion to the weight gain and the LH responsiveness returning only after the individual reaches about 85% of ideal body weight. These progressive endocrine responses are also similar to those occurring during puberty, indicating the importance of body weight in causing maturation of the CNS-hypothalamic-pituitary axis and providing additional information as to why girls who exercise strenuously before menarche and have less body fat also have a delayed onset of menstruation. Frisch and Revelle reported that undernourished girls reach menarche at an older age but at the same mean weight as well-nourished girls. Treasure et al., using ultrasound scanning, showed that as women with anorexia nervosa gained weight, changes occurred in ovarian morphology. These changes progressed from small ovaries without follicles, to ovaries of normal size and multiple small follicles and finally to the appearance of a dominant follicle. These changes are similar to the changes in ovarian morphology that occur during normal pubertal development.

Anorexia nervosa is a psychiatric disorder, and women with this disease should receive appropriate psychiatric treatment. These individuals, as well as those with dietary weight loss, usually resume ovulatory menstrual cycles when they gain weight and approach their ideal body weight.

POLYCYSTIC OVARY SYNDROME. Polycystic ovary syndrome (PCOS) is a CNS-hypothalamic disorder that usually produces tonically elevated LH levels. Most of the women with these disorders have elevated androgen levels, but not all have clinical evidence of androgen excess (hirsutism). Thus the presence of PCOS must be considered in the differential diagnosis of both primary and secondary amenorrhea even if signs of hyperandrogenism are absent. Because most individuals with PCOS have signs of androgen excess, this subject is discussed in detail in Chapter 40.

FUNCTIONAL HYPOTHALAMIC AMENORRHEA. There is a group of individuals with secondary amenorrhea who do not ingest drugs, do not engage in strenuous exercise, are not undergoing environmental stress, and have not lost weight. No pituitary, ovarian, or uterine abnormalities are present in these individuals. The general term *functional hypothalamic amenorrhea* (FHA) has been used to characterize this disorder. During normal ovulatory cycles, LH is secreted in a pulsatile manner that varies in frequency and amplitude at different times of the cycle, being more rapid in the follicular phase than in the luteal phase (Figure 38-10). Women with amenorrhea due to hypothalamic dysfunction do not exhibit these characteristic cyclic alterations in LH pulsatility. They either have no pulses (Figure 38-11) or have a persistent pattern of pulsatility that is normally found in only one portion of the ovulatory cycle, usually the slow frequency normally found in the luteal phase, despite having a steroid milieu similar to the follicular phase (Figure 38-12). Since each LH pulse represents a response to a pulse of GnRH, it appears that individuals with FHA have an abnormality in the normal cyclic variations of GnRH pulsatility, probably due to an abnormality in the CNS neurotransmitters and possibly produced by increased opioid activity. As reported by Ferin et al., Quigley et al., and Wildt and Leyendecker, administration of the opioid antagonists naloxone and naltrexone to women with FHA is followed

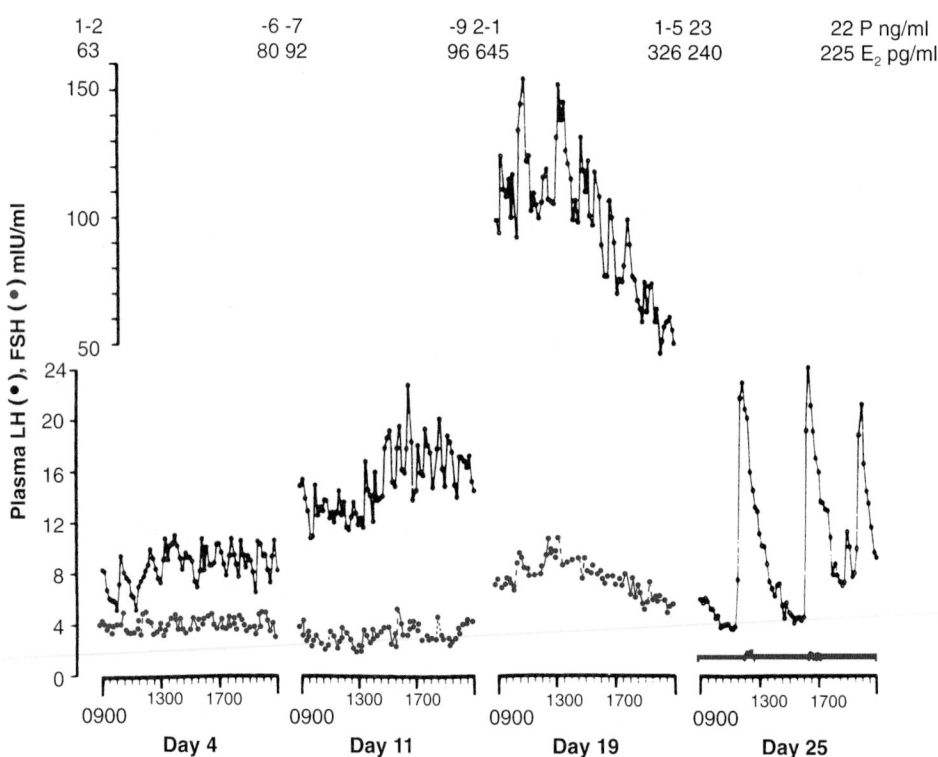

FIGURE 38-10 Serial measurements of plasma LH and FSH in two subjects sampled every 10 minutes at weekly intervals during cycles in which LH surge was observed on one of sampling days. (From Reame NE, Sauder SE, Kelch RP, et al: J Clin Endocrinol Metab 59:328, 1984. Copyright 1984 by The Endocrine Society.)

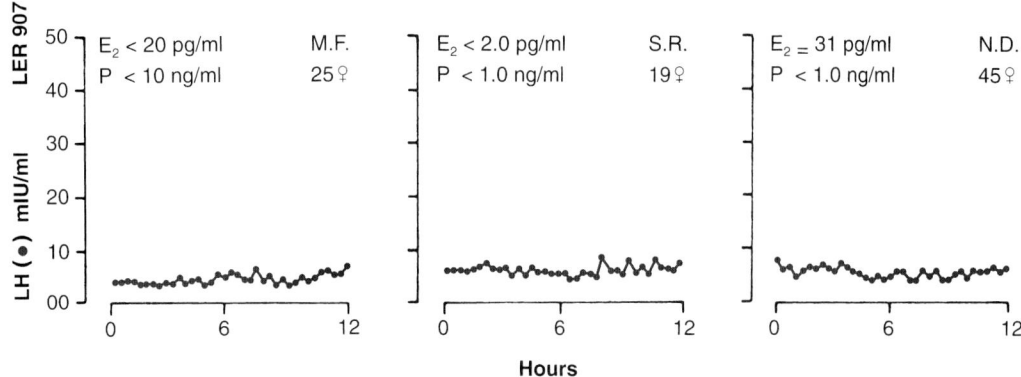

FIGURE 38-11 A pulsatile pattern of LH secretion in women with hypogonadotrophic hypogonadism and hypothalamic amenorrhea. (From Crowley WF Jr, Filicori M, Spratt DI, et al: Rec Prog Hormone Res 41:473, 1985.)

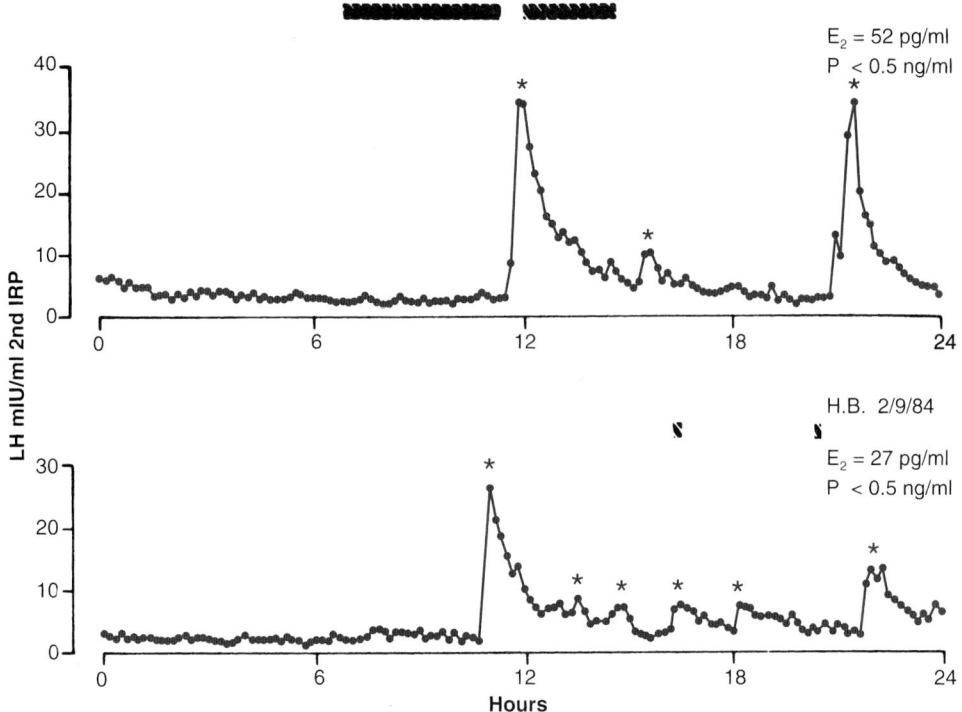

FIGURE 38-12 Defects in frequency of LH secretion episodes in subjects with hypothalamic amenorrhea. Asterisks indicate LH pulses. (From Crowley WF Jr, Filicori M, Spratt DI, et al: Rec Prog Hormone Res 41:473, 1985.)

by an increase in frequency of LH pulses as well as induction of ovulation.

Berga et al. measured several pituitary hormones at frequent intervals in a 24-hour period in 10 women with FHA and 10 women with normal cycles. As also reported by others, they found a 53% reduction in LH pulse frequency among the women with FHA; however, the LH pulse amplitude was similar in the two groups. In addition to reduced secretion of LH, there was reduced secretion of FSH, prolactin, and thyroid-stimulating hormone (TSH), as well as altered rhythms of growth hormone (GH) and cortisol with elevated cortisol levels. However, the pituitary response to releasing hormones was unchanged. Thus multiple hormonal alterations occur in FHA as an adaptive central neuroendocrine event.

When sufficient GnRH is produced to stimulate sufficient gonadotrophin production to maintain circulating estradiol levels above 40 pg/ml, the term *hypothalamic-pituitary dysfunction* is used to characterize this disorder. However, when the estradiol levels fall below 40 pg/ml, the term *hypothalamic-pituitary failure* has been used, indicating a more serious disorder. Serum estradiol levels above 40 pg/ml are usually sufficient to stimulate endometrial growth to an extent that sloughing occurs when progesterone levels fall several days after exogenous progestins are last administered. The withdrawal bleeding response to progesterone administration has also been used to differentiate between these two diagnostic categories.

Pituitary Causes
(Hypoestrogenic Amenorrhea)

NEOPLASMS. Although most pituitary tumors secrete prolactin, some do not and may be associated with the onset of secondary amenorrhea without hyperprolactinemia. Chromophobe adenomas are the most common non–prolactin-secreting pituitary tumors; however, both basophilic (ACTH secreting) and acidophilic (GH secreting) adenomas may be incapable of secreting prolactin. Individuals with the latter types of tumor, although having secondary amenorrhea, frequently have other symptoms produced by these lesions and present to the clinician with symptoms of acromegaly, or Cushing syndrome.

NONNEOPLASTIC LESIONS. Pituitary cells can also become damaged or necrotic as a result of anoxia, thrombosis, or hemorrhage. When pituitary cell destruction occurs as a result of a hypotensive episode during pregnancy, the disorder is called *Sheehan syndrome.* When the disorder is unrelated to pregnancy, it is called *Simmond disease.* It is important to diagnose this cause of secondary amenorrhea, because in contrast to the hypothalamic disorders, pituitary damage can be associated with decreased secretion of other pituitary hormones, particularly ACTH and TSH, in addition to LH and FSH. Thus these individuals may have secondary hypothyroidism or adrenal insufficiency that may seriously impair their health, in addition to their decreased estrogen levels.

Ovarian Causes
(Hypogonadotrophic Hypogonadism)

The ovaries may fail to secrete sufficient estrogen to produce endometrial growth if the follicles are damaged as a result of infection, interference with blood supply, or depletion of follicles caused by bilateral cystectomies. These individuals may become amenorrheic after a variable period of time has elapsed following medical treatment of bilateral tuboovarian abscess, after bilateral cystectomy for benign ovarian neoplasms, or sometimes after a hysterectomy during which the vascular supply to the ovaries is compromised (sometimes called *cystic degeneration of the ovaries*).

Occasionally the ovaries cease to produce sufficient estrogen to stimulate endometrial growth several years before the age of the physiologic menopause. When this condition occurs before the age of 40, the term *premature ovarian failure* (POF) instead of premature menopause is best used to describe the clinical entity. Coulam et al. estimated that as many as 1% of women under age 40 have hypergonadotrophic amenorrhea, with the incidence

steadily increasing from ages 15 to 39. Frequently the condition of POF is transient before permanent ovarian failure occurs; occasionally, individuals with a diagnoses of POF may ovulate and conceive during this transition period. POF frequently occurs after gonadal irradiation or systemic chemotherapy. POF has also been reported in individuals with steroid hormonal enzyme deficiencies who menstruate temporarily and then have secondary amenorrhea.

Histologically, individuals with POF have two types of ovarian pathologic findings. In the majority there is generalized sclerosis similar to the findings of a normal postmenopausal ovary (Figure 38-13), whereas in about 30% numerous primordial follicles with no progression past the antrum stage are seen (Figure 38-14). The latter condition has been called the *gonadotrophin-resistant ovary syndrome* or *ovarian hypofolliculogenesis* and is histologically different from the gonadal streak, in which no follicles are seen. Women with this condition may have primary amenorrhea, but usually sufficient estrogen is produced so that they menstruate for several months or even years. Many individuals with POF, particularly those with primordial follicles that appear normal, also have an autoimmune disease such as hypoparathyroidism, Hashimoto's thyroiditis, or Addison's disease. Many individuals with POF who do not have clinical evidence of an autoimmune disease have antibodies to gonadotrophins as well as to several other endocrine organs such as the thyroid and adrenal glands, suggesting an autoimmune etiology.

Alper and Garner estimated that about 30% to 50% of individuals with chromosomally normal POF without a history of irradiation or chemotherapy have an associated autoimmune disease, most commonly thyroid disease, which was present in 85% of the group with an autoimmune disorder. Mignot et al., using sophisticated immunofluorescence techniques, demonstrated that 92% of women with POF had laboratory evidence of autosensitization. About two thirds of these were positive for nonorgan-specific antibodies, mainly antinuclear antibodies and rheumatoid factors. Fifty percent had organ-specific antibodies. Although the majority of these women had no evidence of autoimmune disease, it is recommended that immunologic screening be performed on all individuals under age 35 who have POF.

Diagnostic Evaluation and Management

All women who consult a clinician for the symptom of secondary amenorrhea should have a diagnostic evaluation initiated at that visit, even though 6 months may not have elapsed since the last menstrual period. Amenorrhea is a source of concern to the woman, and it will relieve her concern if attempts are made to find the cause of the symptom. The clinician first should perform a detailed history and physical examination to rule out pregnancy as a cause of the amenorrhea. In addition, he

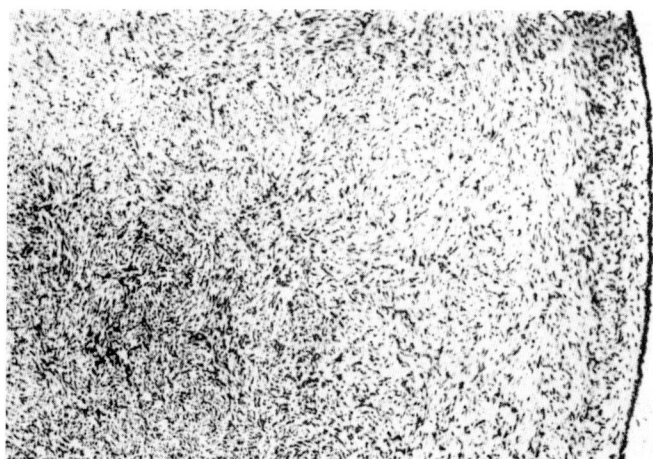

FIGURE 38-13 Representative section of ovary from patient with premature ovarian failure (POF). Cortex of ovary is devoid of follicles. (From Tulandi T and Kinch RAH: Obstet Gynecol Surv 35:521, 1981.)

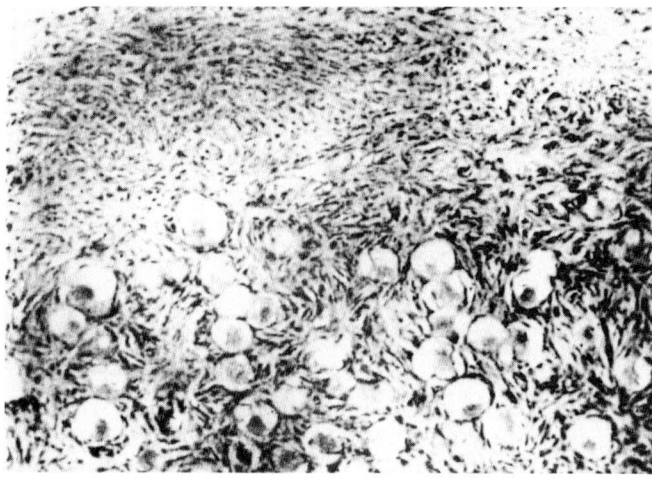

FIGURE 38-14 Representative section of ovary from patient with insensitive ovary syndrome. Numerous primordial follicles are seen. (From Tulandi T and Kinch RAH: Obstet Gynecol Surv 35:521, 1981.)

or she should determine whether there is the possibility of IUA. Any instrumentation of the endometrial cavity, particularly temporally related to pregnancy, should alert the clinician to the possibility that IUA are present. The initial diagnostic evaluation to determine if IUA are present is placement of a uterine sound into the uterine cavity followed by a hysterography or hysteroscopy. The diagnosis can also be confirmed by detecting presumptive evidence of ovulation by means of either a biphasic basal temperature or an elevated serum progesterone level. If IUA are ruled out, the history should disclose whether medications are currently being used or if oral contraceptives have been recently discontinued. In addition, questions regarding diet, weight loss, stress, and strenuous exercise are pertinent. A history of hot flushes, decreasing breast size, or vaginal dryness and physical examination of these organs are helpful in estimating the degree of estrogen deficiency. If the history and physical examination fail to reveal the cause of the amenorrhea, a complete blood count, urinalysis, and serum chemistries should be measured to rule out systemic disease. A sensitive TSH assay should also be performed to rule out the uncommon asymptomatic thyroid disorders that produce secondary amenorrhea, and serum estradiol, FSH, and prolactin levels should be measured (Figure 38-15). If prolactin levels are elevated, a diagnostic evaluation for the etiology of this problem should be undertaken, as discussed in Chapter 39. Administration of injectable progesterone or oral progestins are an indirect means to determine if sufficient estrogen is present to produce endometrial growth that will slough after the progesterone levels fall (progesterone challenge test). Before estradiol assays became generally available for clinical use, this procedure was widely used to provide a rough estimate of circulating estrogen levels.

Currently there is little need for this procedure except to reassure the woman that she can menstruate. In addition the observation of withdrawal bleeding after progesterone indicates that estradiol secretion is not markedly decreased (usually above 40 pg/ml) and the cause of the amenorrhea is not as serious as if bleeding had not occurred. Women with PCOS, moderate stress, exercise, weight loss, or hypothalamic-pituitary dysfunction will usually have estradiol levels above 40 pg/ml, and withdrawal bleeding after progestins usually occurs. Individuals with pituitary tumors, ovarian failure, severe dietary weight loss or anorexia nervosa, severe stress, or the rare hypothalamic lesions will usually have low estradiol levels (less than 40 pg/ml), and they will not have withdrawal bleeding after progesterone administration.

If the estradiol level is above 40 pg/ml, a diagnosis of PCOS is confirmed by finding sonographic evidence of more than 10 follicles in each ovary. Even if hirsutism is absent, when there is sonographic evidence of PCOS, serum testosterone and DHEA-S should be measured to determine if either or both are elevated. If estradiol levels are above 40 pg/ml and there is no sonographic evidence of polycystic ovaries, and a history of drug ingestion, stress, weight loss, or strenuous exercise is not obtained, the woman should be told that hypothalamic-pituitary dysfunction is present and the exact etiology cannot be determined with current technology, as frequent LH sampling is costly and impractical. She should also be informed that hypothalamic-pituitary dysfunction is usually a self-limiting disorder and not a serious threat to health or a cause of untreatable infertility.

Women with low estradiol and low FSH levels have either a CNS lesion or hypothalamic pituitary failure. Women with low estradiol and elevated FSH levels (>30

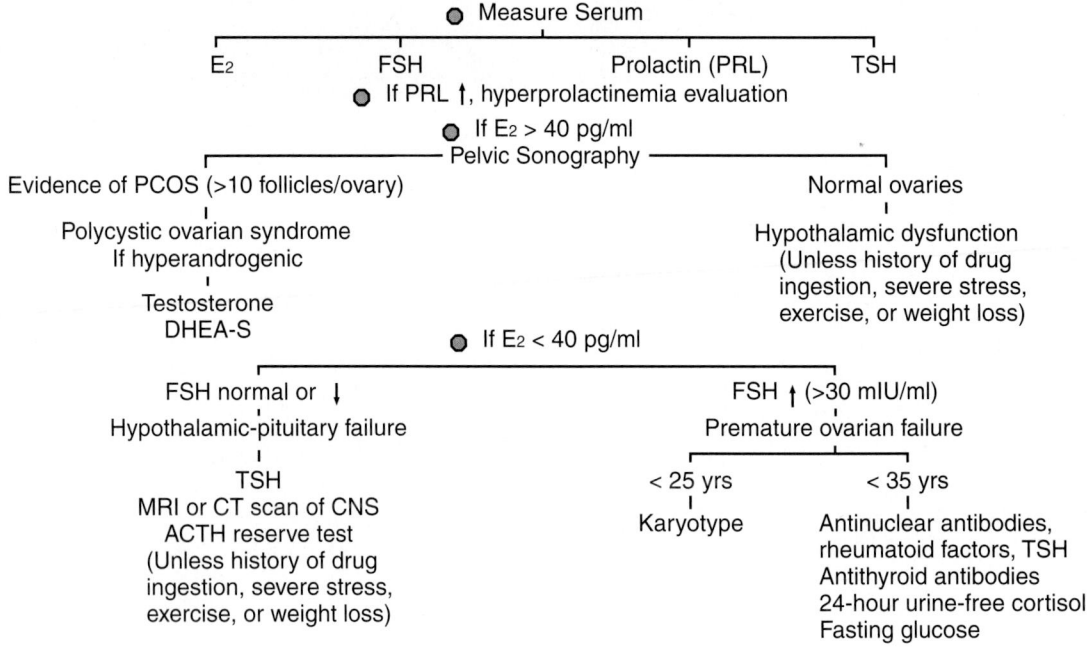

FIGURE 38-15 Diagnostic evaluation of secondary amenorrhea.

mIU/ml) have POF. If severe weight loss, strenuous exercise, or severe stress is not present, and FSH and estradiol levels are low, a CT scan of the hypothalamic-pituitary region should be performed to rule out a lesion, even if the prolactin level is normal. If a lesion is seen or if there is a history compatible with possible pituitary destruction (hypotension during pregnancy), a test of ACTH reserve should be performed. An insulin tolerance test in which hypoglycemia is induced should normally cause a cortisol increase of 6 μg/100 ml within 120 minutes and is a satisfactory test of ACTH function. If no lesion is identified, the term *hypothalamic-pituitary failure* may be used as a nonspecific diagnosis. Frequently individuals with this diagnosis resume normal ovarian function without treatment.

If POF is diagnosed because of an elevated FSH level and no cause of ovarian destruction is elicited, the possibility of autoimmune disease should be considered if the woman is less than 35 years of age. Therefore antithyroid antibodies and antinuclear antibodies should be measured and a 24-hour urine-free cortisol level measured to detect possible Addison disease. In addition, tests to detect rheumatoid factors should be performed, and fasting blood sugar, serum calcium, phosphorus, and a sensitive TSH measurement should also be undertaken. To rule out mosaicism, a karyotype should be obtained in women with POF who are 25 or younger. Biopsy of the gonads by laparoscopy or laparotomy is not indicated as individuals with POF are usually sterile, although occasionally a follicle may ovulate. Suppression of gonadotrophin levels with estrogen, oral contraceptives, and GnRH analogues has

been advocated to induce rebound ovulation following their withdrawal. Although gonadotrophins are suppressed by these agents, these techniques are usually ineffective for inducing ovulation. If ovulation occurs following such treatment, it is a sporadic event and not a result of the therapy.

The appropriate treatment depends upon the diagnosis and on whether conception is desired. Non–prolactin-secreting pituitary tumors should be surgically excised if possible. Individuals with weight loss should be advised to gain weight. If strenuous exercise results in low estrogen levels (<30 pg/ml), the amount of exercise should be reduced or estrogen supplementation administered to prevent possible development of osteoporosis. Several investigators have shown that amenorrheic as well as oligomenorrheic athletes with decreased estradiol levels have decreased density of trabecular bone in the lumbar spine (Figure 38-16). Klibanski et al. also have shown that women with low estradiol levels caused by hypothalamic amenorrhea who have normal nutrition and activity levels have a profound reduction in spinal bone density. In contrast to an earlier report by Schlechte et al., who postulated that individuals with hypoestrogenic amenorrhea did not have decreased bone loss unless they had hyperprolactinemia, Klibanski et al. reported that hyperprolactinemia by itself did not influence the degree of bone loss. In their study bone loss was similar in hyperprolactinemic amenorrheic women with low estrogen levels and women with normal prolactin and low estrogen levels (Figure 38-17). A group of women with hyperprolactinemia and regular menses did not have bone loss. Thus

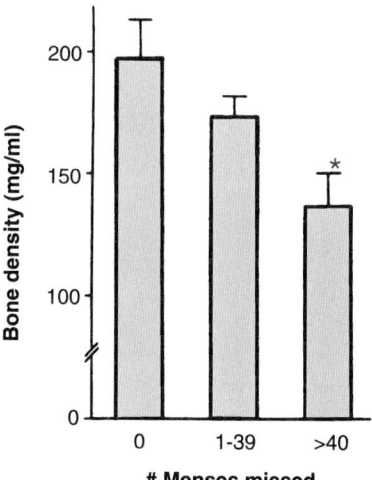

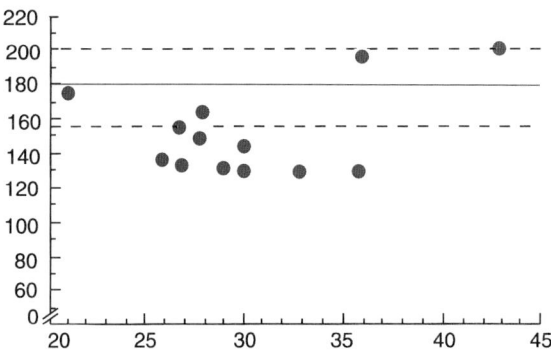

FIGURE 38-16 Relationship between bone density and number of missed menses in collegiate women athletes. For each subject, number of missed menses was determined from her menarche to age 19. Asterisk indicates significantly different from control group. (From Lloyd T and Myers C, et al: Obstet Gynecol 72:639, 1988.)

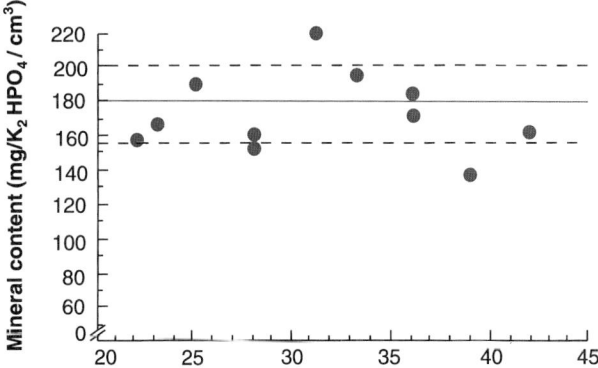

bone loss is directly related to decreased endogenous serum estradiol levels without being affected by hyperprolactinemia.

If women with PCOS or hypothalamic-pituitary dysfunction desire conception, clomiphene citrate administration is very successful in inducing ovulation. If pregnancy is not desired, monthly progestin administration (medroxyprogesterone acetate 10 mg/day for the first 12 days of each month) should be given to reduce the increased risk of endometrial cancer associated with unopposed estrogen. If women with hypothalamic-pituitary failure desire fertility, ovulation can be induced with human menopausal gonadotrophin (HMG) or intermittent GnRH. Clomiphene is not successful if the estrogen levels are low. If pregnancy is not desired, then estrogen-progestogen replacement is indicated for all amenorrheic women with low estradiol levels (<40 pg/ml), including those with POF, to reduce the risk of osteoporosis and atherosclerosis. Women with POF may become pregnant with the use of exogenous steroid stimulation of the endometrium and transfer of donor embryos.

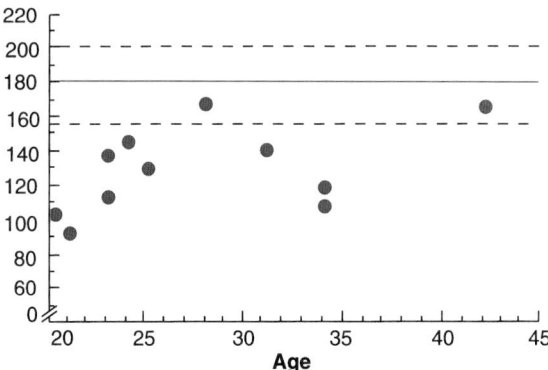

FIGURE 38-17 Spinal bone density in 13 women with hyperprolactinemic amenorrhea *(top panel)*, 12 eumenorrheic hyperprolactinemic women *(middle panel)*, and 11 women with hypothalamic amenorrhea *(bottom panel)*. Mean *(solid lines)* and standard deviation (± SD, *dashed lines*) for 19 normal women are shown. (From Klibanski A, Biller BMK, Rosenthal DI, et al: J Clin Endocrinol Metab 67:124, 1988.)

KEY POINTS

- The incidence of secondary amenorrhea of more than 6 months' duration in the general population is 0.7%.

- The incidence of amenorrhea lasting more than 6 months after discontinuation of oral contraceptives is 0.8%.

- The most important and probably most common cause of amenorrhea in adolescent girls is anorexia nervosa.

- A woman 13 years of age or older without any breast development has estrogen deficiency due to a severe abnormality and needs a diagnostic evaluation.

- Menarche is delayed about 0.4 year for each year of premenarcheal athletic training.

- Gonadal failure is the most common cause of primary amenorrhea, accounting for nearly half the patients with this syndrome.

- Individuals with gonadal failure and an X chromosome abnormality are less than 63 inches in height.

- The testes of individuals with androgen resistance have about a 20% chance of becoming malignant after age 20 years.

- Uterovaginal agenesis is the second most common cause of primary amenorrhea, with an incidence of about 15% of individuals with this symptom.

- About one third of individuals with gonadal failure have major cardiovascular or renal abnormalities.

- Congenital renal abnormalities occur in about one third of women with uterovaginal agenesis.

- The differential diagnosis between estrogen deficiency caused by gonadal failure and hypogonadotrophic hypogonadism is best established with measurement of serum follicle-stimulating hormone (FSH).

- The diagnosis of gonadal failure, or hypergonadotrophic hypogonadism, can be established if the FSH levels exceed 30 mIU/ml.

- Individuals with gonadal failure should have a peripheral karyotype performed to determine if a Y chromosome is present. If it is present, or signs of hyperandrogenism are present, the gonads should be excised to prevent development of malignancy, mainly a gonadoblastoma.

- Individuals with primary amenorrhea and hypogonatrophic hypogonadism do not need karyotyping but need a cranial computed tomography (CT) scan to rule out a central nervous system (CNS) tumor.

- The most frequent cause of intrauterine adhesions (IUA) is curettage performed during pregnancy or shortly thereafter.

- The amenorrhea associated with strenuous exercise is related to stress, not weight loss, and is most probably caused by an increase in CNS opioids (beta-endorphin) and catechol estrogens, both of which interfere with gonadotrophin-releasing hormone (GnRH) release.

- When women lose 15% below ideal body weight, amenorrhea can occur due to CNS-hypothalamic dysfunction. When weight loss decreases below 25% of ideal body weight, pituitary gonadotrophin function can also become abnormal.

- Anorexia nervosa occurs in about 1 in 1000 white women. It is uncommon in men and women older than 25 and rare in blacks and Asians.

- Individuals with anorexia nervosa have impaired peripheral conversion of thyroxine (T_4) to triiodothyronine (T_3), resulting in normal T_4 levels, decreased T_3 levels, and increased reverse T_3 levels.

- The normal cyclic pattern of luteinizing hormone (LH) pulsatility is not present in individuals with functional hypothalamic amenorrhea. Either no pulse or pulses of slow frequency, similar to those in the normal luteal phase, are usually observed.

- The GnRH alterations as reflected in LH pulsatility in persons with severe weight loss and anorexia nervosa are similar to those seen in normal prepubertal girls. When such individuals gain weight, GnRH changes similar to those occurring during puberty take place.

- When uterine bleeding fails to occur after progestin is administered, estradiol levels are usually lower than 40 pg/ml.

- In contrast to hypothalamic disorders, pituitary causes of amenorrhea can be associated with ACTH and TSH deficiency.

- Individuals with premature ovarian failure have two different histologic findings: generalized sclerosis or primordial follicles scattered through the stroma.

- Individuals with premature ovarian failure frequently have antibodies to gonadotrophins and other endocrine organs, indicating an autoimmune etiology.

- A karyotype should be obtained in women with premature ovarian failure younger than 25 but not in those who are older.

- Amenorrhea with low estrogen levels is associated with decreased density of trabecular bone.

- The most frequent cause of secondary amenorrhea is hypothalamic dysfunction.

BIBLIOGRAPHY

Adashi EY, Casper RF, Fishman J, et al: Stimulatory effect of 2-hydroxyestradiol on prolactin release in hypogonadal women, J Clin Endocrinol Metab 51:413, 1980.

Adashi EY, Rakoff J, Divers W, et al: The effect of acutely administered 2-hydroxyestrone on the release of gonadotropins and prolactin before and after estrogen priming in hypogonadal women, Obstet Gynecol Surv 35:363, 1980.

Alper MM and Garner PR: Premature ovarian failure: its relationship to autoimmune disease, Obstet Gynecol 66:27, 1985.

Berga SL, Mortola JF, Girton BS, et al: Neuroendocrine aberrations in women with functional hypothalamic amenorrhea, J Clin Endocrinol Metab 68:301, 1989.

Beumont PJV, George GCW, Pimstone BL, et al: Body weight and the pituitary response to hypothalamic releasing hormones in patients with anorexia nervosa, J Clin Endocrinol Metab 43:487, 1976.

Boyar RM, Katz J, Finkelstein JW, et al: Anorexia nervosa: immaturity of the 24-hour luteinizing hormone secretory pattern, N Engl J Med 291:861, 1974.

Carr DB, Bullen BA, Skrinar GS, et al: Physical conditioning facilitates the exercise-induced secretion of beta-endorphin and beta-lipotropin in women, N Engl J Med 305:560, 1981.

Coulam CB, Adamson SC, and Annegers JF: Incidence of premature ovarian failure, Obstet Gynecol 67:604, 1986.

Crowley WF Jr, Filicori M, Spratt DI, et al: The physiology of gonadotropin-releasing hormone (GnRH) secretion in men and women, Rec Prog Hormone Res 41:473, 1985.

Drinkwater BL, Nilson K, Chestnut CH III, et al: Bone mineral content of amenorrheic and eumenorrheic athletes, N Engl J Med 322:277, 1984.

Feicht CB, Johnson TS, and Matrin BJ: Secondary amenorrhea in athletes, Lancet 1:1145, 1978.

Ferin M, Van Vugt D, and Wardlaw S: The hypothalamic control of the menstrual cycle and the role of endogenous opioid peptides, Recent Prog Horm Res 40:441, 1984.

Friedman CI, Barrows H, and Kim MH: Hypergonadotropic hypogonadism, Am J Obstet Gynecol 145:360, 1983.

Fries H, Nillius SJ, and Pettersson F: Epidemiology of secondary amenorrhea, Am J Obstet Gynecol 118:473, 1974.

Frisch RE, Gotz-Welbergen AV, McArthur JW, et al: Delayed menarche and amenorrhea of college athletes in relation to onset of training, JAMA 246:1559, 1981.

Frisch RE and Revelle R: Height and weight at menarche and a hypothesis of critical body weights and adolescent events, Science 169:397, 1970.

Frisch RE and Revelle R: Height and weight at menarche and a hypothesis of menarche, Arch Dis Child 46:695, 1971.

Frisch RE, Rose E, Wyshak G, et al: Delayed menarche and amenorrhea in ballet dancers, N Engl J Med 303:17, 1980.

Goldenberg RL, Grodin JM, Aodbard D, and Ross GT: Gonadotropins in women with amenorrhea, Am J Obstet Gynecol 116:1003, 1973.

Griffin JE, Edwards C, Madden JD, et al: Congenital absence of the vagina, Ann Intern Med 85:224, 1976.

Ingram JM: The bicycle stool in the treatment of vaginal agenesis and stenosis: a preliminary report, Am J Obstet Gynecol 140:867, 1981.

Kletzky OA, Davajan V, Nakamura RM, et al: Clinical categorization of patients with secondary amenorrhea using progesterone-induced uterine bleeding and measurement of serum gonadotropin levels, Am J Obstet Gynecol 121:695, 1975.

Klibanski A, Biller BMK, Rosenthal DI, et al: Effects of prolactin and estrogen deficiency in amenorrheic bone loss, J Clin Endocrinol Metab 67:124, 1988.

LaBarbera AR, Miller MM, Ober C, et al: Autoimmune etiology in premature ovarian failure, Am J Reprod Immunol Microbiol 16:115, 1988.

Ledger WL, Thomas EJ, Browning D, et al: Suppression of gonadotrophin secretion does not reverse premature ovarian failure, Br J Obstet Gynaecol 96:196, 1989.

Lieblich JM, Rogol AD, White BJ, et al: Syndrome of anosmia with hypogonadotropic hypogonadism (Kallmann syndrome): clinical laboratory studies in 23 cases, Am J Med 73:506, 1982.

Lloyd T, Myers C, Buchanan JR, et al: Collegiate women athletes with irregular menses during adolescence have decreased bone density, Obstet Gynecol 72:639, 1988.

Marshall WA and Tanner JM: Variations in pattern of pubertal changes in girls, Arch Dis Child 44:291, 1969.

Maschchak CA, Kletzky OA, Davajan V, et al: Clinical and laboratory evaluation of patients with primary amenorrhea, Obstet Gynecol 57:715, 1981.

Mason HD and Sagle M: Reduced frequency of luteinizing hormone pulses in women with weight loss–related amenorrhea and multifollicular ovaries, Clin Endocrinol 280:611, 1988.

McArthur JW, Bullen BA, Beitins IZ, et al: Hypothalamic amenorrhea in runners of normal body composition, Endocr Res Commun 7:13, 1980.

Mignot MH, Schoemaker J, Kleingeld M, et al: Premature ovarian failure. I. The association with autoimmunity, Eur J Obstet Gynecol Reprod Biol 30:59, 1989.

Moraes-Ruehsen M de, Blizzard RM, Garcia-Bunuel R, et al: Autoimmunity and ovarian failure, Am J Obstet Gynecol 112:693, 1972.

Nappi RE, DÁmbrogio G, Petragglia F, et al: Hypothalamic amenorrhea: evidence for a central derangement of hypothalamic-pituitary-adrenal cortex axis activity, Fertil Steril 59:571, 1993.

Penny R, Goldstein IP, and Frasier SD: Gonadotropin excretion and body composition, Pediatrics 61:294, 1978.

Pettersson F, Fries H, and Nillius SJ: Epidemiology of secondary amenorrhea, Am J Obstet Gynecol 117:80, 1973.

Quigley ME, Sheehan KL, Casper RF, and Yen SSC: Evidence for increased dopaminergic and opioid activity in patients with hypothalamic hypogonadotropic hypogonadism, J Clin Endocrinol Metab 50:949, 1980.

Reame NE, Sauder SE, Case GD, et al: Pulsatile gonadotropin secretion in women with hypothalamic amenorrhea: evidence that reduced frequency of gonadotropin-releasing hormone secretion is the mechanism of persistent anovulation, J Clin Endocrinol Metab 61:851, 1985.

Reame NE, Sauder SE, Kelch RP, et al: Pulsatile gonadotropin secretion during the human menstrual cycle: evidence for altered frequency of gonadotropin-releasing hormone secretion, J Clin Endocrinol Metab 59:328, 1984.

Rebar RW and Connolly HV: Clinical features of young women with hypergonadotropic amenorrhea, Fertil Steril 53:804, 1990.

Rebar RW, Erickson GF, and Yen SSC: Idiopathic premature ovarian failure: clinical and endocrine characteristics, Fertil Steril 137:35, 1982.

Reid RL, Hoff JD, Yen SSC, et al: Effects of exogenous β-endorphin on pituitary hormone secretion and its disappearance rate in normal human subjects, J Clin Endocrinol Metab 52:1179, 1981.

Reindollar RH, Byrd JR, and McDonough PG: Delayed sexual development: a study of 252 patients, Am J Obstet Gynecol 140:371, 1981.

Reindollar RH, Novak M, Tho SPT, and McDonough PG: Adult-onset amenorrhea: a study of 262 patients, Am J Obstet Gynecol 155:531, 1986.

Rosen GF, Vermesh M, dÁblaing G, et al: The endocrinologic evaluation of a 45,X true hermaphrodite, Am J Obstet Gynecol 157:1272, 1987.

Russell JB, DeCherney AH, and Collins DC: The effect of naloxone and metoclopramide on the hypothalamic pituitary axis in oligomenorrheic and eumenorrheic swimmers, Fertil Steril 52:583, 1989.

Russell JB, Mitchell D, Musey PI, et al: The relationship of exercise to anovulatory cycles in female athletes: hormonal and physical characteristics, Obstet Gynecol 63:452, 1984.

Russell JB, Mitchell DE, Musey PI, et al: The role of β-endorphins and catechol estrogens on the hypothalamic-pituitary axis in female athletes, Fertil Steril 42:690, 1984.

Schenker JG and Margalioth EJ: Intrauterine adhesions: an updated appraisal, Fertil Steril 37:593, 1982.

Schlechte JA, Sherman B, and Martin R: Bone density in amenorrheic women with and without hyperprolactinemia, J Clin Endocrinol Metab 56:1120, 1983.

Sherman BM, Halmi KA, and Zamudio R: LH and FSH response to gonadotropin-releasing hormone in anorexia nervosa: effect of nutritional rehabilitation, J Clin Endocrinol Metab 41:135, 1975.

Treasure JL, King EA, Gordon PAL, et al: Cystic ovaries: a phase of anorexia nervosa, Lancet 28:1379, 1985.

Tulandi T and Finch RA: Premature ovarian failure, Obstet Gynecol Surv 36:521, 1981.

Vigersky RA, Andersen AF, Thompson RG, et al: Hypothalamic dysfunction in secondary amenorrhea associated with simple weight loss, N Engl J Med 297:1141, 1977.

Vigersky RA, Loriaux DL, Andersen AE, et al: Delayed pituitary hormone response to LRF and TRF in patients with secondary amenorrhea associated with simple weight loss, J Clin Endocrinol Metab 43:893, 1976.

Warren MP: The effects of exercise on pubertal progression and reproductive function in girls, J Clin Endocrinol Metab 51:1150, 1980.

Warren MP, Jewelwicz R, Dyrenfurth I, et al: The significance of weight loss in the evaluation of pituitary response to LH-RH in women with secondary amenorrhea, J Clin Endocrinol Metab 40:601, 1975.

Wildt L and Leyendecker G: Indication of ovulation by the chronic administration of naltrexone in hypothalamic amenorrhea, J Clin Endocrinol Metab 64:1334, 1987.

Hyperprolactinemia, Galactorrhea, and Pituitary Adenomas

Etiology, Differential Diagnosis, Natural History, Management

KEY TERMS

Bromocriptine (2-Br-Alpha-Ergocryptine Mesylate). Semisynthetic ergot alkaloid that is a dopamine receptor agonist and is used to treat hyperprolactinemia.

Cabergoline. A long-acting dopamine receptor agonist that directly inhibits secretion of prolactin from the pituitary and is an effective treatment for hyperprolactinemia.

Computed Tomography (CT). An imaging technique to detect soft tissue abnormalities that uses a computer to integrate differences in x-ray beam attenuation resulting from varying densities in adjacent tissue.

Craniopharyngioma. A rare hypothalamic tumor that can produce hyperprolactinemia.

Empty Sella Syndrome. An intrasellar extension of the subarachnoid space resulting in compression of the pituitary gland and an enlarged sella turcica that may be associated with galactorrhea and hyperprolactinemia.

Galactorrhea. Nonpuerperal secretion from the breast of watery or milky fluid that contains neither pus nor blood.

Hyperprolactinemia. Levels of circulating prolactin above normal (greater than 20 to 25 ng/ml) that can cause galactorrhea or amenorrhea or both.

Hypocycloidal Tomography. Multiple radiographs of the sella turcica at intervals of 2 to 3 mm with a hypocycloidal movement.

Macroadenoma. An uncommon type of prolactin-secreting pituitary adenoma (prolactinoma) greater than 1 cm in diameter, usually with extrasellar extension.

Magnetic Resonance Imaging (MRI). Technique of soft tissue imagery using resonance of hydrogen nuclei in static magnetic field exposed to low-frequency radiowaves.

Microadenoma. The common type of prolactinoma less than 1 cm in diameter.

Prolactin. Polypeptide hormone secreted by anterior pituitary lactotrophs that has mammotrophic and lactogenic functions.

Prolactin-Inhibiting Factor. The neurotransmitter (believed to be dopamine) that inhibits prolactin synthesis and release.

Prolactinoma. The most common pituitary tumor arising from chromophobic cells that secrete prolactin.

Prolactin is a polypeptide hormone containing 198 amino acids and having a molecular weight of 22,000 daltons. It circulates in different molecular sizes—a monomeric (small) form (mol wt 22,000), a polymeric (big) form (mol wt 50,000), and an even larger polymeric (big-big) form (mol wt >100,000). Big prolactin is presumed to be a dimer, and big-big prolactin may represent an aggregation of monomeric molecules. The small form is biologically active, and about 80% of the hormone secreted is in this form. Most immunoassayable prolactin is also in this form; however, the larger forms are also immunoreactive and thus are measurable in prolactin radioimmunoassays.

The biologic effects of the polymeric forms are unclear, but in some bioassays the forms are inactive, as they have reduced binding to mammary tissue membranes. Prolactin is synthesized and stored in the pituitary gland in chromophobe cells called *lactotrophs*, which are located mainly in the lateral areas of the gland. In addition, prolactin is synthesized in decidual and endometrial tissue. From these tissues prolactin is secreted into the circulation and, in the event of pregnancy, into the amniotic fluid. Prolactin is normally present in measurable amounts in serum, with mean levels of about 8 ng/ml in adult women. It circulates in an unbound form, has a 20-minute half-life, and is cleared by the liver and kidney. The main function of prolactin is to stimulate the growth of mammary tissue as well as to produce and secrete milk into the alveoli. Thus it has both mammogenic and lactogenic functions. Specific receptors for prolactin are present in the plasma membrane of mammary cells as well as many other tissues.

PHYSIOLOGY

Prolactin synthesis and release from the lactotrophs are controlled by central nervous system neurotransmitters, which act on the pituitary via the hypothalamus. The major control mechanism is inhibition, as pituitary stalk section results in increased prolactin secretion. It appears that the major physiologic inhibitor of prolactin release is the neurotransmitter dopamine, which acts directly on the pituitary gland. There are specific dopamine receptors on the lactotrophs, and dopamine inhibits prolactin synthesis and release in pituitary cell cultures. Thus dopamine appears to be the prolactin-inhibiting factor (PIF). Although a hypothalamic prolactin releasing factor (PRF) has not been isolated, it is known that both the neurotransmitter serotonin and thyrotropin-releasing factor stimulate prolactin release. Since the latter stimulates prolactin release only minimally unless infused, it appears that serotonin is PRF or is responsible for its secretion. The rise in prolactin levels during sleep appears to be controlled by serotonin.

Prolactin is secreted episodically, and serum levels fluctuate throughout the day and throughout the menstrual cycle, with peak levels occurring at midcycle. Although changes in prolactin levels are not as marked as the pulsatile episodes of luteinizing hormone (LH), Bäckström et al. reported a decline in both basal concentration and pulse frequency of prolactin in the luteal phase of the cycle. Estrogen stimulates prolactin production and release. Under the influence of estrogen, prolactin levels increase in females at the time of puberty.

During pregnancy, as estrogen levels increase, there is a concomitant hypertrophy and hyperplasia of the lactotrophs. The maternal increase in prolactin occurs soon after implantation, concomitant with the increase in circulating estrogen. Circulating levels of prolactin steadily

increase throughout pregnancy, reaching about 200 ng/ml in the third trimester, and the rise is directly related to the increase in circulating levels of estrogen. Despite the elevated prolactin levels during pregnancy, lactation does not occur because estrogen inhibits the action of prolactin on the breast, most likely blocking prolactin's interaction with its receptor. A day or two following delivery of the placenta, both estrogen levels and prolactin levels decline rapidly and lactation is initiated. Prolactin levels reach basal levels in nonnursing women in 2 to 3 weeks. Although basal levels of circulating prolactin decline to the nonpregnant range about 6 months after parturition in nursing women, following each act of suckling, prolactin levels increase markedly and stimulate milk production for the next feeding.

Nipple and breast stimulation also increase prolactin levels in the nonpregnant female. Other physiologic stimuli that increase prolactin release are exercise, sleep, and stress. In addition, prolactin levels normally rise following ingestion of the noonday meal. For these reasons prolactin levels normally fluctuate throughout the day, with maximal levels observed during nighttime while asleep and a smaller increase occurring in the early afternoon (Figure 39-1). When the amount measured in the circulation in

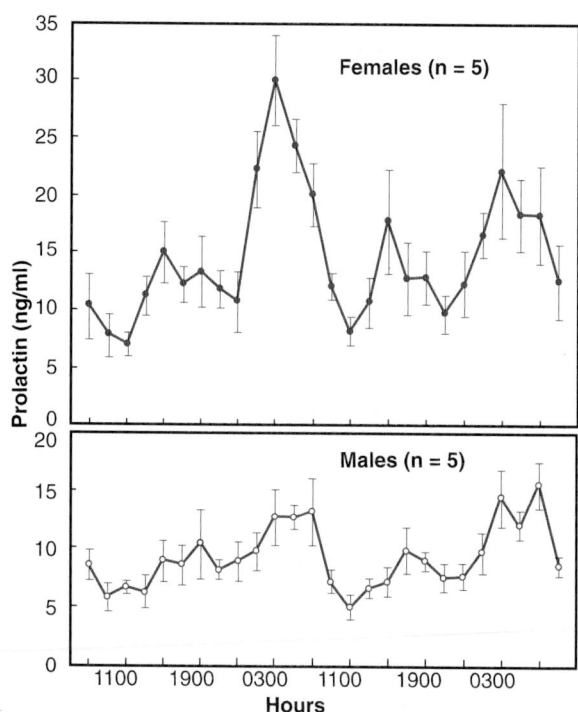

DIURNAL VARIATION OF PROLACTIN

FIGURE 39-1 Hour-to-hour variation of serum prolactin concentration in normal women and men studied throughout 48 consecutive hours. (From Kletzky OA and Davajan V: Hyperprolactinemia: diagnosis and treatment. Reproduced with permission from Infertility, contraception and reproductive endocrinology, ed 4, by Daniel R. Mishell, Jr., M.D., and Val Davajan, M.D. Copyright 1997 by Blackwell Scientific Publications, Malden, Mass. All rights reserved.)

the nonpregnant woman exceeds a certain level, usually 20 to 25 ng/ml, the condition is called *hyperprolactinemia*. The optimal time to obtain a blood sample for assay to diagnose hyperprolactinemia is during the morning hours. Increases in prolactin levels above the normal range can occur without a pathologic condition if the serum sample is drawn from a patient who has recently awakened, has exercised, or has had recent breast stimulation, such as breast palpation, during a physical examination.

The most frequent cause of slightly elevated prolactin levels is stress, particularly the stress caused by visiting the physician's office. An excellent study demonstrating that most mildly elevated prolactin levels are not caused by pathologic hyperprolactinemia was performed by Muneyyirci-Delale et al. These investigators studied 50 women without radiologic evidence of a prolactinoma who had elevated prolactin levels (23 to 156 ng/ml) measured in two consecutive blood samples obtained 1 to 2 weeks apart. When these women had serial blood sampling subsequently performed in a quiet room, 20 had normal prolactin levels in the 1-hour blood sample (Figure 39-2). The initial prolactin levels in these 20 women ranged from 26 to 69 ng/ml. The results of this study indicate that stress-related hyperprolactinemia is a common cause of a mild increase in prolactin. All women with initial prolactin levels less than 70 mIU/ml should have subsequent samples drawn 60 minutes after resting in a quiet room to determine whether true pathologic hyperprolactinemia is present.

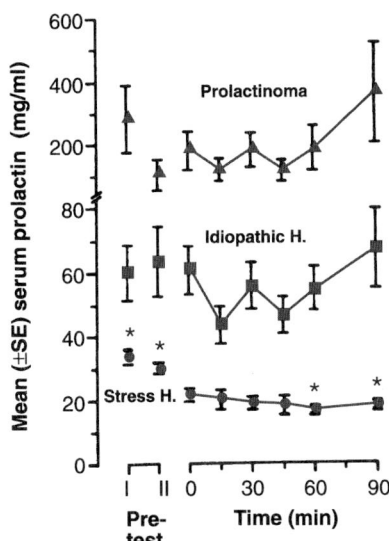

FIGURE 39-2 Mean plus or minus standard error (± SE) serum prolactin levels in women with prolactinoma (N = 20) and idiopathic (N = 30) and stress-related (N = 20) hyperprolactinemia before (pretest I and II) and during hyperprolactinemia test. Differences (* P < 0.01) are in relation to time zero values. (Mean prolactin values among groups were also significantly different—P < 0.01—at all times.) (From Muneyyirci-Delale O, Goldstein D, Reyes FI, et al: NY State J Med 89:205, 1989.)

Hyperprolactinemia can produce disorders of gonadotrophin–sex steroid function, resulting in menstrual cycle derangement (oligomenorrhea and amenorrhea) and anovulation, as well as inappropriate lactation or galactorrhea. The mechanism whereby elevated prolactin levels interfere with gonadotrophin release has not been completely elucidated, but the major factor appears to be alterations in normal gonadotrophin-releasing hormone (GnRH) release. Women with hyperprolactinemia have abnormalities in the frequency and amplitude of LH pulsations, with a normal or increased gonadotrophin response following GnRH infusion.

This abnormality of normal GnRH cyclicity thus inhibits gonadotrophin release but not synthesis. The reason for the abnormal secretion of GnRH has not been completely elucidated, but it is hypothesized that the elevated prolactin levels produce a rise in hypothalamic dopamine levels by a short-loop feedback that fails to suppress prolactin but interferes with normal GnRH release, perhaps by altering norepinephrine secretion. In addition, elevated prolactin levels have been shown to interfere with the positive estrogen effect on midcycle LH release. It has also been shown that elevated levels of prolactin directly inhibit basal as well as gonadotrophin-stimulated ovarian secretion of both estradiol and progesterone. However, this mechanism is probably not the primary cause of anovulation, because women with hyperprolactinemia can have ovulation induced with various agents, including pulsatile GnRH. Some women with moderate hyperprolactinemia as determined by radioimmunoassay have a greater than normal proportion of the big-big forms. Because of the reduced bioactivity of this form of prolactin, these individuals can have normal pituitary and ovarian function.

The clinician should measure serum prolactin levels in all women with galactorrhea, as well as those with oligomenorrhea and amenorrhea without the presence of an elevated level of follicle-stimulating hormone (FSH). Hyperprolactinemia has been reported to be present in 15% of all anovulatory women and 20% of women with amenorrhea of undetermined cause. Galactorrhea is defined as the nonpuerperal secretion from the breast of watery or milky fluid that contains neither pus nor blood. The fluid may appear spontaneously or after palpation. To determine if galactorrhea is present, the clinician should palpate the breast, moving from the periphery toward the nipple in an attempt to express any secretion. The diagnosis of galactorrhea can be confirmed by observing multiple fat droplets in the fluid when it is examined under low-power magnification (Figure 39-3). The incidence of galactorrhea in women with hyperprolactinemia has been reported to range from 30% to 80%, and these differences probably reflect variations in the techniques used to detect mammary excretion. Unless there has been continued breast stimulation after a pregnancy, the presence of galactorrhea serves as a biologic indicator that the prolactin

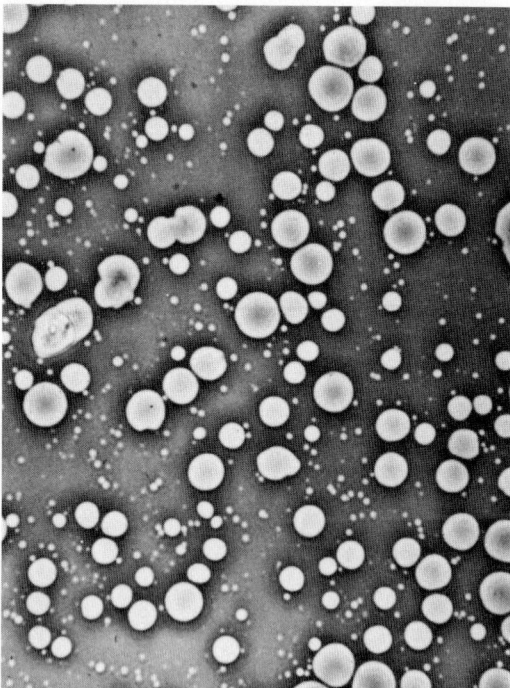

FIGURE 39-3 Fat droplets seen under microscope from a patient with galactorrhea. (From Kletzky OA and Davajan V: Hyperprolactinemia: diagnosis and treatment. In Mishell DR, Davajan V, and Lobo RA, editors: Infertility, contraception and reproductive endocrinology, ed 3, Cambridge, Mass, 1991, Blackwell Scientific Publications.)

Pharmacologic Agents Affecting Prolactin Concentrations

Stimulators
Anesthetics
Psychoactive
  Phenothiazines
  Tricyclic antidepressants
  Opiates
  Chlordiazepoxide
  Amphetamines
  Diazepams
  Haloperidol
  Fluphenazine
  Chlorpromazine
Hormones
  Estrogen
  Oral-steroid contraceptives
  Thyrotropin-releasing hormone
Antihypertensives
  α-Methyldopa
  Reserpine
  Verapamil
Dopamine receptor antagonists
  Metoclopramide
Antiemetics
  Sulpride
  Promazine
  Perphenazine
Others
  Cimetidine
  Cyproheptiadine

Inhibitors
L-Dopa
Dopamine
Bromocriptine
Pergolide
Cabergoline
Depot bromocriptine

From Shoupe D and Mishell DR Jr: Hyperprolactinemia: diagnosis and treatment. In Mishell's textbook of infertility, contraception and reproductive endocrinology, ed 4, Lobo RA, Mishell DR Jr, Paulson RJ, Shoupe D, editors: Blackwell Scientific Publications, Cambridge, Mass, 1997.

level is abnormally elevated. Davajan et al. reported that 62% of women with galactorrhea have hyperprolactinemia, and some individuals with galactorrhea have normal immunoassayable prolactin levels, indicating they may have elevated levels of biologically active prolactin. The incidence of hyperprolactinemia is higher (88%) in those women with galactorrhea who have amenorrhea and low estrogen levels than in those women with galactorrhea and normal menses, oligomenorrhea, or amenorrhea with normal estrogen levels (49%).

ETIOLOGY

Pathologic causes of hyperprolactinemia, in addition to a prolactin-secreting pituitary adenoma (prolactinoma) and other pituitary tumors that produce acromegaly and Cushing's disease, include hypothalamic disease, various pharmacologic agents, hypothyroidism, chronic renal disease, or any chronic type of breast nerve stimulation, such as may occur with thoracic operation, herpes zoster, or chest trauma.

One of the most frequent causes of galactorrhea and hyperprolactinemia is the ingestion of pharmacologic agents, particularly tranquilizers, narcotics, and antihypertensive agents (see box). Of the tranquilizers, the phenothiazines and diazepam can produce hyperprolactinemia

either by depleting the hypothalamic circulation of dopamine or by blocking its binding sites and thus decreasing dopamine action (Figure 39-4). The tricyclic antidepressants block dopamine uptake, and propranolol, haloperidol, phentolamine, and cyproheptadine block hypothalamic dopamine receptors. The antihypertensive agent reserpine depletes catecholamines, and methyldopa blocks the conversion of tyrosine to dihydroxyphenylalanine (dopa). Ingestion of oral contraceptive steroids can also increase prolactin levels, with a greater incidence of hyperprolactinemia occurring with higher estrogen formulations. Nevertheless, galactorrhea does not usually occur during oral contraceptive ingestion because the exogenous estrogen blocks the binding of prolactin to its receptors.

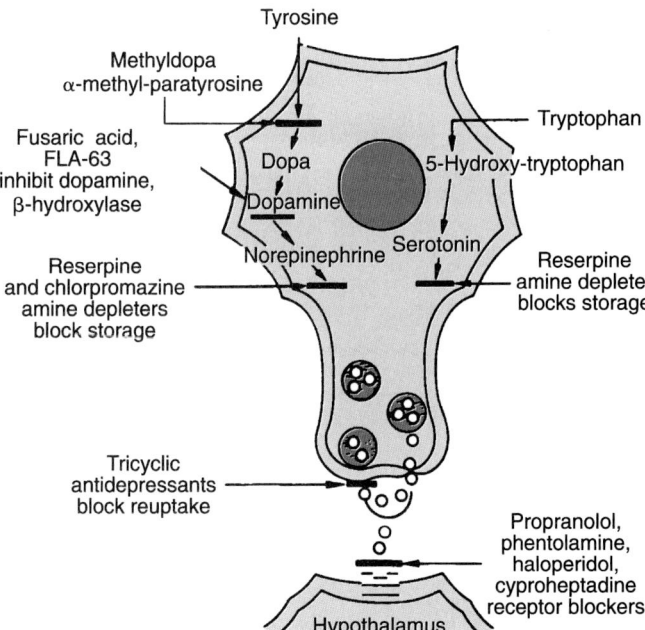

FIGURE 39-4 Schematic representation of inhibitory effects of drugs on synthesis and release of neurotransmitters. (From Kletzky OA and Davajan V: Hyperprolactinemia. In Mishell DR, Davajan V, and Lobo RA, editors: Infertility, contraception and reproductive endocrinology, ed 3, Cambridge, Mass, 1991, Blackwell Scientific Publications.)

Women who develop galactorrhea while ingesting oral contraceptives or any of the other drugs just listed should ideally discontinue the medication, and prolactin should be measured 1 month thereafter to determine if the level has returned to normal. If the medication cannot be discontinued, the prolactin level should be measured, and if it is elevated above 100 ng/ml, imaging of the sella turcica should be performed to determine whether a macroadenoma is present.

Primary hypothyroidism can also produce hyperprolactinemia and galactorrhea because of decreased negative feedback of thyroxine (T_4) on the hypothalamic-pituitary axis. The resulting increase in thyrotropin-releasing hormone (TRH) stimulates prolactin secretion as well as thyroid-stimulating hormone (TSH) secretion from the pituitary. About 3% to 5% of individuals with hyperprolactinemia have hypothyroidism, and thus TSH, the most sensitive indicator of hypothyroidism, should be measured in all individuals with hyperprolactinemia. If the TSH level is elevated, triiodothyronine (T_3) and T_4 should be measured to confirm the diagnosis of primary hypothyroidism, as occasionally a TSH-secreting pituitary adenoma will be present. Treatment with appropriate thyroid replacement usually returns the TSH and prolactin levels to normal within a short time.

Hyperprolactinemia can occur in those individuals with abnormal renal disease resulting from decreased metabolic clearance as well as increased production rate. The cause of the latter is not known.

Central Nervous System Disorders

Hypothalamic Causes

Diseases of the hypothalamus that produce alterations in the normal portal circulation of dopamine can result in hyperprolactinemia. Such diseases include craniopharyngioma and infiltration of the hypothalamus by sarcoidosis, histiocytosis, leukemia, or carcinoma. All these conditions are rare, with craniopharyngioma being the most common. These tumors arise from remnants of Rathke's pouch along the pituitary stalk. Grossly they can be cystic, solid, or mixed, and calcification is usually visible on x-ray examination. They are most frequently diagnosed during the second and third decades of life and usually result in impairment of secretion of several pituitary hormones.

Pituitary Causes

Various types of pituitary tumors, lactotroph hyperplasia, and the empty sella syndrome can be associated with hyperprolactinemia. It has been estimated that as many as 80% of all pituitary adenomas secrete prolactin. The most common pituitary tumor associated with hyperprolactinemia is the prolactinoma, arbitrarily defined as a microadenoma if its diameter is less than 1 cm and as a macroadenoma if it is larger. Hyperprolactinemia has been reported to occur in about 25% of individuals with acromegaly and 10% of those with Cushing disease, indicating that these pituitary adenomas, which mainly secrete growth hormone and adrenocorticotropic hormone (ACTH), frequently also secrete prolactin. Hyperplasia of lactotrophs has been reported to occur in about 8% of pituitary glands examined at autopsy. Individuals with hyperplasia of the lactotrophs cannot be distinguished from those having a microadenoma by any clinical, laboratory, or radiologic method. It is a diagnosis that can be made only at the time of surgical exploration of the pituitary gland. Pituitary enlargement with suprasellar extension caused by lactotroph hyperplasia has been reported. *Functional hyperprolactinemia* is the term used for the clinical diagnosis of women with elevated prolactin levels without evidence of an adenoma. This condition may occur because of decreased dopamine inhibition.

Another cause of hyperprolactinemia is the primary empty sella syndrome. The term *primary empty sella syndrome* describes a clinical situation in which an intrasellar extension of the subarachnoid space results in compression of the pituitary gland and an enlarged sella turcica. The etiology is believed to result from a congenital or acquired (by radiation or surgery) defect in the sella

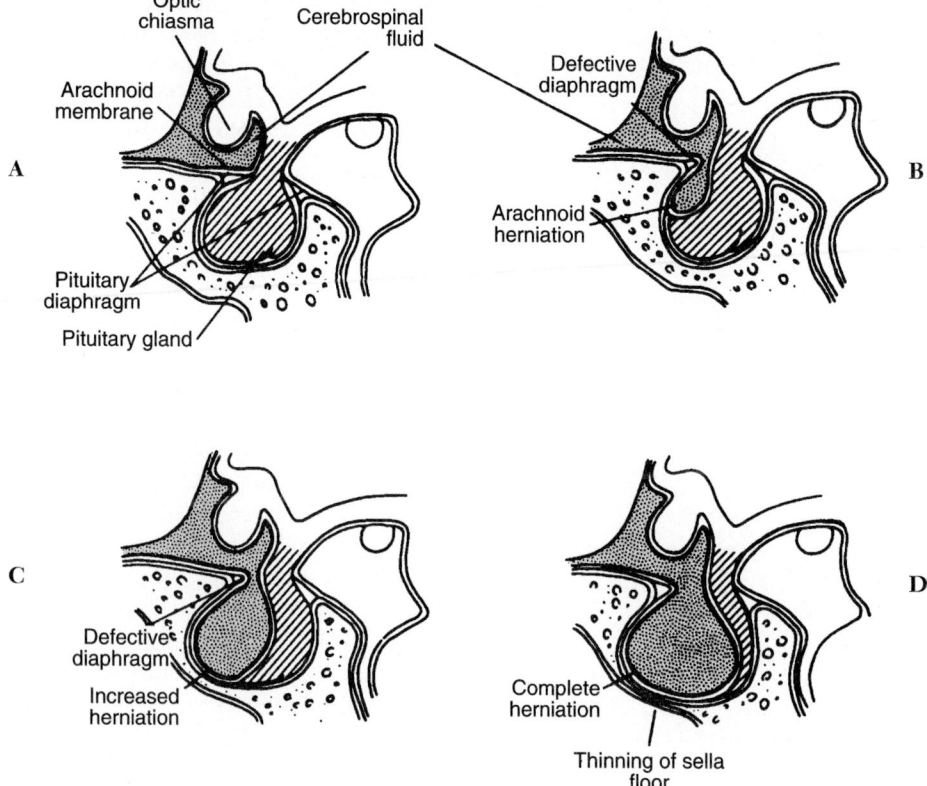

FIGURE 39-5 Diagrammatic representation of empty sella syndrome. **A,** Normal anatomic relationship. **B, C,** and **D,** Progression in development of empty sella syndrome. Note thinning of floor and symmetric enlargement of sella turcica. (From Kletzky OA and Davajan V: Hyperprolactinemia. In Mishell DR, Davajan V, and Lobo RA, editors: Infertility, contraception and reproductive endocrinology, ed 3, Cambridge, Mass, 1991, Blackwell Scientific Publications.)

diaphragm that allows the subarachnoid membrane to herniate into the sella turcica (Figure 39-5). The syndrome is usually associated with normal pituitary function except for hyperprolactinemia. Although some individuals with primary empty sella syndrome have a coexistent prolactinoma, Gharib et al. reported a series of 11 persons with an empty sella and hyperprolactinemia who had no histologic evidence of a prolactinoma or hyperplasia of the lactotrophs. They stated that about 5% of individuals with the empty sella have hyperprolactinemia or amenorrhea-galactorrhea or both. It is theorized that with this syndrome distortion of the infundibular stalk results in decreased levels of dopamine reaching the pituitary to inhibit prolactin. Serum prolactin levels are usually less than 100 ng/ml with the empty sella syndrome, and some women with this syndrome have galactorrhea with normal prolactin levels. Kleinberg et al. reported that about 10% of all individuals with an enlarged sella turcica have the empty sella syndrome. The best modality to diagnose this condition is magnetic resonance imaging (MRI). Computed tomographic (CT) scanning with intrathecal injection of metrizamide can also be used. It is important to establish the diagnosis because the syndrome has a benign course.

Prolactinomas

In an unselected series of 120 autopsies of persons who had had no clinical evidence of pituitary disease, Burrow et al. found pituitary microadenomas to be present in 32 (27%). More recently, Abd El-Hamid et al. reported that adenomas were found in 78 of 486 (16%) pituitary glands examined after unselected autopsies. In both series prolactin was found in about half the glands, indicating that more than 1 in 10 individuals in the general population have a prolactinoma.

Overall about 50% of women with hyperprolactinemia have a prolactinoma. The incidence is higher when the prolactin levels exceed 100 ng/ml, and nearly all individuals with prolactin levels greater than 200 ng/ml have a prolactinoma. The vast majority of prolactinomas in women are microadenomas. Kleinberg et al. reported that overall 20% of individuals with galactorrhea and 35% of women with amenorrhea-galactorrhea had radiologic evidence of pituitary tumors. Tumors are also present in about 20% of women with hyperprolactinemia and menstrual irregularities without galactorrhea. The incidence of prolactinoma is greater in those individuals with a more profound disturbance of normal hypothalamic-pituitary-ovarian function. Davajan et al. reported that 70% of women with hyperprolactinemia, galactorrhea, and secondary amenorrhea with low estrogen levels had radiologic evidence of a pituitary adenoma. Evidence of a tumor occurred in only 20% to 30% of those with hyperprolactinemia and normal menses, oligomenorrhea, or secondary amenorrhea who had sufficient estrogen to undergo withdrawal bleeding after progesterone administration. In both these studies no evidence of tumor was found in individuals with normal menses, galactorrhea, and normal prolactin levels. Therefore radiologic studies do not need to be performed if galactorrhea is present and prolactin levels are normal.

Because prolactinomas develop in the lateral areas of the pituitary gland, it was originally hypothesized that decreased blood supply to these regions resulted in less dopamine being delivered and resultant increased size and number of lactotrophs. Recently studies of dopamine response by a variety of tests indicate that when prolactinomas are present there is a defect in dopamine regulation of prolactin secretion that persists even after surgical removal of the adenoma. This loss of dopaminergic inhibition of prolactin that persists for years after tumor removal is thought to explain the high rate of recurrence of tumors.

Long-term studies of individuals with microadenomas demonstrate that enlargement is uncommon and that many of these tumors regress spontaneously. In a longitudinal retrospective study of 43 women with hyperprolactinemia and a radiologic diagnosis of microadenoma, March et al. found that only 2 women had evidence of enlargement of the adenoma, with a mean duration of follow-up of 5 years. Of these 43 women, 3 had spontaneous regression of their hyperprolactinemia and resumption of normal menses. Koppelman et al. reported similar results. Of 25 women with prolactinomas (18 with microadenomas and 7 with minimally enlarged sella) followed up for a mean duration of 11 years without treatment, only 1 woman had slight progression of a sella abnormality. None had visual field or other pituitary function changes, seven resumed normal menses spontaneously, and galactorrhea spontaneously resolved in six.

The results of these retrospective studies have been confirmed by two prospective studies of untreated microprolactinomas. In a 3- to 7-year prospective longitudinal study of 30 hyperprolactinemic women, Schlechte et al. found that of 13 women with initially abnormal radiographic findings, 4 became normal, 7 did not change, and 2 had evidence of tumor growth. Of 17 women with initially normal radiographic findings, 4 became minimally abnormal. None of the 30 developed a macroadenoma or pituitary hypofunction. In this study, as in the two retrospective studies just reported, more sensitive radiographic techniques (tomograms, followed by CT) were used as the study progressed and could account for the minimal evidence of tumor growth. Sisam et al. overcame this problem

by prospectively following a group of 38 women with hyperprolactinemia and microprolactinomas by serial CT scans for a mean duration of 50 months. None of these women had evidence of tumor progression, even the 2 who had a marked increase in prolactin levels. In this group, nine (25%) had spontaneous improvement of their symptoms. Martin et al. followed the natural history of 41 women with idiopathic hyperprolactinemia and amenorrhea-galactorrhea for up to 11 years. During this time, 9 women conceived spontaneously, and 16 have resumed spontaneous menses with cessation of galactorrhea. Only one woman developed a microadenoma. Thus hyperprolactinemia with or without a microadenoma follows a benign clinical course in most women, and therapy is unnecessary unless pregnancy is desired or estrogen levels are low. Several studies have reported that pregnancy is beneficial for women with functional hyperprolactinemia or prolactin-secreting microadenomas. Following pregnancy, PRL levels decrease in about half the women. Crosignani et al. reported that prolactin levels became normal in about 30% of 176 hyperprolactinemic women after pregnancy. Prolactin levels decreased to normal in 36% of women with functional hyperprolactinemia and 17% of those with adenomas. Therefore if women with hyperprolactinemia desire to become pregnant they should be encouraged to do so, as pregnancy is likely to result in normal or lowered prolactin levels.

DIAGNOSTIC TECHNIQUES

Because most prolactinomas are microadenomas that do not cause enlargement of the sella turcica, the diagnosis usually cannot be made by ordinary anteroposterior and lateral coned x-ray examination of the sella turcica. With the development of more precise radiologic methods of detecting soft tissue pituitary abnormalities, it is now possible to detect even small adenomas.

Initially detection of microadenomas was accomplished by obtaining tomographic radiographic examination of the sella turcica at intervals of 2 to 3 mm in the anteroposterior and lateral projections with a hypocycloidal movement. These are called *hypocycloidal tomograms*. Comparing the results of tomograms with the findings of microadenoma at autopsy, Burrow et al. found that the incidence of both false positive and false negative tomographic findings was about 20% each, with an overall accuracy rate of 61%. Furthermore, radiation exposure with polytomography may be in excess of 20 rads.

Since about 1980 a more accurate diagnostic technique, CT imagery, has been available. After infusion of at least 200 ml of 30% iodinated contrast medium, CT imagery is performed in coronal sections of 1.5 mm. The typical appearance of an adenoma is a region of diminished enhancement in the pituitary gland with a convex upper surface and an abnormal height of 8 mm or greater. With

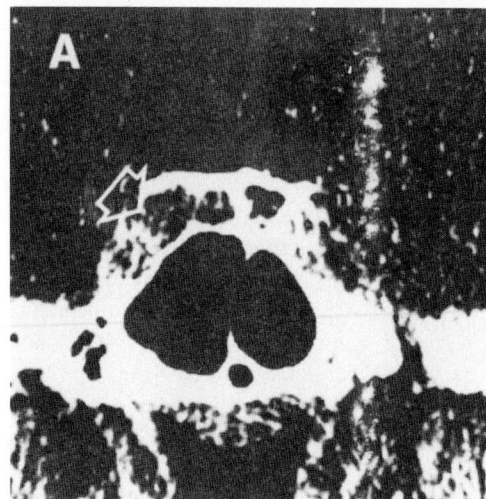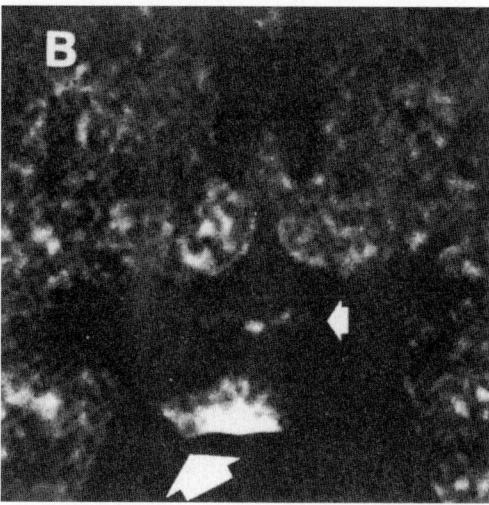

FIGURE 39-6 Images were selected to best demonstrate pathology and do not exactly correspond in level of section through sella turcica. **A,** CT scan (coronal section) showing bony erosion of right sella turcica *(arrow)* with possible soft tissue extension into right cavernous sinus. Height of pituitary gland (not shown) is 9 mm. **B,** MRI (coronal section) showing soft tissue mass extending into right cavernous sinus near carotid artery *(large arrow)*. Height of pituitary gland is 9 mm. Normal optic chiasm is seen *(small arrow)*. (From Stein AL, Levenick MN, and Kletzky OA: Obstet Gynecol 73:996, 1989.)

this technique it is possible to assess accurately the presence of a microadenoma 2 mm in diameter or larger as well as the suprasellar and other extrasellar extensions. This technique also will indicate the presence of an empty sella. Radiation exposure in a CT scan is about 3 rads, significantly less than with polytomography. However, this technique mainly provides information about the bony structure of the sella turcica, not the soft tissue lesions, the adenomas themselves.

Recently the technique of MRI has been developed. With this technique accurate soft tissue imagery is obtained without radiation. Instead, hydrogen nuclei in static magnetic fields exposed to radiowaves of specific frequency resonate and depict tissue hydrogen density. This technique provides 1 mm resolution and thus should be able to detect all microadenomas. Stein et al. compared results of CT and MRI in 22 individuals with suspected pituitary adenomas. MRI was found to be the superior diagnostic modality because of its greater soft tissue contrast (Figure 39-6). Thus MRI should be the diagnostic technique of choice. If MRI or CT are not available, hypocycloidal tomography can be used.

Recommended Diagnostic Evaluation

It is currently recommended that prolactin levels be measured in all women with either galactorrhea, oligomenorrhea, or amenorrhea who do not have an elevated FSH level. If prolactin is elevated, a TSH assay should be performed to rule out the presence of primary hypothyroidism. If TSH is elevated, T_3 and T_4 should be measured to rule out the rare possibility of a TSH-secreting pitu-

itary adenoma. If TSH is elevated and hypothyroidism is present, appropriate thyroid replacement should begin, and the prolactin level will usually return to normal. If TSH is normal and the woman has a normal prolactin level with galactorrhea, no further tests are necessary if she has regular menses. Because some women with galactorrhea, abnormal menstrual function, and normal prolactin levels have been found to have the empty sella syndrome, an MRI or a CT scan should be obtained to establish the diagnosis in women with these findings.

If prolactin levels are elevated and the TSH is normal, an MRI if available or CT scan should be obtained to detect a microadenoma or macroadenoma. Macroadenomas are uncommon and rarely are present with a prolactin level less than 100 ng/ml. If the prolactin level is more than 100 ng/ml or the woman complains of headaches or visual changes, the likelihood of a tumor extending beyond the sella turcica is increased (Figure 39-7). Microadenomas are a common cause of hyperprolactinemia, but rarely enlarge. Neither pregnancy, oral contraceptives, nor hormone replacement therapy stimulates the growth of these small tumors, and therapy is unnecessary unless ovulation induction is desired or hypoestrogenism is present. Follow-up of women with both functional hyperprolactinemia and prolactin-secreting microadenomas should be the measurement of prolactin levels annually.

Visual field determination and tests of adrenocorticotropic hormone (ACTH) and thyroid function are not necessary if a microadenoma is present, as these small tumors do not interfere with overall pituitary function and do not extend beyond the sella. However, these evaluations should be performed in individuals with macroade-

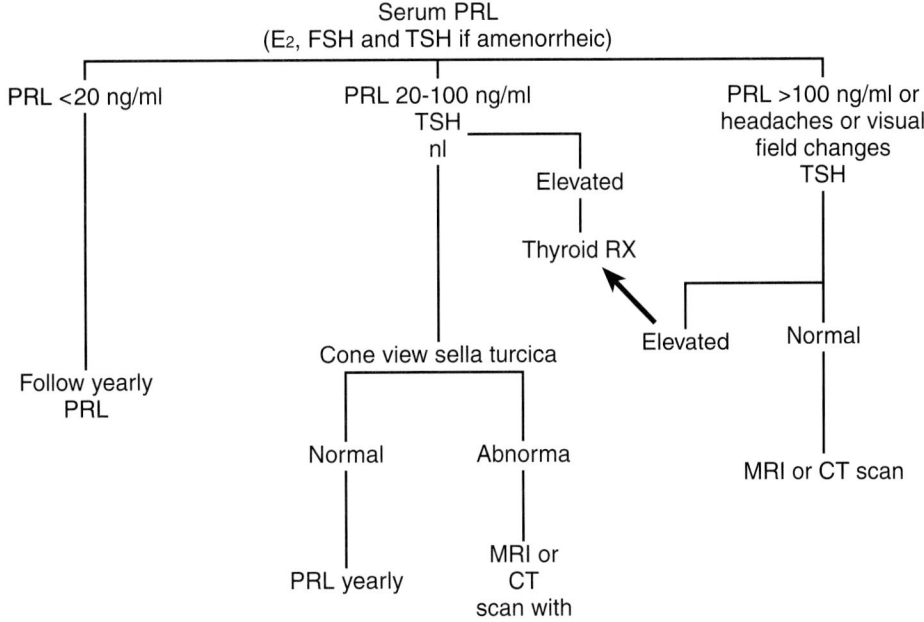

Serum PRL
(E₂, FSH and TSH if amenorrheic)

PRL <20 ng/ml

PRL 20-100 ng/ml
TSH
nl

Elevated

Thyroid RX

PRL >100 ng/ml or
headaches or visual
field changes
TSH

Elevated   Normal

Follow yearly
PRL

Cone view sella turcica

Normal   Abnorma

PRL yearly

MRI or
CT
scan with

MRI or CT scan

FIGURE 39-7   Diagnostic evaluation of galactorrhea, amenorrhea, and oligomenorrhea.

nomas because suprasellar extension of the tumor may exert pressure on the optic chiasm, resulting in bitemporal visual field defects and interference with vision. The size of these tumors may also affect other aspects of pituitary function. Thus a test of ACTH reserve, such as insulin-induced hypoglycemia (insulin tolerance test), as well as tests of thyroid function, should be performed on all individuals with a macroadenoma.

MANAGEMENT

Expectant Treatment

Women with radiologic evidence of a microadenoma or functional hyperprolactinemia who do not wish to conceive may be followed without treatment by measuring prolactin levels once yearly. Many of these women have deficient estrogen, and low estrogen levels in combination with hyperprolactinemia have been shown to be associated with the early onset of osteoporosis. If the woman has low estrogen levels, exogenous estrogen should be administered. Either replacement estrogen-progestin therapy, as is used for postmenopausal women, or oral contraceptives can be utilized. Corenblum and Donovan reported that a group of women with both functional hyperprolactinemia and prolactin-secreting pituitary microadenomas who were treated with either cyclic estrogen and progestin or oral contraceptives for several years did not have an increase in the size of the adenomas or a marked increase in prolactin levels. Mean prolactin levels actually declined with both treatment regimens. Testa reported that 2 years of OC use in a group of women with hyperprolactinemia

with microadenoma did not alter the size of the adenoma. Since side effects and cost are less and compliance is better with exogenous estrogen than with bromocriptine, it is not necessary to use the latter agent unless ovulation and pregnancy are desired. Individuals with hyperprolactinemia with or without microadenomas who have adequate estrogen levels as shown by the presence of oligomenorrhea or amenorrhea with estradiol levels above 40 pg/ml who do not wish to conceive should be treated with periodic progestin withdrawal (medroxyprogesterone acetate 10 mg per day for 10 days each month) or combination oral contraceptives to prevent endometrial hyperplasia.

Medical Therapy

The initial treatment for macroadenomas, as well as for women with hyperprolactinemia who are anovulatory and wish to conceive, should be a dopamine receptor agonist. Bromocriptine, methysergide, metergoline, and cabergoline have been used with success, but only bromocriptine (2-Br-alpha-ergocryptine mesylate) and cabergoline are approved for use in the United States (Figure 39-8). The greatest amount of clinical experience has been with use of bromocriptine. This semisynthetic ergot alkaloid was developed in 1967 to inhibit prolactin secretion. It directly stimulates dopamine receptors, and as a dopamine receptor agonist it inhibits prolactin secretion both in vitro and in vivo. After ingestion, bromocriptine is rapidly absorbed, with peak blood levels reached 1 to 3 hours later. Serum prolactin levels remain depressed for about 14 hours after ingestion of a single dose, after which time the drug is not detectable in the circulation. For this reason

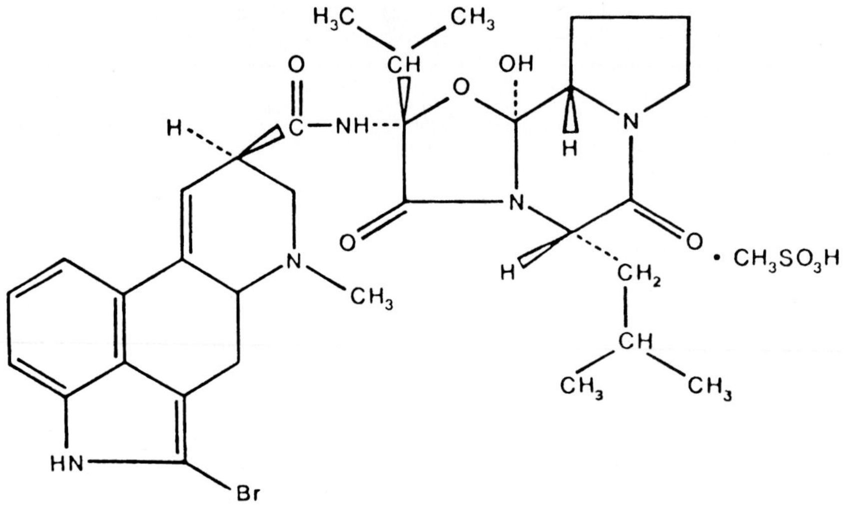

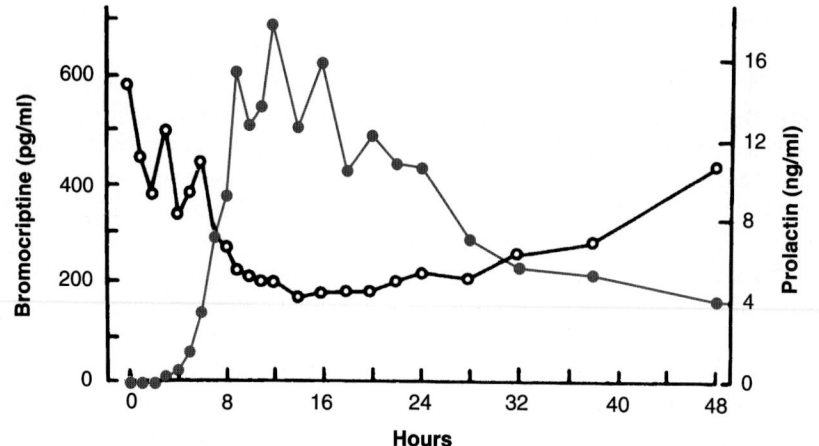

FIGURE 39-8 Formula of bromocriptine.

the drug is usually given at least twice daily, with initial therapy being started at one half of the 2.5-mg tablet to minimize side effects. The most frequent side effects are orthostatic hypotension (with an incidence of 15%), which can produce fainting and dizziness as well as nausea and vomiting. To minimize these symptoms the initial dose should be taken in bed and with food at nighttime. Less frequent adverse symptoms include headache, nasal congestion, fatigue, constipation, and diarrhea. Most of these reactions are mild, occur early in the course of treatment, and are transient. To reduce the adverse symptoms, the dose should be gradually increased every 1 to 2 weeks until prolactin levels fall to normal. The usual therapeutic dose is 2.5 mg twice or three times a day, but larger doses are sometimes used when a macroadenoma is present.

Adverse effects, such as nausea, vomiting, and nasal congestion, occur in about half the women taking oral bromocriptine and may cause them to discontinue treat-ment. Vermesh et al. reported that the drug was very well absorbed vaginally without the presence of side effects. Furthermore, when a single tablet was placed deep in the posterior vaginal fornix, therapeutic blood levels persisted for more than 24 hours, during which time prolactin levels remained suppressed (Figure 39-9). Ginsburg et al. subsequently reported that this method of bromocriptine administration was well accepted, effective, and well tolerated in a group of 31 hyperprolactinemic women, 17 of whom could not tolerate oral bromocriptine. Minor side effects occurred in only three women. The tablet is placed digitally deep in the vagina nightly at bedtime. A single 2.5-mg dose reduced prolactin concentrations in 90% of patients treated and brought the levels to normal in one third of women. Higher doses do not appear to be more effective. Ginsburg et al. recommended that the drug be administered vaginally instead of orally for all women as a smaller

FIGURE 39-9 Mean (± SEM) plasma levels of bromocriptine *(blue circles)* and prolactin *(open circles)* in a single study, extended to 48 hours, after vaginal bromocriptine (2.5 mg). (From Vermesh M, Fossum GT, and Kletzky OA: Obstet Gynecol 72:693, 1988.)

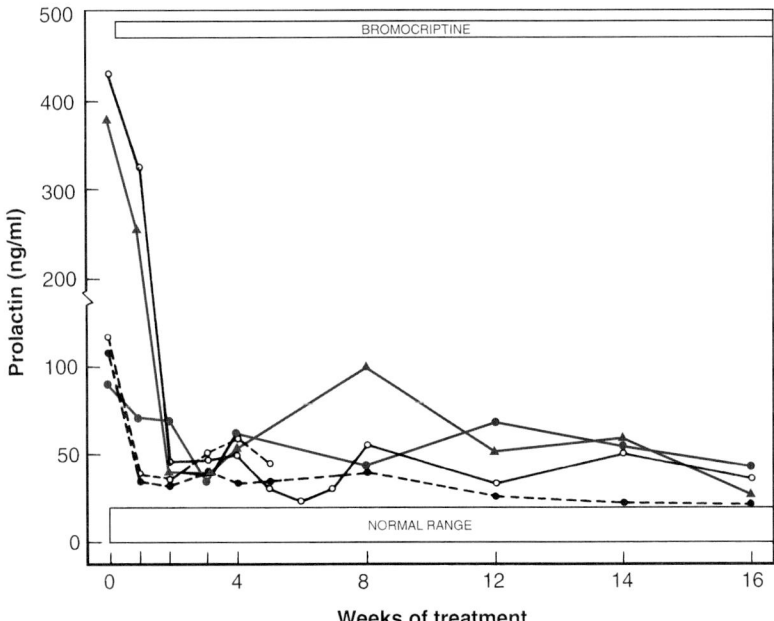

FIGURE 39-10 Mean serum prolactin response to bromocriptine therapy in five patients with radiographic evidence of pituitary adenoma and residual hyperprolactinemia. All five ovulated, and four conceived. (From Kletzky OA, Marrs RP, and Davajan V: Am J Obstet Gynecol 147:528, 1983.)

dose of drug can be used, once-daily administration is more convenient, and side effects are fewer.

Bromocriptine is approved for treatment of adverse symptoms associated with hyperprolactinemia, such as galactorrhea, as well as anovulatory infertility with and without the presence of a prolactin-secreting adenoma. In hyperprolactinemic women without adenomas, prolactin levels return to normal in more than 90%, fertility is restored in 80%, and galactorrhea is eradicated in 60% with bromocriptine therapy. In women with hyperprolactinemia and a microadenoma, similar rates of success have been reported. Therefore bromocriptine is the treatment of choice for women with prolactin-secreting microadenomas who wish to ovulate or are bothered by galactorrhea.

Despite administration of up to 20 mg of bromocriptine per day orally, about 10% of individuals with microadenomas fail to have prolactin levels return to normal, probably because of individual differences in the sensitivity of lactotrophs to bromocriptine. Nevertheless, despite the persistently elevated prolactin levels, many of these women ovulate and conceive (Figure 39-10).

If pregnancy occurs after ovulation is induced with bromocriptine, therapy is usually discontinued, although there is no evidence that the drug is teratogenic or adversely affects pregnancy outcome. If pregnancy is not desired but bromocriptine is used to treat galactorrhea, therapy is usually continued for at least 12 months, after which it should be discontinued for a few weeks. Most women with microadenomas have recurrence of hyperprolactinemia, amenorrhea, and galactorrhea, although

about 10% to 20% have permanent remission after discontinuing bromocriptine treatment. Moriondo et al. reported that after 1 year of bromocriptine treatment, 11% of women with microadenomas had persistent normalization of prolactin, with return of regular menses after the drug was discontinued (Figure 39-11). This incidence of permanent remission reached 22% after 2 years of treatment. A higher rate of permanent remission occurred in women treated with 10 mg per day than with lower dosages, but higher doses of drug increase the incidence of adverse reactions and cause discontinuation of treatment. These investigators found that after bromocriptine was discontinued, there was a 40% reduction in mean prolactin levels in all women treated, and about 60% had a greater than 30% reduction from pretreatment prolactin levels after the drug was discontinued. Rasmussen et al. reported the results of discontinuation of long-term (median of 2 years) bromocriptine therapy in 75 hyperprolactinemic women. In about half the women it was necessary to reinstate treatment because prolactin levels rose. However, in the other half further treatment was unnecessary because mean prolactin levels decreased more than 60% and either returned to normal or were only slightly elevated (Figure 39-12). More than half of these 33 women resumed regular menses without further treatment. These data indicate that the remissions were drug related and not spontaneous. Using CT scans before and during bromocriptine therapy, Bonneville et al. found that about 75% of individuals with microadenomas had reduction in tumor size during bromocriptine treatment, and in 40% the tumor had disappeared (Figure 39-13). To deter-

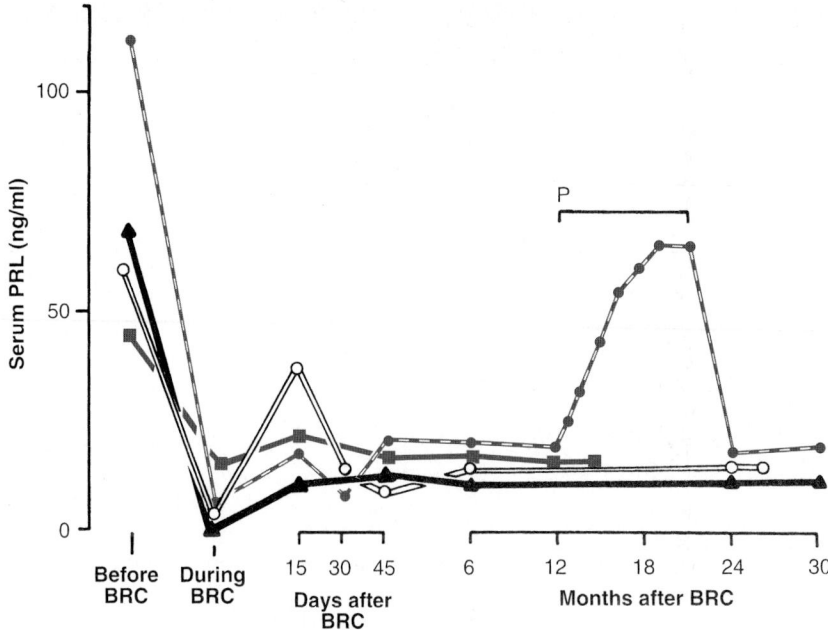

FIGURE 39-11 Serum prolactin levels in four patients who had persistently normal prolactin levels after bromocriptine *(BRC)* treatment for 12 months. *P,* Pregnancy. (From Moriondo P, Travaglini P, Nissim M, et al: J Clin Endocrinol Metab 60:764, 1985. Copyright 1985 by The Endocrine Society.)

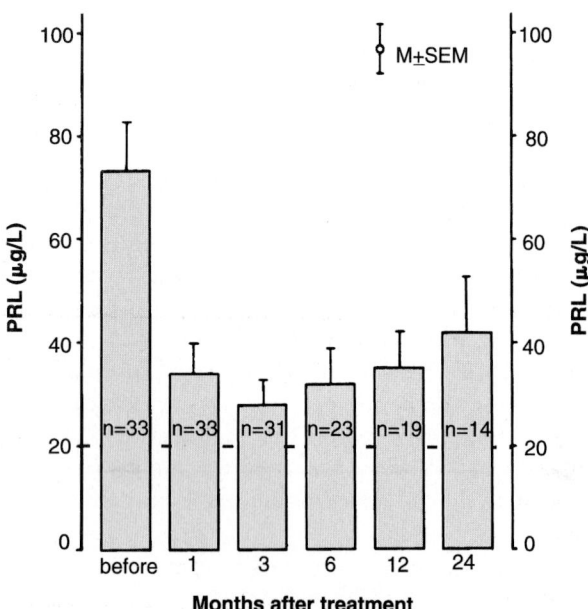

FIGURE 39-12 Geometric mean serum prolactin levels before and after discontinuation of bromocriptine treatment in 33 women with hyperprolactinemic amenorrhea. (From Rasmussen C, Bergh T, and Wide L: Fertil Steril 48:550, 1987.)

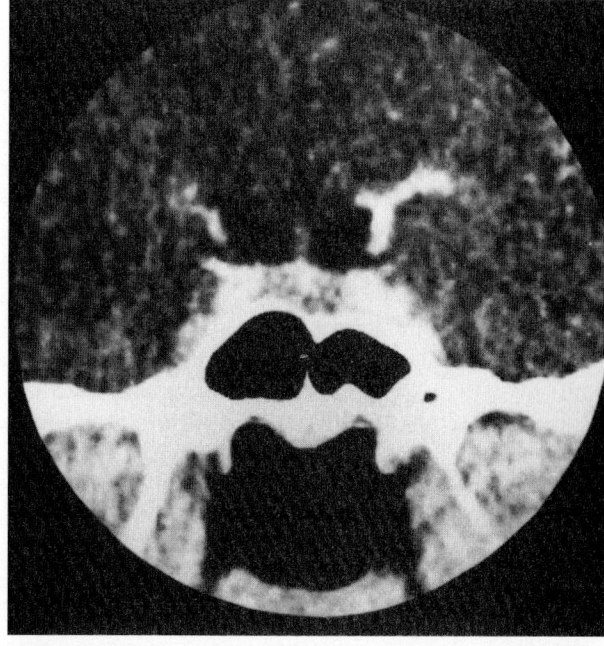

FIGURE 39-13 Coronal CT scan of a woman with microadenoma 4 months after bromocriptine therapy (5 mg per day). Clinical and biologic results were excellent; pituitary gland is nearly normal, with reconstruction of sellar floor. (From Bonneville JF, Poulignot D, Cattin F, et al: Radiology 143:451, 1982.)

mine if permanent remission has occurred, the prolactin level should be measured about 6 weeks after discontinuation of treatment because the levels plateau at this time.

Bromocriptine treatment has also been shown to reduce tumor mass in 80% to 90% of individuals with macroadenomas. In addition, visual disturbances, if present, are usually promptly relieved. Following subsequent surgical removal of these bromocriptine-treated tumors, histologic examination revealed a reduction of tumor cell size, with shrinkage of the cytoplasm being greater than the nucleus. In addition, there are modifications of cell structure and morphology as compared with tumors removed without prior medical treatment. The organelles responsible for prolactin synthesis shrink, indicating that bromocriptine impairs prolactin synthesis as well as release. The reduction in size of macroadenomas usually occurs rapidly, within a few weeks after starting treatment, but following withdrawal of drug the tumor size may increase just as rapidly; thus the drug should be withdrawn cautiously. In contrast to the frequent occurrence of pituitary insufficiency, including diabetes insipidus, after surgical or radiologic treatment of large tumors, bromocriptine treatment is not accompanied by any type of pituitary insufficiency.

Because permanent remission rarely occurs following withdrawal of bromocriptine treatment from individuals with large tumors, long-term treatment is usually necessary. The drug has been administered in some individuals for up to 12 years without problems, and once biochemical, radiologic, and clinical responses to treatment are established, they are generally maintained over a long-term period. Bromocriptine has also been successfully used to treat individuals with failure of, or recurrence after, operation or irradiation therapy.

Molitch et al. reported the results of a 1-year prospective multicenter study of the use of bromocriptine as primary therapy for prolactin-secreting macroadenomas in 27 individuals. Bromocriptine dosage ranged from 5 to 12.5 mg daily, with 7.5 mg being the most frequent dose. Prolactin levels fell in all individuals, and to 11% or less of pretreatment values in all but one. Of this group, two thirds had prolactin levels decrease to normal during treatment. Tumor shrinkage was observed in all individuals, being reduced by more than 50% in half the patients and by about 50% in an additional 20% of the study group. Visual field impairment disappeared in 9 of the 10 individuals with abnormalities. In two thirds of the individuals reduction in tumor size occurred by 6 weeks, but in one third it was not evident until 6 months, indicating there were both rapid and slow responses of tumor to drug treatment. Therefore at least a 6-month trial of medical therapy is warranted for individuals with a macroadenoma.

Because of these excellent results, the poor initial results of operation, and the high recurrence rates, these investigators concluded that bromocriptine should be used as the initial management of individuals with prolactin-secreting macroadenomas. After maximal shrinkage of tumor, medical therapy can be continued or operative treatment used. The cost of continuing bromocriptine treatment is considerable; it is inconvenient to take medication several times a day, and some individuals have unpleasant side effects with the higher dosages that may be necessary. Therefore some individuals prefer operative treatment. If they elect to have an operation, the drug should be continued until the time of operation to prevent tumor expansion. The rates of success after operation are no different among individuals who received or did not receive bromocriptine before the operation.

Cabergoline is a long-acting dopamine receptor agonist. This agent has a direct inhibitory effect on pituitary lactotrophs to decrease prolactin secretion. It is given orally in doses of 0.25 to 1.0 mg twice a week. Peak plasma levels occur in 2 to 3 hours and this drug has a half-life of 65 hours. Its slow elimination and long half-life produces a prolonged prolactin-lowering effect. The initial dose is 0.25 mg twice weekly and the dosage may be increased at intervals of 4 weeks to achieve a satisfactory response. In a randomized trial with bromocryptine, cabergoline lowered prolactin levels to normal in 83% of women, induced ovulation in 72%, and eliminated galactorrhea in 90%. The effectiveness of cabergoline was greater than bromocryptine. Adverse effects, particularly nausea, headaches, and dizziness, occurred with both agents but were less frequent, less severe, and of shorter duration with cabergoline. Therefore cabergoline is better tolerated than bromocryptine and has higher continuation rates. In contrast to the numerous clinical studies performed with bromocryptine there are very few reports of the effects of carbergoline when it is used to treat hyperprolactinemia in women. It is recommended that after serum prolactin levels have remained normal for 6 months carbogoline be discontinued to determine if the prolactin levels stay low without therapy.

Operative Approaches

Transsphenoidal microsurgical resection of prolactinoma has been widely used for therapy, and numerous reports of large series of individuals treated by this technique have been published. In a review of these studies Randall et al. concluded that transsphenoidal operations have minimal risk with a mortality of less than 0.5%, all deaths being reported to occur after treatment of macroadenomas. The risk of temporary postoperative diabetes insipidus is 10% to 40%, but the risk of permanent diabetes insipidus and iatrogenic hypopituitarism is less than 2%. The initial cure rate, with normalization of prolactin levels and return of ovulation, is relatively high for microadenomas (65% to 85%) and less so with macroadenomas (20% to 40%). Vision can return to normal in 85% of patients with loss of acuity and visual field defects.

The initial cure rate is related to the pretreatment prolactin levels. Those tumors with levels less than 100 ng/ml have an excellent prognosis (85%), and those with levels greater than 200 ng/ml have a poor prognosis (35%). Operative treatment of tumors in individuals older than 26 with amenorrhea for more than 6 months carries a poorer prognosis than tumors in younger women with a shorter duration of amenorrhea. Nevertheless, long-term follow-up of patients after operation indicates that late recurrence of hyperprolactinemia is common. Serri et al.

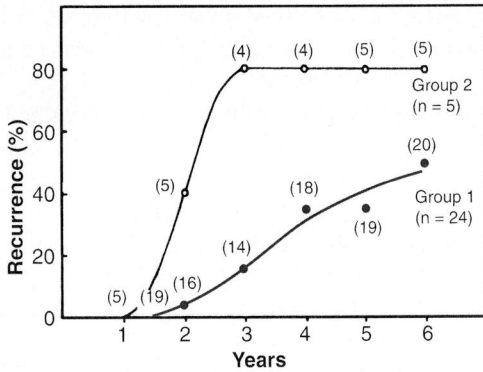

FIGURE 39-14 Cumulative recurrence rate in patients with microprolactinoma (group 1) or macroprolactinoma (group 2) after initially successful operation. Figures in parentheses indicate numbers of patients who were seen at each yearly interval. (From Serri O, Rasio E, Beauregard H, et al: N Engl J Med 309:280, 1983. Reprinted by permission of The New England Journal of Medicine.)

followed 28 women with microadenomas and 16 with macroadenomas for 6 years after operation. Although prolactin levels normalized and menses resumed in 24 (85%) of those with microadenomas and 5 (31%) of those with macroadenomas who had a good initial postoperative response, hyperprolactinemia recurred in half of those with microadenoma and 4 of the 5 with macroadenomas after a mean period of 4 and 2.5 years, respectively (Figure 39-14). There was no significant difference in recurrence rates for those who conceived and those who did not. Rodman et al. reported a lower postoperative recurrence rate (about 20% for both microadenomas and macroadenomas) following initial cure rates of 85% and 37%, respectively. The risk of recurrence in both series appeared to be related to the immediate postoperative prolactin levels, being greater in persons with a prolactin level greater than 10 ng/ml.

The relatively high rates of late recurrence indicate that these individuals have an underlying hypothalamic defect in dopamine regulation that continues after operative removal of the adenoma.

Because of the good results with medical therapy, surgery is recommended only for women with macroadenoma who fail to respond to medical therapy or have poor compliance with this regimen. It is best to reduce the size of macroadenomas maximally with bromocriptine before surgical removal of these extrasellar tumors.

Radiation Therapy

External radiation with cobalt, proton beam, or heavy particle therapy and brachytherapy with yttrium-90 rods implanted in the pituitary have all been used to treat macroadenomas but are not the primary mode of treatment. Results of such therapy have been inconsistent, and there is a delay of several months between treatment and resumption of ovulation. Furthermore, damage to normal pituitary tissue occurs, frequently leading to abnormal anterior pituitary function as well as diabetes insipidus. Damage to the optic nerves may also occur. Thus radiation therapy should be used only as adjunctive management following incomplete operative removal of large tumors.

Pregnancy

Many women with hyperprolactinemia with or without adenomas wish to become pregnant. A small percentage conceive spontaneously, while most require treatment to induce ovulation. Barbieri and Ryan compiled a literature review of the pregnancy courses of 275 women with adenomas, the majority of whose conceptions had been induced by bromocriptine. They reported that of 215 women with microprolactinomas, less than 1% had changes in visual fields, radiologic evidence of tumor enlargement, or neurologic signs. About 5% developed headaches during pregnancy. Of 60 women with macroprolactinomas, 20% developed adverse changes in visual fields and polytomographic or neurologic signs during pregnancy, and some of them required bromocriptine or operative treatment during pregnancy or shortly postpartum. For this reason excision of macroprolactinomas before pregnancy is attempted has been recommended. Nevertheless, because pituitary function is usually diminished after operation, induction of ovulation must be performed with complicated and expensive gonadotrophin treatment. Bromocriptine treatment does not interfere with pituitary function and is thus the therapy of choice for women with macroadenomas who wish to conceive. Continuous bromocriptine treatment throughout pregnancy for women with macroadenomas has been recommended by some, because with this therapy visual disturbances are rare. Despite a lowering of prolactin levels, there is no effect on placental hormone production, and pregnancy outcome does not appear to be affected.

Nevertheless, since bromocriptine crosses the placenta and suppresses fetal prolactin levels, its long-term effects on the newborn are unknown. Therefore it is now advised that women with macroadenomas discontinue the drug after conception, as do those with microadenomas, and have therapy reinitiated if and when symptoms of visual disturbance or severe headaches occur. Most women who conceive after bromocriptine treatment have ingested the drug for a few weeks after conception. In a review of 1410 such pregnancies compiled by Turkalj et al. there was a spontaneous abortion rate of 11%, ectopic pregnancy rate of 0.7%, and twin pregnancy rate of 1.8%. The incidence of minor (2.5%) and major (1%) congenital defects was similar to pregnancy outcomes in untreated populations of women. The mean amount of drug ingested and duration of postconception treatment were similar in mothers who had normal children and those with defects. Thus ingestion of bromocriptine during pregnancy does not appear to increase the risk of congenital abnormalities, spontaneous abortion, or multiple gestation. Postnatal surveillance of more than 200 children born in this series has revealed no adverse effects to date.

Ruiz-Velasco and Tolis compiled the obstetric histories of nearly 2000 pregnancies occurring in hyperprolactinemic women that have been reported in the literature. Most of these pregnancies were induced with bromocriptine. There was a term delivery rate of 85%, an abortion rate of 11%, a prematurity rate of 2%, and a multiple pregnancy rate of 1.2%. Although prolactin levels increased during pregnancy, after delivery the levels returned to pretreatment values in about 85%. A postpartum increase over pretreatment levels was uncommon (3%), while prolactin levels returned to normal in 13%. Likewise, among women who had postpartum radiologic sellar examination, 84% showed no change, 9% improved, and 7% worsened. Thus stopping treatment during pregnancy only occasionally results in tumor growth. It is advised that women with macroadenomas have monthly visual field examination and neurologic testing during pregnancy, but this is probably unnecessary for women with microadenomas unless they develop symptoms of headache or visual disturbances.

Following delivery, breast-feeding may be initiated without adverse effects on the tumors. Godo et al. reported that use of bromocriptine before conception and during pregnancy did not affect the incidence of persistent lactation following discontinuation of nursing. The incidence of menstrual abnormalities and degree of galactorrhea were usually similar to the state that existed before starting bromocriptine therapy. Therefore, following completion of nursing, as well as for women who do not breast-feed at all, bromocriptine should be ingested for 2 to 3 weeks and then discontinued. At that time serum prolactin measurement should be performed and treatment reinstituted according to the findings.

Women with Hyperprolactinemia Who Do Not Wish to Conceive

For women who do not wish to conceive and for whom galactorrhea is not a problem, no therapy is necessary unless estrogen levels are low. Thus to prevent osteoporosis in this clinical situation, estrogen-progestin hormone replacement or oral contraceptives should be given regardless of whether an adenoma is present. Long-term evaluation of all women with hyperprolactinemia should be performed. Unless a macroadenoma is present, measurement of prolactin levels once a year is advisable. Repeat imaging studies are unnecessary unless symptoms of headaches or visual disturbances occur or prolactin levels increase substantially. If bromocriptine therapy is used, temporary discontinuation of medication every year is advisable, with prolactin measurement 6 weeks later. If the level is normal, repeat prolactin measurements should be made semiannually. If the level is increased, therapy may be reinitiated. During medical treatment of macroadenomas, MRI or CT and visual field examination should be performed every 6 months to determine the effect of medication on the tumor. At these intervals a decision about whether to continue long-term bromocriptine treatment or remove the tumor surgically can be made.

KEY POINTS

- Estrogen stimulates prolactin release but blocks its action at the receptor in the breast.

- Physiologic stimuli for prolactin release include breast and nipple palpation, exercise, stress, sleep, and the noonday meal.

- The main symptoms of hyperprolactinemia are galactorrhea and amenorrhea, the latter caused by alterations in normal gonadotrophin-releasing hormone (GnRH) release.

- Hyperprolactinemia is present in 15% of all anovulatory women and 20% of women with amenorrhea of undetermined cause.

- About 60% of all women with galactorrhea have hyperprolactinemia, but almost 90% of women with galactorrhea, amenorrhea, and low estrogen levels have hyperprolactinemia.

- Pathologic causes of hyperprolactinemia include pharmacologic agents (tranquilizers, narcotics, and antihypertensive drugs), hypothyroidism, chronic renal disease, chronic neurostimulation of the breast, hypothalamic disease, and pituitary tumors (prolactinoma, acromegaly, Cushing's disease).

- About 3% to 5% of individuals with hyperprolactinemia have hypothyroidism.

- About 80% of all pituitary tumors secrete prolactin.

- About 25% of individuals with acromegaly and 10% of those with Cushing's disease have hyperprolactinemia.

- About 10% of individuals with an enlarged sella have the empty sella syndrome.

- Autopsy studies reveal that prolactinomas are present in about 10% of the population.

- About 50% of women with hyperprolactinemia will have a prolactinoma, as will nearly all of those with prolactin levels greater than 200 ng/ml.

- About 20% of women with galactorrhea and 35% of those with amenorrhea and galactorrhea have prolactinomas.

- About 70% of women with hyperprolactinemia, galactorrhea, and amenorrhea with low estrogen levels will have a prolactinoma.

- Women with regular menses, galactorrhea, and normal prolactin levels do not have prolactinomas.

- About 13% of women with prolactinomas do not have galactorrhea.

- Most macroadenomas enlarge with time; nearly all microadenomas do not.

- The initial operative cure rate for microadenomas is about 80% and for macroadenomas 30%, but the long-term recurrence rate is at least 20% for each.

- Most frequent side effects of bromocriptine are orthostatic hypotension, nausea, and vomiting.

- In women with hyperprolactinemia and no macroadenoma, bromocriptine treatment returns prolactin levels to normal in 90%, induces ovulatory cycles in 80%, and eradicates galactorrhea in 60%.

- After 1 year of bromocriptine treatment, prolactin levels remain normal in 11% of women with microadenomas; after 2 years permanent remission reaches 22%. After longer use, remissions of 50% have been reported.

- Bromocriptine shrinks 80% to 90% of macroadenomas.

- When pregnancy occurs in women with microadenomas, less than 1% have visual field changes, tumor enlargement, or neurologic signs; about 20% of women with macroadenomas have such adverse changes.

- Pregnancy increases the likelihood that prolactin levels will decrease or become normal over time.

- Estrogen replacement therapy or oral contraceptives will not stimulate growth of prolactin-secreting microadenomas and can be used for therapy of hyperprolactinemia and hypoestrogenism.

- Bromocriptine induction of pregnancy is not associated with an increased risk of congenital abnormalities, spontaneous abortion, or multiple gestation.

- About 85% of patients with prolactinomas have no change in prolactin levels or tumor size after delivery, 10% improve, and 5% worsen.

- The most frequent cause of mildly elevated prolactin levels is stress.

- The best modality to diagnose pituitary adenomas or empty sella syndrome is magnetic resonance imaging (MRI).

- The natural history of nearly all microprolactinomas is to stay the same size, with adverse menstrual problems resolving spontaneously in about one fourth of patients.

- Surgical treatment of prolactinomas is recommended only for patients who fail to respond or do not comply with medical management.

- For women who develop side effects with oral bromocriptine, vaginal administration usually alleviates the problem.

- Cabergoline appears to be more effective and better tolerated than bromocriptine.

BIBLIOGRAPHY

Abd El-Hamid MW, Joplin EF, and Lewis PD: Incidentally found small pituitary adenomas may have no effect on fertility, Acta Endocrinol (Copenh) 117:361, 1988.

Ampudia X, Pulig-Domingo M, Schwarzstein D, et al: Outcome and long-term effects of pregnancy in women with hyperprolactinaemia, Eur J Obstet Gynecol Reprod Biol 46:101, 1992.

Bäckström CT, McNeilly AS, Leash RM, et al: Pulsatile secretion of LH, FSH, prolactin oestradiol and progesterone during the human menstrual cycle, Clin Endocrinol 17:29, 1982.

Barbieri RL and Ryan KJ: Bromocriptine: endocrine pharmacology and therapeutic applications, Fertil Steril 39:727, 1983.

Biller BMK, Molitch ME, Vance ML, Cannistraro KB, et al: Treatment of prolactin-secreting macroadenomas with the once-weekly dopamine agonist cabergoline, J Clin Endocrinol Metab 81:2338, 1996.

Bonneville JF, Poulignot D, Cattin F, et al: Computed tomographic demonstration of the effects of bromocriptine on pituitary microadenoma size, Radiology 143:451, 1982.

Burrow GN, Wortzman G, Rewcastle NB, et al: Microadenomas of the pituitary and abnormal sellar tomograms in an unselected autopsy series, N Engl J Med 304:156, 1981.

Ciccarelli E, Giusti M, Miola C, et al: Effectiveness and tolerability of long-term treatment with cabergoline, a new long-lasting ergoline derivative, in hyperprolactinemic patients, J Clin Endocrinol Metab 69:725, 1989.

Ciccarelli E, Miola C, Avateneo T, et al: Long-term treatment with a new repeatable injectable form of bromocriptine, Parlodel LAR, in patients with tumorous hyperprolactinemia, Fertil Steril 52:930, 1989.

Corenblum B and Donovan L: The safety of physiological estrogen plus progestin replacement therapy and with oral contraceptive therapy in women with pathological hyperprolactinemia, Fertil Steril 59:671, 1993.

Corenblum B and Taylor PJ: Long-term follow-up of hyperprolactinemic women treated with bromocriptine, Fertil Steril 40:596, 1983.

Crosignani PG, Mattei AM, Scarduelli C, et al: Is pregnancy the best treatment for hyperprolactinemia? Hum Reprod 4:910, 1989.

Crosignani PG, Mattei AM, Severini V, et al: Long-term effects of time, medical treatment and pregnancy in 176 hyperprolactinemic women, Eur J Obstet Gynecol Reprod Biol 44:175, 1992.

Davajan V, Kletzky O, March CM, et al: The significance of galactorrhea in patients with normal menses, oligomenorrhea, and secondary amenorrhea, Am J Obstet Gynecol 130:894, 1978.

Fahy UM, Foster PA, Torode HW, et al: The effect of combined estrogen/progestogen treatment in women with hyperprolactinemic amenorrhea, Gynecol Endocrinol 6:183, 1992.

Gharib H, Frey HM, Laws ER Jr, et al: Coexistent primary empty sella syndrome and hyperprolactinemia: report of 11 cases, Arch Intern Med 143:1383, 1983.

Ginsburg J, Hardiman P, and Thomas M: Vaginal bromocriptine: clinical and biochemical effects, Gynecol Endocrinol 6:119, 1992.

Godo G, Kolosziar S, Szilagyi I, et al: Experience related to pregnancy, lactation, and the after-weaning condition of hyperprolactinemic patients treated with bromocriptine, Fertil Steril 51:529, 1989.

Kleinberg DL, Noel GL, and Frantz AG: Galactorrhea: a study of 235 cases, including 48 with pituitary tumors, N Engl J Med 296:589, 1977.

Kletsky OA and Vermesh M: Effectiveness of vaginal bromocriptine in treating women with hyperprolactinemia, Fertil Steril 51:269, 1989.

Koppelman MCS, Jaffe MJ, Rieth KG, et al: Hyperprolactinemia, amenorrhea, and galactorrhea: a retrospective assessment of 25 cases, Ann Intern Med 100:115, 1984.

March CM, Kletzky OA, Davajan V, et al: Longitudinal evaluation of patients with untreated prolactin-secreting pituitary adenomas, Am J Obstet Gynecol 139:835, 1981.

Martin TL, Kim M, and Malarkey WB: The natural history of idiopathic hyperprolactinemia, J Clin Endocrinol Metab 60:855, 1985.

Molitch ME, Elton RL, Blackwell RE, et al: Bromocriptine as primary therapy for prolactin-secreting macroadenomas: results of a prospective multicenter study, J Clin Endocrinol Metab 60:698, 1985.

Moriondo P, Travaglini P, Nissim M, et al: Bromocriptine treatment of microprolactinomas: evidence of stable prolactin decrease after drug withdrawal, J Clin Endocrinol Metab 60:764, 1985.

Mornex R and Hugues B: Remission of hyperprolactinemia after pregnancy, N Engl J Med 324:60, 1991.

Muneyyirci-Delale O, Goldstein D, Reyes FI, et al: Diagnosis of stress-related hyperprolactinemia: evaluation of the hyperprolactinemia rest test, NY State J Med 89:205, 1989.

Rasmussen C, Bergh T, and Wide L: Prolactin secretion and menstrual function after long-term bromocriptine treatment, Fertil Steril 48:550, 1987.

Rasmussen C, Bergh T, Nillius SJ, and Wide L: Return of menstruation and normalization of prolactin in hyperprolactinemic women with bromocriptine-induced pregnancy, Fertil Steril 44:31, 1985.

Rodman EF, Molitch ME, Post KD, et al: Long-term follow-up of transsphenoidal selective adenomectomy for prolactinoma, JAMA 252:921, 1984.

Ruiz-Velasco V and Tolis G: Pregnancy in hyperprolactinemic women, Fertil Steril 41:793, 1984.

Schlechte J, Dolan K, Sherman B, et al: The natural history of untreated hyperprolactinemia: a prospective analysis, J Clin Endocrinol Metab 68:412, 1989.

Serri O, Rasio E, Beauregard H, et al: Recurrence of hyperprolactinemia after selective transsphenoidal adenomectomy in women with prolactinoma, N Engl J Med 309:280, 1983.

Shoupe D and Mishell DR Jr: Hyperprolactinemia: diagnosis and treatment. In: Lobo RA, Mishell DR Jr, Paulson RJ, Shoupe D, editors: Mishell's textbook of infertility, contraception and reproductive endocrinology, ed 4, Blackwell Scientific Publications, Cambridge, Mass, 1997.

Sisam DA, Sheehan JP, and Sheeler LR: The natural history of untreated microprolactinomas, Fertil Steril 48:67, 1987.

Slujmer AV and Lappohn RE: Clinical history and outcome of 59 patients with idiopathic hyperprolactinemia, Fertil Steril 50:72, 1992.

Stein AL, Levenick MN, and Kletzky OA: Computer tomography versus magnetic resonance imaging for the evaluation of suspected pituitary adenomas, Obstet Gynecol 73:996, 1989.

Testa G, Vegetti W, Motta T, et al: Two-year treatment with oral contraceptives in hyperprolactinemic patients, Contraception 58:69, 1998.

Turkalj I, Brain P, and Krupp P: Surveillance of bromocriptine in pregnancy, JAMA 247:1589, 1982.

Vermesh M, Fossum GT, and Kletzky OA: Vaginal bromocriptine: pharmacology and effect on serum prolactin in normal women, Obstet Gynecol 72:693, 1988.

Webster J, Piscitelli G, Polli A, Ferrari CI, et al: A comparison of cabergoline and bromocriptine in the treatment of hyperprolactinemic amenorrhea, N Engl J Med 331:904, 1994.

Hyperandrogenism

Physiology, Etiology, Differential Diagnosis, Management

KEY TERMS AND DEFINITIONS

Acanthosis Nigricans. Dark, raised hyperpigmentation of the skin, found particularly on the nape of the neck and axilla.

5α-Androstane-3α,17β-diol Glucuronide (3α-diol-G). A metabolite of 5α-reductase conversion of testosterone (T) to dihydrotestosterone (DHT) that can be measured in serum and is the most accurate indicator of peripheral androgen metabolism.

Cryptic Hyperandrogenism. Elevated levels of circulatory androgens without clinical manifestations of hirsutism or acne. It is usually accompanied by anovulation.

Dehydroepiandrosterone Sulfate (DHEA-S). An androgen secreted nearly exclusively by the adrenal gland. Serum levels are used as a marker of adrenal androgen activity.

Free Androgen Index (ng/nmol). Measurement of biologically active testosterone, calculated as follows: total testosterone (ng/ml) times 1000 divided by sex hormone–binding globulin (SHBG) (nmols/L).

Free Testosterone. Small portion of circulating testosterone that is not bound to sex hormone–binding globulin or albumin.

Hilus Cell Tumor. Small testosterone-secreting ovarian tumors that most frequently develop after menopause.

Hirsutism. Presence of hair in locations where it is not normally found in a woman, specifically in the midline of the body (upper lip, chin, back, and intermammary region).

Hyperandrogenic Chronic Anovulation. A syndrome consisting of the endocrinologic findings found in polycystic ovarian syndrome without the morphologic and sonographic findings of polycystic ovaries.

Hypertrichosis. A generalized increase in the amount of body hair in its normal location.

Idiopathic Hirsutism (Constitutional or Familial Hirsutism). The most common disorder associated with androgen excess. It is due to increased peripheral androgen metabolism and is associated with normal circulating levels of testosterone and DHEA-S but increased levels of 3α-diol-G.

17-Ketosteroids. Urinary metabolites of DHEA, DHEA-S, androstenedione, and testosterone. They consist of DHEA, androsterone, and etiocholanolone.

Late-Onset Congenital Adrenal Hyperplasia/Late-Onset 21-Hydroxylase Deficiency (LOHD). Also called *late-onset hyperplasia, nonclassic congenital adrenal hyperplasia attenuated,* or *acquired adrenal hyperplasia.* Mild degree of enzymatic 21-hydroxylase deficiency of cortisol biosynthesis that produces signs of androgen excess after puberty without external sexual ambiguity being present at birth. This genetically acquired entity can be present in both severe (homozygous) and mild (heterozygous) forms.

Metformin. An oral antihyperglycemic agent that improves glucose tolerance by increasing the action of insulin and by decreasing hepatic glucose production and intestinal glucose absorption. This agent induces ovulation in some women with polycystic ovarian syndrome whether or not they have glucose intolerance.

Non-Sex Hormone–Binding Globulin Bound Testosterone. Biologically active component of circulatory testosterone, consisting of free testosterone and albumin-bound testosterone.

Pilosebaceous Unit. Structure in skin from which sebaceous glands and hair are derived. Found in the skin in every area of the body except the palms and soles.

Polycystic Ovarian Syndrome (PCOS). An endocrinologic disorder characterized by excessive ovarian androgen production, abnormal gonadotrophin secretion, and chronic anovulation with morphologic changes in the ovary consisting of multiple small subcapsular follicles, increased amounts of stromal tissue, and ovarian enlargement. This disorder begins perimenarcheally, and its clinical manifestations include hirsutism, menstrual irregularity (oligomenorrhea or amenorrhea), and obesity. Findings upon sonographic visualization of the ovaries include multiple (>10) small (2- to 10-mm diameter) follicles in the periphery, increased echogenicity of the stroma, and ovarian enlargement.

5α-Reductase. The enzyme that converts testosterone to its more active metabolite, dihydrotestosterone (DHT).

Sertoli-Leydig Cell Tumor. Testosterone-secreting ovarian tumor that usually is unilateral and palpably enlarged and occurs most frequently in the second to fourth decades of life. It was previously termed *arrhenoblastoma*.

Spironolactone. An aldosterone antagonist that acts as an antiandrogen by binding to the peripheral androgen receptor without inducing androgenic activity. It also inhibits steroidogenesis by interfering with ovarian enzymatic activity as well as inhibiting 5α-reductase activity in the pilosebaceous unit.

Stromal Hyperthecosis. An ovarian disorder characterized by nests of luteinized theca cells within the stroma of bilaterally enlarged ovaries. Clinically this condition is associated with slowly but progressively increasing signs of virilization.

Virilization. Presence of signs of masculinization in a woman. These signs include temporal balding, voice deepening, clitoral enlargement, and increased muscle mass.

The clinical signs associated with excessive androgen production in women are hirsutism and virilization, with hirsutism being much more common.

The pilosebaceous unit is composed of a sebaceous component and a pilary component from which the hair shaft arises. There are two types of hair; vellus hair is soft, fine, and unpigmented, whereas the terminal hair is coarse, thick, pigmented, and undergoes cyclic changes. *Anagen* is the growth phase of hair. It is followed by the transitional *catagen* phase and finally by a resting, or *telogen* phase, after which the hair sheds. Androgen is necessary to produce development of terminal hair, and the duration of the anagen phase is directly related to the levels of circulating androgen.

The level of activity of the enzyme 5α-reductase in the hair follicle directly influences the level of androgenic effect on hair growth. With elevated levels of circulating androgen or increased activity of 5α-reductase, terminal hair appears where normally only vellus hair is present. With these alterations the length of the anagen phase is prolonged and the hair becomes thicker.

The presence of hirsutism without other signs of virilization is associated with relatively mild disorders of androgen production or increased 5α-reductase activity, and circulating testosterone levels are either normal or mildly to moderately elevated (less than 1.5 ng/ml). Hirsutism usually has a gradual onset and if unaccompanied by signs of virilization is not caused by a severe enzymatic defect or a neoplasm. The amount and location of the central hair growth found in women with hirsutism vary. In the milder forms hair is found only on the upper lip and chin, whereas with increasing severity it appears on the cheeks, chest (intermammary), abdomen (superior to the umbilicus), inner aspects of thighs, and lower back and intergluteal areas. The severity of the hirsutism can be roughly quantified by means of the scoring system of Ferriman and Gallwey (Figure 40-1 and Table 40-1). Increased hair growth only on the extremities (hypertrichosis) should not be considered hirsutism, as terminal hair is normally found in this location in women. Women with hirsutism can have normal ovulatory menstrual cycles, oligomenorrhea, or amenorrhea.

Virilization is a relatively uncommon clinical finding, and its presence is usually associated with markedly elevated levels of circulating testosterone (2 ng/ml or greater). In contrast to the gradual development of hirsutism, signs of virilization usually occur over a relatively short time. These signs are due to both the masculinizing and the defeminizing (antiestrogenic) action of testosterone and include temporal balding, clitoral hypertrophy, decreased breast size, dryness of the vagina, and increased muscle mass. Women with virilization are nearly always amenorrheic. The presence of androgen-secreting neoplasms should always be suspected in any woman who develops signs of virilization, particularly if the onset is rapid.

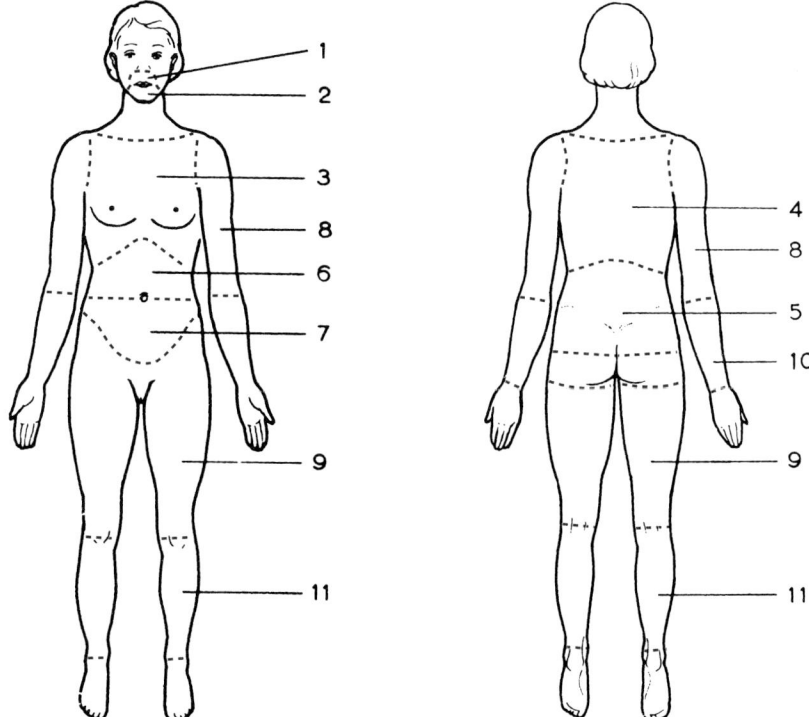

FIGURE 40-1 Demarcation of 11 sites used for numerically grading amount of hair growth—anterior and posterior views. (From Ferriman D and Gallwey JD: J Clin Endocrinol Metab 21:1440, 1961. Copyright 1961 by The Endocrine Society.)

PHYSIOLOGY

The sources of androgen production in the human female are the ovaries and the adrenal glands. The major androgen produced by the ovaries is testosterone and that of the adrenal glands is dehydroepiandrosterone sulfate (DHEA-S). Measurement of the amount of these two steroids in the circulation provides clinically relevant information regarding the presence and source of increased androgen production. In addition to glandular production of androgens, conversion of androstenedione and DHEA to testosterone occurs in peripheral tissue.

The ovaries secrete only about 0.1 mg of testosterone each day, mainly from the theca-stroma cells. Other androgens secreted by the ovary are androstenedione (1 to 2 mg/day) and DHEA (<1 mg/day). The adrenal glands, in addition to secreting large quantities of DHEA-S (6 to 24 mg/day), secrete about the same daily amount of androstenedione (1 mg/day) as the ovaries and less than 1 mg of DHEA per day. The normal adrenal gland secretes little testosterone, although some uncommon adrenal tumors may secrete testosterone directly.

Androstenedione and DHEA do not have androgenic activity but are peripherally converted at a slow rate to the biologically active androgen, testosterone. Only about 5% of androstenedione and a smaller percentage of DHEA are converted to testosterone. The total daily production of testosterone in women is normally about 0.35 mg. Of this, 0.1 mg comes from direct ovarian secretion, 0.2 mg from peripheral conversion of androstenedione, and 0.05 mg from peripheral conversion of DHEA (Table 40-2). Since the ovary and adrenal gland secrete about equal amounts of androstenedione and DHEA, about two thirds (0.22 mg) of the daily testosterone produced in a woman originates from the ovaries. Thus increased circulating levels of testosterone usually indicate abnormal ovarian androgen production. Normal circulating levels of these androgens in women of reproductive age are shown in Table 40-3. Only a small amount of testosterone is metabolized to testosterone glucuronide and then excreted in the urine. Testosterone, which is not a 17-ketosteroid (17-KS), is mainly metabolized to androstenedione and then excreted as androsterone and etiocholanolone, both of which are 17-KS. DHEA, DHEA-S, and androstenedione are excreted as DHEA, androsterone, and etiocholanolone, all of which are 17-KS. The origin of the major amount of urinary 17-KS is the precursor androgen produced in the greatest amounts, DHEA-S. Because DHEA-S has a long half-life in serum, serum levels of DHEA-S correlate well with amounts of 17-KS excreted in the urine. Urinary 17-KS levels were previously measured to assess adrenal androgenic activity. Now DHEA-S levels are measured directly in the serum.

TABLE 40-1
Definition of Hair Gradings at 11 Sites*

Site	Grade	Definition
Upper lip	1	Few hairs at outer margin
	2	Small moustache at outer margin
	3	Moustache extending halfway from outer margin
	4	Moustache extending to midline
Chin	1	Few scattered hairs
	2	Scattered hairs with small concentrations
	3 & 4	Complete cover, light and heavy
Chest	1	Circumareolar hairs
	2	With midline hair in addition
	3	Fusion of these areas, with three-quarters cover
	4	Complete cover
Upper back	1	Few scattered hairs
	2	Rather more, still scattered
	3 & 4	Complete cover, light and heavy
Lower back	1	Sacral tuft of hair
	2	With some lateral extension
	3	Three-quarters cover
	4	Complete cover
Upper abdomen	1	Few midline hairs
	2	Rather more, still midline
	3 & 4	Half and full cover
Lower abdomen	1	Few midline hairs
	2	Midline streak of hair
	3	Midline band of hair
	4	Inverted V-shaped growth
Arm	1	Sparse growth affecting not more than one quarter of limb surface
	2	More than this; cover still incomplete
	3 & 4	Complete cover, light and heavy
Forearm	1,2,3,4	Complete cover of dorsal surface; 2 grades of light and 2 of heavy growth
Thigh	1,2,3,4	As for arm
Leg	1,2,3,4	As for arm

From Ferriman D and Gallwey JD: J Clin Endocrinol Metab 21:1440, 1961. Copyright 1961 by The Endocrine Society.

*Grade 0 at all sites indicates absence of terminal hair.

TABLE 40-2
Origin of Testosterone in Women

Origin	Amount
Ovarian secretion	0–1 mg/day
Peripheral conversion	
Androstenedione → testosterone	0.2 mg/day
Dehydroepiandrosterone → testosterone	0.05 mg/day
Total testosterone production	0.35 mg/day

From Lobo RA: Androgen excess. In Mishell DR Jr, Davajan V, and Lobo RA, editors: Infertility, contraception and reproductive endocrinology, ed 3, Cambridge, Mass, 1991, Blackwell Scientific Publications.

TABLE 40-3
Plasma Concentrations of Androgens During Menstrual Cycle

Steroid Hormone	Phase of Cycle	Plasma Concentration	
		Mean	Range
Androstenedione (ng/ml)	*	1.4	0.7–3.1
Testosterone (ng/ml)	*	0.35	0.15–0.55
Dehydroepiandrosterone (ng/ml)	*	4.2	2.7–7.8
Dehydroepiandrosterone sulfate (μg/ml)	*	1.6	0.8–3.4

From Goebelsmann U: Steroid hormones. In Mishell DR Jr and Davajan V, editors: Infertility, contraception and reproductive endocrinology, ed 2, Oradell, NJ, 1986, Medical Economics Books.

*Unspecified; no major changes during menstrual cycle.

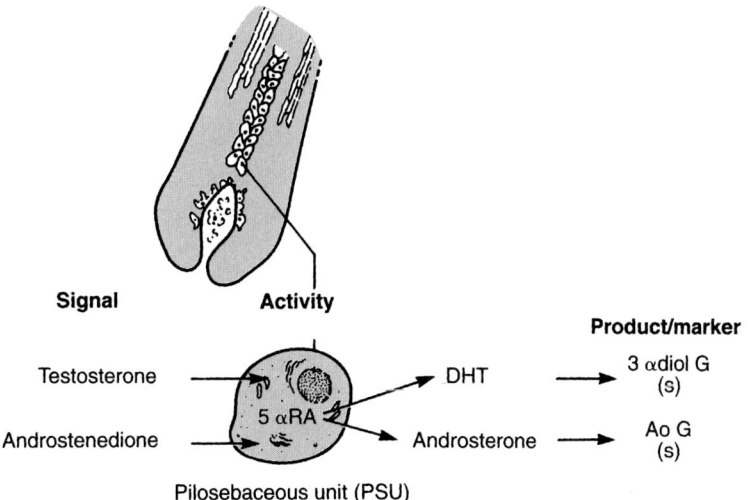

FIGURE 40-2   Peripheral androgen metabolism and markers of this activity. *5α RA*, 5α-Reductase; *DHT*, dihydrotestosterone; 3α-diol-G, 3α-androstanediol glucuronide; Ao G, androsterone glucuronide; (s), serum. (From Lobo RA: Androgen excess. In Mishell DR Jr, Davajan V, and Lobo RA, editors: Infertility, contraception and reproductive endocrinology, ed 3, Cambridge, Mass, 1991, Blackwell Scientific Publications.)

Most testosterone in the circulation (about 85%) is tightly bound to sex hormone–binding globulin (SHBG) and is believed to be biologically inactive. An additional 10% to 15% is loosely bound to albumin, with only about 1% to 2% not bound to any protein (free testosterone). Both the free and albumin-bound fractions are biologically active. Serum testosterone can be measured either as the total amount, the amount that is believed to be biologically active (non-SHBG bound), and as the free form.

To exert a biologic effect, testosterone is metabolized peripherally in target tissues to the more potent androgen 5α-dihydrotestosterone (DHT) by the enzyme 5α-reductase. After further 3-keto reduction, DHT is converted to its distal metabolite, 5α-androstane-3α,17β-diol (3α-diol). 3α-diol is conjugated to 5α-androstane-3α,17β-diol glucuronide (3α-diol-G), which is a stable, irreversible product of intracellular 5α-reductase activity (Figure 40-2).

Even with normal circulatory levels of androgen, increased 5α-reductase activity in the pilosebaceous unit will result in increased androgenic activity, producing hirsutism (Figure 40-3). Serafini et al. measured 5α-reductase activity in skin biopsies and found the level of activity correlated very well with the degree of hirsutism present.

The degree of 5α-reductase activity can be measured in skin biopsies by polymerase chain reaction. Currently this technique is only used for investigational purposes; if necessary for diagnostic reasons, 3-α-diol-G levels can be directly measured in serum. Lobo et al. have shown measurement of this metabolite to be the most accurate indicator of the degree of peripheral androgen metabolism in women. Horton et al. have shown that although serum levels of total testosterone are similar in normal and hirsute women, there are significant differences in the amounts of non-SHBG bound testosterone as well as 3α-diol-G (Figure 40-4). Non-SHBG bound testosterone is elevated in about 60% to 70% of hirsute women, but 3α-diol-G is elevated in more than 80% of such individuals. Thus increased levels of non-SHBG bound testosterone indicate increased ovarian production. If levels of non-SHBG bound testosterone are normal and levels of 3α-diol-G are elevated, testosterone production is not increased, but peripheral conversion of testosterone to its active metabolite (DHT) is increased above normal. Either of these processes can cause symptoms and signs of androgen excess. Thus there are three markers of androgen production in serum, one for each compartment where androgens are produced (Table 40-4).

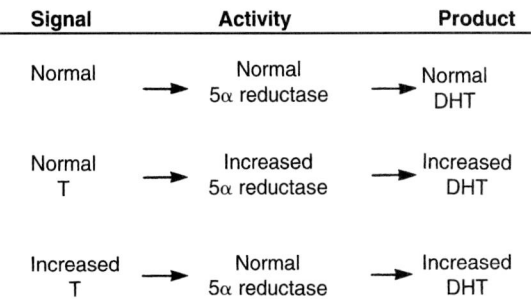

Signal	Activity	Product
Normal	Normal 5α reductase	Normal DHT
Normal T	Increased 5α reductase	Increased DHT
Increased T	Normal 5α reductase	Increased DHT

FIGURE 40-3   Influence of androgen substrate (signal, e.g., testosterone or androstenedione) and 5α-reductase activity (in pilosebaceous units) on local production of biologically active androgens. *T*, Testosterone; *DHT*, dihydrotestosterone. (From Lobo RA: Androgen excess. In Mishell DR Jr, Davajan V, and Lobo RA, editors: Infertility, contraception and reproductive endocrinology, ed 3, Cambridge, Mass, 1991, Blackwell Scientific Publications.)

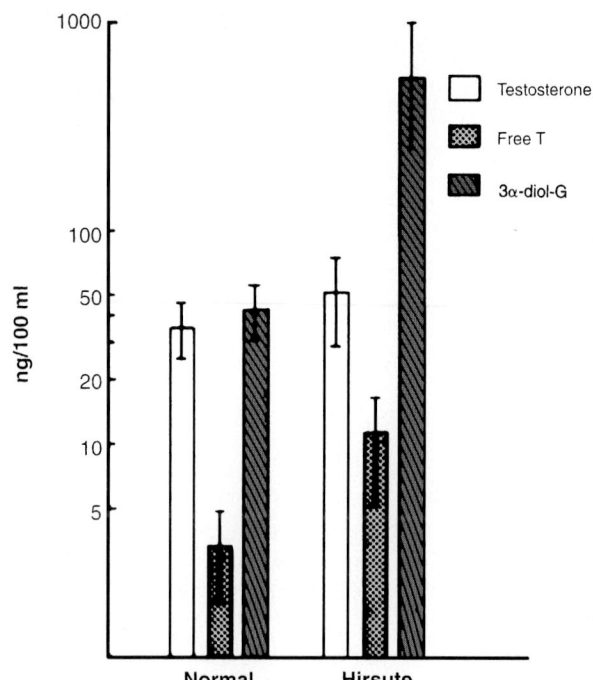

FIGURE 40-4 Plasma total testosterone, unbound testosterone *(free T)* and 5α-androstane-3α, 17β-diol glucuronide *(3α-diol-G)* in normal and hirsute women. Note insignificant elevation with overlap for testosterone and free T testosterone and highly significant increase in *3α-diol-G* without overlap between two groups of women. (Reproduced from Horton R, Hawks D, and Lobo RA: J Clin Invest 69:1203, 1982. By copyright permission of The American Society for Clinical Investigation.)

TABLE 40-4
Markers of Androgen Production

Source	Marker
Ovary	Testosterone
Adrenal gland	DHEA-S
Periphery	3α-diol-G

From Lobo RA: Androgen excess. In Mishell DR Jr, Davajan V, and Lobo RA editors: Infertility, contraception and reproductive endocrinology, ed 3, Cambridge, Mass, 1991, Blackwell Scientific Publications.

ETIOLOGY

There are 10 currently recognized causes of androgen excess in women. One frequent cause is administration of androgenic medication. In addition to testosterone itself, various anabolic steroids, 19-norprogestins, and danazol have androgenic effects. Thus a careful history of medication intake is important for all women with hirsutism.

Hirsutism or virilization can also be associated with some forms of abnormal gonad development. With this etiology, individuals have signs of either external sexual ambiguity or primary amenorrhea, in addition to findings of androgen excess and a Y chromosome present in the gonad. These conditions are discussed in Chapter 38 and will not be further described in the discussion of the differential diagnosis of androgen excess in this chapter.

Signs of androgen excess during pregnancy can be caused by increased ovarian testosterone production. This is usually caused by either a luteoma of pregnancy or hyperreactio luteinalis. The former is a unilateral or bilateral solid ovarian enlargement, whereas the latter is bilateral cystic ovarian enlargement. After pregnancy is completed, the excessive ovarian androgenic production resolves spontaneously and the androgenic signs regress.

A diagnosis of these three causes of androgen excess can usually be easily made by means of a careful history and physical examination. The remaining causes of androgen excess, together with the origin of hyperandrogenism, are listed in Table 40-5. Details of each of these etiologies will be described in decreasing order of their frequency.

Idiopathic Hirsutism (Peripheral Disorder of Androgen Metabolism)

The most common cause of androgen excess in women is manifested by signs of hirsutism and regular menstrual cycles in conjunction with normal circulatory levels of androgens (both testosterone and DHEA-S). Because this type of disorder is frequently present in several individuals in the same family, particularly those of Mediterranean descent, it has also been called *familial* or *constitutional hirsutism*. Since neither ovarian nor adrenal androgen production is increased in these individuals, the cause of the androgen excess was not determined until recently, hence the term *idiopathic hirsutism*. Paulson et al. have

TABLE 40-5
Differential Diagnosis of Hirsutism and Virilization*

Source	Diagnosis
Nonspecific	Exogenous/iatrogenic Abnormal gonadal or sexual development
Pregnancy	Androgen excess in pregnancy: luteoma or hyperreactio luteinalis
Periphery	Idiopathic hirsutism
Ovary	Polycystic ovary syndrome Stromal hyperthecosis Ovarian tumors
Adrenal gland	Adrenal tumors Cushing syndrome Adult-onset congenital adrenal hyperplasia

*Idiopathic hirsutism and polycystic ovary syndrome do not present with virilizations.

shown that about 80% of these individuals have increased levels of 3α-diol-G, indirectly indicating that the cause of hirsutism is increased 5α-reductase activity (Figure 40-5). These investigators directly measured the percent conversion of testosterone to DHT in genital skin as an assessment of 5α-reductase activity in the skin of women with idiopathic hirsutism. The amount of 5α-reductase activity was increased in hirsute women as compared with normal women and correlated well with both the degree of hirsutism and serum levels of 3α-diol-G. Thus idiopathic hirsutism is actually a disorder of peripheral androgen metabolism in the pilosebaceous apparatus of the skin and is possibly genetically determined. The condition should probably be renamed *abnormal peripheral androgen metabolism*. Antiandrogens that block peripheral testosterone action or interfere with 5α-reductase activity are effective therapeutic agents for this disorder. The antiandrogens most commonly used clinically are spironolactone and cyproterone acetate.

Polycystic Ovarian Syndrome

Polycystic ovarian syndrome (PCOS) was originally described in 1935 by Stein and Leventhal as a syndrome consisting of amenorrhea, hirsutism, and obesity in association with enlarged polycystic ovaries. There is not a universally accepted definition of PCOS. Most believe that PCOS should be defined by the presence of ovulatory dysfunction, clinical evidence of hyperandrogenism and/or hyperandrogenemia, and exclusion of related disorders such as late-onset hydroxylase deficiency. Controversy exists as to whether the presence of the morphologic changes of polycystic ovaries need to be present in order to establish the diagnosis of PCOS. The incidence of PCOS in the population has been reported to range between 3% and 5%. The ovaries of most women with PCOS are enlarged, being as much as 5 cm in diameter. The capsules are smooth and white (Figure 40-6). Beneath the capsules are numerous small cysts (Figure 40-7). These anatomic findings are not pathognomonic for PCOS, because they also have been noted in some women with Cushing syn-

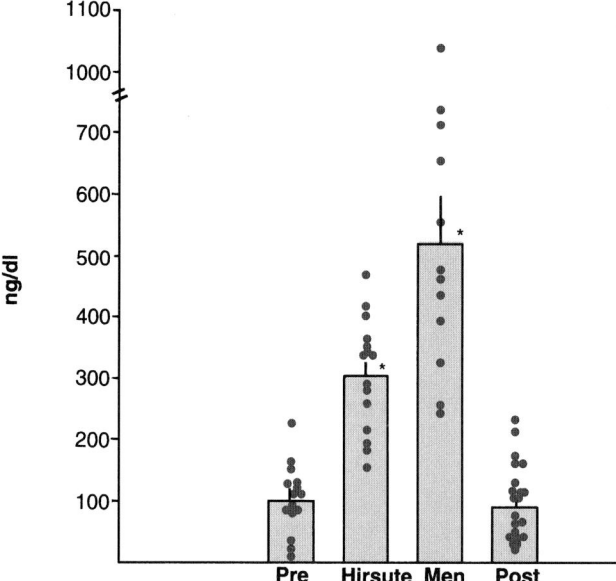

FIGURE 40-5 Serum 3α-diol-G in premenopausal nonhirsute women *(PRE)*, hirsute women, normal men, and postmenopausal nonhirsute women *(POST)*. The *asterisks* denote $P < 0.05$, as compared with PRE. (From Paulson RJ, Serafini PC, Catalino JA, and Lobo RA: Fertil Steril 42:422, 1986.)

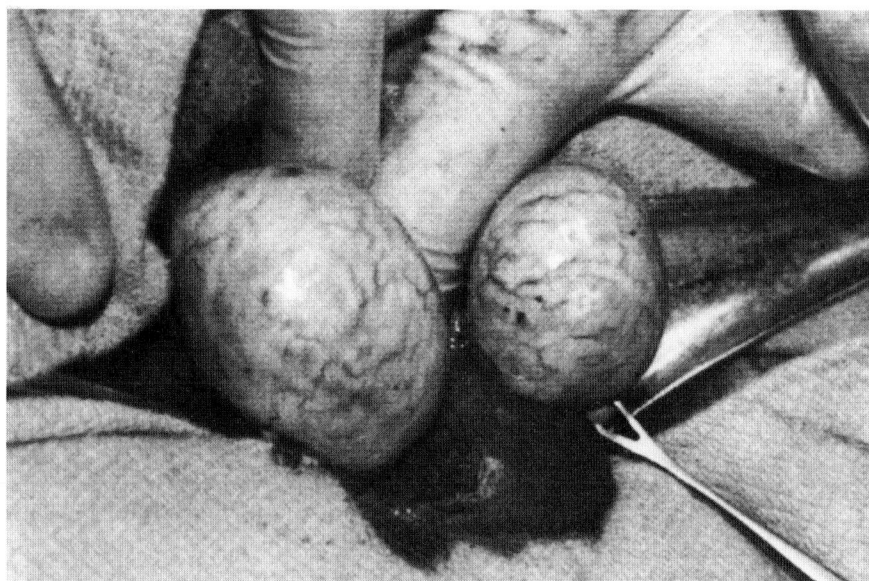

FIGURE 40-6 Gross characteristics of polycystic ovaries. Bilateral enlarged ovaries with smooth and thickened capsule. (From Yen SSC: Chronic anovulation caused by peripheral endocrine disorders. In Yen SSC and Jaffe RB, editors: Reproductive endocrinology, ed 2, Philadelphia, 1986, WB Saunders Co.)

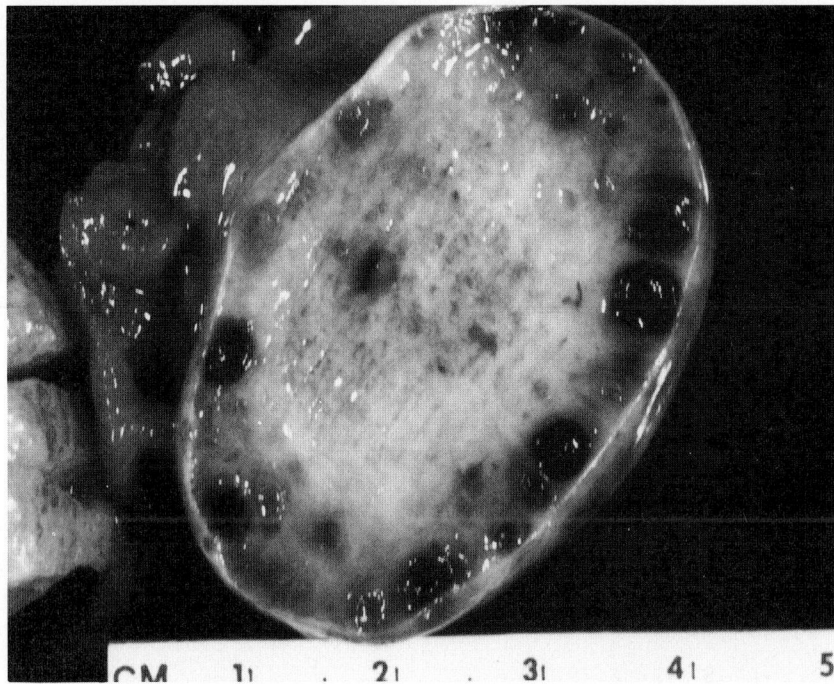

FIGURE 40-7 Sagittal section of a polycystic ovary illustrating large number of follicular cysts and thickened stroma.

drome or congenital adrenal hyperplasia and in association with certain adrenal tumors, and many normal ovulatory women have polycystic ovaries.

Women with PCOS exhibit a variety of clinical presentations. Signs of hyperandrogenism range from mild acne to severe hirsutism. Menstrual irregularities range from oligomenorrhea to amenorrhea. Obesity is not always present. However the presence of obesity in women with PCOS is correlated with a greater incidence of menstrual irregularity and hyperandrogenism than in non-obese women. Weight reduction by means of caloric restriction and exercise improves these symptoms. About 70% of women with this syndrome have enlarged polycystic ovaries that can be visualized sonographically. Sonographically, polycystic ovaries are usually characterized as enlarged ovaries having multiple (>10) subcapsular small follicles (2 to 10 mm in diameter) in the periphery in one plane and increased stromal echogenicity. In contrast to the mean ovarian volume of normal women (4.7 to 5.2 cm³), that of women with PCOS usually is greater than 10 cm³. Many women with the clinical and endocrinologic findings consistent with PCOS do not have sonographic findings of polycystic ovaries. These women are more appropriately characterized as having hyperandrogenic chronic anovulation, not PCOS, as they do not have polycystic ovaries. As many as 25% of normal ovulating women without hyperandrogenism also have polycystic-appearing ovaries seen sonographically. Thus polycystic-appearing ovaries frequently occur in

women without the clinical and endocrinologic features of this syndrome.

This abnormal endocrinologic disorder begins soon after menarche and consists of abnormal gonadotrophin secretion caused by either increased gonadotrophin-releasing hormone (GnRH) pulse amplitude or increased pituitary sensitivity to GnRH. These abnormalities result in tonically elevated levels of luteinizing hormone (LH) in about two thirds of the women with this syndrome (Figure 40-8). After a bolus of GnRH, there is usually an exaggerated response of LH, but not of follicle-stimulating hormone (FSH) (Figure 40-9). In addition, there are increased circulating levels of androgens produced by both the ovaries and the adrenal glands (Figure 40-10). Serum testosterone levels usually range between 0.7 to 1.2 ng/ml, and androstenedione levels are usually between 3 and 5 ng/ml. Koskinen et al. reported that the finding of an elevated LH level, a low FSH level, and an elevated androstenedione level had a high sensitivity and specificity for the diagnosis of PCOS. In addition, about half the women with this syndrome have elevated levels of DHEA-S. Although nearly all women with PCOS have elevated levels of circulating androgens, Lobo et al. found that the presence or absence of hirsutism depends on whether those androgens are converted peripherally by 5α-reductase to the more potent androgen DHT, as reflected by increased circulating levels of 3α-diol-G. Nonhirsute women with PCOS have elevated circulatory levels of testosterone or DHEA-S or both but not 3α-diol-

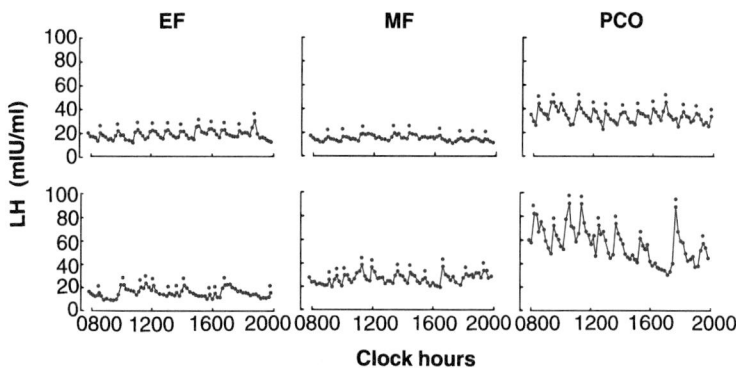

FIGURE 40-8   Patterns of pulsatile luteinizing hormone *(LH)* secretion in patients with polycystic ovarian syndrome *(PCO)* and in control subjects with normal early follicular *(EF)* and midfollicular *(MF)* phases. The *asterisks* indicate significant pulses. (From Kazer AR, Kessel B, and Yen SSC: J Clin Endocrinol Metab 65:233, 1987.)

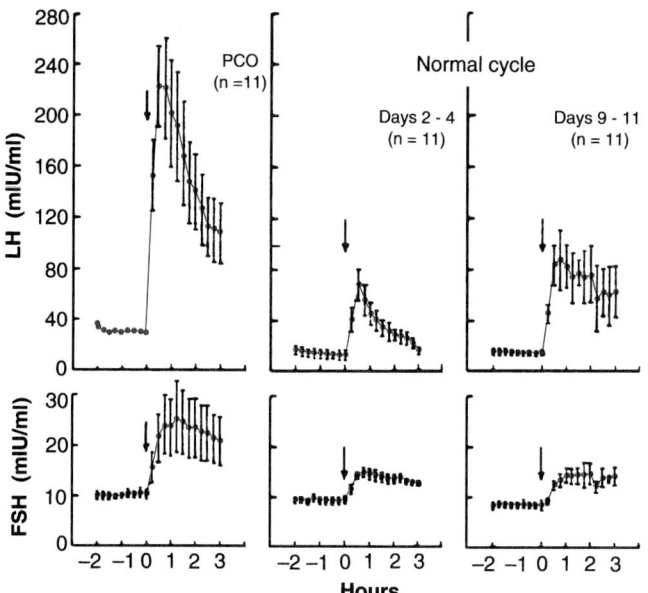

FIGURE 40-9   Comparison of quantitative luteinizing hormone *(LH)* and follicle-stimulating hormone *(FSH)* release in response to a single bolus of 150 μg of GnRH in patients with polycystic ovarian syndrome *(PCO)* and in normal women during low-estrogen (early follicular) and high-estrogen (late follicular) phases of their cycles. (From Rebar R, Judd HL, Yen SSC, et al: J Clin Invest 57:1320, 1976.)

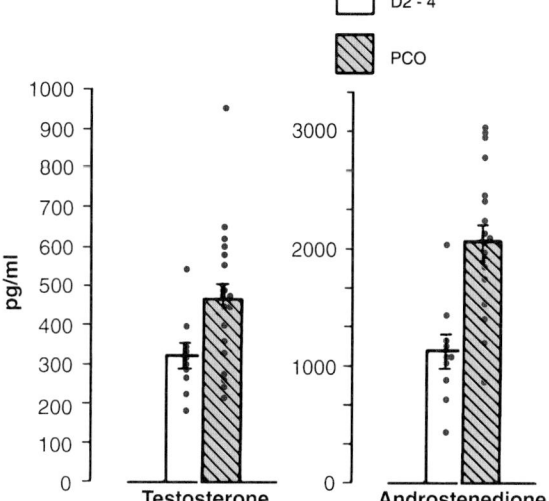

FIGURE 40-10   Mean (±SD) concentrations of testosterone and Δ[4]-androstenedione in 19 patients with polycystic ovarian syndrome *(PCO)* and 10 normal subjects between days 2 and 4 *(D2-4)* of their menstrual cycles. (From DeVane GW, Czekala NM, Judd HL, et al: Am J Obstet Gynecol 121:496, 1975.)

G. The tonically elevated levels of LH are usually above 15 mIU/ml.

Because FSH levels in women with PCOS are normal or low, an LH-FSH ratio greater than 3, provided the LH level is not lower than 8 mIU/ml, is frequently found in women with clinical features of the syndrome. Lobo et al. reported that about 70% of women with PCOS had either an elevated level of immunoreactive LH or an immunologic LH-FSH ratio greater than 3 but that all but one woman with PCOS had elevated serum levels of biologically active LH (Figure 40-11).

Hoffman et al. reported that about half the women

with PCOS have elevated levels of DHEA-S, with one third of them having levels greater than 4 μg/ml. Although Chang et al. have shown that adrenocorticotropic hormone (ACTH) levels in these women are normal, they found that infusions of ACTH produce an exaggerated response of DHEA-S, indicating that the zona reticularis of the adrenal gland in some women with PCOS has increased sensitivity to ACTH and that the adrenal gland may be involved in the pathogenesis of this syndrome.

In addition to increased levels of circulatory androgens, Lobo et al. found that women with PCOS had increased levels of biologically active (non-SHBG bound) estradiol, although total circulating levels of estradiol were not

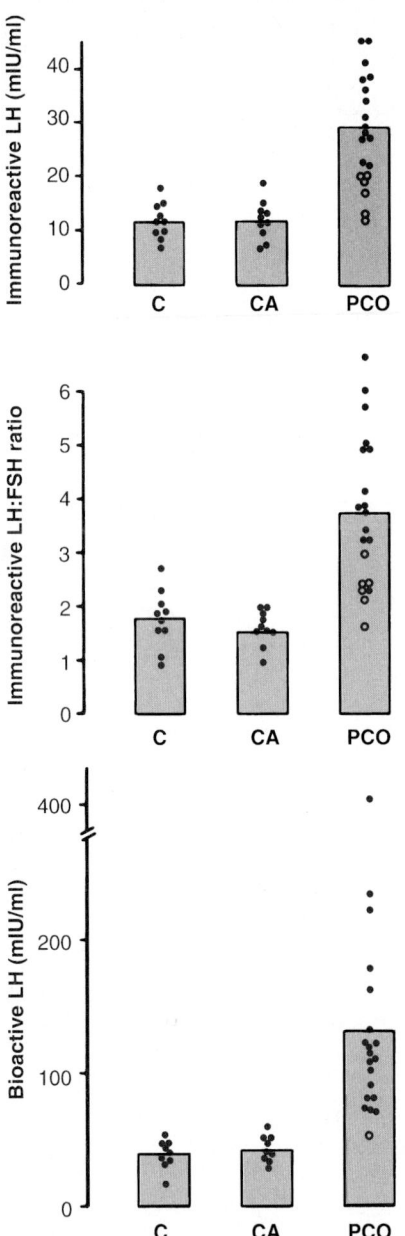

FIGURE 40-11 Serum measurements of immunoreactive LH, immunoreactive LH:FSH ratios, and bioactive LH in control subjects (C), women with chronic anovulation (CA), and women with PCOS (PCO). Boxes represent the mean ±3 standard deviation (SD) of control levels. (From Lobo RA, Kletzky OA, Campeau JD, et al: Fertil Steril 39:674, 1983. Reproduced with permission of the publisher, The American Fertility Society.)

increased (Figure 40-12). The increased amount of non-SHBG bound estradiol is caused by a decrease in SHBG levels, which is produced primarily by the increased levels of androgens and secondarily by the obesity present in many of these women. The tonically increased levels of biologically active estradiol may stimulate increased GnRH pulsatility and produce tonically elevated LH levels and anovulation. In addition, the lowered SHBG level increases the biologically active fractions of the elevated androgens

in the circulation. The importance of the decreased levels of SHBG is shown schematically in Figure 40-13.

About 20% of women with PCOS also have mildly elevated levels of prolactin (20 to 30 ng/ml), possibly related to increased pulsatility of GnRH or to a relative dopamine deficiency or to both.

It is well established that some degree of insulin resistance occurs in most women with PCOS. Insulin and insulin-like growth factor-I (IGF-I) enhance ovarian androgen production by potentiating the stimulatory action of LH on ovarian androstenedione and testosterone secretion. High levels of insulin bind with the receptor for IGF-I as a result of the significant homology of the IGF-I receptor with the insulin receptor. The granulosa cells also produce IGF-I and IGF binding proteins (IGFBP). This local production of IGF-I and IGFBP may result in paracrine control and enhancement of LH stimulation and production of androgens by the theca cells in women with PCOS. Since IGFBP levels are lower in women with PCOS, this leads to increased bioavailable IGF-I, which increases stimulation of the theca cells in combination with LH to produce higher levels of androgen production. Insulin resistance and the resultant hyperinsulinemia stimulate ovarian androgen production. Studies in monkeys have demonstrated that androgen excess does not result in abnormal insulin secretion. It is not clear why women with PCOS have insulin resistance, while age-matched and weight-matched controls who do not have PCOS do not exhibit insulin resistance.

Dunaif et al. studied a group of hyperandrogenic women with and without PCOS and obesity with glucose tolerance tests and insulin levels. They found that hyperinsulinemia occurred only in the women with PCOS, whether or not they were obese, but only the obese women with PCOS had impaired glucose tolerance. In a subsequent study they found that nonobese women with PCOS also had glucose intolerance, but the incidence was less than in the obese women. In a prospective evaluation of 254 women with PCOS who had an oral glucose tolerance test, they found that 31% had impaired glucose tolerance and 7.5% undiagnosed diabetes. In nonobese women with PCOS 10% had impaired glucose tolerance and 1.5% had diabetes. Thus the negative impact of obesity and PCOS on insulin resistance is additive. Fasting glucose levels were poor predictors of diabetes in these women. It would appear advisable to perform an oral glucose tolerance test at the time of diagnosis of PCOS and periodically thereafter. If abnormalities in glucose metabolism are found, appropriate interventions, such as diet and exercise, should be recommended as they may prevent or delay the conversion of impaired glucose tolerance for diabetes. Acanthosis nigricans (AN) was found in about 30% of the hyperandrogenic women. About half of the hyperandrogenic women who had PCOS and were obese had AN. Although it has been suggested that the presence of *h*yperandrogenism *i*nsulin *r*esistance, and *AN* constitute a

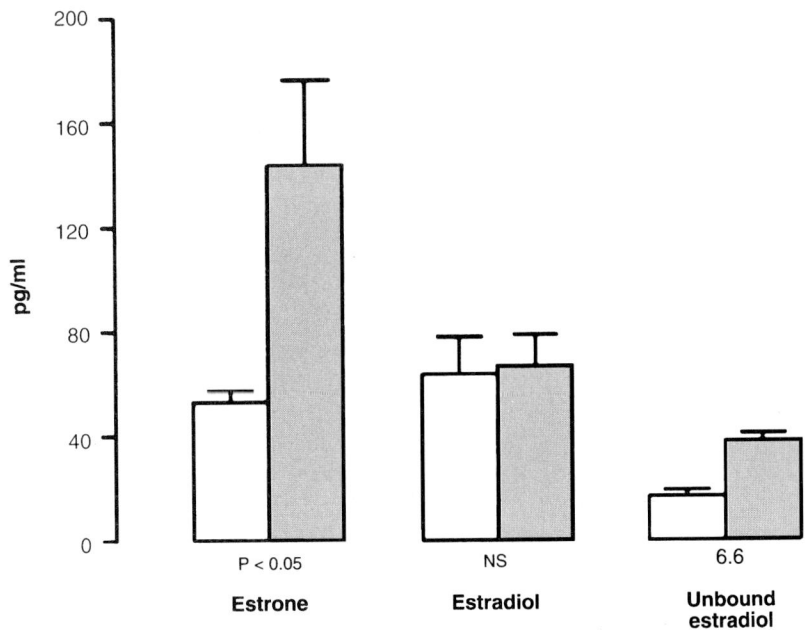

FIGURE 40-12 Serum estrogen concentrations in 13 normal women and 22 PCOS patients *(shaded areas).* (From Lobo RA, Granger L, Goebelsmann U, et al: J Clin Endocrinol Metab 52:156, 1981. Copyright 1981 by The Endocrine Society.)

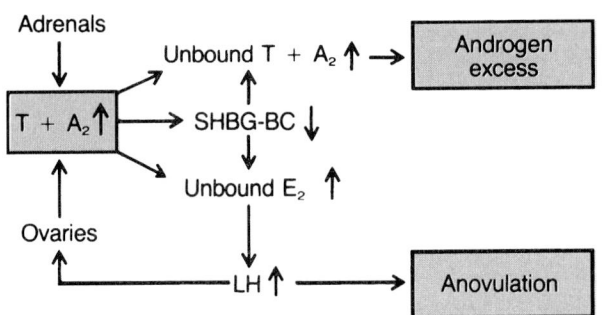

FIGURE 40-13 Scheme depicting the possible role of adrenal-derived androgen (*T*, testosterone; A_2, androstanediol) in initiating androgen excess and anovulation. (From Lobo RA and Goebelsmann U: Am J Obstet Gynecol 142:394, 1982.)

special syndrome, the HAIR-AN syndrome, most investigators believe women with PCOS who have AN are a subgroup of those with PCOS and do not have a distinct endocrine disorder. No causal relation among PCOS, obesity, insulin resistance, and hyperandrogenism has been elucidated to date. Although some investigators have suggested that hyperandrogenism causes insulin resistance, Lobo et al. have presented data indicating that the reverse is true: hyperinsulinemia produces hyperandrogenism in women with PCOS. Administration of the antihyperglycemic agent metformin decreases insulin levels and also lowers serum androgen levels.

Although the ovaries of women with PCOS produce excessive amounts of androgen, particularly androstene-dione, there is no inherent endocrinologic abnormality in the ovaries. The tonically elevated levels of LH cause the stromal tissue to produce more androstenedione and other androgens, which in turn produces premature follicular atresia. Furthermore, the ovaries are deficient in aromatase, and this deficiency results in less conversion of androstenedione to estrogen in the ovary. The polycystic ovary does not secrete increased amounts of estrone or estradiol, but the increased levels of androstenedione are peripherally converted to estrone, causing increased circulating estrone levels.

The etiology of this endocrinologic abnormality has not been determined. It has been suggested that heredity, central catecholamine abnormalities, psychologic stress, insulin resistance, and obesity may be involved. The evidence for a genetic cause is suggestive but not clearly established. Data suggesting an abnormality in central nervous system catecholamine metabolism are more convincing but not yet conclusive. Although women with PCOS have more psychologic stress than do control subjects, the stress may be a result, not the cause, of the syndrome. Obesity probably enhances the syndrome because of the decrease in SHBG levels but is probably not important in the pathogenesis. The syndrome of PCOS also occurs in some thin women, and many obese women do not have PCOS.

Whatever the etiology, the endocrinologic effects of PCOS produce a vicious cycle of events, as shown by Yen et al. (Figure 40-14). The increased pulsatility of GnRH produces tonically elevated LH levels and increased ovarian androgen production. Peripheral conversion of

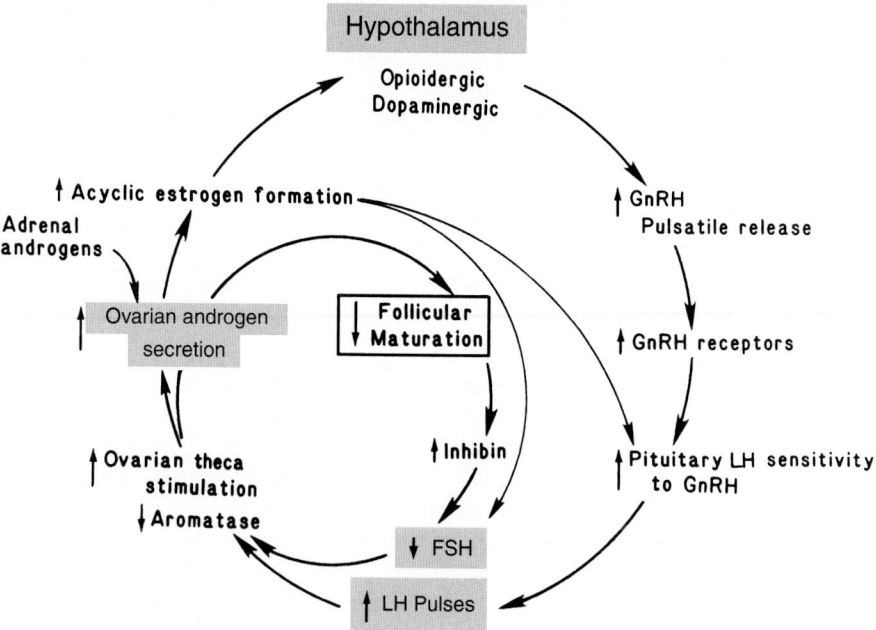

FIGURE 40-14 The interdependent event of high LH-FSH ratio occasioned by an increased GnRH secretion as a consequence of reduced hypothalamic inhibition. This setting induces an increased ovarian androgen production by the theca cells and acyclic estrogen feedback system in maintenance of chronic anovulation in PCOS. (Modified from Yen SSC, Chaney C, and Judd HL: Functional aberrations of the hypothalamic-pituitary system in polycystic ovary syndrome: a consideration of the pathogenesis. In James VHT, Serio M, and Guisti G, editors: The endocrine function of the human ovary, New York, 1976, Academic Press.)

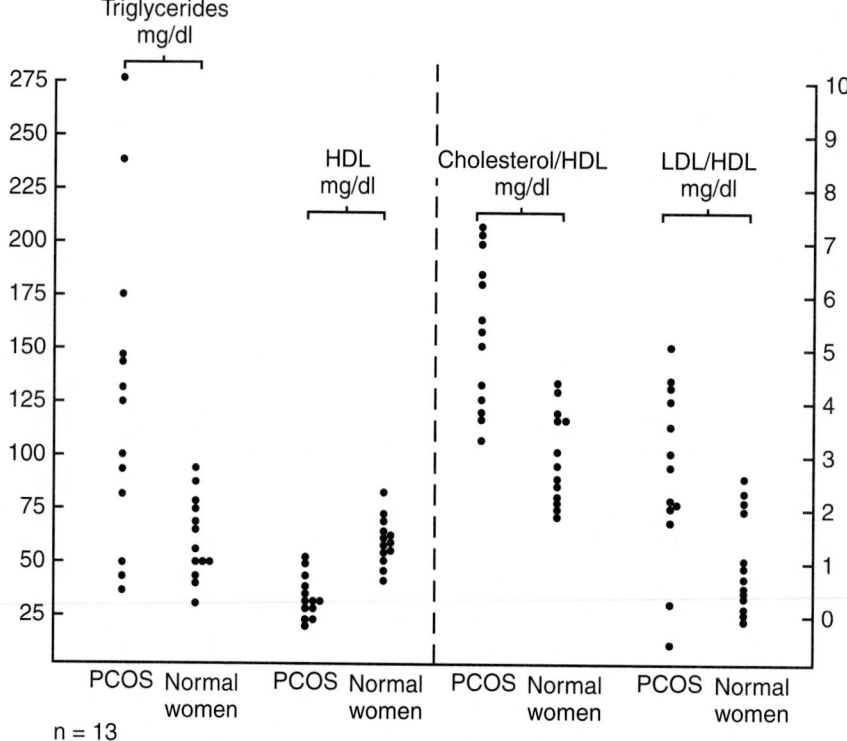

FIGURE 40-15 Lipid and lipoprotein profiles in 13 women with polycystic ovary syndrome (PCOS) versus control group when matched for percent ideal body weight. Differences are evident in all measures ($p < 0.01$). (From Wild RA and Bartholomew MJ: Am J Obstet Gynecol 159:423, 1988.)

androstenedione to estrone in conjunction with the decreased SHBG levels causes tonic hyperestrogenism, which increases the pituitary sensitivity to GnRH and leads to increased LH release.

Because of hyperandrogenism and obesity, women with PCOS have abnormal lipoprotein profiles. The increase in triglycerides and the decrease in LDL cholesterol and HDL may be related to the increased body weight and/or hyperandrogenism (Figure 40-15). If PCOS is not treated, the endocrinologic abnormalities persist and gradually worsen until the ovary stops functioning at the menopause. Longterm sequelae of PCOS were examined in 33 women aged 40 to 59 who had undergone ovarian wedge resection 22 to 31 years previously. Compared with age-matched controls, they had a significantly greater incidence of hypertension and diabetes mellitus (Figure 40-16). Using multiple logistic regression analysis it was predicted that women with PCOS have an increased risk of developing cardiovascular disease compared with controls, but one long-term follow-up study by Pierpont et al. reported that women with PCOS do not have an increased risk of death due to cardiovascular disease.

Stromal Hyperthecosis

Stromal hyperthecosis is an uncommon benign ovarian disorder in which the ovaries are bilaterally enlarged to about 5 to 7 cm in diameter. Histologically there are nests of luteinized theca cells within the stroma (Figure 40-17). The capsules of these ovaries are thick, similar to those found in PCOS, but unlike PCOS, subcapsular cysts are uncommon. The theca cells produce large amounts of testosterone as

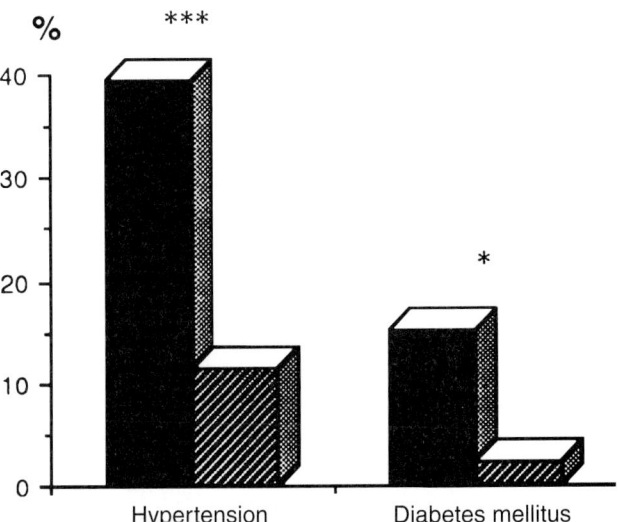

FIGURE 40-16 Prevalence of hypertension (medically treated) and manifest diabetes mellitus in 33 PCOS subjects and 132 referents. *Filled bars* illustrate the PCOS subjects. *Striped bars* illustrate the referents. Statistical comparisons were made between the women with PCOS and referents. Differences were considered significant at $*P \leq 0.05$ and $***\times P \leq 0.001$. (From Dahlgren E, Janson PO, Johansson S, et al: Fertil Steril 57:505, 1992.)

determined by retrograde ovarian vein catheterization. Like PCOS, this disorder has a gradual onset and is initially associated with anovulation or amenorrhea and hirsutism. However, unlike PCOS, with increasing age the ovaries secrete steadily increasing amounts of testosterone. Thus when women with this disorder reach the fourth decade of life, the severity of the hirsutism increases and signs of virilization, such as temporal balding, clitoral enlargement, deepening of the voice, and decreased breast size, appear and gradually increase in severity. By this time serum testosterone levels are usually greater than 2 ng/ml, similar to levels found in ovarian and adrenal testosterone-producing tumors. However, with the latter conditions the symptoms of virilization appear and progress much more rapidly than with ovarian hyperthecosis, in which symptoms progress gradually over many years.

Androgen-Producing Tumors

Ovarian Neoplasms

It is possible for nearly every type of ovarian neoplasm to have stromal cells that secrete excessive amounts of testosterone and cause signs of androgen excess. Thus on rare occasions excess testosterone produced by both benign and malignant cystadenomas, Brenner tumors, and Krukenberg tumors has caused hirsutism or virilization or both. Certain germ cell tumors contain many testosterone-producing cells. The testosterone produced by two of these neoplasms—Sertoli-Leydig cell tumors and hilus cell tumors—nearly always causes virilization. In addition, lipoid cell (adrenal rest) tumors can produce increased amounts of testosterone or DHEA-S or both. Rarely granulosa-theca cell tumors can also produce testosterone in addition to increased levels of estradiol.

Androgen-producing ovarian tumors usually produce rapidly progressive signs of virilization. Sertoli-Leydig cell tumors usually develop during the reproductive age (second to fourth decades), and by the time they produce detectable signs of androgen excess, the tumor is nearly always (more than 85% of the time) palpable during bimanual examination. These tumors are uncommon. Less than 1% of solid ovarian neoplasms are Sertoli-Leydig cell tumors. Hilus cell tumors most often occur after menopause. They are usually small and not palpable during bimanual examination; however, the history of rapid development of signs of virilization and the presence of markedly elevated levels of testosterone (more than 2½ times the upper limits of the normal range) with normal levels of DHEA-S usually facilitate the diagnosis.

Adrenal Tumors

Nearly all the androgen-producing adrenal tumors are adenomas or carcinomas that generate large amounts of the C_{19} steroids normally produced by the adrenal gland:

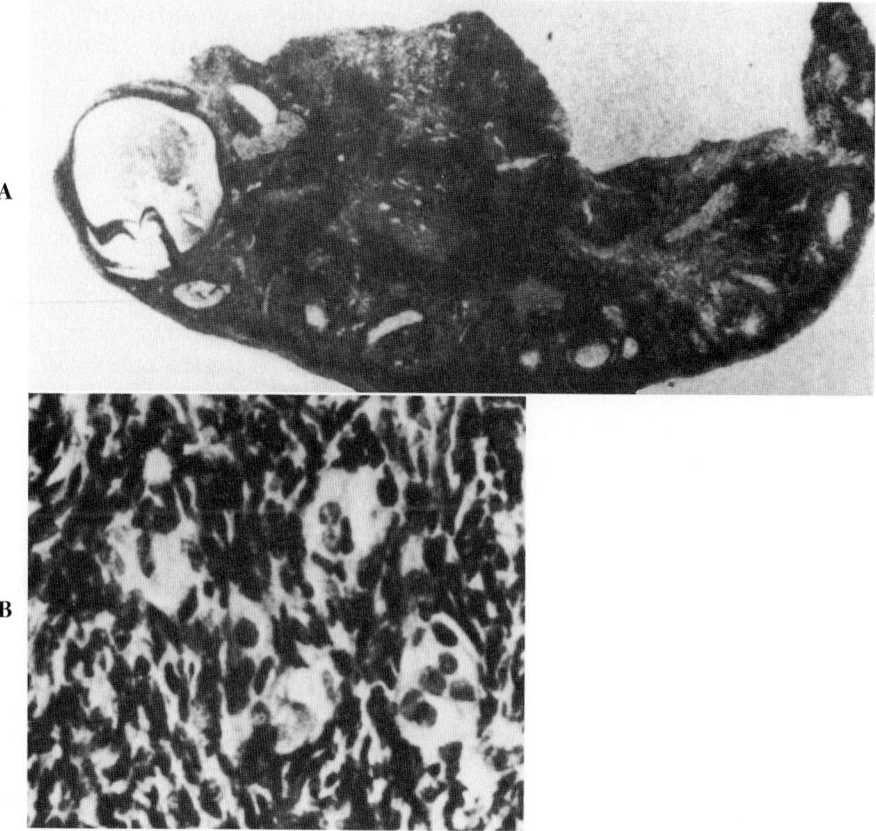

FIGURE 40-17 **A,** Sagittal section of typical hyperthecotic ovary illustrating small number of follicular cysts and massive amount of stromal hyperplasia. **B,** Islands of luteinized thecalike cells deep in stroma of ovary in hyperthecosis. (From Wilroy RS Jr, Givens JR, Wiser WL, et al: Hyperthecosis: an inheritable form of polycystic ovarian disease. In Bergsma D, editor: Genetic forms of hypogonadism, Miami: Symposia Specialists for the National Foundation-March of Dimes, BD:OAS XI(4):81, 1975, with permission.)

DHEA-S, DHEA, and androstenedione. Although these tumors do not usually directly secrete testosterone, testosterone is produced by extraglandular conversion of DHEA and androstenedione. Women with these tumors usually have markedly elevated serum levels of DHEA-S (>8 μg/ml). Women with these laboratory findings and a history of rapid onset of signs of androgen excess should undergo a computerized tomography (CT) scan or magnetic resonance imaging (MRI) of the adrenal glands to confirm the diagnosis. In addition to these uncommon tumors, a few testosterone-producing adrenal adenomas have been reported. The cellular patterns of these tumors resemble those of ovarian hilus cells, and the tumors secrete large amounts of testosterone. Because adrenal adenomas also secrete DHEA-S, a high likelihood of their presence exists when DHEA-S levels are greater than 8 μg/ml and testosterone levels are more than 1.5 ng/ml.

Late-Onset 21-Hydroxylase Deficiency

Congenital adrenal hyperplasia (CAH) is an inherited disorder caused by an enzymatic defect (usually 21-hydroxylase [21-OHase] or less often 11β-hydroxylase), resulting in decreased cortisol biosynthesis. As a consequence,

ACTH secretion increases and adrenal cortisol precursors produced proximal to the enzymatic block accumulate and are converted mainly to DHEA and androstenedione. These C_{19} steroids are in turn peripherally converted to testosterone, which produces signs of androgen excess.

Because the enzymatic defects are congenital, the classic severe form (complete block) usually becomes clinically apparent in fetal life by producing masculinization of the female external genitalia. The severe form of CAH is the most common cause of sexual ambiguity in the newborn. The more attenuated (mild) block of 21-OHase activity usually does not produce physical signs associated with increased androgen production until after puberty. Thus this entity, termed late-onset 21-hydroxylase deficiency (LOHD) or late-onset congenital adrenal hyperplasia, is associated with the development of signs of hyperandrogenism in a woman in the second or early third decade of life.

Although the incidence of classic CAH is only 1 per 14,500 live births worldwide, Speiser et al., using HLA-B genotyping of families with LOHD-affected individuals, concluded that the incidence of LOHD varied among different ethnic groups but overall was probably the most frequent autosomal genetic disorder in humans. The incidence of LOHD was estimated to be 0.1% among a diverse white population; among Yugoslavians, Hispanics, and Ashkenazi Jews, however, the incidence was 1.6%, 1.9%, and 3.7%, respectively (Figure 40-18). Both classic CAH and LOHD are transmitted in an autosomal recessive manner at the CYP21B locus and are linked to the HLA-B locus.

The molecular basis of the disease is complex. Depending on the population, one fourth to one fifth of individuals with classic CAH have a deletion of the CYP21B locus, as detected by restriction endonuclease digestion and the Southern blot test. In other families the gene defect is caused by a point or frame shift mutation that alters the protein product, greatly impairing its function. Thus a spectrum of mutations results in the enzymatic defects, as shown in Table 40-6.

LOHD is a phenotype that is symptomatic after adolescence and does not define the genotype. Affected individuals may be homozygous for alleles, yielding mildly abnormal enzymatic activity, or compound heterozygotes with a combination of defective alleles. The so-called cryptic 21-OHase deficiency, on the other hand, represents mild or asymptomatic individuals with biochemically identified defects that, with the advent of molecular diagnostic techniques, have been redefined as belonging to several different clinical presentations.

New et al. have proposed a schema for identifying and classifying the clinical spectrum of disease shown in Table 40-6. Since there are three possible manifestations of CYP21Y alleles (normal, mildly defective, or severely defective), there are six possible genotypes representing three clinical phenotypes (asymptomatic, LOHD, and classic CAH).

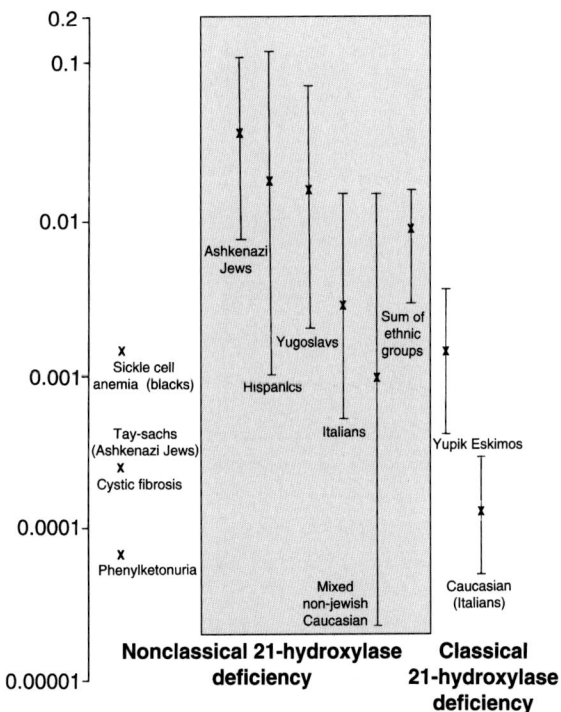

FIGURE 40-18 Relative frequencies of nonclassic 21-hydroxylase deficiency, classic 21-hydroxylase deficiency, and other autosomal recessive disorders. (From Speiser PW, Dupont B, Rubenstein P, et al: Am J Hum Genet 37:650, 1985.)

TABLE 40-6
Genotypic Characterization of the Forms of 21-Hydroxylase Deficiency

Form of 21-Hydroxylase Deficiency	Clinical Phenotype	Hormonal Phenotype (in Response to ACTH)	Genotype
Classic (CAH)	Prenatal virilization, fully symptomatic	Marked elevation of precursors (serum 17-hydroxyprogesterone and Δ-androstenedione)	21-OH-def^{severe} / 21-OH-def^{severe}
Nonclassic (LOHD)	Symptomatic: later development of virilization; milder symptoms Asymptomatic: no virilization or other symptoms	Moderate elevation of precursors	21-OH-def^{severe} / 21-OH-def^{mild} 21-OH-def^{mild} / 21-OH-def^{mild}
Carrier	Asymptomatic	Precursor level greater than normal	21-OH-def^{severe} / 21-OHase (normal) 21-OH-def^{mild} / 21-OHase (normal)
Normal	Asymptomatic	Lowest levels—some overlap seen with carriers	21-OHase (normal) / 21-OHase (normal)

From New MI, White PC, Pang S, et al: The adrenal hyperplasias. In Scriver CR, Beaudet AL, Sly S, and Valle D: Metabolic basis of inherited diseases, ed 6, New York, 1989, McGraw-Hill Book Co.

Individuals with LOHD may be compound heterozygotes, with one mildly and one severely defective allele, or homozygous, with two mildly defective alleles. Although biochemical differences in the hormonal response to ACTH have been shown between these two genotypes, their phenotypes are similar. Carriers can be identified among family members who are heterozygous with one normal allele. These individuals have normal basal 17-hydroxyprogesterone (17-OHP) levels, a mild degree of hirsutism, if present, and smaller increases of 17-OHP after ACTH stimulation, usually between 3.5 and 10 ng/ml.

LOHD is also usually associated with menstrual irregularity. It has been hypothesized that the mechanism for anovulation is similar to that which occurs with PCOS. The increased levels of androgen lower SHBG levels, thus increasing the amount of biologically active circulating estradiol. The increased estradiol stimulates tonic LH release, which increases ovarian androgen production and locally inhibits follicular growth and ovulation. Thus women with this disorder present with postpubertal onset of hirsutism and oligomenorrhea or amenorrhea, similar to women with PCOS. However, women with LOHD, unlike those with PCOS, commonly have a history of prepubertal accelerated growth (ages 6 to 8 years) with later decreased growth and a short ultimate height. A history of this growth pattern, a family history of postpubertal onset of hirsutism, findings of mild virilization, and DHEA-S levels greater than 5 μg/ml are indicators of the presence of CAH.

To differentiate LOHD from PCOS, measurement of basal (early morning) serum 17-OHP levels should be performed. This assay has replaced the less precise measurement of the 17-OHP urinary metabolite, pregnanetriol. If basal levels of 17-OHP are greater than 8 ng/ml, the diagnosis of LOHD is established. If 17-OHP is above normal (2.5 to 3.3 ng/ml) but less than 8 ng/ml, an ACTH stimulation test should be performed. A baseline 17-OHP should be measured and 0.25 μg of synthetic ACTH infused as a single bolus. One hour later another serum sample of 17-OHP should be measured. If the level of 17-OHP increases more than 10 ng/ml, the diagnosis of LOHD is established (Figure 40-19). Individuals with LOHD should be treated with continuous corticosteroids to arrest the signs of androgenicity and restore ovulatory menstrual cycles.

Cushing Syndrome

Excessive adrenal production of glucocorticoids due to increased ACTH secretion (Cushing disease) or adrenal tumors produces the signs and symptoms of Cushing syndrome. These findings include hirsutism and menstrual irregularity in addition to the classic findings of central obesity, dorsal neck fat pads, abdominal striae, and muscle wasting and weakness. The latter catabolic effect of glucocorticoid excess differs from the anabolic effects

of testosterone excess, but some women with PCOS may have other clinical findings that are similar to those found with Cushing syndrome. In such instances Cushing syndrome can be easily excluded by performing an overnight dexamethasone suppression test. To perform this test, dexamethasone, 1 mg, should be ingested at 11 PM, and plasma cortisol is measured the following morning at 8 AM (Figure 40-20). If the cortisol level is less than 5 μg/100 ml, Cushing syndrome is ruled out. If the cortisol level fails to suppress to this degree, the diagnosis of Cushing syndrome is not established. It is necessary to perform a complete dexamethasone suppression test (Liddle's test) or measurement of urinary free cortisol and plasma ACTH to determine whether Cushing syndrome exists.

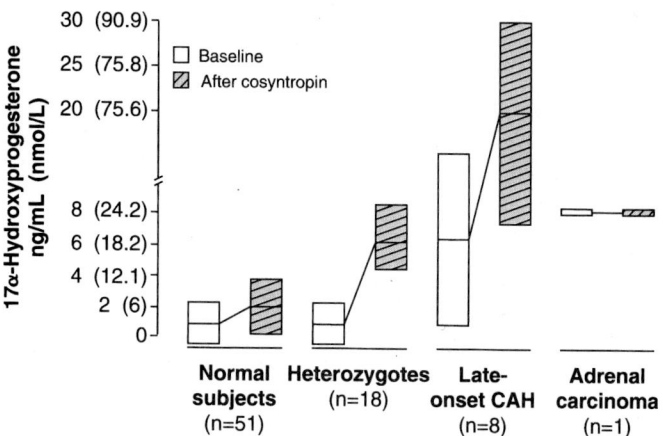

FIGURE 40-19 Means and ranges of 17α-hydroxyprogesterone levels before and after cosyntropin administered intramuscularly in normal subjects, suspected heterozygotes, patients with late-onset congenital adrenal hyperplasia *(CAH)*, and one patient with adrenal carcinoma. (From Baskin HJ: Arch Intern Med 147:847, 1987.)

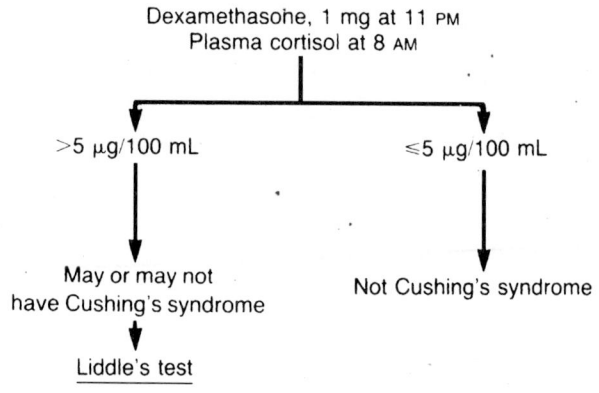

FIGURE 40-20 Outline of overnight dexamethasone suppression test. (From Goebelsmann U and Lobo RA: Androgen excess. In Mishell DR Jr, Davajan V, and Lobo RA, editors: Infertility, contraception and reproductive endocrinology, ed 2, Cambridge, Mass, 1986, Blackwell Scientific Publications.)

DIFFERENTIAL DIAGNOSIS

The differential diagnosis of the various causes of androgen excess can usually be made without difficulty by means of a complete history, a careful physical examination, and measurement of serum levels of testosterone and DHEA-S to determine if there is an ovarian or adrenal source of excess androgen production.

Measurement of total testosterone, free testosterone, the free androgen index, and non-SHBG bound testosterone (unbound testosterone) have all been advocated to assist in the diagnosis of hyperandrogenism. Loric et al. measured all these serum parameters in a group of hirsute women and age-matched control subjects. Slopes of the first two of these parameters overlapped between the two groups, whereas no overlap of values occurred with the last two assays. It has been suggested by these and other investigators that measurement of the free androgen index or non-SHBG bound testosterone is a more specific discriminator of hyperandrogenism than total or free testosterone. Clinically, however, measurement of total testosterone is all that is necessary. It is not clinically important whether a hirsute woman has a total testosterone level in the highest portion of the normal range or a mildly elevated level of non-SHBG bound testosterone. Schwartz et al. reported that when total testosterone levels are elevated, there is an excellent correlation with free testosterone levels. Thus, to determine the magnitude of elevated androgens, as well as their source, measurement of total testosterone is more cost-effective than the other assays and provides the clinician with the information necessary to establish the diagnosis.

As mentioned, androgen excess due to iatrogenic causes, sexual ambiguity, or pregnancy-associated ovarian tumors can usually be easily determined by the history and physical examination. Masculinizing ovarian or adrenal tumors are associated with rapidly progressive signs of hirsutism and virilization. Serum testosterone levels greater than 2 ng/ml with normal DHEA-S levels indicate the probable presence of an ovarian tumor. The diagnosis can be confirmed by bimanual pelvic examination and ultrasonography, CT scan, or MRI. Women with a rapid progression of virilization and DHEA-S levels greater than 8 μg/ml most likely have an androgen-producing adrenal adenoma, and the diagnosis can be confirmed by CT scan or MRI. A long history of gradually increasing hirsutism, even if accompanied by virilization, is not consistent with the diagnosis of adrenal or ovarian tumors. The diagnosis of ovarian stromal hyperthecosis should be suspected for individuals with these signs and testosterone levels greater than 1.5 ng/ml. Women with physical findings consistent with Cushing syndrome should have the diagnosis ruled out or confirmed by an overnight dexamethasone suppression test followed by Liddle's test if necessary. PCOS, LOHD, and idiopathic hirsutism may be associated with a similar history and findings at physical examination. Menstrual irregularity, however, is uncommon among women with idiopathic hirsutism, and testosterone and DHEA-S levels are normal. Women with LOHD commonly have a family history of androgen excess, early onset of rapid growth, and short stature, as well as signs of mild virilization. The diagnosis of LOHD is established by measurement of 17-OHP either by an early-morning serum sample or following ACTH stimulation. Women with PCOS commonly have elevated LH levels, low FSH levels, elevated androstenedione levels, and mildly increased testosterone or DHEA-S levels, with sonographic findings of polycystic ovaries, whereas women with idiopathic hirsutism have normal levels of these hormones and normal ovarian morphology. Treatment of hirsutism depends on whether the androgen excess is ovarian, adrenal, or peripheral.

MANAGEMENT

Ovarian and Adrenal Tumors

Nearly all Sertoli-Leydig cell tumors are unilateral. If the woman desires further reproduction and these tumors are well differentiated and confined to the ovary, the tumors may be treated by unilateral salpingo-oophorectomy. Since most hilus cell tumors occur after menopause, they are best treated by bilateral salpingo-oophorectomy and total abdominal hysterectomy. Adrenal adenomas and carcinomas also should be treated by operative removal. Adrenal carcinomas frequently have metastasized to the liver by the time the androgenic signs have developed. Despite chemotherapy the prognosis is poor after metastases have occurred. Stromal hyperthecosis is also best treated by bilateral salpingo-oophorectomy together with total abdominal hysterectomy. After removal of the ovaries of women with stromal hyperthecosis or any of the androgen-producing tumors, the acne and oiliness of the skin disappear, breast size increases, and clitoral size decreases. The excess central hair becomes finer and grows less rapidly but does not disappear. Electrolysis can remove the facial hair, and depilatories, bleaches, or shaving can be used to treat the body hair.

Late-Onset 21-Hydrolase Deficiency

Individuals with late-onset of CAH (LOHD) should be treated daily with glucocorticoids such as hydrocortisone (15 to 20 mg), prednisone (5 to 7.5 mg), or dexamethasone (0.5 to 0.75 mg) in divided doses. Sometimes lower doses of these agents may be sufficient to suppress ACTH and decrease adrenal androgen production. The aim of treatment is to suppress androstenedione and 17-OHP levels to the normal range. Signs of androgen excess lessen over a few months. Ovulation usually resumes within a few weeks.

Polycystic Ovarian Syndrome

The treatment of PCOS depends on which aspect of the disorder—hirsutism, infertility, or irregular, prolonged menses (dysfunctional uterine bleeding)—is of greatest concern to the woman. The best treatment for PCOS, unless pregnancy is desired, is oral steroid contraceptives, because these agents inhibit LH, decrease circulating testosterone levels, and increase levels of SHBG and thus bind and inactivate more of the testosterone in the circulation (Figure 40-21). It is best to use a low–estrogen-dose oral contraceptive formulation containing a low androgenic progestin. Oral contraceptives also decrease serum DHEA-S levels. If the levels are only mildly elevated (<4 µg/ml), oral contraceptives alone will usually reduce them

to normal. If DHEA-S levels are moderately elevated (>4 µg/ml), dexamethasone (0.25 to 0.5 mg at bedtime) should be given together with the oral contraceptive. If hirsutism continues to be a problem, spironolactone (50 to 100 mg twice daily) can be administered to decrease androgenic action in the target organs. Several investigators have shown that administration of the oral antihyperglycemic agent metformin to women with PCOS increases insulin sensitivity and lowers free testosterone levels and in many women induces ovulation.

GnRH analogues have also been shown to inhibit ovarian androgen production. When given in combination with oral contraceptives, the latter will reduce adrenal androgen production and increase SHBG, as well as prevent hypoestrogenic side effects associated with GnRH

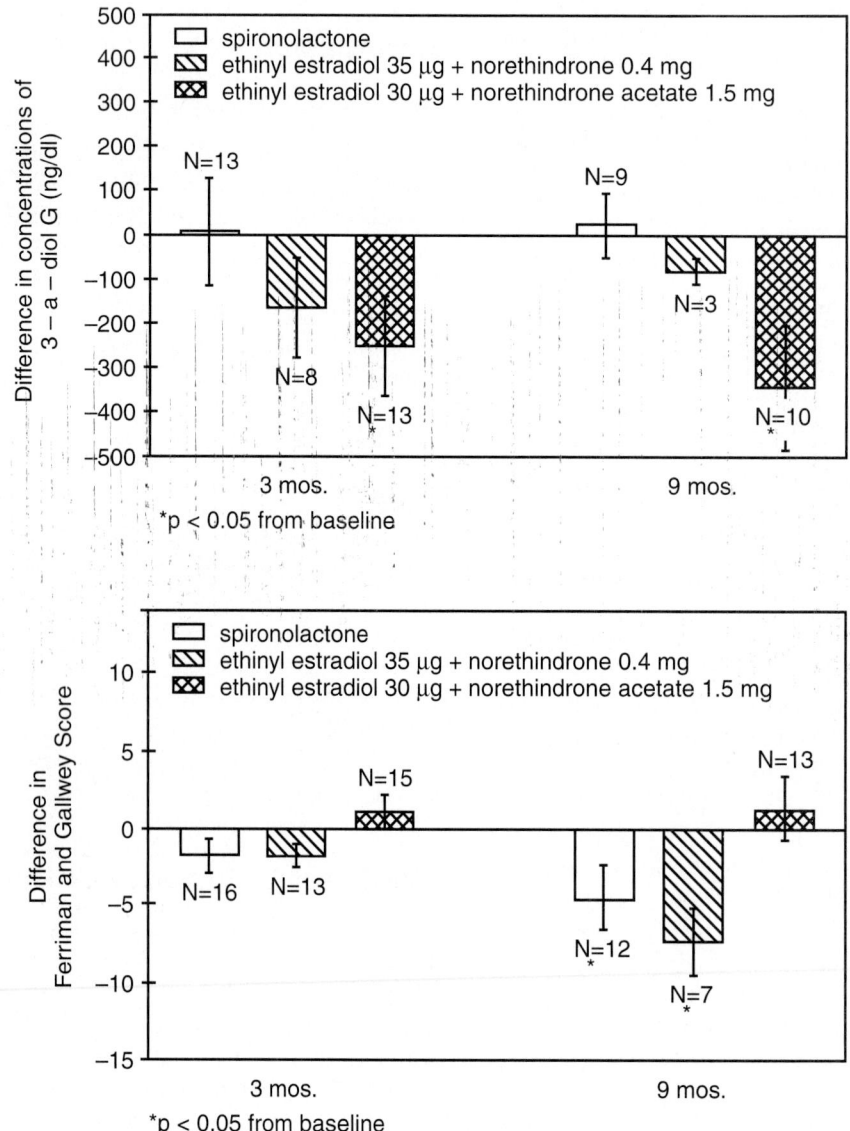

FIGURE 40-21 The effect of spironolactone, ethinyl estradiol 35 µg plus norethindrone 0.4 mg and ethinyl estradiol 30 µg plus norethindrone acetate 1.5 mg on mean ± SEM 3—diol concentrations and Ferriman-Gallwey scores at 3 months and 9 months of treatment in hirsute women. (From Wild RA, Demers LM, Applebaum-Bowden D, and Lenker R: Contraception 44:113, 1991.)

agonist therapy. GnRH agonists are expensive, and their use should be reserved for women whose hirsutism is not sufficiently improved with a combination of oral contraceptives and spironolactone and wish to preserve ovarian function. Treatment with GnRH analogues does not permanently alter the pathophysiology of PCOS. A few months after this analogue treatment is discontinued, gonadotrophin and androgen levels return to pretreatment levels.

Rittmaster and Thompson suppressed ovarian function with a GnRH analogue in a group of moderately or severely hirsute women with PCOS and another hirsute group without evidence of PCOS. After 6 months of ovarian suppression, adrenal suppression with dexamethasone was added. Measurement of androgens before and after these treatment regimens indicated that the ovary was the major source of testosterone and androstenedione in the women with PCOS but that a substantial adrenal contribution also was present (Figure 40-22). Adrenal production was the major source of circulating androgens in the women without PCOS.

Women with PCOS who desire fertility should be treated with ovulation-inducing agents. Clomiphene cit-

rate should be used initially. If ovulation does not occur with this agent, human menopausal gonadotrophin (hMG) can be administered with or without GnRH. If DHEA-S levels are elevated the combination of administering dexamethasone 0.5 mg each night together with cyclic clomiphene citrate has been reported to induce ovulation in women who do not respond to clomiphene citrate alone.

Nestler et al. demonstrated that the frequency of spontaneous ovulation as well as ovulation induction with clomiphene citrate was increased in obese women with PCOS following treatment with metformin 500 mg three times a day. In this randomized trial 90% of women treated with metformin plus clomiphene citrate ovulated compared to 8% treated with clomiphene citrate alone. Thus this therapy can be utilized in obese women with PCOS who fail to ovulate with clomiphene citrate alone.

Ovarian wedge resection was the original treatment for PCOS. However, this therapy was associated with a high incidence of postoperative adhesion formation. When ovulation-inducing agents were developed, they replaced ovarian wedge resection as the primary form of treatment. In the past 15 years, surgical treatment of PCOS with partial ovarian destruction utilizing electrocautery or laser is again being performed with success. This technique, also called *laparoscopic ovarian drilling*, is mainly used for women with PCOS in whom clomiphene citrate has failed to induce ovulation. Approximately 10 to 15 punctures are made through the surface of each ovary with a needle inserted about 8 mm and activated with a coagulating current for 2 seconds. In these clomiphene-resistant women, ovulatory cycles have been reported to occur in 70% to 90% of those treated (Table 40-7). If ovulation does not occur spontaneously, most of the remaining anovulatory women will ovulate when treated with clomiphene citrate. After partial ovarian destruction, androgen levels usually become normal. Gjønnaess reported that two thirds of women treated with ovarian electrocautery were still ovulating 18 to 20 years after the procedure and androgen levels remained decreased for this length of time. If women with PCOS do not have hirsutism but have dysfunctional bleeding or oligomenorrhea, oral contraceptive therapy should be used. For women with contraindications to combined oral contraceptives, withdrawal bleeding should be induced with monthly progestins such as oral medroxyprogesterone acetate 10 mg daily for the first 10 days of the month. These agents should be administered to prevent development of endometrial hyperplasia due to unopposed estrogen. Prolonged endometrial hyperplasia is a risk factor for adenocarcinoma of the endometrium, and women with untreated PCOS have an increased risk of developing this disease. Dahlgren et al. have reported that the incidence of endometrial cancer in women with hirsutism, obesity, and infertility was greater than in controls.

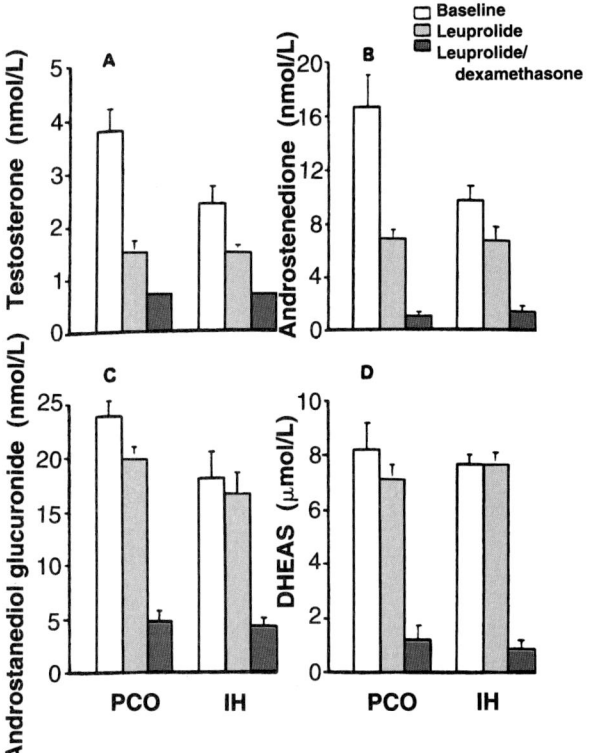

FIGURE 40-22 Hormone levels in women with polycystic ovary syndrome *(PCO)* and idiopathic hirsutism *(IH)* at baseline, after leuprolide alone, and after the combination of leuprolide and dexamethasone. Testosterone levels **(A)** after leuprolide and dexamethasone were undetectable; the detection limit of the assay is shown. (From Rittmaster RS and Thompson DL: J Clin Endocrinol Metab 70:1096, 1990.)

TABLE 40-7
Ovulation and Pregnancy After Electrocautery and Laser Treatment of Polycystic Ovaries

N	Ovulation %	Pregnancy %	Authors and year of publication
Electrocautery			
35	92	69*	Gjønnaess (1984)
6	83	67	Greenblatt and Casper (1987)
14	64	36	v.d. Weiden et al. (1989)
21	81	52	Armar et al. 1990
29	71	52	Abdel Gadir (1990)
7	71	57	Gürgan et al. (1991)
10	70		Kovacs et al. (1991)
22		86	Armar and Lachelin (1993)
104	76	70	Naether et al. (1993)
10	70		Tiitinen et al. (1993)
Laser vaporization			
85	53	56	Daniell and Miller (1989)
19	80	37	Keckstein et al. (1990)
10	70		Gürgan et al. (1991)
Wedge resection			
8	65	0	Huber et al. (1988)
12	83	58	Kojima et al. (1989)

From Gjønnaess H: Acta Obstet Gynecol Scand 73:407, 1994.

*Before laparoscopy, some patients had been resistant to hormonal stimulation therapy. After inclusion of patients made responsive to clomiphene citrate (CC) by electrocautery, the pregnancy rate increased to 80%.

TABLE 40-8
Treatment of Hirsutism According to Source of Androgen Excess

Androgen	Treatment
↑ Testosterone	Oral contraceptives
↑ DHEA-S (<5 µg/ml)	Oral contraceptives
↑ DHEA-S (>5 µg/ml)	Dexamethasone
↑ Testosterone, DHEA-S (7 µg/ml)	Oral contraceptives + dexamethasone
↑ 3α-diol G, normal T, normal DHEA-S	Sprionolactone*

From Lobo RA: Androgen excess. In Mishell DR Jr, Davajan V, and Lobo RA, editors: Infertility, contraception and reproductive endocrinology, ed 3, Cambridge, Mass, 1991, Blackwell Scientific Publications.

*Spironolactone may also be substituted for any of the above regimens if no improvement is noted after 3 to 4 months of treatment.

For the woman over age 35 with excessive ovarian androgen production caused by PCOS who does not desire future fertility and does not desire to continue medication, bilateral salpingo-oophorectomy and hysterectomy may be utilized to permanently remove the ovarian source of androgen and eliminate the possibility of developing endometrial cancer.

Idiopathic Hirsutism

Although hirsutism is a benign condition, it is frequently of great concern to the woman. Women with idiopathic hirsutism have normal circulating levels of testosterone and DHEA-S. Nearly all individuals with symptomatic hirsutism who have normal testosterone and DHEA-S levels have elevated levels of 3α-diol-G indicative of increased peripheral androgen activity. It is not necessary to measure 3α-diol-G in women with hirsutism without elevated circulating androgen levels, because the presence of hirsutism is itself evidence of increased peripheral androgen activity. An agent that inhibits peripheral androgen activity should be administered to women with these findings.

Because of the length of the hair growth cycle, responses

to treatment should not be expected to occur within the first 3 months of therapy. Objective methods of assessing changes of hair growth, such as photographs, are useful. With use of the agents listed in Table 40-8, a successful response should occur in about 70% of women with 1 year of therapy. Remaining excess hair can be removed by electrolysis. Treatment should be continued for 4 years and then stopped to determine if hirsutism recurs. If so, therapy can be reinitiated.

Many agents are available to inhibit the various sources of androgen production that may lead to hirsutism (Table 40-8). Oral contraceptives (OCs) suppress LH and ovarian testosterone production by the inhibitory action of the progestational component. The estrogenic component in OCs increases SHBG levels in the circulation, which decreases free testosterone levels. The progestins in the OCs also inhibit 5α-reductase activity in the skin. Women in whom OCs are contraindicated or produce side effects may be treated with medroxyprogesterone acetate. This agent also inhibits LH, which causes decreased testosterone production, although to a lesser extent than occurs with combined oral contraceptives. Treatment with GnRH agonists is expensive and reserved for severe clinical manifestations of ovarian hyperandrogenism, not hirsutism alone.

Ketoconazole, which blocks adrenal and gonadal steroidogenesis by inhibiting cytochrome P-450–dependent enzyme pathways, has been used in dosages of 200 mg twice a day to treat women with hyperandrogenism associated with PCOS and idiopathic hirsutism. This potent drug effectively decreases hair growth and acne, but major side effects and complications (including hepatitis) occur in the majority of women treated. These problems limit the use of ketoconazole to very select women, who require careful monitoring.

Antiandrogens include spironolactone, an aldosterone antagonist, C_{21} progestins, such as medroxyprogesterone acetate, and cyproterone acetate. The latter agent is available in Europe but not in the United States. Spironolactone has been used and studied extensively and should be considered the treatment of choice in the United States for women with idiopathic hirsutism as well as many with PCOS. This agent, in addition to being an androgen receptor blocker, also decreases ovarian testosterone production and inhibits 5α-reductase activity. Various dosages from 50 to 200 mg daily have been used. Lobo et al. reported that a dose of 200 mg/day of spironolactone is more effective than 100 mg/day. Barth et al. found a clinically evident response of decreased hair after 3 months of 200 mg spironolactone daily. After 1 year of treatment a 15% to 25% reduction occurred in both hair shaft diameter and linear growth rate at all body sites. With the higher dose of spironolactone, liver function tests and plasma electrolytes are usually unchanged, and side effects occur infrequently except for irregular uterine bleeding. The latter can be controlled with concomitant use of oral contraceptives. Electrolytes and blood pressure should be monitored for the first few weeks of therapy to be certain hypotension and hyperkalemia do not occur. Finisteride, a 5α-reductase inhibitor, at a dose of 5 mg/day, and flutamide, a nonsteroidal antiandrogen at a dose of 250 mg/day, have also been used to treat hirsutism and have a similar level of effectiveness as spironolactone 100 mg/day. None of these agents are approved for the treatment of hirsutism, but most information has been accumulated with spironolactone.

In summary, the treatment of hirsutism should depend on the source of the excess androgens. If testosterone levels are elevated, indicating excess ovarian androgen production, oral contraceptive therapy should be instituted. If DHEA-S levels are increased, indicating excess adrenal androgen secretion, dexamethasone therapy should be used. If neither is elevated, spironolactone should be administered. Lobo has developed an outline for the treatment of hirsutism according to the source of the androgen excess that can be used as a guide for therapy (Table 40-9).

TABLE 40-9
Agents Available to Inhibit Various Sources of Androgen Production

Ovarian

Oral contraceptives
Progestins including depo-medroxyprogesterone acetate
Gonadotrophin-releasing hormone agonist
Antiandrogenism (cyproterone acetate, spironolactone)
Ketoconazole
Corticosteroids

Adrenal

Corticosteroids
Oral contraceptives
Spironolactone
Ketoconazole

Peripheral

Cyproterone acetate
Spironolactone
Progesterone (topical)
Oral contraceptives
5α-reductase inhibitors

Modified from Lobo RA: Androgen excess. In Mishell DR Jr, Davajan V, and Lobo RA, editors: Infertility, contraception and reproductive endocrinology, ed 3, Cambridge, Mass, 1991, Blackwell Scientific Publications.

KEY POINTS

- The three cyclic changes of hair development include a growth phase called anagen, followed by a transitional phase called catagen and a resting phase called telogen.

- Testosterone levels in women with hirsutism without virilization are lower than 1.5 ng/ml.

- Circulating testosterone levels in the presence of virilization are usually greater than 2 ng/ml.

- The major androgen provided by the ovaries is testosterone and that of the adrenal glands, DHEA-S.

- Total daily testosterone production is 0.35 mg: 0.1 mg from ovarian secretion, 0.2 mg from peripheral conversion of androstenedione, and 0.05 mg from peripheral conversion of DHEA.

- About two thirds of the daily testosterone production in a woman originates in the ovaries.

- There are three markers of androgen production, one for each compartment where androgens are produced. In the ovary it is testosterone; in the adrenal gland, DHEA-S; and in the periphery, 3α-diol-G.

- About 85% of testosterone is bound to SHBG and is biologically inactive, 10% to 15% is bound to albumin, and 1% to 2% is not bound. Both of the latter fractions are biologically active.

- Non-SHBG bound testosterone is elevated in about 60% to 70% of women with hirsutism, and 3α-diol-G is elevated in about 98%.

- About 80% of individuals with idiopathic hirsutism have elevated levels of 3α-diol-G.

- Individuals with idiopathic hirsutism have increased 5α-reductase activity.

- Women with PCOS usually have testosterone levels between 0.7 and 1.2 ng/ml and androstenedione levels of 3 to 5 ng/ml; about half have elevated levels of DHEA-S.

- About 30% of women with PCOS do not have hirsutism.

- About 70% of women with PCOS have elevated levels of immunologic LH or an immunologic LH-FSH ratio greater than 3, and nearly all have elevated levels of biologically active LH and biologically active estradiol and increased amplitude of LH pulse.

- About 40% of women with PCOS have hyperinsulinemia and impaired glucose tolerance.

- Acanthosis nigricans is a common finding in obese women who have PCOS. It is generally unnecessary to measure free testosterone, free androgen, free androgen index, or non-SHBG bound testosterone. Only total testosterone needs to be measured.

- If untreated, women with PCOS have an increased risk of developing diabetes mellitus and hypertension after menopause.

- Women with ovarian neoplasms have testosterone levels more than 2½ times the upper limits of the normal range.

- The diagnosis of LOHD is established if the basal (early morning) serum 17-hydroxyprogesterone (17-OHP) levels are greater than 8 ng/ml or if the level at 1 hour after infusion of 0.25 μg ACTH is more than 10 ng/ml.

- About 40% of women with PCOS have impaired glucose tolerance (30%) or undiagnosed noninsulin dependent diabetes mellitus (10%).

- Metformin given to women with PCOS decreases insulin sensitivity and lowers free testosterone levels. It frequently causes ovulation to occur and increases the frequency of ovulation when clomiphene citrate is given to women with PCOS.

- Women with LOHD have a block in cortisol biosynthesis of 11β-hydroxylase or 21-hydroxylase resulting in increased circulating levels of 17-OHP.

- Because of the length of the hair growth cycle, response should not be expected until after 3 months of therapy has been used. Successful responses should occur in about 70% of those patients treated.

- If after an overnight dexamethasone suppression test serum cortisol levels are lower than 5 µg/100 ml, Cushing syndrome is ruled out.

- The best treatment for hirsutism due to increased peripheral androgen metabolism is the antiandrogen spironolactone.

- Women with PCOS who desire fertility should be treated with agents that stimulate ovulation, starting with clomiphene citrate and, if the condition is unresponsive, proceeding to hMG with or without GnRH agonists or metformin. An alternative treatment is partial ovarian destruction (ovarian drilling).

- The treatment of hirsutism should depend on the source of the excess androgens. If testosterone levels are elevated, indicating excess ovarian androgen production, oral contraceptive therapy should be instituted. If DHEA-S is increased, indicating excess adrenal androgen secretion, dexamethasone therapy should be used. If neither is elevated, spironolactone should be administered.

- Spironolactone, an aldosterone antagonist, is the most effective treatment for idiopathic hirsutism. The major side effect is abnormal bleeding, which can be controlled with use of oral contraceptives. Spironolactone should be administered in a dose of 100 to 200 mg/day.

BIBLIOGRAPHY

Andreyko JL, Monroe SE, Jaffe RB, et al: Treatment of hirsutism with a gonadotrophin-releasing hormone agonist (nafarelin), J Clin Endocrinol Metab 63:854, 1986.

Ardaens Y, Robert Y, Leemaitre L, et al: Polycystic ovarian disease: contribution of vaginal endosonography and reassessment of ultrasonic diagnosis, Fertil Steril 55:1062, 1991.

Azziz R and Zacur HA: 21-Hydroxylase deficiency in female hyperandrogenism: screening and diagnosis, J Clin Endocrinol Metab 69:577, 1989.

Balen AH, Conway GS, Kaltsas G, et al: Polycystic ovary syndrome: the spectrum of the disorder in 1741 patients, Hum Reprod 10:2107, 1995.

Barth JH, Cherry CA, Wojnarowska F, and Dawber RPR: Spironolactone is an effective and well tolerated systematic antiandrogen therapy for hirsute women, J Clin Endocrinol Metab 68:966, 1989.

Baskin HJ: Screening for late-onset congenital adrenal hyperplasia in hirsutism or amenorrhea, Arch Intern Med 147:847, 1987.

Boyers P, Buster JE, and Marshall JR: Hypothalamic-pituitary-adrenocortical function during long-term low-dose dexamethasone therapy in hyperandrogenized women, Am J Obstet Gynecol 142:330, 1982.

Burger CW, Korsen T, van Kessel H, et al: Pulsatile luteinizing hormone patterns in the follicular phase of the menstrual cycle, polycystic ovarian disease (PCOD) and non-PCOD secondary amenorrhea, J Clin Endocrinol Metab 61:1126, 1985.

Carlstrom K, Gershagen S, Marcolin G, et al: Free testosterone and testosterone/SHBG index in hirsute women: a comparison of diagnostic accuracy, Gynecol Obstet Invest 24:256, 1987.

Chang RJ, Mandel FP, Wolfsen AR, et al: Circulating levels of plasma adrenocorticotropin in polycystic ovary disease, J Clin Endocrinol Metab 54:1265, 1982.

Chapman AJ, Wilson M, Obhrai M, et al: Effect of bromocriptine on pulsatility in the polycystic ovary syndrome, Clin Endocrinol 27:571, 1987.

Chapman G, Dowsett M, Dewhurst CJ, and Jeffocate SL: Spironolactone in combination with an oral contraceptive: an alternative treatment for hirsutism, Br J Obstet Gynaecol 92:983, 1985.

Chez RA: Clinical aspects of three new progestogens: desogestrel, gestodene, and norgestimate, Am J Obstet Gynecol 160:1296, 1989.

Conway GS and Jacobs HS: Clinical implications of hyperinsulinemia in women, Clin Endocrinol 39:623, 1993.

Cumming DC and Wall SR: Non–sex hormone–binding globulin–bound testosterone is a marker for hyperandrogenism, J Clin Endocrinol Metab 61:873, 1985.

Cumming D, Yang JC, Rebar RW, et al: Treatment of hirsutism with spironolactone, JAMA 247:1295, 1982.

Dahlgren E, Janson PO, Johansson S, et al: Women with polycystic ovary syndrome wedge resected in 1956 to 1965: a long-term follow-up focusing on natural history and circulating hormones, Fertil Steril 57:505, 1992.

DeVane GW, Czekala NM, Judd HL, et al: Circulating gonadotropins, estrogens, and androgens in polycystic ovarian disease, Am J Obstet Gynecol 121:496, 1975.

Dewailly D, Vantyghem-Haudiquet MC, Sainsard C, et al: Clinical and biological phenotypes in late-onset 21-hydroxylase deficiency, J Clin Endocrinol Metab 63:418, 1986.

Dibbelt L, Knuppen R, Jutting G, et al: Group comparison of serum ethinyl estradiol, SHGB and CBG levels in 83 women using 2 low-dose combination oral contraceptives for 3 months, Contraception 43:1, 1991.

Dunaif A, Graf M, Mandeli J, et al: Characterization of groups of hyperandrogenic women with acanthosis nigricans, impaired glucose tolerance, and/or hyperinsulinemia, J Clin Endocrinol Metab 65:499, 1987.

Ehrmann DA, Cavaghan MK, and Barnes RB: Prevalence of impaired glucose tolerance and diabetes in women with polycystic ovary syndrome, Diabetes Care 22:141, 1999.

Felemban A, Tan SL, and Tulandi T: Laparoscopic treatment of polycystic ovaries with insulated needle cautery: a reappraisal, Fertil Steril 73:266, 2000.

Ferriman D and Gallwey JD: Clinical assessment of body hair growth in women, J Clin Endocrinol Metab 21:1440, 1961.

Filicori M, Flamigni C, Campaniello E, et al: The abnormal response of polycystic ovarian disease patients to exogenous pulsatile gonadotropin-releasing hormone: characterization and management, J Clin Endocrinol Metab 69:825, 1989.

Fox R, Corrigan E, Thomas PA, and Hull MGR: The diagnosis of polycystic ovaries in women with oligo-amenorrhoea: predictive power of endocrine tests, Clin Endocrinol (Oxf) 34:127, 1991.

Givens JR, Andersen RN, Wiser WL, et al: A gonadotropin responsive adrenocortical adenoma, J Clin Endocrinol Metab 38:126, 1974.

Gjønnaess H: Late endocrine effects of ovarian electrocautery in women with polycystic ovary syndrome, Fertil Steril 69:697, 1998.

Gjønnaess H: Ovarian electrocautery in the treatment of women with polycystic ovary syndrome (PCOS): factors affecting the results, Acta Obstet Gynecol Scand 73:407, 1994.

Goldzieher JW: Polycystic ovarian syndrome, Fertil Steril 35:371, 1981.

Goldzieher JW and Axelrod LR: Clinical and biochemical features of polycystic ovarian disease, Fertil Steril 14:631, 1963.

Hann LE, Hall DA, McArdle CR, and Seibel M: Polycystic ovarian disease: sonographic spectrum, Radiology 150:531, 1984.

Helfer EL, Miller JL, and Rose LI: Side effects of spironolactone therapy in the hirsute woman, J Clin Endocrinol Metab 66:208, 1988.

Hensleigh PA and Woodruff JD: Differential maternal-fetal response to androgenizing luteoma or hyperreactio luteinalis, Obstet Gynecol Surv 33:262, 1978.

Hoffman D, Klove K, and Lobo RA: The prevalence and significance of elevated dehydroepiandrosterone sulfate levels in anovulatory women, Fertil Steril 42:76, 1984.

Horton R, Hawks D, and Lobo RA: 3α,17β-androstanediol glucuronide in plasma: a marker of androgen action in idiopathic hirsutism, J Clin Invest 69:1203, 1982.

Horton R and Lobo RA: Peripheral androgens and the role of androstanediol glucuronide, Clin Endocrinol Metab 15:293, 1986.

Hull MGR: Epidemiology of infertility and polycystic ovarian disease: endocrinological and demographic studies, Gynecol Endocrinol 1:235, 1987.

Ireland K and Woodruff JD: Masculinizing ovarian tumors, Obstet Gynecol Surv 31:83, 1976.

Judd HL, Rigg LA, Anderson DC, et al: The effects of ovarian wedge resection on circulating gonadotropin and ovarian steroid levels in patients with polycystic ovary syndrome, J Clin Endocrinol Metab 43:347, 1976.

Judd HL, Scully RE, Herbst AL, et al: Familial hyperthecosis: comparison of endocrinologic and histologic findings with polycystic ovarian disease, Am J Obstet Gynecol 117:976, 1973.

Kazer AR, Kessel B, and Yen SSC: Circulating luteinizing hormone pulse frequency in women with polycystic ovary syndrome, J Clin Endocrinol Metab 65:233, 1987.

Kirschner MA, Samojlik E, and Szmal E: Clinical usefulness of plasma androstanediol glucuronide measurements in women with idiopathic hirsutism, J Clin Endocrinol Metab 65:597, 1987.

Klove KL, Roy S, and Lobo RA: The effect of different contraceptive treatments on the serum concentration of dehydroepiandrosterone sulfate, Contraception 29:319, 1984.

Knochenhauer ES, Key TJ, Kahsar-Miller, et al: Prevalence of the polycystic ovary syndrome in unselected black and white women of the southeastern United States: a prospective study, J Clin Endocrinol Metab 83:3078, 1998.

Kohn B, Levine MS, Pollack MS, et al: Late-onset steroid 21-hydroxylase deficiency: a variant of classical congenital adrenal hyperplasia, J Clin Endocrinol Metab 55:817, 1982.

Koivunen R, Laatikainen T, Tomas C, et al: The prevalence of polycystic ovaries in healthy women, Acta Obstet Gynecol Scand 78:137, 1999.

Kokaly W and McKenna TJ: Relapse of hirsutism following a long-term successful treatment with oestrogen, Clin Endocrinol 52:379, 2000.

Koskinen P, Erkkota R, Penttila T-A, et al: Optimal use of hormone determinations in the biochemical diagnosis of the polycystic ovary syndrome, Fertil Steril 65:517, 1996.

Kuttenn F, Couillin P, Girard F, et al: Late-onset adrenal hyperplasia in hirsutism, N Engl J Med 313:224, 1985.

Legro RS, Kunselman AR, Dodson WC, and Dunaif A: Prevalence and predictors of risk for type 2 diabetes mellitus and impaired glucose tolerance in polycystic ovary syndrome: a prospective controlled study in 254 affected women, J Clin Endocrinol Metab 84:165, 1999.

Li TC, Saravelos H, Chow MS, et al: Factors affecting the outcome of laparoscopic ovarian drilling for polycystic ovarian syndrome in women with anovulatory infertility, Br J Obstet Gynaecol 105:338, 1998.

Lobo RA and Goebelsmann U: Adult manifestation of congenital adrenal hyperplasia due to incomplete 21-hydroxylase deficiency mimicking polycystic ovarian disease, Am J Obstet Gynecol 138:720, 1980.

Lobo RA and Goebelsmann U: Evidence for reduced 3β-ol-hydroxysteroid dehydrogenase activity in some hirsute women thought to have polycystic ovary syndrome, J Clin Endocrinol Metab 53:394, 1981.

Lobo RA and Goebelsmann U: Effect of androgen excess on inappropriate gonadotropin secretion as found in polycystic ovary syndrome, Am J Obstet Gynecol 142:394, 1982.

Lobo RA, Goebelsmann U, and Horton R: Evidence for the importance of peripheral tissue events in the development of hirsutism in polycystic ovary syndrome, J Clin Endocrinol Metab 57:393, 1983.

Lobo RA, Granger L, Goebelsmann U, et al: Elevation in unbound serum estradiol as a possible mechanism for inappropriate gonadotropin secretion in women with PCO, J Clin Endocrinol Metab 52:156, 1981.

Lobo RA, Granger LR, Paul WL, et al: Psychological stress and increases in urinary norepinephrine metabolites, platelet serotonin and adrenal androgens in women with polycystic ovary syndrome, Am J Obstet Gynecol 145:496, 1983.

Lobo RA, Kletzky OA, Campeau JD, et al: Elevated bioactive luteinizing hormone in women with the polycystic ovary syndrome, Fertil Steril 39:674, 1983.

Lobo RA, Paul WL, and Goebelsmann U: Dehydroepiandrosterone sulfate as an indicator of adrenal androgen function, Obstet Gynecol 57:69, 1981.

Lobo RA, Paul WL, and Goebelsmann U: Serum levels of DHEA-S in gynecologic endocrinopathy and infertility, Obstet Gynecol 57:607, 1981.

Lobo RA, Shoupe D, Serafini P, et al: The effects of two doses of spironolactone on serum androgens and anagen hair in hirsute women, Fertil Steril 43:200, 1985.

Loric S, Guechot J, Duron F, et al: Determination of testosterone in serum not bound by sex-hormone–binding globulin: diagnostic value in hirsute women, Clin Chem 34:1826, 1988.

Mandel FP, Chang RJ, Dupont B, et al: HLA genotyping in family members and patients with familial polycystic ovarian disease, J Clin Endocrinol Metab 56:862, 1983.

Michelmore KF, Balen AH, Dunger DB, and Vessey MP: Polycystic ovaries and associated clinical and biochemical features in young women, Clin Endocrinol 51:779, 1999.

Milewicz A, Silber D, and Kirschner MA: Therapeutic effects of spironolactone in polycystic ovary syndrome, Obstet Gynecol 61:429, 1983.

Moghetti P, Castello R, Negri C, et al: Metformin effects on clinical features, endocrine and metabolic profiles, and insulin sensitivity in polycystic ovary syndrome: a randomized, double-blind, placebo-controlled 6-month trial, followed by open, long-term clinical evaluation, J Clin Endocrinol Metab 85:139, 2000.

Mornet E, Crete P, Kuttenn F, et al: Distribution of deletions and seven point mutations on CYP21-genes in three clinical forms of steroid 21-hydroxylase deficiency, Am J Hum Genet 48:79, 1991.

Murdoch AP, McClean KG, Watson MJ, et al: Treatment of hirsutism in polycystic ovary syndrome with bromocriptine, Br J Obstet Gynaecol 94:358, 1987.

Nestler JE, Jakubowicz DJ, Evans WS, et al: Effects of metformin on spontaneous and clomiphene-induced ovulation in the polycystic ovary syndrome, N Engl J Med 338:1876, 1998.

New MI, Lorenzen F, Lerner AJ, et al: Genotyping steroid 21-hydroxylase deficiency: hormonal reference data, J Clin Endocrinol Metab 57:320, 1983.

New MI, White PC, Pang S, et al: The adrenal hyperplasias. In Scriver CR, Beaudet AL, Sly S, and Valle D, editors: Metabolic basis of inherited diseases, ed 6, New York, 1989, McGraw-Hill Book Co.

Nicolini U, Ferrazzi E, Bellotti M, et al: The contribution of sonographic evaluation of ovarian size in patients with polycystic ovarian disease, J Ultrasound Med 4:342, 1985.

Pache TD, Wladimiroff JW, Hop WCJ, and Fauser BCJM: How to discriminate between normal and polycystic ovaries: transvaginal US study, Radiology 183:421, 1992.

Pang S, Wallace MA, Hofman L, et al: Worldwide experience in newborn screening for classical congenital adrenal hyperplasia due to 21-hydroxylase deficiency, Pediatrics 81:866, 1988.

Parisi L, Tramonti M, Casciano S, et al: The role of ultrasound in the study of polycystic ovarian disease, J Clin Ultrasound 10:167, 1982.

Paulson RJ, Serafini PC, Catalino JA, and Lobo RA: Measurements of 3α,17β-androstanediol glucuronide in serum and urine and the correlation with skin 5α-reductase activity, Fertil Steril 46:222, 1986.

Phocas I, Chryssikopoulos A, Sarandakou A, et al: A contribution to the classification of cases of non-classic 21-hydroxylase-deficient congenital adrenal hyperplasia, Gynecol Endocrinol 9:229, 1995.

Plymate SR, Fariss BL, Bassett ML, et al: Obesity and its role in polycystic ovary syndrome, J Clin Endocrinol Metab 52:1246, 1981.

Polson DW, Adams J, Wadsworth J, and Franks S: Polycystic ovaries: a common finding in normal women, Lancet I:870, 1988.

Raj SG, Thompson IE, Berger MJ, et al: Clinical aspects of the polycystic ovary syndrome, Obstet Gynecol 49:552, 1977.

Rebar R, Judd HL, Yen SSC, et al: Characterization of the inappropriate gonadotropin secretion in polycystic ovary syndrome, J Clin Invest 57:1320, 1976.

Rittmaster RS: Differential suppression of testosterone and estradiol in hirsute women with the superactive gonadotropin-releasing hormone agonist leuprolide, J Clin Endocrinol Metab 67:651, 1988.

Rittmaster RS, Loriaux DL, and Cutler GB: Sensitivity of cortisol and adrenal androgens to dexamethasone suppression in hirsute women, J Clin Endocrinol Metab 61:462, 1985.

Rittmaster RS and Thompson DL: Effect of leuprolide and dexamethasone on hair growth and hormone levels in hirsute women: the relative importance of the ovary and the adrenal in the pathogenesis of hirsutism, J Clin Endocrinol Metab 70:1096, 1990.

Schwartz U, Moltz L, Brotherton J, and Hammerstein J: The diagnostic value of plasma free testosterone in non-tumorous and tumorous hyperandrogenism, Fertil Steril 40:66, 1983.

Serafini P, Ablan R, and Lobo RA: 5α-reductase activity in the genital skin of hirsute women, J Clin Endocrinol Metab 60:349, 1985.

Speiser PW, Dupont B, Rubenstein P, et al: High frequency of nonclassical steroid 21-hydroxylase deficiency, Am J Hum Genet 37:650, 1985.

Speiser PW, New MI, and White PC: Molecular genetic analysis of nonclassic steroid 21-hydroxylase deficiency associated with HLA-B14, DR1, N Engl J Med 319:19, 1988.

Stein IF and Leventhal ML: Amenorrhea associated with bilateral polycystic ovaries, Am J Obstet Gynecol 29:181, 1935.

Swanson M, Sauerbrei EE, and Cooperberg PL: Medical implications of ultrasonically detected polycystic ovaries, J Clin Ultrasound 9:219, 1981.

Velazquez E, Acosta A, and Mendoza SG: Menstrual cyclicity after metformin therapy in polycystic ovary syndrome, Obstet Gynecol 90:392, 1997.

Venturoli S, Fabbri R, Dal Prato L, et al: Ketoconazole therapy for women with acne and/or hirsutism, J Clin Endocrinol Metab 71:335, 1990.

Wild RA and Bartholomew MJ: The influence of body weight on lipoprotein lipids in patients with polycystic ovary syndrome, Am J Obstet Gynecol 159:423, 1988.

Wild RA, Demers LM, Applebaum-Bowden D, and Lenker R: Hirsutism: metabolic effects of two commonly used oral contraceptives and spironolactone, Contraception 44:113, 1991.

Wild RA, Umstot ES, Andersen RN, et al: Adrenal function in hirsutism. II. Effect of an oral contraceptive, J Clin Endocrinol Metab 54:676, 1981.

Williams IA, Shaw RW, and Burford G: An attempt to alter the pathophysiology of polycystic ovary syndrome using a gonadotrophin hormone releasing hormone agonist—nafarelin, Clin Endocrinol 31:345, 1989.

Wilroy RS Jr, Givens JR, Wiser WL, et al: Genetic forms of hypogonadism, Birth Defects 11(4), 1975.

Yeh HC, Futterweit W, and Thornton JC: Polycystic ovarian disease: US features in 104 patients, Radiology 163:111, 1987.

Yen SSC: Chronic anovulation caused by peripheral endocrine disorders. In Yen SSC and Jaffe RB, editors: Reproductive endocrinology, ed 2, Philadelphia, 1986, WB Saunders Co.

Yen SSC, Chaney C, and Judd HL: Functional aberrations of the hypothalamic-pituitary system in polycystic ovary syndrome: a consideration of the pathogenesis. In James VHT, Serio M, and Guisti G, editors: The endocrine function of the human ovary, New York, 1976, Academic Press.

Infertility

Etiology, Diagnostic Evaluation, Management, Prognosis

KEY TERMS AND DEFINITIONS

Artificial Insemination. Method to place sperm in the female reproductive tract by means other than sexual intercourse. If the sperm are from the husband, the technique is called *artificial insemination husband* (AIH). If the sperm are from another man, the method has been called *artificial insemination donor* (AID). Other terms are *donor insemination* and *therapeutic donor insemination* (TDI).

Assisted Reproductive Technology. Various techniques utilized to increase fecundability by nonphysiologic methods of enhancing probability of fertilization. Categories include in vitro fertilization, gamete intrafallopian tube transfer, zygote intrafallopian tube transfer, and tubal embryo transfer.

Asthenospermia. Loss or reduction of the motility of the spermatozoa.

Azoospermia. Absence of sperm in the semen.

Clomiphene Citrate. A weak synthetic estrogenic compound with three benzene rings given orally to induce ovulation in anovulatory women with circulating estradiol levels more than 40 pg/ml.

Controlled Ovarian Hyperstimulation (COH). Inducing development of more than one dominant follicle with pharmacologic agents, usually clomiphene citrate or human menopausal gonadotrophin, also called *superovulation* or *multiple follicular recruitment* (MFR). COH is usually combined with intrauterine insemination to treat unexplained infertility.

Fecundability. Probability of conception occurring in a population of couples in a given period of time, usually 1 month.

Fimbrioplasty. Surgical technique of removing adhesions between fimbrial fronds of the partially occluded distal end of the oviduct.

Gamete Intrafallopian Transfer (GIFT). Placement of human ova and sperm into the distal end of the oviduct.

Hamster Egg Penetration Assay (Sperm Penetration Assay). Test of the fertilizing ability of human sperm based on their ability to penetrate zona-free hamster ova.

Human Menopausal Gonadotrophin (HMG). Formulation made up of equal amounts of follicle-stimulating hormone (FSH) and luteinizing hormone (LH) derived from urine obtained from postmenopausal women. The injectable agent is used to stimulate follicular development in both anovulatory and ovulatory women.

Hysterosalpingogram (HSG). Fluoroscopic and radiographic visualization of the interior of the female upper genital tract after instillation of radiopaque dye.

Intracytoplasmic Sperm Injection (ICSI). Technique by which a single spermatozoon is injected into the cytoplasm of an ovum.

Infertility. Inability of couples of reproductive age to establish a pregnancy by having sexual intercourse within a certain period of time, usually 1 year. Infertility is considered primary if the woman has never been pregnant and secondary if it occurs after one or more pregnancies.

Intrauterine Insemination. Placement of spermatozoa that have been separated from the seminal fluid into the endometrial cavity through a small catheter.

In Vitro Fertilization. Fertilization of human ova by sperm in a laboratory environment.

Luteal Phase Deficiency (Inadequate Luteal Phase). Deficient progesterone secretion or action resulting in a delay of normal endometrial development.

Microsurgery. Operative technique using magnification and fine, nonreactive suture material.

Oligozoospermia (Oligospermia). Presence of fewer than 20 million sperm per milliliter of semen.

Ovarian Hyperstimulation Syndrome (OHSS). Ovarian enlargement to a diameter of more than 6 cm as a result of stimulation of multiple follicles. In the mild form there is abdominal pain, distention, and weight gain. In the moderate form ovarian enlargement is more than 10 cm in diameter with ascites, nausea, and vomiting. Severe OHSS is associated with hemoconcentration, oliguria, and elevated serum creatine. Pleural effusions and ascites can be present; OHSS becomes critical when hypercoagulability and hypotension occurs. This condition may be fatal.

Postcoital Test. Examination of the cervical mucus to evaluate the presence of sperm several hours after sexual intercourse.

Pronuclear Stage Tubal Transfer (PROST) or Zygote Intrafallopian Transfer (ZIFT). In vitro fertilization with transfer of the zygote to the oviducts by transabdominal cannulation.

Salpingitis Isthmica Nodosa. Diverticula of the endosalpinx in the muscularis of the isthmic portion of the oviduct.

Salpingolysis. Removal of adhesions attached to an oviduct that appears normal on gross inspection.

Salpingostomy. Surgical creation of a new opening of a completely occluded distal end of the oviduct.

Semen Analysis. Quantitation of various parameters of a recently ejaculated semen specimen analyzed after liquefaction has occurred.

Spinnbarkeit. Property of elasticity (distensibility) of cervical mucus.

Teratozoospermia. Greater-than-normal (50%) incidence of abnormal forms of sperm in semen analysis.

Treatment-Independent Pregnancy. Infertile women conceiving without use of infertility therapy.

Tubal Embryo Transfer (TET) or Tubal Embryo Stage Transfer (TEST). Same as ZIFT, except additional incubation to embryo stage occurs before transfer to the oviducts.

Unexplained Infertility. The diagnosis of an infertile couple when ovulation and tubal patency, as well as a normal semen analysis, are all present.

Testicular Sperm Extraction. Retrieval of sperm from the testis by biopsy or aspiration from men with azoospermia due to obstruction of the vas deferens or epididymis (obstructive azoospermia) or without such obstruction (nonobstructive azoospermia). The sperm are injected into ova retrieved by follicle aspiration by the ICSI procedure.

The term *infertility* is generally used to indicate that a couple has a reduced capacity to conceive as compared with the mean capacity of the general population. In a group of normal fertile couples, the monthly conception rate, or fecundability, is about 20%. Couples with infertility are grouped into two categories: (1) those with low fecundability who are hypofertile and eventually are able to conceive without treatment and (2) those who are never able to conceive without therapy and are therefore sterile. Examples of the first group include couples whose male partner has oligospermia or female partner has mild endometriosis. Examples of the second group include couples with male partners who have azoospermia and those with female partners who have complete occlusion of the oviducts.

INCIDENCE OF INFERTILITY

Results from the three U.S. National Surveys of Family Growth performed under the direction of U.S. governmental agencies provide information about infertility in this country. Analysis of the data obtained from the surveys performed in 1982, 1988, and 1995 indicate that the proportion of U.S. women aged 15 to 44 with impaired fecundity increased from 8% in 1982 and 1988 to 10% in 1995, a 20% rise. It was estimated that the number of women with impaired fecundity in the United States increased from 4.6 million to 6.2 million between 1982 and 1995, a 35% rise. Most of this increase occurred among nulliparous women in the oldest age group (35 to 44) due to women of the baby-boom group reaching this age. Many in this age group had delayed childbearing. The percentage of women with impaired fecundability seeking medical assistance for this problem remained stable, about 44% between 1988 and 1995. However because more women had impaired fecundability there was a 30% increase in women who utilized medical help for this problem in the United States, an increase from 2.1 to 2.7 million women.

INFERTILITY AND AGE

Data from both older and more recent studies indicate that the percentage of infertile couples increases with increasing age of the female partner. Analysis of data from three national surveys in the United States revealed that the percentage of presumably fertile married women not using contraception who failed to conceive in 1 year steadily increased from ages 25 to 44 (Table 41-1). Data from a study of presumably fertile nulliparous women married to husbands with azoospermia who underwent donor artificial insemination revealed that the percentage who conceived after 12 cycles of insemination declined substantially after age 30 (Table 41-2). In general terms, about one in seven couples are infertile if the wife is 30 to 34 years of age, one in five are infertile if she is 35 to 40, and one in four are infertile if she is 40 to 44. Another way to interpret these data is to state that as compared with women aged 20 to 24, fertility is reduced by 6% in the next 5 years, by 14% between ages 30 and 34, by 31% between ages 35 and 39, and to a much greater extent after age 40.

Because human reproduction is an inefficient process, it takes time to become pregnant. Therefore, because a woman's reproductive life span is limited to a certain number of years, if couples intend to have children, they should be counseled to maximize the length of time during which they attempt to conceive. Because the percentage of couples with decreased rates of fecundability increases with age of the female partner, couples should be informed that the probability of conception is substantially reduced by delaying childbearing until later in life. This reduction is caused by two factors: (1) the incidence of infertility increases with increasing age of the woman and (2) the total length of time during which conception is possible is less in older women. Because the occurrence of monthly ovulation decreases greatly after age 45, as a woman becomes older, a corresponding decrease occurs in the total duration of time during which she may conceive.

FECUNDABILITY

Analysis of data from presumably fertile couples who stop using contraception in order to conceive reveals that about only half the couples will conceive in 3 months, three fourths will conceive in 6 months, and by 1 year about 90% will have conceived (Figure 41-1). Statistical analysis of these data indicate that the normal monthly fecundability rate is about 0.2.

This information is extremely important when analyzing data concerning the results of various treatment methods applied to a group of infertile couples. This group includes those with hypofertility due to presumed causes (e.g., mild endometriosis) as well as those with idiopathic (unexplained) infertility. For example, Leridon and Spira estimated that if the mean fecundability of the population is 0.2, 14% of the couples will not have conceived after 12 months; during the following year, however, 69% of the nonsterile couples in this population will conceive without treatment (Table 41-3). Analysis of these statistical tables reveals that after 2 years of trying to conceive, about 4% of these couples will not have done so. Their mean monthly fecundability is about 0.08, and 57% will conceive in the next year. Of the 2% still not pregnant at this time, 3 years after trying to conceive, the monthly fecundability rate drops to about 0.06, 0.05, and 0.04 in the next 3 years, respectively. Thus in the fourth, fifth, and sixth years of attempting to conceive, 48%, 42%, and 37% of the nonpregnant women should conceive without treatment. Infertility is usually defined as inability to conceive in 1 year. When so defined, the group of infertile couples includes those who have difficulty in conceiving quickly (hypofertile) as well as those who will never be able to conceive (sterile).

TABLE 41-1
Percentage of Married Women Who Are Infertile, by Age, from Three National U.S. Surveys

Age	Infertile (%)
20–24	7.0
25–29	8.9
30–34	14.6
35–39	21.9
40–44	28.7

From Menken J, Trussell IJ, and Larsen U: Science 23:1389, 1986.

TABLE 41-2
Percentage of Pregnancy Rates by Age at 1 Year in Normal Women with Azoospermatic Husbands After Donor Insemination

Age	Pregnancy Rate (%)
<25	73.0
26–30	74.1
31–35	61.5
36–40	55.8

From Schwartz D and Mayaux MJ: N Engl J Med 306:404, 1982.

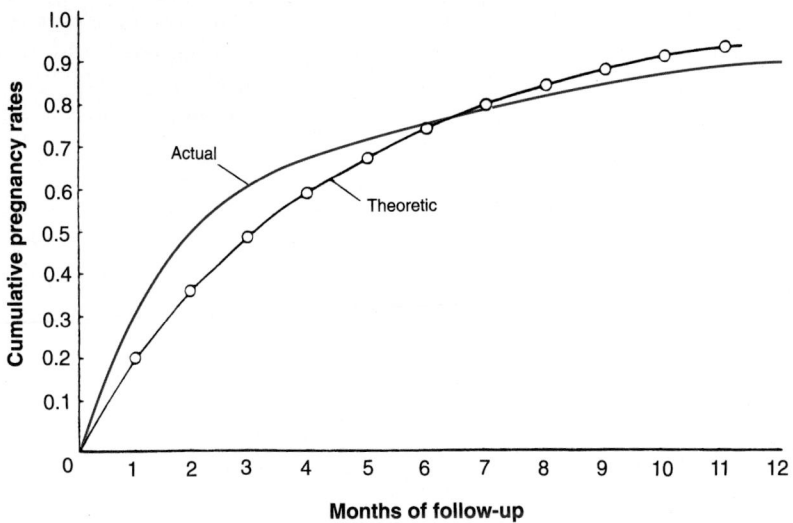

FIGURE 41-1 Curve of theoretic time to pregnancy in women with a monthly fecundability rate of 0.2 *(open circles)* and curve of actual time to pregnancy in fertile women discontinuing contraception *(solid line)*. (Open-circle data from Hull MGR, Glazener CMA, Kelly NJ, et al: Br Med J 291:1693, 1985; and solid-line data from Murray DL, Reich L, and Adashi EY: Fertil Steril 51:35, 1989.)

TABLE 41-3
Incidence of Conception over Time Among Nonsterile Couples with Mean Fecundability of 0.2

No. of Months Without Conception	Proportion (%) of Couples Not Yet Having Conceived	Mean Fecundability of Couples Not Yet Having Conceived	Proportion (%) of Couples Who Will Conceive Within 12 Months Among Couples Not Yet Having Conceived
0	100.0	0.20	86.0
6	31.9	0.14	77.0
12	14.0	0.11	69.2
24	4.3	0.08	57.0
36	1.9	0.06	48.2
48	1.0	0.05	41.7
60	0.6	0.04	36.7

Adapted from Leridon H and Spira A: Fertil Steril 41:580, 1984.

Several studies have reported the incidence of spontaneous conception among infertile couples without a specifically diagnosed cause of infertility (unexplained infertility). Four long-term studies have reported fecundity rates in couples with unexplained infertility of at least 1 year's duration without treatment. In all four studies there was indirect documentation of ovulation, evidence of fallopian tubal patency, and the presence of a normal semen analysis. In three of the four studies a normal postcoital test and normal laparoscopic evaluation of the pelvis were also present. Thus the most meaningful diagnostic tests of the infertility evaluation were normal in the couples studied. The cumulative pregnancy rates at the end of 2 to 7 years without any treatment ranged from 43% to 87% (Figure 41-2). Collins et al. reported that the live-birth rate of 873 infertile couples in several Canadian centers observed without treatment for 18,364 months steadily rose to more than 35% at 3 years and 45% after 7 years (Figure 41-3). Of the 562 couples in this group with unexplained infertility who received no treatment, one third had a live birth during the first 3 years of observation without treatment.

Thus, in order to determine that any method of treatment of infertility is superior to no treatment, statistical analysis of the treatment results on the incidence of pregnancy over time needs to be performed. Ideally, these results should be compared with a nontreated control group. At the least, these pregnancy rates should be compared with the rates of the nontreated women with a normal diagnostic evaluation reported in the four studies mentioned. Various statistical formulas for performing such analyses based on life-table analysis have been described. This statistical approach is necessary to determine if treat-

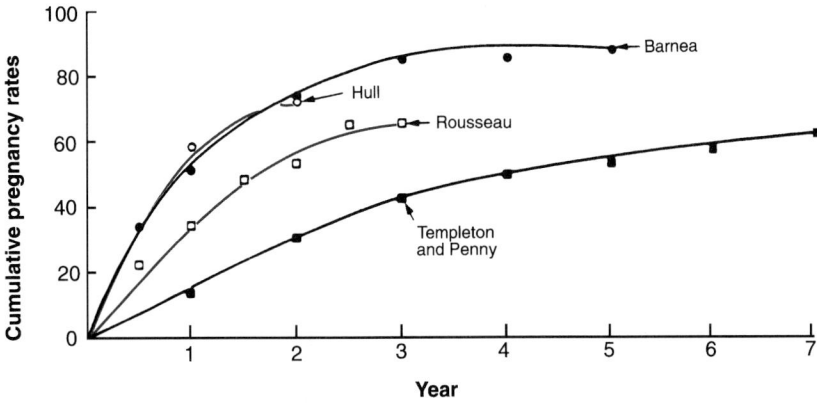

FIGURE 41-2 Pregnancy rates over time in untreated couples with normal basic (five-step) infertility investigation—results of four studies. (Adapted from Barnea ER, Holford TR, and McInnes DRA: Obstet Gynecol 66:24, 1985; Hull MGR, Glazener CMA, Kelly NJ, et al: Br Med J 291:1963, 1985; Rousseau S, Lora J, Lepage Y, and Van Campenhout J: Fertil Steril 40:768, 1983; and Templeton AA and Penney GC: Fertil Steril 37:175, 1982.)

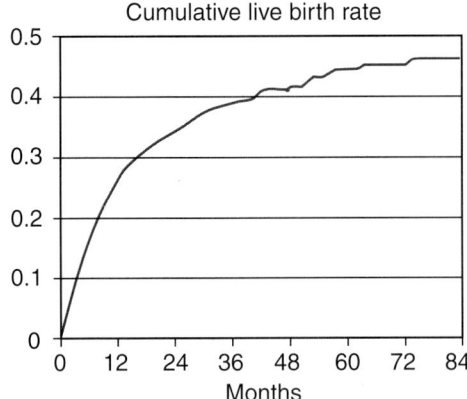

FIGURE 41-3 Cumulative rate of conceptions leading to live birth. Couples (873) who remained untreated throughout follow-up; cumulative rate of live birth conception at 36 months was 38.2% (95% CI 34.2, 42.3). (Modified from Collins JA, Burrows EA, and Willan AR: Fertil Steril 64:22, 1996.)

CAUSES OF INFERTILITY

The exact incidence of the various factors causing infertility varies among different populations and cannot be precisely determined. In general, however, 10% to 15% of infertility results from anovulation; 30% to 40% is caused by pelvic factors, such as adhesions from endometriosis or infection, or tubal occlusion that interferes with normal ovum transport; about 30% to 40% is associated with abnormalities in the male reproductive system, which are associated with either oligozoospermia, high viscosity of semen, low sperm motility, or low volume of semen (male factor); and an additional 10% to 15% of infertility is associated with abnormal sperm-cervical mucus penetration (cervical factor). It has not been shown that the presence of other abnormalities, such as antisperm antibodies, luteal phase deficiency, subclinical genital infection, or subclinical endocrine abnormalities such as hypothyroidism or hyperprolactinemia in ovulatory women are actual causes of infertility. There are no prospective randomized studies that demonstrate that treatment of these latter entities results in greater fecundability than occurs without treatment. If any of these entities do cause infertility, they do so infrequently. With current techniques of investigation, it is impossible to diagnose the cause of infertility in about 25% of couples, and they are considered to have idiopathic or unexplained infertility. However, as explained earlier, most of these couples are hypofertile and eventually are able to conceive without treatment.

DIAGNOSTIC EVALUATION

The diagnostic evaluation of infertility should be thorough and completed as rapidly as possible. During the initial interview the couple should be informed about the rates of normal human fecundability and how these rates are decreased by increasing age of the female partner over

ment methods are indeed beneficial, since data from uncontrolled studies can be erroneous. These formulas provide mathematical techniques to determine the monthly probability of conception and the cumulative conception rate.

After using these techniques of analysis, therapy should be offered to the couple only if it is found that such therapy hastens the time in which conception will take place as compared with untreated controls or couples with a similar duration of infertility and a normal diagnostic infertility evaluation. Furthermore, couples should be counseled that with sufficient time the likelihood of eventually conceiving without empiric treatment (and its associated expense) may be similar to that occurring in a shorter time period with use of certain therapies. For couples with unexplained infertility, treatment with controlled ovarian hyperstimulation and intrauterine insemination, as well as in vitro fertilization, have both been shown to increase fecundability rates compared with no treatment.

age 30 and duration of infertility for more than 3 years. The various tests in the diagnostic evaluation and the reasons why they are performed should be thoroughly explained. In addition, the sequence of performing these tests, their degree of discomfort, cost, and time in the cycle at which they should be performed should also be discussed. The available therapies and the prognosis for treatment of the various causes of infertility should also be included in the dialogue. The couple should be informed that after a complete diagnostic infertility evaluation, the cause for the infertility will not be able to be determined in about 25% of couples. Methods to increase the fecundability rates of couples with a normal diagnostic evaluation such as controlled ovarian hyperstimulation and intrauterine insemination, as well as assisted reproductive techniques, should also be mentioned.

Each couple should be instructed about the optimal time in the cycle for conception to occur and should be encouraged to have coitus on the day before ovulation.

Unless the husband has oligospermia, daily intercourse for 3 consecutive days at midcycle should be encouraged. Since the egg disintegrates within a few hours after it reaches the ampulla of the oviduct, it is best that sperm be present in this area when the egg arrives so that fertilization can occur. Therefore coitus should occur before ovulation.

A study was performed by Wilcox et al. among fertile couples who stopped contraception in order to conceive and recorded the cycle day when they had sexual intercourse. Hormone analysis was performed to determine the day of ovulation. All the couples who had intercourse after ovulation occurred did not become pregnant. The pregnancy rate was about 30% if intercourse occurred on the day of ovulation as well as 1 and 2 days prior to ovulation. The pregnancy rate was about 10% if coitus occurred 3, 4, or 5 days before ovulation. No pregnancies occurred when intercourse took place 6 days or more before ovulation (Figure 41-4). It is therefore considered optimal to perform insemination or have sexual intercourse on the day prior to ovulation. Sperm retain their viability and fertilizing capacity for a longer time period than the ovum is capable of being fertilized after ovulation occurs. Therefore it is best to have the sperm in the oviduct awaiting the release of the egg and its transport into the tubal ampulla. Since peak levels of LH occur 1 day prior to ovulation, measurement of LH by urinary LH immunoassays is the best way to determine the optimal time to have intercourse or insemination. Tests that measure LH in a random daily urine specimen are usually more convenient for planning natural or artificial insemination than the tests that detect LH in the first morning urine specimen. Ovulation most commonly occurs on the day following the detection of LH in a random specimen, and it occurs on the day when LH is detected in the first morning specimen, which contains urine formed during the prior night.

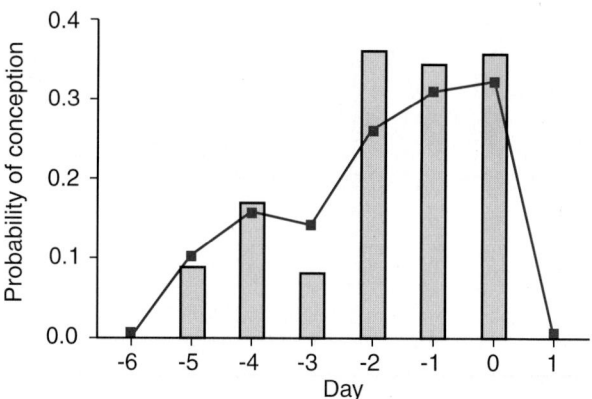

FIGURE 41-4 Probability of conception on specific days near the day of ovulation. The *bars* represent probabilities calculated from data on 129 menstrual cycles in which sexual intercourse was recorded to have occurred on only a single day during the 6-day interval ending on the day of ovulation (day 0). The *solid line* shows daily probabilities based on all 625 cycles, as estimated by the statistical model. (From Wilcox AJ, Weinberg CR, and Baird DD: N Engl J Med 333:1517, 1995.)

In some instances, women produce less-than-adequate amounts of vaginal lubricant. Various vaginal lubricants and chemicals, as well as saliva, used to improve coital satisfaction may interfere with sperm transport. Some men experience midcycle impotence because of the pressure of performing intercourse on demand. In such cases the intercourse schedule should be less rigorous. The couple should also be told that among fertile couples there is only about a 20% chance of conceiving in each ovulatory cycle even with optimally timed coitus, and that it takes time to become pregnant. Thus the two terms *time* and *timing* should be emphasized during the initial counseling session. Couples should also be advised to cease smoking cigarettes and drinking caffeinated beverages, if they do so, since both cigarette smoking and caffeine consumption have been shown independently in several studies to decrease the chances of conception. Baird et al. reported that the common practice of vaginal douching also reduces the chance of conception by about 30%. Therefore infertile women should be advised to discontinue all vaginal douching.

All couples should have a complete history taken, including a sexual history, and a physical examination. After this initial evaluation, tests should be undertaken to determine if the woman is ovulating and has patent oviducts, and if a semen sample of the male partner is normal.

Documentation of Ovulation

Preliminary information that the woman is ovulatory is provided by a history of regular menstrual cycles. If the woman is having regular menstrual cycles, a serum progesterone level should be measured in the midluteal phase to provide indirect evidence of ovulation as well as normal luteal function. Although in the normal luteal phase progesterone levels in blood vary in a pulsatile manner, a serum progesterone level above 10 ng/ml is indicative of adequate luteal function. Progesterone levels of 10 ng/ml or higher are found during at least 1 day of the luteal phase of normal ovulatory cycles in which conception occurred. Measurement of daily BBT also provides indirect evidence that ovulation has taken place. The BBT graph also provides information concerning the approximate day of ovulation and duration of the luteal phase. The BBT should be taken shortly after awakening only after at least 6 hours of sleep and prior to ambulating, with oral sublingual placement of a special thermometer with gradients between 96° and 100° F.

Women with oligomenorrhea (menses at intervals of 35 days or longer) or amenorrhea who wish to conceive should be treated with agents that induce ovulation regardless of whether they have occasional ovulatory cycles. Therefore for such women direct or indirect measurement of progesterone is unnecessary until after therapy is initiated.

Semen Analysis

While information about ovulation is being obtained, the male partner's reproductive system should be evaluated by means of semen analysis. The male partner should be advised to abstain from coitus for 2 to 3 days before collection of the semen sample, because frequent ejaculation lowers the sperm count in some individuals. It is best to collect the specimen in a clean (not necessarily sterile), wide-mouthed jar after masturbation. It is important that the entire specimen be collected, because the initial fraction contains the greatest density of sperm. Ideally, collection should take place in the location where the analysis will be performed. The degree of sperm motility should be determined as soon as possible after liquefaction, which usually occurs 15 to 20 minutes after ejaculation. Sperm motility begins to decline 2 hours after ejaculation, and it is best to examine the specimen within this time period. Semen should not be exposed to marked changes in temperature, and if collected at home during cold weather, the specimen should be kept warm during transport to the laboratory.

Parameters of semen that should be evaluated include volume, viscosity, sperm density, sperm morphology, and sperm motility. The last parameter should be evaluated in terms of percentage of total motile sperm as well as quality of motility (rapidity of movement and amount of progressive motility). There are no absolute standards for determining the normality of a semen sample, but recommended guidelines are shown in Table 41-4. It is beyond the scope of this text to fully discuss the etiology and diagnostic evaluation of men with semen abnormalities. The various etiologies of semen abnormalities are cited in Table 41-5. However, as reported by Barratt et al., when semen analyses were performed on a group of men whose wives had conceived within the past 4 months, about 75% had at least one abnormal characteristic and 25% had two abnormalities. These results indicate that there is normally a wide variability in the parameters used to characterize semen. Second, the criteria used to establish morphology may be too stringent. Third, it is probably more important to consider the number of abnormal parameters instead of an abnormality in a single parameter when interpreting a semen analysis. Finally, because the characteristics of semen analysis will vary over time, if an abnormality is found, it is best to repeat the test on two or three occasions at least a month apart.

Laboratory Tests

The initial laboratory tests performed on the female partner should include a complete blood count, urine analysis, cervical cytology, and a fasting blood-glucose determination. If the woman is over age 35, a serum FSH and estradiol level should be measured on cycle day 2, 3, or 4. An elevated FSH level (more than 20 mIU/ml) in a normally cycling woman provides indirect evidence of impending ovulatory failure. In one study of in vitro fertilization all eggs aspirated from ovarian follicles of women with FSH levels more than 24 mIU/ml in that cycle were not able to be fertilized when incubated with sperm. If the FSH is in the normal range and the estradiol is elevated, more than 100 pg/ml, it is also indirect evidence of impending ovulatory failure. It is also worthwhile to determine if antibodies to *Chlamydia trachomatis* are present in the serum by measuring IgG antibodies to this organism. There is a good correlation between the titer of antibodies to this organism and the presence of tubal adhesions and/or obstruction. Thomas et al. reported that if the antibody

---

TABLE 41-4
Recommended Standards for Semen Analysis

Parameter	Recommended Normal Value
Volume	≥2.0 ml
pH	7.2–7.8
Sperm density	$\geq 20 \times 10^6$/ml
Total sperm count	$\geq 40 \times 10^6$/ml
Sperm motility	≥50% with progressive motility
Vital staining	≥50% live (exclude dye)
Sperm morphology	≥50%
White cell count	$< 10^6$/ml

Modified from Aitken RJ, Comhaire FH, Eliasson R, et al: WHO laboratory manual for the examination of human semen and semen–cervical mucus interaction, Cambridge, 1987, Cambridge University Press.

titer was 1 in 32 or less there was a 5% incidence of tubal damage, but if the titer was greater than 1 in 32, tubal damage was present in 35% of patients. Finally a serum CA-125 level should be measured to indirectly assess the likelihood that endometriosis is present. Pelvic sonography should be undertaken to assess the possible presence of an ovarian endometrioma. Routine measurement of thyroid-stimulating hormone (TSH) and prolactin in

women with regular ovulatory cycles at the time of the initial visit is not cost effective. These tests are usually normal, and even if abnormalities are present in women with regular ovulatory cycles, they are not associated with infertility. Treatment with thyroid replacement and bromocriptine has not been shown to increase the chance of conception in women with ovulatory cycles compared with no therapy.

If an abnormality is found in one of the first two non-invasive diagnostic procedures (documentation of ovulation and semen analysis), that abnormality should be treated before proceeding with the more costly and invasive procedures, unless there is a history or laboratory findings (elevated *Chlamydia* antibody titer) suggestive of tubal disease. For example, if the woman has oligomenorrhea and does not ovulate each month, after a normal semen analysis is observed, ovulation should be induced with clomiphene citrate before performing the other diagnostic measures. Provided no other infertility factors are present, most anovulatory women (80% to 90%) conceive after induction of ovulation with therapeutic agents and half the couples will conceive during the first three ovulatory cycles.

If these initial diagnostic tests are normal, the more uncomfortable and costly hysterosalpingogram (HSG) should be performed in the follicular phase of the next cycle.

Hysterosalpingogram

It is best to schedule the hysterosalpingogram during the week following the end of menses to avoid irradiating a possible pregnancy. Before the procedure a bimanual pelvic examination should be performed, and if adnexal tenderness is present the procedure should be postponed until antibiotic therapy has been administered and the tenderness has resolved. This technique reduces the risk of causing an episode of acute recurrent salpingitis. Some authorities recommend that antibiotic prophylaxis (such as doxycycline 100 mg twice a day for 5 days starting 2 days before the procedure) be given to all women who have an HSG, but this recommendation is not universally performed. The examination should be performed with use of a water-soluble contrast medium and image-intensified fluoroscopy. A water-soluble contrast medium enables better visualization of the tubal mucosal folds and vaginal markings than does an oil-based medium. It is important to be able to evaluate the appearance of the intratubal architecture to determine the extent of damage to the oviduct. A meta-analysis by Watson et al. of clinical studies, including four randomized trials, indicated that a therapeutic benefit is more likely to occur when oil-soluble contrast media are used in a hysterosalpingogram performed for the diagnostic evaluation of infertility. The odds of pregnancy occurring after the procedure were twofold higher when oil-soluble media were used com-

TABLE 41-5
Causes of Semen Abnormalities

Finding	Etiology
Abnormal count	
Azoospermia	Klinefelter's syndrome or other genetic disorders
	Sertoli-cell-only syndrome
	Seminiferous tubule or Leydig cell failure
	Hypogonadotrophic hypogonadism
	Ductal obstruction, including Young's syndrome
	Varicocele
	Exogenous factors
Oligozoospermia	Genetic disorder
	Endocrinopathies, including androgen receptor defects
	Varicocele and other anatomic disorders
	Maturation arrest
	Hypospermatogenesis
	Exogenous factors
Abnormal volume	
No ejaculate	Ductal obstruction
	Retrograde ejaculation
	Ejaculatory failure
	Hypogonadism
Low volume	Obstruction of ejaculatory ducts
	Absence of seminal vesicles and vas deferens
	Partial retrograde ejaculation
	Infection
High volume	Unknown factors
Abnormal motility	Immunologic factors
	Infection
	Varicocele
	Defects in sperm structure
	Metabolic or anatomic abnormalities of sperm
	Poor liquefaction of semen
Abnormal viscosity	Etiology unknown
Abnormal morphology	Varicocele
	Stress
	Infection
	Exogenous factors
	Unknown factors
Extraneous cells	Infection or inflammation
	Shedding of immature sperm

From Bernstein GS and Siegel MS: Male factor in infertility. In Mishell DR Jr, Davajan V, and Lobo RA, editors: Infertility, contraception and reproductive endocrinology, ed 3, Cambridge, Mass, 1991, Blackwell Scientific Publications.

pared with water-soluble media. These results differ from those of a recently published large randomized trial by Spring et al. that found no difference in pregnancy rates when the hysterosalpingogram was performed with oil-soluble or water-soluble contrast media. Thus the therapeutic benefit of oil-soluble contrast media remains inconclusive. Because oil-soluble contrast media have a greater number of complications, including pain resulting from peritoneal irritation and formation of granulomas than do water-soluble media, it is probably best to perform routine hysterosalpingograms with water-based media. The diagnostic HSG will not only determine whether the tubes are patent but also, if disease is present, will help to determine the magnitude of the disease process as well as provide information about the lining of the oviduct and uterine cavity that cannot be obtained by laparoscopic visualization. The procedure can also determine whether salpingitis isthmica nodosa is present in the interstitial portion of the oviduct. Mol et al. reported that if one oviduct is patent, fecundability is only minimally reduced compared with two patent oviducts. Therefore it is not necessary to perform tubal reconstructive surgery on a woman with one patent oviduct. However a diagnostic laparoscopy should be performed to detect the presence of peritubal adhesions. The finding of a normal endometrial cavity at the time of HSG obviates the need for hysteroscopy. Fayes et al. reported that women with infertility and a normal HSG had no abnormalities of the uterine cavity when subsequently examined by hysteroscopy.

If severe tubal disease, such as a large hydrosalpinx, is found at the time of HSG, and the couple wishes to attempt in vitro fertilization, it is recommended to perform a salpingectomy in order to increase the incidence of pregnancy. However, if the disease process is not too extensive, surgical tubal reconstruction may be advised, and then a diagnostic laparoscopic examination should precede the scheduled tubal operation to determine the extent of the disease process throughout the pelvis. Most tubal reconstructive surgical procedures can be performed endoscopically. If extensive disease is present that requires a laparotomy, laparoscopy may be performed immediately before laparotomy, and the two procedures can be performed sequentially with the same anesthetic or separately to allow time to explain the prognosis of reconstructive surgery to the patient.

It was previously advised to routinely perform a postcoital test and a laparoscopy as part of the initial infertility evaluation. The treatment of an abnormal postcoital test is controlled ovarian hyperstimulation and intrauterine insemination. Since this is the same therapy for infertile couples with a normal postcoital test and tubal patency, it does not appear to be cost effective or necessary to continue to perform a postcoital test. A diagnostic laparoscopy was also previously advised to be performed routinely as part of the diagnostic evaluation of all women with infertility. Since this invasive procedure usually requires general anesthesia and is costly, it should only be performed if there is a likelihood of visualizing peritubal adhesions or pelvic endometriosis. Ovarian endometriomas can usually be visualized by pelvic sonography. If the sonographic appearance of the ovaries is normal and the hysterosalpingogram is normal, it is unlikely that peritubal adhesions that restrict ovarian pickup are present in a woman who also has a negative *Chlamydia* antibody titer and a normal CA-125 level. Meikle et al. reported that only 4 of 74 infertile women with a normal HSG and a negative *Chlamydia* antibody titer had evidence of tubal disease at the time of diagnostic laparoscopy. The probability that peritubal adhesions of sufficient severity to cause infertility will be found at the time of laparoscopy is therefore much less than 5% in a woman with no history of salpingitis or symptoms of dysmenorrhea, a normal bimanual pelvic examination, a normal CA-125 level, and absence of antibodies to *Chlamydia trachomatis*. Therefore it is not cost effective to perform a diagnostic laparoscopy as part of the initial infertility evaluation in women in whom these laboratory tests, pelvic sonogram, hysterosalpingogram, history, and physical examination are all normal. Provided the woman is under age 40 and having ovulatory cycles and there are more than 5 million motile sperm in the ejaculate of the male partner, several cycles of controlled ovarian hyperstimulation and intrauterine insemination should be undertaken before performing a diagnostic laparoscopy. This therapy has been shown to increase fecundability rates to 10% to 25% per cycle and is thus useful initial therapy for hypofertile couples.

Diagnostic Laparoscopy

If a diagnostic laparoscopy is performed because endometriomas are visualized sonographically or there is radiographic evidence of peritubal adhesions, it should be scheduled to take place in the follicular phase of the menstrual cycle. At the time of laparoscopy following a normal HSG, neither a dilation and curettage nor hysteroscopy should be routinely performed. Neither procedure will provide additional information or therapy, and the curettage may further impede future fertility by producing intrauterine adhesions. At the time of laparoscopy, indigo carmine should be introduced through the cervix into the peritoneal cavity to confirm tubal patency. Performing the laparoscopy in the follicular phase of the cycle before maximal endometrial growth enables the dye to pass into the oviducts with less chance of obstruction.

The following additional laboratory procedures have been advocated by some to assist in determining the cause of the infertility: (1) measurement of serum TSH and prolactin in ovulatory women, (2) luteal phase endometrial biopsy, (3) measurement of antisperm antibodies in both the male and female partner, (4) bacteriologic cultures of the cervical mucus and semen, and (5) hamster egg penetration test.

If abnormalities are discovered in any of the initial three steps of the infertility evaluation, treatment has been found to increase the incidence of pregnancy significantly as compared with no treatment, particularly treatment of anovulation or total tubal obstruction. Treatment of abnormalities found in the five diagnostic procedures just mentioned has not been documented to be more effective than withholding therapy. Therefore the necessity and cost effectiveness of performing these additional tests and correcting the abnormalities found by them have not been demonstrated. Until it is demonstrated conclusively that treatment of abnormalities diagnosed by these additional tests of the infertility investigation results in a significantly better pregnancy rate than placebo or no treatment, the advisability of continuing the diagnostic evaluation beyond the initial three diagnostic steps remains unproven and should not be performed.

Data supporting this statement will now be summarized.

Measurement of TSH and Prolactin in Ovulatory Women

If women with anovulation have hypothyroidism or hyperprolactinemia, treatment with thyroid replacement or bromocriptine, respectively, has been shown to cause resumption of ovulation and enhanced fecundity. However, if women with regular ovulatory cycles have hyperprolactinemia, Glazener et al. reported that pregnancy rates 1 year after the diagnostic evaluation without treatment were similar to those of ovulatory women without hypoprolactinemia. Several investigators have performed randomized clinical trials with bromocriptine and placebo that have shown that treatment with bromocriptine does not increase fecundity rates in ovulatory infertile women. Lincoln et al. reported that less than 1% of women with infertility and normal ovulatory cycles had elevated TSH levels. None of these women became pregnant when treated with thyroxine.

Luteal Deficiency

It has never been established that luteal phase defects of progesterone production or action cause infertility. The diagnosis of luteal deficiency can be determined by finding serum progesterone levels consistently below 10 ng/ml in the luteal phase of several cycles, indicating a deficit in progesterone production, or finding consistent histologic evidence of a delay in development of the normal secretory endometrial pattern, indicating an inadequate effect of normal progesterone production on the endometrium. To establish the diagnosis histologically the normal secretory endometrial development must lag *3 days* or more behind the expected pattern for the time of the cycle originally described by Noyes et al. Furthermore, this finding must be consistent and found in *at least two cycles*. Dat-

ing needs to be calculated by use of indicators that will detect the day of ovulation, optimally by use of serial pelvic sonography, not by subtracting 14 days from the onset of the next menses.

Because the onset of the next menses is the least accurate parameter to determine if luteal deficiency exists, the diagnosis of this entity occurs more frequently when this technique is used to establish the diagnosis than when pelvic sonography is used (Figure 41-5). Peterson et al. reported that the percentage of out-of-phase endometrial biopsies among both fertile and infertile women was similar, being nearly 50% when dating from the day of onset of last menses was used, about 30% when subtracting 14 days from the onset of the next menses was used, and about 25% when the urinary LH peak was used to estimate the day of ovulation (Figure 41-6 and Figure 41-7). When the most precise method of detecting ovulation—pelvic sonography—was used, out-of-phase endometrial biopsies occurred in 3.5% of infertile women and 10% of fertile women.

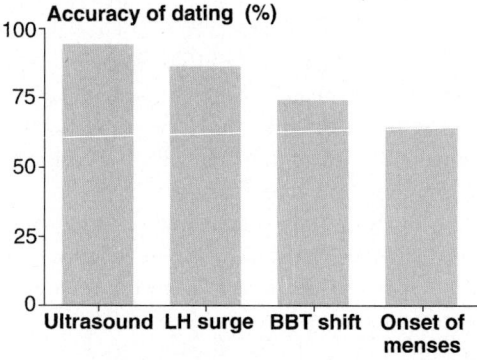

FIGURE 41-5 Percentage of endometrial biopsy interpretations that correlated within 2 days using four different methods of ovulation prediction. Onset of menses: $P < 0.05$ compared with ultrasonography. (From Shoupe D, Mishell DR Jr, LaCarra M, et al: Obstet Gynecol 73:88, 1988.)

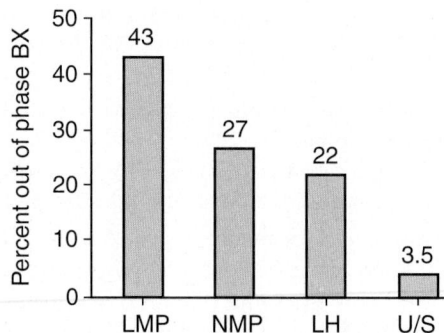

FIGURE 41-6 Prevalence of out-of-phase endometrial biopsy specimens among 340 infertile women: biopsies are on basis of onset of LMP, next menstrual period (NMP), urinary LH testing, and documentation of follicle rupture by ultrasonographic examination (U/S). (From Peters AJ, Lloyd RP, and Coulam CB: Am J Obstet Gynecol 166:1738, 1992.)

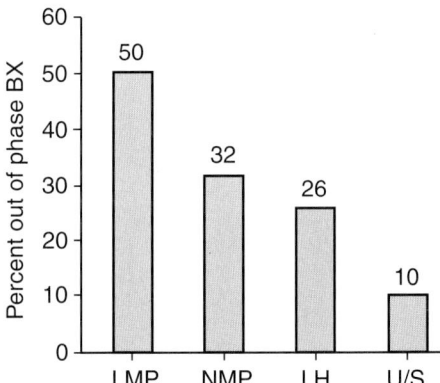

FIGURE 41-7 *Prevalence of out-of-phase endometrial biopsy specimens among 30 fertile women on basis of onset of LMP, next menstrual period (NMP), urinary testing, and documentation of follicle rupture by ultrasonography examination (U/S). (From Peters AJ, Lloyd RP, and Coulam CB: Am J Obstet Gynecol 166:1738, 1992.)*

Erroneous diagnosis of this entity also occurs because of the subjective interpretation of histologic dating criteria. Li et al. reported that a 10% disagreement of more than 2 days occurred when the same observer dated the specimens on two separate occasions. Scott et al. reported that there was great interobserver variation in dating endometrial biopsy specimens, even when performed by five experienced pathologists. Davis et al. reported that the incidence of luteal phase defect in normal fertile women, as determined by serial endometrial biopsies, was 31.4% if a single biopsy was 3 or more days out of phase and 6.6% if sequential biopsies were analyzed.

The data from these and other studies indicate that the diagnosis of luteal phase inadequacy by the use of subjective histologic observations of endometrial biopsy specimens is imprecise, and when used, the incidence of this entity is similar in fertile and infertile populations. These results indicate that luteal phase deficiency, when diagnosed by the currently used imprecise criterion of histologic maturation of the endometrium, is probably a normal biologic variant and not a true cause of infertility. Accordingly, this entity is diagnosed and treated much more often than it actually exists.

Conception rates as high as 75% with the use of progestins, clomiphene citrate, and hCG have been reported by certain investigators, but as summarized by Karamardian and Grimes there are no randomized, placebo-controlled trials that demonstrate a significantly greater conception rate of women with luteal deficiency as a result of treatment. Similar conception rates have been observed among infertile couples without treatment.

Immunologic Causes of Infertility

Substantial evidence from animal studies indicate that antibodies can be induced in females from antigens obtained from organs in the male reproductive tract and that the presence of these antibodies interferes with normal reproduction. Both sperm-agglutinating antibodies and sperm-immobilizing antibodies have been found in the serum of some infertile women, but they have also been found in the serum of fertile control subjects. The agglutinating antibodies are found more frequently than immobilizing antibodies in most series, and in some series the incidence of sperm-agglutinating antibodies in infertile women is similar to that of the control group. Even with the finding of sperm agglutination or immobilization in serum, it has not been demonstrated that a similar degree of sperm inactivation occurs in the lower genital tract. Thus there is no definitive evidence that sperm agglutination or immobilization in the serum of infertile women is the cause of their infertility. One of the reasons for this discrepancy is the fact that both the serum assays—agglutination and immobilization—measure mainly IgM and IgG antibodies while the antibodies locally produced in the genital tract are mainly IgA. For this reason some investigators have measured antisperm antibodies in cervical mucus and found a correlation between the presence of such antibodies and infertility.

No data have shown that the finding of antibodies against sperm in either the male or the female partner is a cause of infertility. A retrospective analysis of corticosteroid therapy and no treatment was performed by Smarr and Hammond in women with high titers of antisperm antibodies. Even though the analysis was retrospective and therapy was administered in a nonrandomized manner, the results are in agreement with those of a randomized study in males indicating that corticosteroid treatment of either the male or female partner does not produce a significantly increased pregnancy rate compared with no therapy.

Autoimmunity to sperm in both semen and serum has been found in some infertile men, particularly those who have had testicular infection, injury, or a surgical procedure such as vasectomy reversal. Men with these antibodies have been treated with corticosteroid therapy and sperm-washing techniques. The effectiveness of such treatment remains to be established, since a study by Haas and Beer failed to show that corticosteroid therapy given to men with antisperm antibodies resulted in significantly greater pregnancy rates than occurred when the men were not given such treatment.

In 1993 results of four prospective studies were published that reported the incidence of fertility occurring after a diagnostic infertility evaluation was performed in which the presence of antisperm antibodies was documented. These studies were performed in four different laboratories in three different countries. Several different techniques for immunoassay were used. All four studies showed there was no correlation between the presence of antisperm antibodies in either member of the couples and the chance of conception. Pregnancy rates over time were similar in couples who had or did not have antisperm antibodies. Therefore it is not justified to perform tests to detect these antibodies as part of the diagnostic infertility evaluation since their presence does not affect fecundability.

Infection

Some researchers have suggested that asymptomatic, or occult, infection of the upper female genital tract and the male genital tract is a cause of infertility. Friberg and Gnarpe suggested in 1973 that infection with what was then called *T. mycoplasma* in the male could interfere with normal sperm function, and infection of the female reproductive tract could interfere with normal sperm transport. The current name now used for those organisms is *Ureaplasma urealyticum.* Two other microorganisms of the genus *Mycoplasma* that are found in the female genital tract are *Mycoplasma hominis* and *Mycoplasma fermentans.* Although Friberg and Gnarpe and others have reported that treatment of infertile couples with antibiotics, such as tetracycline or doxycycline, that eradicate these organisms resulted in high pregnancy rates, controlled studies have reported no difference in pregnancy rates between couples treated with antibiotics and those not treated. Harrison et al. studied 88 infertile couples with no demonstrable cause of infertility. One third were treated with doxycycline, one third received placebo, and one third received no treatment. *T. mycoplasma* was isolated from about two thirds of the couples in each group and was eradicated only in the group treated with doxycycline. Nevertheless, conception rates were similar in each group (Table 41-6). Matthews et al. performed a similar study and obtained similar results. Other investigators have suggested that asymptomatic *C. trachomatis* infection may also cause infertility, but the dosage of doxycycline used in these randomized studies would also have eradicated these organisms. Thus there is no evidence that asymptomatic infection of the genital tract of the human male or female can cause infertility.

TABLE 41-6
Controlled Studies of Outcome of Therapy of Couples with Unexplained Infertility and *U. urealyticum* Infections

Authors	Treatment	No. of Couples	No. of Pregnancies	Conceptions (%)
Harrison et al.	Doxycycline	30	5	17
	Placebo	28	4	14
	None	30	5	17
Matthews et al.	Treated	51	10	20
	None	18	4	22

From Bernstein GS: Occult genital infection and infertility. In Mishell DR Jr, Davajan V, and Lobo RA, editors: Infertility, contraception and reproductive endocrinology, ed 3, Cambridge, Mass, 1991, Blackwell Scientific Publications.

Fertilization Abnormality: Zona-Free Hamster Egg Penetration Test

The zona-free hamster egg penetration test originally described by Yanagimachi et al. is a test developed to predict the fertilizing ability of sperm and provides an additional, more sensitive parameter to assess sperm function than the routine semen analysis. Many variable factors affect the test results.

Vazquez-Levin et al. reported that this test did not correlate well with in vitro fertilization of human eggs. Mao and Grimes surveyed the literature written about this test and concluded the sensitivity and specificity of the sperm penetration assay was too low to justify its routine use as part of the infertility investigation.

O'Shea et al. reported that 6-month fecundity rates were not statistically different among couples whose male partner had a normal amount of motile sperm but different percentages of hamster egg penetration. Even couples with penetration scores of zero did not conceive significantly less often than those with higher percentages of penetration. Therefore the value of performing the zona-free hamster egg–human sperm penetration test as part of the evaluation of the infertile couple has not been satisfactorily demonstrated, and this expensive assay should not be used as part of the infertility diagnostic evaluation.

PROGNOSIS

All infertile couples should be informed of the prognosis for pregnancy associated with treatment of their particular cause of infertility. The highest probability of conception with treatment other than assisted reproductive techniques occurs among couples in whom anovulation is the only abnormality, with a substantially lower probability of pregnancy following tubal disease or sperm abnormalities (Figure 41-8). Among a group of infertile couples with unexplained infertility who were followed for 2 years without treatment after the evaluation was completed, it was found that the chances of becoming pregnant were greater in women younger than 35 (about 75%) than in women older than 35 (50%) (Figure 41-9). The cumulative conception rate at the end of 2 years without therapy for those couples was much greater for those who had tried to conceive for less than 3 years before evaluation (about 75%) than in those who had tried to conceive for more than 3 years (about 30%) (Figure 41-10). In three of the four studies of infertile couples who received no therapy mentioned earlier, more than half the couples that eventually conceived did so in the first year after completing the infertility evaluation, and the vast majority of those who conceived, which was greater than 50% of the entire group, who did conceive without treatment, did so within 2 years (see Figure 41-2). Thus infertile couples with no demonstrable cause of infertility have their best prognosis for conception without treatment forabout 2 years after

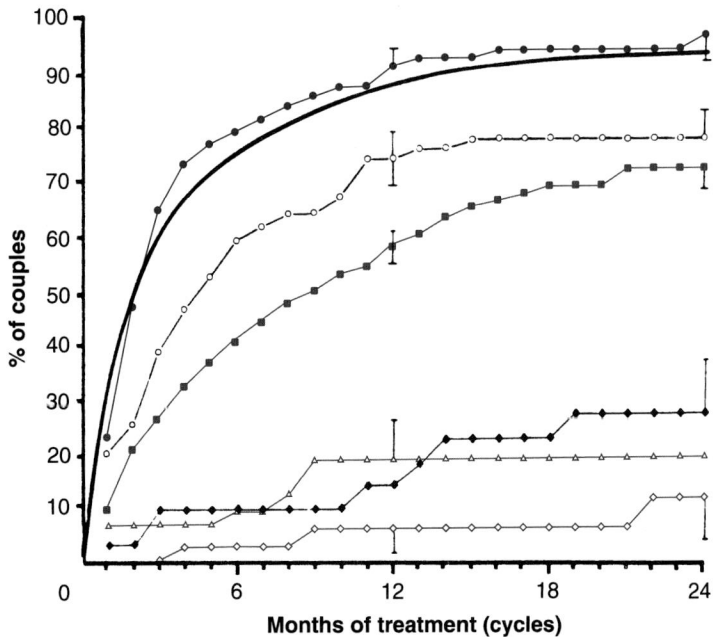

FIGURE 41-8 Cumulative rates of conception in couples with a single cause of infertility treated appropriately, excluding use of donor insemination or in vitro fertilization, as compared with normal rates (highest rates reported in couples with proved fertility). Rates for couples with each cause shown as *solid line*, normal; *blue circles*, amenorrhea; *open circles*, oligomenorrhea; *blue squares*, unexplained infertility; *open triangles*, tubal damage (moderate or severe); *black diamonds*, failure of sperm penetration of mucus (normal semen); *open diamonds*, oligospermia and failure to penetrate mucus. Standard errors of proportions are given at 12 and 24 months. (From Hull MGR, Glazener CMA, Kelly NJ, et al: Br Med J 291:1693, 1985.)

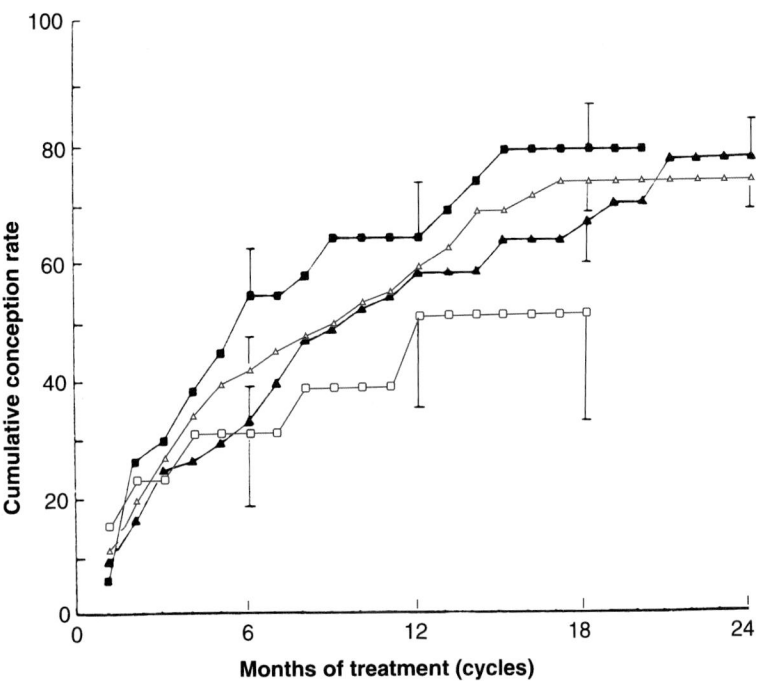

FIGURE 41-9 Cumulative rates of conception from first attendance at clinic in couples with unexplained infertility related to age of woman. Rates for each age group are shown as *solid squares*, <25 years; *blue triangles*, 25-29 years; *solid triangles*, 30-34 years; *blue squares*, >35 years. Standard errors of proportions are given at 6, 12, 18, and 24 months. (From Hull MGR, Glazener CMA, Kelly NJ, et al: Br Med J 291:1693, 1985.)

the initial infertility evaluation is completed, and a poor prognosis thereafter. To increase their chances of conception or to shorten the time interval until conception takes place, various treatment methods have been advocated.

The assisted reproductive techniques of both in vitro fertilization (IVF) and gamete intrafallopian tube transfer (GIFT) have been used to treat couples with unexplained infertility. Although with each of these techniques monthly fecundability rates equal or exceed the normal level of 0.20, these therapies are invasive, time consuming, costly, and uncomfortable.

Controlled ovarian hyperstimulation (COH) with either clomiphene citrate or hMG followed by intrauterine insemination (IUI) also increase pregnancy rates compared with no treatment during short time intervals. Chaffkin et al. reported that treatment with hMG plus IUI enhanced fecundability rates to a greater degree than treatment with hMG or IUI alone (Figure 41-11).

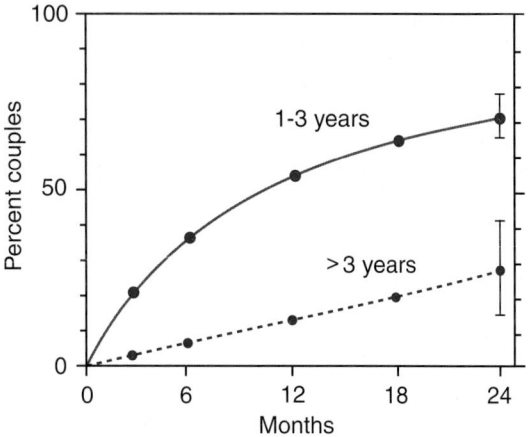

FIGURE 41-10 Cumulative pregnancy rates in unexplained infertility without treatment related to duration of infertility. (From Hull MGR: Int J Gynaecol Obstet 47:99, 1994.)

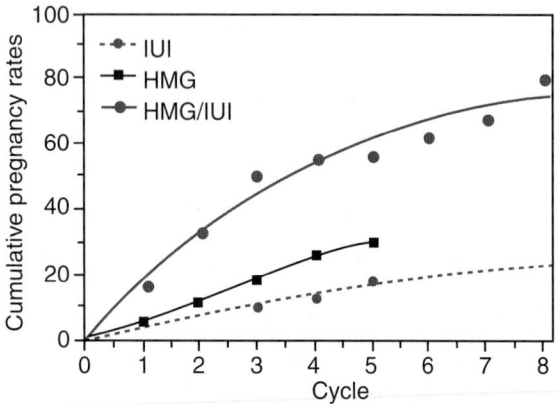

FIGURE 41-11 Overall cumulative proportion of pregnant patients comparing hMG, IUI, and combined hMG/IUI therapies. Life-table analysis was calculated by the method of Cramer et al., and the curves were fitted by computer analysis of the individual data points. (From Chaffkin LM, Nulsen JC, Luciano AA, and Metzger DA: Fertil Steril 55:252, 1991.)

Most series report cycle fecundability rates with the various techniques of COH and IUI to be in the range of 10% to 25% if the woman is under age 40 and the man has a normal semen analysis. Following four to six cycles of this type of therapy in couples with these characteristics, the cumulative pregnancy rate is about 50% in couples with unexplained infertility.

Because cycle fecundability and cumulative pregnancy rates are enhanced with COH and IUI this therapy should be tried for several cycles in couples with unexplained infertility prior to initiating some form of assisted reproductive technique. However, if the age of the woman is more than 40 or there are marked abnormalities in the semen analysis, an attempt at in vitro fertilization should probably be tried initially to determine whether fertilization occurs.

OUTCOME OF PREGNANCY

Several studies have reported the pregnancy outcome of women with long-standing infertility who conceive after treatment. The use of ovulation-inducing drugs, as well as reconstructive tubal surgery, have each independently been shown to be associated with an increased incidence of ectopic pregnancy as compared with the normal population. Use of ovulation-inducing drugs alone, as well as when combined with IVF and GIFT, has been shown to increase the incidence of multiple gestations. Therefore, if conception occurs after treatment with either ovulation induction or tubal reconstructive surgery, monitoring of the early gestation with serial hCG measurements and ultrasonography assists in determining whether or not the pregnancy is intrauterine and how many gestational sacs are present. Varma et al. reported that infertile couples who conceive do not have a higher rate of spontaneous abortion or perinatal mortality than occurs in normal couples.

MANAGEMENT OF THE CAUSES OF INFERTILITY

The management of the various causes of infertility will be presented in the order generally followed in an infertility investigation. Management of primary infertility factors, such as anovulation, sperm abnormalities, and tubal obstruction, will be presented first, followed by treatment of unexplained infertility.

Anovulation

Therapeutic agents currently available to induce ovulation are clomiphene citrate, hMG, pure follicle-stimulating hormone (FSH) and GnRH. In addition, as discussed in Chapter 39, if anovulation is due to hyperprolactinemia, bromocriptine is an effective means to induce ovulation. Also, as noted in Chapter 40, women with congenital adrenal hyperplasia or anovulation accompanied by excessive production of adrenal androgens resulting from other causes can have ovulation induced by corticosteroid therapy.

Clomiphene Citrate

Clomiphene citrate is the pharmacologic agent of choice for women with oligomenorrhea as well as those with amenorrhea who have sufficient ovarian estradiol production to have circulating estradiol levels above 40 pg/ml. This synthetic, weak estrogen acts by competing with endogenous circulating estrogens for estrogen-binding sites on the hypothalamus and thereby blocking the negative feedback of endogenous estrogen. GnRH is then released in a normal manner, stimulating FSH and LH, which in turn cause oocyte maturation with increased estradiol production. The drug is usually given daily for 5 days beginning 5 days after the onset of spontaneous menses or withdrawal bleeding induced with progesterone in oil or an oral progestin.

During the days the drug is ingested, serum levels of LH and FSH rise, accompanied by a steady increase in serum estradiol (Figure 41-12). After ingestion of clomiphene citrate is discontinued, estradiol levels continue to increase, and the negative feedback on the hypothalamic-pituitary axis causes a decrease in FSH and LH, similar to the change seen in the late follicular phase of a normal ovulatory cycle. About 5 to 9 days (mean 7 days) after the last clomiphene citrate tablet has been ingested, the expo-

nentially rising level of estradiol from the dominant follicle has a positive feedback effect on the pituitary or hypothalamus, producing a surge in LH and FSH, which usually results in ovulation and luteinization of the follicle.

Presumptive evidence of ovulation can be obtained by observation of a sustained rise in BBT or measurement of an elevation of serum progesterone. It is best to obtain the serum sample for progesterone measurement about 2 weeks after the last clomiphene tablet has been ingested, because this will usually be in the middle of the luteal phase, about 1 week after ovulation. A rise in serum progesterone level above 3 ng/ml correlates well with the finding of secretory endometrium on an endometrial biopsy sample, but Hull et al. have reported that maximal midluteal progesterone levels in clomiphene citrate-induced ovulatory conception cycles are consistently above 15 ng/ml. These levels are higher than the 10 ng/ml level, which is the minimum concentration of progesterone found in spontaneous ovulatory conception cycles because following pharmacologic ovulation induction, more than one follicle usually matures and undergoes luteinization.

Various treatment regimens have been advocated for the use of clomiphene citrate. Most start with an initial dosage of 50 mg per day for 5 days beginning on the fifth day of spontaneous or induced menses. If presumptive evidence of ovulation occurs with this dosage, the same dosage of clomiphene citrate is ingested in subsequent cycles until conception occurs. If ovulation fails to occur with the initial dosage, a sequential, graduated, increasing dosage regimen has proven to be effective

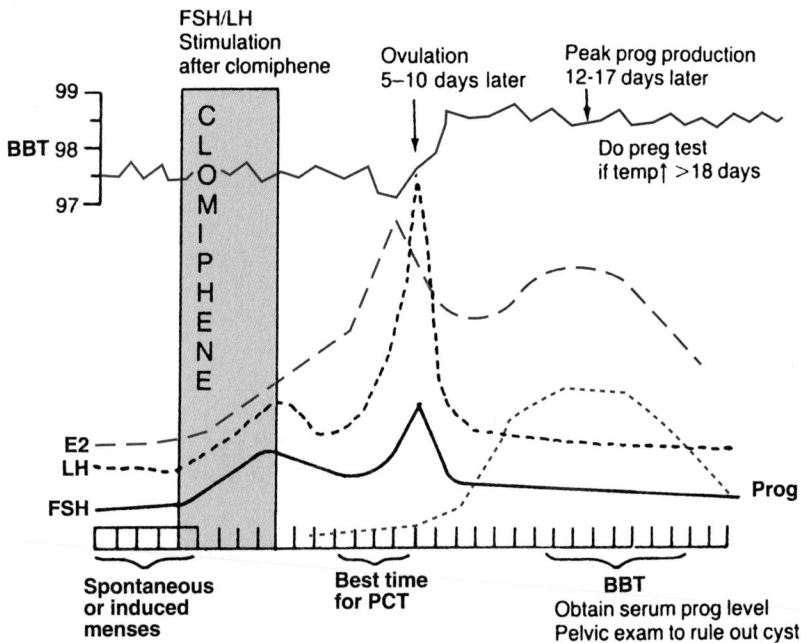

FIGURE 41-12 LH, FSH, estradiol (E₂), and progesterone (prog) levels before, during, and after successful treatment with clomiphene citrate. (From March CM and Mishell DR Jr: Induction of ovulation. In Mishell DR Jr, Davajan V, and Lobo RA, editors: Infertility, contraception and reproductive endocrinology, ed 3, Cambridge, Mass, 1991, Blackwell Scientific Publications.)

with a minimum of side effects. With this regimen if ovulation does not occur with the 50-mg dosage, the dosage of drug is increased in the next treatment cycle to 100 mg per day for 5 days. If ovulation does not occur with 100 mg per day in subsequent cycles, the dosage is sequentially increased to 150 mg, 200 mg, and finally 250 mg for 5 days. If ovulation is induced with any of these dosages, the woman is maintained on her individualized ovulatory dosage until conception occurs. If ovulation does not occur with 250 mg, in the next cycle 250 mg is given daily for 5 days, and 1 week after the last tablet has been ingested, 5000 IU of human chorionic gonadotrophin (hCG) is given to increase the chances of inducing ovulation by simulating the LH surge. In the 10 years' experience with this treatment regimen reported by Gysler et al. about half the women who ovulated and half those who conceived did so following treatment with the 50 mg per day regimen, and an additional one fifth did so with the 100 mg per day dosage. However, about one fourth of all women who ovulated or conceived did so following treatment with a higher dosage regimen, indicating the value of the individualized sequential treatment regimen.

With this dosage regimen of clomiphene citrate more than 90% of women with oligomenorrhea and 66% with secondary amenorrhea and estradiol levels of 40 pg/ml or higher will have presumptive evidence of ovulation. Although only about half the patients who ovulate with this treatment will conceive, Gysler et al. reported that 85% of those with no other causes of infertility conceived after such treatment. Hammond et al., by calculating the rate of fecundability during several months of treatment, reported that if ovulation is induced with clomiphene citrate and no other causes of infertility are present, conception rates over time are similar to those of a normal fertile population who stop using barrier methods of contraception in order to conceive (Figure 41-13). Using life-table analysis these investigators reported that the monthly pregnancy rate (fecundability) of women treated with clomiphene citrate who had no other infertility factor was 22%, compared with a rate of 25% calculated for women discontinuing diaphragm use. The monthly fecundability remained constant throughout nearly 1 year of treatment. Nearly all of the anovulatory women without other infertility factors in this series, as well as other women with correctable infertility factors, had conceived after 10 cycles of treatment. Therefore therapy should be continued for at least 10 to 12 cycles to improve the chance of conception. These data indicate that discontinuation of therapy is the major reason for the reported difference in ovulation and conception rates in anovulatory women treated with clomiphene citrate. Clomiphene citrate does not itself cause infertility, as has been stated in some reports. If other causes of infertility are found, they should be treated and induction of ovulation with clomiphene citrate continued.

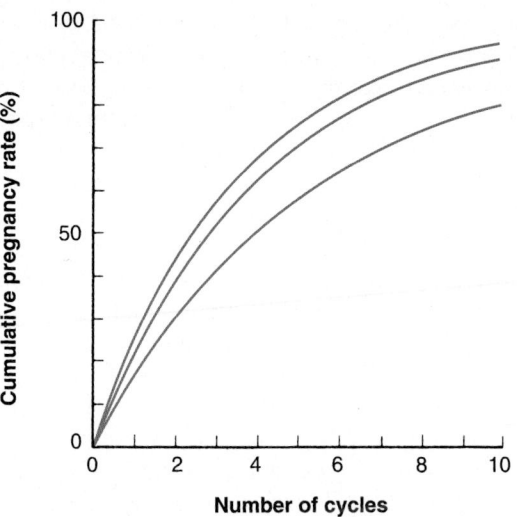

FIGURE 41-13 Cumulative pregnancy rates in patients undergoing ovulation induction compared with patients discontinuing diaphragm use. Top curve: diaphragm (monthly fecundability = 0.247); middle curve: clomiphene, pure (monthly fecundability = 0.22); bottom curve: clomiphene, all (monthly fecundability = 0.157). (Modified from Hammond G, Halme JK, and Talbert LM: Obstet Gynecol 62:196, 1983.)

When conception occurs after ovulation has been induced with this drug, the incidence of multiple gestation is increased to about 5%, with nearly all being twin gestations. The incidence of clinical spontaneous abortion ranges between 15% and 20%, similar to the rate in the general population. The rates of ectopic gestation, intrauterine fetal death, and congenital malformation are also not significantly increased. Animal data indicate that if the drug is given in high dosages during the time of embryogenesis, there is an increased incidence of fetal anomalies. However, limited human data indicate that if the drug is ingested during the first 6 weeks after conception has occurred, the incidence of fetal malformation, although higher (5.1%) than normal, is not significantly increased. Although no definitive data show that the drug is teratogenic in humans, it is best that the woman be reexamined before each course of treatment to be certain that she is not pregnant. It is also important to determine that the ovaries have not become enlarged, because formation of ovarian cysts is the major side effect of clomiphene treatment.

If cysts are present, they will regress spontaneously without therapy, but if additional clomiphene citrate is given and further gonadotrophin release is induced, stimulation and further enlargement of the cyst may occur. Clinically palpable ovarian cysts occur in about 5% of women treated with clomiphene citrate but in less than 1% of treatment cycles. The cysts usually range in size from 5 to 10 cm and do not require surgical excision as they nearly always regress spontaneously. Cysts can occur in any treatment cycle with any dosage, and the incidence is not increased with the higher dosages of drug. Recurrence of cyst formation with the same dosage is uncommon. Other side effects, which occur in less than 10% of women treated with this drug, include vasomotor flushes, blurring of vision, abdominal pain or bloating, urticaria, and a slight degree of hair loss.

About 5% to 10% of women treated with the individually graduated, sequential regimen of clomiphene citrate fail to ovulate with the highest dosage. Because treatment with hMG and GnRH is expensive and time consuming, other treatment regimens have been used with success. For the woman with evidence of some amount of adrenal hyperactivity as determined by the finding of an elevation of dehydroepiandrosterone sulfate (DHEA-S) (>2.8 μg/ml), Lobo et al. reported an ovulation rate of approximately 50% when clomiphene was given after adrenal suppression has been achieved by administration of 0.5 mg dexamethasone nightly for 2 weeks. Withdrawal bleeding was then induced with 100 mg progesterone in oil given intramuscularly. Dexamethasone was continued nightly, and the high dose of clomiphene (250 mg per day) was given for 5 days, followed 1 week later by 5000 IU of hCG. Daly et al. reported that when DHEA-S levels were more than 200 μg/dl a significantly greater number of women ovulated when they were treated with clomiphene citrate plus 0.5 mg dexamethasone than with clomiphene citrate alone. In some women with normal DHEA-S levels who failed to ovulate with 5 days of high dosages of clomiphene citrate, Lobo et al. reported that ovulation can sometimes be induced if clomiphene is given at a dosage of 250 mg per day for 8 days instead of 5 days, followed 1 week later by hCG. Fluker reported that of 30 women who failed to ovulate when given 150 mg or 200 mg of clomiphene for 5 days, 14 ovulated and 5 conceived when given 100 mg of clomiphene daily for 10 days. Others, such as O'Herlihy et al., have recommended that the higher dosage of clomiphene be administered daily until the diameter of the largest follicle measured by ultrasound reaches 1.8 cm, at which time hCG is given. The overall results achieved with clomiphene citrate therapy are shown in Table 41-7.

hMG and FSH

Amenorrheic women with low estrogen levels will not ovulate when clomiphene citrate is given and need to be treated with either hMG or FSH. These agents can also be given to anovulatory women with adequate levels of estrogen who fail to ovulate with clomiphene citrate. Formulations of hMG are derived from extracts of urine of postmenopausal women and contain an equal amount of LH and FSH. HMG needs to be given by intramuscular or subcutaneous injection. Formulations of FSH are derived from extracts of urine from postmenopausal women or recombinant DNA. These formulations are administered by subcutaneous injection. The use of these agents for ovulation induction is more complicated, time consuming,

TABLE 41-7
Typical Overall Results After Clomiphene Citrate Therapy

Result	Percentage
Ovulation	
Oligomenorrhea	>90
Secondary amenorrhea	67
Pregnancy (overall)	50
Pregnancy (no other infertility factors)	85
Twins	5
Abortion	20
Other side effects	13
Teratogenicity	No increase

From March CM and Mishell Dr Jr: Induction of ovulation. In Mishell DR Jr, Davajan V, and Lobo RA, editors: Infertility, contraception and reproductive endocrinology, ed 3, Cambridge, Mass, Blackwell Scientific Publications.

and expensive than treatment with clomiphene citrate. The incidence of side effects is greater and the type of side effect is more serious than occurs with clomiphene citrate. These side effects are the consequences of stimulation of multiple follicles and include multiple gestations and the ovarian hyperstimulation syndrome, which can produce ascites, pleural effusion, oliguria, and hemoconcentration with thromboembolism.

Because each woman responds individually to the dosage of hMG or FSH—even the same woman in different treatment cycles—it is essential to monitor treatment carefully with frequent measurement of estrogen levels and ovarian ultrasonography. Monitoring needs to take place frequently, because there is little difference between the minimal degree of ovarian follicular development necessary to induce ovulation and the amount of follicular development that results in hyperstimulation. When urinary estrogen alone was used to determine the optimal time to induce ovulation with hCG, a level between 50 and 100 mg per day was used, equivalent to serum estrogen levels of 500 to 1000 pg/ml. With ultrasound monitoring, hCG is administered when the follicle reaches a diameter of at least 1.6 cm. A treatment protocol for hMG monitoring is shown in the box on p. 1186.

This regimen should be able to consistently induce ovulation with an overall pregnancy rate of about 60%. The pregnancy rate per cycle is similar to that following clomiphene therapy—22%. Therefore, with sufficient duration of treatment and no other infertility factors, cumulative pregnancy rates should be greater than 90%. Lam et al. reported that the cumulative pregnancy rate after nine cycles of hMG therapy was 77%. The incidence of spontaneous abortion after hMG therapy is high (25% to 35%), and despite monitoring, clinically detectable ovarian enlargement occurs in about 5% to 10% of treatment cycles.

"Step-up" Treatment Protocol with Human Menopausal Gonadotropin (hMG)

1. Perform baseline ultrasonography of ovaries.
2. Administer hMG, 150 IU/day for 3 to 5 days.
3. Repeat estradiol measurement. If level has doubled, continue same hMG dosage; if not, increase hMG by 50% for 3 days.
4. Repeat step 3 until estradiol doubles.
5. Perform ovarian scan every 2 to 3 days until the dominant follicle is ≥14 mm.
6. Perform daily ultrasonography until the follicle is ≥ 18 mm.
7. Stop hMG and perform postcoital test.
8. Twenty-four hours later give 10,000 IU of hCG. If the postcoital test result is poor, perform intrauterine insemination.

From March CM: Induction of ovulation. In Lobo RA, Mishell DR, Jr, Paulson RJ, and Shoupe D, editors: Mishell's textbook of infertility, contraception, and reproductive endocrinology, ed 4, Malden, Mass, 1997, Blackwell Scientific Publications.

However, the incidence of severe ovarian hyperstimulation syndrome (OHSS) should be less than 0.1% of properly monitored cycles. OHSS usually occurs 3 to 7 days after hCG administration and can usually be prevented by withholding the hCG injection when the serum E_2 level is above 3000 pg/ml and there are more than 4 mature follicles or more than a total of 20 sonographically visualized follicles. There is no evidence of an increase in fetal malformation rates after hMG treatment.

Although two epidemiologic studies have suggested that there may be an association between the use of ovulation-inducing agents and an increased risk of developing ovarian cancer later in life, other studies have reported no change in the risk. Because of methodologic problems in the two observational studies that showed an association, there is no firm evidence that the association was causally related to the use of ovulation-inducing agents, and women contemplating their use should be so informed.

Gonadotrophin-Releasing Hormone

An alternative to administration of hMG is GnRH treatment. Because continuous administration of GnRH will saturate the receptors and thus inhibit gonadotrophin release to induce ovulation, GnRH needs to be administered in a pulsatile manner at intervals of 1 to 2 hours. Because GnRH is a peptide, it cannot be administered orally, and the two routes of administration in current use are intravenous and subcutaneous. A greater amount of drug must be administered by the subcutaneous route than by the intravenous route; however, the subcutaneous route avoids use of an intravenous catheter with its accompanying problems. The medication is administered by means of a small portable pump, which is usually worn attached to an article of clothing. Ovulation rates of about

75% to 85% per treatment cycle have been reported. Kovacs et al. and Braat et al. administered pulsatile GnRH by the subcutaneous route and intravenous route to 41 and 49 anovulatory women, respectively. Each reported that the conception rate per cycle of treatment was 22%. The cumulative pregnancy rate at the end of six cycles of treatment was 85% in the first study and 78% in the second. These pregnancy rates are similar to that reported with use of hMG (Figure 41-14). One advantage of GnRH is that hyperstimulation occurs less often with it than with hMG and therefore less monitoring is required. However, many women find wearing the pump, which is needed for intermittent pulsing, to be inconvenient. Therefore the woman can choose whether she wishes to receive hMG or GnRH.

In 1985 Hull et al. reported that of all the causes of infertility, treatment of anovulation results in the greatest success. In their study treatment of women with anovulation accompanied by amenorrhea (excluding ovarian failure) by one of the agents just discussed resulted in a 96% pregnancy rate after 2 years, with a fecundability curve nearly identical to the rates of normal fertile couples (see Figure 41-8). In a group of women with oligomenorrhea the 2-year pregnancy rate was 78%—significantly lower, mainly because of failure of ovulation induction in some women with polycystic ovarian syndrome (PCOS). Gonadotrophin preparations that contain 3 to 9 times as much FSH as LH have not proved to be more successful

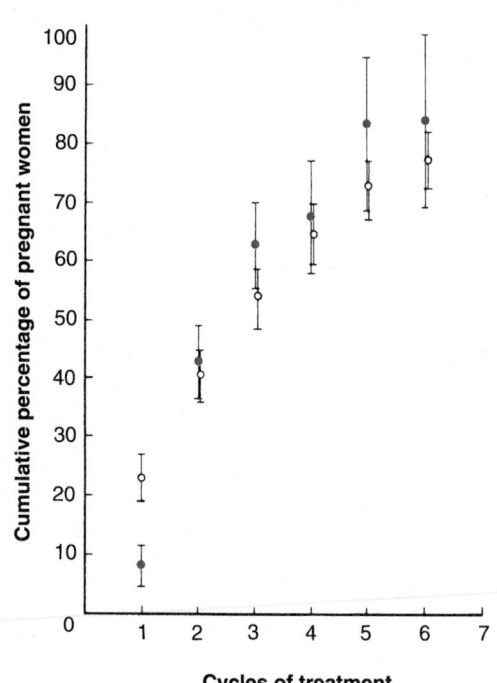

FIGURE 41-14 Comparison of therapy with gonadotrophin-releasing hormone (●) to that with human pituitary gonadotrophin (○) (mean ± SE). (From Kovacs GT, Phillips S, Healy DL, and Burger HG: Med J Aust 151:21, 1989.)

than hMG for inducing ovulation in women with PCOS. Preparations containing pure FSH have also been used, but there are no randomized studies that indicate that pure FSH is more effective than hMG to induce ovulation in women with PCOS. However, pretreatment with GnRH analogues followed by either hMG or GnRH has resulted in higher pregnancy rates than when GnRH analogues are not administered.

Fleming et al. reported that use of this combination treatment in women with polycystic ovaries who had not ovulated after treatment with clomiphene citrate or hMG resulted in a cumulative pregnancy rate of 77% after six cycles of treatment (Figure 41-15). Dodson et al. reported that in a small group of anovulatory women with polycystic ovaries use of hMG alone resulted in a cycle fecundity of 0.16, but with a GnRH agonist together with hMG the cycle fecundity was 0.27. Thus use of a GnRH agonist together with hMG may result in conception in those women with polycystic ovary syndrome who fail to respond to hMG alone. Also as discussed in Chapter 40 use of metformin can induce ovulation in women with PCOS.

Because these medications are expensive, endoscopic partial ovarian destruction with electrocautery or laser has also been used by several groups to treat women with polycystic ovaries who do not ovulate with clomiphene citrate. Ovarian wedge resection was previously used to induce ovulation in women with PCOS before ovulatory-inducing drugs became available. However, severe postoperative adhesion formation often occurred, and this technique should no longer be used. To avoid this problem, partial ovarian destruction with electrocau-

terization or laser ablation of multiple sites has been performed. This laparoscopic technique has resulted in a high rate of spontaneous ovulation and pregnancy. Even the women who do not ovulate spontaneously after this therapy usually ovulate when treated with clomiphene citrate, which was ineffective before partial ovarian destruction. Gjønnaess, who initially described this technique in 1984, reported that after treating 252 women with PCOS with ovarian electrocautery during a 12-year period, 92% ovulated and 89% conceived. The ovulation rate after treatment was influenced by body weight, being 97% in slim women and only 70% in obese women. If the treatment results in ovulatory cycles only about 4% of the women cease having ovulatory cycles in each of the first 3 years after treatment, and 10 or more years after ovarian electrocautery 80% of the women who initially ovulated were still having regular ovulatory cycles. Gjønnaess summarized the results of several investigators who have reported ovulation and pregnancy rates after electrocautery and laser treatment of PCOS (Table 41-8).

Male Cause of Infertility

Most gynecologists who care for infertile couples should understand how to interpret a semen analysis as well as how to offer a prognosis for a disorder of abnormal semen. Although gynecologists usually do not perform a diagnostic evaluation or treat the male with a reproductive disorder, they should be able to provide counsel regarding the use of intrauterine insemination with either the husband's or a donor's semen, as well as with treatment by intracytoplasmic sperm injection (ICSI), testicular sperm extraction (TESE), or microsurgical epididymal serum aspiration (MESA).

Intrauterine insemination has been used to treat oligospermia, as well as abnormalities of semen volume or viscosity, with pregnancy rates in the 25% to 35% range in various series. Cruz et al. reported that in a group of infertile couples whose male partner had oligoasthenospermia, the pregnancy rate was significantly greater with intrauterine inseminations, 14.3%, than with intracervical inseminations, 2.0%, of their husband's semen.

McGovern et al. reported that the prognosis for pregnancy after intrauterine insemination was significantly greater if the original semen analysis had greater than 30% motility and after swim-up there was a motility rate greater than 70% than for samples with lower percentages of motility. Berg et al. reported that if more than 800,000 motile sperm are present after swim-up separation, the pregnancy rate following intrauterine insemination in couples with unexplained infertility treated with controlled ovarian hyperstimulation was about 10% per cycle, but if fewer than this number of sperm was present, the pregnancy rate was only 1% per cycle.

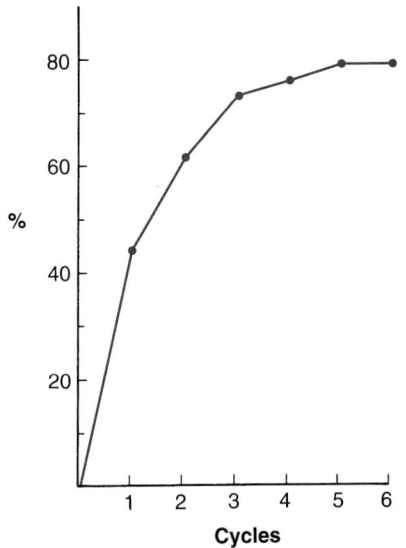

FIGURE 41-15 Cumulative pregnancy rates in patients with polycystic ovary syndrome receiving combined gonadotrophin agonist and hMG therapy. (Modified from Fleming R, Haxton MJ, Hamilton MPR, et al: Am J Obstet Gynecol 159:376, 1988.)

TABLE 41-8
Ovulation and Pregnancy After Electrocautery and Laser Treatment of Polycystic Ovaries

N	Ovulation (%)	Pregnancy (%)	Authors and Year of Publication	Ref.
Electrocautery				
35	92	69	Gjønnaess (1984)	(1)*
6	83	67	Greenblatt and Casper (1987)	(16)
14	64	36	v.d. Weiden et al. (1989)	(2)
21	81	52	Armar et al. 1990	(17)
29	71	52	Abdel Gadir (1990)	(4)
7	71	57	Gürgan et al. (1991)	(18)
10	70		Kovacs et al. (1991)	(5)
22	86		Armar and Lachelin (1993)	(7)
104	76	70	Naether et al. (1993)	(19)
10	70		Tirtinen et al. (1993)	(20)
Laser vaporization				
85	53	56	Daniell and Miller (1989)	(21)
19	80	37	Keckstein et al. (1990)	(22)
10	70		Gürgan et al. (1991)	(18)
Wedge resection				
8	65	0	Huber et al. (1988)	(23)
12	83	58	Kojima et al. (1989)	(24)

From Gjønnaess H: Acta Obstet Gynecol Scand 73:407, 1993.

*Before the laparoscopy, some of the patients had been resistant to hormonal stimulation therapy. After inclusion of patients made responsive to CC by the electrocautery, the pregnancy rate increased to 80% (1).

The technique of intrauterine insemination of sperm following their separation from the semen by centrifugation should be used to treat mild to moderate abnormalities in the semen analysis and unexplained infertility. This procedure is associated with higher pregnancy rates if it is combined with controlled ovarian hyperstimulation than when used in natural ovulatory cycles. Intrauterine insemination is also of benefit to women with cervical stenosis, such as that sometimes found following cervical conization. Ideally, insemination should take place on the day of or 1 day before ovulation. It is advisable to utilize urinary LH enzyme-linked immunosorbent assay (ELISA) kits to determine the optimal date to perform insemination since the urinary LH peak occurs on the day prior to ovulation. Insemination should be scheduled the morning after LH is initially detected in an afternoon urine specimen.

Separation of sperm from the seminal fluid by double centrifugation, the swim-up technique, or use of a density gradient should be performed before intrauterine insemination. Intrauterine insemination of seminal fluid can produce severe uterine cramps as a result of prostaglandin release. To separate the sperm from the semen, the semen specimen is placed in a centrifuge tube and the volume is tripled with an electrolyte and amino acid solution such as Ham's F-10. After being mixed on a vortex mixer, the specimen is centrifuged twice, discarding the supernatant each time and subsequently adding more diluent. After the final centrifuge the sperm pellet is placed in a small amount of solution (0.3 to 0.5 ml), withdrawn into a small catheter, and directly placed high into the endometrial cavity.

Other techniques have been used to separate the sperm with the greatest motility from the remainder of sperm in the specimen, so that only the highest quality sperm are used for insemination. Layering a solution of Ham's F-10 over the sperm pellet, incubating the mixture for 30 minutes to 2 hours, and inseminating the supernate (the swim-up technique) has been utilized (Figure 41-16). Separation of the most motile sperm with use of various density gradients such as Percoll can be performed more rapidly than the swim-up technique and has a similar efficacy. The original density gradient, Percoll, is no longer available for human use. Several other gradients are available and yield similar rates of sperm recovery as Percoll. If pregnancy fails to occur after several cycles of intrauterine insemination with the husband's sperm or there are marked abnormalities in the semen analysis with less than 1 million motile sperm after separation, the technique of IVF plus ICSI or insemination with donor sperm can be utilized.

Until a few years ago, if there were severe abnormalities in the semen analysis, the prognosis for fertility was less than that for any other cause of infertility, even with the use of in vitro fertilization techniques. Attempts to enhance fertilization rates of aspirated oocytes with the technique of subzonal insemination of sperm were unsuccessful because fertilization rates remained low, about 15%. After Van Steirteghem et al. developed the tech-

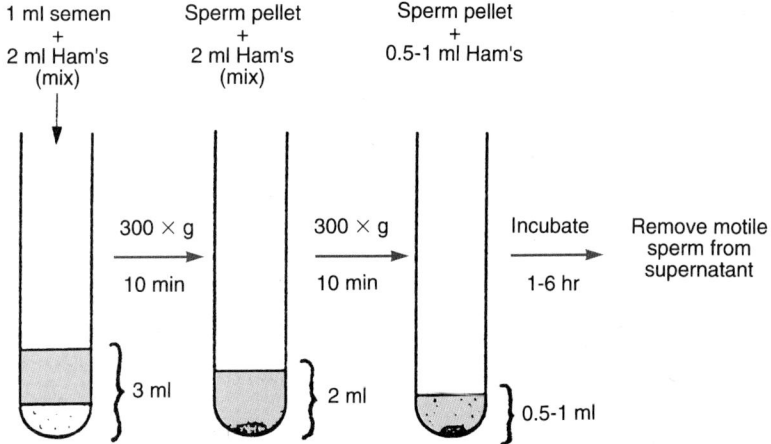

1 ml semen
+
2 ml Ham's
(mix)

Sperm pellet
+
2 ml Ham's
(mix)

Sperm pellet
+
0.5-1 ml Ham's

300 × g

10 min

300 × g

10 min

Incubate

1-6 hr

Remove motile
sperm from
supernatant

} 3 ml

} 2 ml

} 0.5-1 ml

FIGURE 41-16 Standard method of sperm preparation for IVF: two-step wash plus swim-up technique. (From Paulson RJ: Human in vitro fertilization and related assisted reproductive techniques. In Mishell DR Jr, Davajan V, and Lobo RA, editors: Infertility, contraception and reproductive endocrinology, ed 3, Cambridge, Mass, 1991, Blackwell Scientific Publications.)

nique of intracytoplasmic sperm injection, fertilization rates of oocytes injected with a single spermatozoon that was obtained from men with severe abnormalities in the semen analysis were increased to about 50%. Pregnancy rates per embryo transfer were about 35%, significantly greater than the 16% rate of pregnancy with embryos fertilized by subzonal insemination techniques.

In a study by Palermo et al. similar fertilization rates of about 60% of the oocytes injected were achieved with sperm from semen samples containing no motile sperm, few motile sperm, and high numbers of motile sperm. In addition, a fertilization rate of about 60% was obtained whether the sperm were freshly obtained by masturbation, by electroejaculation, or were previously frozen. Nearly a 50% fertilization rate of oocytes was also achieved when the sperm were aspirated directly from the epididymal fluid.

In this study fewer than 1% of the couples studied failed to achieve fertilization of at least one oocyte with this technique. High ongoing pregnancy rates of 30% or more were also achieved, regardless of the number of motile sperm identified in the original semen analysis.

The excellent results obtained with intracytoplasmic sperm injection by the group that originally described the technique has now been replicated in other centers. By using this technique, the pregnancy rate of couples whose male partner has an extremely low concentration of motile sperm in the semen samples, less than 100,000 per ml, can reach 35% per treatment cycle. With a loss rate of 25%, the live-birth rate of 27% is similar to that of other causes of infertility that are treated by in vitro fertilization. Studies of pregnancies resulting from ICSI and standard in vitro fertilization (IVF) reveal a similar rate of pregnancy loss and multiple gestation. Therefore intracytoplasmic sperm injection is now the assisted reproductive technique of choice for all causes of male infertility, as

well as for those couples with no known cause of infertility in whom fertilization does not occur with standard IVF procedures. Questions remain as to whether ICSI should be tried before or after an attempt of regular in vitro fertilization if severe abnormalities of sperm number and function exist. It also remains to be determined what is the magnitude of sperm abnormalities that would indicate that the initial fertilization attempt should be performed by ICSI. It has been suggested that a sperm concentration of less than 2 million sperm per ml of semen is an indicator for initial use of ICSI. With the technique of ICSI the probability of achieving a viable pregnancy is inversely correlated with the age of the woman. Oehninger et al. reported that the fertilizability of human ova with ICSI remained constant, at about 60%, in women in different age groups, but ongoing pregnancy rates decreased from about 50% when the woman was less than 35 years old to 23% among women aged 35 to 40 to less than 6% for women over age 40. Use of donor eggs should be considered in women over age 40 and/or elevated circulating levels of FSH who are candidates for ICSI. A few years ago, the finding of azoospermia in seminal fluid was considered an untreatable cause of infertility. After development of the techniques of ICSI as an adjunct to in vitro fertilization, it was found that spermatozoa retrieved from the testes of azoospermic men could fertilize ova retrieved from their partner's ovaries. Palermo et al. reported that the clinical pregnancy rate is higher when testicular or epididymal sperm is retrieved from men with obstruction in their vas deferens (obstructive azoospermia) than when testicular sperm is retrieved from men with azoospermia without reproductive tract obstruction (nonobstructive azoospermia). The rates were 57% and 49%, respectively. Shulman et al. reported that even if the sperm retrieved from the testes remains immotile, the pregnancy rate after ICSI is about 16% per cycle of oocyte retrieval. Jezek et al.

reported that the likelihood of retrieval of spermatozoa from testicular tissue of men with azoospermia and normal FSH levels is nearly 100%. Even if the FSH levels are markedly elevated, there is at least a 50% likelihood that spermatozoa can be retrieved from the testes and used to perform an intracytoplasmic sperm injection procedure. Thus the presence of a combination of azoospermia and an elevated FSH level is not a contraindication for performing a testicular sperm extraction procedure. There has been concern that infants born after ICSI may have a greater number of chromosomal abnormalities and/or birth defects. The results of a large survey of 730 infants born after ICSI by Loft et al. reported the incidence of clinical abnormalities and major birth defects was not significantly greater than the occurrence in the general population. The results of two other studies of about 1000 infants born after conception by ICSI indicate that the rate of major malformations, 3.3%, is similar to that found in national registries or surveys of pregnancies after in vitro fertilization. The rate of chromosomal abnormalities in the infants was also not above the expected levels. Although more data need to be accumulated, the reassuring information in these reports can be used to counsel the steadily increasing numbers of infertile couples who are considering the use of ICSI.

Some couples, particularly those whose male partner has azoospermia, may choose to utilize donor sperm insemination. If they do so, the attitudes of both partners regarding the use of donor semen and the stability of the marriage need to be thoroughly discussed before the procedure is performed. Donors must be carefully screened to be certain that they are in good health, do not have a potentially inherited disorder, and will not transmit an infectious agent in the semen. Thus screening for syphilis, hepatitis B and C, *Neisseria gonorrhoeae*, and *Chlamydia trachomatis* must be performed. Since tests to determine the presence of antibodies for the AIDS retrovirus (human immunodeficiency virus [HIV]) may not become positive for several months after the disease has been acquired, it is now recommended that only semen that has been frozen for at least 6 months' storage be used for donor insemination, at which time an antibody test for the AIDS virus can be performed on the donor. A set of guidelines for semen donor insemination has been published by the Association for Reproductive Medicine. These guidelines provide information regarding indications for donor insemination, as well as suggested procedures for selection and screening of possible semen donors.

Most centers using frozen semen for insemination have reported that the pregnancy rate per cycle is less than with fresh semen. Hammond et al. reported that a 50% cumulative pregnancy rate after insemination with previously frozen sperm was only reached after 6 months of treatment, and the monthly fecundity rate was only 9% (Figure 41-17). However, in the study by Gillett et al. with use of frozen semen from donors the monthly fecundity

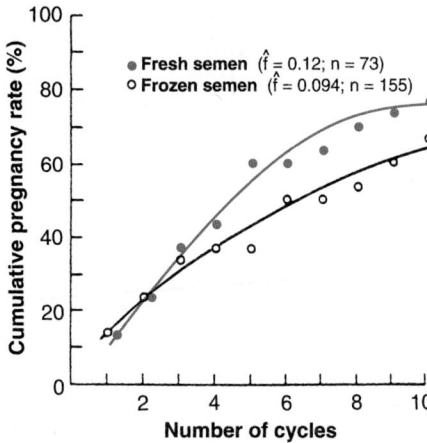

FIGURE 41-17 Cumulative fecundability curves for fresh or frozen semen (fresh: f = 0.12, n = 73; frozen: f = 0.094, n = 155). (From Hammond MG, Jordan S, and Sloan CS: Am J Obstet Gynecol 155:480, 1986.)

rate was 18%, with a 45% cumulative pregnancy rate at 3 months. Thus the pregnancy rate with frozen sperm varies from center to center, and the couple should be appropriately counseled.

Uterine Causes of Infertility

Intrauterine Adhesions

In addition to menstrual abnormalities and recurrent abortion, some women may not be able to conceive because of the presence of intrauterine adhesions (IUA). As mentioned in Chapter 16, most women with IUA have had a previous curettage of the uterine cavity, most often during or shortly following a pregnancy. If the only abnormal finding in the infertility investigation is the presence of IUA, the prognosis for conception after hysteroscopic lysis of the adhesions is good. March reported that of 69 infertile women with IUA and no other infertility factors, 52 (75%) conceived after hysteroscopic treatment.

Leiomyoma

Congenital uterine defects rarely cause infertility, and the uterine anomalies associated with maternal ingestion of DES have not been shown in randomized studies to be a cause of infertility. It is also difficult to assess the effect of leiomyomas on conception, since so many women with leiomyomas have no difficulty conceiving. Nevertheless, it is plausible that cervical myomas could cause distortion of the endocervix, interfering with normal sperm transport, and that some submucous leiomyomas may interfere with sperm transport or normal implantation of the blastocyst. Large intrauterine leiomyomas can also occlude the interstitial portion of the oviduct and prevent normal sperm transport. If no other cause of infertility is found and myomas of moderate size and position that may interfere with sperm transport are present, then a myomectomy is justified. Vercellini et al. reviewed all studies published about the effect of myomectomy on infertility between 1982 and 1996. The overall conception rate after myomectomy among seven prospective studies of women with no other causes of infertility was 61%. However no study included a comparison group of infertile women with leiomyomas treated expectantly.

Tuberculosis

If the HSG reveals findings consistent with pelvic tuberculosis, then endometrial biopsy and culture should be performed to confirm the diagnosis. The radiographic features of pelvic tuberculosis that are virtually diagnostic of the disease include (1) calcified lymph nodes or granulomas in the pelvis, (2) tubal obstruction in the distal isthmus or proximal ampulla, sometimes resulting in a "pipe-stem" configuration of the tube proximal to the obstruction, (3) multiple strictures along the course of the tube, (4) irregularity to the contour of the ampulla, and (5) deformity or obliteration of the endometrial cavity without a previous curettage (Figure 41-18). Appropriate antituberculosis medication should be initiated, but women with pelvic tuberculosis should be considered sterile, as pregnancies after therapy are rare. Therefore no tubal reconstructive surgical procedures should be attempted. If tuberculosis is present in the oviduct but not the uterus, pregnancies have been reported following in vitro fertilization.

Tubal Causes of Infertility

During the past two decades the incidence of infertility caused by damage to the oviduct has increased because of an increased incidence of salpingitis. Obstructions occur at either the distal or proximal portion of the oviduct and sometimes in both regions. Distal obstruction is much more common than proximal obstruction. In a Swedish study only 15% of the women with tubal disease had proximal tubal obstruction. The prognosis for fertility after surgical tubal reconstruction depends on the amount of damage to the oviduct as well as the location of the obstruction. If there is extensive damage, the chances for conception after tubal reconstruction are very unlikely. Women with extensive tubal disease have a greater chance of conceiving with an in vitro fertilization procedure, and thus the extent and location of the intrinsic and extrinsic tubal disease should be ascertained by hysterosalpingography and possibly laparoscopy in an effort to determine whether tubal reconstruction or in vitro fertilization offers the better prognosis. Whether laparoscopic visualization of the oviduct is necessary to determine the extent of tubal damage or whether this can be determined by a hysterosalpingogram alone has not been established. Nevertheless, if large hydrosalpinges are seen at the time of the hys-

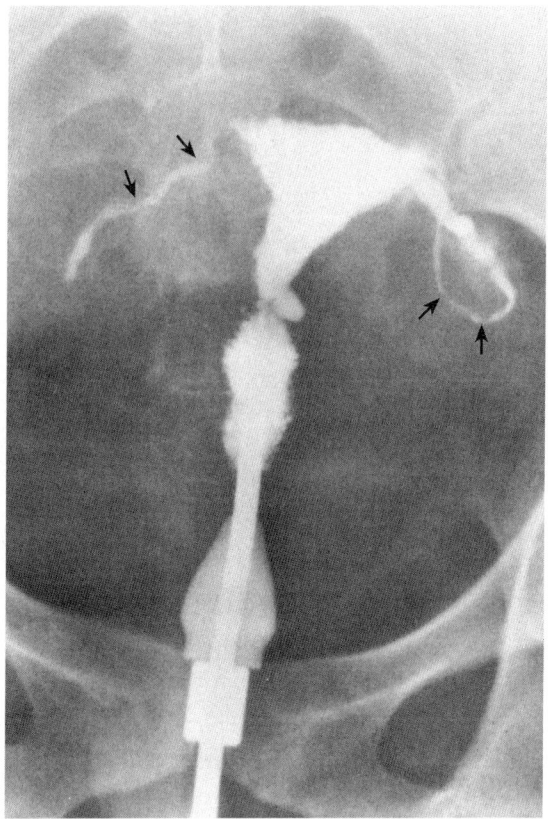

FIGURE 41-18 Tuberculous salpingitis in 37-year-old nulligravida with primary infertility for 15 years. Right tube is obstructed in zone of transition between isthmus and ampulla. *Arrows* indicate multiple strictures in both tubes. Nodular contour of endometrial cavity may also be related to tuberculosis and is analogous to pattern that has been found in ampulla in other cases. Small diverticulum near internal os probably represents adenomyosis. Diagnosis of tuberculosis was confirmed by endometrial culture. (From Richmond JA: Hysterosalpingography. In Mishell DR Jr, Davajan V, and Lobo RA, editors: Infertility, contraception and reproductive endocrinology, ed 3, Cambridge, Mass, 1991, Blackwell Scientific Publications.)

terosalpingogram, it is best to suggest that the woman have in vitro fertilization rather than undergo tubal reconstructive surgery. It is recommended that hydrosalpinges be excised before in vitro fertilization. If both proximal and distal obstructions of the oviduct exist, the damage to the oviduct is usually so extensive that the oviduct cannot function normally. Therefore, although it is possible to achieve tubal patency after surgical repair of a tube with both proximal and distal blockage, subsequent intrauterine pregnancy is uncommon. Therefore, surgical reconstruction should not be performed in such instances.

Distal Tubal Disease

The HSG will determine whether the tubal obstruction is complete or partial, the size of the distal sacculation, and the appearance of the mucosal folds and rugal pattern of the endosalpinx (Figure 41-19). Laparoscopy will assist in

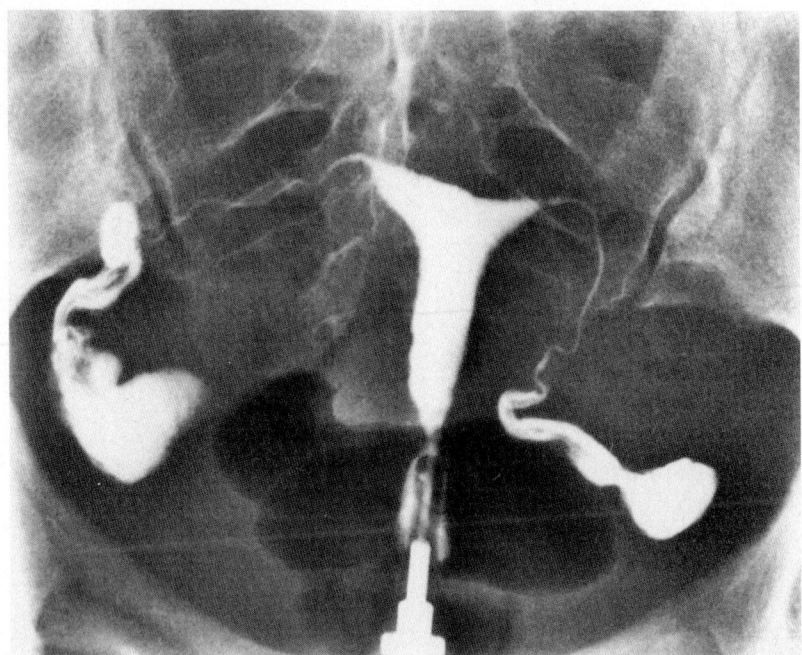

FIGURE 41-19 HSG showing bilateral hydrosalpinges with dilation, clubbing, and obstruction at fimbriated ends. Patient was 32-year-old woman with 10-year history of primary infertility. (From Richmond JA: Hysterosalpingography. In Mishell DR Jr, Davajan V, and Lobo RA, editors: Infertility, contraception and reproductive endocrinology, ed 3, Cambridge, Mass, 1991, Blackwell Scientific Publications.)

determining the size of the hydrosalpinx, the amount of muscularis, and the thickness of the wall of the oviduct after distention with dye. Laparoscopic examination will determine whether pelvic adhesions are present and the extent of such adhesions. Women with fimbrial obstruction are not a homogeneous group, and the prognosis for intrauterine pregnancy following distal tubal reconstruction is related to the extent of the disease process. Therefore, it is important to perform both hysterosalpingography and laparoscopy before surgical reconstruction to provide an individualized prognosis.

If the fimbriae of the distal end of the oviduct are relatively normal with only partial occlusion by adhesions or fimbrial bridges, removal of these adhesions by means of a fimbrioplasty procedure will result in higher conception rates (in the range of 60%) than if the distal end is completely occluded and a cuff salpingostomy procedure is required. Overall conception rates following salpingostomy are in the 30% range, with a high percentage (about one fourth) being tubal pregnancies. As reported by Schlaff et al., with the use of microsurgical techniques for the treatment of distal tubal disease the intrauterine pregnancy rate has not increased when compared with the results following conventional macrosurgery, but the rate of ectopic pregnancy appears to be somewhat greater following microsurgery (Table 41-9). The incidence of ectopic pregnancy after surgical reconstruction for distal tubal disease is directly related to the amount of tubal damage existing before the operative procedure.

TABLE 41-9

Comparison of Pregnancy Outcome After Terminal Neosalpingostomy Using Careful Conventional Techniques (1978) Versus Microsurgical Techniques (1989)

	1978	1989
Mild	15	10
Pregnant*	13 (86)	7 (70)
Ectopic†	1 (7/8)	1 (10/14)
Moderate	30	29
Pregnant*	9 (30)	9 (31)
Ectopic†	4 (13/44)	4 (14/44)
Severe	42	56
Pregnant*	2 (5)	9 (16)
Ectopic†	0 (0/0)	2 (4/22)
Total	87	95
Pregnant*	24 (28)	26 (27)
Ectopic†	5 (6/21)	7 (7/27)

From Schlaff WD, Hassiakos DK, Damewood MD, and Rock JA: Fertil Steril 54:984, 1990.

*Values in parentheses are percentages.

†Values in parentheses are percentages of total patients in the category/percentages of only those patients in the category who became pregnant.

Boer-Meisel et al. correlated the results of tubal reconstruction with the degree of tubal damage according to the severity of five factors: (1) extent of adhesions, (2) nature of adhesions, (3) diameter of the hydrosalpinx, (4) appearance of the endosalpinx, and (5) thickness of the tubal wall. Utilizing these criteria they developed three prognostic categories: good—with a cumulative pregnancy rate of about 75%; intermediate—about 20%; and poor—less than 5%. In the good category, only 1 of 22 pregnancies was ectopic, but in the intermediate group half the pregnancies were tubal, and in the poor prognostic group six of seven pregnancies were ectopic. They concluded that if there were fixed adhesions with absent rugal folds and a thick, fixed tubal wall, distal tubal reconstructive surgery should not be performed.

Donnez and Casanas-Roux classified the degree of distal tubal occlusion into four categories on the basis of hysterosalpingography (Figure 41-20). Following microscopic tubal reconstruction the cumulative pregnancy rate was directly related to the degree of occlusion. If the distal tubal ostium was completely normal but peritubal adhesions were present, lysis of these adhesions by a procedure called salpingolysis resulted in a 64% intrauterine pregnancy rate, similar to that obtained with a fimbrioplasty for partial obstruction. About half the women who underwent salpingostomy for degree II occlusion conceived, with no ectopic pregnancies, but only about one fourth of those with degree III or IV occlusions had subsequent intrauterine pregnancies, and the ectopic pregnancy rate was about 10% (Figure 41-21 and Table 41-10). Thus fol-

lowing operation for more extensive distal tubal disease, nearly one third of the pregnancies that occurred were ectopic.

In both these studies the best prognostic factor was thickness of the tubal wall. If there was a hydrosalpinx greater than 2 cm in diameter with a thick tubal wall, the prognosis for a term pregnancy following distal tubal reconstruction was extremely poor. Hulka reported that when more than one half of the ovary was involved with adhesions, no woman had a term pregnancy following salpingostomy.

Rock et al. classified women with distal fimbrial occlusion into three categories based on the extent of tubal disease (see the box on p. 1195). Schlaff et al. then performed a life-table analysis of couples in these three categories with no other causes of infertility after the female partner underwent neosalpingostomy. They found that 80% of those women with mild tubal disease conceived, whereas only 31% of those with moderate disease and 16% of those with severe disease conceived (Figure 41-22). The ectopic pregnancy rate was higher in the latter two categories. Thus this information should be presented to the woman when she is counseled, and if the prognosis for term pregnancy is poor, she should be advised to undergo in vitro fertilization instead of surgical tubal reconstruction.

It is now possible to perform distal tubal reconstructive surgery by operative laparoscopy. Dubuisson et al. reported the results of a series of 65 consecutive distal tuboplasties, both fimbrioplasties and neosalpingostomies

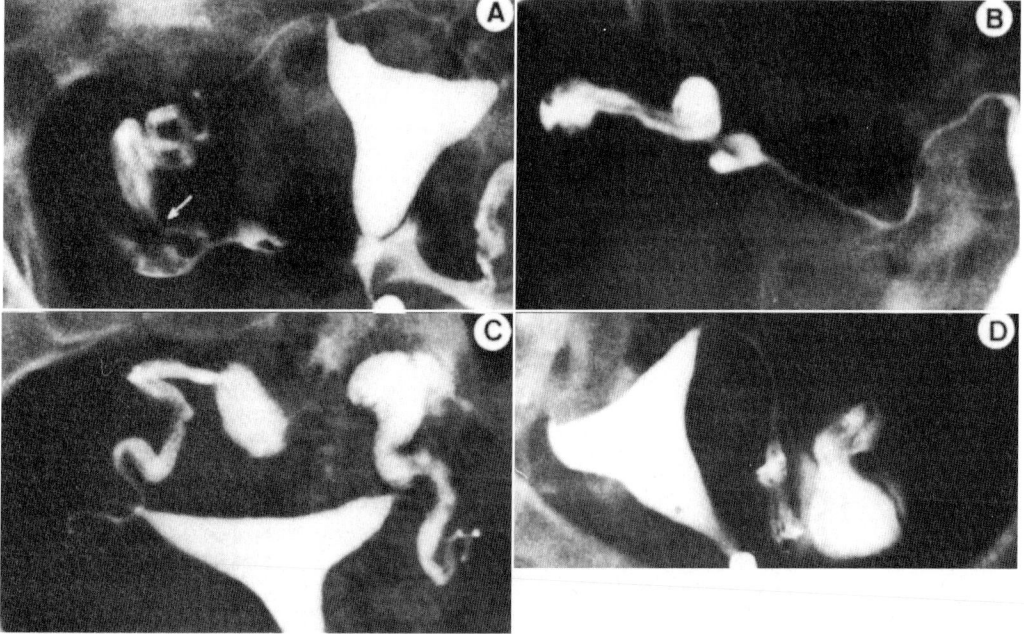

FIGURE 41-20 Classification of distal tubal occlusion based on degree of dilation seen on HSG. **A,** Degree I—conglutination of the fimbrial folds *(arrow)* with tubal patency. **B,** Degree II—complete distal occlusion with normal ampullary diameter. **C,** Degree III—complete distal occlusion with ampullary dilation 15 to 25 mm in diameter. **D,** Degree IV—occlusion with ampullary distention greater than 25 mm. (From Donnez J and Casanas-Roux F: Fertil Steril 46:200, 1986.)

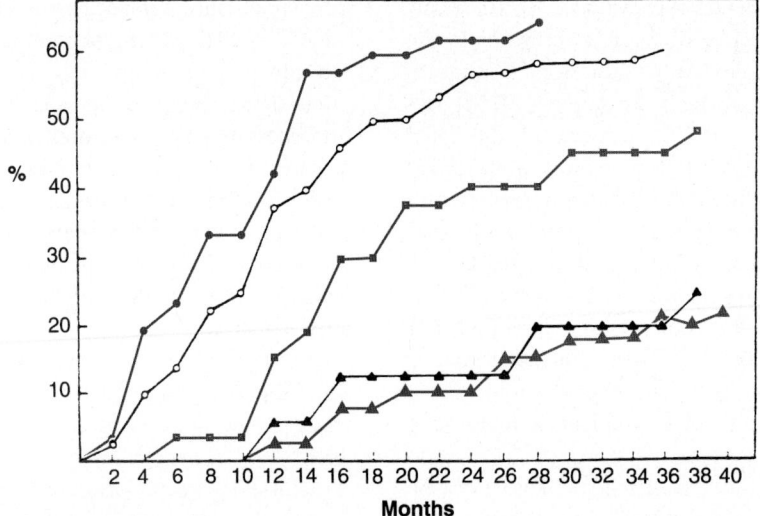

FIGURE 41-21 Cumulative pregnancy rates following microsurgical repair of these lesions are depicted. (● = salpingolysis; ◯) = fimbrioplasty; ▣ = salpingostomy [degree II]; ▲ = salpingostomy [degree III]; ▲ = salpingostomy [degree IV]). (From Donnez J and Casanas-Roux F: Fertil Steril 46:200, 1986.)

TABLE 41-10
Pregnancy Rate After Microsurgery and Ciliated Cell Percentage in Cases of Distal Tubal Occlusion

Type of Operation	No. Patients	No. Intrauterine Pregnancies	No. Ectopic Pregnancies
Fimbrioplasty			
Occlusion of degree I	132	79 (60%)	2 (2%)
Salpingostomy			
Occlusion of degree II	27	13 (48%)	0
Occlusion of degree III	16	4 (25%)	1 (6%)
Occlusion of degree IV	40	9 (22%)	5 (12%)
TOTAL	83	26 (31%)	6 (7%)
Salpingolysis	42	27 (64%)	1 (2%)

Modified from Donnez J and Casanas-Roux F: Fertil Steril 46:200, 1986.

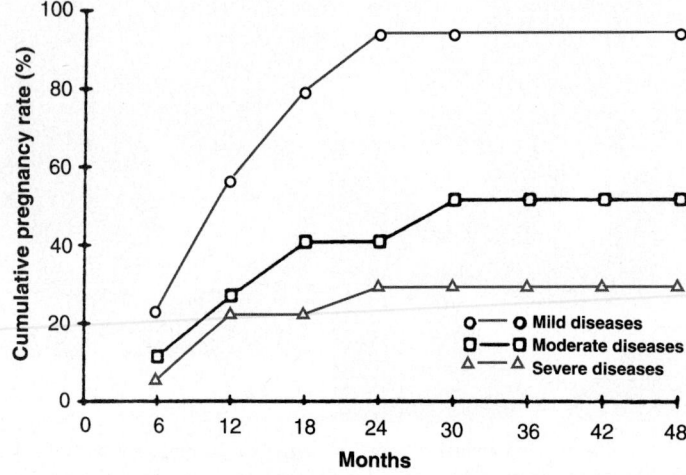

FIGURE 41-22 Life-table analysis of pregnancy outcome after neosalpingostomy by extent of disease. (From Schlaff WD, Hassiakos DK, Damewood MD, and Rock JA: Fertil Steril 54:984, 1990.)

ference in the pregnancy rates between the two treatment modalities. It appears that the prognoses for fertility after salpingostomy by any operative technique is correlated more with the extent of disease than with the type of surgical procedure. Because laparoscopic salpingostomy results in less morbidity, length of hospitalization, and cost than performing the procedure by laparotomy, the former technique should become the procedure of choice to treat distal tubal disease.

An argument can be made that if the extent of tubal disease is so severe that it cannot be treated by laparoscopic surgery on an outpatient basis, then the woman should not have a laparotomy but be treated by one or more cycles of in vitro fertilization.

Proximal Tubal Blockage

If no dye reaches the oviduct during an HSG, the diagnosis of proximal tubal blockage is likely. However, since spasm of the intrauterine portion of the oviduct can occur, the diagnosis cannot be confirmed unless laparoscopy is performed with general anesthesia. Laparoscopy also allows examination of the distal portion of the oviduct, which cannot be visualized radiographically if there is proximal blockage. Proximal tubal blockage is most commonly due to residual damage after infection, but it can be due to plugs of material or endometriosis. Frequently, tubal diverticula, also called *salpingitis isthmica nodosa (SIN)*, are present.

Unlike the results of distal tubal reconstruction, the use of microsurgery has improved intrauterine rates for proximal tubal disease. Before the use of microsurgery, tubal intrauterine blockage was treated by reimplantation of the patent portion of the oviduct into the endometrial cavity. Term pregnancy rates following tubocornual implantation were in the 30% range. This procedure has now been replaced by a microsurgical tubocornual reanastomosis procedure in which the diseased portion of oviduct is excised and the patent distal oviduct is reanastomosed to the portion of the interstitial segment of the oviduct that is patent. With this technique various authors have reported term pregnancy rates of about 50%, with ectopic pregnancy rates of less than 10%.

Donnez and Casanas-Roux reported that the pregnancy rate following tubocornual reanastomosis was related to the extent of preexisting disease as determined at the time of HSG (Figure 41-24). The best pregnancy rate—55%—was obtained when the interstitial portion of the oviduct was not damaged and less than 1.5 cm of occluded tube needed to be removed. The pregnancy rate declined to 33% when the interstitial portion of the tube was occluded and still further with the presence of some (25%) or numerous (16%) diverticular lesions. The ectopic pregnancy rate of all women treated was 7%, but of those who conceived, 15% had an ectopic pregnancy.

performed endoscopically. The intrauterine pregnancy rate was 26% after fimbrioplasty and 29% after neosalpingostomy, similar to the success rate after microsurgery. Canis et al. reported similar results. Of 87 women who had a distal tuboplasty performed by laparoscopy, one third had intrauterine pregnancies, nearly all of whom had mild or moderate disease (Figure 41-23). A comparison of the pregnancy rates obtained after laparoscopic surgery with those obtained in an earlier series by the same investigators after laser microsurgical distal tuboplasty performed through a laparotomy incision revealed no statistical dif-

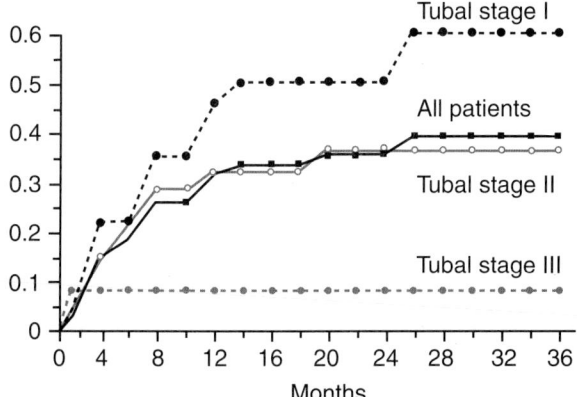

FIGURE 41-23 Cumulative pregnancy rates with laparoscopic distal tuboplasty after 4 years. (From Canis M, Manhes H, Mage G, et al: Fertil Steril 56:616, 1991.)

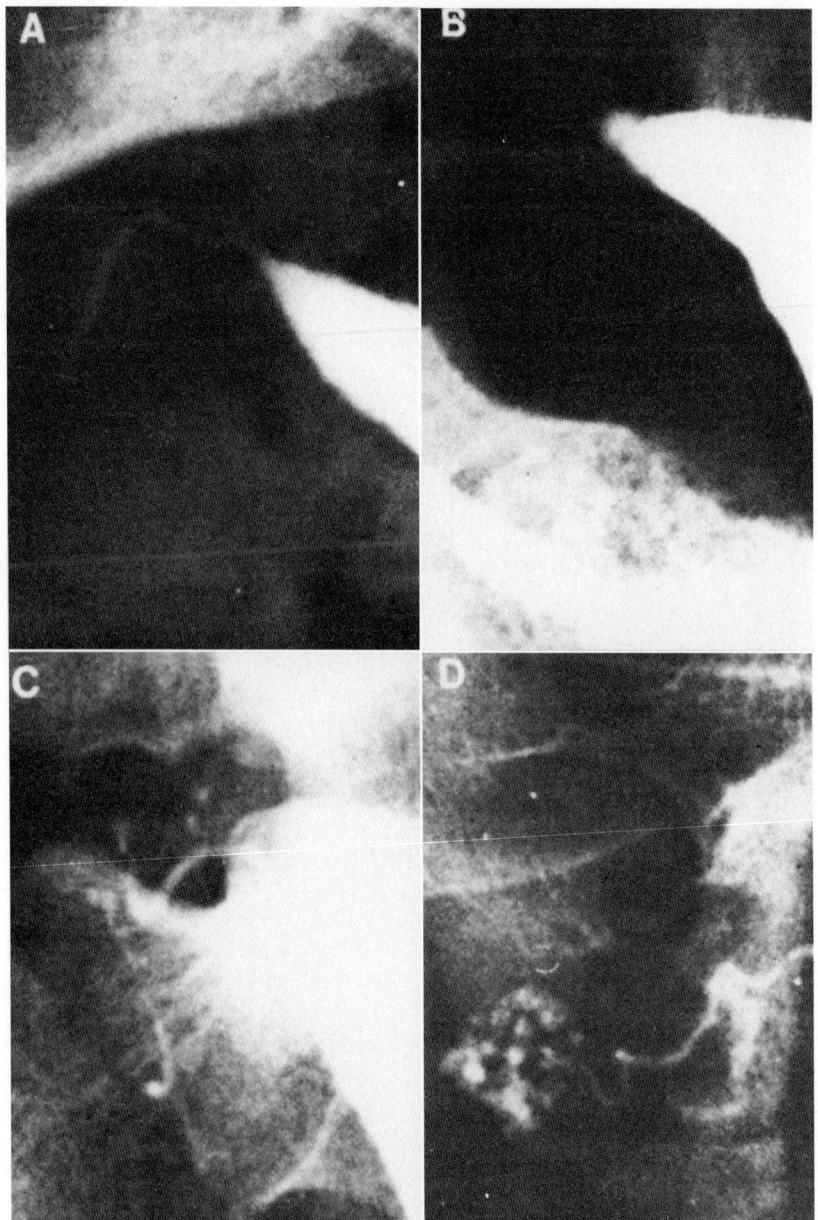

FIGURE 41-24   Types of occlusion following HSG. **A,** Undamaged intramural portion. **B,** Occluded intramural portion. **C,** Cornual occlusion with contrast extravasation in tubal wall. **D,** Occlusion with numerous diverticular lesions. (From Donnez J and Casanas-Roux F: Fertil Steril 46:1089, 1986.)

The surgical treatment of a proximal tubal blockage has now been replaced in most centers by the use of transcervically placed probes, catheters, or balloons, which are placed under fluoroscopic or hysteroscopic guidance in an outpatient setting with local anesthesia and sedation (Figure 41-25). After a canula is placed at the tubal ostium, radiographic dye is injected through the oviduct. This technique is called selective salpingography. If this technique does not produce tubal patency then a catheter is inserted into the interstitial portion of the oviduct to achieve patency. Results from several centers indicate that this outpatient procedure of selective salpingography and tubal cannulation, provided it is performed by well-trained, capable individuals, yields patency and pregnancy rates similar to those achieved by microsurgical reanastomosis (Table 41-11). Patency rates after these procedures range from 60% to 85%, with subsequent pregnancy rates in the 20% to 50% range in different series of small numbers of women. These relatively easy outpatient procedures, whether performed under fluoroscopic or hysteroscopic visualization, should now be considered the initial treatment of choice for proximal tubal obstruction.

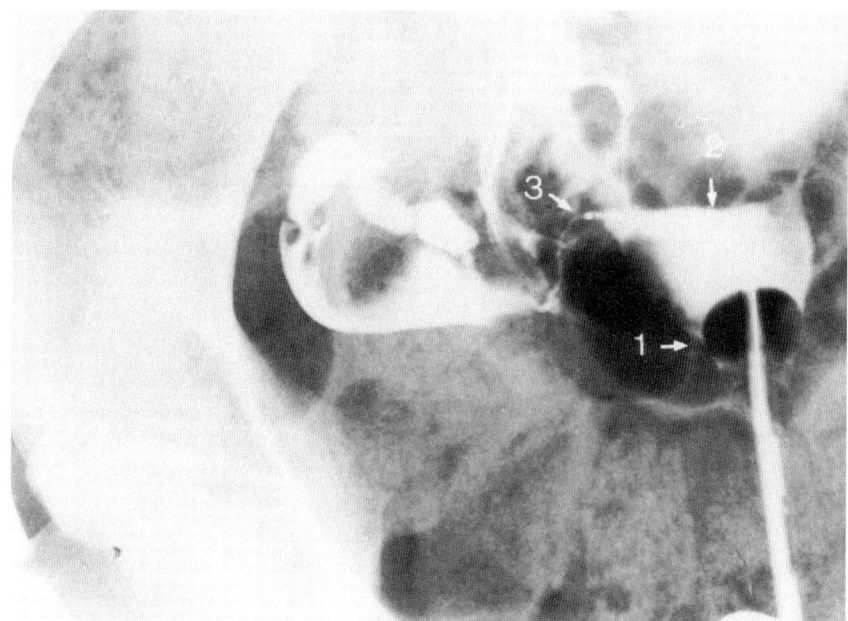

FIGURE 41-25 Hysterosalpingogram demonstrating transcervical balloon tuboplasty system in place following successful balloon dilation of a cornual occlusion. Two tandem balloons of the introductory catheter are inflated in lower uterine segment and in the endocervical canal *(1)*. The selective salpingography catheter is wedged into the cornual angle *(2)*. Balloon marker of the transcervical balloon tuboplasty catheter is shown *(3)*. Injection of contrast medium through transcervical balloon tuboplasty catheter demonstrates tubal patency and peritoneal spillage. (From Confino E, Tur-Kaspa I, DeCherney A, et al: JAMA 264:2079, 1990.)

TABLE 41-11
Review of Pregnancy Rates and Outcomes After Hysteroscopic Cannulation

Author and Year of Publication	No. Patients	No. Pregnancies (%)			
		Total	Ongoing*	SAB	Ectopic
Ransom, et al, 1997	17†	10 (59)	8 (47)	1 (5.9)	1 (5.9)
Das, et al, 1995	21	15 (71.4)	12 (57)	2 (9.5)	1 (3.6)
Sakumoto, et al, 1993	88	38 (43)	NA	NA	NA
Deaton, et al, 1990	7	2 (29)	2 (29)	0	0
SUBTOTAL	133	65 (48.9)	22 (48.9)	3 (6.7)	2 (4.4)
Excluded (small series)					
Sulak, et al, 1987	2	1 (50)	1 (50)	0	0
Daniell, et al, 1987	1	1 (100)	1 (100)	0	0

Note: NA = not available; SAB = spontaneous abortion.

*Ongoing pregnancies are all those of >20 weeks' gestation. Some investigators reported term pregnancies.

†Seventeen patients in this study had bilateral occlusion; five others had unilateral blockage.

Modified from Honoré GM, Holden AEC, and Schenken RS: Pathophysiology and management of proximal tubal blockage. Fertil Steril 71:785,1999

Adjunctive Therapy

Adjunctive procedures for surgical tubal reconstruction previously included prophylactic antibiotics, intraperitoneal corticosteroids, postoperative hydrotubation, and placement of tubal stents. Prospective studies have not demonstrated postoperative hydrotubation to have any benefit, and tubal stents should not be used because they may cause mucosal damage. Recent data from the Nordic

Adhesion Prevention Study Group reported that intraperitoneal corticosteroids failed to reduce adhesion scores in infertility patients. Currently, the most widely used method to reduce postoperative adhesion formation is the postoperative use of intraperitoneal barriers. Intraperitoneal barriers reduce adhesion formation by preventing the formation of fibrin bridges between healing tissues. These devices, available in both liquid and solid forms, provide the surgeon with the option of general peritoneal coverage or site-specific application. Barriers currently in use include liquids (Dextran, crystalloid) and solids that are both absorbable (Interceed Absorbable Adhesion Barrier, Johnson & Johnson) and artificial nonabsorbable membranes (Polytetrafluoroethylene, Gore-Tex Surgical Membrane, W.L. Gore Co.). The most commonly used adjuvant to reduce postoperative adhesion formation is crystalloid solutions, such as lactated Ringer's, phosphate-buffered saline, or normal saline, which are administered as an instillate at the end of the surgical procedure, despite a substantial body of clinical data demonstrating an adhesion reformation rate of approximately 80%. Dextran is a water-soluble glucose polymer originally used as a plasma expander. Most of the research in adhesion prevention has focused on a 32% solution of dextran 70 suspended in 10% dextrose (Hyskon). Initial data with the use of Hyskon was very promising. However, its adhesion reduction effects were largely limited to "dependent" portions of the pelvis. A prospective, randomized study from Scandinavia demonstrated no benefit from the instillation of 100 to 200 ml of Hyskon on adhesion scores at follow-up laparoscopy. A prospective, multicenter, randomized study conducted to assess the efficacy of Interceed demonstrated that the postsurgical placement of Interceed significantly reduced adhesion formation after endometriosis and ovarian and tubal surgery. Interceed does not require suturing

and is spontaneously absorbed in 3 to 4 weeks. However, complete hemostasis needs to be accomplished before its placement to maintain its maximal adhesion prevention benefit. Placement of artificial, nonabsorbable barriers has also been demonstrated to reduce postoperative adhesion scores in women undergoing adhesiolysis and myomectomy. This artificial membrane requires suturing in place with nonabsorbable suture. Although there is concern regarding leaving this nonabsorbable barrier in place permanently, histologic analysis of the retrieved barrier showed no tissue adherence to the material and mild to no foreign body response. Although both absorbable and nonabsorbable barriers have been shown to be safe and effective in all human clinical trials, their use does not eliminate adhesion formation. Efficacy of the barriers is limited to surgical situations in which the area in question can be completely covered. Techniques operators can use to minimize adhesions include fine-caliber suture material of low tissue reactivity, meticulous hemostasis, minimalization of tissue handling and desiccation, in addition to the use of absorbable or nonabsorbable barriers.

Tulandi et al., in a randomized prospective study, demonstrated that second-look laparoscopy 1 year after failure of terminal salpingostomy or salpingo-ovariolysis to achieve pregnancy was not beneficial in achieving higher pregnancy rates. The benefit of second-look laparo-

Patient's Name _____ Date _____

Stage I (Minimal) · 1-5
Stage II (Mild) · 6-15
Stage III (Moderate) · 16-40
Stage IV (Severe) · >40
Total _____

Laparoscopy _____ Laparotomy _____ Photography _____
Recommended Treatment _____

Prognosis _____

PERITONEUM	ENDOMETRIOSIS	<1cm	1-3cm	>3cm
	Superficial	1	2	4
	Deep	2	4	6
OVARY	R Superficial	1	2	4
	Deep	4	16	20
	L Superficial	1	2	4
	Deep	4	16	20

	POSTERIOR CULDESAC OBLITERATION	Partial	Complete
		4	40

	ADHESIONS	<1/3 Enclosure	1/3-2/3 Enclosure	>2/3 Enclosure
OVARY	R Filmy	1	2	4
	Dense	4	8	16
	L Filmy	1	2	4
	Dense	4	8	16
TUBE	R Filmy	1	2	4
	Dense	4*	8*	16
	L Filmy	1	2	4
	Dense	4*	8*	16

*If the fimbriated end of the fallopian tube is completely enclosed, change the point assignment to 16.

FIGURE 41-26 American Fertility Society classification of endometriosis. (From Andrews WC, Buttram VC, Behrman SJ, et al: Fertil Steril 43:351, 1985.)

scopy performed within a few weeks or months after tubal reconstructive surgery has also not been demonstrated in a prospective randomized trial. Thus a second-look laparoscopy performed at some time interval after tubal reconstructive surgery is not cost effective.

If pregnancy does not occur within 6 to 12 months after tubal reconstruction, another HSG should be performed. If tubal obstruction has recurred, a repeat surgical procedure is not advised because pregnancy rates are less than 10%.

Endometriosis

Some investigators have estimated that as many as 40% of infertile women have endometriosis. If endometriosis is found at the time of laparoscopy, the extent of the disease should be classified according to the stages recommended by the American Society of Reproductive Medicine (Figure 41-26). The etiology, diagnosis, and treatment of endometriosis are presented in detail in Chapter 19.

Olive et al. reported that about 65% of women with mild endometriosis and no other cause of infertility conceived without treatment. With moderate or severe disease these authors reported that pregnancy rates with expectant management were much lower—25% and 0%, respectively. Thus a causal relationship between endometriosis and infertility is present when there is moderate or severe disease with extensive adhesions involving the oviducts and interfering with their normal motility. However, it has not been shown that minimal or mild endometriosis that does not involve the oviducts or ovaries is a cause of infertility. It is more likely that pelvic endometriosis is a result of infertility with many years of retrograde menstruation. No medical therapy has been shown to increase fertility rates in women with endometriosis and if tubal adhesions or endometriomas are not present, surgical treatment of pelvic endometriosis has also not resulted in improved fertility rates compared with no therapy. Inoue et al. analyzed conception rates in a group of 2080 infertile women who had a diagnostic laparoscopy. Of this group 1263 had endometriosis and 817 did not. The two groups had a similar mean age and duration of infertility. After various types of therapy the conception rates in the two groups were similar, 30.7% and 30.0%, respectively. Among those women treated with in vitro fertilization conception, rates were also similar whether or not endometriosis was present.

Mild Endometriosis

It has been postulated that there is an increase in intraperitoneal macrophages in women with mild endometriosis, and these cells may enter the lumen of the oviducts and phagocytose sperm. However, with the exception of one randomized trial from Canada, medical or surgical treatment of mild endometriosis does not result in signifi-

cantly increased pregnancy rates as compared with no treatment. Overall pregnancy rates for women with mild endometriosis, with or without treatment, are in the 60% to 75% range. In a prospective randomized study, Bayer et al. reported that the pregnancy rate of a group of women with mild endometriosis was not increased following a course of danazol therapy as compared with those receiving no medical treatment (Figure 41-27). Schenken and Malinak, as well as Garcia and David, reported that pregnancy rates following conservative surgical treatment of mild endometriosis were nearly identical to the rates of groups of women in the same institution who had no surgical corrective treatment. Inoue et al. reported that if electrocoagulation of mild or moderate endometriosis was performed at the time of diagnostic laparoscopy, then conception rates were slightly lower in women in whom the endometriotic lesions were not coagulated. In the Canadian study by Marcoux et al. twice as many women conceived when the endometrial implants were resected or ablated compared with no therapy of implants, but in the treated group the fecundity rate was only 6% per cycle. A subsequent and smaller clinical trial from Italy reported no difference in pregnancy rate whether minimal to mild endometriosis was ablated or not. Thus, with one exception, these studies indicate that mild endometriosis most likely is not a cause of infertility, and there is no proven efficacy of therapy. Endometriosis may be a result of infertility, and women with endometriosis are a subfertile population. Thus if only mild endometriosis is found at the time of laparoscopy and no other cause of infertility is present, then it is advisable to treat these individuals with controlled ovarian hyperstimulation and intrauterine

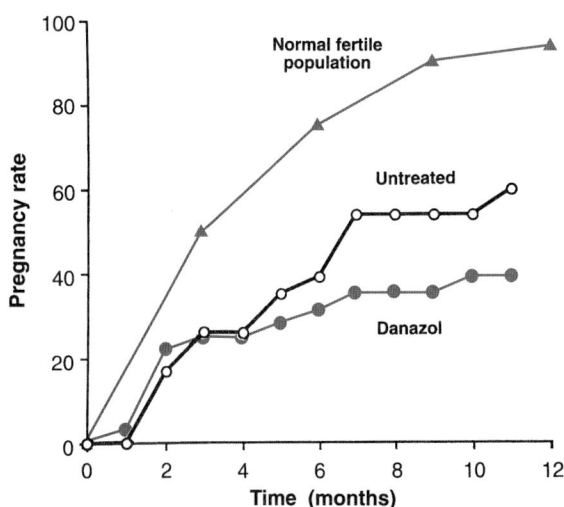

FIGURE 41-27 Cumulative pregnancy rates in danazol-treated and untreated groups over a 12-month period. Cumulative pregnancy rate in an ideal fertile population is also shown for comparison. (Adapted from Cooke ID, Sulaiman RA, Lenton EA, and Parsonos RJ: Clin Obstet Gynecol 8:531, 1981; and Bayer SR, Seibel MM, Saffan DS, et al: J Reprod Med 33:179, 1988.)

insemination similar to the treatment of unexplained infertility. Simpson et al. reported results of a nonrandomized, prospective, multicenter cohort analysis in Canada that analyzed results of different therapies of 297 women with endometriosis and regular cycles and patent oviducts whose partners had more than 5 million motile sperm in their ejaculate. They found that the relative likelihood of pregnancy with the use of clomiphene citrate supraovulation was 2.9 times that of women who received no treatment. Use of danazol was associated with the same likelihood of pregnancy as occurred with no treatment.

Moderate Endometriosis

If pelvic adhesions that cannot be lysed at the time of laparoscopy or ovarian endometriomas larger than 1 cm in diameter are present, medical therapy will not cause sufficient regression to improve fertility rates, and surgical treatment should be undertaken. For women with moderate disease without ovarian endometriomas and minimal adhesions that can be cut at the time of laparoscopy, no evidence indicates that medical treatment improves fertility rates compared with no treatment.

The use of danazol, GnRH agonists, progestins, or oral contraceptives has not been shown to increase fertility rates compared with observation without treatment.

Hughes et al. performed a meta-analysis of four randomized clinical trials and five cohort studies of women who had mild or moderate endometriosis treated with either danazol or progestins compared with a control group who received a placebo or no therapy. No individual study showed a significantly greater pregnancy rate with treatment, and the common odds ratio for pregnancy occurring with treatment compared with no treatment was 0.85 (Figure 41-28). They also performed a meta-analysis of six randomized clinical trials in which ovulation suppression with GnRH agonists or progestins was compared with danazol. The common odds ratio was 1.07, an insignificant difference.

The results of these studies provide additional evidence for the belief that unless the extent of the endometrial disease is severe enough to produce adhesions that interfere with oviduct motility, endometriosis itself is a result and not a cause of infertility. In these studies all women with tubal occlusion were excluded. However, the low cumulative fertility rates 30 months after laparoscopic diagnosis of endometriosis in treated or untreated women indicate that women with endometriosis have impaired fertility.

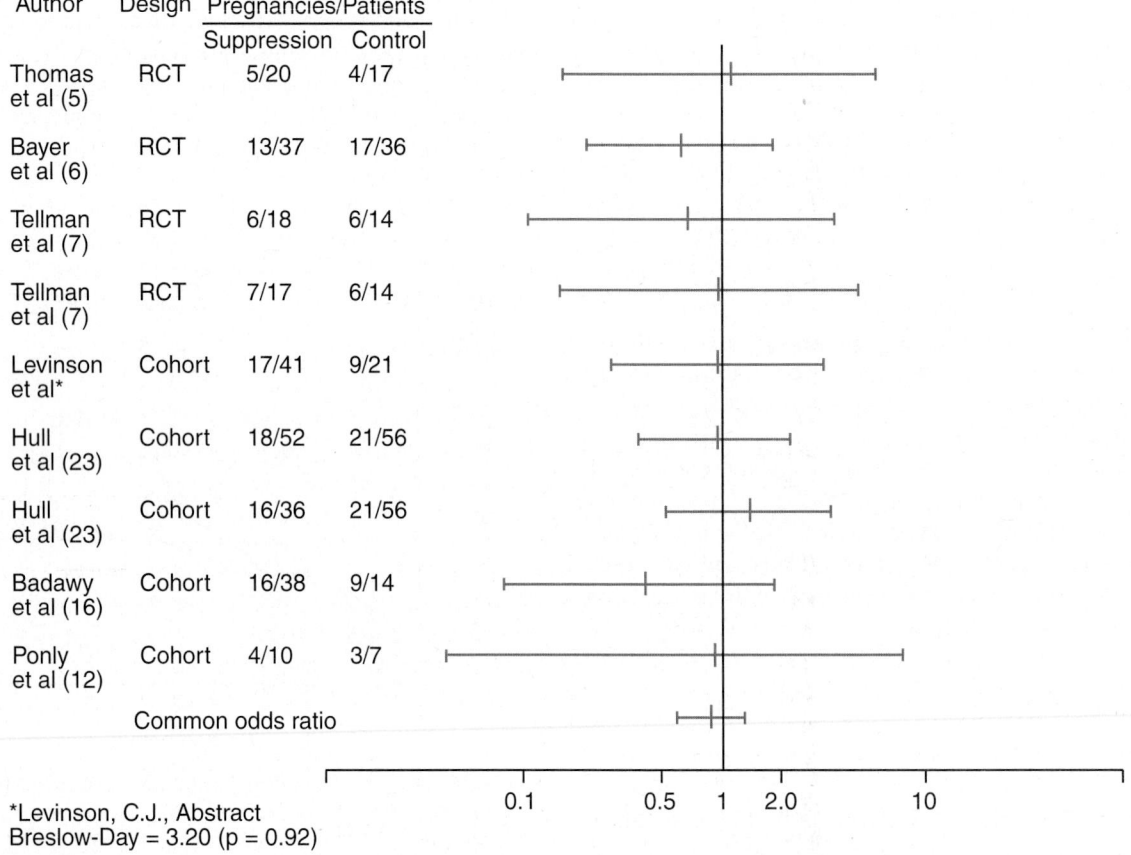

FIGURE 41-28 Controlled studies comparing ovulation suppression versus no treatment in women with endometriosis-associated infertility: Ors for pregnancy. (From Hughes EG, Fedorkow DM, and Collins JA: Fertil Steril 59:963, 1993.)

Furthermore, because danazol, MPA, or a GnRH agonist each causes regression of endometriosis, the fact that pregnancy rates are no greater in women receiving treatment than in those receiving no therapy confirms the belief that the residual endometriosis does not cause infertility.

Severe Endometriosis

Conservative operative resection of endometriosis should be performed for women with infertility and moderate or severe disease with adhesions that cannot be cauterized or lysed at the time of laparoscopy or those with endometriomas more than 1 cm in diameter. Preoperative treatment with danazol or GnRH agonists for 6 weeks to 3 months is advised by some authorities to facilitate the surgical resection, but there appears to be no benefit from postoperative danazol or GnRH agonist treatment. Conception rates for women treated operatively have been reported to be in the 50% to 60% range for those with moderate disease and 30% to 40% for those with severe disease. These rates are better than those reported for expectant management. Three of five cohort studies reported that pregnancy rates following laparoscopic surgical treatment of endometriosis was significantly greater than use of danazol or no treatment. The common odds ratio for pregnancy was 2.67 times greater with use of laparoscopic surgery.

Of the women who do conceive after surgical resection, about half will do so in the first 6 months, and nearly all in the first 15 months after the operative procedure, similar to what occurs after discontinuation of medical therapy.

Olive and Martin reported that women with severe endometriosis had a 50% pregnancy rate after being treated with carbon dioxide laser laparoscopy, similar to the rates of those treated with laparotomy (Figure 41-29). If women have such severe disease that it cannot be treated by endoscopic surgery, perhaps in vitro fertilization should be utilized instead of performing a laparotomy, similar to the approach proposed for severe distal tubal disease. Pregnancy rates following in vitro fertilization for endometriosis are about 20% per treatment cycle. Therefore both treatment options should be offered to individual women with severe endometriosis.

Operative treatment of endometriosis has for many years included the use of electrocautery as well as microsurgical techniques. In the past 15 years argon and carbon dioxide lasers have been used to vaporize adhesions and endometrial implants. Studies in animals and humans have shown no difference in the results of treatment of periadnexal adhesions with carbon dioxide laser or electrocautery. In a prospective randomized study Tulandi reported that pregnancy rates were similar following the use of each of these two techniques for lysis of periadnexal adhesions. The duration of operating time may be reduced with the laser, but the technique has the disadvantages of higher cost and necessity for additional training, because it is more difficult to use the laser than electrocautery.

Unexplained Infertility

For couples in whom the female member is ovulatory and has patent oviducts and the male member has at least 20 million motile sperm in the ejaculate, the diagnosis of unexplained infertility should be made and treatment ini-

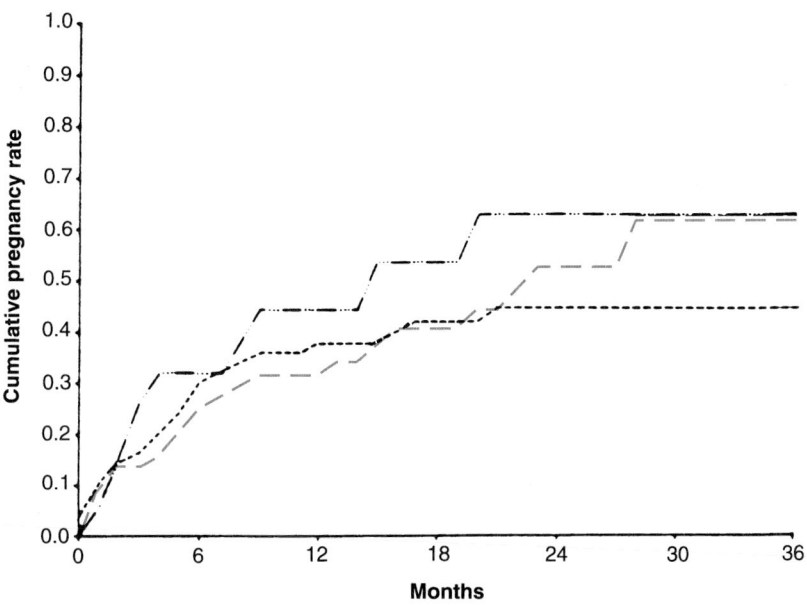

FIGURE 41-29 Cumulative pregnancy rates for women with endometriosis using life-table analysis. The – – – line indicates patients with stage I endometriosis, - - - - indicates patients with stage II endometriosis, and –. . .– indicates those with stage III disease. (From Olive DL and Martin DC: Fertil Steril 48:18, 1987.)

tiated with controlled ovarian hyperstimulation (COH) and appropriately timed preovulatory IUI with a sample of freshly prepared, recently ejaculated sperm or in vitro fertilization. COH should be performed with either clomiphene citrate or hMG. Insemination is best performed on the day prior to spontaneous ovulation, on the morning following the day that LH is initially detected in a random urine specimen, or 36 hours after intramuscular hCG is given to induce ovulation. A meta-analysis of several randomized trials by Zeyneloglu et al. comparing IUI with timed intercourse after COH in couples with unexplained infertility revealed that the pregnancy rate per cycle with IUI is about 20%, whereas with timed intercourse it is about 11% (Figure 41-30). The sperm to be inseminated can be separated from the semen by a two-step centrifuge procedure with addition of a buffered electrolyte solution with or without removing the most motile sperm by the swim-up technique. Alternatively the sperm can be separated by placing them in a density gradient medium for a short time and retrieving the most motile sperm from the densest portion of the medium. Dodson et al. reported results of a randomized trial of COH and IUI using these three methods of sperm separation. There were no significant differences in per cycle pregnancy rates with any of the methods. Clinicians can therefore use whichever of the three techniques of sperm separation is most convenient for their practice site before performing IUI.

It is much easier for the clinician and woman to undergo ovarian stimulation with clomiphene citrate than with hMG because use of the former drug is less expensive and requires less monitoring. Monitoring is necessary with hMG to reduce the possibility of developing the ovarian hyperstimulation syndrome and/or multiple gestations. When clomiphene citrate is used to cause ovarian

hyperstimulation in ovulatory women, treatment should be initiated on cycle day 2 to 3 before the dominant follicle is recruited. A dose of 100 mg/day for 5 days usually results in the development of 2 to 3 dominant follicles, which release eggs shortly after the endogenous LH surge or after giving exogenous hCG.

Deaton et al. performed a prospective, randomized, clinical trial comparing the use of clomiphene citrate and timed intrauterine insemination with timed periovulatory sexual intercourse in an unstimulated cycle in 67 couples with unexplained infertility or mild endometriosis. The monthly fecundity rate in the treatment cycles was 0.095 compared with 0.033 in the control cycles, a significant difference.

In 1998 Guzick et al. published a review of data from 45 published studies of various therapies of unexplained infertility including mild endometriosis. After adjustment for study quality pregnancy rates per initiated treatment cycle were 1.3% to 4.1% for no treatment, 8.3% for clomiphene citrate plus IUI, 17.1% for hMG plus IUI, and 20.7% for IVF (Table 41-12). Although the pregnancy rate in this analysis of nonrandomized studies was higher with hMG plus IUI than with clomiphene citrate plus IUI, use of hMG is more costly, requires frequent sonographic and hormone monitoring, and has a higher complication rate than clomiphene citrate. In a prospective randomized trial comparing hMG plus IUI with hMG and intracervical insemination, and intracervical or intrauterine insertion without hMG Guzick et al. found the pregnancy rate per treatment cycle with hMG plus IUI was 9%, about twice as high as the other three treatment regimens. One third of the couples treated with hMG plus IUI conceived after four treatment cycles (Table 41-13). Unfortunately, even with monitoring, 20% of the pregnancies that occurred

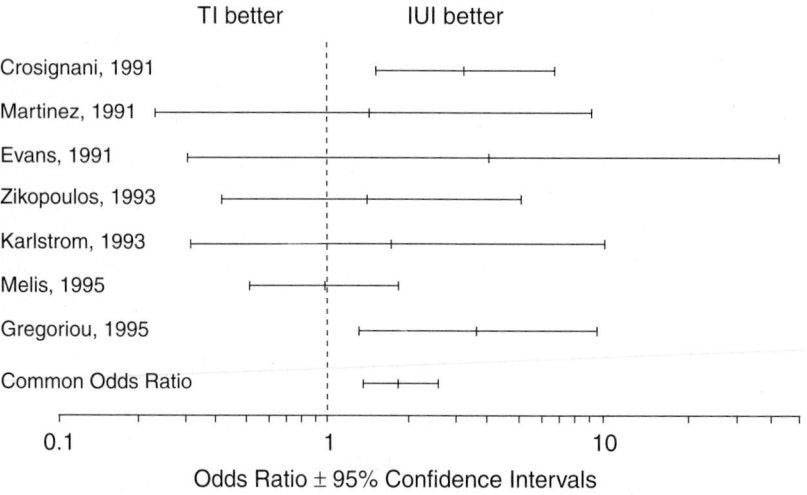

FIGURE 41-30 The odds ratio of the studies included in the meta-analysis. (From Zeyneloglu HB, Arici A, Olive DL, et al: Comparison of intrauterine insemination with timed intercourse in superovulated cycles with gonadotropins: a meta-analysis, Fertil Steril 69:486, 1998.)

TABLE 41-12
Aggregate Data for Each Treatment

Treatment	No. Studies	No. (%) Pregnancies Per Initiated Cycle	Percentage of Quality-Adjusted Pregnacies Per Initiated Cycle
Control groups	11	64/3539 (1.8)	1.3
Control groups, randomized studies	6	23/597 (3.8)	4.1
IUI	9	15/378 (4)	3.8
CC	3	37/617 (6)	5.6
CC + IUI	5	21/315 (6.7)	8.3
hMG	13	139/1806 (7.7)	7.7
hMG + IUI	14	207/1133 (18)	17.1
IVF	9	378/683 (22.5)	20.7
GIFT	9	158/607 (26.0)	27.0

*Many studies appear in more than 1 row if they reported on more than 1 treatment.

Abbreviations: CC, Clomiphene citrate; *IUI*, intrauterine insemination; *hMG*, gonadotropins; *IVF*, in vitro fertilization; *GIFT*, gamete intrafallopian transfer.

Modified from Guzick DS, Sullivan MW, Adamson GD, et al: Efficacy of treatment for unexplained infertility. Fertil Steril 70:207, 1998.

TABLE 41-13
Pregnancy Rates Per Couple

Treatment Group	No. Couples	No. Insemination Cycles	No. Pregnancies	Pregnancy Rate Per Couple* (%)	Pregnancies During Insemination Cycle[†] No Pregnancies/No. Insemination Cycles (%)
Intracervical insemination	233	706	23	10	14/706 (2)
Intrauterine insemination	234	717	42	18	35/717 (5)
Superovulation and intracervical insemination	234	637	44	19	26/637 (4)
Superovulation and intrauterine insemination	231	618	77	33	54/618 (9)

*The results of chi-square tests of a priori comparison, adjusted for center, are as follows: intracervical insemination as compared with super-ovulation and intracervical insemination, $P = .006$; intracervical insemination as compared with intrauterine insemination, $P = .01$; intracervical insemination as compared with superovulation and intrauterine insemination: P less than .001; intrauterine insemination as compared with superovulation and intrauterine insemination, P less than .001; superovulation and intracervical insemination as compared with superovulation and intrauterine insemination, P less than .001. The P value that indicates statistical significance after the Bonferroni correction is .01.

†The results of chi-square tests of a priori comparison, adjusted for center, are as follows: intracervical insemination as compared with super-ovulation and intracervical insemination, $P = .024$; intracervical insemination as compared with intrauterine insemination, $P = .003$; intracervical insemination as compared with superovulation and intrauterine insemination, P less than .001; intrauterine insemination as compared with superovulation and intrauterine insemination, P less than .001; superovulation and intracervical insemination as compared with superovulation and intrauterine insemination, $P = .005$. The P value that indicates statistical significance after the Bonferroni correction is .01.

Modified from Guzick DS, for the National Cooperative Reproductive Medicine Network: Efficacy of superovulation and intrauterine insemination in the treatment of infertility. N Engl J Med 340:177,1999.

with use of hMG were multiple gestations. It therefore appears best to initially treat unexplained infertility in a woman younger than age 40 with clomiphene citrate and IUI for four to six cycles. If pregnancy fails to occur then referral to an infertility specialist for treatment with hMG plus IUI or IVF is advisable.

Several authors have reported that with the use of COH and IUI fecundability rates decline dramatically after age 40. Pregnancy rates with in vitro fertilization also decrease substantially after age 40. In several reports, the pregnancy rate per cycle with COH and IUI in women older than age 40 was only 5% compared with 10% to 15% in younger women. Some studies report no pregnancies in women older than 42 treated with COH plus IUI. Even if pregnancy occurs the pregnancy loss rate doubles in conceptions occurring in women older than 40, compared to younger women. The more expensive in vitro fertilization procedure in women over age 40 is also not as effective as it is in younger women. Live birth rates of about 10% per cycle with in vitro fertilization have been reported in women of this age with use of their own oocytes. With the use of donor oocytes live birth rates increase to about 45% per IVF embryo transfer cycle.

Thus in infertile women older than age 40 treated by in vitro fertilization the use of donor eggs is advisable. This informative data should be used to counsel infertile couples when the female partner is older than age 40, because the various treatments differ in respect to cost and chance of successful live birth.

In Vitro Fertilization

The technique of in vitro fertilization (IVF) with embryo transfer is now being widely used to treat infertile couples. Although the method was originally restricted to women who had no functioning oviducts as a result of severe tubal disease, it is now being used for women with severe endometriosis and couples with male factor or unexplained infertility. Since the rate of pregnancy following IVF is directly related to the number of embryos placed in the uterine cavity, nearly all IVF clinics currently utilize some form of ovarian hyperstimulation to increase the number of oocytes obtained at the time of follicle aspiration. Stimulation protocols utilizing clomiphene citrate, hMG or FSH, or a combination of agents are being used. These agents are usually given after a period of suppression with a GnRH agonist. Monitoring of follicle growth is usually performed by both daily ultrasonography and estrogen measurement.

Some centers perform in vitro fertilization with a single ovum retrieved from an unstimulated follicle. There are two main advantages for performing IVF with eggs collected from the dominant follicle in a normal, unstimulated ovulatory cycle. First, the substantial cost of administering hMG and additional days of monitoring that are necessary in stimulated cycles are avoided. Second, more aspiration cycles can be performed in the same time period. Thus aspirating eggs from unstimulated cycles is both cost effective and time efficient. In addition, the problems associated with multiple gestation and cryopreservation of excess embryos are avoided. Foulet et al. reported a similar pregnancy rate, 22.5% per cycle, with this technique as others have with hyperstimulation. However, the pregnancy rate per cycle reported by most others is in the 15% range.

Originally, oocyte retrieval was done by laparoscopic visualization. Follicle aspiration is now being performed routinely through the vagina into the cul-de-sac with sonographic guidance of needle placement.

Following aspiration of the oocytes they are cultured in a rigidly controlled, sterile laboratory environment. Various culture media are used in different clinics. The media are freshly prepared at frequent intervals, and sterility is ensured. The eggs are incubated in an atmosphere of 5% carbon dioxide and high humidity.

A few hours after egg retrieval, sperm that has been separated from semen are added to the culture medium. About 18 hours later the oocytes are observed to determine if fertilization has occurred. The oocytes that are fertilized are then cultured for an additional 48 to 96 hours, and from one to four normally cleaving embryos are then placed into the uterus of the patient in a sterile environment without the use of general anesthesia. Embryo placement is performed through a small catheter placed through the cervical canal. With the development of sequential culture media it has become possible to allow embryos to develop in vitro to the blastocyst stage, 5 days after fertilization, prior to transfer into the endometrial cavity. Several centers report per cycle pregnancy rates of 40% to 60% with blastocyst culture and transfer. Most centers are freezing the embryos not utilized and transferring them in subsequent spontaneous ovulatory cycles, if pregnancy does not occur in the initial treatment cycle. Since women over age 40 have decreased implantation rates compared with younger women, most centers transfer four or more embryos to those women unless donor oocytes are used.

Pregnancy rates with IVF vary among different centers, and one of the reasons for the variability is the lack of standardization of the definition of the term *pregnancy rate*. If women who exhibit a transitory rise of hCG following embryo transfer but who have no clinical or ultrasound-demonstrated evidence of pregnancy are defined as pregnant, then the size of the numerator will be increased. The denominator will be highest if all women starting the process are included, but most centers report pregnancy rates per number of women with follicle aspiration or number of women with embryo transfer. Use of the latter two categories will decrease the size of the denominator and thus increase the pregnancy rates reported.

A modification of in vitro fertilization, called *gamete intrafallopian transfer (GIFT)*, can be used if the infertile woman has functioning oviducts. With this technique both oocytes and sperm are placed into the oviduct through a catheter at the time of laparoscopy or minilaparotomy. Although in vitro fertilization, embryo culturing, and embryo transfer into the uterus are avoided by this technique, ovarian hyperstimulation and laparoscopy are still required. Modifications of GIFT include *zygote intrafallopian transfer (ZIFT)* and *tubal embryo stage transfer (TEST)*. With ZIFT the oocytes are fertilized in vitro and transferred 24 hours later. Tubal embryo transfer (TET) is similar to ZIFT except the embryos are transferred 8 to 72 hours after fertilization. The Society for Assisted Reproductive Technology (SART) performs annual surveys of the various techniques of assisted reproduction. These annual surveys provide useful information for infertile couples who wish to consider use of assisted reproductive technology to conceive. The data from the most recent survey can be used to counsel women about the expected outcomes of pregnancy. The 1996 SART survey reported that the live-delivery rate per cycle in which ova were

TABLE 41-14

Comparison of Reported Outcomes for All Assisted Reproductive Technology Procedures

	Standard IVF	IVF+ICSI	GIFT	ZIFT	Donor*	CPE†	CPE-DO	Host Uterus
No. cycles or procedures‡	30,598	14,049	2879	1200	3768	9610	1096	688
Cancellations (%)	20.3	NA	16.3	11.3	6.6	6.6	4.7	0
No. retrievals	24,383	14,049	2409	1065	NA	NA	NA	688
No. transfers	22,664	13,195	2379	996	3345	8661	1027	597
No transfers/no. retrievals (%)	93.0	93.9	98.8	93.5	NA	NA	NA	86.8
No. pregnancies	7581	4357	834	399	1510	1783	274	217
Pregnancy loss (%)	15.9	16.6	16.3	17.5	13.3	18.3	21.9	13.8
No. deliveries	6379	3632	698	329	1309	1457	214	187
No. deliveries/no. retrievals (%)	26.2	25.9	29.0	30.9	NA	NA	NA	27.2
Percentage singleton pregnancies	60.3	62.2	66.0	64.1	59.7	72.6	74.3	61.5
No. ectopic pregnancies	35	18	3	1	4	10	1	1
No. ectopic pregnancies/no. transfers (%)	0.1	0.2	0.1	0.1	0.1	0.1	0.1	0.2
No. birth defects/no. neonates (%)§	1.8	1.8	1.3	0.9	1.3	1.9	4.2	1.6

*Donor includes known or anonymous but not surrogate.

†Cryopreserved embryo transfer cycles not done in combination with fresh embryo transfers and not with donor egg-embryo.

‡Includes all cycles regardless of age and diagnosis.

§Birth defect reporting did not account for all neonatal outcomes.

Abbreviations: IVF, In vitro fertilization; *ICSI,* intracytoplasmic sperm injection; *GIFT,* gamete intrafallopian transfer; *ZIFT,* zygote intrafallopian transfer; *CPE,* cryopreserved embryos; *CPE-DO,* cryopreserved embryo from donor egg; *NA,* not applicable.

Modified from American Society for Reproductive Medicine: Assisted reproductive technology in the United States: 1996 results generated from the American Society for Reproductive Medine/Society for Assisted Reproductive Technology Registry. Fertil Steril 71:798,1999.

retrieved was 26.2% for IVF and 25.9% for IVF plus ICSI (Table 41-14). The rate of deliveries per IVF embryo transfer cycle has been steadily increasing each year.

In 1996 about one third of the IVF cycles in the United States were accompanied by an ICSI procedure. With all techniques of assisted reproduction about 60% of the pregnancies are singleton gestations, 32% twins, 6% triplets, and the rest higher-order births. Schieve et al. analyzed data from 300 U.S. clinics who reported data about IVF to the Centers for Disease Control and Prevention in 1991. The risk of multiple birth varied directly with the number of embryos transferred and inversely with maternal age. The analysis indicated that it is not beneficial in terms of greater pregnancy rates to transfer more than two embryos after IVF if the woman is less than 35 years of age. In this age group the multiple birth rate increased to 40% or more when three or more embryos were transferred. When two embryos were transferred in this age group, the twin rate was still 20%. Transfer of three embryos in women age 35 to 39 increased the multiple birth rate from 11.6% to 29.4%. It would appear best to limit the number of embryos transferred to two for women less than age 35 and three for women 35 to 39. No limit of numbers of embryos transferred should be undertaken for women over age 40 because the multiple birth rate was less than 25% even if five embryos were transferred.

Data from several large centers in three different countries indicate that the pregnancy rate per IVF treatment cycle remains relatively constant for about six cycles. After six cycles the cumulative pregnancy rate is about 60% (Figure 41-31). After six cycles of IVF the procedure is associated with a significant decrease in pregnancy rates. Women should be counseled that chances of pregnancy occurring with IVF after six failed cycles of IVF are very low.

An important factor when counseling couples about any assisted reproductive technique (ART) concerns the pregnancy outcome. With any form of ART resulting in a singleton gestation advancing to the second trimester, perinatal outcome, gestational age, mean birth weight, congenital malformations, and complications of pregnancy or labor are no different than in the normal fertile population. Therefore viable singleton pregnancies occurring after ART should not be considered high-risk pregnancies. However, there is an increased risk of spontaneous abortion and preterm delivery among women with multiple gestations conceived by ART. All types of ART with ovarian stimulation are followed by about 40% incidence of multiple gestations. The majority of these pregnancies are twins (25%), with 5% being higher-order gestations. Furthermore about 4% of all pregnancies with IVF are tubal pregnancies, with 1% being combined ectopic and intrauterine pregnancies. Therefore these pregnancies need to be closely monitored, as described in Chapter 17.

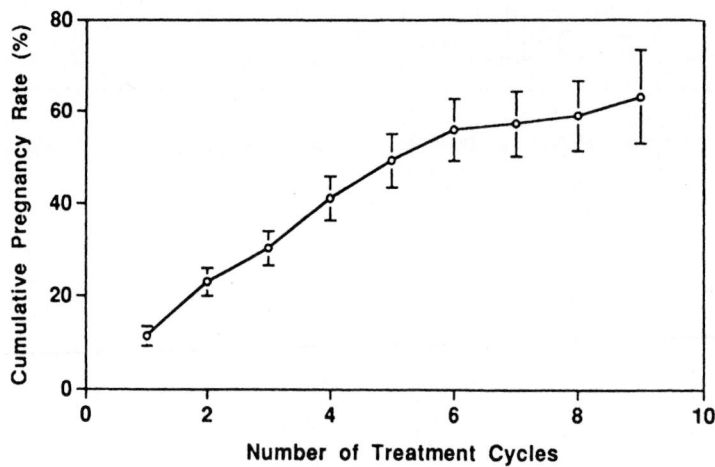

FIGURE 41-31 Overall cumulative pregnancy rate in IVF treatment (with 95% confidence interval). (From Dor J, Seidman DS, Ben-Shlomo I, et al: Cumulative pregnancy rate following in-vitro fertilization: the significance of age and infertility aetiology, Hum Reprod 11:425, 1996.)

Cryopreservation of embryos that have undergone IVF is being used in most assisted reproductive centers. Cryopreservation allows embryos that cannot be immediately transferred to the woman to be stored for future use. If more than four eggs are fertilized in a given cycle, the excess embryos can be frozen. In addition, if there are indications that the woman is at risk of developing ovarian hyperstimulation syndrome, which would be enhanced by endogenous hCG production from pregnancy, the fertilized embryos can be frozen and transferred to the endometrial cavity at a later date.

Wada et al. studied the outcome of 283 infants conceived from cryopreserved embryos. If a pregnancy takes place after a transfer of a frozen embryo, there is no evidence of a deleterious effect on the fetus. As a matter of fact, the incidence of fetal malformations appears to be significantly reduced compared with the normal IVF process. Furthermore, there is no increased risk of perinatal mortality or preterm delivery. Even in twin gestations after cryopreservation, the incidence of preterm birth was significantly lower than in twin gestations resulting from the normal IVF process. This reassuring information should be conveyed to those infertile couples undergoing IVF with cryopreservation of the fertilized embryo.

FINAL COUNSELING

If treatment of the infertile couple fails to result in conception after 2 years, the couple should be informed that the chances for conception are remote. It is best to inform the couple of the prognosis for fertility and the duration beyond which conception should not be expected at the time of the initial consultation, and this information should be restated at subsequent visits. When the period during which conception should be expected has been exceeded, the couple should be informed that further testing and treatment are not warranted and other alternatives such as adoption should be considered.

Finally, it is important for the couple to consider psychologic counseling, because the prospect of permanent infertility can cause severe mental trauma.

KEY POINTS

- In 1995 about 10% of all U.S. couples with wives in the reproductive age group were infertile. This group included 6.2 million women.

- The incidence of infertility steadily increases in women after age 30.

- Among fertile couples who have coitus in the week before ovulation, there is only about a 20% (monthly fecundability rate of 0.2) chance of developing a clinical pregnancy in each ovulatory cycle.

- About half of fertile couples attempting to conceive will become pregnant in 3 months, 75% in 6 months, and 90% at the end of 1 year.

- Infertile couples who conceive do not have higher rates of spontaneous abortion or perinatal mortality than age-matched control subjects.

- In the United States approximately 10% to 15% of cases of infertility are caused by anovulation, 30% to 40% by an abnormality of semen production, 30% to 40% by pelvic disease, and 10% to 15% by abnormalities of sperm transport through the cervical canal. About 10% to 20% of cases are unexplained.

- The primary diagnostic tests for infertility are documentation of ovulation, semen analysis, and hysterosalpingogram.

- The basal body temperature (BBT) increases when circulating levels of progesterone increase, and a sustained increase of BBT occurs following ovulation.

- A sustained rise in BBT or a serum progesterone level greater than 5 ng/ml is presumptive evidence of ovulation.

- A midluteal phase serum progesterone level above 10 ng/ml is an indication of adequate luteal function.

- A high percentage of fertile men will have at least one abnormal parameter in their semen analysis.

- In women with a normal hysterosalpingogram, a hysteroscopy is unnecessary because it will not detect additional abnormality.

- Other diagnostic tests for infertility, including (1) measurement of serum prolactin and TSH in ovulatory women, (2) a late luteal phase endometrial biopsy, (3) immunologic tests to detect sperm antibodies, (4) bacterial culture of cervical mucus and semen, and (5) zona-free hamster egg penetration test by husband's sperm have not been proven to be beneficial in determining a cause of infertility.

- There is no evidence that treatment of an abnormality in the tests just listed significantly improves pregnancy rates compared with withholding therapy.

- Of all the causes of infertility, treatment of anovulation results in the greatest success.

- When ovulation is induced with clomiphene citrate and no other causes of infertility are present, conception rates over time are similar to those of a normal fertile population.

- Discontinuation of therapy is the major reason for the reported difference in ovulation and conception rates in anovulatory women treated with clomiphene.

- More than 90% of women with oligomenorrhea and 66% with secondary amenorrhea and estradiol levels of 40 pg/ml or higher will have presumptive evidence of ovulation following clomiphene therapy.

- When conception occurs after clomiphene treatment, the incidence of multiple gestation is increased to about 5%, with nearly all of them being twin gestations. The incidences of clinical spontaneous abortion, ectopic gestation, intrauterine fetal death, and congenital malformation are not significantly increased.

- Formation of ovarian cysts is the major side effect of clomiphene treatment.

- About 5% to 10% of women treated with the individualized, graduated, sequential regimen of clomiphene citrate fail to ovulate with the highest dosage.

- Treatment of anovulation with hMG effects an ovulatory rate of about 100%.

- The pregnancy rate per cycle with hMG treatment is similar to that following clomiphene therapy—22%.

- The incidence of spontaneous abortion after hMG therapy is high—25% to 35%—and clinically detectable ovarian enlargement occurs in about 5% to 10% of treatment cycles.

- If GnRH is used for ovulation induction it needs to be administered in a pulsatile manner at intervals of 1 to 2 hours.

- For women with polycystic ovaries who do not ovulate following administration of clomiphene citrate, partial ovarian destruction by electrocautery or laser through the laparoscope is effective in inducing ovulation.

- Pregnancy rates for oligospermia following intrauterine insemination are in the 25% to 35% range.

- Semen donors need to be carefully screened to be certain that they are in good health, do not have a potentially inherited disorder, and will not transmit an infectious agent in the semen.

- Because antibodies to HIV may not develop for several months after infection, it is recommended that all donor insemination be performed with frozen sperm that has been stored for at least 6 months at which time negative antibodies to HIV should be observed in the donor before the sperm is used for insemination.

- The prognosis for fertility after tubal reconstruction depends on the amount of damage to the oviduct as well as the location of the obstruction.

- If both proximal and distal obstructions of the oviduct exist, intrauterine pregnancy is uncommon, and operative reconstruction should not be performed, IVF is the best therapy.

- Women with pelvic tuberculosis should be considered sterile, and no tubal reconstructive procedures should be attempted. IVF may be attemped if the endometrial cavity is not infected.

- Overall conception rates following salpingostomy are in the 30% range with a high percentage—about one fourth—being tubal pregnancies.

- The pregnancy rate after salpingolysis and fimbrioplasty for partial distal obstruction is about 65%.

- Unlike the results of distal tubal reconstruction, the use of microsurgery has improved intrauterine pregnancy rates for proximal tubal disease.

- Proximal tubal obstruction is now usually treated by cannulation of the oviducts with catheters or balloons placed under hysteroscopic visualization.

- The benefit of second-look laparoscopy after tubal surgery has not been established.

- Evidence that minimal or mild endometriosis is a *cause* of infertility has not been established.

- No medical therapy for endometriosis has proved to increase pregnancy rates compared with no treatment.

- Pregnancy rates for women with mild endometriosis can be increased with the use of controlled ovarian hyperstimulation and intrauterine insemination but not with danazol.

- About 65% of women with mild endometriosis and no other cause of infertility conceive without treatment. With moderate or severe disease, pregnancy rates with expectant management are 25% and 0%, respectively.

- Conception rates for women treated surgically have been reported to be in the 50% to 60% range for those with moderate endometriosis and 30% to 40% for those with severe endometriosis.

- About half of infertile women with myomas conceive after myomectomy.

- Luteal phase deficiency, as currently diagnosed histologically, is probably a normal biologic variant and not a true cause of infertility.

- No data conclusively demonstrate that the finding of antisperm antibodies in either member of the couple is a cause of infertility.

- In women with unexplained infertility the use of controlled ovarian hyperstimulation (COH) and intrauterine insemination (IUI) yields monthly fecundability rates of 10% to 15%. Therefore COH and IUI should be the initial treatment for women who ovulate, have patent oviducts, and whose male partner has at least 5 million motile sperm in the ejaculate.

- For IVF with and without ICSI the delivery rate per cycle in which ova are retrieved is about 25%.

- The rate of pregnancy following in vitro fertilization is directly related to the number of embryos placed in the uterine cavity.

- The pregnancy rate per cycle of in vitro fertilization remains relatively constant for about six cycles after which it declines. After six cycles the cumulative pregnancy rate is about 60%.

- There is a high spontaneous abortion rate (about 30%) for pregnancies after in vitro fertilization.

- If an infertile couple fails to conceive after 2 years of therapy, they should be informed the chances for conception are remote.

- The optimal treatment for all causes of sperm abnormalities is intracytoplasmic sperm injection (ICSI). With this technique, pregnancy rates per cycle are similar to that of IVF performed for other causes of infertility.

BIBLIOGRAPHY

Ahmed Ebbiary NA, Llenton EA, Salt C, et al: The significance of elevated basal follicle stimulating hormone in regularly menstruating infertile women, Hum Reprod 9:245, 1994.

Aitken RJ, Comhaire FH, Eliasson R, et al: WHO laboratory manual for the examination of human semen and semen-cervical mucus interaction, Cambridge, 1987, Cambridge University Press.

Alper MM, Garner PR, Spence JEH, et al: Pregnancy rates after hysterosalpingography with oil- and water-soluble contrast media, Obstet Gynecol 68:6, 1986.

American Society for Reproductive Medicine: Assisted reproductive technology in the United States: 1996 results generated from the American Society for Reproductive Medicine/Society for Assisted Reproductive Technology Registry, Fertil Steril 71:798, 1999.

Andrews WC, Buttram VC, Behrman SJ, et al: Revised American Fertility Society classification of endometriosis: 1985, Fertil Steril 43:351, 1985.

Argawal SK and Buyalos RP: Clomiphene citrate with intrauterine insemination: is it effective therapy in women above the age of 35 years? Fertil Steril 65:759, 1996.

Armar NA, McGarrible HHG, Honour J, et al: Laparoscopic ovarian diathermy in the management of anovulatory infertility in women with polycystic ovaries: endocrine changes and clinical outcome, Fertil Steril 53:45, 1990.

Artini PG, Fasciani A, Cela V, et al: Fertility drugs and ovarian cancer, Gynecol Endocrinol 11:59, 1997.

Baird DD, Weinberg CR, Voigt LF, et al: Vaginal douching and reduced fertility, Am J Public Health 86:844, 1996.

Balash J, Fabregues F, Creus M, and Vanrell JA: The usefulness of endometrial biopsy for luteal phase evaluation in infertility, Hum Reprod 7:973, 1992.

Barnea ER, Holford TR, and McInnes DRA: Long-term prognosis of infertile couples with normal basic investigations: a life-table analysis, Obstet Gynecol 66:24, 1985.

Bayer SR, Seibel MM, Saffan DS, et al: Efficacy of danazol treatment for minimal endometriosis infertile women: a prospective randomized study, J Reprod Med 33:179, 1988.

Berg U, Brucker C, Berg FD: Effect of motile sperm count after

swim-up on outcome of intrauterine insemination, Fertil Steril 67:747, 1997.

Boer-Meisel ME, te Velde ER, Habbema JDF, et al: Predicting the pregnancy outcome in patients treated for hydrosalpinx: a prospective study, Fertil Steril 45:23, 1986.

Bolumar F, and the European Study Group on Infertility and Subfecundity: Caffeine intake and delayed conception: a European multicenter study on infertility and subfecundity, Am J Epidemiol 145:324, 1997.

Bonduelle M, Legein J, Buysse A, et al: Prospective follow-up study of 423 children born after intracytoplasmic sperm injection, Hum Reprod 11:1558, 1996.

Bongain A, Castillon JM, Isnard V, et al: In vitro fertilization in women over 40 years of age: a study on retrospective data for eight years, Eur J Obstet Gynecol Reprod Biol 76:225, 1998.

Canis M, Manhes H, Mage G, et al: Laparoscopic distal tuboplasty: report of 87 cases and a 4-year experience, Fertil Steril 56:616, 1991.

Chaffkin LM, Nulsen JC, Luciano AA, and Metzger DA: A comparative analysis of the cycle fecundity rates associated with combined human menopausal gonadotropin (hMG) and intrauterine insemination (IUI) versus either hMG or IUI alone, Fertil Steril 55:252, 1991.

Chandra A and Stephen EH: Impaired fecundity in the United States: 1982-1995, Fam Plann Perspect 30:34, 1998.

Chung CC, Fleming R, Jamieson ME, et al: Randomized comparison of ovulation induction with and without intrauterine insemination in the treatment of unexplained infertility, Hum Reprod 10:3139, 1995.

Collins JA, Burrows EA, and Willan AR: The prognosis for live birth among untreated infertile couples, Fertil Steril 64:22, 1995.

Collins JA, Burrows EA, Yeo J, and Young LAI EV: Frequency and predictive value of antisperm antibodies among infertile couples, Hum Reprod 8:592, 1993.

Collins JA, Wrixon W, Janes LB, et al: Treatment-independent pregnancy among infertile couples, N Engl J Med 309:1201, 1983.

Confino E, Tur-Kaspa I, DeCherney A, et al: Transcervical balloon tuboplasty: a multicenter study, JAMA 264:2079, 1990.

Corson G, Trias A, Trout S, et al: Ovulation induction combined with intrauterine insemination in women 40 years of age and older: is it worthwhile? Hum Reprod 11:1109, 1996.

Cramer DW, Walker AM, and Schiff I: Statistical methods in evaluating the outcome of infertility therapy, Fertil Steril 32:80, 1979.

Cruz JR, Dubey AK, Patel J, et al: Is blastocyst transfer useful as an alternative treatment for patients with multiple in vitro fertilization failures? Fertil Steril 72:218, 1999.

Cruz RI, Kemmann E, Brandeis VT, et al: A prospective study of intrauterine insemination of processed sperm from men with oligoasthenospermia in superovulated women, Fertil Steril 46:673, 1986.

Daly DC, Walters CA, Soto-Albors CE, et al: A randomized study of dexamethasone in ovulation induction with clomiphene citrate, Fertil Steril 41:844, 1984.

Daniell JF and Miller W: Hysteroscopic correction of cornual occlusion with resultant term pregnancy, Fertil Steril 48:490, 1987.

Daniell JF and Miller W: Polycystic ovaries treated by laparoscopic laser vaporization, Fertil Steril 51:232, 1989.

Das K, Nagel TC, and Malo JW: Hysteroscopic cannulation for proximal tubal obstruction: a change for the better? Fertil Steril 63:1009, 1995.

Davis OK, Berkeley AS, Naus GJ, et al: The incidence of luteal phase defect in normal, fertile women, determined by serial endometrial biopsies, Fertil Steril 51:582, 1989.

Deaton JL, Gibson M, Riddick DH, Brumsted JR: Diagnosis and treatment of cornual obstruction using a flexible tip guidewire, Fertil Steril 53:232, 1990.

Deaton JL, Nakajima ST, Gibson M, et al: A randomized, controlled trial of clomiphene citrate and intrauterine insemination in couples with unexplained infertility of surgically corrected endometriosis, Fertil Steril 54:1083, 1990.

Dodson WC, Hughes CL, Yancy SE, and Haney AF: Clinical characteristics of ovulation induction with human menopausal gonadotropins with and without leuprolide acetate in polycystic ovary syndrome, Fertil Steril 42:915, 1989.

Dodson WC, Moessner J, Miller J, et al: A randomized comparison of the methods of sperm preparation for intrauterine insemination, Fertil Steril 70:574, 1998.

Donderwinkel PF, van der Vaart Hester H, Wolters VM, et al: Treatment of patients with long-standing unexplained subfertility with in vitro fertilization, Fertil Steril 73:334, 2000.

Donnez J and Casanas-Roux F: Prognostic factors influencing the pregnancy rate after microsurgical cornual anastomosis, Fertil Steril 46:1089, 1986.

Donnez J and Casanas-Roux F: Prognostic factors of fimbrial microsurgery, Fertil Steril 46:200, 1986.

Dor J, Seidman DS, Ben-Shlomo I, et al: Cumulative pregnancy rate following in-vitro fertilization: the significance of age and infertility aetiology, Hum Reprod 11:425, 1996.

Dubuisson JB, Bouquet de Joliniere J, Zubriot FX, et al: Terminal tuboplasties by laparoscopy: 65 consecutive cases, Fertil Steril 54:401, 1990.

Dubuisson JB, Chapron C, Morice P, et al: Laparoscopic salpingostomy: fertility results according to the tubal mucosal appearance, Hum Reprod 9:334, 1994.

Eggert-Kruse W, Huber K, Rohr G, and Runnebaum B: Determination of antisperm antibodies in serum samples by means of enzyme-linked immunosorbent assay: a procedure to be recommended during infertility investigation? Hum Reprod 8:1405, 1993.

Fayes JA, Mutie G, and Schneider PJ: The diagnostic value of hysterosalpingography and hysteroscopy in infertility investigation, Am J Obstet Gynecol 156:558, 1987.

Fedele L, Bianchi S, Arcaini L, et al: Buserelin versus danazol in the treatment of endometriosis-associated infertility, Am J Obstet Gynecol 161:871, 1989.

Filmar S, Gomel V, and McComb P: The effectiveness of CO_2 laser and electromicrosurgery in adhesiolysis: a comparative study, Fertil Steril 45:407, 1986.

Fisch P, Collins JA, Casper RF, et al: Unexplained infertility: evaluation of treatment with clomiphene citrate and human chorionic gonadotropin, Fertil Steril 51:441, 1987.

Fluker MR, Wang IY, Rowe TC: An extended 10-day course of clomiphene citrate (CC) in women with CC-resistant ovulatory disorders, Fertil Steril 66:761, 1996.

Frederick JL, Denker MS, Rojas A, et al: Is there a role for ovarian stimulation and intra-uterine insemination after age 40? Hum Reprod 9:2284, 1994.

Friberg J and Gnarpe H: *Mycoplasma* and human reproductive failure. III. Pregnancies in "infertile" couples treated with doxycycline for T-mycoplasmas, Am J Obstet Gynecol 116:23, 1973.

Friedler S, Strassburger D, Raziel A, et al: Intracytoplasmic injection of fresh and cryopreserved testicular spermatozoa in patients with nonobstructive azoospermia. A comparative study, Fertil Steril 68:892, 1997.

Gadir AA, Mowafi RS, Alnaser HMI, et al: Ovarian electrocautery versus human menopausal gonadotrophins and pure follicle stimulating hormone therapy in treatment of patients with polycystic ovarian disease, Clin Endocrinol 33:585, 1990.

Geber S, Paraschos T, Atkinson G, et al: Results of IVF in patients with endometriosis: the severity of the disease does not affect outcome, or the incidence of miscarriage, Hum Reprod 10:1507, 1995.

Gil-Salom M, Minguez Y, Rubio C, et al: Intracytoplasmic sperm injection: a treatment for extreme oligospermia, J Urol 156:1001, 1996.

Gjønnaess H: Ovarian electrocautery in the treatment of women with polycystic ovary syndrome (PCOS), Acta Obstet Gynecol Scand 73:407, 1994.

Glazener CMA, Coulson C, Lambert PA, et al: Clomiphene treatment for women with unexplained infertility: placebo-controlled study of hormonal responses and conception rates, Gynecol Endocrinol 4:75, 1990.

Glazener CMA, Kelly NJ, and Hull MGR: Prolactin measurement in the investigation of infertility in women with a normal menstrual cycle, Br J Obstet Gynaecol 94:535, 1987.

Guzick DS, Sullivan MW, Adamson GD, et al: Efficacy of treatment for unexplained infertility, Fertil Steril 70:207, 1998.

Guzick DS, for the National Cooperative Reproductive Medicine Network: Efficacy of superovulation and intrauterine insemination in the treatment of infertility, N Engl J Med 340:177, 1999.

Gysler M, March CM, Mishell DR Jr, et al: A decade's experience with an individualized clomiphene treatment regimen including its effect on the postcoital test, Fertil Steril 37:161, 1982.

Hammond MG, Halme JK, and Talbert LM: Factors affecting the pregnancy rate in clomiphene citrate induction of ovulation, Obstet Gynecol 62:196, 1983.

Hammond MG, Jordan S, and Sloan CS: Factors affecting pregnancy rates in a donor insemination program using frozen semen, Am J Obstet Gynecol 155:480, 1986.

Harrison RF, DeLouvois J, Blades M, et al: Doxycycline treatment and human infertility, Lancet 1:605, 1975.

Hatch EE and Bracken MB: Association of delayed conception with caffeine consumption, Am J Epidemiol 138:1082, 1993.

Hendershot GE, Mosher WD, and Pratt WF: Infertility and age: an unresolved issue, Fam Plann Perspect 14:287, 1982.

Holtz G and Kling OR: Effect of surgical technique on peritoneal adhesion reformation after lysis, Fertil Steril 37:494, 1982.

Homburg R, Eshel A, Kilborn J, et al: Combined luteinizing hormone releasing hormone analogue and exogenous gonadotrophins for the treatment of infertility associated with polycystic ovaries, Hum Reprod 5:32, 1990.

Honoré GM, Holden AEC, and Schenken RS: Pathophysiology and management of proximal tubal blockage, Fertil Steril 71:785, 1999.

Howe G, Westhoff C, Vessey M, et al: Effects of age, cigarette smoking, and other factors on fertility: findings in a large prospective study, Br Med J 290:1697, 1985.

Howe RS, Sayegh RA, Durinzi KL, and Tureck RW: Perinatal outcome of singleton pregnancies conceived by in vitro fertilization: a controlled study, J Perinatol 10:261, 1990.

Hughes EG, Fedorkow DM, and Collins JA: A quantitative overview of controlled trials in endometriosis-associated infertility, Fertil Steril 59:963, 1993.

Hull MGR: Effectiveness of infertility treatments: choice and comparative analysis, Int J Gynaecol Obstet 47:99, 1994.

Hull MGR, Eddowes HA, Fahy U, et al: Expectations of assisted conception for infertility, Br Med J 304:1465, 1992.

Hull MGR, Glazener CMA, Kelly NJ, et al: Population study of causes, treatment, and outcome of infertility, Br Med J 291:1984, 1985.

Hull MGR, Savage PE, Bromham DR, et al: The value of a single serum progesterone measurement in the midluteal phase as a criterion of a potentially fertile cycle ("ovulation") derived from treated and untreated conception cycles, Fertil Steril 37:355, 1982.

Inoue M, Kobayashi Y, Honda I, et al: The impact of endometriosis on the reproductive outcome of infertile patients, Am J Obstet Gynecol 157:278, 1992.

Jansen RPS: Failure of intraperitoneal adjuncts to improve the outcome of pelvic operations in young women, Am J Obstet Gynecol 153:363, 1985.

Jezek D, Knuth UA, and Schulze W: Successful testicular sperm extraction (TESE) in spite of high serum follicle stimulating hormone and azoospermia: correlation between testicular morphology, TESE results, semen analysis and serum hormone values in 103 infertile men, Hum Reprod 13:1230, 1998.

Jones WR: Immunologic infertility: fact or fiction? Fertil Steril 33:577, 1980.

Karamardian LM and Grimes DA: Luteal phase deficiency: effect of treatment on pregnancy rates, Am J Obstet Gynecol 167:1391, 1992.

Kohl B, Kohl H, Krause W, and Deichert U: The clinical significance of antisperm antibodies in infertile couples, Hum Reprod 7:1384, 1992.

Kovacs GT, Phillips S, Healy DL, and Burger HG: Induction of ovulation with gonadotrophin-releasing hormone—life-table analysis of 50 courses of treatment, Med J Aust 151:21, 1989.

Kurachi K, Aono T, Minagawa J, et al: Congenital malformations of newborn infants after clomiphene-induced ovulation, Fertil Steril 40:187, 1983.

Lalich RA, Marut EL, Prins GS, and Scommegna A: Life table analysis of intrauterine insemination pregnancy rates, Am J Obstet Gynecol 158:980, 1988.

Land JA, Evers JLH, and Goossens VJ: How to use chlamydia antibody testing in subfertility patients, Hum Reprod 13:1094, 1998.

Lang EK, Dunaway HE, and Roniger WE: Selective osteal salpingography and transvaginal catheter dilatation in the diagnosis and treatment of fallopian tube obstruction, AJR 154:735, 1990.

Larsen T, Larsen JF, Schioler V, et al: Comparison of urinary human follicle-stimulating hormone and human menopausal gonadotropin for ovarian stimulation in polycystic ovarian syndrome, Fertil Steril 53:426, 1990.

Leeton J, Healy D, Rogers P, et al: A controlled study between the use of gamete intrafallopian transfer (GIFT) and in vitro fertilization and embryo transfer in the management of idiopathic and male infertility, Fertil Steril 48:605, 1987.

Lenton EA, Sobowale OS, and Cooke ID: Prolactin concentrations in ovulatory but infertile women: treatment with bromocriptine, Br Med J 2:1179, 1977.

Leridon H and Spira A: Problems in measuring the effectiveness of infertility therapy, Fertil Steril 41:580, 1984.

Lewin A, Reubinoff B, Poratl-Katz A, et al: Testicular fine needle aspiration: the alternative method for sperm retrieval in non-obstructive azoospermia, Hum Reprod 14:1785, 1999.

Li TC, Dockery P, Rogers AW, and Cooke ID: How precise is histologic dating of endometrium using the standard dating criteria? Fertil Steril 51:759, 1989.

Lincoln SR, Ke RW, Kutteh WH. Screening for hypothyroidism in infertile women, J Reprod Med 44:455, 1999.

Lobo RA, Granger LR, Davajan V, et al: An extended regimen of clomiphene citrate in women unresponsive to standard therapy, Fertil Steril 37:762, 1982.

Lobo RA, Paul W, March CM, et al: Clomiphene and dexamethasone in women unresponsive to clomiphene alone, Obstet Gynecol 60:497, 1982.

Loft A, Peterson K, Erb K, et al: A Danish national cohort of 730 infants born after intracytoplasmic sperm injection (ICSI) 1994-1997, Hum Reprod 14:2143, 1999.

Luciano AA, Hauser KS, and Benda J: Evaluation of commonly used adjuvants in the prevention of postoperative adhesions, Am J Obstet Gynecol 146:88, 1983.

Luciano AA, Turksoy RN, and Carleo J: Evaluation of oral medroxyprogesterone acetate in the treatment of endometriosis, Obstet Gynecol 72:323, 1988.

Mao C and Grimes DA: The sperm penetration assay: can it discriminate between fertile and infertile men? Am J Obstet Gynecol 159:279, 1988.

March CM and Israel R: Gestational outcome following hysteroscopic lysis of adhesions, Fertil Steril 36:455, 1981.

Marcoux S, and the Canadian Collaborative Group on Endometriosis: Laparoscopic surgery in infertile women with minimal or mild endometriosis, N Engl J Med 337:217, 1997.

Martinez AR, Bernardus RE, Vermeiden JPW, and Schoemaker J: Basic questions on intrauterine insemination: an update, Obstet Gynecol 48:811, 1992.

Martinez AR, Bernardus RE, Voorhorst FJ, et al: Intrauterine insemination does and clomiphene citrate does not improve fecundity in couples with infertility due to male or idiopathic factors: a prospective, randomized, controlled study, Fertil Steril 53:847, 1990.

Matthews CD, Clapp KH, Tansing JA, et al: T-mycoplasma genital infection: the effect of doxycycline therapy on human unexplained infertility, Fertil Steril 30:98, 1978.

McFaul PB, Traub AI, and Thompson W: Treatment of clomiphene citrate–resistant polycystic ovarian syndrome with pure follicle-stimulating hormone or human menopausal gonadotropin, Fertil Steril 53:792, 1990.

McGovern P, Quagliarello J, and Arny M: Relationship of within-patient semen variability to outcome of intrauterine insemination, Fertil Steril 51:1019, 1989.

Meikle SF, Zhang X, Marine WM, et al: Chlamydia trachomatis antibody titers and hysterosalpingography in predicting tubal disease in infertility patients, Fertil Steril 62:305, 1994.

Menken J, Trussell IJ, and Larsen U: Age and infertility, Science 23:1389, 1986.

Merek D, Langley M, Gardner DK, et al: Introduction of blastocyst culture and transfer for all patients in an in vitro fertilization program, Fertil Steril 72:1035, 1999.

Milki AA, Fisch JD, and Behr B: Two-blastocyst transfer has similar pregnancy rates and a decreased multiple gestation rate compared with three-blastocyst transfer, Fertil Steril 72:225, 1999.

Milki AA, Hinckley MD, Fisch JD, et al: Comparison of blastocyst transfer with day 3 embryo transfer in similar patient populations, Fertil Steril 73:126, 2000.

Mills MS, Eddowes HA, Cahill DJ, et al: A prospective controlled study of in-vitro fertilization, gamete intrafallopian transfer and intrauterine insemination combined with superovulation, Hum Reprod 7:490, 1992.

Mol BWJ, Swart P, Bossuyt PMM, et al: Is hysterosalpingography an important tool in predicting fertility outcome? Fertil Steril 67:663, 1997.

Mosgaard BJ, Schou G, Lidegaard O, et al: Infertility, fertility drugs, and invasive ovarian cancer: a case-control study, Fertil Steril 67:1005, 1997.

Motta ELA, Nelson J, Batzofin J, and Serafini P: Selective salpingography with an insemination catheter in the treatment of women with cornual fallopian tube obstruction, Hum Reprod 10:1156, 1995.

MRC Working Party on Children Conceived by In Vitro Fertilisation: Births in Great Britain resulting from assisted conception, 1978-1987, Br Med J 300:1299, 1990.

Murray DL, Reich L, and Adashi EY: Oral clomiphene citrate and vaginal progesterone suppositories in the treatment of luteal phase dysfunction: a comparative study, Fertil Steril 51:35, 1989.

Noyes RW, Hertig AT, and Rock J: Dating the endometrial biopsy, Fertil Steril 39:277, 1983.

Oehninger S, Malaoney M, Veeck L, et al: Intracytoplasmic sperm injection: achievement of high pregnancy rates in couples with severe male factor infertility is dependent primarily upon female and not male factors, Fertil Steril 64:977, 1995.

O'Herlihy C, Pepperell JR, Brown JB, et al: Incremental clomiphene therapy: a new method for treating persistent anovulation, Obstet Gynecol 58:535, 1981.

Ombelet W, Vandeput H, Van de Putte G, et al: Intrauterine insemination after ovarian stimulation with clomiphene citrate: predictive potential of inseminating motile count and sperm morphology, Hum Reprod 12:1458, 1997.

Osada H, Fijii I, Tsunoda I, et al: Outpatient evaluation and treatment of tubal obstruction with selective salpingography and balloon tuboplasty, Fertil Steril 73:1032, 2000.

O'Shea DL, Odem RR, Cholewa C, and Gast MJ: Long-term follow-up of couples after hamster egg penetration testing, Fertil Steril 60:1040, 1993.

Osmanagaoglu K, Tournaye H, Camus M, et al: Cumulative delivery rates after intracytoplasmic sperm injection: 5 year follow-up of 498 patients, Hum Reprod 14(10):2651, 1999.

Palermo GD, Adler A, Cohen J, et al: Intracytoplasmic sperm injection: a novel treatment of all forms of male factor infertility, Fertil Steril 63:1231, 1995.

Palermo GD, Schliegel PN, Hariprashad JJ, et al: Fertilization and pregnancy outcome with intracytoplasmic sperm injection for azoospermic men, Hum Reprod 14:741, 1999.

Parazzini F, Negri E, La Vecchia C, et al: Treatment of infertility and risk of invasive epithelial ovarian cancer, Hum Reprod 12:2159, 1997.

Parazzini F, for the Gruppo Italiano per lo Studio dell'Endometriosi: Ablation of lesions or no treatment in minimal-mild endometriosis in infertile women: a randomized trial, Hum Reprod 14:1332, 1999.

Patton GW Jr: Pregnancy outcome following microsurgical fimbrioplasty, Fertil Steril 37:150, 1982.

Patton PE, Williams TJ, and Coulam CB: Microsurgical reconstruction of the proximal oviduct, Fertil Steril 47:35, 1986.

Peters AJ, Lloyd RP, and Coulam CB: Prevalence of out-of-phase endometrial biopsy specimens, Am J Obstet Gynecol 166: 1738, 1992.

Peterson CM, Poulson AM Jr, Hatasaka HH, et al: Ovulation induction with gonadotropins and intrauterine insemination compared with in vitro fertilization and no therapy: a prospective, nonrandomized cohort study and meta-analysis, Fertil Steril 62:535, 1994.

Plosker SM, Jacobson W, and Amato P: Predicting and optimizing success in an intra-uterine insemination programme, Hum Reprod 9:2014, 1994.

Rammar E and Freidrich F: The effectiveness of intrauterine insemination in couples with sterility caused by male infertility with and without a female hormone factor, Fertil Steril 69:31, 1998.

Ranieri M, Beckett VA, Marchant S, et al: Gamete intra-fallopian transfer or in-vitro fertilization after failed ovarian stimulation and intrauterine insemination in unexplained infertility? Hum Reprod 10:2023, 1995.

Ransom M and Garcia A: Surgical management of cornual-isthmic tubal obstruction, Fertil Steril 68:887, 1997.

Rock JA, Katayama P, Martin EJ, et al: Factors influencing the success of salpingostomy techniques for distal fimbrial obstruction, Obstet Gynecol 52:591, 1978.

Rossing MA, Daling JR, Weiss NS, et al: Ovarian tumors in a cohort of infertile women, N Engl J Med 331:771, 1994.

Rousseau S, Lord J, Lepage Y, and Van Campenhout J: The expectancy of pregnancy for "normal" infertile couples, Fertil Steril 40:768, 1983.

Ruiz A, Remohi J, Minguez Y, et al: The role of in vitro fertilization and intracytoplasmic sperm injection in couples with unexplained infertility after failed intrauterine insemination, Fertil Steril 68:171, 1997.

Sahakyan M, Harlow BL, Hornstein MD: Influence of age, diagnosis, and cycle number on pregnancy rates with gonadotropin-induced controlled ovarian hyperstimulation and intrauterine insemination, Fertil Steril 72:500, 1999.

Sakumoto T, Shinkawa T, Izena H, et al: Treatment of infertility associated with endometriosis by selective tubal catheterization under hysteroscopy and laparoscopy, Am J Obstet Gynecol 169:744, 1993.

Schenken RS and Malinak LR: Conservative surgery versus expectant management for the infertile patient with mild endometriosis, Fertil Steril 37:183, 1982.

Schieve LA, Peterson HB, Meikle SF, et al: Live-birth rates and multiple-birth risk using in vitro fertilization, JAMA 282:1832, 1999.

Schlaff WD, Hassiakos DK, Damewood MD, and Rock JA: Neosalpingostomy for distal tubal obstruction: prognostic factors and impact of surgical technique, Fertil Steril 54:984, 1990.

Schoolcraft WB, Gardner DK, Lane M, et al: Blastocyst culture and transfer: analysis of results and parameters affecting outcome in two in vitro fertilization programs, Fertil Steril 72:604, 1999.

Schwarz D and Mayaux MJ: Female fecundity as a function of age: results of artificial insemination in 2193 nulliparous women with azoospermic husbands, Fédération des Centres d'Etude et de Conservation du Sperme Humain, N Engl J Med 306:404, 1982.

Scott RT, Snuder RR, Strickland DM, et al: The effect of interobserver variation in dating and endometrial histology on the diagnosis of luteal phase defects, Fertil Steril 50:888, 1988.

Seiler JC, Gidwani G, and Ballard L: Laparoscopic cauterization of endometriosis for fertility: a controlled study, Fertil Steril 46:1098, 1986.

Sherins RJ, Thorsell LP, Dorfmann A, et al: Intracytoplasmic sperm injection facilitates fertilization even in the most severe forms of male infertility: pregnancy outcome correlates with maternal age and number of eggs available, Fertil Steril 64:369, 1995.

Shoupe D, Mishell DR Jr, LaCarra M, et al: Correlation of endometrial maturation with four methods of estimating day of ovulation, Obstet Gynecol 73:88, 1988.

Shulman A, Feldman B, Madgar I, et al: In-vitro fertilization treatment for severe male factor: the fertilization potential of immotile spermatozoa obtained by testicular extraction, Hum Reprod 14:749, 1999.

Silber SJ, Nagy Z, Devroey P, et al: The effect of female age and ovarian reserve on pregnancy rate in male infertility: treatment of azoospermia with sperm retrieval and intracytoplasmic sperm injection, Hum Reprod 12:2693, 1997.

Simon A, Avidan B, Mordel N, et al: The value of menotrophin treatment for unexplained infertility prior to an in-vitro fertilization attempt, Hum Reprod 6:222, 1991.

Simpson CW, Taylor PJ, and Collins JA: A comparison of ovulation suppression and ovulation stimulation in the treatment of endometriosis-associated infertility, Int J Obstet Gynecol 38:207, 1992.

Smarr SC and Hammond MG: Effect of therapy on infertile couples with antisperm antibodies, Am J Obstet Gynecol 158:969, 1988.

Spring DB, Barka HE, and Pruyn SC: Potential therapeutic effects of contrast materials in hysterosalpingography: a prospective randomized clinical trial, Radiology 214:53, 2000.

Stumpf PG and March CM: Febrile morbidity following hysterosalpingography: identification of risk factors and recommendations for prophylaxis, Fertil Steril 33:487, 1980.

Sulak PJ, Letterie GS, Hayslip CC, et al: Hysteroscopic cannulation and lavage in the treatment of proximal tubal occlusion, Fertil Steril 48:493, 1987.

Telimaa S: Danazol and medroxyprogesterone acetate inefficacious in the treatment of infertility in endometriosis, Fertil Steril 50:872, 1988.

Templeton AA and Penney GC: The incidence, characteristics, and prognosis of patients whose infertility is unexplained, Fertil Steril 37:175, 1982.

Te Velde ER, Van Kooy RJ, and Waterreus JJH: Intrauterine insemination of washed husband's spermatozoa: a controlled study, Fertil Steril 51:182, 1989.

Thomas K, Coughlin L, Mannion PT, and Haddad NG: The value of chlamydia trachomatis antibody testing as part of routine infertility investigations, Hum Reprod 15:1079, 2000.

Thurmond AS and Rosch J: Nonsurgical fallopian tube recanalization for treatment of infertility, Radiology 174:371, 1990.

Tomlinson MJ, Barratt CLR, and Cooke ID: Prospective study of leukocytes and leukocyte subpopulations in semen suggests they are not a cause of male infertility, Fertil Steril 60:1069, 1993.

Tsirgotis M, Nicholson N, Yang D, et al: Assisted fertilization with intracytoplasmic sperm injection, Fertil Steril 62:781, 1994.

Tulandi T: Salpingo-ovariolysis: a comparison between laser surgery and electrosurgery, Fertil Steril 45:489, 1986.

Tulandi T and Guralnick M: Treatment of tubal ectopic pregnancy by salpingotomy with or without tubal suturing and salpingectomy, Fertil Steril 55:53, 1991.

Tummon IS, Asher LJ, Martin JSB, et al: Randomized controlled trial of superovulation and insemination for infertility associated with minimal or mild endometriosis, Fertil Steril 68:8, 1997.

Van Steirteghem AC, Liu J, Joris H, et al: Higher success rate by intracytoplasmic sperm injection than by subzonal insemination: report of a second series of 300 consecutive treatment cycles, Hum Reprod 8:1055, 1993.

Varma TR, Patel RH, and Bhathenia RK: Outcome of pregnancy after infertility, Acta Obstet Gynecol Scand 67:115, 1988.

Vazquez-Levin M, Kaplan P, Sandler B, et al: The predictive value of zona-free hamster egg sperm penetration assay for failure of human in vitro fertilization and subsequent successful zona drilling, Fertil Steril 53:1055, 1990.

Vercellini P, Maddalena S, De Giorgi O, et al: Abdominal myomectomy for infertility: a comprehensive review. Hum Reprod 13(4):873, 1998.

Vermesh M, Kletzky OA, Davajan V, and Israel R: Monitoring techniques to predict and detect ovulation, Fertil Steril 147:259, 1987.

Wada I, Macnamee MCX, Wick K, et al: Birth characteristics and perinatal outcome of babies conceived from cryopreserved embryos, Hum Reprod 9:543, 1994.

Watson A, Vail A, Vandekerckhove P, et al: A meta-analysis of the therapeutic role of oil soluble contrast media at hystersalpingography: a surprising result? Fertil Steril 61:470, 1994.

Weiner S, DeCherney AH, and Polan ML: Human menopausal gonadotropins: a justifiable therapy in ovulatory women with long-standing idiopathic infertility, Am J Obstet Gynecol 158:111, 1988.

Wilcox AJ, Weinberg CR, and Baird DD: Timing of sexual intercourse in relation to ovulation, New Engl J Med 333:1517, 1995.

Wilcox A, Westhoff C, Vessey M, et al: Effects of age, cigarette smoking, and other factors on fertility: findings in a large prospective study, Br Med J 290:1697, 1985.

Winston RM: Microsurgical tubocornual anastomosis for reversal of sterilization, Lancet 1:284, 1977.

Winston RM: Microsurgery of the fallopian tube: from fantasy to reality, Fertil Steril 34:521, 1980.

Yanagimachi R, Yanagimachi H, and Rogers BT: The use of zona-free animal ova as a test system for the assessment of the fertilizing capacity of human spermatozoa, Biol Reprod 15:471, 1976.

Zeyneloglu HB, Arici A, Olive DL, et al: Comparison of intrauterine insemination with timed intercourse in superovulated cycles with gonadotropins: a meta-analysis, Fertil Steril 69: 486, 1998.

Menopause

Endocrinology, Consequences of Estrogen Deficiency, Effects of Hormonal Replacement Therapy, Treatment Regimens

KEY TERMS AND DEFINITIONS

Atrophic Vaginitis. Inflammation of the vaginal epithelium due to atrophy secondary to decreased levels of circulating estrogen.

Bisphosphonates. A new class of compounds characterized by two carbon-phosphorous bonds that inhibit the rate of bone resorption and osteoporotic fractures. Bisphosphonates approved for prevention and treatment of osteoporosis include alendronate and risedronate.

Climacteric. The physiologic period in a woman's life during which there is regression of ovarian function.

Continuous Combined Hormone Replacement. Administration of a small dose of progestin every day together with daily estrogen orally or transdermally to postmenopausal women.

Cortical Bone. Bone in the limbs (axial skeleton). With estrogen deficiency bone density decreases more slowly in cortical than in trabecular bone.

Estrogen Replacement Therapy (ERT). Administration of physiologic doses of estrogen orally or transdermally to postmenopausal women without addition of a progestin (also called unopposed estrogen therapy).

Hormone Replacement Therapy (HRT). Administration of an estrogen and a progestin to postmenopausal women.

Hot Flush. Pathognomonic symptom of the menopause; an abrupt physiologic phenomenon brought about by changes in hypothalamic thermoregulation to induce loss of body heat. Each episode lasts about 3 to 4 minutes and occurs at unpredictable, irregular intervals. During the symptomatic flush there is increased digital perfusion and increased vascular peripheral skin temperature and sweating.

Menopause. Permanent cessation of menstruation caused by failure of ovarian follicular development and estradiol production in the presence of elevated gonadotrophin levels.

Osteopenia. Decreased quantity of bone mass of a lesser amount than osteoporosis. An early state of osteoporosis with a bone mineral density T score between −1 and −2.5.

Osteoporosis. A systematic skeletal disease characterized by low bone mass and microarchitectual deterioration of bone tissue with a consequent increase in bone fragility and susceptibility to fractures. The bone mineral density T score is less than −2.5.

Perimenopausal Transition. The time between the onset of irregular menses and permanent cessation of menstruation. The average duration is about 4 years.

Premature Ovarian Failure. Cessation of menstruation due to depletion of ovarian follicles before the age of 40. It is also called premature menopause.

Raloxifene. A benzothiophene SERM that has an estrogen agonist effect on bone by suppressing bone resorption and an estrogen antagonist effect on the endometrium and breast tissue.

Selective Estrogen Receptor Modulator (SERM). Agents that bind to estrogen receptors and have estrogen agonist effects on certain tissues and estrogen antagonist effects on other tissues. SERM compounds include raloxifene, clomiphene citrate, and tamoxifen.

Sequential Hormone Replacement (also referred to as cyclic hormone replacement). Administration of relatively high daily doses of a progestin for 2 weeks or less per month together with daily estrogen for part or all of the remainder of the month.

Tibolone. A synthetic steroid with estrogenic, progestogenic, and androgenic activity. When given orally this agent reduces hot flushes, increases bone density, and does not stimulate endometrial proliferation.

Trabecular Bone. Bone in the spinal column and distal radius. With estrogen deficiency osteoporosis develops more rapidly in trabecular than in cortical bone.

T score. The difference between bone mineral density of the individual at a specific site and the mean bone density of young adults of the same gender divided by the standard deviation of this mean. The T score is expressed as the difference in standard deviations of the measured bone density from the mean value of young adults.

Unopposed Estrogen Therapy. Postmenopausal estrogen therapy given without the addition of a progestin.

Z Score. The difference between bone mineral density of the individual at a specific site and the mean normal value of adults of the same age and gender divided by the standard deviation of this mean. The Z score is expressed as the difference in standard deviations of the measured bone density from the mean normal value of age- and gender-matched controls.

The decrease in the amount of ovarian follicular estrogen synthesis occurs gradually over several years, and the permanent cessation of menses is only one facet of the climacteric process. In practice the terms *menopause* and *climacteric* are used interchangeably. The mean age of menopause in the United States is between 51 and 52 years, with a normal distribution curve and 95% confidence limits between ages 45 and 55 years (Figure 42-1). The time between the onset of menstrual irregularity and menopause is called the *perimenopause*. The median age of the onset of the perimenopause is 47.5 years, and its median length is about 4 years (Figure 42-2). About 10% of women do not have a perimenopausal transition but have regular cycles until there is an abrupt cessation of menses. Prior to the onset of the perimenopause the mean menstrual cycle length gradually decreases as a result of a shortened duration of the follicular phase (Figure 42-3).

The age at which the menopause occurs is genetically predetermined, unlike the age of menarche, which is related to body mass. The age of menopause is not related to the number of prior ovulations and therefore is not

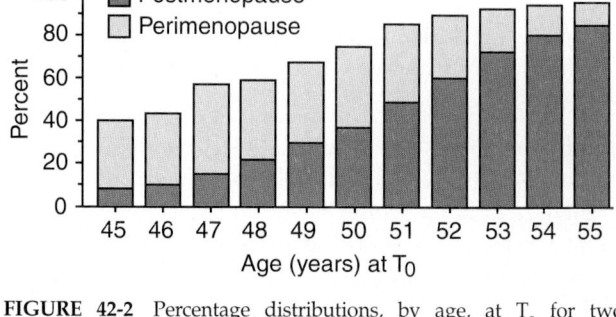

FIGURE 42-2 Percentage distributions, by age, at T_0 for two menopausal transitions, excluding surgical menopause: Massachusetts Women's Health Study 1981-82 ($n = 5547$). Median age at inception of perimenopause, 47.5 years; median age at menopause, 51.3 years. (From McKinlay SM, Brambilla DJ, and Posner JG: Maturitas 14:103, 1992.)

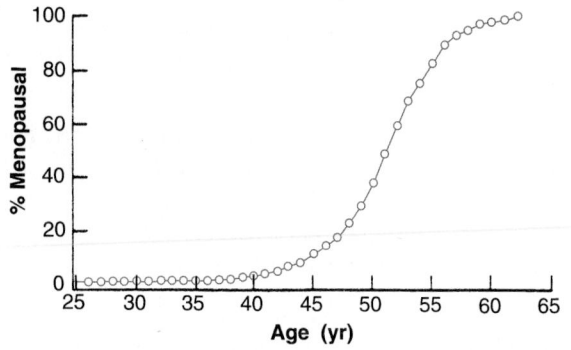

FIGURE 42-1 Cumulative proportion of women experiencing natural menopause, according to age. (From Stanford JL, Hartge P, Brinton LA, et al: J Chronic Dis 40:995, 1987.)

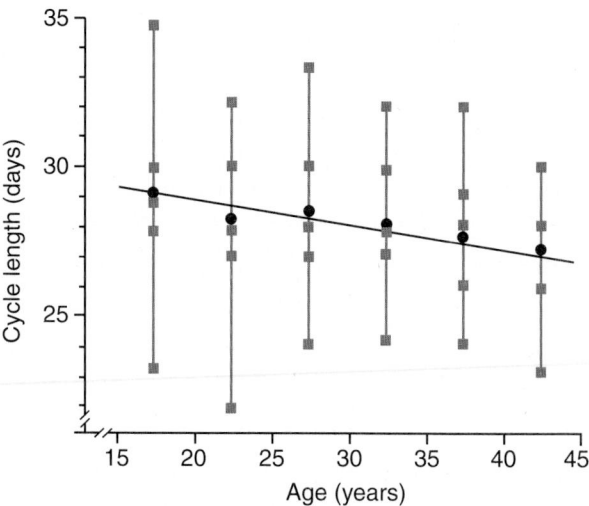

FIGURE 42-3 Usual menstrual cycle length in 1988 by age. ● = mean; ■ = 5th, 25th, 50th, 75th, and 95th percentile. (From Munster K, Schmidt L, and Helm P: Br J Obstet/Gynaecol 99:422, 1992.)

correlated with the number of pregnancies, duration of lactational amenorrhea, use of oral contraceptives, or failure to ovulate spontaneously. Menopausal age is also not related to race, socioeconomic conditions, education, height, weight, age at menarche, or age at the last pregnancy. The age of menopause has been shown to be significantly decreased by about 2 years in women who smoke cigarettes. The mean age of menopause in cigarette smokers is about 50 years. About 100 years ago the mean age of the menopause was approximately 40 years, but now it is about 51 years because women are living longer, and those who genetically would have a later menopause are now living past that age. If a woman stops menstruating before age 40, the condition should be called premature ovarian failure instead of premature menopause because of adverse psychologic connotations associated with the latter term. Menopause prior to age 40 occurs in about 1% of U.S. women, and about 10% undergo menopause before age 46. Genetic abnormalities on the long and short arm of the X chromosome are the probable cause of early menopause, and these genetic abnormalities can be transmitted to female offspring. Cramer et al. reported that early menopause, occurring before age 46, is 6 times more likely to occur in women with a family history of early menopause, and the strongest association with development of early menopause in an individual occurs among women whose mother or sister underwent menopause before age 40. If a woman continues to menstruate after the age of 55, because of a prolonged duration of anovulatory cycles with unopposed estrogen, there is an increased likelihood that the endometrium will be hyperplastic or malignant. For this reason it is advisable to biopsy the endometrium of any woman who continues to menstruate after the age of 55.

In the United States the current average life expectancy for a woman is about 78 years. About 27 years, or more than one third of a woman's average life span, is spent after the menopause during which time endogenous estrogen levels are very low. In 1990 there were 127 million women in the United States, with more than 35 million women over 50 years of age. The population of women overall, as well as that of postmenopausal women, is steadily increasing in the United States and worldwide. In 1998 it was estimated that there were more than 40 million women older than age 50 in the United States, and this number is expected to reach 60 million by the year 2020. It was also estimated that in the United States by the year 2005 25 million women will live more than 30 years after menopause.

ENDOCRINOLOGY

The anatomic and physiologic alterations in the ovary that eventually result in diminished estrogen production begin several years before permanent cessation of menstruation.

The number of ovarian follicles is steadily depleted as a woman ages. The human female has about 6 to 7 million oogonia during the twentieth week of fetal age. At birth this number is reduced to about 100,000. After menarche, as a woman ages, the number of primary follicles in the ovary gradually decreases, with markedly reduced numbers after age 40. After the menopause usually no follicles are present in the ovaries, but on occasion a few follicles may remain. Inhibin is a glycoprotein produced by the granulosa cells of developing follicles during the follicular phase of the cycle. The gonadal production of inhibin is stimulated by FSH, and inhibin suppresses pituitary FSH secretion as part of a closed-loop feedback system. MacNaughton et al. have shown that circulating follicular phase inhibin levels are significantly lower among women aged 45 to 49 than among women younger than age 45 (Table 42-1). The fall in inhibin levels may be due to the decreased number of ovarian follicles or to altered granulosa cell function that accompanies increasing age. Because estradiol levels do not undergo a similar significant decrease between ages 45 and 49, it is possible that synthesis of these two hormones are a result of separate functions of the granulosa cells. As inhibin levels fall there is a concomitant rise in FSH, which initially results in greater secretion of estradiol from the follicle. In contrast to earlier studies performed on a small number of women, which showed a decrease in estradiol levels in the perimenopausal period, more recent studies have shown that when FSH levels initially increase there is a concomitant slight increase in circulating estradiol levels and a more marked increase of urinary excretion of estrogen conjugates (Figure 42-4). About 6 months to 1 year before the menopause, as the number of follicles is further depleted, the elevated FSH levels fail to stimulate sufficient

TABLE 42-1
Mean Hormone Levels in the Follicular Phase

Age Range (Years)	n	FSH (IU/l)	INH (U/l)	E2 (pmol/l)	LH (IU/l)
20–29	9	4.9	239	149	6.1
30–39	10	5.5	235	210	5.8
40–44	9	5.2	207	152	5.3
45–49	9	13.0*	128*	130‡§	7.8†

From MacNaughton J, Banah M, McCloud P, et al: Clin Endocrinol 36:339, 1992.

INH, inhibin.

*Significant, $P < 0.05$, 20–29, 30–39, and 40–44 versus 45–49.

†Not significant, $P < 0.05$, 20–29, 30–39, and 40–44 versus 45–49.

‡Not significant, $P < 0.05$, 20–29 versus 45–49, or 40–44 versus 45–49.

§Significant, $P < 0.05$, 30–39 versus 45–49.

σ, Estimated population standard deviation. FSH, σ = 5.28; INH, σ = 83.07; E2 σ = 73.35; LH, σ = 3.80.

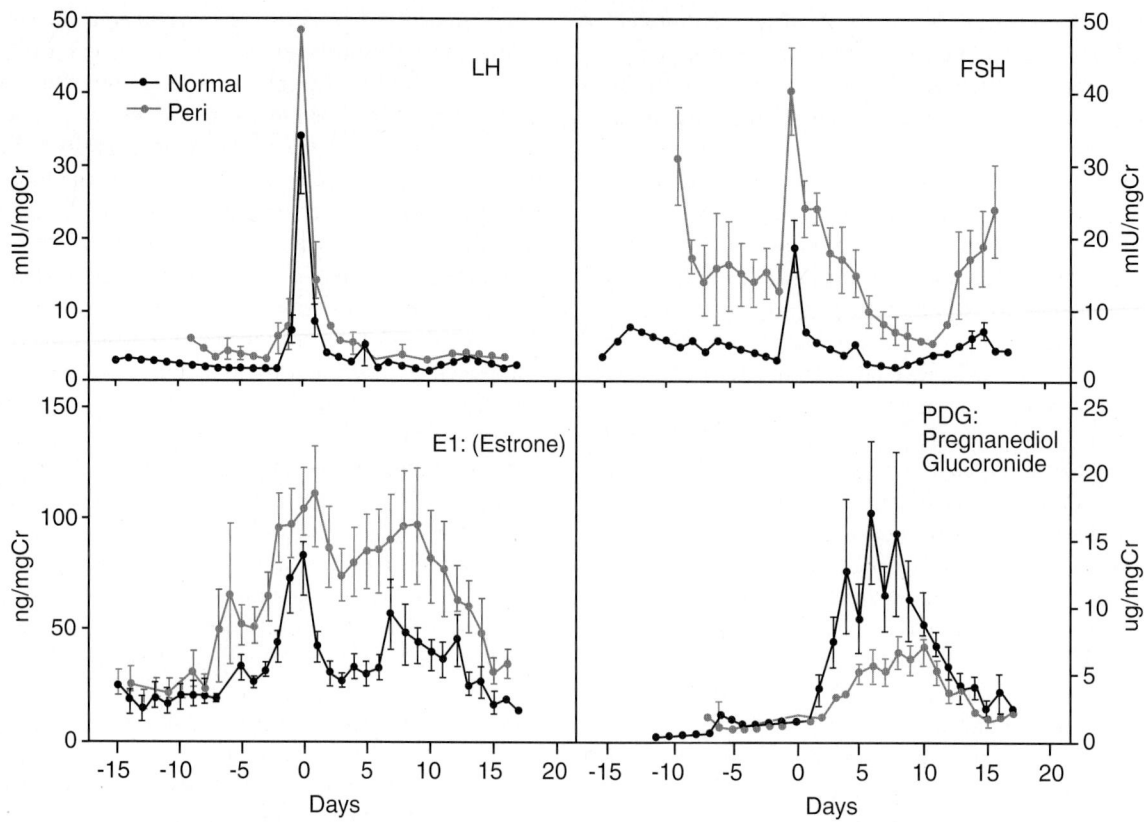

FIGURE 42-4   Mean ± SEM daily urinary gonadotrophin and sex steroid excretion patterns in 11 perimenopausal women, age 43-52. (From Santoro N, Rosenberg Brown J, Adel T, and Skurnick J: J Clin Endocrinol Metab 81:1495, 1996.)

estradiol secretion and estradiol levels steadily decline, eventually leading to failure of endometrial development and absence of uterine bleeding, clinically observed as the menopause. Thus the initial fall in inhibin levels is the first index of declining ovarian function. The accompanying rise in FSH levels, which can be easily measured, can be used as a clinical parameter to indicate that the woman has entered the perimenopausal transition. Since these initial alterations of FSH and inhibin levels are frequently transient and are then followed by a period of normal cyclic endocrinologic function it is important to determine that the increase in FSH, especially if it occurs prior to age 50, is consistently observed and is associated with low estradiol levels to verify that permanent failure of ovarian function has occurred.

Although most studies of the hormonal changes that occur about the time of the menopause are cross-sectional, Rannevik et al. performed a longitudinal study of 160 women over a 12-year period during which the women's menstrual pattern changed from regular cycles to irregular cycles to cessation of menses. These investigators did not measure inhibin but observed that a significant increase in both FSH and LH levels occurred about 5 years before the menopause, with the increase in FSH being more marked than the increase in LH (Figure 42-5).

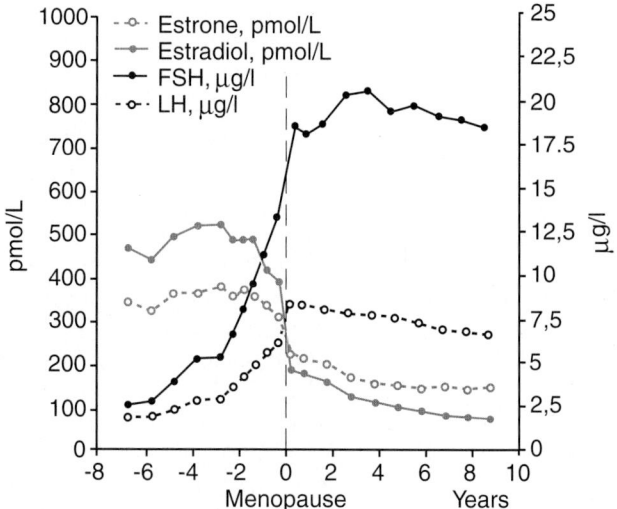

FIGURE 42-5   Mean serum levels of FSH, LH, estradiol, and estrone during the perimenopausal transition. (From Rannevik G, Jeppson S, Johnell O, et al: Maturitas 21:103, 1995.)

Levels of these gonadotrophins increased further about 6 months prior to the menopause and peaked about 1 year postmenopausally for LH and 2 to 3 years postmenopausally for FSH. Shortly after the LH peak occurs LH levels gradually decline during the following 8 years. FSH levels decline slightly from 4 to 9 years postmenopausally. The incidence of ovulatory cycles, as determined by elevated luteal phase progesterone levels, decreased from 60% during the 5 to 6 years before the menopause to 5% in the 6 months before the menopause. During the ovulatory cycles of women in the perimenopausal transition, the amount of urinary pregnanediol secretion is significantly decreased compared with earlier in life (see Figure 42-4). When estrogen levels initially fall during the 6 to 12 months prior to menopause, the estrone to estradiol ratio becomes greater, reflecting a more rapid initial decline in estradiol than estrone levels caused by the continuing formation of estrone from androstenedione in peripheral fat. Postmenopausally there is a parallel moderate decline in both estrone and estradiol levels. Administration of large amounts of oral or parenteral estrogen will not cause FSH levels to return to premenopausal concentrations. Since FSH release is mainly controlled by inhibin and inhibin levels remain low postmenopausally, FSH will remain elevated even when large amounts of exogenous estrogen are administered. Therefore, measurement of FSH cannot be used as a clinical means to determine whether sufficient exogenous estrogen is being given to produce physiologic replacement amounts. Immediately postmenopausally there are slight but significant decreases of circulating testosterone, androstenedione, and sex hormone bonding globulin levels, but between 3 and 8 years postmenopausally, levels of these three substances remain relatively constant (Table 42-2).

One of the consequences of the decrease in the estrogen-androgen ratio is acceleration of growth of facial hair, an event that frequently occurs after menopause. In postmenopausal women about 3000 μg of androstenedione is produced each day—95% of adrenal origin and 5% of ovarian origin. Androstenedione is converted to estrone in the peripheral body fat, and its rate of conversion increases as individuals age.

In a slim postmenopausal woman about 1.5% of androstenedione is converted to estrone, resulting in production of about 40 μg of estrone per day. With a greater amount of body fat, more estrone is produced. An obese woman converts as much as 7% of androstenedione to estrone, producing about 200 μg of estrone per day. For this reason obese women are less likely to develop hot flushes and other symptoms of estrogen deficiency, are less likely to develop osteoporosis, and are more likely to develop endometrial hyperplasia and adenocarcinoma of the endometrium. Slimness, however, is a risk factor for both osteoporosis and hot flushes.

PHYSIOLOGIC ALTERATIONS

Body Mass

The results of two recent longitudinal studies indicate that following menopause both body weight and total body fat increase, with a shift of fat deposition from peripheral sites to the abdomen, resulting in a greater ratio of the waist-to-hip circumference. This shift of fat distribution from a gynecoid to android type is believed to be a risk factor for the development of cardiovascular disease. The Postmenopausal Estrogen/Progestin Interventions (PEPI) Study was a randomized trial comparing effects of estrogen or estrogen plus a progestin or progesterone with placebo. At the end of 3 years women who ingested the hormones gained an average 1 kg less weight than women taking the placebo (Figure 42-6).

TABLE 42-2
Serum Levels of Testosterone, SHBG, and T/SHBG Ratio

Months Pre-/Postmenopause	Testosterone		SHBG		T/SHBG	
	n	nmol/l	*n*	mg/l	*n*	Ratio
Premenopause						
25–30	20	1.5 ± 0.48				
13–18	43	1.7 ± 0.49	17	4.3 ± 1.46	17	0.5 ± 0.22
1–6	42	1.7 ± 0.50	54	4.0 ± 1.64	21	0.4 ± 0.23
Postmenopause						
13–24	47	1.4 ± 0.47	74	3.7 ± 1.75	38	0.4 ± 0.22
37–48	29	1.3 ± 0.50	64	3.4 ± 1.41	26	0.4 ± 0.31
61–72	17	1.3 ± 0.40	42	3.6 ± 1.33	17	0.5 ± 0.35
85–96	17	1.2 ± 0.38	30	3.5 ± 1.55	17	0.4 ± 0.27

From Rannevik G, Jeppsson S, Johnell O, et al: Maturitas 21:103, 1995.

Results are expressed as means ± SD.

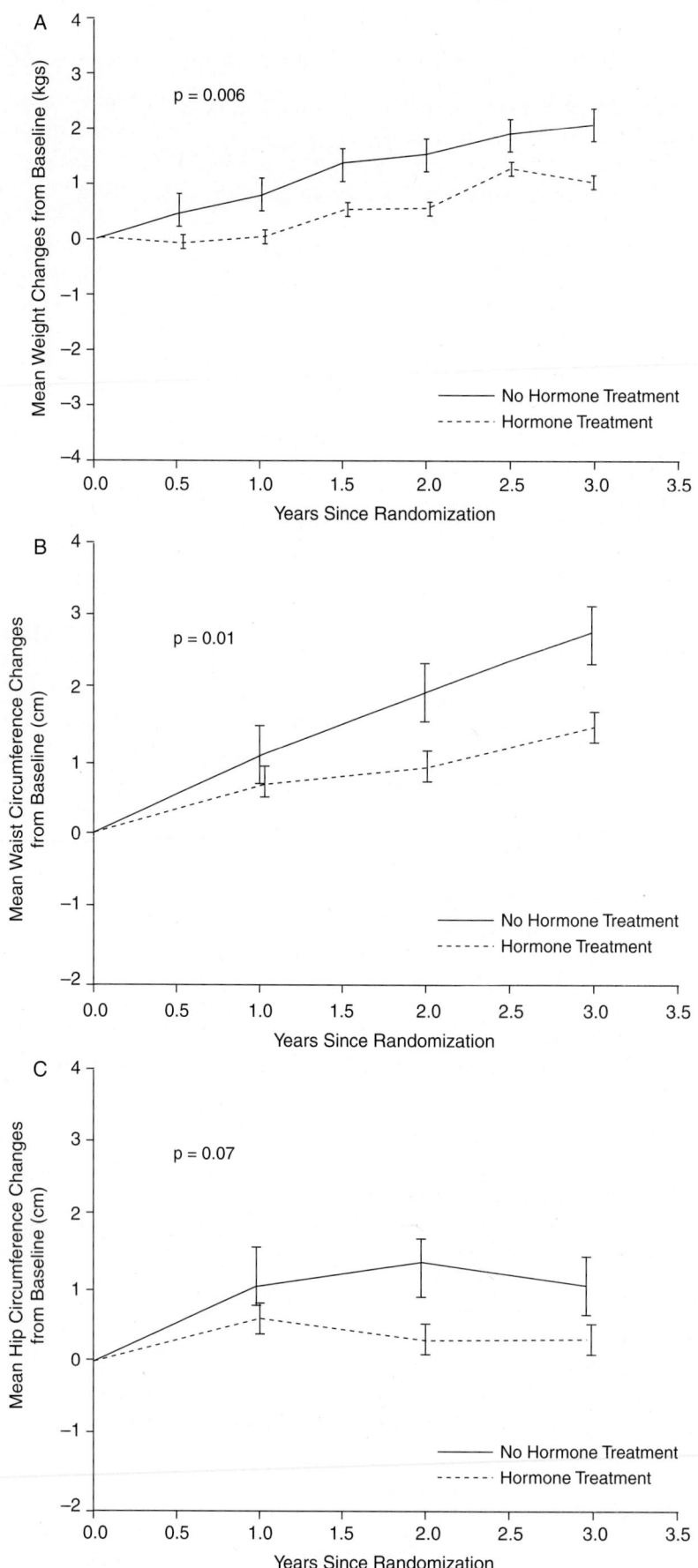

FIGURE 42-6 Changes from baseline in weight and waist and hip circumference (mean ± standard error) across time for all randomized women grouped according to treatment assignment (no significant differences were detectable among active treatment arms, *P* < 0.20. (From Espeland MA, for the Postmenopausal Estrogen/Progestin Interventions Study Investigators: Effect of postmenopausal hormone therapy on body weight and waist and hip girths, J Clin Endocrinol Metab 82:1549, 1997.)

Use of hormone replacement also reduced the shift of body fat to the abdomen with a resultant decrease in waist circumference. Another 1-year randomized trial reported similar results. Thus body weight increases as women age, and use of estrogen with or without a progestin results in significantly less weight gain than occurs without hormone use. Prevention of the shift of body fat to the abdomen may be one mechanism whereby estrogen replacement reduces the risk of cardiovascular disease.

Skin and Teeth

Most of the subepithelial portion of the skin is composed of the protein collagen. With postmenopausal estrogen deficiency the amount of collagen in the dermis progressively diminishes, the skin becomes thin, and wrinkling occurs. An early change is the development of vertical lines on the skin above the upper lip. In a cross-sectional study of the effect of estrogen on skin, Brincat et al. found that postmenopausal women who received exogenous estrogen had significantly thicker skin and a greater amount of collagen in the dermis than those who did not take estrogen (Figure 42-7). The difference became significant more than 3 years after the menopause. Estrogen users maintained their premenopausal skin thickness, whereas the nonusers had progressively thinner skin with less collagen in the dermis as they aged. These findings were also observed in a 1-year randomized clinical trial of conjugated estrogen and placebo performed by Maheux et al. In this study administration of estrogen significantly increased both the skin thickness and amount of collagen in the dermis in postmenopausal women compared with a lack of change with placebo. The results of this study indicate that postmenopausal administration of estrogen maintains the premenopausal levels of synthesis of collagen and thus prevents thinning of the skin and retards the wrinkling process. Results of three cohort studies reported by Paganini-Hill et al., Grodstein et al., and Krall et al. found that women ingesting estrogen postmenopausally are less likely to lose teeth in both the upper and lower jaw and less likely to use dentures than women who do not take estrogen. In the Krall study the number of teeth retained was directly related to the duration of estrogen use, supporting a causal relation between estrogen use and prevention of tooth loss.

Genitourinary Tract

Decreasing estrogen production leads to atrophy of the vaginal epithelium, which can produce the distressful symptoms of senile vaginitis or atrophic vaginitis. This type of vaginitis can cause itching, burning, discomfort, dyspareunia, and, with sufficient thinning of the epithelium, vaginal bleeding may occur. Senile vaginitis is best treated with estrogen replacement therapy. Local therapy can be used for the first few weeks. However, because vaginal administration of estrogen results in irregular systemic absorption as the vaginal epithelium thickens, for long-term prevention of vaginal atrophy, as well as osteoporosis and atherosclerosis, estrogen should be administered systemically. Estrogen deprivation decreases the collagen content of the structures that support the uterus, the cardinal and uterosacral ligaments, causing them to lose their tonicity, and uterine descensus may occur. Decreased collagen in the endopelvic fascial tissue in the vaginal wall may result in the development of a cystocele, rectocele, and/or enterocele. All these conditions are more often found in postmenopausal than in premenopausal women.

The cells lining the trigone of the bladder and the urethra are embryologically derived from tissue in the urogenital sinus, and estrogen stimulates their proliferation.

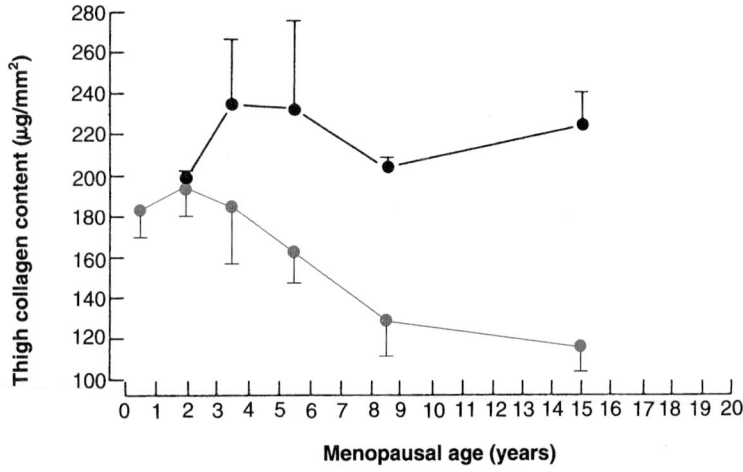

FIGURE 42-7 Relation between thigh skin collagen content and menopausal age in 52 patients treated with sex hormone implants *(black circles)* and in 77 untreated patients *(blue circles)*. (From Brincat M, Moniz CJ, Studd JWW, et al: Br J Obstet Gynaecol 92:256, 1985.)

Estrogen deficiency can lead to atrophic changes in the epithelium of these areas of the urinary tract, producing symptoms of urinary urge incontinence, urinary frequency, dysuria, and nocturia. With the decreased synthesis of collagen in the endopelvic fascia, there is decreased support of the urethrovesical junction, and with increased intraabdominal pressure, urinary stress incontinence can develop. Each of these urinary symptoms can be alleviated or prevented to varying degrees with estrogen replacement therapy. Several groups of investigators have reported that estrogen replacement results in subjective improvement of the symptoms of stress urinary incontinence in more than half the women receiving such therapy. Local and systemic estrogen administration should be the initial treatment of both stress and urgency urinary incontinence when they initially develop postmenopausally. It is also advisable that postmenopausal women perform pelvic floor exercises routinely to reduce their likelihood of developing severe stress urinary incontinence.

Hot Flushes

The pathognomonic symptom of menopause is the hot flush or flash, which is caused by a decrease in circulating estrogen levels. The change in estrogen levels leads to alterations in hypothalamic thermoregulation that are probably mediated through the central nervous system. The frequency and severity of hot flushes is directly correlated with the magnitude of the decrease in estrogen levels over time. With a sudden change in estrogen levels, such as occurs after premenopausal oophorectomy, a woman is more likely to develop symptomatic hot flushes than when there is a gradual decrease in circulating estrogen levels.

In the longitudinal study of Massachusetts women

reported by McKinlay et al., the women self-reported the incidence of hot flushes at periodic intervals as they aged. About 10% of women reported that they experienced hot flushes prior to the onset of the perimenopausal period, after which the frequency increased to about 30%. The incidence of hot flushes peaked at about 50% of women evaluated in the study in the time period just after menses ceased. The incidence of hot flushes declined from the second to fourth year after menopause, with only 20% of women reporting hot flushes 4 years after menopause (Figure 42-8). Because there is no further decline in estrogen levels more than 5 years postmenopausally, hot flushes are uncommon during the late postmenopausal years. Since estrogen levels do not begin to decline in most women until 1 year premenopausally, the development of hot flushes more than 1 year prior to the menopause is probably not due to estrogen deficiency but to other factors such as stress. Therefore exogenous estrogen should not be administered to treat these symptoms if they develop in perimenopausal women with normal circulating estradiol levels.

Obese individuals are less likely to develop hot flushes, as they do not have as great a decrease in estrogen levels postmenopausally. Erlik et al. have shown that postmenopausal women with hot flushes have lower circulating estrone and estradiol levels as well as less sex hormone–binding globulin (SHBG) bound estradiol than postmenopausal women without hot flushes (Figure 42-9). These investigators reported that women with hot flushes had less total body weight and a lower percentage of ideal body weight compared with those without hot flushes. About half of women with flushes have at least one a day, and about 20% have more than one a day. These flushes frequently occur at night, awaken the individual, and then produce insomnia (Figure 42-10).

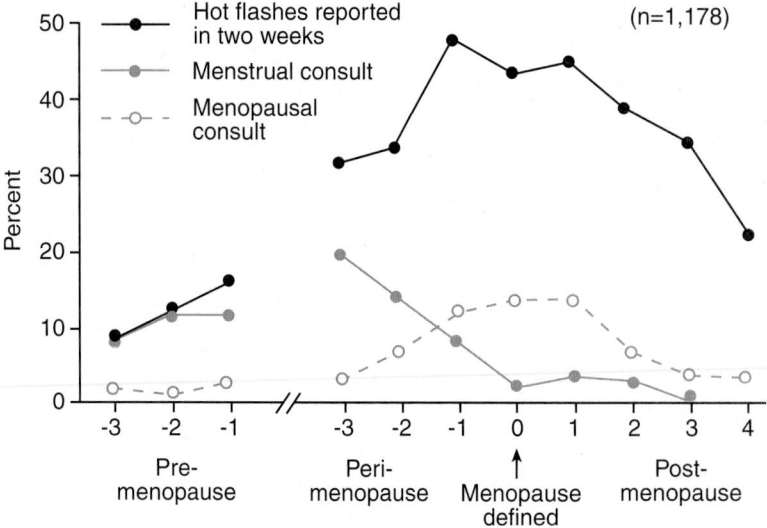

FIGURE 42-8   Relationship between hot flashes reported in 2 weeks and physician contact for menstrual problems or menopause symptoms in 9 months (*n* = 1178). (From McKinlay SM, Brambilla DJ, and Posner JG: Maturitas 14:103, 1992.)

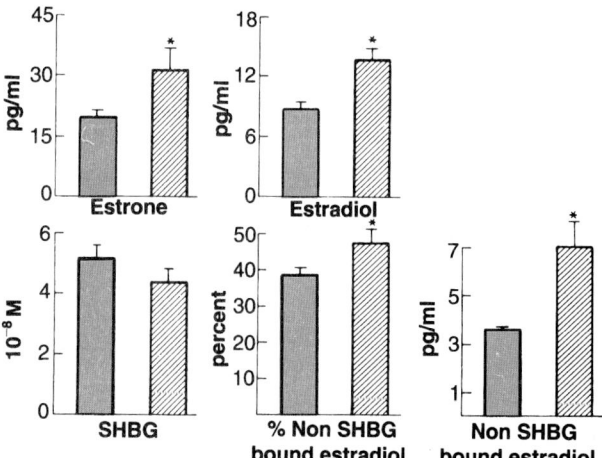

FIGURE 42-9 Mean ± SE levels of estrone, estradiol, sex hormone–binding globulin *(SHBG)*, percent non–SHBG-bound estradiol, and non–SHBG-bound estradiol in 24 women with hot flashes *(blue bars)* as compared with levels in 24 asymptomatic subjects *(striped bars)*. *, Significantly different from asymptomatic subjects. (From Erlik Y, Meldrum DR, and Judd HL: Obstet Gynecol 59:403, 1982. Reprinted with permission from The American College of Obstetricians and Gynecologists.)

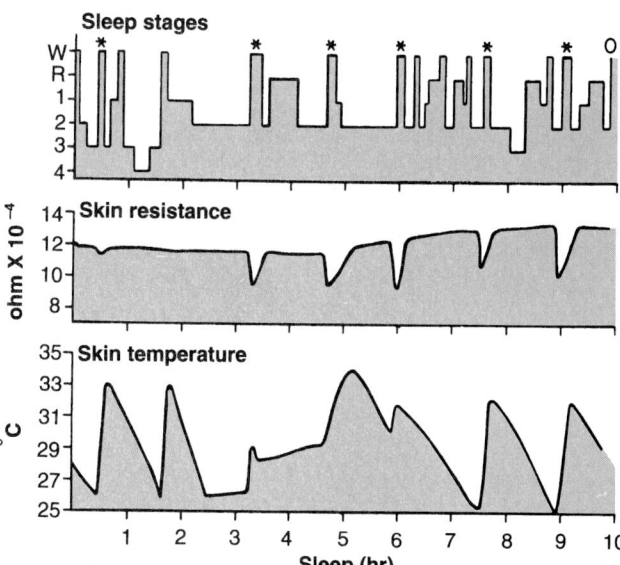

FIGURE 42-10 Sleepgram and recordings of skin resistance and temperature in postmenopausal subject with severe hot flushes. Asterisk indicates an objectively measured hot flush. (From Erlik Y, Tataryn IV, Meldrum DR, et al: JAMA 245:1741, 1981. Copyright 1981, American Medical Association.)

About one third of women with hot flushes have sufficiently severe symptoms to request medical assistance. Hot flushes do not persist in most women for more than 2 to 3 years, and it is uncommon for a woman to have hot flushes that last more than 5 years after menopause. The hot flush is an abrupt, unpredictable systemic physiologic phenomenon that takes place over a period of 30 seconds

to 5 minutes. The flush is preceded by an increase in digital perfusion, which is followed by increases in peripheral skin temperature, circulating norepinephrine and LH levels, and heart rate (Figure 42-11). With each flush there are increases in LH, adrenocorticotropic hormone (ACTH), and cortisol but not FSH or estradiol. The LH increase is an effect of the change in the hypothalamic-pituitary axis and not a cause of the hot flush, because women without a pituitary gland also have hot flushes.

The most effective treatment for the hot flush is estrogen, as Coope demonstrated in a randomized, double-blind, crossover clinical trial with estrogen and placebo. Women with hot flushes initially received either a placebo or estrogen and after 3 months crossed over to the other therapy. Although the placebo diminished the frequency of hot flushes, when the women receiving placebo were crossed over to estrogen therapy, their hot flushes disappeared (Figure 42-12). Those who were treated with estrogen first had a marked diminution of hot flushes, significantly more than with the placebo, and when they were crossed over to placebo, the incidence of hot flushes returned to prestudy levels. Results from the PEPI randomized placebo-controlled trial showed that all treatment arms were associated with a marked statistically significant reduction in vasomotor symptoms compared with placebo. No additional benefit was obtained with estrogen plus a progestin compared with estrogen alone. The results of these and other studies demonstrate that for treatment of hot flushes, estrogen is more effective than placebo but that administration of a placebo also reduces the incidence of hot flushes. Since so many of the hot flushes occur at night if the woman is taking oral estrogen, it is advisable for her to ingest the estrogen tablet before bedtime.

Initially a dose of 0.625 mg of conjugated estrogen or estrone sulfate or 1 mg estradiol should be administered orally or 0.05 mg estradiol transdermally. Frequently a higher dose is needed to relieve the symptoms of hot flushes, especially if the ovaries are removed premenopausally. If the hot flushes are not relieved by large doses of exogenous estrogen, the cause of the flush is probably due to other factors, such as stress, and not estrogen deficiency.

Some women, such as those with a recent history of breast or endometrial cancer, should not take estrogen until it is certain that there is no metastatic disease present that could be stimulated by exogenous estrogen. The best alternative treatment is a progestogen. Schiff et al. showed in a randomized, double-blind, crossover clinical trial that oral medroxyprogesterone acetate (MPA) in a dosage of 20 mg per day relieves hot flushes significantly more effectively than placebo, and Loprinzi et al. reported similar results when 20 mg of megestrol acetate were administered twice a day. Several investigators have shown that injections of depot-MPA (DMPA) in a dosage of 150 mg once every 3 months also reduced the incidence of hot flushes. Lobo et al.

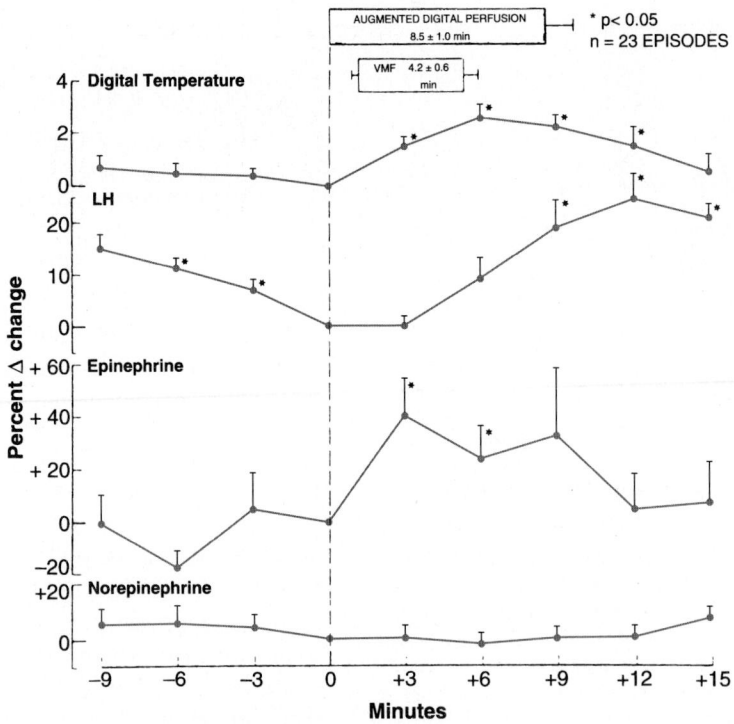

FIGURE 42-11 Composite graph of objective parameters obtained in five symptomatic postmenopausal women. Data are normalized to beginning of augmented digital perfusion *(0 time)*. (From Mashchak CA, Kletzky OA, Artal R, and Mishell DR Jr: Maturitas 6:301, 1984.)

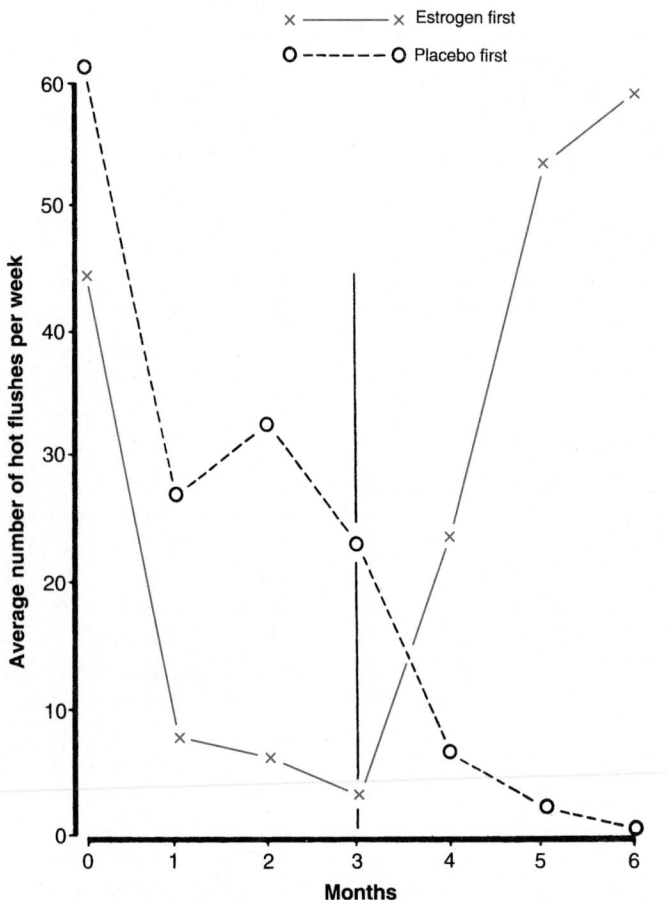

FIGURE 42-12 Average number of hot flushes per week in randomized, double-blind, 6-month crossover study of estrogen and placebo therapy. (From Coope J: Double-blind crossover study of estrogen replacement therapy. In Campbell S, editor: Management of the menopause and post-menopausal years, Lancaster, England, 1976, MTP Press Ltd.)

compared use of 150 mg of DMPA with 0.625 mg of conjugated equine estrogens for the treatment of hot flushes and found that DMPA was as effective as the oral estrogen. Other agents that have been shown to significantly reduce hot flushes more than placebo include clonidine, naloxone, and methyldopa. If there are concerns about administration of progestins to women who had tumors with progesterone receptors, oral clonidine ingested in a dose of 150 µg per day or administered via a skin patch applied once a week may be utilized to alleviate not flushes.

Bellergal, composed of ergotamine tartrate, levorotatory alkaloids, and phenobarbital, has been used to treat women with postmenopausal hot flushes. However, in a double-blind, placebo-controlled study by Bergmans et al., Bellergal was only found to be more effective than a placebo in relieving climacteric complaints for the first 4 weeks of therapy. After 8 weeks of treatment, relief of hot flushes with Bellergal was no better than with the placebo.

Other Systemic Symptoms

Symptoms such as anxiety, depression, irritability, and fatigue increase after menopause. Controversy exists as to whether estrogen relieves these symptoms directly or whether because estrogen prevents hot flushes and allows the woman to sleep better, these symptoms are relieved indirectly.

Several cross-sectional studies, as well as randomized, placebo-controlled clinical trials, demonstrate that estrogen replacement reduces the prevalence of depression symptoms among postmenopausal women. Postmenopausal women have lower levels of plasma β-endorphin (β-EP) and β-lipotrophin (β-LPH) than women of reproductive age. Genazzani et al. reported that estrogen administration to postmenopausal women increased plasma β-EP and β-LPH to normal levels. The modulation of these peptide levels by estrogen may be one mechanism whereby estrogen replacement therapy improves the woman's mood and sense of well-being, since lowered endorphin levels have been associated with symptoms of depression.

Headache is one of the most common complaints of women who seek medical assistance for any type of ailment or for routine care. Results of a cross-sectional, retrospective study by Neri et al. indicated that headaches of the migraine type usually improve or disappear postmenopausally, whereas tension headaches usually worsen or remain unchanged. This information is helpful when counseling perimenopausal women with headaches of these types.

Several studies have recently indicated that estrogen replacement improves cognitive function. Kampen and Sherwin reported that estrogen use was associated with improved performance on specific memory tests. Robinson et al. reported that estrogen use in nondemented, postmenopausal women was associated with enhanced

recall of proper names. Steffens et al. reported that use of estrogen by elderly nondemented women was associated with significantly higher scores on mental state examinations than occurred in women not taking estrogen. These studies indicate that estrogen replacement can produce beneficial effects on cerebral function in elderly women without dementia. Alzheimer's disease is the most common form of dementia. It is more prevalent in women than in men of the same age, and the prevalence doubles every 4.5 years after age 50. Alzheimer's disease, or senile dementia, is the major reason for admission to assisted care facilities. Data from 10 observational studies indicate that estrogen use reduces the incidence of Alzheimer's disease. In the two large longitudinal studies of long duration by Paganini-Hill and Kawas et al. the risk of developing Alzheimer's disease was significantly less in women who received estrogen than those of a similar population who did not take estrogen. In the former study the risk of developing Alzheimer's disease decreased with increasing duration of estrogen use. A cross-sectional study by the same authors in a different population also indicated that the use of estrogen replacement by postmenopausal women not only reduces the risk, but also delays the age of onset of developing Alzheimer's disease.

Decreased libido is a symptom frequently mentioned by postmenopausal women. Sherwin and Gelfand reported that administration of intramuscular testosterone increased both libido and coital activity, although some androgenic side effects such as hirsutism also occurred. A recent clinical trial compared the effect of transdermal testosterone administered by a patch with placebo in women with a prior oophorectomy and hysterectomy who were also ingesting conjugated equine estrogens daily. The women receiving testosterone transdermal patches had a significantly greater increase in libido and frequency of sexual intercourse than those using the placebo patch. Transdermal testosterone did not alter serum lipids or increase acne or hair growth. Myers et al. in a randomized, clinical trial compared the use of an oral estrogen-testosterone combination with a placebo and found that use of the hormonal preparation did not significantly alter sexual activity or measurements of sexual arousal. Watts et al. reported that oral testosterone decreased circulating high density lipoprotein cholesterol levels and significantly increased the incidence of acne and hair growth. Thus, although there is evidence that parenteral testosterone increases libido, data from a randomized trial indicate that oral testosterone does not have a similar effect. In addition, oral testosterone, unlike transdermal testosterone, has adverse metabolic and clinical effects. Parenteral testosterone can also be formulated in a transdermal gel or buccally administered lozenges. When so administered circulating testosterone levels increase. However little information is available regarding clinical and metabolic effects of these types of formations. The use of parenteral testosterone should mainly be used by women who have absent ovaries and complaints of decreased libido. As noted earlier there is only a slight decline in circulating testosterone levels postmenopausally in women who have intact ovaries. Testosterone is produced in the ovarian stroma, and the elevated LH levels present postmenopausally continue to stimulate ovarian testosterone secretion for many years postmenopausally.

OSTEOPOROSIS

Osteoporosis is an asymptomatic disorder, and its presence usually is not detected until a fracture occurs many years after its onset. After menopause in white and Asian women, bone density decreases at the rate of 1% to 2% a year for the first few years after which the rate of bone loss continues at a slightly decreased rate as aging occurs. Bone loss usually occurs to a lesser extent among black women. Postmenopausal bone loss occurs more rapidly in trabecular than in cortical bone, and the rate of fractures begins to increase about age 60 in structures composed mainly of trabecular bone, such as the vertebral spine and distal radius (Figure 42-13). By age 60, 25% of white and Asian women not receiving estrogen replacement develop spinal compression fractures. Postmenopausal loss of bone mass in cortical bone due to estrogen deficiency occurs at a slower rate than in trabecular bone, so osteoporotic fractures of the femoral neck usually do not begin to occur until about age 70 or 75. By age 80, 20% of all white women not receiving estrogen replacement will develop hip fractures, and about 15% of these will die from the fracture itself or from complications within 6 months. In the United States it has been estimated that annually there are about 300,000 hip fractures, about 100,000 radius fractures, and about 400,000 other fractures (mainly thoracic vertebral fractures) in postmenopausal women. Femoral neck fractures and their consequences are the twelfth leading cause of death in women in the United States. The total annual acute health care cost from osteoporosis in the United States exceeds $10 billion. An additional $2 billion is spent for long-term convalescent care for women who have suffered a hip fracture.

Nonmodifiable factors for developing of postmenopausal osteoporosis include the following: white or Asian race, family history of osteoporosis, dementia, and poor general health. Modifiable risk factors include low dietary calcium intake, low vitamin D intake, high caffeine intake, high alcohol intake, cigarette smoking, chronic corticosteroid use, low body weight (less than 127 pounds), early menopause (before age 45), premenopausal amenorrhea (more than 1 year), and a sedentary lifestyle.

Postmenopausal estrogen deficiency results in increased rates of bone resorption, while the rate of bone formation is unchanged. Riggs et al. took biopsy specimens from women with postmenopausal osteoporotic fractures and measured bone resorption and formation before and after estrogen therapy. Individuals with osteoporosis had a higher bone resorption rate than normal (Figure 42-14). With a few months of estrogen treatment, bone resorption rates returned to normal. Bone formation in women with osteoporosis was normal before and after the estrogen therapy.

Although the mechanism whereby estrogen prevents a decrease in bone density is not precisely known, it has been determined that postmenopausal serum levels of calcium and phosphorus are slightly increased and serum levels of parathyroid hormone and the active form of vitamin D (1,25-dihydroxyvitamin D) are decreased, as is calcium absorption. In addition, calcitonin levels are lowered. Serum calcium levels are maintained within a fairly narrow range and regulated in part by parathyroid hormone production. Parathyroid hormone increases serum calcium levels by three mechanisms: bone resorption, renal tubular resorption of calcium in the kidney, and production of an enzyme (1-alpha-hydroxylase) that changes vitamin D from its inactive form (which occurs in the diet or sunlight) to its active form and thereby increases calcium absorption from the gut. It has been postulated that sex steroids, including

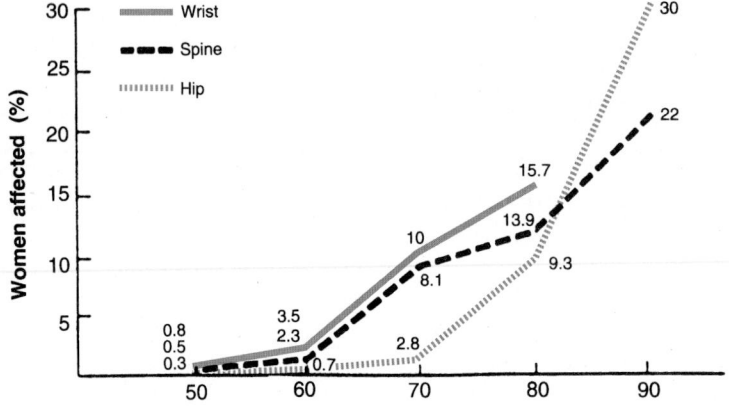

FIGURE 42-13   Cumulative incidence of osteoporosis fractures in women. (From Ettinger B: Symposium proceedings, Int J Fertil, San Francisco, April 1985, p 18.)

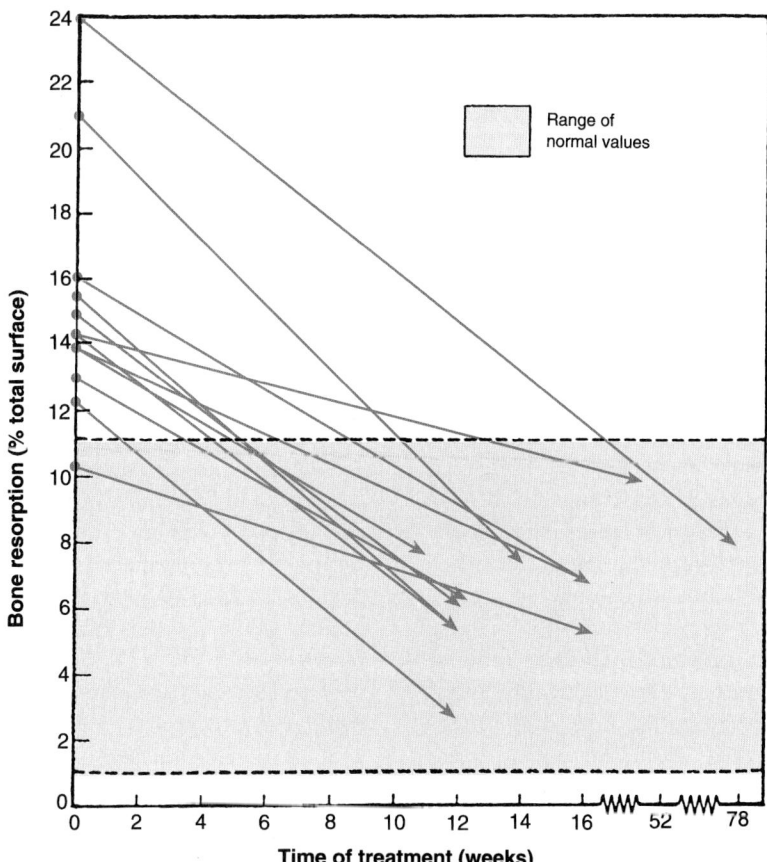

FIGURE 42-14   Effect of sex hormone on bone resorption. (From Riggs BL, Jowsey J, Kelley PJ, et al: J Clin Invest 48:1065, 1969. Copyright 1969, The American Society for Clinical Investigation.)

estrogen, androgens, and progestins, block the action of parathyroid hormone on bone, reducing the amount of calcium reabsorbed from bone. After menopause, as estrogen levels decline, there is less inhibition of the action of parathyroid hormone on bone resorption, so serum calcium levels increase, serum parathyroid hormone levels decrease, and there is less tubular resorption of calcium, resulting in greater urinary excretion of calcium. There is less formation of 1-alpha-hydroxylase, reducing the amount of active vitamin D and leading to less absorption of dietary calcium from the gut. Most of the serum calcium is then derived from bone, which causes the steady loss of about 1.5% of bone mass each year after menopause.

Human osteoblast cells have estrogen receptors, and it is likely that estrogen therapy decreases bone loss by acting directly on these receptors. Estrogen also increases calcitonin levels, and calcitonin prevents bone resorption. Therefore there may be several mechanisms whereby estrogen prevents bone loss.

At least 25% of the bone needs to be lost before osteoporosis is diagnosed by routine x-ray examination. Methods previously used to establish the early diagnosis of osteoporosis in trabecular bone, specifically dual photon absorptiometry and computed tomography (CT) scans, are complicated and expensive. Dual-energy x-ray absorptiometry (DEXA) has greater precision and can be completed in a shorter time than either CT or dual photon absorptiometry. DEXA can measure bone mineral density directly at the sites where fractures usually occur, in the spine and femoral neck, and is now the preferred technique to measure bone mineral density. Results of bone mineral density (BMD) measurements are usually expressed as T scores and Z scores. These values are the difference between the BMD of the individual at a specific site and the mean BMD divided by the standard deviation of the mean of young normal adults of the same gender, T score, or age- and gender-matched controls, Z scores. T scores and Z scores are expressed as the difference in standard deviation of the measured bone density from the mean value of the control group. Osteopenia is present when the T score is between –1 and –2.5. Osteoporosis is present when the T score is less than –2.5. Bone mineral density measurements are indicated only when clinical decisions will be influenced by the information gained, for example, when a woman will only take estrogen if there are objective measurements of bone loss in her skeleton. Bone density measurement should also be determined before initiating treatment with agents other than estrogen, such as alendronate or calcitonin, because of their expense and side effects. The National Osteoporosis Foundation recommends that bone mineral density measurements be performed on all women 65 years or older and all postmenopausal women under age 65 with at least one risk factor for osteoporosis as well as postmenopausal women with fractures and women taking postmenopausal estrogen for prolonged periods of time. Since only about 25% of white and Asian women develop postmenopausal osteoporosis it would be very useful to be able to have a substance that can be measured in blood or urine that would be a sensitive indicator of the magnitude of bone loss and thus the likelihood of developing osteoporosis in an individual woman. Measurement of serum alkaline phosphatase and urinary hydroxyproline have been used in the past to reflect the degree of bone formation or bone resorption. Measurement of these substances is too insensitive to be used as markers for the low rate of bone loss that occurs with postmenopausal osteoporosis. Therefore assays to measure other markers of bone turnover in serum and urine have been developed. Measurements of urinary excretion of two type I collagen degradation products, carboxytelopeptide (C-telopeptide, CTX) and aminotelopeptide (N-telopeptide, NTX), have been used to assess the magnitude of bone resorption in an individual as well as the response to therapies that prevent bone loss. Controversy exists concerning the reliability of measurements of these and other markers of bone turnover as clinical indicators for the development of osteoporosis in an individual woman as well as the response to the treatment. One problem is that the markers reflect the amount of bone turnover in the entire skeleton, not specific sites such as the spine and hip, the most common location of osteoporotic fractures. Furthermore there are substantial degrees of measurement error and a great amount of daily variation in the levels of the markers in urine, resulting in low correlation coefficients and limited predictive values. Therefore measurement of these markers does not provide reliable information for predicting bone mineral density changes in an individual woman. Marcus et al. assessed the association of several markers with changes in bone mineral density in a subset of women enrolled in the randomized PEPI trial. They concluded that bone turnover markers, including urinary C-telopeptide and N-telopeptide, offered little useful information for predicting changes in bone mineral density in individual women whether or not they were treated with hormone replacement therapy. Therefore DEXA measurement of bone density in the spine and hip at intervals of 2 years is considered more reliable than measurement of urinary collagen degradation products or other markers of bone turnover. It has been suggested that indications to start pharmacologic therapy include a T score lower than −2 without risk factors and lower than −1.5 with risk factor(s) or women older than age 70 with multiple risk factors without measurement of bone density.

Both prospective (cohort) and several retrospective (case-control) studies have shown that estrogen therapy reduces the amount of postmenopausal bone loss as well as the incidence of fracture in the hip and spine. Lindsay et al. performed a randomized clinical trial in a group of young women who had undergone oophorectomy. Half of them were treated with 20 μg of the synthetic estrogen mestranol and half with placebo; bone density was measured at yearly intervals. After 10 years the group receiving estrogen had no decrease in mean bone density, whereas those who received the placebo had a steady decline in bone density (Figure 42-15). Some of the placebo group developed loss of anterior vertebral height, indicating that compression fractures had occurred. Al-Azzawi et al. used dual photon absorptiometry to measure bone mass in the lumbar spine and the femoral neck in this group of women 15 years after oophorectomy. Long-term estrogen treatment resulted in greater bone mineral density in these two sites, one cortical and the other trabecular bone, in the estrogen users compared with the placebo group. In addition to this randomized trial of oophorectomized women in the PEPI randomized trial, BMD was measured by DEXA in the hip and spine of 875 healthy postmenopausal women who received either a placebo, estrogen alone, or estrogen plus a progestin cyclically or continuously. At the end of 2 years women in the placebo group lost a mean of 1.8% spine BMD and 1.7% hip BMD. In women receiving hormone therapy there was a mean increase of 3.5% to 5% spine BMD and 1.7% hip BMD. The results of these two randomized trials provide a high level of evidence that estrogen prevents postmenopausal bone loss.

One group of women in the first trial received the estrogen for 4 years and then stopped taking it. Although they did not lose bone mass in the 4 years they took estrogen, once they stopped taking it, they started losing bone at the same rate as initially occurred in the placebo group

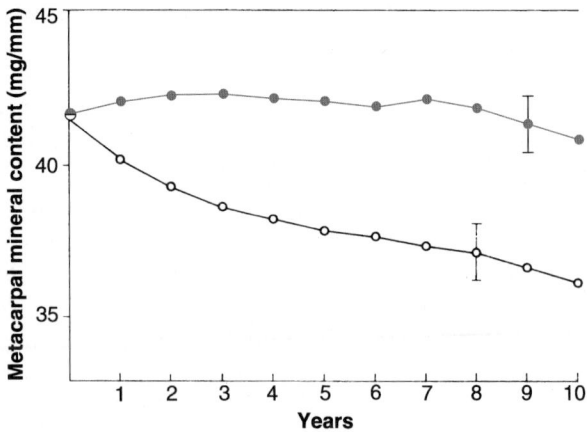

FIGURE 42-15 Bone mineral content (± maximum SE) in those treated with estrogen *(blue line)* and placebo *(black line)*. (From Lindsay R, Hart DM, Forrest C, and Baird C: Lancet 2:1151, 1980.)

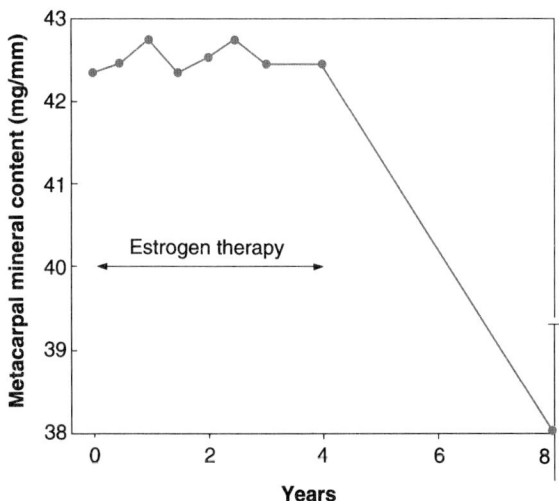

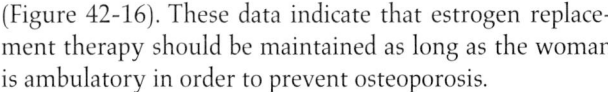

FIGURE 42-16 Effects of withdrawal of estrogen therapy on bone mineral content after 4 years of active treatment. (From Lindsay R, Hart DM, MacLean A, et al: Lancet 1:1325, 1978.)

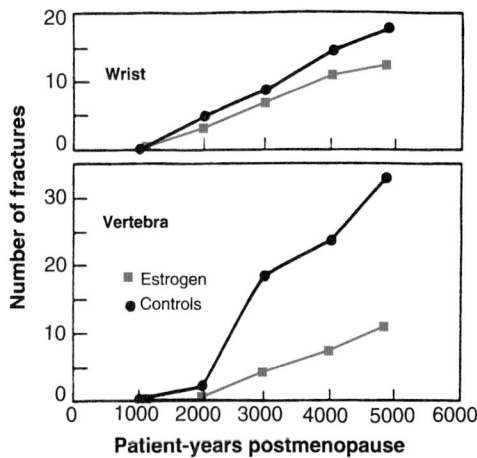

FIGURE 42-17 Cumulative wrist and vertebral fractures according to postmenopausal patient-years at risk. (From Ettinger B: Estrogen replacement therapy. In symposium proceedings, Int J Fertil, San Francisco, April 1985.)

(Figure 42-16). These data indicate that estrogen replacement therapy should be maintained as long as the woman is ambulatory in order to prevent osteoporosis.

Ettinger et al. performed a cohort study among postmenopausal women who used and did not use estrogen and found a significantly reduced risk of wrist and vertebral fractures among the group using estrogen. The number of fractures in both groups increased with the number of postmenopausal years but was significantly less in the estrogen users (Figure 42-17).

Several other observational studies have shown that estrogens reduce the incidence of hip fractures. Weiss et al. reported that a significant reduction in hip and forearm fractures occurred only among those women who had taken estrogen for more than 5 years. In this study, women who took estrogen for more than 5 years had less than half the number of fractures in these sites as the nonusers.

Cauley et al. reported the results of a long-term cohort study of 9704 ambulatory nonblack women. The risk for hip, wrist, or all nonspinal fractures was reduced by 30% to 40% among current estrogen users but not past estrogen users, compared with never users. Women who began estrogen use soon after menopause and continued its use for 10 years or more, but then stopped using it, were no longer protected against nonspinal fractures several years after stopping estrogen treatment. Estrogen alone and estrogen-progestin therapy were equally effective in reducing fracture risk and had similar effects for preserving bone mass. The association between current estrogen and reduced risk of hip fracture only occurred among women over age 75. In long-term current users of estrogen, there was more than an 80% reduction in hip fractures after age 75 compared with women who did not take estrogen replacement. The greatest benefit of estrogen

replacement therapy occurred when it was initiated early in menopause and diminished if it was initiated more than 5 years after menopause. The combination of early initiation and long term use resulted in a 50% reduction in all nonspinal fracture risk. The authors concluded that current use of estrogen reduces the risk of hip, wrist, and all nonspinal fractures and that this benefit is maximized when therapy begins within 5 years of menopause and is continued for more than 10 years. Because the incidence of hip fracture begins to increase at an exponential rate after age 70, this finding has both great public health and clinical significance. In order to provide the greatest reduction in risk of developing hip fractures when elderly, women should start estrogen or estrogen-progestin treatment shortly after the menopause and continue taking it until they are in their 70s. However there are data which indicate that if ERT is started before ages 60 to 70 years and used continuously, there is an increase in BMD. These findings support the belief that it is beneficial to initially start ERT in a woman aged 60 to 70 years to protect the skeleton from further bone loss and, probably, osteoporotic fractures.

Studies in which bone density was measured over time have shown the minimal dosage of estrogen needed to prevent bone loss in most women is 0.625 mg of conjugated equine estrogens or estrone sulfate or 0.5 mg of micronized estradiol. Higher doses of conjugated equine estrogen do not increase bone density, but some studies now show that when women also ingest 1500 mg of calcium daily, bone loss is prevented with only 0.3 mg of conjugated equine estrogen or esterified estrogens. Transdermal administration of 0.05 mg of estradiol daily also prevents bone loss. These dosages of the various types of estrogen replacement therapy should be considered the physiologic replacement doses of estrogen to administer to asymptomatic postmenopausal women at risk for developing postmenopausal osteoporosis.

Indirect evidence suggests that progestins by themselves also reduce the rate of bone reabsorption because they decrease the amount of urinary calcium excretion. Studies by several investigators have demonstrated that both the sequential and the continuous administration of a progestin with an estrogen prevents loss of bone density and may actually increase bone density slightly, suggesting a synergistic action of the progestin with the estrogen. Therefore addition of a progestin to estrogen replacement therapy does not inhibit, and may augment, the beneficial effect of estrogen on reducing the rate of bone resorption.

Several investigators have shown that dietary calcium supplementation without estrogen does not completely prevent postmenopausal bone loss but may decrease the rate that bone density is decreased postmenopausally compared with no calcium supplementation. Riis et al. and Ettinger et al., among others, have shown that 2 years' ingestion of 1500 or 2000 mg calcium daily, without estrogen, by postmenopausal women resulted in a similar decrease in density of trabecular bone as occurred in women receiving no calcium supplementation without estrogen (Figure 42-18). Reid et al. and Prince et al., among others, have shown that large doses of calcium supplementation reduced the amount of bone loss compared with placebo. Aloia et al. reported that 1700 mg of calcium supplementation retarded but did not prevent loss of bone, particularly the trabecular bone in the spine. In contrast, hormone replacement therapy prevented loss of bone for 3 years in both trabecular and cortical bone (Figure 42-19). The results of this study provide additional data indicating that high doses of calcium supplementa-

tion, even with additional supplements of vitamin D and weight-bearing exercise, retard but do not prevent bone loss in postmenopausal women not receiving estrogen replacement.

Ingesting the recommended daily intake of dietary calcium (1200 to 1500 mg/day) during the adolescent years results in greater peak adult bone mass than occurs if insufficient calcium is ingested. Thus postmenopausally, women who have ingested the recommended dietary intake of calcium during their adolescent years are less likely to have sufficient reduction in bone density to cause fractures than those ingesting insufficient calcium during this stage of life (Figure 42-20).

Results of a National Institutes of Health (NIH) consensus panel on optimal calcium intake were published in 1994. This panel recommended that postmenopausal women between ages 50 and 65 taking estrogen ingest 1000 mg of calcium daily while those in this age group not taking estrogen and all women over age 65 ingest 1500 mg of calcium per day (Table 42-3). Published data regarding the need for calcium supplementation in postmenopausal women receiving estrogen replacement do not support these recommendations. Stevenson et al. reported that no significant differences in the changes in bone density occurred among a group of postmenopausal women with and without estrogen treatment who ingested a mean of 500 mg of calcium daily compared with those who ingested a mean of 1600 mg daily. However, Dawson-Hughes et al. reported that postmenopausal women with a daily calcium intake of only 400 mg could significantly reduce bone loss by increasing their calcium intake to 800 mg/day by ingesting 500 mg calcium citrate malate daily. It thus appears that for postmenopausal women ingesting a sufficient amount of calcium in their diet, more than 500 to 800 mg daily, calcium supplementation is unnecessary, if they are also receiving estrogen. Calcium supplementation is mainly of benefit for those women who have an inadequate daily ingestion of less than 500 mg/day

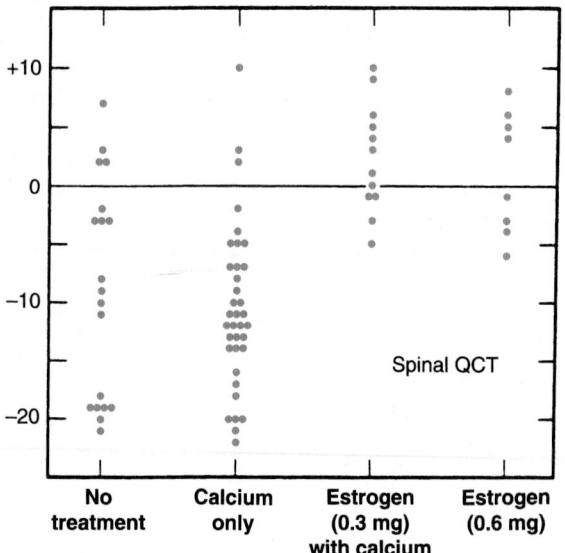

FIGURE 42-18 Skeletal changes in women after 2 years of calcium ingestion, expressed as a percentage of baseline values. (From Ettinger B, Genant HK, and Cann CE: Ann Intern Med 106:40, 1987.)

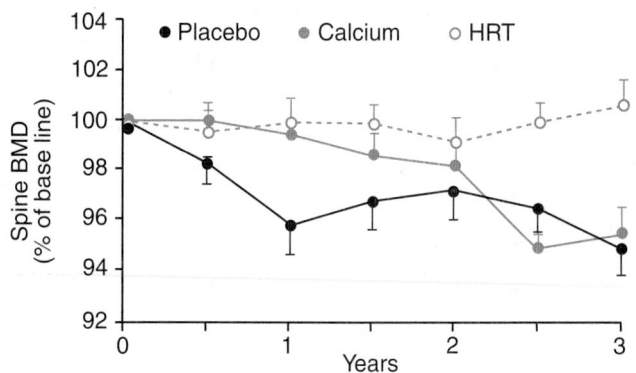

FIGURE 42-19 The biannual rates of change in bone mineral density of the lumbar spine. (From Aloia JF, Vaswani A, Yeh JK, et al: Ann Intern Med 120:97, 1994.)

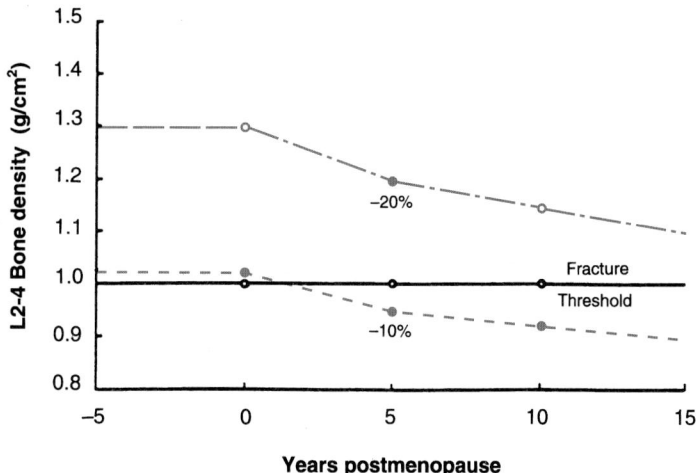

FIGURE 42-20 Effect of peak bone mass. *Upper line* represents bone density in woman with high peak bone mass who loses 20% of bone density after menopause. *Lower line* represents bone density in woman with low peak bone mass who loses only 10% of bone density postmenopausally but becomes osteoporotic. (From Stevenson JC: Obstet Gynecol 175:36S, 1990.)

TABLE 42-3
Optimal Calcium Requirements Recommended by the National Institutes of Health Consensus Panel

Age Group	Optimal Daily Intake of Calcium, mg
Infant	
Birth–6 mo	400
6 mo–1 yr	600
Children	
1–5 yr	800
6–10 yr	800–1200
Adolescents/young adults	
11–24 yr	1200–1500
Men	
25–65 yr	1000
Over 65 yr	1500
Women	
25–50 yr	1000
Over 50 yr (postmenopausal)	
On estrogens	1000
Not on estrogens	1500
Over 65 yr	1500
Pregnant and nursing	1200–1500

From NIH Consensus Development Panel on Optimal Calcium Intake. JAMA 272:1941, 1994.

dietary calcium. It is preferable to maintain adequate intake of calcium by eating foods containing this mineral than by supplemental calcium sources. Curhan et al. reported that women ingesting large amounts of dietary calcium had a reduced incidence of kidney stones, whereas those receiving calcium supplementation had an increased risk of developing renal calculi. Foods rich in calcium are shown in Table 42-4.

All individuals need sufficient amounts of vitamin D, about 400 to 800 IU/daily, to ensure that dietary calcium is absorbed. Individuals with insufficient dietary vitamin D intake or those not exposed to sunlight, such as institutionalized women, should receive supplementary vitamin D to improve calcium balance and possibly reduce fracture risk.

Exercise in the premenopausal years increases bone density. However, weight-bearing exercise alone will not prevent postmenopausal bone loss. Studies by Cavanaugh et al. and Sinaki et al. reported that neither a program of brisk walking nor nonloading back exercise altered the rate of trabecular bone loss postmenopausally. Prince et al. reported that a moderate exercise program with or without dietary calcium supplementation does not prevent the loss of bone mass in the early postmenopausal years, but estrogen plus progestin and exercise prevented loss of bone in the forearm (Figure 42-21). Because exercise is beneficial for a woman's overall health, postmenopausal women should be encouraged to walk daily or do other types of exercise routinely.

In summary, estrogen replacement increases calcium absorption and reduces the rate of bone resorption. Estrogen will not stimulate new bone growth but will stabilize osteoporosis if it is present and, most importantly, will prevent osteoporosis if therapy is started at the time of menopause. For women at the greatest risk to develop osteoporosis, specifically thin white or Asian women, estrogen replacement is the optimal means to prevent postmenopausal bone loss. For women with contraindications for estrogen replacement who are losing bone or already have osteoporosis, the bisphosphates alendronate and risedronate also suppress bone resorption. Both these agents have been shown to prevent bone resorption and reduce the incidence of vertebral and nonvertebral fractures in randomized placebo-controlled trials. The recommended dose of alendronate is 5 mg/day for osteoporosis prevention and 10 mg/day for treatment of osteoporosis. The dose of risedronate is 5 mg/day for both indications. Both agents can produce esophageal irritation and need to be ingested daily with 6 to 8 ounces of plain water at least 30 minutes before ingesting food or other beverage. The subjects need to remain in an upright position for at least 30 minutes after drug ingestion and until they have ingested food to enhance absorption. There are no clinical studies comparing the efficacy and side effects of these two agents, both of which inhibit the increased rate of bone resorption that occurs postmenopausally. Calcitonin administered by a daily nasal spray in a dose of 200 µg is also approved for the treatment of osteoporosis if the patient refuses or cannot tolerate estrogen. Nassal calcitonin has been shown to increase vertebral bone mass compared with placebo.

Selective estrogen receptor modulators (SERMs) are agents that have estrogen agonist effects on certain tissues and estrogen antagonist effects on other tissues. Examples of SERMs include clomiphene citrate, tamoxifen, and raloxifene hCl. Raloxifene has estrogen agonist effects on bone and antagonist effects on the breast, endometrium, vagina, and vasomotor symptoms. When given in a dose of 60 mg daily raloxifene prevents bone loss and also reduces the risk of vertebral fracture in women with and without osteoporotic fractures. There are no data currently available that show a protection against hip fracture with raloxifene as has been observed with estrogen. Furthermore in trials in which estrogen use was compared with alendronate or raloxifene, increases in bone mineral density were greater or similar with estrogen than the use of the other agents.

TABLE 42-4
Sources of High Dietary Calcium

Product	Calcium (mg)	Product	Calcium (mg)
Milk		**Fruit juice**	
Whole (3.3% fat), 1 cup	291	Orange (calcium fortified), 8 oz	300
Low fat (2% fat), 1 cup	297	**Seafood**	
Nonfat (skim), 1 cup	302		
Buttermilk, 1 cup	285	Sardines (with bones), 4 oz	496
Chocolate, 1 cup	284	Salmon (pink, canned), 6 oz	333
Cheese		Oysters (fresh, raw), 8 oz	213
		Shrimp (canned), 3 oz	98
American, 1 oz	163	Lobster, 3 oz	55
Blue, 1 oz	150	**Nuts**	
Cheddar, 1 oz	205		
Swiss, 1 oz	273	Almonds, 1/2 cup	152
Cottage, low fat, 1/2 cup	77	Peanuts (roasted), 1 cup	104
Edam, 1 oz	208	Brazil nuts (shelled), 1/2 cup	130
Feta, 1 oz	140	Soybean nuts, 1/2 cup	75
Gruyere, 1 oz	287	**Vegetables***	
Mozzarella, part skim, 1 oz	183		
Muenster, 1 oz	204	Mustard greens, 1 cup	193
Yogurt		Broccoli, 1 cup	136
		Okra, 1 cup	147
Whole, plain, 8 oz	274	Bok choy, 1/2 cup	126
Low fat, plain, 8 oz	415	Collards (raw), 1/2 cup	179
Nonfat, plain, 8 oz	452	Collards (frozen), 1/2 cup	149
Flavored, low fat, 1 cup	389	Turnip greens (raw), 1/2 cup	126
Frozen dairy			
Ice cream, vanilla, 1 cup	176		
Ice milk, vanilla, 1 cup	176		
Frozen yogurt, vanilla, 1 cup	249		

From Menopause Management 3:15, 1990.

*High calcium foods such as spinach, Swiss chard, and beet greens are not included because they have a high content of oxalic acid, which binds to calcium, making it poorly absorbed by the body.

Lindsey et al. reported that in women with established osteoporosis the combination of estrogen and alendronate increased bone density more than estrogen alone. However there was not a significant difference in new fracture risk between the two regimens in this 1-year clinical trial.

Another agent that prevents osteoporosis and reduces fracture risk is tibolone. This drug has estrogenic, androgenic, and progestogenic action. It is not yet approved for use in the United States but has been available in Europe

for several years. Tibolone reduces vasomotor symptoms but does not stimulate endometrial proliferation.

ATHEROSCLEROSIS

Under the age of 50, men have about a threefold greater incidence of myocardial infarction (MI) than women. In both sexes the incidence increases with age, but the rate of increase is greater in women after age 50 than in men. As a result, the ratio of MI in women to men after age 50 decreases to 2:1 by age 65 and 1:1 by age 80.

Although no randomized clinical trials comparing estrogen with placebo on the risk of MI have been completed, an abundance of observational epidemiologic data indicates that estrogen replacement therapy retards the development of atherosclerosis in postmenopausal women and reduces their risks of developing MI.

Grodstein and Stampfer performed a meta-analysis of 31 observational studies of both case-control and cohort designs. There was approximately a 50% reduction in risk of MI among current estrogen users compared with nonusers (relative risk [RR], 0.5; 95% confidence interval [CI], 0.45 to 0.09) (Figure 42-22). Ever users of estrogen, including current and past users, had about a 36% reduction in risk of MI (RR, 0.64 [CI, 0.69 to 0.68]).

In a prospective cohort study reported by Bush et al. in every 10-year age category over the age of 50 years, the estrogen users had significantly lower cardiovascular mortality rates than nonusers. After adjustment for age, the relative risk of death from cardiovascular disease in the estrogen users compared with the nonusers was 0.34 (95% confidence interval, 0.12 to 0.81) (Table 42-5). The difference in fatal cardiovascular disease was a result of lower rates than expected in the estrogen users rather than higher rates than expected in the nonusers.

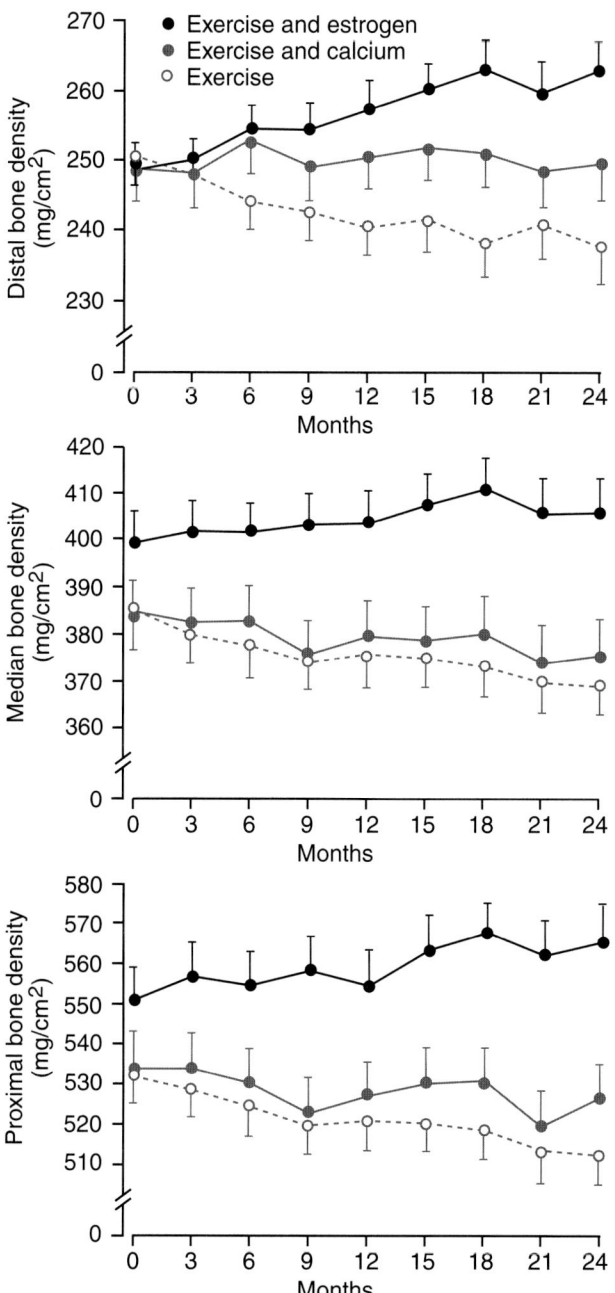

FIGURE 42-21 Effects of the three interventions on bone density at distal, median, and proximal forearm areas during the 2-year study period. (From Prince RL, Smith M, Dick IM, et al: N Engl J Med 325:1189, 1991.)

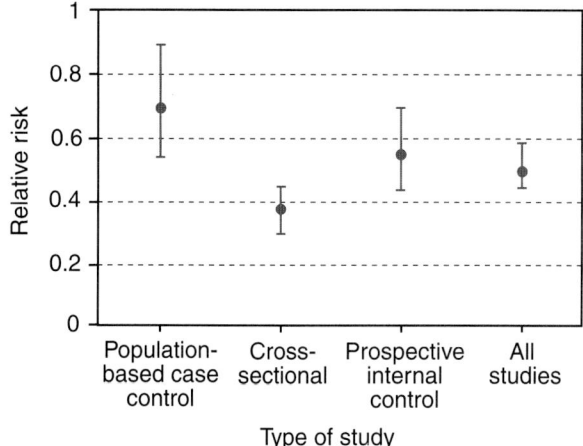

FIGURE 42-22 Summary of studies of heart disease and estrogen in those women currently using estrogen. (From Grodstein F and Stampfer M: Prog Cardiovasc Dis 38(3):199, 1995.)

TABLE 42-5
Cardiovascular Disease Death Rates (per 10,000) According to Estrogen Use

| | Estrogen Use | |
Age at Risk	Nonuser (N = 1677)	User (N = 593)
40–49	0.0	0.0
50–59	16.2	4.5
60–69	39.1	11.8
70–79	150.8	61.7
Crude rate	30.9	11.7
Age-adjusted rate	38.1	13.1
Relative risk (95% confidence interval)		0.34 (0.12–0.81)

From Bush TL, Barrett-Connor E, Cowan LD, et al: Circulation 75:1104, 1987.

Estrogen use also significantly reduced the risk of death from cardiovascular disease in postmenopausal women who were current smokers and in women in whom clinical cardiovascular disease was already present.

Henderson et al. prospectively followed 8841 women residing in a retirement community and found a significant reduction of deaths from acute MI among estrogen users than nonusers (relative risk, 0.59). Current estrogen users had the greatest protection from death from coronary artery disease, with a relative risk of 0.47, and former estrogen recipients had a relative risk of 0.62 when compared with those who had never used estrogen. Adjust-

ment for the presence of known risk factors for cardiovascular disease, including a history of high blood pressure, a history of angina or acute MI, and smoking, did not alter the protection of the cardiovascular system derived from estrogen therapy for postmenopausal women.

The Nurses' Health Study is a cohort study of 59,370 postmenopausal female registered nurses. Although not a randomized clinical trial, this study is the largest and most carefully performed prospective study of the effects of estrogen on postmenopausal women. In 1996 Grodstein et al. published results of an analysis of data from this study and reported that the risk of major coronary disease adjusted for cardiovascular risk factors, such as body mass and smoking, among current estrogen users compared with that of women in this study who had never used estrogen was 0.60. Among women who were using estrogen plus progestins compared with nonhormone users the risk for coronary disease was 0.39 (Table 42-6). Women who had used hormones in the past but had stopped using them had a gradual decrease in their cardiovascular beneficial effect with increasing time since last use (Figure 42-23).

Additional evidence from studies of women undergoing coronary artery angiography supports the belief that estrogen use retards the development of atherosclerosis. In a retrospective study of a large number of women who had coronary angiography for chest pain, Gruchow et al. reported that the mean amount of coronary artery occlusion did not increase after age 60 among estrogen users, compared with younger women (Figure 42-24). Among a group of women not taking estrogen the mean amount of occlusion increased as they aged and was significantly greater than among the women who took estrogen after age 60.

TABLE 42-6
Relative Risk of Cardiovascular Disease among Current Users of Conjugated Estrogen Alone or with Progestin Compared with Nonusers, 1978 to 1992*

| | | | Major Coronary Disease | |
| | | | Relative Risk (95% CI) | |
Hormone Use	Person-Years	No. of Cases	Age Adjusted	Multivariate Adjusted†
Never used	304,744	431		1.0
Currently used				
Estrogen alone	82,626	47	0.45 (0.34–0.60)	0.60 (0.43–0.83)
Estrogen with progestin	27,161	8	0.22 (0.12–0.41)	0.39 (0.19–0.78)

From Grodstein F, Stampfer MJ, Manson JE, et al: N Engl J Med 335:453, 1996.

*CI, confidence interval.

†The analysis was adjusted for age (in 5-year categories), time (in 2-year categories), age at menopause (in 2-year categories), body-mass index (in quintiles), diabetes (yes or no), high blood pressure (yes or no), high cholesterol level (yes or no), cigarette smoking (never, formerly, or currently [1 to 14, 15 to 24, or 25 or more cigarettes per day]) past oral-contraceptive use (yes or no), parental history of myocardial infarction before the age of 60 years (yes or no), and type of menopause (natural or surgical).

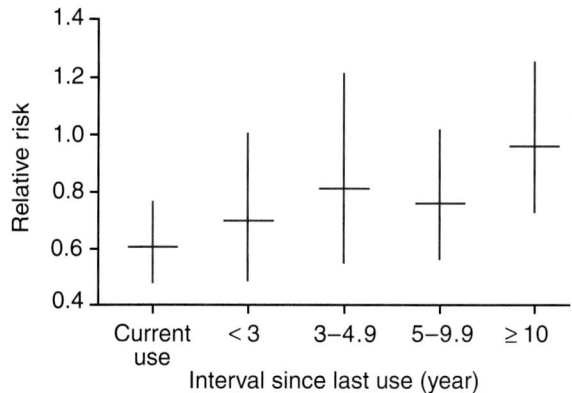

FIGURE 42-23 Relative risk of major coronary heart disease among current hormone users and among past users, according to the interval since last use. Data are for the period from 1976 to 1992. *Horizontal bars* indicate relative risks, and *vertical bars* 95 percent confidence intervals. (From Grodstein F, Stampfer MJ, Manson JE, et al: N Engl J Med 335:453, 1996.)

McFarland et al. reported that among 345 women undergoing coronary artery catheterization for suspected MI, estrogen users were only half as likely as nonusers to have severe coronary artery disease (more than 70% occlusion). Sullivan et al. performed a retrospective 10-year follow-up of 2268 women who had coronary angiography. Survival rates at 10 years were significantly higher among estrogen users with both mild to moderate as well as severe degrees of coronary artery occlusion. In the latter group the 10-year survival rate was only 60% among estrogen nonusers whereas it was 97% among estrogen users (Figure 42-25). After appropriate adjustment for other risk factors, estrogen was found to have a significant

independent effect on survival. Two retrospective observational studies by O'Keefe et al. and Newton et al. reported that among women who had a coronary angioplasty or initial myocardial infarction those who used estrogen after the procedure or event had a lower subsequent rate of mortality than women matched for age and risk factors who were not taking estrogen. These observational data indicate that estrogen prevents worsening of existing atherosclerosis and that prior cardiovascular disease is not a contraindication to estrogen replacement. However the results of a large clinical trial reported by Hulley et al. in which the use of estrogen plus a progestin was compared with placebo in elderly women (mean age 67) with existing cardiovascular disease found there was no difference in the incidence of cardiovascular events between the two arms at the end of the 5-year study. The study found that the incidence of a cardiovascular event was increased during the first year of the study among the hormone users, but was decreased among hormone users during the last 2 study years by 33%. If the study had been continued for a longer duration, a cardiovascular protective effect with hormone use may have been observed. The decision as to whether to initiate HRT in women with existing cardiovascular disease is currently unclear because of the different findings between the randomized clinical trial and the observational studies. However there is no reason to stop hormone replacement in women with cardiovascular disease who have been using hormones for more than 1 year.

Paganini-Hill et al. showed in a cohort study that postmenopausal estrogen use significantly reduced the risk of death from stroke among women 75 to 85 years of age. Other studies, such as the Nurses' Health Study, were unable to demonstrate a protective effect of postmenopausal estrogen use on the risk of stroke.

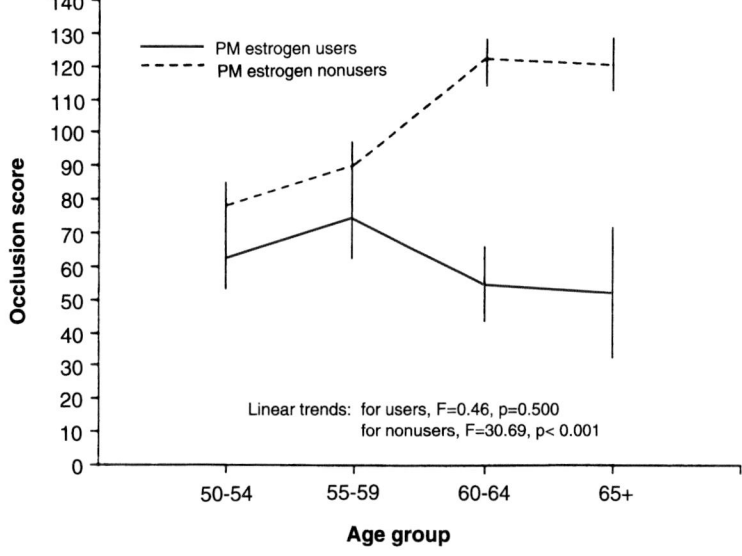

FIGURE 42-24 Occlusion scores by age groups for postmenopausal (PM) estrogen users and nonusers. Numbers of users/nonusers in each age group are 48/174 (50 to 54 years), 47/224 (55 to 59 years), 35/203 (60 to 64 years), and 24/178 (≥65 years). (From Gruchow HW, Anderson AJ, Barboriak JJ, and Sobocinski KA: Am Heart J 115:954, 1988.)

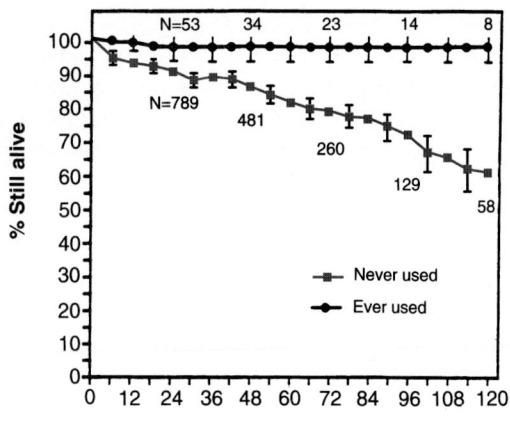

FIGURE 42-25 Ten-year survival of patients with left main coronary stenosis of 50% or greater or other stenosis of 70% or greater. (From Sullivan JM, Vander Zwaag R, Hughes JP, et al: Arch Intern Med 150:2557, 1990.)

TABLE 42-7
Relative Risk Estimates from Cohort Studies of Use of Estrogen Replacement Therapy and All Causes of Mortality

Investigator/Year	Relative Risk AC
Burch et al., 1974	0.4*
Stampfer et al., 1985	0.5†
Wilson et al., 1985	0.97
Henderson et al., and Paganini-Hill et al., 1988	0.8*
Pettiti et al., 1986	0.7*
Bush et al., 1987	0.5*
Hunt et al., 1988	0.6*
Criqui et al., 1988	0.7*
Henderson et al., 1991	0.8*

*$P < 0.05$.

†RR = 0.9 after eliminating that part of the cohort with cancer or coronary heart disease at baseline ($P = 0.42$).

The women in these latter studies were mostly under the age of 70, an age when stroke incidence is less common than over age 70. In 1993 Finucane et al. reported results of a nationwide study of 1910 women initially enrolled in the early 1970s who were followed for an average of 12 years. The population in this study has yielded one of the largest number of women with cardiovascular disease followed in a longitudinal study. The use of hormones postmenopausally was found to be associated with a 30% reduction in stroke incidence and a 65% reduction in stroke morbidity, both figures being statistically significant. The results indicate that estrogen use probably protects against the development of cerebral artery atherosclerosis as well as coronary artery atherosclerosis. Several recent studies using sonography have shown a direct beneficial effect of estrogen on the carotid artery. Punnonen et al. used ultrasonography to detect carotid artery atherosclerosis. They reported that postmenopausal women taking estrogen had significantly less atherosclerosis in their carotid arteries than postmenopausal women matched by age and body mass who were not taking estrogen. Jonas et al. also reported that with use of ultrasonography women taking estrogen or estrogen plus a progestin had less carotid artery atherosclerosis than matched controls not taking estrogen. In a longitudinal study using ultrasound, Espeland et al. reported that use of estrogen replacement halts or even reverses the progression of carotid artery intimal wall thickness over time among postmenopausal women by direct action on the vessels as the effect was independent of changes in lipoprotein concentrations. Akkad et al. reported that estrogen use for 6 months reduced the size of existing atherosclerotic plaque in the carotid arteries.

Since cardiovascular disease is the major cause of death among women over 50, many studies have shown that estrogen reduces the risk of overall mortality among postmenopausal women (Table 42-7).

Henderson et al. reported that the relative risk of overall mortality steadily decreased with increasing duration of estrogen use. Ettinger et al. compared risk of death among women enrolled in a large health maintenance organization who began estrogen replacement within 3 years of menopause and used it for at least 5 years with the risk of death for age-matched nonusers. In this study the mean length of estrogen use was 17 years. The risk of death for all causes was 0.54 among the estrogen users compared with the nonusers, mainly due to a 60% reduction in coronary disease death and a 73% reduction in other cardiovascular disease deaths among the estrogen users (Figure 42-26) Folsom et al. analyzed the association of hormone replacement therapy and mortality, as well as specific disease incidence, in a cohort of 41,070 postmenopausal women in Iowa. They reported that the age-adjusted risk of death was reduced by 22% in the hormone users compared with nonusers, mainly because of a 20% decrease in coronary heart disease. These studies indicate that postmenopausal estrogen replacement increases a woman's life span mainly by reducing death rates from cardiovascular disease, the most common cause in death in women.

It was previously believed that the main mechanism whereby oral estrogen replacement retards atherosclerosis postmenopausally is prevention of the adverse alterations in endogenous circulating lipid levels that normally occur after the menopause. In longitudinal studies, Matthews et al. and Jensen et al. reported that total serum cholesterol, low-density lipoprotein (LDL) cholesterol, and triglyceride levels

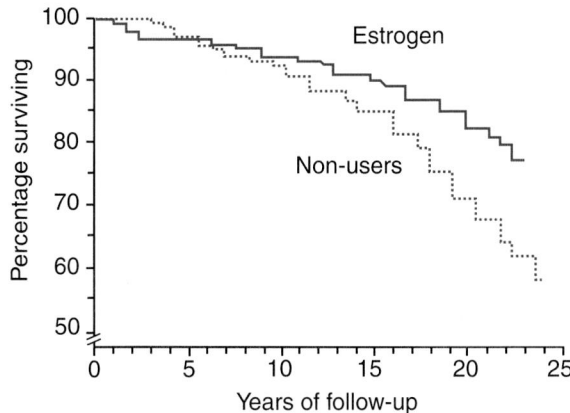

FIGURE 42-26 All-cause mortality in postmenopausal women using estrogen versus that in matched controls. (From Ettinger B, Friedman GD, Bush T, and Quesenberry CP Jr: Obstet Gynecol 87:6, 1996.)

increased postmenopausally, whereas high-density lipoprotein (HDL) cholesterol levels declined (Figure 42-27). Several investigators have reported that ingestion of various oral estrogen formulations postmenopausally prevents some of the unfavorable alterations in the lipid profile. As summarized by Bush and Miller, numerous studies have shown that administration of oral conjugated equine estrogens as well as other oral estrogens raises triglyceride and serum HDL cholesterol levels and lowers LDL cholesterol levels, with minimal changes in total cholesterol levels (Figure 42-28). The majority of studies utilizing parenteral administration of estrogen show similar lipid changes.

The effects of combinations of estrogens and progestins for postmenopausal women on lipid metabolism depend on the doses and the potencies of both the estrogen and the progestin used in the regimen. In the randomized Postmenopausal Estrogen/Progestin Interventions (PEPI) trial, the beneficial changes in lipid metabolism observed with estrogen alone were only slightly reduced with the addition of a synthetic progestin given sequentially or continuously and not changed when micronized progesterone was given sequentially.

It is now believed that altering the concentration of the various cholesterol subfractions in blood with exogenous estrogen is only of minor importance and that the major mechanism whereby estrogen reduces cardiovascular disease is by a direct action on the arterial wall. Lieberman et al. reported that oral estrogen administered for 9 weeks resulted in an improvement in flow-mediated, endothelium-dependent dilatation, probably by increasing the synthesis and release of nitric oxide. Bonilla-Musoles et al. reported that increased arterial blood flow occurs soon after initiation of estrogen replacement and is not altered by the addition of a progestogen. Proudler et al. reported that another mechanism whereby ERT may reduce the risk of coronary heart disease is by decreasing the levels of serum angiotensin-converting enzyme (ACE) activity. The lowering of ACE activity occurred in women given a combination of estrogen and progestogen. Others have reported that estrogen replacement increases vascular antioxidant activity, preventing plaque formation, as well as reverses the constricting effect of acetylcholine on the coronary arteries. Thus exogenous estrogen, with or without progestin, produces these direct protective effects on

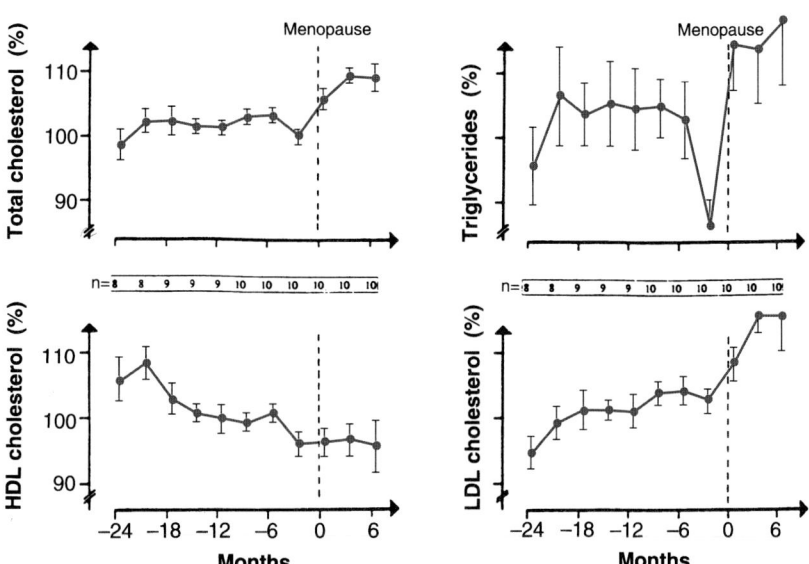

FIGURE 42-27 Time course of menopause-related changes in serum lipids and lipoproteins in 10 women who underwent natural menopause during study and number at each examination. (Values are expressed as percentages of mean during premenopausal period and are given as mean ± SEM for every two examinations performed.) H/LDL, High-low-density lipoprotein. (From Jensen J, Nilas L, and Christiansen C: Maturitas 12:321, 1990.)

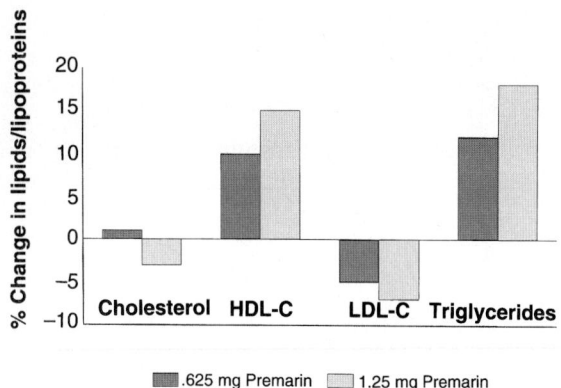

FIGURE 42-28 Percent change in lipid lipoproteins by dose of Premarin. (From Bush TL and Miller VT: Effects of pharmacologic agents used during menopause: impact on lipids and lipoproteins. In Mishell DR Jr, editor: Menopause: physiology and pharmacology, St. Louis, 1987, Mosby–Year Book Inc.)

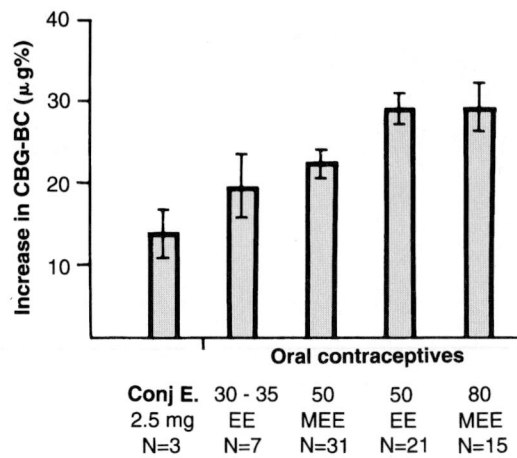

FIGURE 42-29 Increase in corticosteroid-binding globulin–binding capacity (CBG-BC) (mmg/dl) in relation to dose of synthetic estrogen. *Conj E,* Conjugated equine estrogen; *EE,* ethinyl estradiol; *MEE,* mestranol. (From Moore DE, Kawagoe S, Davajan V, et al: Am J Obstet Gynecol 130:482, 1978.)

the arterial wall and accounts for the epidemiologic findings of a similar protective effect with estrogen alone, as well as estrogen plus progestin, as reported in the Nurses' Health Study. In summary estrogen replacement therapy has a cardiovascular protective effect, a cerebrovascular protective effect, and a cardiovascular protective effect in women who smoke. Further, the addition of progestins to estrogen replacement probably does not reduce this protective vascular effect.

ADVERSE EFFECTS OF ESTROGEN REPLACEMENT

Metabolic Effects

With any drug there is a benefit/risk ratio, but the risks of estrogen replacement therapy are minimal. Exogenous estrogen administration produces effects on serum proteins, specifically an increase in serum globulins. One of these globulins, angiotensinogen, can be converted to angiotensin and produce an increase in blood pressure, whereas other globulins may produce a hypercoagulable state and possibly thrombosis. However, these metabolic changes are related to the dosage and type of estrogen administered, and the dose and type of estrogen given for postmenopausal hormone replacement therapy are much less potent than those used in oral contraceptives. For prevention of osteoporosis, bone density studies have shown that the equivalent of 0.625 mg of conjugated equine estrogen needs to be ingested. Women with hot flushes sometimes need to receive a higher dose, the equivalent of 1.25 mg of conjugated equine estrogen or greater, for relief of these symptoms.

However, even 2.5 mg of conjugated equine estrogen causes less of an increase in the liver-binding globulins than does 30 µg of ethinyl estradiol (Figure 42-29), which is the estrogen used in oral contraceptives. Ethinyl estra-

diol, because of the presence of the ethinyl group on the 17 position of the steroid molecule, causes a much greater increase in liver globulin production than does estrone sulfate. Mashchak et al. compared the potency of various doses of three types of natural oral estrogens—estrone sulfate, conjugated equine estrone sulfate, and micronized estradiol—with that of two synthetic estrogens—diethylstilbestrol and ethinyl estradiol. Ethinyl estradiol was much more potent in terms of increasing globulin levels than any of the natural estrogens. In terms of equivalent weight, when an increase in liver globulins was used as the parameter of estrogenic activity, ethinyl estradiol was found to be about 90 times as potent as conjugated equine estrogen and about 200 times as potent as estrone sulfate (Table 42-8). Thus 30 or 35 µg of ethinyl estradiol, which is the dosage of estrogen in most of the currently used oral contraceptive formulations, has the equivalent biologic activity on hepatic globulin synthesis as about 2.5 mg of conjugated equine estrogens. Therefore, although 0.625 mg of conjugated estrogen, the dose usually prescribed, is 20 times greater in amount than the 0.03 mg of ethinyl estradiol, the dose used in most oral contraceptives, the biologic activity of the former estrogen on globulin synthesis is one fifth less than the latter, since equine estrogen has only about one hundredth the potency of an equivalent amount of ethinyl estradiol.

Oral contraceptives with high doses of estrogen were found to increase the blood pressure of some women, but there is no evidence that the doses of oral estrogens used to treat postmenopausal women cause an increase in blood pressure.

In a cross-sectional study reported by Barrett-Connor et al., although mean systolic and diastolic blood pressure increased with age, there was no significant difference between estrogen users and nonusers (Table 42-9). During

TABLE 42-8
Relative Potency According to Four Specific Parameters of Estrogenicity

Estrogen Preparation	Serum FSH	Serum CBG-BC	Serum SHBG-BC	Serum Angiotensinogen
Piperazine estrone sulfate	1.0	1.0	1.0	1.0
Conjugated estrogens	1.4	2.5	3.2	3.5
Micronized estradiol	1.3	1.9	1.0	0.7
Diethylstilbestrol	3.8	70.0	28.0	13.0
Ethinyl estradiol	(80–200)*	(1000)*	614	232

From Mashchak CA, Lobo RA, Dozono-Takano R, et al: Am J Obstet Gynecol 144:511, 1982.

FSH, Follicle-stimulating hormone; *CBG-BC*, corticosteroid-binding globulin-binding capacity; *SHBG-BC*, sex hormone–binding globulin-binding capacity.

*Estimate in absence of parallelism.

TABLE 42-9
Systolic and Diastolic Blood Pressure According to Age and Postmenopausal Estrogen Use*

Age	Systolic Blood Pressure (mm Hg)		Diastolic Blood Pressure (mm Hg)	
	Users	Nonusers	Users	Nonusers
55–59	130.8 ± 18.8	135.0 ± 25.1	79.4 ± 9.6	81.3 ± 12.0
60–64	134.1 ± 18.9	136.5 ± 19.2	79.4 ± 9.4	81.6 ± 9.8†
65–69	139.3 ± 20.3	140.4 ± 21.4	81.9 ± 10.8	82.6 ± 12.2
70–74	147.9 ± 25.9	147.8 ± 20.9	82.0 ± 10.3	83.8 ± 22.7

From Barrett-Connor E, Brown WV, Turner J, et al: JAMA 241:2167, 1979. Copyright 1979, The American Medical Association.

*All data adjusted for obesity. Means and standard deviations are given.

†$P \leq 0.05$.

the 3-year PEPI randomized clinical trial, there was no difference in the mean systolic and diastolic blood pressure among any of the groups of women given estrogen with or without a progestin and those given a placebo (Figure 42-30). The results of a prospective study follow-up, reported by Lip et al., indicate that when hypertensive women were given estrogen replacement, there was no change in mean systolic and diastolic blood pressure or significant increase in need of hypertensive drugs during an average follow-up of more than 1 year, despite an increase in mean body weight. Furthermore, roughly equal numbers of women had an increase or decrease of systolic and diastolic blood pressure of 5 mm Hg or more. These data indicate that existing hypertension is not a contraindication for starting estrogen replacement therapy, and the development of hypertension when taking estrogen replacement therapy should not be a reason for stopping use of these agents.

Aylwood et al. showed that the natural estrogens in the dosages used for hormonal replacement do not increase the circulating levels of various clotting factors, which were observed in women ingesting ethinyl estradiol. Results of the PEPI trial, as well as a study by Scarabin et al., showed that estrogen or estrogen-progestin use was associated with decreased levels of circulating fibrinogen and factor VII, as well as plasminogenic activator inhibitor, compared with levels obtained in postmenopausal women not taking estrogen. Bar et al. reported that estrogen replacement reduced platelet aggregation. These hematologic findings suggest that use of estrogen postmenopausally should not increase the risk of venous thrombosis in postmenopausal women. The results of older epidemiologic studies, including the case-control study by Devor et al., found no significant relationship between estrogen replacement therapy and risk of venous thrombosis, even in the presence of known risk factors for thrombosis. In the study by Devor et al. postmenopausal women with a past history of thrombophlebitis did not have an increased incidence of thrombophlebitis when given estrogen replacement therapy compared with women with a similar history not given these agents. However, results of several more recent case-control studies consistently found that postmenopausal estrogen users were 2 to 4 times more likely to have an episode of venous thromboembolism than women not taking estrogen.

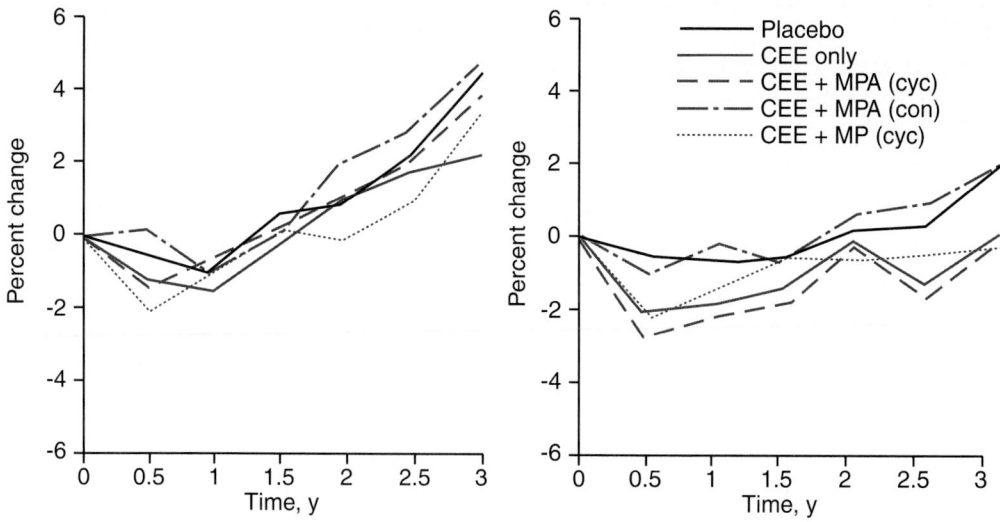

FIGURE 42-30 Mean percent change from baseline by treatment arm for systolic (left) and diastolic (right) blood pressure. See box for explanation of treatment groups. (From the Writing Group for the PEPI Trial: JAMA 273:199, 1995.)

Data from the Nurses' Health Study indicated that postmenopausal estrogen users were twice as likely to experience a pulmonary embolism as nonestrogen users. In most of these studies the increased risk occurred predominantly in the first year of use. In the study by Lowe et al. an increased risk of venous thrombophlebitis was observed in women with postmenopausal hormone use who had and did not have inherited thrombotic abnormalities such as activated protein C resistance. The risk of venous thrombophlebitis was greater with hormone use among women with hereditary thrombophillic disorders than those without. However even in women without inherited thrombophilia taking hormones, the risk of venous thrombophlebitis was increased fourfold compared to women not taking hormone replacement.

Postmenopausal estrogen use has minimal effect on glucose metabolism. Several recent studies including the PEPI randomized trial have shown no alternations in glucose tolerance tests as well as fasting insulin levels in women treated with 0.625 conjugated equine estrogen daily for 3 years. In a large prospective study of more than 21,000 postmenopausal women followed up for 12 years, Manson et al. reported that current users of postmenopausal hormonal replacement had a significantly decreased risk of developing noninsulin-dependent diabetes mellitus (R.R. 0.8) and there was no effect among past hormone users of developing this disorder. In the prospective study of Gabal et al. the risk of developing noninsulin-dependent diabetes mellitus was unchanged in postmenopausal women following the use of estrogen compared with nonusers. Most studies have shown a statistically increased risk of gallbladder disease in postmenopausal estrogen users. The Nurses' Health Study found the risk of cholecystectomy was twofold higher among estrogen users compared with nonusers. An increased risk for gallbladder disease was also found in the PEPI clinical trial. Estrogen use may accelerate the formation of cholelithiasis by increasing biliary cholesterol saturation.

There is no consistent association with a change in risk of osteoarthritis or rheumatoid arthritis with postmenopausal estrogen use. Several studies, including the Nurses' Health Study, reported an increased risk of developing systemic lupus erythematosus with postmenopausal estrogen use, but in women with existing disease use of estrogen did not increase disease activity.

Neoplastic Effects

Much concern has been raised about the neoplastic risks of postmenopausal estrogen replacement therapy, particularly on breast and endometrial cancer, since estrogen causes cells in these tissues to proliferate. The possibility exists that exogenous estrogen can stimulate growth of a nonpalpable breast cancer, and carcinoma of the breast may exist in the preclinical state for as long as 8 years before it is palpable. Therefore it is advisable for all women to have a mammogram to rule out subclinical breast cancer before initiating estrogen therapy and annually thereafter.

Many epidemiologic studies have investigated the relation between exogenous estrogen use and the risk of breast cancer.

To date six meta-analyses have been performed in which the data from 16 to 36 studies were combined to yield a larger data base. Each of these six analyses concluded that the risk of developing breast cancer among women who had ever used estrogen compared with nonusers was not significantly changed, with most summary results of risks being close to 1.0 (Table 42-10).

TABLE 42-10

Meta-Analysis of Overall RR of Estrogen and Breast Cancer in Women Who Had Ever Used Estrogen Compared with Never Used

Author	Year	Studies	Summary RR	CL
Armstrong	1988	23	1.01	(0.95–1.08)
Dupont and Page	1991	28	1.07	NA
Steinberg et al.	1991	16	1.0	NA
Grady and Ernster	1991	37	1.01	(0.98–1.06)
Sillero-Arenas	1992	27	1.06	(1.00–1.12)
Colditz et al.	1993	31	1.02	(0.93–1.12)

In 1997 a collaborative reanalysis of 51 studies of breast cancer and hormone replacement was performed involving almost 53,000 women with breast cancer and 108,000 controls. This study determined that ever-use of hormone replacement was associated with a slight but significantly increased risk of diagnosis of breast cancer, 1.14. Past use of estrogen as well as a family history of breast cancer and estrogen use was not associated with a significantly increased risk of breast cancer diagnosis compared to women not taking hormones postmenopausally. Data from several other cohort studies including the Nurses' Health Study also found no significantly increased risk of breast cancer in past users of estrogen replacement (Table 42-11). Controversy exists about long-term current use of

hormones and the development of breast cancer. Both the Collaborative Study and the Nurses' Health Study found a significantly increased risk of breast cancer diagnosis in long-term current users ranging from 1.24 to 1.46. However, several other studies, including the Iowa Woman's Health Study and two large case-control studies reported by Stanford et al. and Newcomb et al., found no significantly increased risk of diagnosis of breast cancer with current long-term use of estrogen. The Breast Cancer Diagnosis Detection Project found that women using estrogen from 8 to 16 years had a significantly increased risk of diagnosis of breast cancer if their body mass index was less than 24.4 with the risk being 1.5, but there was no increased risk in women with a body mass index above 24.4, the relative risk being 1.0. Several studies of long-term past use of hormone replacement also failed to show an increased risk of invasive breast cancer diagnosis. Two recent studies by Schairer et al. and Ross et al. reported a significantly increased risk of breast cancer diagnosis in women using sequential estrogen-progestin hormone replacement therapy with high doses of progestin for less than 2 weeks per month, but the study by Ross et al. reported no increased risk of invasive breast cancer with use of estrogen alone or with continuous combined estrogen progestin therapy. One large case-control study by Li et al. found an increased risk of lobular invasive breast cancer but not ductal invasive cancer of the breast with long-term use of estrogen plus progestin hormone replacement therapy. There was no significantly increased risk of either type of cancer with use of estrogen alone. Therefore, most epidemiologic studies indicate that ever-use, past use, and use of estrogen alone has no effect on

TABLE 42-11

Duration of Current and Past Postmenopausal Hormone Therapy and Relative Risk of Breast Cancer in the Nurses' Health Study, 1976 to 1992

Hormone Use	Cases of Breast Cancer	Person-Years of Follow-up	Adjusted Relative Risk (95% CI)*
None	972	374,197	1.0
Current			
1–23 mo	82	31,966	1.14 (0.91–1.45)
24–59 mo	140	49,672	1.20 (0.99–1.44)
60–119 mo	150	44,112	1.46 (1.22–1.74)
≥120 mo	141	37,454	1.46 (1.20–1.76)
Past			
1–23 mo	193	81,047	0.90 (0.77–1.05)
24–59 mo	120	54,046	0.86 (0.71–1.05)
60–119 mo	89	34,952	1.00 (0.80–1.26)
≥120 mo	48	18,104	1.03 (0.76–1.41)

From Colditz GA, Hankinson SE, Hunter DJ, et al: N Engl J Med 332:1589, 1995.

*Adjusted for age, type of menopause, age at menopause, parity, age at first delivery, age at menarche, family history of breast cancer, history of benign breast disease, and time period.

CI, confidence interval.

the increase of breast cancer detection. However two studies indicate that estrogen combined with sequential progestins has an increased risk of breast cancer diagnosis, and one study reports that estrogen combined with continuous progestins has no change in risk. The hypothesis that high doses of progestin may be associated with an increased risk of breast cancer diagnosis is supported by the observation that mitotic activity in normal breast tissue increases during the luteal phase of the cycle. Furthermore in vitro studies noted increased mitotic activity in cultures of breast tissue with progestin exposure.

There have been several studies which consistently have found that the risk of mortality for breast cancer when estrogen is taken at the time of diagnosis is significantly reduced compared to age-matched controls who were not taking hormones at the time of diagnosis of breast cancer (Figure 42-31). Gajados et al. reported that tumors diagnosed in estrogen users are smaller, more frequently diagnosed by mammogram, and more likely to be well differentiated and be positive for estrogen and progesterone receptors than breast cancer diagnosed in nonhormone users. It appears that women taking hormone replacement have an earlier diagnosis and subsequent treatment of breast cancer with resultant decreased mortality compared with women not taking hormones at the time of diagnosis.

After review of this large amount of epidemiologic data, some of which is conflicting, it appears reasonable to suggest that the increased risk of breast cancer diagnosis with long-term use of estrogen, which is found to be increased in some, but not all studies in current, not past users, may be due to detection bias because of the more

frequent use of mammograms in women receiving hormone replacement than nonusers. Data from these recent epidemiologic studies do not provide evidence that postmenopausal estrogen use initiates breast cancer by changing normal cells to cancer cells because of the consistent findings of no increased risk of breast cancer in past users of estrogen, even with use for long durations. It is also possible that estrogen, progestins, or both may promote the growth of a small, nonclinically palpable breast carcinoma increasing the likelihood of diagnosis of the cancer. Women should be informed about this interpretation of the data. All postmenopausal women should be advised to have a mammogram annually, whether or not they are receiving postmenopausal hormones.

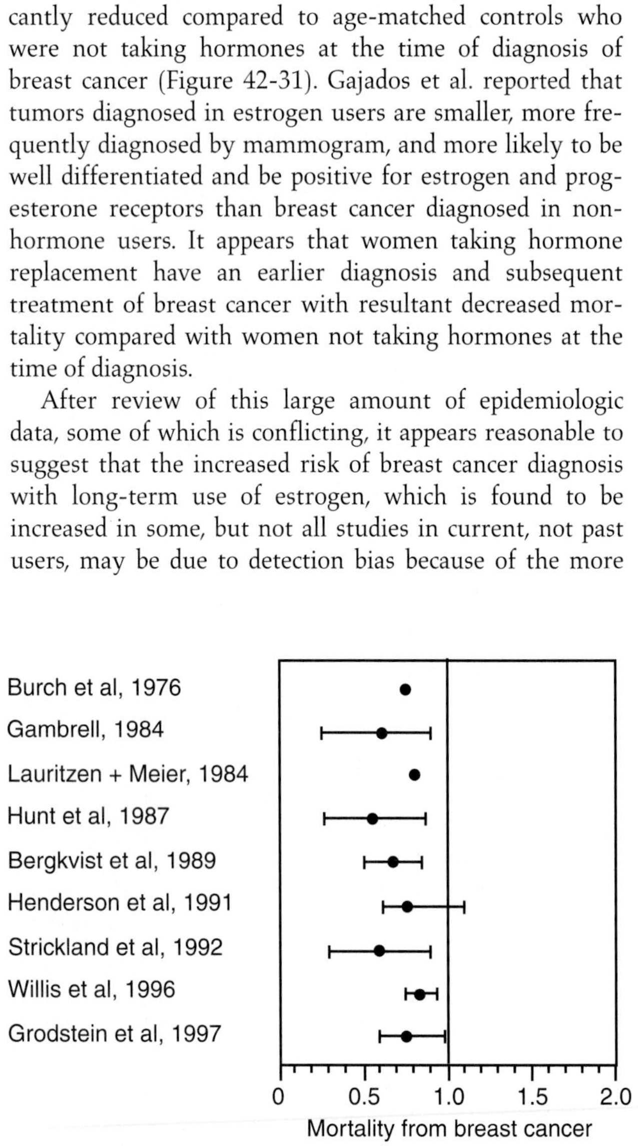

A comprehensive analysis by Colditz et al. showed that the risk of breast cancer in women with a family history of breast cancer who received estrogen replacement was not significantly increased compared with nonusers (RR, 1.07). This survey as well as the results of the collaborative reanalysis of worldwide data, which reached the same conclusion, indicate that clinicians should advise women who have a family history of breast cancer that they can take estrogen replacement without altering their risk of developing breast cancer.

Endometrial Cancer

Many epidemiologic studies have reported that there is a significantly increased risk of developing endometrial cancer in postmenopausal women who are ingesting estrogen without a progestin (unopposed estrogen) compared with nonestrogen users of a similar age. In a 1995 meta-analysis of 37 observational studies, Grady et al. reported that the summary relative risk for developing endometrial cancer among ever users of unopposed estrogen compared with never users was 2.3 (CI, 2.1 to 2.5) (Table 42-12). The risk increased with increasing duration of use of estrogen as well as with increasing dosage. This increased risk persists for several years after this therapy is discontinued. Therefore women who have taken unopposed estrogen need to be carefully monitored for many years after discontinuation or after initiation of additional progestin treatment.

The endometrial cancer that develops in estrogen users is nearly always well differentiated and is usually cured by performing a simple hysterectomy. In Grady's summary the risk of developing stage 0 to 1 endometrial cancer with unopposed estrogen was 4.20 but for stages 2 to 4 it was only 1.4, an insignificant increase. Collins et al. reported that women who had endometrial cancer and were not receiving estrogen had a 10-year survival rate of about 50%, and a control population without cancer matched for age and lack of estrogen had about an 80% survival rate at the end of 10 years (Figure 42-32). A group of women who had endometrial cancer and were also taking estrogen had a survival rate about the

Burch et al, 1976
Gambrell, 1984
Lauritzen + Meier, 1984
Hunt et al, 1987
Bergkvist et al, 1989
Henderson et al, 1991
Strickland et al, 1992
Willis et al, 1996
Grodstein et al, 1997

Mortality from breast cancer

FIGURE 42-31 Mortality from breast cancer in 9 studies. Relative risk of dying when malignancy develops during estrogen use compared with control subjects *(filled circles)*; 95% confidence interval when available or calculable *(horizontal lines)*. (From Natrajan PK, Soumakis K, and Gambrell Jr RD: Estrogen replacement therapy in women with previous breast cancer, AmJ Obstet Gynecol 181:288, 1999.)

TABLE 42-12
Relative Risk from Meta-Analysis: Postmenopausal Estrogen Therapy and Endometrial Cancer

	RR[a]	95% CI[b]	No. of Studies
Ever-users of estrogens			
All eligible studies	2.3[c]	2.1–2.5	29
Cohort studies	1.7[c]	1.3–2.1	4
Case-control studies	2.4[c]	2.2–2.6	25
Hospital controls	2.2[b]	2.0–2.5	10
Gynecologic controls	3.3[d]	2.7–4.0	6
Community controls[e]	2.4[c]	2.0–2.9	10
Conjugated estrogen dose (mg)			
0.3	3.9	1.6–9.5	3
0.625	3.4	2.0–5.6	4
≥1.25	5.8	4.5–7.5	9
Duration of use (y)			
<1	1.4	1.0–1.8	9
1–5	2.8	2.3–3.5	12
5–10	5.9	4.7–7.5	10
>10	9.5[d]	7.4–12.3	10
Regimen			
Intermittent and cyclic	3.0[d]	2.4–3.8	8
Continuous	2.9[d]	2.2–3.8	8
Type of estrogen			
Conjugated	2.5[f]	2.1–2.9	9
Synthetic[g]	1.3[d]	1.1–1.6	7
Time since last use (y)			
≥1	4.1[d]	2.9–5.7	3
1–4	3.7	2.5–5.5	3
≥5	2.3	1.8–3.1	5
Stage/invasiveness			
Stage 0–1	4.2	3.1–5.7	3
Stage 2–4	1.4	0.8–2.4	3
Noninvasive	6.2	4.5–8.4	4
Invasive	3.8[d]	2.9–5.1	6
Death from endometrial cancer	2.7	0.9–8.0	3

From Grady D, Gebretsadik T, Kerlikowske K, et al: Obstet Gynecol 85:304, 1995.

RR, relative risk; *CI,* confidence interval; *NA,* data not available.

[a]Pooled relative risk from meta-analysis.

[b]Pooled 95% CI from meta-analysis.

[c]*P* homogeneity < 0.0001.

[d]*P* homogeneity < 0.01.

[e]Community controls include residential, neighborhood, and population-based controls.

[f]*P* homogeneity < 0.05.

[g]Synthetic estrogens include primarily ethinyl estradiol, estradiol valerate, estriol, and unspecified other estrogens; diethylstilbestrol and estrogen combined with androgen excluded, except in cases where such use was lumped with all synthetic estrogens.

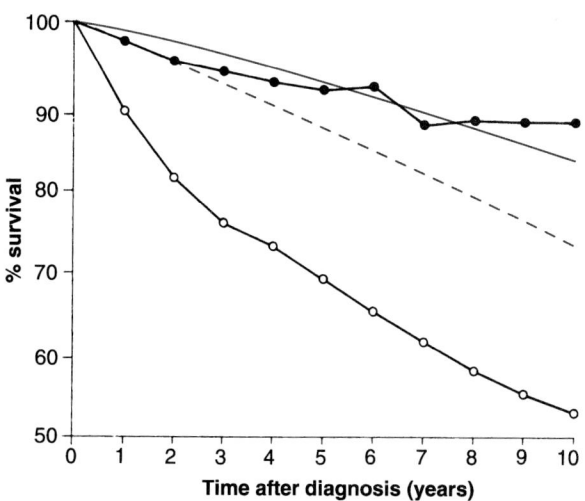

FIGURE 42-32 Survival of women with endometrial cancer and history of estrogen use *(solid circles)* compared with estrogen-user controls (age-adjusted mortality) *(solid blue line),* with women with endometrial cancer who were not estrogen users *(open circles),* and with non–estrogen-user controls (age-adjusted mortality) *(blue dashed line).* (From Collins J, Donner A, Allen LH, and Adams O: Lancet 2:961, 1980.)

same as a control population taking estrogen (90%), indicating that the well-differentiated endometrial carcinoma occurring with estrogen treatment can be adequately treated by performing a hysterectomy and is usually not lethal. The risk of developing endometrial carcinoma for women receiving estrogen replacement can be markedly reduced by administering progestogens. Estrogen acts only if a specific receptor is present within the target cell. The estrogen receptor complex activates messenger RNA, which then changes DNA to produce cell division and also synthesizes new estrogen receptors. Progesterone, which normally is produced in the last half of the normal menstrual cycle, inhibits estrogen receptor synthesis so no new receptors are formed. Therefore the endometrium does not proliferate in the latter half of the menstrual cycle because progesterone prevents estrogen receptor synthesis and further growth and division of the cells despite continued estrogen production. To summarize, estrogen increases the synthesis of both estrogen and progesterone receptors in the endometrium; progesterone and synthetic progestins decrease the synthesis of both these receptors and thus have an antiproliferative action.

In the PEPI study the addition of progestins to estrogen was shown to prevent the increased risk of endometrial hyperplasia associated with estrogen alone. The risk of developing endometrial hyperplasia was reduced when the progestins were administered sequentially or continuously. The epidemiologic data reporting the risk of endometrial cancer developing with estrogen plus progestin therapy compared with a control group not receiving any hormonal replacement are contradictory, with

TABLE 42-13

Odds Ratios (ORs) and 95% Confidence Intervals (CIs) of Invasive Endometrial Cancer in Relation to Use of Medium-Potency Estrogens with Progestins, by Type of Addition of Progestin and Progestin Derivation

| | Addition of Progestins | | | | Progestin Derivation | | | |
| | Cyclic | | Continuous | | Progesterone | | Testosterone | |
Category	No. of Case Patients/ No. of Control Subjects	OR* (95% CI)	No. of Case Patients/ No. of Control Subjects	OR* (95% CI)	No. of Case Patients/ No. of Control Subjects	OR* (95% CI)	No. of Case Patients/ No. of Control Subjects	OR* (95% CI)
Never	597/2963	1.0 (referent)	641/3014	1.0 (referent)	635/3140	1.0 (referent)	604/2871	1.0 (referent)
Ever	90/300	2.0 (1.4–2.7)	41/237	(0.7 (0.4–1.0)	51/216	2.0 (1.3–3.0)	85/398	1.0 (0.8–1.4)
Total†	687/3263		682/3251		686/3266		689/3269	
Duration								
<5 yr	38/191	1.5 (1.0–2.2)	32/162	0.8 (0.5–1.3)	23/87	1.5 (0.9–2.6)	53/268	1.1 (0.7–1.5)
≥5 yr	40/78	2.9 (1.8–4.6)	2/53	0.2 (0.1–0.8)	25/33	3.2 (1.7–6.0)	19/109	0.9 (0.5–1.5)
Per year of use		1.10 (1.06–1.15)		0.86 (0.77–0.97)		1.12 (1.06–1.18)		1.00 (0.95–1.06)
Subtotal†	78/269		34/215		48/120		72/377	

From Weiderpass E, Adami H-O, Baron JA, et al: Risk of endometrial cancer following estrogens replacement with and without progestins, J Natl Cancer Inst 91:1131, 1999.

*Adjusted for age, parity, age at menopause, body mass index (body weight in kg/height in m²), use of oral contraceptives, age at last birth, smoking, and duration of use of estrogens without progestins, progestagens, and orally administered estriol. For the analysis of cyclic addition of progestins, we also adjusted for continuous addition of progestins and vice versa. For the analysis of progesterone-derived progestins, we also adjusted for intake of testosterone-derived progestins and vice versa.

†Differences between total and subtotal numbers are due to missing values for duration of use.

several cohort studies indicating that the risk was decreased and three case-control studies reporting a nonsignificant small increase in endometrial cancer. In a large case-control study by Weiderpass et al. in Sweden the risk of developing endometrial cancer was increased 7.5-fold in women who used estrogen alone for more than 5 years, and increased 3-fold in women who used estrogen plus cyclic progestin for more than 5 years compared to nonhormone users. However women who used estrogen plus continuous progestin for more than 5 years had a significantly reduced risk of developing endometrial cancer, with a relative risk of 0.2 (Table 42-13). The results of this study suggest that it is better to take progestins continuously than cyclically with estrogens to reduce the risk of developing endometrial cancer in women with a uterus.

Colon and Rectal Cancer

In 1999 Nanda et al. performed a meta-analysis of the 27 studies in which a relation of postmenopausal hormone use and colorectal cancer was studied. They found a 33% reduction in the risk of colon cancer with current or recent hormone use but no decrease in risk of rectal cancer. Ever-use of hormones was associated with no change in risk of colon cancer (Table 42-14). Results from the Nurses' Health Study reported by Grodstein et al. also found a reduction in risk of colon cancer as well as rectal cancer with current or recent use of postmenopausal hormones.

Ovarian Cancer

A meta-analysis of the relation of postmenopausal hormone use and the risk of epithelial ovarian cancer was performed by Garg et al. in 1998 in which data from nine published studies were reviewed. The summary odds ratio for the risk of ovarian cancer with ever-use of hormone was 1.15, and with 10 or more years of hormone use increased to 1.27, which was of borderline statistical significance.

However the data are conflicting. Some of these studies found that estrogen has a protective effect against this disease, some showed no association, and others indicated that estrogen is associated with an increased risk of ovarian cancer. Thus a causal relation between estrogen and ovarian cancer risk remains undetermined because of inconsistency of the epidemiologic studies.

TREATMENT REGIMENS

Clinicians are becoming increasingly aware of the health benefits of postmenopausal estrogen replacement and are communicating this information to their patients. As a result, prescription of postmenopausal estrogen replacement, as well as use of progestins, is steadily increasing in the United States. Although the benefits of estrogen replacement therapy far exceed any possible risk, it is estimated that only about 25% of postmenopausal American women have ever taken estrogen replacement. One quarter

TABLE 42-14
Hormone Replacement Therapy and Colorectal Cancer: Summary Risk Estimates

	RR*	95% CI	No. of Studies
Ever-use of HRT			
Including studies not separating colon cancer from rectal cancer	0.89	0.76, 1.05	17†
Colon cancer only	0.92	0.79, 1.08	15†
Colon cancer, excluding Wu-Williams	0.88	0.80, 0.97	14†
Rectal cancer only	0.97	0.85, 1.11	11†
Recency of use and colon cancer			
Recent use	0.67	0.59, 0.77	7†
Former use	0.93	0.82, 1.06	6
Duration of use and colon cancer			4
<5 yr	1.03	0.74, 1.44	
≥5 yr	0.89	0.70, 1.44	
Colon cancer subsite with ever use			10*
Right	0.85	0.65, 1.11	
Left	0.90	0.75, 1.08	

From Nanda K, Bastian LA, Hasselblad V, and Simel DL: Hormone replacement therapy and the risk of colorectal cancer: a meta-analysis, Obstet Gynecol 93:880, 1999.

OR, odds ratio; *RR*, relative risk; *CI*, confidence interval; *NR*, not reported; *BMI*, body mass index.

*Reference group is women who have never used hormone replacement therapy.

†Personal communication, Annlia Paganini-Hill, Ph.D.

of American women who are given prescriptions for estrogen therapy never have them filled, and another quarter start the estrogen therapy but discontinue it within 12 months. Ferguson et al. reported that the primary reason that postmenopausal women decide not to use estrogen or discontinue its use is the occurrence of uterine bleeding. For this reason, continuous combined instead of cyclic estrogen-progestin regimens are being increasingly prescribed for women who are more than a few years postmenopausal.

Estrogen therapy for postmenopausal women should be given in the lowest possible dose that relieves vasomotor symptoms, prevents vaginal and urethral epithelial atrophy, maintains the collagen content of the skin, reduces the rate of bone resorption, and prevents acceleration of atherosclerosis. Postmenopausal estrogen can be ingested orally each day or transdermally once or twice per week. Vaginal estrogen formulations are available in creams, tablets, and within a plastic device. Oral estrogens that are currently available include varying doses of conjugated equine estrogen, esterified estrogens, estrone sulfate, and micronized estradiol. Several types of transdermal estrogen patches that contain varying doses of estradiol are also approved for use. Estrogen therapy given to postmenopausal women should result in physiologic and not pharmacologic circulating levels of estrogen, so that the risk of developing hypertension and venous thrombophlebitis is reduced. Data from the recent report of the Nurses' Health Study indicate that the adjusted relative risk for developing coronary heart disease was significantly reduced only for the women ingesting

0.625 mg of conjugated estrogen, not for those ingesting 1.25 mg or more (Table 42-15). The optimal long-term dose of estrogen that should be given to asymptomatic women to reduce the risk of osteoporosis and cardiovascular disease, termed the *physiologic replacement dose,* is probably 0.625 mg of conjugated equine estrogen or estrone sulfate or 0.5 mg of micronized estradiol. Some studies have shown that doses of 0.3 mg of conjugated equine estrogens or esterified estrogens with calcium supplementation are also protective against bone loss. The long-term effects of transdermal estradiol have not yet been determined, but it appears that a daily dose of 0.05 mg transdermally provides physiologic estrogen replacement. Higher doses of each type of estrogen may be needed for 1 or 2 years to relieve hot flushes. Vaginal administration of estrogen may be used initially to relieve atrophic vaginitis, but it is best to use other routes for long-term use because vaginal estrogen absorption is variable among women.

For postmenopausal women who have a uterus, progestins are usually administered cyclically or continuously to reduce the risk of adenocarcinoma of the endometrium. In the cyclic regimen the estrogen is usually given every day of the month and the progestin given daily for the first 10 to 14 days of the month. With the continuous combined regimen, both the estrogen and the progestin are administered every day of the month except for one formulation in which the progestin is given for 3 out of each 6-day interval. The cyclic regimens produce monthly withdrawal bleeding in about 80% of the women. The

TABLE 42-15

Relative Risk of Cardiovascular Disease among Current Hormone Users as Compared with Women Who Never Used Hormones, According to the Dose of Estrogen, 1980 to 1992*

| | | | Coronary Heart Disease | |
| | | | Relative Risk (95% CI) | |
Dose (mg)	Person-Years	No. of Cases	Age Adjusted†	Multivariate Adjusted†
0.3	13,900	8	0.40 (0.20–0.79)	0.57 (0.28–1.16)
0.625	61,512	29	0.35 (0.25–0.50)	0.53 (0.36–0.78)
1.25	25,895	19	0.62 (0.40–0.98)	0.82 (0.51–1.33)
>1.25	2238	2	0.79 (0.20–3.15)	0.92 (0.23–3.72)
P for trend				0.22

From Grodstein F, Stampfer MJ, Manson JE, et al: N Engl J Med 335:453, 1996.

*CI, confidence interval.

†The analysis was adjusted for age (in 5-year categories), time (in 2-year categories), age at menopause (in 2-year categories), body-mass index (in quintiles), diabetes (yes or no), high blood pressure (yes or no), high cholesterol level (yes or no), cigarette smoking (never, formerly, or currently [1 to 14, 15 to 24, or 25 or more cigarettes per day]), past oral-contraceptive use (yes or no), parental history of myocardial infarction before the age of 60 years (yes or no), and type of menopause (natural or surgical).

continuous regimen usually results in irregular bleeding and spotting during the first 3 to 6 months after initiating therapy in the majority of women, but with longer use nearly all women remain amenorrheic.

In the PEPI trial 0.625 mg of conjugated equine estrogen was given daily in all of the treatment arms. In the cyclic progestin arm 10 mg of medroxyprogesterone acetate was given for the first 12 days of each month and in the continuous progestin arm 2.5 mg of medroxyprogesterone acetate was given daily. Of the 119 women given estrogen alone, 27 developed complex hyperplasia and 14 atypical hyperplasia. None of the women given either of the progestin regimens developed atypical hyperplasia or adenocarcinoma of the endometrium in the 3 years of the trial. Although 2 of 118 women given the cyclic regimen developed complex hyperplasia, none of the women given continuous progestin developed complex hyperplasia (Table 42-16).

Formulations have now been marketed that contain different estrogens (conjugated equine estrogen, estradiol, and ethinyl estradiol) and different progestins (including medroxyprogesterone acetate, norethindrone acetate, and norgestimate) in a single oral tablet as well as a transdermal patch. Each of these agents has been shown to prevent the development of endometrial hyperplasia in clinical studies.

TABLE 42-16

Summary of Endometrial Biopsy Changes Since Normal Baseline to Most Extreme Abnormal Results, by Treatment Regimen*

| | Treatment Regimen | | | | | |
Result	Placebo	CEE Only	CEE + MPA (cyc)	CEE + MPA (con)	CEE + MP	Total (%)
Normal†	116	45	112	119	114	506 (84.9)
Simple (cystic) hyperplasia‡	1	33	4	1	5	44 (7.4)
Complex (adenomatous) hyperplasia‡	1	27	2	0	0	30 (5.0)
Atypia‡	0	14	0	0	1	15 (2.5)
Adenocarcinoma	1	0	0	0	0	l (0.2)
TOTAL	119	119	118	120	120	596 (100)

From the Writing Group for the PEPI Trial: JAMA 273:199, 1995.

*Includes 30 cases in which the diagnosis was assigned by the local gynecologist because the local, central, and arbiter pathologists gave different options. *CEE,* conjugated equine estrogen; *MPA,* medroxyprogesterone acetate.

†*P* = 0.16 (normal versus abnormal) for placebo compared with CEE + MPA (cyc), CEE + MPA (con), and CEE + MP.

‡*P* < 0.001 for placebo compared with CEE only.

If a progestin is added to the regimen to protect the endometrium, it does not negate the beneficial effects of estrogen on vasomotor symptoms or on bone density. The progestin may have an adverse effect on the vaginal, epithelium, and urethral mucosa and may produce undesired central nervous system (CNS) symptoms and adversely affect mood and sense of well-being.

Magos et al., in a double-blind, placebo-controlled study, demonstrated a dose-related deleterious effect of norethindrone on CNS symptoms, especially depression, anxiety, and irritability. Holst et al. reported that fatigue, tension, irritability, and depression were increased during the interval of progestin administration. Women who have undergone a hysterectomy are no longer at risk for endometrial cancer. Therefore administration of estrogen without a progestin is recommended for postmenopausal women who no longer have a uterus. Administrating the estrogen for 5 days each week and not during the weekend may be used for those women who experience breast tenderness with daily estrogen therapy.

For those women with a uterus who have intolerable mental symptoms with progestins, an estrogen-only regimen may be used in conjunction with an annual endometrial biopsy or vaginal ultrasonography to measure the endometrial thickness.

To date 20 studies involving 4759 women with postmenopausal bleeding who were examined by transvaginal sonography have been published. Gull et al. analyzed these studies and reported that if the endometrial echo complex was 4 mm or less only 12 cancers were present, for a incidence of 0.25%. This rate is lower than the false-negative rate of endometrial biopsy or uterine curettage. The results of this large study indicate that when postmenopausal bleeding is present, with or without use of hormones, if the endometrial echo complex is 4 mm or less, it is not necessary to perform a biopsy, since the risk of endometrial cancer being present is remote. If the bleeding persists, then injection of saline into the endometrial cavity, followed by sonography (hydrosonography) or hysteroscopy, should be performed to determine whether an endometrial polyp or submucosal myoma is the cause of the bleeding. If these entities are not present and the bleeding persists, serial sonograms will aid in determining whether hyperplasia is developing. Annual uterine sonography or endometrial biopsy should be performed in women who have a uterus and are receiving unopposed estrogen because they cannot tolerate progestins. If the endometrial thickness remains 4 mm or less, there is no need to do an endometrial biopsy.

A routine pretreatment endometrial biopsy or pelvic sonography is unnecessary because it has not been proven to be cost effective. Also, after initiating combination estrogen-progestin therapy routine annual endometrial biopsies or sonographies are unnecessary. If breakthrough bleeding occurs, but not regular withdrawal bleeding after cyclic use of progestin, a sample of endometrial tissue should be examined histologically if sonography reveals the endometrial echo complex to be thicker than 4 mm. Annual mammography should be recommended for all women aged 50 years or older, regardless of whether or not they are receiving estrogen therapy.

Contraindications to estrogen therapy occur infrequently. These include the presence of breast or endometrial cancer, as well as active thrombophlebitis and undiagnosed abnormal uterine bleeding. Women with active liver disease should avoid the oral administration of estrogen.

Controversy exists as to whether a woman who has had a past history of thrombophlebitis can take postmenopausal estrogen replacement, since there are no randomized clinical trials that have studied this issue. Individuals with an episode of thrombophlebitis of unexplained etiology should have measurement of protein C, protein S, and antithrombin, and a test to detect the presence of activated protein C resistance performed to determine whether one of these thrombophillic conditions exists. If present, prolonged anticoagulant therapy may be advisable. If there is no decrease in these coagulation inhibitors and activated protein C resistance is not present, estrogen replacement may be utilized for its many health benefits, but its use may increase the risk of another episode of thrombophlebitis and the patient should be counseled accordingly.

Controversy also exists regarding administration of estrogen to a woman who has had breast or endometrial cancer but has no evidence of disease at present. No randomized trials have investigated this problem. A committee opinion of the American College of Obstetrics and Gynecologists states, "Because estrogen replacement therapy has well-documented health benefits including prevention of osteoporosis some clinicians may consider it for women who appear to be free from disease." Therefore, if women with a past history of breast or endometrial cancer wish to take estrogen replacement they may do so with appropriate informed consent.

Estrogen is the treatment of choice for the relief of vasomotor symptoms and symptoms caused by vaginal and urethral mucosa atrophy. In addition, estrogen reduces the risk of developing osteoporotic fractures, myocardial infarction, and probably Alzheimer's disease. Nearly all postmenopausal women can derive a substantial benefit from the use of estrogen replacement therapy, but the majority of women do not take estrogen at all or only take it for a short duration to provide symptom relief. Many postmenopausal women do not wish to take estrogen replacement therapy despite its many benefits because they believe that taking supplemental estrogen is not natural and that exogenous estrogen will cause breast cancer. These concerns have led to an increased use of herbal therapies by perimenopausal women to relieve menopausal symptoms and improve mood, the ability to concentrate, and increase libido. These agents have been called "alternative medicines." A recent survey indicated that about 34% of U.S. adults used one or more alternative therapies in the prior year. These herbal products have medical effects and should be considered as drugs even though they are sold in health food and grocery stores. There is a lack of standards and quality control for these agents, and the products may be adulterated. There are little or no scientific studies that have investigated the effects of most of these agents including black cohosh and St. John's wort on the problems associated with estrogen deficiency. A randomized trial by Hirata et al. found that dong quai was no more effective than placebo in relieving hot flashes or changing the vaginal epithelium. Studies have been performed on products containing the isoflavones, a class of phytoestogens found primarily in soybeans. Duncan et al. reported that soy with high doses of isoflavones did not significantly lower FSH levels and had no effect on the vaginal epithelium or endometrial histology. Ingestion of phytoestrogens appears to reduce the frequency of hot flushes but has no proven benefit on genitourinary symptoms, osteoporosis, or cardiovascular disease, as does estrogen. Postmenopausal women need to be advised about these data so they will understand the limited effects of phytoestrogens with soy and herbal therapies compared with the proven benefits of the estrogen products that are approved by the U.S. Food and Drug Administration for prevention of hot flushes, vaginal atrophy, and osteoporosis.

KEY POINTS

- The median age of the onset of perimenopause is 47.5 years, and its median length is about 4 years.

- The initial endocrinologic change signaling the onset of menopause is decreased ovarian inhibin production accompanied by an increase in pituitary FSH release.

- Ovarian estradiol secretion does not begin to significantly diminish until 6 months to 1 year before the menopause.

- There is only a slight decrease in circulating testosterone and androstenedione levels immediately postmenopausally, and between 3 and 8 years postmenopausally levels of these two hormones remain relatively constant.

- Measurement of FSH cannot be used to determine the physiologic amount of estrogen replacement needed.

- Postmenopausally there is an increase in body weight and total body fat that is unaffected by estrogen administration.

- Postmenopausally there is a distribution of fat from peripheral sites to the abdomen. This change of fat distribution is prevented by exogenous estrogen.

- About 50% of postmenopausal women experience hot flushes, and the incidence decreases to 20% 4 years after the menopause.

- Estrogen is the best therapy for the hot flush; other effective therapies are progestins and clonidine.

- Exogenous estrogen in postmenopausal women appears to reduce the incidence of Alzheimer's disease, as well as delay the onset of this problem.

- Parenteral, but not oral, testosterone is effective for the treatment of decreased libido.

- To effectively reduce the incidences of hip fracture estrogen needs to be started soon after the menopause and taken until after age 70.

- Physiologic replacement doses of estrogen include 0.625 mg of conjugated equine estrogen and estrone sulfate, 0.5 mg of micronized estradiol, and transdermal administration of 0.05 mg of estradiol daily. These amounts of estrogen prevent bone loss in most women. The dose of 0.625 mg of conjugated equine estrogen has been shown to significantly reduce the risk of myocardial infarction.

- Exogenous estrogen reduces the overall death rate in postmenopausal women, mainly because of the reduction in risk of death from cardiovascular disease, the major cause of death among women.

- Protection against cardiovascular disease occurs with estrogen-progestin combination, as well as estrogen alone, because the main mechanism whereby estrogen reduces cardiovascular disease is by a direct effect on the arterial wall, which is unaffected by progestins.

- Estrogen replacement therapy has been shown in recent studies to increase the risk of venous thrombosis.

- Ever-use of estrogen does not increase the risk of breast cancer. Long-term use of estrogen may increase the risk of diagnosis of breast cancer in current but not past users, but the data are conflicting.

- Estrogen plus cyclic use of progestins may increase the risk of breast cancer diagnosis more than nonhormone users, but one study has shown no change in risk of breast cancer with estrogen and continuous use of progestin.

- Survival rates of breast cancer are greater among women who have this disease diagnosed while taking estrogen therapy than among age-matched controls who are not taking estrogen therapy.

- Estrogen replacement therapy does not further increase the risk of diagnosis of breast cancer in women with a family history of breast cancer compared with that of nonusers.

- Estrogen replacement therapy appears to reduce the risk of colon cancer and has no effect on the risk of ovarian cancer.

- For women with a uterus who cannot tolerate progestin, estrogen alone can be given and development of hyperplasia monitored by pelvic sonographic measurement of endometrial thickness.

- If sonographic measurement of the endometrial echo complex (thickness) is 4 mm or less, the chance of endometrial cancer being present is about 0.25%.

- Contraindications to estrogen replacement include the presence of breast or endometrial cancer, active thrombophlebitis, and undiagnosed abnormal bleeding.

- The mean age of menopause is about 51 years.

- Age at menopause is genetically predetermined and is not related to the number of ovulations, race, socioeconomic conditions, education, height, weight, age at menarche, or age at last pregnancy.

- The basic feature of menopause is depletion of ovarian follicles with degeneration of the granulosa and theca cells while stromal cells continue to produce the androgens androstenedione and testosterone.

- Androstenedione is converted to estrone in the peripheral body fat, and its rate of conversion increases as women age. Obese postmenopausal women have higher levels of estrone than thin women and are less likely to have hot flushes or osteoporosis and more likely to develop endometrial cancer.

- Postmenopausal women with hot flushes have lower circulating estrone and estradiol levels, less total body weight, and a lower percentage of ideal body weight as compared to those without hot flushes.

- About 1% to 1.5% of bone mass is lost each year after menopause in nonobese white and Asian women. Fractures begin to occur about age 60 to 65 in trabecular bone, such as the vertebral spine, and by age 60, 25% of these women develop spinal compression fractures. Hip fractures begin to increase after age 70.

- By age 80, 20% of all white women will develop hip fractures, and 15% of these fractures are fatal within 6 months. In the United States each year osteoporosis causes about 300,000 hip fractures, 100,000 radius fractures, and 400,000 other fractures.

- Women with postmenopausal osteoporosis have a higher bone resorption rate than normal, while the rate of bone formation with osteoporosis is normal.

- In terms of equivalent weight, when an increase in liver globulins is used as the parameter of estrogenic activity, ethinyl estradiol is about 90 times as potent as conjugated equine estrogen.

- Levels of LDL cholesterol have a positive correlation with coronary heart disease, while levels of HDL cholesterol have an inverse relation to coronary heart disease. Postmenopausal estrogen users have decreased levels of LDL cholesterol as well as increased levels of HDL cholesterol compared with postmenopausal nonestrogen users.

- The risk of developing endometrial cancer is 2 to 10 times greater in postmenopausal women who are ingesting estrogen without progestins compared with nonestrogen users. The risk is increased with higher dosages and prolonged use of estrogen and can be reduced below the incidence in nonusers by the addition of continuous progestins.

- Estrogen increases the synthesis of both estrogen and progesterone receptors in the endometrium; progesterone and synthetic progestins decrease the synthesis of both these receptors and thus have an antimitotic, antiproliferative action.

- Indications for estrogen therapy in menopause include the presence of vasomotor symptoms as well as prevention of atrophic vaginitis, atrophic urethritis, and osteoporosis.

- Before estrogen therapy is instituted, a pretreatment mammogram should be performed and repeated annually thereafter.

- At least 25% of bone needs to be lost before osteoporosis can be diagnosed by routine x-ray examination.

- Dual-energy x-ray absorptiometry (DEXA) is the most accurate method to measure bone density. The bone mineral density is usually expressed as T scores and Z scores.

- Bone mass measurements are indicated only when clinical decisions will be influenced by the information gained.

- Measurement of markers of bone resorption such as urinary excretion of collagen degradation products are of limited clinical use.

- In addition to estrogen, alendronate, risendronate, raloxifene, and calcitonin will reduce postmenopausal bone loss.

- Postmenopausal estrogen use increases the risk of gallbladder disease.

- To prevent development of osteoporosis, estrogen replacement should be given as long as the woman is ambulatory.

- Addition of a progestin to estrogen replacement does not inhibit the beneficial effect of estrogen on reducing the rate of bone reabsorption.

- Estrogen increases calcium absorption and reduces the rate of bone reabsorption postmenopausally. It does not stimulate bone formation.

- Estrogen users have about a 50% reduction in risk of developing myocardial infarction compared with nonusers.

- Angiographic studies indicate estrogen retards the development of coronary atherosclerosis.

- Oral estrogen replacement does not raise systolic or diastolic blood pressure.

- The endometrial cancer that develops among estrogen users is usually well differentiated and nearly always cured by hysterectomy.

- It is estimated that currently only about 20% of postmenopausal American women use estrogen replacement.

- Estrogen without a progestin is recommended for postmenopausal women who have had a hysterectomy.

- Progestins can be given cyclically or continuously with estrogen to reduce the risk of endometrial cancer. When given cyclically about 80% of women have regular withdrawal bleeding. When given continuously most women bleed during the first 6 months but become amenorrheic after 1 year.

- Most herbal products have not been shown to decrease menopausal symptoms.

- Soy extracts help prevent hot flushes but have no effect on the vaginal epithelium or bone.

BIBLIOGRAPHY

Adashi JD, Sargeant EJ, Sagle MA, et al: A double-blind randomized controlled trial of the effects of medroxyprogesterone acetate on bone density of women taking oestrogen replacement therapy, Br J Obstet Gynaecol 104:64, 1997.

Akkad A, Hartshorne T, Bell PR, and Al-Azzawi F: Carotid plaque regression on oestrogen replacement: a pilot study, European J Vasc Endovasc Surg 111:347, 1996.

Al-Azzawi F, Hart DM, and Lindsay R: Long term effect of oestrogen replacement therapy on bone mass as measured by dual photon absorptiometry, Br Med J 294:1261, 1987.

Aloia JF, Vaswani A, Yeh JK, et al: Calcium supplementation with and without hormone replacement therapy to prevent postmenopausal bone loss, Ann Intern Med 120:97, 1994.

Aylwood M, Maddock J, Lewis PA, et al: Oestrogen replacement therapy and blood clotting, Curr Med Res Opin 4(suppl 3):83, 1971.

Bar J, Tepper R, Fuchs J, et al: The effect of estrogen replacement therapy on platelet aggregation and adenosine triphosphate release in postmenopausal women, Obstet Gynecol 81:2621, 1993.

Barrett-Conner E: Postmenopausal estrogen therapy and selected (less-often-considered) disease outcomes, Menopause 6:14, 1999.

Beral V, for the Collaborative Group on Hormonal Factors in Breast Cancer (Radcliffe Infirmary, Oxford, American Cancer Society, Emory Univ, Atlanta, et al: Breast cancer and hormone replacement therapy. Collaborative reanalysis of data from 51 epidemiological studies of 52,705 women with breast cancer and 108,411 women without breast cancer, Lancet 350:1047, 1997.

Beresford SAA, Weiss NS, Voight LF, et al: Risk of endometrial cancer in relation to use of oestrogen combined with cyclic progestagen therapy in postmenopausal women, Lancet 349:458, 1997.

Bergkvist L, Adami H-O, Persson I, Bergstrom R, Kruseemo UB: Prognosis after breast cancer diagnosis in women exposed to estrogen and estrogen-progestogen replacement therapy. Am J Epidemiol 130:221, 1989.

Bergmans MGM, Merkus JMWM, Corbey RS, et al: Effect of Bellergal retard on climacteric complaints: a double-blind, placebo controlled study, Maturitas 9:227, 1987.

Bonilla-Musoles F, Marti MC, Ballester MJ, et al: Normal uterine arterial blood flow in postmenopausal women assessed by transvaginal color Doppler sonography: the effect of hormone replacement therapy, J Ultrasound Med 14:497, 1995.

Brincat M, Moniz CJ, Studd JWW, et al: Long-term effects of the menopause and sex hormones on skin thickness, Br J Obstet Gynaecol 92:256, 1985.

Brinton L and Hoover R: Estrogen replacement therapy and endometrial cancer risk: unresolved issues, Obstet Gynecol 81:265, 1993.

Burch JC, Byrd BF Jr, Vaughn WK: Results of estrogen treatment in one thousand hysterectomized women for 14,318 years. In Van Keep PA, Greenblatt RD, Albeaux-Fernet M, editors: Concensus on menopause research. Lancaster (United Kingdom), 1976, MTP Press.

Bush TL, Barrett-Connor E, Cowan LD, et al: Cardiovascular mortality and noncontraceptive use of estrogen in women: results from the Lipid Research Clinics Program follow-up study, Circulation 75:1102, 1987.

Bush TL and the Writing Group for the PEPI Trial (Parke-Davis, Morris Plains, NJ): Effects of hormone therapy on bone mineral density: results from the postmenopausal estrogen/progestin intervention (PEPI) trial, JAMA 276:1389, 1996.

Calle EE, Miracle-McNahill HL, Thun MJ, and Heath CW Jr: Estrogen replacement therapy and risk of fatal colon cancer in a prospective cohort of postmenopausal women, J Natl Cancer Inst 87:517, 1995.

Cauley JA, Seeley DG, Ensrud K, et al: Estrogen replacement therapy and fractures in older women, Ann Intern Med 122:9, 1995.

Cavanaugh DJ and Cann CE: Brisk walking does not stop bone loss in postmenopausal women, Bone 9(4):201, 1988.

Chesnut CH, McClung MR, Ensrud KER, et al: Alendronate treatment of the postmenopausal osteoporotic woman: effect of multiple dosages on bone mass and bone remodeling, Am J Med 99:144, 1995.

Clarkson TB, Anthony MNS, and Jerome CP: Lack of effect of raloxifene on coronary artery atherosclerosis of postmenopausal monkeys, J Clin Endocrinol Metab 83:721, 1998.

Colditz GA, Egan KM, and Stampfer MJ: Hormone replacement therapy and risk of breast cancer: results from epidemiologic studies, Am J Obstet Gynecol 168:1473, 1993.

Colditz GA, Hankinson SE, Hunter DJ, et al: The use of estrogens and progestins and the risk of breast cancer in postmenopausal women, N Engl J Med 332:1589, 1995.

Collins J, Donner A, Allen LH, and Adams O: Oestrogen use and survival in endometrial cancer, Lancet 2:961, 1980.

Coope J: Double-blind cross-over study of estrogen replacement therapy. In Campbell S, editor: Management of the menopause and post-menopausal years, Lancaster, England, 1976, MTP Press Ltd.

Costa MM, Reus VI, Wolkowitz WM, et al: Estrogen replacement therapy and cognitive decline in memory-impaired post-menopausal women, Biol Psychiatry 46:182, 1999.

Cramer DW, Xu H, and Harlow BL: Family history as a predictor of early menopause, Fertil Steril 64:740, 1995.

Curham GC, Willett WC, Speizer FE, et al: Comparison of dietary calcium with supplemental calcium and other nutrients as factors affecting the risk for kidney stones in women, Ann Intern Med 126:497, 1997.

Daly E, Vessey MP, Hawkins MM, et al: Risk of venous thromboembolism in users of hormone replacement therapy, Lancet 348:977, 1996.

Dawson-Hughes B, Dallal GE, Krall EA, et al: A controlled trial of the effect of calcium supplementation on bone density in postmenopausal women, N Engl J Med 323:878, 1990.

Delmas PD, Bjarnason NH, Mitlak BH, et al: Effects of raloxifene on bone mineral density, serum cholesterol concentrations, and uterine endometrium in postmenopausal women, N Engl J Med 337:1641, 1997.

Devor M, Barrett-Connor E, Renvall M, et al: Estrogen replacement therapy and the risk of venous thrombosis, Am J Med 92:275, 1992.

Dummings SR, for the Fracture Intervention Trial Research Group (Univ of Calif, San Francisco; Merck Research Labs, Rahway, NJ; Univ of Tenn, Memphis; et al): Effects of alendronate on risk of fracture in women with bone density but without vertebral fractures: results from the Fracture Intervention Trial, JAMA 280:2077, 1998.

Egeland GM, Kuller LH, Matthews KA, et al: Hormone replacement therapy and lipoprotein changes during early menopause, Obstet Gynecol 76:776, 1990.

Erlik Y, Meldrum DR, and Judd HL: Estrogen levels in postmenopausal women with hot flashes, Obstet Gynecol 59:403, 1982.

Erlik Y, Tataryn IV, Meldrum DR, et al: Association of waking episodes with menopausal hot flushes, JAMA 245:1741, 1981.

Espeland MA, for the Postmenopausal Estrogen/Progestin Interventions Study Investigators: Effect of postmenopausal hormone therapy on body weight and waist and hip girths, J Clin Endocrinol Metab 82:1549, 1997.

Espeland MA, Applegate W, Furberg CD, et al: Estrogen replacement therapy and progression of intimal-medial thickness in the carotid arteries of postmenopausal women, Am J Epidemiol 142:1011, 1995.

Espeland MA, for the ACAPS Investigators (Bowman Gray School of Medicine, Winston-Salem, NC; Univ of Tennessee, Memphis; Univ of Kentucky, Lexington; et al): Estrogen replacement therapy and progression of intimal-medial thickness in the carotid arteries of postmenopausal women, Am J Epidemiol 142:1011, 1995.

Ettinger B, Friedman GD, Bush T, and Quesenberry CP Jr: Reduced mortality associated with long-term postmenopausal estrogen therapy, Obstet Gynecol 87:6, 1996.

Ettinger B, Genant HK, and Cann CE: Long-term estrogen replacement therapy prevents bone loss and fractures, Ann Intern Med 102:319, 1985.

Ettinger B, Genant HK, and Cann CE: Postmenopausal bone loss is prevented by treatment with low-dosage estrogen with calcium, Ann Intern Med 106:40, 1987.

Ferguson KJ, Hoegh C, and Johnson S: Estrogen replacement therapy: a survey of women's knowledge and attitudes, Arch Intern Med 149:133, 1989.

Finucane FF, Madans JH, Bush TL, et al: Decreased risk of stroke among postmenopausal hormone users: results from a national cohort, Arch Intern Med 153:73, 1993.

Folsom AR, Mink PJ, Sellers TA, et al: Hormonal replacement therapy and morbidity and mortality in a prospective study of postmenopausal women, Am J Public Health 85:1128, 1995.

Gabal LL, Godoman-Gruen D, and Barrett-Conner E: The effect of postmenopausal estrogen therapy on the risk of non-insulin-dependent diabetes mellitus, Am J Public Health 87:443, 1997.

Gajdos C, Tartter PI, and Babinszki A: Breast cancer diagnosed during hormone replacement therapy, Obstet Gynecol 95:513, 2000.

Gambacciani M, Ciaponi M, Cappagli B, et al: Body weight, body fat distribution, and hormonal replacement therapy in early postmenopausal women, J Clin Endocrinol Metab 82:414, 1997.

Gambrell RD Jr: Proposal to decrease the risk and improve the prognosis of breast cancer. Am J Obstet Gynecol 150:119, 1984.

Gapstur SM, Morrow M, and Sellers TA: Hormone replacement therapy and risk of breast cancer with a favorable histology: results of the Iowa Women's Health Study, JAMA 281:2091, 1999.

Garg PP, Kerlikowske K, Subak L, et al: Hormone replacement therapy and the risk of epithelial ovarian carcinoma: a meta-analysis, Obstet Gynecol 92:472, 1998.

Garnero P, Sornay-Rendu E, Deboeuf F, and Delmas PD: Markers of bone turnover predict postmenopausal forearm bone loss over 4 years: the OFELY study, J Bone Miner Res 14:1614, 1999.

Genant HK, Baylink DJ, Gallagher JC, et al: Effect of estrone sulfate on postmenopausal bone loss, Am J Obstet Gynecol 76:759, 1990, Fig 1.

Genazzani AR, Petraglia F, Facchinetti F, et al: Steroid replacement treatment increases β-endorphin and β-lipotropin plasma levels in postmenopausal women, Gynecol Obstet Invest 294:1261, 1988.

Grady D, Wenger NK, Herrington D, et al: Postmenopausal hormone therapy increases risk for venous thromboembolic disease, Ann Intern Med 132:689, 2000.

Grady D, Gebretsadik T, Kerlikowske K, et al: Hormone replacement therapy and endometrial cancer risk: a meta-analysis, Obstet Gynecol 85:304, 1995.

Grady D, Rubin SM, Petitti DB, et al: Hormone therapy to prevent disease and prolong life in postmenopausal women, Ann Intern Med 117:1016, 1992.

Greendale GA, for the Postmenopausal Estrogen/Progestin Interventions Trial Investigators (Univ Calif, Los Angeles; Wake Forest Univ, Winston-Salem, NC; George Washington Univ, Washington, DC; et al): Symptom relief and side effects of postmenopausal hormones: results from the postmenopausal estrogen/progestin interventions trial, Obstet Gynecol 92:982, 1998.

Grodstein F, Colditz GA, and Stampfer MJ: Post-menopausal hormone use and tooth loss: a prospective study, J Am Dent Assoc 127:370, 1996.

Grodstein F, Martinez DM, Platz EA, et al: Postmenopausal hormone use and risk for colorectal cancer and adenoma, Ann Intern Med 128:705, 1998.

Grodstein F, Stampfer MJ, Colditz GA, et al: Postmenopausal hormone therapy and mortality, N Engl J Med 336:1769, 1997.

Grodstein F, Stampfer MJ, Goldhaber SZ, et al: Prospective study of exogenous hormones and risk of pulmonary embolism in women, Lancet 348:983, 1996.

Grodstein F, Stampfer MJ, Manson JE, et al: Postmenopausal estrogen and progestin use and the risk of cardiovascular disease, N Engl J Med 335:453, 1996.

Gruchow HW, Anderson AJ, Barboriak JJ, and Sobocinski KA: Postmenopausal use of estrogen and occlusion of coronary arteries, Am Heart J 115:954, 1988.

Gull B, Carlsson SA, Karlsson B, et al: Transvaginal ultrasonography of the endometrium biopsy. Am J Obstet Gynecol 182:509, 2000.

Guttman SP, Rodriguez LAG, Catellsague J, et al: Hormone replacement therapy and risk of venous thromboembolism: population based case-control study, BMJ 314:796, 1997.

Haines CJ, Chung TKH, Lleung PC, et al: Calcium supplementation and bone mineral density in postmenopausal women using estrogen replacement therapy, Bone 16:529, 1995.

Harris ST, Wats NB, Genant HK, McKeever CD, et al: Effects of risedronate treatment on vertebral and nonvertebral fractures in women with postmenopausal osteoporosis. A randomized controlled trial, JAMA 282:1344, 1999.

Heckbert SR, Weiss NS, Koepsell TD, et al: Duration of estrogen replacement therapy in relation to the risk of incident of myocardial infarction in postmenopausal women, Arch Intern Med 157:1330, 1997.

Hempling RE, Wong C, Piver MS, et al: Hormone replacement therapy as a risk factor for epithelial ovarian cancer: results of a case-control study, Obstet Gynecol 89:1012, 1997.

Henderson BE, Paganini-Hill A, and Ross RK: Decreased mortality in users of estrogen replacement therapy, Arch Intern Med 151:75, 1991.

Henderson VW, Paganini-Hill A, Emanuel CK, et al: Estrogen replacement therapy in older women: comparisons between Alzheimer's disease cases and nondemented control subjects, Arch Neurol 51:896, 1994.

Hirata JD, Small R, Sweirsz LM, et al: Does dong quai have estrogenic effects in postmenopausal women? A double-blind, placebo-controlled trial, Fertil Steril 68:981, 1997.

Hoibraaten E, Abdelnoor M, Sandset PM: Hormone replacement therapy with estradiol and risk of venous thromboembolism, Thromb Haemost 82:1218, 1999.

Holst J, Backstrom T, Hammarback S, and von Schoultz B: Progestogen addition during oestrogen replacement therapy—effects on vasomotor symptoms and mood, Maturitas 11:13, 1989.

Hosking D, for the Early Postmenopausal Intervention Cohort Study Group (Univ of Nottingham, England): Prevention of bone loss with alendronate in postmenopausal women under 60 years of age, N Engl J Med 338:485, 1998.

Hovik P, Sundsbak HP, Gaasemyr M, and Sandvik L: Comparison of continuous and sequential oestrogen-progestogen treatment in women with climacteric symptoms, Maturitas 11:75, 1989.

Hunt K, Vessey M, McPherson K, Coleman M: Long-term surveillance of mortality and cancer incidence in women receiving hormone replacement therapy. Br J Obstet Gynecol 94:620, 1987.

Hylley S, Grady D, Bush T, et al: Randomized trial of estrogen plus progestin for secondary prevention of coronary heart disease in postmenopausal women, JAMA 280:605, 1998.

Jick H, Derby LE, Myers MW, et al: Risk of hospital admission for idiopathic venous thromboembolism among users of postmenopausal oestrogens, Lancet 348:981, 1996.

Jick S, Walker A, and Jick H: Estrogens, progesterone, and endometrial cancer, Epidemiology 4:20, 1993.

Jonas HA, Kronmal RA, Psaty BM, et al: Current estrogen-progestin and estrogen replacement therapy in elderly women: association with carotid atherosclerosis, Ann Epidemiol 6:314, 1996.

Kampen DL and Sherwin BB: Estrogen use and verbal memory in healthy postmenopausal women, Obstet Gynecol 83:979, 1994.

Karlsson B, Granberg S, Wikland M, et al: Transvaginal ultrasonography of the endometrium in women with postmenopausal bleeding: a Nordic multicenter study, Am J Obstet Gynecol 172:1488, 1995.

Kawas C, Resnick S, Morrison A, et al: A prospective study of estrogen replacement therapy and the risk of developing Alzheimer's disease: the Baltimore Longitudinal Study of Aging, Neurology 48:1517, 1997.

Krall EA, Dawson-Hughes B, Hannan MT, et al: Postmenopausal estrogen replacement and tooth retention, Am J Med 102:536, 1997.

Kushida K, Takahashi M, Kawana K, and Inoue T: Comparison of markers for bone formation and resorption in premenopausal and postmenopausal subjects, and osteoporosis patients, J Clin Endocrinol Metab 80:2447, 1995.

Lauritzen C, Meier F: Risks of endometrial and mammary cancer morbidity and mortality in long-term oestrogen treatment. In van Herendael HB, Riphagen FE, Goessens L, van de Pas H, editors: The climacteric: an update. Lancaster (United Kingdom), 1984, MTP Press.

Li CI, Weiss NS, Stanford JL, and Daling JR: Hormone replacement therapy in relation to risk of lobular and ductal breast carcinoma in middle-aged women, Cancer 88:2570, 2000.

Lieberman EH, Gerhard MD, Uehata A, et al: Estrogen improves endothelium-dependent, flow-mediated vasodilation in postmenopausal women, Ann Intern Med 121:936, 1993.

Lindsay R, Cosman F, Lobo RA, Walsh BW, et al: Addition of alendronate to ongoing hormone replacement therapy in the treatment of osteoporosis: a randomized controlled clinical trial, J Clin Endocrinol Metab 84:3706, 1999.

Lindsay R, Hart DM, Forrest C, and Baird C: Prevention of spinal osteoporosis in oophorectomized women, Lancet 2:1151, 1980.

Lindsay R, Hart DM, MacLean A, et al: Bone response to termination of oestrogen treatment, Lancet 1:1325, 1978.

Lindsay R and Tohme JF: Estrogen treatment of patients with established postmenopausal osteoporosis, Obstet Gynecol 76:290, 1990.

Lip GYH, Beevers M, Churchill D, and Beevers DG: Hormone replacement therapy and blood pressure in hypertensive women, J Hum Hypertens 8:491, 1994.

Lobo RA, McCormick W, Singer F, et al: Depomedroxyprogesterone acetate compared with conjugated estrogens for the treatment of postmenopausal women, Obstet Gynecol 63:1, 1984.

Loprinzi CL, Michalak JC, Quella SK, et al: Megestrol acetate for the prevention of hot flushes, N Engl J Med 331:347, 1994.

Lowe G, Woodward M, Vessey M, et al: Thrombotic variables and risk of idiopathic venous thromboembolism in women aged 45-64 years, Thromb Haemost 83:530, 2000.

MacNaughton J, Banah M, McCloud P, et al: Age related changes in follicle stimulating hormone, luteinizing hormone, oestradiol and immunoreactive inhibin in women of reproductive age, Clin Endocrinol 36:339, 1992.

Magos AL, Brewster E, Singh R, and O'Dowd T: The effects of norethisterone in postmenopausal women on oestrogen replacement therapy: a model for the premenstrual syndrome, Br J Obstet Gynaecol 93:1290, 1986.

Maheux R, Naud F, Rioux M, et al: A randomized, double-blind, placebo-controlled study on the effect of conjugated estrogens on skin thickness, Am J Obstet Gynecol 170:642, 1994.

Manson JE, Rimm EB, Colditz GA, et al: A prospective study of postmenopausal estrogen therapy and subsequent incidence of non–insulin-dependent diabetes mellitus, Ann Epidemiol 2:665, 1992.

Marcos R, Holloway L, Wells B, et al: The relationship of biochemical markers of bone turnover to bone density changes in postmenopausal women: results from the postmenopausal estrogen/progestin interventions (PEPI) trial, J Bone Miner Res 14:1583, 1999.

Mashchak CA, Lobo RA, Dozono-Takano R, et al: Comparison of pharmacodynamic properties of various estrogen formulations, Am J Obstet Gynecol 144:511, 1982.

McClung M, for the Alendronate Osteoporosis Prevention Study

Group (Providence Health System, Portland, Ore., et al): Alendronate prevents postmenopausal bone loss in women without osteoporosis: a double-blind, randomized, controlled trial, Ann Intern Med 128:253, 1998.

McFarland KF, Boniface ME, Hornung CA, et al: Risk factors and noncontraceptive estrogen use in women with and without coronary disease, Am Heart J 117:1209, 1989.

McKinlay SM, Brambilla DJ, and Posner JG: The normal menopause transition, Maturitas 14:103, 1992.

Meier CR, Sturkenboom MCJM, Cohen AS, et al: Postmenopausal estrogen replacement therapy and the risk of developing systemic lupus erythematosus or discoid lupus, J Rheumatol 25:1515, 1998.

Modena MG, Molinari R, Muia N Jr, et al: Double-blind randomized placebo-controlled study of transdermal estrogen replacement therapy on hypertensive postmenopausal women, Am J Hypertens 12:1000, 1999.

Mulnard RA, Cotman CW, Kawas C, et al: Estrogen replacement therapy for treatment of mild to moderate Alzheimer disease. A randomized controlled trial, JAMA 283:1007, 2000.

Myers LS, Dixen J, Morrissette D, et al: Effects of estrogen, androgen, and progestin and sexual psychophysiology and behavior in postmenopausal women, J Clin Endocrinol Metab 70:1224, 1990.

Nagamani M, Kelver ME, and Smith ER: Treatment of menopausal hot flashes with transdermal administration of clonidine, Am J Obstet Gynecol 156:561, 1987.

Nanda K, Bastian LA, Hasselblad V, et al: Hormone replacement therapy and the risk of colorectal cancer: a meta-analysis, Obstet Gynecol 93:880, 199.

Natrajan PK, Soumakis K, and Gambrell D Jr: Estrogen replacement therapy in women with previous breast cancer, Am J Obstet Gynecol 181:288, 1999.

Neri I, Granella F, Nappi R, et al: Characteristics of headache at menopause: a clinico-epidemiologic study, Maturitas 17:31, 1993.

Newcomb PA, Longnecker MP, Mittendorf J, et al: Long-term hormone replacement therapy and risk of breast cancer in postmenopausal women, Am J Epidemiol 142:788, 1995.

Newton KM, LaCroix AZ, McKnight B, et al: Estrogen replacement therapy and prognosis after first myocardial infarction, Am J Epidemiol 145:269, 1997.

NIH Consensus Development Panel on Optimal Calcium Intake: Optimal calcium intake, JAMA 272:1941, 1994.

O'Keefe JH, Kim SC, Hall RR, et al: Estrogen replacement therapy after coronary angioplasty in women, J Am Coll Cardiol 29:1, 1997.

Paganini-Hill A: The benefits of estrogen replacement therapy on oral health: the Leisure World cohort, Arch Intern Med 155:2325, 1995.

Paganini-Hill A and Henderson VW: Estrogen deficiency and risk of Alzheimer's disease in women, Am J Epidemiol 140: 256, 1994.

Paganini-Hill A, Ross RK, and Hendersen BE: Postmenopausal oestrogen treatment and stroke: a prospective study, Br Med J 297:519, 1988.

Prince RL, Smith M, Dick IM, et al: Prevention of postmenopausal osteoporosis: a comparative study of exercise, calcium supplementation, and hormone-replacement therapy, N Engl J Med 325:1189, 1991.

Proudler AJ, Ahmed AIH, Crook D, et al: Hormone replacement therapy and serum angiotensin-converting–enzyme activity in postmenopausal women, Lancet 346:89, 1995.

Punnonen RH, Jokela HA, Dastidar PS, et al: Combined oestrogen-progestin replacement therapy prevents atherosclerosis in postmenopausal women, Maturitas 21:179, 1995.

Punnonen R, Jokela H, Heinonen PK, et al: Hormone replacement therapy and atherosclerosis, J Reprod Med 40:267, 1995.

Rannevik G, Jeppsson S, Johnell O, et al: A longitudinal study of the perimenopausal transition: altered profiles of steroid and pituitary hormones, SHBG and bone mineral density, Maturitas 21:103, 1995.

Ravn P, Bidstrup M, Wasnich RD, et al: Alendronate and estrogen-progestin in the long-term prevention of bone loss: four-year results from the early postmenopausal intervention cohort study, Ann Intern Med 131:935, 1999.

Reid IR, Ames RW, Evans MC, et al: Effect of calcium supplementation on bone loss in postmenopausal women, N Engl J Med 328:460, 1993.

Reubinoff BE, Stein P, Wurtman J, et al: Effects of hormone replacement therapy on weight, body composition, fat distribution, and food intake in early postmenopausal women: a prospective study, Fertil Steril 64:963, 1995.

Riggs BL, Jowsey J, Kelley IPJ, et al: Effects of sex hormones on bone in primary osteoporosis, J Clin Invest 48:1065, 1969.

Riis B, Thomsen K, and Christiansen C: Does calcium supplementation prevent postmenopausal bone loss? N Engl J Med 326:173, 1987.

Robinson D, Friedman L, Marcus R, et al: Estrogen replacement therapy and memory in older women, J Am Geriatr Soc 42:919, 1994.

Rodriguez C, Calle EE, Coates RJ, et al: Estrogen replacement therapy and fatal ovarian cancer, Am J Epidemiol 141:828, 1995.

Ross RK, Paganini-Hill A, Wan PC, and Pike MC: Effect of hormone replacement therapy on breast cancer risk: estrogen versus estrogen plus progestin, J Natl Cancer Inst 92:328, 2000.

Rubin GL, Peterson HB, Lee NC, et al: Estrogen replacement therapy and the risk of endometrial cancer: remaining controversies, Am J Obstet Gynecol 162:148, 1990.

Sands RH, Studd JWW, Crook D, et al: The effect of estrogen on blood pressure in hypertensive postmenopausal women, J North Am Menopause Soc 4:115, 1997.

Santoro N, Rosenberg Brown J, Adel T, and Skurnick JH: Characterization of reproductive hormonal dynamics in the perimenopause, J Clin Endocrinol Metab 81:1495, 1996.

Scarabin PY, Plu-Bureau G, Bara L, et al: Haemostatic variables and menopausal status: influence of hormone replacement therapy, Thromb Haemost 70:584, 1993.

Schairer C, Byrne C, Keyl PM, et al: Menopausal estrogen and estrogen-progestin replacement therapy and risk of breast cancer (United States), Cancer Causes Control 5:4991, 1994.

Schairer C, Lubin J, Troisi R, et al: Menopausal estrogen and estrogen-progestin replacement therapy and breast cancer risk, JAMA 283:485, 2000.

Schiff I, Tulchinsky D, Cramer D, and Ryan KJ: Oral medroxyprogesterone in the treatment of postmenopausal symptoms, JAMA 224:1443, 1980.

Schneider DL, Barrett-Conner EL, and Morton DJ: Timing of postmenopausal estrogen for optimal bone mineral density: the Rancho Bernardo Study, JAMA 277:543, 1997.

Sellers TA, Mink PJ, Cerhan JR, et al: The role of hormone replacement therapy in the risk for breast cancer and total mortality in women with a family history of breast cancer, Ann Intern Med 127:973, 1997.

Sherwin BB and Gelfand MM: The role of androgen in the maintenance of sexual functioning in oophorectomized women, Psychosom Med 49:397, 1987.

Sherwin BB and Gelfand MM: A prospective one-year study of estrogen and progestin in postmenopausal women: effects on clinical symptoms and lipoprotein lipids, Obstet Gynecol 73:759, 1989.

Sillero-Arenas M and Delgado-Rodriguez M: Menopausal hormone replacement therapy and breast cancer: a meta-analysis, Obstet Gynecol 286:94, 1992.

Slooter AJC, Bronzova J, Witteman CM, et al: Estrogen use and early onset Alzheimer's disease: a population-based study, J Neurol Neurosurg Psychiatry 67:779, 1999.

Smith RNJ, Holland EFN, and Studd JWW: The symptomatology of progestogen intolerance, Maturitas 18:87, 1994.

Stampfer MJ, Colditz GA, Willett WC, et al: Postmenopausal estrogen therapy and cardiovascular disease: ten-year follow-up from the Nurses' Health Study, N Engl J Med 325:756, 1991.

Stanford JL, Hartge P, Brinton LA, et al: Factors influencing the age at natural menopause, J Chron Dis 40:995, 1987.

Stanford JL, Weiss NS, Voigt LF, et al: Combined estrogen and progestin hormone replacement therapy in relation to risk of breast cancer in middle-aged women, JAMA 274:137, 1995.

Steffens DC, Norton MC, Plassman BL, et al: Enhanced cognitive performance with estrogen use in nondemented community-dwelling older women, J Am Geriatr Soc 47:1171, 1999.

Strickland DM, Gambrell RD Jr, Butzin CA, Strickland K: The relationship between breast cancer survival and prior postmenopausal estrogen use. Obstet Gynecol 80:400, 1992.

Sullivan JM, Vander Zwaag R, Hughes JP, et al: Estrogen replacement and coronary artery disease, Arch Intern Med 150:2557, 1990.

Voight L, Weiss N, Chu J, et al: Progestagen supplementation of exogenous oestrogens and risk of endometrial cancer, Lancet 338:274, 1991.

Watts NB, Harris ST, Genant HK, et al: Intermittent cyclical etidronate treatment of postmenopausal osteoporosis, N Engl J Med 323:73, 1990.

Weiderpass E, Adami H-O, Baron JA, et al: Risk of endometrial cancer following estrogen replacement with and without progestins, J Natl Cancer Inst 91:1, 1999.

Weiss NS, Ure CL, Ballard JH, et al: Decreased risk of fractures of the hip and lower forearm with postmenopausal use of estrogen, N Engl J Med 303:1195, 1980.

Westendoorp ICD, Veld BAI, Bots ML, et al: Hormone replacement therapy and intima-media thickness of the common carotid artery. The Rotterdam Study, Stroke 30:2562, 1999.

Willis DB, Calle EE, Miracle-McMahill HL, Heath CW Jr: Estrogen replacement therapy and the risk of fatal breast cancer in a prospective cohort of postmenopausal women in the United States. Cancer Causes Control 7:449, 1996.

Woodruff JD and Pickar JH: Incidence of endometrial hyperplasia in postmenopausal women taking conjugated estrogen (Premarin) with medroxyprogesterone acetate or conjugated estrogens alone, Am J Obstet Gynecol 170:1213, 1994.

The Writing Group for the PEPI Trial (Natl Heart, Lung, and Blood Inst, Bethesda, MD): Effects of hormone replacement therapy on endometrial histology in postmenopausal women: the postmenopausal estrogen; progestin interventions (PEPI) trial, JAMA 275:3760, 1996.

The Writing Group for the PEPI Trial: Effects of estrogen or estrogen/progestin regimens on heart disease risk factors in postmenopausal women: the postmenopausal estrogen/progestin interventions (PEPI) trial, JAMA 273:199, 1995.

Index

Note: Pages in *italics* indicate illustrations; those followed by t refer to tables.